Emergency Medicine
A COMPREHENSIVE STUDY GUIDE

Emergency Medicine

A COMPREHENSIVE STUDY GUIDE

American College of Emergency Physicians

Edited by

Judith E. Tintinalli, M.D.
Clinical Associate Professor of Emergency Medicine
Wayne State University School of Medicine, Detroit
Department of Emergency Medicine
William Beaumont Hospital
Royal Oak, Michigan

Robert J. Rothstein, M.D.
Chairman, Department of Emergency Medicine
Harbor–UCLA Medical Center
Torrance, California

Ronald L. Krome, M.D.
Chief, Department of Emergency Medicine
William Beaumont Hospital
Royal Oak, Michigan

McGRAW-HILL BOOK COMPANY

NEW YORK   ST. LOUIS   SAN FRANCISCO   AUCKLAND   BOGOTÁ   GUATEMALA   HAMBURG

JOHANNESBURG   LISBON   LONDON   MADRID   MEXICO   MONTREAL   NEW DELHI   PANAMA

PARIS   SAN JUAN   SÃO PAULO   SINGAPORE   SYDNEY   TOKYO   TORONTO

NOTICE

Medicine is an ever-changing science. As new research and clinical experience broaden our knowledge, changes in treatment and drug therapy are required. The editors and the publisher of this work have checked with sources believed to be reliable in their efforts to provide drug dosage schedules that are complete and in accord with the standards accepted at the time of publication. However, readers are advised to check the product information sheet included in the package of each drug they plan to administer to be certain that the information contained in these schedules is accurate and that changes have not been made in the recommended dose or in the contraindications for administration. This recommendation is of particular importance in connection with new or infrequently used drugs.

EMERGENCY MEDICINE: A Comprehensive Study Guide

Copyright © 1985 by McGraw-Hill, Inc. All rights reserved. Printed in the United States of America. Except as permitted under the United States Copyright Act of 1976, no part of this publication may be reproduced or distributed in any form or by any means, or stored in a data base or retrieval system, without the prior written permission of the publisher.

4567890HALHAL89876

ISBN 0-07-001439-6

This book was set in Times Roman by Waldman Graphics, Inc.; the designer was Hermann Strohbach.
Halliday Lithograph Corporation was printer and binder.

Library of Congress Cataloging in Publication Data
Main entry under title:

Emergency medicine.

   Rev. ed. of: A Study guide in emergency medicine. c1978.
   Includes bibliographies and index.
   1. Emergency medicine.   I. Tintinalli, Judith E.
II. Rothstein, Robert J., date.   III. Krome,
Ronald L., date.   IV. American College of Emergency
Physicians.   V. Study guide in emergency medicine.
VI. Title.   [DNLM: 1. Emergencies.   2. Emergency
Medicine. WB 105 S933]
RC86.7.E586   1985   616′.025   84-17185
ISBN 0-07-001439-6

CONTENTS

SECTION 6   THE DIGESTIVE SYSTEM

SECTION 7   RENAL AND GENITOURINARY DISORDERS

SECTION 8   GYNECOLOGY AND OBSTETRICS

SECTION 9   PEDIATRICS

SECTION 10   ENDOCRINE EMERGENCIES

SECTION 11   HEMATOLOGIC AND ONCOLOGIC EMERGENCIES

SECTION 12   DERMATOLOGIC EMERGENCIES

SECTION 13   INFECTIONS

SECTION 14   EYE, EAR, NOSE, THROAT—ORAL SURGERY

SECTION 15   NONTRAUMATIC MUSCULOSKELETAL DISORDERS

SECTION 16   TRAUMA

SECTION 17   NEUROLOGY

SECTION 18   PSYCHIATRIC EMERGENCIES

SECTION 19   PHYSICIAN-PATIENT INTERACTIONS

SECTION 20   EMERGENCY MEDICAL SYSTEMS

LIST OF CONTRIBUTORS

Ali Aghamohamadi, M.D.
Attending Otolaryngologist
Griffin Hospital, Derby, Connecticut

James T. Amsterdam, D.M.D., M.D.
Assistant Professor of Surgery, Division of Oral Surgery
  and Dentistry
University of Cincinnati College of Medicine and Hospital
Cincinnati, Ohio
Clinical Instructor of Dental Medicine
Medical College of Pennsylvania
Philadelphia, Pennsylvania

Warren Appleton, M.D., J.D.
Evergreen Hospital
Kirkland, Washington

Frederick A. Arcari, M.B., Ch.B.
Associate Clinical Professor of Surgery
Wayne State University School of Medicine
Detroit, Michigan

Regine Aronow, M.D.
Director, Poison Control Center
Children's Hospital of Michigan
Associate Professor
Wayne State University
  School of Medicine
Detroit, Michigan

Georges C. Benjamin, M.D.
Chief, Emergency Medical Section
Walter Reed Army Medical Center
Washington, D.C.
Assistant Professor of Medicine
Uniformed Services University of the Health Sciences
Bethesda, Maryland

Ramon Berguer, M.D., Ph.D.
Chief, Section of Vascular Surgery
Harper Hospital
Professor of Surgery
Wayne State University School of Medicine
Detroit, Michigan

Carol D. Berkowitz, M.D.
Assistant Professor of Pediatrics
UCLA School of Medicine
Director, Pediatric Clinic and Group Practice
Harbor–UCLA Medical Center
Torrance, California

Howard A. Bessen, M.D.
Assistant Professor of Medicine
Department of Emergency Medicine

Harbor–UCLA Medical Center
Torrance, California

Ruth Beverly, M.S.W.
Rape Counseling Center
Detroit Police Department
Detroit, Michigan

Brooks F. Bock, M.D.
Medical Director, Emergency Department
Seton Medical Center
President, American College of Emergency Physicians
Austin, Texas

Michael Callaham, M.D.
Chief, Division of Emergency Medicine
University of California, S.F.
San Francisco, California

Richard W. Carlson, M.D., Ph.D.
Professor of Medicine
Chief, Division of Pulmonary/Critical Care
Wayne State University School of Medicine
Chief of Medicine
Detroit Receiving Hospital
Detroit, Michigan

Peter Carter, M.D.
Baylor University Medical Center
Dallas, Texas

Eugene E. Cepeda, M.D.
Department of Neonatology
Hutzel Hospital
Detroit, Michigan

Richard Ceyzyk, M.S.W.
Department of Emergency Medicine
Detroit Receiving Hospital
Detroit, Michigan

Thomas A. Chapel, M.D.
Clinical Associate Professor of Dermatology and Syphology
Wayne State University
Detroit, Michigan

Roland Clark, M.D.
San Diego, California

Mary Ann Cooper, M.D.
Director, Emergency Department
St. Francis Hospital and Medical Center
Hartford, Connecticut

Robert H. Dailey, M.D.
Chief, Emergency Department
Highland Hospital
Oakland, California

Daniel F. Danzl, M.D.
Associate Professor
Department of Emergency Medicine
University of Louisville
Louisville, Kentucky

Steven J. Davidson, M.D.
Associate Professor (Emergency Medicine)
Department of Emergency Medicine
The Medical College of Pennsylvania
Philadelphia, Pennsylvania

Michael L. DeMars, M.D.
Emergency Department
William Beaumont Hospital
Royal Oak, Michigan
Clinical Instructor, Section of Emergency Medicine
Wayne State University
Detroit, Michigan

Steven C. Dronen, M.D.
Assistant Professor
Department of Emergency Medicine
University of Cincinnati College of Medicine
Cincinnati, Ohio

Daniel Esposito, M.D.
Clinical Instructor in Medicine
Division of Hematology
Georgetown University Hospital
Washington, D.C.

Beverly Fauman, M.D.
Director of Education
Department of Psychiatry
Sinai Hospital of Detroit
Detroit, Michigan

A. Joel Feldman, M.D.
Assistant Professor of Surgery
Wayne State University School of Medicine
Vice Chief, Section of Vascular Surgery
Harper Hospital
Detroit, Michigan

Claude Frazier, M.D.
Asheville, North Carolina

Scott Freeman, M.D.
Assistant Professor, Section of Emergency Medicine
Department of Surgery
Wayne State University
Detroit, Michigan

Kenneth Frumkin, M.D., Ph.D.
Chief, Department of Emergency Medicine
Madigan Army Medical Center
Tacoma, Washington

Kenneth Gitlin, M.D.
Instructor, Orthopaedic Surgery Resident Training Program
William Beaumont Hospital
Royal Oak, Michigan

B. Ken Gray, M.D.
Director, Department of Emergency and Ambulatory Medicine
William Beaumont Hospital
Royal Oak, Michigan

Lester Haddad, M.D.
Clinical Assistant Professor
National Capital Poison Center
Department of Emergency Medicine
Georgetown University Hospital
Washington, D.C.

Ann L. Harwood, M.D.
Chairman, Department of Emergency Medicine
University Hospital of Jacksonville
Associate Professor, Division of Emergency Medicine
University of Florida
Gainesville, Florida

Marilyn T. Haupt, M.D.
Wayne State University School of Medicine
Detroit, Michigan

Bruce E. Haynes, M.D.
Assistant Professor of Medicine
Department of Emergency Medicine
UCLA School of Medicine
Torrance, California

Barry Heller, M.D.
Clinical Faculty, Department of Emergency Medicine
Harbor–UCLA Medical Center
Torrance, California

Barry H. Hendler, D.D.S., M.D.
Acting Chairman, Department of Oral and Maxillofacial Surgery
University of Pennsylvania School of Dental Medicine
Clinical Professor of Medicine and Surgery (Dental Medicine) and Director of Oral and Maxillofacial Surgery
Medical College of Pennsylvania
Philadelphia, Pennsylvania

Gregory L. Henry, M.D.
Chief, Department of Emergency Medicine
Beyer Memorial Hospital
Clinical Instructor, Section of Emergency Medicine
University of Michigan Medical Center
Ann Arbor, Michigan

Harry Herkowitz, M.D.
William Beaumont Hospital
Royal Oak, Michigan

Robert S. Hockberger, M.D.
Assistant Professor of Medicine
UCLA School of Medicine
Director, Emergency Medicine Residency
Harbor–UCLA Medical Center
Torrance, California

Jerome R. Hoffman, M.D.
Assistant Professor of Medicine
Director, Office of Pre-Hospital Care
Emergency Medicine Center
UCLA Hospital and Clinics
Los Angeles, California

Stanley H. Inkelis, M.D.
Assistant Professor of Pediatrics
Associate Director, Pediatric Emergency
Harbor–UCLA Medical Center
Torrance, California

Raymond E. Jackson, M.D.
Emergency Department
Detroit Receiving Hospital
Detroit, Michigan

Harold A. Jayne, M.D.
Assistant Professor of Clinical Emergency Medicine
Chief of Division
Resident Director of Emergency Medicine
University of Illinois at Chicago
Chicago, Illinois

Carl Jelenko, III, M.D.
Towson, Maryland

Robert C. Jorden, M.D.
Chairman, Division of Emergency Medicine
University of Mississippi Medical Center
Jackson, Mississippi

John F. Keighley, M.D.
St. Joseph Hospital
Syracuse, New York

Kenneth W. Kizer, M.D., M.P.H.
Director, Emergency Medical Services Authority
State of California
Sacramento, California

Robert Knopp, M.D.
Chief of Emergency Medicine
Valley Medical Center
Fresno, California

Ronald L. Krome, M.D.
Chief, Department of Emergency Medicine
William Beaumont Hospital
Royal Oak, Michigan

Richard Levy, M.D.
Professor and Chairman
Department of Emergency Medicine
University of Cincinnati College of Medicine
Cincinnati, Ohio

Christopher H. Linden, M.D.
University of Colorado School of Medicine
Rocky Mountain Poison Center
Denver, Colorado

Toby Litovitz, M.D.
Director, National Capital Poison Center
Assistant Professor of Emergency Medicine
Georgetown University Hospital
Washington, D.C.

Neal Little, M.D.
Emergency Physician
St. Joseph Mercy Hospital
Clinical Instructor
University of Michigan Medical School
Ann Arbor, Michigan

Robert C. Luten, M.D.
Assistant Professor
University of Florida
Director of Pediatric Emergency Services
Department of Emergency Medicine
University Hospital of Jacksonville
Jacksonville, Florida

James R. Mackenzie, M.D.
Head, Section of Emergency Services
Department of Surgery
University of Michigan Hospitals
Ann Arbor, Michigan

Frank I. Marlowe, M.D.
Professor of Surgery
Medical College of Pennsylvania
Chief, Division of Otolaryngology
Presbyterian—University of Pennsylvania Medical Center
Philadelphia, Pennsylvania

James Mathews, M.D.
Chief, Section of Emergency Medicine
Northwestern University Medical School
Chicago, Illinois

Judith B. Matthews, R.N.
Towson, Maryland

James H. McCrory, M.D.
Director, Division of Pediatric Critical Care Medicine
University Hospital of Jacksonville
Assistant Professor of Pediatrics
University of Florida
Gainesville, Florida

Harvey W. Meislin, M.D.
Department of Emergency Medicine
Arizona Health Sciences Center
Tucson, Arizona

Hagop S. Mekhjian, M.D.
Professor of Medicine
Division of Gastroenterology
The Ohio State University College of Medicine
Columbus, Ohio

Vera Morkovin, M.D.
Associate Professor of Emergency Medicine
Michigan State University
East Lansing, Michigan

H. Arnold Muller, M.D.
Associate Professor of Medicine
Emergency Medicine Division
Department of Medicine
Pennsylvania State University College of Medicine
Hershey, Pennsylvania
(Official leave of absence while serving as Secretary of
Health, Commonwealth of Pennsylvania.)

James T. Niemann, M.D.
Assistant Professor of Medicine
UCLA School of Medicine
Associate Chairman
Department of Emergency Medicine
Harbor–UCLA Medical Center
Torrance, California

Michael A. Nigro, D.O.
Glendale Neurological Associates
Birmingham, Michigan

David Nolan, M.D.
Medical Director/Health Officer
Western Michigan Associated Health Departments
Associate Professor of Community Medicine
Wayne State University School of Medicine
Detroit, Michigan

Richard M. Nowak, M.D.
Vice Chairman
Department of Emergency Medicine
Henry Ford Hospital
Detroit, Michigan

Peter Ostrow, M.S.W.
Southwest Detroit Community Mental Health Services
Detroit, Michigan

John W. Packer, M.D.
Raleigh Orthopaedic Clinic
Raleigh, North Carolina

George Podgorny, M.D.
Clinical Professor, Emergency Medicine
East Carolina University School of Medicine
Associate Professor of Clinical Surgery
Bowman Gray School of Medicine of Wake Forest University
Winston-Salem, North Carolina

Paul R. Pomeroy, M.D.
Director, Emergency Department
St. Mary Hospital
Livonia, Michigan

Gene Ragland, M.D.
Staff Physician
St. Joseph Mercy Hospital
Clinical Instructor, Department of Surgery
University of Michigan Medical School
Ann Arbor, Michigan

Nick Relich, M.D.
Codirector, Neonatal Intensive Care Unit and Newborn
  Services
St. John Hospital
Detroit, Michigan

Charles Rennie, III, M.D.
Assistant Professor of Surgery
UCLA School of Medicine
Director, Adult Acute Care
Department of Emergency Medicine
Harbor–UCLA Medical Center
Torrance, California

Roscoe Robinson, M.D.
Professor of Medicine
Vanderbilt University Medical Center
Nashville, Tennessee

Robert J. Rothstein, M.D.
Chairman, Department of Emergency Medicine
Harbor–UCLA Medical Center
Torrance, California

Barry H. Rumack, M.D.
Director
Rocky Mountain Poison Center
Denver, Colorado

Douglas A. Rund, M.D.
Associate Professor and Director
Division of Emergency Medicine
Department of Preventive Medicine
The Ohio State University College of Medicine
Columbus, Ohio

Ronald Sacher, M.B., B.Ch.
Associate Professor of Medicine and Pathology
Georgetown University Medical Center
Washington, D.C.

Carl Sacks, M.D.
Clinical Instructor, Emergency Medicine
Detroit Receiving Hospital
Wayne State University
Detroit, Michigan

James Seidel, M.D., Ph.D.
Associate Professor of Pediatrics
UCLA School of Medicine
Chief of Ambulatory Pediatrics
Harbor–UCLA Medical Center
Torrance, California

Seetha Shankaran, M.D.
Assistant Professor of Pediatrics
Children's Hospital of Michigan
Wayne State University School of Medicine
Detroit, Michigan

Richard Owen Shields Jr., M.D.
Emergency Department
Detroit Receiving Hospital
Detroit, Michigan

Dale Sillix, M.D.
Assistant Professor of Medicine
Department of Medicine—Nephrology Division
Wayne State University
Detroit, Michigan

J. K. Sims, M.D.
Chief, Emergency Medical Services Systems Branch
State of Hawaii Department of Health
Honolulu, Hawaii

J. Stephan Stapczynski, M.D.
St. Mary Medical Center, Long Beach
Assistant Clinical Professor of Medicine
UCLA School of Medicine
Los Angeles, California

Zwi Steiger
Associate Professor of Surgery
Wayne State University
Detroit Receiving Hospital and University Health Center
Detroit, Michigan

George Sternbach, M.D.
Deputy Medical Director, Emergency Medicine
Stanford University Medical Center
Stanford, California

Robert Swetnam, D.O.
Associate Chairman, Department of Emergency Medicine
Providence Hospital
Southfield, Michigan

Anthony J. Thomas Jr., M.D.
Head, Section of Male Infertility
Departments of Urology and Gynecology
Cleveland Clinic Foundation
Cleveland, Ohio

Judith E. Tintinalli, M.D.
Clinical Associate Professor of Emergency Medicine
Wayne State University School of Medicine, Detroit
Department of Emergency Medicine
William Beaumont Hospital
Royal Oak, Michigan

L. Scott Ulin, M.D.
Parkway Regional Medical Center
North Miami Beach, Florida

Michael Vance, M.D.
Department of Emergency Medicine
St. Lukes Medical Center
Phoenix, Arizona

John H. van de Leuv, M.D.
Director, Emergency Medicine and Trauma Center
Methodist Hospital of Indiana, Inc.
Indianapolis, Indiana
Associate Clinical Professor
Department of Emergency Medicine
Wright State School of Medicine
Dayton, Ohio

Joseph F. Waeckerle, M.D.
Chairman, Department of Emergency Medicine
Baptist Medical Center
Clinical Associate Professor
University of Missouri at Kansas City School of Medicine
Kansas City, Missouri

Donald Weaver, M.D.
Assistant Professor of Surgery
Department of Surgery
Wayne State University School of Medicine
Detroit, Michigan

Joseph J. Weiss, M.D.
Consultant, Wayne County General Hospital
Westland, Michigan

Martin Weissman, M.D.
Instructor, Orthopaedic Surgery Resident Training Program

William Beaumont Hospital
Royal Oak, Michigan

Howard A. Werman, M.D.
Division of Emergency Medicine
The Ohio State University College of Medicine
Columbus, Ohio

Blaine C. White, M.D.
Associate Professor, Section of Emergency Medicine
College of Human Medicine
Michigan State University
East Lansing, Michigan

Robert F. Wilson, M.D.
Professor of Surgery
Director, Thoracic and Cardiovascular Surgery
Wayne State University School of Medicine
Chief of Surgery
Detroit Receiving Hospital
Detroit, Michigan

Carleton D. Winegar, M.D.
Instructor of Emergency Medicine
Department of Surgery
Wayne State University School of Medicine
Detroit, Michigan

Joseph Zeccardi, M.D.
Director, Emergency Department
Clinical Associate Professor of Surgery (Emergency Medicine)
Thomas Jefferson University Hospital
Philadelphia, Pennsylvania

PREFACE

EMERGENCY MEDICINE: *A Comprehensive Study Guide* is the second edition of A STUDY GUIDE IN EMERGENCY MEDICINE. The book is intended to combine the comprehensiveness of a textbook and the informal utility of a study guide. The "Study Guide," our predecessor, was the first attempt to formally embody the knowledge reflected in the core content as defined by the American College of Emergency Physicians. In this new edition, we have expanded the number of topics under consideration and we have examined with greater detail the methods of managing emergencies. Our major priority has been to make this a practical text that meets the needs of the student interested in or rotating through emergency medicine, the resident in training, the practitioner, and the board candidate.

JUDITH E. TINTINALLI
ROBERT J. ROTHSTEIN
RONALD L. KROME

SECTION 1
RESUSCITATIVE
PROBLEMS
AND TECHNIQUES

CHAPTER 1
BASIC
CARDIOPULMONARY
RESUSCITATION
AND TECHNIQUES

A. Basic Cardiopulmonary Resuscitation

Raymond E. Jackson

Basic cardiopulmonary resuscitation (CPR) encompasses the concepts and techniques which form the foundation for effective emergency care. It is the responsibility of emergency physicians to direct the resuscitation of patients in the emergency department and often of patients in the field. Teaching nurses, emergency medical technicians, paramedics, and the lay public the basic techniques and principles used in resuscitation is also a duty of the emergency physician.

The purpose of cardiopulmonary resuscitation is to provide artificial circulation of oxygenated blood to the vital organs, especially the heart and brain, in an attempt to halt the degenerative processes associated with ischemia and anoxia until spontaneous circulation can be restored. Guidelines for application of basic cardiopulmonary resuscitation have been established by the American Heart Association and are reviewed in this chapter and elsewhere. Some adjuvant procedures and techniques which may be of future use are also described.

Applying effective cardiopulmonary resuscitation demands a methodical approach to rapidly and adequately assess the patient's condition, and to assure effective delivery of care. The performance of eight maneuvers in a stepwise fashion enables the care provider to quickly assess the patient's responsiveness, airway patency, and presence of spontaneous ventilations and circulation. These steps are as follows:

1. Establish unresponsiveness
2. Obtain assistance
3. Properly position the victim
4. Open the airway
5. Establish breathlessness
6. Ventilate the patient
7. Establish presence or absence of pulse
8. Perform closed-chest compressions

ESTABLISH UNRESPONSIVENESS

The first step in assessing an individual who has collapsed is to establish his or her unresponsiveness. This is done by firmly but gently shaking the patient and providing auditory stimulation such as ''Annie, Annie, are you alright?'' Other noxious stimuli such as ammonia capsules, sternal rubs, or the trapezius pinch can be quickly applied to establish the degree of unresponsiveness. At this point, a rapid general survey of the patient can be made to assess color and general condition of the skin, the presence of any unusual odors, and any evidence of trauma or drug use.

OBTAIN ASSISTANCE

If the victim is outside the hospital and does not respond to these stimuli, call for help immediately. If there are two or more rescuers, one should be immediately sent to call and alert the emergency medical service system, while any others at the scene can help with CPR. In the hospital, the code should be called which activates the cardiopulmonary arrest team. If the victim is indeed in cardiac arrest, it is most imperative that advanced life support be instituted as soon as possible, since the limiting factor to the eventual outcome is the time from the onset of arrest to reestablishment of an effective spontaneous circulation.

PROPERLY POSITION THE VICTIM

For the physician or attendant to effectively perform CPR, the victim must be supine. If not, carefully turn the person flat onto his or her back by kneeling beside him or her, placing one hand on the back of the head and neck, and with the other hand rolling the victim toward you. The concept is to attempt to move the patient's head, neck, and torso as one unit to protect the stability of the cervical spine. If the victim is found in bed, either place the individual on the floor or position a firm support such as a plywood board under the thoracic cage. This will increase the effectiveness of the chest compression's ability to generate intrathoracic pressure.

OPEN THE AIRWAY

In the unconscious patient, the mouth must be opened and the upper airway inspected for any evidence of foreign objects, vomitus, or blood. If any is found, you should turn the victim's head to one side (unless cervical spine injury is suspected) and with

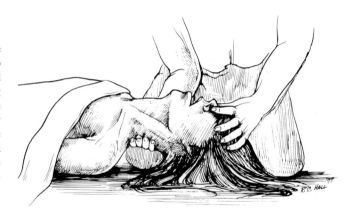

Figure 1-2. The head tilt technique.

your fingers attempt to remove any object from the oropharynx. Be very cautious not to push any object deeper into the airway. In the emergency room, direct visualization with the laryngoscope can be performed, with fluid removed by suction and foreign objects extracted with McGill forceps.

With loss of muscle tone, the tongue may fall back into the oropharynx and cause upper airway obstruction in obtunded individuals. Also, the negative pressure generated during inspiratory efforts can force the tongue back into the posterior oropharynx, creating a one-way valve effect which occludes the airway during inspiration (Fig. 1-1). The head tilt procedure often can alleviate this glossal obstruction if some muscle tone is present. With poor muscle tone, a jaw thrust or a chin lift is needed to remove the tongue from the posterior oropharynx.

Head Tilt

To perform a head tilt, place one hand beneath the victim's neck and the other hand on the forehead (Fig. 1-2). The neck is then flexed in relation to the thorax, and the head extended in relation to the neck (the so-called sniffing position). If this maneuver does not establish a patent airway, the chin lift or jaw thrust maneuver should be attempted.

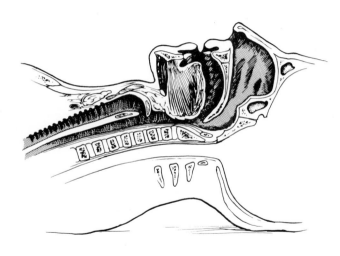

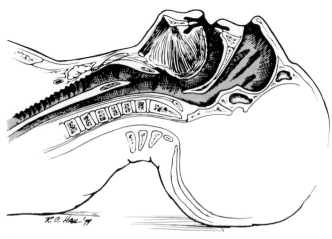

Figure 1-1. An obstructed airway may be relieved by flexing the neck in respect to the torso and hyperextending the head in relation to the neck. This maneuver elevates the tongue from the oropharynx.

Chin Lift

The chin lift is a highly effective maneuver in some patients in which the head tilt maneuver has failed to open the airway. The rescuer lifts the chin by taking the hand that had supported the neck, placing the fingers under the symphysis of the mandible, and lifting the chin forward and up, being careful not to compress the soft tissues under the tongue (Fig. 1-3). The other hand is kept on the forehead. The chin is lifted so that the teeth are barely brought together, but the mouth is not closed completely. If the victim has dentures, the chin lift is more effective if they remain in place.

Jaw Thrust

The jaw thrust maneuver is done in conjunction with the head tilt–neck lift maneuver. The rescuer positions himself or herself at the head of the patient, placing the hands at the sides of the

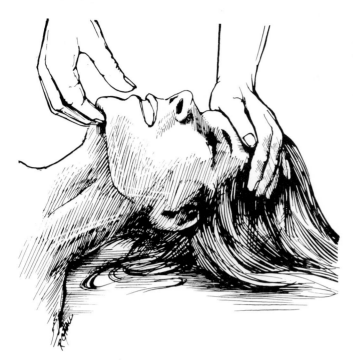

Figure 1-3. The chin lift.

victim's face, grasping the angles of the mandible and lifting the mandible forward (Fig. 1-4). The rescuer may rest his or her elbows on the surface on which the patient is lying. The jaw thrust, without use of the head tilt, is the safest method for opening an obstructed upper airway in a patient while maintaining the integrity of the cervical spine.

Relieving Foreign Body Obstruction

Foreign bodies may cause either partial or complete airway obstruction. With partial airway obstruction, the victim may be capable of good or poor air exchange. With good air exchange, the victim can cough forcefully, although there may be wheezing between coughs. As long as good air exchange continues, encourage the victim to persist with spontaneous coughing and breathing. Do not interfere with his or her attempts to expel the foreign body. The child with partial airway obstruction and good air exchange should not be turned upside down because this may impact the foreign body against the vocal cords.

Poor air exchange is characterized by a weak, ineffective cough, inspiratory stridor, and respiratory distress. If the victim has poor air exchange, the partial obstruction should be managed as though it were a complete airway obstruction. With complete airway obstruction, the victim is unable to speak, breathe, or cough. If still conscious, he or she may clutch the neck (universal distress signal). In an unconscious victim, you can identify airway obstruction by the chest wall's lack of rise with each attempted ventilation.

Maneuvers for Relieving Obstruction

The three maneuvers recommended for relieving foreign body obstruction are back blows, manual abdominal or chest thrusts.

and manually removing the foreign body. Back blows produce an instantaneous increase in airway pressure, which may result in either partial or complete dislodgment of the foreign body. Manual thrusts produce a lower but more sustained increase in pressure than back blows and may further assist in dislodging the foreign body. Combining these techniques appears to be more effective than using one technique alone.

Back Blows

The back blow technique is a series of four rapid, sharp blows delivered over the spine and between the shoulder blades with the heel of the hand. They may be given with the victim standing, sitting, or lying, and should be applied forcefully and rapidly. Whenever possible, the victim's head should be lower than the chest to make good use of the effect of gravity.

Manual Thrusts

The manual thrust technique consists of four thrusts to the upper abdomen or lower chest, which forcibly expel air from the lungs. The low chest thrust develops somewhat higher flows and peak pressure than the abdominal thrust.

The abdominal thrust can be performed with the victim sitting or standing. The rescuer should stand behind the victim and wrap his or her arms around the victim's waist. The rescuer then makes a fist with one hand and places the thumb side of the fist against the victim's epigastric area. Then the rescuer places the free hand around the fist and delivers four quick upward thrusts (Fig. 1-5).

If the victim is lying, he or she must be positioned on the back, and the airway opened. The rescuer can be either astride or alongside the victim. It is preferable to be alongside the victim because the rescuer has more maneuverability. The heel of one hand should be placed against the victim's abdomen between the xiphoid process and the umbilicus, and covered with the heel of the other hand. The rescuer then presses into the victim's abdomen with a quick upward thrust.

A victim can perform this maneuver on himself or herself by delivering a quick upward thrust to the abdomen with the fist, or by leaning forward and compressing the abdomen over any firm object such as the back of a chair, a table, or porch railing. Com-

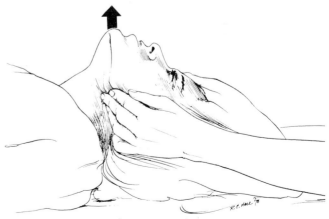

Figure 1-4. Jaw thrust.

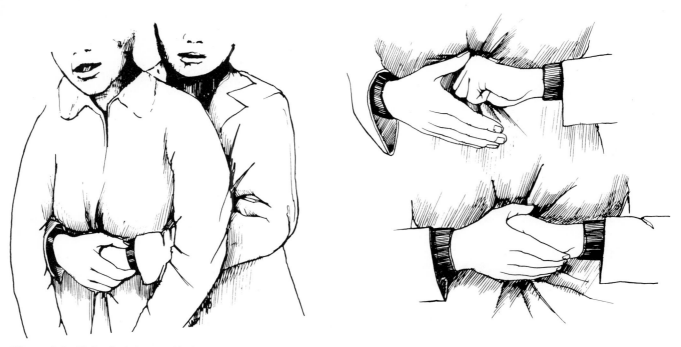

Figure 1-5. Abdominal thrust with the victim standing. Make a fist with one hand and place the thumb side of your fist against the victim's epigastric area. Place your other hand around your fist. Deliver four quick upward thrusts.

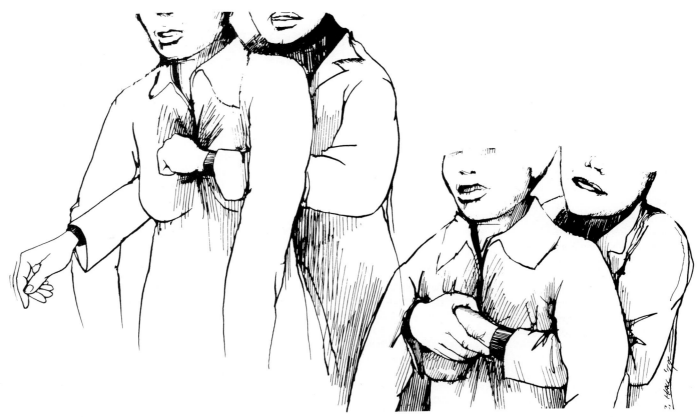

Figure 1-6. Chest thrust with the victim standing. Make a fist with one hand and place the thumb side of your fist against the victim's lower sternum. Deliver four quick upward thrusts.

plications of the abdominal thrust include rupture or laceration of the abdominal viscera.

Chest thrusts are performed in a similar manner when the victim is standing or sitting. The rescuer stands behind the victim and wraps his or her arms around the chest, placing the thumb side of the fist on the sternum (Fig. 1-6). The chest is then forcefully compressed four times. If the victim is supine, he or she should be placed on the back and the airway opened. The rescuer's hands are then placed over the chest as in closed-chest massage, and the chest compressed four times. The chest thrust is useful if the rescuer cannot fully wrap his or her arms around the victim's abdomen, or when direct abdominal pressure is likely to cause complications, as in advanced pregnancy.

The sequence in which these maneuvers should be executed is: Check the oropharynx, apply back blows, and apply manual thrusts; then repeat the cycle until the obstruction is cleared. If at any time the foreign object appears in the oropharynx, it is removed manually.

ESTABLISH BREATHLESSNESS

After efforts have been made to open the upper airway, you can determine the patient's ability to spontaneously breathe by placing an ear over his or her mouth and nose, listening and feeling for the escape of exhaled air. Observe the chest and abdomen for ventilation movements. Occasionally, patients may have agonal respirations despite total cardiovascular collapse. These respirations are characterized by occasional sighing and should not be interpreted as effective ventilatory efforts. If the patient is apneic, or is having agonal respirations, rescue breathing should be established immediately.

VENTILATE THE PATIENT

The mouth-to-mouth method of rescue breathing is initiated by gently pinching the patient's nostrils with the thumb and index finger. Then, after taking a deep breath, the rescuer places his or her open mouth around the outside of the victim's mouth to make an airtight seal, and then forcibly exhales air into the patient's airway. The volume exhaled should be about twice the normal resting tidal volume, or about 1500 mL. Larger tidal volumes should be avoided because of the danger of creating gastric distensions and subsequent regurgitation and aspiration. The first four ventilations are delivered in rapid succession without allowing for passive exhalation from the victim's lungs. These four initial breaths are done not only to increase residual lung volume, thereby opening some alveoli, but also to replace the hypercarbic, hypoxic air with air containing a higher FI_{O_2} and lower FI_{CO_2}. The expired air which is being used to ventilate only has an FI_{O_2} of 16 to 17 percent so that resources able to deliver higher oxygen concentrations are needed as soon as possible. The rescuer should not inhale the victim's expired air because the oxygen delivered will progressively decrease. With these breaths, the rescuer watches the victim's chest to determine if it rises with each forced inhalation, and to make sure it falls with each exhalation. The rescuer should be able to feel any resistance to airflow during inhalation and should listen for the sound of air escaping from the lungs during exhalation. Any observed impairment to airflow during rescue breathing indicates an obstruction in the flow of air through the upper airway, trachea, or major bronchi, or may indicate a physical impairment to lung expansion such as pneumothorax or massive pulmonary effusion. Lungs congested from pulmonary edema or adult respiratory distress syndrome (ARDS) are relatively noncompliant and can offer increased resistance to expansion. If lack of chest wall motion is noted or there is a high amount of resistance to airflow, the oropharynx must be reinspected for an obstruction and efforts to relieve the obstruction should be executed as described above.

Closed-chest massage at this point would be totally ineffective until the patient can be properly ventilated. Once the foreign object is successfully removed, the rescuer checks for spontaneous ventilations and pulse, then proceeds.

With severe maxillofacial trauma, mouth-to-nose ventilations may be more effective than mouth-to-mouth. This is done by using the jaw thrust maneuver in an attempt to pull the tongue from the posterior oropharynx, and sealing the mouth shut with the thumb and forefinger during inhalation. The mouth is opened during exhalation to diminish the resistance to airflow, and because of the possibility of nasopharyngeal obstruction by the soft palate. Patients with stomas or tracheostomies are ventilated by placing the mouth over the stoma or tracheostomy tube.

ESTABLISH PRESENCE OR ABSENCE OF PULSE

After the initial salvo of four ventilations, the presence of a pulse is determined by placing two fingers on the carotid artery, which is located by placing the index and middle fingers on the trachea and then sliding the fingers between the trachea and sternocleidomastoid muscles. A second rescuer may check for the presence of a pulse in the femoral area. Although the presence of a pulse is not a reliable indicator of organ perfusion, its absence indicates cardiac arrest. If there is indeed pulselessness, or if the pulse is weak or very bradycardic, closed-chest massage is begun immediately. If a strong pulse is present but spontaneous ventilations are absent, rescue breathing is continued by ventilating the lungs every 5 s, rechecking the carotid or femoral pulse frequently.

PERFORM CLOSED-CHEST COMPRESSIONS

With evidence of inadequate circulation, closed-chest massage must be initiated. The victim must be supine and should be on a firm surface. The correct position of the hands for chest compressions is found by placing two fingers of one hand over the xiphoid process and the heel of the other hand on the sternum 1 to 2 in cephalad to the xiphoid process. Then remove the first hand from the xiphoid process and place it on top of the hand resting on the sternum (Figs. 1-7 and 1-8). The fingers may or may not be interlocked but they should remain off the chest wall. The rescuer should position himself or herself over the victim, and then straighten and lock the elbows so that the sternum is compressed directly downward 1.5 to 2 in (Fig. 1-9). With two rescuers, the chest can be compressed at a rate of 60 per min with a ventilation interposed after every fifth compression in an adult. The relaxation phase of the cycle is accomplished by relieving the pressure on the chest but never removing the hands from the chest wall. The optimum ratio of compression to relaxation of the chest wall is 1:1, with the rate at which the compressions are performed being a less significant factor in generating a cardiac output. If there is only

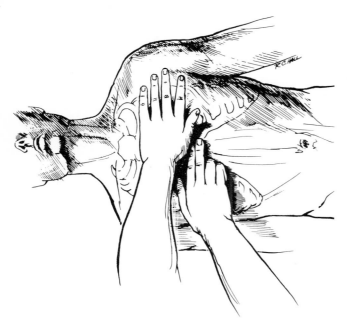

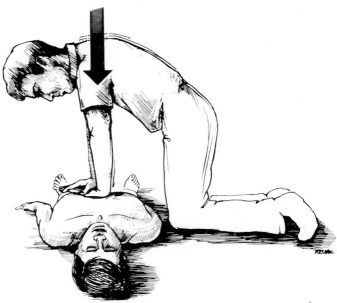

Figure 1-7. Place your index and middle fingers of one hand on the xiphoid process and then the heel of your other hand one fingerbreadth above the distal end of the sternum.

Figure 1-9. During compression, keep your elbows straight and position your shoulders over the victim's sternum.

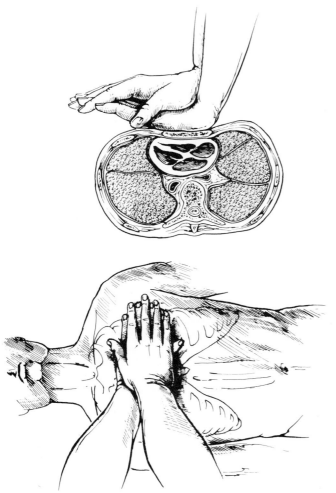

Figure 1-8. Remove your hand from the xiphoid process and place it on top of the sternum.

one rescuer, 15 compressions are carried out at a rate of 80 per min, after which the rescuer repositions himself or herself at the head of the patient and delivers two breaths in rapid succession. The rescuer then returns to the proper position on the chest and repeats the cycle of 15 compressions to two ventilations, rechecking the victim for spontaneous respiration, and the carotid pulse every 4 to 5 min.

RESUSCITATION IN CHILDREN

In children, airway obstruction or anoxia is almost always the etiology for cardiopulmonary arrest. The technique of ventilations and chest compressions in children is similar to that in adults. As in adults, the eight basic steps are performed as outlined above.

The maneuvers of the head and neck used to alleviate upper airway obstruction must be modified in infants and small children, because the trachea of the child under age 2 does not have the cartilaginous support of an adult. If the head should be hyperextended on the neck, the pliable tracheal structures may collapse on themselves to cause obstruction. The infant or small child should be positioned in the sniffing position by placing a towel or a hand under the head. Pulling the mandible forward with the jaw thrust or chin lift maneuver along with proper positioning of the head will often be all that is needed to relieve upper airway obstruction. The airway should then be cleared of any foreign material, either by suction or manual means.

The volume of ventilation in children is smaller than with adults but should be enough just to see the chest rise. In infants and small children, puffs of air are delivered from the mouth. Establishing the presence of a pulse in children is best done in the femoral area. If the pulse is normal and the skin color good, the circulation is most likely adequate. Often, poor circulation and bradycardia are converted by establishing a clear airway and providing adequate ventilation with oxygen.

Only one rescuer is needed to provide CPR for the infant or child. The rate and depth of chest compression in children varies with age. With infants, the thorax is enclosed by the rescuer's hands, with the thumbs over the lower third of the sternum. Compressions are delivered at a rate of 120 to 140 per min at a depth of $\frac{1}{2}$ to $\frac{3}{4}$ in. For children, the sternum is depressed $\frac{3}{4}$ to $1\frac{1}{2}$ in with the heel of one hand at a rate of 100 to 120 per min. The ratio of ventilations to compressions is 5:1, as in adults.

COMPLICATIONS

Complications of basic closed-chest massage include sternal and rib fractures, which may lead to lung contusions and pneumo-hemothoraces. Myocardial contusions, primarily of the right ventricle, have been noted, as well as acute hemorrhagic pericardial effusions. In the abdominal cavity, gastric distension, erosions, and rupture have occurred. The incidence of liver lacerations is approximately 2 percent. Careful performance of basic closed-chest massage can diminish, but not totally abolish, many of these complications.

Late complications include development of pulmonary edema, electrolyte abnormalities, gastrointestinal hemorrhage, pneumonia, recurrent cardiopulmonary arrest, anoxic encephalopathy, acute renal failure, ARDS, and septicemia.

TERMINATING RESUSCITATIVE EFFORTS

Resuscitative efforts should be continued until ventilation and circulation are restored, the patient is transported to a hospital setting, the rescuer himself or herself is near collapse, or until a physician assumes responsibility for the patient.

BIBLIOGRAPHY

Bivins H, Knopp R, Tierman, C, et al: Blood volume displacement with inflation of antishock trousers. *Ann Emerg Med* 11:409, 1982.

Bjork R, Snyder B, Campion B, et al: Medical complication of cardiopulmonary arrest. *Arch Intern Med* 142:500, 1982.

Chandra N, Synder L, Weisfeldt M: Abdominal binding during cardiopulmonary resuscitation in man. *JAMA* 246:351, 1981.

Chandra N, Weisfeldt M, Tsitlik J, et al: Augmentation of carotid blood flow during CPR in dogs by ventilation at high airway pressures simultaneous with chest compression. *Am J Cardiol* 48:1053, 1981.

Criley J, Blaufuss A, Kissel G: Cough induced cardiac compression: Self administered form of cardiopulmonary resuscitation. *JAMA* 136:1246, 1976.

Dohl S: Postcardiopulmonary resuscitation pulmonary edema. *Crit Care Med* 11:434, 1983.

Donegan J: New concepts in cardiopulmonary resuscitation. *Anesth Analg (Cleve)* 60:100, 1981.

Ducas J, Roussas C, Karasrdis C, et al: Factors affecting the intrathoracic pressure during CPR. *Circulation* 64 (suppl. IV):302, 1981.

Eisenberg M, Bergner L, Hallstrom A: Cardiac resuscitation in the community: Importance of rapid provision and implication for program planning. *JAMA* 241:1905, 1979.

Eisenberg M, Copass M. Hallstrom A, et al: Management of out of hospital cardiac arrest: Failure of basic emergency medical technician services. *JAMA* 243:1049, 1980.

Fitzgerald K, Babbs C, Frissura H, et al: Cardiac output during cardiopulmonary resuscitation at various compression rates and durations. *Am J Physiol* 241:H442, 1981.

Gaffney F, Thal E, Taylor W, et al: Hemodynamic effects of medical antishock trousers (MAST garment): *J Trauma* 21:931, 1981.

Gann D: Emergency management of the obstructed airway. *JAMA* 243:1141, 1980.

Guildner C: Resuscitation—opening the airway: A comparative study of techniques for opening the airway obstructed by the tongue. *JACEP* 5:675, 1976.

Jude J, Kouwenhoven W, Knickerbocker G: Cardiac Arrest: Report of application of external cardiac massage on 118 patients. *JAMA* 178:1063, 1961.

Kouwenhoven W, Jude J, Knickerbocker G: Closed chest cardiac massage. *JAMA* 173:1064, 1960.

Luce J, Cary J, Ross B, et al: New developments in cardiopulmonary resuscitation. *JAMA* 244:1366, 1980.

Lund I, Skullberg A: Cardiopulmonary resuscitation by lay people. *Lancet* 2:702, 1976.

MacKenzie G, Taylor S, McDonald A, et al: Hemodynamic effects of external cardiac compression. *Lancet* 1:1342, 1964.

McDonald J: Systolic and mean arterial pressures during manual and mechanical CPR in humans. *Ann Emerg Med* 11:292, 1982.

McIntyre K, Parisi A, Benfari R, et al: Pathophysiologic syndromes of cardiopulmonary resuscitation. *Arch Intern Med* 138:1130, 1978.

Nagel E, Fine E, Krischer J, et al: Complications of CPR. *Crit Care Med* 9:424, 1981.

Ohmoto T, Miura I, Konno S: A new method of external cardiac massage to improve diastolic augmentation and prolonged survival time. *Ann Thorac Surg* 21:284, 1976.

Orlowski J: Pediatric cardiopulmonary resuscitation. *Emerg Med Clin NA* 1:3, 1983.

Ralston S, Babbs C, Niebauer M: Cardiopulmonary resuscitation with interposed abdominal compression in dogs. *Anesth Analg (Cleve)* 61:645, 1982.

Redding J: Abdominal compression in cardiopulmonary resuscitation. *Anesth Analg (Cleve)* 50:668, 1971.

Redding J: The choking controversy. Critique and evidence on the Heimlich maneuver. *Crit Care Med* 7:475, 1979.

Redding J: Cardiopulmonary resuscitation: An algorithm and some pitfalls. *Am Heart J* 98:788, 1979.

Rudikoff M, Maughan W, Effron M, et al: Mechanisms of blood flow during cardiopulmonary resuscitation. *Circulation* 61:345, 1980.

Standards for cardiopulmonary resuscitation (CPR) and emergency cardiac care. *JAMA* (suppl.) 227, 1974.

Standards and guidelines for cardiopulmonary resuscitation and emergency cardiac care. *JAMA* 244:453–512, 1980.

Taylor G, Rubin R, Tucker M, et al: External cardiac compression: A randomized comparison of mechanical and manual techniques. *JAMA* 240:644, 1978.

Thompson R, Hallstrom A, Cobb L: Bystander initiated cardiopulmonary resuscitation in the management of ventricular fibrillation. *Ann Intern Med* 90:737, 1979.

Voorhees W, Niebauer M, Babbs C: Improved oxygen delivery during cardiopulmonary resuscitation with interposed abdominal compressions. *Ann Emerg Med* 12:128, 1983.

B. Adjunctive Techniques

Scott Freeman

Mechanical devices that deliver chest compressions and ventilations are capable of generating comparable systolic and mean blood pressures, and equal resuscitation success rates without an increase in the incidence of complications.

Several alternative methods of performing cardiac massage have developed during experimental attempts to improve upon standard closed-chest massage. These alternatives are based upon the concept that blood flow during closed-chest massage is not the result of squeezing the heart, but results from generalized increases in pressures of all the thoracic vascular compartments, with the heart acting as a passive conduit.

COUGH CPR

In 1976 Criley reported seven patients who were able to maintain consciousness during ventricular fibrillation by coughing every 1 to 3 s. They showed that blood flow can be generated without chest compressions. Cough CPR should be taught to all patients at high risk for developing a lethal arrhythmia.

SIMULTANEOUS VENTILATION AND COMPRESSION CPR

To allow the generation of high intrathoracic pressure during closed-chest massage, the standard CPR method was altered so that high intrathoracic pressures could be generated by inflating the lungs during the compression phase of closed-chest massage. This form of resuscitation is termed simultaneous ventilation and compression CPR (SVC CPR).

ABDOMINAL BINDING

Binding the abdomen during closed-chest massage increases intrathoracic pressure by preventing the descent and inversion of the diaphragm, thereby changing the compliance of the thorax. The military antishock trouser (MAST) may act as an abdominal binder in humans and thus has potential to augment blood flow during CPR. When MAST is applied, the total peripheral vascular resistance increases without a significant autotransfusion or preload effect.

With interposed abdominal counterpulsation (IAC CPR), the abdomen is compressed over an air-filled bladder during the relaxation phase of chest compression.

All these methods, with the exception of cough CPR, are experimental methods that offer hope in improving the eventual outcome of resuscitation, but which have yet to be shown to be either more efficacious or safer in the resuscitation of humans than standard CPR.

MAST

The MAST (military antishock trouser) garment is a one-piece, layered device made of polyvinyl fabric, capable of sustaining internal air pressures of up to 104 torr and is used to reverse the signs of shock. It encloses the body from the lower rib cage to, but not including, the feet. The lower extremities are each enclosed separately, allowing access to the perineal area. Three compartments cover the abdomen and two extremities and are fastened with Velcro fasteners. Some versions of the garment allow separate inflation and deflation of these compartments. Most are inflated with a foot pump and have an interposed inflation pressure-monitoring device. Internal pressures of the suit are limited by a pressure-relief valve and the Velcro's ability to withstand stress.

The device is at least 70 years old, predating blood transfusion. Its invention is attributed to Crile, who reported its use to control intraabdominal hemorrhage in 1903. Out-of-hospital use of the garment appears to have been first suggested by Crile in 1941 after he and other passengers in a plane lost consciousness as they flew into the vortex of a tornado. Once recovered from the experience, he suggested to the military forces that a pneumatic suit would prevent fighter-pilot blackout. This observation led to the use of the G-suit by fliers in World War II.

During 1969 in Vietnam the suit was used on victims of trauma to the lower extremities, pelvis, and perineum by the U.S. Army during evacuation to surgical hospitals. Civilian use of the garment in the prehospital setting was reported in 1973 on 20 patients with hypotension or hypovolemia. In recent years the MAST garment has come into widespread prehospital use and continues to be a focus of clinical and physiologic investigation.

The effect of MAST on hypotension was ascribed to increased peripheral vascular resistance by Crile but this no longer appears to be its sole method of functioning. Factors involved in reversing shock appear to include at least four mechanisms:

1. Tamponade of bleeding in the lower body
2. Increase in peripheral resistance in the lower body
3. Selective perfusion of the upper body
4. An initial increase of venous return (preload) from the lower body

This last mechanism, that of increasing preload, was once proposed to be the major method of action, although this no longer appears to be the case.

Physiologic Effects

Crile in 1903 attributed the suit's effect on hypotension to an increase in peripheral vascular resistance. Although this proposal was made in 1903, it was largely ignored until recently, with the suit's function being explained by an autotransfusion effect, or increase in preload.

In 1955 it was reported that a volume of 250 mL was displaced to the thorax when an anti-G suit was inflated above 75 torr. This figure was derived from an experiment on normal human subjects placed in the MAST device while on a teeterboard. As the MAST garment was inflated the center of gravity shifted toward the head. (This work also appears to have been ignored by those proposing larger amounts of autotransfusion as the mechanism for the garment's function.) The presumed mechanism of action was probably based upon observation of the amount of fluid required to maintain blood pressure as the garment was deflated. In the first (1973) reported civilian use of the MAST device this autotransfusion effect was estimated to be 1000 mL.

More recently, Gaffney et al. (1981) demonstrated marked increases in peripheral vascular resistance when the MAST garment was inflated on normal human volunteers. Included in their observations were decreases in both stroke volume and cardiac output. They concluded that increases in mean arterial pressure were explicable solely on the increase in peripheral vascular resistance. Objections that neither of these experiments realistically reveals the function of MAST have been raised because of the use of normotensive subjects. In an attempt to simulate the usual setting in which the MAST device is used, phlebotomized human volunteers were subjected to blood volume measurements by isotope scanning before and after application of MAST. Isotope scanning allowed evaluation of the blood volume in a compartmental manner. Although the phlebotomy in this experiment amounted to 17 percent of the total blood volume, the amount measured as displaced to the upper body was less than 5 percent. The mean blood volume after phlebotomy was 4434 mL, making the autotransfused amount less than 222 mL for this group.

In an animal experiment shock was induced by phlebotomy and direct measurements of the inferior vena cava flow were obtained as MAST inflation occurred. The volume of autotransfused blood in this setting was about 4 mL/kg which, if extrapolated to humans, agrees with volumes determined to be autotransfused by noninvasive techniques. Total peripheral vascular resistance in this setting was found not to change significantly, and the authors postulated that the major effect of MAST application was attributable to a rise in peripheral vascular resistance in the lower extremities and abdomen, causing redirection of blood flow to supradiaphragmatic vital organs, rather than a significant shift in blood volume from the splanchnic and lower extremity capacitance vessels.

It appears that the subtle distinction between redistribution of blood flow and redistribution of blood volume has confused the understanding of MAST's functioning in the past. When volume expansion is used to elevate the central venous pressure to the same degree as that seen in normal humans who have had the MAST device applied, no change occurs in mean arterial pressure, in contrast to significant elevation of mean arterial pressure when the MAST garment was applied to these subjects. Redistribution of blood flow by the application of MAST was first demonstrated in 1968 during animal experiments. Flows in the carotid artery increased 26 percent while femoral artery blood flow decreased 33 percent in this nonshock model. An attempt to delineate blood flow in a shock model with radioactive microspheres failed to demonstrate changes in the distribution of flow with the use of MAST.

Pulmonary functioning is affected by the MAST garment. This probably occurs because it limits diaphragmatic excursion. In normal human volunteers the effects of two different styles of MAST on vital capacity were examined. With a standard MAST garment, in which the abdomen is only partially covered, inflation to 100 torr failed to significantly alter vital capacity. Using the second style of MAST, in which the abdomen was completely covered by the garment, inflation to 100 torr decreased vital capacity by 13.8 percent. A case report containing respiratory parameters in a patient with traumatic quadriplegia on whom the MAST device was used revealed larger decreases in vital capacity. At 40 torr vital capacity was increased 27 percent; at 100 torr it was decreased 42 percent with preservation of the FEV_1/FVC ratio at both pressures. This indicates that this device causes a restrictive type of lesion. In a retrospective study of 25 patients requiring MAST for shock, only those with head injury (4 out of 5) showed evidence of hypercarbia. In this head-injured group mortality was 80 percent.

The effect of the MAST garment on intracranial pressure has been examined in animal models. Even in the presence of experimentally created intracranial mass lesions the intracranial pressure failed to change significantly when the MAST suit was inflated. Cerebral perfusion pressure in a shock model improved as a result of MAST inflation elevating the mean arterial pressure.

Pressure from pneumatic enclosures is transmitted to the tissues. With an air splint inflated to 40 torr on a human upper extremity, blood flow distal to the splint was "negligible" or undetectable. Measurements of pressure in the perinephric space of dogs with inflated MAST were 80 percent of the suit pressure. This transmitted pressure has been used to explain the apparent ability of MAST to control bleeding from lacerated vessels by decreasing the transmural pressure gradient. Should this pressure decrease the size of an intact vessel, then a dramatic increase in resistance would occur. According to Poiseuille's law, when flow is laminar, the resistance of a vessel is inversely proportional to the fourth power of the vessel's radius. Metabolism in tissues covered by MAST can be affected. In a shock animal model lactate production increases in the structures covered by the suit when it is inflated above the systolic pressure. Centrally obtained lactate levels rose in this setting upon deflation of the garment. These observations help explain the multiple case reports of compartment syndromes in the lower extremities associated with the use of MAST.

Initial attempts to explain the function of MAST focused on a presumed autotransfusion that occurred from the lower extremities to the central circulation. When studied, this autotransfusion effect was too small to fully explain the effectiveness of the device in increasing blood pressure in shock states. It now appears that the major method by which blood pressure is restored is the redistribution of blood flow cephalad secondary to an increased resistance in the lower part of the body.

Benefits and Efficacy

From studies with populations of limited size, the MAST garment appears effective in restoring blood pressure toward normal in the shock state. The garment can be applied in about 1 min and application is an easily reversible maneuver. It is difficult to assess the prevalence rates of complications from most of the literature on MAST because of the small numbers of cases examined.

A study with a large number of cases (1120) has recently been published and attempts to establish the prevalence of complications with the use of the garment as well as its efficacy. Patients included were in shock as defined by systolic pressure below 90 torr with clinical evidence of decreased tissue perfusion or tachycardia. Blood pressure was increased by 20 torr or to normal in 58 percent, heart rate was decreased to 110 per min or less in 17 percent, and improved tissue perfusion was evident in 14 percent of the population; at least one of these indicators improved in 84 percent. The degree to which blood pressure was found to change is presented in Table 1-1 with data from another study. In patients whose initial systolic pressure was less than 60, the mean response was 48 mmHg.

Survival rates reported in studies on MAST are not directly attributable to the use of the garment. The largest study reports a rate of 73 percent when nonsurvival was defined as death within the first 24 h. Another study (N = 66) shows an overall rate of 82 percent and a rate of 89 percent for potentially lethal and serious injuries.

Control of hemorrhage secondary to pelvic fracture and stabilization of fractures of the pelvis and femur are indications for the use of MAST. Although many authors have reported use of the garment for this purpose on a case-by-case basis, little is known about the efficacy of this technique.

Complication rates are best derived from the study of Wayne and MacDonald. The study failed to reveal significant respiratory compromise or metabolic acidosis on deflation nor any cases of compartment syndrome in the lower extremities in 1120 patients. Skin changes were noted in 4 percent (33 out of 1120) but none required grafting. Renal failure requiring hemodialysis occurred in eight (0.97 percent) of this initially hypotensive group.

The only large patient study regarding the use of MAST failed to reveal frequent serious complications. Cases of lower extremity ischemia have been occasionally reported. The potential for the device to diminish vital capacity exists, but this is not a frequent clinical problem.

The MAST garment is an effective tool in restoring blood pressure in the shock state. The garment is easily and rapidly applied. It appears safe and its actions are quickly reversible.

Indications and Contraindications

The MAST garment is now considered essential equipment for ambulances by the American College of Surgeon's Committee on Trauma.

General indications for application are:

1. If systolic blood pressure is below 100 in the presence of clinical shock
2. To control hemorrhage from fractured pelvis or intraabdominal bleeding
3. To stabilize fractured pelvis or femur

Use in cardiogenic shock has been examined and advocated. Increases in systolic blood pressure with decreases in pulse rate have been reported when the MAST garment has been applied in

shock states secondary to sepsis, anaphylaxis, and loss of neurogenic vascular control.

An absolute contraindication for the use of MAST is the presence of pulmonary edema.

Relative contraindications for MAST use are pregnancy, impaled objects, and evisceration of the abdominal contents. During gestation only the leg compartments are recommended for use. The list of contraindications may expand as we reach a better understanding of the garment's effects. The application of the MAST suit results in an increase in the vascular resistance of the lower extremities and this may not be well tolerated by all patients. Multiple case reports of compartment syndromes in the lower extremities have accumulated following MAST application.

In the past, other cautions about the use of MAST have been raised, but have not been proved. Animal studies on the relationship between the application of MAST and intracranial pressure have failed to reveal deleterious effects in the presence of shock. The use of MAST increases cerebral perfusion pressure, thus eliminating some cerebral anoxia by preventing increases in intracranial pressure due to cerebral edema occurring during shock. Vital capacity is measurably decreased when the MAST suit is applied but the amount of decrease is usually well tolerated. Some authorities have feared that emesis might be triggered by application of MAST, but case reports of this are lacking.

Application and Removal

The MAST garment is designed to be applied with the patient supine. The leg compartments are inflated first, then the abdominal compartment. Inflation should stop when systolic blood pressure reaches 100 torr, or when the device itself limits further inflation. Application of the device for more than 2 h should increase one's concern about the development of compartment syndromes in the lower extremities. Deflation should be done in a stepwise manner that is the reverse of the inflation sequence. Deflation should be stopped if blood pressure falls more than 5 torr; volume expansion should be instituted before further deflation. The standard maneuver for maintaining blood pressure upon deflation is increasing preload, with crystalloid or blood. Recently, however, with the thought that the MAST garment acts by increasing afterload, one reviewer of the subject suggested that pharmacologically induced afterload is also an appropriate way to maintain blood pressure upon deflation of the garment. Deflation of MAST is associated with an increase in metabolic acidosis, but this was not a significant clinical problem when large numbers of patients were examined.

The length of time that MAST may safely be applied without contributing to lower extremity ischemia has not been determined. Compartmental syndrome in the absence of trauma to the lower extremity has been reported with as little as 140 min of MAST application. This complication should therefore be weighed against the benefits of the garment. Fortunately, this side effect of MAST appears infrequent, as it failed to appear in a large (1120 subjects) retrospective human study on the use of the garment.

Rapid loss of pressure within the MAST suit can be dangerous. Changes in temperature can cause partial deflation of the garment. For instance, if the garment were applied where the temperature was 38°C (100°F) and the patient was transported in an air-conditioned environment of 24°C (75°F), the suit could lose as much as 28 torr. When the altitude at which the suit is used changes,

Table 1-1. Increase in Systolic Blood Pressure (torr)

0–40		40–80		>80	
(478/821)	58%	(300/821)	37%	(43/821)	5%
(16/38)	42%	(16/38)	42%	(6/38)	16%

the pressure within the suit also varies, rising as altitude increases and decreasing as it falls. Extrapolating from experimental data, MAST pressure changes approximately 1.8 torr for each 1000-ft change in altitude.

BIBLIOGRAPHY

Ashton H: Effect of inflatable plastic splints on blood flow. *Br Med J* 2:1427–1430, 1966.

Bass RR, Allison EJ, Reines HD, et al: Thish compartment syndrome without lower extremity trauma following application of pneumatic antishock trousers. *Ann Emerg Med* 12:382–384, 1983.

Batalden DJ, Wickstrom PH, Ruiz ER, et al: Value of the G suit in patients with severe pelvic fracture—controlling hemorrhagic shock. *Arch Surg* 109:326–328, 1974.

Bivins HG, Knopp R, Tiernan C, et al: Blood volume displacement with inflation of antishock trousers. *Ann Emerg Med* 11:409–412, 1982.

Brotman S, Browner BD, Cox EF: MAS trousers improperly applied causing a compartment syndrome in lower-extremity trauma. *J Trauma* 22:598–599.

Chandra N, Synder L, Weisfeldt M: Abdominal binding during cardiopulmonary resuscitation in man. *JAMA* 246:351, 1981.

Chandra N, Weisfeldt M, Tsitlik J, et al: Augmentation of carotid blood flow during CPR in dogs by ventilation at high airway pressures simultaneous with chest compression. *Am J Cardiol* 48:1053, 1981.

Civetta JM, Nussenfeld SR, Rowe TR, et al: Prehospital use of the military anti-shock trouser (MAST). *JACEP* 5:581–587, 1976.

Cram AE, Davis JW, Kealey GP, et al: Effects of pneumatic antishock trousers on canine intracranial pressure. *Ann Emerg Med* 10:28–31, 1981.

Criley J, Blaufuss A, Kissel G: Cough induced cardiac compression: Self administered form of cardiopulmonary resuscitation. *JAMA* 136:1246, 1976.

Cutler BS, Dassett WM: Application of the G-suit to the control of hemorrhage in massive trauma. *Ann Surg* 173:511–514, 1971.

Dannewitz SR, Lilja GP, Ruiz E: Effect of pneumatic trousers on intracranial pressure in hypovolemic dogs with an intracranial mass. *Ann Emerg Med* 10:176–181, 1981.

Ducas J, Roussas C, Karasrdis C, et al: Factors affecting the intrathoracic pressure during CPR. *Circulation* 64(suppl. IV):302, 1981.

Ferrario CM, Nadzam G, Fernandez LA, et al: Effects of pneumatic compression on the cardiovascular dynamics in the dog after hemorrhage. *Aerosp Med* 41:411–415, 1970.

Gaffney FA, Thal ER, Taylor WF, et al: Hemodynamic effects of medical anti-shock trousers. *J Trauma* 21:931–937, 1981.

Gilbert RD: Depression of respiratory function by pneumatic antishock trousers in traumatic quadriplegia. *Ann Emerg Med* 12:378–381, 1983.

Goldsmith SR: Comparative hemodynamic effects of antishock suit and volume expansion in normal human beings. *Ann Emerg Med* 12:348–350, 1983.

Johnson BE: Anterior tibial compartment syndrome following use of MAST suit. *Ann Emerg Med* 10:209–210, 1981.

Kaplan BC, Civetta JM, Nasel EL, et al: The military anti-shock trouser in civilian pre-hospital emergency care. *J Trauma* 13:843–848, 1973.

Lee HR, Blank WF, Massion WH, et al: Venous return in hemorrhagic shock after application of military anti-shock trousers. *Am J Emerg Med* 1:7–11, 1983.

MacKenzie G, Taylor S, McDonald A, et al: Hemodynamic effects of external cardiac compression. *Lancet* 1:1342, 1964.

Maull KI, Capehart JE, Cardea JA, et al: Limb loss following military anti-shock trousers (MAST) application. *J Trauma* 21:60–62, 1981.

McCabe JB, Seidel DR, Jasser JA: Antishock trouser inflation and pulmonary vital capacity. *Ann Emerg Med* 12:290–293, 1983.

McClaughlin AP, McCullough DL, Kerr WS, et al: The use of external counterpressure (G-suit) in the management of traumatic retroperitoneal hemorrhage. *J Trauma* 107:940–944, 1972.

McSwain NE: Pneumatic trousers and the management of shock. *J Trauma* 17:719–724, 1977.

McSwain NE: Observations on the use of the pneumatic counter-pressure device. American College of Surgeons, Bull 9, October 1979.

Ohmoto T, Miura I, Konno S: A new method of external cardiac massage to improve diastolic augmentation and prolonged survival time. *Ann Thorac Surg* 21:284, 1976.

Palafox BA, Johnson MN, McEwen BS, et al: ICP changes following application of the MAST suit. *J Trauma* 21:55–59, 1981.

Ransom K, McSwain NE: Respiratory function following application of MAST trousers. *JACEP* 7:297–299, 1978.

Ralston S, Babbs C, Niebauer M: Cardiopulmonary resuscitation with interposed abdominal compression in dogs. *Anesth Analg (Cleve)* 61:645, 1982.

Ransom KJ, McSwain NE: Metabolic acidosis with pneumatic trousers in hypovolemic dogs. *JACEP* 8:184–187, 1979.

Redding J: Abdominal compression in cardiopulmonary resuscitation. *Anesth Analg (Cleve)* 50:668, 1971.

Reines HD, Khoury NP: Use of military antishock trousers in the hospital. *Am J Surg* 139:307–309, 1980.

Roth JA, Rutherford RB: Regional blood flow effects of G suit application during hemorrhagic shock. *SG&O* 133:637–643, 1971.

Rudikoff M, Maughan W, Effron M, et al: Mechanisms of blood flow during cardiopulmonary resuscitation. *Circulation* 61:345, 1980.

Sanders AB, Meislin HW: Effect of altitude change on MAST suit pressure. *Ann Emerg Med* 12:140–144, 1983.

Shenasky JH, Gillenwater JY: The renal hemodynamic and functional effects of external counterpressure. *SG&O* 134:253–258, 1972.

Soler J, Muller HA, Kennedy TJ: Clinical use of the G-suit. *JACEP* 5:609–611, 1976.

Stair TO: The mechanism of MAST: Stalking the elusive autotransfusion. *Am J Emerg Med* 1:112–113, 1983.

Taylor G, Rubin R, Tucker M, et al: External cardiac compression: A randomized comparison of mechanical and manual techniques. *JAMA* 240:644, 1978.

Tenney SM, Honig CR: The effect of the anti-G suit on the ballistocardiogram. *J Aviation Med* 26:194–199, 1955.

Voorhees W, Niebauer M, Babbs C: Improved oxygen delivery during cardiopulmonary resuscitation with interposed abdominal compressions. *Ann Emerg Med* 12:128, 1983.

Wansensteen SL, Ludewig RM, Eddy DM: The effect of external counterpressure on the intact circulation. *SG&O* 127:253–258, 1968.

CHAPTER 2
CEREBRAL
RESUSCITATION

Carleton D. Winegar, Blaine C. White

INTRODUCTION

Continuous availability of substrate and oxygen for human cells is mandatory for maintenance of life. The high degree of order present in living tissues can only be maintained by burning fuels and capturing a portion of the energy released as adenosine triphosphate (ATP). The production of ATP by oxidative phosphorylation in mitochondria drives the anabolic reactions necessary to preserve the ordered state of living tissue. Entropy is increased, in accordance with the second law of thermodynamics, because these reactions are not totally efficient. Continued perfusion to deliver fuels and oxygen is essential to maintain these reactions. The inevitable consequence of failure of perfusion or oxygenation is decreased order. Attempts to protect the brain during resuscitation fail when perfusion and high energy metabolism are not maintained during and after ischemic anoxic cerebral insults.

There are over 400,000 cardiac arrests outside hospitals and an estimated 70,000 cardiac resuscitations annually in the United States. Brain death or permanent incapacitating neurological disability occurs in over 50 percent of patients surviving arrest outside the hospital. Only one-third of the survivors are able to return to their previous lifestyles and jobs, and only 10 percent are without evidence of intellectual impairment. Advances in treating these patients are therefore desperately needed.

Clinically, irreversible neuronal damage can occur after 4 to 6 min of complete ischemic anoxia. If cell death itself occurred during this period, the chance of improving neurologic outcome would be remote. It was hoped that rapid application of cardiopulmonary resuscitation (CPR) after cardiac arrest would protect the brain for substantially longer periods of time; however, very little cerebral protection does occur. When defibrillation is delayed more than 6 min after arrest, neurologic outcomes become progressively worse, even with the immediate initiation of CPR.

There is reason for optimism, however. During the last 20 years evidence has accumulated indicating that the final neurologic deficits following ischemic anoxia are not due to immediate neuronal death. Indeed, evidence now suggests the brain can tolerate between 20 and 30 min of complete ischemic anoxia without irreversible injury. This conclusion is supported by evidence of recovery of ATP levels, protein synthetic capability, and action potential generation after these severe insults. Consequently, the final neurologic injury observed may result from mechanisms oc-

curring after resuscitation as the initial insult "matures." Postresuscitation interventions may be possible.

The development and application of effective therapy to preserve neuronal viability in patients who have sustained ischemic anoxic brain insults will be based on a growing understanding of the pathophysiology of these insults. The purpose of this chapter is to review our growing understanding of this pathophysiology and to examine laboratory trials of protective therapies directed at intervening in these processes.

PATHOPHYSIOLOGY OF IRREVERSIBLE BRAIN INJURY

Brain tissue has unusually high energy requirements to maintain its basal metabolic state. Despite this, brain tissue stores of oxygen, substrate, and ATP are small. Consequently, the brain is totally dependent on continuous perfusion to maintain high energy metabolism and functional and structural integrity.

Normally, the cerebral circulation adjusts to the nutritional needs of brain cells via autoregulation. Cerebral blood flow (CBF) remains relatively constant when cerebral perfusion pressure is varied in the range of 60 to 150 mmHg. Beyond this range CBF varies directly with the perfusion pressure. During ischemia, progressive functional and metabolic disturbances are manifested as blood flow diminishes. When flow is more than 30 percent normal, neurons can maintain cellular ATP content by stimulation of anaerobic glycolysis despite compromised oxygen delivery. Restoration of perfusion results in rapid cell revival. Between 15 to 30 percent normal flow, glucose availability becomes rate-limiting and cellular ATP content declines. Neurons subjected to prolonged ischemia of this severity are unable to maintain cell homeostasis, and progression to irreversible injury may occur even after reperfusion.

The No Flow Versus Low Flow Controversy

One would expect that any amount of blood flow would be better than no flow to the brain. However, when CBF is reduced to less than 10 percent normal, a paradoxical finding has been noted. Neuronal recovery is better after complete ischemia than after severe incomplete ischemia. In both these conditions, there is rapid depletion of ATP and membrane depolarization occurs. All anabolic and most catabolic metabolism breaks down. However, if a trickle flow remains, there is continued delivery of enough substrate to maintain anaerobic metabolism, resulting in a marked increase in tissue lactate. Severe cellular acidosis can develop and lead to protein and membrane degeneration which results in an irreversible injury. During severe incomplete ischemia, brain tissue acidosis is three to four times greater than during complete ischemia. Glucose administration concurrent with severe incomplete ischemia worsens neurologic recovery; the fasting state prior to ischemia improves outcome.

Calcium Ion Shifts During Cerebral Insults

Calcium ion balance is actively maintained outside normal cells with a gradient of 10,000 to 1 between the extracellular fluid and the cytosol. Influx of calcium into neurons and vascular smooth muscle cells is documented in all global insults, resulting in permanent brain injury. A precipitous fall in cellular ATP during ischemia, anoxia, or severe hypoglycemia results in the inability to maintain ionic gradients across the cell membrane, and calcium moves intracellularly. There is also an intracellular rise in calcium during status epilepticus by the overloading of the ejection pumps through repeated depolarizations.

Calcium ion influx has been implicated as the final common pathway triggering cell death. This influx may be etiologic in initiating cell death rather than its sequela. Hepatocytes in culture were protected from 12 different membrane-active toxins in the absence of calcium. In the presence of calcium, all cells died. To further understand the pathophysiology of brain damage, the events resulting from this uncontrolled calcium ion influx must be examined (see Fig. 2-1).

The Delayed Hypoperfusion Syndrome

During the past 10 years, studies of cerebral perfusion after complete and incomplete ischemia (less than 30 percent normal CBF), have uniformly provided evidence of greatly reduced CBF following reperfusion. Likewise, CBF is reduced following hypoglycemia and status epilepticus. In spite of an adequate resuscitation, after a 20-min cardiac arrest in dogs, cortical CBF is reduced to less than 20 percent normal after 90 min and remains below 20 percent for the following 18 h (see Fig. 2-2). This hypoperfusion occurs concurrently with cellular postischemic hypermetabolism, allowing continued inequality of blood supply and cellular demand. Thus, the final brain damage seen after brain injury may result in part from failure to perfuse the organ after resuscitation.

Two hypotheses have been excluded from the explanation of this failure of reperfusion. Early intracranial pressure changes are small or absent in ischemic anoxic models when head trauma is not involved, and cannot explain the early perfusion failure. However, a further deterioration in neurologic function may occur 12 to 72 h after resuscitation because of increasing interstitial edema and rises in intracranial pressure, resulting in a secondary perfusion failure. Another hypothesis offered to explain the hypoperfusion phenomenon is that intravascular obstruction occurs. However, there is no evidence of fibrin deposition or platelet thrombi postischemia using light and electron microscopy. The obvious

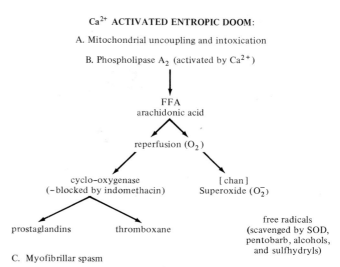

Ca²⁺ ACTIVATED ENTROPIC DOOM:

A. Mitochondrial uncoupling and intoxication

B. Phospholipase A₂ (activated by Ca²⁺)

FFA
arachidonic acid

reperfusion (O₂)

cyclo-oxygenase
(–blocked by indomethacin)

[chan]
Superoxide (O₂⁻)

prostaglandins   thromboxane

free radicals
(scavenged by SOD,
pentobarb, alcohols,
and sulfhydryls)

C. Myofibrillar spasm

Figure 2-1. Injury mechanisms in which high cytoplasmic calcium has been implicated as the triggering factor (FFA = free fatty acids; SOD = superoxide dismutase; CVR = cerebral vascular resistance). (From Winegar CD, Henderson O, White BC, et al. Early amelioration of neurologic deficit by lidoflazine after 15 minutes of cardiopulmonary arrest in dogs. *Ann Emerg Med* 12:471, 1983.)

remaining explanation, suggesting that there is intracerebral vasospasm resulting from calcium entry into vascular smooth muscle, is attractive. Once the actinomyosin complex is formed, the high concentrations of calcium in the cell prevent relaxation.

Mitochondrial Calcium Handling and ATP

The inability of cells to maintain or reestablish cellular ATP following brain insults is a critical event leading to cell death. In-

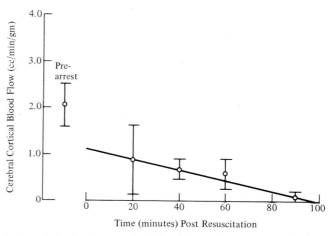

Figure 2-2. Cerebral cortical blood flow after 20 min perfusion arrest (five dogs: Data shown as mean and 1SDU). Cerebral cortical blood flow is reduced progressively during reperfusion following a 20-min cardiac arrest, and approaches zero after 90 min (p < 0.001 compared to prearrest). (From White BC, Gadzinski DS, Hoehner PJ, et al. Correction of canine cerebral cortical blood flow and vascular resistance after cardiac arrest using flunarizine, a calcium antagonist. *Ann Emerg Med* 11:118, 1982.)

creased intracellular calcium results in both an increased utilization of ATP via activation of a number of energy-consuming reactions, and in decreased mitochondrial production of ATP.

Exposure of mitochondria to calcium and metabolic substrate results in a burst of oxygen consumption, accompanied by the pumping of protons out of the mitochondria and the uptake of calcium. The electrochemical gradient established from the energy of oxidation is directly used in mitochondrial uptake of calcium, without the intermediate production of ATP. When there is elevated calcium in the cytosol, mitochondrial calcium pumping is obligatory, energy consuming, and uncouples the use of oxidation-derived energy from the production of ATP. If this process continues, mitochondrial structural and functional integrity is lost.

Oxygen, Calcium, and Membrane Degeneration

A rise in intracellular calcium results in the activation of phospholipase A2, which produces deterioration of membrane structure and function and rapid liberation of free fatty acids, predominantly arachidonic acid, into the cytosol. Free fatty acids increase linearly with time during the insult and are noted in anoxic ischemia, hypoglycemia, and status epilepticus.

With reoxygenation, arachidonic acid is converted in neurons, smooth muscle, and platelets to vasospastic prostaglandins, and a number of other cytotoxic compounds which can result in membrane degeneration through lipid peroxidation. A rapid increase in cellular prostaglandins has been shown to occur in the brain during recirculation following anoxia. Release of these vasospastic agents can perpetuate small-vessel hypoperfusion. Because synthesis of these cytotoxic compounds is determined by substrate availability, the calcium-stimulated rise in arachidonic acid triggers this cascade of reactions. Cell damage continues during and after resuscitation.

CPR Implications

The purpose of CPR is to provide adequate perfusion to vital organs to maintain viability until definitive resuscitation occurs. The clinical outcome data in humans fail to demonstrate protection from early but prolonged CPR. Cerebral flows greater than 30 percent normal are necessary to maintain brain viability. Cerebral flows produced in laboratory studies by basic CPR are uniformly less than 10 percent normal. Theoretically, the severe, incomplete ischemia produced by CPR may even contribute to the brain insult by increasing cerebral acidosis, moving additional calcium into the cerebral microcirculation, and allowing oxidative metabolism of arachidonic acid to various cytotoxic compounds without providing for even marginally adequate high energy metabolism. There is 100 percent functional brain death in experimental animals following 30 min of CPR and resuscitation from cardiac arrest. Clearly, a thorough reevaluation of the indications and methods for out-of-hospital basic CPR must be made.

THERAPY OFFERING CEREBRAL PROTECTION

Proven Therapies Currently Available

To date, there are few proven therapeutic interventions to lessen neurologic damage during and following resuscitation. Because

shortening the duration of entropic decay would be expected to improve neurologic recovery, efforts have been directed to reduce response times and provide definitive care in the prehospital setting. Survival and neurologic recovery are both improved in paramedic systems.

Monitoring and control of intracranial pressure following head trauma can prevent a progressive fall in perfusion pressure produced by cerebral edema and result in improved recovery. After cardiac arrest and other global insults, unfortunately, control of the late rise in intracranial pressure will not protect neurons from the initial hypoperfusion syndrome where severe irreversible cell death can occur.

In the postinsult period, additional secondary damage to the brain can be produced by failure of extracerebral organ systems. Thus, improving postinsult intensive care indirectly can improve the final neurologic deficit. Treating hypoxia, acidosis, anemia, hypotension, seizures, electrolyte imbalance, sepsis, and uremia will minimize this secondary damage.

Experimental Therapies

The newly evolving knowledge of the pathophysiology of cerebral injury has stimulated novel therapeutic approaches of direct intervention in these pathways. Improved cerebral outcome can be expected through maintaining viability during ischemia with new CPR methods, and by blocking the calcium influx–initiated damage after resuscitation.

Improved CPR

New, experimental CPR techniques can achieve CBF greater than 30 percent experimentally, augmenting forward flow by increasing the intrathoracic to extrathoracic pressure gradient. Simultaneous ventilation and compression CPR, and interposed abdominal counterpulsation CPR produce CBF between 30 to 40 percent. However, 30 min of simultaneous ventilation and compression CPR have not improved neurologic outcome when the technique was substituted for conventional CPR in animals. Interposed abdominal counterpulsation has not yet been put to this experimental test.

In the laboratory setting, standard closed-chest massage and concurrent administration of epinephrine to the central circulation produces CBF of 35 percent normal. Interposed abdominal counterpulsation CPR with epinephrine can produce CBF of 100 percent normal. Open-chest massage can maintain CBF greater than normal. There is no detectable neurologic deficit in animals after 30 min of resuscitation with continuous open-chest massage. Thus, until new CPR methods can be utilized, shortening the time to ACLS where pressors can be administered may improve recovery. For prolonged in-hospital resuscitative attempts, open-chest massage may be indicated.

Blocking Calcium Influx

Several experiments now indicate that the postarrest hypoperfusion syndrome can be ameliorated by either pre- or postinsult administration of numerous calcium-blocking agents, or the vasodilatory prostaglindin, prostacyclin. Likewise, pretreatment with indomethacin to block the postischemic vasospastic prostaglandin surge protects against this hypoperfusion. Following a 20-min cardiac arrest and resuscitation, cortical CBF is maintained at or above normal for the next 2 h when the animal is treated post-ischemia with flunarizine (see Fig. 2-3). Thus, the usual postinsult perfusion failure and secondary neuronal damage can be amelio-rated pharmacologically.

Calcium-initiated membrane degeneration can be diminished with therapy. Pentobarbital, which has calcium-blocking proper-ties, and calcium antagonists will suppress the free fatty acid rise in neurons after global ischemia. Decadron blocks calcium acti-vation of phospholipase A2 and would be expected to stabilize membrane structure.

Mitochondrial energy uncoupling produced by increased cal-cium in the cytosol should be improved if calcium antagonists given during resuscitation prevent further influx or increase efflux. In the presence of elevated intracellular calcium, high-dose ste-roids can protect mitochondrial ATP synthesis in vitro.

Functional and histologic neuronal recovery are improved in animals treated prior to anoxic ischemia with calcium antagonists, prostacyclin, or indomethacin. Pretreatment with nimodipine re-sults in preservation of learned avoidance behavior in rats. We have demonstrated amelioration of functional neurologic deficit in dogs treated postresuscitation after a 15-min arrest. In this pro-spective blind study, animals treated with lidoflazine showed in-tact brainstem and beginning higher cortical function 12 h follow-ing arrest. Four of five control dogs were functionally brain dead (see Fig. 2-4). Others have reported similar protection by lido-flazine administered after resuscitation in animals at the end of 4 days. In humans, a small series of patients resuscitated from out-of-hospital arrest and treated with calcium blockers after re-suscitation has been reported. In the treatment group, 33 percent were discharged home and all appeared neurologically intact at discharge and 3 months later. All patients in the control group

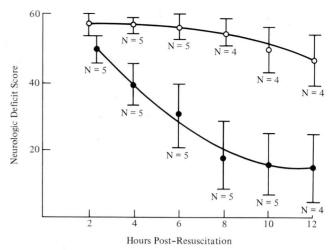

Figure 2-4. Early amelioration of postarrest neurologic deficit by lidoflazine. ○—○: untreated; ●—●: treated. (Data are mean ± 1 SEM.) The calcium antagonist lidoflazine ameliorates early neurologic deficit as determined by repetitive deficit scoring in a blind and prospectively randomized trial. (From Winegar CD, Henderson O, White BC, et al. Early amelioration of neurologic deficit by lidoflazine after 15 minutes of cardiopulmonary arrest in dogs. *Ann Emerg Med* 12:471, 1983.)

receiving standard therapy either died or were severely disabled neurologically.

These early experimental investigations offer promise of major advances in cerebral resuscitation by calcium blockers. Interna-tional multicenter human trials are now being planned. Work is continuing to identify the role of the projects of arachidonic acid oxidation in postischemic brain injury and to develop further in-tervention tools to halt these processes.

CONCLUSION

Current cerebral resuscitation attempts result in poor outcomes. Cerebral hypoperfusion during and after resuscitation cannot maintain viable neurons. After cerebral injury, calcium influx ap-pears to initiate a number of harmful cell processes, including uncoupling of mitochondrial ATP production, progressive cerebral hypoperfusion, membrane degeneration, and the formation of a number of cytotoxic compounds through oxidation of the free fatty acids released. Advances in cerebral resuscitation can be accom-plished by decreasing the duration of the insult, improving CBF during CPR, and by inhibition of calcium-activated injury.

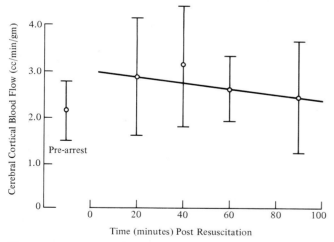

Figure 2-3. Cerebral cortical blood flow treated with flunarizine (6 μg/kg IV) (five dogs: Data shown as mean and 1SDU). Per-fusion of the cerebral cortex is preserved during at least the first 90 min postresuscitation, following a 20-min cardiac arrest, by administration of the calcium antagonist flunarizine (p < 0.001 compared to untreated controls). (From White BC, Gadzinski DS, Hoehner PJ, et al. Correction of canine cerebral cortical blood flow and vascular resistance after cardiac arrest using flunarizine, a calcium antagonist. *Ann Emerg Med* 11:119, 1982.)

BIBLIOGRAPHY

Addonizo VP, Fischer CA, Ecmunds LH: Effects of verapamil and ni-fedipine on platelet activation. *Clin Res* 28:607, 1980.
Altura BM, Altura BT: Pharmacologic inhibition of cerebral vasospasm in ischemia, hallucinogen ingestion, and hypomagnesemia: Barbitu-rates, calcium antagonists, and magnesium. *Am J Emerg Med* 1(2):180, 1983.
Altura BT, Turlpaty PD, Altura BM: Pentobarbital sodium inhibits cal-cium uptake in vascular smooth muscle. *Biochim Biophys Acta* 595:309, 1980.

Ames A III: Earliest irreversible changes during ischemia. *Am J Emerg Med* 1(2):139, 1983.

Ames A III, Guarian BS: Effects of glucose deprivation on function of isolated mammalian retina. *J Neurophysiol* 26:617, 1963.

Babbs CF, Ralston SH, Voorhees WD III: Improved cardiac output during CPR with interposed abdominal compressions. *Ann Emerg Med* (in press).

Bergner L, Eisenberg M, Hallstrom A, et al: Evaluation of paramedic services for cardiac arrest. U.S. Department of Health and Human Services, National Center for Health Services Research Report (HS 02456). December 1981.

Bircher NG, Safar P. Cerebral preservation during cardiopulmonary resuscitation (CPR) in dogs. *Anesthesiology* V59 No 3:A93, 1983.

Bircher NG, Safar P: Comparison of standard and ''new'' closed chest CPR and open-chest CPR in dogs. *Crit Care Med* 9:384, 1981.

Blaustein MP, Ector AC: Barbiturate inhibition of calcium uptake in depolarized nerve terminals in vitro. *Mol Pharmacol* 22:369, 1975.

Borgers, M, Thone F, Van Reempts J, et al: The role of calcium in cellular dysfunction. *Am J Emerg Med* 1(2):154, 1983.

Borle A: Control, modulation, and regulation of cell calcium. *Rev Physiol Biochem Pharmacol* 90:14, 1981.

Braunwald E: Mechanism of action of calcium channel blocking agents. *N Engl J Med* 307:1618, 1982.

Chan PH, Fishman RA: Brain edema: Induction in cortical slices by polyunsaturated fatty acids. *Science* 201:358, 1978.

Chan PH, Fishman RA: Transient formation of superoxide radicals in polyunsaturated fatty acid induced brain swelling. *J Med* 298:659, 1978.

Chiang F, Kowade M, Ames A III, et al: Cerebral ischemia III: Vascular changes. *Am J Pathol* 52:455, 1968.

Dayton WR, Schollmeyer JV: Isolation from porcine cardiac muscle of a calcium-activated protease that partially degrades myofibrils. *J Mol Cell Cardiol* 12:533, 1980.

Earnest MP, Yarnell PR, Merrill SL, et al: Long term survival and neurologic status after resuscitation from out-of-hospital cardiac arrest. *Neurology* 30:1298, 1980.

Edvinsson L, Andersson KE, Brandt L: Effects of calcium antagonists on cerebral blood vessels. *J Cerebral Blood Flow Metabol* 1:S344, 1981.

Eisenberg MS, Bergner L, Hallstrom A: Cardiac resuscitation in the community. Importance of rapid provision and implications for program planning. *JAMA* 241:1905, 1979.

Fiskum G: Involvement of mitochondria in ischemic cell injury and in regulation of intracellular calcium. *Am J Emerg Med* 1(2):147, 1983.

Flower RJ: Drugs which inhibit prostaglandin biosynthesis. *Pharmacol Rev* 23:33, 1974.

Flower RJ, Blackwell GJ: Anti-inflammatory steroids induce biosynthesis of a phospholipase A2 inhibitor which prevents prostaglandin generation. *Nature* 278:456, 1979.

Gadzinski DS, White BC, Hoehner PJ: Alterations in canine cerebral cortical blood flow and vascular resistance post cardiac arrest. *Ann Emerg Med* 11:58, 1982.

Gaudet RJ, Levine L: Transient cerebral ischemia and brain prostaglandins. *Biochem Biophys Res Commun* 6:893, 1979.

Grinwald PM, Nayler WG: Calcium entry in the calcium paradox. *J Mol Cell Cardiol* 13:867, 1981.

Hallenbeck JM, Furlow TW: Prostaglandin I2 and indomethacin prevent impairment of post-ischemic brain reperfusion in the dog. *Stroke* 10:629, 1979.

Harper AM, Craigen L, Kazda S: Effect of the calcium antagonist nimodipine on cerebral blood flow and metabolism in the primate. *J Cerebral Blood Flow Metabol* 1:349, 1981.

Harris RJ, Symon L, Bronston NM, et al: Changes in extracellular calcium activity in cerebral ischemia. *J Cerebral Blood Flow Metabol* 1:203, 1981.

Hass WK: Beyond cerebral blood flow, metabolism, and ischemic thresholds: An examination of the role of calcium in the initiation of cerebral infarction. In Cerebral Vascular Disease, vol. 3, Proceedings of the Salzburg Conference of Cerebral Vascular Disease, Amsterdam, 1981, pp 3–17.

Heymans C: Survival and revival of nervous tissue after arrest of circulation. *Physiol Rev* 30:375, 1950.

Hoffmeister F, Kazda S, Krause HP: Influence of nimodipine on the postischemic changes of brain function. Acta *Neurol Scand* 60(Suppl. 72):358, 1979.

Hossmann KA: Neuronal survival and revival during and after cerebral ischemia. *Am J Emerg Med* 1(2):191, 1983.

Hossmann KA, Kleihues P: Reversibility of ischemic brain damage. *Arch Neurol* 29:375, 1973.

Hossmann V, Hossmann KA, Takagi N: Effect of intravascular platelet aggregation on blood recirculation following prolonged ischemia of the cat brain. *J Neurol* 222:159, 1980.

Johnsson H: Effects of nifedipine on platelet function in vitro and in vivo. *Thromb Res* 21:523, 1981.

Kagstrom E, Smith ML, Siesjo BK: Local cerebral blood flow in the recovery period following complete cerebral ischemia in the rat. *J Cerebral Blood Flow Metabol* 3:170, 1983.

Kagstrom E, Smith ML, Siesjo BK: Recirculation in the rat brain following incomplete ischemia. *J Cerebral Blood Flow Metabol* 3:183, 1983.

Katz AM, Reuter H: Cellular calcium and cardiac cell death. *Am J Cardiol* 44:188, 1979.

Koehler RC, Chandra N, Guerci AD: Augmentation of cerebral perfusion by simultaneous chest compression and lung inflation with abdominal binding following cardiac arrest in dogs. *Circulation* 67:266, 1983.

Koehler RC, Michael JR, Guerci AD: Effect of epinephrine on cerebral blood flow during cardiopulmonary resuscitation in dogs. *Anesthesiology* 59(3):A94, 1983.

Kuwashima J, Nakamura K, Fujitani B: Relationship between cerebral energy failure and free fatty acid accumulation following prolonged brain ischemia. *Jpn J Pharmacol* 28:277, 1978.

Lazarewics JW, Strosznajder J, Gromek A: Effects of ischemia and exogenous fatty acids on the energy metabolism in brain mitochondria. *Bull Acad Pol Sci [Biol]* 29:599, 1972.

Lehninger AL: Role of phosphate and other proton donating cations in respiration-coupled transport of calcium by mitochondria. *Proc Nat Acad Sci USA* 71:1520, 1974.

Mitchell P, Moyle J: Chemiosmotic hypothesis of oxidative phosphorylation. *Nature* 213:137, 1967.

Moncada S, Higgs EA, Vane JR: Human arteries and venous tissues generate prostacyclin—a potent inhibitor of platelet aggregation. *Lancet* 1:18, 1977.

Myerburg RJ, Conde CA, Sung RJ: Clinical, electrophysiologic and hemodynamic profiles of patients resuscitated from prehospital cardiac arrest. *Am J Med* 68:568, 1980.

Nayler WG, Poole-Wilson PA, Williams A: Hypoxia and calcium. *J Mol Cell Cardiol* 11:683, 1979.

Nemoto EM, Hossmann KA, Cooper HK: Post-ischemic hypermetabolism in cat brain. *Stroke* 12:666, 1981.

Nemoto EM, Shiu GK, Nemmer JP, et al: Free fatty acid accumulation in the pathogenesis and therapy of ischemic-anoxic brain injury. *Am J Emerg Med* 1(2):175, 1983.

Nicholson C: Measurement of extracellular ions in the brain. *Trends in Neurosciences* 3:216, 1980.

Pichard JD: Role of prostaglandins and arachidonic acid derivatives in the coupling of cerebral blood flow to cerebral metabolism. *J Cerebral Blood Flow Metabol* 1:361, 1981.

Rehncrona S, Kagstrom E: Tissue lactic acidosis and ischemic brain damage. *Am J Emerg Med* 1(2):168, 1983.

Rehncrona S, Mela L, Siesjo BK: Recovery of brain mitochondrial function in the rat after complete and incomplete cerebral ischemia. *Stroke* 10:437, 1979.

Rogers MC, Weistfeldt ML, Traystan RJ: Cerebral blood flow during CPR. *Anesth Analg (Cleve)* 60:73, 1981.

Schanne FA, Kane AB, Young EE, et al: Calcium dependence of toxic cell death: A final common pathway. *Science* 206:700, 1979.

Schwartz AC: Calcium blockers: Status post cardiac arrest. (abs.) *Ann Emerg Med* 12:137, 1983.

Siesjo BK: Cell damage in the brain: A speculative synthesis. *J Cerebral Blood Flow Metabol* 1:155, 1981.

Snyder JV, Nemoto EM, Carrol RG, et al: Global ischemia in dogs: Intracranial pressure, brain blood flow and metabolism. *Stroke* 6:21, 1975.

Stajduhar K, Steinberg R, Safar P: Cerebral blood flow and common carotid artery blood flow during open chest cardiopulmonary resuscitation in dogs. *Anesthesiology* 59(3):A117, 1983.

Steen PA, Newberg LA, Milde JH, et al: Nimodipine improves cerebral blood flow and neurologic recovery after complete cerebral ischemia in the dog. *J Cerebral Blood Flow Metabol* (in press).

Towart R, Perzborn E: Nimodipine inhibits carboxcylic thromboxane-induced contractions of cerebral arteries. *Eur J Pharmacol* 69:213, 1981.

Vaagenes P, Cantadore R, Safar P, et al: Effect of lidoflazine on neurologic outcome after cardiac arrest in dogs. *Anesthesiology* 59(3):A1000, 1983.

Van Neuten JM, Vanhoutte PM: Improvement of tissue perfusion with inhibitors of calcium ion influx. *Biochem Pharmacol* 29:479, 1980.

Van Reempts J, Borgers M: Brain protection: A histological assessment. *J Cerebral Blood Flow Metabol* 2(Suppl. 1):S57, 1982.

Walker J, Bruestle JC, White BC: Perfusion of the cerebral cortex using abdominal counter-pulsation during CPR. *Ann Emerg Med* (in press).

Weinberger LM, Gibbon MH, Gibbon JH: Temporary arrest of the circulation to the central nervous system: I. Physiologic effects. *Arch Neurol Psychiatr* 43:615, 1940.

White BC, Gadzinski DS, Hoehner PJ: Correction of canine cerebral cortical blood flow and vascular resistance after cardiac arrest using flunarizine, a calcium antagonist. *Ann Emerg Med* 11:119, 1982.

White BC, Hoehner PJ, Wilson RF: Mitochondrial oxygen use and ATP synthesis: Kinetic effects of calcium and phosphate modulated by glucocorticoids. *Ann Emerg Med* 9:396, 1980.

White BC, Jackson RE, Joyce KM: Cerebral cortical perfusion during open and closed CPR in dogs. Augmentation with epinephrine. *Ann Emerg Med* (in press).

White BC, Winegar CD, Henderson O, et al: Prolonged hypoperfusion in the cerebral cortex following cardiac arrest and resuscitation in dogs. *Ann Emerg Med* 12:414, 1983.

White BC, Winegar CD, Jackson RE: Cerebral cortical perfusion during and following resuscitation from cardiac arrest in dogs. *Am J Emerg Med* 1:128, 1983.

Winegar CD, Henderson O, White BC: Early amelioration of neurologic deficit by lidoflazine after fifteen minutes of cardiopulmonary arrest in dogs. *Ann Emerg Med* 12:471, 1983.

Yatsu FM, Moss SA: Brain lipid changes following hypoxia. *Stroke* 2:587, 1971.

CHAPTER 3
ADVANCED
AIRWAY SUPPORT

Daniel F. Danzl

INTRODUCTION

"Advanced airway support" refers to those techniques available to establish an airway and ventilate a patient after basic maneuvers have been utilized. Initial airway establishment may include basic maneuvers such as the head tilt, jaw thrust, and neck or chin lift. Foreign body removal may have been attempted by finger sweep or forceps, back blows, and thoracic or abdominal thrusts. Ventilation can be initiated using mouth-to-mouth or mouth-to-mask techniques.

This chapter will review other methods available to accomplish adequate ventilation. The use of oral and nasal airways, the bag-valve-mask unit, and the esophageal obturator airway are discussed. The techniques of oro- and nasotracheal intubation, translaryngeal insufflation, fiberoptic laryngoscopy, and cricothyroidotomy are presented. Use of neuromuscular blockade in the emergency department is discussed, as well.

Lastly, suctioning, extubation, and the use of ventilators in the emergency department are reviewed.

ORAL AND NASAL AIRWAYS

The oral airway, or oropharyngeal tube, lifts the base of the tongue off the hypopharynx. Adult, child, and infant sizes should be available. The oral airway should only be used in patients without protective airway reflexes since it stimulates the gag reflex. In the emergency department, a shortened oral airway functions as a bite block and helps prevent trismic occlusion of an orotracheal tube.

Two components of the triple airway maneuver, mouth opening and the jaw thrust, are accomplished with the oral airway. The third, head extension, is occasionally necessary to free the base of the tongue from the posterior pharyngeal wall.

The tube is placed over the tongue after the mouth is opened. One technique is to insert it after depressing the tongue with a tongue blade. Another method is to insert the tube with the convexity caudad. It is then rotated back after insertion (Fig. 3-1). Improper insertion will increase airway resistance by pushing the base of the tongue backward.

A variation of the oropharyngeal tube is the S tube (Fig. 3-2). It is inserted like an oral airway, and then the victim's head is extended. Ventilation is initiated after the nose is pinched and the flange sealed against the lips.

Nasal airways, or nasopharyngeal tubes, are easier to insert than oral airways and are better tolerated by patients not deeply comatose and with active gag reflexes. Epistaxis is minimized by using a lubricated soft tube with good technique. Insertion of a nasal airway may be a useful temporizing maneuver in patients with seizures, trismus, or cervical spine injuries prior to nasotracheal intubation.

Plastic or soft rubber nasopharyngeal tubes, lubricated with a vasoconstrictor–anesthetic agent, are inserted parallel to the palate into the hypopharynx (Fig. 3-3). The tube is advanced until maximal airflow is heard. If inserted too deeply, the tip may stimulate laryngospasm or enter the esophagus. Patients can be ventilated by bag and mask with the nasal airway in place.

The Bag-Valve-Mask Unit

The bag-valve-mask (BVM) unit includes a self-inflating bag, a nonrebreathing valve, and a face mask. The unit is not easy to use effectively. Depending on the operator's expertise, mouth-to-mask ventilation may be superior. The BVM can allow oxygen delivery during both artificial and spontaneous ventilation.

To deliver 100 percent oxygen, there needs to be a reservoir as large as the bag volume and an oxygen flow rate equaling the respiratory minute volume. The nonrebreathing valve at the mask or endotracheal (ET) tube allows air entry into the lungs with bag compression, while exhaled air exits through a separate port. Various sizes of transparent masks should be available.

Before ventilating the patient, the operator should insert an oro- or nasopharyngeal tube and extend the stable neck. Then the mask is clamped snugly to the face with the thumb and index finger on the mask, with the other fingers pulling the chin upward.

A major advantage of initially using a bag to ventilate via an ET tube is that the operator can better judge pulmonary compliance. Common errors in technique include allowing air leaks around the mask and inadequate tidal volume delivery.

Esophageal Obturator Airway

The esophageal obturator airway (EOA) is an additional ventilatory adjunct when endotracheal intubation is not a viable prehospital option. It helps prevent gastric insufflation and regurgitation

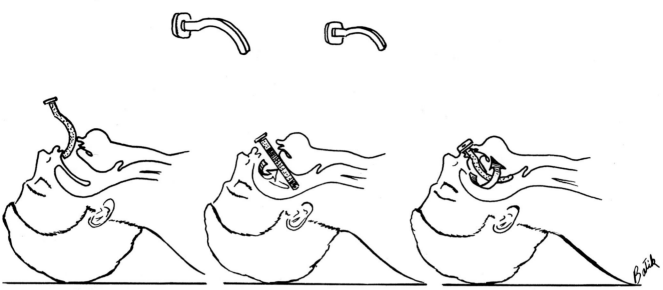

Figure 3-1. Oral airway insertion.

during positive pressure ventilation, but is not a substitute for tracheal intubation.

The major advantage of the EOA is that insertion does not require laryngeal visualization. Thus it can be placed quickly by trained personnel. When necessary, the cervical spine can be held motionless.

The tube should only be inserted in apneic, comatose patients over 16 years of age. Patients with upper airway obstruction,

known esophageal disease, or caustic ingestions require different airway management, as do patients with nasal or intraoral hemorrhage.

The original EOA is a large-bore 34-cm tube with a rounded, occluded distal tip. A snap lock connects the tube through the center of a clear plastic oronasal mask. There are multiple openings in the proximal half of the tube below the mask at the hypopharyngeal level.

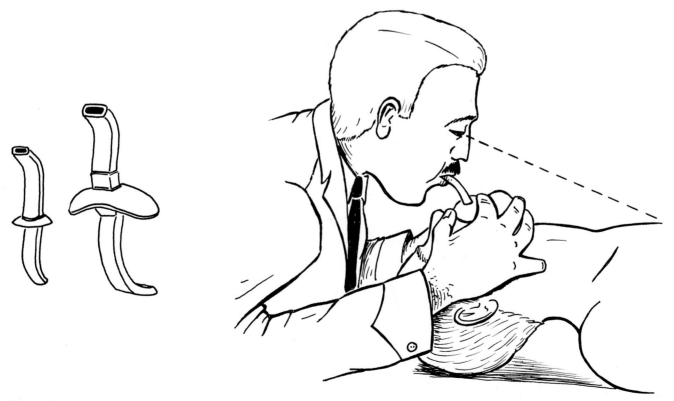

Figure 3-2. Providing ventilation with an S tube.

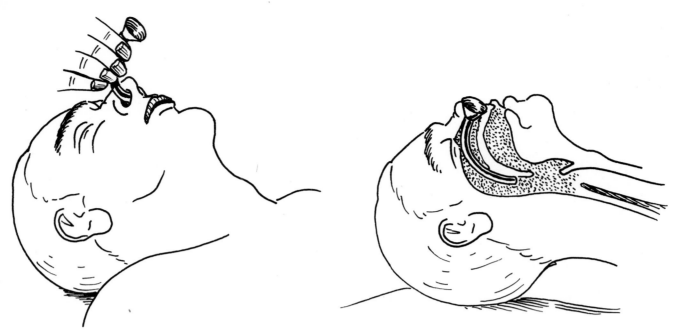

Figure 3-3. Nasopharyngeal tube.

After attaching the mask to the proximal end of the tube, the patient's mandible and tongue are pulled forward with the head held in a neutral position. If a neck injury is excluded, slight neck flexion will decrease the incidence of inadvertent tracheal intubation. The tube is inserted after the distal tip is lubricated (Fig. 3-4). Do not force the tube against an obstruction.

Once the mask is carefully sealed by hand to the patient's face, ventilation is initiated by mouth or bag-valve unit. This forces air into the trachea, the only unobstructed orifice. Auscultation for bilateral breath sounds ensures esophageal placement of the tube. Then the cuff is inflated with 30 mL of air. The cuff must lie below the level of the carina, or partial compression of the trachea will obstruct ventilation.

One variation of Don Michael's original EOA is the esophageal gastric airway. There are two holes in the mask. The esophageal obturator attaches to one, and a nasogastric tube can be passed

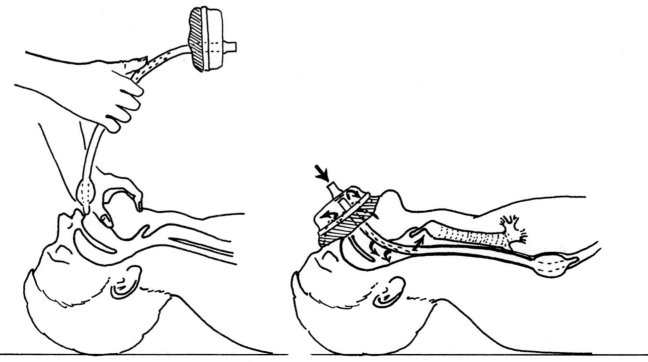

Figure 3-4. Esophageal airway.

down the tube through a valve into the stomach. The unit allows ventilation through the second hole.

Another modification of the EOA, the tracheoesophageal airway, uses a standard ET tube. The ET tube, with a high-volume, low-pressure cuff, is positioned in the esophagus. The modified face mask has two openings, one for the ET tube and the second for oropharyngeal ventilation. The ET tube in the esophagus vents the stomach and facilitates gastric decompression. This should decrease the incidence of esophageal rupture. If the tube is accidentally inserted into the trachea, it is left as a functional ET tube.

The amount of initial oxygenation possible with the EOA using a FI_{O_2} of 100 percent is theoretically similar to that provided with an ET tube. The P_{CO_2}, with EOA ventilation, will be higher. In a field evaluation of EOA, Smith et al. noted a marked improvement in both oxygenation and ventilation after ET intubation.

The most common complication, seen in about 10 percent of EOA insertions, is inadvertent tracheal intubation. Subsequent asphyxia will occur unless this complication is quickly recognized.

The incidence of esophageal rupture is unknown as many of these patients do not receive postmortem examinations. The probable cause of esophageal tears distal to the cuff is increased intragastric pressure against an occluded esophagus during CPR.

Other esophageal injuries may result from direct trauma of the tube, or postemesis (Mallory-Weiss syndrome). If conscious, patients' symptoms may include shortness of breath, chest pain, and dysphagia. Signs include subcutaneous emphysema, pneumomediastinum, Hamman's crunch, and gastrointestinal hemorrhage.

There will be an increased incidence of complications in patients who are not apneic or deeply comatose. They may vomit, aspirate, or develop laryngospasm or supraglottic obstruction.

After the patient arrives in the emergency department, the operator should intubate the trachea with a cuffed ET tube prior to removal of the EOA. Suctioning equipment and assistants should be nearby for the procedure. If a patient with an EOA in place suddenly becomes responsive, with protective airway reflexes, the patient should be rolled on his or her side, the cuff deflated, and the tube removed.

OROTRACHEAL INTUBATION

Introduction

A prerequisite for successful resuscitation is adequate oxygenation. Although adequate oxygenation is obtainable with the preceding techniques, the most reliable means to ensure a patent airway, provide ventilation and oxygenation, and prevent aspiration is endotracheal intubation.

Indications

In the emergency department, endotracheal intubation is indicated in all patients without intact protective airway reflexes. In this clinical setting, attempted continuous monitoring of nonintubated comatose patients is fraught with hazard.

In addition, many conscious patients require emergency intubation. They may be unable to spontaneously clear the airway of secretions, require mechanical ventilation, have aspirated, or have poor laryngeal reflexes.

In apneic or arrested patients with stable cervical spines, orotracheal intubation is the most rapid method to secure the airway.

Technique

While calling for an assistant, the operator should check and arrange the necessary equipment. The appropriate size tube and an additional tube one size smaller should be selected, and the cuff checked for air leaks. Then the distal tube is lubricated with lidocaine jelly. Picking a tube with the proper diameter is essential (see Table 3-1). The typical adult male will require a Magill size 8–10 tube, the female a size 7–9. In children, tube size must be estimated from the diameter of the child's little finger or by checking a chart. Most tubes will require cutting after orotracheal intubation, or they will gradually inch down toward the carina.

Tubes with low-pressure, high-volume cuffs are best for children over 6 years old and adults. Below age 6, the operator should use uncuffed tubes. Thin-walled cuffs may prevent aspiration when properly inflated better than medium-walled cuffs. Since microcirculation to the tracheal mucosa is not impaired until cuff pressures exceed 40 cm water, the operator should attempt to maintain the cuff pressure between 25 to 34 cm water. After nasogastric decompression, the cuff pressure should be deflated to 15 to 20 cm water, or just to the point of eliminating audible air leaks. Cuff overinflation can compromise the ET tube lumen.

The light on the size and type of laryngoscope desired should be tested. The straight Magill blade directly lifts the epiglottis. The curved Macintosh blade rests in the vallecula above the epiglottis, and indirectly lifts it off the larynx by traction on the frenulum (Fig. 3-5). Expertise at intubation with both blades is desirable, since they offer differing advantages, depending on the clinical setting and body habitus. The curved blade may be less traumatic and reflex-stimulating since it does not directly touch the larynx, while allowing more room for adequate visualization during tube placement. The straight blade is mechanically easier in many patients without large central incisors. Selecting the proper size blade greatly facilitates intubation (Table 3-2).

When your equipment is in order, the patient should be placed in the sniffing position. *Note:* The novice laryngoscopist's most common reasons for failure—inadequate equipment preparation and poor patient positioning—occur *prior* to the use of the laryngoscope.

Flexion of the lower neck with extension at the atlantooccipital joint (sniffing position) aligns the oral-pharyngeal-laryngeal axis, allowing a direct view of the larynx. Placing a folded towel or small pillow under the occiput is often helpful (Fig. 3-5).

If possible, the patient should be oxygenated by mask with 100 percent oxygen prior to intubation. The operator begins with the laryngoscope in the left hand and an ET tube or tonsil suction catheter in the right hand. After removal of dentures and any obscuring blood, secretions, or vomitus, the tonsil succor is exchanged for the endotracheal tube and inserted during the same laryngoscopy.

The blade is inserted into the right corner of the patient's mouth. If a curved Macintosh blade is used, the flange will push the tongue to the left side of the oropharynx. If the blade is inserted down the middle, the tongue forces the line of sight posteriorly, resulting in an apparent "anterior larynx."

After visualizing the arytenoids and the epiglottis, the epiglottis

Table 3-1. Approximate Sizes of Endotracheal and Tracheostomy Tubes

Approximate age	Weight (kg)	Orotracheal tubes* ‡ Outside diameter (mm)	French size (Circumference)	Magill sizes	Length of tube (cm)† OT	NT	Suction catheters (French sizes)	‡ Adapters mm ID	Tracheostomy tubes 3 types, sizes Shiley	Aberdeen	Holinger	Approx length (mm)
		14.0	42									
		13.3	40		22–26	29	14					
Adult male		13.0	39									
		12.7	38	10	22–26	29	14					60
(French 34–40)		12.3	37									
		12.0	36		22–26	29	14					
Adult female		11.7	35	9								
		11.3	34		20–24	27	12					60
(French 32–36)		11.0	33									
		10.7	32	8	20–24	27	12					
12–13 yrs.		10.7	32	8	19	25	10	9	6	7.0	6	60
		10.3	31	7	19	25	10	9	6	7.0	6	
10–11 yrs.		10.0	30		18	24	10	9	6	6.0	6	60
		9.7	29	6	18	24	10	9	6	6.0	6	
8–9 yrs.		9.3	28	5½	17	22½	10	8	4	6.0	5	55
		9.0	27	5	17	22½	10	8	4	6.0	5	
6–7 yrs.		8.7	26	4½	15	22	10	7	4	5.0	4	55
		8.3	25	4	15	22	10	7	4	5.0	4	
4–5 yrs.	16–20	8.0	24	3½	14	18½	10	7	4	5.0	·4	50
		7.7	23	3	14	18½	8	7	4	5.0	4	
2–3 yrs.	11–15	7.3	22	2½	13	17	8	6	4	5.0	4	50
		7.0	21	2	13	17	8	6	4	5.0	4	
1–2 yrs.	9–11	6.7	20	1½	12	15½	8	6	3	5.0	3	45
		6.3	19	1	12	15½	8	6	3	5.0	3	
3–12 mos.	5–9	6.0	18		11	14	8	5	2	4.5	3	45
		5.7	17		10	12½	6	5	1	4.0	2	
Newborn–3 mos.	2.5–5	5.3	16	0	10	12	6	5	0	3.5	1	40
		5.0	15		10	11½	6	4	0	3.5	1	
Newborn	2–2.5	4.7	14		9½	10½	6	4	0	3.5	0	30
		4.3	13	00	8	9	6	3	0	3.5	0	
Premature	1–2	4.0	12		8	9	6	3	00		00	<30
		3.7	11		8	9	6	2	00		00	

*For adults and large children, tubes with large-volume soft cuffs are recommended; for children under 6 years of age, uncuffed tubes. For nasotracheal tubes select 1 mm outside diameter (2–3 French size) smaller than for orotracheal intubation.

†The lengths of pediatric orotracheal tubes given here are purposely short, to be used with the adapter within the mouth. OT = orotracheal: NT = nasotracheal.

‡Inside diameter (ID) is 1–4 mm less than outside diameter (OD), depending on wall thickness of tube.

Source: Safar et al: 1981.

is lifted directly with the straight blade or indirectly with the curved blade.

The larynx is exposed by pulling on the handle in the direction it points, that is, 90° to the blade. Cocking the handle back, especially with the straight blade, will fracture incisors.

If the arytenoid cartilages are recognized, one can avoid the most common error, too-deep insertion of the blade. If only the posterior commissure is visible, having an assistant apply pressure on the cricoid (Sellick's maneuver) is helpful. While inserting the

tube, the operator should watch the tip. To avoid esophageal intubation, observe the cuff as it passes completely through the cords.

Attempts at blind passage only invite anoxia. Emergency personnel should always be willing to abort the attempt if visualization of the larynx is not successful, and resume mask ventilation.

With proper technique and practice, malleable blunt-tipped metal or plastic stylets are rarely necessary. If the patient's anatomy requires it, the proximal end of the stylet may be bent 45°, but

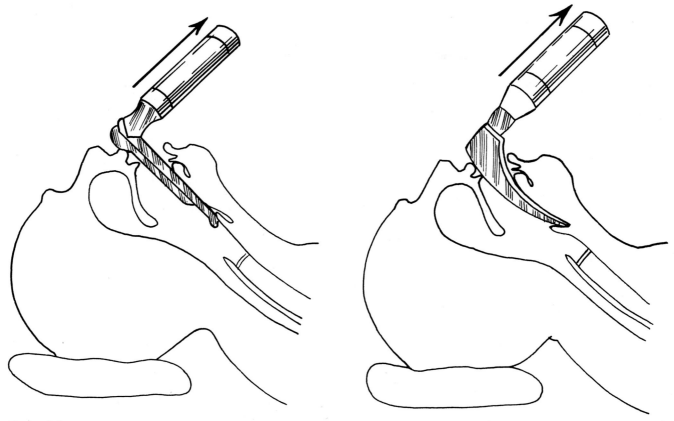

Figure 3-5. Endotracheal intubation using a straight and curved blade.

be certain the tip does not extend beyond the end of the endotracheal tube.

The tube is positioned by palpating its tip at the suprasternal notch, and advancing it 2 to 3 cm. After cuff inflation, the operator inserts an oropharyngeal airway, and auscultates to verify bilateral lung expansion. Inadvertent endobronchial intubation is usually on the right side. The operator then cuts and secures the tube, being careful not to impede cervical venous return with the tape.

Complications

Acute complications, in addition to oral trauma, include lack of recognition of endobronchial or esophageal intubation. The tube may be obstructed by a bulging cuff, secretions, kinking, or biting. The deleterious cardiovascular and intracranial pressure changes occasionally associated with endotracheal intubation may be attenuated with intravenous and topical lidocaine.

While they are uncommon, chronic complications of endotracheal intubations done under emergency conditions do occur, and may be quite debilitating. Arytenoid cartilage displacement, usually on the right, prevents the patient from phonating properly, with a resultant husky voice. Cordal synechiae may develop anteriorly, or commissural stenosis posteriorly. Subglottic stenosis is the most disastrous complication.

Chemical and ischemic mucosal damage may be minimized by using plastic tubes with cuffs properly inflated. Tube motion in the larynx and trachea should be prevented. This usually occurs in combative patients or those on ventilators.

NASOTRACHEAL INTUBATION

Introduction

Nasotracheal intubation is an essential skill allowing a flexible approach to airway management. Prior to the introduction of neuromuscular blockade as an adjunct in anesthesia, difficulties in

Table 3-2. Laryngoscope Blades

| | Straight Blade | | Curved Blade | |
Size	Length (mm)	Example	Length (mm)	Example
Adult (large)	190	Flagg no. 4	158	Macintosh no. 4
Adult (medium)	160	Flagg no. 3	130	Macintosh no. 3
Child (2–9 yrs.)	133	Flagg no. 2	108	Macintosh no. 2
Child (3 mo.–2 yrs.)	115	Wis-Hipple no. 1J	100	Macintosh no. 1
Infant (under 3 mo.)	102	Flagg no. 1, Miller Infant		
Premature	75	Miller Premature		

Source: Safar et al: 1981.

successful and atraumatic visualization of the larynx were overcome by developing expertise in blind nasotracheal intubation.
However, as was noted in a recent editorial, ''Blind nasotracheal
intubation—the lost art,'' it must be practised.

Airway management in the emergency department presents unique
challenges. The success rate for a prospective series of 300 patients by Danzl and Thomas managed with blind nasotracheal
intubation in the emergency department was 92 percent.

Technique

Spray both nares with a topical vasoconstrictor-anesthetic, then
select a cuffed endotracheal tube 1 mm in size smaller than that
optimal for oral intubation. Advance the tube, lubricated with
lidocaine jelly, along the nasal floor on the more patent side. If
the nares appear equal, initially try the right side. Having the bevel
face the septum helps prevent abrasions of Kiesselbach's plexus.
Steady, gentle pressure, or slow rotation of the tube usually by-
passes small obstructions. If the right side is impassible, attempt
the other side before selecting a tube $\frac{1}{2}$ mm in size smaller.

In patients with intact, protective airway reflexes, translaryngeal
anesthesia may facilitate intubation. After palpating the superior
border of the cricoid cartilage in the midline, puncture the cricothyroid membrane with a 22–25 gauge $\frac{1}{2}$ to 1" needle on a 3 to
5 mL syringe (Fig. 3-6). The needle should be perpendicular to
the membrane in the midline, with the point of injection just
cranial to the cricoid cartilage. After aspirating air, swiftly inject
1.5 to 2.0 mL of 4% lidocaine (sterile for injection), and press
the site firmly with a finger for a few seconds.

An assistant can apply cervical traction to the patient's head,
and initially maintain it in a neutral or slightly extended position.
Stand to the side of the patient, with one hand on the tube, and
with the thumb and index finger of the other hand straddling the
larynx. Advance the tube while rotating it medially 15 to 30°,
until you hear maximal airflow through the tube. Then gently but
swiftly advance the tube during early inspiration. Entrance into

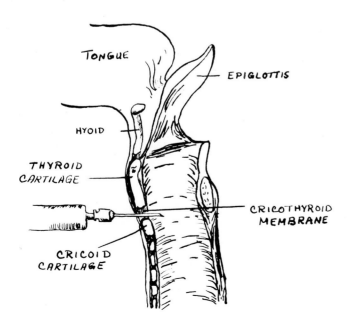

Figure 3-6. Cricothyroid puncture.

the larynx may initiate a slight cough, and most expired air should
exit through the tube despite the cuff being uninflated.

Advancement toward the carina can be observed externally.
Auscultate to verify bilateral lung expansion and cuff inflation.
Secretions in the tube should be removed prior to positive pressure
ventilation. The tube is easily secured and well tolerated.

If you are unsuccessful, carefully inspect the neck to determine
the malposition of the tube. Most commonly, it is in the pyriform
fossa on the same side as the nares used. A bulge will be seen
and palpated laterally. Withdraw the tube into the retropharynx
until breath sounds are again heard. Redirect while manually displacing the larynx toward the bulge. If there is no contraindication,
flexion and rotation of the neck to the ipsilateral side often helps
while rotating the tube medially.

The other common misplacement is posterior in the esophagus.
There will be no breath sounds through the tube, and the trachea
will be elevated slightly. Attempt redirection after extending the
patient's head and performance of Sellick's maneuver. If occult
cervical spine pathology is suspected, use a tube with directional
tip control (Endotrol) or a fiberoptic laryngoscope.

Rarely, the tip of the tube lies anteriorly between the epiglottis
and base of the tongue. A supralaryngeal bulge will be visible.
Redirect after flexing the stable neck. If the tube rests on the vocal
cords, shrill, turbulent air noises will be heard. Rotate the tube
slightly to realign the bevel with the cords, or squirt 4% lidocaine
down the tube onto the cords.

Indications

Nasal intubation is helpful in situations where laryngoscopy is
difficult, neuromuscular blockade hazardous, or cricothyroidotomy unnecessary.

Emergency department patients may present with trismus from
seizures, facial trauma, infection, tetanus, or decorticate-decere-
brate rigidity. It may be impossible to align the oral-pharyngeal-
laryngeal axis in patients with arthritis, masseter spasm, temporomandibular dislocation, or prior oral surgical procedures. Agitated
patients, or those with a peculiar body habitus may be impossible
to intubate orally.

Nasal intubation with a fiberoptic laryngoscope may be required
for neoplastic lesions obstructing the pharynx, Ludwig's angina,
peritonsillar abscess, and epiglottitis. If the radiographic status of
the neck in a traumatized patient is unknown, the nasal route is
an alternative to cricothyroidotomy or translaryngeal insufflation.

Nasotracheal tubes, in addition to being better tolerated by patients than oral tubes, are less traumatic to the tracheal mucosa
since there is less intratracheal tube movement when the head
moves.

Contraindications

Nasal and some midface fractures and hemostatic disorders are
relative contraindications to nasotracheal intubation. Patients with
basilar skull fractures should have the tube removed electively
after the patient is stabilized, since it may contribute to the later
development of meningitis or sinusitis.

Severe traumatic intraoral hemorrhage may necessitate orotracheal intubation or cricothyroidotomy. Nasotracheal intubation
should not be done blindly in patients with acute epiglottitis. If
the nares will only accommodate a 7-mm tube, traumatized pa-

tients requiring fiberoptic bronchoscopy will require reintubation in the operating room.

Translaryngeal anesthesia is contraindicated if the landmarks are obscured by thyroid or tumor impingement on the cricothyroid membrane, or in obese or combative patients.

Complications

Serious complications of nasotracheal intubation are quite rare. In the Deane series of 1187 patients, there was no permanent laryngeal damage.

Epistaxis is seen with inadequate topical vasoconstriction, excessive tube size, poor technique, or anatomic defects. Excessive force can damage the nasal septum or turbinates. The tube should be suctioned to avoid thrombotic occlusion, and the cuff rechecked for a potential puncture by a turbinate.

There are unusual reports of retropharyngeal lacerations, nasal necrosis, and maxillary sinusitis. With any route of intubation, one may see stridor on extubation, tube obstruction or displacement, subglottic stenosis or edema, cuff overinflation, or tracheobronchitis.

TRANSLARYNGEAL INSUFFLATION

Translaryngeal positive pressure ventilation offers a temporizing, alternative approach to airway obstruction when surgical cricothy-

roidotomy is not feasible. It is not a substitute for airway control with a cuffed tube.

The equipment required for this technique is readily available in emergency departments. The high-pressure oxygen source is provided by either a 50-psi wall source coupled to a flow meter, or an oxygen tank with high-pressure tubing and a push button release valve. The pop-off valve should be set at 50 cm water for adults, and 25 to 30 cm water for small children to avoid barotrauma.

The technique in adults involves puncturing the inferior aspect of the cricothyroid membrane at a caudal angle with a 12–14 gauge over-the-needle plastic catheter. After removing the needle and advancing the catheter toward the carina, the catheter is attached via high-pressure tubing to a high-pressure oxygen source (25 to 50 psi) (Fig. 3-7). The patient is ventilated for approximately 1 to 2 full seconds, or until the chest begins to rise. The valve is then released for 4 to 5 s to allow exhalation. If exhalation is inadequate, as will occur with complete glottic obstruction, a second catheter with a three-way stopcock should be inserted next to the first one. The stopcock is closed during inspiration, and open during exhalation. A technically easier alternative is to intermittently cover one of the two catheters with a finger. Begin ventilation with the oxygen source set at 25 psi until correct catheter placement is assured. Then turn it up to 50 psi.

Any material obstructing the airway might be disimpacted by the positive airway pressure from below. Translaryngeal catheter ventilation is also a temporizing maneuver to consider in cervically traumatized patients who cannot be intubated nasotracheally.

Figure 3-7. Translaryngeal ventilation.

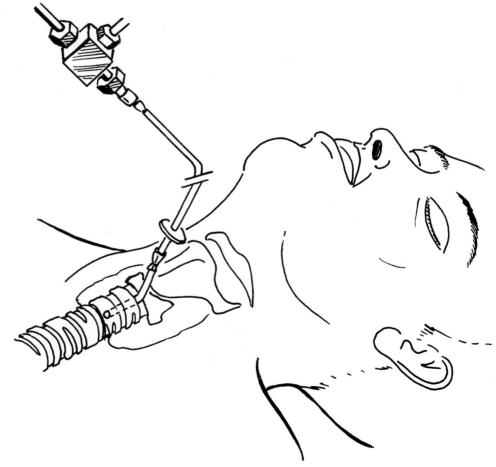

Complications

The complications of this technique include those mentioned occurring with puncture of the cricothyroid membrane. In addition, interstitial oxygen insufflation into tissue planes is possible if the catheter is misplaced or after lung barotrauma. Tearing the anterior wall of the esophagus, or pneumothorax with overzealous insufflation is possible. It is not known if jet ventilation is harmful to tracheobronchial mucosa. Upper airway secretions can be exsufflated, but direct suctioning is not possible.

High-frequency jet ventilation via percutaneous translaryngeal catheters has also been reported for emergency ventilation. The frequencies are 100 to 500 per minute, using tidal volumes less than the dead space. The advantages of this approach are that the jet ventilators are compact and portable, there is no need to synchronize respirations, and the low airway pressure is unlikely to induce barotrauma. Double-lumen tubes reaching variable distances from the carina are being developed to facilitate exhalation.

FIBEROPTIC LARYNGOSCOPE

The flexible fiberoptic laryngoscope is a valuable adjunct in airway management (Fig. 3-8). It is designed to allow direct visualization of laryngeal structures and possible obstructions or injuries during difficult intubations.

Begin by focusing the eyepiece and lubricating the flexible shaft. Immerse the lens at the tip of the laryngoscope in warm water to prevent fogging.

Remove the adaptor for an ET tube size 7.0 mm or larger. Then slip the ET tube over the shaft up to the handle. The distal end of the laryngoscope must extend beyond the end of the ET tube. Hold the laryngoscope with the left hand, and control the tip

deflection while advancing it through the cords. The laryngoscope will function as a stylet for the tube. After the laryngoscope is in the trachea, advance the ET tube and remove the laryngoscope.

CRICOTHYROIDOTOMY

Cricothyroidotomy is an emergency procedure which may be lifesaving as a last resort in establishing an airway. It is an essential psychomotor skill, with far fewer and less serious complications than emergency tracheostomy.

Cricothyroidotomy was initially condemned in 1921 by Chevalier Jackson for its allegedly high incidence of subglottic stenosis. Most of the patients in this preantibiotic era study had high-pressure tubes placed in the setting of acute laryngeal disease. Unfortunately, the technique was not reevaluated until recently. In Brantigan and Grow's series of 655 patients with cricothyroidotomy for respiratory management, the complication rate was 6.1 percent. Chronic subglottic stenosis did not occur.

The complication rate for patients with emergency cricothyroidotomies varies widely. In Boyd's series of 147 patients undergoing the procedure, the complication rate was 8.6 percent. In McGill's series of 38 cricothyroidotomies performed in the emergency department, the complication rate was 32 percent. Nevertheless, in several large series of tracheostomies, the complication rate ranges from 28 to 65 percent, and they are of greater severity.

Indications

Indications for immediate cricothyroidotomy include severe, ongoing tracheobronchial hemorrhage, massive midfacial trauma, and inability to control the airway with the usual less invasive

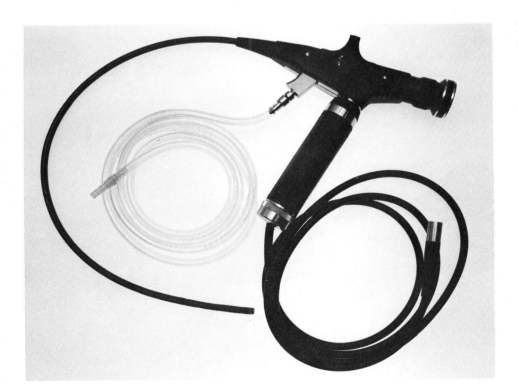

Figure 3-8. Fiberoptic laryngoscope.

maneuvers. (Less invasive procedures may be contraindicated or impossible with mechanical upper airway obstruction, facial or cervical trauma, uncontrollable oral hemorrhage, or for no obvious reason.)

Further clinical situations requiring cricothyroidotomy include oral or pharyngeal edema from infection, anaphylaxis, or chemical inhalation injuries. Patients with anatomical variants, occult foreign bodies, or obstructing lesions may be impossible to intubate.

Removal of blood or vomitus may not be possible in patients with trismus or masseter spasm. In addition, cricothyroidotomy may be required if blind or fiberoptic nasotracheal intubation is unsuccessful. Lastly, prolonged unsuccessful attempts at nasotracheal intubation may lead to progressive hypoxia.

Contraindications

This technique should not be used on patients who can be safely intubated orally or nasally.

Emergency cricothyroidotomy is relatively contraindicated in the presence of acute laryngeal disease due to trauma or infection. Tracheostomy may be required in patients who develop airway obstruction after removal of an endotracheal tube in place over 72 h.

In small children under 10 years of age, a 12–14 gauge catheter over the needle is safer than a formal cricothyroidotomy or tracheostomy.

Since this is a technique of last resort, a hemorrhagic disorder is not an absolute contraindication. Hemostatis is certainly easier to achieve than with a tracheostomy.

The patient must be completely immobilized because the incision site is just below the vocal cords and above the thyroid isthmus. The esophagus is posterior, and the carotid and jugular vessels lateral to the incision.

Technique

Instruments required for emergency cricothyroidotomy include a curved Mayo scissors, a dilator, a tracheal hook, and a no. 15 scalpel blade.

Manual cervical traction is applied to the immobilized patient by an assistant. After identifying the anatomical landmarks and palpating the cricothyroid membrane, a vertical 2-cm incision is made through the skin with the blade. Some authors recommend puncturing the membrane with just a needle, which may provide a temporizing airway and guide for the incision. The blade is then rotated to make a horizontal stab through the inferior aspect of the membrane, after it has been repalpated. With the blade left in the larynx, scissors points are inserted beside the blade and spread horizontally. Then the scalpel is removed, and a dilator or hemostat inserted and opened (Fig. 3-9). If blunt scissors are unavailable, use the blunt end of the scalpel. The scissors are then removed. The largest tracheotomy tube which doesn't injure the larynx is placed, usually a no. 4 Shiley in adults (outer diameter 8.5 mm).

The cuff is then inflated, and the tube securely tied. Alternatively, a small cuffed (size 5) endotracheal tube may be inserted. It should be removed after locating a curved tracheotomy tube, which is less traumatic to the posterior tracheal wall.

Vertical skin incisions decrease the incidence of marginal vessel hemorrhage. The cricothyroid membrane should be punctured inferiorly and at a caudal angle, since the cricothyroid arteries anastamose superiorly over the membrane. A tracheal hook helps stabilize the larynx in some patients. Several ''can-opener'' cricothyroidotomy devices are available, but there is insufficient clinical experience reported to comment on their safety.

In patients with massive neck swelling, the hemorrhage, subcutaneous emphysema, edema, or fat may make identification of normal landmarks impossible. In such cases, a more formal cutdown or tracheostomy may be necessary.

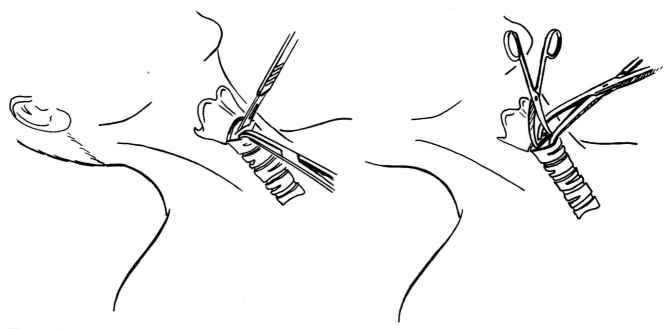

Figure 3-9. Emergency cricothyroidotomy.

Complications

Immediate complications of emergency cricothyroidotomy include prolonged execution time, excessive hemorrhage, aspiration, and unsuccessful or incorrect tube placement. The most common misplacement is superior to the thyroid cartilage through the thyrohyoid membrane. Inferior tracheotomy placement has also been reported.

Other potential complications include mediastinal or subcutaneous emphysema, or creation of a false passage into the trachea. Adjacent vascular, neural, endocrine, esophageal, or pulmonary structures may be injured.

Long-term complications include dysphonia from thyroid cartilage fractures, transient dysphagia, or voice changes. Infection and perichondritis may occur. Innominate artery erosion or pneumothorax, serious complications of tracheostomy, have not been reported with this technique.

NEUROMUSCULAR BLOCKADE

The use of muscle relaxants to facilitate endotracheal intubation in the emergency department should generally be avoided. Usually the airway can be secured with the previously mentioned techniques.

Neuromuscular blockade should never be attempted unless personnel experienced in its use and the equipment necessary for rapid sequence induction ("crash intubation") are available.

However, there are patients whose clinical conditions require neuromuscular blockade to facilitate mechanical ventilation. Patients with status asthmaticus or status epilepticus, drug-induced seizures, or tetanic spasms from clostridial infection or strychnine may require blockade. Patients ventilated with positive end-expiratory pressure for adult respiratory distress syndrome or pulmonary edema may benefit from paralysis.

The three most commonly used agents are succinylcholine (Anectine), curare, and pancuronium bromide (Pavulon). Agents such as succinylcholine mimic acetylcholine, allowing persistent depolarization at the neuromuscular end plate. Nondepolarizing agents including curare and pancuronium compete with acetylcholine at the end plate.

The dose of succinylcholine is 1.0 mg/kg intravenously for patients over 12 years old, and 2.0 mg/kg for younger children. Repetitive doses with half that amount are given every 5 min if necessary. When the patient is alert, presedation is advised. Atropine 0.5 to 1.0 mg IV can be given a few minutes prior to injection of succinylcholine to attenuate its vagal side effects. After prolonged depolarization, a desensitization block may develop, requiring treatment with neostigmine.

Because of its rapid onset and short duration of action, succinylcholine is preferable when the indication for paralysis is inability to secure the airway.

There are many potential complications when using succinylcholine. Initial muscle fasciculations, with a resultant increase in intragastric pressure, may result in aspiration. Pretreatment with a subparalytic dose of pancuronium can prevent fasciculations. Vagal stimulation and its sequelae occur.

The serum potassium will rise an average 0.5 mEq/L in normal patients. However, those patients with muscle trauma, burns, central nervous or upper motor neuron disorders, renal failure, or hyperkalemia from any cause are at greater risk. Rarely, prolonged apnea will be seen in patients with an atypical pseudocholinesterase. Acute malignant hyperthermia can be precipitated in genetically susceptible patients.

Curare and pancuronium are the nondepolarizing agents which compete with acetylcholine at the motor end plate. Pancuronium is given at a dose of 0.05 mg/kg IV. Its onset of action is delayed for several minutes. The blockade is reversible with neostigmine (maximum dose 2.5 mg), but should not be attempted for approximately 30 min when some recovery from paralysis is seen.

For prolonged paralysis to facilitate ventilation, pancuronium is superior to succinylcholine because it has fewer cardiovascular side effects.

Emergency physicians using muscle relaxants must be aware of their complex pharmacology, and have the equipment and expertise to deal with potential side effects.

SUCTIONING

Numerous conditions render patients unable to clear tracheal secretions. A rigid-tip plastic tonsil succor should be used for large quantities of oropharyngeal secretions, including blood and vomitus. To suction the nasopharynx and tracheobronchial tree, use a well-lubricated, soft, curved-tip catheter. Straight catheters will usually pass into the right mainstem bronchus. If a curved-tip catheter is available, turning the head to the right in addition to catheter rotation will facilitate passage into the left bronchus.

Select a suction catheter of a size no larger than half the diameter of the tube to be suctioned. This will prevent pulmonic collapse from insufficient ventilation during suctioning. Oxygenate the patient before and after suctioning. Insert the catheter without suctioning, and then remove, suctioning with rotation, over 10 to 15 s.

Complications of suctioning include hypoxia, cardiac arrhythmias, hypotension, pulmonic collapse, and direct mucosal injury. The magnitude of the intracranial pressure increase during endotracheal suctioning may be related to the increase in intrathoracic pressure with coughing. Topical laryngotracheal or translaryngeal lidocaine may be helpful. In a study of nonparalyzed head-injured patients, IV lidocaine did not block the increase in intracranial pressure with tracheal stimulation.

EXTUBATION

Emergency department extubations are potentially hazardous. While patients are recovering their protective airway reflexes, they may "fight" the tube. Occasionally squirting 1 to 2 mL of 4% lidocaine (sterile for injection) down the endotracheal tube will decrease bucking. Absorption of lidocaine via the airway yields sustained levels, while the maximum serum level is lower than that from an equivalent intravenous dose.

Prior to extubation, rule out metabolic or circulatory abnormalities. Check for respiratory insufficiency. On command, the patient should have an inspiratory capacity of 15 mL/kg. There should be no retractions, and the grip firm. Prior nasogastric decompression is advised.

Arrange all necessary equipment and personnel to treat any acute complications. After suctioning secretions, assure adequate oxygenation of the patient with 100 percent oxygen. Explain the procedure to the patient. Ventilate with positive pressure using the bag-valve-mask unit to exsufflate secretions while the cuff is deflated. At the end of a deep inspiration, remove the tube and oxygenate by mask.

Observe the patient closely for stridor. Postextubation laryngospasm is initially treated with oxygen by positive pressure. If necessary, nebulized racemic epinephrine (0.5 mL 2.25% in 4 mL saline) often helps. Rarely, neuromuscular blockade to facilitate reintubation or cricothyroidotomy is necessary.

VENTILATORS

Pressure-cycled mechanical ventilators perform very poorly during resuscitations. When the chest is compressed, the inspiratory cycle is terminated before an adequate tidal volume has been delivered. Volume-cycled mechanical ventilators are often difficult to coordinate with chest compressions.

However, manually triggered oxygen-powered breathing devices with valves (Flynn, Elder, or Robertshaw) allow coordinated immediate positive pressure ventilation. The valve should have a safety pop-off, which is usually set at 50 cm water for adults and 25 to 30 cm water for children over 12. The high pressure may be hazardous to smaller children. These devices have a manual trigger button, which is released after the chest rises. The oxygen source should be capable of immediately delivering a flow rate of 100 liters per minute. Although the oxygen is not humidified, it is intended for short-term use only.

Spontaneously breathing patients can trigger the sensitive demand valve by inhaling. The FI_{O_2} is adjustable by way of the flow rates delivered despite the respiratory rate. Some devices can be set on an inhalation mode, constantly delivering the flow rate desired. This is not affected by the patient's spontaneous inspirations.

SUMMARY

Emergency physicians should be experts in the knowledge and performance of the psychomotor skills reviewed in this chapter.

Advanced airway support is the initial and critical step in all resuscitations. Mastery of these techniques allows a successful flexible approach to airway management.

BIBLIOGRAPHY

American College of Surgeons Committee on Trauma: Advanced Trauma Life Support Course. Lincoln, Neb., American College of Surgeons, 1980.

Baraka A: Blind nasotracheal intubation—the lost art. *MEJ Anaesth* 5:3, 1978.

Bernhard WN, Cottrell JE, Sivakumaranc C, et al: Adjustment of intracuff pressure to prevent aspiration. *Anesthesiology* 50:363–366, 1979.

Boster SR, Danzl DF, Madden RJ, et al: Translaryngeal adsorption of lidocaine. *Ann Emerg Med* 11:461–64, 1982.

Boyd AD, Conlan AA, Spencer FC: A clinical evaluation of cricothyroidotomy. *Surg Gynecol Obstet* 149:365–368, 1979.

Brantigan CO, Grow JB: Cricothyroidotomy: Elective use in respiratory problems requiring tracheotomy. *J Thorac Cardiovasc Surg* 71:72–80, 1976.

Danzl DF, Thomas DM: Nasotracheal intubations in the emergency department. *Crit Care Med* 8:677–682, 1980.

Deane RS, Shinozaki T, Morgan JG: An evaluation of the cuff characteristics and incidence of laryngeal complications using a new nasotracheal tube in prolonged intubations. *J Trauma* 17:311–314, 1977.

DeGarmo BH, Dronen S: Pharmacology and clinical use of neuromuscular blocking agents. *Ann Emerg Med* 12:48–55, 1983.

Don Michael TA, Lambert EH, Mehran A: Mouth to lung airway for cardiac resuscitation. *Lancet* 2:1329, 1968.

Gallagher TJ, Klain MM, Carlon GC: Present status of high frequency ventilation. *Crit Care Med* 10:613–617, 1982.

Greisz H, Qvarntrom O, Willen R: Elective cricothyroidotomy: A clinical and histopathological study. *Crit Care Med* 10:387–389, 1982.

Klain M, Smith RB: High frequency percutaneous translaryngeal jet ventilation. *Crit Care Med* 5:280–287, 1977.

Kress TD, Balasubranmaniam S: Cricothyroidotomy. *Ann Emerg Med* 11:197–201, 1982.

McGill J, Clinton JE, Ruiz E: Cricothyrotomy in the emergency department. *Ann Emerg Med* 11:361–364, 1982.

Meislin HW: The esophageal obturator airway: A study of respiratory effectiveness. *Ann Emerg Med* 9:54–59, 1980.

Pilcher DB, DeMeules JE: Esophageal perforation following use of esophageal airway. *Chest* 69:377–380, 1976.

Roizen MF, Feeley TW: Pancuronium bromide. *Ann Intern Med* 88:64–68, 1978.

Safar P, Asmund A, Leardal S: *Cardiopulmonary Cerebral Resuscitation.* Philadelphia, Saunders, 1981.

Simon RR, Brenner BE, Rosen MA: Emergency cricothyroidotomy in the patient with massive neck swelling. Part 2: Clinical aspects. *Crit Care Med* 11:119–123, 1983.

Smith JP, Bodai BI, Aubourg R, et al: A field evaluation of the esophageal obturator airway. *J Trauma* 23:317–321, 1983.

White PF, Schlobohm RM, Pitts LH, et al: A randomized study of drugs for preventing increases in intracranial pressure during endotracheal suctioning. *Anesthesiology* 57:242–244, 1982.

CHAPTER 4
VENOUS ACCESS

Robert H. Dailey

The ability to quickly establish access to the venous circulation is one of the single most crucial abilities needed by the emergency physician for administration of drugs, restoration of blood volume, or for monitoring central venous pressure. The successful accomplishment of these goals is the objective of this chapter.

Sites (Figs. 4-1 and 4-2)

The body abounds with accessible veins. Those of the arms are generally most convenient and easily catheterized. The veins in the legs are generally avoided because of greater technical difficulty and the chance of producing dangerous phlebitis. Deep vein cannulations of the trunk are invasive and generally reserved for central venous pressure (CVP) monitoring. A brief commentary on advantages and disadvantages of each is warranted here.

The cephalic vein, both in the forearm and upper arm, is large, constant, and straight; it is thus easily catheterized and does not need armboard stabilization thereafter; it is the vein of choice for routine circumstances. Veins of the hand are usually accessible even in obese persons but are short, tortuous, and more painful to catheterize and difficult to stabilize. Veins other than the cephalic in the forearm are often convenient. Veins in the antecubital fossa are excellent in emergency situations because of their large size and ease of catheterization. However, an armboard is necessary to prevent catheter kinking or dislodgment from normal elbow mobility. The basilic vein in the upper arm is most often not visible but is large-bore, and with practice can often be successfully catheterized blindly. However, there is a high incidence of accidental puncture of the brachial artery by the inexperienced operator.

Veins in the leg are more often accessed by cutdown. Most common is the superficial saphenous vein at the ankle: a large, constant, and superficial vein easily isolated and cannulated. The proximal (great) saphenous vein in the thigh is a good alternative for a cutdown. It is best cut down upon 2 in below the inguinal ligament at the junction of the medial and middle third of the thigh with the patient lying supine. The deep femoral vein is accessed percutaneously, immediately medial to the femoral artery, or in the pulseless patient, again at approximately the junction of the median and middle third of the inguinal ligament. Catheters can be advanced from both the proximal saphenous and the femoral vein into the right atrium for central venous pressure monitoring.

The external jugular vein is very constant in both adults and children. It is easily distended with Valsalva or Trendelenburg maneuvers, but because of poor subcutaneous support it is often technically difficult to catheterize. Internal jugular and subclavian catheterizations are used for central venous pressure monitoring and will be discussed in that section. Veins of the superficial abdomen, the scalp, the penis, and other unusual sites may be attempted under difficult circumstances when invasive procedures are not warranted and time permits.

Technique Considerations

Venous access, whether percutaneous or cutdown, is a surgical procedure and carries with it a high risk of infection which can be fatal (septic thrombophlebitis). Accordingly, insertion of catheters should always be preceded by a surgical prep, preferably with Betadine. When considering venous access, a brief survey of all the patient's veins should be made, and the one most appropriate and easily accessible chosen. Materials should be readied beforehand and necessary help available. If the veins are generally poor, they can often be enlarged and made more visible by 5 min of hot, moist compresses; this time delay is often well repaid by forestalling multiple unsuccessful and painful punctures. A little Betadine ointment should be placed at the skin puncture site, and a surgical dressing applied. If the patient is uncooperative or if the stability of the site otherwise endangered, a gentle circumferential occlusive taping may be necessary, with the intravenous line looped through the dressing in such a fashion as to avoid direct tugging on the IV site itself. When pertinent (as with gastrointestinal bleeding), the size of the IV catheter should be written on the tape dressing.

Equipment is all-important in venous access. Formerly, steel needles, both disposable and nondisposable, were used; however, their inevitable infiltration has led to the common acceptance of catheters for any but the shortest term therapy, despite the danger of infection. Catheters should be chosen for their ease of insertion, flow rate, and cost. The most commonly used catheters are those placed over needles. These are used for routine extremity intravenous therapy and are adequate for 90 percent of situations.

Flow Rates

In resuscitation of severely hypovolemic patients, flow rates become all-important. Flow is a function of the fourth power of the radius of the tube lumen, and thus the internal diameter of any

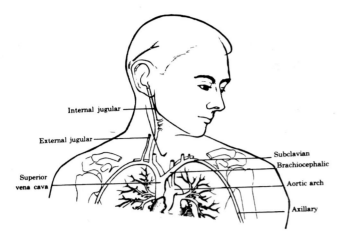

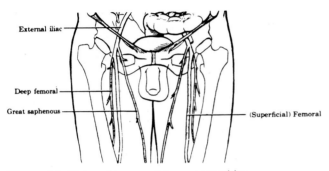

Figure 4-1. Veins of torso and lower extremities.

cells. The resultant decreased viscosity of the blood cells markedly increases flow. For high volume of either blood or crystalloid only blood administration set tubing should be used, since online micropore filters, stopcocks, and one-way valves on intravenous tubing will severely decrease flow rate.

CENTRAL VENOUS PRESSURE CATHETERIZATION AND MONITORING

The use of CVP catheters and monitoring is now a well-established practice in emergency medicine. Indications include monitoring of rapidly changing intravascular volume (e.g., gastrointestinal bleeding, major trauma, etc.), rapid delivery of drugs to the heart (e.g., CPR), monitoring fluid administration in severe closed head injuries, and venous access when peripheral veins are not available (secondary to drug abuse, old cutdowns, or severe peripheral vascular constriction).

catheter is the single most crucial factor. In the past, recommendations for intravenous therapy of exsanguinating patients have been vague, e.g., "large-bore IVs should be started at multiple sites." We need no longer be vague. The now-standard no. 8 French catheter sheath (see below) used with a pressure infusion cuff (Fig. 4-3) around the intravenous bag can deliver almost a liter of crystalloid per minute. Recently a no. 14 French catheter (4.5-mm internal diameter) has been devised which can deliver up to 2 liters a minute! Thus a single such catheter can provide for all but the most exceptional exsanguinating circumstance. Care must be exercised to simultaneously monitor central venous pressure when using such a high-flow device to avoid acute volume overload!

Both functions (volume repletion and CVP monitoring) can be served by a Y-arm catheter sheath inserted percutaneously into the femoral vein; with the no. 8 French catheter the patient can be volume repleted from pulselessness to a palpable pulse and blood pressure. Then a smaller monitoring catheter can be inserted through the catheter diaphragm into the right atrium for CVP measurement (with continued volume repletion still possible through the Y arm). *Note:* Femoral catheters should be left in place no longer than 48 h, since infection can and will produce catastrophic iliofemoral thrombophlebitis. (With proper sterile precautions and the use of silastic catheters, the deep femoral system has been successfully used on a long-term basis.)

The use of the pressure infusion cuff has been shown to increase flow 2 to 3 times and is superior to online hand-pumped bulbs (Fig. 4-4). For administration of packed cells, speed of delivery is enhanced by rapid addition of saline solution to the packed

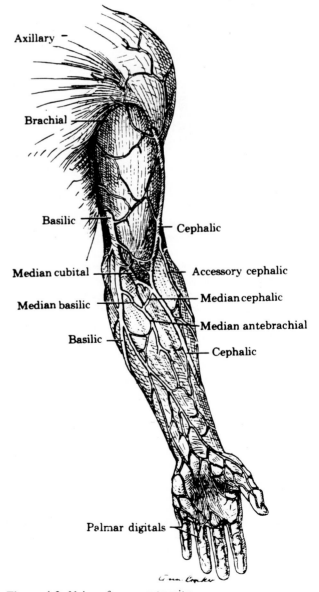

Figure 4-2. Veins of upper extremity.

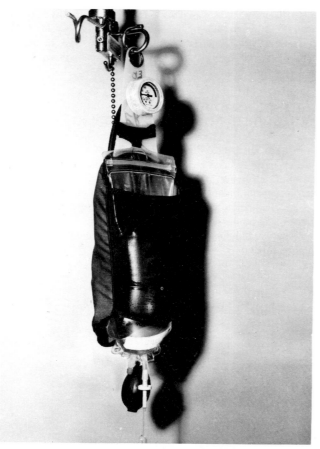

Figure 4-3. Pressure infusion cuff.

Central venous pressure is a dynamic reflection of several factors: (1) right ventricular function, (2) circulating blood volume, (3) total venous resistance, and (4) intrathoracic pressure. It is thus basically *a guide to right ventricular capacity and need for volume replacement* and gives only inferential evidence for each of the above four factors. With acute changes in left ventricular function, measurements of pulmonary wedge pressure (by Swan-Ganz catheter) are mandatory.

Sites and Techniques for Central Venous Pressure Catheter Insertion

Peripheral Sites

Peripheral sites are noninvasive and thus safe; however, they often require cutdowns, and deliver a low flow with normal-sized catheters due to the catheter's considerable length. Peripheral sites also have a frequent failure rate due to catheter malposition and kinking. In the arm the brachial-basilic system must be used since catheters inserted into the cephalic system consistently become "lost" in a plexus of veins at the shoulder, and so will not commonly pass into the central circulation. Smooth passage and correct tip positioning are aided if the patient is in the sitting position with the head angulated sharply toward the catheterized arm, abduction of that arm, and wire-guiding of the catheter (see below). The external jugular vein is becoming increasingly popular now,

since J wire-guided catheters pass centrally in 75 to 90 percent of cases.

The femoral vein has been mentioned above.

Central Sites

Central sites are not as safe as peripheral sites since the techniques are blind and invasive. Complications or failure increase in direct proportion to the inexperience of the operator, lack of direct supervision, and ignorance of anatomy. Strict aseptic surgical technique will considerably lower incidence of sepsis. No single technique is superior in all cases. When severe hypovolemia is suspected, volume repletion should precede these invasive techniques, since the central veins will be collapsed; under these circumstances complications such as pneumothorax most frequently occur.

Anatomy

A brief review of anatomy is warranted (Figs. 4-1 and 4-5). The major veins of the upper thorax are deeply and centrally placed and well protected by clavicles, sternum, and strap muscles. The internal jugular veins join the subclavian veins to form the brachiocephalics (innominates), which in turn join to become the superior vena cava. The sternocleidomastoid muscle attaches by two heads to both the sternum and clavicle, and the triangle formed by these two heads and the clavicle directly overlies the internal jugular vein. The right internal jugular has a straight course into

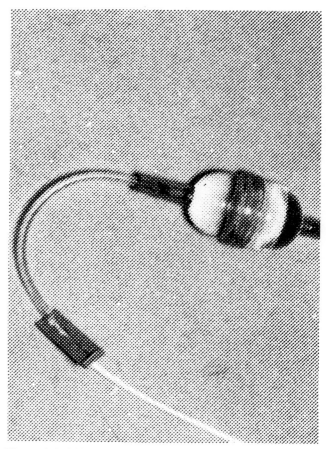

Figure 4-4. Abbott online hand pump bulb. (From Dula et al.)

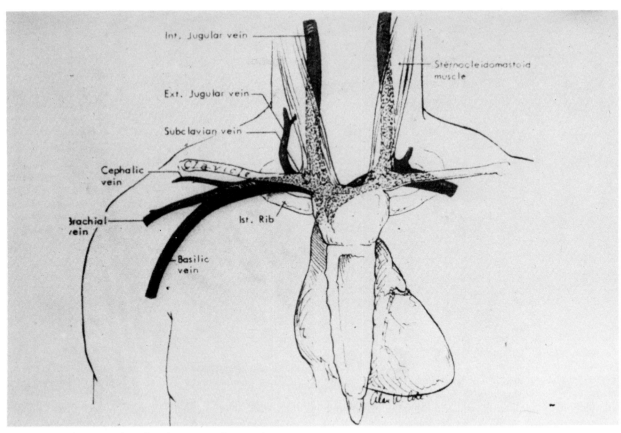

Figure 4-5. Relationships of major torso veins to other anatomy.

the superior vena cava, whereas all the major tributaries curve. Both external jugular veins enter the subclavian vein at almost right angles. The subclavian veins lie immediately posterior to the junction of the medial and middle third of the clavicle, and are anterior and inferior to the artery; the pleura is immediately posterior and inferior to the subclavian vessels (Fig. 4-6). The internal jugular vein generally lies anterolateral to the carotid (the opposite of the femoral relationship of vein and artery).

Equipment

A host of equipment has been used for CVP catheter placement. These warrant a very practical discussion. The catheter-through-needle has been the traditional method of invasive access of central veins until recently. But there are numerous problems associated with it. The commonly used insertion needle is large (14 gauge) and dangerous (5-mm bevel); its catheter is smaller (16 gauge), but the cutdown hub used is smaller still (18 gauge), limiting gravity flow to less than 50 mL per minute. Thus, it cannot be used as a volume resuscitation catheter.

A long ($5\frac{1}{4}$-in) catheter-over-needle has been used, especially in internal jugular cannulation. But the long bevel often frustrates advancing the catheter, despite free blood return.

These two types of catheters are steadily being replaced by wire-guided (Seldinger) catheters. These must now be considered the equipment of first choice for invasive, blind techniques, and so will be detailed here. A hollow-bore (thin-walled) needle is inserted into the vein (Fig. 4-7a). A flexible wire is inserted (Fig. 4-7b) and the needle removed (Fig. 4-7c), leaving just the wire

in the vein. The catheter is then threaded over the wire and into the vein with a twisting motion (Fig. 4-7d). The wire is then removed, leaving only the catheter in place. If a large-bore catheter is necessary, the apparatus is used with a venodilator, which necessitates a stab (no. 11 blade) for smooth skin penetration (Fig. 4-7e). In this situation the venodilator is removed with the wire, leaving the large-bore catheter sheath in place (Fig. 4-7f).

The principal advantages of wire-guided catheters are (1) the small (thus safer) needle for insertion, (2) the step-up capability with a venodilator allowing high flow rates, (3) the use of J wires to access the central circulation from the external jugular vein, and (4) the flexibility of exchanging standard intravenous catheters, central venous catheters, and Swan-Ganz catheters without repeated stabs (the reader is directed to the recent literature for more detailed explanations than can be provided here).

Techniques

The internal jugular and subclavian veins may be cannulated by several common techniques. Use of the *internal jugular vein* in the last few years has become preferred over the subclavian approach since, performed correctly, the incidence of pneumothorax is lessened. Two approaches are commonly used.

In the *anterior approach* (Fig. 4-8), the needle is directed into the top of the apex of a triangle formed by the tendinous and muscular heads of the sternocleidomastoid muscle and directed slightly laterally to the axis of the body. Blood return should be obtained within 3 cm since the internal jugular vein is very superficial here.

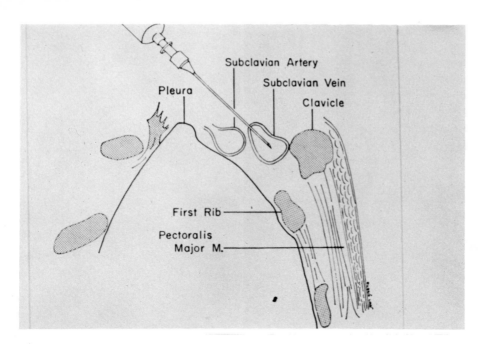

Figure 4-6. Coronal section through midclavicle.

In the *lateral* or *posterior approach* (Fig. 4-9) the head is turned slightly away from the involved side and the needle inserted at the posterior margin of the sternocleidomastoid muscle, 2 to 3 fingerbreadths above the clavicle, and directed toward the suprasternal notch. Blood should be aspirated within 4 to 5 cm.

The widely used *infraclavicular subclavian* (Fig. 4-10) technique necessitates that the shoulders be thrown back to avoid pneumothorax. This can best be accomplished with an IV bag or rolled towel placed axially beneath the high thoracic spine. The needle is inserted beneath the clavicle at about the midclavicle, and directed toward the suprasternal notch. The needle should be advanced parallel to the gurney (posterior direction will result in pneumothorax) to a distance of no more than 6 cm.

The *supraclavicular subclavian* (Fig. 4-11) technique is not as popular in the United States but is quite acceptable. Here, the patient's head is again turned slightly away from the involved side. The needle enters just above the clavicle, 1 cm lateral to the insertion of the muscular head of the sternocleidomastoid muscle, and directed so as to bisect the angle formed between the sternocleidomastoid and the clavicle, and about 10° anteriorly to a depth of no more than 2 to 3 cm. This technique is also called the "junctional" technique, as the needle will enter the subclavian vein at its junction with the internal jugular vein.

Preparation—General Aspects

Before performing central catheterization the physician should first consider whether the patient *really* needs the technique or whether peripheral technique could not be performed just as well. Once embarked upon, the technique most suiting the anatomy of the patient should be performed with all equipment ready beforehand, including the CVP manometer setup.

The patient should be placed in Trendelenburg's position, then perform the Valsalva maneuver; the entire route of the neck should be prepped so that all three approaches are possible. The right side is slightly preferred over the left, since (1) the lung apex is slightly lower, (2) there is a straight relationship between the right internal jugular vein and the superior vena cava, and (3) the thoracic duct cannot be injured. In cases of chest injury the injured side should be catheterized so the uninjured side will not be threatened with pneumothorax. A local anesthetic should be used when time and the patient's consciousness permit.

After landmarks are identified, a 5- to 10-mL syringe attached to a hollow-bore needle appropriate to the size of the guide wire should be inserted. Since an 18-gauge needle is most commonly used, the use of an exploratory small-bore needle is unnecessary. Gentle, continuous negative pressure on the syringe should be maintained. When free flow of blood is obtained, the syringe is removed and the fingertip occludes the hub before wire insertion. When the catheter has been advanced over the wire to the proper depth and the wire removed, the catheter should be sutured to the chest wall, a little Betadine ointment placed at the needle puncture site, and a surgical dressing applied. If one approach fails, another technique should be performed on the *same* side, since use of the other side places the patient at risk for bilateral pneumothorax. A chest film should be performed immediately and 6 h after the procedure to assure proper placement and absence of pneumothorax or hydrothorax.

Central Venous Pressure Measurement

Measurement of CVP should always be performed. First, the point of reference equivalent to the right atrium—"zero point"—must be determined and marked on the patient's chest wall. This point has been determined to be just 1 to 3 cm anterior to the midaxillary line at the level of the fourth costochondral junction. The three-way stopcock on the manometer should be manipulated to fill the manometer with IV solution. Then, with the patient level, supine, and breathing easily, fluid from the manometer should be run into the patient until it reaches a steady state. With the zero of the manometer apposing the zero reference point on the chest wall, the meniscus at end expiration gives the correct reading.

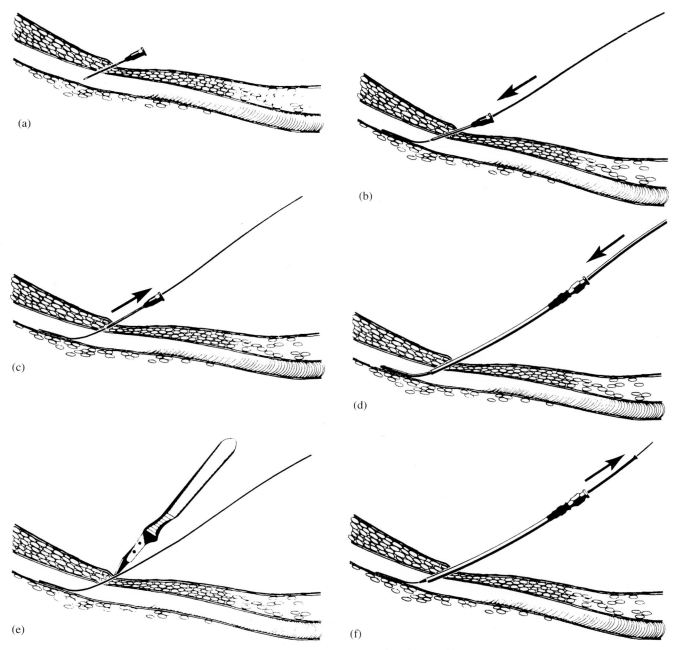

(a)

(b)

(c)

(d)

(e)

(f)

Figure 4-7. Seldinger technique of catheter insertion (wire-guided). (From Conahan et al.)

Interpretation of Central Venous Pressure Measurement

First, the change in CVP over time or with fluid challenge is more valuable than absolute values. However, the first value is a guide to diagnosis, further volume repletion, and/or other modes of therapy. If a high CVP is obtained (greater than 12 to 15 cm), certain artifacts should be ruled out. These include: continued Trendelenburg position; external zero reference point is too low on the chest wall; catheter tip is outside the thorax (e.g., in the internal jugular, axillary vein, etc.); catheter is kinked or semioccluded by vein wall; catheter is across tricuspid valve into right ventricle; catheter

is in artery; patient is breathing against resistance (e.g., ventilator, respiratory distress, etc.) and finally, stopcock malposition, that is, IV fluid running into the manometer.

Once these artifacts have been ruled out, the most common causes of high CVP are, in rough order of frequency, right ventricular failure secondary to left ventricular failure, corpulmonale, pulmonary embolism, right ventricular infarct, pericardial tamponade, tension pneumothorax, and superior vena cava obstruction. With an initial CVP reading greater than 15, fluid challenge is seldom warranted.

A low CVP is more commonly obtained; that is, below 5 to 6 cm. Artifacts to be ruled out are: patient in a thorax-elevated

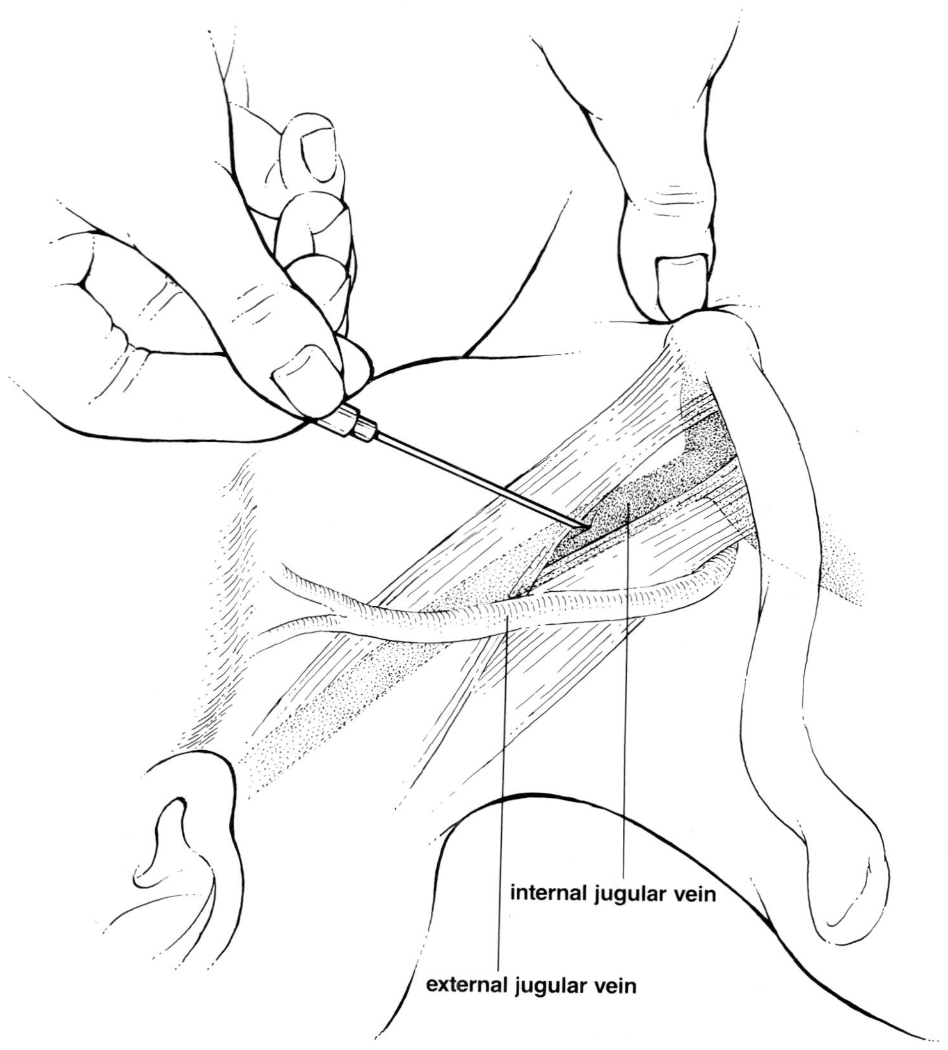

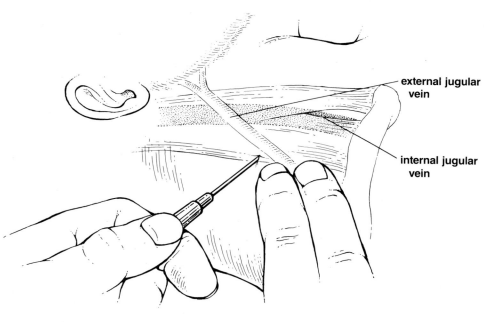

Figure 4-8. Anterior approach to internal jugular vein.

internal jugular vein

external jugular vein

Figure 4-9. Posterolateral approach to internal jugular vein.

external jugular vein

internal jugular vein

Figure 4-10. Infraclavicular approach to subclavian vein.

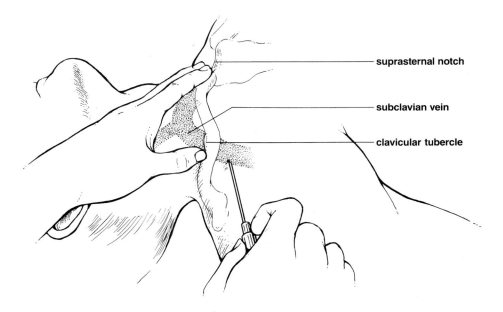

suprasternal notch

subclavian vein

clavicular tubercle

position (sitting), or the external zero reference point is too high on the chest wall. A low CVP is generally due to low circulating blood volume or decreased splanchnic venous tone (e.g., anaphylaxis, spinal shock, fear, pain, etc.). Low CVP demands rapid infusion of crystalloids with continued monitoring, while pursuing a diagnosis.

Patients with normal CVPs (5 to 10 cm) are usually fluid challenged; that is, 50- to 100-mL infusions of crystalloid, followed by a minute or two of equilibrium, and then remeasurement. This technique is particularly useful in hypotensive patients in whom optimum heart-filling pressures are desired.

Complications

There is a large literature on complications of invasive CVP techniques. The three most common and devastating are pneumothorax, arterial puncture, and infection. Others, in roughly decreasing order, are hydrothorax, hydromediastinum, air or catheter embolism, thrombosis, arrhythmias, nerve injuries, osteomyelitis of the clavicle, erosion and perforation of the superior vena cava (giving rise to hydromediastium or hydrothorax), or right atrium (resulting in hydropericardium), knotting with other catheters, and puncture of endotracheal tube cuffs. The list goes on, but once

Figure 4-11. Supraclavicular approach to subclavian vein.

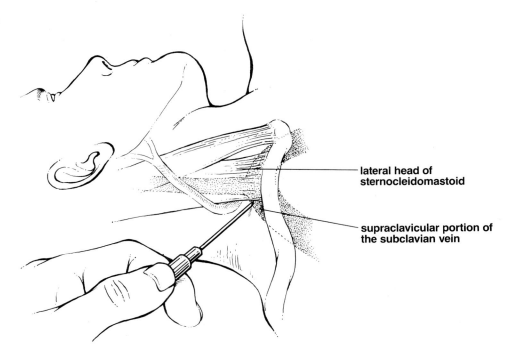

lateral head of sternocleidomastoid

supraclavicular portion of the subclavian vein

again, knowledge of anatomy, careful technique, and aseptic preparation will make such complications rare.

VENOUS CUTDOWN

Surgical access to veins is indicated only when percutaneous puncture is impossible. Favorite sites are the basilic vein in the antecubital fossa and the saphenous vein at the ankle.

The basilic vein is located 2 fingerbreadths above and 2 fingerbreadths medial to the olecranon. The saphenous vein is just anterior to the medial malleolus. Additionally, the saphenous vein is accessible in the proximal thigh 3 fingerbreadths below the midpoint of the inguinal ligament.

To avoid cannulating the artery, identify the artery and the vein before ligating or nicking a vessel. Slip a forceps or hemostat under the vessel and apply pressure. Pulsatile flow will be evident in the artery. Unfortunately, no technique is reliable in the patient without circulation. Careless technique can produce tendon or nerve injury, or extensive soft tissue bleeding. The technique is as follows:

1. Prepare and anesthetize the skin.
2. Make a transverse skin incision, and by blunt dissection, separate the subcutaneous tissue until the vein is exposed.
3. After freeing the vein from the surrounding tissues, pass two separate sutures beneath the vein—one proximal and one distal. Leave the proximal suture untied. Tie the distal suture to occlude the vein, but keep the ends of the suture long so they can be used for applying traction to the vein.
4. Make a nick in the vein between the proximal and distal suture.
5. While applying traction on the vein, insert the catheter into the vein. Tie the proximal suture to secure the catheter in the vein.
6. Suture the cutaneous incision.

PULMONARY CAPILLARY WEDGE PRESSURE

In certain circumstances, fluid administration in critically ill patients is monitored most effectively by following changes in the pulmonary capillary wedge pressure. In addition, specific diseases can be diagnosed by comparing pressures in the pulmonary artery and pulmonary capillaries.

A Swan-Ganz balloon-tipped catheter is most frequently employed for this purpose. The triple-lumen catheter can be used to measure pulmonary artery, pulmonary wedge, and central venous pressures; to withdraw blood from the pulmonary artery; and to determine cardiac output by the thermodilution technique.

The catheter is inserted into the central venous circulation by the internal jugular or subclavian technique. When the right atrium is entered, the balloon is inflated and the catheter is carried by the blood flow into the pulmonary circulation where it is advanced to the smaller arteries. The balloon is then deflated. It is reinflated only during recording of the capillary wedge pressure. Pressures are measured on a pressure transducer and displayed on an oscilloscope monitor or recorder. A water manometer or sphygmomanometer is not useful for monitoring pulmonary wedge pressures because these devices are not sensitive enough to accurately reflect small, but significant pressure changes.

Pulmonary wedge pressure is essentially identical to the pressure in the pulmonary veins, and as such is a precise indicator of pulmonary congestion and pulmonary edema. The normal pulmonary capillary wedge pressure is about 10 mmHg. Pulmonary edema generally results with a pulmonary capillary wedge pressure of about 30 mmHg.

The pulmonary capillary wedge pressure is closely related to the mean left atrial pressure, but it may not reflect the left ventricular end-diastolic pressure when ventricular compliance is markedly reduced, as in acute myocardial infarction.

Pulmonary artery systolic and diastolic pressures reflect the force generated by right ventricular contraction and the resistance to flow offered by the pulmonary arterioles and capillaries. A pulmonary diastolic pressure greater than the capillary wedge pressure may be present in disorders such as pulmonary embolism, pulmonary fibrosis, or chronic cor pulmonale.

Complications of balloon catheter monitoring include cardiac arrhythmias, balloon-induced pulmonary capillary rupture, pulmonary infarction, and pulmonary thromboembolism.

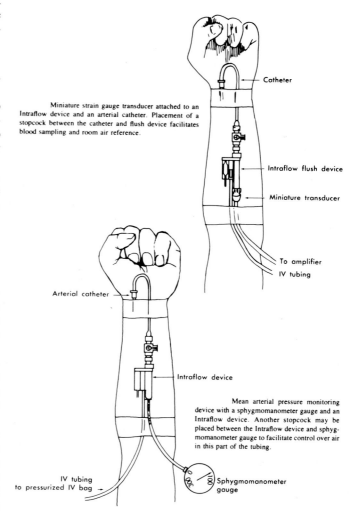

Miniature strain gauge transducer attached to an Intraflow device and an arterial catheter. Placement of a stopcock between the catheter and flush device facilitates blood sampling and room air reference.

Catheter

Intraflow flush device

Miniature transducer

To amplifier
IV tubing

Arterial catheter

Intraflow device

Mean arterial pressure monitoring device with a sphygmomanometer gauge and an Intraflow device. Another stopcock may be placed between the Intraflow device and sphygmomanometer gauge to facilitate control over air in this part of the tubing.

IV tubing
to pressurized IV bag

Sphygmomanometer gauge

Figure 4-12. An intraarterial pressure-monitoring system consists of an indwelling arterial catheter, pressure-monitoring system, and a heparin infusion system. Arterial pressure is recorded by connecting the system to a water manometer, sphygmomanometer gauge, or pressure transducer. (From Schroeder JS, Daily EK: *Techniques in Bedside Hemodynamic Monitoring.* St. Louis, Mosby, 1976, p. 101. Used by permission.)

ARTERIAL CANNULATION

Arterial cannulation can be performed for direct measurement of intraarterial pressure and for frequent arterial blood sampling. In conditions such as marked vasoconstriction and low cardiac output states, or in premature or newborn infants, substantial discrepancy can exist between the intraarterial blood pressure and blood pressure readings determined by sphygmomanometry. Cardiac output can vary significantly from beat to beat in atrial fibrillation or if there are premature ventricular contractions. Using the cuff method, one records the systolic pressure occurring over several systoles. In contrast, intraarterial pressure monitoring can indicate average pressures as well as pressure extremes.

An intraarterial pressure-monitoring system consists of an indwelling arterial catheter, a pressure-monitoring system, and a heparin infusion system.

The radial, brachial, and femoral arteries are sites commonly chosen for indwelling arterial catheters. The radial artery is generally the preferred site for intraarterial monitoring. Although the brachial artery is easily cannulated, it is the sole source of blood to the hand, and thrombosis can lead to serious complications. The femoral artery is easily identified and punctured, but it can be difficult to detect or control bleeding in the soft tissues of the groin resulting from arterial puncture. In addition, thrombosis of the femoral artery can lead to loss of the extremity.

An indwelling needle or Teflon catheter is inserted into the artery directly or by the Seldinger technique. Once the arterial line is established, patency can be maintained by infusing a heparin solution, either as a continuous or intermittent infusion. Arterial pressure is recorded by connecting the system to a water manometer, sphygmomanometer gauge, or pressure transducer (Fig. 4-12). A water manometer is an inexpensive device for measuring intraarterial pressure. Each 13.6 cm the column rises above the midaxillary line is equivalent to 10 mmHg mean arterial pressure. If a sphygmomanometer gauge is used, it is connected to the intraarterial line and arterial pressures are read directly from the height of the mercury column. A strain gauge pressure transducer provides the most accurate recording, and the pressure curve can then be recorded or displayed on an oscilloscope monitor.

BIBLIOGRAPHY

Anderson HW, Benumof JL, Trousdale FR, et al: Increasing the functional gauge of the side port of large catheter sheath introducers. *Anesthesiology* 56:57, 1982.

Blitt CD, Wright WA, Petty WC, et al: Central venous catheterization via the external jugular vein: A technique employing the J-wire. *JAMA* 229(7):817, 1974.

Conahan TJ III, Schwartz AJ, Geer RT: Percutaneous catheter introduction: The Seldinger technique. *JAMA* 237(5):446, 1977.

Costin BS, Harris JH: Complications of tubes and catheters. *South Med J* 76(2):218, 1983.

Dailey RH: Use of wire-guided catheters in the emergency department. *Ann Emerg Med* 12:489, 1983.

Daily PO, Griepp RB, Shumway NE: Percutaneous internal jugular vein cannulation. *Arch Surg* 101:534, 1970.

Dronen SC, Yee AS, Tomlanovich MC: Proximal saphenous vein cutdown. *Ann Emerg Med* 10(6):328, 1981.

Dula DJ, Muller HA, Donovan JW: Flow rate variance of commonly used IV infusion techniques. *J Trauma* 21(6):480, 1981.

Forrester JS, Diamond GA, Swan HJC: Bedside diagnosis of latent cardiac complications in acutely ill patients. *JAMA* 222:59, 1972.

Getzen LC, Pollak EW: Short-term femoral vein catheterization: a safe alternative venous access? *Am J Surg* 138:875, 1979.

Guyton AC, Jones CE: Central venous pressure: Physiological significance and clinical implications. *Am Heart J* 86:431, 1973.

Iverson KV, Reeter A: Rapid fluid replacement: A new methodology. *Ann Emerg Med* (abs) 12(4):238, 1983.

Joyce SM, Barsan WG, Hedges JR, et al: PASG-aided peripheral venous access vs central venous access for delivery of drugs using a radioisotope technique during normal perfusion and CPR. *Ann Emerg Med* (abs) 12(4):238, 1983.

Knopp R, Dailey RH: Central venous cannulation and pressure monitoring. *JACEP* 6(8):358, 1977.

Kramer DA, Staten-McCormick M, Freeman SB: Percutaneous brachial vein catheterization: An alternate site for IV access. *Ann Emerg Med* (abs) 12(4):238, 1983.

Lasala PA, Starker PM, Askanazi J: The saphenous system for long-term parenteral nutrition. *Crit Care Med* 11(5):378, 1983.

Magil RA, Delaurentis DA, Rosemond GP: The infraclavicular venipuncture. *Arch Surg* 95:320, 1967.

Maki DG, Goldman DA, Rhame FS: Infection control in intravenous therapy. *Ann Intern Med* 79:867, 1973.

Mateer Jr, Thompson BM, Aprahamian C, et al: Rapid fluid resuscitation with central venous catheters. *Ann Emerg Med* 12(3):149, 1983.

Robson MC: Technique for obtaining accurate reproducible central venous pressure. *Johns Hopkins Med J* 122(4):232, 1968.

Schwartz AJ, Jobes DR, Levy WJ, et al: Intrathoracic vascular catheterization via the external jugular vein. *Anesthesiology* 56:400, 1982.

Seldinger SI: Catheter Replacement of the Needle in percutaneous arteriography. *Acta Radiol* 39:368, 1953.

Tucker JF, Danzl DF, Teague E, et al: Feasibility of infusion of intravenous fluids distal to military anti-shock trousers. *Ann Emerg Med* (abs) 12(4):238, 1983.

Van Bergern FH, Weatherhead DS, Treloar AE, et al: Comparison of indirect and direct methods of measuring arterial blood pressure. *Circulation* 10:481, 1954.

Weil MH, Shubin H: The "VIP" approach to the bedside management of shock. *JAMA* 207(2):337, 1969.

Weil MH, Shubin H, Rosoff L: Fluid repletion in circulatory shock. *JAMA* 192(8):84, 1965.

Yoffa D, Melb MB: Supraclavicular subclavian venipuncture and catheterization. *Lancet* 2:614, 1965.

CHAPTER 5
ACID-BASE BALANCE

Robert F. Wilson

INTRODUCTION

Defining Terms

The Latin *acidus,* meaning sour-tasting, refers to the sour taste of acid substances such as vinegar. The term *base* was introduced in 1774 by Rouelle, who defined it as a substance that reacts with an acid to form a salt. Bronsted defined an acid as any substance that could apply a hydrogen ion; a base was any substance that could accept a hydrogen ion.

pH

The concentration of hydrogen ions, even in a very acid solution, is extremely low. In a so-called neutral solution, the number of hydrogen (H^+) ions equals the number of hydroxyl (OH^-) ions; in water at 25°C the number is 1/10,000,000 or 10^{-7} mol per liter. The term pH refers to the negative logarithm of the hydrogen ion concentration. Hasselbalch coined the term after Sorensen referred to a hydrogen ion concentration of 10^{-7} as "7 puissance hydrogen." Thus, a solution with a pH of 1 has a hydrogen ion concentration of 1×10^{-1} and is extremely acidic, whereas a solution with a pH of 13 has a hydrogen ion concentration of 1×10^{-13} and is extremely alkaline.

Henderson-Hasselbalch Equation

$$pH = pK + \log \frac{\text{proton acceptor (base)}}{\text{proton donor (acid)}}$$

The Henderson-Hasselbalch equation relates the pH to the pK (the negative log of the dissociation constant) plus the log of the ratio of the concentration of a base to its related acid.

About 80 percent of the buffering for the extracellular fluid is the bicarbonate-carbonic acid system. The average normal concentration of bicarbonate is 24 mEq per liter; the average normal concentration of carbonic acid is 1.2 mEq per liter. Thus, the ratio of bicarbonate to carbonic acid is normally 20:1. The log is 1.3; adding 1.3 to 6.1 (the pK of the bicarbonate-carbonic acid system) results in 7.4—the normal pH. Various compensatory mechanisms try to keep the bicarbonate-acid ratio at 20:1. If the plasma bicarbonate level falls, the body attempts to decrease carbonic acid

by hyperventilating, and vice versa.

$$pH = 6.1 + \frac{\log HCO_3}{\log H_2CO_3}$$

$$pH = 6.1 + \log \frac{24}{1.2}$$

$$pH = 6.1 + 1.3 = 7.4$$

Buffers

Although the pK for the bicarbonate-carbonic acid system is usually considered to be quite constant, it may vary quite a bit in acutely ill patients. A wide variety of metabolic and respiratory factors produce or take up hydrogen ions. These could cause wide swings in the pH if it were not for a group of substances referred to as *buffers,* which are capable of at least partially neutralizing acids and bases. The acid-buffering capacity of any agent or solution is determined by the number of hydrogen ions that the agent can take up for each unit change in pH.

The average adult man has a total buffer base, or buffering capacity, of about 1000 mEq. Chief buffers in blood are hemoglobin within the red cells and bicarbonate and protein in the plasma. Most of the buffering against carbon dioxide is provided by hemoglobin, but the bicarbonate-carbonic acid system is primarily responsible for moment-to-moment buffering of the blood and interstitial fluid. The most important intracellular buffers are phosphate and protein. Patients with anemia, low plasma protein levels, or decreased muscle mass have a reduced buffering capacity and are apt to have wide swings in pH when they become ill or injured. In such individuals, impaired tissue perfusion of relatively short duration may cause severe acidosis.

Most of the body's buffer systems primarily neutralize acid. As a consequence, the body generally tolerates an acid load much better than a base excess.

Carbon Dioxide Content

Carbon dioxide content refers to the total of all the carbon dioxide present in the blood, normally 24 to 31 mEq/L. In the plasma, CO_2 content includes carbonic acid, bicarbonate, and the carbamino compounds. The amount of carbonic acid present averaging about 1.2 mEq/L can be estimated by multiplying the P_{CO_2} by 0.03. The arterial bicarbonate concentration normally averages about 24 mEq/L. The concentration of the carbamino compounds, CO_2 combined with amino groups on proteins, averages about 0.5 to 1.5 mEq/L. Thus, under ordinary circumstances, the arterial bicarbonate concentration is approximately 1.5 to 2.0 mEq/L less than the arterial CO_2 content. Since the venous P_{CO_2} is normally about 6 to 7 torr higher than the arterial P_{CO_2} and the venous bicarbonate is about 1.0 mEq/L higher than arterial bicarbonate, the venous CO_2 content is usually about 2.5 to 3.0 mEq/L higher than the arterial bicarbonate. Estimating arterial bicarbonate from the arterial or venous CO_2 content may be more accurate at times than calculating it from the arterial P_{CO_2} and pH. Bicarbonate concentrations cannot be reliably calculated from pH and P_{CO_2} measurements in acutely ill patients because of changes in the pK.

ACID PRODUCTION, TRANSPORT, AND EXCRETION

Carbon Dioxide (Volatile Acid) Production and Transport

About 12,000 to 20,000 mEq of CO_2, or volatile acid, is produced by the body each day from the metabolism of carbohydrate, protein, and fat, and is excreted by the lungs. Most carbon dioxide transport to the lungs from peripheral tissues is provided by plasma bicarbonate and red cell hemoglobin. Carbon dioxide present as carbonic acid in arterial blood averages about 1.2 mEq/L, equivalent to a P_{CO_2} of 40 torr.

Ordinarily the kidney excretes about 70 mEq of acid each day, but in acidotic patients, excretion may be increased fourfold. Renal tubular excretion of acid normally is accomplished by three mechanisms: (1) direct excretion of hydrogen, which accounts for only about 0.1 mEq of acid per day; (2) excretion with urine buffers, including Na_2HPO_4, which accounts for about 20 mEq of acid per day; and (3) excretion with ammonia (produced in the distal tubular cells from glutamine and other precursors), which accounts for about 50 mEq of hydrogen ions per day.

In the proximal tubule, sodium and bicarbonate are absorbed independently of the direct effects of aldosterone, and hydrogen ion is secreted into the tubular lumen in exchange for sodium ion. If the extracellular fluid is reduced, or if there is a sodium deficiency, increased amounts of sodium and bicarbonate are absorbed in the proximal tubule. If saline solution is given, expanding the extracellular fluid, proximal tubular absorption of sodium and bicarbonate is decreased.

In the distal tubule, H_2CO_3 is dissociated into H^+ and HCO_3^-. Here H^+ and K^+ are excreted into the urine in exchange for Na^+. HCO_3^- formed in the cell and Na^+ absorbed out of the tubule lumen move out the other side of the tubule cell into the bloodstream.

Anything that increases intracellular concentration of hydrogen ion also increases the secretion of hydrogen ion into the distal tubular lumen and increases sodium reabsorption. When a potassium deficiency develops in the extracellular fluid, potassium ions leave tissue cells in exchange for hydrogen, resulting in an intracellular acidosis. Increased potassium is also absorbed in the distal tubule in exchange for hydrogen ions, which are excreted and may cause a paradoxical acidosis. Conversely, hyperkalemia causes an intracellular alkalosis that decreases bicarbonate reabsorption.

EVALUATING ACID-BASE ABNORMALITIES

Categorizing the Abnormality

Acid-base abnormalities are defined in terms of the pH and the relative amounts of arterial bicarbonate and carbonic acid or P_{CO_2}. The normal concentration of bicarbonate in blood is 21 to 26 mEq/L. If the P_{CO_2} is normal and the bicarbonate concentration is greater than 26 mEq/L, the patient has a metabolic alkalosis.

The P_{CO_2} is normally 35 to 45 mmHg. If the P_{CO_2} is lower than 35 mmHg, the patient has a respiratory alkalosis. In contrast, if the P_{CO_2} is greater than 45 mmHg, the patient has a respiratory acidosis.

The acid-base situations that are possible using these definitions can be tabulated into nine simple categories (Table 5-1).

Effect of P_{CO_2} and HCO_3 on pH

The pH which results from various combinations of P_{CO_2} and bicarbonate is listed in Table 5-2.

At the most frequent P_{CO_2} and bicarbonate levels, a 10-torr change in the P_{CO_2} produces a change of about 0.10 in pH while a 5 mEq/L change in bicarbonate also produces a pH change of about 0.10.

Compensatory Changes

Any abnormality that disturbs the normal ratio between arterial bicarbonate and carbonic acid tends to immediately stimulate a compensating metabolic or respiratory response to try to bring the ratio back to normal. To have complete compensation, the bicarbonate would have to change by about 5mEq/L for each 10-mmHg change in the P_{CO_2}. However, the acute response in bicarbonate is usually very slow and partial (20 percent). Even chronically, the compensation is only about 70 to 80 percent. The reverse is true for primary metabolic problems. For example, if a patient develops a metabolic acidosis with a low bicarbonate, he or she will tend to hyperventilate, producing a compensatory respiratory alkalosis. If bicarbonate fell by 10 mEq/L, the P_{CO_2} would fall

Table 5-1. Simplified Acid-Base Categories as Defined by The P_{CO_2} and Bicarbonate Levels

P_{CO_2} mmHg	Bicarbonate (mEq per liter)		
	Less than 21	**21 to 26**	**More than 26**
More than 45	Combined metabolic and respiratory acidosis	Respiratory acidosis	Metabolic alkalosis and respiratory acidosis
35 to 45	Metabolic acidosis	Normal	Metabolic alkalosis
Less than 35	Metabolic acidosis and respiratory alkalosis	Respiratory alkalosis	Combined metabolic and respiratory alkalosis

Table 5-2. HCO_3 (mEq per liter)

P_{CO_2} (torr)	14	19	24	29
60	6.99	7.12	7.22	7.31
50	7.07	7.20	7.30	7.39
40	7.17	7.30	7.40	7.48
30	7.29	7.42	7.52	7.61

about 20 mmHg to produce complete compensation; however, the acute compensation (minutes) may be only about 25 to 50 percent of that, and the compensation over several hours may be only about 50 to 75 percent complete.

In general, respiratory compensations can occur very rapidly. In contrast, metabolic compensatory responses by the kidney, and to a certain small extent by other tissue cells, takes much longer. In addition, the compensatory respiratory response to a metabolic alkalosis is restricted somewhat by the hypoxemia that develops with respiratory acidosis, unless oxygen is given.

If a combined acidosis or alkalosis develops and persists, the prognosis for the patient is greatly reduced. Inability to compensate usually means a severe disturbance of ventilation or of renal function and cell metabolism.

Laboratory Report Consistency

Correlating Carbon Dioxide Content and Bicarbonate

When drawing blood for blood gas studies in patients with complicated acute problems, additional blood for electrolyte determinations should be drawn. The bicarbonate present can then be estimated from the CO_2 content. Ordinarily, the arterial bicarbonate estimated from the arterial pH and P_{CO_2} should be approximately 1.5 to 2.0 mEq/L less than the arterial CO_2 content, and 2.5 to 3.0 mEq/L less than the venous CO_2 content.

Correlating pH and Electrolyte

Correlating pH and potassium and other electrolyte values also helps estimate the acid-base status of the patient. Patients with an acidosis tend to have higher potassium levels than patients with an alkalosis. In general, a rise or fall in pH of 0.10 is associated with a corresponding fall or rise of about 0.5 mEq/L in plasma potassium. Thus, a patient with a pH of 7.30 and a plasma potassium of 4.8 mEq/L would tend to have a plasma potassium level of 3.8 if his or her pH were raised to 7.50. The potassium level in serum is slightly higher than that in plasma, because the clotting process releases some potassium.

Correlating Chloride and Bicarbonate Levels

Plasma chloride and bicarbonate concentrations tend to move in opposite directions. Thus, patients who have a metabolic alkalosis (and high plasma bicarbonate levels) tend to have low plasma chloride levels, whereas those with metabolic acidosis (and low plasma bicarbonate levels) tend to have normal or elevated chloride levels. However, if there are increased amounts of unmeasured anions present (causing an increased anion gap), bicarbonate may be very low and chloride may be normal or even low.

Anion Gap

The anion gap is defined as the difference between the serum sodium concentration and the sum of the bicarbonate (or CO_2 content) and chloride ions. Therefore,

$$Anion\ gap = Na - (Cl + CO_2\ content)$$

The "anion gap" supposedly represents the sum of the "unmeasured" serum anions, including sulfates, phosphates, proteins, and organic acids, such as lactate acid. Ordinarily the sodium concentration is 138 to 142 mEq/L and the sum of the CO_2 content and chloride anions is 124 to 131 mEq/L. Thus, the difference (or anion gap) between the sodium concentration and the sum of these two anions is 8 to 16 mEq/L. In patients with excessive acid production, the anion gap tends to be increased. On the other hand, in patients with metabolic acidosis due to loss of bicarbonate, the anion gap usually stays relatively normal.

In the absence of renal failure or in the presence of intoxication with methanol or ethylene glycol, an increased anion gap is usually due to keto anions or lactate accumulation. In alcoholic patients, an increased anion gap is largely 3-hydroxybutyrate. In uncontrolled diabetes, the increased anion gap is assumed to be due to increased 3-hydroxybutyrate and acetoacetate. In patients without uremia, alcoholic intoxication, or diabetes, an increased anion gap is usually due to lactate accumulation.

An anion gap of 30 mEq/L or more indicates an organic acidosis, even in the presence of uremia. With anion gaps of 20 to 29 mEq/L, 75 percent of patients have an identified organic acidosis. Of those with no identified organic acidosis, changes in total proteins, phosphate, potassium, or calcium account for about 50 percent of the increased anion gap. The etiology of the other 50 percent of the anion gap is usually not apparent.

In general, if the anion gap exceeds 0.5 times the serum bicarbonate concentration plus 16.0 mEq/L, the diagnosis of an organic acidosis is justified. Thus, a patient with a HCO_3 of 6 mEq/L and an anion gap of 30 mEq/L probably has a fairly severe organic acidosis, because $HCO_3 \times 0.5 = 3$ and $16 + 3 = 19$, which is much less than the anion gap of 30.

There may be a wide spectrum of acid-base patterns in diabetic ketoacidosis ranging from pure anion gap acidosis to pure hyperchloremic acidosis. Severe dehydration tends to result in increased retention of ketones and an increased anion gap. Although only a few patients with diabetic ketoacidosis have a hyperchloremic acidosis on admission, after 4 to 8 h of therapy with saline solution most patients developed a hyperchloremic acidosis because of retention of chloride in excess of sodium and because of excretion of ketones by the kidney.

In general, however, we have found that changes in the anion gap are far more important than actual anion gap levels.

Venous Studies

If, for some reason, it is difficult to obtain arterial blood or if a percutaneous sample is obtained and it is not clear whether the sample is arterial or venous, central venous blood from a subclavian or pulmonary artery catheter can be used to advantage. Normally the arterial values can be obtained by adding 0.05 to the pH, subtracting 6 to 7 torr from the P_{CO_2}, and 1.0 mEq/liter from the bicarbonate. During shock, with moderate hypothermia, the correction factor for pH is 0.15; during recovery from shock, the pH correction is 0.08.

CLINICAL ACID-BASE ABNORMALITIES

Metabolic Acidosis

Etiology

Causes of metabolic acidosis are divided into two main groups: those associated with increased production of organic acids, and those associated with a loss of bicarbonate. The most frequent causes of increased production of organic acids include shock, ketoacidosis, and uremia, and toxicity due to salicylates, methanol, ethylene glycol, or paraldehyde. Ketoacidosis may be diabetic or alcoholic (nondiabetic) in origin. The most frequent causes of bicarbonate loss (usually resulting in hyperchloremia) include severe diarrhea, pancreatic fistulas, renal tubular acidosis, adrenal insufficiency, ureterosigmoidostomy, and therapy with acetazolamide (Diamox), ammonium chloride, arginine hydrochloride, or amino acid hydrochlorides (as in TPN). These two situations can often be differentiated by the "anion gap." In patients with excessive acid production (such as lactic acidosis), the anion gap tends to be increased. On the other hand, in patients with "hyperchloremic" metabolic acidosis due to loss of bicarbonate (such as with diarrhea), the anion gap will usually stay relatively normal.

The most frequent cause of an organic acidosis in critically ill or injured patients, especially those with impaired blood flow or sepsis, is lactic acidosis. If inadequate oxygen is available for proper aerobic cell metabolism, hydrogen ions build up. The resultant acidosis could rapidly destroy the cell and stop all metabolism unless some of the hydrogen ions were used to convert pyruvate to lactate and then to lactic acid. Thus, although excess lactic acid is considered dangerous, it is often forgotten that it represents an important compensation for acidosis.

Pathophysiology

Any increase in the quantity of hydrogen ions in the bloodstream almost immediately results in an increase in alveolar ventilation. As a general rule, each mEq/L fall in bicarbonate tends to cause a 1.0- to 1.3-mmHg fall in the P_{CO_2}. Thus, if the bicarbonate falls to 9 mEq/L, the P_{CO_2} would be expected to fall to 20 to 25 mmHg. In general, however, the P_{CO_2} can seldom be driven below 15 mmHg. If the fall in P_{CO_2} is less than 1.0 mmHg per mEq fall in bicarbonate, respiratory compensation is inadequate or abnormal. Further compensation is provided during the next several days by increased renal excretion of acid. Recent data suggest that patients with lactic acidosis hyperventilate comparably to patients with other types of metabolic acidosis.

In general, mild to moderate acidosis can increase the strength of muscular contraction (as in the phenomenon treppe). However, a pH of less than 7.10 to 7.15 can impair muscular and cardiovascular function. Furthermore, if the bicarbonate is less than 5.0 mEq/L, any further reduction in bicarbonate can markedly reduce pH.

Acidosis increases the secretion of catecholamines but, if severe, it decreases the end organ response in a variety of systems. Severe acidosis tends to cause arterial vasodilation and venous constriction, increasing the tendency to capillary stasis. Severe acidosis also tends to cause pulmonary vasoconstriction with increased strain on the right heart. However, acidosis shifts the oxygen dissociation curve to the right, releasing more oxygen to the tissues.

Diagnosis

Diagnosis is based on the finding of a low pH with low bicarbonate levels. Calculation of the anion gap can help differentiate the cause of the metabolic acidosis. Screening for various toxins may be necessary in severe acidosis of obscure etiology. Types of renal tubular acidosis may sometimes be differentiated by bone and kidney x-rays.

Treatment

Treatment of metabolic acidosis is aimed primarily at correcting the underlying problem. For shock, this would include improvement of tissue perfusion, and for diabetes mellitus, administration of insulin. If a metabolic acidosis persists after such efforts, particularly if the pH is less than 7.15, sodium bicarbonate therapy should be considered. Sodium bicarbonate should probably be given if the arterial bicarbonate remains 5 mEq/L or less; any additional decrease in bicarbonate could cause a precipitous fall in pH. However, the amount of bicarbonate given should probably not exceed 1 mEq/kg at a time so as to prevent alkaline overshoot. For each 0.1 pH rise, oxygen availability to tissue drops by about 10 percent because of the shift of the oxygen dissociation curve. Giving bicarbonate to patients with hypoxemia due to a right-to-left shunt (as in ARDS) may rapidly lower the arterial P_{O_2} to dangerous levels.

Bicarbonate deficits are generally calculated using 30 to 50 percent of the body weight as the bicarbonate space. In patients with acute mild to moderate bicarbonate deficits of less than 10 mEq/L, calculations using a 30 percent bicarbonate space seem to provide adequate correction. For bicarbonate deficits of 10 to 15 mEq/L, 40 percent of the body weight can be used as the bicarbonate space. However, in patients with severe acidosis with base deficits exceeding 15 mEq/L, the bicarbonate space involves almost the entire total body water and should be considered equal to 50 percent of the body weight.

For example, in an acutely ill 80-kg man, with a bicarbonate concentration of 10 mEq/L (i.e., a deficit of 14 mEq/L), we would assume he has a bicarbonate space of 40 percent, or 32 L. As a consequence, he would have a total bicarbonate deficit of (80 kg × 40%) × 14 mEq/L = 448 mEq. However, we would only give about 1 mEq/kg (80 mEq) at a time (over 15 to 30 min). If the patient were hemodynamically unstable, we might give bicarbonate faster.

If bicarbonate is given too rapidly, it can cause a paradoxical cerebral acidosis. The increased CO_2 generated by the bicarbonate readily crosses the blood-brain barrier while bicarbonate itself crosses the blood-brain barrier very slowly. The increased cerebrospinal fluid CO_2 generates carbonic acid which causes a cerebrospinal fluid acidosis in spite of an increasing blood alkalemia. Raising the pH from 7.00 to 7.40 with alkali therapy can raise plasma lactate concentrations by almost 50 percent because of shifts of lactate from the intracellular fluid to the extracellular fluid.

Metabolic Alkalosis

Etiology

The two most frequent causes of metabolic alkalosis are excessive diuresis (with loss of potassium and chloride) and excessive loss of gastric secretions (with loss of hydrogen and chloride). Normally the stomach makes 2 to 5 mEq of free acid per hour. Thus, in a 24-h period a patient who is vomiting excessively due to pyloric stenosis from peptic ulcer disease and increased acid secretion is particularly apt to develop a severe metabolic alkalosis.

Hypokalemia due to excess diuresis with excessive loss of potassium in the urine may cause a metabolic alkalosis. Potassium will tend to come out of tissue cells to correct the hypokalemia, and hydrogen ions go in. In addition the kidney will tend to conserve potassium and excrete hydrogen ions. Since potassium loss in urine is proportional to the volume of urine, use of large quantities of diuretics can easily produce a severe hypokalemia along with an excessive loss of chloride. Diarrhea or excessive colostomy or ileostomy drainage may also cause severe hypokalemia.

Mineralocorticoids tend to cause metabolic alkalosis by promoting the absorption of bicarbonate and sodium and by increasing the excretion of potassium, hydrogen, and chloride ions. The depletion of potassium causes even more excretion of hydrogen ions, aggravating the metabolic alkalosis. Reabsorption of potassium appears to be independent of aldosterone, but an aldosterone deficiency markedly reduces the ability of the distal tubule to secrete hydrogen ion and thus regenerate or reabsorb bicarbonate.

Massive transfusions of bank blood can greatly increase the quantity of citrate in the body (17 mEq from each unit of whole blood and 5 mEq from each unit of red blood cells). As this citrate is metabolized over the next 24 to 48 h, plasma bicarbonate levels rise proportionally, producing an increasing alkalosis. Ringer's lactate has a pH of about 5.5 or lower. However, after it is given, about half of it (L-lactate) is metabolized in the liver into bicarbonate, which tends to cause a metabolic alkalosis. The D-lactate is excreted in the urine.

There is an increasing tendency to attempt to prevent stress gastric ulceration and bleeding by maintaining a pH inside the stomach of 5.0 or higher with antacids and/or cimetidine. In some instances, large quantities of antacid are required. Absorption of these antacids and/or removal of the excess acid that they neutralize may significantly contribute to alkalosis.

Patients with severe sepsis not infrequently develop a metabolic alkalosis (in spite of the respiratory alkalosis that is often already present). In about half these patients, the metabolic alkalosis appears to be iatrogenic. In the other half the cause for the metabolic alkalosis may be related to septic inhibition of anaerobic metabolism and reduced lactate formation.

Dehydration which is not severe enough to interfere with tissue perfusion may cause a "contraction alkalosis." When the extracellular fluid and the urine output are large, sodium and bicarbonate reabsorption in the kidney is reduced. In contrast, when the extracellular fluid is contracted, sodium and bicarbonate absorption in the kidney is increased.

Physiological Effects

Alkalosis increases endogenous catecholamine release. However, it inhibits sympathetic nervous system activity, decreases α-adrenergic effects and accentuates β-adrenergic vasodilator effects.

Severe metabolic alkalosis also reduces the amount of ionized calcium present in the plasma, increasing neuromuscular irritability and impairing cardiovascular function. Alkalosis may also cause tachyarrhythmias, probably due to certain ion changes. The hypokalemia which develops secondary to an alkalosis may also interfere with striated and smooth muscle function, causing weakness and/or ileus.

If the metabolic alkalosis is combined with or develops in addition to a respiratory alkalosis, the pH can rise rapidly to above 7.55. In a study at Detroit General Hospital we found that the mortality rate of critically ill or injured patients was increased if their pH rose above 7.55. Patients maintaining an arterial pH above 7.70 almost invariably died.

The usual pulmonary compensation for a metabolic alkalosis is hypoventilation with slow, shallow breathing. As the P_{CO_2} rises because of hypoventilation, the P_{O_2} falls, but the chemoreceptors will not allow the arterial P_{O_2} to fall much below 60 mmHg. Thus the arterial P_{CO_2} will not usually rise above 55 to 60 mmHg unless the associated hypoxia is corrected by giving oxygen.

Diagnosis

The diagnosis of a metabolic alkalosis is made from laboratory studies revealing a bicarbonate level exceeding 26 mEq/L and pH above 7.45. In most instances, there is also an associated hypokalemia and hypochloremia. Clinically, metabolic alkalosis is characterized by slow, shallow respiration (in contrast to the hyperventilation generally seen with metabolic acidosis).

Treatment

Some investigators have divided metabolic alkalosis into two types: "chloride-responsive alkalosis" (in which the urine chloride concentration is less than 10 to 20 mEq/L) and "chloride-resistant alkalosis" (in which the urine chloride concentration is greater than 20 mEq/L). Chloride-responsive alkalosis, such as that caused by vomiting or excessive nasogastric suction, is due to a chloride deficit which in turn results in decreased sodium reabsorption in the proximal tubule. An increased sodium concentration in the distal tubule causes increased exchange of H^+ and K^+ for Na^+. The sodium is absorbed and the H^+ and K^+ are excreted. Coincident with the increased H^+ excretion there is increased "absorption" or retention of HCO_3^- perpetuating the alkalosis.

If there is a deficiency of K^+, there is an even greater excretion of H^+ and retention of HCO_3^- which may result in a paradoxical aciduria (excretion of acid urine in the presence of an alkalemia). If adequate chloride is administered to patients with chloride-responsive alkalosis, the increased chloride in the glomerular filtrate allows increased sodium absorption in the proximal tubule. As less sodium is presented to the distal tubule, less H^+ is excreted, less HCO_3^- is absorbed and the metabolic alkalosis begins to resolve.

If the patient is adequately hydrated, chloride deficit is calculated on the basis of 20 percent of the body weight. If the patient is severely dehydrated, one can use 60 percent of the body weight to calculate the chloride deficit. Half the chloride deficit is corrected at a time. Approximately one-fourth of the chloride is given as potassium chloride and three-fourths as sodium chloride. Normally the potassium is not given faster than 20 mEq per hour and is not given if the serum potassium levels exceed 5.0 mEq per liter.

If the alkalosis is very severe (the CO_2 content exceeds 40 mEq/L, the pH exceeds 7.55, or the patient has tetany) one-half is given as sodium chloride, and one-fourth as 1% NH_4Cl, arginine hydrochloride, or hydrochloric acid. Ammonium chloride theoretically should be helpful, but many of these patients have renal or hepatic problems which increase the risk of giving ammonium compounds. If hydrochloric acid (0.10 or 0.15 normal) is used, it must be given by slow infusion into a large vein at approximately 25 to 50 mL/hr. Arginine hydrochloride, which was used primarily to treat hepatic failure in the past, is effective and safe for treating these problems. In some instances, Diamox (acetazolamide), which increases renal bicarbonate excretion, may be used to correct a mild to moderate metabolic alkalosis. However, these patients are often too sick to take oral medications.

Chloride-resistant alkalosis is usually not associated with hypovolemia. Consequently, relatively large quantities of Na^+ and Cl are filtered, and increased H^+ and K^+ are excreted as the Na^+ is reabsorbed in the distal tubule. These patients are apt to require large quantities of potassium to correct the alkalosis.

Respiratory Alkalosis

Etiology

In stressful situations such as shock, sepsis, or trauma, there is a tendency to hyperventilate and develop respiratory alkalosis with a P_{CO_2} of about 25 to 35 mmHg or less. If hypoxia or metabolic acidosis develops, the patient tends to hyperventilate even more, causing a more severe respiratory alkalosis. Other causes of respiratory alkalosis include pulmonary embolism, asthma, and hepatic failure.

Physiological Effects

Alkalosis shifts the oxyhemoglobin dissociation curve to the left, causing hemoglobin to hold its oxygen more tightly. This lowers the P_{O_2} and reduces oxygen availability to tissues by about 10 percent for each pH increase of 0.10.

One of the main determinants of cerebral blood flow is the arterial P_{CO_2}. A P_{CO_2} of 25 to 30 torr is used to treat or prevent cerebral swelling and decrease cerebrospinal fluid pressure due to trauma or subarachnoid hemorrhage. However, a very severe respiratory alkalosis with P_{CO_2} less than 20 to 25 torr can reduce cerebral blood flow enough to cause cerebral metabolic acidosis. This intracerebral metabolic acidosis will then cause the respiratory center to increase ventilation even more, producing a progressively more severe respiratory alkalosis.

Occasionally, it may be difficult to differentiate hyperventilation of psychogenic origin from hyperventilation due to sepsis or pulmonary emboli. In such patients, careful continued observation of the patient and his or her blood gases is essential. Other tests such as lung scans and blood cultures may be helpful.

Treatment

Treatment of respiratory alkalosis due to hysterical hyperventilation is best accomplished by having the patient rebreathe his or her expired air, which has a P_{CO_2} about two-thirds that in arterial blood. Not infrequently, the most convenient rebreathing device is a paper bag. Once the P_{CO_2} begins to rise toward normal, the cerebral blood flow usually improves enough to correct the intracerebral acidosis and return the pattern of ventilation toward normal.

In critically ill patients who have moderate to severe respiratory alkalosis and are not on a ventilator, sedation may be given, but very cautiously, and one must be sure that the patient does not begin to hypoventilate and develop a severe hypoxia. If the patient is on a ventilator, he or she may be placed on I.M.V. and the respirator rate progressively reduced as long as (1) the P_{CO_2} is less than 45 mmHg, (2) the pH is above 7.35, and (3) the patient's respiratory rate is less than 30 to 35 per min. In some instances, 60 to 300 mL of dead space may also be added to the endotracheal tube or tracheostomy to raise the P_{CO_2}.

Respiratory Acidosis

Etiology

A P_{CO_2} elevated above 45 mmHg is usually due to inadequate minute ventilation and/or increased dead space. Inadequate minute ventilation is most frequently due to head or chest trauma or excess sedation. Patients with chronic obstructive pulmonary disease (COPD) have increased dead space and may also have decreased alveolar ventilation. In general, a rise in the P_{CO_2} stimulates the respiratory center to increase the respiratory rate and minute ventilation. However, when the arterial P_{CO_2} begins to exceed 60 to 70 mmHg, as may occur in some 5 to 10 percent of patients with severe chronic emphysema, the respiratory acidosis may depress the respiratory center. Under such circumstances, the stimulus for ventilation is provided primarily by hypoxemia acting on the chemoreceptors in the carotid and aortic bodies. In patients with chronic hypercarbia, administration of high concentrations of oxygen may severely depress or arrest ventilation and cause an abrupt and dangerous further increase in the respiratory acidosis.

In patients on IV hyperalimentation, metabolism of large quantities of carbohydrate may cause hypercarbia by increasing the body's production of CO_2 beyond the ability of the lungs to eliminate it. This is most apt to occur in patients who have impaired ventilatory function and are receiving 3 L or more of 20 to 25% glucose per day.

Diagnosis

Respiratory acidosis, by definition, is present when the arterial P_{CO_2} exceeds 45 mmHg. If the pH is less than 7.40, respiratory acidosis is presumably the primary problem and not a compensatory response to a metabolic alkalosis. With a sudden severe decrease in minute ventilation, the P_{CO_2} rises rapidly and the pH may fall abruptly because bicarbonate compensation by the kidney is very slow. A rapid increase of the arterial P_{CO_2} to 60 mmHg can cause the pH to fall to about 7.22. However, over the next few hours or days, a rise in bicarbonate will gradually restore the pH to about 7.35.

Treatment

Treatment of respiratory acidosis is primarily designed to improve alveolar ventilation. In patients with COPD, bronchodilators such as aminophylline or various sympathomimetic agents, such as iso-proterenol or Adrenalin, together with careful administration of small amounts of oxygen, may be helpful. However, ventilator assistance may be required in some patients who do not respond adequately to lesser measures. Unfortunately, it may be difficult to extubate such patients later.

In patients with a chronic respiratory acidosis, reduction of the P_{CO_2} should generally proceed relatively slowly. Minute ventilation for a 70-kg man is normally about 6 L. In a patient with COPD and severe hypercarbia, it may be wise to start with a minute ventilation of about 5 L/min and then gradually increase it according to the clinical response and changes in P_{CO_2}. Rapid correction of a chronic respiratory acidosis, after a compensatory metabolic alkalosis has developed, can cause sudden development of a severe combined metabolic and respiratory alkalosis. The resultant abrupt rise in pH and fall in ionized calcium can result in dangerous arrhythmias or seizures. In patients with a chronic respiratory acidosis, the arterial P_{CO_2} should probably not be reduced by more than 5.0 mEq/h.

More recently the problems with ventilation in malnourished individuals has been explored in depth. Increased carbohydrate intake increases CO_2 production and may contribute to respiratory failure. However, administration of glucose may enable previously exhausted subjects to continue work. This may be important in patients with impaired ventilation because a minute ventilation of more than 60 percent of maximum cannot be sustained for prolonged periods. In malnourished individuals, however, increased protein intake can increase the ventilatory response to increased CO_2.

BIBLIOGRAPHY

Adrogue HJ, Wilson H, Boyd AE III: Plasma acid-base patterns in diabetic ketoacidosis. *N Engl J Med* 307:1603, 1982.

Askanazi J, Nordenstrom J, Rosenbaum SH, et al: Nutrition for the patient with respiratory failure: Glucose vs fat. *Anesthesiology* 54:373, 1981.

Askanazi J, Rosenbaum SH, Hyman AI, et al: Effects of parenteral nutrition on ventilatory drive. *Anesthesiology* 53:5185, 1980.

Askanazi J, Weissman C, Rosenbaum SH, et al: Nutrition and the respiratory system. *Crit Care Med* 10:163, 1982.

Barton M, Lake R, Rainey TG, et al: Is Catecholamine release pH mediated? *Crit Care Med* 10:751, 1982.

Brenner RJ, Spring, DB, Sebastian A, et al: Incidence of radiologically evident bone disease, nephrocalcinosis and nephrolithiasis in various types of renal tubular acidosis. *N Engl J Med* 307:217, 1982.

Fulop M: Ventilatory response in patients with acute lactic acidosis. *Crit Care Med* 10:173, 1982.

Gabow PA, Kaehny WD, Fennessey PV, et al: Diagnostic importance of an increased serum anion gap. *N Engl J Med* 303:854, 1980.

Hood I, Campbell ENM: Is pK ok? *N Engl J Med* 306:864, 1982.

Moore SE, Good JT: Mixed venous and arterial pH: A comparison during hemorrhagic shock and hypothermia. *Ann Emerg Med* 11:300, 1982.

Narins RG, Emmet M: Simple and mixed acid-base disorders: A practical approach.

Natelson S, Nobel D: Effect of the variation of pK of the Henderson-Hasselbach equation on values obtained for total CO_2 calculated from P_{CO_2} and pH values. *Clin Chem* 23:767, 1977.

Pichette C, Bercovich M, Goldstein M, et al: Elevation of the blood lactate concentration by alkali therapy without requiring additional lactic acid accumulation: Theoretical considerations. *Crit Care Med* 10:323, 1982.

Settergren G, Soderland S, Eklof A: Blood oxygen tension and oxyhemoglobin saturation in hypoxemia due to right-to-left shunt or low inspired oxygen concentration. *Crit Care Med* 10:163, 1982.

Tenney SM, Reese, RE: The ability to sustain great breathing efforts. *Respir Physiol* 5:187, 1968.

Wahren J, Felig P, Ahlborg G, et al: Glucose metabolism during leg exercise in man. *J Clin Invest* 50:2715, 1971.

Wilson RF, Gibson DR, Percinel AK, et al: Severe alkalosis in critically ill patients. *Arch Surg* 104:551, 1972.

CHAPTER 6
FLUID AND
ELECTROLYTE
PROBLEMS

Robert F. Wilson

Fluid and electrolyte and acid-base problems occur frequently in critically ill and injured patients. Unfortunately, management of these problems in the emergency department may be difficult because of the urgency of the situation and the lack of baseline laboratory tests. We have developed a series of axioms which should help the practitioner approach these patients.

AXIOMS

1. Never completely trust the laboratory
   Some of the greatest problems in fluid and electrolyte or acid-base management have occurred when aggressive therapy was started because of an erroneous laboratory result. Laboratory errors do occur, especially at night and on weekends. Not only are there errors in obtaining the sample and labeling it, but also in performing the test and reporting the result. Consequently, the physician should try to decide what each test will probably show each time a test is requested, before the result comes back. If the laboratory result does not seem to correlate well with the patient's condition or any other data, three things should be done:
   a. The patient and his or her record should be carefully reexamined.
   b. If the laboratory result still does not seem to fit, the test should be repeated.
   c. If there is still a question about the validity of the laboratory result, a sample from a normal individual should be submitted for analysis.
   In some instances an abnormal result on an apparently normal "control" provides the first evidence that a laboratory error exists and may have existed for some time. Occasionally, laboratory errors are suspected because all the results of a certain test are higher or lower than expected.
2. Abnormalities should be treated at approximately the rate at which they developed
   Biologic systems react primarily to rate of change and not to absolute concentrations. If a patient gradually develops an abnormality, he or she progressively adapts to that abnormality to some extent so that it becomes increasingly "normal." Attempts to rapidly correct such values (to those generally accepted as normal) may cause more harm than good.

   A not infrequent example of this is the patient who has been on a low-salt diet and diuretics for years. A serum sodium concentration of less than 110 mEq/L may be well tolerated and is now relatively "normal" for this patient. Administration of normal saline solution in an attempt to return the patient's serum sodium levels rapidly to 135 to 142 mEq/L is likely to cause severe congestive heart failure. On the other hand, if a patient has a cardiac arrest, the metabolic acidosis which develops within a few minutes can and should be corrected rapidly with sodium bicarbonate.

   In general, if a patient is hemodynamically stable, there is no urgency to rapidly correct an abnormal laboratory result. Even when an abnormality has developed rather rapidly and it is tolerated well, we correct only half the calculated deficit at a time. We then reevaluate the patient and repeat the laboratory test to determine the rate and amount of correction still required.
3. The highest priority in treatment is maintenance of intravascular volume and tissue perfusion
   In correcting multiple fluid, electrolyte, and acid-base abnormalities, the highest priority should generally be given to correction of fluid volume and perfusion deficits; second priority to correction of pH; third priority to potassium, calcium, and magnesium abnormalities; and fourth priority to correction of sodium and chloride abnormalities. If blood volume and tissue perfusion are restored to normal, many electrolyte and acid-base abnormalities will correct themselves spontaneously.

   Changes in pH and potassium, calcium, and magnesium levels are generally closely related. In no instance should one be corrected without considering the effect that it may have on the others. For example, acidosis is usually associated with hyperkalemia and increased levels of ionized calcium and magnesium. In contrast, alkalosis tends to be associated with low levels of potassium and ionized calcium and magnesium. If a severely acidotic patient has a low serum potassium level, one should suspect that a laboratory error has occurred or that the patient has a severe potassium deficiency. If calcium,

Table 6-1. Atomic and Equivalent Weights

Element	Symbol	Atomic Weight	Equivalent Weight
Calcium	Ca	40	20
Carbon	C	12	3
Chlorine	Cl	35.5	35.5
Hydrogen	H	1	1
Magnesium	Mg	24	12
Oxygen	O	16	8
Phosphorus	P	31	6.2
Potassium	K	39	39
Sodium	Na	23	23
Sulfur	S	32	5.3

Table 6-2. Size and Sodium and Potassium Content of Various Fluid Spaces

	% of Body Weight	% of Total Body Na	% of Total Body K
Plasma	4.5	11.2	0.4
Interstitial fluid (lymph)	12.0	20.0	1.0
Dense connective tissue and cartilage	4.5	11.7	0.4
Bone	4.5	43.1	7.6
Transcellular	1.5	2.6	1.0
Total extracellular	27.0	97.6	10.4
Total intracellular	33.0	2.4	89.6
Total body	60.0	100.0	100.0

potassium, and magnesium levels are all very low, symptoms are apt to be less severe than if only one were decreased.

Proper correction of abnormalities also requires some knowledge of the atomic weights of the elements most likely to be involved in fluid and electrolyte problems (Table 6-1).

WATER

Fluid Spaces

Normally about 55 to 60 percent of the body weight of an adult is water. In the newborn, there is more water, usually equivalent to 70 to 80 percent of the body weight. Fat is relatively anhydrous, and muscle is about 77 percent water. Consequently, obese adult women may have less than 50 percent of their weight as water while muscular men may have 60 to 65 percent of their weight as water.

The total body water is normally divided into the intracellular fluid (ICF) and extracellular fluid (ECF). Classically it has been taught that the ICF is 40 percent of the body weight and the ECF (which includes interstitial fluid, plasma, bone, connective tissue, and transcellular fluid) is equal to about 20 percent of the body weight. It is now clear, however, that the ECF is about 25 to 30 percent of the body weight and the ICF is equal to about 30 to 35 percent of the body weight (Table 6-2).

The electrolyte concentrations in the plasma and interstitial fluid are approximately the same except for protein-bound electrolytes such as calcium and magnesium. Cellular fluid has much more potassium, magnesium, phosphate, and proteinate than the ECF, but it has relatively little sodium and virtually no calcium or chloride (Table 6-3).

Fluid Requirements

Daily fluid requirements include (1) *basic needs* for urine and insensible water loss; (2) *current losses* for gastrointestinal loss,

sweat, or increased loss of insensible water; and (3) *correction* for any defects or excesses.

Basic needs include urine loss of about 600 to 1000 mL/($m^2 \cdot$ day) and an insensible water loss of about 350 to 700 mL/($m^2 \cdot$ day) on an average-sized adult man. This amounts to about 1500 mL of urine and 1000 mL of insensible water loss per day. Insensible water loss includes about 300 mL from the skin and 700 mL from the lungs.

Current losses for fever are about 500 mL of increased insensible water loss per 1° above 98.6°F(37°C), 500 to 1500 mL extra for sweating, and milliliter-for-milliliter loss of gastrointestinal fluid. The electrolyte contents of various fluids that may be lost can vary greatly, but certain average values can be used (Table 6-4).

Water deficits can be estimated from weight loss, thirst, and physical signs. Severe thirst usually indicates fluid deficit of at least 3 percent of the body weight. Soft eyes, tachycardia, severe oliguria, or organ dysfunction usually indicate severe dehydration. If an adult patient appears slightly, moderately, or severely dehydrated, he or she has lost fluid equal to 6, 8, or 10 percent of the body weight, respectively.

ELECTROLYTE ABNORMALITIES

Sodium

The total body sodium normally is about 40 to 45 mEq/kg or about 3000 mEq in an average normal 80-kg man. Almost 98 percent is present in extracellular fluid which is about 25 to 30 percent of the body weight (contrary to the 20 percent figure classically used). Intracellular sodium levels are usually less than 10 to 12 mEq/L.

Table 6-3. Electrolyte Concentration of Fluid Spaces (mEq/L)

Cations	Plasma	Interstitial Fluid	Cellular Fluid	Anions	Plasma	Interstitial Fluid	Cellular Fluid
Na	142	145	10	Chloride	102	114	0
K	4.2	5.0	150	Bicarbonate	26	30	10
Ca	4.7	2.5	0	Proteinate	16	1	40
Mg	2.1	1.5	40	Sulfate	1	1	10
				Phosphate	2	2	140
				Organic acids	6	6	0
Total	153	154	200		153	154	200

Table 6-4. Average Electrolyte Contents of Various Body Fluids (mEq/L)

	Sodium	Potassium	Chloride	Bicarbonate
Stomach	60–80	5–10	80–120	—
Bile	130–140	4–6	95–105	30–40
Pancreas	130–140	4–6	40–60	80–100
Small intestine	130–140	4–6	80–100	20–30
Colon	80–140	25–45	80–100	30–50
Sweat	40–50	5–10	45–60	

Note: Water deficits can be estimated from weight loss, thirst, and physical signs. Severe thirst usually indicates fluid deficit of at least 3 percent of body weight.

Hyponatremia

Etiology

The total body sodium tends to be quite constant, and the most frequent cause of hyponatremia is too much total body water, producing a dilutional hyponatremia. In patients with severe trauma, sepsis, cardiac failure, cirrhosis, renal failure, or chronic malnutrition, there is a tendency to retain excessive amounts of water, even with careful fluid management.

Occasionally hyponatremia is due to sodium loss. Some of the more frequent causes of sodium loss include excessive vomiting, diarrhea, and sweating. Hyponatremia is apt to develop if these losses are replaced with fluids that do not contain adequate sodium. Sodium losses also occur with adrenal insufficiency and salt-losing nephritis, especially with cystic disease of the renal medulla, the postoliguric phase of acute vasomotor nephropathy, and after renal transplantation or relief of urinary obstruction. Factitious hyponatremia may occur because of severe hyperglycemia or hyperlipidemia. Because glucose tends to stay in extracellular fluid, hyperglycemia tends to draw water out of cells into the ECF. Each 100 mg/dL in plasma glucose levels decreases the serum sodium concentration by almost 1.6 to 2.0 mEq/L. Thus, a patient who had a serum concentration of 150 mEq/L when his or her glucose level was 100 mg/100 ml would probably have a serum sodium concentration of about 120 mEq/L if his or her blood glucose levels rapidly rose to 1100 mg/100 mL. In "true" hyponatremia, plasma osmolarity is reduced; in factitious hyponatremia, plasma osmolarity is normal or increased.

Physiologic Effects

Many of the physiologic changes and signs and symptoms seen with hyponatremia are due to associated cerebral edema or increased total body water. This may contribute to the headache, anorexia, irritability, and personality changes often seen with mild to moderate hyponatremia. Rapid falls in serum sodium levels below 125 mEq/L can increase neuromuscular irritability and can cause nausea, vomiting, and occasional convulsions and death.

One of the major effects of sodium is related to the osmolarity of the ECF. Serum osmolarity can be measured directly by determining the freezing point of the serum or it can be calculated from the sodium, glucose, and blood urea nitrogen levels using the following formula:

$$\text{Osmolarity} = 2\text{Na} + \frac{\text{glucose}}{18} + \frac{\text{BUN}}{2.8}$$

Normal serum osmolarity is about 270 to 295 mOsm/L, i.e.,

$$\text{Osm} = 2(140) + \frac{90}{18} + \frac{14}{2.8}$$
$$= 280 + 5 + 5 = 290$$

If the osmolar discriminant or osmolar gap (measured serum osmolarity minus calculated osmolarity) is more than 10 mOsm/L there are usually significant amounts of osmotically active substances, such as alcohol or lactate, present. An osmolar discriminant greater than 50 may be fatal.

Diagnosis

Most hyponatremia is due to dilution (a relative excess of total body water) which may be iatrogenic or due to disease (prolonged shock, congestive heart failure, hepatic failure, or nephrotic syndrome). A decrease in the total body sodium due to excess diuresis, vomiting, diarrhea, or sweating is less common. The importance of each factor can usually be determined by careful review of the patient's intake and output. Additional information can be obtained by comparing the sodium concentration and osmolarity of the serum and urine. A urine sodium less than 10 to 20 mEq/L suggests that the body content of sodium is low (if renal perfusion is adequate). If the urine sodium concentration is high, the patient usually has a water overload.

Rarely, the patient may have the syndrome of inappropriate antidiuretic hormone secretion (SIADH). SIADH may be idiopathic, drug-induced (thiazides), or due to head trauma, tumors (lung, brain or ovary), or infection (especially meningitis). Characteristics of SIADH include (1) hyponatremia, (2) increased urine sodium, (3) polyuria, and (4) urine osmolarity greater than plasma osmolarity. Whenever hyponatremia is associated with a urinary sodium excretion which equals or exceeds dietary intake, SIADH or adrenal insufficiency should be suspected.

Treatment

If hyponatremia is due to hemodilution, fluid restriction is usually the best treatment. However, if the hyponatremia develops rapidly and the patient is very restless, administration of 3% saline solution may be necessary. The 3% saline solution (which contains 0.5 mEq of sodium per milliliter) is given at 50 to 100 mL per hour, with careful watching for fluid overload. Close attention is also given to changes in blood and urine sodium levels. Unfortunately, hypertonic saline solution often only increases the serum sodium concentration transiently because most of the administered sodium is rapidly excreted. Consequently it may be wise to give some furosemide to reduce the amount of water present in the body. One method of therapy involves giving furosemide and then replacing urinary electrolyte losses.

Methods of calculating sodium deficits are controversial. We correct sodium deficits using a sodium space equivalent to 20 percent of the body weight. Thus, an 80-kg man with a serum sodium of 120 mEq/L and normal hydration would be assumed to have a sodium deficit equal to (20% of 80 kg) × (140 − 120) or (16) (20) = 320 mEq.

Some feel that sodium levels equilibrate with the total body water, and consequently that total sodium deficits should be calculated using 60 percent of the body weight. In chronically ill or malnourished patients who have an increased ECF space, sodium corrections based on 60 percent of body weight can overload the patient with sodium. In dehydrated patients, using 60 percent of the body weight for calculating sodium deficits is less of a problem.

Treatment of pseudohyponatremia, such as that due to hyperglycemia, is directed at its cause. Once adequate urine output is obtained and insulin becomes effective, glucose levels fall and the serum sodium levels will usually correct spontaneously.

Hypernatremia

Hypernatremia is usually due to a decrease in total body water because of excessive losses of water or inadequate intake. An increased serum concentration of sodium causes few symptoms except lassitude, weakness, and fatigue. The associated decrease in total body water, which is the most frequent cause of hypernatremia, may cause problems due to decreased perfusion of vital organs.

If excessive sodium is given, the kidney will excrete it. However, if renal function or perfusion is impaired, a dangerous expansion of the ECF may occur. One source of excessive sodium administration is the use of carbenicillin. Each gram of carbenicillin has 4.7 mEq of sodium. Ticarcillin averages 5.2 mEq of sodium per gram but may be as high as 6.5 mEq/g in the vial. Thus, if 30 to 40 g of carbenicillin are given daily, the patient will receive 141 to 188 mEq of sodium.

Hypernatremia can be corrected by careful administration of water. If there is any evidence of cardiac failure, this must be done slowly to prevent a sudden increase in intravascular volume. In addition, administration of large quantities of water to hyperosmolar patients, especially if done rapidly, can cause cerebral edema.

Potassium

Chemical analysis of cadavers with ^{40}K reveals a total body potassium content of about 53 mEq/kg. However, "exchangeable potassium" measured by dilution of ^{42}K in a period of 48 h provides values averaging about 45 mEq/kg. In women with severe muscle wasting, the total exchangeable body potassium content may be as low as 20 to 25 mEq/kg. Almost 98 percent of the total body potassium is within cells where the average concentration may be 120 to 150 mEq/L. Over 70 to 75 percent of the total body potassium is in muscle. Thus, severe protein malnutrition may be associated with severe total body deficiencies in potassium as well as the other main intracellular electrolytes, magnesium and phosphorus.

Hypokalemia

Etiology

Hypokalemia may be caused by metabolic alkalosis or increased potassium losses from the body. A rise in the pH of 0.10 due to increased plasma bicarbonate levels generally causes a 0.5 (0.3 to 0.8) mEq/L fall in serum potassium levels. Thus, if a patient with a serum potassium level of 4.2 mEq/L and a pH of 7.40 is given bicarbonate and his or her pH is raised to 7.60, the serum potassium level will fall to about 3.2 mEq/L. Interestingly, immediately after an elevation in the P_{CO_2}, plasma potassium levels rise transiently and then return to baseline values.

Hypokalemia seen with excessive vomiting is due primarily to the metabolic alkalosis which develops. The alkalosis in turn causes increased renal excretion of potassium. Hypercalcemia can also cause increased potassium loss in the urine.

Although normal kidneys can conserve sodium well, potassium losses in the urine are almost "obligatory" and are usually directly proportional to the volume of urine. Urine potassium averages about 40 to 50 mEq/L. Even with severe acute potassium deficits, urine potassium losses will generally exceed 30 mEq/L for at least several days. Heavy use of loop diuretics such as furosemide (Lasix) may cause urine potassium losses to exceed 100 mEq/L. Diarrhea, particularly from an inflamed bowel or a villous adenoma, usually contains at least 25 mEq of potassium per liter. Adrenal corticosteroids and hyperaldosteronism cause the kidneys to excrete potassium and retain sodium and bicarbonate. This can cause a significant hypokalemic metabolic alkalosis.

During the treatment of severe diabetic ketoacidosis, a very dangerous hypokalemia may develop rapidly when blood glucose levels begin to fall, unless potassium is given. As the pH rises toward normal and blood and urine volumes increase, potassium levels can fall precipitously. In addition, as insulin becomes effective and glucose begins to enter tissue cells, potassium, magnesium, and phosphate move intracellularly with it.

Physiologic Effects

Severe hypokalemia with levels below 2.5 mEq/L may cause muscle weakness and may increase the tendency to ileus in the intestinal tract. Hypokalemia also tends to cause a metabolic alkalemia with increased acid excretion in the urine (paradoxical aciduria). It may also impair the ability of the kidneys to concentrate urine, and it increases the tendency to glycosuria. The sensitivity of the heart to digitalis and the likelihood of digitalis toxicity with arrhythmias or an AV block is increased in the presence of hypokalemia. Administration of potassium and magnesium are often important parts of the treatment of arrhythmias due to digitalis toxicity.

Diagnosis

The diagnosis of hypokalemia is made primarily on serum electrolyte studies. Urine potassium levels can give some indication of the duration of hypokalemia and total body deficit. Urine potassium levels that are normal (30 to 50 mEq/L) suggest the presence of an acute potassium deficit. Urine potassium levels less than 10 mEq/L suggest a more chronic and more severe potassium deficit. However, if the hypokalemia is due to metabolic alkalosis or primary aldosteronism, urine potassium levels may be high despite severe chronic hypokalemia.

Whenever possible, serum potassium levels should be interpreted relative to the arterial pH. A low serum potassium level may be expected in an alkalotic patient, but hypokalemia in an acidotic patient is either a laboratory error or evidence of a very severe potassium deficit. In some instances, the patient can act as if he or she is hypokalemic even with normal blood levels, particularly after cardiopulmonary bypass and when he or she has metabolic alkalosis. In patients with metabolic alkalosis, paradoxical aciduria suggests a functional hypokalemia. On ECG, hypokalemia less than 3.0 mEq/L may cause low voltage QRS complexes, flattened T waves, depressed ST segments, prominent P and U waves, and prolonged QT intervals. The U wave can be seen in many normal individuals in the early precordial leads (V_1–V_3) but it is more prominent with hypokalemia, diastolic hypertension, and coronary artery disease.

Treatment

Acute severe hypokalemia is treated by infusing 10 to 20 mEq of KCl in 50 to 100 mL of 5% dextrose in water (D_5W) or 0.9% saline per hour by IV piggyback. Potassium equilibrates in the total body water, and it generally takes 40 to 50 mEq to raise the serum potassium level by 1.0 mEq/L. Chronic deficits may require larger amounts of potassium to maintain any increase in potassium levels. If serum potassium levels do not respond to potassium infusion, the patient may be losing excessive quantities of potassium. As a rule no more than 40 mEq/kg should be put in a liter of IV fluids (except by careful IV piggyback) and no more than 40 mEq should be given per hour.

Chronic hypokalemia may be associated with very severe potassium deficits, which often total 300 to 500 mEq or more. The percentage by which serum levels (corrected for pH) are below 4.2 mEq/L, is double the percentage of total body potassium deficit. Thus, a serum potassium level of 2.1 mEq/L at a pH of 7.4 indicates a 50 percent reduction in serum potassium and a 25 percent reduction in total body potassium. Total body potassium ranges between 20 mEq/kg in a markedly wasted woman to 45 mEq/kg in a normal muscular man.

Hyperkalemia

Etiology

Normally, 90 to 95 percent of the potassium taken in is excreted in the urine. Thus, anuria may cause a progressive rise in serum potassium levels. Since each kilogram of lean muscle tissue contains about 90 to 100 mEq of potassium, breakdown of tissue from trauma or sepsis may release large quantities of potassium into the bloodstream. If the patient is oliguric, serum potassium levels may rise abruptly, particularly if the patient is sodium-restricted. A similar problem may develop with hemolysis due to transfusion reactions.

Excessive intake of potassium is an infrequent cause of hyperkalemia, but can occur with IV administration of potassium-containing drugs. Aqueous (potassium) penicillin, for example, contains about 1.7 mEq of potassium per million units. Laboratory errors can also easily cause a factitious hyperkalemia. Hemolysis of blood specimens will release potassium from red blood cells. Metabolic acidosis tends to cause hyperkalemia. Each 0.1 pH decrease in arterial pH increases serum potassium levels by about 0.5 mEq/L.

Physiologic Effects

As potassium levels rise above 6.0 mEq/L, cardiac conductivity and contractility may be impaired. As serum potassium levels rise above 6.5 to 7.0 mEq/L, an intracardiac block is produced, first in the atria, then in the AV node, and finally in the ventricles, with the heart finally stopping in diastole. Occasionally, hyperkalemia may cause such weakness that ventilatory failure may develop. The effects of hyperkalemia are increased if the patient has hyponatremia and hypocalcemia.

Diagnosis

One should suspect hyperkalemia in patients with oliguric renal failure, severe hemolysis or excessive tissue breakdown. On ECG one may see high, peaked (steeple) T waves and depressed ST segments. With increasing hyperkalemia the P waves may disappear and the QRS complexes widen.

Treatment

Emergency treatment of hyperkalemia with arrhythmias or cardiovascular instability includes IV administration of 10mL of $CaCl_2$ in 5 to 10 min, 1 ampule (45 to 50 mEq) of sodium bicarbonate in 10 to 20 min, and 50 mL of 50% glucose with 5 to 10 units of insulin over 5 to 10 min. These may be repeated once or twice as needed over 30 to 60 min. Calcium directly antagonizes the effects of potassium on the heart of the cell membrane. Sodium bicarbonate causes an alkalosis which tends to reduce serum potassium levels. It also increases the serum concentration of sodium, which helps oppose the potassium effects. As glucose enters cells, it pulls potassium, magnesium, and phosphorus in with it. After the initial 50% glucose, 20% glucose with 40 units of insulin may be given slowly.

Kayexalate (sodium polystyrene sulfonate), which may be administered by mouth or by retention enemas, pulls potassium from the body by an ion exchange mechanism. Each gram of sodium resin eliminates about 2 mEq of potassium. Orally, 15 g of Kayexalate are given with 15 g of sorbital two to four times a day. Rectal administration is 50 g of Kayexalate in 150 mL of water with 50 g of sorbitol. The enema should be retained at least 30 min. The sorbitol increases evacuation of bowel contents. If a patient is in acute renal failure, hemodialysis and/or peritoneal dialysis should be set up while the above measures are being used.

If serum potassium levels are less than 6.5 mEq/L and there are no ECG changes due to the hyperkalemia, treatment may be slower. Wherever possible, all potassium-containing solutions should be discontinued or given as a sodium salt of the same agent. Diuresis is extremely helpful. Even when renal function is severely impaired, each liter of urine contains at least 20 to 30 mEq of potassium per liter.

Calcium

The total body calcium content is about 15 to 20 g/kg with about 99 percent in bone as mineral apatite. The normal total daily intake orally is about 30 to 40 mEq (600 to 800 mg) of which only 15 percent is absorbed and excreted in the urine.

Hypocalcemia

Total plasma calcium levels average 8.5 to 10.5 mg/dL. The calcium present in the plasma is in three forms: protein-bound calcium (normally 4.0 to 4.5 mg/dL), complexed (nonprotein-bound, nonionized) calcium (normally 0.5 to 1.0 mg/dL), and ionized calcium (normally 4.2 to 4.8 mg/dL). Increasingly, calcium levels are being reported as mEq/L, which is half of the number expressed as milligrams per deciliter. Thus, 10 mg/dL of calcium is the same as 5.0 mEq/L or 2.5 mOsm/L. The ionized calcium fraction is responsible for virtually all the physiologic effects of calcium, of which the neuromuscular changes are the most obvious.

Etiology

Hypocalcemia is an important and frequent metabolic problem in critically ill patients. One of the commonest causes of hypocalcemia is hypoproteinemia. Each gram of albumin binds approximately 0.8 to 0.9 mg of calcium and each gram of globulin binds approximately 0.1 to 0.2 mg of calcium. Therefore, if the plasma albumin level is 3 g/100 mL and the globulin level is 2 g/100 mL, it may be assumed that the albumin is binding about 2.4 to 2.7 mg/100 mL calcium and that the globulin is binding about 0.2 to 0.4 mg/100 mL calcium. If there is a normal concentration of ionized and complexed calcium, one would expect a total calcium in the blood of about 8.3 mg/dL. One can also use a standard table to estimate the ionized calcium from the total protein and total calcium levels (Table 6-5).

Any process which interferes with cell metabolism such as shock, sepsis, or cardiopulmonary bypass, may reduce ionized calcium levels. This is apparently due to movement of calcium across the cell membrane into the cytoplasm of poorly functioning cells. Following trauma, serum calcium levels may be low, especially with the fat embolism syndrome, not only because of cell damage but also because of fatty acid inhibition of the plasma membrane calcium pump.

Acute pancreatitis is an important cause of hypocalcemia. Pancreatic lipase breaks down fat into fatty acids and glycerol. The fatty acids combine with calcium to form calcium soaps and reduce serum calcium levels. In addition, as protein moves into the inflammatory exudate, the resultant hypoproteinemia may cause ionized calcium levels to fall precipitously. Pancreatitis may somehow reduce parathormone secretion and the response of tissues to it. If total calcium levels fall below 7 mg/100 mL, the prognosis is guarded.

Cimetidine, a histamine (H_2) receptor-blocking agent used to treat peptic ulcer, may also decrease the synthesis or secretion of parathyroid hormone and reduce serum calcium levels.

Hypocalcemia is occasionally due to hypoparathyroidism, which is most frequently due to surgical removal or damage of the parathyroid glands. Parathormone increases serum calcium levels by increased calcium absorption from the intestine and renal tubes.

Physiologic Effects

Although normal ionized calcium levels are 2.1 to 2.4 mEq/L, serious changes do not usually occur until the ionized calcium

levels in serum are less than 1.6 to 1.7 mEq/L. Proper levels of ionized calcium are important for optimal cardiac and neuromuscular function. Decreased ionized calcium levels increase neuromuscular excitability and may thereby cause carpopedal spasm and cramps. Decreased ionized calcium levels also reduce the strength of contraction of muscle and the sensitivity of the heart to digitalis. Hypocalcemia should be looked for in patients with refractory heart failure.

Low ionized calcium levels increase parathormone (PTH) secretion which mobilizes calcium from bone and decreases renal tubular absorption of phosphate and bicarbonate. This, in turn, may cause an increased absorption of chloride, producing a tendency to hyperchloremic hypophosphatemic renal tubular acidosis.

The ECF concentration of calcium per liter is about 10^{-3} mol, whereas the concentration inside cytoplasm is about 10^{-7} mol. This 10,000:1 gradient is maintained by active cell metabolism. Ischemia, hypoxia, and sepsis interfere with cell membrane function and allow calcium to move into the cytoplasm. The increased cytoplasmic calcium further interferes with cell metabolism. In addition, efforts by mitochondria to pump the excess calcium out of the cytoplasm into the mitochondrial matrix greatly reduce adenosine triphosphate (ATP) formation. Consequently, giving calcium during shock or sepsis may transiently improve hemodynamics but, if cell metabolism does not also improve, the additional calcium moves into the cytoplasm and further impairs cell metabolism.

Movement of calcium into ischemic cerebral vascular smooth muscle cells may cause failure of cerebral reperfusion after strokes or cardiac arrest and may be a major cause of the poor results in management of these problems. Recently, there has been an increased interest in the use of calcium blockers for cerebral resuscitation and their mechanisms of action.

Diagnosis

Initial symptoms of hypocalcemia include paresthesias around the mouth or in the fingertips. Hypocalcemia should be suspected in patients who are irritable or who have hyperactive deep tendon reflexes. It should also be suspected in those who have seizures, particularly if they have ever had thyroid surgery, even if many years previously. A positive Chvostek's or Trousseau's sign is generally considered clinical evidence of hypocalcemia. A positive Chvostek's sign is a twitching at the corner of the mouth which occurs when the examiner taps over the facial nerve just in front of the patient's ear. Trousseau's sign, which is generally a more reliable indicator of hypocalcemia, is positive if carpal spasm is produced when the examiner applies a blood pressure cuff to the upper arm and maintains a pressure halfway between systolic and diastolic for 3 min. These signs may also be found with normal total serum calcium if the patient is very alkalotic (i.e., has a low ionized calcium level) or if the patient is hypomagnesemic. Similar signs and symptoms also may be caused by strychnine or tetanus toxin. Hypocalcemia may occasionally be diagnosed on ECG by prolonged QT intervals.

Decreased plasma levels of ionized calcium or decreased levels of total calcium in the presence of normal plasma protein concentrations are diagnostic.

Treatment

Treatment includes correction of the underlying cause and administration of calcium salts. Ten mL of a 10% $CaCl_2$ solution may

Table 6-5. Ionized Calcium (mEq/L) at Various Total Calcium and Total Protein Levels

Total Calcium (mg/dL)	Total Protein (g/dL)			
	4.0	5.0	6.0	7.0
12.0	3.6	3.3	3.0	2.6
11.0	3.3	3.0	2.7	2.4
10.0	3.0	2.6	2.4	2.2
9.0	2.7	2.4	2.2	1.9
8.0	2.4	2.1	1.9	1.6
7.0	2.0	1.8	1.6	1.5
6.0	1.6	1.5	1.4	1.3

be given slowly intravenously followed by a continuous IV drip providing a gram of $CaCl_2$ every 8 to 12 h. Calcium is generally not given after thyroid and parathyroid resections unless the patient is symptomatic, or the hypocalcemia is severe and prolonged for more than 10 to 14 days.

During massive transfusions, if the patient is in severe, persistent shock in spite of adequate volume replacement therapy, 10 mL of 10% $CaCl_2$ given after every 4 units of blood may dramatically improve cardiovascular function. Calcium is seldom required during transfusions for elective surgery.

Although the use of calcium has been advocated for the resuscitation of patients with asystole or electromechanical dissociation, it has recently been shown that the chances of a successful resuscitation with prehospital arrest is significantly reduced by using calcium. On the other hand, patients with bradyasystolic arrest and chronic renal failure are apt to have hyperkalemia and hypocalcemia and may benefit from calcium administration.

Hypercalcemia

Etiology

In hospitalized patients, the most frequent cause of hypercalcemia is metastatic malignancies, particularly from the lung and breast. Primary hyperparathyroidism accounts for most of the remaining cases. In general, the higher the serum calcium level, especially about 14.0 mg/dL, the more likely the hypercalcemia is due to malignancy. With very high calcium levels and no obvious evidence of a malignancy, an enlarged parathyroid gland can sometimes be palpated in the neck.

In patients who are immobilized, calcium may leave bone rapidly, producing hypercalcemia, at least temporarily. Urinary excretion of calcium in such patients may exceed 200 to 300 mg/day, and there is an increased tendency to nephrolithiasis. In these patients the parathyroid vitamin D axis is suppressed.

Physiologic Effects

Total calcium levels above 12.0 mg/dL cause symptoms, and levels above 14 to 16 mg/dL have a poor prognosis unless treated aggressively. These patients are weak, lethargic, and confused. Frank coma is uncommon, but calcium levels should be drawn in any patient with coma of unknown etiology. Vomiting and polyuria (due to hypercalcemic impairment of ADH function) may also be present, causing increasing dehydration. Hypercalcemia increases the sensitivity of the heart to digitalis and may precipitate digitalis toxicity. If the calcium levels become very high, the heart may stop in systole.

Diagnosis

Hypercalcemia should be suspected in patients with extensive metastatic bone disease and in individuals with clinical problems such as renal calculi, pancreatitis, or ulcer disease. As with hypocalcemia, total calcium level in hypercalcemic patients should be correlated with serum proteins. If the patient is hypoproteinemic, total calcium levels may be normally low in spite of increased ionized calcium levels. On ECG, hypercalcemia may be associated with a decreased ST segment and QT interval. However, hypercalcemia does not cause an abnormally short QT interval when the interval is corrected for rate.

Treatment

Treatment involves giving large quantities of fluid (dilution), reducing ionized calcium levels by making the patient alkalotic (deacidifying), and giving furosemide or ethacrinic acid to increase the renal excretion of calcium (diuresis). However, up to a third of patients with hypercalcemia will also have hypokalemia. If hypercalcemia is due to malignant disease, over half the patients may have hypokalemia. Use of diuretics may aggravate this hypokalemia.

Steroids may be of some benefit, probably by causing calcium to shift inside the cell where it may be bound to mitochondria. Mithramycin (15 to 25 μg/kg by IV bolus) is used occasionally, especially with metastatic bone disease. Intravenous phosphates are rarely used now because of the rapid fall in calcium that may occur, along with tissue position of calcium phosphate, renal cortical necrosis, and even shock.

If a parathyroid adenoma is present, it should be removed as soon as possible. An adenoma large enough to cause symptoms may even be palpable in the neck. If the hypercalcemia appears to be due to a large carcinoma of the lung, the lung lesion should be resected or irradiated.

Magnesium

Magnesium is vital in all biologic systems and is the key element in chlorophyll, the basic producer of the world's food chain. The total body content of magnesium averages about 2000 mEq, with about 60 to 70 percent present in bone. The majority of the remaining magnesium is intracellular. The serum concentration of magnesium is about 1.8 to 2.4 mEq/L and a third of the magnesium present in the blood is protein-bound. The usual daily requirement is about 24 to 28 mEq per day.

Hypomagnesemia

Etiology

In adults, deficiencies are most frequently seen in patients with cirrhosis, malnutrition, pancreatitis, or excessive gastrointestinal fluid losses. Diarrhea is more of a problem (Mg^{2+} content of 10 to 14 mEq/L) than upper gastrointestinal loss (1 to 2 mEq/L). Chronic hyperparathyroidism increases urinary losses of magnesium and will eventually also cause hypomagnesemia. Intravenous hyperalimentation without adequate magnesium can cause an abrupt fall in plasma magnesium levels as magnesium is "pulled" into cells with glucose. Hypophosphatemia, which can also develop with IV hyperalimentation, by itself can also cause hypomagnesemia. Patients with severe diabetic ketoacidosis may develop hypomagnesemia as treatment begins to be effective and tissue cells begin to take up glucose along with potassium and phosphate.

Physiologic Effects

Magnesium is essential for many vital enzymes, including the activation of membrane-bound adenosine triphosphatase (ATPase). Hypomagnesemia may be associated with increased muscular irritability similar to that seen with hypocalcemia. Magnesium is an important mediator of neural transmission in the central nervous system, and hypomagnesemia may cause many central nervous system signs and symptoms, including depression, vertigo, ataxia, and seizures. In severe chronic alcoholics, delirium tremens may be caused by or associated with moderate to severe magnesium deficiencies. Cardiac arrhythmias may be due to magnesium deficiency, and the arrhythmias of digitalis toxicity may be due to both potassium and magnesium deficiencies. Magnesium may also be valuable in normomagnesic tachyarrhythmias.

Some metabolic manifestations of magnesium deficiency may include impaired therapy of hypokalemia, impaired PTH, decreased response to thiamine, and vitamin-D resistant hypocalcemia. Other manifestations include hypothermia, hypotension, nephropathy, incomplete distal renal tubular acidosis, dysphagia, and anemia due to shortened red blood cell survival.

Diagnosis

Diagnosis is suggested by evidence of increased neuromuscular irritability in the presence of normal serum calcium levels. Hypomagnesemia should be suspected in alcoholics, cirrhotics, and patients on IV fluids for prolonged periods. Hypomagnesemia may develop rapidly during IV hyperalimentation, especially when anabolism begins. Total body magnesium may fall to rather low levels before the plasma concentration falls below normal. The ECG changes include PR and QT interval prolongation, widened QRS complexes, depression of the ST segments, and inversion of the T waves in the precordial leads. These changes are similar to those caused by hypokalemia, and Mg^{2+} deficiency may alter cardiac intracellular potassium content.

Treatment

In chronic alcoholics with delirium tremens and in patients with proven hypomagnesemia, 6 to 8 g of magnesium may be given intramuscularly or slowly intravenously the first day, followed by 4 to 6 g (16 to 32 mEq) per day thereafter. If IV alimentation is being given, 12 to 16 mEq (1.5 to 2.0 g) should be added to each liter if the patient is hypomagnesemic.

If magnesium is being given rapidly, as with eclampsia, deep tendon reflexes should be checked frequently and blood levels should be measured, at least daily. If deep tendon reflexes decrease or are absent, magnesium administration should stop, at least temporarily.

Hypermagnesemia

Etiology

Hypermagnesemia occurs rather infrequently, except in patients with renal failure who are given magnesium-containing drugs, particularly antacids such as Maalox. Other (rare) causes include untreated diabetic acidosis or adrenal insufficiency.

Physiologic Effects

Progressively increasing magnesium levels above 3.0 to 4.0 mEq/L will initially reduce neuromuscular irritability and then cause deep tendon reflexes to disappear. Continued rise in magnesium levels above 5.0 mEq/L may cause severe vasodilation and hypotension. Levels above 10 mEq/L may cause neuromuscular paralysis with ventilatory failure.

Diagnosis

Serum magnesium levels are usually diagnostic. However, the possibility of hypermagnesemia should be considered in patients with renal failure, particularly those who are on magnesium-containing antacids such as Maalox.

Treatment

Initial treatment includes dilution by administering IV fluids and using diuretics, especially furosemide, as needed. Peritoneal and hemodialysis may be tried but are ineffective with divalent cations.

Chloride

Chloride is largely extracellular where its concentration is usually about five-sevenths of that seen with sodium. Unlike sodium, there is little chloride in bone, and virtually all chloride is diffusible and metabolically active.

Hypochloremia

Etiology

The most frequent causes of hypochloremia are excessive diuresis, especially after administration of loop diuretics, or loss of gastric secretions through vomiting or nasogastric suction.

Physiologic Effects

The most frequent physiologic effects are those due to the metabolic alkalosis usually seen with hypochloremia.

Diagnosis

Low serum chloride levels are diagnostic, but may be partly due to dilution. If urinary chloride levels are low (less than 10 to 20 mEq/L, the patient usually has a severe chloride deficit. If urine chloride levels are 60 mEq/L or higher, the hypochloremia is probably due to hemodilution.

Treatment

Chloride-responsive metabolic alkalosis will usually respond to IV administration of chloride alone. Chloride-resistant alkalosis usually requires potassium and chloride and may also require hydrogen ions. Hypochloremia due to dilution from excess total body water is usually best treated by cautious dehydration.

Deficits in total body chloride content are best treated by giving one-fourth of the calculated chloride deficit as KCl and three-fourths as NaCl. The total body chloride deficit can be estimated fairly accurately by multiplying 20 percent of the body weight by the serum chloride deficit. An 80 kg patient with a serum chloride of 60 mEq/L has a total deficit of (80 kg × 20%) (100 − 60) = 16 × 40 or 640 mEq. If the patient is severely dehydrated, the total chloride deficit may be estimated by assuming that mild, moderate, or severe dehydration involves a 6, 8, or 10 percent loss respectively of body weight as ECF containing 100 mEq of chloride per liter.

Hyperchloremia

Hyperchloremia is usually due to dehydration, and under such circumstances it is usually associated with hypernatremia. Excess administration of chloride as saline, KCl, and amino acid hydrochlorides can also cause hyperchloremia. The most frequent acid-base problem seen with IV hyperalimentation is a hyperchloremic metabolic acidosis (due to the amino acid hydrochlorides).

The physiological effects of hyperchloremia are due primarily to the underlying dehydration or metabolic acidosis. Elevated serum chloride and sodium levels indicate dehydration. Elevated chloride levels with normal or low serum sodium levels usually indicate excess chloride administration as KCl or amino acid hydrochlorides.

Hyperchloremia due to dehydration is best treated by slowly administering increased water without chloride. High chloride levels due to excess chloride administration can be corrected by giving the needed sodium and potassium as lactate, acetate, or phosphate salts.

Phosphorus (Phosphate)

The normal adult man contains about 700 g of phosphorus, of which about 80 percent is present in bones. Serum phosphorus levels drop with age from a high of 7.0 mg/dL in the newborn, to 5.0 mg/dL in adults. Serum calcium and phosphorus levels are inverse to each other, and the product of their two concentrations in milligrams per deciliter usually averages about 30 to 40. The normal oral intake is about 10 to 12 mOsm with urinary excretion largely regulated by PTH.

Hypophosphatemia

Etiology

Hypophosphatemia is being increasingly recognized, especially with IV hyperalimentation which increases phosphate movement into cells for phosphorylation of various carbohydrate compounds. Hypophosphatemia may also be seen with metabolic alkalosis, especially after prolonged antacid therapy. Respiratory alkalosis may also cause a rapid and abrupt hypophosphatemia. Impaired intestinal absorption of phosphate may be due to antacids. Sustained vomiting or diarrhea can greatly increase phosphate losses from the body. Potassium and magnesium deficiencies also increase phosphate loss in the urine. Hyperparathyroidism and alcoholism are additional causes of hypophosphatemia.

Physiologic Effects

Progressive weakness and tremors may be noted as blood phosphate levels fall below 0.5 to 1.0 mg/dL. Circumoral and fingertip paresthesias may be present along with absent deep tendon reflexes. Mental obtundation, anorexia, and hyperventilation may also occur. Severe long bone pain and symptoms of various rheumatic syndromes may be present.

Hypophosphatemia may be associated with depletion of ATP in red blood cells and platelets, reducing their survival time. Associated membrane changes may result in a bleeding tendency due to impaired platelet function and a tendency for red blood cells to become rigid spherocytes, thereby impairing capillary perfusion. In addition, the decreased 2,3-diphosphoglycerate (2,3-DPG) associated with hypophosphatemia increases the affinity of hemoglobin for oxygen, thereby reducing the arterial P_{O_2} and decreasing oxygen availability to tissues.

Phosphate depletion in macrophages may impair chemotaxis and phagocytosis, resulting in decreased resistance to infection. This may be a particular problem in patients who have been on antibiotics for prolonged periods and require IV hyperalimentation.

Muscle function impairment with hypophosphatemia may cause so much weakness that the patient cannot be properly weaned from a ventilator or ambulated. Even myocardial function, as measured by left ventricular stroke work, may be impaired.

Diagnosis

Any evidence of malnutrition should arouse suspicion of hypophosphatemia. This problem should be looked for with particular care when IV hyperalimentation is begun.

Treatment

Treatment of hypophosphatemia should be primarily preventive and must be an integral part of any nutrition program. At least 7 to 9 mOsm of phosphate, usually as a combination of KH_2PO_4 and K_2HPO_4, should be given with each 1000 calories. In some instances, more than double that amount of phosphate may be required to bring phosphate levels up to normal. Because phosphate administration may cause a precipitous fall in serum calcium levels, calcium should also be given, usually as 0.2 to 0.3 mEq/(kg · day) of calcium gluconate.

In many textbooks, phosphate is given intravenously in terms of milliequivalents. This can create some problems because serum phosphorus exists in various proportions of phosphate (PO_4^{-3}), monohydrogen phosphate (HPO_4^{-2}) and dihydrogen phosphate ($H_2PO_4^{-1}$). Thus, no valence can be applied consistently to "phosphate." Nevertheless, there is a tendency to treat phosphate administration as if each mOsm were equal to 3 mEq.

Hyperphosphatemia

Hyperphosphatemia is most apt to be seen with renal dysfunction. It may also be seen with hypoparathyroidism, or any problem associated with hypocalcemia or hypomagnesemia. Problems due to hyperphosphatemia are probably not nearly as important as those due to the associated renal failure, hypocalcemia, or hypomagnesemia which is usually present. Hyperphosphatemia is best managed by improvement of urine output and renal function. Any associated electrolyte problem should be corrected simultaneously.

BIBLIOGRAPHY

Aldinger KA, Samaan NA: Hypokalemia with hypercalcemia, prevalence and significance of treatment. *Ann Intern Med* 87:571–573, 1977.

Auffant RA, Dunns JG, Amicte R: Iodized calcium concentration and cardiovascular function after cardiopulmonary bypass. *Arch Surg* 116:1072–1076, 1981.

Barker GL: Hyperkalemia presenting as ventilatory failure. *Anesthesia* 35:885–886, 1980.

Bartter FC, Schwartz WB: The syndrome of inappropriate secretion of antidiuretic hormone. *Am J Med* 42:790, 1967.

Braunwald E: The mechanism of action of calcium-channel blocking agents *N Engl J Med* 307:1611, 1982.

Carddock PR, Yawata Y, Van Santen, et al: Acquired phagocytic dysfunction. A complication of the hypophosphatemia of parenteral hyperalimentation. *N Engl J Med* 290:1403, 1974.

Chernow B, Smith J, Rainey TG, et al: Hypomagnesemia with implications for the critical care specialist. *Crit Care Med* 10:193, 1982.

Chernow B, Zaloga G, McFadden E, et al: Hypocalcemia in critically ill patients. *Crit Care Med* 10:848, 1982.

Connor TB, Rosen BL, Blanstein MP, et al: Hypocalcemia precipitating congestive heart failure. *N Engl J Med* 307:869, 1982.

Cox RE: Hypoparathyroidism, an unusual case of seizures. *Ann Emerg Med* 12:314, 1983.

Edwards H, Zinberg J, King TC: Effect of cimetidine on serum calcium levels in an elderly patient. *Arch Surg* 116:10–8–1089, 1981.

Ellman H, Dembin H, Seriff N: The rarity of shortening of the Q-T interval in patients with hypercalcemia. *Crit Care Med* 10:320, 1982.

Ferris TF, Levintin H, Phillips ET, et al: Renal potassium induced by vitamin D. *J Clin Invest* 41:1222, 1962.

Fiskin RA, Heath DA, Bold AM: Hypercalcemia—a hospital survey. *Q J Med* 49:405–418, 1980.

Fitzgerald F: Clinical Hypophosphatemia. *Ann Rev Med* 29:177–189, 1978.

Harrington JT, Cohen JJ: Measurements of urinary electrolytes—indications and limitations. *N Engl J Med* 293:1241, 1975.

Hartman F, Russier B, Zohlman R, et al: Rapid correction of hyponatremia in the syndrome of inappropriate secretion of antidiuretic hormone. *Ann Intern Med* 78:870, 1973.

Iseri LT, Freed J, Bures AR: Magnesium deficiency and cardiac disorders. *Am J Med* 58:837–846, 1975.

Kassirer JP, Schwartz WB: The response of normal man to selective depletion of hypochloric acid. *Am J Med* 40:10–18, 1966.

Katz MD: Hyperglycemia-induced hyponatremia—calculation of the expected serum sodium depression. *N Engl J Med* 289:843, 1973.

Kreusser W, Kurakawa K. Aznar E, et al: Effects of phosphate depletion on magnesium metabolism in rates. *J Clin Invest* 61:573, 1978.

Leibman J, Edelman IS: Inter-relations of plasma potassium concentration, plasma sodium concentration, arterial pH and total exchangeable potassium. *J Clin Invest* 38:2176–2188, 1959.

Lim M, Linton RAF, Band DM: Early changes in plasma potassium after acute alterations in $PaCO_2$ in anesthetized dogs, monitored continuously with intravascular potassium selective electrodes. *Crit Care Med* 10:747, 1982.

McMahon MJ, Woodhead JS, Hayward RD: The nature of hypocalcemia in acute pancreatitis. *Br J Surg* 65:216, 1978.

Miller CE, Remenchik AP: Problems involved in accurately measuring the K content of the human body. *Ann NY Acad Sci,* 110:175, 1965.

Pine RW, Vincenzi FF, Larrico CJ: Apparent inhibition of the plasma membrane Ca^{2+} pump by oleic acid. *J Trauma* 23:366, 1983.

Robertson GJ Jr., Moore EW, Suitz DM, et al: Inadequate parathyroid response in acute pancreatitis. *N Engl J Med* 294:512, 1976.

Scribner BH, Burnell JH: Interpretation of the serum potassium concentration. *Metabolism* 5:468–479, 1956.

Seller RH, Langiano J, Kim KE, et al: Digitalis toxicity and hypomagnesemia. *Am Heart J* 79:57, 1970.

Stenven H, Thompson BM, Aprahamian C, et al: Use of calcium in prehospital cardiac arrest. *Ann Emerg Med* 12:136, 1983.

Stewart AF, Adler M, Byers C, et al: Calcium homeostasis in immobilization, an example of reportive hypercalciuria. *N Engl J Med* 306:1136, 1982.

Surawicz B: Relationship between electrocardiogram and electrolytes. *Am Heart J* 73:814, 1967.

Swaminathan R, Bradley R, Morgan DB, et al: Hypophosphatemia in surgical patients. *Surg Gynecol Obstet* 148:448–454, 1979.

Vann PW, Coulter M, Wasserberger JS: Use of calcium in brady-asystolic arrest. *Ann Emerg Med* 11:590, 1982.

White BC, Winegar CD, Wilson RF, et al: The possible role of calcium blockers in cerebral resuscitation: A review of the literature and synthesis for future studies. *Crit Care Med* 11:202, 1983.

Wilson RF, Soullier G. Antonenko D: Ionized calcium levels in critically ill surgical patients. *Am Surg* 45(8):485–490, 1979.

CHAPTER 7
SHOCK

Robert C. Jorden

GENERAL

Shock is the common denominator of a large variety of disease processes seen in the emergency department. Shock as a diagnosis never stands on its own, since an underlying process is always present. Nevertheless, shock represents a life-threatening decompensation of vital functions and, as such, demands immediate recognition and specific intervention. As is true in most disease processes, the sound treatment of shock is based on a thorough understanding of pathophysiology. This chapter reviews the pathophysiology of shock from several different perspectives. Initially we will discuss elements common to all forms of shock. Specific types of shock will then be explored in detail.

Inadequate tissue perfusion is still an accurate definition of shock. The cell, which is the ultimate target of compromised perfusion, will eventually die if deprived of oxygen and energy sources for a long enough time. At some point, when enough cells in vital organs are disrupted, shock becomes irreversible; that is, death of the organism is inevitable even if vital signs are restored. Prior to reaching this final state, however, several compensatory mechanisms are involved and exhausted.

In the early stages of shock, compensation is geared toward preserving cardiac output. Catecholamine release provides a chronotropic and inotropic effect on the heart, resulting in an increased pulse and enhanced contractility. Blood pressure is maintained by increasing peripheral vascular resistance, largely due to sympathetic nervous system stimulation and circulating catecholamines. Preload is also enhanced by contraction of the capacitance veins. As shock progresses, blood flow is redistributed to vital organs at the expense of less vital tissues such as skin, gut, and muscles.

In the later stages of shock, compensatory measures begin to fail. Blood pressure and cardiac output drop and flow to vital organs becomes compromised. Changes occur in the microcirculation which further impede oxygen delivery to cells. Precapillary sphincters relax while postcapillary sphincters remain intact. The result is stagnation of flow and sludging. Rheological abnormalities further contribute to sludging. The laminar flow, in part due to the driving pressure propelling the blood, is altered. Shear stress, which is normally able to bend red cells, thus enhancing their flow through capillaries, is lost. The result is rouleaux formation, and further stagnation of flow in the microcirculation.

The cell, which has been the benefactor of all the body's efforts at compensation, will begin to show signs of altered function as compensatory measures fail. A stepwise progression of cellular events has been described by Baue. The first effects of shock involve the cell membrane. There is a decrease in the membrane potential as sodium enters the cell while potassium leaves it. Stimulation of the ATPase-dependent Na-K pump then occurs. Adenosine triphosphate (ATP) is utilized and mitochondria are stimulated. Cellular cyclic adenosine monophosphate (cAMP) decreases and the ATP level further decreases. As the energy supply deteriorates, more sodium enters the cell and swelling occurs in the cell, the mitochondria, and the endoplasmic reticulum. Eventually lysosomes leak and autolysis occurs. Trump has demonstrated several stages characterized by morphologic changes in the cell subjected to shock. The observed alterations are reversible until stage 5 is reached, at which point resuscitation is of no benefit (see Table 7-1).

As the supply of oxygen and energy substrates diminishes, the cells revert to anaerobic metabolism to generate ATP. This grossly inefficient pathway also results in the formation of lactic acid. The net effect is an intracellular acid buildup and, ultimately, systemic acidemia. The acidotic state has a depressant effect on myocardial contractility and vascular smooth muscle.

There appears to be a point of no return for individual cells as well as for the overall organism in shock. Although this point is well defined for the cell, the clinician caring for patients in shock is less able to identify this landmark. Schwartz suggests that a sudden and substantial decrease in oxygen consumption may be the marker of irreversible shock. Animal studies support this hypothesis but clinical verification is not yet available.

The sum of all the natural compensatory measures called into action in shock are designed to preserve cellular perfusion and thus prevent death. In addition to hemodynamic compensation, a number of neuroendocrine responses occur which are aimed at optimizing blood flow and delivering adequate nutrients to the cells. The hormonal response to shock is mediated primarily through the hypothalamus. The latter is indirectly responsible for the release of glucocorticoids, growth hormone, and aldosterone. These hormones, along with insulin and glucagon, ensure adequate supply and utilization of glucose by cells. Likewise, catecholamines elevate serum glucose in addition to mediating their hemodynamic effects. Antidiuretic hormone (ADH), renin, and angiotensin release are also stimulated by shock. They have a salutary effect on hemodynamics and blood volume.

The role of the physician in the management of shock is to supplement the body's response to shock by providing supportive care and eradicating the cause of the shock state. In carrying out this role, it is helpful to monitor a number of parameters which

Table 7-1. Morphologic Changes in the Cell Subjected to Shock

Stage	Normal
Stages 1a and 2	Swelling of cytoplasm and endoplasmic reticulum
Stage 3	Mitochondria shrink, inner compartment gets smaller and more dense
Stage 4	Mitochondrial swelling
Stage 5	Continued swelling of mitochondria, clumps of flocculent, dense material appear
Stage 6	Interruptions of cell membrane; lysosomes disappear
Stage 7	Cell becomes a mass of debris

measure hemodynamic function and provide a measure of patient response. Although obvious clinical parameters such as mentation and urine output are nevertheless important bedside indicators of vital organ perfusion, other routine measurements of obvious value in shock are blood pressure, pulse, and pulse pressure. More sophisticated measurements requiring invasive procedures can also be obtained. Other than the central venous pressure (CVP), these parameters are not often followed in the emergency department. They do, however, provide important information diagnostically and therapeutically for critically ill patients. These determinations, along with their derivations and normal values, are listed in Table 7.2.

Table 7-2. Additional Indicators of Vital Organ Perfusion

Parameter	Derivation	Normal Values
CVP	Measured	5–12 cm H_2O
PAP	Measured	9–19 mmHg
PAEDP	Measured	4–13 mmHg
PCWP	Measured	4.5–13 mmHg
MAP	$DP + \frac{1}{3}(SP - DP)$	80–90 mmHg
CO	$SV \times HR$	4–8 L/min
CI	CO/BSA	2.8–3.8 L/(m² · min)
LVSW	$SV \times (MAP - PCWP) \times .0136$	60–130 gm · meter/beat
LVSWI	LVSW/BSA	40–80 gm · meter/(m² · beat)
SVR	$\dfrac{(MAP - CVP) \times 80}{CO}$	800–1400 dyn/(s · cm⁵)
SVRI	$SVR \times BSA$	1600–2200 dyn/(s · cm⁵m²)
PVR	$\dfrac{(MPA - PCWP) \times 80}{CO}$	100–300 dyn/(s · cm⁵)
PVRI	$PVR \times BSA$	200–450 dyn/(s · cm⁵m²)
O_2 Consumption	$(CaO_2 - CVO_2) \times CO \times 10$	150–300 mL/min
O_2 Delivery	$CaO_2 \times CO \times 10$	800–1200 mL/min

Note: Abbreviations

CVP: Central venous pressure
PAP: Mean pulmonary artery pressure
PAEDP: Pulmonary artery end-diastolic pressure
CO: Cardiac output
CI: Cardiac index
MAP: Mean arterial pressure
DP: Diastolic pressure
SP: Systolic pressure
LVSW: Left ventricular stroke work
MPA: Mean pulmonary artery pressure

LVSWI: Left ventricular stroke work index
SVR: Systemic vascular resistance
SVRI: Systemic vascular resistance index
PVR: Pulmonary vascular resistance
PVRI: Pulmonary vascular resistance index
O_2 Consumption: Oxygen consumption
O_2 Delivery: Oxygen delivery
BSA: Body surface area
SV: Stroke volume

HEMORRHAGIC SHOCK

Pathophysiology

The etiology of hemorrhagic shock, of course, is blood loss. Regardless of whether the loss is external or internal, or due to trauma, gastrointestinal hemorrhage, or a ruptured aortic aneurysm, the basic pathophysiology is the same. Blood pressure and cardiac output drop due to the decrease in circulating blood volume. The volume deficit is detected by carotid and cardiac receptors which in turn provide the centrally mediated neurohumoral compensatory response already discussed.

Another compensatory mechanism operating in hemorrhagic shock is an autotransfusion of interstitial fluid into the vascular space. The Starling forces, which explain this flow of interstitial fluid, are the colloid osmotic pressure and the hydrostatic pressure of both the vascular compartment and the interstitium. These pressures are normally balanced in a dynamic equilibrium. With blood loss, this balance is altered. Hydrostatic pressure is lowered, and a pressure gradient from the interstitium to the vascular space is produced. The interstitial fluid replenishes the intravascular volume over a period of hours, providing the hemorrhage is not overwhelming.

Clinical Presentation

The clinical manifestations of hemorrhagic shock are familiar to all. In the early stage the patient may appear relatively normal, but will have a resting tachycardia and a narrowed pulse pressure and may demonstrate orthostatic changes in the pulse and blood pressure. The skin may be cool and moist if blood loss is large enough to cause a shift in circulation toward more vital organs. Young, healthy patients may exhibit no other signs of shock despite a 25 to 30 percent volume deficit. Beyond this point, or at an earlier stage in blood loss for less healthy patients, rapid deterioration in blood pressure and cardiac output occur. It is therefore important to recognize early signs of shock and treat them aggressively to prevent this decompensation.

Management

The goal of management of hemorrhagic shock is rapid restoration of the intravascular volume and identification and correction of the bleeding source. Intravenous access is prerequisite to volume replacement, but while this is being secured, the patient can be put in the Trendelenburg position and the military antishock trouser (MAST) suit applied. These two maneuvers help shift volume from the body's periphery to the central circulation. The MAST suit creates a small autotransfusion and increases vascular resistance and thus, by increasing systemic blood pressure, enhances blood flow to vital organs.

The number, types, and location of intravenous lines necessary for a given resuscitation is at the discretion of the treating physician. Generally, large-bore peripheral lines provide the most rapid rate of fluid infusion and are the mainstay of treatment. The use of central lines is controversial since measurement of the central venous pressure (CVP) is not always informative or necessary in obvious blood loss. In addition, the insertion of these lines does result in significant complications. On the other hand, in unstable patients, victims of penetrating chest trauma, and patients with less cardiovascular reserve, CVP monitoring may be helpful in tailoring the resuscitative effort.

The number of lines inserted depends on the amount of blood loss and the severity of the patient's condition. In the absence of a specific formula for the correct number of lines, the guiding principle is to err on the side of placing too many rather than too few. The use of cutdowns is usually reserved for those patients with poor peripheral veins or the critically ill patient with massive blood loss who requires a maximum initial resuscitative effort. If a cutdown is needed, the distal saphenous vein offers several advantages. It is constant in its anatomy, is superficial, will accept large-bore cannulas and can be used in conjunction with the MAST suit, provided blood pumps are utilized.

The amount and type of fluid utilized for hemorrhagic shock depends on the amount of blood lost and whether hemorrhage is ongoing. Except in massive bleeding, blood products are not usually necessary intially. Initial management consists of sending blood for type and cross match and initiation of fluid resuscitation with crystalloid or colloid. Although still controversial, most centers use Ringer's lactate or normal saline, not colloid as the initial IV fluid. Given the effectiveness of both types of fluid, the lack of added risk for adult respiratory distress syndrome (ARDS) with crystalloid and the marked difference in cost, crystalloid appears to be the initial fluid of choice. Other fluids such as dextran and hetastarch currently are not routinely used as resuscitation fluids.

The decision to initiate transfusion is a clinical one which depends on the initial presentation of the patient, response to crystalloid, and whether the hemorrhage has been controlled. If the patient is moribund on arrival, O-negative blood should be started immediately. Most often, however, blood is started after 2 to 4 L of crystalloid have been given and the patient is still showing signs of hypovolemia or has continued blood loss. Type-specific blood can be given safely in this situation and is usually available in 10 to 15 min.

Another factor in deciding to start blood is the hematocrit. Because it takes time for the interstitial fluid to enter the vascular space, dilution of the hematocrit does not occur initially and it is therefore not an accurate reflection of blood volume. The exception to this rule is the victim of massive blood loss who will present with a low initial hematocrit. Although this hematocrit is not an accurate reflection of blood volume, it is an indicator of severe blood loss and the need for transfusion. The other function of an initial hematocrit is the need to establish a baseline value. Repeat hematocrits can then be used as a rough measure of blood loss and can help in making the decision concerning transfusion (see Fig. 7-1).

The remainder of the management of hemorrhagic shock entails monitoring vital signs, urine output, and hematocrit. More invasive monitoring with CVP catheters, intraarterial lines, or Swan-Ganz catheters may be indicated eventually in the unstable patient. The insertion of these lines can usually wait until the patient is transferred to an ICU setting. Other measures which should be performed include obtaining blood for baseline clotting functions, platelet count, and electrolytes, and cardiac monitoring and application of supplemental oxygen.

CARDIOGENIC SHOCK

Pathophysiology

Cardiogenic shock is a clinical syndrome of hypotension with evidence of compromised perfusion in the presence of an acute myocardial infarction. Although the syndrome may develop on the basis of myocardial trauma, it is almost exclusively due to coronary atherosclerosis. Ten to 15 percent of all patients admitted with acute myocardial infarction develop cardiogenic shock. A small percentage of these patients do so on the basis of rupture of the ventricular septum or a papillary muscle but the majority

Figure 7-1. Fluid resuscitation after hemorrhage.

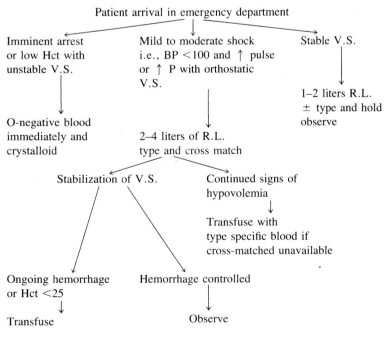

(R.L. = Ringer's lactate; V.S. = vital signs.)

go into shock due to the amount of damaged myocardium. Autopsies of patients dying of cardiogenic shock demonstrate infarction of 35 to 75 percent of their left ventricle. It is generally agreed that 35 to 40 percent of the left ventricular myocardium must be damaged before shock will ensue. It has also been determined that all patients dying of the syndrome have apical involvement and that 84 percent have severe disease of the left anterior descending coronary artery. The majority of patients who develop cardiogenic shock have had a previous infarction but some patients do present in shock with the initial infarction.

Despite aggressive therapy, cardiogenic shock still has a mortality rate in excess of 80 percent. Because treatment is so unsatisfactory, the optimal treatment of the disease is prevention, as will be discussed later.

When 35 to 40 percent of the left ventricle is infarcted, its function is compromised to the extent that arterial pressure cannot be maintained. In this case, the normal compensatory measures mediated by the autonomic nervous system and circulating catecholamines can be deleterious. Increased peripheral vascular resistance increases afterload and thus the oxygen demand of the ventricle. Reflex tachycardia likewise increases oxygen demand. Venoconstriction results in an increased preload, further accentuating failure. A vicious cycle is thus established. Increased oxygen demand results in increased damage and less functioning myocardium. Blood pressure and cardiac output continue to fall. When mean arterial pressure falls below 70, coronary perfusion is inadequate, which further extends the area of infarction.

Two other parameters frequently measured in cardiogenic shock, cardiac index and left ventricular filling pressure [as approximated by pulmonary capillary wedge pressure (PCWP) or pulmonary artery end-diastolic pressure (PAEDP)], provide both diagnostic and prognostic information (see Table 7-3). As reported by Rackley et al., a cardiac index above 2 L/(m² · min) and a PAEDP less than 29 carry the best prognosis.

Clinical Presentation

The clinical presentation of cardiogenic shock depends on how severely decompensated the patient is. Patients may present with little evidence of compromise, only to deteriorate rapidly and expire while still in the emergency department. The clinical picture of cardiac decompensation includes hypotension (blood pressure less than 80 or a decrease of 90 mmHg in a normally hypertensive patient); cool, diaphoretic skin; cyanosis; dyspnea; clouded sensorium; and a decreased urine output. Pulmonary edema is usually evident on chest examination.

Management

An important role of the emergency physician in managing cardiogenic shock is attempting to prevent it. Aggressive management of patients with acute myocardial infarction should help prevent infarct extension and therefore cardiogenic shock. Early recognition and prompt management of those conditions which increase myocardial demand are the principles of management (see Table 7-4).

Once the full picture of cardiogenic shock is present, an aggressive supportive approach is in order. Intubation to ensure adequate ventilation and oxygenation is essential. Hemodynamic manipulations are best done under the guidance of Swan-Ganz catheter monitoring. If unavailable in the emergency department, an expedited trip to an ICU should be undertaken. While the patient awaits transfer, Lasix should be given for its venodilatory effect and consequent decrease in preload and in an attempt to initiate diuresis. Dopamine should also be started in an effort to improve the blood pressure. A combination of dopamine and dobutamine may be beneficial. Approximately 20 percent of patients in cardiogenic shock present with normal or nearly normal left ventricular filling pressures. Only one-third of these patients respond to volume expansion. Given these data, it may not be wise to attempt a blind fluid challenge in the emergency department without knowing the wedge pressure.

Once the Swan-Ganz catheter is in position, hemodynamic measurements can be obtained which will specifically define the patient's status and further dictate therapy. The goal is to improve cardiac output by optimizing the filling pressure (18 to 24 in cardiogenic shock), improve myocardial contractility with pressors, and improve perfusion and decrease afterload with vasodilators.

If pharmacologic manipulations do not improve the clinical situation, counterpulsation with an intraaortic balloon pump may prove beneficial. Immediate hemodynamic improvement usually occurs with the balloon. Long-term survival has been variously reported from minimal up to greater than 50 percent. Early revascularization in conjunction with aortic balloon pumping has also been investigated. These data are also less than clear-cut. Timing of this emergency surgery does have bearing on survival. Some feel that if the procedure cannot be performed in 12 to 16 h after infarction, survival is adversely affected.

One last intervention undergoing investigation is the intracorporeal left ventricular assist device. This partial mechanical heart is reportedly ten times more effective than the intraaortic balloon pump. It is suggested that this device may be of value in those patients not helped by the intraaortic balloon pump.

SEPTIC SHOCK

Pathophysiology

Septic shock is a form of distributive shock initially, in that blood volume is dispersed into a greatly dilated peripheral circulation. Other causes of such a maldistribution of circulating blood volume

Table 7-4. Signs of Increased Myocardial Demand

Sign	Rx
Tachycardia (without CHF)	Pain relief
	Small doses of Inderal IV
Bradycardia (with hypotension)	Atropine 0.6 mg IV
Arrhythmias	Specific Rx
Hypertension with normal pulse	Nitroglycerin, nitroprusside
Pulmonary congestion	Lasix

Table 7-3. Additional Parameters Providing Diagnostic and Prognostic Information

Group	PAEDP, mmHg	CI, L/(m² · min)	Mortality, %
I	>29		100
II	<29 + >15	<2	92
III	<15	<2	63
IV	<29	>2	13

include anaphylaxis, spinal cord injury, and vasovagal reactions. This section will concentrate on the more common and usually more serious septic shock.

Septic shock is caused by bacteria and their products circulating in the blood. Although both gram-positive and gram-negative organisms are capable of producing shock, the gram-negative bacteria and in particular gram-negative rods are by far the most common etiologic agent. The bulk of this section will therefore deal with gram-negative rod bacteremia and the resultant shock which occurs in approximately 40 percent of cases.

Although the importance of gram-negative bacteremia has been appreciated since the early 1950s, it still remains a very serious disease with a mortality of 25 percent. If shock complicates the picture, the mortality is variously stated as 35 to 50 percent. Since the 1950s there has been a steady increase in the incidence of this syndrome and it now has a prevalence of 12.75 cases per 1000 hospital admissions. This translates into an annual incidence of 330,000 cases. The syndrome occurs in all age groups but is more common in the elderly, with a peak incidence during the seventh decade of life. Several factors can predispose an individual to gram-negative bacteremia, including immunocompromise from chemotherapy or immunosuppressant drugs, underlying malignancy, genitourinary tract manipulations, and respiratory tract manipulations, including tracheostomy and biopsy. The most common source of infection resulting in gram-negative bacteremia is the urinary tract, which accounts for 34 percent of cases. The next largest source of infection is the unknown category, which comprises 30 percent of all cases. Sources of bacteremia and their incidences are listed in Table 7-5.

Infections arising in the biliary, genitourinary, and reproductive tracts and other sites result in a more benign course (mortality 15 percent). This figure contrasts with a mortality rate of 30 percent when the source of infection is in the respiratory or gastrointestinal tract or when the source is unknown. As mentioned, underlying disease predisposes one to bacteremia; it also results in a higher mortality resulting from the bacteremia. Underlying diseases are categorized as rapidly fatal, ultimately fatal, or nonfatal. The mortality rates of gram-negative bacteremia in these three groups are 40, 31, and 15 percent, respectively.

The infecting organism in gram-negative bacteremia is most often *Escherichia coli,* which causes 31 percent of all cases. Many other gram-negative organisms can result in bacteremia and shock. The more common of these are listed in Table 7-6.

Although it is controversial, most feel that the pathophysiologic effects of septic shock are due to endotoxin. Endotoxin is a lipopolysaccharide in the cell wall of gram-negative rods. More specifically, endotoxins have three component parts: oligosaccharide side chains, a core polysaccharide, and lipid A, which is responsible for the toxic effects of endotoxins. The side chains

Table 7-5. Sources and Incidence of Bacteremia

Source of Infection	% of Incidence
Urinary tract	34
Unknown	30
GI tract	14
Respiratory tract	9
Skin and soft tissue	7
Other	3
Biliary tract	2
Reproductive system	1

Table 7-6. Organism Causing Gram-Negative Bacteremia

Source	Percentage
Escherichia coli	31
Klebsiella pneumoniae	12
Pseudomonas spp.	10
Enterobacter spp.	8
Proteus and *Providencia*	8
Bacteroides spp.	7
Other gram-negative bacilli	6
Serratia marcescens	2
More than one species	16

vary from species to species, whereas the core polysaccharide–lipid A complex is relatively constant regardless of bacterial species.

Experimental endotoxin shock may not be identical to gram-negative bacteremic shock but striking similarities are present. Fever, shock, disseminated intravascular coagulation (DIC), complement activation, and transient leukopenia followed by leukocytosis are features of both entities. With such evidence, it is hard to refute an important if not a primary role of endotoxin in producing the symptoms of septic shock.

Precisely how the bacteria or their endotoxins result in the clinical picture of septic shock is not known. The complexity of the primary and secondary effects of bacteremia make it difficult to arrive at a simple unifying theory. Some of the pathophysiologic mechanisms that have been demonstrated will be reviewed.

At the cellular level there is evidence of impaired energy utilization. Animal studies have documented a reduced transmembrane potential with concomitant increase in cellular Na, Cl, and water, presumably due to failure of the Na-K pump. A similar situation exists in severe hemorrhagic shock. In the latter situation, however, these changes are due to an exhaustion of ATP supply. In endotoxic shock, even just prior to death, cellular ATP levels are normal. This finding suggests the possibility of inhibition of ATPase, the enzyme needed to utilize ATP for the Na-K pump.

In addition to impaired energy utilization, there is also evidence for faulty cellular ATP production via the Krebs cycle in septic shock. This suboptimal energy production is reflected in a decreased oxygen consumption which is seen in the early phases of septic shock. In late septic shock, mitochondrial damage and ultimately cell autolysis is due to impaired oxygen delivery and subsequent cellular acidosis.

On a more macroscopic level, McCabe has popularized a pathophysiologic theory based on simultaneous stimulation of fibrinolysis and activation of the intrinsic clotting system. The theory postulates complex alterations and interactions between the coagulation, fibrinolytic, kinin, and complement systems. The entire process starts with the activation of Hageman factor (factor XII) by endotoxin. Activated Hageman factor activates the intrinsic clotting system and converts plasminogen to plasmin. Plasmin stimulates fibrinolysis and also digests activated Hageman factor. Fragments of the Hageman factor then activate the kinin system, resulting in bradykinin release. The latter is a potent vasodilator. Finally, the complement system is activated both by gram-negative bacteria directly and by plasmin. Complement activation results in the production of anaphylatoxin, chemotactic factors, and histamine. The net result of complement activation is an increased capillary permeability.

Hence many of the clinical findings of septic shock, including hypotension, vasodilation, transudation of fluid across capillary membranes, and DIC, can be explained by McCabe's theory. The theory is not without experimental support. Clinical studies have documented Hageman factor activation, bradykinin production and release, and depletion of the third component of complement in gram-negative bacteremia.

There is also evidence to suggest that endotoxin can alter the microcirculation, resulting in fluid loss across capillary membranes. Such studies have demonstrated endothelial cell thickening and red blood cell extravasation after infusion of endotoxin. It is postulated that capillary leak results from endothelial cell hydration and swelling, which produce gaps between cells.

Other factors which may contribute to the pathophysiology of septic shock include endorphins, vasopressin, prostaglandins, and myocardial depression. Beta endorphins are endogenous opiates secreted by the same cells in the hypothalamus that secrete ACTH. Hence, any stimulus such as shock which causes ACTH release will also cause β endorphin release. Opiates can cause hypotension through myocardial depression and lowered peripheral vascular resistance. The hypotensive effects of endogenous opiates may therefore contribute to the clinical picture of septic shock. Reversal of hypotension by naloxone, particularly in early septic shock, lends support to the theory that β endorphins may partially mediate the hypotension of septic shock.

Recent studies have documented very high levels of vasopressin during septic shock. Previous investigations have demonstrated that vasopressin causes intestinal smooth muscle constriction, vasoconstriction, reduced superior mesenteric artery flow, and myocardial depression. Again, some of these effects may contribute to the signs and symptoms of septic shock.

There is growing evidence that prostaglandins may play a role in the pathophysiology of septic shock. Thromboxane A_2 (TXA$_2$) is a potent vasoconstrictor and platelet aggregator, while prostacyclin (PGI$_2$) causes vasodilatation and prevents platelet aggregation. These combined effects may result in pulmonary hypertension, systemic hypotension, and DIC, all of which can be seen in septic shock.

Prostaglandins are formed from arachidonic acid by the enzyme cyclooxygenase. Several studies have shown that both TXA$_2$ and PGI$_2$ are elevated in septic shock. These studies have also shown that administration of indomethacin, which inhibits cyclooxygenase, prevents these elevations. Likewise, those animals pretreated with indomethacin or given indomethacin after the onset of shock have less hypotension and an improved survival compared to controls. Other studies confirm the deleterious effect of thromboxane but show no increase in PGI$_2$ levels and, in fact, document a beneficial effect from administering PGI$_2$. Even though the data conflict, it is apparent that at least one prostaglandin contributes to the pathophysiology of septic shock. Future treatment of this disease may therefore include inhibition of prostaglandin formation.

A decreased myocardial contractility has been demonstrated during septic shock. Exactly how much of this alteration affects cardiac output and contributes to the shock state is unknown. Likewise, the etiology of the altered contractility is unknown, although postulated to be a direct effect of the endotoxin. There is evidence for global subendocardial ischemia during septic shock, but again whether this abnormality is the cause of reduced contractility is undetermined.

Clinical Presentation

Typically, the clinical features of septic shock can be divided into two phases. In the early phase, vasodilatation predominates; patients are warm and flushed, and are hyperdynamic, usually with a normal or elevated cardiac output. Agitation or confusion are frequently present, as is temperature elevation and hyperventilation. In fact, fever and hyperventilation are often the earliest signs of septic shock and should be acted upon promptly to enhance final patient outcome. At this stage, hypotension may not be present, depending on the degree of compensation.

In the late phase of this syndrome, a more typical shock state prevails. Peripheral perfusion as well as vital organ perfusion is impaired. In its most severe form, patients are obtunded, urine output is reduced, cardiac output and blood pressure are diminished, and peripheral vasoconstriction is apparent. There may also be signs of severe DIC, including ecchymoses or frank bleeding.

The above description represents a typical presentation and course of septic shock. Unfortunately, when the patient is first seen, he or she may be anywhere in this course, or may present in an atypical fashion. Less typical presentations of septic shock include fever alone, unexplained respiratory alkalosis, confusion, acidosis, or hypotension. Any of these findings should alert one to the possibility of a septic etiology, especially in the elderly or debilitated patient.

In addition to the history and physical examination, laboratory data are helpful in establishing the diagnosis of septic shock. Transient, initial leukopenia followed by leukocytosis with a leftward shift is the rule with bacteremia. The degree of leukocytosis is variable.

Arterial blood gases may reflect a respiratory alkalosis initially due to a central stimulation of the respiratory center. As frank shock develops, lactic acidosis ensues due to inadequate tissue perfusion and a reversion to anaerobic metabolism.

Coagulation defects are common in the setting of gram-negative bacteremia. In a retrospective review of 222 patients, Kreger observed some defect in 64 percent of the patients. These defects can be divided into three groups: thrombocytopenia, DIC, and other defects with or without thrombocytopenia. Thrombocytopenia alone or with other defects occurred in 56 percent of the patients. The converse, other defects with or without thrombocytopenia, was seen in 31 percent of the patients. Although DIC was seen in 11 percent of patients, only 3 percent had clinical evidence of bleeding. Other authors have quoted a 5 percent incidence of DIC in gram-negative bacteremia. In Kreger's series, the incidence of coagulation defects was higher in patients with rapidly fatal underlying disease. He also demonstrated a higher incidence of shock and death in patients with coagulation defects compared to those with no defects. Likewise, patients with DIC more often had shock or a fatal outcome than those patients with other coagulation defects.

Blood cultures are the ultimate method by which bacteremia is confirmed. Unfortunately, blood cultures are not positive 100 percent of the time in bacteremia, suggesting that some cases of bacteremia may escape identification by blood culture. Again, in Kreger's review, 69 percent of the 1258 cultures obtained from 404 patients were positive.

The technique of culture collection, especially the number of cultures taken, has bearing on the percent of recovery of the organism. Except in neonates, multiple cultures should be obtained.

Washington found that the yield increased from 80 percent, to 89 percent, to 99 percent if one, two, or three sets of cultures were obtained, respectively. The timing of cultures in this study was over a 24-h period. Unfortunately, this is not always possible in clinical practice, when the patient's condition requires prompt administration of antibiotics. Under such circumstances, Martin recommends that three cultures be drawn, but does not specify the time interval between cultures.

Management

Treatment of septic shock of any etiology can be divided into three modes of therapy: supportive care, drainage of pus, and

administration of antibiotics. Supportive care is geared to the severity of the patient's condition and may include fluid resuscitation, administration of pressor agents, and active airway management in the critically ill patient. The treatment of shock initially consists of giving adequate amounts of crystalloid. In less critical patients, fluid resuscitation can be gauged by the response in vital signs. More seriously ill patients and those patients needing vasopressors should undergo central venous pressure monitoring or left atrial pressure monitoring. Patients in whom the blood pressure does not respond, despite restoration of adequate filling pressures, require vasopressor support. Dopamine is most commonly recommended as the agent of choice. Purely α-adrenergic drugs should be avoided since they elevate blood pressure at the expense of peripheral perfusion and may therefore be damaging at the

Table 7-7. Antibiotic Regimens*

Source of Infection	Probable Bacteria	Antibiotics
Biliary system	Coliforms, *Enterococcus, Bacteroides, C. perfringens*	AG & cefoxitin (AG & chloramphenicol)
Peritonitis of GI origin	Coliforms, *Enterococcus, Bacteroides*	Cefoxitin & amikacin (Pen + Clin + gentamicin)
Brain abscess		
(acute)	*S. aureus, Streptococcus, Pneumococcus*	Nafcillin & chloramphenicol (ceph 1 or 2)
(chronic)	*Bacteroides,* anaerobic *Streptococcus, Actinomyces*	Pen G + metronidazole (ceph 1 or 2 + metronidazole)
Osteomyelitis (postoperative)	*S. aureus,* coliforms, *Pseudomonas*	P-Pen (ceph 1) add an AG
Perirectal abscess	Coliforms, *Bacteroides, Enterococcus, Proteus*	Cefoxitin (PCN + clin + AG)
PID	*Gonococcus, Chlamydia, Bacteroides* coliforms, *Streptococcus, Mycoplasma*	Cefoxitin + doxycycline (clin + Pen G)
Pneumonia		
lobar, CA without UD	*Pneumococcus,* Group A *Streptococcus*	Pen G (erythro)
lobar CA with UD	*Pneumococcus, H. influenzae,* Group A *Streptococcus, Klebsiella,* coliforms, *S. aureus*	AG + ceph 1 or 2
Bronchopneumonia CA without UD	*Pneumonococcus, Mycoplasma,* Legionnaires' disease	Erythromycin (tetracycline)
Bronchopneumonia CA with UD	*Pneumococcus, H. influenzae,* Group A *Streptococcus, Klebsiella,* coliforms, *S. aureus, Mycoplasma,* Legionnaires' disease	AG + ceph 1 or 2 + erythromycin
Bronchopneumonia HA	*Pseudomonas, Klebsiella, Enterobacter, Serratia, Proteus, Providencia, Acinetobacter, S. aureus*	Pen-AP + AG (AG + ceph 3)
Meningitis		
Adult without compromise	*Meningococcus, Pneumococcus,* Group A *Streptococcus*	Pen G (chloramphenicol)
Adult with immunosuppression or alcoholism	*Meningococcus, Pneumococcus,* Group A *Streptococcus,* coliforms, *Pseudomonas, H. influenza*	Moxalactam (only if gram − seen on smear) (cefotaxime)
Child <10 years old	*H. influenzae, Pneumococcus, Meningococcus*	Chloramphenicol + ampicillin (cefotaxime)
Infant <1 month	Group B or D *Streptococcus,* coliforms, *Listeria, H. influenzae, Meningococcus, Pneumococcus*	Ampicillin + gentamicin
Toxic shock	*S. aureus*	P-Pen (ceph 1)
Source unknown		
Uncompromised	Coliforms, *Proteus, S. aureus,* Group A or D *Streptococcus*	Ceph 1 + AG (P-Pen + AG)
Compromised	Coliforms, *Pseudomonas, Proteus, S. aureus*	AG + Pen-AP + ceph 1 (AG + vancomycin)

*Adapted from Sanford JP Guidelines to Antimicrobial Therapy, 1983.   Drugs in parentheses indicate alternative therapy.
Note: Abbreviations:

AG: Aminoglycosides
Pen-G: Aqueous penicillin G
P-Pen: Synthetic penicillinase-resistant penicillin
Pen-AP: Anti-pseudomonas penicillin (ticarcillin, carbenicillin, piperacillin)
Ceph: Cephalosporins
Ceph 1: 1st generation (cephalothin, cefazolin, cephradine)

Ceph 2: 2d generation (cefamandule, cefoxitin, cefuroxime)
Ceph 3: 3d generation (cefotaxime, cefoperazone, moxalactam)
Clin: Clindamycin
CA: Community-acquired
HA: Hospital-acquired
UD: Underlying disease

cellular level. Dopamine has the advantages of being a positive inotropic agent at the lower dose range and of sparing renal perfusion, and is therefore the preferred drug.

The remainder of supportive care is just that. Whatever support the patient's condition merits should be undertaken. At the same time that supportive measures are instituted, one must make a thorough search for the etiology of the septicemia. Physical examination coupled with laboratory investigation will establish the proper diagnosis in the majority of cases. Establishing the source of infection cannot be overemphasized, since appropriate initial antibiotic therapy depends on accurate prediction of what organisms are likely to be involved.

The second form of therapy employs surgical drainage. In most instances of abscess formation, recovery will not occur until the lesion is drained or excised. Such surgery may take the form of evacuation of pus, as in the case of a perirectal abscess or the removal of an infected organ, for example a gangrenous gallbladder.

The final phase of treatment of septic shock is the prompt and appropriate use of antibiotics. No one disputes the beneficial effects of antibiotics in sepsis, but the choice of antibiotics is often less than unanimous. One point of controversy is the use of multiple antibiotic regimens. Some feel that the synergistic effects of certain antibiotic combinations warrant their use, while others feel there is no advantage and potential detriment in such combinations. A logical approach to antibiotic choice is to establish the source of the infection, consider the organisms known to occur in a given instance, and employ the antibiotic(s) which provide specific coverage. Unfortunately, in 30 percent of cases, a specific source of infection is not apparent. In such a circumstance, broad-spectrum coverage with two or three antibiotics may be necessary, since both gram-positive and gram-negative coverage may be mandatory. Table 7-7 lists various sites of infection, probable organisms, and at least one antibiotic regimen.

The use of steroids in the management of septic shock remains controversial. Several investigations reveal no benefit from steroids and Kreger's retrospective study indicated a detrimental effect of steroids. If steroids are utilized, they should be given in large doses (30 mg per kilogram methylprednisolone or greater than 1 g of hydrocortisone). Based on studies to date, however, there is no strong evidence in support of steroids and they should probably not be used in septic shock.

The use of antiserum to endotoxin has recently been investigated by Ziegler et al. in a prospective study of 212 patients with gram-negative sepsis. The antiserum utilized was developed against the J-5 mutant strain of *E. coli,* which contains only core determinants. Results indicate a beneficial effect of the antiserum. The mortality rate of the control group was 39 percent, compared to 22 percent in the antiserum group. In the critically ill patient with profound shock, the respective mortality rates were 77 percent compared to 44 percent. Though not presently available to practitioners, antiserum may play a significant role in the management of gram-negative bacteremia in the future.

SUMMARY

Although the clinical entity of shock has been known to physicians for centuries, there remain many unanswered questions concerning the pathophysiology and treatment of shock. Though different mechanisms are at work in the various forms of shock, all these types of shock result in injury to a common target, the cell. Continued research regarding what happens to the cell in shock and what can be done to prevent such changes may provide the key to the successful management of shock in the future. The material reviewed in this section touches on the macroscopic management of shock. In the future this therapy may be combined with measures directed at the cell itself. Hopefully, such measures will result in an improved outlook for an entity which currently exhibits a high morbidity and mortality.

BIBLIOGRAPHY

Altura BM: Reticuloendothelial system and neuro-endocrine stimulation in shock therapy. *Adv Shock Res* 3:3–25, 1980.

Baue AE: Mitochondrial function in shock, in The cell in shock. Proceedings of a symposium on recent research developments and current clinical practice in shock. Scope Publ., 11–15, 1974.

Baue AE, Chaudry I: Some clinical adventures and misadventures. *Adv Shock Res* 3:67–75, 1980.

Butler RR Jr, Wise WC, Halushka PV, et al: Thromboxane and prostacyclin production during septic shock. *Adv Shock Res* 7:133–145, 1982.

Chaudry IH, Baue AE: The use of substrates and energy in the treatment of shock. *Adv Shock Res* 3:27–46, 1980.

Chaudry IH, Clemens MG, Baue AE: Alterations in cell function with ischemia and shock and their correction. *Arch Surg* 116:1309–1317, 1981.

Chien S: Rheology in the microcirculation in normal and low flow states. *Adv Shock Res* 8:71–80, 1982.

Dewood MA, Notske RN, Hensley GR, et al: Intraaortic balloon counterpulsation with and without reperfusion for myocardial infarction shock. *Circulation* 61(6):1105–1112, 1980.

Drucker WR, Chadwick CDJ, Gann DS: Transcapillary refill in hemorrhage and shock. *Arch Surg* 116:1344–1353, 1981.

Fletcher JR, Ramwell PW: Indomethacin treatment following baboon endotoxin shock improves survival. *Adv Shock Res* 4:103–111, 1981.

Gaffney FA, Thal ER, Taylor WF, et al: Hemodynamic effects of medical anti-shock trousers (Mast garment). *J Trauma* 21:931–937, 1981.

Gahhos FN, Chiu RC, Hinchey EJ, et al: Endorphins in septic shock. *Arch Surg* 117:1053–1057, 1982.

Geddes JS, Adgey AAJ, Pantridge JF: Prevention of cardiogenic shock, *Am Heart J* 99:244–253, 1980.

Guntheroth WG, Jacky JP, Kawabori I, et al: Left ventricular performance in endotoxin shock in dogs. *Am J Physiol* 242:172–176, 1982.

Hagemeijer F, Laird JD, Haalebos M, et al: Effectiveness of intraaortic balloon pumping without cardiac surgery for patients with severe heart failure secondary to a recent myocardial infarction. *Am J Cardiol* 40:951–956, 1977.

Illner H, Shires GT: Membrane defect and energy status of rabbit skeletal muscle cells in sepsis and septic shock. *Arch Surg* 116:1302–1305, 1981.

Keung EC, Ribner HS, Schwartz W, et al: Effects of combined dopamine and nitroprusside therapy in patients with severe pump failure and hypotension complicating acute myocardial infarction. *J Cardiovasc Pharmacol* 2:113–119, 1980.

Klastersky J, Cappel R, Debusscher L: Effectiveness of betamethasone in management of severe infections. *N Engl J Med* 284:1248–1250, 1971.

Kleinman WM, Krause SM, Hess ML: Differential subendocardial perfusion and injury during the course of gram-negative endotoxemia. *Adv Shock Res* 4:139–152, 1980.

Kreger BE, Craven DE, Carling PC, et al: Gram-negative bacteremia, reassessment of etiology, epidemiology and ecology in 612 patients. *Am J Med* 68:332–343, 1980.

Kreger BE, Craven DE, McCabe WR: Gram-negative bacteremia, re-evaluation of clinical features and treatment in 612 patients. *Am J Med* 68:344–355, 1980.

Luderitz O, Galanos C, Lehmann V, et al: Lipid A: Chemical structure and biological activity. *J Infect Dis* 128:17–29, 1973.

McCabe WR: Gram-negative bacteremia. Diseases-a-month. Chicago, Year Book Medical Publ., 3–38, 1973.

Monafo WW: Volume replacement in hemorrhagic shock, and burns. *Adv Shock Res* 3:47–56, 1980.

Muller-Eberhard HJ: The significance of complement activity in shock, in The cell in shock. Proceedings of a symposium on recent research developments and current clinical practice in shock. Scope Publ., 35–38, 1974.

Norman JC, Duncan M, Frazier OH, et al: Intracorporeal (abdominal) left ventricular assist devices or partial artificial hearts. *Arch Surg* 116:1441–1445, 1981.

Pae WE, Pierce WS: Temporary left ventricular assistance in acute myocardial infarction and cardiogenic shock. *Chest* 79:692–695, June 1981.

Perkin RM, Levin DL: Shock in the pediatric patient. *J. Pediatr* 101:163–169, 1982.

Peters RM, Hargens AR: Protein vs electrolytes and all of the Starling forces. *Arch Surg* 116:1293–1298, 1981.

Puri VK, Paidipaty B, White L: Hydroxyethyl starch for resuscitation of patients with hypovolemia and shock. *Crit Care Med* 9:833–837, 1981.

Rackely CE, Russell RO, Mantle JA, et al: Cardiogenic shock. *Cardiovasc Clin* 11:15–24, 1981.

Scheidt S, Wilner G, Mueller H, et al: Intraaortic balloon counterpulsation in cardiogenic shock. *N Engl J Med* 288:979–984, 1973.

Schumer W: Modern concepts of treatment of septic shock. *Curr Surg* 1–4, 1982.

Schwartz S, Frantz RA, Shoemaker WC: Sequential hemodynamic and oxygen transport responses in hypovolemia, anemia, and hypoxia. *Am J Physiol* 241:864–871, 1981.

Shah DM, Newell JC, Saba TM: Defects in peripheral oxygen utilization following trauma and shock. *Arch Surg* 116:1277–1281, 1981.

Sheagren J: Septic shock and corticosteroids (editorial). *N Engl J Med* 305:456–457, 1980.

Terradellas JB, Bellot JF, Saris AB, et al: Acute and transient ST segment elevation during bacterial shock in seven patients without apparent heart disease. *Chest* 81:4, 1982.

Trump BF: The role of cellular membrane systems in shock, in The cell in shock. Proceedings of a symposium on recent research developments and current clinical practice in shock. Scope Publ. 16–29, 1974.

Webb PJ, Westwick J, Scully MF, et al: Do prostacyclin and thromboxane play a role in endotoxic shock? *Br J Surg* 68:720–724, 1981.

Weissglas IS, Hinchey EJ, Chiu RC: Naloxone and methylprednisolone in the treatment of experimental septic shock. *J Surg Res* 33:131–135, 1982.

Wilson MF, Brackett DJ, Tompkins P, et al: Elevated plasma vasopressin concentrations during endotoxin and *E. coli* shock. *Adv Shock Res* 6:15–26, 1981.

Wise WC, Cook JA, Halushka PV: Implications for thromboxane A in the pathogenesis of endotoxic shock. *Adv Shock Res* 6:83–91, 1981.

Young LS, Martin WJ, Meyer RD, et al: Gram-negative rod bacteremia: Microbiologic, immunologic, and therapeutic considerations. *Ann Intern Med* 86:456–471, 1977.

Ziegler EJ, McCutchan A, Fierer J, et al: Treatment of gram-negative bacteremia and shock with human antiserum to a mutant *Escherichia coli*. *N Engl J Med* 307:1225–1268, 1982.

CHAPTER 8
DISTURBANCES OF
CARDIAC RHYTHM
AND CONDUCTION

J. Stephan Stapczynski

The interpretation and treatment of cardiac arrhythmias is basic to the practice of emergency medicine. This chapter reviews the important cardiac rhythm and conduction disturbances, their clinical significance, and emergency treatment. Discussions of defibrillation, cardioversion, and artificial cardiac pacemakers are also included.

Although emphasis is appropriately placed on drug treatment of these arrhythmias, it is also important that underlying and reversible causes of rhythm and conduction disturbances—such as hypoxia, alkalosis, electrolyte abnormalities, or drug toxicity—be recognized and treated.

THE NORMAL CARDIAC CONDUCTING SYSTEM

The heart consists of three types of specialized tissue: (1) pacemaker cells that undergo spontaneous depolarization and can initiate an electric impulse, (2) conducting cells that form the specialized conducting system and rapidly propagate an electric impulse throughout the heart, and (3) contractile cells which contract when electrically depolarized.

The sinus node is normally the dominant cardiac pacemaker unless its activity is depressed by disease or drugs. The sinus node is located near the junction of the superior vena cava and right atrium. Blood supply is from the sinus node artery which arises from either the proximal few centimeters of the right coronary artery in about 55 percent of individuals, or from the proximal few millimeters of the left circumflex artery in the other 45 percent. The sinus node is innervated by both sympathetic and parasympathetic nerve endings which can greatly modify the discharge rate. The intrinsic sinus node discharge rate is between 90 to 100 in middle-aged adults; the usual resting heart rate is lower, reflecting the predominance of parasympathetic activity at rest.

The electric impulse generated by the sinus node spreads like ripples throughout the right and then the left atrium, activating atrial contraction. Additionally, specialized atrial conduction tracts (anterior, middle, and posterior internodal tracts) serve to propagate the electric impulse through the atria and between the sinus node and the atrioventricular (AV) node.

The atria and ventricles are electrically insulated from each other by the fibrous connective tissue of the atrioventricular ring (annulus fibrosis). Normally, electric impulses from the atria can only reach the ventricles by passing through the AV node and infranodal conducting system.

The AV node is just beneath the right atrial endocardium and directly above the insertion of the septal leaflet of the tricuspid valve. The blood supply to the AV node in 90 percent of humans is by way of a branch off the right coronary artery as it turns to form the posterior descending artery, and in the other 10 percent, comes off the left circumflex artery. This accounts for the common occurrence of AV conduction disturbances with acute inferior myocardial infarctions. The AV node is innervated by both sympathetic and parasympathetic fibers. It has two important electrophysiologic characteristics: a slow conduction velocity and a long refractory period. The slow conduction velocity through the AV node allows time for atrial contraction to give an extra boost to ventricular filling which increases stroke volume according to the Frank-Starling principle. This "atrial kick" is most important in patients with ventricular failure. The long refractory period of the AV node protects the ventricles from excessively rapid stimulation; very rapid heart rates have a reduced cardiac output and may deteriorate into ventricular fibrillation. Cells around the AV node have pacemaker potential and can pace the heart should discharges from the sinus node fail or fall below a certain rate.

Electric impulses leave the inferior pole of the AV node along the bundle of His, which travels downward along the posterior margin of the membranous portion of the interventricular septum to reach the top of the muscular portion. The common bundle is only 1 to 2 cm in length before it divides at the crest of the muscular interventricular septum into the right and left bundle branches (RBB and LBB). The RBB is a compact group of fibers that travels down to the apex of the right ventricle before separating into smaller branches. The LBB travels 2 to 3 cm before fanning out into a virtual sheet of fibers to cover the left ventricle. There are two relatively distinct pathways to the base of the papillary muscles, the left anterior superior fascicle (LASF) and left posterior inferior fascicle (LPIF).

The blood supply to the RBB and LASF is from the same sources: about half the time from both the AV nodal artery and branches from the left anterior descending coronary artery, and the other half from the left anterior descending artery alone. The LPIF is supplied about half the time from the AV nodal artery and the other half by both the AV nodal artery and left anterior descending artery. Infarction in the region supplied by the left anterior descending artery is capable of affecting the RBB and LASF but very rarely the LPIF.

Accessory tracts are embryologic remnants of myocardium found in the AV annulus that can transmit electric impulses between the atria and ventricles, bypassing all or part of the AV node and infranodal system. These bypass tracts are the anatomic basis for the preexcitation syndrome.

THE NORMAL ECG

The clinical surface ECG records the potential (voltage) differences between "neutral" ground and recording electrodes. The ECG is generated by the electrical activity of the heart and depicts the net sum of this activity recorded over time. By convention, a potential difference that points toward a recording electrode is assigned a positive deflection on the ECG, and a potential that points away from the recording electrode is assigned a negative deflection. Also by convention, routine ECG recordings are obtained with paper speed at 25 mm/s (2.5 cm/s) and signal calibration of 1.0 mV/10 mm (1.0 cm).

In Figure 8-1, depolarization starts on the left side of the ventricular septum and initially proceeds to the right; this is recorded as a small negative deflection in the recording electrode. Subsequent depolarization involves the free walls of both ventricles, and since the left side has a much larger mass, the net sum of electrical activity is directed toward the recording electrode and a tall, positive deflection is recorded.

The P-QRS-T complex of the normal ECG represents electrical activity over one cardiac cycle (Fig. 8-2).

The P wave indicates atrial depolarization; atrial repolarization is usually obscured by the QRS complex. The normal P wave duration is less than 0.10 s (2.5 mm) and normal amplitude is less than 0.3 mV (3 mm). A P wave originating from the sinus node is directed inferiorly and to the left on the frontal plane.

The PR interval is the time between the onset of depolarization in the atria and ventricles, and is commonly used as an estimation of AV nodal conduction time. For adults in sinus rhythm, the PR interval is 0.12 to 0.20 s (3 to 5 mm).

The QRS complex indicates ventricular depolarization. In general, depolarization starts on the endocardium and spreads outward to the epicardium. Despite the large amount of myocardium that must be depolarized, the specialized conducting system makes this a rapid process and the normal QRS duration is 0.06 to 0.10 s (1.5 to 2.5 mm). Any delay in conduction (such as bundle branch blocks) results in a wide QRS. Depolarizations which originate in the ventricles or from a portion of the conducting system below the bifurcation of the bundle of His also have a wide QRS complex because of the slow cell-to-cell transmission (as opposed to propagation over the faster conduction system) of the electric impulse required to activate all the ventricular myocardium.

While small negative initial deflections (Q waves) are normal, large Q waves can be due to an electrically unexcitable area just under the recording electrode. An abnormal Q wave has a width of 0.04 s or greater and a height one-third that of the QRS complex.

The ST segment represents the plateau phase of ventricular

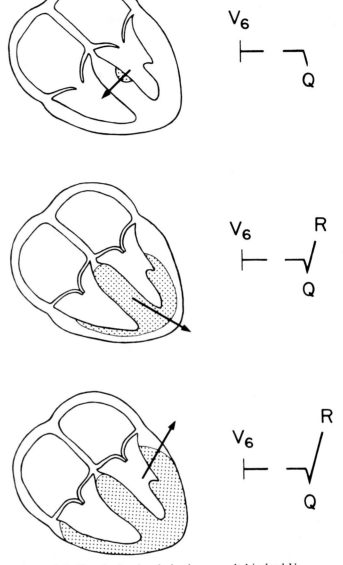

Figure 8-1. Ventricular depolarization recorded in lead V_6.

depolarization. While the ST segment is usually isoelectric, small deviations, less than 0.1 mV (1 mm), are not always pathologic.

The T wave indicates ventricular repolarization. Whereas depolarization is a rapid, near-simultaneous release of stored energy (like the release of a compressed spring), repolarization is a slow, asynchronous event where the metabolic machinery of each individual cell restores the transmembrane potential. Therefore, the T wave duration is much longer and the amplitude much lower than those of the QRS complex. In general, repolarization starts on the epicardium and spreads to the endocardium. Many factors can influence this normal repolarization sequence: (1) metabolic (hypoxia, fever, drugs), (2) autonomic stimuli (abdominal pain, hyperventilation), (3) myocardial hypertrophy, (4) myocardial ischemia or inflammation, and (5) abnormal depolarization.

The QT interval represents the total duration of ventricular depolarization. While QT duration is commonly between 0.33 and 0.42 s, it does vary inversely with heart rate. The corrected

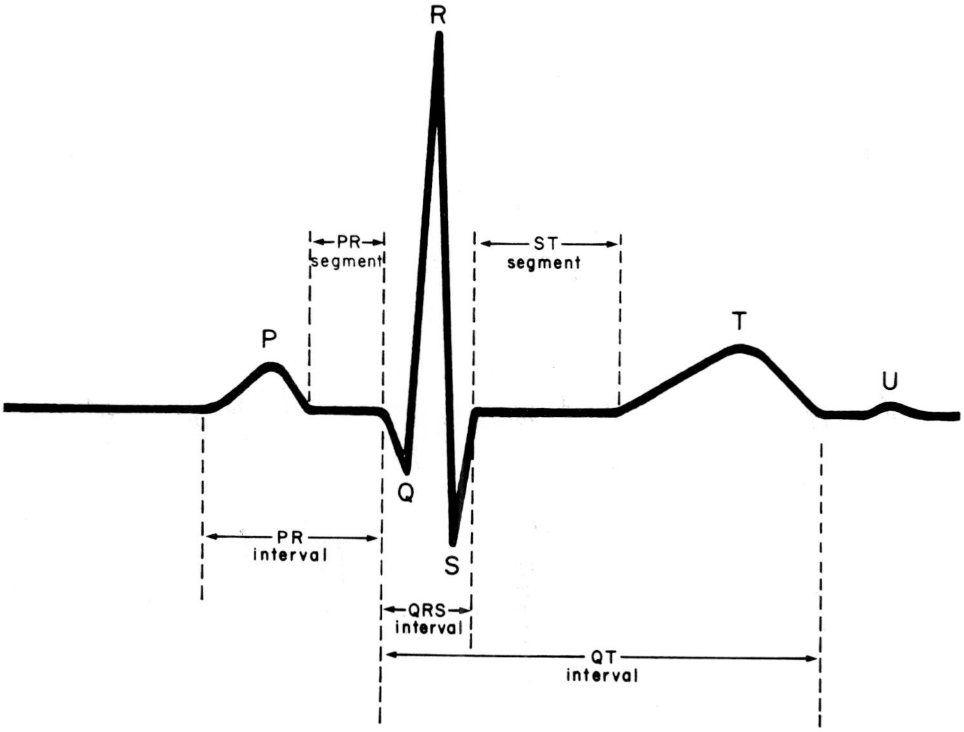

R

Figure 8-2. Normal P-QRS-T ECG pattern.

interval is obtained by dividing the measured QT interval (in seconds) by the square root of the R-R interval (in seconds). The normal corrected QT interval is less than 0.47 s.

The U wave indicates poorly understood ventricular afterpotentials and can be seen as a normal component of the surface ECG, especially in leads V_1 and V_2. Prominent U waves may occur with hypokalemia or ischemia.

CARDIAC ARRHYTHMIAS

Cardiac arrhythmias and conduction disturbances can be classified according to a number of methods: (1) heart rate; (2) site of origin, delay, or block; (3) mechanism; or (4) ratio of atrial to ventricular depolarizations (P waves to QRS complexes). For the cardiac arrhythmias, this chapter separates them into the site of origin.

Cardiac arrhythmias may decrease cardiac output if the ventricular rate is too fast or too slow. In the normal resting adult, heart rates between 40 to 160 are usually well tolerated as physiologic adaptations are able to maintain an adequate cardiac output and blood pressure. However, in adults with significant heart or peripheral arterial disease, rates below 50 or above 120 may produce ischemia in susceptible organs.

Mechanisms of Tachyarrhythmias

Cardiac tachyarrhythmias are presumed to be caused by one of two mechanisms: ectopic focus or reentry. While this concept can be used to direct therapy, uncertainty still exists over the precise mechanism of many arrhythmias, and therapy is still often empirical.

An ectopic focus is an area of the heart, away from the normal sinus node pacemaker, that acquires independent pacemaker activity and usurps the pacemaking role, resulting in single or multiple extra depolarizations.

Reentry occurs when a closed loop of conducting tissue transmits an electrical impulse around the loop, either once or repeatedly, and stimulates an atrial and/or ventricular depolarization with each pass around the circuit. Electrophysiologically, reentry requires a temporary or permanent unidirectional block in one limb of the circuit and slower-than-normal conduction around the entire circuit. Both these conditions occur when cardiac conducting tissue is stimulated during the partial refractory period (before full repolarization).

For example, the inciting impulse traveling in the normal downward direction encounters the two limbs of the reentry circuit, finds limb a blocked, and travels down limb b (Fig. 8-3). Upon reaching the bottom portion of the circuit where the two limbs rejoin, the impulse can then travel retrograde up limb a and reach the upper connection of the circuit. Normally, conduction is so rapid that the impulse would encounter limb b still refractory to stimulation and no further propagation would occur. However, if conduction around the circuit is slow enough, limb b would be able to conduct the impulse again in the antegrade direction. With the right size circuit and conduction velocity, an electric impulse can be maintained traveling around the circuit in a cyclical manner. Each time the impulse passes the upper and lower limb connections, a signal can be sent out stimulating atrial and ventricular depolarizations.

Supraventricular Arrhythmias

Sinus Arrhythmia

Some variation in the sinus node discharge rate is common, but if the variation exceeds 0.12 s between the longest and shortest

Figure 8-3. Reentry circuit.

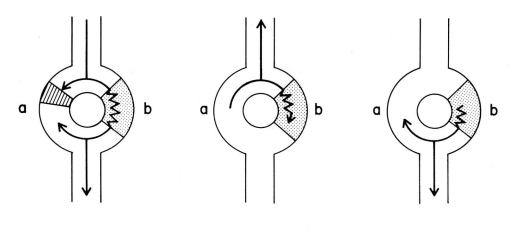

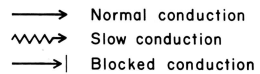

→ Normal conduction

〜〜〜➤ Slow conduction

→| Blocked conduction

intervals, sinus arrhythmia is present. The ECG characteristics of sinus arrhythmia are: (1) normal sinus P waves and PR intervals, (2) 1:1 AV conduction, and (3) variation of at least 0.12 s between the shortest and longest P-P interval (Fig. 8-4).

Clinical Significance

Sinus arrhythmia is most commonly found in children and young adults, disappearing with advancing age. Sinus arrhythmia varies in two manners: the more common phasic (respiratory) variety and the less common nonphasic variety. In the phasic variety, the sinus node rate accelerates during inspiration and decelerates during expiration due to changes in vagal tone occurring with respiration (Bainbridge reflex). The irregularity in either the phasic or nonphasic varieties can be exaggerated by conditions which increase vagal tone. During the long intervals of sinus arrhythmia, junctional escape beats may be seen.

Treatment

None is required.

Sinus Bradycardia

Sinus bradycardia occurs when the sinus node rate falls below 60. The ECG characteristics of sinus bradycardia are: (1) normal sinus

P waves and PR intervals, (2) 1:1 AV conduction, and (3) atrial rate below 60 (Fig. 8-5).

Clinical Significance

Sinus bradycardia represents a suppression of the sinus node discharge rate, usually in response to three categories of stimuli: (1) physiologic (well-conditioned athletes, during sleep, with vagal stimulation), (2) pharmacologic (digitalis, narcotics, reserpine, β-adrenergic antagonists, quinidine), or (3) pathologic (acute inferior myocardial infarction, increased intracranial pressure, carotid sinus hypersensitivity, hypothyroidism).

Treatment

1. Treatment depends on the cause, the heart rate, and whether there are symptoms of hypoperfusion. In general, bradycardias do not require treatment unless the rate is below 50 and there is clinical evidence of hypoperfusion.
2. Initial drug treatment is atropine 0.5 mg IV, given as needed every 5 min until the desired response is achieved or a total vagolytic dose (about 0.05 mg/kg in humans) is given. Usually, if no response is seen by a dose of 2.0 mg, further doses are not effective.
3. If atropine is ineffective, isoproterenol can be infused at rates starting at 0.5 μg/min and increased as required to maintain a heart rate of 60. This concentration can be obtained by diluting

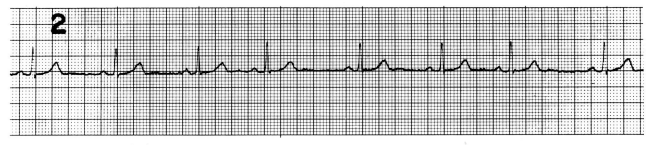

Figure 8-4. Sinus arrhythmia.

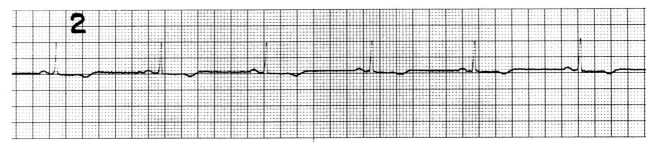

Figure 8-5. Sinus bradycardia, rate 44.

1 mg of isoproterenol in 500 mL of 5% dextrose in water (D_5W) and starting the infusion at 1 mL/min. Isoproterenol is a less attractive agent than atropine because it greatly increases myocardial oxygen consumption and stimulates ventricular ectopy.
4. A ventricular demand pacemaker is required when atropine or isoproterenol is not effective.

Sinus Tachycardia

Sinus tachycardia originates from acceleration of the sinus node discharge rate. The ECG characteristics of sinus tachycardia are: (1) normal sinus P waves and PR intervals, (2) an atrial rate usually between 100 and 160, and (3) normally there is 1:1 conduction between the atria and ventricles, although with rapid rates, AV blocks can occur (Fig. 8-6).

Clinical Significance

Sinus tachycardia represents an acceleration of the sinus node discharge rate, usually in response to three categories of stimuli: (1) physiologic (infants and children, exertion, anxiety, emotions), (2) pharmacologic (atropine, epinephrine and other sympathomimetics, alcohol, nicotine, caffeine), or (3) pathologic (fever, hypoxia, anemia, hypovolemia, pulmonary embolism). In many of these conditions, the increased heart rate is an effort to increase cardiac output to match increased circulatory needs.

Treatment

1. No specific treatment is usually required, but any underlying conditions should be investigated and treated.
2. Some patients with acute myocardial infarction have an "in-

appropriate" tachycardia and may benefit from slowing the heart rate with β-adrenergic antagonists.

Premature Atrial Contractions (PACs)

PACs originate from ectopic pacemakers anywhere in the atrium other than the sinus node. The ECG characteristics of PACs are: (1) ectopic P′ wave appearing sooner (premature) than the next expected sinus beat, (2) the ectopic P′ wave has a different shape and direction, and (3) the ectopic P′ wave may or may not be conducted through the AV node (Fig. 8-7). A PAC is not conducted through the AV node if it reaches the AV node during the absolute refractory period and is conducted with a delay (longer PR interval) during the relative refractory period. Most PACs are conducted with typical QRS complexes, but some may be aberrantly conducted through the infranodal system. The sinus node is often depolarized and "reset" so that while the interval following the PAC is often slightly longer than the previous cycle length, the pause is less than fully compensatory.

Clinical Significance

PACs are common in all ages and often seen in the absence of heart disease. Stress, fatigue, alcohol, tobacco, or coffee may precipitate PACs. Frequent PACs may also be seen in chronic lung disease, ischemic heart disease, or digitalis toxicity. PACs may trigger sustained atrial tachycardia, flutter, or fibrillation.

Treatment

1. Any precipitating drugs or toxins should be discontinued.
2. Underlying disorders should be treated.

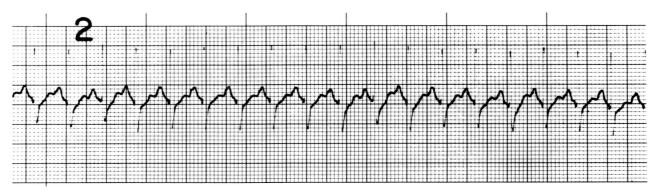

Figure 8-6. Sinus tachycardia, rate 176.

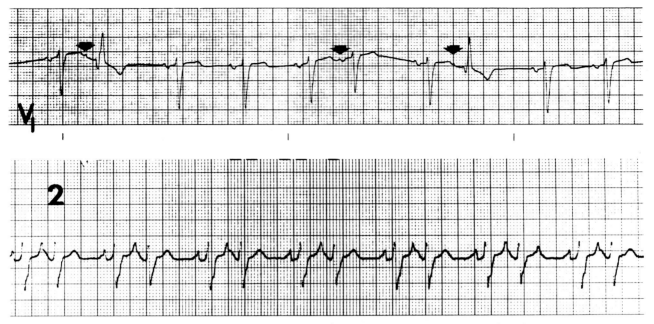

Figure 8-7. Premature atrial contractions (PACs). Top: Ectopic P′ waves (arrows). Bottom: Atrial bigeminy.

3. PACs that produce symptoms can be suppressed with quinidine, procainamide, or β-adrenergic antagonists.

Multifocal Atrial Tachycardia (MFAT)

Multifocal atrial tachycardia (MFAT, also known as chaotic atrial rhythm or wandering atrial pacemaker) is an irregular rhythm caused by at least two different sites of atrial ectopy. The ECG characteristics of MFAT are: (1) three or more types of P waves (sinus and at least two different ectopic atrial foci) in one lead, (2) varying PR intervals, (3) atrial rhythm usually between 100 to 180, and (4) nonconducted ectopic P′ waves (Fig. 8-8). MFAT can be confused with atrial flutter or fibrillation.

Clinical Significance

MFAT is most often found in elderly patients with decompensated chronic lung disease, but also may complicate congestive heart failure, sepsis, or be caused by methylxanthine toxicity. Digitalis toxicity is an unlikely cause of MFAT.

Treatment

1. Treatment is directed toward the underlying disorder. With decompensated lung disease, oxygen and bronchodilators improve pulmonary function, arterial oxygenation, and decrease atrial ectopy.
2. Specific antiarrhythmic therapy is rarely indicated. However, ventricular rate control with digoxin is occasionally needed when atrial ectopy cannot be adequately controlled.
3. Cardioversion has little effect on these multiple sites of atrial ectopy.

Atrial Flutter

Atrial flutter is a rhythm that originates from a small area within the atria. The exact mechanism—whether reentry, automatic focus, or other—is not yet known. As studied with intracardiac electrodes, electric activity usually begins in the inferior right atrium and propagates upward and to the left. ECG characteristics of atrial flutter are: (1) regular atrial rate between 250 to 350 (most

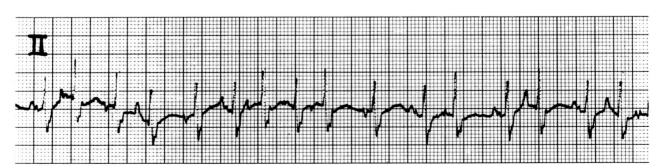

Figure 8-8. Multifocal atrial tachycardia (MFAT).

commonly 280 to 320); (2) sawtooth flutter waves directed superiorly and most visible in leads II, III, aV_F; and (3) AV block, usually 2:1, but occasionally greater or irregular (Fig. 8-9). One-to-one AV conduction may occur in patients with bypass tracts or when AV nodal conduction is enhanced by quinidine. Aberrant conduction may occur and cause atrial flutter to resemble ventricular tachycardia. Carotid sinus massage is a useful technique to slow ventricular response and unmask flutter waves.

Clinical Significance

Atrial flutter rarely occurs in patients without heart disease. It is most commonly seen in patients with ischemic heart disease or acute myocardial infarction. Less common causes include congestive cardiomyopathy, pulmonary embolus, myocarditis, blunt chest trauma, and, rarely, digitalis toxicity. Atrial flutter may be a transitional arrhythmia between sinus rhythm and atrial fibrillation.

Treatment

1. Low energy cardioversion (25 to 50 J) is very successful in converting more than 90 percent of cases of atrial flutter into sinus rhythm. Energies less than 10 J should be avoided as they are more likely to convert atrial flutter into atrial fibrillation than into sinus rhythm.
2. If cardioversion is contraindicated, ventricular rate control can be achieved with digoxin, verapamil, or propranolol.
3. Quinidine or procainamide can be used after ventricular rate control is achieved to chemically slow or convert the atrial arrhythmia, or prevent recurrence of the arrhythmia.

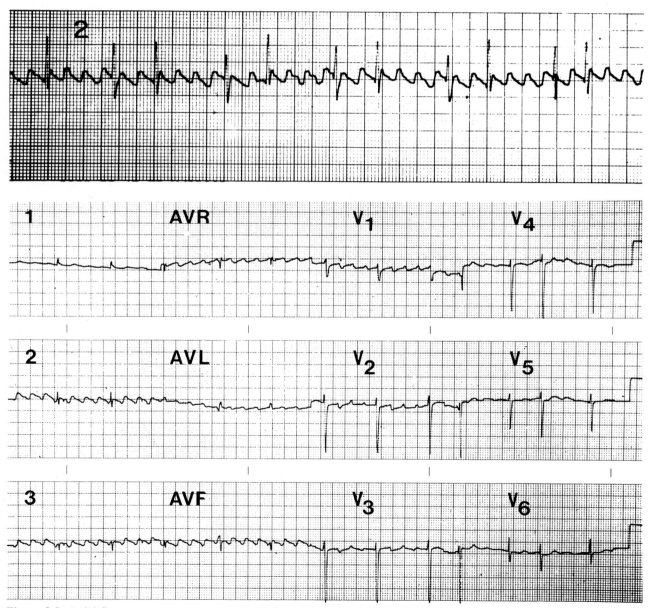

Figure 8-9. Atrial flutter.

4. Intravenous verapamil will occasionally convert atrial flutter into sinus rhythm (about 30 percent) or atrial fibrillation (about 20 percent).

Atrial Fibrillation

Atrial fibrillation occurs when there are multiple small areas of atrial myocardium continuously discharging and contracting. There is no uniform atrial depolarization and contraction, but instead, only a quivering of the atrial wall. While the atrial rate is usually above 400, the ventricular rate is limited by the refractory period of the AV node. The ECG characteristics of atrial fibrillation are: (1) fibrillatory waves of atrial activity, best seen in leads V_1, V_2, V_3, and aV_F; and (2) irregular ventricular response, usually around 170 to 180 in patients with a healthy AV node (Fig. 8-10). Disease or drugs (especially digitalis) may reduce AV node conduction and markedly slow ventricular response. A more rapid ventricular response may be seen in patients with bypass tracts; rates above 200 are possible. In this case, since ventricular activation occurs by way of the bypass tract, the QRS complex is usually wide. In addition, aberrancy—usually with a right bundle branch block configuration—is possible with rapid rates alone.

Clinical Significance

Atrial fibrillation can occur in a paroxysmal or sustained manner. Predisposing factors for atrial fibrillation are increased atrial size and mass, increased vagal tone, and variation in refractory periods between different parts of atrial myocardium. Atrial fibrillation is usually found in association with four disorders: rheumatic heart disease, hypertension, ischemic heart disease, and thyrotoxicosis. Less common causes are chronic lung disease, pericarditis, acute alcoholic intoxication, or atrial septal defect.

In patients with left ventricular failure, left atrial contraction makes an important contribution to cardiac output. The loss of effective atrial contraction, as in atrial fibrillation, may produce heart failure in these patients. Atrial fibrillation also predisposes to peripheral venous and atrial emboli, with the risk of pulmonary and systemic arterial embolism. Up to 30 percent of patients in chronic atrial fibrillation have at least one embolic episode. Conversion from chronic atrial fibrillation to sinus rhythm also carries up to a 1.5 percent risk of arterial embolism.

Treatment

1. Atrial fibrillation with a rapid ventricular response and acute hemodynamic deterioration should be treated with synchronized cardioversion. Over 60 percent can be converted with 100 J and over 80 percent with 200 J. Conversion to and retention in sinus rhythm is more likely when atrial fibrillation is of short duration and the atria are not greatly dilated. If initial cardioversion is unsuccessful, procainamide IV should be given to facilitate further cardioversion attempts.
2. In more stable patients, the first goal is to achieve ventricular rate control with either propranolol IV, most effective in patients with rheumatic mitral stenosis; digoxin IV, or verapamil IV—a small percentage (less than 10 percent) will convert from atrial fibrillation to sinus rhythm.
3. Patients with a slow ventricular response not due to digitalis have AV node disease and probably a more generalized disorder of cardiac conduction (sick sinus syndrome). These patients are at increased risk for profound bradycardias or asystole following cardioversion or antiarrhythmic drug therapy.

Supraventricular Tachycardia (SVT)

Supraventricular tachycardia is a regular, rapid rhythm that arises from either reentry or an ectopic pacemaker in areas above the bifurcation of the bundle of His. The reentrant variety is clinically the most common. These patients often present with acute, symptomatic episodes termed paroxysmal supraventricular tachycardia (PSVT).

Ectopic SVT usually originates in the atria with an atrial rate of 100 to 250 (most commonly 140 to 200) (Fig. 8-11). The regular P waves can be mistaken for atrial flutter or, if there is a 2:1 AV block, sinus rhythm.

Reentrant SVT constitutes the majority of patients with SVT: about two-thirds of these patients have reentry within the AV node and the other third have reentry involving a bypass tract. Much smaller numbers of patients have reentry in other sites. In the normal heart, reentrant SVT at the typical rates of 160 to 200 is often tolerated for hours or days. However, cardiac output is always depressed—regardless of the blood pressure—and rapid rates may produce heart failure.

Reentrant SVT within the AV node is usually initiated when an

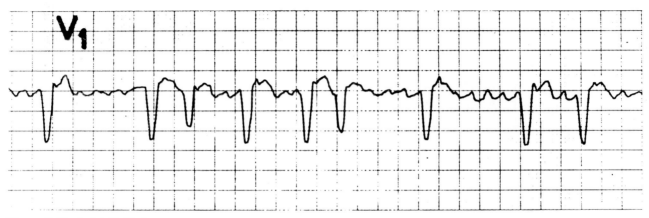

Figure 8-10. Atrial fibrillation.

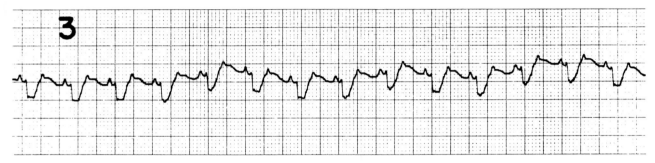

Figure 8-11. Ectopic supraventricular tachycardia (SVT) with 2:1 AV conduction.

ectopic atrial impulse encounters the AV node during the partially refractory period (Fig. 8-12). There are two functionally different parallel conducting limbs within the AV node that are connected above at the atrial end and below at the ventricular end of the node. This circuit is capable of sustained reentry when properly stimulated. AV conduction is usually 1:1 and the QRS complex is usually normal, unless there is aberrant infranodal conduction.

In patients with bypass tracts, the two parallel limbs of the reentry circuit are the AV node and the bypass tract, with connections at the atrial and ventricular ends by myocardial cells. While reentry can occur in either direction, it usually occurs in a direction that goes down the AV node and up the bypass tract, producing a narrow QRS complex. In the Wolff-Parkinson-White syndrome, about 85 percent of the reentrant SVTs have narrow QRS complexes.

Clinical Significance

Ectopic SVT may be seen in patients with acute myocardial infarction, chronic lung disease, pneumonia, alcoholic intoxication, and digitalis toxicity [where it is often associated with AV block and termed paroxysmal atrial tachycardia (PAT) with block]. It is commonly held that a high percentage of SVT with block, as much as 75 percent, is due to digitalis toxicity. However, not all studies have found this to be the case. The common arrhythmias of digitalis toxicity are listed in Table 8-1.

Reentrant SVT can occur in a normal heart, or in association with rheumatic heart disease, acute pericarditis, myocardial infarction, mitral valve prolapse, or one of the preexcitation syndromes.

SVT often causes a sensation of palpitations and lightheaded-

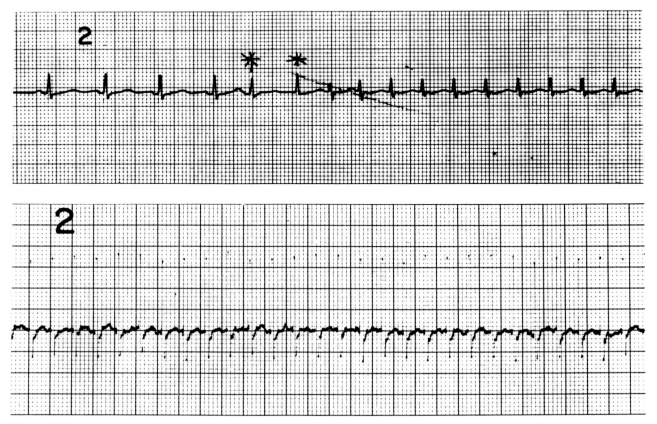

Figure 8-12. Reentrant supraventricular tachycardia (SVT). Top: 2d PAD (*) initiates run of PAT. Bottom: SVT, rate 286.

Table 8-1. Common Arrhythmias of Digitalis Toxicity (Approximate Incidence)

PVCs (60%)
  Unifocal, multifocal, bigeminy, or trigeminy

AV block (20%)
  Second-degree
    Mobitz I, Mobitz II
  Third-degree

Ectopic SVT (20–30%)
  Rate 70–130
  Gradual appearance and disappearance
  AV dissociation and/or block

Junctional escape beats (10%)

Ventricular tachycardia (10%)
  Bidirectional ventricular tachycardia associated with high mortality

Sinus bradycardia, SA block, and sinus pause (1–10%)

ness. In patients with coronary artery disease, anginal chest pain and dyspnea may occur from the rapid heart rate. Frank heart failure and pulmonary edema may occur in patients with poor left ventricular function. The loss of atrial contribution to cardiac output is often poorly tolerated in patients with left ventricular failure.

Treatment

Ectopic SVT due to digitalis toxicity is treated by:

1. Discontinuing the digitalis.
2. As long as there is not a high-grade AV block, correcting any existing hypokalemia to bring serum potassium into the high-normal range in an effort to reduce atrial ectopy.
3. Reducing atrial ectopy by phenytoin infused intravenously at a rate less than 50 mg/min until the desired response is achieved, the total dose reaches 15 to 18 mg/kg, or early signs of toxicity develop, with nystagmus or ataxia. Propranolol is also useful to reduce atrial ectopy although more risks are associated with its acute use.
4. Cardioversion is not effective and is potentially hazardous.

Ectopic SVT not due to digitalis toxicity is treated by:

1. Digoxin to slow and control ventricular response.
2. Antiarrhythmic therapy with quinidine or procainamide to reduce atrial ectopy once ventricular rate control is achieved.

Reentrant SVT can be converted by impeding conduction through one limb of the reentry circuit; sustained reentry is then impossible and sinus rhythm resumes.

1. Maneuvers which increase vagal tone, slow conduction, and prolong the refractory period in the AV node. These maneuvers can be done by themselves or after administration of drugs.
   a. Carotid sinus massage attempts to massage the carotid sinus and its baroreceptors against the transverse process of C6. Massage should be done for 10 s at a time, first attempted on the side of the nondominant cerebral hemisphere, and should never be done simultaneously on both sides. Prolonged AV block during carotid massage may occur in patients with AV node disease or who are on digitalis. Patients with carotid artery stenosis may develop cerebral ischemia or infarction from over-vigorous carotid massage.
   b. Facial immersion in cold water ("diving reflex") for 30 s.
   c. Gagging.
2. Verapamil is the drug of choice, 0.075 to 0.15 mg/kg (3 to 10 mg) IV over 15 to 60 s, with a repeat dose in 30 min if necessary. Studies have found that more than 90 percent of adults with reentrant SVT will respond within 1 to 2 min to verapamil.
3. Parasympathetic tone can be increased with edrophonium, a 1 mg IV test dose, a wait of 3 to 5 min, followed by 5 to 10 mg IV over 60 s. Historically, edrophonium did not have the 90 percent response rate seen with verapamil.
4. Vagal tone can be enhanced by pharmacologically elevating blood pressure with a pure peripheral vasoconstrictor; do not use agents with β-adrenergic activity. This method should be combined with carotid sinus massage. Blood pressure should be monitored frequently and diastolic pressure should not be allowed to exceed 130 mmHg. This method should not be used if hypertension is already present.
   a. Metaraminol 200 mg/500 mL D_5W or norepinephrine 4 mg/500 mL D_5W can be infused at rates of 1 to 2 mL/min and titrated until the rhythm converts.
   b. Methoxamine or phenylephrine 0.5 to 1.0 mg IV over 2 to 3 min, with repeat doses as required.
5. Propranolol 0.5 to 1.0 mg IV slowly over 60 s, repeated every 5 min, until the rhythm converts or the total dose reaches 0.1 mg/kg. Historically, propranolol has about a 50 percent success rate in converting reentrant SVT.
6. Digoxin 0.5 mg IV with repeat doses of 0.25 mg in 30 to 60 min until a response occurs or the total dose reaches 0.02 mg/kg. The chief drawback of digoxin has been its long onset of action and potential hazard in patients with accessory (bypass) tracts.
7. Synchronized cardioversion should be done in any unstable patient with hypotension, pulmonary edema, or severe chest pain. The dose required is usually small, less than 50 J.

Junctional Arrhythmias

Traditionally, a junctional impulse is considered to be one that arises from the AV node or bundle of His above the bifurcation. While pacemaker tissue cannot be found in the AV node itself in experimental animals, the matter is not settled in humans. From its source, the impulse spreads retrograde toward the atria and antegrade toward the ventricles. Depending on the site of origin, conduction velocity, and refractory periods, the atria may be activated before, during, or after ventricular depolarization. Atrial depolarization may not be visible if retrograde conduction is blocked or atrial activation occurs simultaneously with ventricular activation and the P′ waves are obscured by the QRS complex. AV dissociation may occur if the rate of discharge from the junctional pacemaker is faster than the sinus node rate and the junctional impulse is blocked from retrograde conduction toward the atria.

Junctional Premature Contractions (JPCs)

Junctional premature contractions are due to an ectopic pacemaker within the AV node or common AV bundle. The ECG characteristics of JPCs are: (1) the ectopic QRS complex is premature, (2) the ectopic P′ wave has a different shape and direction (usually

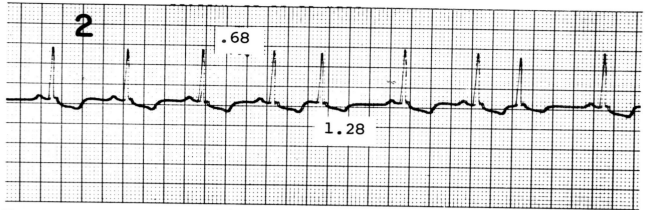

Figure 8-13. Junctional premature contractions (JPCs).

inverted in leads II, III, and aV$_F$), (3) the ectopic P$'$ wave may occur before or after the QRS complex, (4) the PR interval of the ectopic beat is shorter than normal, (5) the QRS complex is usually of normal shape, unless there is aberrant conduction, and (6) the sinus node is usually not affected and the postectopic pause is fully compensatory (Fig. 8-13). JPCs may be isolated, multiple (as in bigeminy or trigeminy), or multifocal.

Clinical Significance

JPCs are uncommon in healthy hearts. They occur in congestive heart failure, digitalis toxicity, ischemic heart disease, or acute myocardial infarctions (especially of the inferior wall).

Treatment

1. No specific treatment is usually required.
2. Treat the underlying disorder.
3. Antiarrhythmic therapy with quinidine or procainamide may be useful if JPCs are frequent, symptomatic, or initiating more serious arrhythmias.

Junctional Rhythms

Under normal circumstances, the sinus node discharges at a faster rate than the AV junction, so the pacemaker function of the AV junction is overridden. If sinus node discharges slow or fail to reach the AV junction, then junctional escape beats may occur, usually at a rate between 40 to 60, depending on the level of the pacemaker. Generally, junctional escape beats do not conduct

retrograde into the atria so a QRS complex without a P$'$ wave is usually seen (Fig. 8-14).

Under other circumstances, enhanced junctional automaticity may override the sinus node and produce either an accelerated junctional rhythm (rate 60 to 100) or junctional tachycardia (rate greater than 100). Usually, both the atria and ventricles are captured by the enhanced junctional pacemaker (Fig. 8-15).

Clinical Significance

Junctional escape beats may occur whenever there is a long enough pause in the impulses reaching the AV junction: sinus bradycardia, slow phase of sinus arrhythmia, AV block, or during the pause following premature beats. Sustained junctional escape rhythms may be seen with congestive heart failure, myocarditis, hyperkalemia, or digitalis toxicity. If the ventricular rate is too slow, myocardial or cerebral ischemia may develop.

Accelerated junctional rhythm and junctional tachycardia may occur from digitalis toxicity, acute rheumatic fever, or inferior myocardial infarction. With digitalis toxicity, the rate is usually between 70 to 130. If this rhythm develops in a patient being treated with digoxin for atrial fibrillation, the ECG is characterized by regular QRS complexes superimposed on atrial fibrillatory waves. Regularization of ventricular response during digitalis therapy in a patient with atrial fibrillation should raise the suspicion of digitalis toxicity.

Treatment

1. Isolated, infrequent junctional escape beats usually do not require specific treatment.

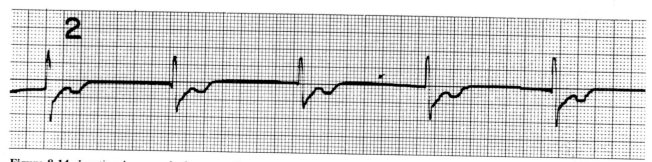

Figure 8-14. Junctional escape rhythm, rate 42.

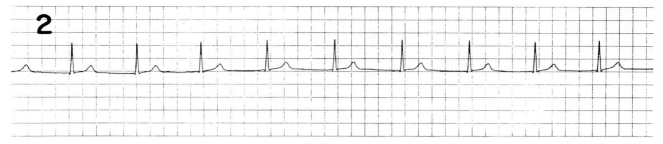

Figure 8-15. Accelerated junctional rhythm, rate 61.

2. If sustained junctional escape rhythms are producing symptoms, the underlying cause should be treated. Atropine can be used to temporarily accelerate sinus node discharge rate and enhance AV nodal conduction.
3. Accelerated junctional rhythm and junctional tachycardia usually do not produce significant symptoms. If the cause is digitalis toxicity, the drug should be discontinued. If the rate is fast and producing symptoms, it can be decreased by giving supplemental potassium to increase the serum level into the high-normal range.

Ventricular Arrhythmias

Premature Ventricular Contractions (PVCs)

Premature ventricular contractions are due to impulses originating from single or multiple areas in the ventricles. The ECG characteristics of PVCs are: (1) a premature and wide QRS complex, (2) lack of a preceding P wave, (3) the ST segment and T wave of the PVC are directed opposite the major QRS deflection, (4) most PVCs do not affect the sinus node so there is usually a fully compensatory postectopic pause or the PVC may be interpolated between two sinus beats, (5) many PVCs have a fixed coupling interval (within 0.04 s) from the preceding sinus beat, and (6) many PVCs are conducted into the atria, producing a retrograde P wave (Fig. 8-16).

Occasionally, a ventricular fusion beat occurs when a supraventricular and ventricular impulse nearly simultaneously depolarize the ventricles. The QRS configuration of a fusion beat contains features of the individual components (Fig. 8-17).

A PVC may be confused with an aberrantly conducted supraventricular beat. Aberration versus ventricular origin can be suspected from several ECG findings; this is discussed in a separate section.

Clinical Significance

PVCs are very common, even in patients without evidence of heart disease. They occur in most patients with ischemic heart disease and are universally found in patients with acute myocardial infarction. Other common causes of PVCs include digitalis toxicity, congestive heart failure, hypokalemia, alkalosis, hypoxia, and sympathomimetic drugs.

While there is a correlation between the severity of underlying coronary artery disease and the degree of ventricular ectopy, it is not known whether ventricular ectopy itself is an independent risk factor for future morbidity or mortality. Lown has made an attempt with his classification to quantitate the risks associated with chronic ventricular ectopy, but his classification is not universally accepted (Table 8-2).

In the setting of an acute myocardial infarction, PVCs indicate the underlying electrical instability of the heart. These patients are at increased risk for the development of primary ventricular fibrillation. Current work indicates that various degrees of PVCs ("warning arrhythmias") are not reliable predictors of subsequent ventricular fibrillation.

Although it is experimentally established that electric impulses, such as PVCs, that occur during or soon after repolarization (the so-called "vulnerable period") can initiate ventricular tachycardia or fibrillation, clinical studies have found that more paroxysms of ventricular tachycardia are initiated by late-coupled PVCs than early-coupled PVCs (R-on-T phenomenon).

Treatment

1. In the setting of possible or definitive acute myocardial infarction, most physicians would treat PVCs with intravenous lidocaine. Many physicians would also treat the same group of patients prophylactically with lidocaine. Further discussion on this concept is in the chapter on myocardial infarction.
2. In patients with chronic ectopy, there is no current satisfactory method of identifying those who would benefit from oral antiarrhythmic therapy. It does seem reasonable to treat those patients having PVCs that are (1) multifocal, (2) short-coupled (R-on-T), (3) that occur back-to-back (two PVCs in a row), or (4) that occur as short runs of ventricular tachycardia (three or more PVCs in a row). Quinidine, disopyramide, procainamide, or propranolol are usually used. Oral antiarrhythmic therapy should be carefully monitored.

Ventricular Parasystole

Parasystole occurs when an independent ectopic pacemaker is protected from the influence of outside impulses ("entrance block"). A parasystolic pacemaker can arise anywhere in the heart, but is

Table 8-2. Lown Grading System for Ventricular Ectopy

Grade	
1	Uniform PVCs <30/h
2	Uniform PVCs >30/h
3	Multiform PVCs
4A	Couplets (2 consecutive PVCs)
4B	Triplets (3 or more consecutive PVCs)
5	R-on-T PVCs

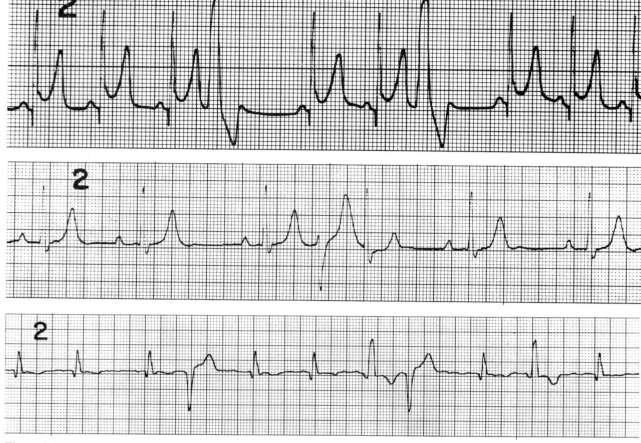

Figure 8-16. Premature ventricular contractions (PVCs). Top: Unifocal PVC. Center: Interpolated PVC. Bottom: Multifocal PVCs.

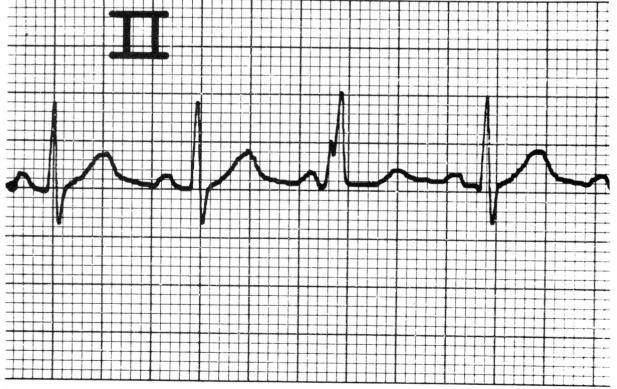

Figure 8-17. Fusion beats.

Figure 8-18. The fifth and eighth ventricular complexes are premature and of similar morphology but have different coupling intervals. The second complex (marked "F") represents a fusion beat. The interectopic interval is 2.36 s. (From Heger JW, Niemann JT, Boman KG, et al: *Cardiology for the House Officer.* Baltimore, Williams & Wilkins, © 1982.)

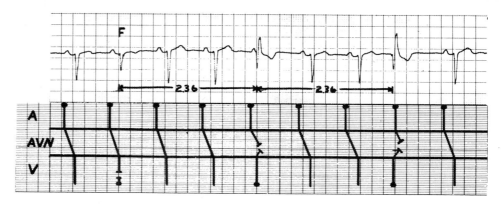

most often located in the ventricles where it produces a rhythm that operates alongside of and is independent of the sinus node.

The ECG characteristics of ventricular parasystole are (1) variation in the coupling interval between the preceding sinus beat and the ectopic beat, (2) common relation between the interectopic beat intervals, and (3) occurrence of fusion beats (Fig. 8-18). Usually, long rhythm strips are necessary to establish that the interectopic intervals are multiples of a common parasystolic rate.

Clinical Significance

Ventricular parasystole is most often associated with severe ischemic heart disease, acute myocardial infarction, hypertensive heart disease, or electrolyte imbalance. While parasystole is often self-limited and benign, it may lead to ventricular tachycardia or fibrillation.

Treatment

1. The underlying disease should be treated.
2. Antiarrhythmics are indicated in patients with symptomatic episodes or beats which initiate ventricular tachycardia.

Accelerated Idioventricular Tachycardia (AIVR)

Accelerated idioventricular tachycardia is an ectopic rhythm of ventricular origin occurring at rates of 40 to 100. Even though AIVR is not a tachycardia, such terms as idioventricular tachycardia, nonparoxysmal ventricular tachycardia, or slow ventricular tachycardia have been applied.

The ECG characteristics of AIVR are: (1) wide and regular QRS complexes, (2) rate between 40 to 100 that is often close to the preceding sinus rate, (3) most runs of short duration (3 to

30 beats), and (4) an AIVR often beginning with a fusion beat (Fig. 8-19).

Clinical Significance

This condition is most commonly found in the setting of an acute myocardial infarction, but may also be seen in patients without heart disease. While there is some variable association with ventricular tachycardia, there is no apparent association with ventricular fibrillation. AIVR usually produces no symptoms itself. Sometimes the loss of atrial contraction and subsequent fall in cardiac output may produce hemodynamic deterioration.

Treatment

1. Treatment is not necessary. On occasion, AIVR may be the only functioning pacemaker and suppression with lidocaine can lead to cardiac asystole.
2. If sustained AIVR produces symptoms secondary to a decrease in cardiac output, treatment with atrial pacing may be required.

Ventricular Tachycardia

Ventricular tachycardia is the occurrence of three or more beats from a ventricular ectopic pacemaker at a rate greater than 100. The ECG characteristics of ventricular tachycardia are (1) wide QRS complexes; (2) rate greater than 100 (most commonly 150 to 200); (3) the rhythm is usually regular, although there may be some beat-to-beat variation; and (4) the QRS axis is usually constant (Fig. 8-20).

There are several variants of ventricular tachycardia. *Ventricular flutter* is the phrase used for a regular zigzag pattern without distinguishable QRS complexes or T waves. In *bidirectional*

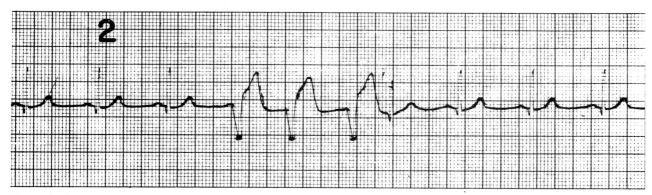

Figure 8-19. Accelerated idioventricular rhythms (AIVR).

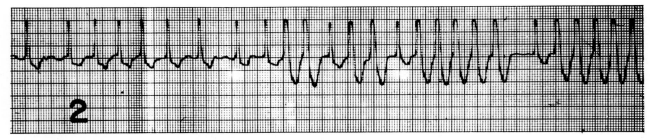

Figure 8-20. Ventricular tachycardia.

ventricular tachycardia the QRS complexes alternate polarity as recorded in a single lead. In *alternating ventricular tachycardia* the QRS complexes alternate in height (but not polarity) in a single lead. (Both bidirectional alternating ventricular tachycardia indicate serious myocardial disease and are often due to digitalis toxicity.) In *polymorphous ventricular tachycardia* the QRS complexes have many different shapes in one lead. *Atypical ventricular tachycardia* (torsades de pointes, or "twisting of the points") is where the QRS axis swings from a positive to negative direction in a single lead (Fig. 8-21). Despite the appearance, this rhythm originates from a single focus. Atypical ventricular tachycardia usually occurs in short runs of 5 to 15 s at a rate of 200 to 240. This form of ventricular tachycardia generally occurs in patients with serious myocardial disease who have a prolonged and uneven ventricular repolarization (prolonged QT interval). Drugs which further prolong repolarization—quinidine, disopyramide, procainamide, phenothiazines, tricyclic antidepressants—exacerbate this arrhythmia. Conventional treatment with lidocaine is often ineffective. Effective treatment usually involves accelerating the heart rate (thereby shortening ventricular repolarization) with isoproterenol (2 to 8 µg/min) or overdrive ventricular pacing (rate 120 to 140).

Clinical Significance

Ventricular tachycardia is very rare in patients without underlying heart disease. The most common causes of ventricular tachycardia are ischemic heart disease and acute myocardial infarction. Less common causes include hypertrophic cardiomyopathy, mitral valve prolapse, and toxicity from many drugs (digitalis, quinidine, procainamide, sympathomimetics). Hypoxia, alkalosis, and electrolyte abnormalities exacerbate the tendency toward ventricular ectopy and tachycardia.

Some patients with ventricular tachycardia may still be able to maintain an effective cardiac output with a reasonable blood pressure while others may be in cardiac arrest.

Treatment

1. Unstable patients or those in cardiac arrest should be treated with synchronized cardioversion. Ventricular tachycardia can be converted with energies as low as 1 J and over 90 percent can be converted with less than 10 J. Rarely is more than 100 J needed.

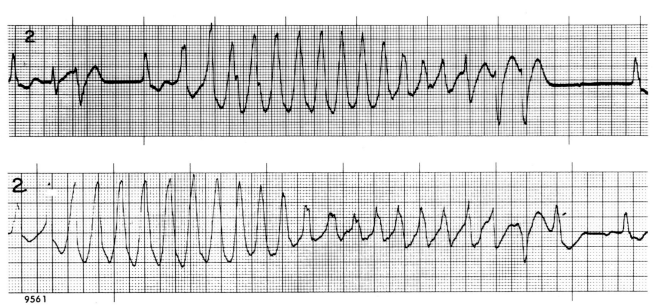

9561

Figure 8-21. Two examples of short runs of atypical ventricular tachycardia showing sinusoidal variation in amplitude and direction of the QRS complexes: "Les Torsades de Pointes" (twisting of the points). Note that the top example is initiated by a late occurring PVC (lead II).

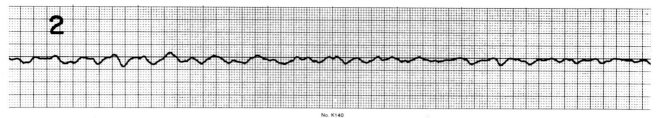

Figure 8-22. Ventricular fibrillation.

2. Clinically stable patients should be treated with intravenous antiarrhythmics.
   a. 75 mg of lidocaine (1.0 to 1.5 mg/kg) is given IV over 60 to 90 s, followed by a constant infusion at 1 to 4 mg/min [10 to 40 μg/(kg · min)]. A repeat bolus dose of 50 mg lidocaine may be required during the first 20 min to avoid a subtherapeutic dip in serum level due to the early distribution phase.
   b. 500 mg of bretylium (5 to 10 mg/kg) is given IV over 10 min.
   c. Procainamide is infused IV at a rate of less than 50 mg/min until the arrhythmia converts, the total dose reaches 15 to 17 mg/kg in normals (12 mg/kg in patients with congestive heart failure), or early signs of toxicity develop with hypotension or QRS prolongation. The loading dose should be followed by a maintenance infusion of 2.8 mg/(kg · h) in normal subjects [1.4 mg/(kg · h) in patients with renal insufficiency].

Ventricular Fibrillation

Ventricular fibrillation is the totally disorganized depolarization and contraction of small areas of ventricular myocardium—there is no effective ventricular pumping activity. The ECG of ventricular fibrillation shows a fine to coarse zigzag pattern without discernible P waves or QRS complexes (Fig. 8-22).

Ventricular fibrillation is never accompanied by a pulse or blood pressure. In patients who are awake and responsive, the ECG pattern of ventricular fibrillation is caused by a loose lead artifact or electrical interference.

Clinical Significance

Ventricular fibrillation is most commonly seen in patients with severe ischemic heart disease, with or without an acute myocardial infarction. Primary ventricular fibrillation occurs suddenly, without preceding hemodynamic deterioration, while secondary ventricular fibrillation occurs after a prolonged period of left ventricular failure and/or circulatory shock. Ventricular fibrillation may also occur from digitalis toxicity, quinidine toxicity, hypothermia, blunt chest trauma, severe electrolyte abnormality, or from myocardial irritation caused by an intracardiac catheter or pacemaker electrode.

Treatment

1. Treatment consists of immediate electrical defibrillation with 200 J. If the first attempt is unsuccessful, defibrillation should be repeated immediately.
2. If the initial two attempts are unsuccessful, CPR should be initiated and further electrical defibrillations done after the administration of various intravenous drugs:
   a. Epinephrine
   b. Sodium bicarbonate
   c. Antiarrhythmics: lidocaine, bretylium, or procainamide.

ABERRANT VERSUS VENTRICULAR TACHYARRHYTHMIAS

Differentiation between ectopic beats of ventricular origin and those of supraventricular origin but conducted aberrantly can be difficult, especially in sustained tachycardias with wide QRS complexes. Several guidelines might help in this distinction.

1. A preceding ectopic P′ wave is good evidence favoring aberrancy, although coincidental atrial and ventricular ectopic beats or retrograde conduction can occur. AV dissociation suggests ventricular origin.
2. Postectopic pause: A fully compensatory pause is more likely after a ventricular beat, but exceptions do occur.
3. Fusion beats are good evidence for ventricular origin, but again exceptions do occur.
4. A varying bundle branch block pattern suggests aberrancy.
5. Coupling intervals are usually constant with ventricular ectopic beats, unless parasystole is present. Varying coupling intervals suggest aberrancy.
6. Response to carotid sinus massage will slow conduction through the AV node and may abolish reentrant SVT and slow the ventricular response in other supraventricular tachyarrhythmias. This has essentially no effect on ventricular ectopy.
7. A QRS duration of longer than 0.14 s is usually only found in ventricular ectopy.
8. QRS morphology: Wellens et al. have studied patients with both ventricular tachycardia and SVT with aberrancy using His bundle electrocardiography. Several morphologic ECG criteria were found useful in differentiating between the two (Table 8-3).

Table 8-3. Aberrancy versus Ventricular Ectopy*

QRS Pattern in V_1	Favors	QRS Pattern in V_6	Favors
rSR′ (RBBB pattern) rR′	Aberrancy	qRS	Aberrancy
R qR RS Slurred downslope R	Ventricular	rS S qR or QR R qQ′	Ventricular
Slurred upstroke R	Either	RS Slurred R	Either

*Source: Am J Med 64:27, 1978.

CONDUCTION DISTURBANCES

Sinoatrial (SA) Block

The sinus node discharge must be conducted into the atria to pace the heart during sinus rhythm. If sinus node discharges are delayed or blocked in their outward propagation, then sinoatrial block is present. Sinoatrial block is divided into first-, second-, and third-degree varieties.

First-degree SA block means that the impulse is delayed in its conduction out of the sinus node into the atria—a condition that cannot be recognized on the clinical ECG.

Second-degree SA block means that some impulses get through and some are blocked. Second-degree SA block can be suspected whenever an expected P wave and the corresponding QRS complex are absent. In the variable (Wenckebach) type of second-degree SA block, the missing P wave would come after a period of progressive prolongation of the sinus node to atrium conduction time, again something undetectable on the clinical ECG. However, another ECG finding common to the Wenckebach phenomenon can be seen—progressive shortening of the P-P intervals prior to the missing P wave (Fig. 8-23). In the constant type of second-degree SA block, the sinoatrial conduction time remains constant before and after the blocked impulses. In this situation, the interval encompassing the missing beat is an exact or near-exact multiple of the cycle length (Fig. 8-24).

Third-degree SA block occurs when the sinus node discharge is completely blocked and no P wave originating from the sinus node is seen. There are three other causes of absent sinus P waves in addition to third-degree SA block: (1) sinus node failure, (2) a sinus node stimulus inadequate to activate the atria, and (3) atrial unresponsiveness.

Clinical Significance

Sinoatrial block usually arises from myocardial disease (acute rheumatic fever, acute inferior myocardial infarction, other causes of myocarditis) or drug toxicity (digitalis, atropine, quinidine, salicylates, propranolol). In rare individuals, vagal stimulation can produce SA block.

Treatment

1. Treatment depends on the underlying cause, associated arrhythmias, and whether symptoms of hypoperfusion are present.
2. Sinus node discharge rate and sinoatrial conduction can be facilitated by atropine or isoproterenol when clinically required.
3. Cardiac pacing is indicated when symptomatic bradycardia is unresponsive to atropine or isoproterenol.

Sinus Arrest (Pause)

Sinus pause is a failure of impulse formation within the sinus node. In sinus arrest, the P-P interval has no mathematical relation to the basic sinus node discharge rate (Fig. 8-25).

Clinical Significance

The same conditions which produce SA block can also produce sinus arrest, especially digitalis toxicity. The combination of digitalis and carotid sinus massage is well known to be able to produce prolonged sinus arrest. Brief periods of sinus arrest may occur in healthy individuals from increased vagal tone. If sinus arrest is prolonged, AV junctional escape beats often occur.

Treatment

1. Treatment depends on the underlying cause, heart rate, and presence of symptoms.
2. If sinus arrest is symptomatic, atropine or isoproterenol will increase sinus node discharge rate.
3. Cardiac pacing is indicated when symptomatic bradycardia is unresponsive to atropine or isoproterenol.

Atrioventricular (AV) Dissociation

Atrioventricular dissociation is a condition in which the atria and ventricles are driven by separate and independent pacemakers. It is not a primary rhythm disturbance, but is secondary to another conduction or rhythm abnormality. There are two varieties of AV dissociation: passive (default or "escape"), and active (usurpation).

Passive AV dissociation occurs when an impulse fails to reach the AV node due to sinus node failure or block. Usually an escape rhythm takes over and paces the ventricles. When the sinus node recovers, atrial activity resumes but there may be a period during which the ventricles are still driven by the escape pacemaker, and the P waves and QRS complexes occur independent of each other (Fig. 8-26).

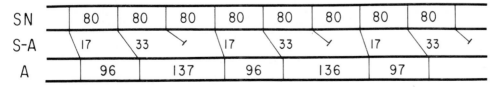

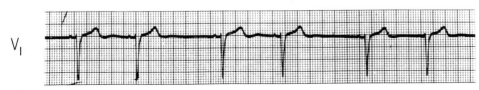

Figure 8-23. Second-degree SA block type I (Wenckebach). (From Braunwald E: *Heart Disease. A Textbook of Cardiovascular Medicine.* Philadelphia, Saunders, 1980.)

Figure 8-24. Second-degree constant SA block type II (lead V₄).

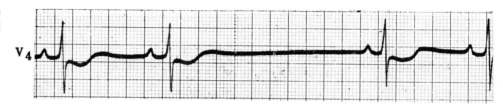

Active AV dissociation occurs when a lower pacemaker accelerates to usurp the sinus node and captures the ventricles but the atria are still paced as before (Fig. 8-27).

In both varieties of AV dissociation, fusion beats are common. It is also common for the two pacemakers to operate with nearly identical rates, possibly due to mechanical or electrical influences which tend to keep them in phase with each other—a condition termed isorhythmic dissociation.

Clinical Significance

Passive AV dissociation occurs when the sinus node discharge rate is slowed by sinus bradycardia, sinus arrhythmia, SA block, or sinus pause. Common causes of this include: (1) ischemic heart disease (especially acute inferior myocardial infarction), (2) myocarditis (especially acute rheumatic fever), (3) drug toxicity (especially digitalis), and (4) vagal reflexes. It may also be seen in well-conditioned athletes.

Active AV dissociation occurs when the automaticity of lower pacemakers is enhanced. Common causes include myocardial ischemia and drug toxicity (especially digitalis).

Treatment

1. Most occurrences of AV dissociation have an acceptable heart rate and are well tolerated.
2. Therapy, if any, is directed toward the underlying cause.

Atrioventricular (AV) Block

Clinical classification of AV block was done before modern understanding of the sites and mechanisms involved in impairing conduction between the atria and ventricles. This is unfortunate because this classification is too simple to categorize all the problems that may occur with AV conduction. However, this system is almost universally used.

First-degree AV block is characterized by a delay in AV conduction, manifested by a prolonged PR interval. Second-degree AV block is characterized by intermittent AV conduction—some atrial impulses reach the ventricles and others are blocked. Third-

degree AV block is characterized by complete interruption in AV conduction.

Precise localization of AV conduction blocks can be made with His bundle electrocardiography. Although this method is not available for use in the emergency department, correlations can be made between the clinical ECG, the approximate location of the block, and the risk of future progression.

Atrioventricular blocks can also be divided into nodal and infranodal blocks, an important distinction because the clinical significance and prognosis vary with the site. Atrioventricular nodal blocks are usually due to reversible depression of conduction, often self-limited, generally have a stable infranodal escape pacemaker pacing the ventricles, and therefore do not have a serious prognosis. Infranodal blocks are usually due to organic disease of the His bundle or bundle branches, often the damage is irreversible, they generally have a slow and unstable ventricular escape rhythm pacing the ventricles, and they may have a serious prognosis depending on the clinical circumstance.

First-Degree AV Block

In first-degree AV block, each atrial impulse is conducted into the ventricles, but more slowly than normal. This is recognized by a PR interval of greater than 0.20 s (Fig. 8-28). The AV node is usually the site of conduction delay, although it may occur at any infranodal level.

Clinical Significance

First-degree AV block is occasionally found in normal hearts. Other common causes include increased vagal tone (whatever the cause), digitalis toxicity, acute inferior myocardial infarction, and myocarditis.

Treatment

1. None is usually required.
2. Prophylactic pacing in acute myocardial infarction is not indicated unless more serious infranodal conduction disturbances are present.

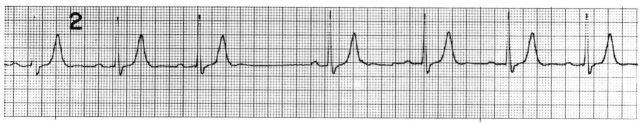

Figure 8-25. Sinus pause.

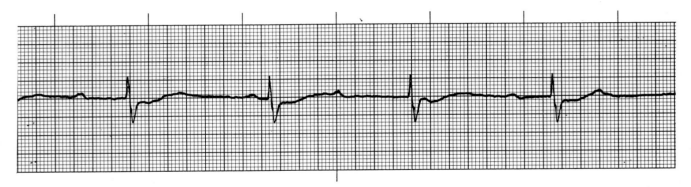

Figure 8-26. Passive AV dissociation, secondary to 3d degree AV block.

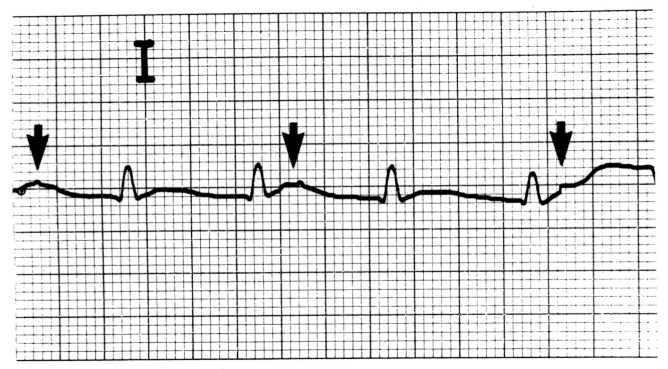

Figure 8-27. Active AV dissociation. (Arrows indicate P waves.)

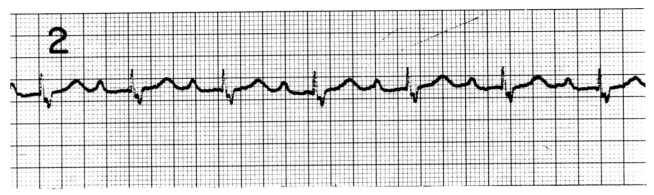

Figure 8-28. First-degree AV block (PR interval = 0.3 s).

Second-Degree Mobitz I (Wenckebach) AV Block

In this block there is progressive prolongation of AV conduction (and the PR interval) until an atrial impulse is completely blocked (Fig. 8-29). Conduction ratios are used to indicate the ratio of atrial to ventricular depolarizations: 3:2 indicates 2 out of 3 atrial impulses are conducted into the ventricles. Usually, only a single atrial impulse is blocked. After the dropped beat, the AV conduction returns to normal and the cycle usually repeats itself with either the same conduction ratio (fixed ratio) or a different conduction ratio (variable ratio). This type of block almost always occurs at the level of the AV node and is often due to reversible depression of AV nodal conduction.

The Wenckebach phenomenon has a seeming paradox. Even though the PR intervals progressively lengthen prior to the dropped beat, the increments by which they lengthen decrease with successive beats; this produces a progressive shortening of the R-R interval prior to the dropped beat (Fig. 8-29). This sign can be used to indicate that a Wenckebach phenomenon is occurring, even when the conduction delay cannot be seen, as in SA Wenckebach block.

Wenckebach block is believed to occur because each successive depolarization produces prolongation of the refractory period of the AV node. When the next atrial impulse comes upon the node, it is earlier in the relative refractory period and conduction occurs more slowly relative to the previous stimulus. This process is progressive until an atrial impulse reaches the AV node during the absolute refractory period and conduction is blocked altogether. The pause allows the AV node to recover and the process can resume.

Clinical Significance

This block is often transient and usually associated with an acute inferior myocardial infarction, digitalis toxicity, myocarditis, or is seen after cardiac surgery. Wenckebach block may also occur when a normal AV node is exposed to very rapid atrial rates.

Treatment

1. Specific treatment is not necessary unless slow ventricular rates produce signs of hypoperfusion.
2. 0.5 mg of atropine IV is given, repeated every 5 min as necessary, titrated to the desired effect, or until the total dose reaches 2.0 mg.
3. Isoproterenol is hazardous in the setting of acute myocardial infarction or digitalis toxicity and its use should be avoided.

4. Transvenous ventricular demand pacing should be initiated if atropine is unsuccessful.

Second-Degree Mobitz II AV Block

In this block, the PR interval remains constant before and after the nonconducted atrial beats (Fig. 8-30). One or more beats may be nonconducted at a single time.

Mobitz II blocks usually occur in the infranodal conducting system, often with coexistent fascicular or bundle branch blocks, and the QRS complexes are therefore usually wide. Even if the QRS complexes are narrow, the block is generally in the infranodal system.

When second-degree AV block occurs with a fixed conduction ratio of 2:1, it is not possible to differentiate between a Mobitz type I (Wenckebach) or Mobitz type II block. If the QRS complex is narrow, then the block is in the AV node or infranodal system with about equal incidence. If the QRS complex is wide, the block is more likely to be in the infranodal system.

Clinical Significance

Type II blocks imply structural damage to the infranodal conducting system, are usually permanent, and may progress suddenly to complete heart block—especially in the setting of an acute myocardial infarction.

Treatment

1. Atropine or isoproterenol may be tried, but are often unsuccessful and do not provide a long-term solution to the problem.
2. Most cases will require a transvenous ventricular demand pacemaker.

Third-Degree (Complete) AV Block

In third-degree AV block, there is no atrioventricular conduction. The ventricles are paced by an escape pacemaker at a rate slower than the atrial rate (Fig. 8-31). Third-degree AV block can occur either at nodal or infranodal levels.

When third-degree AV block occurs at the AV node, a junctional escape pacemaker takes over with a ventricular rate of 40 to 60 and, since the rhythm originates above the bifurcation of the bundle of His, the QRS complexes are narrow.

When third-degree AV block occurs at the infranodal level, the

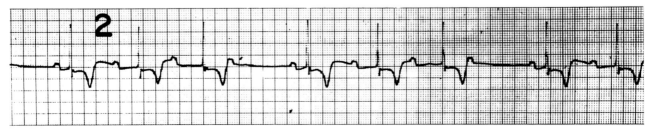

Figure 8-29. Second-degree Mobitz I (Wenckebach) AV block with 4:3 AV conduction.

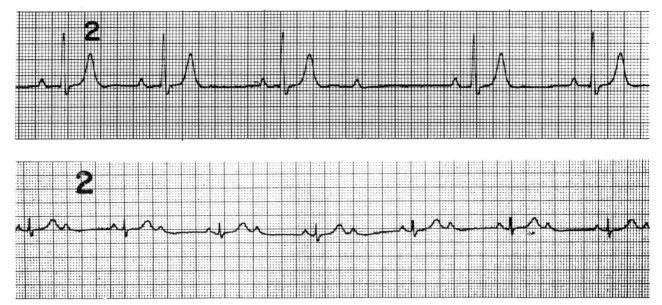

Figure 8-30. Top: Second-degree Mobitz II AV block. Bottom: Second degree AV block with 2:1 AV conduction.

ventricles are driven by a ventricular escape rhythm at a rate less than 40.

Clinical Significance

Nodal third-degree AV blocks may develop in up to 8 percent of acute inferior myocardial infarctions where it is usually transient, although it may last for several days.

Infranodal third-degree AV blocks indicate structural damage to the infranodal conducting system, as seen with an extensive acute anterior myocardial infarction. The ventricular escape pacemaker is usually inadequate to maintain cardiac output and is unstable with periods of ventricular asystole.

Treatment

1. Nodal third-degree AV blocks should be treated like second-degree Mobitz I AV blocks with atropine or ventricular demand pacemaker as required.
2. Infranodal third-degree AV blocks require a ventricular demand pacemaker. Isoproterenol can be used to temporarily accelerate the ventricular escape rhythm before pacemaker placement.

FASCICULAR BLOCKS

Unifascicular Block

Unifascicular block is a conduction block that affects one of the three major infranodal conduction pathways: right bundle branch (RBB), left anterior superior fascicle (LASF), and left posterior inferior fascicle (LPIF). A wide variety of disease processes can produce conduction block in the fascicles: ischemia, cardiomyopathies, valvular (especially aortic), myocarditis, cardiac surgery, congenital, and degenerative processes affecting the conduction tissue (Lenegre's or Lev's diseases).

In LASF block, left ventricular activation is by way of the LPIF and proceeds in an inferior-to-superior and right-to-left direction. The ECG characteristics of LASF block are: (1) normal QRS duration, (2) frontal plane mean QRS axis of less than −45°, (3) R wave in lead I greater than the R waves in leads II or III, and (4) deep S wave in leads II, III, and aV$_F$ (Fig. 8-32). The LASF is small and easily affected by focal lesions. Other causes of left axis deviation should be excluded—inferior myocardial infarction, hyperkalemia, preexcitation syndromes, or body habitus. Left ventricular hypertrophy itself does not cause such an extensive left axis deviation as seen with LASF block.

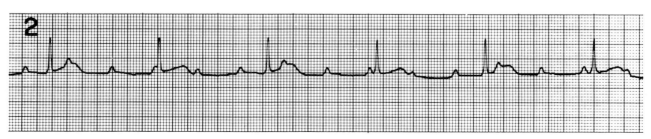

Figure 8-31. Third-degree AV block.

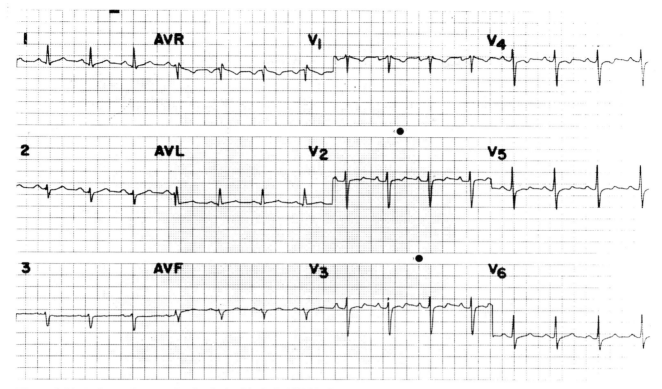

Figure 8-32. Left anterior superior fascicular block (LASF block).

In LPIF block, left ventricular activation is by way of the LASF and proceeds in a superior-to-inferior and left-to-right direction. The ECG characteristics of LPIF block are: (1) normal QRS duration, (2) frontal plane mean QRS axis greater than 110°, (3) small r and deep S wave in lead I, and (4) small q and large R wave in lead III (Fig. 8-33). The LPIF is broad and not affected by focal lesions; its presence indicates widespread organic heart disease. Other causes of right axis deviation are chronic cor pulmonale, right ventricular hypertrophy, and lateral myocardial infarction.

In RBB block, ventricular activation is by way of the left bundle branch, proceeding from the left to the right ventricle. The ECG characteristics of RBB block are: (1) prolonged QRS duration (greater than 0.12 s); (2) triphasic QRS complexes (RSR′) in lead V_1; (3) wide S waves in the lateral leads I, V_5, and V_6; and (4) normal onset of ventricular activation in lead V_6 (Fig. 8-34). The frontal plane mean QRS axis is usually not deviated to the right unless there is associated right ventricular hypertrophy.

Bifascicular Block

Bifascicular block refers to conduction blocks over two fascicles: (1) RBB and LASF, (2) RBB and LPIF, or (3) left bundle branch (LBB) block.

In LBB block, ventricular activation is by way of the RBB and proceeds from right to left and inferior to superior. The ECG characteristics of LBB block are: (1) prolonged QRS duration (greater than 0.12 s); (2) large and wide R waves in leads I, aV_L, V_5, and V_6; (3) small r wave followed by deep S wave in leads II, III, aV_F, and V_1 to V_3; and (4) no q waves in leads I, aV_F, V_5, and V_6 (Fig. 8-35).

Trifascicular Block

Trifascicular block refers to a combination of conduction blocks in all three fascicles, either permanent or transient: (1) RBB and LASF with first-degree AV block, (2) RBB and LPIF with first-degree AV block; (3) LBB with first-degree AV block, or (4) alternating RBB and LBB block.

While bi- and trifascicular conduction blocks indicate advanced organic heart disease, long-term follow-up studies of ambulatory patients indicate that the risk of sudden progression to complete heart block and sudden death due to ventricular asystole is not high. Placement of a ventricular demand pacemaker is indicated only for symptoms due to documented bradyarrhythmias.

However, in the face of an acute myocardial infarction, the risks of complete heart block are much greater when new or preexistent bi- or trifascicular conduction blocks are present. In this setting, prophylactic placement of a ventricular demand pacemaker is indicated. This is further discussed in the chapter on acute myocardial infarction.

PRETERMINAL RHYTHMS

Several arrhythmias may be seen during cardiac resuscitation. Ventricular tachycardia and fibrillation are readily treatable and resuscitation often results in a functional survivor. The four other arrhythmias included here have a low successful resuscitation rate and are much less likely to yield a functional survivor. Further discussion on this is included in the chapter on cardiac resuscitation.

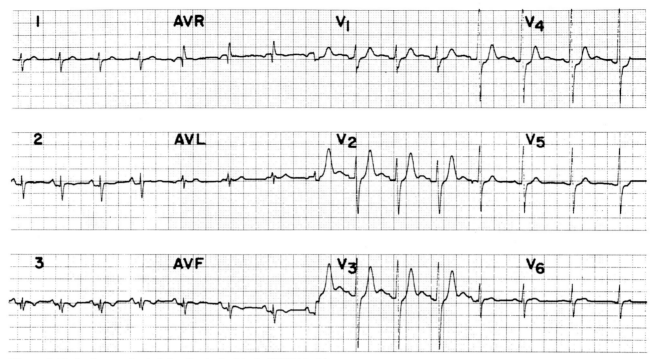

Figure 8-33. Left posterior inferior fascicular block (LPIF block).

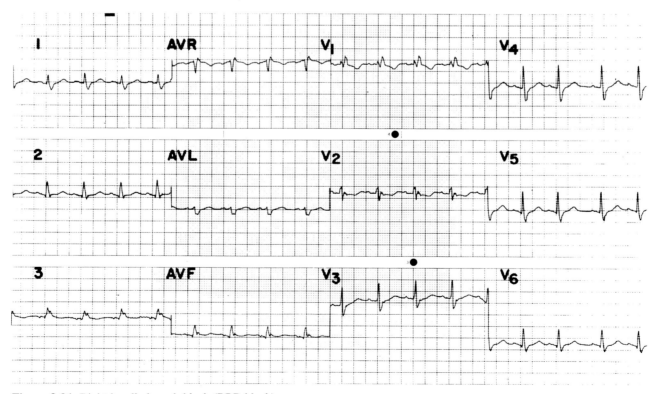

Figure 8-34. Right bundle branch block (RBB block).

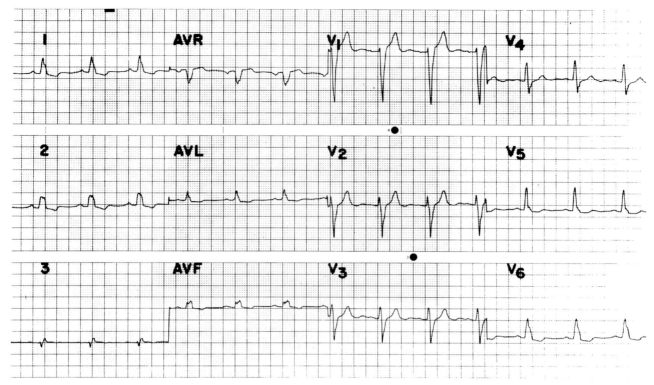

Figure 8-35. Left bundle branch block (LBB block).

Electromechanical Dissociation (EMD)

Electromechanical dissociation is the presence of electrical complexes without accompanying mechanical contraction of the heart (Fig. 8-36). In the setting of a cardiac arrest, EMD is due to a profound metabolic abnormality of the myocardium, rendering it noncontractile. At this time, there is no proven therapy. Although calcium has been the traditional agent, recent studies question its efficacy in EMD. Electrical pacing is, of course, not effective.

Other conditions which may mimic EMD are (1) severe hypovolemia, (2) cardiac tamponade, (3) tension pneumothorax, (4) massive pulmonary embolus, and (5) rupture of the ventricular wall. The first three conditions are potentially treatable if recognized early.

Idioventricular Rhythm (IVR)

An IVR is an escape rhythm of ventricular origin with very wide QRS complexes (more than 0.16 s) and a rate less than 40 (Fig. 8-37). Effective cardiac contractions and pulses may or may not be present. Idioventricular rhythm may occur as the result of complete infranodal AV block, acute myocardial infarction, cardiac tamponade, or exsanguinating hemorrhage. Treatment consists of attempting to accelerate the heart rate with atropine or isoproterenol. Large doses of corticosteroids have had anecdotal success.

Agonal Ventricular Rhythm

Agonal rhythm is the occurrence of very broad and irregular ventricular complexes at a slow rate, usually without associated ventricular contractions (Fig. 8-38).

Cardiac Asystole (Cardiac Standstill)

Asystole is complete absence of any cardiac electrical activity. Treatment consists of attempting to stimulate electrical activity with intravenous drugs such as atropine, epinephrine, or isoproterenol. Transthoracic or transvenous ventricular pacing may occasionally produce electrical capture but rarely yields effective pumping action if prior agents were unsuccessful.

TACHYCARDIA-BRADYCARDIA SYNDROME (SICK SINUS SYNDROME)

Sick sinus syndrome (SSS) is a heterogeneous disorder consisting of abnormalities of supraventricular impulse generation and conduction which produce a wide variety of intermittent supraventricular tachy- and bradyarrhythmias. The tachyarrhythmias are usually atrial fibrillation, junctional tachycardia, reentrant SVT, and atrial flutter. The bradyarrhythmias are marked sinus bradycardia, prolonged sinus arrest, and sinoatrial block usually associated with AV nodal conduction abnormalities and inadequate AV junctional escape rhythms.

Clinical Significance

Symptoms of SSS are due to the effects of either fast or slow heart rate. Common symptoms include syncope or near-syncope, palpitations, dyspnea, chest pain, and cerebrovascular accidents.

A wide variety of cardiac disease can affect the sinus and AV node, producing the arrhythmias of SSS: ischemic, rheumatic, myocarditis and pericarditis, rheumatologic diseases, metastatic tumors, surgical damage, or cardiomyopathies.

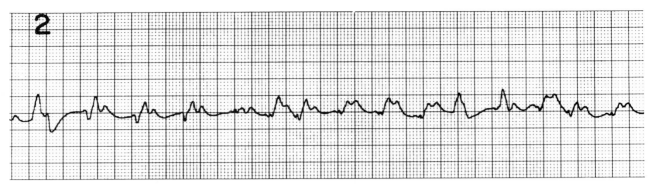

Figure 8-36. Electromechanical dissociation (EMD).

Conditions such as abdominal pain, increased intracranial pressure, thyrotoxicosis, and hyperkalemia which increase vagal tone may exacerbate the abnormalities of SSS and cause increased symptoms. Drugs such as digitalis, quinidine, procaminamide, disopyramide, nicotine, and β-adrenergic antagonists also cause increased symptoms.

Ambulatory ECG monitoring is usually necessary for the diagnosis of SSS since a routine ECG cannot be expected to show the intermittent arrhythmias common in this syndrome. The demonstration of increased sensitivity of the sinus node to carotid sinus massage, Valsalva's maneuver, or atropine suggests sinus node dysfunction but is not conclusive proof for the diagnosis of SSS.

Treatment

1. Symptomatic bradycardias require a permanent ventricular demand pacemaker. Because of the frequent association of AV conduction abnormalities, ventricular pacing is usually done, although atrial pacing is reasonable in selected patients.
2. Treatment of atrial tachyarrhythmias with digitalis, quinidine, disopyramide, procainamide, or propranolol carries the risk of aggravating preexisting AV block or sinus arrest. Therefore, most patients should have pacemaker implantation before drug therapy is begun.

PREEXCITATION SYNDROMES

Preexcitation occurs when some portion of the ventricles are activated by an impulse from the atria sooner than would be expected if the impulse were transmitted down the normal conducting pathway. Several different forms of preexcitation have been described, based on anatomic, clinical, electrocardiographic, and electrophysiologic abnormalities. All forms of preexcitation are felt to be due to accessory tracts that bypass all or part of the normal conducting system. These bypass tracts have specific names (Fig. 8-39).

James fibers are a continuation of the posterior internodal tract and connect the atrium and proximal His bundle. Atrial impulses can therefore completely bypass the AV node to activate the ventricles. On ECG, this appears as (1) a short PR interval because the usual delay in the AV node is bypassed, and (2) a normal QRS because James fibers insert directly into the infranodal conducting system and the ventricles are activated normally. When this is associated with reentrant SVT, the clinical condition is termed the Lown-Ganong-Levine (LGL) syndrome.

Mahaim bundles are composed of myogenic tissue, originate from either the AV node, His bundle, or bundle branches, and insert into the ventricles in the septal region. Atrial impulses pass through the AV node but then bypass all or part of the infranodal conducting system to activate the ventricles. Ventricular activation then occurs from two sources, the bypass tract and the normal conducting system, and the QRS complex represents a fusion of the two. The initial depolarization starts at the ventricular insertion of the bypass tract and is spread slowly by cell-to-cell transmission of the impulse. Subsequent depolarization by way of the faster normal conducting system then overtakes the initial depolarization and activates the bulk of ventricular myocardium. The QRS complex is basically normal with a slurred and distorted initial portion termed a delta wave. On ECG, this appears as a normal PR in-

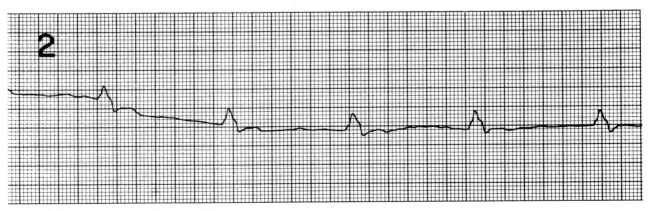

Figure 8-37. Idioventricular rhythm (IVR).

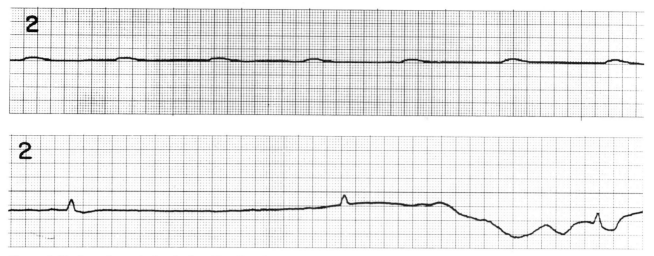

Figure 8-38. Agonal ventricular rhythm. Top: Regular. Bottom: Irregular.

terval, and an initial distortion of ventricular depolarization (delta wave).

Kent bundles are composed of myogenic tissue and directly link the atria to the ventricles, completely bypassing the AV node and infranodal system. This is the most common form of preexcitation and is the anatomic basis for the Wolff-Parkinson-White (WPW) syndrome. On ECG, this appears as a shortened PR interval and an initial distortion of ventricular activation (delta wave). Sometimes the bypass tract does not conduct an atrial impulse in the antegrade direction and the QRS complex is entirely normal. However, these concealed bypass tracts may conduct retrograde and be able to sustain reentrant SVT.

The WPW syndrome has been divided into types, depending on the direction of the initial delta wave on the surface ECG. This in turn is determined by where the bypass tract (bundle of Kent) inserts into the ventricles and which portion of the ventricles is activated first. In reality, accessory tracts can insert anywhere around the AV annulus; the three types are just the most common locations.

In type A WPW, ventricular activation first occurs in the inferior-posterior region of the left ventricle and the delta wave is directed anteriorly. A positive initial deflection with a dominant R wave is seen in lead V_1. Q waves in leads II, III, and AV_F are common (Fig. 8-40).

In type B WPW, ventricular activation first occurs in the inferior-posterior region of the right ventricle and the delta wave is directed posteriorly and to the left. A negative initial deflection and rS or QS pattern are seen in lead V_1 (Fig. 8-41).

In type C WPW, ventricular activation first occurs in the posterior-lateral region of the left ventricle and the delta wave is directed to the right, superiorly, and anteriorly. A positive delta wave is seen in lead V_1 with a negative or isoelectric delta wave in leads V_5 and V_6.

Because there is altered depolarization, repolarization is often

Figure 8-39. Anatomic sites of bypass tracts.

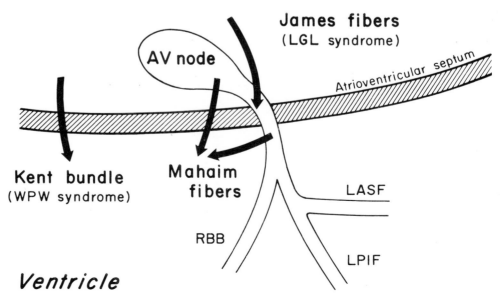

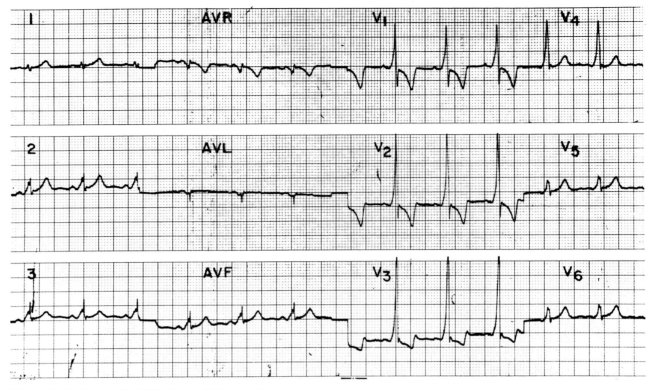

Figure 8-40. Type A Wolff-Parkinson-White syndrome.

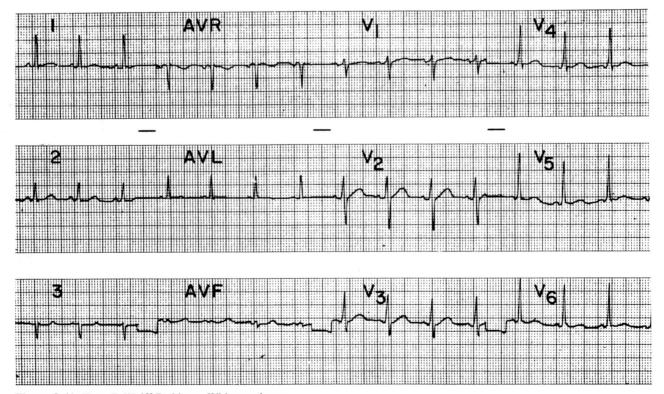

Figure 8-41. Type B Wolff-Parkinson-White syndrome.

abnormal with changes in the ST segments and T waves. The ECG changes of WPW may mimic changes seen with myocardial ischemia or infarction. Type A WPW may appear as an inferior-posterior myocardial infarction, and type B WPW may appear as an anterior myocardial infarction.

Clinical Significance

There is a high incidence of tachyarrhythmias in patients with WPW—atrial flutter (about 5 percent), atrial fibrillation (10 to 20 percent), and paroxysmal reentrant SVT (40 to 80 percent).

Reentrant SVT occurs when an impulse is sustained around a loop composed of the bypass tract and the AV conducting system, the impulse traveling down one and up the other. Whether the QRS complex is wide or narrow depends on which limb of the circuit is used as the downward pathway to activate the ventricles. In about 85 percent of the time, reentrant SVT occurs with the impulse being conducted down the normal AV conducting system and up the bypass tract. In this situation, ventricular activation occurs entirely over the normal system, the QRS complex is normal, and no delta wave is seen. Reentry is usually initiated by a premature atrial contraction which encounters a bypass tract which is still refractory from the previous sinus beat, but the AV node has partially recovered and conducts the impulse more slowly than normal (Fig. 8-42). In some patients the bypass tract does not conduct antegrade during sinus rhythm and so no delta wave is seen, but it does conduct retrograde so reentrant SVT occurs. Patients with concealed bypass tracts account for about 20 percent of all patients with reentrant SVT.

If patients with WPW develop atrial flutter or fibrillation, im-

pulses can reach the ventricles via the accessory tract, the normal conducting system, or both. Which pathway is used depends on the refractory periods of each. Most patients with WPW have longer refractory periods in their accessory tracts than in the AV node, but a minority have the opposite. In patients with short refractory periods in their accessory tracts, more atrial impulses can be conducted through the accessory tract than the AV node, so most of the QRS complexes will be wide. In atrial flutter, 1:1 AV conduction is possible with ventricular rates of 300 (Fig. 8-43). In atrial fibrillation, very rapid and irregular ventricular rates are possible. These rapid rhythms may resemble ventricular tachycardia, and excessive stimulation of the ventricles may precipitate ventricular fibrillation.

Treatment

1. Reentrant SVT in the WPW syndrome can be treated like other cases of reentrant SVT. Since the AV node is involved in the reentry circuit, any maneuver or drug (verapamil, propranolol, digitalis) that slows conduction through the AV node will be effective.
2. Atrial flutter or fibrillation with a rapid ventricular response is best treated with cardioversion. As an alternative, agents which prolong the refractory period of the accessory tract—such as lidocaine or procainamide—can be used. In general, phenytoin, propranolol, or verapamil have a variable effect on accessory conduction and should not be used. Digitalis is contraindicated as it may shorten the refractory period and enhance conduction over the bypass tract.

DEFIBRILLATION AND SYNCHRONIZED CARDIOVERSION

Defibrillation and cardioversion is the technique of passing a short burst (about 5 ms) of direct electric current across the thorax to terminate tachyarrhythmias. The electric current simultaneously depolarizes all excitable cardiac tissue and terminates any areas of reentry by halting further propagation of the impulse around the reentry loop. This places all cardiac cells in the same depolarized state, and following repolarization a dominant pacemaker (usually the sinus node) paces the heart in a regular manner.

Defibrillation or cardioversion uses the same type of equipment. A device stores a known quantity of electric energy in a storage capacitor and on command, discharges it through two paddles placed on the chest wall. Usually, a rhythm monitor and a synchronizer circuit are built into the device. Paddle placement can be either anterior-posterior or apex-right parasternal. While some authors have found a lower energy requirement for conversion using anterior-posterior paddles, others have not. For emergency situations, paddle placement probably doesn't matter.

To reduce transthorax electrical impedance and increase the amount of current passing through the heart, certain techniques are important at the paddle–chest wall interface. Electrode paste, gel, or saline pads are applied to the surface of the paddles. Firm pressure of 10 to 12.5 kg/cm² (20 to 25 lb/in²) is used to achieve good electrical contact. Larger paddles, within reason, have a reduced impedance, but this does not appear to significantly influence the energy required for conversion.

Older devices had significant internal energy losses and delivered as little as 40 percent of the stored energy to the patient. This

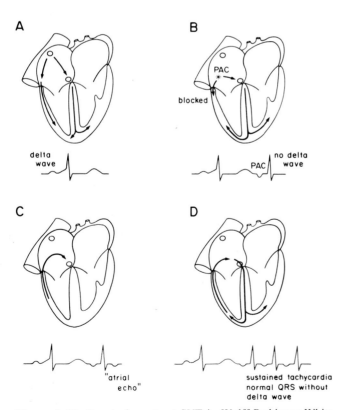

Figure 8-42. Onset of reentrant SVT in Wolff-Parkinson-White syndrome.

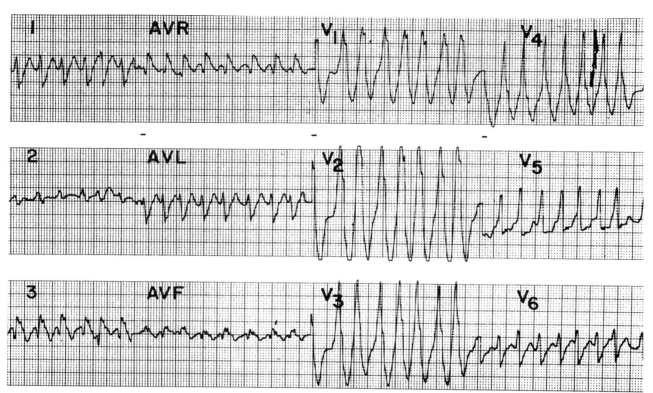

Figure 8-43. Atrial fibrillation in Wolff-Parkinson-White syndrome.

is not a problem with modern defibrillators as they deliver very close to the stored amount.

Defibrillation should be done as soon as ventricular fibrillation is diagnosed. The longer ventricular fibrillation persists, the less likely resuscitation will be successful. Current ACLS guidelines recommend 200 to 300 J for the initial two defibrillation attempts with a maximum of 360 J for later attempts. Several studies have found that most patients can be defibrillated with 160 to 200 J. Recommendations for children are for 2 J/kg (1 J/lb) in the initial attempt and 4 J/kg on subsequent attempts.

Synchronized cardioversion applies the electric current at a time during the cardiac cycle well away from the vulnerable period when there is little chance of inducing ventricular fibrillation—usually about 10 ms after the peak of the R wave. On most machines, the synchronizer circuit must be turned on each time an impulse is desired. Many devices also display by the monitor screen or a flashing light that the synchronizer circuit is properly detecting the QRS complex. Cable leads, rather than the paddles, should be used to monitor the cardiac rhythm to avoid any movement artifact that could be misinterpreted by the synchronizer circuit as the QRS complex.

Complications of defibrillation include:

1. Direct myocardial damage: unusual unless there are repeated shocks at high energy (more than 325 J).
2. Ventricular fibrillation: incidence is less than 5 percent with a synchronized discharge but probably greater in the presence of digitalis or quinidine toxicity, hypokalemia, or acute myocardial infarction. However, patients on maintenance digoxin therapy can be safely cardioverted using low energies (less than 50 J).

3. Systemic emboli: about 1.2 to 1.5 percent in patients with chronic atrial fibrillation.
4. Atrial, junctional, or ventricular ectopy: usually transient and benign.
5. Pulmonary edema: usually occurs in patients with mitral or aortic valvular disease or left ventricular failure.
6. Hypotension: rare, inexplicable, and may last for several hours before spontaneously resolving.
7. Muscle damage: elevated levels of creatine phosphokinase (CPK) and lactic dehydrogenase (LDH) are common but the myocardial fractions [CPK-MB, LDH1, LDH2, and α-hydroxybutyric dehydrogenase (HBD)] are rarely abnormal.

CARDIAC PACEMAKERS

Artificial cardiac pacemakers have two components: a power source (battery with pulse generator) and an electrode inserted into the heart (transvenous, transthoracic, or epicardial).

The pulse generator can be designated to operate in either a fixed rate mode (asynchronous or competitive) or a demand mode (synchronous or noncompetitive).

In the fixed rate mode, the pulse generator produces an electrical signal at the preset rate regardless of the patient's own intrinsic cardiac rhythm. Serious arrhythmias or ventricular fibrillation may occur if the pacemaker discharges during the vulnerable period (T wave) and for this reason, fixed rate pacing is rarely done.

In the demand mode, the pulse generator has a sensing circuit which detects spontaneous cardiac activity and will discharge only if no cardiac depolarization is detected for a preset interval. Demand pacemakers may have two response modes, either inhibited or triggered. In the inhibited response mode (most commonly used), the pulse generator is inhibited by the sensed cardiac activity and does not generate an impulse. In the triggered response mode, the pacemaker detects the patient's intrinsic cardiac activity and then discharges during the absolute refractory period. On ECG, this appears as pacing spikes following each intrinsic QRS complex.

A three-letter code system is beginning to be used for pacemaker designation (see Table 8-4). The most common type of pacemaker used—the ventricular demand inhibited response pacemaker—would be designated as VVI.

Permanent pacemakers are powered by mercury-zinc or lithium batteries which have approximate lifetimes of 5 to 6 and 8 to 12 years, respectively. Most units are preset for rates around 70 with a pacing interval of 0.84 s. The demand pacemaker has a built-in refractory period (0.2 to 0.4 s) during which it will not sense; this prevents it from being inhibited by its own stimulus. Most demand pacemakers have a magnetic switch which temporarily converts the pulse generator from the demand mode to the fixed rate mode when a magnet is held over the unit. In this way the pacing rate can be quickly determined, but the magnet should be applied for only short periods to avoid initiating tachyarrhythmias. There are new programmable pacemakers in which the rate and stimulus strength can be reset by noninvasive means. Since pacemaker complexity varies, the manufacturer supplies with each unit identification cards which patients should carry with them.

Temporary pacemakers are powered by 9-V radio-type batteries. On these pacemakers, there are settings for the mode (fixed or demand), rate (40 to 140), and stimulus strength (0.2 to 20 mA). During emergency pacing, initial settings should be in the demand mode with a rate around 70 and stimulus strength around 3.0 mA. The negative terminal should be connected to the distal electrode.

The electrode may be either unipolar or bipolar. The unipolar setup has the negative electrode within the heart and the positive electrode in the chest wall. Permanent pacemakers using the unipolar setup have the positive electrode on their surface covering while temporary pacemakers use a needle implanted in the skin of the anterior thorax. The bipolar setup has both electrodes within a few millimeters of each other and both lie within the heart.

The most frequent electrode placement is into the apex of the right ventricle using a transvenous approach. Different catheters used depend on the clinical situation. Rigid or semirigid catheters (6F or 7F) are inserted through a venous puncture or cutdown and usually require fluoroscopy for correct placement. Semifloating (3F or 4F) or flexible balloon-tipped catheters (3F or 5F) can be introduced and directed into the right ventricle without fluoroscopy using blood flow. Flexible catheters can become dislodged by the

Table 8-4. Coding System for Permanent Pacemakers

First Letter	Second Letter	Third Letter
Chamber Paced	**Chamber Sensed**	**Mode of Response**
A = Atrium		I = Inhibited
V = Ventricle		T = Triggered
D = Double (both)		O = Not applicable

patient or cardiac movement and are usually replaced with semi-rigid catheters within 24 h.

Transthoracic electrodes are inserted into the right ventricle through a left parasternal or subxiphoid intracardiac puncture. They are used in cardiac resuscitation when rapid placement is essential. The major disadvantage of transthoracic electrodes is that they can become dislodged with closed-chest compression. In addition, coronary artery laceration or pericardial tamponade is a hazard of percutaneous cardiac puncture. While electrical capture may be obtained in an occasional patient, it is rare to produce effective cardiac contractions with transthoracic pacing (Fig. 8-44).

Indications for Emergency Pacing

Emergency cardiac pacing is indicated either therapeutically (for symptomatic bradyarrhythmias) or prophylactically (for conduction defects which have a high risk of developing sudden complete heart block or asystole).

As noted before, symptomatic bradyarrhythmias should be treated with atropine and/or isoproterenol as a temporary measure to support cardiac rhythm prior to pacemaker placement. Some patients may respond adequately to atropine alone and do not require pacemaker insertion.

Most authors would recommend prophylactic placement of a pacemaker in any patient with acute myocardial infarction who has a new or age-indeterminant bi- or trifascicular block. In addition, second-degree Mobitz II and, of course, third-degree AV blocks are also indications for pacemaker insertion. Despite successful pacing, many patients with acute myocardial infarction and these serious conduction blocks have extensive left ventricular damage and a high mortality from pump failure.

Pacemaker Malfunction

Pacemaker malfunction can result from a failure to properly sense the intrinsic cardiac rhythm, a failure to effectively pace, or both. While the problem can be in the pulse generator, most acute pacemaker malfunctions are due to problems with the electrodes.

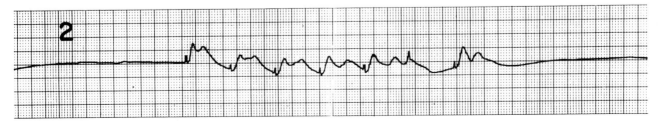

Figure 8-44. Ventricular capture with transthoracic pacing.

Failure to sense may occur when the voltage of the patient's own intrinsic QRS complex is too low to be detected by the sensing circuit of the pacemaker. Changing from a bipolar to unipolar setup (if possible) may help the pacemaker sense the intrinsic cardiac activity. Failure to sense may cause the pacemaker to discharge during the T wave and trigger serious arrhythmias.

Failure to pace may occur when tissue reaction around the electrode makes the myocardium insensitive to the electric discharge generated by the pacemaker. It is common for the pacing threshold to increase during the first few weeks after insertion, but further rises are infrequent.

Failure to both sense and pace may be due to battery exhaustion, fracture of the wires in the catheter, or displacement of the electrodes. Battery exhaustion is indicated when the pacing rate slowly decreases. Greater than a 10 percent change from the initial rate is an urgent indication for replacement. Catheter wire fracture may cause either sustained or intermittent interruption in electrical conductivity. Sudden onset of symptoms and/or bradyarrhythmias suggests catheter fracture. Catheter fractures are rarely seen on routine chest radiographs. The transvenous electrode is usually positioned in the right ventricular apex, with a characteristic appearance on chest radiograph and ECG. Displacement can be suggested when changes on radiographs or ECG occur.

Unipolar electrodes are more sensitive to electric interference from muscle activity or external electric equipment. Such interference will inhibit the pacemaker and suppress impulse formation.

BIBLIOGRAPHY

Ali N, Dais K, Banks T, et al: Titrated electrical cardioversion in patients on digoxin. *Clin Cardiol* 5:417, 1982.

Antman EM, Stone PH, Muller JE, et al: Calcium channel blocking agents in the treatment of cardiovascular disorders. Part I. Basic and clinical electrophysiologic effects. Part II. Hemodynamic effects and clinical applications. *Ann Intern Med* 93:886, 1980.

Barold SS, Coumel P: Mechanisms of atrioventricular junctional tachycardia. Role of reentry and concealed accessory bypass tracts. *Am J Cardiol* 39:97, 1977.

Bauernfeind RA, Amat-Y-Leon F, Dhingra RC, et al: Chronic nonparoxysmal sinus tachycardia in otherwise healthy persons. *Ann Intern Med* 91:702, 1979.

Bower PJ: Sick sinus syndrome. *Arch Intern Med* 138:133, 1978.

Brodsky M, Wu D, Denes P, et al: Arrhythmias documented by 24 hour continuous electrocardiographic monitoring in 50 male medical students without apparent heart disease. *Am J Cardiol* 39:390, 1977.

Cabeen WR, Roberts NK, Child JS: Recognition of the Wenckebach phenomenon. *West J Med* 129:521, 1978.

Calvert A, Lown B, Gorlin R: Ventricular premature beats and anatomically defined coronary heart disease. *Am J Cardiol* 39:627, 1977.

Chung EK: Wolff-Parkinson-White syndrome—current views. *Am J Med* 62:252, 1977.

Del Negro AA, Fletcher RD: Indications for and use of artificial cardiac pacemakers. Parts I and II. *Curr Probl Cardiol* Oct and Nov 1978.

Ditchey RV, Karliner JS: Safety of electrical cardioversion in patients without digitalis toxicity. *Ann Intern Med* 95:676, 1981.

Engel TR, Meister SG, Frankel WS: The "R-on-T" phenomenon. An update and critical review. *Ann Intern Med* 88:221, 1978.

Ewy GA: Cardiac arrest and resuscitation: Defibrillators and defibrillation. *Curr Probl Cardiol* Feb 1978.

Ferrer MI: Preexcitation. *Am J Med* 62:715, 1977.

Gallagher JJ, Pritchett ELC, Sealy WC, et al: The preexcitation syndromes. *Prog Cardiovasc Dis* 20:285, 1978.

Heissenbuttel RH, Bigger JT: Bretylium tosylate: A new available antiarrhythmic drug for ventricular arrhythmias. *Ann Intern Med* 91:229, 1979.

Hinton RC, Kistler JP, Fallon JT, et al: Influence of etiology of atrial fibrillation on incidence of systemic embolism. *Am J Cardiol* 40:509, 1977.

Horowitz LN, Josephson ME: Diagnosis and evaluation of concealed accessory atrioventricular pathways. *Pract Cardiol* 6:129, 1980.

Josephson ME, Kastor JA: Supraventricular tachycardia: Mechanisms and management. *Ann Intern Med* 87:346, 1977.

Josephson ME, Spielman SR, Greenspan AM, et al: Mechanisms of ventricular fibrillation in man. Observations based on electrode catheter recordings. *Am J Cardiol* 44:623, 1979.

Kastor JA: Atrioventricular block. *N Engl J Med* 292:462, 572, 1975.

Kastor JA, Horowitz LN, Harken AH, et al: Clinical electrophysiology of ventricular tachycardia. *N Engl J Med* 304:1004, 1981.

Kaul TK, Macfarlane PW, Thomson RM, et al: An analysis of electrocardiographic, radiographic, and vectorcardiographic findings in patients with implanted cardiac pacemakers. *Am Heart J* 99:686, 1980.

Kerber RE, Jensen SR, Grayzel J, et al: Elective cardioversion: Influence of paddle-electrode location and size on success rates and energy requirements. *N Engl J Med* 305:658, 1981.

Kuhn M: Verapamil in the treatment of PSVT. *Ann Emerg Med* 10:538, 1981.

Lange WR, Kennedy HL: The ECG recognition of atrioventricular junctional rhythm. *Pract Cardiol* 5:49, 1979.

Lichstein E, Ribas-Meneclier C, Gupta PK, et al: Incidence and description of accelerated ventricular rhythm complicating acute myocardial infarction. *Am J Med* 58:192, 1975.

Lima JJ, Goldfarb AL, Conti DR, et al: Safety and efficacy of procainamide infusions. *Am J Cardiol* 43:98, 1979.

McAnulty JH, Rahimtoola SH, Murphy E, et al: Natural history of "high risk" bundle branch-block. Final report of a prospective study. *N Engl J Med* 307:137, 1982.

Morris DC, Hurst JW: Atrial fibrillation. *Curr Probl Cardiol* Aug 1980.

Rosen KM: Junctional tachycardia. Mechanisms, diagnosis, differential diagnosis, and management. *Circulation* 47:654, 1973.

Schneider JF, Thomas HE, Kreger BE, et al: New acquired left bundle-branch block: The Framingham study. *Ann Intern Med* 90:303, 1979.

Schneider JF, Thomas HE, Kreger BE, et al: New acquired right bundle-branch block. The Framingham study. *Ann Intern Med* 92:37, 1980.

Sclarovksy S, Strasberg B, Lewin RF, et al: Polymorphous ventricular tachycardia: Clinical features and treatment. *Am J Cardiol* 44:339, 1979.

Shine KI, Kastor JA, Yurchak PM: Multifocal atrial tachycardia. Clinical and electrocardiographic features in 32 patients. *N Engl J Med* 279:344, 1968.

Smith WM, Gallagher JJ: "Les Torsades de Pointes": An unusual ventricular arrhythmia. *Ann Intern Med* 93:578, 1980.

Stargel WW, Shand DG, Routledge PA, et al: Clinical comparison of rapid infusion and multiple injection methods for lidocaine loading. *Am Heart J* 102:872, 1981.

Stemple DR, Fitzgerald JW, Winkle RA: Benign slow paroxysmal atrial tachycardia. *Ann Intern Med* 87:44, 1977.

Swerdlow CD, Winkle RA, Mason JW: Determinants of survival in patients with ventricular tachyarrhythmias. *N Engl J Med* 308:1436, 1983.

Talano JV, Euler D, Randall WC, et al: Sinus node dysfunction. An overview with emphasis on anatomic and pharmacologic considerations. *Am J Med* 64:773, 1978.

Tye KH, Samant A, Desser KB, et al: R on T or R on P phenomenon? Relation to the genesis of ventricular tachycardia. *Am J Cardiol* 44:632, 1979.

Vera Z, Klein RC, Mason DT: Recent advances in programmable pacemakers. Consideration of advantages, longevity and future expectations. *Am J Med* 66:473, 1979.

Vlay SC, Reid PR: Ventricular ectopy: Etiology, evaluation, and therapy. *Am J Med* 73:899, 1982.

Wang K, Goldfarb BL, Gobel FL, et al: Multifocal atrial tachycardia. A clinical analysis in 41 cases. *Arch Intern Med* 137:161, 1977.

Waxman HC, Myerburg RJ, Appel R, et al: Verapamil for control of ventricular rate in paroxysmal supraventricular tachycardia and atrial fibrillation or flutter. *Ann Intern Med* 94:1, 1981.

Weaver WD, Cobb LA, Copass MK, et al: Ventricular defibrillation—a comparative trial using 175–J and 320–J shocks. *N Engl J Med* 307:1101, 1982.

Wellens HJT, Frits WHMB, Lie KI: The value of the electrocardiogram in the differential diagnosis of a tachycardia with widened QRS complexes. *Am J Med* 64:27, 1978.

Wells JL, MacLean WAH, James TN, et al: Characterization of atrial flutter. Studies in man after open heart surgery using fixed atrial electrodes. *Circulation* 60:665, 1979.

Wu D, Denes P, Amat-Y-Leon F, et al: Clinical, electrocardiographic and electrophysiologic observations in patients with paroxysmal supraventricular tachycardia. *Am J Cardiol* 41:1045, 1978.

Zipes DA: Second-degree atrioventricular block. *Circulation* 60:465, 1979.

Zipes DA, Fisch C: Atrioventricular dissociation. *Arch Intern Med* 131:593, 1973.

CHAPTER 9
PHARMACOLOGY OF
CARDIOVASCULAR
DRUGS

Jerome R. Hoffman

ANTIARRHYTHMICS

Electrophysiology

To best understand the action of antiarrhythmic agents, it is worthwhile to review the basic electrophysiology of cardiac cells. All cardiac cells have the potential to act as spontaneous electrical pacemakers; this potential is present to a variable degree in different cardiac tissue, and greatest in the sinoatrial (SA) node. Normal cardiac rhythm is maintained by the dominance of this single pacemaker (which is capable of discharging at a greater frequency than any other cell), the presence of a conduction system which allows for fast and generally uniform conduction along predetermined pathways of impulse transmission, and the existence of long and uniform duration of action potentials, as well as refractory periods, in cardiac cells. The SA node is generally responsible for routine pacemaker activity in the heart, and conduction through the atrium to the atrioventricular (AV) node, with subsequent propagation of the impulse along the bundle of His and into the ventricular Purkinje fibers, allows for regular and orderly transmission of cardiac impulses. The prolonged duration of Purkinje fiber action potential, lasting even longer than that of ventricular muscle fibers, assures orderly conduction of impulses under normal circumstances.

Arrhythmias generally occur because of alterations in normal impulse formation or conduction. Abnormalities of impulse propagation in the face of enhanced automaticity can lead to reentry phenomena. Altered cardiac excitability may present a separate mechanism not entirely subsumed by the previous two categories.

Certain characteristics of the normal action potential in cardiac cells are important to understand. In the resting cell, the interior of the cell is negatively charged compared to the cell's exterior. This electrical difference, called the resting membrane potential, generally ranges from -60 to -90 mV, depending upon the specific cell involved. There is a high potassium concentration inside the cell, with the intracellular sodium concentration being low, while the reverse is true on the exterior of the cell membrane. This ionic gradient is maintained by an active sodium-potassium transmembrane pump which is ATP energy-dependent. Each cell has a threshold potential as well, which is that level of transmembrane electrical negativity at which the cell will be depolarized. When this happens, a series of regular transmembrane permeability changes takes place, and the action potential is initiated (Fig. 9-1). The cell reaches its threshold potential either spontaneously, because of a decrease in its negativity brought about by phase 4 (see below), or because of electrical conduction from neighboring depolarized cells.

Phase 4 is the normal change in resting membrane potential that allows pacemaker cells to reach their threshold for spontaneous depolarization. In the normal heart, phase 4 has a more rapid upslope in the sinus node than anywhere else in the heart, and thus the sinus node reaches its threshold more rapidly and regularly than any other cardiac tissue. An increase in the slope of phase 4 in other cardiac tissue, or a decrease in phase 4 slope in the sinus node, may account for the generation of some arrhythmias. When the threshold potential is reached, phase 0 begins. During phase 0, which lasts only a few milliseconds and whose upslope is dependent upon intrinsic properties of the particular cell membrane involved, there is rapid influx of sodium into those cells which contain the so-called "sodium-dependent fast channel." There is also slow calcium influx by way of the "calcium-dependent slow channel." All myocardial cells contain slow response channels, but fast response channels are absent in the AV node and SA node, accounting for the increased importance of calcium channel activity in these two regions. Sodium movement into the cell is fostered by the extreme concentration gradient of sodium extracellularly, and continues while the transmembrane electrical potential actually becomes positive intracellularly. The presence of this increasing intracellular positivity produces a resistance to further influx of sodium, despite the presence of a continued sodium concentration gradient.

In phase 1, which is generally thought to represent a rapid repolarization phase, there is inactivation of further sodium influx, and a current of chloride influx has also been described. In phase 2, which represents the plateau phase of the cardiac action potential, there is little current flow, other than that which is dependent upon the slow calcium channels. Repolarization occurs primarily during phase 3, during which time potassium outflow from the cell occurs to a limited extent. At this time, the baseline concentration gradients and transmembrane electrical gradients are re-

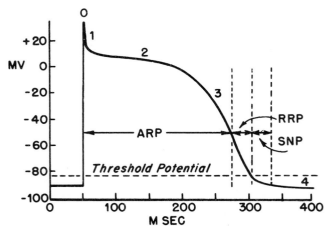

Figure 9-1. Action potential of a Purkinje fiber. Phase O represents depolarization; phases 1, 2, 3, repolarization; and phase 4, the resting potential.

established, via the energy-dependent ATP pump, and phase 4 begins again.

During repolarization normal cardiac cells are resistant to further depolarization, regardless of the excitatory stimulus applied, until they have reached a critical negative transmembrane electrical potential. In Purkinje fibers, for example, the membrane must be repolarized to at least -50 to -55 mV before depolarization can be restimulated. This level of repolarization defines the end of the absolute refractory period (ARP), which in turn is dependent on the length of the entire action potential duration (APD). Thus, underlying conditions which shorten the APD, such as anoxia or acetylcholine, may increase the risk of arrhythmias by shortening the ARP, thus facilitating reentry phenomena. Conversely, certain drugs (class III agents such as amiodarone) and electrolyte abnormalities (such as hypocalcemia) which lengthen the APD can decrease the incidence of arrhythmias by uniformly prolonging the ARP.

Once the absolute refractory period is over, the cell still is relatively less responsive to normal stimuli than it is at its resting membrane potential. This so-called effective refractory period (ERP) mandates that a supernormal stimulus must be applied before the cell can be depolarized again. The ERP also varies directly with the length of the entire action potential duration.

Changes in the refractory periods of specific cardiac tissue are very important in the generation of reentrant arrhythmias in particular. Reentry phenomena occur when two electrical pathways are joined both proximally and distally, and one is relatively more refractory than the other (Fig. 9-2). Therefore, when an impulse reaches both pathways simultaneously, at the point of their proximal meeting (point A), it may be conducted adequately down one of the pathways (1) while continued refractoriness in the other pathway (2) produces a block in antegrade conduction. When the conducted impulse reaches the point where the two pathways are jointed distally (point B), it may be conducted retrograde back up the second pathway (2), if this pathway is now no longer refractory, and may generate a cyclical flow of current as this retrograde conduction once again stimulates the point of proximal union.

In order for this circus current to be generated, therefore, there must be variable degrees of refractoriness in the two pathways. This so-called ''dispersion of refractoriness'' most commonly occurs at the interface of normal and ischemic tissue, because is-

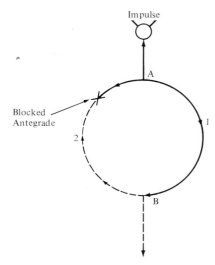

Figure 9-2. Mechanism of a reentrant arrhythmia. Point A is the point of proximal branching of two pathways (1 and 2). Point B is their distal meeting point.

chemia itself generally increases the length of both the absolute refractory period and the effective refractory period. Antiarrhythmic agents which either lengthen refractoriness in normal tissue, or shorten refractoriness in ischemic tissue, can therefore be effective in interrupting such reentry arrhythmias.

Most antiarrhythmic agents are now understood on the basis of their effect on the cardiac action potential. These agents are generally classified into four classes, with class I having two important subgroups, according to the electrophysiologic mechanism of their antiarrhythmic effects (Table 9-1). All class I agents are local anesthetics with depressant effects on myocardial cell membranes. Their major antiarrhythmic effect is based on their slowing of the rate of rise of the fast inward sodium current, which in turn lengthens the ERP and delays the return of excitability. These agents thus depress conduction velocity, prolong the ERP, and inhibit spontaneous diastolic depolarization. Their effect on the total APD, however, is variable. Class Ia agents depress phase 0 and prolong the APD; class 1b drugs depress phase 0 only slightly and are associated with shortening of the APD.

Alterations in the transmembrane potential will affect the

Table 9-1. Classification of Antiarrhythmic Drugs

Class	Standard Drugs	New and Investigational Agents
Ia	Quinidine Procainamide Diisopyramide	Tricyclic antidepressants Flecainide Ajmaline Ethmozin Encainide
Ib	Lidocaine Phenytoin	Mexiletine Tocainide
II	Propranolol	Metoprolol Pindolol Timolol Atenolol
III	Bretylium	Amiodarone
IV	Verapamil Nifedipine	Diltiazem

activity of class I agents. In the presence of increased negative transmembrane potential produced, for example, by hypokalemia, these agents would be expected to have less efficacy, which has been corroborated clinically. Conversely, in the presence of myocardial ischemia, where transmembrane potential is less negative, their effects are, not surprisingly, increased.

Class II antiarrhythmics are defined by their antisympathetic activity. These agents, which consist currently of β-blockers, work by blocking phase 4 depolarization, which is normally augmented by catecholamines. The antiarrhythmic spectrum of these agents is relatively narrow.

Class III agents work by uniformly prolonging the action potential duration throughout myocardial tissue. This allows these drugs to have a wide spectrum of potential activity, and a significant effect on arrhythmias not only independent of their location of origin but independent of the pathophysiologic basis of their production (i.e., enhanced automaticity, reentry, or altered excitability) as well. By prolonging the APD, these agents also significantly prolong the ARP.

Class IV agents exert their effect on the slow response calcium channels, and are thus particularly effective in arrhythmias that either originate in or are transmitted through the SA node and (most particularly) the AV node. All myocardial cells contain these slow channels, which allow for transport of both calcium and sodium during phases 0, 1, and 2 of the action potential. At the same time, most myocardial cells also have sodium-dependent fast channels, which allow for rapid sodium influx during phase 0. Fast channel activity is predominantly responsible for the shape of the action potential in cells in which it is contained, while the configuration of the action potential is very different in those which only contain slow channels. For this reason, action potentials generated in the AV and SA nodes appear with a different configuration than those elsewhere in the heart, and not surprisingly calcium channel-blocking agents, which diminish calcium entry into myocardial cells through these slow channels, have by far their greatest effect on the slow channel-dependent SA and AV nodes.

As with other types of drugs, specific activity of the various members of this group vary significantly, and thus certain agents have much greater clinical antiarrhythmic activity than others, while separate effects of these drugs, on arterial muscle relaxation, for example, may be more pronounced in agents with little or no antiarrhythmic effect.

We will now discuss specific, commonly used agents from each of these groups. Experimental and new agents with significant promise are listed in Table 9-1. We will also discuss epinephrine, which, while not an antiarrhythmic per se, has received widespread attention and use in the arrhythmias associated with cardiac arrest; atropine, which is a first-line drug in the treatment of certain conduction disturbances; electrical cardioversion, which is the treatment of choice for most hemodynamically unstable tachyarrhythmias; and defibrillation.

Specific Agents

Lidocaine

Lidocaine is a class Ib antiarrhythmic. Its effect is based on its local anesthetic properties on cell membranes. Lidocaine is widely used in the treatment of ventricular arrhythmias associated with myocardial ischemia, and has received much attention in regard to its potential use as a prophylactic agent against tachyarrhythmias in the same setting.

Lidocaine increases the ventricular fibrillation threshold. It also may be useful in both preventing and treating reentrant arrhythmias by decreasing dispersion of refractoriness between normal and ischemic tissues. Lidocaine shortens action potential duration in ischemic tissue more than in normal tissue, thus tending to equalize conditions in both, which in turn favors the elimination of reentrant arrhythmias.

Indications. Lidocaine remains the drug of first choice in the treatment of ventricular arrhythmias in the setting of acute myocardial ischemia. It is also widely recommended in the management of ventricular tachycardia, as well as ventricular fibrillation unresponsive to early defibrillation. Lidocaine should always be given following successful conversion of ventricular tachyarrhythmias as well. In addition, lidocaine, along with procainamide, is one of the most reasonable currently available drugs for the treatment of atrial flutter and fibrillation and/or wide, complex supraventricular tachycardias seen in the Wolff-Parkinson-White (WPW) syndrome. Finally, it has received much attention as a prophylactic agent in the presence of acute myocardial ischemia. While no studies have documented a clear-cut decrease in mortality from tachyarrhythmias with the use of prophylactic lidocaine, the absence of so-called "warning arrhythmias" prior to the development of potentially fatal tachyarrhythmias has led to widespread adoption of prophylactic lidocaine in this setting.

Dose. Therapeutic lidocaine levels can be achieved following the administration of 1.5 mg/kg intravenously, given slowly at a rate of no more than 50 mg/min. This should be followed by a continuous intravenous infusion at a rate of 2 to 4 mg/min, with serially decreasing infusion rates over the first 24 h as tissue compartments become saturated. A second bolus of approximately half the initial amount should be administered 5 to 10 min after the initial bolus, to avoid the development of a subtherapeutic trough. In prehospital settings, where no accurate infusion system may be available, repeat boluses of one-half the initial dose every 10 min may be given to a total dose of 225 mg. Infusion rates should be decreased in the presence of decreased lidocaine metabolism, as occurs with heart failure, hypotension, or severe liver disease. Continuous oscilloscope monitoring should be provided while the drug is being administered.

Adverse effects. Lidocaine is generally a very safe drug when given at appropriate rates in appropriate doses. Adverse effects of lidocaine are generally produced by either too rapid administration or an excessive total dose. These adverse effects primarily impact upon central nervous system function, producing lightheadedness, confusion, paresthesias, coma, and seizures. Such effects are generally responsive to withdrawal of further medication. Adverse cardiovascular effects are rare, and generally occur only in the presence of major overdose. Instances of high-degree SA or AV block, including complete heart block and asystole, have been described in such circumstances; negative inotropic effects have also been reported, but again seem to occur only in the setting of major overdose. Lidocaine should nevertheless be used with great caution in patients with significant underlying conduction system disease.

Methemoglobinemia has been reported in association with lidocaine use in a very small number of patients, and true allergic reactions to lidocaine and other amide-type local anesthetics are rare.

Procainamide (Pronestyl)

Action. Procainamide is a class Ia agent, which increases the duration of the action potential, elevates the threshold of ventricular muscle to electrical stimulation, and reduces automaticity by decreasing the slope of phase 4. It can directly depress normal myocardial conduction, as well as suppress an ectopic or reentrant focus.

Indications. Procainamide is generally used for ventricular arrhythmias resistant to lidocaine. It is effective in treating supraventricular arrhythmias, although it may not necessarily be the drug of choice. It is favored for the treatment of atrial flutter and fibrillation in the WPW syndrome. Procainamide is contraindicated in second- or third-degree AV conduction defects and should not be given to persons who are sensitive to amide (—CONH—) anesthetics.

Dose. The dose of procainamide is 100 mg in an intravenous bolus at 25 to 50 mg/min; repeated every 5 min until the arrhythmia is converted, QRS or QT prolongation develops, or a total dose of 1 g has been given.

Adverse effects. The most serious adverse effects of procainamide are its cardiovascular depressant effects, which are dose-related. Prolongation of the QRS and QT interval may occur, followed by progressive impairment of AV conduction, and finally by ventricular fibrillation. Hypotension can occur if the dose is excessive or if the drug is given too rapidly. Patients receiving intravenous bolus procainamide should be placed on continuous cardiac monitoring to facilitate recognition of early QRS-QT changes, and have their blood pressure checked while the infusion is being given.

Quinidine (Gluconate or Sulfate)

Action. Quinidine, like procainamide, is a class Ia agent with essentially the same mechanism of action. Large doses of quinidine produce peripheral vasodilation so that hypotension and cardiovascular collapse can occur if it is administered parenterally. Quinidine depresses SA and ectopic pacemakers. If AV conduction is normal, the vagolytic action of quinidine causes a reduction in the refractory period of the AV junction and may facilitate AV conduction. If AV conduction is depressed, quinidine may depress it further.

Indications. Quinidine is useful for the management of supraventricular and ventricular arrhythmias. It is used for the treatment of premature atrial contractions (PACs), for the conversion of atrial flutter or fibrillation, and for the maintenance of normal sinus rhythm. If used to treat atrial flutter or fibrillation without digitalis, quinidine may decrease the degree of AV block and thus facilitate the development of a dangerous, rapid ventricular response.

Quinidine is also occasionally used for the chronic treatment of premature ventricular contractions (PVCs) or recurrent ventricular tachycardia. It should not be given in the presence of second- or third-degree AV conduction disturbances.

Dose. For oral administration, a test dose of 200 mg of quinidine sulfate should be administered to ascertain the presence of hypersensitivity or idiosyncracy.

A number of methods have been described for quinidization. One currently recommended method is the administration of quinidine sulfate, 300 to 400 mg orally, every 6 h. Careful ECG monitoring is necessary and quinidine blood levels should be obtained to guide efficacy of treatment.

Intravenous administration of quinidine is extremely dangerous. Intravenous quinidine gluconate can produce severe hypotension or cardiac standstill. Peak action with the intravenous route occurs in about 1 h. We repeat, the intravenous administration of quinidine is extremely dangerous.

Adverse effects. The most common adverse effects of quinidine are headache, nausea, vomiting, tinnitus, vertigo, and visual disturbances. Mild prolongation of the QT interval and ST-T wave depression are usually therapeutic effects, but excessive QT changes may initiate ventricular tachycardia of the torsades de pointes variety and has been associated with sudden death.

Widening of the QRS complex (50 percent) is an early sign of toxicity. Other toxic effects include SA and AV block, PVCs, ventricular tachycardia, and ventricular fibrillation.

Idiosyncratic reactions to quinidine include urticaria, fever, maculopapular eruptions, and thrombocytopenia.

Phenytoin (Dilantin)

Action. Phenytoin is similar to lidocaine (class Ib) in that it enhances conduction at the Purkinje–myocardial junction and shortens the duration of the action potential in injured tissues. It raises the threshold for ventricular fibrillation.

Indications. Phenytoin is theoretically effective in the management of digitalis toxicity, but is not uniformly effective in abolishing ventricular arrhythmias due to ischemic heart disease.

Dose. Phenytoin is given intravenously at a dose of 18 mg/kg, with onset of clinical action occurring at blood levels produced by one-third to one-half of the total dose. Intravenous phenytoin should only be given in the presence of continuous ECG monitoring, and at a maximal rate of 50 mg/min, to avoid hypotension or major conduction abnormalities. Infusion should be discontinued if hypotension or QRS widening occur.

Adverse effects. Hypotension can occur when the diluent for phenytoin, propylene glycol, is given as a bolus infusion. Hypotension, asystole, or ventricular fibrillation also can be produced by the administration of large, rapid bolus doses of phenytoin. Other adverse effects include urticaria, purpura, maculopapular eruptions, and bradycardia. Sinoatrial or AV conduction disturbances may occur but are unusual if phenytoin is administered slowly. Phenytoin should be given with caution in the presence of nodal or infranodal conduction defects.

Propranolol (Inderal)

Action. Propranolol has a quinidine-like effect on the action potential. In therapeutic doses, its major effect is its β-adrenergic blocking activity (i.e., class II agent). It blocks the effects of catecholamines on β receptors, thus decreasing heart rate and depressing myocardial contractility.

Indications. Propranolol is potentially effective for supraventricular and ventricular arrhythmias, although it is most often used when other drugs have failed. It can convert paroxysmal supraventricular tachycardia (PSVT) to normal sinus rhythm and can decrease the ventricular response in atrial fibrillation. It is useful in the management of PSVT in the WPW syndrome, when QRS complexes are narrow. It may be effective in the conversion of ventricular tachycardia and ventricular fibrillation when lidocaine and procainamide are ineffective.

Other common uses of propranolol include the management of myocardial ischemia or infarction because it decreases myocardial oxygen demands; management of all chronic types of hypertension, and especially high renin hypertension; and for the treatment of idiopathic hypertrophic subaortic stenosis (IHSS). Intravenous propranolol can be lifesaving in thyroid storm and (in conjunction with an arteriodilator) in acute aortic dissection.

Dose. For urgent situations, the dose is 0.5 to 1.0 mg given as an intravenous bolus at a rate not to exceed 1 mg/min. The dose may be repeated in 2 to 5 min. Significant myocardial depression can occur once a total dosage of 2 to 5 mg is exceeded; therefore, doses in excess of this should be given with caution and should never exceed 10 mg intravenously.

Adverse effects. Adverse effects include nausea, vomiting, lightheadedness, mental depression, bradycardia, hypotension, bronchospasm, hyperglycemia, and pulmonary edema. Propranolol is generally not administered to patients with asthma or allergic rhinitis. It is contraindicated in serious sinus bradycardia, advanced SA and AV conduction abnormalities, and in congestive heart failure and cardiogenic shock, unless the latter are the result of tachyarrhythmias.

Bretylium Tosylate

Action. Bretylium is a class III antiarrhythmic which prolongs action potential duration throughout myocardial tissue but more so in normal than ischemic tissue. Bretylium also raises the ventricular fibrillation threshold, and has been reported to facilitate defibrillation by decreasing the so-called defibrillation threshold.

Indications. Bretylium has been reported to be effective in facilitating conversion of ventricular tachycardia and ventricular fibrillation refractory to other agents, as well as in stabilizing recurrent ventricular tachyarrhythmias. It recently has been elevated to the level of a first-line agent in the treatment of ventricular fibrillation by the American Heart Association, although many authorities continue to use lidocaine as the first-line agent in this situation, and reserve bretylium for patients in whom lidocaine, and perhaps procainamide, have failed. The ultimate role of bretylium in the treatment of cardiac arrest secondary to ventricular tachyarrhythmias remains to be determined. Bretylium does not appear to have any use in the treatment of premature ventricular contractions, and any potential role in the prophylaxis of ventricular tachyarrhythmias during ischemic episodes must be moderated by concern about its potential for adverse effects.

Dose. Bretylium is currently given as an intravenous bolus of 5 to 10 mg/kg, which can be repeated every 6 to 8 h. Bretylium's onset of action may be delayed, so evaluation of its efficacy should not be made until at least 15 min after it has been given.

Adverse effects. Significant hypotension, which is predominantly orthostatic but may have a nonorthostatic component, is not uncommon following the administration of bretylium. Bretylium may cause an initial increase in premature ventricular complexes, because of its effect on norepinephrine release and uptake, and isolated case reports of development of ventricular tachyarrhythmias following its use have been published. Nausea and vomiting may also be produced in conscious patients being treated for ventricular tachycardia.

Verapamil

Verapamil (class III) is one of three calcium channel-blocking agents currently available in the United States, and has received the greatest attention of any of these agents regarding antiarrhythmic activity. Like the other calcium channel blockers, verapamil's greatest antiarrhythmic potential relates to arrhythmias which involve the AV node. Suppression of sinus node activity is not clinically useful (and in certain instances it is clinically dangerous), and calcium channel blockers have little or no direct electrophysiologic effect on the ventricles. The calcium channel blockers may affect ventricular arrhythmias indirectly when their hemodynamic effects improve underlying metabolic conditions responsible for specific ventricular arrhythmias, such as can be seen in the presence of coronary artery spasm.

Verapamil is the drug of choice in the treatment of PSVT in almost all instances. Most PSVT involves a reentrant circuit in the AV node, and verapamil's profound effect in delaying antegrade conduction through the AV node has made it extremely effective in terminating such reentrant arrhythmias. Verapamil successfully converts upward of 90 percent of PSVT, and successfully slows the ventricular response in most other instances. Its onset of action is rapid and is, in fact, immediate in a large percentage of cases. Rate-related hemodynamic instability is routinely reversed in such circumstances, and thus verapamil generally is safe and effective in PSVT, even in the presence of mild congestive heart failure or slight degrees of hypotension (systolic blood pressure between 90 and 100 mmHg).

Verapamil also is effective in slowing ventricular response in atrial fibrillation and atrial flutter in most cases. Because of its very rapid onset of action, it can be used to quickly ameliorate the hemodynamic consequences of an excessively fast ventricular response in these conditions when cardioversion is contraindicated. This can be extremely important, since the onset of action of intravenous digoxin, the other standard alternative, may be delayed as long as 30 min.

Most patients with WPW and PSVT demonstrate narrow QRS complexes during their episodes of tachycardia. This indicates antegrade conduction through the AV node, with retrograde conduction over the bypass tract completing the circuit. Occasionally, antegrade conduction occurs over the accessory pathway, which results in widened QRS complexes. Verapamil is safe and effective in patients with narrow-complex tachycardia, even in the presence of WPW, because of its pronounced negative dromotropic effect on the AV node. On the other hand, patients with wide-complex tachycardia should not receive verapamil. This is true when the wide-complex tachycardia represents antegrade conduction through the accessory pathway in WPW because of the potential for increased ventricular rate secondary to possible diminution of conduction time over the accessory pathway. Wide-complex tachycardia may of course also represent true ventricular tachycardia, in which case verapamil is also relatively contraindicated, as it can be expected to have no general positive effect in such circumstances, and its vasodilatory and negative inotropic effects could significantly exacerbate hemodynamic consequences in this situation.

Verapamil is also contraindicated in atrial fibrillation or atrial flutter associated with WPW. In these circumstances, antegrade conduction to the ventricles can proceed either over the accessory pathway or through the AV node. By decreasing conduction through the AV node, verapamil would favor conduction through the accessory pathway, thus potentially increasing ventricular response even if conduction time through the accessory pathway is not independently changed. In those patients in whom conduction is facilitated through the accessory pathway, ventricular response rate will be even further increased, and thus the number of cases reported in which WPW patients deteriorated into ventricular fibrillation following the administration of verapamil for atrial fibrillation or atrial flutter is not particularly surprising.

It is reasonable and proper to use verapamil in PSVT where the QRS complexes are narrow, as it is both safe and extremely effective. This efficacy holds for infants and children as well as for adults, and applies to patients with WPW as well as those with purely AV nodal reentry mechanisms, as long as there is antegrade conduction through the AV node. Electrical cardioversion is indicated in these patients when there is gross hemodynamic instability, but verapamil should be used in the absence of such decompensation. In atrial fibrillation or atrial flutter, verapamil may be helpful because of its capacity to rapidly slow ventricular response, but should be avoided when wide and bizarre QRS complexes suggest the possibility of antegrade conduction over an accessory pathway. If all QRS complexes are narrow, suggesting antegrade conduction through the AV node, verapamil may be helpful.

Dose. Verapamil is generally given at a dose of 0.075 to 0.15 mg/kg intravenously. It can be delivered as a rapid bolus, and the initial dose may be repeated in approximately 10 min. Verapamil can be combined with normal doses of edrophonium in PSVT, which may be particularly useful if the initial dose of verapamil has been unsuccessful. It may likewise be combined with an α-adrenergic agonist, such as phenylephrine, when a patient presents with PSVT and relative hypotension. In this circumstance, it may be reasonable to elevate blood pressure with the α agent, and then use verapamil to help convert the arrhythmia back to normal sinus rhythm. (Patients with significant hypotension should be immediately cardioverted electrically.)

Verapamil may also be given as an intravenous infusion at a rate of 0.015 mg/(kg · h). In the case of atrial fibrillation or atrial flutter, once the ventricular response has been slowed, consideration should be given to digitalization of the patient as the effects of verapamil will dissipate over 1 to 6 h.

Adverse effects. Verapamil is a relatively safe drug when given to appropriate patients. Side effects, whether given intravenously or orally, are generally very limited, and include most predominantly constipation, and to a lesser extent nausea and vomiting. Cardiovascular side effects are related to the drug's intrinsic pharmacologic properties, and can generally be avoided if the drug is not given to patients in whom such predictable effects may be expected to exacerbate underlying problems. Thus, verapamil should not be given to patients with significant congestive heart failure or severe hypotension, as its negative inotropic effects can cause deterioration in these circumstances. Once again, when these problems are secondary to excessive ventricular rate because of tachyarrhythmias which are responsive to verapamil, they may in fact be reversed by the administration of verapamil; in most such instances, however, verapamil should be avoided, unless there are no other therapeutic modalities available.

Verapamil should also be avoided in patients with high-degree AV nodal block, as it can produce complete heart block in such a circumstance. Patients with sinus node disease should likewise not receive verapamil or any other calcium channel-blocking agent, as complete sinus arrest can be produced in such a circumstance. Finally, verapamil should not be used in patients with WPW and PSVT or atrial fibrillation or atrial flutter, when antegrade conduction over the accessory pathway results in wide QRS complexes.

Oral verapamil, when given to patients on chronic, stable doses of digitalis, has been shown to decrease digitalis clearance by 50 percent in the first week. Thus, patients with such a history should be monitored for signs of digitalis toxicity, and may require a reduction in digitalis dose.

Epinephrine

Epinephrine exerts both α- and β-adrenergic agonist effects, in relatively equal degrees. Thus, epinephrine clinically increases heart rate, mildly increases cardiac inotropic tone, and increases peripheral vascular resistance. Since all these can contribute to an increase in blood pressure, epinephrine has in the past been used as a vasopressor. Currently, epinephrine is widely used as a cardiac stimulant in circumstances of cardiac arrest.

Indications. Epinephrine is considered a first-line agent in the treatment of cardiac arrest, and has been used as such in cases of ventricular fibrillation, asystole, and electromechanical dissociation (EMD). During cardiac arrest and artificial external cardiopulmonary resuscitation (CPR), epinephrine redistributes blood flow away from skin and mesentery, toward the heart and brain. This effect is related to α-adrenergic-mediated increases in systemic vascular resistance.

Epinephrine has been purported to "coarsen fine ventricular fibrillation"; there is, however, no clear experimental evidence that this is true, or that, if true, it would facilitate successful defibrillation. In fact, there is a significant amount of animal evidence suggesting that epinephrine does not clinically increase the likelihood of successful defibrillation. However, epinephrine does increase the likelihood of continued hemodynamic stability in animals which have been successfully defibrillated. This likewise has been shown to be due to epinephrine's effect on systemic vascular resistance, and can be duplicated by other α-adrenergic agents. It is not clear if this beneficial effect, seen in relatively healthy animals which have been subjected to ventricular fibrillation, would be equally beneficial in relatively unhealthy human hearts. Nevertheless, epinephrine remains a widely used and recommended agent following initially unsuccessful defibrillation attempts for ventricular fibrillation.

Epinephrine is also considered a first-line agent in the treatment of asystole and EMD, although outcome in both these conditions is uniformly poor despite use of the entire current pharmacopeia. Thus, it is not clear whether epinephrine, or any of the other drugs used in these circumstances, is truly beneficial for such patients.

Dose. Epinephrine is given in a dose of 0.5 to 1.0 mg, as 5 to 10 mL of a 1:10,000 solution. The drug should be given in a peripheral vein, and circulated with CPR for 90 s. Epinephrine conceivably may be given in a central vein or as an intracardiac injection, but there is significant concern regarding increased toxicity with either of these techniques.

Side effects. Side effects are, of course, of relatively minor consequence in the setting of cardiac arrest, which is the only "antiarrhythmic" indication for epinephrine. Epinephrine does increase myocardial oxygen consumption significantly, and thus can exacerbate ventricular irritability in the setting of myocardial ischemia. Epinephrine's α-adrenergic activity produces increases in systemic vascular resistance, which could conceivably be detrimental to a failing myocardium in that increased afterload might significantly decrease cardiac output.

Atropine

Action. Atropine is a vagolytic drug which has its greatest effects on the heart in those areas influenced by parasympathetic tone, most particularly the SA node and the AV node.

Indications. Atropine is extremely useful in situations of symptomatic bradycardia associated with hypotension, signs of decreased end-organ perfusion such as chest pain, pulmonary edema, altered mental status, or decreased urine output, and the presence of "escape" ventricular beats. In the presence of these signs and symptoms, atropine should be used if the underlying heart rate is suspected as the cause of the patient's hemodynamic instability. If heart rate is speeded to the range of 70 per minute or more, and symptoms do not regress, other causes should be sought.

Atropine also has been used, in higher than normal doses, in patients with bradyasystolic arrest. Despite initial enthusiasm regarding its use in this circumstance, subsequent experience has suggested that high-dose atropine does not significantly influence the dismal prognosis in such patients.

Dose. Atropine should be given in doses of 0.5 mg intravenously, repeated every 5 min, to a total dose of 2 to 3 mg. "High"-dose atropine, for asystole only, is given in doses of 1 mg, repeated every 5 min, to a total of 2 to 4 mg.

Adverse effects. Tachycardia produced by atropine can cause marked increases in myocardial oxygen demand, and thus produce ventricular tachyarrhythmias. This is particularly true when high doses of atropine are given, and thus any use of high-dose atropine should be restricted to patients with asystole. Patients with symptomatic bradycardia should be given appropriate normal doses of atropine.

Electrical Cardioversion and Defibrillation

Electrical cardioversion is the treatment of choice for patients with either supraventricular or ventricular tachyarrhythmias who are unable to sustain adequate end-organ perfusion because of increased ventricular rate. Such patients should not wait for the delay in onset of pharmacologic agents.

Unconscious patients can be cardioverted without any sedation. On the other hand, conscious patients should be premedicated prior to electrical cardioversion. Small doses of intravenous valium, possibly combined with small doses of an intravenous opiate, are highly useful premedication for cardioversion.

Patients with identifiable R waves, such as those with atrial fibrillation, atrial flutter, and PSVT should be electrically cardioverted with the machine in the synchronized mode, which allows the defibrillator to sense the onset of the patient's own QRS complex and deliver the electrical energy at a time in the cardiac cycle distant from the period of repolarization. This avoids triggering an R-on-T phenomenon, which can result in ventricular tachycardia (VT) or ventricular fibrillation (VF). VF should be defibrillated with the machine out of the synchronized mode, because the lack of an R wave will prevent the machine from ever sensing an appropriate time to deliver the stored energy. VT can be converted in either manner, as there are R waves present for sensing, while at the same time there is little likelihood of detrimental effect from unsynchronized cardioversions. Most author-

ities, however, recommend synchronized cardioversion in the presence of VT.

Atrial Fibrillation

Atrial fibrillation (AF) may be associated with a broad range of ventricular response rates. Therefore, there may be significant hemodynamic compromise in the face of extremely rapid ventricular rates, little hemodynamic instability with relatively controlled ventricular rates, and anything in between. There may, of course, be hemodynamic instability unrelated to the ventricular rate in such patients, not only because of other unassociated conditions but also because of the approximately 15 percent decrease in cardiac output brought about by the lack of atrial systole. Nevertheless, in many cases the rate of ventricular response will significantly determine the patient's ability to maintain a stable circulation during AF.

Patients with rapid AF who are hemodynamically unstable should be electrically cardioverted. Patients with acute AF, who generally do not have an extremely enlarged left atrium and who have not had a long history of previous episodes of AF, usually manifest fairly large, coarse *a* waves on their electrocardiogram. These patients are relatively easy to electrically convert into sinus rhythm, and tend to remain in sinus rhythm following such therapy. Most such patients will be successfully cardioverted with 100 J of stored energy. Patients who have been in chronic AF, for periods of time in excess of perhaps 3 years, usually have very large left atria, manifest small, fine *a* waves on electrocardiogram, and are notoriously difficult to convert to sinus rhythm or maintain in sinus rhythm following occasionally successful conversion. If such patients present with significant hemodynamic instability in the face of a very rapid heart rate, they may deserve attempted cardioversion, with the knowledge that these attempts are not likely to be particularly successful. There may possibly be an increased incidence of success with higher energies, in the range of 200 J, but this is not clear; neither is it clear that patients successfully converted with higher energies will be any more likely to continue in sinus rhythm. Therefore, these patients are more likely to benefit from pharmacologic therapy which produces some degree of AV nodal block and therefore decreases ventricular response. Such therapy is certainly the treatment of choice in the absence of acute hemodynamic decompensation, such that there is time to effect rate control with intravenous medications.

Atrial Flutter

Atrial flutter is a notoriously electrosensitive supraventricular rhythm, which can almost always be successfully cardioverted with small amounts of delivered energy. Probably more than 90 percent of patients with atrial flutter will be successfully cardioverted with as low as 10 to 20 J of stored energy, although some of these patients may convert into AF rather than sinus rhythm. There is little reason to believe that higher amounts of delivered energy are particularly necessary in most cases.

Paroxysmal Supraventricular Tachycardia

Paroxysmal supraventricular tachycardia (PSVT) is also fairly easy to convert with relatively small amounts of electrical energy. Most patients with PSVT who require emergent cardioversion, because of inability to maintain adequate perfusion in face of their tachycardia, will respond successfully to anywhere between 10 and 50 J of stored energy.

Ventricular Fibrillation and Ventricular Tachycardia

There has been a substantial amount of data generated in both animal and human studies to suggest that electrical defibrillation from ventricular fibrillation (VF) can be accomplished with far lower amounts of electrical energy than has been previously thought necessary. It has been well demonstrated that the critical element in successful defibrillation is rapid availability of defibrillation, rather than any particular amount of energy delivered to the myocardium. Furthermore, there is little reason to believe that high amounts of energy, in the range of 350 to 400 J, are any more likely to successfully defibrillate a patient than are lower amounts of energy (in the range of 150 to 200 J).

Although major morphologic cardiac damage is probably rare at any of the energies currently used in clinical practice, there is reason to believe that there is increased damage on a cellular level following delivery of higher amounts of energy. For this reason there has been an increasing trend toward the use of lower amounts of energy, approximating 200 J of stored energy, as the treatment of choice for VF. There is no evidence to suggest that increasing the amount of energy delivered following an initially unsuccessful defibrillation is likely to produce greater success, nor is there evidence that such techniques as "double defibrillation" have any particular clinical value. The subject remains somewhat controversial, in the absence of definitive data, but the best current evidence seems to suggest that there may be significant advantages in using smaller amounts of energy, while there do not seem to be any clear advantages to using larger amounts of energy.

Time to defibrillation is critically important, and early defibrillation is the single dominant element in generating survival following cardiac arrest (in adults). In fact, almost all successful resuscitations from VF occur in patients who respond to initial defibrillation attempts, regardless of other pharmacologic therapy.

Ventricular tachycardia (VT) is generally easier to convert electrically than is VF, and may well respond to as little stored energy as 10 to 20 J. Many authorities recommend beginning cardioversion attempts for VT at higher levels, in the range of 100 J, to avoid the necessity of repetitive cardioversions, but once again it is not clear that the use of such higher energies is particularly more likely to be successful.

VASOACTIVE AGENTS

Vasoactive agents exert their effect directly through their action on either the myocardium or on the vascular tree. We will discuss positive inotropic agents, which increase myocardial contractility; vasopressors, which increase systemic vascular resistance and thus blood pressure; and vasodilators, which have the potential to improve cardiac performance by decreasing the resistance against which the myocardium must pump.

Sympathomimetic Drugs—Pharmacology

Norepinephrine is stored in the sympathetic nerve. When sympathetic stimulation occurs, norepinephrine is released and diffuses to the sympathetic receptor site, where it activates the receptor cell. Once its function is completed, it returns to the cytoplasm of the nerve cell. The enzyme monamine oxidase destroys excess amounts of norepinephrine. Another enzyme, catechol-O-methyltransferase (COMT), inactivates excess norepinephrine.

Sympathomimetic drugs are pharmacologic agents which affect sympathetic activity by stimulating the receptors directly or by altering the synthesis, release, or uptake of norepinephrine. Levarterenol or L-norepinephrine, epinephrine, and isoproterenol affect sympathetic receptors directly. Amphetamine enters the nerve cell and causes the release of norepinephrine. Other agents, such as ephedrine, metaraminol bitartrate, and mephentermine act by both mechanisms. Cocaine, ephedrine, and the tricyclic antidepressants prevent the reuptake of norepinephrine into the cytoplasm and thus prolong its action. This is why a patient receiving a tricyclic antidepressant such as imipramine may develop a heightened response to exogenously administered catecholamines.

Drugs such as ephedrine and metaraminol are characterized by an initial strong vasopressor response, followed by a diminishing response. The initial pressor response is due to the fact that they prevent reuptake of norepinephrine. Once norepinephrine is degraded and depleted, the pressor response declines. However, a mild pressor response is maintained due to the direct yet weaker action of ephedrine or metaraminol on the sympathetic receptor.

Sympathetic receptors are of three types: α, β_1, and β_2. Stimulation of α receptors causes vasoconstriction, stimulation of β_1 receptors causes tachycardia and an increased force of myocardial contraction, and stimulation of β_2 receptors causes vasodilation and bronchodilation. Many β agents affect both β_1 and β_2 receptors. For the purposes of this discussion we have subdivided the sympathetic agents into vasopressors, which are primarily α agents, and inotropic agents, which are generally β agents.

Vasopressors

Vasopressors currently in use are α-adrenergic agonists, which exert their effect by raising systemic vascular resistance. This in turn generally tends to raise blood pressure (unless it causes a simultaneous significant decrease in cardiac output). Vasopressors, therefore, have been used extensively in the treatment of shock states, but concern regarding their effect on the pumping ability of the heart (and particularly of a sick heart) has limited their use in recent years.

Vasopressors clearly have a role in situations where hypotension is related to large decreases in systemic vascular resistance. Many vasodilatory shock states, such as sepsis or drug overdose, however, have a significant venous component that may not be reversed by the pressors. Vasopressors also increase myocardial oxygen consumption directly, which can decrease the efficiency of myocardial contractility, as can the increased resistance caused by the increase in afterload; these effects can also attenuate possible benefits of α agents.

Norepinephrine

Action. See previous discussion.

Indications. Norepinephrine has traditionally been used primarily for its effect on systemic vascular resistance. Norepinephrine increases arterial constriction and, therefore, can elevate blood pressure. It may be particularly useful in situations of hypotension secondary to α-adrenergic blockade, but the value of vasopressors in other forms of shock, and particularly cardiogenic shock, is highly uncertain. Like other α-adrenergic agents, norepinephrine could conceivably be useful in maintaining hemodynamic tone following defibrillation from VF, but this is unclear (see earlier discussion).

Dose. One ampoule (4 mL containing 4 mg of levarterenol base) is diluted in 500 mL of 5% dextrose in water (D_5W) and infused to maintain the systolic blood pressure at a desired level. If this is unsatisfactory, up to 16 mL in 500 mL of D_5W can be used. If such high doses are necessary, the blood pressure may rise but tissue perfusion may decrease because of intense vasoconstriction. One ampoule (5 mg) of phentolamine hydrochloride is generally added for every two ampoules of levarterenol to minimize local vasoconstriction.

Adverse effects. Cardiac arrhythmias can occur, especially if hypoxia is present. Blood pressure elevation is due to peripheral vasoconstriction and cardiac output generally remains unchanged.

Venoconstriction can cause an increase in venous return so that in the presence of heart failure, pulmonary edema can result. This occurs more often after prolonged administration of L-norepinephrine. The use of L-norepinephrine in hypovolemic or hemorrhagic shock, especially where fluid and blood are inadequately replaced, increases mortality and morbidity.

Epinephrine

Action. See section on antiarrhythmics.

Indications. Epinephrine is used in cardiac arrest (see section on antiarrhythmics). It is not commonly used as a vasopressor because it dramatically increases myocardial oxygen consumption, and thus has a marked potential to produce arrhythmias. (Epinephrine is used in other circumstances, including acute allergic reactions and anaphylaxis, and acute asthmatic exacerbations, as well as in combination with local anesthetics to prolong their actions. These indications for epinephrine are outside the scope of this discussion.)

Dose. See section on antiarrhythmics.

Adverse effects. Epinephrine can produce tachyarrhythmias, particularly in the setting of hypoxia or acidosis. Its activity is impaired by acidemia, and it is inactivated by a bicarbonate solution. Epinephrine can cause myocardial or vessel wall necrosis if injected directly intramyocardially or intraarterially.

Inotropic Agents

Most clinically useful inotropic agents work by stimulating β-adrenergic receptors, although some, such as digitalis, exert direct effects on the heart independently of sympathetic receptors. Clinically, inotropic agents are used in situations of depressed myocardial contractility, whether manifested as forward pump failure (shock) or backward failure (congestive heart failure).

Inotropic agents stimulate the heart to pump more effectively. For this reason they can directly increase cardiac output, blood pressure, and perfusion pressure. In the setting of congestive heart failure inotropic agents may secondarily decrease preload and pulmonary wedge pressure by the same mechanism. Inotropic agents are thus useful when intrinsic heart disease or extrinsic factors (drugs, toxins, etc.) result in decreased myocardial contractility.

Unfortunately, increased inotropy is associated with increases in myocardial oxygen demand, and this can limit the efficacy of these agents in many circumstances. For example, in patients with cardiogenic shock secondary to acute myocardial ischemia, inotropic agents may be beneficial if they increase coronary perfusion to a degree sufficient to offset increases in myocardial oxygen consumption. On the other hand, they may actually be detrimental if their effect on oxygen consumption outweighs their contribution to increased diastolic perfusion.

Dopamine

Action. Dopamine is an inotropic agent with special dopaminergic effects when given in low doses. It causes vasodilation of the renal and mesenteric arteries, as well as the coronary and cerebral arterial beds, in this "low"-dose range. Intermediate doses produce primarily β_1 stimulation, while high doses cause generalized vasoconstriction through α stimulation.

Dopamine can increase myocardial oxygen consumption, particularly when it produces significant increases in peripheral vascular resistance and heart rate as well as inotropy. Dopaminergic doses produce diuresis by significantly increasing renal blood flow.

Indications. Dopamine is indicated in the treatment of hypotension unrelated to hypovolemia. It may be particularly useful in cardiogenic or septic shock, especially where reasonably long periods of inotropic support are needed, and thus maintenance of adequate renal blood flow is mandatory. Dopamine can sometimes be given in conjunction with vasodilators such as nitroprusside in selected patients with cardiogenic shock, or it can be combined with vasodilators such as isoproterenol, or β-adrenergic blocking agents such as phentolamine, to prevent α receptor-induced vasoconstriction. In experimental animals, this combination can increase cardiac output and renal blood flow. In clinical situations, the major problem with such a combined regimen is severe hypotension.

Dose.

Low dose: 1 to 5 μg/(kg · min)
Intermediate dose: 5 to 15 μg/(kg · min)
High dose: 15 to 30 μg/(kg · min)

Adverse effects. Dopamine increases myocardial oxygen consumption, and thus can produce ventricular arrhythmias, particularly in patients with underlying tachycardia. When given in high doses, it increases the resistance against which the heart must pump, and this can be deleterious in some patients with myocardial failure. Diabetics are especially prone to early vasoconstriction, and gangrene has been reported in some patients in shock even with intermediate doses. The cardiovascular effects of dopamine are potentiated in patients receiving monoamine oxidase inhibitors.

Digitalis

Action. Digitalis has long been used for treatment of congestive heart failure, as well as to reduce ventricular response in certain supraventricular tachyarrhythmias by slowing AV nodal conduction. Digitalis inhibits the ATP-dependent sodium-potassium transmembrane pump, thus decreasing transport of sodium and potassium across myocardial cell membranes. It increases the refractory period and diminishes the conduction velocity of both SA and AV nodes, but shortens the refractory period of atrial muscle (including atrial bypass tracts found in WPW). In the setting of congestive heart failure, the inotropic effects of digitalis may significantly reduce ventricular chamber size by increasing stroke volume and thus reducing preload. This decreases myocardial oxygen consumption sufficiently to offset the increase in oxygen demand produced by the inotropy itself, resulting in a net favorable effect.

Indications. Digitalis is indicated in the treatment of congestive heart failure unresponsive to fluid restriction and appropriate diuretic therapy. Digitalis is not indicated in the treatment of acute pulmonary edema, and is also inappropriate in patients with subaortic stenosis. Recent interest in the use of vasodilators in similar patients has led some physicians to contend that digitalis is hardly ever a first-line agent, but most experts continue to feel it has a substantial role in many cases. Digitalis is also useful in atrial fibrillation, atrial flutter, or PSVT, when there is a rapid ventricular response. Digitalis slows ventricular response in these circumstances, and can also produce conversion to normal sinus rhythm.

Dose. Digitalis should be given intravenously for initial control of new-onset supraventricular tachyarrhythmias, with a first dose of 0.25 to 0.5 mg. Subsequent repeat doses of 0.25 mg can be given each hour until an appropriate response has been achieved. In general, total doses of greater than 1.0 mg should be given with great caution. Doses must be decreased in the presence of renal failure. Several other cardiac drugs, such as quinidine and calcium channel blockers, decrease digitalis clearance, and should thus effect chronic therapy accordingly.

Adverse effects. Digitalis toxicity can occur when the total dose of digitalis is inappropriately high for the patient in question. Decreased renal function, hypokalemia, hypercalcemia, and hypomagnesemia increase the risk of digitalis toxicity, as does dehydration, and the cardiac drugs mentioned above. Symptoms of digitalis toxicity include anorexia, nausea, vomiting, and changes in visual acuity and color perception. Digitalis toxicity can be manifested by almost any type of arrhythmia, with increased numbers of premature ventricular contractions, ventricular tachycardia, junctional tachycardia, high-degree AV block, PSVT with block, and sinus arrest being among the more common arrhythmias seen in this condition. While hypokalemia increases the risk of digitalis toxicity, significant toxicity itself may produce hyperkalemia, as a result of paralysis of the transmembrane sodium-potassium pump. Milder degrees of toxicity, in which levels of potassium in the serum tend to be low, can be treated with intravenous infusions of potassium if there is no evidence of high-degree AV conduction block. When digitalis toxicity is associated with frank hyperkalemia, there is nevertheless an intracellular deficiency of potassium, which may, in fact, be responsible for the subsequent arrhythmias. Treatment in this circumstance is somewhat controversial, as it is not clear whether methods should be taken to decrease the total body potassium, at the risk of increasing intracellular hypokalemia; to increase the total body potassium, in the face of extracellular hyperkalemia; or to use measures which would ordinarily encourage movement of potassium back into cells (such as bicarbonate, calcium, or glucose/insulin therapy), for these may be fruitless in the absence of a functioning transmembrane sodium-potassium pump.

Lidocaine and phenytoin are antiarrhythmics that have classically been used in digitalis toxicity, but their efficacy is not proven. Atropine and electrical pacing have been tried in cases of bradycardia, but these too have not met with a great deal of success. Hemodialysis and resin hemoperfusion have been attempted in some cases of severe digitalis poisoning, but have generally been unsuccessful in light of digitalis' very large volume of distribution. Evidence is currently available to show extraordinary efficacy of digitalis antibody fragments, in the setting of both routine digitalis intoxication and severe digitalis overdose. The value of this treatment is, however, limited by the relative unavailability of such antibodies at the present time.

Dobutamine

Action. Dobutamine is a synthetic β-adrenergic agonist whose primary effect is to increase myocardial contractility. It produces very little effect on systemic vascular resistance, and produces less tachycardia than dopamine or other β agents. It does not share dopamine's specific effect of increasing renal blood flow. It may be particularly useful in patients who require increased inotropic state but cannot tolerate large increases in heart rate, or the increases in systemic vascular resistance often produced by effective inotropic doses of dopamine.

Indications. Dobutamine is useful in selected instances of cardiogenic shock, particularly when depression of ventricular function is associated with increases in heart rate and/or systemic vascular resistance.

Dose. Dobutamine should be used at the lowest possible effective dose. Low doses of dobutamine begin at 0.5 μg/(kg · min), while the usual dose range is between 2.5 to 10 μg/(kg · min).

Adverse effects. As with other β agents, dobutamine may directly increase myocardial oxygen demand, and thus facilitate or exacerbate arrhythmias.

Isoproterenol

Action. Isoproterenol is a combined β_1 and β_2 stimulant. It increases the force and rate of myocardial contraction, while lowering peripheral vascular resistance and decreasing diastolic blood pressure. Isoproterenol dramatically increases myocardial oxygen demand.

Indications. Isoproterenol is indicated for the treatment of symptomatic bradycardia, when initial attempts to increase heart rate with atropine have been ineffective. Isoproterenol has also been used in cardiac asystole, but there is little evidence of clinical efficacy in this circumstance.

Dose. One to two mg of isoproterenol should be mixed in 500 mL D_5W, and infused at a rate titrated to produce the appropriate effect on heart rate. The drug should be given cautiously as tachyarrhythmias may supravene. Intravenous boluses of 0.2-mg isoproterenol have been tried in patients with asystole, but there is little evidence that this is clinically effective.

Adverse effects. Isoproterenol markedly increases myocardial oxygen demands, and may therefore produce or exacerbate angina and/or myocardial infarction in a previously ischemic patient. Tachyarrhythmias, as well as hypotension secondary to vasodilation, can also occur.

Calcium

Action. Calcium regulates cell permeability to sodium and potassium. An increase in calcium diminishes membrane permeability and a decrease increases permeability. The lower the calcium, the closer the cell resting potential approaches threshold.

During depolarization, calcium is displaced from the binding sites on the sarcoplasmic reticulum. It enters the muscle cytoplasm where it facilitates the development of cross-linkages between contractile proteins, thus facilitating muscle contraction. Calcium also affects cellular action potential in the SA and AV nodes (see previous discussion). Hydrogen ion appears to interfere with this function; this may be one reason acidosis causes a decrease in myocardial contractility.

Indications. Calcium is clearly indicated in situations of hypocalcemia and severe hyperkalemia, as well as in a variety of unusual situations including black widow spider bites with hypotension, fluoride poisoning, and overdose with calcium channel-blocking agents. It should be strongly considered in patients who suffer cardiac arrest while on renal dialysis, since these patients are prone to severe hyperkalemia. Calcium has also been used in other patients with cardiac arrest who present with asystole or electromechanical dissociation, but there is little reason to believe that it is actually helpful in these situations. Several recent reviews suggest that use of calcium may in fact be deleterious in such patients, although the consistently poor outcome with such rhythms makes such an analysis difficult.

Dose. 5 mL of calcium chloride or 10 mL of calcium gluconate is given intravenously at a rate of approximately 1 to 2 mL/min.

Adverse effects. Calcium is a tremendous myocardial irritant which produces significant increases in myocardial oxygen demand. For this reason, while it may transiently induce the heart to contract more forcefully, even in the presence of true electromechanical dissociation, it is often more toxic than helpful to a severely hypoxic and failing myocardium. Calcium is particularly contraindicated in patients with digitalis toxicity, and rapid bolus injection can cause cardiac standstill. Early studies suggesting that calcium channel-blocking agents may have significant protective value in the face of both myocardial and cerebral ischemia provide further reason for concern regarding regular use of calcium itself.

Vasodilators

Systemic vasodilators, or unloading agents, recently have received a great deal of attention in the treatment of a variety of cardiac conditions. These include, most importantly, acute congestive heart failure and pulmonary edema, and cardiogenic shock. These agents also have been used both acutely and chronically in patients with symptoms of myocardial ischemia. Vasodilators can exert their effects on either the arterial or venous system, or in some circumstances, on both circulations.

Venodilators such as nitroglycerin, morphine sulfate, and furosemide, have traditionally been used in the setting of pulmonary edema. These drugs effectively decrease circulating blood volume, thus decreasing preload delivered to the left ventricle, and decrease pulmonary capillary wedge pressure.

Arteriodilators such as hydralazine, trimethaphan, and α-adrenergic blocking agents, have traditionally been used in the treatment of hypertensive crisis or ongoing hypertensive disease. Nitroprusside exerts significant vasodilatory effects on both the arterial and venous circulation. By decreasing preload through its actions on the venous system and by decreasing afterload through its actions on the arterial circuit, thus allowing a failing myocardium to pump more effectively, it can be tremendously beneficial in patients with severe pulmonary edema, most of whom have increases in systemic vascular resistance as well as increased pulmonary capillary wedge pressure. Mixed vasodilators are also par-

ticularly valuable in patients with decreases in cardiac output and hypotension, in the face of elevated systemic vascular resistance.

While the rationale for the use of vasodilators in congestive heart failure is fairly clear, their place in the treatment of some hypotensive patients may seem somewhat paradoxical. Systemic vascular resistance is elevated in many patients with significantly decreased myocardial contractility, as a reflex effort to maintain adequate blood pressure. Nevertheless, this increase in afterload places a severe further burden on a failing myocardium, which may not be able to pump effectively against this increased resistance. Critical organ perfusion can be severely decreased. Afterload-reducing agents, such as nitroprusside or the arteriodilators, can be beneficial in this situation by altering the environment in which the failing myocardium has to work. If a decrease in afterload allows for improved performance, cardiac output will rise; if, on the other hand, the decrease in systemic vascular resistance brings about a further decrease in coronary perfusion pressure, results can be catastrophic. Such agents therefore must be used with great caution and intensive monitoring in hypotensive patients, but their efficacy can be dramatic. This is enhanced, in fact, by their ability to concomitantly reduce myocardial oxygen demand in this circumstance, and therefore perhaps provide another mechanism whereby the ischemic myocardium can begin to function more normally.

Vasodilators can be used in conjunction with other agents to increase their usefulness while decreasing their potential hazards. Concomitant use of inotropic agents allows some patients to maintain and improve blood pressure despite large decreases in systemic vascular resistance produced by unloading. Venodilators, which can effectively treat acute pulmonary edema, in which baseline pulmonary wedge pressure is markedly elevated, can nevertheless interfere with optimum cardiac pumping if preload is too vigorously diminished (by way of the Frank-Starling mechanism). In such circumstances, Swan-Ganz catheterization can allow rational titration of vasodilator therapy, which can sometimes be combined with judicious fluid infusion to maximize effective preload while at the same time decreasing outflow resistance and thus allowing for improved myocardial function.

Nitroprusside

Action. Nitroprusside is a systemic vasodilator with approximately equal effects on the venous and arterial circulations. It is extremely rapidly acting, very potent, and has a very short half-life when given intravenously, so that its effects are virtually immediately terminated when infusion of the drug is stopped.

Indications. Nitroprusside is the drug of choice in patients with hypertensive crisis. It has also received increasing attention and use in some patients with cardiogenic shock, in whom elevated systemic vascular resistance is contributing to pump failure. This is particularly true in patients with dilated hearts in the setting of congestive heart failure, where simultaneous decreases in both preload and afterload may enable the heart to function far more efficiently while consuming less oxygen. In this circumstance nitroprusside may be combined with either fluids, to maximize preload (and thus to allow for optimum pumping according to the Frank-Starling mechanism), or with inotropic agents such as dopamine. Nitroprusside has the added advantage in these circumstances of directly decreasing myocardial oxygen demands and, in fact, may prevent or ameliorate ongoing ischemia or infarction.

Dose. Nitroprusside should be given as an intravenous infusion; 100 mg of nitroprusside can be mixed in 1 L of D_5W, and titrated to effect. Average initial dosage ranges between 0.5 and 1.0 μg/(kg · min), with the dose increased if necessary. Much lower doses may be effective in long-term infusions for pump failure.

Adverse effects. While nitroprusside favorably alters the demand for oxygen consumption by the myocardium, it can unfavorably affect oxygen supply if the decrease in systemic vascular resistance is large enough to significantly lower diastolic filling of the coronary arteries. Therefore, it should be used with caution in patients with underlying hypotension, and in such circumstances should never be used without available hemodynamic monitoring. Overly rapid infusion of nitroprusside can produce dramatic falls in blood pressure, with severe consequences to sensitive organs (especially brain, heart, and kidneys).

Nitroprusside should generally not be used without hemodynamic monitoring, although initial infusion in the emergency department for hypertensive crisis can be accomplished for a short period of time with very careful blood pressure monitoring at the bedside. This requires constant titration according to ongoing blood pressure measurements taken every 15 s initially, until a stable blood pressure is reached. Long-term infusions, and initial infusions for pump failure, should always be accompanied by arterial pressure monitors and Swan-Ganz catheterization.

Nitroglycerin

Action. Nitroglycerin is a direct vasodilator which acts principally on the venous system, although it also produces direct coronary artery vasodilation. Nitroglycerin is used sublingually (and transcutaneously) in the treatment of acute myocardial ischemia, while intravenous nitroglycerin has received increasing attention in the treatment of congestive heart failure and pulmonary edema, especially in association with acute ischemic episodes. Both sublingual and intravenous nitroglycerin may decrease infarct size in many patients with acute myocardial infarction.

Doses. Sublingual nitroglycerin can be given as individual tablets titrated to effect, with total dose limited primarily by changes in blood pressure and symptomatic response. Nitroglycerin intravenous infusion should be started at 10 to 20 μg/min and increased by 5 to 10 μg/min every 5 to 10 min until there is a desired clinical response.

Adverse effects. Nitroglycerin can cause hypotension as a result of relative hypovolemia, brought about by venous dilatation. This is particularly likely to occur in patients with low underlying blood pressures, and in those patients who may be compensating for decreases in cardiac output by large increases in systemic vascular resistance. Occasionally nitroglycerin also can cause large increases in vagal tone, thus leading to hypotension on this basis. These two separate reactions can be distinguished because the latter is associated with bradycardia while the former is associated with tachycardia. Vagal responses are generally transient, but can be treated with small doses of atropine if necessary. Excessive venodilation should be treated by putting the patient in Trendelenburg's position or with small infusions of fluids as necessary. Nitroglycerin commonly produces symptoms of headache, particularly in patients who are not used to this drug.

BIBLIOGRAPHY

Braunwald E: Mechanism of action of calcium channel blocking agents. *N Engl JM* 307:1618–1627, 1982.

Coon GA, Clinton JE, Ruiz E: Use of atropine for bradyasystolic prehospital cardiac arrest. *Ann Emerg Med* 10:462–467, 1981.

Goldstein RA, Passamani ER, Roberts R: A comparison of digoxin and dobutamine in patients with acute infarction and cardiac failure. *N Engl JM* 303:846–850, 1980.

Haynes RE, Chinn TL, Copass MK, et al: Comparison of bretylium tosylate and lidocaine in management of out-of-hospital ventricular fibrillation: A randomized clinical trial. *Am J Cardiol* 48:353–356, 1981.

Holmes HR, Babbs CF, Voorhees WD, et al: Influence of adrenergic drugs upon vital organ perfusion during CPR. *Crit Care Med* 8:137–140, 1980.

Kuhn M: Verapamil in the treatment of PSVT. *Ann Emerg Med* 10:538–544, 1981.

Lie KI, Wellens HJ, VanCapelle FJ, et al: Lidocaine in the prevention of primary ventricular fibrillation—a double blind, randomized study of 212 consecutive patients. *N Engl JM* 291:1324–1326, 1974.

Nademanee K, Singh BN: Advances in antiarrhythmic therapy—the role of newer antiarrythmic drugs. *JAMA* 247:217–222, 1982.

Noneman JW, Rogers JF: Lidocaine prophylaxis in acute myocardial infarction. *Medicine* 57:501–515, 1978.

Opie LH. Vasodilating drugs. *Lancet* 1:966–972, 1980.

Otto CW, Yakaitis RW, Redding JS, et al: Comparison of dopamine, dobutamine, and epinephrine in CPR. *Crit Care Med* 9:366, 1981.

Singh BN, Collett JT, Chew CYC: New perspectives in the pharmacologic therapy of cardiac arrhythmias. *Prog Cardiovasc Dis* 22:243–301, 1980.

Standards and guidelines for cardiopulmonary resuscitation (CPR) and emergency cardiac care (ECC). *JAMA* 244:453–512, 1980.

Weaver WD, Cobb LA, Copass MK, et al: Ventricular defibrillation—a comparative trial using 175–J and 320–J shocks. *N Engl JM* 307:1101–1106, 1982.

CHAPTER 10
LIFE-THREATENING
SIGNS AND SYMPTOMS

A. Chest Pain

J. Stephan Stapczynski

Chest pain is a common presenting complaint in the emergency department and represents a diagnostic challenge for several reasons: (1) There is always the possibility of heart disease in every complaint of chest pain; (2) accurate diagnosis requires interpreting the patient's subjective perception of pain; (3) diagnosis is based primarily on history; physical findings and diagnostic tests are not specific or sensitive enough; and (4) pain from visceral organs can be referred to almost anywhere in the chest or abdomen. If serious or life-threatening causes of acute chest pain can be excluded in the emergency department, then the patient can be discharged for further outpatient evaluation. The examiner's immediate concerns are the potentially life-threatening causes of acute chest pain: unstable angina, acute myocardial infarction (AMI), aortic dissection, pulmonary embolus, spontaneous pneumothorax, and esophageal rupture (Boerhaave's syndrome).

When peripheral nerve endings are stimulated, pain is perceived by the brain and its location interpreted by the parietal cortex. There are two categories of pain sensation: somatic and visceral. Somatic sensation results from irritation of fine pain fibers in the dermis. These nerves enter the spinal cord at a single level. Because of the high concentration of these fibers in the skin and their exact mapping onto the parietal cortex, somatic pain is usually perceived as sharp, piercing, and precisely located. Visceral pain results from stimulation of pain fibers located in internal organs. These nerves enter the spinal cord at multiple adjacent cord levels along with somatic pain nerves. There are connections between visceral and somatic fibers, which is why visceral pain is felt on some part of the body surface. Visceral pain is perceived when impulses from the internal organs and the resting potential from the somatic nerves summate in the spinal cord to reach a pain perception threshold level. This threshold is not reached and pain is not felt if the impulses of the somatic resting potential are blocked by subcutaneous local anesthesia. Visceral pain is less distinct, usually dull or aching in quality, and less precisely located. Visceral pain nerves from the thorax and upper abdomen enter the spinal cord at the level of T1 to T6.

A useful classification of chest pain is based on this distinction between somatic and visceral pain. Superficial chest wall pain is a somatic type of pain. It is usually described as sharp or piercing, can be precisely localized, and is exacerbated by palpation. Respiratory (or pleuritic) pain is a somatic type of pain, but its main characteristic is a distinct accentuation by respiratory motion. It is important to remember that more than the pleura moves with respiration. Deep visceral pain is usually dull, aching, or pressure-like, but its distinguishing characteristic is its poor localization anywhere within the T1 to T6 dermatome range.

TREATMENT PRIORITY

Patients with acute chest pain should be given evaluation and treatment priority; certain steps should be done even before a complete history and physical examination. A principle used in the First Hour program of the American Heart Association is to approach every patient with acute chest pain as a possible AMI. Any patient in obvious distress and with abnormal vital signs or deep visceral pain should have oxygen administered, a cardiac monitor applied, and an intravenous line established as soon as possible. Obviously, such generalizations should be applied with common sense, but it is better to err on the side of caution.

INITIAL EVALUATION

History

A careful, accurate history is the most important tool in the diagnosis of chest pain. However, recent work has pointed out the many pitfalls involved in relying on isolated factors in the history. No one part of the history can stand by itself; accurate diagnosis requires a composite picture. It is important to remember that a patient may have more than one cause of pain—coronary artery disease and hiatal hernia with reflux are very common in the middle-aged population.

Onset and Duration

Typical angina pectoris is episodic, usually lasts between 5 and 15 min, is induced by exertion, and relieved within 3 to 5 min by rest or sublingual nitroglycerin. Unstable angina may occur at rest (angina decubitus), last longer, and not be relieved as readily. Variant (Prinzmetal's) angina occurs without provocation, often at rest or at night, but is usually relieved with nitroglycerin. Patients with variant angina can usually exercise to a moderate degree without difficulty. The pain of AMI generally lasts longer than 15 to 30 min. Pain from myocardial ischemia typically builds up to reach its maximum, whereas pain from aortic dissection or pulmonary embolus is usually severe at onset. Pain from the gastrointestinal tract or chest wall is more variable, lasting from seconds to hours to days, and may be associated with swallowing or body movement.

Quality

Sharp, piercing, stabbing pain is typical of musculoskeletal chest wall origin. One large study of patients with documented pulmonary emboli found that 74 percent had pleuritic chest pain and an additional 14 percent had nonpleuritic pain. In differentiating between the various etiologies of visceral chest pain, the quality of the pain is not helpful; patients with AMI can have a burning type of pain and patients with esophageal reflux can have a pressure type of pain.

Location and Radiation

The specific location of deep visceral pain within the T1 to T6 dermatome range cannot be relied upon as diagnostic, but certain locations are classic. Angina almost always has a retrosternal component, as do most other causes of deep visceral pain. Angina often radiates to the neck, shoulders, and down the inside of the left or both arms. Patients with aortic dissection typically have radiation of the pain to the back and upper abdomen as the dissection progresses over time. Patients with esophageal reflux almost always have both retrosternal and epigastric pain. Pain frequently radiates to the back and, with severe episodes, into the arms.

Relief of Symptoms

A clear history of relieving factors is helpful, but diagnostic tests in the emergency department are inaccurate, as pointed out in several articles from a recent symposium on the differential diagnostic aspects of chest pain. As with any cause of pain, a number of patients with chest pain will respond to the "placebo nature" of a therapeutic trial. Studies have found that about three-fourths of patients with coronary artery disease respond to sublingual nitroglycerin with complete relief within 3 min, although there is also a high false-positive rate. When a patient with prior stable angina presents to the emergency department with acute chest pain, less than half respond to nitroglycerin. Up to 90 percent of

patients with diffuse esophageal spasm report relief with nitroglycerin; almost half within 5 min. While 70 percent of patients with a prior history of esophageal reflux give a history of moderate to good relief with antacids, only 25 percent respond while in the emergency department with acute chest pain. Pain caused by acid infusion of the lower esophagus (Bernstein test) is not relieved by local anesthetics, suggesting that a positive response to oral viscous lidocaine should not be considered significant.

PHYSICAL EXAMINATION

Observation of the patient is important. General signs of tachypnea, diaphoresis, cyanosis, or pallor are significant. The vital signs should be obtained and recorded. Tachycardia is nonspecific but should never be disregarded entirely. Blood pressure should be checked in both arms, as a systolic pressure difference greater than 20 mmHg indicates arterial obstruction.

The chest wall should be palpated, and areas of point tenderness noted. The apical impulse is usually a small area (less than 2 cm or 2 fingerwidths) at or medial to the midclavicular line. Lateral displacement or enlargement of the apical impulse indicates cardiomegaly.

The heart should be auscultated carefully for heart sounds, murmurs, and rubs. The loudness of the first heart sound is due to the vigor of mitral valve closure and left ventricular contraction. A soft S_1 indicates preclosure of the mitral valve (severe aortic regurgitation) or weak left ventricular contraction. The second heart sound has two components, the first and second components due to aortic and pulmonary valve closure, respectively. Splitting normally increases during inspiration. With advancing age, splitting narrows and many patients over 50 have a single S_2. Wide splitting is most commonly caused by a right bundle branch block and occasionally heard when an inferior myocardial infarction affects the right ventricle. Fixed splitting is usually due to an atrial septal defect and, occasionally, severe heart failure. Paradoxical splitting is most commonly due to a left bundle branch block, and, rarely, aortic stenosis, aortic regurgitation, and AMI. The third heart sound is caused by the sudden deceleration of blood flow from the atria into the ventricle when the limits of ventricular distensibility are approached. The fourth heart sound is caused by atrial contractions strong enough to distend the left ventricle and produce vibrations. Physiologic S_3s or S_4s can be heard in normal or hyperactive hearts in patients under 40. Pathologic S_3s are accompanied by symptoms and signs of heart failure. Pathologic S_4s are seen when left ventricular compliance is reduced, as occurs with acute ischemia. The key to classifying murmurs is their timing: systolic ejection, holosystolic, late systolic, diastolic decrescendo, or diastolic rumble. Most elderly patients have systolic ejection murmurs due to degenerative changes in the aortic valve leaflets (aortic sclerosis).

ANCILLARY STUDIES

An ECG should be done on all patients with acute chest pain, except for those with trivial chest wall pain. An ECG characteristic of ischemic changes (new Q waves, ST segment elevation, ST segment depression, or symmetric T wave inversions) is helpful but a normal ECG does not exclude myocardial ischemia. Only about half of patients with spontaneous angina have ECG changes. A slightly higher percentage of patients with AMI will have changes on the initial ECG done in the emergency department. ECG changes of pericarditis or pulmonary embolism are relatively nonspecific and not pathognomonic. Acute pain from the upper gastrointestinal tract or hyperventilation may cause ECG changes, typically ST segment depressions and T wave inversions.

Measurement of total serum creatine kinase (CK) is not helpful in the emergency department. In patients with AMI, 4 to 8 h is required before total CK exceeds the upper limits of normal. One study concerning the use of total CK in the emergency department found that less than 25 percent of the patients with AMI had elevated levels in the emergency department. Another major problem with total CK is the incidence of false positives; many causes of skeletal damage elevate serum CK. The major helpfulness of serum enzyme measurement would be in the patient with an equivocal history and normal ECG. Unfortunately, the low sensitivity and specificity of total CK make the results of this test unreliable in the emergency department. The MB isoenzyme of CK (CK-MB) is highly specific for myocardium and elevated levels can be detected as little as 3 h after the onset of pain in AMI. Even then, the sensitivity of an elevated CK-MB for a patient with AMI while in the emergency department is only about 60 percent if obtained during the first 8 h after onset of pain. Further studies will be necessary to evaluate the usefulness of CK-MB measurement in the emergency department.

The chest x-ray rarely provides diagnostic information. With pulmonary emboli, various combinations of infiltrates, atelectasis, pleural effusions, focal oligemia, and/or lung volume loss is seen in most patients. In aortic dissection, a widened mediastinum is seen in about 40 to 50 percent of cases. A more specific sign is separation of greater than 4 to 5 mm between the intimal calcium and edge of the aortic silhouette in the region of the aortic knob but, unfortunately, this is found in less than 10 percent of cases. Most patients with acute chest pain have a normal chest x-ray or one with only incidental findings.

MAJOR CAUSES OF CHEST PAIN

Angina Pectoris

Typical angina is episodic, lasts 5 to 15 min, is provoked and reproducible by exertion, and relieved by rest or sublingual nitroglycerin. There is almost always some retrosternal component, and radiation to the neck, shoulders, or arms is common. In individual patients, the character of each attack varies little with recurrent episodes. With angina, it is very unusual for a patient to feel better when recumbent.

Variant (Prinzmetal's) Angina

This form of angina occurs without provocation, often while the patient is at rest or during a similar time each day. With acute attacks, there is ST segment elevation on the ECG representing transmural myocardial ischemia. Variant angina is thought to be caused by spasm of the epicardial coronary arteries, either in normal vessels (about one-third of these patients) or in vessels with atherosclerotic lesions (about two-thirds).

Unstable (Crescendo or Preinfarction) Angina

Unstable angina is the clinical syndrome between angina and AMI. The natural history of untreated unstable angina is a high early infarction and death rate. Modern medical therapy greatly reduces this risk so it is very important to recognize and hospitalize these patients. Three subgroups are recognized as unstable angina: (1) angina of recent onset—4 to 8 weeks; (2) angina of changing character—becoming more frequent, severe, or resistant to nitroglycerin; and (3) angina at rest—angina decubitus.

Acute Myocardial Infarction

Anginal pain that lasts longer than 15 min, is not relieved by nitroglycerin, or is accompanied by diaphoresis, dyspnea, nausea, or vomiting suggests an AMI. About 20 percent of acute infarctions are not accompanied by chest pain, especially in diabetic patients.

Aortic Dissection

Abrupt onset of tearing chest pain or interscapular back pain is the most common symptom of aortic dissection. The frequency of various signs and symptoms varies according to whether the ascending and/or descending aorta is affected (Table 10A-1). About 30 percent of these patients will have neurologic symptoms.

Pericarditis

The pain of pericarditis is often acute, steady, and severe with a retrosternal location and radiation to the back, neck, or jaw. Pain may be pronounced with each cardiac systole, chest motion, or respiration and is relieved by sitting up and leaning forward. If there is associated pleuritis (pleuropericarditis), pain may be predominantly pleuritic. The diagnosis of pericarditis is confirmed by the presence of a pericardial friction rub, which can have one to three components: presystolic, systolic, and early diastolic. However, rubs may be only intermittently detectable clinically. The ECG can show ST segment elevation or T-wave inversion depending upon the stage of the disease process; serial ECGs best illustrate these changes. A small pericardial effusion is often present but can only be detected by echocardiogram.

Other Cardiac Conditions

Hypertrophic cardiomyopathy (idiopathic hypertrophic subaortic stenosis) and valvular aortic stenosis may cause anginal pain, pre-

Table 10A-1. Signs and Symptoms of Aortic Dissection

	Aortic Involvement, %	
	Ascending	Descending
Location of pain:		
Anterior	45	17
Back	5	28
Both	38	45
None	12	10
Systolic BP >160 mmHg	30	55
History of hypertension	50	70
Aortic regurgitation	65	7
Heart failure	20	3
Alteration of peripheral pulses	65	10

Source: Prog Cardiovasc Dis 23:237, 1980.

sumably because of inadequate blood supply to the hypertrophied myocardium. Mitral valve prolapse and mitral stenosis also have occasional chest pain. Generally, these disorders are not responsive to nitroglycerin.

Pulmonary Embolism

Pleuritic chest pain, dyspnea, and tachypnea are the most common symptoms of pulmonary embolism. As mentioned before, some patients have nonpleuritic chest pain. Almost all patients with documented pulmonary emboli have known risk factors for thromboembolism.

Mediastinitis

Mediastinitis usually follows spontaneous or traumatic esophageal perforation and is characterized by retrosternal pain, fever, and luekocytosis. A chest x-ray may show widening of the mediastinum or mediastinal emphysema due to infection with gas-producing organisms. Mediastinal emphysema may also occur from rupture of alveoli or bronchioles and most commonly occurs during an acute asthmatic attack. Severe substernal pain and an audible mediastinal crunch suggest this diagnosis.

Other Pleuropulmonary Disorders

A wide variety of pleuritic or pulmonary disorders can produce chest pain. Spontaneous pneumothorax usually presents with sudden onset of sharp pleuritic chest pain and dyspnea. Pneumonia or other respiratory infections present with productive cough, fever, and pleuritic or constant chest pain.

Esophageal Disorders

A variety of esophageal disorders, occurring singly or in combination, may cause acute chest pain: gastroesophageal reflux, hiatal hernia, achalasia, diffuse esophageal spasm, and esophageal dysmotility. Several studies have shown that determining the presence of the following factors is most helpful in establishing a history of esophageal disease: (1) frequent heartburn; (2) symptoms of acid regurgitation; (3) dysphagia; (4) globus sensation; (5) patient is easily surfeited after meals; (6) pain with eating acid, spicy, or fried foods; (7) pain onset occurs several minutes *after* stopping exercise; and (8) there is a background ache for several minutes after an acute attack.

Musculoskeletal Chest Pain

Musculoskeletal causes of chest pain were first appreciated in the 1920s. There are several specific syndromes that commonly cause chest pain.

The *costosternal syndrome* is localized to the parasternal area, often the left third or fourth intercostal spaces, and occasionally radiates to the left arm or shoulder. It frequently occurs at rest, may be exacerbated with exercise, changes in body position, or other stresses imposed on the chest wall. It has a variable duration, lasting seconds to minutes to hours. The specific cause is un-

known, perhaps due to spasm or cramping of intercostal muscles. Tietze's syndrome (costochondritis) refers to pain *and* swelling confined to the second costal or sternoclavicular cartilages. Both syndromes are self-limited and treated with heat, antiinflammatory agents, analgesics, and rest.

The *thoracic outlet syndrome* can cause chest, neck, and shoulder pain. A careful history usually elicits occasional paresthesias of the upper extremities. Tenderness is common in the supraclavicular fossa. Hyperabduction and external rotation of the arms can reproduce symptoms and diminish radial pulses. Elevation and exercise of both arms cause paresthesias and weakness in both hands.

Radicular pain, caused by osteoarthritis or other spondyloarthropathies, may present as chest pain. Dorsal root pain is sharp and piercing in character with superficial paresthesias, whereas ventral root pain is deep, dull, and boring. Symptoms are usually bilateral and may occur over any area of the chest, axilla, shoulders, or arms. Pain may occur with movement, coughing or sneezing (Déjerine's sign), or after prolonged recumbency.

Hyperventilation

Hyperventilation can cause chest pain with many different qualities and locations. There is generally an inconsistent relationship to the onset or cessation of exercise. Pain may last for hours or days with episodes of sharp, stabbing pain superimposed upon a constant, dull ache. Hyperventilation may be obvious with increased rate and depth of respirations or may be subtle with frequent sighs interposed on a normal ventilatory pattern. The ECG may have nonspecific ST-T changes.

SUMMARY

Certain patients with chest pain have an indefinable look or attitude that suggests serious illness and they deserve priority for evaluation and treatment. Others, despite loud and repeated outcry, can be relegated to waiting because the physician or triage nurse is certain that their chest pain is not life-threatening. The physician must rely on his or her analytical and interrogative skills to arrive at the diagnosis. A careful history and physical examination are the physician's most important tools. Ancillary tests may support the diagnosis but cannot be expected to confirm it. The diagnosis of myocardial ischemia or infarction should never be excluded simply because the ECG is normal or unchanged from previous tracings.

BIBLIOGRAPHY

Areskog NH, Tibbling L (eds.): Differential diagnostic aspects of chest pain. *Acta Med Scand Suppl* 644:1, 1981.

Bell WR, Simon TL, Memets DL: The clinical features of submassive and massive pulmonary emboli. *Am J Med* 62:355, 1977.

Dalen JE, Pape LA, Cohn LH, et al: Dissection of the aorta: Pathogenesis, diagnosis, and treatment. *Prog Cardiovasc Dis* 23:237, 1980.

Davis HA, Jones DB, Rhodes J: "Esophageal angina" as the cause of chest pain. *JAMA* 248:2274, 1982.

Epstein SE, Gerber LH, Borer JS: Chest wall syndrome. A common cause of unexplained cardiac pain. *JAMA* 241:2793, 1979.

Evens DW, Lum LC: Hyperventilation: An important cause of pseudoangina. *Lancet* 1:155, 1977.

Finlayson JK, Short D: Is it a coronary? *Br Med J* 284:87, 1982.

Goldman L, Weinberg M, Weisberg M, et al: A computer-derived protocol to aid in the diagnosis of emergency room patients with acute chest pain. *N Engl J Med* 307:588, 1982.

Horwitz LD: The diagnostic significance of anginal symptoms. *JAMA* 229:1196, 1974.

Levine HJ: Difficult problems in the diagnosis of chest pain. *Am Heart J* 100:108, 1980.

Nattel S, Warnica JW, Ogilvie RI: Indications for admission to a coronary care unit in patients with unstable angina. *Can Med Assoc J* 26:180, 1980.

Reese L, Vksik P: Radioimmunoassay of serum myoglobin in screening for acute myocardial infarction. *Can Med Assoc J* 124:1585, 1981.

Richter JE, Castell DO: Gastroesophageal reflux. Pathogenesis, diagnosis, and therapy. *Ann Intern Med* 97:93, 1982.

Walker WJ: Changing US lifestyle and declining vascular mortality—a retrospective. *N Engl J Med* 303:649, 1983.

B. Respiratory Failure

I. General Approach to Respiratory Failure
Judith E. Tintinalli

PATHOPHYSIOLOGY

Respiration is the exchange of oxygen and carbon dioxide between the environment and tissues. It consists of ventilation, diffusion of gases across the alveolocapillary membrane, transfer of oxygen and carbon dioxide to and from the tissues, and cellular utilization of oxygen. Respiratory failure is the failure to maintain adequate oxygen–carbon dioxide exchange in body tissues.

Ventilation is the movement of gas from one space to another. Systems that provide ventilation are the upper and lower airways, alveoli, and the bellows apparatus consisting of the diaphragm, chest wall, and its neurogenic controls.

Compliance is the change of unit volume per change in unit pressure. Pulmonary compliance is determined by the elastic properties of the lung parenchyma and chest wall, including the pleural space. A decrease in compliance results in an increase in the work of breathing. Examples of chest wall or pleural space factors that decrease compliance are obesity, limitation of diaphragmatic movement by ascites or bowel distension, hemothorax or pneumothorax, or pleural effusion. Pulmonary parenchymal processes such as pneumonia, pulmonary edema, or adult respiratory distress syndrome (ARDS) can also decrease compliance.

Airway resistance is the rate of pressure drop across the airway per rate of flow of air. Devices commonly used to measure airflow (which therefore measure airway resistance) are the forced expiratory volume (FEV/1 s), and the peak expiratory flow rate. At rest conditions the upper airways contribute 20 to 30 percent of airway resistance, and the small peripheral airways 10 to 20 percent. With exercise, the upper airways may contribute 50 percent of the airway resistance.

Neuromuscular control of respiration is by the medullary and carotid chemoreceptors, by the peripheral neural connections to the chest muscles and diaphragm, and by muscular contractions of the bellows mechanism itself. The brainstem medullary chemoreceptor is sensitive to small changes in hydrogen ion concentration in the cerebrospinal fluid, brought about by diffusion of carbon dioxide across the blood-brain barrier. Therefore, a peripheral increase in arterial P_{CO_2} causes an increase in ventilation mediated by the medullary chemoreceptor. The carotid bodies are sensitive to arterial P_{O_2}, so that hypoxemia can also result in hyperventilation, though not as prominently as hypercapnia can. Interruption of nerve pathways to the chest wall muscles or diaphragm, or muscular disease will affect ventilation by impairment of the bellows mechanism.

Environmental gases reach the alveoli through the process of ventilation. Deoxygenated blood is pumped to the alveolar capillaries by the right ventricle. At the alveolocapillary membrane, oxygen is released from hemoglobin and diffuses across the membrane, and carbon dioxide diffuses in the reverse direction. Oxygenated blood is then pumped out of the lungs and to the tissues by the left ventricle. Finally, oxygen is released from hemoglobin at the tissue level, and is utilized in cellular metabolism.

Diffusion is the movement of gases from an area of high concentration to an area of low concentration. Oxygen diffusion is affected by the pressure change in oxygen, blood flow through the alveolar capillaries, and the thickness of the alveolocapillary membrane. An increase in thickness of the alveolocapillary membrane, as in fibrosis, pulmonary edema, or inflammation, will decrease the diffusion of oxygen across the membrane.

The appropriate exchange of oxygen and carbon dioxide across the alveolocapillary membrane involves not only the ability of gases to diffuse but is dependent upon an appropriate flow of blood through the alveolar capillaries. Ventilation of areas that are not perfused, or perfusion of areas that are not ventilated, will result in hypoxemia because of ventilation-perfusion mismatch (shunting).

A simple way to measure the severity and cause of hypoxemia is by determining the alveolar to arterial difference of oxygen (AaD_{O_2}). This can be calculated from the following formula using arterial blood gases with the patient breathing room air:

$$AaD_{O_2} = \text{alveolar } P_{O_2} - \text{arterial } P_{O_2}$$

where, at sea level, and breathing room air,

$$P_{O_2} = (760 - 47)(0.21) - \text{arterial } P_{CO_2}/0.8$$

in which 760 = barometric pressure at sea level

47 = partial pressure of water vapor at sea level

0.21 = % O_2 in room air

0.8 = constant

arterial P_{O_2} = patient's values at room air

arterial P_{CO_2} = patient's values at room air

Normal AaD_{O_2} is 5 to 20 mmHg. In patients with preexisting lung disease, an increase in AaD_{O_2} from previous determinations, coupled with clinical evaluation, is more important than a single AaD_{O_2} calculation.

Based upon arterial blood gas analysis, respiratory failure is divided into three categories:

1. Type I: Hypoxemia with eucarbia or hypocarbia. This responds poorly to oxygen because the primary mechanism is shunting.
2. Type II: Hypoxemia with hypercarbia. This type responds to improved ventilation and low flow oxygen so the hypoxic drive to respiration will not be eliminated.
3. Type III: Normal oxygen with hypercarbia. This type responds to improved ventilation alone.

CLINICAL SIGNS AND SYMPTOMS

In view of the complex physiology of respiration, the causes of respiratory failure are numerous (Table 10BI-1), and emergency diagnosis requires a rapid yet organized evaluation. Often, respiratory function deteriorates so quickly that the first step is intubation and assisted ventilation. In this situation there are no objective laboratory criteria that can determine the decision to intubate for the physician. Rather, a clinical judgment of the severity of respiratory distress, or of the patient's inability to sustain the work of breathing, must lead to intubation. "If you think of it, do it" is a phrase that is especially applicable to the need for intubation.

Signs and symptoms of respiratory failure include dyspnea, tachypnea, and tachycardia. Cyanosis may or may not be present, depending on the amount of unsaturated hemoglobin present. The most accepted definition of dyspnea is "the unpleasant sensation of difficulty in breathing." The lack of specificity to the definition occurs because a number of physiologic mechanisms or disorders can cause dyspnea, and because the patient's perception and interpretation of discomfort are totally subjective. In some patients, dyspnea, especially exercise-induced dyspnea, may be due to intercostal and diaphragmatic muscle fatigue. In others, dyspnea is reported where the patient perceives that the effort exerted to achieve a given increase in chest volume is greater than previously for the same intensity of exertion.

Patients present for an evaluation and treatment of dyspnea if it is acute, occurs at rest, or develops at a lower level of effort than previously. Clinical evaluation begins with history. The examiner must determine in detail the circumstances under which dyspnea develops; whether it occurs at exertion or rest, what type of exertion produces it, and whether the symptoms are acute or chronic. Also to be noted are such factors as the occurrence of trauma, the inhalation of toxic gases, the existence of cardiopulmonary disease, or the possibility of foreign-body obstruction. Is the patient comfortable supine, or must he or she sit upright or be bolstered by pillows to breathe comfortably? The patient may already carry a diagnosis such as asthma, emphysema, or heart

Table 10BI-1. Some Causes of Respiratory Failure

Medullary respiratory center
  Drug overdose
  Central alveolar hypoventilation
  Organic lesions of the respiratory center
Neuromuscular connections
  Guillain-Barre syndrome
  Myasthenia gravis
  Tetanus
  Cervical cord injury
  Pharmacologic neuromuscular blockade
  Botulism
Chest bellows
  Kyphoscoliosis
  Massive obesity
  Flail chest
  Muscular dystrophies
  Myopathies
  Myxedema
  Pleural disease
  Diaphragmatic dysfunction
Upper airway
  Foreign body
  Trachael stenosis
  Carcinoma
  Hematoma
  Vocal cord paralysis
  Inflammation
Lower airway
  Asthma
  COPD
Alveoli
  ARDS
  Pulmonary embolism
  Pulmonary edema
  Pneumonia
  Emphysema
  Pneumothorax
  Interstitial fibrosis

failure, which makes evaluation more straightforward. Current medication history should also be reviewed.

On physical examination, the examiner should observe the patient's respirations, noting the presence of inspiratory or expiratory stridor, intercostal or suprasternal retractions, and confirm the rate and depth of respirations which may have been previously recorded by nursing personnel. Palpation of normal chest respiratory movement can allow a better assessment of the depth of respiration than can visual assessment alone. If the examiner places one hand on the front of the patient's chest and one hand on the back, and then has the patient inspire deeply and exhale forcefully and rapidly, an increase in the expiratory phase can easily be identified. The examiner must check for pulsus paradoxus, jugular venous distension, peripheral or central cyanosis, and the presence of neck scars, especially from tracheotomy or thyroidectomy. The examiner palpates for a right ventricular heave, the point of maximum cardiac impulse, and cardiac thrills. If blunt chest trauma occurred in the recent past, observe chest inspiration and expiration anteriorly, laterally, and tangentially for flail movements. The examiner then palpates the ribs and sternum to detect point tenderness, crepitus, or rib mobility due to fracture. Chest auscultation must be carefully done to determine if breath sounds are present bilaterally, to detect wheezes, rales, rhonchi, and areas of consolidation or effusion. If tidal volume is poor, air exchange, especially at the bases, may be too poor to result in rales or rhonchi even if pathology is present.

The initial history and physical examination should narrow diagnostic possibilities. Where organic pathology, as opposed to functional hyperventilation, is likely, minimum initial screening studies of complete blood count, chest x-ray, electrocardiogram, and arterial blood gases are generally in order. In patients with asthma or chronic obstructive pulmonary disease, use of a peak expiratory flowmeter can provide objective assessment of initial lung function, and can be repeated to check response to therapy in the emergency department.

SOME CONSIDERATIONS IN DIFFERENTIAL DIAGNOSIS (TABLE 10BI-2)

An important cause of acute dyspnea is upper airway obstruction. The presence of inspiratory or expiratory stridor should direct immediate attention to the upper airway. The fact that upper airway obstruction can be misdiagnosed as "asthma" has led to the term "pseudoasthma" being applied to this diagnosis. The stridorous neck sounds of airway obstruction can be transmitted to the lung bases and be misinterpreted as the wheezes of asthma.

PULMONARY DYSPNEA

Asthma

The diagnosis of bronchial asthma is usually made without difficulty because of the presence of end-expiratory wheezes on auscultation. Patients with asthma may complain of dyspnea out of proportion to arterial blood gas findings, possibly because large lung volumes produce excessive stretching of pulmonary receptors. As air exchange decreases, wheezes may decrease in intensity so that the most severe asthmatic may not wheeze. In such a case the presence of labored respirations, low tidal volume, and an increased expiratory phase should suggest the diagnosis. Wheezing can also occur with pulmonary emboli, cardiac failure, and carcinoid syndrome.

Pneumothorax

Spontaneous pneumothorax in young individuals is probably due to a defect in the alveolar wall. It can also occur in pulmonary conditions such as asthma, tuberculosis, or bullous emphysema. Unless the degree of lung collapse is substantial, or unless there is an easily detectable difference in breath sounds on both sides of the chest, the diagnosis can easily be missed.

The diagnosis of pneumothorax in the patient with emphysema and acute dyspnea should always be considered. An individual

Table 10BI-2. Dyspnea: Immediate Concerns

Upper airway obstruction
Tension pneumothorax
Pulmonary embolism
Pulmonary edema
Pulmonary failure
Asthma and emphysema

with normal pulmonary function can tolerate a sudden pneumothorax fairly well but the patient with emphysema and minimal pulmonary reserve can deteriorate rapidly, even with a small pneumothorax. The increased lung volumes and markedly prolonged expiratory phase of patients with chronic obstructive pulmonary disease can result in a marked diminution of breath sounds, so that a unilateral decrease in breath sounds from pneumothorax can be difficult or impossible to detect on clinical grounds alone. The only way to make a certain diagnosis is by immediate chest roentgenogram.

Iatrogenic pneumothorax can occur as a result of subclavian venipuncture, or in a patient with emphysema who is receiving mechanical ventilation with high airway pressure. The possibility of pneumothorax should always be considered if such patients develop sudden respiratory deterioration. The diagnosis of pneumothorax is important to make because it can develop quickly into tension pneumothorax.

The patient with thoracic trauma can develop dyspnea from any number of causes, for example, hemothorax or pneumothorax, pulmonary contusion, pericardial tamponade, or bronchial rupture. These will be discussed in the section on trauma.

Pulmonary Embolism

Pulmonary embolism should be a diagnostic consideration in the patient with acute dyspnea. Common predisposing factors are oral contraceptives, heart failure, recent hospitalization or immobilization, carcinoma, and peripheral venous insufficiency. Signs of acute right ventricular strain, such as a sternal heave or an accentuated pulmonic closure sound, are important clues to the diagnosis. Dyspnea may be due to a decrease in lung compliance caused by atelectasis and vascular volume changes in the lung. In a recent series, of 327 patients with proven pulmonary emboli, dyspnea was present in 84 percent and tachypnea in 92 percent.

Chronic Obstructive Pulmonary Disease

Patients with this disorder complain of chronic productive cough, wheezing, and dyspnea on exertion. On physical examination a prolonged expiratory phase is evident. Scattered rhonchi, wheezes, and coarse rales may also be detectable on auscultation.

Pneumonia

Fever, purulent sputum production, tachypnea, and often pleuritic chest pain are common signs of pneumonia. Chest x-ray is needed to confirm the diagnosis. If the patient appears toxic, is immunosuppressed, very young or elderly, or if involvement is multilobar, admission and careful treatment and observation are in order. Calculation of the AaD_{O_2} in such patients is helpful because it may indicate much more shunting than would be suspected from the x-ray, or by arterial blood gas determination alone. More detailed discussion is provided in the chapter on pneumonia.

Cardiac Dyspnea

When the left ventricular end-diastolic pressure rises, that pressure is reflected backward through the left atrium to the pulmonary capillary bed. A rise of the pulmonary capillary wedge (PCW) pressure to critical levels is reflected in the sensation of dyspnea. If the PCW pressure continues to rise, plasma exudes into the pulmonary interstitium and alveoli, resulting in pulmonary edema. Pulmonary vascular engorgement decreases pulmonary compliance, increases the resistance to airflow, and increases the work of breathing. Engorgement of the bronchial wall and its vessels will result in narrowing of the airways. Pulmonary edema and vascular congestion reduce the volume of alveolar air exchange, and cause restrictive ventilatory insufficiency. This is reflected by a decrease in vital capacity in patients with cardiac failure. Interstitial and alveolar edema impedes oxygen diffusion across the alveolocapillary membrane as well.

The patient with cardiac failure will exhibit dyspnea initially with exertion, then with rest, and finally will develop orthopnea and paroxysmal nocturnal dyspnea. During recumbency, fluid is reabsorbed from edematous extremities. Total blood volume as well as the intrathoracic volume increase, causing relative fluid overload of the left ventricle. As myocardial failure progresses, jugular venous distension, tachycardia, presystolic gallop, peripheral edema, and crepitant basilar rales will develop.

Differentiation between Pulmonary and Cardiac Dyspnea

Symptoms such as cough, chest pain, and dyspnea can occur with either respiratory or cardiac failure, and can develop acutely with either disease. Blood gas abnormalities such as hypoxia and hypercarbia can occur with both cardiac and respiratory failure. The basilar rales of pulmonary edema may be mimicked by chronic obstructive pulmonary disease with basilar fibrosis. Finally, both cardiac and pulmonary failure may coexist. A chest film may aid in the differential diagnosis, although clinical symptoms of cardiac failure usually appear before radiologic changes. In chronological order, radiologic changes of heart failure are: redistribution of flow to the upper lobes of the lung, development of a perihilar haze, development of an alveolar infiltrate, and flagrant pulmonary edema. Auscultation of a cardiac gallop confirms the diagnosis of cardiac failure, but may not be readily distinguishable in the presence of tachycardia and noisy respirations. Intravenous aminophylline may improve clinical signs and symptoms in both pulmonary and cardiac disease. Diuretic administration will produce a prompt response in cardiac failure. In severe or unstable cases, advanced hemodynamic monitoring is necessary for appropriate diagnosis and management.

Simple Hyperventilation

Acute or chronic anxiety can produce complaints of dyspnea. Frequent sighing or an irregular respiratory pattern is commonly observed in anxious patients. Dyspnea may occur because such patients have an increased awareness of their ventilatory pattern and ventilatory work. In hyperventilation, the minute ventilation is out of proportion to metabolic requirements. Abnormal psychogenic, chemical, or muscular stimuli are responsible for the increased ventilation. The time-honored treatment is having the patient rebreathe into a paper bag. Occasionally, sedatives may be necessary.

Metabolic Acidosis

Hydrogen ion in the spinal fluid stimulates the medullary respiratory center so that patients with metabolic acidosis due to causes such as uremia or ketoacidosis exhibit hyperventilation or Kussmaul's respirations. Arterial blood gases are needed to distinguish between primary hyperventilation, central neurogenic hyperventilation, and metabolic acidosis. Although the clinical circumstances in which these disorders occur are usually distinct, this is not always the case.

TREATMENT

Treatment involves a number of modalities that vary with the clinical setting and the condition of the patient. In the emergency department, the most critical issues are to recognize impending or progressive respiratory failure, and to intubate and provide mechanical ventilation when needed.

The physician must insert an intravenous line, obtain an electrocardiogram and chest x-ray, and institute cardiac monitoring. Arterial blood gases must be obtained immediately. At this point, avoid administering sedatives, especially if the patient is combative, agitated, restless, or confused, since these may be signs of hypoxia.

Do not leave a patient in respiratory difficulty unattended. Position the patient upright and give oxygen by nasal cannula, face mask, nonrebreathing mask, or Venturi mask. Avoid high concentrations of oxygen in patients with chronic obstructive lung disease. (Indications and uses for various oxygen delivery devices are discussed in another chapter.) Examine the patient to ensure that upper airway obstruction is not present. Check for pneumothorax, pleural effusion, pulmonary edema, or pulmonary consolidation. If the patient appears to be deteriorating, perform endotracheal or nasotracheal intubation without delay. Other indications for emergency intubation and ventilation include inability to relieve severe hypoxemia with the use of face mask, and shock or metabolic acidosis due to persistent hypoxemia.

Early use of positive end-expiratory pressure (PEEP) may be beneficial in acute respiratory failure characterized by a low functional residual capacity, such as in smoke inhalation, aspiration pneumonia, near-drowning, or pulmonary edema. However, PEEP may not be as helpful in treating patients with a high functional residual capacity, such as in emphysema. Application of PEEP increases the functional residual capacity, prevents alveolar collapse, and improves the distribution of gas and blood within the lungs. When given, PEEP is usually adjusted to provide 5 to 15 cm of H_2O pressure. Complications of PEEP include a decrease in cardiac output due to a decrease in venous return, hypercapnea, failure to improve hypoxemia, and pneumothorax.

BIBLIOGRAPHY

Fahey PJ, Hyde RW: Won't breathe vs. can't breathe. *Chest* 84:19–25, 1983.

Fisher CJ: Physiology of respiration, in Tomlanovich M, Nowak R (eds): Adult Respiratory Emergencies. *Med Clin North Am* 1(2):223–240, 1983.

Scharf S, Bye P, Pardy R, et al: Dyspnea, fatigue, and second wind. *Am Rev Respir Dis* 129:588–589, 1984.

Wasserman, K: Exercise testing in the dyspneic patient. *Am Rev Respir Dis* 129(Suppl 2) S1–S100, Feb. 1984.

Zema MJ, et al: Dyspnea: The heart or the lungs. *Chest* 85:59–64, 1984.

II. Permeability Pulmonary Edema and the Adult Respiratory Distress Syndrome

Marilyn T. Haupt, Richard W. Carlson

INTRODUCTION

Permeability pulmonary edema is a distinct form of edema which is frequently fulminant and leads to severe hypoxemia, intrapulmonary shunting, reduced lung compliance, and, in some cases, irreversible parenchymal lung damage. When these features develop, they are usually termed the "adult respiratory distress syndrome" (ARDS). This syndrome may be associated with a variety of diseases and injuries and it is not clear if the mechanisms of lung injury are similar for each disorder.

Permeability edema differs from the more commonly encountered "cardiac," "high-pressure," or "hemodynamic" edema with respect to the characteristics of the volume and the composition of the fluid which escapes the pulmonary microcirculation, as well as the associated conditions that precipitate edema (Table 10BII-1). In turn, the therapeutic approach for permeability edema differs from high-pressure edema.

PATHOPHYSIOLOGY

The easiest formulation to analyze pulmonary edemagenesis is the Starling equation which quantitates fluid movement across the pulmonary microvascular membrane in relation to the microvascular and perimicrovascular hydrostatic and oncotic forces:

$$\dot{Q}_f = K_f [(P_{mv} - P_{pmv}) - \delta(\pi_{mv} - \pi_{pmv})]$$

in which $\dot{Q}_f$ = fluid flow across pulmonary microvascular membrane

K_f = hydraulic filtration coefficient

P_{mv}, P_{pmv} = hydrostatic pressures on microvascular and perimicrovascular sides of the microvascular membrane, respectively

π_{mv}, π_{pmv} = corresponding oncotic pressures

δ = reflection coefficient and represents degree to which membrane presents a physical barrier to protein molecules.

It is the factor δ that can be used to distinguish high pressure from permeability edema. In high-pressure edema, the membrane remains an effective barrier to protein equilibrium and δ approaches 1. In high-pressure edema the primary forces which lead to an increase in fluid flux are thus the hydrostatic and oncotic pressure differences and the filtration coefficient K_f. In permeability edema, the microvascular membrane is no longer an effective barrier to protein flux. In this condition δ approaches zero and the oncotic pressure difference ($\pi_{mv} - \pi_{pmv}$) therefore influences fluid flux minimally. Hydrostatic pressure thus assumes an even greater importance in edema formation, and an increase in hydrostatic pressure will accelerate fluid flux into the lung to a far

greater extent than in hemodynamic edema. Assessment or estimation of pulmonary hydrostatic pressure therefore has major therapeutic implications in the management of permeability pulmonary edema.

Central to the pathogenesis of permeability pulmonary edema is the involvement of a variety of biochemical mediators that typify an inflammatory response. Some of these mediators are the result of a series of reactions facilitated by enzyme systems. Therefore, in many of the disorders associated with permeability edema activation of these enzyme cascades can be demonstrated. One of these is the complement system, which may be triggered by a variety of substances (Fig. 10BII-1), including antibody-antigen complexes (classical pathway), endotoxin, exposure to cell surfaces (bacteria, fungi), and to complex polysaccharides. The intermediate products C3a and C5a lead to neutrophil aggregation and the release of proteases and superoxide radicals which damage the pulmonary vascular endothelium (Table 10BII-2). In addition, metabolism of membrane-bound phospholipid on cell membranes leads to the formation of arachidonic acid. In turn, this compound is the parent for a host of leukotrienes and prostaglandins (Fig. 10BII-2), which contribute to further endothelial and alveolar injury.

Another enzyme cascade involves the coagulation pathways. Collagen in the subendothelial basement membrane will activate

Table 10BII-1. Clinical Causes of Pulmonary Edema

Hemodynamic edema (high pressure, cardiogenic)
  Left ventricular failure
    Acute myocardial infarction
    Cardiomyopathies
    Valvular heart disease
  Volume overload
    Crystalloid
    Colloid
    Blood and/or blood products
Permeability edema (low pressure, noncardiogenic)
  Bacterial and other types of shock
  Drug use and overdose—heroin, aspirin, ethchlorvynol
  Gastric aspiration
  Near-drowning
  Thromboembolism and microembolism
  Fat embolization
  Amniotic fluid embolization
  Smoke inhalation
  Bacterial and viral pneumonias
  Disseminated intravascular coagulation
  Multiple trauma
  Pancreatitis
  Multiple transfusions
  Eclampsia (pregnancy-induced hypertension)
  Acute neurologic crises

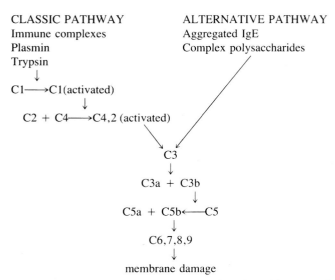

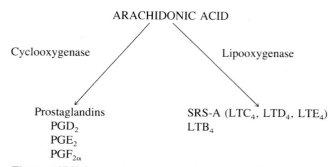

CLASSIC PATHWAY
Immune complexes
Plasmin
Trypsin

ALTERNATIVE PATHWAY
Aggregated IgE
Complex polysaccharides

Figure 10BII-1. The complement system is activated in many of the conditions associated with ARDS. C3a and C5a have a variety of physiologic actions including membrane damage and chemotaxis of neutrophils. Additional membrane damage is produced by activation of the C6–C7 components.

ARACHIDONIC ACID

Cyclooxygenase

Lipooxygenase

Prostaglandins
PGD_2
PGE_2
$PGF_{2\alpha}$

SRS-A (LTC_4, LTD_4, LTE_4)
LTB_4

Figure 10BII-2. Metabolism of arachidonic acid through major biochemical pathways leads to a variety of physiologically active mediators.

DIAGNOSIS

The clinical features of ARDS may present within a variable interval, usually 12 to 72 h after the initial injury or medical crisis. Tachypnea, labored breathing, and impaired gas exchange (arterial P_{O_2} less than 50 torr with an FI_{O_2} of more than 0.5) are characteristic of this stage of the syndrome. The chest radiograph will demonstrate progressive alveolar infiltrates which are usually bilateral. Pulmonary compliance is reduced. Accordingly, airway pressures are high when the patient is placed on mechanical ventilation.

The diagnosis of a permeability lesion may be facilitated by sampling and analysis of pulmonary edema fluid suctioned from the trachea. However, fluid in sufficient quantities for analysis may not be available from all patients. Sampling may be performed by suctioning fluid from the endotracheal tube with a soft plastic catheter; the fluid is subsequently collected in a Lukens trap (Fig. 10BII-4). The fluid should be rejected if it is contaminated with mucus, sputum, or other debris. Colloid osmotic pressure and/or total protein is measured on the simultaneous edema fluid and plasma samples. In permeability edema, the edema fluid-to-plasma protein ratio or colloid osmotic pressure ratio will exceed

Hageman factor (factor XII) when exposed to plasma. The components of the coagulation system, the fibrinolytic system, and kinin system are activated and result in additional mediator release and endothelial damage (Fig. 10BII-3).

To complicate this process, the mechanical properties of the lung are adversely affected. Surfactant is inactivated or reduced with consequent destabilization of lung units. The lung becomes stiffer, and greater pressure is required to inflate it to a given volume. This may be quantitated as a reduction in pulmonary compliance. When pulmonary edema is observed in a critically ill or injured patient with reduced lung compliance and severe hypoxemia refractory to supplemental oxygen, the criteria for the diagnosis of ARDS are met. A vicious cycle of ongoing pulmonary destruction and continued interaction of the enzymatic and biochemical cascading reactions develops. This process is frequently irreversible (approximately 50 percent of cases are fatal) unless the inciting event is controlled.

Table 10BII-2. Substances Released by Neutrophils Implicated in Lung Injury

Collagenase
Fibrinolysins
Plasminogen
Elastase
Histamine
Kininogenases
Leukotrienes
Prostaglandins
Oxygen radicals
   Superoxide anion
   Hydrogen peroxide
   Hydroxyl radical

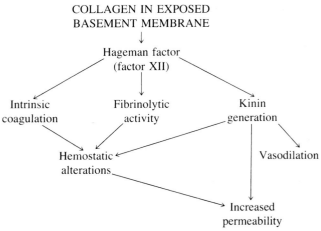

COLLAGEN IN EXPOSED
BASEMENT MEMBRANE

Hageman factor
(factor XII)

Intrinsic
coagulation

Fibrinolytic
activity

Kinin
generation

Hemostatic
alterations

Vasodilation

Increased
permeability

Figure 10BII-3. Activation of Hageman factor can be triggered by subendothelial collagen, leading to involvement of the coagulation system, the fibrinolytic system, and the kinin system. Thus, cascading secondary reactions amplify membrane damage and increase vascular permeability.

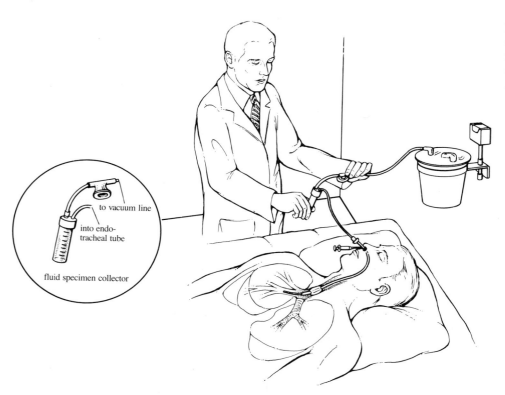

Figure 10BII-4. Technique of suctioning pulmonary edema fluid. (Reproduced with permission from *Curr Rev Respir Ther*, 5:36, 1982.)

to vacuum line

into endo-
tracheal tube

fluid specimen collector

60 percent; whereas for high-pressure edema the ratio is less than 60 percent. Other substances such as collagenase, elastinase, and angiotensin-converting enzyme may be detected in increased quantities in edema fluid.

MANAGEMENT

Since most instances of permeability pulmonary edema are associated with other disorders (e.g., bacterial infection, gastric aspiration, trauma, drug intoxication), therapy should be primarily directed to treating the underlying insult. However, supportive therapy to maintain acceptable oxygenation and hemodynamic competence must be assured.

Mechanical ventilatory support will be required for most patients with moderate to severe edema. Incremental supplementation with oxygen to increase arterial P_{O_2} is likely to be of limited effectiveness in ARDS, even with the use of mechanical ventilation. Accordingly, the physician must use other techniques to improve oxygenation. The use of positive end-expiratory pressure (PEEP) has virtually revolutionized the treatment of oxygenation deficits. PEEP recruits and helps stabilize lung units that may be filled with fluid and susceptible to collapse. Therefore, an increased number of lung units participate in gas exchange when PEEP is used. Because elevated inspired oxygen fractions (FI_{O_2}) may contribute to additional lung injury, the use of PEEP allows the reduction of FI_{O_2} to safer levels. As the level of PEEP increases, however, close attention must be directed to possible adverse circulatory effects, including the reduction of venous return, and therefore cardiac output and oxygen delivery. PEEP may also lead to detrimental effects related to pulmonary barotrauma (pneumothorax, pneumomediastinum).

Invasive hemodynamic monitoring allows the measurement of cardiac output, arterial and mixed venous oxygen tensions, pulmonary artery pressures, including the wedge or occluded pressure (PAWP). This serves as a clinical index of pulmonary microvascular hydrostatic pressure (P_{mv}) as well as left ventricular volume and compliance. Because P_{mv} plays a major role in transcapillary fluid flux in permeability pulmonary edema, PAWP should be maintained at levels as low as possible—provided that peripheral perfusion is maintained. Judicious use of diuretics or vasodilators may be required when PAWP is elevated, and there is progressive pulmonary edema or worsening of gas exchange.

Adequacy of peripheral perfusion can be assessed, not only by bedside guides (blood pressure, sensorium, urine output, etc.) but also by the measurement of cardiac output and the determination of systemic oxygen delivery and oxygen consumption. These values are dependent upon cardiac output and hemoglobin, as well as arterial and mixed venous oxygen tensions and saturations. The level of blood lactic acid will reflect the adequacy of oxygen transport and utilization.

Fluid infusion may be required to maintain cardiac output and peripheral perfusion, particularly in the face of the decreased venous return that may be produced by sudden increases of PEEP. The choice of fluid in this setting remains controversial (crystalloid or colloid), but the goal of fluid therapy should be to augment intravascular and intracardiac volumes with improvement of cardiac output and consequently oxygen transport to the systemic tissues. Careful hemodynamic assessment before and after a fluid challenge is necessary to interpret the response.

Current experimental studies are directed to analyzing the role of anticoagulants, antihistamines, and cyclooxygenase and oxygen radical inhibitors, as well as corticosteroids in reducing permeability damage. To date, however, the effectiveness of these agents in humans is unproven.

SUMMARY

Permeability edema may be distinguished from the more common cardiogenic or hemodynamic edema on the basis of associated clinical conditions, pathophysiology, and if available, analysis of pulmonary edema fluid. This distinction has important therapeutic implications. The goals of successful management of permeability edema and ARDS include treatment of the underlying condition and maintenance of adequate pulmonary oxygen loading with mechanical ventilation and PEEP, while assuring adequate circulatory function and tissue oxygen delivery.

BIBLIOGRAPHY

Carlson RW, Schaeffer RC, Michaels SG, et al: Pulmonary edema fluid. Spectrum of features in 37 patients. *Circulation* 60:1161–1169, 1979.

McGuire WW, Spragg RG, Cohen AB, et al: Studies on the pathogenesis of the adult respiratory distress syndrome. *J Clin Invest* 69:543–553, 1982.

Rinaldo JE, Rogers RM: Adult respiratory distress syndrome. Changing concepts of lung injury and repair. *New Engl J Med* 306:900–909, 1982.

Petty TL, Fowler AA: Another look at ARDS. *Chest* 82:98–104, 1982.

C. Cyanosis

Ann L. Harwood

DEFINITION

Cyanosis refers to that bluish color of the skin and mucous membranes which results from an increased amount of reduced hemoglobin or hemoglobin derivatives. The detection of cyanosis can be highly subjective and is not considered a sensitive indicator of the state of arterial oxygenation. In fact, cyanosis is determined by the absolute amount of reduced hemoglobin in the blood; the amount of oxygenated hemoglobin present is of little influence. Cyanosis is usually present when there are 5 g or more of reduced hemoglobin in 100 mL of capillary blood. The increase in the amount of reduced hemoglobin in the cutaneous vessels can result from either an increase in the quantity of venous blood in the skin, a result of dilatation of the venules, or from a decrease in the oxygen saturation in the capillary blood. In some instances, cyanosis can be detected when the arterial saturation has fallen to 85 percent; in others, cyanosis may not be detected until the saturation is 75 percent. Of importance is the fact that it is the absolute rather than the relative amount of reduced hemoglobin which produces cyanosis. It was Stadie who first demonstrated the relationship between cyanosis and arterial hypoxemia.

Factors which are felt to influence detection of cyanosis include the rate of blood flow through the capillaries, the types of light conditions under which the patient is examined, and the skill of the individual observer. The degree of cyanosis is modified by the quality of cutaneous pigment, the color of the blood plasma, thickness of skin, and state of the cutaneous capillaries. Many consider the tongue as one of the most sensitive sites for observing central cyanosis. The earlobes, conjuctivae, and nail beds are not considered reliable.

Additional factors which affect the detection of cyanosis include the complexities of the microcirculation. The amount of reduced hemoglobin in the capillaries will be affected by blood flow, oxygen content, tissue oxygen, tension, oxygen extraction, and the hemoglobin dissociation curve. It is apparent that accurate clinical detection of the presence and degree of cyanosis is often difficult.

Clinically, the presence of cyanosis must suggest the possibility of tissue hypoxia. However, it is important to note that the absence of cyanosis does not mean that there is no tissue hypoxia; severe states of tissue hypoxia are possible without the presence of cyanosis. Cyanosis demands a thorough clinical evaluation for possible tissue hypoxia. Additionally, unexplained cyanosis, particularly in association with normal arterial oxygen tension, should prompt a search for an abnormal hemoglobin.

CENTRAL AND PERIPHERAL CYANOSIS

Cyanosis can be divided into two categories, central and peripheral. The central type is seen under conditions where arterial blood is unsaturated or an abnormal hemoglobin derivative exists. In central cyanosis, the mucous membranes and skin are both affected. In contrast, peripheral cyanosis is due to the slowing of blood flow to an area and abnormally great extraction of oxygen from normally saturated arterial blood. Congestive failure, peripheral vascular disease, shock states, and cold exposure all create states of vasoconstriction and decrease peripheral blood flow. The differentiation between central and peripheral cyanosis may not be possible in conditions where there may be an admixture of mechanisms (see Table 10C-1).

THE ROLE OF ARTERIAL BLOOD GAS DETERMINATION

To the clinician, the presence of cyanosis most often suggests the possibility of tissue hypoxia. Arterial blood gases are necessary for the further assessment of the cyanotic patient. Arterial oxygen saturation will be normal in peripheral cyanosis if cardiopulmonary function is normal. It will be decreased if cyanosis is due to hypoxia. Of note, the presence of an abnormal hemoglobin derivative is not detected by routine arterial blood gases.

Table 10C-1. Causes of Cyanosis

Central cyanosis
  Decreased arterial oxygen saturation
    Decreased atmospheric pressure—high altitude
    Impaired pulmonary function
      Alveolar hypoventilation
      Uneven relationships between pulmonary ventilation and
        perfusion
      Impaired oxygen diffusion
    Anatomic shunts
      Certain types of congenital heart disease
      Pulmonary arteriovenous fistulas
      Multiple small intrapulmonary shunts
    Hemoglobin with low affinity for oxygen
  Hemoglobin abnormalities
    Methemoglobinemia—hereditary, acquired
    Sulfhemoglobinemia—acquired
    Carboxyhemoglobinemia (not true cyanosis)
Peripheral cyanosis
  Reduced cardiac output
  Cold exposure
  Redistribution of blood flow from extremities
  Arterial obstruction
  Venous obstruction

Source: Braunwald E: Cyanosis, hypoxia and polycythemia, in Petersdorf RG, Adams RD, Braunwald E, et al (eds): *Harrison's Principles of Internal Medicine,* ed 10. New York, McGraw-Hill, 1983, pp 1881–1882.

Spectrophotometry will be necessary to determine the presence of a hemoglobin derivative.

Few tests are as vulnerable to errors introduced by improper sampling, handling, and storage as are blood gas analyses. One study reports a 15.8 percent incidence of preanalytic error for arterial blood gas samples from emergency departments. In contrast, a 0.1 percent incidence of error exists from samples obtained from an indwelling arterial catheter.

Special attention should be given to the following sources of preanalytic error for arterial blood gas samples:

1. Heparin is the anticoagulant of choice, but one must be cautious that the syringe be flushed with heparin and then emptied thoroughly. This will allow adequate anticoagulation of a 2-to-4-mL blood sample with assurance that the results will not be altered by the anticoagulant. Excessive heparin affects the pH, P_{CO_2} and P_{O_2}, as well as the hemoglobin determination.

2. Air bubbles that mix with the blood sample will result in gas equilibration, thus significantly lowering the P_{CO_2} values with an increase in pH and P_{O_2}. It is recommended that any sample obtained with more than minor air bubbles be discarded.

3. Reducing the temperature of the blood by placing the sample immediately in an ice slush will significantly deter changes in the P_{CO_2} and pH for a period of several hours. If the sample is not iced immediately, changes can be significant. As a general rule, arterial blood samples should be analyzed within 10 min or cooled immediately. A delay up to 1 h for running a cool sample will have no significant effect on the results. Failure to properly cool the sample is a common source of preanalytic error.

DIFFERENTIAL DIAGNOSIS OF CYANOSIS

Hypoxia, anemia, and polycythemia can be diagnosed by means of hemoglobin, hematocrit, and arterial blood gas determination. The red cyanosis of polycythemia vera occurs because the increase in number of red blood cells and hemoglobin concentration results in sludging of blood flow in cutaneous capillaries and venules. Similarly, cyanosis is enhanced in chronic hypoxemia accompanied by polycythemia.

If arterial gases, hematocrit, and hemoglobin are normal, the cause of cyanosis may be due to abnormal skin pigmentation or an abnormal hemoglobin. Argyria is a slate blue to gray coloration of the skin resulting from either chronic ingestion or chronic local application of silver salts or colloidal silver. The color does not blanch with pressure, in contrast to true cyanotic skin, which will blanch. Skin biopsy confirms the diagnosis. Carboxyhemoglobinemia does not cause cyanosis. Occasionally, however, carboxyhemoglobinemia does produce a cherry-red flush of the skin, retina, or mucous membranes.

Cyanosis can be caused by methemoglobinemia and sulfhemoglobinemia. Most cases are due to acquired states secondary to chemicals or medications. Benzocaine, nitrates, and nitrites may produce methemoglobinemia. The sulfonamides, phenacetin, acetanilid, and aniline may produce sulfhemoglobinemia or methemoglobinemia. The incidence of acquired methemoglobinemia secondary to industrial exposure to aniline dyes and aromatic amino and nitro compounds has decreased with improvement in occupational health standards. Hereditary methemoglobinemia is a genetic disorder affecting the enzyme methemoglobin reductase, resulting in structural alterations of the hemoglobin molecule. Patients afflicted with this deficiency have cyanosis but tend to be asymptomatic.

Although there exist a wide number of drugs which can produce methemoglobinemia, no currently used drug does so at therapeutic dose levels. Acetanilid and phenacetin are aniline derivatives and frequent causes of methemoglobinemia and sulfhemoglobinemia. Certain sulfonamides and local anesthetics may produce methemoglobinemia. Methemoglobinemia is manifested clinically by cyanosis with as little as 1.5 g of methemoglobin present in 100 mL of blood. Since methemoglobin is incapable of binding with oxygen, the symptoms of methemoglobinemia are secondary to hypoxia. The severity is related to the quantity of methemoglobin present, the rapidity of onset, and the patient's own cardiopulmonary system. Cyanotic patients without cardiovascular or pulmonary disease should be suspected of having methemoglobinemia, especially if cyanosis is not relieved by oxygen administration. Further, the venous blood will appear chocolate brown. Spectrophotometry is required for identification of the pigment and its quantity. In acquired methemoglobinemia, no treatment is necessary unless stupor or coma is present. Methylene blue in a dose of 1 to 2 mg per kilogram of body weight given intravenously over 5 min in a 1% solution is the agent of choice.

Sulfhemoglobinemia may result from one of the oxidizing drugs. Phenacetin (APC, Empirin compound) and acetanilid (Bromo Seltzer) are the most common causative agents. Sulfhemoglobin is inert as an oxygen carrier and when present can produce deep cyanosis at a level of less than 0.5 g of sulfhemoglobin per 100 mL of blood. Once formed, there is no way of converting sulfhemoglobin to hemoglobin and the treatment calls for the removal of the causative agent.

BIBLIOGRAPHY

Blount SG: Cyanosis: Pathophysiology and differential diagnosis. *Prog Cardiovasc Dis* 13:595, 1971.

Drysdale HC, Hunton J: Methaemalbuminaemia as a cause of cyanosis. *Br Med J* 6118:962, 1978.

Lavorgna L: Neonatal cardiology. *Pediatr Ann* 8(2):65–83, 1979.

Lin YT, Yen LC, Oka Y: Pathophysiology of general cyanosis. *NY State J Med* 77(9):1393–1396, 1977.

Parker WA: Argyria and cyanotic. *Am J Hosp Pharm* 34:287–289, 1977.

Schmitter CR: Sulfhemoglobinemia and methemoglobinemia—Uncommon causes of Cyanosis. *Anesthesiology* 43(5):586–587, 1975.

Spagnolo SV: Cyanosis of cirrhosis. *Med Clin North Am* 59(4):983–987, 1975.

Sprout WL, Neeld WE, Woessner WW: Management of chemical cyanosis. *Arch Environ Health* 30:302–306, 1975.

Winslow EH: Visual inspection of the patient with cardiopulmonary disease. *Heart and Lung* 4(3):421–429, 1975.

D. Coma and Altered States of Consciousness

Gregory L. Henry

Although coma is the most dramatic of the disorders of consciousness, it is only the end point in a continuum. Any disease process which can cause coma may initially present with mild alterations of, and progressively decreasing, mental status. It is often difficult or impossible to determine the direction and final outcome of a change in mental status until the most important test, time, has been applied.

In severe nervous system disease, a change in mental status is often the first sign of a severe pathologic process. It is a well-recognized rule within the neurosciences that functional change is always greater and always precedes structural change in the brain and spinal cord. Of all the central nervous system functions, mental status is the most delicate and the most sensitive early bellwether of advancing disease.

It is important for any health professional dealing with altered mental status to realize that nothing replaces our standard approach to all emergency patients, namely, "A, B, C3." Airway management and *breathing* should be the first priorities of the evaluation of any patient in the emergency department. *Cardiac* status is next assessed and supported as necessary. The other two Cs stand for *cervical* spine immobilization and *compression* of obvious hemorrhage. It will be of little benefit to the patient or to society to have properly diagnosed a subdural hematoma if you have missed a fourth cervical vertebrae fracture and created a quadriplegic. The basic rule is that a comatose patient has suffered a cervical spine injury until proven otherwise.

The principal function of this chapter will be to review classification systems for patients with altered mental status and to provide a framework for evaluating such patients in the emergency setting. The immediate duty of the emergency department, with regard to patients with altered mental status, is to divide the potentially exhaustive list of disease entities into two major groups. The first and most common subset is that of diffuse metabolic and toxic disease. The second major group is that of structural, focal, and central nervous system disease. Since the management of toxic and metabolic disease is principally medical and the management of focal disease is frequently surgical, it is important that these differentiations be made early so that correct treatment can be initiated. To delay making this important differential can mean severe disability and even death to the patient.

The determination of structural neurologic disease is based on a focal neurologic examination. Those patients who are developing discrete, isolated lesions of motor or sensory function or specific cortical defects will have structural or anatomic damage most of the time. This is the group of patients in whom immediate surgical therapy is most beneficial in salvaging meaningful life.

DEFINITIONS

A clear understanding of the terminology of altered mental status is necessary before classifying various disease entities. The physician is better served by describing in the body of the chart exactly what he or she sees. Nonspecific terms are often misleading and not helpful for further examiners who must reassess the patient on an ongoing basis. It is much more useful to record in the chart objective findings such as the patient's ability to handle three-object retention and mathematical calculations as opposed to using terms such as "stuporous" or "lethargic." But since the following terminology has become universal in medical literature, some general understanding of the terms is needed. "Consciousness" is defined as an awareness of self and the environment. Disorders of consciousness can be divided into states where the patient appears asleep and states where the patient appears awake but is unresponsive.

Patients Who Appear Asleep

Sleep. A state of nonpathologic decreased mental status from which the patient can be easily aroused to full consciousness.

Lethargy. Depressed mental status in which the patient may appear wakeful but has depressed awareness of self and environment globally.

Stupor. Unresponsiveness from which the patient can be aroused with vigorous noxious stimuli. The stuporous patient, however, does not return to a normal baseline of awareness of self or environment.

Coma. A state of unresponsiveness from which the patient is unarousable to both verbal and physical stimuli to a level from which he or she can make any meaningful response.

Psychogenic coma. A state of unresponsiveness, either voluntary or involuntary, from which the patient cannot be brought to reasonable cortical response by noxious verbal or physical stimuli. These patients do, however, have normal physiologic testing and EEG responses.

Patients who Appear Awake but are Unresponsive

Abulic state (akinetic mutism) (coma vigil). The patient is awake with eyes open but extremely slow to respond to questions asked. The patient's frontal lobe function is so depressed, from any number of processes, that he or she is unable to respond meaningfully in a normal time frame. It should be noted that these patients often do have reasonable mental status but because of the huge delays in their ability to process information and answer they are often misdiagnosed in the emergency department. These patients may take several minutes to respond to any problem or question posed.

Locked-in syndrome (Count of Monte Cristo syndrome) (M. Nortier de Villefort). Patients who appear absolutely motionless but with eyes open. The lesion in the locked-in syndrome is the destruction of the ventral pontine motor tracts. The only function these patients maintain is vertical eye movement. It is important, in all unresponsive patients who appear awake, that the examiner ask them to look up. If a patient can look up but cannot move his or her eyes from side to side, the diagnosis of locked-in syndrome is secured.

Psychogenic unresponsiveness (the catatonic state). A level of unresponsiveness in which the patient appears awake and may maintain normal motor posturing and neurologic testing, but who, for voluntary or involuntary reasons, is not able to communicate with the examiner.

Confusional States

This category covers a series of disorders in which the patient's mental status is not depressed, but in which he or she misinterprets external stimuli. These states may overlap with causes of depressed mental status and may be extremely difficult to differentiate in an emergency setting. The hallmarks of these conditions are global confusion, inability to appropriately process stimuli, or inability to make meaningful responses. Such findings are characteristic of a toxic ingestion, metabolic encephalopathy, or central nervous system infection.

THE PATHOPHYSIOLOGY OF ALTERED MENTAL STATUS

Although the specific causes of altered mental status are legion, the pathophysiology is either bilateral cerebral cortical disease or

suppression of the brainstem reticular activating formation (RAF). Cellular disorders such as lipid storage disease or neuronal degeneration rarely present as acute changes in mental status.

Bilateral Cortical Disease

Focal lesions in one cerebral cortex cause neurologic findings specific to that region but do not cause alteration of mental status. If the altered mental status is thought to be based on cortical disease both cortices should be involved. For example, patients who have had large sections of the cerebral cortex removed by surgery can still be awake and alert. The most common causes of bilateral cortical disease altering mental status are toxins such as alcohol and illicit drugs, and deficiencies of the metabolic substrates oxygen and glucose.

If the brain is deprived of its normal supply of oxygen, either by impairment of systemic oxygen uptake or distribution, for more than about 10 s, loss of consciousness ensues. A marked decrease or increase of serum glucose can rapidly lead to changes in mental status.

Reticular Activating System Lesions

The other principal mechanism by which altered mental status is produced is through involvement of the reticular activating formation, a small grouping of fibers which traverses the brainstem and thalamus. Through continuous stimulation of the cortex, the RAF maintains the state of wakefulness. Any sudden interruption of RAF activity affects alertness. For example, the mechanism by which a boxer's blow to the chin causes sudden coma is not through damage to the cortical structures but rather through torque forces on the brainstem which interrupt RAF activity.

The reticular activating formation can be affected in three principal ways: by supratentorial pressure, infratentorial pressure, and intrinsic brainstem lesions.

Supratentorial pressure. The manner in which supratentorial lesions produce coma is by enlarging and displacing tissue. This causes compression of the opposite hemisphere, as well as deeper diencephalic and brainstem structures. By pressing on the brainstem through this remote mechanism, the RAF is also compressed. The skull is a limited area and the brain and its protective and supporting structures occupy the entire intracranial space. When additional volume accumulates in the skull, either as a discrete mass or from generalized edema, pressure is directed to the point of least resistance. The temporal lobes, which rest on the tentorium cerebelli, may be forced through the tentorial notch, compressing brainstem structures and cranial nerves. Therefore, the mechanism of coma in patients with acute supratentorial lesions such as epidural, subdural, or intraparenchymal bleeding is not due to destruction of specific cortex but rather from pressure directed toward deeper brainstem structures.

Infratentorial pressure. The brainstem lies below the tentorium cerebelli and is anatomically distinct from the great mass of cerebral tissue which lies above. The brainstem shares the posterior fossa with the ventricular aqueduct of Sylvius, the fourth ventricle, and the cerebellum. An increase in pressure in this area may be accompanied by movement of the posterior fossa contents upward through the tentorial notch or downward through the foramen magnum. For example, tumors involving the meninges, brainstem, and cerebellum, or acute cerebellar hemorrhage can increase pressure. This causes compression on the reticular activating formation and resultant coma.

Intrinsic brainstem lesion. Lesions intrinsic to the brainstem itself, such as traumatic or hypertensive pontine hemorrhage, may also compress the reticular activating formation directly.

In summary, severely depressed mental status is due to either bilateral cortical disease or involvement of the reticular activating formation. Bilateral cortical disease is almost always due to metabolic or toxic causes and generally shows no focal neurologic findings. Reticular activating formation dysfunction, on the other hand, is more likely the result of structural disease and will most frequently have focal neurologic findings.

GENERAL APPROACH TO THE PATIENT WITH ALTERED MENTAL STATUS

Initial Management

In the usual clinical approach to a patient, the examiner first obtains a history, then performs a physical examination and laboratory studies, and finally administers treatment. However, this sequence is not correct for patients in a coma. Coma is such a major variance from normal neurologic functioning that immediate supportive efforts are required. The "A, B, C3" approach must be activated. For patients who do not have an active gag reflex, positive airway control is urgently needed to prevent aspiration. If cervical spinal fracture is suspected, or if the mechanism of coma is unknown, the neck must be stabilized while the airway is secured, and endotracheal intubation should be avoided. For patients in whom there is no obvious facial trauma and who are actively breathing, nasotracheal intubation is an excellent alternative. In patients who have had severe midfacial and oral trauma and in whom the standard approaches are contraindicated, a cricothyroidotomy may be necessary.

Once airway control is established, oxygenation and hyperventilation are necessary. Mild hyperventilation corrects acidosis and lowering the P_{CO_2} reduces intracranial pressure. The P_{CO_2} should be lowered to approximately 25 torr. This level can usually be obtained by ventilating the patient approximately 20 to 25 times per minute.

Cardiac status should be assessed to make certain that the patient has reasonable cardiac output and that there is no reason to begin cardiac pulmonary resuscitation.

Immobilization of the cervical spine, as has been previously mentioned, is mandatory in patients in whom the cause of coma is unknown. Without a definite history the possibility of trauma always exists. The mere smell of alcohol on the breath of the patient does not constitute a definite cause for his or her altered mental status. It is the general rule that all alcoholics fall and hit their head. Encounters where the alcoholic is both intoxicated and suffering from an intracranial lesion *and* a cervical spine fracture are well within the experience of emergency physicians. Aggressive neck immobilization and restraints to the body so the head and body function as a unit is the most effective way to anticipate cervical spine injury.

Finally, obvious hemorrhage should be stopped before detailed neurologic examination is begun. One of the earliest signs of shock is apprehension and confusion. As shock worsens, mental status quickly deteriorates, and thus the patient in hemorrhagic shock may well be lethargic or comatose. Vital signs should be obtained and recorded at this point if not already done.

Initial Treatment

As an intravenous line is being inserted, blood should be removed for laboratory analysis. Generally, enough blood should be drawn to allow for CBC, glucose, BUN, creatinine, and electrolyte analyses. It is generally standard to administer intravenously thiamine, 100 mg; glucose, 25 to 50 g; and naloxone, 2 to 4 ampoules of 0.4 mg each. Newer thiamine derivatives do not produce anaphylactoid reactions when given intravenously. Nutritionally deficient patients such as alcoholics or patients receiving cancer chemotherapy should receive thiamine prior to glucose administration. Thiamine is given to facilitate carbohydrate metabolism and to prevent the unwanted complication of Wernicke's syndrome.

The standard dose of glucose is 25 to 50 g as a 50% solution. In the patient with an intracranial mass lesion glucose increases the osmotic load and is potentially beneficial in reducing intracranial pressure. In the patient who is comatose because of hyperglycemia, the recommended dose of glucose is inconsequential. Dextrostik determination of blood glucose could be done prior to glucose administration, but this is not necessary.

Generally, two 0.4-mg ampoules of naloxone are given intravenously, and followed by two more ampoules if no response is seen. There are no dose-related adverse affects of naloxone reported, although the possibility of an acute opiate withdrawal syndrome increases along with the dose of naloxone. Unlike its predecessor, nalorphine, naloxone does not produce respiratory depression. Naloxone is an effective antagonist of opiates and synthetic narcotics such as propoxyphene and pentazocine. A very large dose of naloxone may be required to overcome the endorphin receptor effects of the synthetic narcotics. Any patient who can be aroused with naloxone may become combative and disoriented, so patients should be properly restrained before naloxone is given.

Obtaining the History

The patient may not be a reliable source of information, so other sources must be sought. One of the great mysteries in emergency medicine is the appearance of a comatose patient in the emergency department, without evident means of arrival. This defiance of the laws of physics is accomplished many times each week in any busy emergency department. Some data may be obtained from the patient's personal effects such as medical alert tags, wallet, purse, or pill containers.

Family and friends should be contacted to provide a history. They may be able to describe previous episodes or an event that led up to the current episode. Specific questions about abnormal motor movements, food or drug ingestions, trauma, and underlying diseases should be asked. It is important to provide reassurance that the medical history obtained will remain part of the medical record and will not be inappropriately given to law enforcement officials.

General Physical Examination

Vital signs should be constantly monitored. Arrhythmias should be monitored and treated as clinically indicated. Tachypnea should be considered a sign of inadequate oxygenation and not a sign of central nervous damage. Oxygenation and ventilation should be corrected and then mental status reevaluated. Both hypertension and hypotension should be considered to have a nonneurologic cause in a patient with shock until proved otherwise. Although systemic hypertension can be caused by an elevation in intracranial pressure, systemic hypertension should not initially be ascribed to a primary neurologic event. Constant cardiac monitoring of the comatose patient is useful to check for intermittent cardiac problems such as fluctuating bradycardias or ventricular arrhythmias. Although these are unusual causes of coma, they represent treatable entities from which a patient may have an excellent neurologic recovery.

As the patient is examined, signs of trauma should be carefully sought. Blood behind the tympanic membranes as well as ecchymoses in the mastoid area should be particularly noted. Any patient with these findings should be considered to have a basilar skull fracture. Careful palpation of the head may reveal cephalohematomas which are not visible at first glance. Palpation of the neck, although often advocated, is generally nonproductive in the comatose patient. It is best to assume that there is a cervical spine fracture, and immobilize the neck and perform necessary x-rays. Other general signs of trauma such as contusions, fractures, lacerations, and abrasions, should also be noted.

Skin

Needle tracts suggest IV drug use. Cyanosis suggests hypoxemia, polycythemia, or an abnormal hemoglobin. Pallor likewise may be an early indication that the patient has inadequate oxygen-carrying capacity due to blood loss or anemia. Carbon monoxide poisoning may produce a cherry-red glow of the mucous membranes. Other more generalized skin findings such as multiple abscesses, cellulitis, uremic frost, or icterus may point to underlying conditions which affect mental status.

Breath

One should never assume that coma is due to alcohol merely because the odor of alcohol is detectable. The fruity fragrance of acetone or the distinct odor of anaerobic infection should be noted. Fetor hepaticus indicates advanced liver disease. A feculent odor suggests bowel obstruction, while the distinctive odor of almonds indicates cyanide poisoning.

Cardiac Examination

Tachyarrhythmias or bradyarrhythmias can alter mental status because of decreased cardiac output. Endocarditis or arrhythmias which dislodge mural thrombi can produce cerebral emboli. Acute myocardial infarction may reduce cardiac output enough to depress consciousness. An intracranial lesion can result in static ECG changes, such as prolongation of the QT interval or ST-T changes, as well as arrhythmias. The mechanism is probably massive sympathetic outflow resulting in coronary spasm.

Abdominal Examination

Organomegaly, ascites, bruits, and pulsatile masses should be noted to detect conditions that are causative, or present but unassociated with a decrease in mental status. For example, hepatomegaly and ascites may be present in hepatic encephalopathy. The presence of an abdominal aortic aneurysm is consistent with advanced atherosclerotic disease. Grey Turner's sign (periumbilical ecchymoses) suggests retroperitoneal hemorrhage. A pelvic rectal examination should be performed in all comatose patients to detect bleeding, masses, infection, or foreign bodies.

Neurologic Examination

The patient should be observed for involuntary movement of all four extremities and abnormal posturing. The patient who is agitated and yet has decreased mental status may have a toxic encephalopathy. Opisthotonic contractions may be due to tetanus, strychnine poisoning, dystonic reactions, or decerebration. Seizures should be observed to determine if they are focal or generalized.

Respiratory Pattern

The pattern and rate of respiration should be noted and recorded, as it may indicate the level of neurologic injury in the patient.

An awake patient at rest generally breathes about 18 times per minute, and has occasional sighing or deeper respirations as demanded by carbon dioxide levels. When the cortex is no longer functioning and the nervous system is relying on diencephalic control of breathing, *Cheyne-Stokes respirations* occur. This is a type of breathing characterized by periodic, regularly increasing breaths alternating with short periods of apnea. The breathing crescendoes to a peak and then ceases suddenly. The apneic phase is usually short. The most frequent causes for Cheyne-Stokes respirations are bilateral metabolic hemispheric disease or structural disease of the bilateral cerebral hemispheres and basal ganglia. The principal mechanism underlying Cheyne-Stokes respirations has to do with loss of forebrain control of ventilatory stimulation.

Hyperventilation in the stuporous or comatose patient may be from a variety of causes. Attempts to correct hypoxia, compensation for metabolic acidosis, and brain injury itself all cause hyperventilation. Central neurogenic hyperventilation is frequently seen with midbrain involvement with destruction of those areas which normally monitor ventilatory patterns. When hyperventilation is caused by central nervous system disease it indicates upper brainstem damage.

Apneustic breathing is characterized by a prolonged pause at the end of inspiration, much like breath-holding. It is seen with lesions about the fifth cranial nerve. *Cluster breathing* is breathing in short bursts and is almost always associated with lesions at the level of the pons. *Ataxic breathing,* irregular breathing without pattern or regularity, is a forerunner of agonal respirations and death.

Autisms are involuntary neurologic acts carried out for maintenance and protection of the body. Yawning, although its mechanism is not well understood, frequently accompanies expanding lesions of the posterior fossa.

The autisms of vomiting, hiccuping, and coughing have neurogenic centers involved in their control. In the face of altered mental status, hiccuping, coughing, and vomiting may be indications of lesions involving lower brainstem centers.

Mental Status

Mental status may be the most sensitive early indicator of nervous system disease and is the first function to be affected in a variety of lesions. The ability to respond to voice and follow commands should be recorded. If the patient cannot respond to voice, then response to firm but gentle touch must be assessed. Finally, response to noxious stimuli is recorded. There is no need to inflict pain upon a patient suspected of feigning coma, since there are other more humane techniques for detecting functional disease.

Cranial Nerves

Visual threat is an unreliable test in unresponsive patients, since reactions can be checked voluntarily in certain awake patients. Lack of response to visual threat is not certain evidence for coma. Conversely, during visual threat, when air is moved toward the cornea, a blink response can result in a comatose patient.

Inspection of the ocular fundi gives the examiner the only opportunity to actually view the brain. Evidence of papilledema, hemorrhage, and spontaneous venous pulsations should be sought. Spontaneous venous pulsations in erect patients indicate normal intracranial pressure. This is often difficult to assess with comatose patients since they are recumbent. If spontaneous venous pulsations are seen when the patient is in the recumbent position, however, they clearly indicate that there is not increased intracranial pressure.

Pupils

The size, shape, and reactivity, both direct and consensual, of each pupil should be recorded. The pupillary pathways are relatively resistant to metabolic insult. They receive their parasympathetic supply from the thalamic pretectal region and their sympathetic supply from the superior cervical ganglion which courses along the carotid artery.

Pupillary findings must be interpreted along with the neurologic examination. As a general rule hemispheric disease has very little influence on pupillary function. Usually patients who are comatose from metabolic involvement of the cerebral hemispheres will have small to midrange pupils which are reactive to light. Structural lesions involving the diencephalon may cause small but reactive pupils.

Disparities in pupil size and reactivity can occur with eye trauma, ocular drugs, or previous eye surgery.

A unilateral fixed and dilated pupil should not necessarily be equated with an intracranial mass lesion. It may be the result of a cycloplegic agent instilled in one eye. An expanding aneurysm which compresses the third cranial nerve may cause an ipsilateral fixed and dilated pupil, but does not affect mental status. The general rule is that if a patient is alert, a dilated pupil is most likely not the result of increasing intracranial pressure. The mechanism for the fixed and dilated pupil seen with severe head injury is herniation of the uncus of the temporal lobe through the tentorial notch, which compresses the third cranial nerve. No patient with this degree of increased intracranial pressure will exhibit normal mental status.

Lesions which involve the midbrain tectal regions may cause midsized to large pupils which may respond poorly to light. Pontine lesions frequently cause fixed pinpoint pupils which are not affected by naloxone. Anoxia, atropine, and cycloplegics may all cause dilated pupils. Pinpoint pupils, which are reversible with naloxone, result from narcotics. Certain narcotics, however, such as propoxyphene, may leave the pupils intact and reactive. One cannot rule out a narcotic overdose strictly on the basis of pupillary size and reactivity.

Ocular Movements

In the awake patient, eye movements are directed by both anterior frontal lobe and posterior occipital lobe control centers which are connected to the pontine gaze centers. These gaze centers lie adjacent to the sixth cranial nerve, and in turn direct eye movements by way of the medial longitudinal fasciculus (MLF). The MLF, which runs from the upper cervical spine through the area of the third cranial nerve, is the principal interconnection for all conjugate eye movements. Because it extends over a considerable length into the brainstem itself, testing of the MLF is the best single method for judging intactness of the brainstem.

Without cortical control, most comatose patients will have roving eye movements, assuming the brainstem is intact. Eye movements may be disconjugate or conjugate, but as long as both eyes cross the midline there is no evidence of damage at the brainstem level.

The eyes may be abnormally deviated due to injury involving cortical gaze centers or pontine gaze centers. A general rule regarding cortical injuries is that the eyes will look toward a physiologically inactive lesion and away from an irritative, or active focus. For example, during a seizure the eyes will look away from the side of the seizure focus.

To decide whether the cause of coma is a cortical or brainstem lesion, oculocephalic mechanisms must be tested. The presence of oculocephalic reflexes depends on the fact that the MLF receives constant information as to the position of the patient's head through the output of the semicircular canals. Without cortical influences, an intact brainstem maintains the eyes forward or upward when the patient is supine. This is the basis of the ''doll's eye maneuver,'' the involuntary movement of the eyes upward and downward upon passive flexion and extension of the head. In a comatose patient in whom a cervical spine injury is suspected, the test is contraindicated.

Oculovestibular or cold caloric testing is a more sophisticated method to test the integrity of the brainstem (Table 10D-1). To perform the test, the examiner injects 50 mL of ice-cold water against the tympanic membrane. Countercurrent flow is set up in the semicircular canals and information is transmitted to pontine gaze centers near the ipsilateral sixth nerve nucleus. The altered endolymphatic flow allows the centers to believe that the head has

Table 10D-1. Oculovestibular Testing for Brainstem Integrity

Ice Water Effect	Interpretation
Both eyes deviate and good nystagmus produced	Patient is not comatose
Both eyes deviate toward cold water—bilateral—no fast phase	Coma, but intact brainstem function
No eye movement despite cold stimuli to both sides—indirectly	Brainstem—complete structure metabolic—drop—hypothermia
Movement of only eye ipsilateral to side stimulant but no opposite eye	Intranuclear ophthalmoplegia

been rapidly turned in the opposite direction. There are only four clinical responses possible:

1. Bilateral nystagmus
2. Bilateral fixed conjugate deviation
3. No response
4. Unilateral eye deviation

For the sake of the following discussion, we will assume that 50 mL of ice water has just been instilled in the right ear of a patient. If cold caloric stimulation of the right ear produces prominent nystagmus of both eyes, the cerebral cortex, MLF, and brainstem are intact. If both eyes move conjugately toward the side irrigated with cold water, and if they remain deviated in that direction, the midbrain and its brainstem reflexes are intact on that side. When cold water is instilled into the other ear, both eyes should again move conjugately toward the side of the cold water irrigation. This assures that the entire brainstem reflex system is intact, that the pontine and midbrain structures are functioning normally.

If the eyes simply do not move in any direction despite bilateral testing, the brainstem is structurally or physiologically functionless. For example, severe hypothermia, drug overdose, or brainstem herniation can all result in absence of oculovestibular reflexes. Therefore, lack of response to cold caloric testing does not necessarily signify an irreversible process.

Finally, cold water stimulation may produce an ipsilateral ocular response only.

If the right ear is irrigated and the right eye moves but the left does not, an intranuclear ophthalmoplegia is present. That is, the sixth cranial nerve on the side tested is functioning, but it is not able to transmit information to the opposite side of the brainstem. The opposite third cranial nerve which would cause the conjugate medial movement of the left eye has not been stimulated. Such a situation almost always indicates structural damage of the brainstem. This finding necessitates a rapid evaluation to determine if there is a structural problem which can be surgically corrected.

Other Cranial Nerves

Other useful tests of the cranial nerves involve the corneal reflex and the facial muscles. The sensory portion of the corneal reflex is mediated through the fifth cranial nerve. Its efferent motor reaction is processed through the seventh cranial nerve. One must look for both the direct and consensual response to determine if the reflex is working properly.

Facial asymmetry can only be judged in active motion. Particularly below the level of the nose, many normal people have mildly asymmetric faces. One cannot rule in or out a seventh-nerve lesion on the basis of a mild lower facial asymmetry at rest.

The eighth cranial nerve is of little localizing value in stuporous and comatose patients. Its fibers cross through the trapezoid body at the level of the lower pons and are therefore not strictly isolated to a particular side of the brainstem. Examination of the ninth, tenth, eleventh, and twelfth cranial nerves in comatose patients is likewise of little value in determining the level of functioning or underlying mechanism. Documentation of the gag response, however, is important to evaluate the risk of aspiration.

Motor Testing

The first part of the motor examination, observation, should have already been completed. Spontaneous motor movements are gen-

erally a good sign. The ability of the muscles to move without external stimuli indicates the patient is sending some cortical instructions down the motor pathway. Any patient who can follow a command or move a body part on command is showing high-level motor system function. Such a patient is not comatose.

Responses to stimuli help to isolate the level at which the nervous system is functioning. Abduction of the limbs or movements toward the site of noxious stimulation show motor system involvement, at least at diencephalic levels.

Decorticate posturing is hyperextension in the legs, and flexion at the arms and the elbows with the hands coming in toward the center of the body. Such posturing can occur with lesions of the internal capsule and upper midbrain which interfere with the corticospinal pathways.

Decerebrate rigidity, in which the teeth are clenched and the arms and legs extended, is seen in only a few situations. It usually is caused by severe disease involving the central midbrain, leaving the lower brainstem below the central midbrain regions intact. Posterior fossa lesions causing pressure against the brainstem may also cause this type of posturing. Decerebrate posturing can also accompany postanoxic cerebral demyelinization.

Total paralysis in the comatose patient with no posturing despite the application of noxious stimuli should be considered a grave finding. This indicates that no protective brainstem mechanisms are functioning. This can be seen in severe, deep, metabolic and toxic comas but is more likely in structural lesions which affect the brainstem nuclei. To be certain that no movement is possible, stimuli must be given both above and below the foramen magnum. Patients with cervical spinal injuries may only be able to grimace or move facial musculature if their motor tracts have been severed in the cervical cord region.

Sensory Examination

Sensory examination of the comatose patient essentially parallels the motor examination. Both the sensory or afferent fibers and the motor or efferent fibers should be tested. Hemisensory lesions as well as specific sensory levels should be sought.

Reflex Status

Reflexes in comatose patients may be sensitive but not terribly specific. An upgoing toe can indicate lesions along the cortical spinal tract all the way from the cerebral cortex down to the motor neuron. The importance of reflex testing in the comatose patient, as in the awake patient, lies in determining the general level of the lesion by comparing responses side to side and top to bottom. Abdominal reflexes are of extremely low value and not worth testing in comatose patients.

In summary, the neurologic examination (see Table 10D-2) of the patient with altered mental status has only a few areas of vital importance. Correct assessment of the level of mental status is paramount. Examination of respiratory pattern, extraocular movements, pupils, and motor function all need to be simultaneously integrated to determine the level of neurologic function. The principal goal of the neurologic examination is to distinguish structural, localized lesions from diffuse metabolic disease.

LABORATORY AND X-RAY EVALUATION

The selection of laboratory and radiographic tests is guided by the history and initial evaluation. However, initial supportive therapy

Table 10D-2. Rostrocaudal Brainstem Deterioration Secondary to Expanding Right Supratentorial Mass

Anatomic Level	Consciousness	Respiration	Pupils	Oculovestibular	Motor
Upper diencephalon	Drowsy (dull)	Eupnea with yawns and sighs	Small, reactive	Depression of ocular checking and fast component of nystagmus	Left hemiparesis, bilat. paratonia
Lower diencephalon	Coma	Cheyne-Stokes (CSR)	Small, reactive	Loss of above	Left hemiparesis, decorticate
Mesencephalon	Coma	CSR Central Neurogenic Hyperventilation (CNH)	Midposition fixed (MPF)	Dysconjugate response (loss of medial rectus function on horizontal gaze)	Decerebrate
Upper pons	Coma	CNH: ataxic	MPF	As above	Weak decerebrate
Lower pons	Coma	Ataxic; eupnea	MPF	None	Flaccid; areflexic
Medulla	Coma	Apnea	MPF	None	Same

for the comatose patient must be done first, and an orderly approach to the laboratory can then follow.

A complete blood count is generally routine. Severe anemia or leukemias may be of diagnostic importance in coma.

Alterations in serum electrolytes, such as hyper- or hyponatremia or hypercalcemia, can cause altered mental status. Coma can result from sudden shifts in serum osmolality below 260 mOsm/L, and above 330 mOsm/L. Glucose, sodium, and the alcohols are the most potent osmotically active substances generally encountered in clinical medicine. Hypoglycemia has been previously discussed.

Blood urea nitrogen (BUN), if it rises slowly, is usually not a cause of coma. Patients in whom there has been a sudden increase in BUN above 60 mg/100 mL may suffer significant alterations in mental status.

Arterial blood gases must be determined in all comatose patients. Hypoxia and hypercarbia can cause coma, and alkalosis and acidosis can change mental status.

Toxic drug screening should be ordered for those patients who have a nonfocal cause for coma and in whom no other discernible abnormal laboratory studies are found. However, toxic screens usually take several hours to complete and basic treatment decisions must be made before results are obtained.

The indication for emergency lumbar puncture is a strong suspicion of a nonfocal infection of the central nervous system. Lumbar puncture is contraindicated in the presence of a mass lesion. In all other circumstances lumbar puncture is at least relatively contraindicated until a CT scan is performed.

The EEG evaluation should be reserved for in-hospital patients who have been properly stabilized and where the usual causes of coma are ruled out. Its basic function at that point is to document lack of cortical activity.

The most important radiologic study is that of the cervical spine, to rule out fracture. A cross-table lateral view, followed by anteroposterior and odontoid views, are the minimum views needed. Even if the cervical spine films are found to be normal, if cervical cord injury is suspected, the neck must remain immobilized.

The CT scan has become the definitive test in the management of focal neurologic disease. In coma patients, the CT scan can detect not only intracranial lesions but fractures of the skull as well. It can detect amounts of blood as minute as 5 mL. Cervical spine films must be done before a CT scan as it is impossible to position the patient in the scanner without flexing the neck. If an emergency department does not have access within its hospital to CT scanning it should have transfer arrangements available to obtain the study when focal neurologic disease entities are suspected.

SPECIFIC CAUSES OF STUPOR AND COMA

There are literally hundreds of chemical agents and disease entities which can alter mental status. Before individual entities can be discussed it is necessary to review the most common general categories which cause coma. Two mnemonics can be useful: the word TIPS and the vowels A, E, I, O, U (Table 10D-3). By considering these disease entities important causes of coma will not be overlooked.

From an operational standpoint, the neurologic examination and laboratory studies divide the causes of altered mental status into toxic metabolic diseases and supratentorial and infratentorial structural lesions which affect the reticular activating formation. It is useful, therefore, to review some specific disease entities based on this categorization. The following etiologies of coma represent a review of the more common causes encountered in the emergency department.

Toxic and Metabolic Disorders

In most hospital emergency departments, metabolic causes dominate as the principal mechanism of coma. When toxic ingestions of drugs or other chemicals are included in this group, it is clearly the leading cause of coma in the United States. Intrinsic neurologic diseases such as Schelder's leukodystrophy and other intrinsic nervous system diseases can cause coma but they develop over a long period of time, and will not usually be confused with acute decreases in mental status.

10D-3. Mnemonic Aid for Coma Causes

TIPS	Vowels
T—Trauma; all types, temperature I—Infection—neurologic and systemic P—Psychiatric and porphyria S—Space-occupying lesions, stroke, subarachnoid hemorrhage, shock	A—Alcohol and ingested drugs and toxins E—Endocrine—all types exocrine, liver, electrolytes I—Insulin—diabetes mellitus O—Oxygen and opiates U—Uremia, renal causes including hypertensive problems

Glucose metabolism. In many series, the most common cause of altered mental status in the emergency department is hypoglycemia. Both hyper- and hypoglycemia may cause alterations of mental status. Diabetics are at high risk for altered mental status, not only because of abnormal glucose metabolism but because of infection and other metabolic derangements. Hypoglycemia is not only seen in diabetics. Patients with pancreatic tumors, retroperitoneal sarcomas, and chronic alcoholics with liver disese may also present in a hypoglycemic state. Severe hypoglycemia can be induced with oral hypoglycemic agents.

Liver disease. In advanced stages of cirrhosis and other degenerative liver diseases, cellular changes are seen in the brain. These abnormal cells probably contribute to decreased mentation but have an unknown affect on the actual level of consciousness. Rapid elevations of serum ammonia levels may contribute to depressed mental status. Patients with advanced liver disease frequently have decreased liver glycogen stores, predisposing to hypoglycemia.

Uremia. Uremic patients basically have no pathologic changes in the cells of their brain. The coma of uremia is related to changes in osmolality as the BUN rises. Cerebral water content will adjust to very gradual changes in BUN, but coma may develop with a rapid rise in the BUN.

Oxygen. All portions of the cardiorespiratory system can be involved as causes of coma. Severe anemia decreases oxygen delivered to the brain. Low cardiac output due to arrhythmias or loss of myocardial contractility can cause decreased cerebral perfusion. Occasionally, older patients placed on antihypertensive medications will become lethargic. Blood pressure may have been reduced too rapidly, causing cerebral hypoperfusion. A rapid increase in P_{CO_2}, as with pulmonary disease, correlates closely with neurologic symptoms. With chronic hypercarbia, however, mental status does not deteriorate because the brain can become adjusted to higher levels of P_{CO_2}.

Endocrine disorders. Alterations in serum sodium affect the central nervous system by changing the serum osmolality and causing shifts in intracellular brain fluid. Extreme hypothyroidism can likewise cause metabolic shifts which result in depressed mental status or even coma. Hyperthyroidism, on the other hand, usually causes an agitated and tremulous state, and coma is not seen until the patient is in severe thyroid storm or suffers a cerebral vascular accident.

Carcinoma. Coma can be caused by the remote effects of cancer. Hyponatremia due to inappropriate antidiuretic hormone (ADH) secretion in carcinoma of the lung, pancreas, ovary, and prostate are well recognized. Metabolic alkalosis in association with Cushing's syndrome may become severe enough to alter mental status. The progressive multifocal leukoencephalopathies seen with lymphomas may first present with a depression of consciousness. Hyper- or hypocalcemia may also cause alterations in mental status.

Poisons and toxins. Alcohol is still the most widely used and most popular metabolic poison. Its effects are usually short-lived and it is metabolized within a matter of hours. Barbiturate comas, on the other hand, may be of extremely long duration, depending on the type of barbiturate ingested. Cases of barbiturate coma lasting several weeks followed by the return of normal mental status have been recorded. Severe metabolic acidosis from drugs such as methyl alcohol, ethylene glycol, and paraldehyde can be seen in patients who readily abuse the more traditional ethanol.

Central nervous system infections. Central nervous system infections and septicemia can be included in the toxic metabolic causes of coma. Meningitis can cause alterations in mental status.

In bacterial meningitis, most notably tuberculous meningitis, the infecting organisms can compete with the brain itself for glucose. Viral encephalitis may markedly alter consciousness and may at first present as an acute encephalopathy, followed by a rapid downhill course with depressed mental status. It should not be forgotten that severe infection anywhere in the body can produce little-understood substances which can cause depressed mental status.

Subarachnoid hemorrhage. Subarachnoid hemorrhage is the only intracranial hemorrhage which is not focal in nature. Bleeding into the subarachnoid space quickly spreads throughout the cerebral spinal fluid. The resultant vasospasm is an initial homeostatic attempt to stop subarachnoid bleeding. This vasospasm may be partially responsible for the rapid decrease in mental status. Subarachnoid hemorrhage should be considered high on the list of diagnostic possibilities in all patients who experience headache with decreasing mental status.

Epilepsy. A general rule is "all that seizes is not epilepsy." A patient who has had a seizure may present to the emergency department in postictal coma. If the underlying disease is truly idiopathic epilepsy, the patient usually has a rapid return to normal mental status without residual focal deficits. Seizures lasting more than 15 min should be suspected to be structural in nature. It is always important to check for underlying causes of seizures such as encephalitis, meningitis, metabolic abnormalities, and trauma.

Disorders of temperature regulation. Hypothermia below the level of 32°C can in and of itself depress neurologic functioning enough to cause coma. Hypothermia may result from underlying diseases such as myxedema or hypopituitarism, or ingested toxins. Hyperthermia above the level of 42°C may also depress mental status to the point of coma. Patients with severe hyper- or hypothermia frequently have underlying neurovascular disease and are often left with severe neurologic residues.

Cofactor disease. Wernicke's encephalopathy due to carbohydrate overload and lack of thiamine can cause coma. Also, in rare instances of severe nutritional deprivation, altered mental status may be seen as the result of other minor cofactor deficiencies such as cobalt, manganese, or zinc.

Supratentorial Focal Lesions

These are localized anatomic lesions lying wholly or partially in the area above the tentorium cerebelli. They affect mental status principally by increased pressure, which compromises the reticular activating formation, and by bilateral cerebral hemisphere involvement. Such focal pressure may cause herniation of the temporal lobe (uncus) into the infratentorial space. This compresses the ipsilateral third cranial nerve, causing the uncal syndrome, with ataxic respirations, contralateral hemiparesis, and ipsilateral pupillary dilatation being the most common manifestations.

Subdural hematoma. In older patients, trauma victims, alcoholics, and those patients on anticoagulants, subdural hematoma is always a consideration. Even if focal neurologic findings are not present, if the patient belongs to one of these groups and has an acute change in mental status, subdural hematoma should still be considered. Subdural hematomas may compress supratentorial structures bilaterally and thus present much like dementia or progressive encephalopathy. A history of trauma, although helpful, is certainly not necessary to entertain the diagnosis of subdural hematoma. In chronic subdural hematomas, symptoms can fluctuate mildly from day to day. Laboratory tests, EEGs, and skull x-rays are of little value in diagnosis. The test of choice if this lesion is suspected is the enhanced CT scan.

Acute epidural hematoma. Acute epidural hematomas are almost always related to major trauma. The bleeding is usually the result of tearing of the middle meningeal artery due to skull fracture. Unlike subdural bleeding which is venous, epidural bleeding is arterial in nature and therefore progresses rapidly. The suspected epidural hematoma must be treated aggressively if the patient is to be salvaged.

Subdural empyema. This is a relatively rare cause of coma but must be considered in patients who have recently undergone otolaryngologic surgery, particularly related to acute sinusitis. It is occasionally seen in conjunction with acute meningitis when *Streptococcus* is the offending organism. Meningitis is not associated with focal neurologic signs. If a patient has symptoms of meningitis plus focal findings, a subdural empyema or brain abscess should be considered. Herpes simplex encephalitis, although a diffuse disease, tends to have a particular predilection for the temporal lobes. These patients thus present with temporal lobe-type syndromes and may appear to have a focal neurologic process.

Cerebral vascular accidents. The majority of thrombotic and embolic cerebral vascular accidents are not associated with coma or even significant decreased mental status. However, hemorrhagic cerebral vascular accidents are commonly associated with unconsciousness. Bleeding may be from a ruptured artery, aneurysm, or arterial venous malformation. When bleeding is the result of a hypertensive crisis, the exact site of the lesion is rarely found. If patients with severe hypertension become progressively obtunded, it is wise to stabilize the patient completely and reduce pressure to reasonable levels before attempting to localize the bleeding site.

Intraventricular hemorrhage is a particular subset of cerebral vascular accident. It is associated with an extremely poor prognosis, and death occurs within minutes to hours after pontine and medullary findings appear. The intraventricular hemorrhage does not, per se, harm brain tissue, but blood in the cerebrospinal fluid causes considerable increase in intracranial pressure. It is often very difficult to clinically differentiate intraventricular hemorrhage from pontine bleeding without the benefit of a CT scan. It is important to identify patients with acute cerebellar hemorrhage because this represents the most treatable of the intraparenchymal processes.

Cerebral neoplasms. It would be unusual for coma to be the first presenting sign of a cerebral neoplasm. More likely, the patient may present with a seizure followed by a prolonged postictal state. Bleeding into the tumor itself may cause symptoms indistinguishable from other types of cerebral vascular accidents. The slow enlargement of a supratentorial tumor produces brain swelling which can, over a period of time, dull mental status. Tumors in the lateral or third ventricles may obstruct outflow of cerebral fluid and cause acute downward pressure and displacement of the brainstem. In rare instances neoplasms directly infiltrate or destroy the cerebral connections of the reticular activating formation, causing irreversible coma. Almost all the findings in cerebral neoplasms, however, develop over an extended period of time.

Infratentorial Compressive Syndromes

The infratentorial compressive causes of coma are lesions which do not originate within the brainstem itself, but which by their proximity may compress the brainstem.

Basilar artery occlusion. The entire brainstem is supplied continuously by the vertebral basilar system. The reticular activating formation in particular receives paramedian branches off the basilar artery. Anything which interferes with the blood supply through the vertebral basilar system can cause alteration of consciousness. Posterior circulation transient ischemic episodes are often characterized as ''drop-like'' attacks in which there may be a total loss of muscular tone with or without a loss of consciousness. Problems involving the posterior circulation are extremely difficult to treat but need to be separated from other entities.

Traumatic posterior fossa hemorrhage. Severe trauma may result in bleeding below the tentorium cerebelli but without destruction of the brainstem itself. A hematoma in the posterior fossa can compress the brainstem and may be life-threatening. It is impossible to distinguish this type of hematoma from several other posterior fossa lesions on a physical examination basis alone. Since it represents a surgically correctable cause of coma it is imperative that it be diagnosed.

Acute cerebellar hemorrhage. Bleeding into the cerebellum is usually the result of a nontraumatic rupture of an arteriovenous malformation. Head pain and the onset of sudden vertigo with conjugate deviation of the eyes away to the opposite side of the cerebellar lesion are signs which strongly suggest acute cerebellar hemorrhage. This is the most treatable of the interparenchymal hemorrhages, and if relieved promptly, the possibility exists for good return of neurologic function.

Pontine hemorrhage. Pontine hemorrhage is a devastating, acute brainstem parenchymal lesion which produces coma. It is often difficult to differentiate acute pontine hemorrhage from acute cerebellar hemorrhage. These two lesions are both associated with sudden decreases in consciousness and ataxic breathing, pinpoint pupils, absent or abnormal ocular vestibular responses, and meningismus. Although there are some reports of successful drainage of intrapontine hematomas, the prognosis remains grave. Rapid diagnosis is crucial to separate this problem from an acute cerebellar hemorrhage, which is a surgically treatable disease.

Brainstem tumors. Actual parenchymal lesions of the brainstem, including angiomas, gliomas, and ependymomas, can cause brainstem compression syndromes. Most of these, however, progress slowly over a period of time and present with other localized neurologic findings before mental status is affected. Other posterior fossa tumors such as meningiomas and acoustic neuromas almost always present with cranial nerve findings before mental status is affected.

PRACTICAL ASSESSMENT AND MANAGEMENT GUIDELINES

Up to this point we have attempted to review the basic mechanisms and etiologies of decreased mental status. Translating this into action in the emergency department should now represent little problem. The following is a sample assessment checklist to be used for the patient with severely depressed mental status.

Airway established
Breathing checked (including auscultation to rule out pneumothorax)
Cardiac output assessed
Cervical spine immobilized
Obvious hemorrhage compressed
IV line started
Vital signs (full set)

Thiamine 100 mg IV

Glucose 50 mL 50% IV

Naloxone 2 ampoules IV, repeated if no response

The stable patient—historical features obtained including rate of onset, drugs, trauma, fever, prior episodes

General physical examination—signs of trauma; i.e.,

Battle's sign, hemotympanium, scalp hematomas and lacerations, subcutaneous emphysema of the chest, etc.

Obvious lesions of the abdomen, lesions of the pelvis, and long bone injuries

Skin

Needle marks, cyanosis, pallor, rashes, dehydration

Breath and odors

Alcohol, acetone, fecal material, fetor hepaticus

Cardiac examination

Rhythm, signs of decreased output, see auscultation—endocarditis, valvular disease

Abdominal findings

Organomegaly, ascites, bruits, flank echymoses (Grey Turner's sign), rectal and pelvic exam as time permits

Neurologic examination

Observation

Respiratory pattern

normal

Cheyne-Stokes

hyperventilation

apneustic breathing

ataxic breathing

agonal breathing

Autisms

yawning

coughing

hiccuping

vomiting

Mental status

responds to voice

responds to touch

responds to noxious stimuli

Cranial nerves

visual threat

inspection of fundi for papilledema and hemorrhages

Pupils

size

reactions—direct and consensual

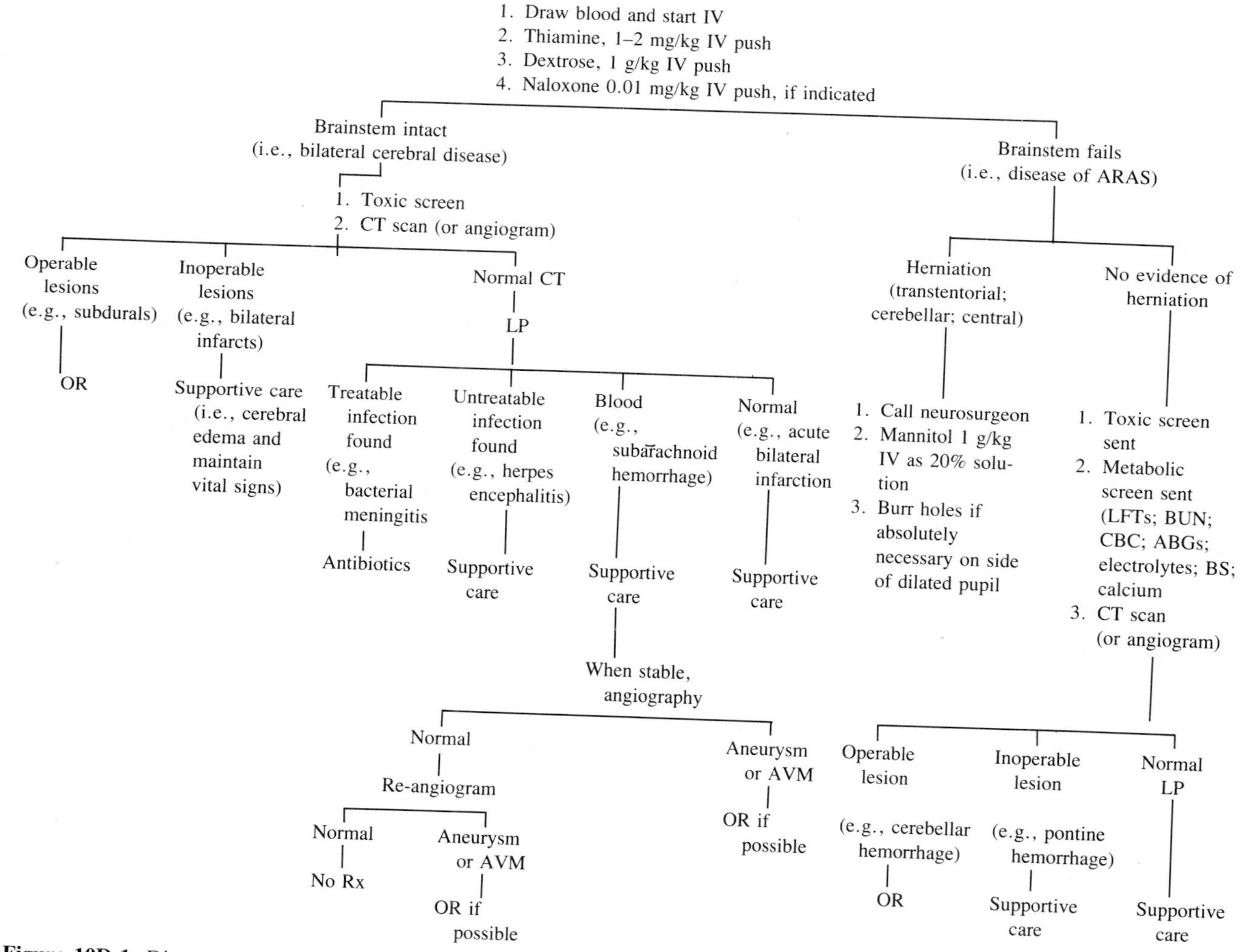

Figure 10D-1. Diagnosis and Treatment Protocol in the Comatose Patient (From Samuels MA: *Manual of Neurologic Therapeutics.* Boston, Little, Brown and Company, 1982, p. 13.)

Extraocular movements
   oculovestibular testing
   oculocephalic testing (if appropriate)
Corneal reflex
Facial asymmetry
Motor system
   posturing
   ability of the limbs to move
   stimuli
Decerebration, decortication, or true abduction by high-level
   centers
Pathologic reflexes

X-rays and laboratory studies. The need for all x-ray and laboratory studies is relative. The need for the following tests will be guided by initial examination and patient's intitial response to therapy.

CBC
BUN
Electrolytes
Glucose
Calcium
Toxic screen for drugs

Arterial blood gses
Cervical spine x-rays
Skull x-rays
CT scan
Lumbar puncture

Treatment Algorithm

Figure 10D-1 illustrates an excellent decision tree algorithm for the management of the comatose patient.

BIBLIOGRAPHY

Barr M: *The Human Nervous System,* ed 2. New York, Harper & Row, 1972.
De Jong R: *The Neurological Examination,* ed 4. New York, Harper & Row, 1979.
Fisher CM: The neurological examination of the comatose patient. *Acta Neurol Scand [Suppl]* 45(36):56, 1969.
Plum F, Posner J: *Diagnosis of Stupor and Coma,* ed 3. Philadelphia, Davis, 1980.

E. Headache

Carl Sacks

Headache is the phenomenon that ensues when the signals coming from the nociceptors, located in the head and parts of the neck, exceed the threshold for pain. Extracranially, all the soft tissue envelopes—skin, fat, muscle, blood vessels, and periosteum contain nociceptors, while the bony skull itself is devoid of them. Intracranially, nociceptors are found in the great venous sinus, its tributaries, the dura at the base of the skull, the dural arteries, the falx cerebri, and the proximal parts of the large arteries at the base of the brain. Signals from the nociceptors are sent through the A, delta, and C fibers of the Vth, IXth, Xth, and XIth cranial nerves, as well as by branches of the second and third cervical nerves. Extracranially, the fifth cranial serves the nociceptors of the face, most of the scalp, as well as the respiratory pathways and sinuses. Intracranially, it serves the nociceptors above the tentorium cerebri. The IXth, Xth, and XIth cranial nerves annex the intracranial nociceptors below the tentorium. Cranial nerves II and III annex the nociceptors of the occipital skull and the neck. Some fibers of these cervical nerves converge on the spinal nucleus of the trigeminal nerve. It is therefore possible for pain of nuchal origin to be interpreted as head pain. The afferent fibers synapse at their respective nuclei, with many of the postsynaptic fibers projecting to the nucleus gigantocellularis of the bulbar reticular formation, and the periaqueductal gray matter. Many adjacent groups of cells have functions akin to those of the substantia gelatinosa of the spinal cord, and inhibit the pre- and postsynaptic impulses, and thus block pain reception. There are also many areas, especially in the frontal cortex, that when stimulated inhibit the appreciation of pain.

There are only a limited number of mechanisms for producing pain. There must either be displacement of, distension of, traction on, or direct pressure upon either one of the aforementioned pain-sensitive structures, or upon a nerve itself that conducts pain. Finally, certain chemical structures can themselves lower the pain threshold.

Although much headache information may be gleaned from chemical and radiologic examinations, most useful information comes from a carefully taken history and the physical examination. The physician should seek answers to the following questions: What are the temporal relationships of the pain? What are the spatial relationships of the pain? What are the innate qualities of the pain? In short, the examiner must determine time, place, and quality of the pain.

Time. What events preceded the headache? How long does it last? What phenomena are associated with it? What are, and how long do sequelae of the headache last?

Place. Where does it hurt? Stimulation of extracranial pain receptors causes pain that is, in general, either felt at the site of stimulation, or it may be referred to a frontal area of the head.

Intracranial pain-sensitive structures above the tentorium are conducted by the Vth cranial nerve, and are felt in that part of the head anterior to a frontal plane that passes through each external auditory meatus. Intracranial pain of infratentorial origin is conducted by cranial nerves IX, X, and XI, and is felt in the part of the head posterior to this plane.

Quality. Pain of vascular origin tends to be throbbing in nature. Pulsating pain corresponds to distension of the pain-sensitive vessels by systole. It is aggravated by the recumbent position, which increases intravascular pressure and distension of vessels. One-sided vascular pain is often ameliorated by ipsilateral common carotid pressure, and aggravated by contralateral carotid compression. It must be noted that this procedure should be carried out only with great caution in patients with either a focal neurological deficit, or carotid bruits.

Pain of extracranial origin is often altered—either made better or worse—by direct pressure on the pain site. Pain of intracranial origin is often exacerbated by rapid, shaking head movements, which cause inertial displacement and increased traction on already irritated pain-sensitive structures. Finally, as we now understand the basic causal mechanisms of headache, we may infer that pain will be stopped or alleviated by reversing the basic etiologies: Stop the displacement, traction, distension, or direct pressure on the pain-sensitive structures; raise the threshold of the pain receptors; or prevent the brain itself from interpreting the incoming signals as pain.

The purpose of the emergency examination is to uncover any life-threatening manifestations concomitant with the headache, and any localizing or lateralizing neurologic signs that may further define the level of intracranial pathology.

As chemical causes of headache are legion, for example, hypoxia, hypoglycemia, uremia, or anemia, relevant radiologic and laboratory examinations are determined by a careful history and physical examination.

The basic and most important radiologic examination is, without doubt, the CT scan, which is without risk, and will discover, define, and locate all but the smallest intracranial lesion.

The electroencephalogram (EEG) is also a secondary tool. Slow-wave activity may be associated with an area of ischemia, a space-occupying lesion, or occasionally a migraine headache. Increased EEG response to photic stimulation may also be associated with some migraine headaches, especially if the subject has an associated history of travel sickness.

Following is a discussion of the pathophysiology, clinical features, diagnosis, and treatment of migraine headache, cluster headache, trigeminal neuralgia, subarachnoid hemorrhage, traumatic and posttraumatic headache, hypertensive headache, toxic metabolic headache, ocular headache, postlumbar puncture headache, and cranial arteritis.

THE VASCULAR HEADACHE

Migraine Headache

Classic migraine is a stellar example of a headache defined by temporal, spatial, and qualitative characteristics of pain. Although timing of attacks varies widely from one subject to another, it is characteristically constant for the individual, who usually can tell how many headaches he or she will have per month or per week, the times or seasons of the year when headaches occur more fre-

quently, the usual duration of the individual attack, and what may provoke or precede it. The prodome is a phenomenon that starts days to hours before the actual onset of pain, and is characterized by such variable emotions as elation, depression, hunger, or thirst. The headache itself may be immediately preceded by the aura, an ischemic phenomenon caused by vasconstriction of intracranial arteries. The nature of the aura is dictated by the site of ischemia. For example, ischemia of the retina or the occipital cortex may cause scintillating scotoma, or visual field defects. Vasospasm and ischemia of branches of the middle cerebral artery can result in contralateral hemiplegia or hemiparesis. Spasm of the vertebrobasilar vessels that supply the occipital cortex, cerebellum, and brainstem, can cause scotoma or blindness, ataxia, nausea, and even loss of consciousness.

The typical throbbing pain that succeeds the aura is due to arterial vasodilation and the effects of substances such as histamine, serotonin, prostaglandins, slow-reacting substance A, and some of the bradykinins. These substances set up a sterile inflammation, lower the pain threshold in the regional nociceptors and potentiate vasodilation.

Pain usually starts on one side of the head and not unusually becomes bilateral as the headache progresses. The site of onset may vary from one attack to another. The duration of pain may be from hours to even days in the rare cases of migraine status. Initially, the pain is throbbing amd more severe when the subject lies down. Throbbing may be ameliorated by direct digital compression of the painful area, or by pressure on the ipsilateral common carotid. A dilated, edematous artery may occasionally compress the third cranial nerve or its nucleus, causing a transient ophthalmoplegia or mydriasis—the well-known ophthalmoplegic migraine. With vasodilatation the vessels become more permeable, resulting in perivascular edema which tamponades the throbbing blood vessel. The pain then gradually loses its pulsatile nature and becomes dull and nagging. Sometimes during the pain interval there will be associated unilateral or bilateral parasympathetic manifestations such as lacrimation, rhinorrhea, facial flushing, and edema. Nausea and vomiting are invariably present. Although common migraine retains the characteristic periodicity, throbbing headache, nausea and vomiting of classic migraine, the aura is absent as is the prodrome.

Although migraine may occur at any age, it often begins in childhood or at puberty. With increasing age, the pain component of the syndrome may abort, leaving only a periodic prodrome aura or parasympathetic manifestations—the so-called equivalent. The logical specific therapy for migraine pain is to reverse vasodilatation and block the elaboration or action of the vasoactive substances that induce inflammation and lower the pain threshold. Raising the pain threshold directly, or dulling the cerebral appreciation of pain by nonspecific analgesics, is a purely nonspecific symptomatic but often necessary approach. The most frequently used vasoconstrictors are the ergotamine compounds and the β blockers. Methysergide is a potent antagonist of serotonin. Cyproheptadine is an antagonist of both serotonin and histamine, as is the new medication BC105.

The temporal pattern of a patient's migraine attacks will determine if therapy will be directed solely against each individual attack, or if continuous long-term prophylactic therapy must be added. If migraine attacks are less than once a week, therapy is directed at terminating the acute attack only. Here, ergotamines are the principal therapy. The sooner after the onset of symptoms they are started, the more effective they will be. They are ideally taken upon the appearance of the aura. The ergotamines are uniquely effective against the pulsatile characteristics of the migraine headache. As the headache progresses and the arterial walls become edematous, they are less responsive to vasoconstrictors. When the migraine passes from the throbbing to the constant, dull headache, the ergots and other vasoconstrictors are minimally effective. This phase is best treated with aspirin, acetaminophen, codeine, and other relatively nonspecific analgesics.

More frequent attacks call for a combination of daily prophylaxis to reduce the frequency and intensity of attacks, along with the aforementioned drugs for the acute exacerbations. The simplest and most benign preventive therapy consists essentially in avoiding red wines, ripe cheeses, and other foods rich in vasoactive amines. A time-release combination of ergotamine, belladonna, and phenobarbital is often used, either by itself or in combination with a β-blocking agent, such as propranolol, at the starting dose of 20 mg three times a day. Methysergide maleate, 2 mg twice a day, is also effective. Amitriptyline has been found to be occasionally useful in a combination of migraine and depression that has been unresponsive to usual therapy.

Ergotamine can cause a feeling of lightheadedness and drowsiness. Its action as a potent smooth-muscle constrictor can cause peripheral ischemia and necrosis. It is contraindicated in pregnancy, hypertension, and coronary or other vascular insufficiency. Propranolol can aggravate asthma or other forms of respiratory insufficiency. It is equally contraindicated in sinus bradycardia, advanced heart block, cardiogenic shock, and congestive heart failure. Propranolol may cause a warning tachycardia secondary to hypovolemia, hypoxia, or hypoglycemia. Methysergide maleate can induce nausea, vomiting, diarrhea, drowsiness, and ataxia. Prolonged uninterrupted therapy has been associated with retroperitoneal fibrosis leading to hydronephrosis, and Leriche syndrome. Associated pulmonary fibrosis has been alluded to in the literature. In view of its potential for major disaster, methysergide maleate should not be given for prolonged periods, and the prescribing physician is obligated to keep constant vigil for the first signs of major complications.

Cluster Headache

The cluster headache is another example of a recurrent headache with a pathognomonic time and place profile. The patient is more likely to be male than female, and age of onset is from the mid-thirties to midforties. Unlike migraine, there is no prodrome or aura, and pain is not associated with nausea or vomiting. There is a marked but not exclusive tendency for the attacks to be nocturnal, often arousing the subject from sleep. With rare exceptions, the attacks occur at the same time of the year, and at the same time of the day. Each individual attack seems to be of the same length, usually ½ to 2 h; and each daily attack or cluster seems to have the same number of small individual attacks. Each individual attack is invariably in the same side of the face, lasts for several minutes, and is described as intensely burning and boring. It is frontal in origin, and does not extend back into the scalp, as does migraine. It is always accompanied by intense ipsilateral vasodilatation, facial flushing, lacrimation, and rhinorrhea, and there may be an associated Horner's syndrome in up to one-third of all cases. There are no trigger zones as in trigeminal neuralgia. The whole series of clusters last from 1 to 3 months.

Postulated etiologies are the unilateral elaboration of a vaso-dilator substance such as a histamine, or a unilateral seventh-nerve parasympathetic stimulation, or sympathetic inhibition. An unfamiliar variation of the above is the chronic cluster headache, which commences as above, but with time, intervals between headaches diminish, and the duration of headaches increases, culminating in a prolonged hemifacial pain and associated parasympathetic symptoms.

Treatment is similar to that of migraine, only interval treatment is now obligatory. Intramuscular, oral, or sublingual ergotamine counteract the acute attack. Interval, oral ergotamine and propranolol may also help, but not infrequently must be combined with methysergide maleate. Recently, fair to excellent results have been reported with prednisone, indomethacin, and lithium carbonate.

Trigeminal Neuralgia

Trigeminal neuralgia can be considered as epilepsy of the fifth cranial nerve. The patient is usually middle-aged, in the fifth decade, and twice as likely to be female as male. The pain, which is almost exclusively unilateral in distribution, presents as an incredibly painful series of paroxysms, which follow the distribution of a branch of the trigeminal nerve. The second and third branches are affected with approximately equal frequency. Pain occurring simultaneously in both the second and third branches is not exceptional; pain in the first branch of the trigeminal nerve is rare, and pain in all three branches should make one contemplate an alternative diagnosis. The character of the pain is searing and electrical, not unlike the sensation evoked by a dental drill on a live nerve. Each paroxysm lasts from seconds to a few minutes, and is followed by a minute or so of remission before the onslaught of the next attack. The whole series of electrical volleys may last for minutes to several hours. With time, the periods of absolute remission between series of attacks decreases, with the untreated subject often contemplating suicide as a legitimate alternative to agony. Unlike migraine, the pain comes without warning. There is no accompanying facial flushing, lacrimation, or rhinorrhea. Nausea and vomiting are not sequelae.

"Trigger zones" are the pathognomonic feature of trigeminal neuralgia. These are small areas around the lips, on the gums, and just below the nose that, when touched, will evoke an attack. They can be ignited by such proletarian acts as shaving, brushing the teeth, washing the face, eating, or drinking. There is often a latent period of a minute or more between stimulation and attack. There also seems to be a temporal summation phenomenon. A series of repeated stimuli of low amplitude, such as chewing, is usually much more provocative than a single one of higher intensity. Just as a seizure is the result of an aberrant electrical discharge of the cerebral cortex, the painful ictus of trigeminal neuralgia is the result of an aberrant electrical discharge through the fifth cranial nerve. The irritative lesion may be either in the nerve itself, or in its Gasserian or spinal nucleus.

In a 20- or 30-year-old patient, the examiner must consider multiple sclerosis, the demyelination process causing electrical instability. More commonly in the middle-aged patient the irritation may be secondary to infarction, ischemia, infection, or pressure of a space-occupying lesion. Not unexpectedly, selected antiepileptic drugs are the mainstays of nonsurgical therapy. Anticonvulsants which inhibit polysynaptic transmission and post-tetanic potentiation are most effective. The most frequently used drug, carbanazepine, is given in doses of 100 mg twice a day, to 200 mg three times per day. It can cause severe bone marrow depression, and has been less frequently associated with hepatic, neurologic, and dermatologic disorders, among others.

Phenytoin, the well-known anticonvulsant, has been used in doses ranging from 200 mg to 400 mg per day. It can cause dizziness, ataxia, confusion, gingival hypertrophy, skin rash, thrombocytopenia, megaloblastic anemia, and pseudolymphoma.

Chlorphenesin is a muscle relaxant with strong anticonvulsant properties. It is the least toxic of all current therapies for trigeminal neuralgia, but because of limited medical experience, it is used as a secondary drug. The starting dose is 400 mg twice a day, with the maximum dose being 2400 mg per day. Its major side effect is drowsiness.

Failure of medical therapy is the prime indication for neurosurgical elimination of trigeminal pain. The old and often unsuccessful alcohol injection of the Gasserian ganglion has been largely replaced by a progressive sectioning of the sensory roots only, accomplished with the aid of the operating microscope. Serious complications of the procedure are homolateral keratitis, facial numbness, and paresthesias. A small percent of patients have a postoperative facial paralysis that reverses in 4 to 6 months. Some experts have tried alcohol injection of trigger zones before definitive trigeminal surgery.

Subarachnoid Hemorrhage

The vast majority of subarachnoid hemorrhages are due either to direct trauma, with bleeding from small, broken vessels; or to rupture of a congenital aneurysm. Pain may be due to sterile inflammation, resulting from chemical mediators such as bradykinin, released during bleeding, or to traction, displacement, or direct pressure on pain-sensitive structures by a resulting intracranial hematoma and coexisting cerebral edema. Neurologic folk law alleges that the patient hears a sudden snapping sound in his or her head as the aneurysm ruptures. There follows a pain more intense and agonizing than the victim has ever known. In spite of this, he or she tends to hold very still, as the smallest head movement aggravates the suffering, as does the recumbent position.

The original site of pain varies, with a tendency for it to be frontal if the rupture is in the anterior part of the circle of Willis, or occipital if from basilar artery bleeding. In a short time, however, there is almost always a significant occipital pain component due to inflammation of the roots of the second and third cervical nerves as well as from downward displacement of the tentorium by cerebral edema. The neck becomes stiff to flexion and signs of cerebral edema such as projectile vomiting can develop. Papilledema is a latent sign and can appear 16 to 18 h after the onset of intracranial hypertension. Seizures, a sign of cortical irritation, occur in 10 percent or more of patients, and the development of a focal neurologic deficit manifested by anisocoria, hemiparesis, or hemiplegia often contributes to the picture. Alternating lethargy, agitation, and confusion are indicative of the accompanying encephalitis. Diplopia, secondary to the third, fourth, or sixth cranial nerve, and paresis, may also be present.

The single most important diagnostic study to obtain is the CT scan. It will demonstrate subarachnoid blood, the ruptured aneurysm, and any associated subdural hematoma. A lumbar puncture may confirm the diagnosis, but it will not localize the site of bleeding and could contribute to brainstem herniation. An arteriogram will show the exact architecture of an aneurysm or arteriovenous malformation, and confirm any associated vasospasm. It may be a high-risk procedure and is generally indicated if neurosurgical intervention is likely or if the diagnosis cannot be established by other means.

In a salvageable patient, an associated subdural hematoma is evacuated immediately. Most surgeons will not operate immediately upon the aneurysm or arteriovenous malformation itself unless there is no vasospasm, the patient is alert, and has no focal neurologic deficit. When faced with stupor, coma, or focal neurologic deficit, the neurosurgeon will equivocate until clinical improvement or death occurs.

Cerebral edema is minimized by restricting fluid intake, giving IV dexamethasone, 4 to 10 mg 6 h, and by inducing hyperventilation and hypocapnia. As a last resort, osmotic diuretics such as mannitol may be given intravenously at a dose of 1 mg/kg. Vasospasm has been treated with isoproterenol, aminophylline, lidocaine, and an assortment of slow channel calcium blockers with highly variable results. An intravenous continuous drip of ε-aminocaproic acid is used to minimize rebleeding. The dose is usually 4 g the first hour and 1 g per hour thereafter.

MUSCLE TENSION HEADACHE

Sustained contraction of the deep neck muscles and the muscles of mastication can cause pain, both by irritation of nociceptors in the muscle itself and in its richly innervated tendinous insertions onto the skull. Intense muscle spasm is often a primitive response to fear, depression, anxiety, or hostility; or may be a response to primary organic pain of cerebral or nuchal origin such as brain tumor, trauma, migraine, or cervical spondylosis. The pain is constant and nonthrobbing; it is not aggravated by the recumbent position. The muscle spasm is often palpable, and pain may be made worse by direct pressure or pinching of the muscle itself, or of its tendinous insertions. If the neck is stiff and painful, it is equally so in all directions of motion; and unlike meningismus, there is no differential stiffness or aggravation of pain on flexion. The head pain is often described as band-like or bitemporal, following the insertions of the frontalis, temporalis, and deep neck muscles. The most satisfactory and efficient means of curing muscle spasm headache is to discover and cure its primary cause. Failing that, the symptom itself may be treated with analgesics and muscle relaxants.

HEADACHE DUE TO INTRACRANIAL SPACE-OCCUPYING LESION

The headache of an intracranial space-occupying lesion is secondary to direct pressure, traction, or displacement of pain-sensitive structures—essentially the blood vessels on the surface of the brain, the blood vessels at the base of the brain, the falx, the tentorium, the dural vessels, and the great venous sinuses. If a space-occupying lesion develops in the profundity of the brain, away from these structures, headache may be a very latent sign, coming only when a pain-sensitive structure is irritated, either primarily by direct extension, or secondarily after formation of obstructive hydrocephalus and cerebral edema. In these cases, the headache is often preceded by focal or nonfocal neurologic deficits.

The patient complains of a headache unlike any he or she has ever had before. It is usually nonthrobbing, prolonged, and constant. The intensity may wax and wane during the time of day, possibly secondary to changes in the pain threshold. The patient may feel better lying down. At the beginning, there is relief with minor analgesics. The pain may be made worse by head movement. It is generally not affected by pressure on the headache site, unless a secondary muscle spasm headache coexists. Because of the complex sensory innervation, the pain site does not always correspond to the tumor site. However, a few generalizations can be made. A tumor below the tentorium is felt below the occipital area. A tumor above the tentorium is felt in that part of the head anterior to a frontal plane through each external auditory meatus. The pain is usually on the same side of the head as the tumor. Midline pain does not necessarily mean midline tumor, and midline tumor may give unilateral pain. Eventually, a careful neurologic examination will show a focal deficit. The radiologic examination of choice is the CT scan. Indeed, it is wise to obtain a CT scan in any patient suffering from prolonged or progressive headache of undetermined etiology, even when localizing or lateralizing signs, or signs of trauma are completely absent.

TRAUMATIC AND POSTTRAUMATIC HEADACHE

Head trauma plus lateralizing signs mean intracranial hematoma until proved otherwise. The approach is to make the diagnosis by CT scan and refer the patient to neurosurgery immediately.

Because the periostium and the dural vessels are richly endowed with pain receptors, headache is an early sign of an epidural hematoma. The headache is aggravated by head movement. Pain produced by palpation along a linear distribution should make one suspect a corresponding line of fracture. If the painful palpation traverses the path of the meningeal groove, epidural hematoma must be suspected. Ninety percent of all confirmed epidural hematomas have a fracture line traversing the meningeal groove on the initial skull x-ray. Another 5 percent will demonstrate fracture on repeat x-ray, and the last 5 percent are never associated with a radiologically demonstrated skull fracture. The absolute diagnosis is made by finding a biconvex lenticular displacement of the surface of the brain on the CT scan.

The diagnosis of acute posttraumatic subdural hematoma is made by demonstrating a crescent-moon-shaped displacement of the brain away from the inner table of the skull on the CT scan. As with any intracranial space-occupying lesion, pain is aggravated by head movement. And as with any head trauma, there will be pain upon palpation of the injury site, and pain with head movement. To ascertain whether the pain of head movement is due to a space-occupying lesion or muscle spasm, first, before the head is shaken, the examiner should squeeze the deep neck muscles and palpate the head around the insertions of the frontalis, temporalis, and deep neck strap muscles. Determine whether there is muscle spasm, and what sort of pain pattern manipulation elicits. Then have the patient gently shake the head. If the quality and distribution of pain is exactly the same as before, it is probable that the head maneuver is just activating the muscle spasm headache. However, especially in the case of trauma, if this head maneuver evokes an entirely new sort of pain, an intracranial space-occupying lesion

is to be feared. However, the stuporous, agitated, or fearful patient may not be able to distinguish different types of pain.

An atraumatic subdural hematoma may arise, especially in a subject with marked cerebral atrophy. Signs and symptoms are similar to those of intracranial malignancy or abscess. However, because there is significant free space between the inner table of the skull and the outer surface of the brain, there can be extraordinary expansion of the hematoma before it becomes symptomatic.

If a person suffering from documented head trauma returns to an emergency room because of new, more severe, or unremitting headache, it is wise to obtain a CT scan, even in the absence of localizing or lateralizing signs, to search for a post-traumatic space-occupying lesion.

THE HYPERTENSIVE HEADACHE

There are three basic headache and hypertension association patterns: vascular, cerebral edema, and muscle contraction. These patterns may either exist independently of one another, or gradually blend, or they may be commingled from the onset. Of course, headache and hypertension can coexist but be related.

The Vascular Pattern

If an increase in blood pressure causes a vasodilatation of pain-sensitive arteries, the typical vascular pattern of throbbing pain, aggravated by lying down and ameliorated by digital carotid compression, usually results. If there is a coexistent vasospasm, or if for any reason the hypertension is not accompanied by vascular dilatation, the vascular pulsatile headache pattern will not appear.

Cerebral Edema Pattern

The headache is now due to displacement of pain-sensitive structures and is akin to the space-occupying lesion pattern. It is constant, nonpulsatile, may be worse in the recumbent position, and often has a marked occipital pain component due to downward displacement of the tentorium and irritation of infratentorial pain receptors. Sudden head movement often augments pain. Projectile vomiting and papilledema can develop, as can diplopia and alternating lethargy and irritative behavior. It may be that the cerebral edema and the hypertension are two partially independent manifestations of a single cause, as in renal failure, with uremia. The hypertension may cause the cerebral edema directly or by stretching and irritating the frontohypothalamic loop, causing reflex hypertension.

Muscle Contraction Pattern

The pain from each of the two previous headache and hypertension associations can induce a reflex spasm of the neck, brow, and muscles of mastication. To review, pain is constant in the muscles, or at their origins and insertions. The muscles feel contracted and are painful to palpation. In addition, the same fear and anxiety-provoking situation that causes muscle spasm may also engender an adrenal-inspired hypertension, but this is almost always transient in nature.

TOXIC METABOLIC HEADACHES

The pain is, as we remember, constant, nonpulsatile, aggravated by head movement, and often with a pronounced occipital component. The vast majority of toxic metabolic headaches are vascular in nature and caused by a sudden vasodilation of the pain-sensitive arteries, often combined with a lowering of the pain threshold by the toxic metabolic substance. The culprit is a substance that is either taken into or made by the body itself during a pathologic process. The headache is pulsatile, made worse by lying down, and ameliorated by ipsilateral digital vascular compression. Foods containing tyramine, such as ripe cheeses, chicken liver, and pickled herring can cause headache in susceptible people, as does histamine. Nitrates, often found in preserved meats, and monosodium glutamate, the popular food additive, have similar properties.

The characteristic morning-after drinker's headache, or the disulfiram-related headache, is a consequence of breakdown of ethanol to acetaldehyde, a potent vasodilator. Some of the heavier alcohols found in wine and whisky have similar vasoactive properties. Withdrawal from vasoconstrictor, such as caffeine, can cause rebound vasodilation headache. Withdrawal from a substance such as aspirin, which raises the pain threshold, can occasionally cause a rebound, lowering the threshold and resulting in headache. Hypoxia and hypercapnia are both potent cerebral vasodilators. The latter, along with muscle pain, are commonest causes of postseizure headaches. Hypoglycemia and anemia cause vasodilation. It is currently postulated that the vascular headaches accompanying fever and infection are caused by released chemical substances similar to those implicated in migraine, and those accompanying the inflammatory process. Analgesics are only moderately effective; the definitive treatment is that of the cause itself.

A few toxic metabolic headaches, such as those associated with uremia and water intoxication, or vitamin A intoxication, are caused by cerebral edema and displacement of pain-sensitive structures.

OCULAR HEADACHE

Inflammation of the conjunctiva, cornea, or eyelids produces pain at a site of pathology and does not directly cause headache. However, there is often an accompanying spasm of the muscles of the iris and ciliary body, with induced miosis, myopia, and irritation of endogenous pain receptors. Iris and ciliary body irritation is not felt directly in the eye, but is referred to the ipsilateral supraorbital nerve. The pain is intense and throbbing. It is made worse when a bright light is shone in either the affected or contralateral eye. Analogously, the only refractive error that induces this particular head pain is hyperopia, where the ciliary body is in a continuous state of accommodation and muscle spasm. Mydriatics relieve this pain. A muscle contraction headache often coexists.

POST-LUMBAR PUNCTURE HEADACHE

The post-lumbar puncture headache is characteristically intense and throbbing, and unlike vascular headaches of other etiologies, it is worse in the standing position, and better when the patient reclines in a head-down position. After lumbar puncture, cerebrospinal fluid is lost from the cerebral ventricles. There is a subsequent loss of intracranial and perivascular pressure, causing increased pulsation of arteries. The headache can be minimized by withdrawing the smallest amount of cerebrospinal fluid, and by using a small-caliber spinal needle, so as to minimize post-tap leakage through the dural puncture site. Resting in a head-down position, augmented fluid intake, and nonspecific analgesics are also helpful. The use of a blood patch to seal the dural puncture site has met with variable success.

CRANIAL ARTERITIS

Cranial arteritis is an inflammatory process of the cranial arteries caused by diseases such as temporal arteritis, polyarteritis nodosa, the collagen diseases, and hypersensitivity angiitis. All these are associated with a sterile inflammation of the arteries and release of chemical substances that vasodilate and lower the pain threshold. The involved visible blood vessels are swollen, red, and tortuous in appearance. Pain is throbbing and usually burning, and aggravated in recumbency. Compression of the involved blood vessels will always worsen the burning sensation, but lessen the throbbing component. Involvement of intracranial vessels may produce blindness, cerebrovascular accident, or seizure. Treatment is with steroids and occasionally antimitotics.

In summary, a headache is only an epiphenomenon, a sign of stimulation of cranial receptors. By examining the innate qualities of the pain, as well as its temporal and spatial associations, one can define the origin as intracranial or extracranial, and determine if its origins are vascular, muscular, or associated with an intracranial traction and displacement. By combining these observations with a complete history and physical examination, the true etiology of the pain is discovered. Treatment is first and foremost etiologic and only secondarily symptomatic.

BIBLIOGRAPHY

Adams CGM, Ortron CC, et al: Catecholamines and enzyme histochemistry in migrainous arteries: Background to migraine. Second Migrainic Symposium, London, William Heinemann, pp. 19–29, 1967.

Alpers BJ, Yaskin HE: Pathogenesis of ophthalmoplegic migraine. *Arch Ophthalmol* 45:555, 1951.

Anthony M: Plasma-free fatty acids and prostaglandins in migraine and stress. *Headache* 16:58, 1976.

Anthony M, Lance JW: Histamine and serotonin in cluster headache. *Arch Neurol* 25:225, 1971.

Appenzeller O: Altitude headache. *Headache* 12:126–130, 1972.

Atkinson R, Appengeller O: Headache in small vessel disease of the brain—a study of patients with SLE. *Headache* 15:198, 1975.

Behrens MM: Headaches and head pains associated with diseases of the eye. *Med Clin North Am* 621:507–521, 1978.

Christie JH, Hirofumi TG, et al: Computed tomography and radionucleotide studies in the diagnosis of intracranial disease. *Am J Roentgenol* 127:171–174, 1976.

Davis KR, Taveres JM, et al: Computed tomography in head trauma. *Semin Roentgenol* XII(1):53–62, 1977.

Diamond S: Recurrent exertional headache. *JAMA* 237:580, 1977.

Dow DJ, Whitty CM: Electroencephalographic changes in migraine. *Lancet* 2:52, 1947.

Famis E, Haningtor E: A possible pharmacological approach to migraine. *Lancet* 2:298, 1969.

Graham JR: Cluster headache. *Headache* 11:175, 1972.

Hollenhoret RW, Brown JR, et al: Neurological aspects of temporal arteritis. *Neurolio,* :490, 1960.

Hortov BT: Histamine Cephalgia—differential diagnosis and treatment. *Mayo Clin Proc* 31:325, 1956.

Jane JA, Winn HR, et al: The natural history in intracranial aneurysms—rebleeding rates during the acute and long-term period, and implications for surgical management. *Clin Neurosurg* 24:176–184, 1974.

Janetta PJ: Structural mechanisms of trigeminal neuralgia. *J Neurosurg* 26:159, 1967.

Kadrow L: Lithium prophylaxis for chronic cluster headache. *Headache* 13:197–202, 1977.

Kankle EL, Ray BS, et al: Studies on headache—the mechanisms and significance of headache associated with brain tumor. *Bull NY Acad Med* 18:400, 1982.

Ken FWL: Evidence for a peripheral etiology of trigeminal neuralgia. *J Neurosurg* 26(suppl):264, 1967.

Maroon JC: Hemifacial spasm. *Arch Neurol* 35:481–483, 1978.

Matthews WB: Footballers' migraine. *Br Med J* 2:326–327, 1972.

Medina JL, Diamond S: The role of diet in migraine. *Headache* 18:31–35, 1978.

Parker HL: Trigeminal neuralgia associated with multiple sclerosis. *Brain* 51:46, 1978.

Pickering GW: Lumbar puncture headache. *Brain* 71:274, 1984.

Pozniak-Patewicz E: "Cephalic" spasm of head and neck muscles. *Headache* 15:261–266, 1976.

Ray BS, Wolff HG: Experimental studies on headache. Pain-sensitive structures of the head and their significance in headache. *Arch Sun* 41:813, 1949.

Sakai F, Meyer JJ: Regional cerebral hemodynamics during migraine and cluster headaches, measured by the 133 Xe inhalation method. *Headache* 18:169–175, 1978.

Sicuteric F, Franchi G, et al: An anti-aminic drug, BL-105, in the prophylaxis of migraine. *Int Arch Allergy Immunol* 31:78, 1976.

Simons DJ, Day E, et al: Experimental studies on headache. Muscles of the scalp and neck as forces of pain. *Assoc Res Nerv Dis Proc* 3:569–570, 1943.

Traub VM, Korzzyn AD: Headache in patients with hypertension. *Headache* 16:245–247, 1978.

Wadman B, Wermer I: Observations in temporal arteritis. *Acta Med Scand* 192:377–383, 1972.

F. Syncope

Richard Levy

INTRODUCTION

Syncope is a common disorder caused by a multitude of clinical entities (Table 10F-1). The broadest definition of syncope includes all symptom complexes characterized by a temporary loss of consciousness secondary to cerebral ischemia. The duration of unconsciousness and the resulting cerebral dysfunction are transient. Once the circulatory status of the brain returns to normal, the patient makes a rapid recovery and has no sequelae. Many disorders cause loss of consciousness but are not true syncope. For example, seizures produce abnormal electrical discharges and loss of consciousness, but cerebral hypoperfusion does not occur. Similarly, hypoglycemic loss of consciousness is not due to a reduction in cerebral blood flow.

The exact incidence of syncope is unknown, although it is a common presenting complaint in the practice of emergency medicine. The frequency grows proportionally with the age of the patient group, and is a harbinger of more serious diseases in the later decades. Not every case of syncope implies significant disease, but in some instances the symptom is premonitory to a major life threat. Consequently, the patient with syncope must be approached in an orderly fashion to ensure that important clinical entities are not overlooked while at the same time expensive workups of benign disorders are avoided.

DIAGNOSIS

Establishing an etiologic diagnosis of syncope is of considerable importance. Some causes are readily diagnosed, and because of their benign course require little follow-up. Others may be life-threatening, and must be identified before the patient leaves the emergency department. If the syncopal episode is thought to be due to cardiac or obstructive vascular disease, hospitalization is required to assess the underlying disease process and to prescribe treatment.

A careful history and physical examination should be performed on all patients with syncopal attacks. Precipitating events, the patient's position, frequency of attacks, and use of medications are keys to the diagnosis. Cardiovascular and neurologic systems deserve special attention. Patients who are elderly, debilitated, or already known to have underlying cardiovascular disease are at higher risk. These patients require a thorough examination of pulses, heart sounds, and vessels of the neck and abdomen. Checking for orthostatic changes in blood pressure and occult blood in the stool is essential to rule out acute blood loss. A complete blood count, electrolyte panel, blood sugar, blood urea nitrogen (BUN), electrocardiogram, and chest radiograph may be helpful in establishing the diagnosis. Further evaluation may require prolonged rhythm monitoring, exercise testing, echocardiography, or angiography.

Table 10F-1. Causes of Syncope

Cardiac:
  Rhythm disturbances
    Atrial arrhythmias
    Ventricular arrhythmias
    Pacemaker dysfunction
  Outflow obstruction
    Aortic stenosis
    Mitral stenosis
    Pulmonary hypertension
    Congenital lesions with right-to-left shunt
    Atrial myxoma
    Idiopathic hypertrophic subaortic stenosis
Vascular:
  Obstructive
    Transient ischemic attack
    Subclavian steal
    Pulseless disease
  Nonobstructive
    Orthostatic hypotension
    Vasovagal
    Hyperventilation
Reflex:
  Micturition
  Carotid sinus
  Posttussive
  Breath holding

Patients with a history compatible with one of the nonobstructive vascular or reflex causes of syncope usually provide a graphic explanation of their episode. In these patients, the physical examination is confirmatory, but other etiologies must be assiduously pursued. Treatment is individualized and further consultation depends upon the confidence of the physician.

SYNCOPAL ETIOLOGIES

More often than not syncope is due to a combination of abnormal processes. For ease of presentation, common causes of syncope are divided into three categories: cardiac, vascular, and reflex. However, this arbitrary division of etiologies does not infer that each entity can be easily confined to a single explanation.

Cardiac Syncope

Rhythm Disturbances

Bradycardia or tachycardia can produce syncope if cardiac output is reduced to the point of global cerebral hypoxia. Elderly patients with first-time syncope are often suffering from Stokes-Adams attacks. Electrocardiographic evidence of conduction system pathology should be sought in these patients. Other transient arrhythmias causing syncope include paroxysmal atrial tachycardia, atrial fibrillation with a rapid ventricular response, ventricular tachycardia, ventricular fibrillation, and atrioventricular blocks. Pacemaker failure is another cause of syncope and should be considered when evaluating elderly patients.

Transient rhythm disturbances are best detected using a portable electrocardiographic monitoring system (Holter monitor). However, this approach may take longer to detect the rhythm disturbance than is practical.

Outflow Obstruction

Syncope may occur as a result of obstructive lesions on either side of the heart. The most common left-sided lesion is aortic stenosis. With exertion, the narrowed orifice does not permit cardiac output to increase in proportion to increased oxygen demands. Transient arrhythmias may also occur in patients with aortic stenosis. Both these mechanisms cause reduced cerebral blood flow and then syncope. Other left-sided lesions include mitral valve prolapse, atrial myxomas, mitral stenosis, and idiopathic hypertrophic subaortic stenosis. These lesions rarely result in syncope, but should be considered if suggestive murmurs are present.

The major right-sided cause of syncope is pulmonary hypertension. Similar to aortic stenosis, exercise in patients with primary pulmonary hypertension requires additional cardiac output. However, the blood flow through the pulmonary bed is unable to keep up with additional requirements, and syncope may result. A similar picture may occur with pulmonary emboli, and is a result of circulatory inadequacy. Other right-sided causes of syncope include pulmonary stenosis and some congenital heart lesions.

Vascular Syncope

Vascular failure results in inadequate blood flow to the brain. Normally, the vascular bed is autoregulated and constricts following vasodilatation. Occasionally the vascular bed does not respond, and is coupled with little or no increase in heart rate. This combination results in reduced cardiac output, and global cerebral ischemia.

Obstructive Syncope

Syncope may follow an anatomical block to one of the vessels supplying the brain. Although Transient Ischemic Attacks (TIAs) may occur in concert with syncope, they are infrequently the sole reason for syncope. The presence of anatomic blocks may exacerbate the loss of cerebral blood flow while another physiologic event reduces the total peripheral vascular resistance or cardiac output. TIAs should be considered when syncope and reversible neurologic findings are seen concurrently.

The Subclavian Steal Syndrome may produce syncope secondary to significant obstruction of the subclavian or brachiocephalic artery. Blood is shunted through the contralateral vertebral artery and the circle of Willis down the ipsilateral vertebral vessel to resupply blood distal to the obstruction. Syncope may occur following upper extremity exercise when enough blood is diverted away from the brain to produce global ischemia. This TIA-like syndrome should be suspected if one arm has an abnormally low arterial pressure, a bruit is present over the affected vessel, or symptoms can be reproduced by exercising the upper extremities.

Another rare form of vascular obstruction causing syncope is Takayasu's syndrome, or pulseless disease. It is characterized by a segmental panarteritis of the vessels originating from the aortic arch or thoracic artery. The illness is usually limited to young women, especially Asians.

Nonobstructive Syncope

Orthostatic Hypotension is a collection of disease states which have in common the cardiovascular system's inability to adequately respond to assuming the erect position. In the recumbent position, less vascular tone is required to maintain cerebral perfusion. Normally the cardiovascular system responds to sitting or standing with a slight increase in heart rate and vasoconstriction. However, a person suffering from orthostatic hypotension is unable to compensate in this way. Satisfactory vasoconstriction on the venous and arterial side does not occur and the heart rate does not accelerate to the degree necessary to avoid a decrease in cardiac output. If the decrease is severe, syncope ensues.

The most common cause of orthostatic hypotension is volume depletion. The elderly are especially sensitive to volume depletion as compensatory mechanisms diminish with age. Diuretics, dehydration, or blood loss may induce this malady. Varicose veins and prolonged standing result in venous pooling, and produce relative forms of volume depletion.

Many types of drugs can cause orthostatic syncope. Antihypertensives which inhibit the sympathetic nervous system (e.g., α-methyldopa) or which act directly on vascular smooth muscle (e.g., hydralazine) are common offenders. Calcium channel blockers, nitrate, and phenothiazine preparations can cause peripheral vasodilatation.

If postural syncope cannot be explained on the basis of volume depletion or drug use, a neurogenic cause should be sought. Many diseases may damage the autonomic nervous system, producing a dysfunction at the level of the peripheral vascular smooth muscle. Diabetic and alcoholic neuropathies, tabes dorsalis, and syringomyelia are examples. A surgical sympathectomy has a similar effect on the vessel wall. Idiopathic orthostatic hypotension occurs rarely, and should be considered only when all other explanations fail.

Vasovagal syncope (fainting) is the most commonly encountered form of syncope, and is seen in both the healthy and unhealthy patient. The term *vasovagal* has been used to describe this occurrence because of the presence of arterial vasodilatation in combination with increased vagal tone. The attack typically follows exposure to a psychologically unpleasant and anxiety-provoking event. Pain, instrumentation, fright, or the sight of one's blood are common precipitants while fatigue and environmental temperature extremes increase the likelihood of the event. Vasovagal syncope does not occur in the recumbent position, and this information is important in formulating the diagnosis.

Initially, the arterial vasodilation produces a drop in diastolic pressure. With the onset of vagal hyperexcitation, the heart rate decreases, followed by a fall in cardiac output. In addition to bradycardia and hypotension, the patient experiences diaphoresis, loss of color, restlessness, and transient unconsciousness. Upon assuming the recumbent position, the symptoms usually subside rapidly.

Hyperventilation, a condition usually due to an anxiety attack, may produce another form of nonobstructive vascular syncope. The clinical picture includes numbness and tingling of the distal extremities and circumoral area, and can be terminated by slowing the rate of breathing or providing a rebreathing bag. Syncope occurs as a result of hypocapnia producing a transient cerebral vasoconstriction and concurrent peripheral vasodilatation.

Reflex and Miscellaneous Syncope

Syncope may occur as the result of a number of abnormal reflexes. All these causes are neurogenically mediated, and are produced by a decrease in cerebral blood flow.

Carotid Sinus Syncope

Syncope induced by stimulation of the carotid sinus occurs primarily in elderly patients, and has a higher incidence among those suffering from atherosclerosis. It follows internal or external compression of the carotid sinus, and may be produced by rotating or hyperextending the neck. Carotid sinus syncope occurs because of vagus-mediated cardioinhibition, sympatholytic vasodepression, or a central effect directly producing unconsciousness. The diagnosis can be made by electrocardiographically monitoring a patient during carotid sinus massage, but care must be exercised to avoid unintended occlusion of the carotid artery.

Micturition Syncope

This condition occurs in men of all ages and usually follows a period of sleep or recumbency. The event may occur during or immediately after urination. The episodes are brief, and full recovery is the rule. The explanation for this form of syncope is not known.

Posttussive Syncope

Vigorous coughing may provoke syncopal episodes. Transient loss of consciousness has been reported most frequently in bronchitic men. The physiologic mechanism is unclear but is thought to be related to a marked increase in intrathoracic and cerebrospinal pressure with subsequent fall in cardiac output, increase in peripheral pooling, and decrease in cerebral blood flow. Treatment should be aimed at preventing further coughing.

Breath-Holding Syncope

Breath-holding episodes are usually limited to the first two years of life. The child is usually responding to adverse circumstances, and familial relationships should be explored. Syncope may be due to the cerebral anoxia associated with respiratory cessations, or to carotid sinus hypersensitivity. Even though brief seizures may occur anticonvulsants are rarely required.

BIBLIOGRAPHY

Boudoulas H, Weissler AM, Lewis RP, et al: The clinical diagnosis of syncope. *Curr Probl Cardiol* 7:1–40, 1982.

Day SC, Cook EF, Funkenstein H, et al: Evaluation of emergency room patients with transient loss of consciousness. *Am J Med* 73:15–23, 1982.

Freidburg CF: Syncope. *Mod Concepts Cardiovasc Dis* 40:55–63, 1971.

Hess DS, Morady F, Scheinman MM: Electrophysiologic testing in the evaluation of patients with syncope of undetermined etiology. *Am J Cardiol* 50:1309–1315, 1982.

Noble RJ: Syncope. *Cardiovasc Clin* 12:119–129, 1981.

Wright KE, McIntosh HD: Syncope: A review of pathophysiological mechanisms. *Prog Cardiovasc Dis* 13:580–594, 1971.

G. Abdominal Pain

Judith E. Tintinalli

IMMEDIATE CONCERNS
- Ruptured abdominal aortic aneurysm
- Splenic rupture
- Ruptured ectopic pregnancy
- Bowel infarction
- Perforated viscus
- Acute myocardial infarction

''The general rule can be laid down that the majority of ['progressively'] severe abdominal pains which ensue in patients who have been previously fairly well, and which last as long as six hours, are caused by conditions of surgical import.''

Zachary Cope, *The Early Diagnosis of Acute Abdomen*

In adults with severe, acute abdominal pain, the most likely diagnoses are acute appendicitis, acute diverticulitis, perforated peptic ulcer, acute cholecystitis, small bowel obstruction, and acute pancreatitis. In females, acute salpingitis and pyelonephritis may be added to the list.

Despite the characteristic symptom complexes of most of these diseases, Staniland suggests that misdiagnosis may occur in about 30 percent of cases because the disease entity does not fit the accepted symptom pattern. A careful history and initial physical examination, repeat examination when the diagnosis is in doubt, and a high degree of suspicion for the less common causes of acute abdominal pain are the most important factors for accurate diagnosis.

Abdominal pain can be classified as originating in the abdomen, arising from extraabdominal sources, or due to metabolic and neurogenic disorders (Table 10G-1).

PAIN OF INTRAABDOMINAL ORIGIN

Intraabdominal sources of pain include peritoneal inflammation, obstruction of hollow viscera, and vascular disorders.

Peritoneal inflammation. The intestinal tract is colonized by many types of bacteria and the intact mucous membrane of the gastrointestinal tract forms a barrier to the development of infection. Disruption of the mucous membrane by disease or trauma can permit the development of infection involving the peritoneal cavity, viscera, retroperitoneum, or bloodstream.

Peritonitis is the inflammation of the peritoneum due to the action of an irritant. Aseptic peritonitis can be caused by substances such as gastric juice, bile, urine, blood, or pancreatic juice. Aseptic peritonitis may be a precursor of septic peritonitis.

The surface area of the peritoneum is equivalent to about 50 percent of the body surface area, so that peritoneal inflammation can lead to the exudation or transudation of large volumes of fluid, resulting in severe fluid and electrolyte disorders, and shock. Inflammation of the visceral peritoneum results in paralytic ileus, with bowel distension, and fluid accumulation.

There are two main types of peritonitis: primary and secondary. Primary peritonitis is uncommon and is chiefly caused by *Pneumococcus, Streptococcus, Escherichia coli*, or *Mycobacterium tuberculosis*. Secondary peritonitis is caused by disease or injury of the abdominal or pelvic viscera. It may involve aerobes or anaerobes and is often polymicrobial. Common causes of peritonitis

Table 10G-1. Classification of Abdominal Pain

Pain originating in the abdomen
    Peritoneal inflammation
    Obstruction of hollow viscera
    Vascular catastrophe
Pain referred from the abdomen
Metabolic disorders
Neurogenic disorders

are perforation of the appendix, diverticula, peptic ulcer, or gallbladder; gangrene of the bowel wall due to mesenteric vascular occlusion; intestinal obstruction, volvulus, or intussusception; pancreatitis; and pelvic infections such as endometritis or salpingitis. Rarely, infection involving male genitourinary tract may extend to produce peritonitis.

Signs and symptoms of peritonitis are abdominal pain and rigidity, fever, rebound tenderness, vomiting, decreased or absent bowel sounds, and abdominal distension. The quality of pain varies with the type and amount of irritant. For example, a small amount of gastric acid released into the peritoneal cavity as a result of a perforated duodenal ulcer usually produces acute, intense pain, whereas extravasation of urine may initially produce few signs or symptoms, unless the urine is infected.

Reflex spasm of the abdominal or pelvic musculature often develops in the area overlying inflammation. The intensity of the spasm varies with the location and severity of the inflammatory process. For example, an abscessed appendix that directly irritates the iliopsoas or obturator internus muscles will cause pain when these muscles are moved. Muscular rigidity may be firm and continuous, as in perforated peptic ulcer, or rigidity may develop when the abdomen is palpated over the inflamed area. Muscular rigidity may be absent even in the presence of peritonitis if it is due to pelvic inflammatory disease, if the patient has weak and flabby abdominal muscles, or if the patient is in deep coma.

Obstruction of hollow viscera. Obstruction or inflammation of the intestines, ureters, or biliary tree may produce intermittent or continuous abdominal pain.

Pain and abdominal tenderness, vomiting, and distension are symptoms of acute intestinal obstruction. Common causes of intestinal obstruction are adhesions secondary to previous abdominal surgery, carcinoma, incarcerated hernia, and volvulus.

Pain due to small intestinal obstruction is usually localized to the periumbilical area, whereas pain due to colonic obstruction is usually referred to the hypogastrium. Distension may at first be localized and detectable only on radiologic examination. As the obstruction progresses, distension becomes generalized and clinically apparent. The patient may be unable to pass rectal gas. Tenderness on palpation develops as bowel loops distend, but abdominal rigidity is not present unless peritonitis develops.

Vascular disorders. Bowel infarction, aortic dissection, or a leaking or ruptured aortic aneurysm are the major vascular disorders that can produce an acute abdomen.

The major symptom of bowel infarction is severe central abdominal pain followed by rapidly progressing signs of toxicity such as fever, leukocytosis, and hypotension. Hematemesis, loose, bloody, mucoid stools, and eventually, bowel obstruction develop. Abdominal pain is so severe that it is usually poorly controlled even with large doses of narcotics.

Aortic dissection is characterized by tearing pain originating in the chest or abdomen and radiating to the back. Depending on the site of dissection, focal neurologic signs or loss of pulses in an extremity may occur. Mesenteric or renal arterial occlusion may develop.

Intraperitoneal rupture of an abdominal aortic aneurysm is characterized by sudden cardiovascular collapse. But a leaking or expanding aortic aneurysm may produce abdominal and back pain and abdominal rigidity, and should be suspected if the back pain radiates to the sacrum, flank, or genitalia.

PAIN OF EXTRAABDOMINAL ORIGIN

The many extraabdominal sources of abdominal pain can generally be described as originating from the abdominal wall, pelvic disease, or referred from areas such as the chest. However, pain localized to the abdomen is usually caused by intraabdominal disease.

Abdominal wall pain. Pain due to myositis, or a contusion or hematoma of the abdominal musculature is accentuated by movement or pressure and may be described as superficial in nature.

Pelvic disease. In the female, acute hypogastric or pelvic pain may be caused by torsion or rupture of an ovarian cyst, salpingitis or pyosalpinx, ruptured ectopic pregnancy, torsion of the uterine fibroid, mittelschmerz, or septic abortion.

Acute salpingitis, especially if it is unilateral, may be difficult to distinguish from appendicitis. Onset of symptoms just after menses, presence of a vaginal discharge, and cervical tenderness (Chandelier sign) are characteristic of salpingitis.

Rupture of an ectopic pregnancy is characterized by sudden abdominal pain, hypotension or cardiovascular collapse, vaginal bleeding, and the presence of an abdominal mass and tenderness. The pain is generally hypogastric, but it can be epigastric or referred to the neck or shoulder.

Referred pain. Intrathoracic disease should always be suspected in a patient with upper abdominal pain. Pneumothorax, pneumonia, pulmonary or myocardial infarction, pleural effusion, esophagitis, or esophageal rupture can be associated with upper quadrant or epigastric pain.

Metabolic Disorders

Diabetic ketoacidosis and hyperlipidemia may produce acute abdominal pain in association with pancreatitis. Porphyria may produce severe pain and mimic intestinal obstruction, although muscle rigidity is absent and bowel sounds are normal or hyperactive. Black widow spider bites and scorpion bites can also cause severe abdominal pain. Generally, abdominal pain due to sickle cell crisis is accompanied by normal bowel sounds and rebound tenderness is absent.

Neurogenic Causes

Disorders such as herpes zoster or spinal disk disease can produce abdominal pain by compressing or irritating the spinal nerves or roots. A tabetic crisis consists of severe vomiting and abdominal pain, but abdominal rigidity is absent.

EVALUATION OF ABDOMINAL PAIN

History. A detailed, careful history is the first step in diagnosis. Questions about the pain should be directed to determine the time and mode of onset; character; location, shifting, or radiation; factors that relieve or intensify the pain; and the presence of associated symptoms such as dysuria, vaginal discharge, and nausea or vomiting.

The onset of pain is likely to be acute in disorders such as acute pancreatitis, ruptured ectopic pregnancy, or perforated duodenal ulcer. In the case of intestinal obstruction, symptoms usually are gradually progressive.

A perforated peptic ulcer may be associated with a sudden, severe, burning pain, whereas an aortic dissection is characterized by tearing pain. Pain associated with obstruction of a hollow viscera can be constant or colicky but is generally unaffected by movement. Pressure or movement accentuate the pain of peritoneal inflammation.

The localization and shifting of pain is a most important feature in diagnosis. Pain can be localized to the epigastrium, periumbilical area, hypogastrium, or a specific quadrant, or it can affect the entire abdomen. Table 10G-2 lists some conditions suggested by specific quadrant pain.

Diseases of viscera such as the gallbladder, appendix, stomach, and duodenum usually produce rather specific localized pain, whereas disorders of the small and large intestine may have less distinct localization of pain. Localized pain that becomes generalized throughout the abdomen usually indicates perforation and dissemination of contaminated material. Distension of the gallbladder or bile ducts generally produces steady right upper quadrant pain, often radiating to the neck or subscapular region.

In appendicitis, pain is due to obstruction and distension of the appendix by inflammation and is generally first noted in the epigastrium or periumbilical area. Some hours later, it shifts to the right lower quadrant. Shifting of pain to the right lower quadrant occurs most often with appendicitis but it can also occur with perforated duodenal ulcer or acute pancreatitis.

Pancreatitis may produce a variable picture but is most com-

Table 10G-2. Differential Diagnosis of Acute Abdominal Pain by Location

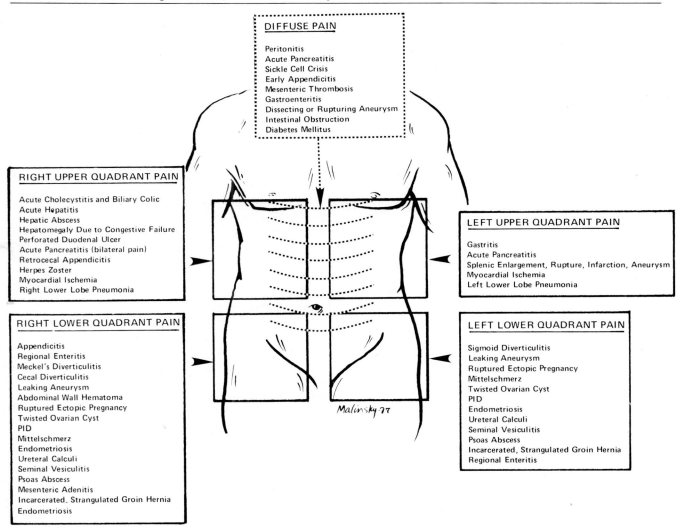

DIFFUSE PAIN

Peritonitis
Acute Pancreatitis
Sickle Cell Crisis
Early Appendicitis
Mesenteric Thrombosis
Gastroenteritis
Dissecting or Rupturing Aneurysm
Intestinal Obstruction
Diabetes Mellitus

RIGHT UPPER QUADRANT PAIN

Acute Cholecystitis and Biliary Colic
Acute Hepatitis
Hepatic Abscess
Hepatomegaly Due to Congestive Failure
Perforated Duodenal Ulcer
Acute Pancreatitis (bilateral pain)
Retrocecal Appendicitis
Herpes Zoster
Myocardial Ischemia
Right Lower Lobe Pneumonia

LEFT UPPER QUADRANT PAIN

Gastritis
Acute Pancreatitis
Splenic Enlargement, Rupture, Infarction, Aneurysm
Myocardial Ischemia
Left Lower Lobe Pneumonia

RIGHT LOWER QUADRANT PAIN

Appendicitis
Regional Enteritis
Meckel's Diverticulitis
Cecal Diverticulitis
Leaking Aneurysm
Abdominal Wall Hematoma
Ruptured Ectopic Pregnancy
Twisted Ovarian Cyst
PID
Mittelschmerz
Endometriosis
Ureteral Calculi
Seminal Vesiculitis
Psoas Abscess
Mesenteric Adenitis
Incarcerated, Strangulated Groin Hernia
Endometriosis

LEFT LOWER QUADRANT PAIN

Sigmoid Diverticulitis
Leaking Aneurysm
Ruptured Ectopic Pregnancy
Mittelschmerz
Twisted Ovarian Cyst
PID
Endometriosis
Ureteral Calculi
Seminal Vesiculitis
Psoas Abscess
Incarcerated, Strangulated Groin Hernia
Regional Enteritis

Malinsky-77

From Wagner DK: Approaches to the patient with acute abdominal pain. *Current Topics* (a program of the Medical College of Pennsylvania). 1:3, 1978, Used by permission.

monly characterized by severe epigastric pain radiating to the flanks or back.

Diaphragmatic irritation may cause pain in the area of distribution of the fourth cervical nerve with the result that pain in the neck or top of the shoulder may be due to conditions as diverse as perforated gastric ulcer, liver abscess, pancreatitis, cholecystitis, or ruptured ectopic pregnancy.

Ureteral obstruction can produce flank pain that radiates to the testicle or vulva or inner aspect of the thigh. However, pain due to inflammation of the appendix can also radiate to the testicle.

Vomiting can be caused by dilation of the nerves of the peritoneum or mesentery, obstruction of a hollow viscera, or direct medullary stimulation. Acute pancreatitis results in marked stimulation of the celiac plexus with severe vomiting. Vomiting can also be seen with disorders such as biliary and renal colic, pyelonephritis, and small intestinal obstruction.

In general, the higher the level of intestinal obstruction, the more frequent and intense the vomiting. At first, vomiting may be a reflex response, but later it occurs because of reflux of gastrointestinal contents into the stomach. Bilious vomiting implies that the irritation or obstruction is distal to the second portion of the duodenum. In a patient with a peptic ulcer, bilious vomiting implies that there is no pyloric obstruction. Feculent vomiting indicates that a large bowel obstruction with an incompetent ileocecal valve, or a lower small bowel obstruction may be present. Occasionally, vomiting may be absent with a large bowel obstruction.

Direct stimulation of the medulla by drugs or toxins can also cause vomiting, but in such a case, abdominal pain is absent.

The correct diagnosis can often be made by noting other symptoms associated with abdominal pain. For example, the association of abdominal pain with dysuria suggests pyelonephritis or cystitis, although a genitourinary infection can be present without urinary tract symptoms. The converse can also occur. For instance, an inflamed appendix lying in close proximity to the ureter may cause ureteral irritation with the appearance of a few white cells in the urine. The presence of a vaginal discharge and the development of pain at the end of menses should cause one to suspect a pelvic inflammatory disease. In the case of sudden, sharp, unilateral lower quadrant pain occurring at the middle of the menstrual cycle, mittelschmerz should be considered.

Physical examination. Physical examination begins with inspection of the abdomen for distension, localized swelling, or visible peristalsis. Muscular rigidity or tenderness will cause limitation of movement with each respiration.

Abdominal tenderness, guarding, or rigidity may be detected by palpation. If abdominal pain is due to intrathoracic disease, deep, continuous palpation may not increase the pain and may overcome any guarding that is present. Hepatosplenomegaly, a distended urinary bladder or gallbladder, a pelvic or abdominal mass, or ovarian or uterine enlargement may be detected. In all patients with abdominal pain, the inguinal and femoral canals should be examined for evidence of a strangulated or incarcerated hernia.

High-pitched tinkling bowel sounds may be present over an area of obstruction. These sounds are usually associated with colicky abdominal pain and are alternated with periods of silence. In the patient with diffuse, mild peritoneal irritation, continuous hyperactive bowel sounds are consistent with gastroenteritis. Bowel sounds are absent in severe ileus.

A pelvic examination should be performed on every female with acute abdominal pain, although even then it may be difficult to distinguish such disorders as unilateral salpingitis from appendicitis.

Prostatic or uterine hypertrophy and rectal bleeding, masses, or strictures can be detected by rectal examination. Tenderness elicited when pressure is exerted on the pelvic peritoneum suggests the presence of appendicitis or a pelvic abscess.

Laboratory studies. Leukocytosis is expected in acute abdominal states; this in itself is of no aid in the differential diagnosis. Vomiting and diarrhea may produce dehydration of electrolyte disturbances, so that serum electrolytes, glucose, and BUN or creatinine levels should be obtained.

A serum amylase level can aid in the differential diagnosis, although it may be elevated in many disease states such as biliary obstruction, pancreatitis, bowel obstruction or infarction, salpingitis, or ruptured ectopic pregnancy, as well as other conditions such as mumps or renal failure. The ratio of amylase clearance to creatinine clearance can be helpful in the diagnosis of acute pancreatitis, for the amylase clearance is increased in pancreatitis. A ratio of 5 percent or greater suggests acute pancreatitis, although an elevated amylase clearance has also been reported in burns and diabetic ketoacidosis.

A clean catch or catheterized sample of urine should be sent for analysis. Pyelonephritis or cystitis can mimic disorders such as salpingitis, cholecystitis, or even appendicitis.

Chest and abdominal roentgenograms are necessary for the evaluation of acute abdominal pain. Upright films of the chest, both posteroanterior and lateral, are desirable to detect free peritoneal air (Fig. 10G-1 and 10G-2). A plain film of the abdomen may demonstrate findings such as renal or biliary calculi, air in the biliary tree (Fig. 10G-3), free intraperitoneal air, an appendicolith (Fig. 10G-4), large or small bowel obstruction (Fig. 10G-5), or volvulus. An upright film of the abdomen should also be obtained to detect the presence of air fluid levels.

If the diagnosis is not clear, barium studies may be helpful as long as perforation is not present. A barium enema may be performed to demonstrate colonic obstruction. Generally, barium is not administered orally if bowel obstruction is suspected.

Abdominal paracentesis or lavage can be performed to detect the presence of pus, blood, bowel, or biliary contents in the peritoneal cavity.

CAUSES OF ACUTE ABDOMINAL PAIN

Common causes of abdominal pain include appendicitis, diverticulitis, perforated viscus, cholecystitis, small bowel obstruction, and acute pancreatitis (Table 10G-3).

Appendicitis. Acute appendicitis is the most common cause of the acute abdomen in the United States and Great Britain. It is

Table 10G-3. Common Causes of Acute Abdominal Pain

Appendicitis
Diverticulitis
Perforated peptic ulcer
Cholecystitis
Small bowel obstruction
Pancreatitis
Salpingitis
Pyelonephritis
Sickle cell crisis

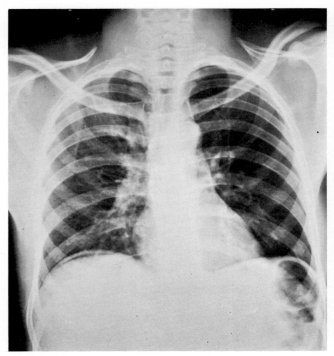

Figure 10G-1. This patient complained of severe upper abdominal pain the night before admission. On physical examination, the abdomen was rigid, and there was hyperresonance to percussion over the right upper quadrant. An upright film of the chest confirmed the clinical impression of a perforated viscus, probably perforated peptic ulcer.

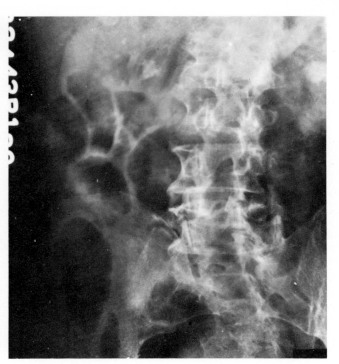

Figure 10G-3. Plain film of the abdomen in a patient with right upper quadrant pain. Note the presence of air in the biliary tree.

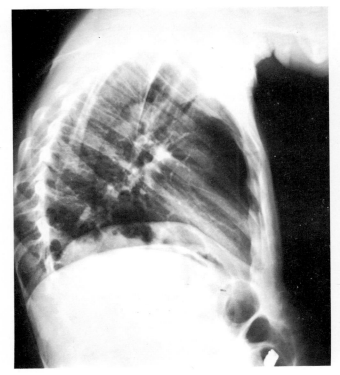

Figure 10G-2. Free air is easily seen under the right diaphragm on the lateral chest projection as well. The patient is somewhat tilted so that the left diaphragm appears much higher than the right.

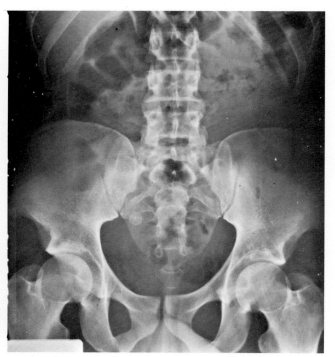

Figure 10G-4. This 25-year-old man had symptoms compatible with acute pancreatitis. A fecalith was evident on this plain film of the abdomen. Twelve hours after the film was taken, the patient developed physical findings compatible with acute appendicitis.

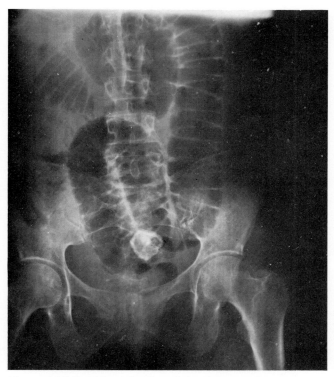

Figure 10G-5. This plain film of the abdomen demonstrates a classic picture of small bowel obstruction. Valvulae conniventes are clearly seen throughout.

essentially a clinical diagnosis with laboratory or radiographic data contributing little to the diagnosis. A careful history and physical examination, including pelvic and rectal examination, are necessary.

It is more difficult to make a diagnosis of acute appendicitis in females than in males. Disorders that can mimic appendicitis include bleeding or torsion of ovarian cysts, salpingitis, retrograde menstrual bleeding, fibroid uterus, and round ligament strain of pregnancy.

In patients over 50, acute sigmoid diverticulitis is the disorder most likely to be confused with appendicitis. In adults, cholecystitis and pyelonephritis should also be considered in the differential diagnosis.

Mesenteric adenitis may mimic the symptoms of acute appendicitis, especially in children, but it may also occur in young adults.

Diverticulitis. About one-half of the population over the age of 40 and about two-thirds over 80 have diverticulosis. Clinical manifestations of the disease range from an absence of symptoms, to mild symptoms such as flatulence or lower abdominal discomfort, to severe disorders such as hemorrhage and peritonitis.

Perforated viscus. Perforations of the stomach and duodenum are most often secondary to a benign ulcer, but malignant ulcers, infections, and penetrating trauma can also result in perforation. In the first 6 to 8 h, chemical peritonitis is produced by gastric and intestinal juices. Sepsis and bacterial peritonitis follow if leakage continues. An increase in capillary permeability results in fluid shifts from the intravascular space into the lumen of the gut, interstitial tissues, and peritoneal cavity. Hypovolemic shock and oliguria result.

A perforated peptic ulcer should be distinguished from a per-

forated appendix, ruptured esophagus, generalized peritonitis secondary to any etiology, and acute pancreatitis.

Cholecystitis. Right upper quadrant tenderness, fever, and leukocytosis suggest the diagnosis of acute cholecystitis. The diagnosis is virtually certain if the patient has a tender, palpable gallbladder. Pyelonephritis can be present with identical symptoms. In patients with pain radiating to the back, pyelonephritis may be a more likely diagnosis than cholecystitis. Of a number of patients with cholecystitis, the greatest percentage will be females over 40, but younger persons in their late teens or early 20s can also develop the disease even in the absence of predisposing factors such as sickle cell anemia. The diagnosis is more likely to be unsuspected in the younger age group.

Cholecystitis can be mistaken for pancreatitis and the differential diagnosis can be difficult if the serum amylase is normal. The serum bilirubin, alkaline phosphatase, and serum glutamic-oxaloacetic transaminase (SGOT) levels may be elevated in either condition. The amylase/creatinine clearance ratio may be diagnostic of pancreatitis. Back pain, especially bilateral back pain, is more suggestive of pancreatitis than cholecystitis. If common duct obstruction is present, pancreatitis may coexist with cholecystitis.

Small bowel obstruction. Intraabdominal adhesions resulting from previous abdominal surgery are the cause of small bowel obstruction in more than half the cases. External hernia, malignant obstruction, and volvulus are less common but important causes of mechanical obstruction in adults. Paralytic ileus or adynamic obstruction can result from a number of causes such as peritonitis, pancreatitis, electrolyte disorders, pyelonephritis, pneumonia or retroperitoneal hemorrhage. All patients with midabdominal pain should be suspected of having small bowel obstruction. The character of the pain may at first be intermittent and colicky, then become severe, constant, and accentuated by movement.

In the majority of patients, physical examination, laboratory studies, and abdominal films should establish an accurate diagnosis. Where the diagnosis is unclear, reevaluation including repeat abdominal films should be done in about 4 h.

Acute pancreatitis. Acute pancreatitis is characterized by severe acute midepigastric pain radiating to the back. Left flank tenderness may also be present; in this case, pyelonephritis should also be considered.

An elevated amylase or lipase level, or an elevated amylase/creatinine clearance ratio suggests pancreatitis. An extremely high serum amylase level, over 1000 Somogyi units, suggests biliary tract obstruction. Otherwise, the level of amylase has little relationship to the severity of the condition. Hypocalcemia may also be present and is usually associated with severe edematous or hemorrhagic pancreatitis. A perforated viscus or intestinal obstruction can be mistaken for acute pancreatitis, for some degree of ileus is associated with all these conditions. True boardlike rigidity is not generally a feature of acute pancreatitis.

A plain film of the abdomen may demonstrate pancreatic calcification or a sentinel loop of dilated jejunum. In some cases, a small left pleural effusion may be present.

SUMMARY

Acute, progressively worsening abdominal pain of 6 h duration suggests a surgical abdomen. The most common causes of an acute abdomen are acute appendicitis, acute diverticulitis, perforated peptic ulcer, and acute pancreatitis. In the majority of cases, synthesizing data from the symptom complex and physical examination leads to the correct diagnosis, but the physician should maintain a high degree of suspicion for less common causes of acute abdominal pain.

BIBLIOGRAPHY

Acute appendicitis in pregnancy. *Br Med J* 4:668–669, 1975.
Crow HC, Bartrum RJ: Ultrasound in diagnosis of acute cholecystitis. *JAMA* 235:2389, 1976.
DeLacey GJ, Wignall BK, Bradbrooke S, et al: Rationalizing abdominal radiography in the accident and emergency departments. *Clin Radiol* 31:453–455, 1980.
Gilmore OJA, Browett JP, Griffin PH, et al: Appendicitis and mimicking conditions. *Lancet* 2:421–424, 1975.
Goodwin WE, Fonkalsrud EW, Goldman R, et al: Diagnostic problems in retroperitoneal disease. *Ann Intern Med* 65:160–189, 1966.
Halasz NA: Counterfeit cholecystitis: A common diagnostic dilemma. *Am J Surg* 130:189–193, 1975.
Hermann RE: Acute cholecystitis. *JAMA* 234:1261–1262, 1975.

Law D, Law R, Eiseman B: The continuing challenge of acute and perforated appendicitis. *Am J Surg* 131:533–535, 1976.
Laws HL, Aldrete JS: Small-bowel obstruction: A review of 465 cases. *South Med J* 69:732–734, 1976.
Levine RI, Glauser FL, Berk JE: Enhancement of the amylase-creatinine clearance ratio in disorders other than acute pancreatitis. *N Engl J Med* 292:329–332, 1975.
McCook TA, Ravin CE, Rice RP: Abdominal radiographs in the emergency department: A prospective analysis. *Ann Emerg Med* 11:7–8, 1982.
Ottinger LW: Acute mesenteric ischemia. *N Engl J Med* 307:535–537, 1982.
Salt WB, Schenker S: Amylase—its clinical significance: A review of the literature. *Medicine* 55:269–281, 1976.
Staniland JR, Ditchburn J, deDombal FT: Clinical presentation of acute abdomen: Study of 600 patients. *Br Med J* 3:393–298, 1972.
Steinheber FU: Medical conditions mimicking the acute surgical abdomen. *Med Clin North Am* 57:1559–1567, 1973.
Wagner DK: Approach to the patient with acute abdominal pain. *Current Topics* (A program of the Medical College of Pennsylvania) 1:1–4, 1978.
Zizic TM, Classen JN, Stevens MB: Acute abdominal complications of systemic lupus erythematosus and polyarteritis nodosa. *Am J Med* 73:525–531, 1982.

H. Gastrointestinal Bleeding

Judith E. Tintinalli

The diagnosis is obvious when a patient has hematemesis or hematochezia, but gastrointestinal (GI) bleeding may also be manifested as unexplained hypotension and tachycardia. In such cases, melena or hematochezia is present or blood will be present in the gastric aspirate.

INITIAL MANAGEMENT

History. The history should be obtained as quickly and briefly as possible. Document the ingestion of alcohol or the administration of aspirin, phenylbutazone, or anticoagulants. Even though a patient may have a previous diagnosis of a potential bleeding upper GI lesion, acute bleeding will be from another source in about one-third to one-half of patients.

Physical examination. On physical examination, the presence of ascites, edema, spider angiomata, and palmar erythema indicates cirrhosis. A coagulation disorder is suggested by ecchymoses, petechiae, or profuse bleeding from venipuncture sites.

Fluid administration. Once the presence of active GI bleeding is confirmed, rapid and aggressive fluid replacement is necessary to prevent exsanguination. For massive bleeding, insert at least two large-bore intravenous lines (one may be a central venous pressure line). The infusion of crystalloid solution and whole blood is generally accepted as the treatment for hemorrhagic shock. Colloid does not seem to provide a clear advantage over crystalloid, and low molecular weight dextran has many disadvantages. The hemodynamic response to crystalloid solution will usually be transient if there is severe active bleeding or if blood loss is substantial. The appropriate use of a balanced electrolyte solution appears to reduce the requirement for whole blood. Lactated Ringer's solution is an appropriate choice in nearly all situations of hemorrhagic shock except in the occasional patient with cirrhosis or lactic acidosis. If possible, lactated Ringer's solution should be avoided in these patients because it may increase the lactate load.

A Foley catheter should be inserted to monitor urine output, which is an indicator of adequate fluid replacement.

Nasogastric irrigation. A large lumen nasogastric tube should be inserted. If there is difficulty passing the nasogastric tube through the nose, 2% phenylephrine drops can be instilled to shrink the mucosa.

A grossly deviated septum may prevent passage of the tube through either nare. In this case, it can be passed orally. A topical anesthetic spray, or lidocaine jelly, or both, can minimize discomfort to the patient.

Complications of nasogastric tube insertion include induction of nasal bleeding, retropharyngeal perforation, and passage into the trachea. The latter can cause laryngospasm, and the stimulation of carinal reflexes can cause hypotension and bradycardia or even asystole. Stimulation of a paroxysm of coughing can cause further hypotension because the Valsalva maneuver impairs venous return. In a patient with head and facial trauma, if the cribriform plate is fractured, the tube can be inadvertently inserted into the cranium.

The gastric aspirate should be tested for the presence of blood if the specimen is not grossly bloody, since blood can be rapidly evacuated from the stomach. It should be noted that guaiac slide tests are associated with false-negative results in the presence of unbuffered gastric juice.

If there is evidence of bleeding, the traditional approach has been to irrigate with iced saline. In fact, there have been no controlled clinical trials which clearly demonstrate the superiority of iced saline vs saline at 37°C for lavage. A recent animal study by Gilbert and Saunders demonstrates no difference in control of bleeding whether or not iced saline or saline at 37°C is used. Whether saline or water is used for lavage appears to be a matter of personal preference. Water intoxication is a theoretical hazard of the use of water for lavage, whereas sodium overload is a potential problem with saline lavage.

Laboratory data. Depending on the clinical situation, a complete blood count, type and cross match, routine electrolytes, blood glucose, BUN, creatinine, prothrombin time, and platelet count should generally be obtained initially.

The initial hemoglobin or hematocrit is no guide to the amount of blood lost. In the acute stages of hemorrhage, vasoconstriction and hemoconcentration will maintain the hematocrit higher than one would expect for the degree of hemorrhage that has occurred. Transcapillary refill, the movement of interstitial fluid into the vascular compartment, may not lower the hematocrit for several hours.

Hyperglycemia may be present in a patient with previously undetected diabetes because of endogenous catecholamine release due to stress. Treatment is generally not necessary unless the blood glucose level is elevated significantly or there are symptoms of hyperglycemia.

The BUN may rise because of the protein overload caused by blood in the gut. Therefore, a serum creatinine is also needed to evaluate renal function. Coagulation abnormalities may be a cause or result of GI bleeding. For instance, if large amounts of blood are given, thrombocytopenia may develop. Unless there is evidence of a coagulopathy such as prolonged oozing from venipuncture sites, ecchymoses or petechiae, or bleeding from multiple anatomic sites (gastrointestinal and genitourinary tracts, for example), the prothrombin time and a platelet count should be sufficient for an initial coagulation survey.

In the elderly or in patients with coronary artery disease, initial and serial ECGs are indicated to rule out the development of a silent myocardial infarction. Especially in the elderly patient with preexisting coronary artery disease, even transient hypotension and anemia may precipitate a myocardial infarction.

Ventilation. In the patient who is comatose, obtunded, or who is weakened so that tracheobronchial aspiration is possible, every effort must be made to ensure an adequate airway. In this situation, nasotracheal intubation should be considered early, before aspiration occurs. Endotracheal intubation is more difficult if the patient is responsive.

Blood administration. If massive active bleeding continues despite iced saline lavage, more aggressive maneuvers must be initiated to prevent exsanguination. Typed and cross-matched blood can be given if bleeding continues or if the vital signs cannot be stabilized with crystalloid solution alone. Occasionally, blood loss may be so extreme that type-specific, uncross-matched blood or O negative blood must be used. The use of uncross-matched or O negative blood in women of childbearing age should be carefully scrutinized. Massive transfusions may be necessary to keep up with active blood loss. Although bank blood up to 3 or 4 weeks old can be used, the older the blood, the less red cell 2,3-diphosphoglycerate (2,3-DPG) it contains. A red cell enzyme, 2,3-DPG increases oxygen delivery to the tissues.

Bleeding tendencies may develop as a consequence of massive transfusion due to depletion of platelets and some clotting factors in bank blood. Fresh frozen plasma and platelet concentrates can be administered as the need arises.

If massive volumes of bank blood are given, multiple pulmonary microemboli can be produced by fat, leukocyte and platelet aggregates, and atheromatous debris present in the blood. Infusing blood through ultrapore filters prevents microembolization, but can also result in thrombocytopenia, since these filters remove 20 percent to 40 percent of blood platelets.

Metabolic effects of massive transfusions are hyperkalemia, metabolic alkalosis, hypocalcemia, and hypothermia. Potassium overload can occur when patients with hyperkalemia or renal failure are given large amounts of bank blood. If large amounts of blood are administered, metabolic alkalosis can result when the citrate preservative is metabolized to bicarbonate. Since tetany could theoretically occur due to a fall in ionized calcium caused by alkalosis and the binding of calcium by citrate, some authorities advocate the administration of 10 mL of 10% calcium gluconate for every 2 to 4 units of blood given.

Infusion of large amounts of cold blood may result in hypothermia, so that if possible, blood should be warmed before it is infused.

Febrile reactions may occur because of sensitivity to donor white cells, platelets, or plasma proteins. These occur most commonly in patients who have had multiple blood transfusions. Pyrogens in donor blood may also cause febrile reactions. Allergic reactions characterized by itching and urticaria can usually be controlled by antihistamines. Hemolytic reactions may occur as a result of red cell incompatibility. Immediate symptoms include severe back pain, chest pain, dyspnea, and headache. If the transfusion is not stopped, disseminated intravascular coagulation and renal failure may follow. Delayed hemolytic reactions are characterized by jaundice, hemoglobinemia, and acute renal failure.

If a transfusion reaction is suspected, stop the transfusion immediately and return the donor blood to the blood bank for analysis. Obtain a sample of the recipient's blood in an oxalated tube and send it to the blood bank. A sample of the patient's plasma should be centrifuged and the supernatant examined for free hemoglobin. The urine should be checked for hemoglobin as well. The renal threshold of free hemoglobin is about 120 mg/100 mL, so that free hemoglobin is invariably present in the plasma before it is detected in the urine. After the transfusion is stopped, 25 g of mannitol should be given intravenously. Fluids should be administered to maintain a urine flow of at least 100 mL/per hour. Diuretics, such as furosemide, can also be given but only after adequate volume replacement.

Balloon tamponade. Indications for use of balloon tamponade in acute upper GI bleeding seem to vary from institution to institution and depend on the availability of endoscopy and angiography, and the capability for emergency surgery. Balloon tamponade can be applied in a situation where esophageal varices appear to be the cause of acute bleeding and where circumstances do not allow for immediate diagnosis by endoscopy or arteriography.

In patients with bleeding esophageal varices it may be possible to arrest bleeding by balloon tamponade. The Sengstaken-Blakemore tube, which is commonly used for this purpose, consists of an esophageal and gastric balloon. The esophageal balloon directly compresses bleeding varices and the gastric balloon acts as an anchor. A third lumen is provided so that nasogastric suction can be performed with the balloon in place.

Before insertion, test the balloons to make sure they are intact. Comatose or obtunded patients should be tracheally intubated before a Sengstaken-Blakemore tube is inserted. The inflated balloon of an endotracheal or nasotracheal tube can sometimes compress the esophagus so that a balloon tube cannot be passed. In such a case, temporary deflation of the tracheal cuff balloon may be necessary.

Once the tube is in place, the patient should be observed closely for the development of complications related to use of the balloon. These include compression of the trachea by the esophageal balloon; esophageal or gastric rupture; mucosal necrosis if the balloon is inflated for more than 24 to 48 h; or dislodgment of the tube so that the balloon obstructs the airway.

Use of the Sengstaken-Blakemore tube is contraindicated in a patient who has a hiatal hernia because when the gastric balloon is inflated, it will be in the chest.

The Sengstaken-Blakemore tube can also be used as a diagnostic tool. Cessation of bleeding after the gastric balloon has been inflated and pulled up snugly suggests a lesion at the esophagogastric junction. If bleeding stops after inflation of the esophageal balloon, varices are the likely source. Persistent bleeding after the inflation of both balloons points to a gastric source.

Drug therapy. Although older studies seemed to demonstrate potential benefit from systemic infusion of aqueous vasopressin, more recent studies do not demonstrate benefit in the management of upper gastrointestinal bleeding. Especially in the elderly, side effects of generalized arteriolar vasoconstriction, tachyphylaxis, and antidiuresis can occur. In some situations, better results are obtained by selective mesenteric arterial vasopressin infusion.

Kiselow and Wagner have reported that levarterenol (8 mg in 100 mL saline) instilled into the stomach can arrest upper GI hemorrhage, but studies using this technique on large numbers of patients are not currently available.

Diagnosis. Procedures for diagnosis can be begun once the patient is stabilized. The initial step is to obtain chest and abdominal roentgenograms.

Barium contrast studies are widely available and are associated with little morbidity, but as initial studies, they are not as satisfactory as arteriography or endoscopy. A barium study can identify lesions that can produce bleeding, such as a peptic ulcer or esophageal varices, but it cannot determine if a particular lesion is actively bleeding. In addition, the coating of the gastric mucosa by barium prevents accurate diagnosis by endoscopy and interferes with visualization of the bleeding site by angiography.

Endoscopic examination is a necessary procedure in the diagnosis of upper gastrointestinal bleeding. Besides identifying active bleeding lesions, topical hemostasis using alcohol or microcrystalline collagen can be applied through the endoscope.

If available, angiography can be used following endoscopy to further delineate sites of active bleeding as long as the rate of bleeding is 0.5 mL/min or greater. At the same time, it provides a route for mesenteric artery vasopressin infusion, or for thrombotic therapy.

CAUSES OF UPPER GI BLEEDING

The most common causes of upper GI bleeding originating above the ligament of Treitz are peptic ulcer, esophagitis and gastritis, and esophageal varices. Uncommon, but other important causes are the Mallory-Weiss syndrome, bleeding disorders, oropharyngeal bleeding, and head injury. Regardless of etiology, the mortality rate seems to be related to the nature of the underlying disease and concomitant medical problems, rather than to the severity of the bleeding. Thus, the importance of appropriate initial emergency department management of upper GI bleeding cannot be overstressed.

Peptic ulcer. About 40 percent to 70 percent of upper GI hemorrhage is due to bleeding peptic ulcer, including duodenal, gastric, and stomal ulcers. About 25 percent of upper GI hemorrhage is due to duodenal ulcer. With conservative management, about 10 percent of duodenal ulcers will rebleed, usually within 24 h. Gastric ulcers are two to three times more likely to rebleed than duodenal ulcers. An anastomotic ulcer is responsible for upper GI bleeding in less than 5 percent of patients. In Palmer's study, two-thirds of patients with a prior gastric surgical procedure bled from a lesion other than an anastomotic ulcer.

Esophagitis and gastritis. In one large series, erosive esophagitis and gastritis were responsible for nearly 20 percent of acute upper GI bleeding. The mortality rate, however, is considerably higher than that of duodenal ulcer. Erosive esophagitis and gastritis are common causes of upper GI bleeding in patients with hiatal hernia.

Esophageal varices. Bleeding varices can account for up to 20 percent of patients with acute upper GI hemorrhage. However, even in patients with known cirrhosis, nearly one-third will bleed from lesions other than varices. Since esophageal varices are highly likely to rebleed (70 percent), accurate diagnosis and effective treatment are mandatory. Interim treatment can be in the form of balloon tamponade or mesenteric artery vasopressin infusion. Portacaval or splenorenal shunting can be performed as an emergency or elective procedure depending on the patient's underlying condition and the clinical situation.

LESS COMMON CAUSES

Swallowed blood. Vomiting of swallowed blood from the nasopharynx or oropharynx can be mistaken for upper GI bleeding. A careful history and physical examination should delineate the source of bleeding and appropriate therapeutic measures can be taken.

Coagulation disorders. Coagulation disorders should be suspected if there are petechiae, ecchymoses, and prolonged oozing from venipuncture sites, or if there is bleeding from multiple anatomic sources. In such cases, a coagulation survey should be obtained before transfused blood is given. Treatment must be directed at the underlying cause.

Mallory-Weiss syndrome. Mallory-Weiss syndrome is massive hematemesis due to a longitudinal laceration of the mucosa in the cardioesophageal region. Severe vomiting is most often the cause, although protracted coughing, seizures, or acute strain have also been implicated.

Stress ulcers. Gastrointestinal bleeding can also occur in association with burns, sepsis, and head injury, and is most often due to erosions of the esophagus, stomach, and duodenum (stress or Curling's ulcers). In such situations, the frequency of massive upper GI bleeding is variable, but most often develops 24 to 48 h after the initial insult.

Occult bleeding. Initially, patients with a history of hematemesis but no active bleeding, or those with coffee-ground vomitus are managed similarly to patients with massive GI bleeding, with modification for the acuteness of the situation. Since acute rebleeding is likely to a varying degree depending on the lesion, these patients should not be discharged from the emergency department. When admitted for observation, diagnosis can be done in a more leisurely fashion. In this instance, barium contrast studies, rather then endoscopy or arteriography, are usually performed first.

LOWER GI BLEEDING

If the upper GI tract has been ruled out as the source, the patient with massive rectal bleeding can be assumed to be bleeding from somewhere below the ligament of Treitz.

Initial Management

With obvious massive rectal bleeding, detailed history taking is impossible. However, the development of severe weakness or dizziness or syncope after a bloody stool suggests serious blood loss, perhaps 1000 mL.

Physical examination. On physical examination, check the skin and mucosal surfaces for evidence of multiple telangiectasia or pigmentation suggestive of Peutz-Jeghers syndrome. Palpation of the abdomen may reveal a mass that may be due to carcinoma or diverticulitis with abscess. Since the majority of colorectal carcinomas are detectable on digital examination, rectal examination is essential in all patients.

Management. Initial management of massive lower GI bleeding is essentially the same as for upper GI bleeding, that is, fluid and blood replacement.

A nasogastric tube should be inserted in the case of massive rectal bleeding to rule out the upper GI tract as the source. The gastric aspirate should be checked for blood if the specimen is not grossly bloody. Proctoscopy and sigmoidoscopy are generally performed next to rule out bleeding from hemorrhoids or another rectosigmoid lesion.

Where available, intestinal angiography is performed to identify the lesion. In the majority of patients bleeding from diverticulosis, an intraarterial infusion of vasopressin can control the bleeding, at least initially. If vasopressin is unavailable or unsuccessful, emergency colectomy may be necessary.

Causes of Massive Lower GI Bleeding

Diverticulosis. From 5 percent to 25 percent of patients with diverticulosis develop serious rectal bleeding. Bleeding is caused by mucosal ulceration and erosion into the wall of the penetrating artery of the diverticulum.

Diverticulosis is the most common cause of massive rectal bleeding in the elderly, and the severity of bleeding increases with age and in the presence of underlying disease. Bleeding occurs abruptly, and is generally not accompanied by abdominal pain, nausea, or vomiting. Bleeding from diverticula appears to be more common in the right side of the colon.

Conservative management with blood transfusion is generally the initial treatment of choice.

Mesenteric arteriography can localize the lesion, and mesenteric arterial vasopressin infusion can control active bleeding in a large number of patients. Otherwise, emergency colectomy with its associated high mortality and morbidity may be necessary in severe hemorrhage. Even after conservative treatment, resection may be necessary because massive bleeding recurs in a substantial number of patients.

Other causes. Hemorrhoids and colonic carcinoma are uncommon causes of massive rectal bleeding. Ulcerative colitis, Crohn's disease, and polyps are other uncommon causes of massive rectal bleeding.

SUMMARY

Vigorous management is necessary for successful resuscitation in the emergency department. Diagnostic studies should be deferred until the patient has been stabilized with fluid and blood replacement. Common causes of upper GI hemorrhage include peptic ulcer, esophagitis and gastritis, and esophageal varices. In the elderly, diverticulosis is the most common cause of massive lower GI bleeding.

BIBLIOGRAPHY

Athanasoulis CA, Waltman AC, Novelline RA, et al: Angiography: Its contribution to the emergency management of gastrointestinal hemorrhage. *Radiol Clin North Am* 11:265–280, 1976.

Deveney CW, Thomas AN: Diagnosis and treatment of hemorrhage in patients with hiatal hernia. *J Thorac Cardiovasc Surg* 73:497–503, 1977.

Fogel MR, Knauer M, Andres LL, et al: Continuous intravenous vasopressin in active upper gastrointestinal bleeding. *Ann Intern Med* 96:565–569, 1982.

Gilbert DA, Saunders DR: Iced saline lavage does not slow bleeding from experimental canine gastric ulcers. *Dig Dis & Sci* 26:1065–1068, 1981.

Heald RJ: Defining the clinical problem of massive rectal bleeding. *Dis Colon Rectum* 17:432–438, 1974.

Johnson WE, Widrich WC, Ansell JE, et al: Control of bleeding varices by vasopressin. *Ann Surg* 186(3):369–376, 1977.

Kamada T, Fusamoto H, Kawano S, et al: Gastrointestinal bleeding following head injury: A clinical study of 433 cases. *J Trauma* 17:44–47, 1977.

Kiselow MC, Wagner M: Intragastric installation of levarterenol. *Arch Surg* 107:387–389, 1973.

Klein FA, Drueck C, Breuer RI, et al: Control of upper gastrointestinal bleeding with a microcrystalline collagen hemostat. *Dig Dis & Sci* 27:981–985, 1982.

Larson DE, Farnell MB: Upper gastrointestinal hemorrhage. *Mayo Clin Proc* 58:371–387, 1983.

Malt RA: Control of massive upper gastrointestinal hemorrhage. *N Engl J Med* 286:1043–1047, 1972.

Layne EA, Mellow MH, Lipman TO: Insensitivity of guaiac slide tests for detection of blood in gastric juice. *Ann Intern Med* 94:774–776, 1981.

Long PC, Wilentz KV, Sudlow G, et al: Modification of the hemoccult slide test for occult blood in gastric juice. *Crit Care Med* 10:692–693, 1982.

Moody F: Rectal Bleeding. *N Engl J Med* 290:839–841, 1974.

Palmer ED: The vigorous diagnostic approach to upper gastrointestinal tract hemorrhage. *JAMA* 207:1477–1480, 1969.

Sedgwick CE, Reale VF: Upper gastrointestinal hemorrhage. *Surg Clin North Am* 56:695–707, 1976.

Spechler SJ, Schimmell EM: Gastrointestinal tract bleeding of unknown origin. *Arch Intern Med* 142:236–240, 1982.

Webb WA, McDaniel L, Johnson RC, et al: Endoscopic evaluation of 125 cases of upper gastrointestinal bleeding. *Ann Surg* 193:624–627, 1981.

Wyler AR, Reynolds AF: An intracranial complication of nasogastric intubation: Case report. *J Neurosurg* 47:297–298, 1977.

SECTION 2
CARDIOVASCULAR
DISEASE

CHAPTER 11
MYOCARDIAL ISCHEMIA,
AND INFARCTION;
HEART FAILURE

J. Stephan Stapczynski

ISCHEMIC HEART DISEASE

Ischemic heart disease and its complications are the most common cause of mortality in the United States, responsible for about 600,000 deaths each year. Nearly 50 percent of these deaths occur prior to arrival at the hospital. In the overwhelming majority of cases, ischemic heart disease is caused by atherosclerosis, an intimal disease of the epicardial coronary arteries. This process, often termed *coronary artery disease* (CAD), is a multifactorial disorder. Epidemiologic research has identified seven major risk factors for CAD: age, male sex, family history, cigarette smoking, hypertension, hyperlipidemia, and diabetes mellitus. Since 1968, there has been a decline in the annual incidence of CAD in the United States, believed due to modification of risk factors in the general population.

Pathophysiology of Myocardial Ischemia

Myocardial ischemia results from imbalance between myocardial oxygen supply and demand. One or both abnormalities may be present in the individual patient (Table 11-1). While the overwhelming majority of patients have fixed arterial obstruction due to atherosclerotic lesions, recent work has documented a greater incidence of coronary artery spasm than was previously appreciated. There are three major determinants of myocardial oxygen supply and three of myocardial oxygen demand (Table 11-2).

Ischemia produces major changes in two of the important functions of myocardial cells, electrical activity and contraction. The ischemic cell has a drastically altered transmembrane action potential. As an example, the ischemic ventricular myocardial cell has an action potential at which the resting potential is elevated, the rate of rise is slower, and the plateau phase is shorter (Fig. 11-1). Between normal and ischemic myocardial tissues, an electrical potential difference exists which generates many of the arrhythmias seen with angina or acute myocardial infarction (AMI). Impaired myocardial contractility most importantly affects left ventricular function. Initially, there is a loss in normal diastolic relaxation, producing a decrease in ventricular distensibility and clinically manifested by an audible S_4. If ischemia becomes more profound, systolic contraction is lost and the affected area becomes hypokinetic or akinetic. If infarction develops, the area rapidly loses stiffness within minutes to hours and the area becomes dyskinetic, moving paradoxically with systolic contractions. All this results in a decreased ejection fraction. To maintain cardiac output, the cardiovascular system often compensates by increasing the filling pressure to maintain an adequate stroke volume, by the Frank-Starling principle.

Natural History of Ischemic Heart Disease

The studies of the natural history of CAD done prior to 1970 cannot be applied to contemporary patients because of limitations of study design. Without coronary arteriography, there was no certainty about the specific diagnosis. There was no specific treatment protocol for all patients: some had no therapy, some had treatment with different medications, and some had surgery. Recent studies have consistently shown that the natural history of CAD is primarily determined by two pathophysiologic factors: (1) the extent of arterial obstruction (one, two, or three vessels obstructed); and (2) the status of left ventricular function. Clinical factors—such as severity of angina, history of infarction, presence of heart failure, or arrhythmias—are closely correlated with the extent of arterial obstruction and left ventricular function. The influence of these clinical factors on the natural history can be accounted for by considering these two pathophysiologic changes. Over the years, the prognosis of CAD treated with medical measures has been improving and the grim prognosis previously given to patients can no longer be applied.

ANGINA PECTORIS

Clinical Features

Stable angina is characterized by episodic chest pain, lasting minutes (usually 5 to 15 min), provoked by exertion or stress, and relieved by rest or sublingual nitroglycerin. The pain almost always has a retrosternal component and commonly radiates to the

Table 11-1. Etiology of Myocardial Ischemia

Decreased myocardial oxygen supply
  Coronary artery obstruction
    Fixed obstruction
      Atherosclerosis
      Miscellaneous causes
    Arterial spasm
  Systemic hypotension
  Severe anemia
Increased myocardial oxygen demand
  Myocardial hypertrophy
  Tachycardia

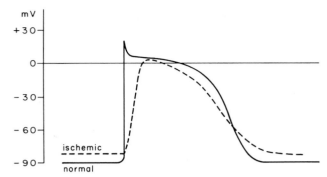

Figure 11-1. Ventricular myocardial cell transmembrane action potential.

neck, jaw, and shoulders, or down the inside of the left or both arms. Secondary symptoms—lightheadedness, palpitations, diaphoresis, dyspnea, nausea, or vomiting—may accompany the pain. Auscultation of the heart may find a transient S_4 or apical systolic murmur. An ECG taken during an acute attack will show ST segment depression or, less commonly, elevation about half the time. Of course, serum creatine kinase (CK) will be normal.

Unstable (crescendo or preinfarction) angina represents a clinical state between stable angina and acute myocardial infarction. If untreated, patients with unstable angina are at high risk for myocardial infarction (21 to 80 percent) and death (1 to 60 percent) during the first month. Medical therapy drastically reduces this risk and so it becomes important to recognize, hospitalize, and treat these patients. Coronary angiography of patients with unstable angina has demonstrated about the same degree of coronary disease as found in patients with stable angina. It is not known what causes the instability of this syndrome. Three clinical subgroups are included in unstable angina: (1) angina of recent onset, usually defined as within 4 to 8 weeks; (2) angina of worsening character, characterized by increasing severity, duration, or requirement for nitroglycerin; and (3) angina at rest, or angina decubitus. When obtaining a history of angina less responsive to nitroglycerin, it is important to inquire about the potency of the tablets, since nitroglycerin degrades over several months. If the patient has taken several tablets without the development of a headache, the nitroglycerin is most likely old and ineffective. In unstable angina, ST-segment or T-wave changes may persist up to several hours after the pain episode, but there is no ECG evidence of new transmural infarction (new Q waves). Serum enzymes may show minor elevations without definite serial changes.

Variant (Prinzmetal's) angina occurs primarily at rest and without provocation. There is a tendency for attacks to recur at similar times of the day. Pain is associated with ST segment elevation that represents transmural myocardial ischemia. Painless episodes may also occur with ST segment elevation. Attacks may be as-

Table 11-2. Major Determinants of Myocardial Oxygen Supply and Demand

Supply
  Aortic diastolic pressure
  Coronary vascular resistance
  Diastolic duration
Demand
  Heart rate
  Wall tension
    Preload—PAWP
    Afterload—mean aortic pressure
  Contractility

sociated with tachyarrhythmias, bundle branch blocks, or atrioventricular block. The current thought is that variant angina is due to spasm of the epicardial coronary arteries. When these patients are studied by coronary angiography, about one-third have no or insignificant atherosclerosis and about two-thirds have CAD in addition to spasm. The latter patients may have exertional angina in addition to variant angina. Spasm is not unique to variant angina; it has been found in patients with typical angina or AMI.

Treatment of Angina

For patients with ischemic heart disease, it is most important for the emergency physician to recognize and admit those patients with AMI and unstable angina. The emergency physician is less likely to become involved in the long-term treatment of patients. Occasionally a patient with stable angina may present with a typical acute attack. The most important concerns for the emergency physician are: (1) Is there a new medical problem causing exacerbation of the angina? (2) Is this unstable angina? (3) Has the patient discontinued the prescribed medications? or (4) Are the medications ineffective? Many times, these patients can be managed by adjusting or refilling their medications. Ideally, this should be done with consultation of the patient's physician and close follow-up should be arranged.

Treatment of angina should start with correction of modifiable risk factors: discontinuing smoking, controlling hypertension and diabetes, and lowering blood lipids by diet. Coexisting disorders that place stress upon the heart should be treated. Medications that increase myocardial oxygen demand, such as sympathomimetics and methylxanthine derivatives, should be discontinued if possible.

Drug treatment is usually started with nitrates (Table 11-3). Sublingual nitroglycerin (NTG) is most effective for acute attacks; relief is usually felt within 3 min. Several long-acting forms are available to prevent anginal attacks: sublingual or oral long-acting nitrates, topical 2 percent nitroglycerin ointment, and prepackaged transdermal nitroglycerin delivery systems. Therapy with long-acting nitrates should be discontinued slowly to avoid exacerbation of symptoms when this medication is withdrawn.

β-Adrenergic blocking agents are used when nitrates are contraindicated or ineffective (Table 11-4). Nonselective agents such as propranolol, nadolol, or pindolol block receptors in the heart and blood vessels. Selective agents, such as metoprolol or atenolol, preferentially inhibit the β_1-receptors of the heart at low or intermediate doses. β-Blockers are absolutely contraindicated in pa-

Table 11-3. Nitrates in the Treatment of Angina

Agent	Dosage Size	Typical Dose	Duration of Action
Nitroglycerin (NTG)	0.2 mg (1/400) 0.3 mg (1/200) 0.4 mg (1/150)	1 SL q 5 min	Up to 30 min
2% NTG ointment		$\frac{1}{2}$–2 in q 4–6 h	3–6 h
Isosorbide dinitrate	SL 2.5,5.0 mg PO 5,10,20 mg	2.5–10.0 mg SL q 2–4 h 5–40 mg PO q 4–6 h	SL 1.5–3.0 h PO 4–6 h
Transdermal NTG	2.5–22.4 mg released over 24 h	1 per day	24 h

tients with severe heart failure and relatively contraindicated in those with insulin-dependent diabetes mellitus. Nonselective blockers are also contraindicated in patients with severe bronchospasm or variant angina. Selective blockers may be used with caution in these patients.

Calcium channel antagonists have shown considerable promise for relief and prevention of typical and variant anginal attacks (Table 11-5). They are too new to fully assess their precise role in the treatment of angina.

ACUTE MYOCARDIAL INFARCTION

Pathogenesis of Acute Myocardial Infarction (AMI)

While the large majority of patients with AMI have coronary artery disease, there is no universal agreement about the exact process that precipitates the acute event. Current concepts concerning the immediate cause of AMI include the interaction of multiple factors: progression of the atherosclerotic process to the point of total occlusion, subintimal hemorrhage at the site of an existing narrowing, coronary artery embolism, coronary artery spasm, and thrombosis at the site of an intimal plaque. Depending on the study, these factors are found in different percentages of patients with AMI. Recent studies strongly support the view that acute intracoronary thrombosis and, to a lesser extent, arterial spasm play frequent and important roles. These two processes are potentially reversible and this has led to renewed interest in ag-

gressive early intervention in AMI. The previous approach of resting the cardiovascular system while monitoring and treating only complications of AMI has been replaced by an approach that directly treats the cause.

Pathophysiology of Acute Myocardial Infarction

As with ischemia, infarction produces major changes in two important myocardial cell functions: electrical depolarization and contractility. The complications of AMI are caused by one or both of these events. During the first few hours, infarction is not a completed process; areas of infarction are interspersed or surrounded by areas of ischemia or injury. The amount of infarcted tissue is a critical factor in determining prognosis, morbidity, and mortality. These ischemic areas are potentially salvageable through medical and surgical therapy.

Arrhythmias are frequent in acute infarction. Tachyarrhythmias and ventricular ectopy are usually caused by the electrical differences between adjacent areas of normal and ischemic myocardium. Bradyarrhythmias and atrioventricular blocks are due to either increased vagal tone or infarction directly affecting the conducting system.

The major result of impaired contractility is left ventricular (LV) pump failure. If 25 percent of the LV myocardium is impaired, heart failure usually develops, and if 40 percent is affected, cardiogenic shock is common. Recent studies have also led to a greater appreciation of the effect of AMI on right ventricular (RV) pump function. If the papillary muscles of the mitral valve are

Table 11-4. Beta-Adrenergic Antagonists in Treatment of Angina

Agent	Tablet Size	Typical Initial Dose	Usual Maximal Total Daily Dose
Propranolol (NS)* (Inderal)	10, 20, 40, 80 mg	10–20 mg qid	640 mg
Nadolol (NS) (Corgard)	40, 80, 120, 160 mg	40 mg qd	240 mg
Metoprolol (S)† (Lopressor)	50, 100 mg	50 mg bid	400 mg
Pindolol (NS) (Vioken)	5, 10 mg	10 mg bid	60 mg
Atenolol (S) (Tenormin)	50, 100 mg	50 mg qd	200 mg
Timolol (NS) (Blocadren)	10, 20 mg	10 mg bid	60 mg

*(NS) = nonselective agent

†(S) = selective agent

Table 11-5. Calcium Channel Antagonists in Treatment of Angina

Agent	Tablet Size	Typical Initial Dose	Usual Maximal Total Daily Dose
Nifedipine (Procardia)	10 mg	10 mg tid	120 mg
Verapamil (Calan)	80, 120 mg	80 mg tid	360 mg
Diltiazem (Cardizem)	30, 60 mg	30 mg qid	240 mg

impaired, acute mitral regurgitation may develop and cause acute pulmonary edema and hypotension.

The infarcted area can undergo autolysis, with distinct clinical syndromes resulting from rupture of the ventricular free wall, ventricular septum, or papillary muscle.

Stasis of the circulation can lead to venous thrombosis and pulmonary embolism. Stasis of blood within the ventricular cavity and exposure of collagen at the site of infarction can lead to development of mural thrombosis and systemic arterial embolism.

Clinical Features of Acute Myocardial Infarction

The classic symptom is severe anginal pain, lasting longer than 15 to 30 min. As with angina, the pain may be atypical but accompanied by other symptoms such as lightheadedness, dyspnea, diaphoresis, palpitations, nausea, or vomiting. The Framingham study found that only about one in four infarctions was preceded by a history of angina and one in five infarctions was clinically unrecognized. Silent infarctions are more frequent in diabetics and the elderly.

The physical examination may be deceptively normal. Commonly, there is a mild to moderate increase in pulse rate although inferior infarctions frequently cause bradycardia. Depending on the degree of pain and sympathetic activation, blood pressure is elevated. Mild fever is common but rarely exceeds 39.5°C (103° F). Palpation of the apical pulse may show it to be diffuse or bulging. The loudness of S_1 may diminish as LV contraction is impaired. Uncommonly, the S_2 is paradoxically split owing to prolonged LV ejection. An S_4 is very common owing to decreased ventricular compliance and a soft S_3 is occasionally heard. New systolic murmurs should be carefully examined. They may indicate: (1) mitral regurgitation due to papillary muscle dysfunction or rupture; (2) ventricular septal rupture; or (3) friction rub of pericarditis.

Ancillary Tests in Acute Myocardial Infarction

Electrocardiography (ECG)

The electrocardiographic diagnosis of AMI requires serial recordings; at most, only about half of the patients with AMI have definitive changes on the initial ECG. The ECG changes of AMI may be obscured or mimicked by many conditions. AMI produces changes in depolarization and repolarization manifested by changes in the QRS complex and T waves, respectively. Transmural infarction produces an electrically dead area of muscle, detected by a Q wave of >0.03 s duration in an overlying electrode. T waves become inverted because ischemia or infarction reverses the sequence of repolarization, causing it to occur in the endocardial to epicardial rather than the normal epicardial to endocardial direc-

tion. In addition, an injury current between normal and ischemic tissue can be detected by ST segment changes. Generally, injury current during systole points away from a normal area and to an ischemic area. As recorded on the surface ECG, ST segment depression reflects subendocardial injury and ST segment elevation indicates subepicardial and/or transmural injury. In transmural infarction, ST segment elevation occurs almost immediately and Q waves usually require several hours to become evident. T-wave inversions generally appear after the Q waves, although this is not invariable. Nontransmural (or subendocardial) infarction produces ST depression and T wave inversion without Q-wave development. Since many other conditions can cause ST-T changes, "ischemic" subendocardial changes are considered to be (1) horizontal or downsloping ST segments of at least 1.0 mm and (2) deep, symmetrical T-wave inversions (Fig. 11-2).

Using abnormal Q waves and ST segment elevation, the ECG is able to localize the area of infarction (Fig. 11-3):

II, III, aV_F: inferior
V_1-V_3: anteroseptal
I, aV_L, V_4-V_6: lateral
V_1-V_6: anterolateral

The one exception is a true posterior infarction, which produces a large R wave and ST segment depression in V_1 and V_2. Localization of AMI is important because the incidence and significance of complications vary with the site. For example, inferior wall infarctions may affect autonomic fibers in the atrial septum, resulting in increased vagal tone as manifested by sinus bradycardia, first degree, or Mobitz I (Wenckebach) atrioventricular block (AVB). These blocks are generally benign and nonprogressive and respond readily to pharmacologic intervention if that becomes necessary. On the other hand, anterior wall infarction may directly damage the conducting system, producing Mobitz II second-degree or third-degree AVB. This is more grave and an indication for placement of a ventricular pacemaker.

Cardiac Enzymes

When myocardial cells are irreversibly injured, they release enzymes into the serum. As discussed in the chapter on chest pain, the commonly available cardiac enzymes should not be used as a criterion in deciding whether to admit patients. The enzymes commonly measured in the coronary care unit are listed in Table 11-6.

Creatine kinase (CK) is found in high concentrations in skeletal muscle, myocardial muscle, and brain tissue. Unfortunately, total serum CK is elevated by many disorders that affect skeletal muscle. The MB isoenzyme (CK-MB) is found primarily in myocardial cells, and elevated serum levels of this enzyme are more specific for myocardial injury. Serum glutamic oxaloacetic trans-

Table 11-6. Serum Enzymes in Diagnosis of Acute Myocardial Infarction

Enzyme	Earliest Rise	Peak	Normalize
CK	6–8 h	24–30 h	3–4 days
CK-MB	3–4 h	18–24 h	2 days
SGOT	8–12 h	36–48 h	3–5 days
LDH	12–24 h	48–96 h	7–10 days
HBD	12 h	72 h	10–14 days

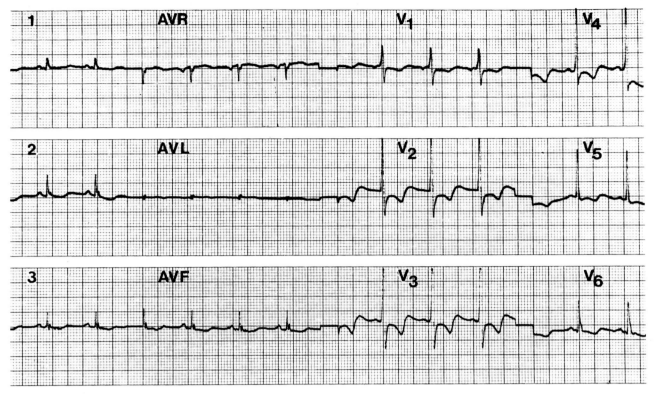

Figure 11-2. Subendocardial ischemic ST-T changes.

aminase (SGOT) is found in many organs, and an elevated level is too nonspecific to be useful. Lactic dehydrogenase (LDH) is likewise found in many organs of the body, but two isoenzymes, LDH_1 and LDH_2, are confined primarily to the heart and their serum concentration or ratio can be separately measured. These isoenzymes also have greater ability to dehydrogenate hydroxybutyric acid than other LDH isoenzymes. So while hydroxybutyrate dehydrogenase (HBD) is not a distinct enzyme, a measure of LDH_1 and LDH_2 concentration can be obtained by measuring serum HBD activity.

Radionuclide Scans

Radionuclide scanning is not commonly available to evaluate patients in the emergency department nor should it be recommended at this time for use in the decision-making process. In certain situations, the radionuclide scan is helpful in evaluating inpatients. Two radionuclides, technetium 99 and thallium 201, are commonly used.

Technetium 99 pyrophosphate is deposited irreversibly in infarcted myocardial tissue, producing a "hot spot" on nuclear imaging. Scans first become positive within 10 to 12 h and become increasingly positive up to 24 to 72 h after onset of chest pain. Sensitivity is highest with transmural infarctions (85 + percent) and less with nontransmural infarctions (50 percent).

Thallium 201 is reversibly taken up by normally perfused myocardial cells; the infarcted or ischemic area appears as a "cold spot" on nuclear imaging. The thallium scan cannot differentiate between ischemia, old infarction, or new infarction and therefore has little diagnostic utility in AMI.

Nontransmural versus Transmural Infarction

Once thought to be more benign, nontransmural (subendocardial) infarction may have about the same incidence of in-hospital complications and mortality as transmural infarction; it all depends on the extent of the myocardial damage and not on whether it is transmural. Additionally, patients with first-time nontransmural infarction have about the same incidence of angina, recurrent infarction, and sudden death after discharge as those with first-time transmural infarctions.

Complications of Acute Myocardial Infarction

Arrhythmias

The out-of-hospital mortality in AMI is almost entirely due to arrhythmias; early assessment and treatment of these arrhythmias must first depend on their detection. All patients should be on continuous cardiac monitoring and, equally important, the monitor must be watched by qualified personnel. The incidence of lethal arrhythmias is greatest in the prehospital phase. The site of infarction does not appear to influence the incidence of arrhythmias (Table 11-7).

Sinus tachycardia is potentially detrimental because of increased myocardial oxygen demand. Diagnosis and therapy should be directed towards the underlying cause: increased sympathetic activity, hypovolemia, hypoxia, etc.

Sinus bradycardia is usually due to increased vagal tone and common with inferior AMIs. Treatment with atropine is usually not required unless the bradycardia is complicated by hypotension

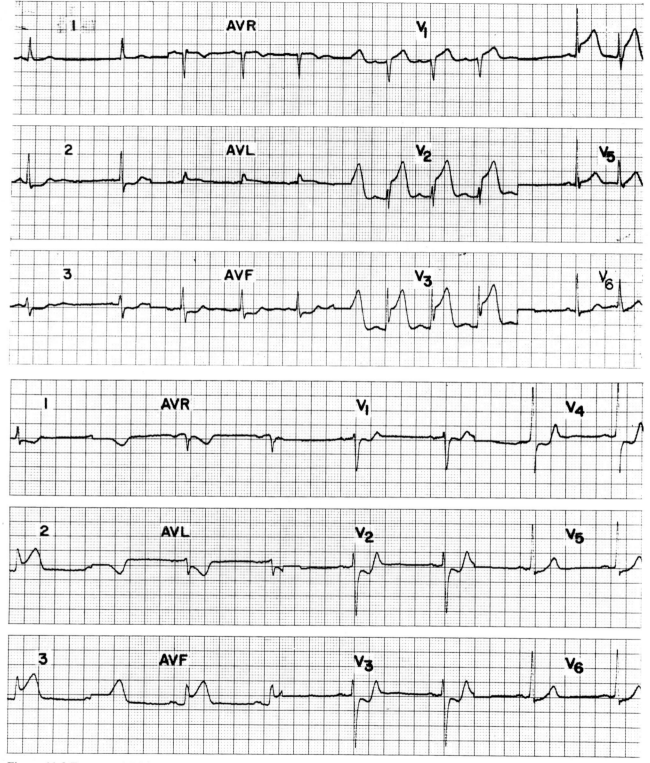

Figure 11.3 Transmural ECG changes of acute myocardial infarction. Top: acute anterior MI; bottom: acute inferior MI.

or premature ventricular contractions (PVCs). Premature atrial contractions (PACs) are common but generally are of no significance unless they initiate more serious arrhythmias, like paroxysmal supraventricular tachycardia (PSVT).

PSVT should be treated because the rapid rate increases oxygen demand and reduces cardiac output. The reentrant variety of PSVT should be treated with vagal maneuvers or cardioversion. Drugs that directly affect the conduction system (e.g., verapamil), parasympathomimetics (e.g., edrophonium) or β-adrenergic blockers (e.g., propranolol) may have significant risk in the potentially unstable hemodynamics of AMI and should be used with caution.

Atrial fibrillation usually occurs within the first 48 h and often

Table 11-7. Approximate Incidence of Arrhythmias in Acute Myocardial Infarction

Sinus tachycardia	40–60%
Sinus bradycardia	3–10%
Premature atrial contractions	15–40%
Paroxysmal supraventricular tachycardia	2–7%
Atrial fibrillation	10%
Atrial flutter	5%
Junctional tachycardia	5–10%
Premature ventricular contractions	100%
Ventricular tachycardia	10%
Accelerated idioventricular rhythm	8–23%
Primary ventricular fibrillation	5–6%

in association with pericarditis. The ventricular rate can be controlled with digoxin or propranolol. Cardioversion is effective if the patient is hemodynamically compromised. Recurrences are common and therapy with procainamide may be required. Atrial flutter responds readily to cardioversion, which is the treatment of choice.

Junctional tachycardia is caused by enhanced automaticity of the junctional pacemaker due to infarction or digoxin toxicity. Treatment is not necessary unless the rapid rate produces hemodynamic deterioration.

Prophylactic lidocaine therapy is recommended by many physicians in all patients with definite or possible AMI during the first 24 to 48 h of hospitalization. Prophylactic lidocaine has been shown to be effective in reducing the risk of primary ventricular fibrillation while the patient with AMI is in the cardiac care unit. The benefits of prophylactic lidocaine during the prehospital and emergency department setting are not proved or universally accepted. Careful studies with large numbers of patients will be needed to determine its value.

PVCs occur in nearly all patients with AMI. The frequency or severity of PVCs is no longer felt to be a reliable predictor of more serious ventricular arrhythmias. However, most physicians would consider the presence of PVCs an indicator of ventricular irritability and recommend treatment with lidocaine, procainamide, or bretylium.

Ventricular tachycardia should be treated according to the hemodynamic status of the patient: if the patient is stable, intravenous lidocaine should be used, and if the patient is unstable, immediate synchronized cardioversion should be done.

Accelerated idioventricular rhythm (AIVR) is usually a transient arrhythmia, with wide QRS complexes, occurring at a rate of 60 to 90 per min. It is thought to arise from a number of causes. While it is usually benign, there is some variable association with ventricular tachycardia but no apparent association with ventricular fibrillation. Close monitoring is advised but specific therapy is usually not indicated for AIVR.

Primary ventricular fibrillation (VF) is the sudden development of VF in the absence of shock or pump failure. The peak incidence is early in the course: 60 percent within 4 h and 80 percent within 12 h. Primary VF is easily prevented and treated. Secondary VF occurs as a terminal event after a progressive course of left ventricular pump failure. Treatment of secondary VF rarely produces long-term success.

Conduction Disturbances

The risk of progression to complete heart block (CHB) during an AMI depends on two major factors: (1) site of the infarction and

(2) the presence of new or indeterminant conduction defects (Table 11-8).

First-degree atrioventricular block (AVB) and Mobitz I (Wenckebach) second-degree AVB are usually due to increased vagal tone, impairing AV node conduction. Progression to CHB is infrequent, rarely occurs suddenly, and if it occurs, a stable infranodal pacemaker with narrow QRS complexes and a reasonable rate around 50 usually takes over. Stable patients can be observed and unstable patients can be treated with atropine.

Mobitz II second-degree AVB is usually seen with anterior ischemia or infarction which affects the infranodal conducting system. CHB may occur suddenly, with only a slow, unstable ventricular pacemaker available for cardiac activity. Infarctions that cause Mobitz II blocks are usually large and, even with pacemaker treatment, many patients die from pump failure.

Left Ventricular Pump Failure and Cardiogenic Shock

AMI nearly always produces impairment of LV pump function; whether this is clinically manifest depends on the extent of damage. Several classifications have been developed to correlate the extent of pump dysfunction with acute in-hospital mortality. The Killip classification is based on clinical criteria and the Forrester-Diamond-Swan classification is based on hemodynamic measurements (Tables 11-9 and 11-10A and B). A rough, imprecise correlation exists between clinical and hemodynamic findings. Pulmonary vascular congestion occurs when pulmonary artery wedge pressure (PAWP) rises above 18 to 20 mmHg and is manifested by dyspnea and rales. Peripheral hypoperfusion occurs when the cardiac index falls below 2.2 to 2.5 L/(min·m²) and is manifested by hypotension, oliguria, mental obtundation, peripheral vasoconstriction, and tachycardia.

Current management of LV pump dysfunction is to treat the underlying hemodynamic derangement. Pulmonary vascular congestion can be relieved by reducing preload with nitrates, morphine, or diuretics. Of the three modalities, nitrates produce the most predictable decrease in PAWP. Many patients with LV failure have a fall in PAWP, presumably due to increased venous capacitance, within minutes after intravenous administration of furosemide. Within 1 h, PAWP further decreases, owing to diuresis. Much of the clinical effect of morphine in LV pump failure is due to its general sedative effect rather than to a direct effect on PAWP. Peripheral vasodilators such as nitroprusside decrease peripheral vascular resistance and increase venous capacitance. This combination lowers systemic vascular resistance and PAWP and, in patients with cardiac failure, usually increases cardiac output. Patients not in heart failure usually have a fall in cardiac output with vasodilator therapy.

Table 11-8. Approximate Incidence of Complete Heart Block in Acute Myocardial Infarction

New or Age-Indeterminant Conduction Defect	
LASFB	4%
LPIFB	8%
First-degree AVB	13%
Left bundle branch block (LBBB)	14%
Right bundle branch block (RBBB)	21%
RBBB and LASFB	30%
RBBB and LPIFB	37%
RBBB and LPIFB or LASFB and first-degree AVB	43%

Table 11-9. Killip-Kimball Classification

Class		Approximate Incidence	Approximate Mortality
I	No failure	30%	5%
II	Mild failure: bibasilar rales and S_3	40%	15–20%
III	Frank pulmonary edema	10%	40%
IV	Cardiogenic shock: Systolic BP < 90 mmHg Peripheral vasoconstriction Oliguria Pulmonary vascular congestion	20%	80%

Depressed cardiac output should be treated by first optimizing preload, although most patients with cardiogenic shock already have a very high PAWP. Further therapy will usually be dictated by the systolic blood pressure (BP). If systolic BP is above 100 mmHg, cardiac output can be increased by afterload reduction with nitroprusside. If systolic BP is below 100 mmHg, afterload reduction should be undertaken cautiously. With mild hypotension (systolic BP 75 to 90 mmHg), an inotropic agent such as dopamine or dobutamine usually is effective. With severe hypotension (systolic BP below 75 mmHg), a vasopressor agent such as norepinephrine should be used to increase BP above 90 mmHg to maintain vital organ perfusion. If inotropic agents are ineffective or required for longer than a few hours, the intraaortic balloon pump (IABP) can be used to mechanically support the circulation.

Mechanical Defects

Cardiac rupture is a catastrophic event that presents with sudden recurrence of chest pain, hypotension, pericardial tamponade, cardiac arrest with electromechanical dissociation, and death. Patients at increased risk are those with first infarction, sustained hypertension after infarction, and the elderly; 50 percent of such events occur within the first 5 days and 90 percent within the first 14 days after infarction. Mortality is 95 percent; a few patients

Table 11-10A. Forrester-Swan-Diamond Classification

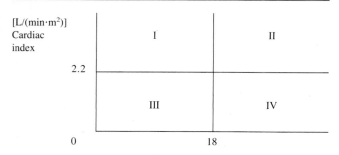

Pulmonary artery wedge pressure (mmHg)

Table 11-10B. Approximate Mortality Rates

Class	Approximate Mortality
I	3%
II	9%
III	23%
IV	51%

survive with volume replacement, pericardiocentesis for treatment of tamponade, and immediate surgery.

Ventricular septal rupture presents with sudden onset of pulmonary edema and a new harsh systolic murmur along the left sternal border. Septal rupture occurs about equally in anterior and inferior infarctions and is located in the muscular portion of the intraventricular septum. Clinical diagnosis may be difficult; often requiring the measurement of P_{O_2} in right ventricular blood obtained via a Swan-Ganz catheter. Therapy should be initiated with afterload reduction by nitroprusside or, if this is ineffective, by the IABP.

Papillary muscle dysfunction is common, especially with inferior infarctions. The clinical presentation is usually mild, with only a transient systolic murmur, but may become severe, with florid pulmonary edema. Treatment of the ischemia and afterload reduction is usually effective. Prognosis of mild dysfunction is very good.

Papillary muscle rupture is more serious and the outcome depends on whether the whole muscle body is ruptured or only the head. Rupture of an entire muscle body is associated with a high mortality rate, up to 50 percent within 24 h. Rupture is usually associated with an inferior-posterior infarction and involves the posterior papillary muscle. Clinical diagnosis of papillary muscle dysfunction or rupture can be difficult and require a Swan-Ganz catheter to measure large V waves in the PAWP.

Thromboembolism

Prolonged bed rest and generalized circulatory stasis predispose the patient with AMI to venous thrombosis and pulmonary embolism. Other predisposing factors include: previous thromboembolism, atrial fibrillation, old age, and obesity. Early ambulation and low-dose subcutaneous heparin (5000 units bid) have reduced the incidence of deep venous thrombosis.

A mural thrombosis can develop at the site of an infarction and later embolize to the carotid, renal, splenic, mesenteric, or peripheral arteries. The clinical incidence is less than 2 to 4 percent. Patients with transmural infarctions and large akinetic or dyskinetic segments are at special risk.

Pericarditis

An acute form of pericarditis, manifested by pain and friction rub, can develop during the first 7 days postinfarction. The cause is the inflammation associated with necrosis of the myocardium adjacent to the pericardium. The postmyocardial infarction (Dressler's) syndrome generally occurs later and is characterized by chest pain, fever, pleuropericarditis, and pleural effusion. The cause is an immunologic reaction to myocardial antigens exposed by the AMI.

Right Ventricular Infarction

Previously thought to be rare, RV infarction is now recognized to occur in 19 to 43 percent of inferior infarctions. However, clinical recognition occurs only 3 to 8 percent of the time. RV infarction is due to right coronary artery obstruction and almost always in association with LV damage. The damage to the right ventricle is nearly always transmural. It was previously held that the right ventricle serves as a volume conduit and that pump dysfunction is not clinically significant. However, severe RV pump dysfunction can present with hypotension and elevated right atrial–jugular venous pressures. It is important to differentiate this from predominant LV dysfunction, constrictive pericarditis, pericardial tamponade, and restrictive cardiomyopathy. Correct diagnosis usually requires simultaneous measurement of PAWP and right atrial pressures or visualization of poor RV contractions on radionuclide scanning. With RV pump dysfunction, it is important to avoid decreases in filling pressure by use of diuretics or nitrates. With hypotension, cautious volume expansion is indicated but should be done with cardiac output and PAWP monitoring. Dobutamine provides good inotropic stimulation when volume expansion is ineffective. Afterload reduction with a predominantly arteriolar vasodilator such as hydralazine is also effective.

Treatment of Acute Myocardial Infarction

All patients with documented or suspected AMI should have an intravenous line established; a D_5W solution is generally used and saline solutions are avoided to prevent sodium overload and pulmonary congestion. In AMI the central venous pressure (CVP) is not a reliable measure of volume status or cardiac dysfunction. The cardiac monitor should be applied and observed by qualified personnel. Supplemental oxygen should be administered to all patients. Patients with a history of oxygen sensitivity or chronic obstructive pulmonary disease (COPD) should be given low concentrations (2 L/min or 24 percent) and all other patients given higher concentrations (4 to 6 L/min or 40 percent). Experimentally, supplemental oxygen at an FI_{O_2} of 40 percent reduces the degree of ST segmental elevation and size of the infarction. Severe hypoxemia or hypercapnia will often require endotracheal intubation and mechanical ventilation, preferably with a volume-cycled respirator, since changes in lung compliance can make pressure-cycled ventilators unreliable. Underlying acid-base disorders, especially alkalosis, should be corrected since they contribute to arrhythmias.

Arrhythmias should be treated as described above. The optimal heart rate during the early phase of AMI is believed to be between 60 and 90. Many physicians recommend prophylaxis with lidocaine for all suspected AMI patients during the prehospital and emergency department phases of treatment. However, the benefit of prophylactic lidocaine in these settings is not proven.

Pain relief is important in the emergency department. Intravenous morphine sulfate is the traditional treatment for the pain of AMI. Sequential small doses (4 to 6 mg) every 10 to 15 min should be used; however, complete pain relief may require up to 15 to 20 mg of morphine. Morphine should be used with caution in patients with severe hypotension (systolic BP < 80 mmHg) or COPD. In the setting of AMI, the beneficial action of morphine is predominantly sedative and analgesic, which reduces oxygen demand. Morphine produces no consistent effect on preload and may actually decrease cardiac output. Meperidine hydochloride has effects similar to those of morphine and can also be used. Pentazocine elevates preload and afterload, decreases contractility, and increases myocardial oxygen demand; it should not be used.

Nitroglycerin (NTG) has traditionally been avoided in AMI for fear of inducing hypotension and tachycardia. However, recent studies have found that sublingual or intravenous NTG is both effective and safe in AMI. Additionally, NTG reduces the degree of injury as measured by ST segment elevation and probably reduces infarct size as detected by Q-wave development. Repetitive small doses (0.4 to 1.6 mg) should be given sublingually at 3- to 5-min intervals as long as systolic BP remains adequate (i.e., > 100 mmHg in most patients or > 120 mmHg in patients with a prior history of hypertension). The response of individual patients is quite variable and may require a total NTG dose of about 20 to 30 mg for complete pain control. Nitroglycerin should be avoided in patients with hypotension. Occasionally patients with AMI have what appears to be a vasovagal reaction, marked by bradycardia and hypotension, to NTG. This is usually transient and responds to elevating the legs and, if required, atropine.

Nitrous oxide 35 to 50 percent is safe and effective in relieving pain and can be used as an alternative to morphine or NTG. The chief benefit of nitrous oxide is that it does not produce myocardial depression or decrease blood pressure. However, it requires constant inhalation to provide continuous pain control.

Several experimental regimens are currently being studied which may play a role in the future. Some of them are potentially applicable to patients in the emergency department and will be discussed here.

Some, but not all studies, indicate that β-adrenergic blockers given early in the course of AMI may limit infarct size, especially in patients with increased sympathetic activity. More significant is the finding that β-blockers improve survival when given on a long-term basis after the AMI. The studies with propranolol, timolol, and metoprolol are significant enough to routinely recommend their use.

Preliminary studies with calcium channel antagonists have shown they reduce infarct size in experimental animals and humans.

Several studies have shown that administration of glucose-insulin-potassium solution within 12 h after the onset of AMI has beneficial effects on myocardial metabolism, cardiac rhythm, pump function, infarct size, and in-hospital mortality. The solution is composed of 300 g glucose, 50 units regular insulin, and 80 mEq potassium in 1 L water and infused at a rate of 1.5 mL/(kg·h) for 48 h via the right atrial port of the Swan-Ganz catheter.

Impressive anecdotal results have been achieved with intracoronary infusion of very low dose streptokinase to dissolve coronary arterial thrombi and restore perfusion during the first few hours of AMI. This technique involves cardiac catheterization with the associated risks, and the long-term benefits have not been fully identified. Intravenous administration of larger doses of streptokinase can be carried out as soon as the patient has been determined to be eligible for thrombolytic therapy in the emergency department. The results of several randomized studies suggest that intravenous streptokinase reduces mortality during the first weeks after AMI by about 20 percent. The use of thrombolytic therapy for AMI is still experimental, and to use it there should be a protocol with definite eligibility and exclusion criteria along with the necessary laboratory monitoring.

Prostaglandins possess several actions that would theoretically be beneficial in AMI and appear to be effective in animal studies. No controlled studies in humans have been published to date.

CONGESTIVE HEART FAILURE

Heart failure is the clinical syndrome that occurs when cardiac pump function is inadequate at normal filling pressures to meet the circulatory demands of the body. Much of the time heart failure is characterized by retention of fluid within many parts of the body (''congestion'' or edema), and the term *congestive heart failure* (CHF) is commonly used. Heart failure can be divided into several categories: (1) whether it is acute or chronic; (2) which chamber of the heart, the right or left ventricle, is more impaired; and (3) whether cardiac output is low or high. CHF occurs as the result of many different diseases; appropriate therapy consists of identifying the primary cause as well as contributing causes.

Etiology

The clinical characteristics of right- and left-sided CHF are often separated for the purposes of discussion but heart failure is most commonly biventricular. Right-sided CHF is most commonly caused by left-sided heart failure. Isolated right-sided failure may occur as the result of cor pulmonale, mitral or tricuspid valvular disease, cardiomyopathy, myocarditis, or congenital heart disease. Right-sided CHF differs from left-sided CHF in several important ways: (1) cardiac output and blood pressure are usually decreased; (2) fluid accumulation occurs primarily in the dependent parts of the body and not the lungs; and (3) if the cause is cor pulmonale, the associated hypoxemia and hypercapnia are potentially treatable. The common causes of LV failure depress cardiac output: hypertension, coronary artery disease, aortic or mitral valve disease, and cardiomyopathies. Left heart failure may occur when exceedingly high circulatory demands are unable to be met even from an elevated cardiac output, as in cases of hyperthyroidism, septic shock, arteriovenous fistula, or Paget's disease.

The most common precipitating factors in heart failure are: (1) cardiac tachyarrhythmias, such as atrial fibrillation; (2) acute myocardial infarction; (3) discontinuation of medication such as diuretics; (4) increased sodium ingestion; (5) administration of drugs that impair myocardial performance, such as propranolol; and (6) physical overexertion.

Acute left-sided heart failure is usually manifested by pulmonary edema. However, pulmonary edema can occur as the result of noncardiac processes. The causes of noncardiogenic pulmonary edema are considered in other sections of this study guide.

Pathophysiology of Congestive Heart Failure

The fluid retention and peripheral edema of CHF are due to several factors. As RV volume and pressure increase the systemic venous and capillary pressure rise and cause transudation of fluid from the vascular compartment into the interstitial space. As cardiac contractility and output decline, compensatory arteriolar vasoconstriction redistributes blood flow so that the brain and heart remain well perfused at the expense of flow to the bowel, kidneys, and muscle. The drop in renal blood flow activates the renin-angiotensin-aldosterone system, causing increased sodium retention. The hepatic metabolism of aldosterone is also impaired, so that the hormone remains active longer in the circulation.

Pulmonary vascular congestion and edema are due to a rise in left atrial pressure, which in turn elevates pulmonary capillary pressure. The major forces involved in the production of pulmonary edema are expressed in the Starling equation as the difference between pulmonary capillary hydrostatic pressure and plasma oncotic pressure. However, important roles are also played by interstitial-fluid hydrostatic and oncotic pressure, alveolar surface tension, and the pulmonary lymphatics. Pulmonary edema does not always occur when capillary hydrostatic pressure exceeds plasma oncotic pressure; the precise mechanisms involved in the production of pulmonary edema are still not understood.

During the phase of interstitial edema, pulmonary resistance rises and lung compliance decreases. The increase in pulmonary vascular resistance redistributes blood flow from the bases to the apices of the lungs. The increase in lung stiffness produces the sensation of dyspnea. When the patient becomes supine for a period of time, fluid present in lower extremity edema can slowly be redistributed to other areas of the body, including the lungs, producing pulmonary edema in the supine position; this is termed *paroxysmal nocturnal dyspnea*. When heart failure is even more severe, the patient cannot even tolerate the slight rise in venous return associated with the supine position; this is *orthopnea*. Fluid is removed from the interstitial space by the pulmonary lymphatics but, when the system is overburdened, fluid spills over into the alveolar spaces. Severe pulmonary edema irritates the bronchioles and they often go into reflex spasm. Alveolar edema is clinically detected by rales and when there is associated bronchospasm, by wheezes. There are regional differences in accumulation of fluid, so that ventilation perfusion inequality results, leading to variable degrees of arterial hypoxemia. In many patients respiratory stimulation produces alveolar hyperventilation and a lowered Pa_{CO_2}, while in others the alveolar edema is so severe that alveolar hypoventilation occurs with an elevated Pa_{CO_2}.

As heart failure develops, three major compensatory mechanisms initially help maintain cardiac output, but they have effects that become deleterious in time. The first compensation is through the Frank-Starling mechanism, by which a myocardial cell contracts with greater force as the precontraction length is increased. Clinically the force of contraction is approximated by the stroke volume or cardiac output and the precontraction length by the LV end diastolic volume or pressure (clinically measured as the PAWP). Unfortunately, a rising filling pressure may exceed plasma oncotic pressure and cause pulmonary edema. An increased preload also increases myocardial oxygen demand. The second compensation is the stimulation of myocardial hypertrophy by pressure or volume overloads. Although potentially beneficial, hypertrophy entails the costs of decreased ventricular compliance and increased myocardial oxygen demand. The third compensation is stimulation of the sympathetic nervous system by a falling cardiac output, causing peripheral vasoconstriction, increased cardiac contractility, and increased heart rate. Many patients with CHF are dependent on catecholamine stimulation to maintain cardiac output and perfusion pressure. This also extracts a cost on myocardial oxygen demand.

Clinical Features of Congestive Heart Failure

Edema, the classic sign of right-sided heart failure, generally occurs in dependent parts of the body such as the feet, ankles, and pretibial region. In bedridden patients sacral edema is prominent. Anasarca, or massive edema, may affect the genitalia, trunk, and upper extremities. If predominantly right-sided CHF is present, the patient can generally lie flat without dyspnea. Ascites is not common in right-sided CHF, although it is somewhat more prominent in patients with tricuspid valvular disease or constrictive pericarditis. Other causes of edema and ascites such as cirrhosis, nephrotic syndrome, protein-losing enteropathy, inferior vena cava obstruction, and venous insufficiency should be excluded.

Transudative pleural effusion can occur in both right- and left-sided CHF because the pleura is perfused by both the systemic and pulmonic circulation. In CHF the pleural effusion is usually more prominent on the right side.

A positive hepatojugular reflux is an early sign of right-sided CHF and, if failure progresses, jugular venous distention will appear.

Hepatic tenderness and enlargement are generally present with moderate to severe right-sided CHF. Liver function tests are compatible with hepatocellular dysfunction; the most frequently abnormal test is the prothrombin time, and jaundice is unusual. With severe failure or tricuspid regurgitation, the liver may be pulsatile.

Nocturia is a common symptom, as patient's extremities are dependent-edema mobilized while in the supine position. Patients usually have an impaired ability to excrete sodium and water. Hyponatremia is common.

LV failure usually first becomes evident with the symptom of exertional dyspnea during activity. As CHF progresses, PND followed by orthopnea develops. Interstitial edema often produces a dry cough while alveolar edema causes coughing of frothy, pink sputum as fluid and red cells exude into the alveolar spaces. Some patients with pulmonary edema, especially the elderly, have Cheyne-Stokes respirations because the prolonged circulatory time between the lungs and brain slows the ventilatory response to alterations in Pa_{O_2}.

On auscultation, moist pulmonary rales and an S_3 or S_4 are detectable. Pulsus alternans, or alternating weak and strong pulses, may be detected by palpation or sphygmomanometry.

The ECG will show the underlying cardiac rhythm and electrical activity but there are no specific findings for pulmonary edema.

Three progressive chest radiographic stages of CHF have been described; however, there may be as much as a 12-h delay in visible radiographic changes after the onset of acute heart failure and up to a 4-day delay in resolution of radiographic changes after clinical improvement. The first stage occurs during chronic elevation in left atrial pressure, which causes reflex pulmonary vasoconstriction and redistribution of blood flow to the upper lung fields. This usually occurs when PAWP is elevated above 12 to 18 mmHg. The second stage occurs when further elevations in left atrial pressure produce interstitial edema, visible as blurred edges of blood vessels, and Kerley A and B lines. The PAWP is typically 18 to 25 mmHg. The third stage occurs when fluid exudes into the alveoli and is characterized by the classic bilateral hazy perihilar infiltrates ("butterfly"). The PAWP is usually above 25 mmHg.

The acid-base derangements in pulmonary edema cannot be predicted from the patient's clinical condition; arterial blood gases should be routinely obtained. The most common abnormalities are hypoxia and acidosis. The acidosis is usually metabolic and may have a respiratory component.

Treatment of Chronic Congestive Heart Failure

Treatment of chronic CHF consists of reducing circulatory demands, increasing myocardial contractility, correcting any precipitating causes, and treating the underlying disease if possible.

The volume overload can be reduced by restricting sodium intake and promoting diuresis with thiazide or loop diuretics. In severe or resistant cases, loop diuretics, such as furosemide, are more effective.

Digitalis has been traditionally used to improve myocardial contractility in CHF. Recent studies on the efficacy of long-term digitalis therapy for CHF have yielded variable results. Digitalis is most effective as a ventricular rate-controlling agent in atrial fibrillation.

As cardiac output falls in CHF, the systemic vascular resistance rises, which has a further deleterious effect on the heart by increasing afterload and wall tension. Vasodilator therapy lowers systemic vascular resistance and improves cardiac output. Several agents have been used, some predominantly affecting the venous system and reducing preload, some affecting predominantly the arterioles and reducing afterload, and some with both actions. Sublingual or oral NTG affects preload almost exclusively, and intravenous NTG affects preload somewhat more than afterload. Intravenous nitroprusside affects afterload more than preload, oral prazosin affects preload and afterload about equally, and oral hydralazine affects afterload almost exclusively. Vasodilator therapy is very effective at producing sustained relief of symptoms at rest; however, its role in improving exercise tolerance is unclear.

Treatment of Acute Pulmonary Edema

Treatment of acute pulmonary edema consists of improving tissue oxygenation, reducing pulmonary congestion, and improving myocardial contractility.

Oxygen is the most important agent for treating acute pulmonary edema; it should be given at high concentrations by mask or nasal cannula. Large numbers of collapsed and fluid-filled alveoli make some patients unresponsive to supplemental oxygen. In this situation *positive end expiratory pressure* (PEEP) can be used to prevent alveolar collapse and improve gas exchange. PEEP can be applied during spontaneous respirations with a tight-fitting mask or endotracheal tube, a method termed *continuous positive airway pressure*. If hypercapnea is present, then positive pressure ventilation, usually through an endotracheal tube, is required. Positive pressure ventilation may adversely affect cardiac output and it is important to provide adequate oxygenation and ventilation at the lowest possible airway pressure.

Sodium bicarbonate should be used for severe metabolic acidosis (pH < 7.10) and *not* for respiratory acidosis. The high sodium content may aggravate the volume overload problem in CHF.

The circulatory demands placed upon the heart can be reduced by decreasing both the preload and afterload. Preload can be reduced by intravenous furosemide 40 to 80 mg. A rapid reduction due to venous dilation is seen, and a further reduction is seen when diuresis develops. If no response occurs within 30 min, furosemide should be repeated at double the initial dose. Preload can also be reduced by sublingual, oral, or topical nitrates, sublingual being the most rapid. The dose of sublingual NTG required in usually more than that used to treat angina, namely 0.8 to 2.4 mg as a single dose. Sodium nitroprusside, 0.5 to 10 μg/(kg·min), can be used to rapidly reduce afterload and preload but requires close hemodynamic monitoring, usually with an intraarterial pressure monitoring line. The goal of afterload reduction is resolution of symptoms without undue systemic hypotension, i.e., systolic BP < 100 mmHg.

Morphine has been a traditional and effective agent in the treatment of acute pulmonary edema. Its major effect is sedative and analgesic; little reduction in preload is seen when closely studied. Sequential small doses (2 to 5 mg IV) should be used.

Rotating tourniquets are traditional but of absolutely no benefit and complications do occur from venous stasis. They should not be used.

Aminophylline is primarily a bronchodilator, but also a weak inotrope, diuretic, and vasodilator. It is useful for treating the reflex bronchospasm of pulmonary edema, or "cardiac asthma." The drug should not be given through a central venous line. The loading dose is 5 to 6 mg/kg IV over 20 to 30 min and a maintenance dose of 0.2 to 0.5 mg/(kg·h) IV.

Digitalis is not generally useful in acute pulmonary edema. It may be more useful in the long-term management of CHF. Inotropic agents may be required when moderate to severe hypotension is present, but unfortunately the heart is often maximally stimulated by endogenous catecholamines and not responsive to parenterally administered agents.

BIBLIOGRAPHY

Angina

Abrams J: Nitroglycerin and long-acting nitrates. *N Engl J Med* 302:1234, 1980.

Antman EM, Stone PH, Muller JE, et al: Calcium channel blocking agents in the treatment of cardiovascular disorders. *Ann Intern Med* 93:875, 886, 1980.

Brown BG, Dodge HJ: Unstable angina: Guidelines for therapy based on the last decade of clinical observations (editorial). *Ann Intern Med* 97:921, 1982.

Cairns JA, Fantus IG, Klassen GA: Unstable angina pectoris. *Am Heart J* 92:373, 1976.

Diamond GA, Forrester JS: Analysis of probability as an aid in the clinical diagnosis of coronary artery disease. *N Engl J Med* 300:1350, 1979.

Fishman WH: Beta-adrenoceptor anatagonists: New drugs and new indications. *N Engl J Med* 305:500, 1981.

Fishman WH: Atenolol and timolol: two new systemic beta-adrenoceptor antagonists. *N Engl J Med* 306:1456, 1982.

Fishman WH: Pindolol: a new beta-adrenoceptor antagonist with partial agonist activity. *N Engl J Med* 308:940, 1983.

Fuch R, Scheidt S: Improved criteria for admission to cardiac care units. *JAMA* 246:2037, 1981.

Hillis LD, Braunwald E: Myocardial ischemia. *N Engl J Med* 296:971, 1034, 1093, 1977.

Luchi RJ, Chahine RA, Raizner AE: Coronary artery spasm. *Ann Intern Med* 91:441, 1979.

Nattel S, Warnica JW, Ogilvie RI: Indications for admission to a coronary care unit in patients with unstable angina. *Can Med Assoc J* 26:180, 1980.

Proudfit WL, Bruschke AVG, Sones FM: Natural history of obstructive coronary artery disease: Ten-year study of 601 nonsurgical cases. *Prog Cardiovasc Dis* 21:53, 1978.

Selzer A, Langston M, Ruggeroli C, et al: Clinical syndrome of variant angina and normal coronary arteriorgram. *N Engl J Med* 295:1343, 1976.

Stern MP: The recent decline in ischemic heart disease mortality. *Ann Intern Med* 91:630, 1979.

Thadani V, Davidson C, Singleton W, et al: Comparison of five beta-adrenoceptor antagonists with different ancillary properties during sustained twice daily therapy in angina pectoris. *Am J Med* 68:243, 1980.

Warren SE, Francis GS: Nitroglycerin and nitrate esters. *Am J Med* 65:53, 1978.

Myocardial Infarction

Anderson JL, Marshall HW, Bray BE, et al: A randomized trial of intracoronary streptokinase in the treatment of acute myocardial infarction. *N Engl J Med* 308:1312, 1983.

Bates RJ, Beutler S, Resnekov L, et al: Cardiac rupture—challenge in diagnosis and management. *Am J Cardiol* 40:429, 1977.

Borak J, Veilleux S: Prophylactic lidocaine: Uncertain benefits in emergency settings. *Ann Emerg Med* 11:493, 1982.

Braunwald E, Muller JE, Kloner RA, et al: Role of beta-adrenergic blockade in the therapy of patients with myocardial infarction. *Am J Med* 74:113, 1983.

Bussman WD: Nitroglycerin in the treatment of acute myocardial infarction. *Acta Med Scand [Suppl]* 651:165, 1981.

Daluz PL, Weil MH, Shubin H: Current concepts on mechanics and treatment of cardiogenic shock. *Am Heart J* 92:103, 1976.

Forrester JS, Diamond G, Chatterjee K, et al: Medical therapy of acute myocardial infarction by application of hemodynamic subsets. *N Engl J Med* 295:1356, 1404, 1976.

Forrester JS, Diamond G, Swan HJC: Correlative classification of clinical and hemodynamic function after acute myocardial infarction. *Am J Cardiol* 39:137, 1977.

Frishman WH, Ribner HS: Anticoagulation in myocardial infarction: Modern approach to an old problem. *Am J Cardiol* 43:1207, 1979.

Grande P, Christiansen C, Pedersen A, et al: Optimal diagnosis of acute myocardial infarction. A cost-effective study. *Circulation* 61:723, 1980.

Hindman MC, Wagner GS, Jaro M, et al: The clinical significance of bundle branch block complicating acute myocardial infarction. *Circulation* 58:679, 689, 1978.

Johnson CC, Bolton EC: Cardiac enzymes. *Ann Emerg Med* 11:27, 1982.

Kahn AH: Pericarditis of myocardial infarction: Review of the literature with case presentation. *Am Heart J* 90:788, 1974.

Kaplan K, Talano JV: Systolic murmurs following myocardial infarction. *Pract Cardiol* 5:25, 1979.

Khaja F, Walton JA, Brymer JF, et al: Intracoronary fibrinolytic therapy in acute myocardial infarction. Report of a prospective randomized trial. *N Engl J Med* 308:1305, 1983.

Killip T, Kimball JT: Treatment of myocardial infarction in a coronary care unit. *Am J Cardiol* 20:457, 1967.

Kim Yi, Williams JF: Large dose sublingual nitroglycerin in acute myocardial infarction: Relief of chest pain and reduction of Q wave evolution. *Am J Cardiol* 49:842, 1982.

Lee G, DeMaria AN, Amsterdam EA, et al: Comparative effects of morphine, meperidine and pentazocine on cardiocirculatory dynamics in patients with acute myocardial infarction. *Am J Med* 60:949, 1976.

Lessem J: Myocardial scintigraphy in an emergency room. *Acta Med Scand [Suppl]* 623:57, 1978.

Mahony C, Hindman MC, Aronin N, et al: Prognostic differences in subgroups of patients with electrocardiographic evidence of subendocardial or transmural myocardial infarction. *Am J Med* 69:183, 1980.

Markis JE, Malagold M, Parker JA, et al: Myocardial salvage after intracoronary thrombolysis with streptokinase in acute myocardial infarction. *N Engl J Med* 305:777, 1981.

Mulholland HC, Pantridge JF: Heart-rate changes during movement in patients with acute myocardial infarction. *Lancet* 1:1244, 1974.

Noneman JW, Rodgers JF: Lidocaine prophylaxis in acute myocardial infarction. *Medicine* 57:501, 1978.

Oliva PB: Pathophysiology of acute myocardial infarction, 1981. *Ann Intern Med* 94:236, 1981.

Rackley CE, Russel RO, Rogers WT, et al: Glucose-insulin-potassium administration in acute myocardial infarction. *Ann Rev Med* 33:375, 1982.

Reese L, Uksik P: Radioimmunoassay of serum myoglobin in screening for acute myocardial infarction. *Can Med Assoc J* 124:1585, 1981.

Spann JF: Changing concepts of pathophysiology, prognosis, and therapy in acute myocardial infarction. *Am J Med* 74:877, 1983.

Stampfer MJ, Goldhaber SZ, Yusuf S, et al: Effect of intravenous strep-tokinase on acute myocardial infarction. Pooled results from random-ized trials. *N Engl J Med* 307:1180, 1982.

Willerson JT, Buja WM: Cause and course of acute myocardial infarction. *Am J Med* 69:903, 1980.

Congestive Heart Failure

Bertel O, Steiner A: Rotating tourniquets do not work in acute congestive heart failure and pulmonary edema. *Lancet* 1:762, 1980.

Biddle TL, Yu PN: Effect of furosemide on hemodynamic and lung water in acute pulmonary edema secondary to myocardial infarction. *Am J Cardiol* 43:86, 1979.

Bussman WD, Schupp D: Effect of sublingual nitroglycerin in emergency treatment of severe pulmonary edema. *Am J Cardiol* 41:931, 1978.

Cohn JN, Franciosa JA: Vasodilator therapy of cardiac failure. *N Engl J Med* 297:27, 254, 1977.

Fleg JL, Gottleib SH, Lakatta EG: Is digoxin really important in treatment of compensated heart failure? A placebo-controlled crossover study in patients with sinus rhythm. *Am J Med* 73:244, 1982.

Heinemann HO: Right-sided heart failure and the use of diuretics. *Am J Med* 64:367, 1978.

Lee DC, Johnson RA, Bingham JB, et al: Heart failure in outpatients. A randomized trial of digoxin versus placebo. *N Engl J Med* 306:699, 1982.

Staub NC: The pathogenesis of pulmonary edema. *Prog Cardiovasc Dis* 23:53, 1980.

Timmis AD, Rothman MT, Henderson MA, et al: Hemodynamic effects of intravenous morphine in patients with acute myocardial infarction complicated by severe left heart failure. *Br Med J* 1:980, 1980.

CHAPTER 12
VALVULAR
HEART DISEASE

J. Stephan Stapczynski

The four heart valves function to force blood to flow in the forward direction only as the ventricles contract. Valvular heart disease may either be stenotic, causing obstruction to flow when the valve should be open, or incompetent, allowing backward regurgitation of blood when the valve should normally be closed. While cardiac catheterization and echocardiography have immensely increased our understanding of valvular heart disease, the emergency physician should remember that the ability to recognize and manage these disorders requires correlating clinical history and physical examination at the bedside. The ancillary tests of chest radiography and electrocardiography usually provide only confirmatory information.

The cardiovascular adaptations to valvular heart disease are complex and varied, depending on whether this disease is acute, subacute, or chronic. Most acute and subacute adaptations persist in the chronic state. The acute adaptations are primarily tachycardia, increased myocardial contractility, and arteriolar vasoconstriction—all in an attempt to maintain cardiac output and perfusion pressure to vital organs. A subacute adaptation is fluid retention producing an increase in venous volume and ventricular filling pressures. This attempts to maintain effective stroke volume by the Frank-Starling principle. Myocardial hypertrophy and cardiac dilatation develop in response to chronic pressure or volume overload. Ventricular hypertrophy and dilatation are seen when either the outflow valve is stenotic or incompetent or the inflow valve is incompetent. Atrial dilatation occurs when the atrioventricular valve is stenotic or incompetent.

Chronic adaptations are able to preserve cardiac output and prevent pulmonary congestion for many years. However, these processes cause myocardial injury that eventually becomes irreversible, and once clinical symptoms of heart failure develop, progressive clinical deterioration is common. Aortic stenosis has a rapid rate of progression, with average survival less than 5 years once symptoms develop, and up to 20 percent of these patients die suddenly. Other chronic valvular lesions are better tolerated. Medical treatment is only effective for the side effects such as systemic and pulmonary venous congestion, and does not affect the underlying mechanical problem. For this reason surgery is often recommended, even when symptoms are absent or mild, to prevent irreversible myocardial injury. There are extensive current studies attempting to determine the best time for surgical intervention in individual patients.

The effects of aortic or mitral valvular disease on the pulmonary vascular bed are significant. As left ventricular diastolic pressure rises, pulmonary venous pressure also rises, causing interstitial pulmonary edema and reflex pulmonary arteriolar vasoconstriction. Initially the vasoconstriction and pulmonary artery hypertension are reversible, but persistence leads to irreversible pulmonary arteriolar changes and pulmonary artery hypertension becomes fixed. Pulmonary hypertension places a pressure overload on the right ventricle and may result in right-sided heart failure with venous engorgement and peripheral edema.

MITRAL STENOSIS

Valvular mitral stenosis is nearly always the result of rheumatic heart disease, usually requiring years of progressive damage to become clinically manifest. The murmur of mitral stenosis is usually detected in the third or fourth decade of life, with symptoms developing 10 to 15 years later. The significant hemodynamic abnormality is an elevated diastolic pressure gradient across the mitral valve. The normal mitral valve area is 4 to 6 cm^2. A diastolic pressure gradient is usually found when the orifice size decreases below 2.5 cm^2; pulmonary congestion is seen below 1.5 cm^2; and right heart failure is found below 1.0 cm^2.

Clinical Features

The most common early sympton is dyspnea, which is precipitated by exertion, tachycardia, anemia, pregnancy, or infection. Attempts to increase blood flow are resisted by the stenotic mitral valve, which produces an increase in left atrial pressure and pulmonary venous pressure. These patients need a slow heart rate and long diastole to keep left atrial pressure and pulmonary venous pressure as low as possible. Eventually, paroxysmal nocturnal dyspnea and orthopnea develop. The enlarged and irritable left atrium commonly produces premature atrial contractions, atrial fibrillation, and, rarely, atrial flutter.

Patients with mitral stenosis are susceptible to pulmonary infections because of sustained vascular congestion. Circulatory stasis predisposes to deep venous thrombosis, pulmonary embolism, and pulmonary infarction. Chronic interstitial edema and pulmonary hypertension can lead to pulmonary interstitial fibrosis and restrictive lung disease. Hemoptysis due to rupture of distended pulmonary-bronchial venous anastomoses is rare but potentially life-threatening. Thrombi may form in the atria or on the valve leaflets, especially in patients in atrial fibrillation, and may embolize to arteries supplying the brain, kidneys, spleen, or extremities.

There are several important physical signs of mitral stenosis. A prominent *a* wave in the jugular veins and an early-systolic left parasternal lift are signs of right ventricular pressure overload. The apical impulse is typically small and tapping in quality, indicating an underfilled left ventricle. The first heart sound is loud and snapping unless the valve is heavily scarred and immobile. An early diastolic opening snap and a following low-pitched, mid-diastolic rumble that crescendos into S_1 is typical. The closer an opening snap occurs to S_2 and the longer the duration of the murmur during diastole, the greater is the severity of obstruction.

Pulmonary hypertension can be suspected from several possible physical signs: (1) an increase in the normal splitting of the two components of S_2 and an accentuation of the second component (pulmonic); (2) a pulmonary ejection click; (3) an early-diastolic blow along the left second or third intercostal spaces (Graham Steell murmur), indicating pulmonary regurgitation; and (4) a holosystolic murmur of tricuspid regurgitation with severe pulmonary hypertension.

Two other conditions may also produce a middiastolic murmur. The Austin-Flint murmur is a middiastolic rumble associated with aortic regurgitation, but there is no accentuation of S_1 and no opening snap. A left atrial myxoma may obstruct flow across the mitral valve and produce a middiastolic murmur. Movement of the tumor may produce a loud sound ("tumor plop") and there are often signs of pulmonary hypertension. Systemic symptoms, such as fever, weight loss, anemia, embolic phenomena, and "pneumonia," are common.

The earliest radiographic change of mitral stenosis is straightening of the left heart border due to left atrial enlargement. Further left atrial enlargement can be recognized as a double density behind the heart. Pulmonary congestion is manifested by an increase in vascular markings, redistribution of flow to the upper lung fields, and Kerley B lines at the bases.

The ECG may show notched or diphasic P waves, indicating left atrial enlargement, and pulmonary hypertension may cause right axis deviation or right ventricular hypertrophy.

Treatment

The treatment of mitral stenosis as it relates to the emergency physician depends primarily on the recognition and initial management of acute complications. The development of fever in a patient with rheumatic heart disease should raise the suspicion of endocarditis. Sustained tachycardias are poorly tolerated by patients with mitral stenosis, atrial fibrillation with a rapid ventricular response being most common in this situation. Digoxin should be used to control ventricular rate and propranolol can be added if digoxin alone is inadequate. Occasionally, synchronized cardioversion may convert atrial fibrillation into sinus rhythm, but recurrences of the arrhythmia are common. Systemic arterial embolism may occur with electrical cardioversion, and a period of anticoagulation is necessary prior to treating chronic atrial fibrillation in this manner. Propranolol is effective in preventing an exaggerated heart rate increase with exercise. Oral anticoagulation

is indicated for patients in sustained atrial fibrillation to prevent systemic arterial emboli. Mild hemoptysis may occur secondary to a temporary rise in pulmonary venous pressure such as can be produced by exercise. Rarely, massive hemoptysis may require blood transfusion and emergency surgery. Pulmonary infarction should be considered in the differential diagnosis of hemoptysis. Bacterial endocarditis prophylaxis should be kept in mind for all procedures that may cause a bacteremia. Rheumatic fever prophylaxis is also recommended for children and young adults still at risk for acute rheumatic fever. Surgical treatment is advised for symptoms that interfere with the patient's pattern of living.

MITRAL REGURGITATION

The mitral valve may be incompetent from disease affecting any portion of the functional mitral valve apparatus: left atrial wall, mitral annulus, mitral valve leaflets, chordae tendineae, papillary muscles, and left ventricular wall. Mitral regurgitation may be acute, intermittent, or chronic, with corresponding clinical presentations.

Acute, severe mitral regurgitation is usually due to rupture of the chordae tendineae, rupture of the papillary muscles, or perforation of the valve leaflets, usually secondary to infective endocarditis or acute myocardial infarction. As blood attempts to regurgitate into the noncompliant left atrium, pressure rises to very high levels and acute pulmonary edema quickly develops. Reflex pulmonary vasoconstriction and signs of acute cor pulmonale may be present.

Intermittent mitral regurgitation is usually due to ischemia, which produces papillary muscle dysfunction or changes in left ventricular compliance. The papillary muscles are sensitive to coronary artery disease because they are the last portion of the ventricle perfused by the coronary arteries. The inferior papillary muscle is most commonly affected by ischemia.

There are many causes of chronic mitral regurgitation: rheumatic heart disease, congenital heart disease, many connective tissue and rheumatologic disorders, hypertrophic and congestive cardiomyopathies, calcified mitral annulus, and complications of infective endocarditis or acute myocardial infarction. With chronic regurgitation, the left atrium dilates so that left atrial pressure rises little, even with large regurgitant flow. As an adaptation, the total stroke volume of the left ventricle increases so that effective forward flow into the aorta is maintained despite the large regurgitant volume across the mitral valve.

Clinical Features

Acute mitral regurgitation presents with dyspnea, tachypnea, and, eventually, pulmonary edema. The apical impulse is usually active, with prominent thrusts and a systolic thrill. Both an S_3 and an S_4 may be heard. The harsh, apical regurgitant murmur starts with S_1 and may end before S_2 because left ventricular and atrial pressures equalize before the end of systole. Acute right ventricular pressure overload may cause jugular venous distention, with a prominent *a* wave and a left parasternal lift.

Patients with intermittent mitral regurgitation usually present with acute episodes of respiratory distress due to pulmonary edema and are relatively asymptomatic between episodes. The predominant symptom of dyspnea may mask the anginal pain of ischemia.

The murmur is usually a soft apical systolic murmur, which increases in intensity with acute episodes, often with S_3 and S_4 gallops. Auscultatory signs may also be obscured by the pulmonary edema signs.

Chronic mitral regurgitation is often well tolerated for years, the earliest signs being exertional dyspnea and fatigue, especially if atrial fibrillation develops. The jugular venous pressure is often normal. The large regurgitant flow into the left atrium may push the entire heart forward and produce a late systolic left parasternal lift. The high-pitched apical holosystolic murmur usually radiates to the axilla. The first heart sound is generally soft and obscured by the murmur. There is usually an S_3 followed by a short diastolic rumble indicating increased flow into the left ventricle. Chronic mitral regurgitation produces left ventricular and atrial enlargement, which is usually detected by chest radiography or electrocardiography.

Treatment

Patients with acute, severe mitral regurgitation need rapid treatment for cardiogenic pulmonary edema with oxygen, afterload reduction (even with normal blood pressure), diuretics, etc. The intraaortic balloon pump can be used to support the circulatory system prior to cardiac catheterization and surgery. Papillary muscle or chordae tendineae rupture entails a high mortality and emergency surgery is often required.

Intermittent mitral regurgitation usually responds to treatment for myocardial ischemia with nitrates. Diuretics are sometimes needed. Some patients achieve relief with the Valsalva maneuver.

Patients with chronic mitral regurgitation who develop congestive heart failure should be treated with digoxin and diuretics. In cases of onset of atrial fibrillation with a rapid ventricular response, the ventricular rate should be controlled with digoxin. Afterload reduction can be used to decrease the percentage of regurgitation and increase forward cardiac output. Oral anticoagulation is occasionally needed to prevent development of atrial thrombi and systemic arterial embolism. Bacterial endocarditis and rheumatic fever prophylaxis are indicated for populations at risk.

MITRAL VALVE PROLAPSE

Mitral valve prolapse is due to a mismatch between the size of the left ventricular cavity and the mitral valve apparatus. Prolapse occurs when the "redundant" mitral valve prolapses into the left atrium as the left ventricle shrinks past a critical volume during systole. Prolapse usually involves a portion of the posterior mitral valve leaflet and occurs during mid to late systole. Often, the tricuspid valve may also prolapse, indicating a more generalized cardiac pathology.

Many disorders have a ventriculovalvular mismatch allowing mitral valve prolapse ("secondary" prolapse): connective tissue diseases (Marfan's syndrome), hypertrophic cardiomyopathy, atrial septal defect, Ebstein's anomaly, ischemic heart disease, rheumatic heart disease, trauma, etc. However, many patients have no discernible underlying cause ("primary" or idiopathic mitral valve prolapse). The incidence of auscultatory and/or echocardiographic evidence of primary mitral valve prolapse in studies of asymptomatic young adults has been found to be between 0.3 and 12 percent. A good estimate for the prevalence of mitral valve prolapse in the general population is about 4 percent, which suggests that this disorder represents more a variation than a disease. Even so, there appear to be certain clinical features associated with mitral valve prolapse.

Clinical Features

Many patients are asymptomatic and are diagnosed on the basis of incidental findings during routine physical examination. Some patients have chest pain (presumably due to tension on the papillary muscles) and palpitations (due to atrial or ventricular tachyarrhythmias). Patients may have syncope from tachyarrhythmias or orthostatic hypotension. Other symptoms, such as anxiety or fatigue, are poorly understood.

Patients with mitral valve prolapse are at increased risk for bacterial endocarditis. Rarely, thrombi may form on the redundant leaflets and embolize to the ophthalmic or cerebral circulation, presenting as amaurosis fugax or transient ischemic attacks. Sudden death, perhaps due to ventricular fibrillation, has been reported in a few patients.

The classic auscultatory findings are a mid- to late-systolic click followed by a late-systolic murmur. The click is caused by the sudden tensing of the loose chordae tendineae as the leaflet reaches the maximal prolapsed position. At this point the valve is often slightly incompetent, allowing for a small amount of mitral regurgitation. The timing of the click and murmur is established by when the critical ventricular volume is reached during systole. Maneuvers which decrease left ventricular volume (strain phase of the Valsalva maneuver, tachycardia, sudden standing, or use of amyl nitrate) allow prolapse to occur sooner in systole and the click-murmur moves closer to S_1. Maneuvers which increase left ventricular volume (squatting, maximal isometric handgrip, bradycardia, passive leg raising, or β-adrenergic blockers) prevent prolapse until late in systole and the click-murmur moves away from S_1. Clicks and murmurs commonly vary in intensity and may not be heard all the time.

The ECG may have nonspecific flattened or inverted T waves, especially in leads II, III, aV_F, and V_4 to V_6. The QT interval may be prolonged. Certain arrhythmias are common: marked sinus arrhythmia, premature atrial contractions, premature ventricular contractions, paroxysmal supraventricular tachycardia, and, in older patients, atrial fibrillation. Some patients with these arrhythmias have no auscultatory findings but do have echocardiographic evidence of mitral valve prolapse.

Heart size and shape are usually normal on chest radiograph. Rare cases with severe mitral regurgitation will show left ventricular and atrial enlargement.

Diagnosis of mitral valve prolapse is generally confirmed by echocardiography or, if necessary, cardiac catheterization.

Treatment

β-Adrenergic antagonists are effective in suppressing arrhythmias and, to some extent, chest pain, presumably by increasing left ventricular size, reducing the ventriculovalvular mismatch, and lessening tension on the papillary muscles. Some patients may require additional antiarrhythmic therapy. Prophylaxis for bacterial endocarditis is indicated. Oral anticoagulation is indicated in patients with a history of systemic embolism.

VALVULAR AORTIC STENOSIS

Valvular aortic stenosis develops primarily from rheumatic heart disease, a congenitally bicuspid aortic valve, or, rarely, idiopathic sclerosis. Rheumatic inflammation of the aortic valve leaflets causes fusion at the commissures, which may be followed by progressive fibrosis and varying degrees of calcification, producing a valve that is usually both stenotic and incompetent. A bicuspid aortic valve is a common congenital abnormality (found in up to 2 percent of the general population) that may, but does not invariably, undergo fibrosis and calcification from a lifetime of hemodynamic stress. Patients with rheumatic or bicuspid aortic stenosis usually present with symptoms at ages between 40 and 60 years. Idiopathic sclerosis of the aortic valve leaflets is common in the elderly and often produces a hemodynamically insignificant systolic ejection murmur. Rarely, calcification of aortic valve sclerosis produces significant stenosis.

The principal hemodynamic abnormality in aortic stenosis is obstruction to left ventricular outflow. The normal aortic valve area is 2 to 3 cm^2, and in general stenosis does not produce significant impairment to forward flow until the orifice has become narrowed to less than 0.8 cm^2, in which case the systolic pressure gradient across the valve usually exceeds 50 mmHg. Cardiac output can be maintained for many years by hypertrophy of left ventricular myocardium. With severe obstruction, stroke volume is partially dependent on adequate filling pressure, which is augmented by an effective left atrial contraction just before ventricular systole ("left atrial kick"). Conversion from sinus rhythm to atrial fibrillation can markedly reduce stroke volume and exacerbate left heart failure.

Clinical Features

The patient with aortic stenosis may remain asymptomatic for many years, but once symptoms occur, average life expectancy is less than 5 years. The characteristic symptoms of aortic stenosis are angina pectoris, syncope, and left heart failure. Exertional dyspnea and other symptoms of left heart failure result from an elevated left ventricular end-diastolic pressure that is transmitted to the pulmonary venous bed and causes pulmonary congestion. Angina pectoris occurs because of the markedly increased oxygen demand of the hypertrophied myocardium and, to some extent, decreased blood flow to the subendocardium due to increased wall tension compressing small arterioles. However, coronary artery disease is also common in these middle-aged patients. Exertional syncope may result when a stenotic valve prevents cardiac output from increasing during exercise. Congestive heart failure indicates advanced disease, with average survival estimated to be less than 2 years after its onset. Atrial fibrillation or sustained tachycardias are poorly tolerated and often produce symptoms.

Initially blood pressure is normal, but as disease progresses, systolic blood pressure falls and pulse pressure narrows. However, elderly patients have a loss in aortic compliance and may have systolic hypertension despite significant aortic stenosis. The carotid pulse has a slow upstroke (often with a "shuttering" feeling), diminished amplitude, and slow downstroke. The apical im-

pulse is enlarged, sustained, and laterally displaced owing to left ventricular hypertrophy and dilatation. An S$_4$ is usually prominent. Aortic stenosis produces a coarse, low-pitched systolic ejection murmur, loudest at the right second intercostal space, with radiation to the carotids and to some extent the apex. The later the murmur peaks in systole, the more severe the obstruction. As stenosis increases in severity, the splitting of S$_2$ becomes narrowed and occasionally reversed (paradoxical splitting). Aortic valve leaflets that are still mobile may have an early systolic ejection click, but increasing age, fibrosis, and calcification usually reduce this finding. The ECG usually shows left ventricular hypertrophy and secondary repolarization changes ("strain pattern").

Aortic stenosis usually produces left ventricular hypertrophy, which causes little cardiac enlargement on chest radiograph. Poststenotic dilatation of the ascending aorta is common. Calcification of the aortic valve leaflets indicates severe aortic stenosis.

Treatment

Strenuous physical exertion should be avoided. Prophylaxis for bacterial endocarditis is indicated. Symptoms of congestive heart failure can be treated with salt restriction, diuretics, and digoxin. However, these patients are partially dependent on an adequate left ventricular filling pressure to maintain cardiac output, and hypovolemia may be life-threatening. Nitrates may be cautiously tried for treatment of chest pain, although they may exacerbate syncope and orthostatic hypotension. Prosthetic replacement of the aortic valve is strongly advised in most patients who develop symptoms of angina, syncope, or heart failure.

AORTIC REGURGITATION

Aortic regurgitation may be acute or chronic, with correspondingly different pathophysiology, clinical features, and treatment.

Acute aortic regurgitation may result from destruction of valve leaflets (due to infective endocarditis, acute rheumatic fever, trauma, or spontaneous rupture) or from sudden dilatation of the aortic root (due to aortic dissection). With acute aortic regurgitation, left ventricular diastolic pressure rises rapidly to very high levels as blood regurgitates into the noncompliant left ventricle, producing acute left ventricular failure and pulmonary edema. Effective stroke volume and cardiac output fall and heart rate increases. The systolic blood pressure does not increase and the diastolic blood pressure cannot fall below the very high left ventricular end-diastolic pressure so that pulse pressure does not increase substantially.

Chronic aortic regurgitation can occur from processes which slowly destroy the valve leaflets (rheumatic heart disease or myxomatous degeneration) or dilate the aortic root (cystic medionecrosis of the aorta, Marfan's syndrome, tertiary syphilis, ankylosing spondylitis, or Reiter's syndrome). With chronic aortic regurgitation, the left ventricle dilates and hypertrophies so that end-diastolic volume markedly increases with little change in end-diastolic pressure. The ejection fraction increases so that effective stroke volume and cardiac output are maintained despite a large regurgitant volume. Heart rate remains unchanged and systolic blood pressure rises while diastolic blood pressure falls, producing an increased pulse pressure. If unchecked, chronic aortic regurgitation will ultimately result in heart failure.

Clinical Features

Acute Aortic Regurgitation

Acute aortic regurgitation is characterized by the sudden onset of dyspnea, tachypnea, tachycardia, and chest pain. Signs of specific causes, such as bacterial endocarditis, aortic dissection, or trauma, may be present. Low cardiac output and vasoconstriction produce pale extremities and sometimes peripheral cyanosis. Heart rate is increased. Systolic and diastolic blood pressures are normal or decreased and pulse pressure widens little. Pulse signs of chronic aortic regurgitation are absent.

The apical impulse is usually normal in position and quality. Auscultation may be difficult because of marked tachycardia and respiratory distress. An important diagnostic feature is a diminished S_1 because the rapidly rising left ventricular diastolic pressure closes the mitral valve before the onset of systole. If the aortic valve leaflets are also destroyed, the aortic component of S_2 is soft. An S_3 is common. The murmur of acute aortic regurgitation is medium-pitched, soft, and of short duration because the early equalization of pressures in the aorta and left ventricle diminishes regurgitant flow. There may be a soft systolic ejection murmur due to increased flow across the aortic valve during systole.

The ECG is generally characterized by nonspecific ST-T changes without evidence of left ventricular hypertrophy. Infectious endocarditis may cause various conduction disturbances as the infection spreads to the nodal and infranodal conducting system.

The chest radiograph will show a normal cardiac size but pulmonary venous congestion and edema. Special attention should be directed to aortic and mediastinal contours in a search for evidence of aortic dissection.

Chronic Aortic Regurgitation

A patient with chronic aortic regurgitation may relate a history of specific causes: rheumatic fever, syphilis, infective endocarditis, different varieties of arthritis, or Marfanoid habitus.

Compensatory mechanisms enable the patient with chronic aortic regurgitation to remain asymptomatic for many years. Characteristic symptoms include chest pain (typical or atypical angina), palpitations, awareness of the heart beat, and symptoms of left heart failure. Chest wall pain may also occur, presumably owing to excessive force of cardiac contractions against the thorax. Patients with severe chronic aortic regurgitation may exhibit bobbing of the head with each systole. Severe aortic regurgitation may cause neck and abdominal pain, presumably due to stretching of the carotid artery or aorta from the large stroke volume. Postural dizziness may occur from a low diastolic pressure inadequate to maintain cerebral circulation.

The carotid pulse is pounding, rapidly rising and falling (water-hammer or Corrigan's pulse). A pistol shot sound or a to-and-fro murmur (Duroziez's sign) may be heard over the femoral artery. Capillary pulsations (Quincke's sign) can be seen in the nailbeds. The pulse pressure is usually widened, and a rough guide to the severity of regurgitation can be obtained from the ratio of pulse pressure to systolic pressure, which in mild disease is usually < 0.5, in moderate disease between 0.5 and 0.7, and in severe disease > 0.7. These pulse signs are not pathognomonic for aortic regurgitation as they may be seen in other hyperdynamic states, such as fever, sepsis, or thyrotoxicosis.

Significant aortic regurgitation will displace the apical impulse laterally owing to left ventricular dilatation. A diastolic thrill may be palpable along the left sternal border and, rarely, a systolic thrill may be felt in the second right intercostal space. The first heart sound is preserved. The aortic component of S_2 is usually normal but may be diminished or absent. A third heart sound is occasionally present. With advanced scarring of the valve leaflets, a systolic ejection sound may be heard, which is presumably due to sudden aortic dilatation at the onset of systole.

The classic murmur of rheumatic aortic regurgitation is a high-pitched, blowing, decrescendo diastolic murmur best heard along the left sternal border. If the murmur is more audible along the right sternal border, a nonrheumatic cause is more likely. The regurgitant stream may cause posterior displacement of the anterior mitral valve leaflet, partially narrow the mitral valve orifice during diastole, and cause a middiastolic to presystolic rumble (Austin Flint murmur).

Mild aortic regurgitation may cause no ECG abnormalities, but severe disease produces left ventricular hypertrophy and secondary repolarization changes (''strain pattern''). The chief radiographic feature of chronic aortic regurgitation is left ventricular enlargement. Dilatation of the ascending aorta is typical in Marfan's syndrome and tertiary syphilis.

Treatment

Acute aortic regurgitation is a medical emergency which causes rapid clinical deterioration and has a high mortality without surgical treatment. Prompt diagnosis is essential. Medical stabilization should be done with oxygen, diuretics, afterload reduction, and the intraaortic balloon pump prior to cardiac catheterization and surgery.

The heart failure of chronic aortic regurgitation is treated with sodium restriction, diuretics, and digoxin. Afterload reduction is helpful in increasing effective stroke volume, especially if hypertension is present. Cardiac arrhythmias and infections may exacerbate the left heart failure. Nitrates have had variable success in treating the associated chest pain. Prophylaxis for bacterial endocarditis is indicated. Ideally, patients with chronic aortic regurgitation should have prosthetic valve replacement before irreversible myocardial damage and symptoms of heart failure develop. Repeat evaluations every 6 to 12 months are advised, even in asymptomatic patients.

TRICUSPID STENOSIS

Tricuspid stenosis is an uncommon valvular disease, which is most often due to rheumatic heart disease and associated with some tricuspid regurgitation, mitral stenosis, and, occasionally, aortic stenosis. In patients with rheumatic tricuspid stenosis, the symptoms are primarily due to left heart valvular damage and/or the resulting pulmonary hypertension. Rare causes of tricuspid stenosis include the carcinoid syndrome, endomyocardial fibroelastosis, endomyocardial fibrosis, and systemic lupus erythematosus. The most significant hemodynamic abnormality is an increased diastolic gradient across the tricuspid valve. The normal tricuspid valve has a diastolic area about 7 cm², and significant obstruction occurs when the orifice size narrows below 1.5 cm².

Clinical Features

While dyspnea and fatigue are common symptoms of rheumatic tricuspid and mitral stenosis, significant obstruction at the tricuspid level prevents the development of pulmonary congestion with exertion. Severe tricuspid stenosis is characterized by signs of increased systemic venous pressure such as hepatomegaly, splenomegaly, ascites, and peripheral edema. Pulmonary congestion is absent and cardiac output is usually diminished, especially with exertion.

The jugular venous pressure is elevated, with a prominent a wave and decreased y descent. The first heart sound is accentuated and often split; both findings are enhanced by inspiration. A tricuspid opening snap is rarely audible at the bedside. The rumbling diastolic murmur is best heard along the lower left sternal border or over the xyphoid process. The murmur characteristically increases in intensity with inspiration and decreases with expiration; this is Carvallo's sign, a useful sign in detecting a tricuspid murmur.

Characteristic ECG changes are tall, peaked P waves in lead II, indicating right atrial enlargement. The chest radiograph demonstrates an enlarged right atrium and dilated superior vena cava without pulmonary artery enlargement or signs of pulmonary hypertension.

Treatment

Medical therapy is directed towards relief of systemic venous congestion. Prophylaxis for bacterial endocarditis and rheumatic fever is indicated. Severe cases may require valve replacement.

TRICUSPID REGURGITATION

Right ventricular failure and dilatation constitute the most common cause of tricuspid regurgitation. Combined tricuspid stenosis and regurgitation may result from rheumatic heart disease. Less common causes of isolated tricuspid regurgitation include infective endocarditis, congenital abnormalities of the valve leaflets, endocardial cushion defects, Ebstein's anomaly, prolapsed leaflet syndrome, blunt chest trauma, and papillary muscle damage.

Clinical Features

Since tricuspid regurgitation is most often caused by right ventricular failure secondary to left-sided failure or mitral stenosis, the common symptoms are dyspnea, orthopnea, and peripheral edema. However, tricuspid regurgitation may protect the patient against symptoms of augmented venous return, and paroxysmal nocturnal dyspnea is uncommon. The clinical features of isolated tricuspid regurgitation are the result of increased systemic venous pressure and decreased cardiac output. Patients with advanced cases have peripheral edema, pulsatile hepatomegaly, splenomegaly, and ascites. The jugular veins are distended, with a large v

wave and rapid y descent. The murmur is soft, blowing, holosystolic, and best heard over the lower sternal border or xyphoid. The murmur often increases in intensity with inspiration (Carvallo's sign).

The ECG findings include tall, peaked P waves of right atrial enlargement but these may be masked by the common occurrence of atrial fibrillation. The chest radiograph usually shows enlargement of both the right atrium and ventricle.

Treatment

Treatment for the systemic venous congestion and right-sided heart failure consists of salt restriction, diuretics, and digoxin. Functional tricuspid regurgitation due to pulmonary hypertension will often improve with attempts to lower pulmonary artery pressure. If right ventricular failure is due to mitral stenosis, prosthetic replacement of the mitral valve is indicated.

PULMONARY STENOSIS

Right ventricular outflow obstruction may result from infundibular, valvular, or supravalvular stenosis. The most common cause of valvular pulmonary stenosis is congenital and the most common cause of infundibular obstruction is the tetralogy of Fallot. The significant hemodynamic abnormality is a systolic pressure gradient across the pulmonary valve. Stenosis can be graded by the peak right ventricular systolic pressure: mild, < 65 mmHg; moderate, between 65 to 120 mmHg, and severe, > 120 mmHg.

Clinical Features

Many patients remain asymptomatic for years. Severe pulmonary stenosis causes external dyspnea and signs of right heart failure. Syncope and sudden death can occur. The jugular veins have a prominent a wave. A right parasternal lift is usually present and a systolic thrill may be felt in the second left intercostal space or suprasternal notch. The second heart sound is widely split. A systolic ejection click followed by a harsh systolic ejection murmur, which increases with inspiration, is usually heard in the left second intercostal space and radiates to the left clavicle.

The ECG findings of severe pulmonary stenosis are right atrial enlargement, right axis deviation, and right ventricular hypertrophy with secondary repolarization changes ("strain pattern"). The chest radiograph usually shows poststenotic dilatation of the main pulmonary artery and evidence of right ventricular enlargement. Pulmonary blood flow is normal in the absence of a right-to-left shunt.

Treatment

Medical management consists of treating the symptoms of venous congestion. Prophylaxis for bacterial endocarditis is indicated. Pulmonary valve surgery is recommended when the peak right ventricular systolic pressure is over 70 mmHg or the peak systolic gradient across the pulmonary valve is over 50 mmHg.

PULMONARY REGURGITATION

Pulmonary regurgitation may be secondary to pulmonary hypertension, producing dilatation of the valve ring and resultant valvular incompetence. Symptoms are more likely to be due to the pulmonary hypertension than to the regurgitation itself. Isolated pulmonary regurgitation may result from a congenital lesion, acute rheumatic fever, or infective endocarditis.

Clinical Features

Isolated pulmonary regurgitation is tolerated for many years. The characteristic symptoms of severe pulmonary hypertension are dyspnea, fatigue, and syncope. The classic murmur of pulmonary regurgitation is a high-pitched, blowing, diastolic murmur at the second left intercostal space. The murmur starts with the pulmonic component of S_2 and has a brief crescendo, followed by a longer decrescendo. A brief midsystolic ejection murmur, reflecting increased flow across the pulmonary valve, is typical.

Treatment

Treatment of pulmonary hypertension, if present, with diuretics, digoxin, vasodilating agents, and mitral valve replacement is the first step. Isolated pulmonary regurgitation is often well tolerated and valve replacement is indicated in only severe cases.

PROSTHETIC VALVE COMPLICATIONS

Complications of prosthetic valves may occur early after surgery or be delayed for years after implantation. The type and incidence of the different complications depend on such factors as: (1) the underlying heart disease, (2) the specific valve replaced; (3) the type of prosthetic valve; and (4) the need for anticoagulation.

Prosthetic valves can be divided into four main types (Table 12-1). The valves themselves can be covered with a variety of materials, such as cloth, Silastic, or Teflon.

Table 12-1. Four Varieties of Prosthetic Valves

Caged-ball
Starr-Edwards (aortic and mitral)
Smeloff-Cutter (aortic and mitral)
Braunwald-Cutter (mitral and tricuspid)
Magovern-Cromie (aortic only)
DeBakey-Surgitool (aortic only)
Disk
Central occluder disk
Beall-Surgitool (mitral and tricuspid)
Kay-Shiley (mitral and tricuspid)
Starr-Edwards (mitral and tricuspid)
Cooley-Cutter
Tilting Disk
Bjork-Shiley
Lillihei-Kaster
Porcine heterograft
Hancock
Carpentier-Edwards
Bileaflet
St. Jude's

A normally functioning prosthetic valve can have distinctive auscultatory features: (1) audible opening and closing sounds; (2) a murmur during normal forward flow of blood through the prosthesis; and (3) a murmur caused by turbulence of blood around the metal portions of the prosthesis. Most prosthetic valves produce systolic ejection murmurs in both the mitral and aortic position. Disk and porcine valves produce diastolic murmurs in the mitral position. Opening sounds in the aortic position are common with ball and bileaflet valves. Opening sounds in the mitral position are common with ball and porcine valves.

Thromboembolism is a major problem with the completely artificial valves, its prevention usually requiring lifelong anticoagulation. Although less of a problem, thrombosis may also occur on the porcine heterograft, especially in the mitral position. Most patients who have an aortic porcine heterograft or a mitral porcine heterograft and stay in sinus rhythm do not need chronic anticoagulation. The presentation of aortic or mitral prosthetic valve thrombosis is usually acute, with obvious development of left heart failure. The presentation of tricuspid prosthetic valve thrombosis is much more insidious.

Mechanical hemolysis of red cells by the prosthetic valve can occur from either a normally functioning or an incompetent valve. Bacterial endocarditis soon after implantation is most commonly caused by staphylococci or gram-negative rods. Delayed endocarditis is most often due to viridans streptococci or *Staphylococcus epidermidis*.

Valvular incompetence can develop from leakage around the valve or, in the case of a porcine heterograft, from cusp rupture. Symptoms suggestive of prosthetic valve dysfunction are increased angina, heart failure, and syncope.

A change in murmurs or muffled valve sounds suggest prosthetic valve dysfunction. Chest radiographs should be done to confirm correct position of the prosthesis. Blurring of the prosthetic valve margins may be secondary to normal valve motion or respiration as well as dysfunction. Cinefluoroscopy, angiography, or echocardiography is necessary to confirm the diagnosis of dysfunction.

Sudden cardiovascular collapse may occur as a result of sticking of the valve in one position or, rarely, catastrophic embolization of the ball portion of a ball-in-cage valve.

BIBLIOGRAPHY

Bardy GH, Talano JV, Meyers S, et al: Acquired cyanotic heart disease secondary to traumatic tricuspid regurgitation. Case report and review of the literature. *Am J Cardiol* 44:1401, 1979.

Barnett HJM, Boughner DR, Taylor DW, et al.: Further evidence relating mitral-valve prolapse to cerebral ischemic events. *N Engl J Med* 302:139, 1980.

Bonchek LI: Indications for surgery of the mitral valve. *Am J Cardiol* 46:155, 1980.

Chizner MA, Pearle DL, DeLeon AC: Natural history of aortic stenosis in adults. *Am Heart J* 99:419, 1980.

Clemens JD, Horwitz RI, Jaffe CC, et al.: A controlled evaluation of the risk of bacterial endocarditis in persons with mitral valve prolapse. *N Engl J Med* 307:776, 1982.

Corrigall D, Bolen J, Hancock EW, et al: Mitral valve prolapse and infective endocarditis. *Am J Med* 63:215, 1977.

Darsee JR, Mikolich JR, Nicoloff NB, et al: Prevalence of mitral valve prolapse in presumably healthy young men. *Circulation* 56:619, 1979.

DeMaria AN, Amsterdam EA, Vismara LA, et al: Arrhythmias in the mitral valve prolapse syndrome. Prevalence, nature, and frequency. *Ann Intern Med* 84:656, 1976.

Edwards JE: The spectrum and clinical significance of tricuspid regurgitation. *Pract Cardiol* 6:86, 1980.

Fenoglio JJ, McAllister HA, DeCastro CM, et al.: Congenital bicuspid aortic valve after age 20. *Am J Cardiol* 39:164, 1977.

Fowler NO, Van der Bel-Kahn JM: Operations on the mitral valve: A time for weighing the issues. *Am J Cardiol* 46:159, 1980.

Fulkerson PK, Beaver BM, Auseon JC, et al: Calcification of the mitral annulus. Etiology, clinical associations, complications and therapy. *Am J Med* 66:967, 1979.

Goldschlager N, Pfeifer J, Cohn K, et al: The natural history of aortic regurgitation: A clinical and hemodynamic study. *Am J Med* 54:577, 1973.

Harrison DC, Isaeff DM, DeBusk RF: Papillary muscle syndromes. *DM*, Jan 1972.

Holmes JC, Fowler NO, Kaplan S: Pulmonary valvular insufficiency. *Am J Med* 44:851, 1968.

Johnson AD, Engler RL, LeWinter M, et al.: The medical and surgical management of patients with aortic valve disease–a symposium. *West J Med* 126:460, 1977.

Kloster FE, Morris CD: Key references. Natural history of valvular heart disease. *Circulation* 65:1283, 1982.

Luisada AA, Portaluppi F, Knighten V: Evaluation of aortic systolic murmur in the aged. *Pract Cardiol* 6(11):61, 1980.

McAllister RG, Friesinger GC, Sinclair-Smith BC: Tricuspid regurgitation following inferior myocardial infarction. *Arch Intern Med* 136:95, 1976.

Mills P, Rose J, Hollingsworth J, et al.: Long-term prognosis of mitral-valve prolapse. *N Engl J Med* 297:13, 1977.

Morganroth J, Perloff JK, Zeldis SM, et al: Acute severe aortic regurgitation. Pathophysiology, clinical recognition, and management. *Ann Intern Med* 87:223, 1977.

Perloff JK: Auscultatory and phonocardiographic manifestations of pulmonary hypertension. *Prog Cardiovasc Dis* 9:303, 1967.

Peters MN, Hall JR, Cooley DA, et al.: The clinical syndrome of atrial myxoma. *JAMA* 230:695, 1974.

Procacci PM, Savran SV, Schreiter SL, et al: Prevalence of clinical mitral-valve prolapse in 1169 women. *N Engl J Med* 294:1986, 1976.

Roberts WC, Perloff JK: Mitral valvular disease. A clinicopathologic survey of conditions causing the mitral valve to function abnormally. *Ann Intern Med* 77:939, 1972.

Ronan JA, Steelman RB, Deleon AC, et al.: The clinical diagnosis of acute severe mitral insufficiency. *Am J Cardiol* 27:284, 1971.

Santos AD, Mathew PK, Hila LA, et al: Orthostatic hypotension: A commonly unrecognized cause of symptoms in mitral valve prolapse. *Am J Med* 71:746, 1981.

Schlant RC: Calcific aortic stenosis. *Am J Cardiol* 27:531, 1971.

Seymour J, Emanuel R, Pattinson N: Acquired pulmonary stenosis. *Br Heart J* 30:776, 1968.

Smith ND, Raizada V, Abrams J: Auscultation of the normally functioning prosthetic valve. *Ann Intern Med* 95:594, 1981.

Stein PD, Sabbah HN: Aortic origin of innocent murmurs. *Am J Cardiol* 39:665, 1977.

CHAPTER 13
THE CARDIOMYOPATHIES, MYOCARDITIS, AND PERICARDIAL DISEASE

James T. Niemann

THE CARDIOMYOPATHIES

Classification and Definition

A cardiomyopathy is currently defined as a heart muscle disorder of unknown cause or association. This definition effectively excludes disorders of myocardial function secondary to systemic arterial hypertension, coronary atherosclerosis, syphilis, valvular heart disease, congenital heart disease, and other structural disorders. For the sake of classification, heart muscle disorders are still frequently divided into primary cardiomyopathies, those of unknown etiology, and secondary cardiomyopathies, those of known etiology or associated with a systemic disease that involves the heart as part of a recognized disease process (Table 13-1). The cardiomyopathies can thus be classified according to etiology or pathology. The cardiomyopathies have also been classified according to clinical presentation: congestive or "dilated," hypertrophic, and restrictive (Table 13-2). A third proposed functional classification highlights the hemodynamic fault responsible for clinical manifestations: systolic pump failure or diastolic compliance failure. A common language or classification is clearly needed, not only for communication but also to serve as a common denominator for clinical investigation. For the sake of clarity, the broad descriptive classification of the cardiomyopathies (congestive, hypertrophic, and restrictive) will be used in the following discussion and functional abnormalities will be highlighted where appropriate to provide a hemodynamic background.

Congestive Cardiomyopathy

This subgroup is characterized hemodynamically by depressed myocardial systolic function or *systolic pump failure*. Left ventricular (LV) contractile force is diminished, resulting in a low cardiac output and increased end-systolic and end-diastolic ventricular volumes and intracavitary pressures. Cardiomegaly results from both dilatation and hypertrophy. Patients with significant hypertrophy appear to survive longer than those with predominant

dilatation. Systemic diseases that may involve the heart and produce a congestive cardiomyopathy as part of a recognized disease process are shown in Table 13-1. A specific etiology or associated disease will be found in fewer than 10 percent of patients.

Clinical Profile

Owing to systolic pump failure, the patient presents with signs and symptoms of congestive heart failure: dyspnea on exertion, orthopnea, and paroxysmal nocturnal dyspnea. Depressed ventricular contractile function and dilatation may also provide an environment for the formation of mural thrombi, and the patient not uncommonly presents with manifestations of peripheral embolization, e.g., an acute neurologic deficit, flank pain and hematuria, or a pulseless, cyanotic extremity.

Murmurs are frequently heard during cardiac auscultation and are not necessarily indicative of primary valvular disease. Ventricular dilatation and resultant lateral displacement of the papillary muscles of the atrioventricular valves inhibit leaflet coaptation and complete valve closure. Holosystolic regurgitant murmurs of mitral and tricuspid valve origin are frequently heard at the apex or lower left sternal border in the patient with biventricular failure. Ventricular dilatation does not produce significant annular dilatation of the atrioventricular valves. On occasion an apical "diastolic rumble" may be heard and is due either to accentuated, early-diastolic atrial-to-ventricular flow, the result of mitral regurgitation and left atrial overload, or to a loud summation gallop. An enlarged, pulsatile liver may be found if tricuspid insufficiency is present. Bibasilar rales and dependent edema are common additional findings.

The posteroanterior (PA) and lateral chest x-ray invariably show an enlarged cardiac silhouette and increased cardiothoracic ratio; biventricular enlargement is common. Evidence of pulmonary venous hypertension ("cephalization" of flow, enlarged hila) is also frequent and may serve to differentiate cardiac enlargement due to myocardial failure from that due to a large pericardial effusion.

The electrocardiogram is almost always abnormal. Left ven-

Table 13-1. Secondary Cardiomyopathies: Heart Muscle Disease of Known Cause or Association

1. Infectious
   Viral
   Protozoal (Chagas' disease)
2. Metabolic
   Thyrotoxicosis
   Myxedema
   Acromegaly
   Hemachromatosis
   Glycogen storage disease
   Thiamine deficiency (beriberi)
   Hypophosphatemia
3. Peripartum
4. Amyloidosis
5. Associated with neuromuscular disorders
   (the muscular dystrophies)
6. Associated with collagen vascular diseases
7. Sarcoidosis
8. Myocardial toxins
   Ethanol
   Heavy metals
   Emetine
   Adriamycin
   Cobalt
9. Physical agents
   Ionizing radiation
   Heat stroke

tricular hypertrophy and left atrial enlargement are the most common findings. Q or QS waves and poor R-wave progression across the anterior precordium may produce a ''pseudoinfarction'' pattern.

Echocardiography in the symptomatic patient demonstrates a decreased ejection fraction, increased systolic and diastolic volumes, and ventricular and atrial enlargement.

Therapy

Management of the patient with idiopathic congestive cardiomyopathy is symptom-directed, and the prescribed therapeutic regimen almost always employs the digitalis glycosides and diuretics. Patients unresponsive to these agents may respond to preload and afterload reduction with nitrates and hydralazine, prazosin, or captopril. A thorough diagnostic evaluation should be undertaken for all patients with unexplained heart failure or cardiomegaly. Such an evaluation may reveal an underlying disease which is amenable to specific therapy in patients with secondary forms of congestive cardiomyopathy.

Hypertrophic Cardiomyopathy

Hypertrophic cardiomyopathy (HCM) is a familial (autosomal dominant) or sporadic cardiac muscle disorder characterized by

Table 13-2. Primary (Idiopathic) Cardiomyopathy

1. Systolic pump failure
   Congestive (dilated) cardiomyopathy
2. Diastolic compliance failure
   Hypertrophic cardiomyopathy
   Restrictive cardiomyopathy

increased left ventricular muscle mass without associated ventricular dilatation. The diagnostic hallmarks of the disease are echocardiographic asymmetric septal hypertrophy and histologic myocardial fiber disarray. This primary myocardial disorder has also been called *hypertrophic obstructive cardiomyopathy, idiopathic hypertrophic subaortic stenosis,* and *muscular subaortic stenosis.*

Former names for this disease emphasized a hemodynamic finding noted during early descriptions of the disease, namely, a pressure gradient between the body of the left ventricle and the subvalvular outflow tract. This finding suggested outflow tract obstruction, since pressure differences between the left ventricle and aorta are also seen in valvular aortic stenosis. More recent data employing sophisticated measurement techniques suggest that the powerful systolic contraction of the hypertrophic left ventricle, rather than true obstruction, is responsible for the observed gradients. The fact that the left ventricle of the typical HCM patient ejects its contents in the first half of systole and that no consistent correlation is found between prognosis and the presence and magnitude or the absence of an outflow gradient lend further support to the current belief that HCM is a heart muscle disease rather than a result of LV outflow obstruction.

Hemodynamically HCM is characterized by abnormal LV diastolic function due to reduced compliance of the hypertrophied left ventricle. This decreased compliance is reflected by an increase in LV filling pressure. Cardiac output, ejection fraction, and end-systolic and diastolic volumes are usually normal. A systolic pressure gradient between the body of the left ventricle and the subvalvular outflow tract can be recorded in some patients at rest or after provocation (exercise, isoproterenol infusion). As previously noted, this recorded gradient has been ascribed to dynamic outflow obstruction by the hypertrophied septum or forceful systolic isometric ventricular contraction. Angiographic and echocardiographic studies have suggested an additional but questioned mechanism, namely, systolic motion of the anterior leaflet of the mitral valve, leading to outflow obstruction. Regardless of the cause of the measured systolic gradient, the major hemodynamic fault and the majority of clinical symptoms in this heart muscle disease are the result of impaired diastolic relaxation and restricted LV filling.

Clinical Profile

Severity of symptoms in most instances is related to patient age, i.e., the older the patient, the more severe the symptoms. Dyspnea on exertion is the most frequent initial complaint and is due to elevated LV diastolic pressure accentuated by exercise. Additional symptoms include chest pain, palpitations, and syncope. A family history of death due to cardiac disease, frequently described as ''massive heart attack'' or ''heart failure,'' is not uncommon. In younger patients, HCM may initially be diagnosed after sudden cardiac death related to an episode of exertion. Complaints of paroxysmal nocturnal dyspnea and pedal edema are uncommon.

Chest pain in HCM patients is due to an imbalance between the oxygen demand of the hypertrophied left ventricle and available myocardial blood flow. In older patients, associated atherosclerotic coronary artery disease may further limit myocardial perfusion. Precordial or retrosternal chest discomfort in HCM may mimic angina pectoris or be ''atypical.'' Response to nitroglycerin administration is poor and highly variable.

The HCM patient may be aware of forceful ventricular contraction and complain of an abnormal heart beat or "palpitations." Atrial and ventricular arrhythmias are not uncommon in these patients but may not be related to symptoms or predictive of sudden death. Rapid atrial arrhythmias, especially atrial fibrillation, are particularly poorly tolerated owing to the increased importance of the atrial contribution to LV filling in the poorly compliant heart.

Twenty to thirty percent of patients will complain of syncope or lightheadedness during or after physical exertion. These symptoms are not related to the magnitude of the gradient and are not of ominous prognostic import.

Jugular venous pressure is usually not elevated; however, a prominent *a* wave may be noted on close inspection of the neck veins. The upstroke of the carotid arterial pulse is rapid and frequently biphasic or bifid (pulsus bisferiens). The apical impulse is sustained and hyperdynamic and a presystolic lift is common.

The first and second heart sounds are usually normal and a fourth sound (S_4) will be heard in most patients. The characteristic systolic ejection-type murmur of HCM is heard best at the lower left sternal border or at the apex and rarely radiates to the carotid arteries. Easily performed bedside maneuvers can be used to increase the intensity and duration of the murmur (Table 13-3). Interventions that decrease LV filling and the distending pressure in the LV outflow tract or that increase the force of myocardial contraction accentuate the murmur of HCM. Such interventions include standing, the Valsalva maneuver, amyl nitrate inhalation, and isoproterenol infusion. The murmur will also be louder with the first sinus beat following a premature ventricular contraction. Maneuvers that increase LV filling (squatting, passive leg elevation, handgrip) have an opposite effect on murmur characteristics.

ECG findings of LV hypertrophy and left atrial enlargement are found in 30 percent and 25 to 50 percent, respectively, of HCM patients. Evidence of chamber enlargement is most common in patients with large gradients across the LV outflow tract. Q waves of considerable amplitude (>0.3 mV), termed *septal Q waves*, are seen in about 25 percent of patients and may be encountered in the anterior, lateral, or inferior leads. These Q waves may mimic those seen following myocardial infarction (*pseudoinfarction pattern*). The polarity of the T wave serves as a diagnostic clue in the separation of HCM septal Q waves from Q waves due to myocardial infarction. Upright T waves in those leads with QS or QR complexes are usually found in HCM; T-wave inversion in such leads is highly suggestive of ischemic heart disease.

PA and lateral chest x-rays are frequently normal and identifiable abnormalities are largely nonspecific. Many patients do not show radiographic evidence of LV or left atrial enlargement. Evidence of pulmonary venous congestion is unusual but has been reported.

Echocardiography has played a substantial role in the diagnosis of HCM, in the correlation of the auscultatory and hemodynamic events with LV anatomic changes, and in defining inheritance patterns. The characteristic echocardiographic finding is disproportionate septal hypertrophy; the ratio of the thickness of the septum to the thickness of the posterior free wall of the left ventricle usually exceeds 1.5. Additional described echocardiographic abnormalities include normal or reduced LV end-diastolic dimensions, systolic anterior motion of the mitral valve, and midsystolic closure of the aortic valve.

Natural History and Therapy

The clinical course of patients with HCM is highly variable and not well correlated with the magnitude of the gradient across the LV outflow tract. In a minority of patients (less than 5 percent) the heart dilates and a clinical picture like that of a congestive cardiomyopathy develops. The onset of paroxysmal or sustained atrial and ventricular tachyarrhythmias may result in an abrupt deterioration of functional status. Bacterial endocarditis occurs in a small number of patients and may likewise result in a sudden change in clinical status. Sudden cardiac death, presumably due to cardiac arrhythmias, occurs at a rate of 4 percent per year. The HCM patient population at risk cannot be predicted on the basis of symptoms or hemodynamic findings.

The mainstay of medical therapy for the symptomatic patient, specifically the patient with chest pain, has been the liberal use of β-blockers (propranolol, usual dose 120 to 320 mg/day in divided doses). Recent studies have demonstrated that calcium blocking agents may be of value in a carefully defined population of HCM patients who do respond to β-blockade. Surgical therapy (septal muscle excision or mitral valve replacement) has not been conclusively shown to offer advantages over medical therapy. Antibiotic prophylaxis is recommended for dental procedures and potentially unsterile surgery. Several authorities discourage competitive athletics of any type, since sudden death following vigorous exertion is not infrequent in patients with HCM.

Restrictive Cardiomyopathy

This is the least common of the clinically recognized and described cardiomyopathies. The hemodynamic characteristics of a restrictive cardiomyopathy include: (1) elevated left and right ventricular end-diastolic pressures; (2) normal LV systolic function (ejection fraction > 50 percent); and (3) an abrupt and rapid rise in early-diastolic ventricular pressure following a marked decline at the onset of diastole. The rapid rise and abrupt plateau in the early-diastolic ventricular pressure tracing results in a characteristic (but not diagnostic) "square-root sign" or "dip-and-plateau" filling pattern. Simultaneously recorded left and right ventricular diastolic pressures are frequently mirror images, varying by only a few millimeters of mercury. These hemodynamic findings are similar to those reported in constrictive pericarditis, and differentiation at times may require surgical biopsy.

Causes of restrictive cardiomyopathy are listed in Table 13-4. In the vast majority of cases, no specific etiology can be defined. Recent data suggest that the idiopathic variety is a more "stable"

Table 13-3. Effect of Bedside Interventions on Murmur Intensity and Duration in HCM

Increase	Decrease
Valsalva maneuver	Passive leg elevation in the supine patient
Standing	
Amyl nitrate inhalation	Handgrip
β-Agonists (isoproterenol infusion)	Squatting
	α-Agonists (phenylephrine infusion)

Table 13-4. Causes of Restrictive Cardiomyopathy

Idiopathic (includes endomyocardial fibrosis and Loeffler's eosinophilic endomyocardial disease)
Secondary (associated with systemic disease)
  Hemachromatosis
  Amyloidosis
  Sarcoidosis
  Progressive systemic sclerosis (scleroderma)

or less progressive disease than the myocardial disease associated with a specific etiology or systemic disease process.

Clinical Profile

In patients with advanced cardiac disease of known etiology, clinical symptoms are similar to those noted in patients with congestive or dilated cardiomyopathy, namely, pedal edema and decreased exercise tolerance or other evidence of pulmonary venous hypertension. Chest pain, either typical for angina or atypical, is also a frequent presenting complaint and its cause is unexplained. Patients with the idiopathic variety or with early secondary forms may be asymptomatic, but are referred for evaluation of an abnormal auscultatory finding (murmur or gallop) or abnormal ECG (abnormal QRS voltage, nonspecific ST-T wave changes, prolonged QRS duration, bundle branch blocks, or an arrhythmia).

Findings on physical examination depend upon the stage or severity of myocardial involvement. An S_3 and/or S_4 is commonly heard in the asymptomatic or minimally symptomatic patient. Gallop rhythms and systolic murmurs (due to mitral regurgitation) are usually heard in advanced cases, as are pulmonary rales, and pedal edema is present.

The routine chest x-ray may be normal and, combined with symptoms and physical findings, may suggest constrictive pericarditis. In advanced cases, enlargement of the cardiac silhouette and pulmonary vascular redistribution are seen.

The ECG is frequently abnormal, but "diagnostic" changes have not been described. The most frequently reported ECG changes include chamber enlargement (ventricular and atrial) and repolarization abnormalities (nonspecific ST-T wave changes). Low-voltage QRS complexes (<0.7 mV) have been frequently reported in patients with restrictive cardiomyopathy secondary to amyloidosis and hemochromatosis complicated by congestive heart failure and radiographic and echocardiographic evidence of cardiac enlargement.

Right and left heart catheterization should be performed in all patients with suspected restrictive cardiomyopathy. Hemodynamic findings are similar to those noted in constrictive pericarditis (dip-and-plateau configuration of ventricular pressure trace). However, there are differences that allow hemodynamic differentiation. The most important of these is that LV diastolic pressure usually exceeds right ventricular diastolic pressure owing to the fact that restrictive cardiomyopathy is largely an LV disease with only secondary right-sided involvement. In some instances, transvenous myocardial biopsy or surgical pericardial biopsy may be required for definitive diagnosis.

Recent observations suggest that myocardial scintigraphy [technetium-99-m-pyrophosphate (^{99m}Tc PYP) scanning] may be of value in the diagnosis of cardiac amyloidosis, the most common of the secondary restrictive cardiomyopathies. Patients with cardiac amyloidosis have been shown to exhibit intense *diffuse* uptake of ^{99m}Tc PYP.

Therapy

With the exception of hemachromatosis (variably responsive to chelation therapy with desferroxamine), therapy for restrictive cardiomyopathy is symptom-directed and consists mainly of diuretics, digoxin, and class I antiarrhythmic agents for complicating rhythm disturbances. However, patients with amyloid cardiomyopathy may be "sensitive to digoxin" (prone to toxicity) owing to amyloid fibril binding of digoxin, and this medication should be used with caution and close follow-up in such patients.

MYOCARDITIS

Definition

Myocarditis is broadly but nonspecifically defined as inflammation of the heart muscle and is most frequently characterized pathologically by focal infiltration of the myocardium by lymphocytes, plasma cells, and histiocytes. Varying amounts of myocytolysis and destruction of the interstitial reticulin network are also seen. The pathologic changes have been ascribed to a number of disease entities (Table 13-5), some of which involve the myocardium secondarily as part of a systemic disease process. Myocarditis is frequently accompanied by pericarditis.

Clinical criteria for the diagnosis of myocarditis include sinus tachycardia or other abnormal rhythm, faint S_1, apical systolic murmur, evidence of cardiac insufficiency, cardiomegaly, fever, leukocytosis, and ECG evidence of repolarization and conduction (atrioventricular or intraventricular) abnormalities.

Clinical Profile

Fever is a common feature, as is sinus tachycardia, usually "out of proportion" with respect to the extent of temperature elevation. Signs and symptoms are dependent upon the extent of myocardial involvement and resultant depression of myocardial systolic function. In severe cases, progressive heart failure with its associated symptoms may be seen. With less extensive myocardial involvement, pericarditis and the clinical manifestations of systemic

Table 13-5. Common Infectious Causes of Myocarditis

Viral Agents
  Coxsackie B virus
  Echovirus
  Influenza virus
  Parainfluenza virus
  Epstein-Barr virus
  Hepatitis B virus
Bacteria
  Corynebacterium diphtheriae
  Neisseria meningitidis
  Mycoplasma pneumoniae
  β-Hemolytic streptococci (rheumatic fever)

illness (fever, myalgias, headache, rigors) may overshadow clinical signs of myocardial dysfunction. Retrosternal or precordial chest pain is a frequent presenting complaint and is most commonly secondary to associated pericardial inflammation (myopericarditis). This chest pain may mimic angina in its character. A pericardial friction rub is commonly heard in patients with myopericarditis.

The chest roentgenogram is usually normal and reported abnormalities (cardiomegaly and pulmonary venous hypertension and/or pulmonary edema) vary with disease severity and are nondiagnostic. Reported ECG changes include nonspecific ST-T wave changes, ST segment elevation (due to associated pericarditis), atrioventricular block, and prolonged QRS duration.

Echocardiography may reveal depressed systolic function in severe cases. Recent clinical and animal investigations with myocardial scintigraphy have demonstrated that ^{99m}Tc-PYP and gallium 67 citrate are avidly accumulated by the inflamed myocardium in a diffuse pattern. An etiologic diagnosis can frequently be confirmed with characteristic acute and convalescent phase viral antibody titers or with transvenous biotomic endomyocardial biopsy.

Treatment

Current therapy in cases of idiopathic or viral myocarditis is largely supportive and symptom-directed. Myocarditis in rheumatic fever and complicating diphtheria or meningococcemia necessitates directed antibiotic therapy.

UNEXPLAINED HEART FAILURE OR CARDIOMEGALY: DIFFERENTIAL DIAGNOSIS AND WORK-UP

Symptoms of congestive heart failure and associated cardiomegaly or evidence of cardiomegaly in the asymptomatic patient necessitates a directed evaluation. In the vast majority of instances, one of the following seven disease entities will eventually be diagnosed. Where appropriate, recognized diagnostic clues are noted.

1. Hypertensive Heart Disease
   Systemic arterial hypertension affects 10 to 20 percent of the adult population. This is a disease with a high prevalence which may be diagnosed at a number of stages. The patient with idiopathic congestive cardiomyopathy and untreated cardiac failure will frequently present with an elevated blood pressure due to autonomically mediated compensatory reflexes. Isolated involvement of the myocardium as the major manifestation of systemic arterial hypertension is rare. A careful search for evidence of other end-organ damage due to arterial hypertension should be undertaken (examination of fundi, assessment of renal function, evaluation for focal neurologic changes or history of such).
2. Ischemic Heart Disease (Ischemic Cardiomyopathy)
   Most patients with clinical signs of biventricular heart failure and cardiomegaly due to obstructive coronary arterial disease will relate a history of typical anginal pain or documented myocardial infarction(s). A few will not, and clinical presentation and physical findings in these cases will mimic those of an idiopathic congestive cardiomyopathy.

3. Valvular Heart Disease
   Although the incidence of rheumatic heart disease in the United States is low, it remains a prevalent disease in underdeveloped countries and is frequently first diagnosed in recent immigrants. The growing ''geriatric'' population is prone to calcific aortic stenosis and mitral annular calcification. In addition, bicuspid or unicuspid aortic valve abnormalities remain as the most common congenital heart disease. All may present with congestive heart failure or incidental cardiac enlargement and systolic and diastolic murmurs may be noted. Echocardiography is the diagnostic test of choice in the patient with suspected valvular heart disease. Hemodynamic and angiographic studies may be confirmatory.
4. Constrictive Pericardial Disease
   Constrictive pericarditis frequently presents with clinical manifestations that mimic right-sided failure. A past history of pericarditis and minimal cardiac enlargement, clear lung fields, and pericardial calcification on chest x-ray are diagnostic clues.
5. Myocarditis
   The patient with severe myocarditis may present with signs and symptoms of cardiac insufficiency. Such patients are usually young, have no significant past cardiac history, have few risk factors for atherosclerotic coronary arterial disease, and present with a recent, abrupt onset of symptoms during or immediately following a systemic or viral illness.
6. Hypertrophic Cardiomyopathy
   The patient with hypertrophic cardiomyopathy may present with a history of shortness of breath or decreased exercise tolerance. Symptoms thus mimic left heart failure. Echocardiography and, if necessary, left heart catheterization are critical diagnostic aids.
7. Congestive Cardiomyopathy
   This diagnosis should be considered only if the first six disease entities have been excluded. A careful search for potential etiologic causes should then be undertaken.

PERICARDIAL HEART DISEASE

The pericardium consists of a serous or loose fibrous membrane (visceral pericardium) overlying the epicardium and a dense collagenous sac (parietal pericardium) which surrounds the heart. The space between the visceral and parietal pericardium may contain up to 50 mL of fluid under normal conditions and intrapericardial pressure is normally subatmospheric. Because its layers are serosal surfaces and owing to its proximity and attachments to other structures, the pericardium may be involved in a number of systemic or localized disease processes (Table 13-6). The clinical presentation of pericardial heart disease is variable and dependent upon the pericardium's response to injury and how this response affects cardiac function. In this section the clinical manifestations and evaluation of acute and constrictive pericarditis are discussed.

Acute Pericarditis

Symptoms and Signs

The most common symptom is precordial or retrosternal chest pain, which is most frequently described as sharp or stabbing. It

Table 13-6. Common Causes of Acute Pericarditis

Idiopathic
Infectious
   Viral (especially Coxsackie virus and echovirus)
   Bacterial [especially staphylococcus, *streptococcus pneumoniae*,
     β-hemolytic streptococci (acute rheumatic fever), *Mycobacterium*
     tuberculosis]
   Fungal (especially *Histoplasma capsulatum*)
Malignancy (leukemia, lymphoma, metastatic breast and lung
   carcinoma, and melanoma)
Drug-induced (procainamide, hydralazine)
Connective tissue disease
Radiation-induced
Postmyocardial infarction (Dressler's syndrome)
Uremia
Myxedema

may be of sudden or gradual onset and radiate to the back, neck, left shoulder, or arm; referral to the left trapezial ridge (due to inflammation of the adjoining diaphragmatic pleura) is a particular distinguishing feature. Chest pain due to acute pericarditis may be aggravated by inspiration or movement. It may be most severe when the patient is supine and is often relieved when the patient sits up and leans forward. In most instances, these characteristics allow the pain of acute pericarditis to be distinguished from the ischemic pain of angina or acute myocardial infarction.

Associated symptoms include: (1) low-grade, intermittent fever, particularly if pericarditis is infectious in origin or of the idiopathic type; (2) dyspnea, due to accentuated pain with inspiration; and (3) dysphagia, ascribed to irritation of the esophagus by the posterior pericardium.

A pericardial friction rub is the most common and important physical finding in pericarditis. A pericardial rub most closely resembles a superficial grating or scratching sound. It is best heard with the diaphragm of the stethoscope at the lower left sternal border or apex when the patient is sitting and leaning forward or in the hands-and-knees position. It may be audible only during a certain phase of respiration and characteristically is transient, i.e., heard one hour and not the next. No inference as to the amount of pericardial fluid should be drawn from the presence or absence of a pericardial friction rub.

A pericardial rub is most often triphasic in character, consisting of a systolic component, an early diastolic component occurring during the early phase of ventricular filling, and a presystolic component synchronous with atrial systole. It is less commonly biphasic, i.e., a systolic component with either an early diastolic or presystolic component. A monophasic rub is unusual (18 percent of cases) but is most often systolic.

Other common associated physical findings include fever and resting sinus tachycardia. Additional signs (paradoxical pulse, venous distention, Kussmaul's sign) may result from the effects of an expanding pericardial effusion on ventricular filling.

Diagnostic Findings

The Electrocardiogram (ECG) in Acute Pericarditis

Serial ECGs recorded over a number of days may be diagnostic in acute pericarditis. The evolutionary ECG changes during acute pericarditis and convalescence have been divided into four stages. During stage 1 or the acute phase, ST segment elevation (reflecting associated subepicardial inflammation and/or injury) is prominent in the precordial leads, especially V_5 and V_6, and in standard lead I. PR segment depression may be noted in leads II, aV_F, and V_4 to V_6 (Fig. 13-1). In stage 2, the ST segment begins returning to the isoelectric line and T wave amplitude decreases. T-wave inversion is rarely seen until stage 3. Stage 3 is characterized by an isoelectric ST segment and T-wave inversion in those leads previously showing ST segment elevation. Resolution of repolarization abnormalities is the hallmark of stage 4.

If a large pericardial effusion develops during the course of acute pericarditis, additional ECG abnormalities may be noted, and include low-voltage QRS complexes and electrical alternans. These phenomena are due to the "insulating" effect of pericardial fluid, which attenuates electrical signals of myocardial origin, and the pendular motion of the heart within the fluid-filled pericardial space.

Although serial ECG tracings are of diagnostic value in acute pericarditis, sequential ECG assessment is not a "diagnostic luxury" afforded the emergency physician. Differentiating pericarditis from the normal variant with "early repolarization" is a common problem and can be difficult when only a single 12-lead ECG is available. Acute pericarditis is a common cause of chest pain and abnormal ECGs in young adults. The ST-T wave changes present in the early repolarization or normal variant ECG mimic those of pericarditis and have been reported in 2 percent of healthy young adults. Investigations attempting to distinguish these two conditions have yielded conflicting results. However, a recently described simple criterion offers considerable diagnostic utility, namely, the ST segment/T-wave amplitude ratio in leads V_5, V_6, or I. Using the end of the PR segment as baseline, or 0 mV, the amplitude or height of the ST segment at its onset is measured in one of the above leads and recorded in millivolts. The height of the T wave in the same lead is measured from the baseline to the T-wave peak. If the ratio of ST amplitude (in millivolts) to T-wave amplitude (in millivolts) is <0.25, a normal variant or early repolarization is most probable. If the ratio is >0.25, acute pericarditis is likely. This criterion may allow differentiation of acute pericarditis (stage 1) from early repolarization during emergency department evaluation (Fig. 13-1).

Radiographic Assessment

Conventional PA and lateral chest x-rays are of limited value in the diagnosis of acute pericarditis and pericardial effusion. The cardiac silhouette may be of normal size and contour in acute pericarditis and, in some instances, the setting of cardiac tamponade. If previous chest x-rays are available for comparison, a recent increase in the size of the cardiac silhouette or an increase in the cardiothoracic ratio without radiographic evidence of pulmonary venous hypertension aids in distinguishing an expanding pericardial effusion from left heart failure. The epicardial "fat pad sign" is rarely seen on the lateral chest x-ray and has been reported in only 15 percent of cases of acute pericarditis during fluoroscopy with image intensification. If acute pericarditis is suspected on the basis of history, physical examination, or ECG, PA and lateral chest x-rays, which demonstrate a pleuropulmonary or mediastinal abnormality, may assist in establishing an etiology, e.g., neoplastic or infectious.

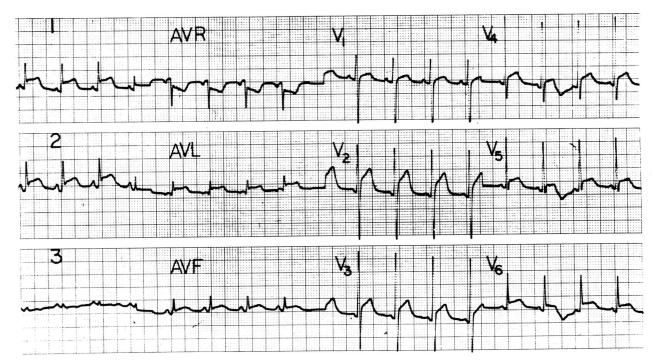

Figure 13-1. This ECG was obtained from a 24-year-old male complaining of retrosternal pleuritic chest pain. A three-component pericardial friction rub was heard on examination. ECG abnormalities consistent with pericarditis are present. There is diffuse ST segment elevation, and PR interval depression is evident in the standard limb leads (PR interval below the isoelectric TP segment). The ST segment/T wave amplitude ratio in V_6 is approximately 0.75. (From Ginzton LE, Laks MM: The differential diagnosis of acute pericarditis from the normal variant: New electrocardiographic criteria. *Circulation* 65: 1004, 1982.)

Echocardiography

Echocardiography has become the procedure of choice for the detection, confirmation, and serial follow-up of patients with acute pericarditis and a pericardial effusion.

Normally, the pericardial sac is only a "potential" space and the myocardium is echocardiographically in direct contact with surrounding thoracic structures. The anterior right ventricular wall is in contact with the chest wall and the posterior LV wall is in contact with the posterior pericardium and adjacent pleura. When a pericardial effusion is present, the pericardial space fills with echo-free fluid. Echocardiographically, a separation is seen between the right ventricle and chest wall and between the left ventricle and posterior pericardium. Quantitation of the size of the effusion is arbitrary and is determined by where the echo-free space is seen (anterior or posterior) and when in the cardiac cycle it occurs, e.g., a small effusion is said to present when an echo-free space is seen only posteriorly and only during systole.

Ancillary Laboratory Evaluation

The laboratory studies listed in Table 13-7 may be of value in establishing an etiologic diagnosis.

Summary

A confident diagnosis of acute pericarditis or pericardial effusion is largely based on sequential or evolutionary ECG changes and a compatible echocardiogram. However, these diagnostic aids are rarely available to the emergency physician. Emergency department diagnosis is, for the most part, dependent upon patient history (pleuritic chest pain), physical examination (pericardial friction rub), compatible ECG abnormalities (ST segment elevation), and a high index of suspicion. All patients with suspected pericarditis should be admitted to the hospital. Although the vast majority of cases will prove to be of idiopathic or viral origin (usually hemodynamically benign and managed conservatively), in-hospital evaluation and observation are required to exclude more life-threatening etiologies amenable to specific therapy.

Table 13-7. Ancillary Diagnostic Studies in Acute Pericarditis

1. CBC and differential WBC count: may suggest infection or leukemia
2. BUN/creatinine: may suggest a diagnosis of uremic pericarditis
3. Streptococcal serology (anti-streptolysin O, anti-DNAse, antihyaluronidase): of particular value in the patient with an antecedent history of rheumatic heart disease or history of pharyngitis
4. Blood cultures (if bacterial infection suspected)
5. Acute and convalescent viral titers
6. Serologic studies: antinuclear antibodies, anti-DNA titers, or RA latex fixation in the patient with systemic symptoms
7. Thyroid function studies
8. Erythrocyte sedimentation rate: will not facilitate an etiologic diagnosis, but can be followed serially to assess response to therapy

Constrictive Pericarditis

Pathology

Constrictive pericarditis is pathologically distinct from acute pericarditis. Following pericardial injury and the resultant inflammatory and reparative process, fibrous thickening of the layers of the pericardium may occur. This fibrous reparative process is most commonly encountered after cardiac trauma with intrapericardial hemorrhage, after pericardiotomy (open-heart surgery, including coronary revascularization), in fungal or tuberculous pericarditis, and in chronic renal failure (uremic pericarditis). When the fibrous and/or collagenous response prevents passive diastolic filling of the normally distensible cardiac chambers, constriction is said to be present. Intrapericardial fluid is not required to produce such a hemodynamic effect. By its nature, constrictive pericarditis is most commonly a clinically chronic process. However, clinical manifestations may occur early if fluid also accumulates within the thickened, noncompliant pericardial sac (so-called effusive constrictive pericarditis). In the vast majority of cases of constrictive pericarditis, proven by hemodynamic assessment (see below), a specific etiology is never determined.

Symptoms and Signs

The symptoms of constrictive pericarditis usually develop gradually and may mimic those of congestive heart failure (CHF). If symptoms develop within months of a pericardial injury, a combination of pericardial effusion and constriction should be suspected. Exertional dyspnea and decreased exercise tolerance are common patient complaints; however, orthopnea, paroxysmal nocturnal dyspnea, and chest pain are unusual. Lower extremity swelling (pedal edema) and increasing abdominal girth (ascites) are also common complaints and are the result of decreased right ventricular diastolic compliance and resultant increase in systemic venous pressure.

In most instances, physical findings and their correct interpretation will lead the clinician to suspect constrictive pericarditis. Examination of the neck veins with the torso of the patient at a 45° angle from the horizontal will reveal jugular venous distention and a rapid y descent of the cervical venous pulse. Elevated venous pressure is also seen in CHF but a rapid y descent is infrequently encountered. Kussmaul's sign (inspiratory neck vein distention) is frequently but not invariably noted in constrictive pericarditis but rarely noted in uncompensated CHF. A paradoxical pulse is found in a minority of patients and thus its absence does not exclude a diagnosis of constrictive pericarditis. On cardiac auscultation, an early diastolic sound, a pericardial "knock," may be heard at the apex 60 to 120 ms after the second heart sound. The pericardial knock sounds like a ventricular gallop but occurs earlier than the S_3 of CHF, which it may mimic. The knock is due to accelerated right ventricular inflow in early diastole and early myocardial distention, followed by an abrupt slowing of further ventricular expansion. There is usually no pericardial friction rub.

Hepatomegaly, ascites, and dependent edema of varying severities are usually found.

Diagnostic Findings

The Electrocardiogram

Diagnostic ECG changes have not been described in constrictive pericarditis. However, low-voltage QRS complexes and inverted T waves are common.

Radiographic Assessment

Conventional PA and lateral chest x-rays most commonly demonstrate a normal or slightly enlarged cardiac silhouette, clear lung fields, and little or no evidence of pulmonary venous congestion. Pericardial calcification, which may be evident in up to 50 percent of patients with constrictive pericarditis, is seen best on the lateral chest x-ray but is not diagnostic of constrictive pericarditis.

Echocardiography

On occasion, echocardiography may demonstrate pericardial thickening and abnormal ventricular septal motion in the patient with suspected constrictive pericarditis. However, its diagnostic utility is much less than in the patient with acute pericarditis.

Cardiac Catheterization

Right heart catheterization will demonstrate typical or characteristic hemodynamic findings. The absence of these typical abnormalities is strong evidence against constrictive pericarditis; however, their presence is not diagnostic, as similar hemodynamic changes have been described in patients with restrictive cardiomyopathies, e.g., amyloid heart disease and hemochromatosis.

Equalization of increased (10 to 25 mmHg) diastolic pressures in the right atrium, right ventricle, and pulmonary artery is typical in constrictive pericarditis. A similar hemodynamic profile is seen in cardiac tamponade. However, in constrictive pericarditis a rapid x and y descent are recorded in the right atrial pressure tracing and an early diastolic dip-and-plateau configuration is recorded during right ventricular pressure measurement. These latter two findings are not encountered in cardiac tamponade. Cineangiography may demonstrate straightening of the right border of the right atrium and thickened pericardium. On occasion, surgical exploration may be required to make a diagnosis, especially when a restrictive cardiomyopathy cannot be excluded by less invasive means.

Summary

Constrictive pericarditis is characteristically a chronic disease process which produces a symptom complex and a constellation of physical findings that mimic chronic congestive heart failure. The diagnosis should be considered strongly in the dyspneic patient with systemic venous hypertension, clear lung fields and an early diastolic gallop sound on physical examination, a low-voltage ECG, and a normal or only slightly enlarged cardiac silhouette on chest x-ray. The presence of pericardial calcification in such a patient makes constrictive pericarditis highly likely.

BIBLIOGRAPHY

Agner RC, Gallis HA: Pericarditis: Differential diagnostic considerations. *Arch Intern Med* 139:407, 1979.

Askanas A, Udoshi M, Sadjadi SA: The heart in chronic alcoholism: a noninvasive study. *Am Heart J* 99:9, 1980.

Benjamin IJ, Schuster EH, Bulkley BH: Cardiac hypertrophy in idiopathic dilated congestive cardiomyopathy: A clinico-pathologic study. *Circulation* 64:442, 1981.

Benotti JR, Grossman W, Cohn PF: Clinical profile of restrictive cardiomyopathy. *Circulation* 61:1206, 1980.

Berger M, Bobak L, Jelveh M, et al: Pericardial effusion diagnosed by echocardiography: Clinical and electrocardiographic findings in 171 patients. *Chest* 74:174, 1978.

Chew C, Ziady GM, Raphael MJ, et al: The functional defect in amyloid heart disease: The "stiff heart" syndrome. *Am J Cardiol* 36:438, 1975.

Cutler DJ, Isner JM, Bracey AW, et al: Hemochromatosis heart disease: An unemphasized cause of potentially reversible restrictive cardiomyopathy. *Am J Med* 69:923, 1980.

Engler RL, Smith P, LeWinter M, et al: The electrocardiogram in asymmetric septal hypertrophy. *Chest* 75:167, 1979.

Fowler NO: Diseases of the pericardium. *Curr Probl Cardiol* 2:6, 1978.

Fowler NO, Manitsas GT: Infectious pericarditis. *Prog Cardiovasc Dis* 16:323, 1973.

Gardiner AJS, Short D: Four faces of acute myopericarditis. *Br Heart J* 35:433, 1973.

Ginzton LE, Laks MM: The differential diagnosis of acute pericarditis from the normal variant: New electrocardiographic criteria. *Circulation* 65:1004, 1982.

Goodwin JF: An appreciation of hypertrophic cardiomyopathy. *Am J Med* 68:797, 1980.

Hamby RJ: Primary myocardial disease: A prospective clinical and hemodynamic evaluation in 100 patients. *Medicine (Baltimore)* 49:55, 1970.

Hancock EW: Constrictive pericarditis: Clinical clues to diagnosis. *JAMA* 232:176, 1975.

Kawai C, Takatsu T: Clinical and experimental studies on cardiomyopathy. *N Engl J Med* 293:592, 1975.

Klacsmann PG, Bulkley BH, Hutchin GM: The changed spectrum of purulent pericarditis: An 86 year autopsy experience in 200 patients. *Am J Med* 64:666, 1977.

Kleiman JH, Motta J, London E, et al.: Pericardial effusions in patients with end-stage renal disease. *Br Heart J* 40:190, 1978.

Kutcher MA, King SB, Alimurung BN, et al.: Constrictive pericarditis as a complication of cardiac surgery: Recognition of an entity. *Am J Cardiol* 50:742, 1982.

Levine HD: Virus myocarditis: A critique of the literature from clinical, electrocardiographic, and pathologic standpoints. *Am J Med Sci* 277:132, 1979.

Lichstein E, Arsura E, Hollander G, et al.: Current incidence of post-myocardial infarction (Dressler's syndrome). *Am J Cardiol* 50:1269, 1982.

Mann T, Brodie BR, Grossman W, et al.: Effusive-constrictive hemodynamic pattern due to neoplastic involvement of the pericardium. *Am J Cardiol* 41:781, 1978.

Mitsutake A, Nakamura M, Inou T, et al: Intense, persistent myocardial avid technetium-99m-pyrophosphate scintigraphy in acute myocarditis. *Am Heart J* 101:683, 1981.

Oakley C: Diagnosis and natural history of congested (dilated) cardiomyopathies. *Postgrad Med J* 54:440, 1978.

Oakley CM: Clinical recognition of the cardiomyopathies. *Circ Res (suppl 2)* 34/35:II-152, 1974.

Oakley CM: Clinical definitions and classification of cardiomyopathies. *Postgrad Med J* 48:703, 1972.

Parker RM: Effects of ethyl alcohol on the heart. *JAMA* 228:741, 1974.

Posner MR, Cohen GI, Skarin AT: Pericardial disease in patients with cancer: The differentiation of malignant from idiopathic and radiation-induced pericarditis. *Am J Med* 71:407, 1981.

Roberts WC, McAllister HA, Ferrans VJ: Sarcoidosis of the heart. *Am J Med* 63:86, 1977.

Roberts WC, Spray TL: Pericardial heart disease. *Curr Probl Cardiol* 2:6, 1977.

Rubinow A, Skinner M, Cohen AS: Digoxin sensitivity in amyloid cardiomyopathy. *Circulation* 63:1285, 1981.

Sainani GS, Krompotic E, Slodki SJ: Adult heart disease due to Coxsackie virus B infection. *Medicine (Baltimore)* 47:133, 1968.

Schnittger I, Bowden RE, Abrams J, et al: Echocardiography: Pericardial thickening and constrictive pericarditis. *Am J Cardiol* 42:388, 1978.

Shabetai R, Curtis G, Engler RL, et al: Nonobstructive and obstructive hypertrophic cardiomyopathies. *West J Med* 130:325, 1979.

Shirley EK, Proudfit WL, Hawk WA: Primary myocardial disease: Correlation with clinical findings, angiographic and biopsy diagnosis. *Am Heart J* 99:198, 1980.

Spodick DH: The pericardial rub: A prospective, multiple observer investigation of pericardial friction in 100 patients. *Am J Cardiol* 35:357, 1975.

Spodick DH: Differential characteristics of the electrocardiogram in early repolarization and acute pericarditis. *N Engl J Med* 295:523, 1976.

Surawicz B, Lasseter KC: Electrocardiogram in pericarditis. *Am J Cardiol* 26:471, 1970.

Unverferth DV, Williams TE, Fulkerson PK: Electrocardiographic voltage in pericardial effusion. *Chest* 75:157, 1979.

Wise DE, Conti CR: Constrictive pericarditis. *Cardiovasc Clin* 7:197, 1976.

CHAPTER 14
PULMONARY EMBOLISM

Robert S. Hockberger

INTRODUCTION

Pulmonary embolism (PE) is the third most common cause of death in the United States, with an estimated incidence of approximately 650,000 cases annually. There are no historical, physical, or laboratory findings which are specific for the disease, and it may mimic clinically many other serious and benign medical disorders. If the diagnosis of this disease is missed in the emergency department, the overall mortality of 8 percent increases four- to fivefold.

PREDISPOSING FACTORS

Injury to the vascular endothelium, venous stasis, and alterations in the coagulating system may predispose an individual to significant thromboembolic phenomenon. Table 14-1 lists the most commonly recognized predisposing factors. Less than 6 percent of all PEs occur in the absence of any predisposing factor.

Pulmonary emboli may arise from pelvic vein thrombosis secondary to pelvic trauma or pelvic surgery (including abortion attempts) or occurring during the postpartum period. In more than 90 percent of cases, however, PEs arise from the deep venous system of the lower extremities. The incidence of embolism from popliteal thrombosis is 50 percent, and when the thrombosis extends to involve the femoral vein, it is almost 70 percent. Unfortunately, the clinical diagnosis of deep venous thrombosis of the lower extremities, particularly when isolated in the calf, is extremely difficult and may be missed in up to 50 percent of cases.

CLINICAL FEATURES

It should be noted that a "classic" picture is infrequently seen. PE has been known to mimic many serious and benign medical disorders (see Table 14-2) and must be considered in any patient at risk who experiences any acute nonspecific cardiopulmonary complaint.

The frequencies of various symptoms and signs observed in the largest series of patients with angiographically documented PE are shown in Table 14-3. Chest pain is the most common symptom and occurs in approximately 90 percent of patients. While the pain is usually pleuritic in nature, it may mimic the pressurelike pain of myocardial ischemia as well as the vague discomfort of non-specific chest wall pain. Chest pain is often noted for 3 to 4 days prior to diagnosis.

Once a thromboembolism migrates to the lungs and lodges in the pulmonary vasculature, platelets degranulate and release a wide variety of biologically active substances, including histamine, catecholamines, serotonin, and prostaglandins. These substances act to cause smooth muscle constriction of the bronchi and pulmonary arteries. The increased airway resistance and decreased total lung volume with uneven ventilation contribute to the dyspnea and tachypnea found in the majority of patients with pulmonary embolism. Tachypnea (respiratory rate more than 16 per minute) is found in over 90 percent of patients. Localized rales, rhonchi, wheezes, or a pleural friction rub is often seen.

The hemodynamic reaction to PE depends upon the extent of vascular occlusion as well as on the patient's prior cardiovascular status. The previously healthy patient develops little pulmonary hypertension unless total pulmonary vascular obstruction approaches 40 to 50 percent. Patients with preexisting cardiopulmonary disease, however, may experience life-threatening changes in their hemodynamic status with only a minor insult. Some degree of hypotension is present in up to 25 percent of pulmonary emboli but frank shock occurs in less than 10 percent.

Fever (over 38°C), tachycardia (more than 100 beats per minute), and an increased pulmonic component of the second heart sound are each present in roughly half of all cases. Clinically evident phlebitis is present in less than one-third of cases.

LABORATORY INVESTIGATION

Arterial Blood Gases

Most patients with PE will experience some degree of hypoxemia. This is due to underperfusion of well-aerated segments of lung secondary to the emboli themselves, decrease in total lung volume secondary to diffuse bronchial constriction, inadequate respirations secondary to pain and splinting, and occasionally some degree of cardiac decompensation. The mean P_{O_2} values among patients with documented PE in two large series were 62 and 72 mmHg, respectively, but 10 to 15 percent of patients with PE have a P_{O_2} greater than 80 mmHg and up to 5 percent have a P_{O_2} greater than 90 mmHg. The presence of an increased alveolar-arterial (A-a) gradient of oxygen is more sensitive although

Table 14-1. Factors Predisposing to Thromboembolism

Heart disease, especially:
   Congestive heart failure
   Myocardiopathy
   Atrial fibrillation
   Myocardial infarction
Stasis of blood flow:
   Pregnancy and parturition
   Obesity
   Varicose veins
   Prolonged immobilization (e.g., long-distance travel)
   Prolonged bedrest (with burns or fractures)
Alterations in coagulation:
   Oral contraceptive use
   Neoplastic disease
   Polycythemia
Trauma:
   Postoperative states
   Leg or pelvic trauma

nonspecific. It is calculated simply by the following formula: $140 - (P_{O_2} + P_{CO_2})$ (normal is 5 to 15 mmHg).

Electrocardiogram

The ECG is usually abnormal in pulmonary embolism. A list of the ECG changes seen in pulmonary embolism is shown in Table 14-4.

The following points should be noted: (1) In the clinical setting of suspected pulmonary embolism, the sudden appearance of ECG findings of acute right heart strain correlate very highly with the presence of pulmonary embolism. (2) In the clinical setting of suspected myocardial infarction, an ECG indicating multiple areas

Table 14-2. Diseases in the Differential Diagnosis of PE

Skin—herpes zoster
Muscle
   Myositis
   Muscle strain
Bone
   Rib fracture
   Thoracic vertebral compression fracture
   Costochondritis
Pleura—Pleurisy
Lung
   Emphysema
   Bronchitis
   Asthma
   Carcinoma
   Tuberculosis
   Spontaneous pneumothorax
   Pneumonia
Pericardium—acute pericarditis
Myocardium—myocardial infarction
Intraabdominal disorders
   Splenic flexure syndrome
   Renal colic
   Acute pancreatitis
   Acute cholelithiasis
   Subdiaphragmatic abscess
   Hepatitis
Psychiatric—hyperventilation syndrome

Table 14-3. Incidence of Symptoms and Signs in 327 Patients with Angiographically Proven Pulmonary Emboli

Symptoms and Signs	Total Series N = 327 (%)	Massive Emboli N = 197 (%)	Submassive Emboli N = 130 (%)
Symptoms			
Chest pain	88	85	82
Pleuritic	74	64	85
Nonpleuritic	14	6	8
Dyspnea	84	85	82
Apprehension	59	65	50
Cough	53	53	52
Hemoptysis	30	23	40
Sweats	27	29	23
Syncope	13	20	4
Signs			
Respirations >16/min	92	95	87
Rales	58	57	60
↑ S_2P	53	58	45
Pulse >100/min	44	48	38
Temperature >37.8°C	43	43	42
Phlebitis	32	36	26
Gallop	34	39	25
Diaphoresis	36	42	27
Edema	24	23	25
Murmur	23	27	16
Cyanosis	19	25	9
Predisposing condition			
Current venous disease	49	55	47
Immobilization	55	60	46
Congestive heart failure and chronic lung disease	38	36	40
Malignant neoplasm	6	8	5

From: Bell WR, Simon TL, DeMets DL: The clinical features of submassive and massive pulmonary emboli. *AM J Med* 62:358, 1977. Used by permission.

of infarction is highly suggestive of PE. (3) The most common ECG finding in pulmonary embolism is nonspecific ST-T wave changes that are transient (lasting hours to days). Comparison with previously obtained ECGs or sequential ECGs obtained in the emergency department may be helpful in raising an initial suspicion of PE. (4) A normal ECG argues against, but does not rule out, acute PE.

Chest X-ray

When the chest x-ray is normal in a patient with severe dyspnea, PE should be strongly suspected. Roentgenograms of the chest are, however, most often abnormal in pulmonary embolism. The chest x-ray in nearly half of all patients with acute PE will show an elevated dome of one hemidiaphragm secondary to the aforementioned decrease in lung volume. Other common but nonspecific radiographic findings include pleural effusions, atelectasis, and transient parenchymal infiltrates.

Two radiographic features that are uncommon but specific for pulmonary embolism are Hampton's hump and Westermark's sign. *Hampton's hump* is an area of density or lung consolidation with a rounded border pointing towards the hilus. *Westermark's sign* refers to the presence of a dilated pulmonary outflow tract on the

Table 14-4. Electrocardiographic Manifestations*: Patients Without Prior Cardiac or Pulmonary Disease

Electrocardiogram	50 Pts., Massive Pulmonary Embolism† (%)	40 Pts., Submassive Pulmonary Embolism (%)	90 Pts., Massive or Submassive Pulmonary Embolism (%)
Normal electrocardiogram	6	23	13
Rhythm disturbances			
Premature atrial beats	2	3	2
Premature ventricular beats	4	3	3
Atrio-ventricular conduction disturbances			
First degree A-V block	0	3	1
P pulmonale	6	5	6
QRS abnormalities			
Right axis deviation	8	5	7
Left axis deviation	4	10	7
Clockwise rotation (V_5)	10	3	7
Incomplete right bundle branch block	8	3	6
Complete right bundle branch block	8	10	9
Right ventricular hypertrophy	6	5	6
$S_1S_2S_3$ Pattern	6	8	7
$S_1Q_3T_3$ Pattern	18	5	12
Pseudoinfarction	16	5	11
Low voltage (frontal plane)	8	3	6
Primary RST segment and T-wave abnormalities			
RST segment depression (not reciprocal)	28	23	26
RST segment elevation (not reciprocal)	18	13	16
T-wave inversion	46	38	42

*Some patients had more than one abnormality.

†The prevalence of none of the various electrocardiographic abnormalities differed significantly between patients with massive or submassive pulmonary embolism. (Chi square greater than 0.05.)

Adapted from: Stein PD, Dalen JE, McIntyre KM, et al: The electrocardiogram in acute pulmonary embolism. *Prog Cardiovasc Dis* 17, No 4:247, 1975.

side of embolization with an area of decreased perfusion distal to it.

Ventilation-Perfusion Lung Scan

When the diagnosis of PE cannot be excluded, a radionuclide perfusion lung scan should be employed. This test measures blood flow in pulmonary vessels as small as 50 μm in diameter and is therefore extremely sensitive. A normal perfusion lung scan excludes the diagnosis of PE.

Abnormal perfusion scans are seen in a number of other settings that alter perfusion. In the clinical setting of suspected PE an abnormal perfusion lung scan should be followed by a pulmonary ventilation scan to heighten specificity. The ventilation and perfusion pictures are then compared. PE generally presents as abnormal perfusion in the presence of normal or near normal ventilation. Any abnormality of the perfusion scan necessitates further work-up, i.e., a search for deep venous thrombosis and/or pulmonary angiography.

Pulmonary Angiography

Pulmonary angiography is the "gold standard" for diagnosing PE. Pulmonary vessels as small as 0.5 mm in diameter are visualized. In one recent study of over 800 pulmonary angiograms performed for suspected PE, the morbidity of the test was less than 1 percent and the mortality was less than 0.01 percent. Complications occur

almost exclusively in elderly patients with ventricular aneurysms, cardiomypathies, or severe congestive heart failure.

The following are indications for performing pulmonary angiography for suspected PE: (1) when the ventilation-perfusion lung scan is of intermediate or low probability but the clinical picture is highly suggestive for pulmonary embolism; (2) when patients are at high risk for bleeding complications during anticoagulation because of problems including severe uncontrolled hypertension, actively bleeding gastrointestinal or genitourinary lesions, a craniotomy or cerebrovascular accident within the previous month, or evidence of lesions known to be associated with intracranial hemorrhage; (3) when dealing with unstable patients thought to be suffering from massive PE prior to the use of expensive and potentially hazardous fibrinolytic therapy or surgical embolectomy.

TREATMENT

Stabilization

Most patients with PE suffer from some degree of hypoxemia secondary to ventilation-perfusion imbalance. The administration of oxygen at 4 to 10 L/min by nasal cannula relieves or diminishes the symptoms of hypoxemia in many patients. Early initiation of adequate oxygen therapy may well prevent hypoxemia-induced cardiac arrhythmias and should therefore, not be withheld in the dyspneic patient prior to obtaining blood gases.

The patient with PE is at greatest risk for succumbing to shock or cardiac arrhythmias during the first 2 h. Early initiation of vigilant monitoring of vital signs and cardiac rhythm is essential. Hypotension in the PE patient may be caused by low cardiac output secondary to resistance to right ventricular outflow or to myocardial dysfunction due to ischemia. Initial therapy should include the aggressive administration of crystalloid fluids if the central venous pressure is low or the use of a vasopressor such as dopamine if it is normal to high. The persistently hypotensive patient with suspected PE should be managed with Swan-Ganz catheter placement, immediate pulmonary arteriography, and early consideration of either fibrinolytic therapy or surgical pulmonary embolectomy.

Anticoagulation

Anticoagulation with heparin has been the cornerstone of therapy for venous thrombosis and PE for over 30 years. Heparin acts through inhibition of certain steps of the coagulation system by combining with antithrombin III, a naturally occurring circulating heparin cofactor. Heparin acts to prevent the extension of an existing thrombus and to prevent subsequent pulmonary emboli. One study of 516 patients found survival after diagnosis of pulmonary embolism in 92 percent of anticoagulated patients versus 42 percent in cases where anticoagulants were withheld because of medical contraindications. In addition, pulmonary emboli recurred in only 16 percent of anticoagulated patients but in 55 percent in nonanticoagulated patients.

The continuous intravenous infusion of heparin appears to result in fewer bleeding complications but requires special equipment, experienced and competent nursing care, and frequent laboratory monitoring. When these requirements are met, therapy should be initiated with a 5000-unit intravenous bolus of heparin followed by approximately 25 units/(kg·h) by continuous infusion. If close monitoring of the patient is not possible, intermittent heparin therapy should be considered. In most patients with submassive PE, 5000 units of heparin intravenously every 4 h is adequate. The partial thromboplastin time is the most commonly used test for assessing control of anticoagulation. It should be checked prior to anticoagulation as a baseline, after several hours of therapy, and then as often as necessary to achieve a value of $1\frac{1}{2}$ to 2 times the control value, although rigid control may not be necessary.

Heparinization should not be attempted in patients who are at high risk for bleeding complications. Heparin does not cross the placenta and can therefore be used safely in pregnant women with PE. Peripartum bleeding, however, remains a problem requiring that heparin be stopped just prior to delivery and restarted only after proper postpartum hemostasis has been obtained. All cases of abnormal bleeding caused by heparin may be reversed through administration of protamine sulfate. Each milligram of protamine sulfate neutralizes approximately 100 units of heparin activity.

Thrombolytic Therapy

The thrombolytic agents streptokinase and urokinase activate the body's own fibrinolytic system by converting the normally present proenzyme plasminogen to the proteolytic enzyme plasmin. There is no demonstrable difference in the efficacy of the two drugs; while streptokinase may be antigenic and requires the concomitant use of intravenous hydrocortisone, urokinase is approximately 4 times as expensive. The major indication for the use of fibrinolytic therapy is in hemodynamically unstable patients, i.e., those with acute massive embolization accompanied by shock. Emergency physicians should consider the utilization of thrombolytic therapy for acute PE only when all the following criteria have been fulfilled: (1) the patient with suspected PE is hemodynamically compromised and has not responded to initial stabilization procedures; (2) pulmonary angiography has documented massive pulmonary embolization; and (3) consultation with a pulmonary specialist has been sought.

Vena Caval Interruption

Surgical techniques for vena caval interruption include ligation, clips, intraluminal devices such as umbrella filters, and transvenous balloon occlusion. Interruption of the inferior vena cava should be considered in the following instances: (1) when there is a contraindication to heparin therapy; (2) when pulmonary emboli recur despite adequate anticoagulation; (3) in the presence of multiple small pulmonary emboli that are thought to be causing chronic pulmonary hypertension; (4) following pulmonary embolectomy; and (5) in cases of septic pelvic thrombophlebitis with recurrent PEs.

Pulmonary Embolectomy

The treatment of massive life-threatening PE by directly removing a potentially fatal embolus has been used with some success in patients on cardiopulmonary bypass. However, since such patients are a poor risk for the added stresses of general anesthesia and surgery, fibrinolytic therapy is rapidly supplanting pulmonary embolectomy in such patients; it has been shown that massive embolization with shock can usually be managed with greater success medically. In the case of severe PE accompanied by cardiopulmonary arrest, however, transvenous pulmonary embolectomy, support with the membrane lung, and induced hypothermia should be considered.

PROGNOSIS

Approximately 10 percent of patients with PE die within 1 h of the event. When the diagnosis of PE is made and appropriate therapy instituted, initial survivors have a mortality of approximately 8 percent. Death after 24 h occurs almost exclusively in chronically ill patients, particularly those with congestive heart failure. The recurrence rate of PE in appropriately treated patients has been reported to be 6 to 25 percent. Most experts agree that the prognosis for PE patients ultimately depends on the outlook for any underlying disease that is present as well as upon the rapidity and care with which treatment is initiated.

BIBLIOGRAPHY

Alpert JS, Smith RE, et al: Treatment of massive pulmonary embolism: The role of pulmonary embolectomy. *Am Heart J* 89:413, 1975.

Bell WR, Simon TL: Current status of pulmonary thromboembolic disease. *Am Heart J* 103(2):239, 1982.

Bell WR, Simon TL, DeMets DL: The clinical features of submassive and massive pulmonary emboli. *Am J Med* 62:355–360, 1977.

Biello DR, Mattar AG, McKnight J, et al: Ventilation-perfusion studies in suspected pulmonary embolism. *AJR* 133:1033–1037, 1979.

Coon WW: Risk factors in pulmonary embolism. *Surg Gynecol Obstet* 143:385, 1976.

Gardner AMN: Inferior vena caval interruption in the prevention of fatal pulmonary embolism. *Am Heart J* 95:679, 1978.

Goldstein BA: The varied clinical manifestations of pulmonary embolism. *Ann Intern Med* 47:202, 1957.

Hull RD, Hirsch J, et al: Pulmonary angiography, ventilation lung scanning, and venography for clinically suspected pulmonary embolism with abnormal perfusion lung scan. *Ann Intern Med* 98:891–899, 1983.

Marder VJ: The use of thrombolytic agents: Choice of patient, drug administration, laboratory monitoring. *Ann Intern Med* 90:802–808, 1979.

Moser KM: Pulmonary embolism. *Am Rev Respir Dis* 115:829–852, 1977.

Pollak CW, Sparks FC, Barker WF: Pulmonary embolism: an appraisal of therapy in 516 cases. *Arch Surg* 107:66, 1973.

Robin ED: Overdiagnosis and overtreatment of pulmonary embolism: The emperor may have no clothes. *Ann Intern Med* 87:775, 1977.

Rosenow EC: Pulmonary embolism. *Mayo Clinic Proc* 56:161, 1981.

Szues MM, Brooks HL, Grossman W, et al: Diagnostic sensitivity of laboratory findings in acute pulmonary embolism. *Ann Intern Med* 74:161, 1971.

Wilson JR, Lampman J: Heparin therapy: A randomized prospective study. *Am Heart J* 97:155, 1979.

CHAPTER 15
HYPERTENSION

Paul R. Pomeroy

True hypertensive emergencies are uncommon, and inappropriate drug selection or overly aggressive therapy can be as harmful to the patient as inaction.

The distinction must be made between a hypertensive emergency, hypertensive urgency, and transient blood pressure elevation due to other disorders.

A *hypertensive emergency* is the elevation of the diastolic blood pressure, usually to 130 mmHg or above, in the presence of a systemic complication such as hypertensive encephalopathy, intracerebral or subarachnoid hemorrhage, toxemia of pregnancy, left ventricular failure, or aortic dissection. The rate of rise of blood pressure may be more important than the absolute level of blood pressure in the development of a complication of hypertension. Toxemia of pregnancy and the hypertension associated with acute glomerulonephritis are illustrative examples. In a hypertensive emergency, the blood pressure should be reduced within minutes to a few hours, with the aim of reaching a diastolic pressure of 90 to 100 mmHg.

In a *hypertensive urgency* the diastolic pressure is usually above 130 mmHg, but there are no symptoms or signs of specific end organ compromise as seen in hypertensive emergencies. Malignant hypertension is categorized as a hypertensive urgency. In urgent situations, the blood pressure should be reduced within 24 h or less.

For transient elevations of the blood pressure, lowering is achieved by correction of or improvement in the underlying disorder. Examples of such conditions are delirium tremens, acute hypoxic states, and anxiety states.

Thus, the golden rule of hypertension is: *Treat the patient, not the blood pressure.*

PATHOPHYSIOLOGY

Hypertensive Cerebrovascular Syndromes

No discussion of cerebrovascular syndromes is complete without an understanding of the changes that occur in the cerebral vasculature secondary to hypertension. A physiologic change is the alteration of cerebral autoregulation, which is the maintenance of constant cerebral blood flow throughout a wide range of blood pressures. There are upper and lower limits of the blood pressure beyond which cerebral blood flow cannot be maintained. In hypertensives, the range of autoregulation is shifted upwards. The practical significance of this is that a severe, abrupt blood pressure

reduction in a patient may exceed the lower limit of autoregulation and give rise to ischemic symptoms. On the other hand, a higher blood pressure is required in an established hypertensive to generate encephalopathy.

Hypertensive patients also develop pathologic changes in the cerebral arteries. Large-artery atherosclerosis is found in both normotensive and hypertensive individuals, and hypertension is one of several risk factors that accelerate its development. Thrombotic or embolic infarction may result from atherosclerosis of the major arteries in the neck. Additionally, hypertensive individuals develop degenerative changes as well as microaneurysms in small arteries. It is felt that occlusion of these vessels gives rise to lacunar infarcts, while microaneurysm rupture creates intracerebral hemorrhage. Saccular (berry) aneurysms occur in the circle of Willis, and the view that they are of congenital origin is disputed. What are congenital are defects in the medial layer of the large cerebral vessels at bifurcation sites. In hypertensives, the defects are larger and aneurysm formation is more likely to occur. It is not illogical to assume a cause-effect relationship.

The Framingham study found hypertension to be the biggest risk factor for stroke, the risk being 7 times greater in hypertensives than in normotensives. The risk is in direct proportion to the blood pressure, *even* in the normotensive range. There are multiple studies, the most publicized being the Veterans Administration Cooperative Study, that show reduced cardiovascular morbidity and mortality when hypertension is treated.

Hypertensive Encephalopathy

Hypertensive encephalopathy is characterized by CNS changes such as progressive headache, somnolence, confusion, seizures, and eventually, coma. There may be transient focal neurologic signs. The syndrome develops progressively over 24 to 48 h. Fundoscopic exudates, hemorrhages, or papilledema are likely to be present but are not necessary to establish the diagnosis.

The mechanism of hypertensive encephalopathy appears to be a breakdown in cerebral autoregulation. Strandgaard and Skinhøj have demonstrated that as the blood pressure progressively rises, the cerebral arterioles take on a "sausage link" appearance and the cerebral blood flow becomes higher than normal. As the blood pressure rises further, the sausage link configuration gives way to generalized vasodilation. These authors suggest that the sausage link appearance represents localized arteriolar spasm, which is an attempt to maintain autoregulation, and local dilation, which is a breakdown of autoregulation. Generalized vasodilation represents a total breakthrough, with an increase in vascular permeability leading to cerebral edema. Neurologic symptoms may be related to the presence of arteriolar spasm or cerebral edema or both.

With appropriate treatment, the signs and symptoms of hypertensive encephalopathy usually resolve within a few hours as long as the blood pressure is adequately reduced. If rapid clinical improvement does not occur with adequate blood pressure reduction, another pathophysiologic entity should be suspected.

Cerebral Thrombosis

Cerebral thrombosis results in ischemic infarction in the distribution of the occluded vessel and a corresponding neurologic deficit. The neurologic deficit becomes maximum within a few hours and does not impair consciousness unless there is bilateral hemispheric pathology or brain stem involvement. The event frequently occurs during sleep and the patient awakes with a neurologic deficit.

Edema occurs in the area surrounding infarction over the ensuing several days and resolves over 1 to 2 weeks. If the infarction is sufficiently large, the edema may be sufficient to cause brain herniation and death, but that is unusual in thrombotic infarction.

The widespread availability of computerized tomographic (CT) scanning has revolutionized the evaluation of strokes. Although it should be possible to categorize most cerebral vascular events on clinical grounds based on characteristic onset and manner of progression (Table 15-1), the CT scan serves several purposes:

1. Differentiates ischemic infarction from hemorrhage
2. Localizes the site of the lesion and attendant edema
3. Quantitates the amount of bleeding, the presence of clot, and whether a mass effect is present

Ischemic infarction is seen as a focal, poorly circumscribed hypodense zone on CT scan. As edema develops, the area becomes more sharply delineated; as edema subsides, the area becomes more isodense.

There is a paucity of clinical or experimental data to guide the physician in the management of a patient with a thrombotic stroke or transient ischemic attack (TIA) who has uncontrolled hypertension. It has been suggested that since blood flow to the ischemic area is directly proportional to blood pressure, absolute or relative hypotension may reduce perfusion and jeopardize the marginal

area around the central zone of infarction. Conversely, if ischemia results in breakdown of the blood-brain barrier, excessive blood pressure will contribute to the amount of marginal edema. Most authors advise a gradual lowering of blood pressure to a range of 90 to 100 diastolic.

Meyer measured cerebral hemodynamics before and after antihypertensive therapy in a group of patients at least 4 weeks after a cerebrovascular accident (CVA) or TIA. Cerebral vascular resistance was reduced in all patients and there was an overall significant increase in cerebral blood flow. Others have demonstrated that treatment versus nontreatment of hypertensive patients who have had a thrombotic stroke yields a substantial reduction in future CVAs in the treated group. Thus, there is evidence to show the benefit of antihypertensive treatment even after a stroke has occurred.

Intracerebral Hemorrhage

Intracerebral hemorrhage is an entity seen primarily in association with hypertension. The onset is acute, with a focal neurologic deficit that develops rapidly. Headache and vomiting are common, and with severe hemorrhage there is usually impaired consciousness. Commonly affected areas are the pons, thalamus, putamen, and cerebellum. Hemorrhage frequently extends into an adjacent ventricle but rarely extends directly into the subarachnoid space.

The usual course of intracerebral hemorrhage is as follows:

1. Hemorrhage occurs for 1 to 2 h and reaches maximal size within that period except for unusual instances of acute exacerbation.
2. Cerebral edema appears around the hematoma in 7 to 8 h and progresses for 24 to 48 h.
3. The combination of hematoma and edema may produce cerebral herniation.
4. Degenerative changes and gliosis occur in the areas of hemorrhage and edema.

On CT scan, cerebral hemorrhage appears as an area of increased density. Even with first-generation scanners, CT diagnosis of intracerebral hemorrhage may be 90 percent accurate even without clinical information. The natural course of intracerebral hemorrhage as outlined above has prompted some physicians to operate early to remove the hematoma and in turn reduce the amount

Table 15-1. Differential Diagnosis of Hypertensive Cerebrovascular Events

	Hypertensive Encephalopathy	Cerebral Thrombosis	Intracerebral Hemorrhage	Subarachnoid Hemorrhage	Transient Ischemia
Onset	Gradual, over 24–48 h	Acute, over 1–2 h	Rapid	Rapid	Rapid, may be recurrent
Neurologic progression	Yes, over 24–48 h	May occur over several hours	Over minutes to hours	Rapid, in minutes	No
Impaired consciousness	Late	Not unless bilateral or brain stem	Usual	Usual and predominant	No
Other symptoms	Progressive headache, lethargy, seizures	Possible prior TIA; may occur during sleep	Sudden headache and vomiting initially		No
Focal signs	Transient and migratory	Present and fixed	Present and fixed	Frequently absent	Present but brief
CSF findings	Pressure may be elevated	Normal unless severe edema	Frequently blood, increased pressure	Blood, increased pressure	Normal

of subsequent edema. Their initial success, in comparison with both conservative management and late surgery, shows promise.

In the acute setting, rapid blood pressure control is essential to minimize the amount of hemorrhage since cerebral blood flow is proportional to blood pressure. Thus a rapidly acting agent should be used. As with all hypertensive cerebrovascular syndromes, antihypertensive agents that cause CNS sedation should be avoided as they may interfere with evaluation of the neurologic status. Even in the early days of antihypertensive therapy when drug availability was limited, the beneficial effect of blood pressure reduction could be shown in patients with intracerebral hemorrhage and ruptured cerebral aneurysm.

Ruptured Cerebral Aneurysm

Ruptured cerebral aneurysm, the most frequent cause of subarachnoid hemorrhage, is usually heralded by sudden headache, dizziness, and vomiting. Except for an altered mental status, there is a paucity of focal neurologic abnormalities. Meningeal irritation from blood in the CSF gives rise to nuchal rigidity. Data from a cooperative study reported by Locksley indicate a peak incidence in the 50 to 55 age group and a lack of obvious precipitating factors (contrary to many of our own individual anecdotal experiences).

A currently debated question in the neurosurgical community is early (first 2 to 3 days) versus delayed (1 to 2 weeks) surgery for ruptured aneurysm. The prevailing practice in the United States is to delay surgery in order to avoid vasospasm, which occurs from 4 to 14 days after initial hemorrhage and gives rise to ischemia. Such a delay increases the risk of rebleeding, which usually occurs within 10 days of initial rupture.

The CT scan show promise of resolving the issue. Kistler et al. have shown both retrospectively and prospectively that the presence of subarachnoid clots on CT scan correlates with subsequent vasospasm, while no blood, diffusely distributed blood, and intracerebral or intraventricular clot do not correlate. Early surgery to clip the aneurysm and remove the clots may reduce the incidence of subsequent vasospasm. The delayed surgery approach, while reducing operative morbidity and mortality, has done little to change overall morbidity and mortality. According to Sahs, early surgery is theoretically attractive. It would prevent rebleeding, reduce the incidence of vasospasm, allow vigorous approaches to treatment of vasospasm with the aneurysm safely clipped, avoid the complications of prolonged bed rest, and reduce the length of hospitalization.

As with intracerebral hemorrhage, if ruptured cerebral aneurysm is associated with hypertension, the blood pressure should be rapidly controlled. In addition to the study of Meyer and Bauer, showing the benefit of blood pressure control in ruptured cerebral aneurysm, early data from a cooperative aneurysm project showed that in terms of immediate morbidity and mortality, hypotensive drug therapy is as effective in the management of acute subarachnoid hemorrhage as surgical therapy.

Transient Ischemic Attack

TIA is by definition a self-limited entity, which is most commonly related to fixed vascular disease but on occasion is due to a small embolus or vascular spasm. There is no altered mental status, and

resolution occurs within 24 h. The same considerations apply to blood pressure control, as discussed under cerebral thrombosis.

Another uncommon entity deserves mention before closing this section. An acute CVA in certain patients, presumably by virtue of the anatomic area affected, results in severe elevation of the blood pressure in previously normotensive individuals as well as in hypertensive patients. This phenomenon should not be confused with the systolic blood pressure increase and bradycardia (Cushing reflex) that may occur with brain stem compression from increased intracranial pressure. This blood pressure increase is thought to be due to catecholamine release and, as reported by Feibel et al., was refractory to conventional antihypertensive therapy with nitroprusside and/or hydralazine. These authors detail seven such cases which were responsive to modest doses of propranolol and suggest that a β-blocker be the drug of choice in this setting.

Toxemia

Toxemia is characterized by hypertension, peripheral edema, proteinuria, and in full-blown cases seizures and coma. When the latter symptoms are present, toxemia can be viewed as a hypertensive encephalopathy of pregnancy. Because blood pressure is normally lower throughout pregnancy, eclampsia can occur at diastolic blood pressures of 100 to 110 mmHg. The characteristic renal lesions of toxemia are swelling of the endothelial and epithelial glomerular cells and fibrin deposition within the glomeruli.

Toxemia occurs most commonly in primigravidas and in multigravidas over the age of 35, especially those with prior histories of renal or hypertensive disease; it usually occurs in the third trimester of pregnancy.

Definitive treatment consists of emptying the uterus. Hydralazine and magnesium sulfate are commonly used in the management of this disorder. Diazoxide has been used successfully in eclampsia but a significant side effect is suppression of uterine contractions, which would require the use of oxytocics. Ganglionic blockers should be avoided because they reduce uterine blood flow in a setting where flow is already compromised.

Left Ventricular Failure and Coronary Insufficiency

Hypertension causes an increase in the afterload (resistance against which the heart must pump), leading to an increase in myocardial oxygen demand. The chronic increase in afterload results in left ventricular hypertrophy and further acute myocardial decompensation may result in pulmonary edema, characterized by dyspnea, frothy, blood-tinged sputum, diffuse, moist pulmonary rales, and, in severe cases, bronchospasm. If increased myocardial oxygen demand cannot be met because of coronary artery narrowing, the chest pain of myocardial ischemia or infarction may occur.

Heart failure due to hypertension is best treated by lowering the blood pressure to reduce the excessive afterload. Agents such as hydralazine, diazoxide, or minoxidil, which further increase cardiac work and myocardial oxygen demand, should be avoided in the setting of heart failure as well as in the management of severe hypertension complicated by coronary insufficiency. In cases where heart failure persists despite conventional therapy for pulmonary edema and adequate blood pressure control, cardiac glycosides can be used.

Aortic Dissection

About 90 percent of patients with aortic dissection have a history of hypertension. Aortic dissection is characterized by severe chest or upper abdominal pain, which generally radiates into the back. Physical findings vary depending on the site of the dissection. The patient may have focal neurologic signs, aortic insufficiency, disparity in extremity pulses, or signs of mesenteric or renal artery occlusion. Once aortic dissection occurs, the major factor responsible for the extension of dissection is the pulsatile force of blood flow with systole. Medical therapy consists of lowering the blood pressure in those patients who are hypertensive and reducing the force of the pulse wave with an agent having a negative inotropic effect, such as a β-blocker. Agents that increase the heart rate, such as hydralazine, diazoxide, and minoxidil, should be avoided.

Acute surgical intervention has usually been reserved for those cases involving the ascending aorta, particularly where acute aortic insufficiency is present. However, it has been recognized that there is still considerable subacute mortality with conservative therapy in dissections of the descending aorta. As surgical techniques have improved, surgery has become the optimum treatment for a subset of patients. Thus, a currently advocated approach is:

1. Diagnosis, stabilization, and initiation of antihypertensive therapy during the initial 4 h.
2. Surgery for cases involving the ascending aorta.
3. Monitoring in an intensive care unit of cases involving the descending aorta.
4. Operative intervention if there is:
   a. Continued pain
   b. Inability to control the blood pressure
   c. Expanding or rupturing aneurysm, or
   d. Development of a neurologic deficit or compromise of a major subdiaphragmatic branch of the aorta.

Accelerated (Malignant) Hypertension

Malignant hypertension is characterized by elevation of the diastolic blood pressure (usually to 130 mmHg or above) and papilledema. Retinal hemorrhages and renal dysfunction, manifested by azotemia, proteinuria, and red cells or red cell casts in the urine, are frequently present. Accelerated or malignant hypertension can occur as a result of any cause of hypertension. A postulated pathology is that of a proliferative endarteritis and necrotizing arteriolitis causing small vessel occlusions, particularly in the kidney, which in turn may result in excessive renin secretion. Malignant hypertension by itself is classified as a hypertensive urgency.

Microangiopathic hemolytic anemia is an uncommon but serious complication of malignant hypertension. It is characterized by hemolytic anemia, reticulocytosis, and schistocytes on peripheral smear. The hypertensive process results in direct vascular damage resulting in fibrin deposition in the vessel endothelium. Red cells and platelets become traumatized and fragmented as they pass through, and fibrin deposition is further enhanced.

Catecholamine-Dependent Hypertension

Catecholamine-dependent hypertensive syndromes include pheochromocytoma, clonidine withdrawal hypertension, and mono-amine oxidase (MAO) inhibitor-related hypertension. It is a rare circumstance in which a patient presents with a known pheochromocytoma, but should that occur or be strongly suspected on the basis of the patient's history, the antihypertensive treatment of choice is combined α- and β-adrenergic blockade.

Patients on larger doses of clonidine (usually 1.2 mg/day or more) who abruptly stop that medication may sustain a sudden return to their pretreatment blood pressure levels accompanied by other symptoms mediated by sudden catecholamine release (previously suppressed by clonidine). Prompt resumption of the clonidine is the treatment of choice.

Patients on MAO inhibitors for depression may develop sudden blood pressure elevations when they ingest tyramine-containing substances or receive certain other medication. The mechanism is impaired catecholamine catabolism due to MAO inhibition and the presence of exogenous catecholamine-like substances or precursors and/or the release of endogenous catecholamines. Foods containing such exogenous substances include aged cheeses, beer, Chianti wine, chicken livers, and pickled herring. Medications include amphetamine and its derivatives (which may be found in nonprescription diet pills), peripherally acting sympathomimetics such as ephedrine and phenylephrine (found in many nonprescription decongestants and nasal sprays), reserpine, guanethidine, mephentermine, metaraminol, and methoxamine. The treatment for severe hypertension in such a circumstance is combined α- and β-adrenergic blockade. Incidentally the combination of an MAO inhibitor and a tricyclic antidepressant may result in vascular collapse. Thus, the manufacturers of these products suggest a drug-free interval of 2 weeks when switching from one to the other.

Transient Blood Pressure Elevation

The term *transient blood pressure elevation* is used to describe situations in which there is an elevation of blood pressure, infrequently to levels above 120 mmHG diastolic, related to another acute underlying disorder. Thus, treatment should be directed toward the primary disease state and not toward the elevated blood pressure. Severe anxiety states frequently result in transient blood pressure elevation. Other examples include delirium tremens, acute hypoxic states, and diseases such as acute edematous pancreatitis.

The psychotic patient with acute agitation, including the drug-induced psychoses of phencyclidine and amphetamines, may have severe blood pressure elevation. In most of these cases sedation will lower the blood pressure to acceptable levels.

Delirium tremens is characterized by generalized sympathetic overactivity resulting in agitation, tachycardia, diaphoresis, and elevated blood pressure. Unless the blood pressure rise is extreme, treatment is the use of one of the benzodiazepines.

Acute hypoxic states such as pulmonary edema, acutely decompensated chronic obstructive pulmonary disease, or acute asthma can cause transient elevation of the blood pressure. Initial vigorous efforts to lower the blood pressure without first correcting the underlying abnormality could lead to hypotension.

In the acute stage a majority of patients with edematous pancreatitis develop elevated blood pressure, which gradually resolves as the inflammation abates. Although the blood pressure elevation is usually modest, in a few cases it has been reported to reach severe levels. The etiology is unknown but may be related to release of a vasoactive peptide during the acute phase.

CLINICAL FEATURES

History

A history should be obtained, with particular reference to duration of known hypertension, recent documented blood pressure recordings, current or prior antihypertensive medication, and a description of the present illness. The history of other current conditions (e.g., asthma) and medications (e.g., MAO inhibitor) is also important. The presence or absence of specific end organ symptoms (cerebral, cardiac, and renal) should be elicited. Symptoms such as headache and dizziness are nonspecific unless they can be correlated with grade 3 or 4 fundoscopic changes. It is the historical presentation in combination with specific findings on examination that determines whether hypertensive emergency or urgency is present.

Physical Examination

Auscultation of the blood pressure by the physician and assessment of the peripheral pulses is important and too frequently omitted. It serves both to confirm the blood pressure recording and often to reveal important diagnostic or therapeutic clues. Disparity in blood pressure between the two arms or between the upper and lower extremities may lead to an unsuspected diagnosis of aortic dissection, subclavian steal syndrome, or coarctation of the aorta. The presence of pulsus alternans indicates early heart failure and can only be detected by personal auscultation of the blood pressure. A diminished and delayed femoral pulse is usually present in coarctation of the aorta.

The sine qua non of the physical examination is the fundoscopic examination to determine the presence of papilledema, hemorrhages, exudates, or arteriolar spasm. The latter is a more subtle finding and indicates a more accelerated course of hypertension.

Gross cardiomegaly by physical examination is rare in hypertensive cardiovascular disease but a left ventricular heave or an S_4 gallop may be present. An aortic insufficiency murmur should be specifically sought. Moist rales indicate heart failure, and in acute pulmonary edema diffuse wheezing is frequently present and may be of sufficient magnitude to mask the rales and thereby cloud the correct diagnosis.

The presence of an abdominal bruit, particularly when high-pitched and having a diastolic component, may indicate renal artery stenosis.

Laboratory Studies

A complete blood count, determinations of blood glucose, blood urea nitrogen (BUN), creatinine, and electrolytes, and urinalysis should be obtained in patients with severe hypertension. Hypokalemia may be present in patients with high-renin forms of hypertension, as well as in patients on diuretic therapy, and does not necessarily indicate a diagnosis of primary aldosteronism.

An ECG should be part of the evaluation of a patient with severe hypertension to assess the presence of ECG criteria of left ventricular hypertrophy (LVH) (Table 15-2) and to detect changes of myocardial ischemia or infarction. Similarly, a chest x-ray may provide evidence of LVH, congestive heart failure, aortic aneurysm, or coarctation of the aorta.

Table 15-2. Point Score System for ECG Diagnosis of LVH

1. QRS amplitude
   a. largest R or S in limb leads $\geqq$ 20 mm
   b. largest S in V_1 or V_2 $\geqq$ 30 mm
   c. R in V_5 or V_6 $\geqq$ 30 mm
   Any of the above — 3 points
2. ST-T segment in the opposite direction from the QRS
   Patient not on digitalis — 3 points
   Patient on digitalis — 1 point
3. Left atrial involvement as evidenced by a terminally negative P wave in V_1 $\geqq$ 1 mm and duration $\geqq$ 0.04 s — 3 points
4. Negative QRS axis of $-30°$ or more — 2 points
5. QRS duration $\geqq$ 0.09 s — 1 point
6. Intrinsicoid deflection of the QRS $\geqq$ 0.05 s in V_5 or V_6 — 1 point

Five points or more total = definite LVH
Four points = probable LVH

Source: Romhilt DW, Estes EH: A point score system for the ECG diagnosis of left ventricular hypertrophy. *Am Heart J* 75:752, 1968,

The use of CT scanning is discussed under the section on hypertensive cerebrovascular disorders.

TREATMENT

General Considerations

The choice of antihypertensive therapy should be based on the clinical presentation of the patient and the physician's knowledge of the available drugs. Aggressive therapy, i.e., reduction of the blood pressure over minutes to a few hours, is indicated for hypertensive emergencies, while in a hypertensive urgency the blood pressure can be reduced more gradually over a period of 24 h (see Table 15-3). Treatment of the underlying disorder is indicated for transient blood pressure elevations.

The objective of parenteral antihypertensive therapy is to produce rapid lowering of the blood pressure. In the elderly and other patients who may have fixed arteriosclerosis, rapid reduction of the blood pressure to normal levels may produce signs of cerebral or cardiac ischemia. In those individuals the goal should be a diastolic pressure of 90 to 100 mmHg.

Substantial reductions in blood pressure are accompanied by a reduced glomerular filtration rate and thus an increase in BUN and creatinine levels. These elevations are usually transient and can be minimized by use of antihypertensive agents that help maintain urine output (the diuretics) or maintain a more normal renal blood flow (methyldopa, most vasodilators).

Oral antihypertensive agents should be initiated as soon as is practical after the initiation of parenteral drugs so as to reduce the duration of parenteral therapy and the intensive monitoring that such therapy frequently requires. A minimum of two-drug and usually three-drug therapy will be necessary, a diuretic, vasodilator, and sympathetic inhibitor combination being most commonly used.

The knowledge of a drug's mechanism of action, hemodynamic effects, and side effects is essential in choosing a drug for use in a specific hypertensive emergency or urgency. An understanding of the mechanism of action of these drugs is truly an exercise in the understanding of the workings of the sympathetic nervous system and the hemodynamics and compensatory mechanisms of the cardiovascular system. This is particularly true when trying to differentiate between the newer drugs that are available to treat hypertension, such as prazosin, captopril, and minoxidil, and the calcium channel blockers.

Diuretics

The exact mechanism by which diuretics produce an antihypertensive effect is unknown but their action is not due to plasma volume depletion, which is only a transient effect. The diuretics vary in their site of action, effect on potassium excretion (preserved by spironolactone, amiloride, and triamterene), and effect on calcium excretion. All presently available diuretics in the United States cause increased uric acid retention and thus may be implicated in episodes of acute gout. The parenterally available diuretics are furosemide and ethacrynic acid.[1]

Furosemide (Lasix)

Action. Furosemide is a potent loop diuretic that also increases venous capacitance.

Indications. Furosemide is the adjunctive choice with all other agents in the treatment of hypertensive emergency and urgency, particularly with the vasodilators, which cause sodium and fluid retention.

Dose. The dosage of furosemide is 40 to 80 mg intravenously or orally. There is an unlimited dose-response curve (in contrast to the benzothiadiazines) so that the intravenous dose may be doubled at 30-min intervals if there is insufficient diuretic response. A total dose of 1000 mg should not be exceeded in 24 h and would only be anticipated in the face of severe renal insufficiency.

Adverse effects. Adverse effects of furosemide include hypokalemia, hypovolemia, and thrombocytopenia. Ototoxicity may occur when the megadoses described above are used within short periods of time.

Vasodilators

Regardless of the initiating mechanism, the hemodynamics of most hypertensive patients result in an increased peripheral vascular resistance. Thus, the development of vasodilator drugs was pursued early; troublesome side effects retarded their further development. The advent of β-blocker drugs that counteract those side effects has led to a resurgence in the vasodilator area.

Although one might attempt to categorize the vasodilators as a homogeneous group, they are hemodynamically a heterogeneous group and thus have different clinical indications for usage. Blood pressure reduction by a prototype vasodilator (hydralazine) results in a number of homeostatic mechanisms that occur reflexly. These include increased venous return; increase in heart rate, cardiac output, and cardiac index; increased plasma renin activity; and increased plasma catecholamines, all of which serve to reduce the antihypertensive effect and may result in adverse side effects.

[1]Not approved by the FDA for use as an antihypertensive agent.

With the introduction of newer vasodilators, comparative hemodynamic studies have been performed and reveal differences in the amount of venodilation, the degree of reflex sympathetic stimulation, and their cardiac effects.

Hydralazine (Apresoline)

Action. Hydralazine causes relaxation of arteriolar smooth muscle, resulting in peripheral vasodilation (without venodilation) and reflex tachycardia. It increases renal, coronary, cerebral, and splanchnic blood flow if the blood pressure drop is not extreme. The onset of action is 5 to 10 min after intravenous use and 30 min after intramuscular use.

Indications. Hydralazine is used for moderate blood pressure reduction in patients without coronary artery disease, left ventricular failure, or aortic dissection. It has been particularly favored in eclampsia and renal disorders.

Dose. The intravenous dose is 10 to 20 mg; intramuscularly the range is 10 to 50 mg and dosage may be repeated after 30 min.

Adverse effects. The cardiac effects are a result of β-receptor stimulation by reflex sympathetic discharge response to vasodilation. The increased cardiac work may be hazardous in the presence of coronary insufficiency or left ventricular failure, and the increased aortic blood flow is undesirable in aortic dissection. Headache and flushing may occur. These effects can be counteracted with a β-blocker. Hydralazine causes sodium and water retention; chronic use of large doses may cause a lupus erythematosus-like syndrome. A peripheral neuropathy responsive to pyridoxine may also occur.

Minoxidil (Loniten)

Action. Minoxidil is a potent vasodilator acting by direct effect on arteriolar smooth muscle and has the same hemodynamic pattern as hydralazine. When compared directly with hydralazine, it has been found to have a clearly more potent antihypertensive effect.

Indications. Although predominantly for chronic use in patients resistant to conventional antihypertensive therapy, particularly those with renal function impairment, minoxidil can be used to achieve acute control in hypertensive urgency. Because of the hemodynamic side effects and sodium and water retention, a β-adrenergic blocker and a diuretic should be used concurrently.

Dose. The initial dose for intended chronic use is 2.5 mg orally. Duration of action is sufficiently long that a once or twice daily schedule can be used; the maximum daily dose is 40 mg/day. In initial attempts to demonstrate an acute usefulness, a small (1-mg) initial dose was used with incremental increases at 6-h intervals, but a more aggressive regimen is reported by Alpert and Bauer. They used a 20-mg loading dose with a "booster" dose of up to 20 mg at 4 h if the diastolic pressure was still above 100 mmHg. Significant blood pressure reduction was seen in 1 h and continued to a peak reduction between 8 and 12 h.

Adverse effects. As with hydralazine, symptoms due to the reflex sympathetic effects are common. Hypertrichosis of the face and extremities occurs, is not dose related, and subsides with cessation of the drug. A poorly publicized effect of minoxidil as reported in a single large series is a high incidence of T-wave flattening or inversion on the ECG. These could be mistaken for ischemic changes. They occur within a few days of initiation of therapy, are seen in those leads having an upright QRS, and may persist for up to 2 years.

Diazoxide (Hyperstat)

Action. Diazoxide is a direct vasodilator which does not affect venous capacitance. It has the same reflex sympathetic effects as hydralazine. Blood pressure falls within 1 to 2 min of intravenous bolus injection, and peak effect is seen in 5 to 10 min. The duration of action is quite variable but may be up to 12 h.

Indications. Diazoxide is used to produce a rapid, substantial fall in blood pressure in patients without coronary artery disease or aortic dissection. Use in severe hypertension with acute pulmonary edema is problematic—the beneficial effect of acutely reducing afterload *may* outweigh the deleterious effects of increased heart rate and increased cardiac work.

Dose. Diazoxide was originally reported to be effective only if given in a rapid intravenous bolus of 300 mg or 5 mg/kg. Slower injection would result in drug inactivation. The result of this practice was an inability to control the degree of drop in the blood pressure; numerous instances of excessive hypotension were reported. Alternative methods of administering the drug were sought and succeeded in achieving an acceptable result. Several investigators used a minibolus approach, such as that reported by Velasco et al., who used an initial 25 to 50 mg bolus with subsequent boluses in 25-mg increments at 10-min intervals until a maximum single dose of 200 mg or a normalized blood pressure was achieved.

More recently constant infusion methods have been reported with a similar measure of success. Garrett and Kaplan studied patients at two infusion rates, 15 and 30 mg/min. No additional medications were used and the goal was a diastolic pressure of 100 to 105 on successive readings. Larger total amounts of diazoxide, in the range of 600 mg, were required, but the desired endpoint was reached in both groups; 38 min at the slower rate and 20 min at 30 mg/min.

Adverse effects. Extravasation of the drug causes local pain. In addition to the cardiac effects and sodium and water retention, hyperglycemia may occur, particularly when large or repeated doses are used. If used in eclampsia, diazoxide impairs uterine contractility and oxytocics may be necessary to achieve adequate labor. Fetal hyperbilirubinemia or hyperglycemia may also occur.

Sodium Nitroprusside (Nipride)

Action. Nitroprusside causes relaxation of arteriolar smooth muscle and increases venous capacitance. There is an increase in heart rate, not as great as that seen with hydralazine or diazoxide, but occurring without any increase in cardiac output or cardiac work; coronary vasodilation and reduced myocardial oxygen consumption occur.

Indications. Nitroprusside is the most universal of the antihypertensive medications and may be used for almost all hypertensive emergencies, particularly hypertensive encephalopathy and left ventricular failure. It is even effective in the catecholamine excess states, in which more specific adrenergic blocker therapy is most desirable.

Dose. The dose of nitroprusside is 50 mg dissolved in 500 mL of 5% dextrose in water to provide a concentration of 100 μg/ mL. The dose range is 0.5 to 10 μg/(kg·min) with an average dose of 3 μg/(kg·min). The drug should be administered under conditions of precise flow rate and frequent blood pressure monitoring. The infusion bottle, and optimally the tubing also, should be protected from light and should not be used after 4 h from the time of preparation. The infusion fluid should not be used for simultaneous administration of other medication.

Adverse effects. Hypotension may occur if the dose is not carefully titrated, especially in the elderly. After prolonged or high-dosage use and in patients with renal dysfunction, thiocyanate levels should be monitored and the drug discontinued if the level exceeds 10 mg/100 mL. Psychosis is one of the manifestations of thiocyanate toxicity.

Nitroglycerin (Nitro-Bid IV, Nitrostat IV)

Action. Although thought of as a venodilator, in higher doses nitroglycerin is also an arterial dilator owing to its direct effect on vascular smooth muscle. It reduces both preload and afterload on the left ventricle. Heart rate increases, cardiac index is reduced (in persons with an initially normal cardiac index), and myocardial oxygen consumption is reduced.

When directly compared with nitroprusside in postoperative coronary bypass hypertension, nitroglycerin improved pulmonary shunting while nitroprusside made shunting worse. Greater increase in cardiac output was seen with nitroglycerin, and it improves coronary collateral flow, while nitroprusside reduces coronary perfusion pressure without any increase in collateral flow. Only 3 of 17 patients studied were unable to achieve adequate blood pressure reduction with nitroglycerin; all responded adequately to nitroprusside.

Indications. Nitroglycerin may be the drug of choice for perioperative hypertension associated with cardiovascular surgical procedures and for hypertension in the presence of acute coronary insufficiency.

Dose. One manufacturer provides 5-, 25-, and 50-mg ampoules to allow a variety of concentrations. The drug is diluted in 5% dextrose in a glass bottle (absorbed by plastic) and infused at an initial rate of 5 μg/min.[2] Infusion rate is increased by 5 μg/min increments every 3 to 5 min up to 20 μg/min and thereafter by 10 μg/min increments until the desired effect is achieved. The infusion fluid should not be used for the simultaneous administration of other medication.

Adverse effects. As with other routes of administration, the most frequent side effect is headache. Tachycardia, nausea, vomiting, apprehension, muscle twitching, substernal discomfort, and abdominal pain may be seen.

Nifedipine (Procardia)

Action. The calcium channel blockers have a variety of different actions, the principal ones being (1) coronary artery dilation, (2) peripheral arterial dilation, (3) a negative inotropic effect, (4) a negative chronotropic effect, and (5) a negative dromotropic effect. The net effect of an individual calcium channel blocker depends on the strength of each of these separate actions plus the

---

[2]If manufacturer's special tubing is used. If standard polyvinyl chloride tubing is used, an initial rate of 25 μg/min is suggested.

reflex mechanisms induced by those actions (primarily in response to vasodilation). The relative strength of each of these actions varies with the individual calcium channel blocker. Thus, verapamil has a predominant effect on AV conduction (negative dromotropic) and is used in the treatment of supraventricular tachyarrhythmias. Nifedipine is predominantly a peripheral vasodilator and the reflex β-adrenergic response counteracts its other direct effects. The degree of blood pressure reduction is proportional to the degree of elevation of the pretreatment blood pressure; thus little blood pressure reduction is seen in normotensives.

Indications. Nifedipine has been used successfully as an antihypertensive agent in hypertensive encephalopathy, acute left ventricular failure, and hypertensive urgency. The same group of investigators has also used nifedipine to reduce afterload in patients with acute pulmonary edema of varying etiologies.

Dose. Nifedipine is available in a 10-mg capsule; in Europe a sublingual formulation is also available. Onset of action with sublingual use is 5 min, and with oral use 20 min. The maximum antihypertensive effect occurs within the first hour, declining gradually over several hours; thus a dosage regimen with 6-h intervals is more effective than a single dose. There is an increase in heart rate, which dissipates after 1 h.

Adverse effects. The side effects of nifedipine are similar to those of most vasodilators: headache, sensation of palpitations, and burning sensation in the face or extremities. These tend to subside with continued treatment.

Sympathetic Blockers or Inhibitors

Reserpine (Serpasil)

Action. Reserpine is thought to act by depletion of catecholamines in the brain and at adrenergic nerve endings.

Indications. With the availability of other agents, there are few situations in which reserpine would be the drug of choice. This is because of its relatively slow action, which is of moderate and variable degree. It should be avoided in any setting in which the neurologic status must be followed.

Dose. The dose is 1 to 5 mg intramuscularly; onset of action occurs within 1 to 3 h. The lowest dose should be used initially and the dose increased at 3-h intervals depending on response.

Adverse effects. The commonest side effects are sedation and nasal stuffiness. Exacerbation of peptic ulcer disease may occur. With chronic use, depression is a common side effect.

Methyldopa (Aldomet)

Action. The mechanism of action of methyldopa has still not been definitively established. For many years it was thought to work as a false neurotransmitter, but more recent evidence favors central adrenergic effect by its metabolite α-methylnorepinephrine.

Indications. As with reserpine, a slow onset of action, a moderate antihypertensive effect, and sedation limit the usefulness of methyldopa for hypertensive emergencies. It lowers blood pressure without reducing renal blood flow or glomerular filtration rate and thus is most useful in patients with renal dysfunction and hypertension.

Dose. The intravenous dose is 250 to 500 mg in 100 mL 5% dextrose infused at a rate of 30 to 60 min. The onset of the effect is not seen for 2 to 3 h. The oral dose is 250 to 500 mg 2 to 4 times daily.

Adverse effects. The main side effect with intravenous use is sedation. With chronic use, orthostatic hypotension may be seen, particularly in volume-depleted patients. Other side effects are liver dysfunction, Coombs positivity, which is rarely associated with hemolytic anemia, blood dyscrasias, drug fever, and a lupus erythematosus-like syndrome. Headache and dry mouth are common.

Clonidine (Catapres)

Action. Clonidine is a CNS α-adrenergic stimulator—such stimulation results in a decrease in central sympathetic outflow. The level of circulating catecholamines is reduced, and sudden release of that suppression is an important factor in the clonidine withdrawal hypertension that may occur in some patients.

Indications. Although usually used in the treatment of chronic hypertension, clonidine may be used acutely to reduce blood pressure in hypertensive urgency. It is the drug of choice in clonidine withdrawal hypertension.

Dose. In hypertensive urgency, an initial dose of 0.2 mg is given orally, followed at hourly intervals by doses of 0.1 mg to a total dose of 0.6 to 0.7 mg or until the desired effect is achieved. For chronic use, daily doses of 1.2 mg should rarely be exceeded.

Adverse effects. Hypotension may rarely occur in sensitive individuals and is not postural. Sedation and dry mouth are the commonest side effects. Patients receiving larger doses (0.6 to 1.2 mg/day and higher) are at risk for clonidine withdrawal hypertension.

Prazosin (Minipress)

Action. Originally thought to be a vasodilator by direct effect on vascular smooth muscle, prazosin is now thought to act by competitive blockade of α_1 (postsynaptic) receptors. Because α_2 (presynaptic) receptors are not affected, in contrast to the use of phentolamine and phenoxybenzamine, a reflex activation of the sympathetic nervous system is not seen.

Indications. Usually used for the chronic treatment of hypertension, prazosin may be used for gradual moderate reduction of severe hypertension, particularly in instances in which an increase in heart rate and cardiac work is not desirable.

Dose. the initial dose is 1 mg orally. Blood pressure reduction is usually seen within 30 min, with peak effect at 1 to 2 h. The duration of the effect is sufficiently long that prazosin may be given on a twice daily basis for chronic use.

Adverse effects. A major side effect is postural hypotension, which is dose-related (initial dose 2 mg or more) and more likely to occur in volume-depleted patients. In early use this gave rise to syncope, which was termed a *first dose effect*. Fluid retention occurs and thus combined therapy with a diuretic is usually beneficial.

Phentolamine (Regitine)

Action. Phentolamine is a complete α-adrenergic blocker (α_1 and α_2) for intravenous use. The α-blockade effect in other organ systems has produced sufficient symptoms to preclude its use in ordinary hypertension.

Indications. The use of phentolamine is restricted to catecholamine excess states such as pheochromocytoma and MAO inhibitor–related hypertension. It can be used as a diagnostic agent in suspected pheochromocytoma. Phenoxybenzamine, a comparable oral compound, is also used in vasospastic conditions.

Dose. The initial dose of phentolamine is a 5-mg intravenous bolus. The activity of such a bolus is short-lived, and its use must be followed by a constant infusion prepared by adding 100 mg to 500 or 1000 mL of 5% dextrose in water. The dose of oral phentolamine is 50 mg every 4 to 6 h; that of phenoxybenzamine is 10 mg daily, with slow increments as indicated by the response.

Adverse effects. Adverse effects are related to α-blockade and include orthostatic hypotension, tachycardia, impotence, nasal congestion, miosis, nausea, vomiting, and diarrhea.

Propranolol (Inderal)

Action. Propranolol is a nonselective β-adrenergic blocker useful in a variety of conditions including hypertension. The exact mechanism by which β-blockade produces hypotension is unknown and is not related to suppression of plasma renin activity. The additional effects of β-blockade are bradycardia, negative inotropic, delayed AV node conduction, and bronchial constriction. The latter is an effect of nonselective β-blockade and may not be seen with the newer "selective" β-blockers such as metoprolol and atenolol.

Indications. Propranolol is an adjunct to some of the vasodilators to counteract adverse cardiac effects as well as to provide additional antihypertensive activity. It may be used in addition to α-blockers in the treatment of catecholamine excess states in which signs of excess β-stimulation are present. β-Blockade is the treatment of choice for "hyperkinetic" hypertension manifested by tachycardia and increased cardiac output.

Dose. The initial oral dose of propranolol for hypertension is 20 or 40 mg, with an initial daily dose range of 80 to 160 mg. The literature is sparse in regard to the acute use of β-blockers for severe hypertension. There are reports citing intravenous usage with diazoxide or nifedipine; additive antihypertensive effects were seen and when the β-blocker precedes the vasodilator, a significant antihypertensive effect occurred within 30 to 60 min. Propranolol was used in a dose of 0.2 mg/kg. It should be administered at a rate of 1 mg/min.

Adverse effects. The main side effects are the result of the pharmacologic activity of the drug. The negative inotropic effect may be hazardous with compromised left ventricular function. The presence of bronchospastic disease dictates that a selective β_1-blocker be used. These impair the adrenergic response to hypoglycemia and thus must be used with caution in insulin-dependent diabetics. Vasospastic conditions may be induced or exacerbated. Sudden withdrawal in patients with coronary artery disease may result in angina or infarction.

Trimethaphan (Arfonad)

Action. Trimethaphan is an intravenous ganglionic blocking agent whose antihypertensive effect is greatest in the upright position. It results in both arterial and venous dilation, reduced car-

Table 15-3. Parenteral Drugs for Use In Hypertension

Drug	Advantages	Disadvantages
Reserpine: 1–5 mg IM	Ease of administration	Delayed onset of action; CNS sedation; variably effective
Methyldopa: 250–500 mg by IVPB q 6 h	No decrease in renal perfusion	Delayed onset of action; CNS sedation; variably effective
Hydralazine: 10–50 mg IM 10—20 mg IV	Maintains cerebral, renal, and coronary perfusion	Sl. delay in onset with IM use; increased HR, CO, and cardiac work
Diazoxide: Miniboluses or 15–30-mg/min infusion	Rapid onset of good effectiveness	Increases HR, CO, and cardiac work; hyperglycemia and sodium retention
Nitroprusside: 50 mg in 500 mL D₅W at 0.5–10μg/ (kg·min)	Rapid onset, can titrate dose, useful in almost all emergencies	Need constant BP monitoring; possible thiocyanate toxicity
Nitroglycerin: 25–50 mg in 500 mL D₅W at 5–10 μg/min	Rapid onset, can titrate dose, use with coronary insufficiency	Special tubing needed or must use higher doses. Not as versatile or effective as nitroprusside
Trimethaphan: 500 mg in 500 mL D₅W	Rapid onset, can titrate dose, good effectiveness	Need constant BP monitoring. Autonomic side effects; reduces cerebral, renal, and uterine blood flow. Tachyphylaxis
Phentolamine 5 mg IV bolus 100 mg/L for IV infusion	Rapid onset	Clinical use limited to catecholamine excess states
Propranolol 0.1–0.2 mg/kg at 1 mg/min IV	Use as an adjunct to vasodilators to counteract side effects or for combined α- and β-blockade	Paucity of clinical data for use in acute hypertensive settings; negative inotropic effect

diac output, tachycardia, and symptoms of ganglionic blockade in other organ systems. Renal (and uterine) blood flow is decreased.

Indications. Trimethaphan is indicated for rapid control of severe hypertension, particularly in the presence of left ventricular failure or dissecting aortic aneurysm.

Dose. An infusion is prepared by adding one ampoule (500 mg) to 500 mL of 5% dextrose in water to yield a concentration of 1 mg/mL. An initial infusion rate of 1 to 4 mg/min is recommended, with dose titration according to response. For maximal effect the patient should be sitting upright or have the head of the bed elevated.

Adverse effects. Adverse effects are related to autonomic blockade and include paralytic ileus, urinary retention, and mydriasis. Tachyphylaxis may occur with prolonged use. Rare cases of respiratory arrest have been reported but without a definite causal relationship. Reduced renal blood flow negates use of trimethaphan in the presence of renal insufficiency, and usage in eclampsia is contraindicated because of reduction in uterine blood flow as well as production of meconium ileus in the fetus.

Pentolinium (Ansolysen)

Pentolinium is a ganglionic blocking agent that may be used intramuscularly or intravenously but is no longer marketed in the United States. It was most likely to be used intramuscularly in severe hypertension with left ventricular failure in a setting in which constant monitoring of blood pressure was not feasible.

Renin-Angiotensin Antagonists

Captopril (Capoten)

Action. Captopril is an oral angiotensin-converting enzyme (ACE) inhibitor, impairing conversion of angiotensin I to angiotensin II. Developed for use in high-renin forms of hypertension, particularly renovascular hypertension, its full mechanism of action is unclear; it still has antihypertensive activity regardless of plasma renin levels, although its greatest effect is in patients with high plasma renin. Thus some additional mechanism of action is likely. There is no increase in heart rate or cardiac output with captopril.

Indications. Captopril was designed for use in renal forms, i.e., renovascular or renal parenchymal, of hypertension, where angiotensin II levels are high. Because it reduces afterload without adverse hemodynamic cardiac effect, it has been used in congestive heart failure with and without hypertension. Trial in acute undifferentiated severe hypertension has been limited.

Dose. Investigators have found that single doses above 25 mg do not increase antihypertensive effect in most patients although further dosage increase does increase the duration of action. There is a significant antihypertensive effect within 15 min after an oral dose, with maximum effect at 90 min. Weinberger found that all patients studied required a diuretic and half of them required a β-blocker for adequate blood pressure control on long term captopril therapy.

Adverse effects. The side effects consistently mentioned by most authors are a skin rash associated with eosinophilia, an alteration in taste sensation, and leukopenia.

SUMMARY

True hypertensive emergencies are uncommon even in centers that treat large numbers of hypertensive patients. This is attributable to public awareness of hypertension and its dangers and a more aggressive antihypertensive posture by physicians.

A hypertensive emergency is the development of a diastolic pressure of 130 mmHg or greater in the presence of a condition such as hypertensive encephalopathy, left ventricular failure, aortic dissection, or hypertensive intracranial hemorrhage. It can also develop with a diastolic pressure of less than 130 mmHg, especially if the rate of rise of the blood pressure has been rapid, as in toxemia. The blood pressure should be lowered in minutes to a few hours.

A hypertensive urgency is the elevation of the blood pressure, usually over 130 mmHg, in the absence of findings of severe end-organ compromise. Blood pressure reduction should be achieved within 24 h.

Transient hypertension can be seen resulting from a variety of disorders and treatment of the underlying disorder achieves normalization of the blood pressure.

The choice of a therapeutic agent depends on the patient's clinical status and the physician's familiarity with the available drugs. A knowledge of the mechanism of action, speed of action, hemodynamic effects, and side effects of each of the major antihypertensive agents forms the basis for sound and safe therapy.

BIBLIOGRAPHY

Alpert MA, Bauer JH: Rapid control of severe hypertension with minoxidil. *Arch Intern Med* 142:2099,1982.

Altchek A, Albright NL, Sommers SC: The renal pathology of toxemia of pregnancy. *Obstet Gynecol* 31:595, 1968.

Anderson RJ, Hart GR, Crumpler CP, et al.: Oral clonidine loading in hypertensive urgencies. *JAMA* 246:848, 1981.

Aoki K, Kondo S, Mochizuki A: Antihypertensive effect of cardiovascular calcium antagonist in hypertensive patients in the absence and presence of beta-adrenergic blockade. *Am Heart J* 96:218, 1978.

Beevers DG, Fairman MJ, Hamilton M, et al: Antihypertensive treatment and the course of established cerebral vascular disease. *Lancet* 1:1407, 1973.

Carter AB: Hypotensive therapy in stroke survivors. *Lancet* 1:485, 1970.

Cohen IM, Katz MA: Oral clonidine loading for rapid control of hypertension. *Clin Pharmacol Ther* 24:11, 1978.

Colucci WS: Alpha-adrenergic receptor blockade with prazosin. *Ann Intern Med* 97:67, 1982.

Crompton MR: Pathogenesis of cerebral aneurysms. *Brain* 89:797, 1966.

Feibel FH, Baldwin CA, Joynt RJ: Catecholamine-associated refractory hypertension following acute intracranial hemorrhage: Control with propranolol. *Ann Neurol* 9:340, 1981.

Fisher CM, Kistler JP, Davis JM: Relation of cerebral vasospasm to subarachnoid hemorrhage visualized by computerized tomographic scanning. *Neurosurgery* 6:1, 1980.

Flaherty JT, Magee PB, Gardner TL, et al.: Comparison of intravenous nitroglycerin and sodium nitroprusside for treatment of hypertension after coronary artery bypass surgery. *Circulation* 65:1072, 1982.

Garrett BN, Kaplan NM: Efficacy of slow infusion of diazoxide in the treatment of severe hypertension with organ hypoperfusion. *Am Heart J* 103:390, 1982.

Glorioso N, Fulgheri PD, Madeddu P, et al.: Active and inactive renin after a single dose of captopril in hypertensive patients. *Am J Cardiol* 49:1552, 1982.

Gottlieb TB, Katz FH, Chidsey CA: Combined therapy with vasodilator drugs and beta adrenergic blockade in hypertension: A comparative study of minoxidil and hydralazine. *Circulation* 45:571, 1972.

Graham RM, Thornell IR, Gain RM: Prazosin: the first-dose phenomenon. *Br Med J* 2:1293, 1976.

Grim CE, Luft FC, Grim CM, et al.:Rapid blood pressure control with minoxidil: Acute and chronic effects on blood pressure, sodium excretion and the renin-aldosterone system. *Arch Intern Med* 139:529, 1979.

Guazzi M, Olivari MT, Polese A: Nifedipine, a new antihypertensive with rapid action. *Clin Pharmacol Ther* 22:528, 1977.

Hall D, Charocopos F, Froer K, et al.: Electrocardiogram changes during long-term minoxidil therapy for severe hypertension. *Arch Intern Med* 139:790, 1979.

Hansson L, Hunyor SN, Julius S, et al.: Blood pressure crisis following withdrawal of clonidine (Catapres, Catapresan) with special reference to arterial and urinary catecholamine levels, and suggestions for acute management. *Am Heart J* 85:605, 1973.

Hayward RD, O'Reilly GVA: Intracerebral hemorrhage: Accuracy of computerised transverse axial scanning in predicting the underlying etiology. *Lancet* 1:1, 1976.

Henning M, Rubenson A: Evidence that the hypotensive action of methyldopa is mediated by central actions of methylnoradrenaline. *J Pharm Pharmacol* 23:1, 1971.

Houser OW, Campbell JK, Baker HL, et al.: Radiologic evaluation of ischemic cerebrovascular syndromes with emphasis on computed tomography. *Radiol Clin North Am* 20:123, l982.

Houston MC: Abrupt cessation of treatment in hypertension: Consideration of clinical features, mechanisms, prevention, and management of the discontinuation syndromes. *Am Heart J* 102:415, 1981.

Huysmans FTM, Thieu TA, Koene RAP: Combined intravenous administration of diazoxide and beta-blocking agent in acute treatment of severe hypertension or hypertensive crisis. *Am Heart J* 103:395, 1982.

Kaneko M, Tanaka K, Shimada T, et al.: Long term evaluation of ultra early operation for hypertensive intracerebral hemorrhage in 100 cases. *J Neurosurg* 58:838, 1983.

Kannel WB, Wolf PA, Verter J, et al.: Epidemiologic assessment of the role of blood pressure in stroke: The Framingham study. *JAMA* 214:301, 1970.

Kistler JP, Crowell RM, Davis KR, et al.: The relation of cerebral vasospasm to the extent and location of subarachnoid blood visualized by CT scan: A prospective study. *Neurology* 33:424, 1983.

Linton AL, Gauras H, Gleadle RI, et al.: Microangiopathic hemolytic anemia and the pathogenesis of malignant hypertension. *Lancet* 1:1277, 1969.

Locksley HB: Report on the Cooperative Study of intracranial aneurysms and subarachnoid hemorrhage. Natural history of subarachnoid hemorrhage, intracranial aneurysms and arteriovenous malformations. *J Neurosurg* 25:219, 1966.

Meyer JS, Bauer RB: Medical management of spontaneous intracranial hemorrhage by the use of hypotensive drugs. *Neurology* 12:36, 1962.

Meyer JS, Sawada T, Kitamura A, et al.: Cerebral blood flow after control of hypertension in stroke. *Neurology* 18:772, 1968.

Mrocek WG, Leibel BA, Davidov M, et al.: The importance of rapid intravenous administration of diazoxide in accelerated hypertension. *N Engl J Med* 285:603, 1971.

Olivari MT, Bartorelli C, Polese A, et al.: Treatment of hypertension with nifedipine, a calcium antagonist agent. *Circulation* 59:1056, 1979.

Polese A, Fiorentini C, Olivari MT, et al.: Clinical use of a calcium antagonist agent (nifedipine) in acute pulmonary edema. *Am J Med* 66:825, 1979.

Romhilt DW, Estes EH: A point score system for the ECG diagnosis of left ventricular hypertrophy. *Am Heart J* 75:752, 1968.

Sahs AL: Editorial: Aneurysmal subarachnoid hemorrhage: An appraisal. *Mayo Clinic Proc* 57:529, 1982.

Sankaran S, Lucas C, Walt, AJ: Transient hypertension with acute pancreatitis. *Surg Gynecol Obstet* 138:235, 1974.

Sassano P, Pedrinelli R, Magagna A, et al.: Humoral and hemodynamic effects of increasing doses of captopril in patients with essential hypertension. *Am J Cardiol* 49:1574, 1982.

Stokes GS, Graham RM, Gain JM, et al.: Influence of dosage and dietary sodium on the first dose effect of prazosin. *Br Med J* 1:1507, 1977.

Stone PH, Antman EA, Muller JE, et al.: Calcium channel blocking agents in the treatment of cardiovascular disorders. Part II: Hemodynamic effects and clinical applications. *Ann Intern Med* 93:886, 1980.

Strandgaard S, Skinhøj E: Pathogenesis of hypertensive encephalopathy. *Lancet* 1:461, 1973.

Velasco M, Gallardo E, Plaja J, et al.: A new technique for safe and effective control of hypertension with intravenous diazoxide. *Curr Ther Res* 19:185, 1976.

Veterans Administration Cooperative Study Group on Antihypertensive Agents: Effects of treatment on morbidity in hypertension: Results in patients with diastolic blood pressures averaging 115 through 129 mmHg. *JAMA* 202:1028, 1967.

Veterans Administration Cooperative Study Group on Antihypertensive Agents: Effects of treatment on morbidity in hypertension: Results in patients with diastolic blood pressure 90 through 114 mmHg. *JAMA* 213:1143, 1970.

Weinberger MH: Role of sympathetic nervous system activity in the blood pressure reponse to long-term captopril therapy in severely hypertensive patients. *Am J Cardiol* 49:1542, 1982.

Weiss NJ: Relation of high blood pressure to headache, epistaxis and selected other symptoms. *N Engl J Med* 287:631, 1972.

Whisnant JP, Phillips LH, Sundt TM: Aneurysmal subarachnoid hemorrhage: Timing of surgery and mortality. *Mayo Clinic Proc* 57:471, 1982.

Wolfe WG, Moran JF: Editorial: The evolution of medical and surgical management of acute aortic dissection. *Circulation* 56:503, 1977.

Additional General References

Bhatia SK, Frohlich ED: Hemodynamic comparison of agents useful in hypertensive emergencies. *Am Heart J* 85:367, 1973.

Byrom FB: The pathogenesis of hypertensive encephalopathy and its relation to the malignant phase of hypertension: Experimental evidence from the hypertensive rat. *Lancet* 2:201, 1954.

Keith, NM, Wagener HP, Barker NW: Some different types of essential hypertension: Their course and prognosis. *Am J Med Sci* 197:332, 1937.

Kincaid-Smith P, McMichael J, Murphy EA: The clinical course and pathology of hypertension with papilledema. *Q J Med* 27:117, 1953.

Scheie HG: Evaluation of ophthalmologic changes of hypertension and arteriolar sclerosis. *Arch Ophthalmol* 49:117, 1953.

CHAPTER 16
CAROTID
ARTERY DISEASE

Ramon Berguer

Stroke is one of the three leading causes of death in the United States. The importance of carotid artery disease as a cause of stroke has long been established. The advent of arteriography and of the technique of endarterectomy to ream atheromatous intima and plaques from the inner lining of arteries have resulted in a dramatic reduction of strokes in patients with carotid artery disease who suffer transient ischemic attacks (TIAs).

Before discussing the current management of carotid artery disease in its different clinical presentations, it is important to grasp the peculiar anatomical and physiological facts relevant to carotid disease and to the mechanisms by which it results in TIAs and strokes.

GENERAL OVERVIEW OF CAROTID ARTERY DISEASE AND ITS PATHOLOGICAL EFFECTS

Patterns of Collateral Circulation

The blood supply to the brain is derived pincipally from the paired internal carotid and vertebral arteries. The internal carotid arteries supply what is called the *anterior* circulation, that is, the hemispheres and the eyes. The vertebral arteries supply the *posterior* circulation, that is, the brain stem, cerebellum, and generally the occipital lobes. In general, in the absence of one of these vessels the others can take over to supply its territory owing to an important arrangement of connecting vessels between both systems and between each pair of arteries.

The most important of these is the circle of Willis, which links the terminal portions of the basilar artery and both internal carotid arteries. This intracranial connection is frequently incomplete, with one or more of the small communicating vessels missing or too small to permit adequate cross flow. Those patients with a normal and widely patent circle of Willis are more likely to tolerate the occlusion of one of the vessels feeding into it.

In addition to this very important intracranial anastomosis there are other extracranial connections which offer alternative routes to supply blood to the brain when a carotid or a vertebral artery become occluded. These extracranial arrangements depend principally on the distribution of the external carotid artery.

The external carotid artery communicates with the distal portion of the internal carotid artery through anastomosis across the orbit of the eye (Fig. 16-1). Thus, a patient with an internal carotid occlusion may derive a substantial portion of that hemisphere's blood supply from branches of the external carotid artery that connect with the ophthalmic artery and from there, and in a retrograde fashion, with the distal portion of the internal carotid artery. In the posterior circulation if one vertebral artery occludes, the opposite artery, if normal, can generally take over its function since both empty into the basilar artery. In addition to this obvious alternative to supply the basilar artery, the external carotid artery can also provide flow to the distal vertebral artery when the proximal vertebral artery is occluded. This is done through anastomoses between the occipital artery and the distal portion of the vertebral artery. This secondary pathway is particularly important when both proximal vertebral arteries are occluded (Fig. 16-2).

Localization of Atherosclerotic Lesions and Their Types

Although atherosclerosis affects all extracranial vessels, in general the large build-up of atherosclerotic material tends to occur in specific areas. These areas are fortunately accessible to the surgeon. The most characteristic location for these large accumulations of atherosclerotic material is the origin of the internal carotid artery (Fig. 16-3). Lesions involving the bifurcation of the common carotid artery and origin of the internal carotid artery account for 40 percent of those found in arteriography or in autopsy studies. Another 20 percent are located at the origin of a vertebral artery.

The subclavian arteries are also frequently affected, but the pathological consequences of these lesions are less severe. Innominate artery lesions are not common, although they are physiopathologically important since they are in the pathway of the carotid artery.

Atherosclerotic plaques evolve in different ways. The initial lesion is usually a raised fibrous plaque. As the plaque grows it protrudes inside the lumen and may cause an obstruction to blood flow. Some of these plaques break down in their central portion and present to the flowing blood a cavity containing cholesterol and thrombotic material. Inasmuch as these thrombus and cholesterol particles are in contact with the bloodstream, they may be carried by it to the brain, where they become impacted in the

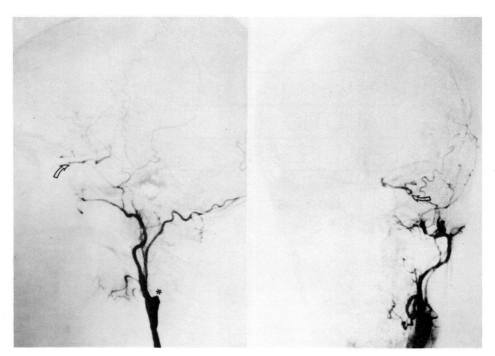

Figure 16-1. Arteriogram, anteroposterior and lateral views, of patients with an occluded internal carotid artery. Note the rich collaterals about the orbit that provide blood from branches of the external carotid artery in a retrograde fashion through the ophthalmic artery into the distal portion of the internal carotid artery.

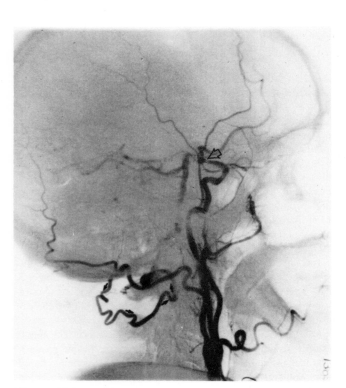

Figure 16-2. Arteriogram of a patient with occluded vertebral arteries and stenosis in the terminal portion of the carotid siphon. Note the large collateral arising from the occipital artery filling the distal vertebral artery and in turn opacifing the basilar artery.

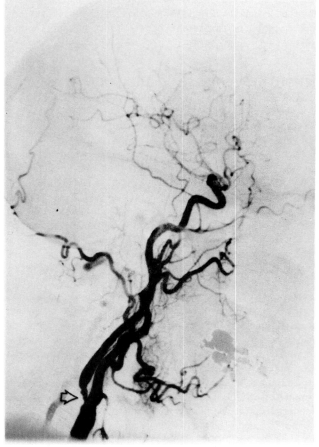

Figure 16-3. A typical atherosclerotic plaque at the origin of the internal carotid artery.

smaller arteries. These small emboli then obstruct blood flow and cause ischemia or death of the tissue supplied by the small vessel in question. This is the mechanism called *microembolization.*

Another mechanism by which disease in the carotid artery affects the brain involves progressive narrowing of the lumen of the artery, causing a severe restriction of blood flow; this, if not compensated by the collateral pathways mentioned above, will result again in either transient or permanent ischemic damage to the brain. It is difficult to assess precisely the proportion of symptomatic carotid artery disease due to microembolization and that due to restriction of blood flow caused by severe stenosis. The prevailing opinion nowadays is that microembolization is a very important pathological mechanism and accounts for a substantial portion of the TIAs seen in these patients. It is pertinent to point out here that a plaque does not need to be large or to cause a serious stenosis to become ulcerated and give symptoms of microembolization.

If a carotid plaque is not causing microembolization but continues to grow, the relative restriction of blood flow imposed in this hemisphere can be compounded by other central causes such as a cardiac arrhythmia or a sudden drop in blood pressure. Eventually, and regardless of whether the plaque is ulcerated or not, its growth will result in a very severe stenosis, whose fate, given enough time, is to become thrombosed. When an internal carotid plaque causes thrombosis of the lumen of this vessel at the stenosis site, the thrombus propagates upwards to near the end of the carotid siphon, since the internal carotid artery has few and exceedingly small branches between its origin and the carotid siphon. Such a sudden thrombosis of the internal carotid artery may cause dramatic effects in an entire hemisphere (stroke) or conversely could have been gradually compensated by the external carotid artery and result in no symptoms at all.

The presence of a severe stenosis in one carotid artery should alert us to the possibility of disease in the opposite carotid artery and in the other vessels of supply, namely, the subclavian and vertebral arteries. If a patient has a severe stenosis in one carotid artery, there is a 60 percent chance that an equally important lesion is present on the opposite side.

The Concept of Bruit

A *bruit,* a noise by another name, is generated by a severely narrowed artery. Narrowing causes turbulence of the stream of blood emerging from the constriction. This turbulence in turn causes the artery walls to vibrate and this vibration, transmitted through the tissues, is heard as a noise. Depending on the degree of turbulence and on the size of the turbulent vortices of blood, the bruit may have a low pitch ("blowy") or a high pitch (squeaky, "seagull cry"). The bruit may also be barely or very clearly audible. Bruits of high intensity can actually be felt as a thrill by palpation.

An understanding of the mechanism of the production of a bruit tells us that the artery has to be severely narrowed before such turbulence and thus a bruit can occur. There is no set figure for the percent of luminal narrowing that will produce a bruit, since its appearance is determined not only by the degree of stenosis but also by the velocity of flow through that particular artery. However, for the particular rate of flow normally occurring in the carotid arteries, a narrowing of over 70 percent of the luminal area will result in a bruit. As the stenosis progresses, the bruit

develops a higher pitch and often a higher intensity. Finally, when the stenosis has narrowed the lumen to a very small orifice, the intensity of the bruit may be so slight that it cannot be heard and the artery is silent again. The next step in the evolution of the lesion is its complete occlusion of the artery by thrombosis.

From what has been said about the production of a bruit, it is obvious that a bruit is only important when it is present or has been present and has since disappeared. The presence of a bruit over the carotid artery generally indicates a severe stenosis of this vessel. The absence of a bruit, on the other hand, could mean that the artery is normal or conversely that the stenosis is so severe that the bruit cannot be heard or that the vessel has thrombosed.

PRESENTATION OF THE PATIENT WITH CAROTID ARTERY DISEASE TO THE EMERGENCY PHYSICIAN

From the point of view of the emergency physician, the encounters with carotid disease in clinical practice take place generally under three conditions. A patient who presents with an unrelated acute problem in the emergency room may be found during physical examination to have a bruit. Examination and interrogation of this patient show no evidence of cerebrovascular disease other than the bruit, which is then called asymptomatic. A patient may also present to the emergency room with symptoms of transient cerebral ischemia, which may or may not be due to carotid disease. This is a more threatening problem since some of these patients will go on and progress to a frank stroke. Finally, a patient may present to the emergency room with a stroke. The management of these different modes of presentation of carotid artery disease will be dealt with separately.

Patient Presenting with an Asymptomatic Bruit

Let us recall that the presence of a neck bruit indicates an underlying stenosis ranging from roughly 70 percent to near total occlusion. Such a severe stenosis, if located in the internal carotid artery, is a threatening lesion and requires the completion of specific diagnostic steps. Furthermore, a severe stenosis in one carotid artery will in many cases be matched by equally serious disease of the opposite carotid. Such a precarious situation if compounded by shock, dehydration, cardiac arrhythmias, etc. that slow the flow of blood across the tight stenosis may result in acute thrombosis and therefore in the possibility of a stroke.

The question has been raised many times in surgical circles of what to do when a patient who is scheduled for an unrelated major surgical operation is found to have an asymptomatic bruit. The concern here is that the decrease in cardiac output and the hypotension that may accompany general anesthesia and intraoperative bleeding may cause the accelerated thrombosis of this already impaired carotid artery and thus result in a stroke in the course of the operation. This hypothesis has been tested in some surgical series. The conclusion is that there is no good evidence to recommend giving priority to a prophylactic endarterectomy before the other planned operation. On the other hand, if the planned procedure is elective and no risk is involved in waiting, most surgeons would first do the carotid endarterectomy provided the carotid lesion in itself justifies an operation.

In an emergency room this situation presents itself when a

patient who has an acute problem of one sort or another is found to have an asymptomatic bruit. In this circumstance, the work-up and treatment of the main problem should proceed normally; the bruit should be worked up later on once the problem that brought the patient to the emergency room is under control.

What then should one recommend to a patient with an asymptomatic bruit? The first thing is to be sure that the patient is indeed asymptomatic. The absence of amaurosis fugax or of transient ischemic attacks causing sensorimotor loss in the face, arm, and leg on one side does not suffice to qualify a bruit as asymptomatic. The patient should be questioned about other signs of cerebrovascular insufficiency, such as dizziness, vertigo, diplopia, blurring of vision, paresthesia, ataxia, or drop attacks.

The first step in the work-up of an asymptomatic bruit is to determine if the source of the bruit is indeed the internal carotid artery. A small percentage of bruits may originate in the aortic valve and be transmitted along the neck. Bruits originating in the subclavian or vertebral arteries, although heard best over the medial half of the clavicle, may be mistaken for carotid bruits. Finally, less than 10 percent of the bruits over the carotid bifurcation will originate in the external carotid artery, which of itself has little pathological relevance. Such bruits do not represent an increased risk of stroke for the patient.

The purpose of the so-called noninvasive evaluation of a neck bruit is to try to identify those bruits not originating in the internal carotid artery and having far less pathological relevance. An arteriogram is too severe and risky a test to diagnose these noncarotid lesions in the absence of symptoms when noninvasive examination can provide the answer. In general, the combination of an oculoplethysmography test with one of the ultrasound imaging techniques permits the separation of patients with a bruit originating in the internal or more rarely the common carotid artery from those in whom the source is an artery (mentioned above) that is unlikely to place the patient at a higher risk for a stroke.

If a patient is asymptomatic but has a neck bruit and the vascular laboratory identifies the bruit as originating in either the subclavian or the external carotid artery, nothing further needs to be done and the patient can be reassured that the stroke risk is not substantially different from that of any other person of the same age group.

Patients with asymptomatic neck bruits in whom the noninvasive examination indicates that the source of the bruit is the internal carotid artery should be advised to undergo arteriography. The reason for this is that, in most circumstances, if a very severe but correctable lesion is found, an endarterectomy may be advisable to decrease the risk of a stroke.

There is no general agreement as to whether asymptomatic bruits originating in a severe stenosis of the internal carotid artery demonstrated by angiography should be treated by prophylactic surgery. There is no doubt either, as mentioned above, that some patients with these lesions will if given enough time, progress to occlusion and many of them will suffer a stroke. The advantage of operating on these patients prophylactically must be measured first against the risk of such an operation, since carotid endarterectomy has as one of its specific complications that of an intraoperative stroke. The combined mortality and morbidity for carotid endarterectomy range roughly between 1 and 5 percent in well-controlled series reported in the medical literature. This is not to say that the mortality and morbidity of carotid endarterectomy in the average hospital achieve these low risk rates. The best evidence at hand suggests that surgeons who are expert in the performance of this operation can by operating decrease very substantially the stroke rate in patients with asymptomatic bruits as compared with patients who are observed instead.

Not all carotid lesions behave in the same manner. Even surgeons who operate on asymptomatic bruits will often decide between operative treatment or observation depending on some specific arteriographic findings. For instance, the patient who is a good surgical risk but has a very severe isolated stenosis (95 percent) of the internal carotid artery is generally an operative candidate. Conversely, a patient with a milder and smoother carotid stenosis who also has diffuse and multiple extra- and intracranial lesions should not have an operation for an asymptomatic carotid bruit because the lesions in the other vessels supplying blood to the brain may not be correctable and yet could be equally threatening. Needless to say, the decision can only be made once an angiogram is obtained. The arteriogram determines the state of the other arteries and rules out the presence of other intracranial lesions, such as aneurysms, which may influence the decision as to whether to operate or not.

In summary, if a patient is seen in an emergency room for an unrelated acute problem and is found to have an asymptomatic bruit, the latter should not delay or change the management of the primary problem. However, once this primary problem is under control, the bruit should be worked up to determine if its origin is in the internal carotid artery.

Patient Presenting with Transient Ischemic Attacks

Transient ischemic attacks are best divided into those of hemispheric origin and those termed *nonhemispheric*. The former are related to the carotid area and consist of symptoms derived from ischemia of the eye or of the hemispheres. Transient ischemia of the eye is usually manifested by complete or partial loss of vision. This is caused by a decrease in blood flow to the entire eye or by embolization of small particles (originating in a carotid plaque) that occlude the blood supply of the optic nerve or of the retina. The most commonly found materials embolizing the eye are cholesterol crystals, which can be identified by ophthalmoscopy as yellow refringent intraarterial bodies, and fibrin-platelet aggregates, which appear as white clumps. If the ischemia of the eye is secondary to a decrease in blood flow but not to embolization, ophthalmic examination will be normal once the transient ischemic attack is over.

When patients report transient visual disturbances of one eye, it is important to verify that the problem is indeed unilateral. Some patients may volunteer that they see well when they cover the problem eye but not at all when they cover the opposite eye. This naturally would indicate ischemia of the problem eye, probably of carotid origin. Sometimes patients report loss of vision "in one eye" when in fact they have a homonymous hemianopsia due to ischemia of the occipital lobe supplied by the posterior cerebral arteries. This is usually the result of vertebrobasilar disease although it can happen also with carotid artery disease in patients whose posterior cerebral arteries take origin from the internal carotid artery.

Other transient ischemic attacks of hemispheric type are aphasia, dysarthria, and paralysis and sensory loss in the face, arm, and leg on the side of the body opposite to that of the involved carotid artery.

Nonhemispheric signs and symptoms are more difficult to detect and elicit; they consist of dizziness, vertigo, diplopia, disorientation, ataxia, blurring of vision, and drop attacks. These symptoms, which are often referred to as *vertebrobasilar insufficiency,* can be due both to carotid and to vertebrobasilar disease.

It has already been said that in the carotid territory the mechanism of TIAs is either poor perfusion, which is usually transitory, or microembolization. There is no evidence that microembolization plays such an important role in the pathological effects of vertebrobasilar arterial disease.

In those patients with symptoms secondary to a severe stenosis rather than to microembolization, the question can be posed as to why the episode happened in a transient manner since the stenosis is stable. It is believed that these patients have a marginal perfusion and that a transient drop in the cardiac output and/or blood pressure results in critical perfusion losses, which in turn cause TIAs.

Therefore, in patients presenting with TIAs the first point to be clarified is whether they are of the hemispheric or nonhemispheric type. In hemispheric TIAs, that is, those of carotid origin, a carotid lesion should be suspected and if found, treated. There is general consensus that in patients with TIAs secondary to carotid artery disease, carotid endarterectomy is the best mode of therapy. Auscultation of the neck will indicate whether there is a bruit. If eye symptoms are present, a fundoscopic examination may reveal the cause of the eye problem to be microembolization. This finding makes the likelihood of carotid disease much higher. One must not forget that conditions resulting in drops in cardiac output and systemic pressure can precipitate TIAs of both the hemispheric and the nonhemispheric type. These conditions include cardiac arrhythmia, orthostatic hypotension, and excessive antihypertensive medication. The presence or absence of arrhythmias should be determined by means of an ECG. Other conditions, such as anemia, dehydration, and polycythemia, that decrease the delivery of oxygen to the brain should be ruled out in the initial examination and, if found, should be corrected.

There is no role for noninvasive examinations in patients with TIAs. The reason is that small plaques not severe enough to cause bruits or restrictions of blood flow can, however, ulcerate and cause microembolization. Patients with such small plaques will frequently have "normal" noninvasive evaluations. The only proper way to evaluate and decide on treatment for a patient with TIAs is by means of an arteriogram provided the patient is an acceptable surgical risk. The arteriogram will identify the most likely source of the TIAs provided such source is an arterial lesion and will add other pertinent information, helpful in deciding whether a carotid endarterectomy should be advised.

Carotid lesions can also cause symptoms of vertebrobasilar insufficiency in the territory of the posterior circulation. This is more likely to happen in those patients with small or occluded vertebral arteries, in whom the flow to the brainstem and to the occipital lobes is supplied principally by the carotid system. In these patients a carotid endarterectomy may also relieve symptoms of vertebrobasilar insufficiency.

In general, then, a patient with TIAs is a candidate for arteriography. Such a patient is likely to be relieved of this problem by a carotid operation and thus decrease substantially the chances of suffering a stroke in the future. In patients with nonhemispheric (vertebrobasilar) TIAs, the arteriogram may reveal the cause of the problem to be either carotid stenosis or vertebral artery disease. Patients with TIAs of vertebrobasilar type have a lesser risk of stroke than those with hemispheric (carotid) TIAs. Vertebrobasilar TIAs, although they represent a lesser risk of stroke, can be incapacitating (diplopia, ataxia, vertigo). If a severe carotid lesion is found in these patients, an operation should be performed. Severe bilateral vertebral artery lesions can also be corrected by vertebral operations, generally a reimplantation or a bypass.

Patient Presenting with an Acute Stroke

By convention a TIA is a neurological deficit that does not last longer than 24 h, while a stroke is a deficit prolonged beyond this time limit. It is assumed that minimal or no permanent neurological damage occurs in the former. A patient with an acute stroke seldom needs an emergency surgical intervention, although in very special circumstances emergency operations may result in the resumption of function.

Treatment of a patient with an acute stroke must ensure homeostasis, proper ventilation, and proper cardiac function. Arteriography during the acute stage of a stroke is attended by an unacceptable rate of complications, including death. The same can be said, in general, of emergency carotid operations for patients with acute strokes. Even if the patient progresses satisfactorily over the ensuing days, arteriography should be delayed for at least 2 weeks and certainly until the patient is neurologically stable. A CT scan provides valuable information as to the extent of the stroke.

Following recovery from the acute period of the stroke, an arteriogram is generally indicated to ascertain if the stroke was due to a carotid lesion and if so, whether the carotid has occluded or is still patent and may cause further deficits in the near future. If the arteriogram shows a lesion that on its own merit is severe and operable, our inclination is to operate on this lesion electively some 3 to 6 weeks following the initial stroke. This is done to prevent further damage in the territory of the involved carotid.

BIBLIOGRAPHY

Berguer R, Feldman AJ: Surgical reconstruction of the vertebral artery. *Surgery,* 93:670–675, 1983.

Fields WS: Aortocranial occlusive vascular disease (stroke) *CIBA Clinical Symposia,* 26:11, 1974.

Thompson JE, Pattman RD, Persson AV: Management of asymptomatic carotid bruits, *AM Surgeon* 42:77, 1976.

CHAPTER 17
MESENTERIC ISCHEMIA

Ramon Berguer

Mesenteric ischemia is a rare condition. Like all vascular syndromes it may present acutely, with perfusion of the bowel ceasing suddenly, or chronically, with symptoms occurring when the demands for blood flow exceed its supply (mesenteric angina).

ANATOMIC AND PHYSIOPATHOLOGICAL BACKGROUND

Blood Supply to the Bowel

The gut has a triple blood supply, which originates from the celiac and the superior and inferior mesenteric arteries. All three are anterior branches of the aorta, and as such they become involved to some degree in atherosclerosis of the aorta, most often at the point where they branch off from the latter. The three main trunks are interconnected not far from their origin. The pancreatico-duodenal arcade connects the hepatic artery (branch of the celiac artery) with the superior mesenteric artery. The meandering artery connects the transverse colic (branch of the superior mesenteric artery) with the left colic (branch of the inferior mesenteric artery). When one of the major trunks becomes occluded at its origin, these connections enlarge and in general are quite able to supply blood to the neighboring territory in an efficient manner. In a few patients these anastomotic connections either are too small or do not exist at all, and these individuals are more liable to ischemic complications following severance or occlusion of one of their major trunks. This anatomical defect is, however, rare.

In addition to being intercommunicated, the arteries supplying the bowel have lesser peripheral connections with other arterial territories: the small branches of the celiac are connected with the esophageal blood supply, and the inferior mesenteric artery territory is also connected to the hypogastric artery supply around the rectum.

Of the three arteries of supply, the celiac and the superior mesenteric artery are the most important. Inferior mesenteric artery occlusion is a common finding in patients with abdominal aortic aneurysms since the artery originates from the aneurysmal sac. As this aneurysmal sac becomes layered with thrombi, the artery often occludes although its territorial supply, the left colon, is usually well provided for by the meandering artery coming from the transverse colic artery (branch of the superior mesenteric artery).

Intestinal Response to Ischemia

From a physiopathological point of view, a segment of bowel might be considered as made of up of two layers: an inner layer of mucosa, of high metabolic requirement owing to the constant shedding and replacement of its epithelium, and a thicker outer layer composed of the muscularis and the serosa, which has a much lesser metabolic rate and on whose function depends the motility and the integrity of the bowel wall.

When a bowel loop becomes ischemic, the mucosa is injured and dies within a very short period of time. As the mucosa sloughs, the submucosa, which is very rich in capillaries, is exposed to the intestinal contents and bleeds. This results in the formation of ulcerations or larger areas of denudation and the loss of microscopic or gross amounts of blood into the bowel wall.

Outside the mucosa layer the musculoserosal coat is also subjected to ischemia. Its initial response to such an insult is spasm. The consequence of this muscle spasm is vomiting and, more frequently, diarrhea. If ischemia persists following this initial bout of hyperactivity, the muscle gradually loses tone, and the bowel becomes paralyzed and dilated.

Up to this point the integrity of the bowel wall has not been lost and, at least in the initial phases, the injury is reversible provided the blood supply is reestablished. Assuming that no muscular damage has been incurred, the mucosa may be restored in 2 to 3 weeks. During this time, of course, the bowel would not be functional.

If on the contrary the ischemic injury persists, the insult to the musculoserosal layers will be compounded by two additional factors: migration of bacteria into the wall originating from the intestinal content and partial digestion of the devitalized wall by intestinal enzymes. This will result eventually in the perforation of the bowel wall and the establishment of a bacterial and chemical peritonitis.

Types of Acute Mesenteric Ischemia

Acute mesenteric ischemia can be due to occlusion of the large arteries and veins supplying and draining the bowel or to thrombosis of the distal vascular bed, an entity called *nonocclusive mesenteric infarction*. The occlusion of the arteries of the bowel can be secondary to an embolus or to thrombosis of an already deteriorated artery. We are dealing with four etiologies for acute mesenteric ischemia: arterial embolus, arterial thrombosis, mesenteric vein thrombosis, and nonocclusive mesenteric infarction. The most common of all these causes is embolism of the blood supply to the bowel, principally of the superior mesenteric artery, followed by thrombosis of the arteries to the bowel and nonocclusive mesenteric infarction, with a similar incidence. Mesenteric venous thrombosis is a diagnosis made in the past quite frequently but is seldom seen nowadays. It is likely that because most of these diagnoses were made at postmortem, the observers were seeing the venous thrombosis that is the end stage of mesenteric infarction.

In nonocclusive mesenteric infarction the thrombosis affects the distal small vessels of the mesenteric bed. It is associated with conditions of low cardiac output, dehydration, shock, and digitalis toxicity. The first three cause considerable slowing of the mesenteric blood flow. Digitalis has been shown to have a direct effect on the mesenteric bed, causing its vasoconstriction. This modality of mesenteric ischemia should be suspected in patients with poor cardiac output, severe hypotension, or shock who develop abdominal pain.

DIAGNOSIS AND TREATMENT

Syndrome of Acute Mesenteric Ischemia

Acute mesenteric ischemia is a disease that affects mostly old people. Clearly, arterial embolization can also be seen in younger individuals with atrial fibrillation or aortic valve prostheses or disease.

All four types of acute ischemia of the bowel have a similar course. It is a dramatic but uncharacteristic clinical picture, which results in the diagnosis being made in too few cases or too late in the course of the disease and in a mortality rate between 50 and 70 percent.

When the diagnosis is made early in the course of the disease, prompt surgical intervention can dramatically change the course of these patients. Since there are no specific findings, awareness of the possibility of this entity remains the best guarantee of an early diagnosis. It should always be kept in mind whenever dealing with sudden abdominal pain in an older patient who has evidence of atherosclerotic arterial disease in the heart or limbs.

The first manifestation of acute bowel ischemia is pain. It is always there though it may be difficult to elicit in a patient who is extremely ill. The pain tends to be diffuse and to have a constant quality, as opposed to the alternation of cramps and relief that is characteristic of intestinal obstruction. The onset of pain is often accompanied by diarrhea and elevation of the white cell count. After a while, the muscular layer of the intestine becomes paralyzed and the patient develops an ileus with decreased or absent bowel sounds and abdominal distension. Later in the course of the disease, perforation and all the classic signs of a full-blown peritonitis appear: massive loss of fluid in the infarcted bowel wall takes place, hypotension develops, metabolic acidosis becomes evident, and eventually shock and death ensue.

Again, as can be inferred from the description of the nonspecific clinical signs and symptoms, awareness of the possibility of this entity is the best help in its early diagnosis. An x-ray of the abdomen will show some nonspecific pattern of dilatation of the bowel loops. A ground glass appearance with absence of bowel gas has been hailed as characteristic but is actually an uncommon finding. Late signs, such as "thumb-printing," which can be seen in plain x-ray or in barium studies as a consequence of hemorrhage in the submucosa, are rare diagnostic signs but particularly useful in ischemia of the left half of the colon.

The most important diagnostic step when the suspicion of mesenteric ischemia is entertained is to obtain an anteriogram. This is done by an initial aortic flood study followed by selective injection of the celiac and superior and inferior mesenteric arteries. The arteriogram will substantiate the diagnosis and often establish the etiology of the condition. A superior mesenteric artery embolus has a characteristic angiographic appearance. In nonocclusive mesenteric infarction the main arteries of supply are patent, but there is spasm of the branches of the main vessels and poor or very late opacification of the fine vessels filling the bowel wall.

In addition to differentiating between arterial embolization, arterial thrombosis, and nonocclusive mesenteric infarction, angiography often permits the selective catheterization of the superior mesenteric artery for infusion of vasodilators, a step that is considered fundamental in the treatment of nonocclusive mesenteric infarction.

Once the angiographic diagnosis is made, the patient is taken to the operating room. Until this time the most important maneuver is maintenance of homeostasis in the patient. Massive losses of plasma and blood into the infarcted intestinal wall must be replaced. Intravenous antibiotics are given. Cardiac function, if poor, should be restored, since this is a most important etiology of nonocclusive mesenteric infarction. The resuscitation of these patients must start at the point that the diagnosis is made and is as important a part in their treatment as the angiogram and the operation.

In the operating room the plan varies according to the etiology as determined by the arteriogram. If we are dealing with an arterial embolus in the superior mesenteric artery, an embolectomy is the treatment of choice. Following the embolectomy the bowel will be assessed for viability, and after appropriate observation the areas that are clearly gangrenous will be resected. If the etiology is an arterial thrombosis, the operation of choice is a graft, which will take origin in the aorta or iliac arteries and will be anastomosed to that portion of the superior mesenteric artery distal to the thrombosis. In nonocclusive mesenteric infarction the infusion of vasodilators through the catheter that was left in the superior mesenteric artery proceeds throughout the operation while the obviously gangrenous portions of bowel are resected.

It is common at operation to find areas of bowel that have questionable viability. It is known that once a proper cardiac output and fluid balance are restored, many of these areas will recover viability. Therefore when doubt exists at the time of operation, it is advisable to leave them intact and come back 6 to 12 h later for what is called a "second look" operation. During this interval the patient should continue to be resuscitated in an intensive manner and to receive antibiotics. The role of anticoagulation at this stage has not been clearly established. It is presumed that after 12 h of resuscitative efforts and during the second look operation all those areas of the bowel that were to recover would have done so. Those that are clearly nonviable are resected.

One of the consequences of mesenteric infarction is often the loss of massive length of bowel, to the extent that in many cases there is no gut left, a situation incompatible with life. Since these mesenteric infarctions tend to damage very substantial lengths of bowel, saving every possible inch of it at operation is very important.

In conclusion, only through early suspicion, angiography, and operation can the appalling mortality of acute mesenteric ischemia be reversed.

Chronic Intestinal Ischemia

This very rare entity seldom presents a problem to the emergency physician. It is a chronic condition, more common in women than in men (which is uncharacteristic for atherosclerotic disease). It is the result of chronic and severe occlusion of the arterial supply to the gut. These patients usually have progressively developed collateral circulation as the arteries have narrowed and eventually occluded. At some point the large demands for increased blood flow that take place during digestion of food cannot be met by this compromised supply and the syndrome develops.

Patients affected with this problem are usually very thin. They have postprandial pain, which they can easily relate to the intake of food as well as to the quantity of food ingested. Because of this many of them develop ''bird'' eating habits, having many very small meals throughout the day, to avoid a sudden large increase in mesenteric blood flow demand. A change in bowel habits, either diarrhea or constipation, is also a common complaint. An abdominal bruit has been hailed as an important physical sign but this is very questionable, since, indeed, occluded arteries do not cause bruits and many of those heard may be secondary to disease of other branches of the aorta and not necessarily from the mesenteric supply.

The disease is rare and the diagnosis is made by exclusion after the common causes of intermittent abdominal pain have been ruled out. The diagnosis is finally established by angiography when disease involving the three mesenteric vessels is shown in a lateral arteriographic view. Given that the anastomoses between the three mesenteric vessels are both constant and efficient, it is widely held that unless two of the three mesenteric vessels of supply are occluded, the diagnosis should not be made.

Once the diagnosis is made, surgical therapy is usually successful in relieving the symptoms. The operation is either a bypass from the aorta to a segment of the vessel beyond the occlusion or a transaortic endarterectomy of the orifices of the vessels involved.

BIBLIOGRAPHY

Boley SJ: Acute mesenteric vascular occlusion. *Contemp Surg* 22:125–161, 1983.

Boley SJ, Sprayregan S, Siegelman SS, et al: Initial results from an aggressive roentgenological and surgical approach to acute mesenteric ischemia. *Surgery* 82:848–855, 1977.

Eklof B, Hoevels J, Ihse I: The surgical treatment of chronic intestinal ischemia. *Ann Surg* 187:318–324, 1978.

Ottinger LW: Nonocclusive mesenteric infarction. *Surg Clin North Am* 54:689–698, 1974.

Stoney RJ, Ehrenfeld WK, Wylie EJ: Revascularization methods in chronic visceral ischemia caused by atherosclerosis. *Ann Surg* 186:468–476, 1977.

CHAPTER 18
THORACIC AND ABDOMINAL AORTIC ANEURYSMS

A. Joel Feldman

Any portion of the aorta may be involved with aneurysmal disease. Although the asymptomatic patient is not a problem for the emergency physician, the symptomatic patient requires prompt, accurate diagnosis and expeditious therapy. Delay, incorrect diagnosis, or improper therapy will frequently cost these patients their lives.

ACUTE DISSECTING ANEURYSM OF THE AORTA

Acute dissection is the most common catastrophe involving the aorta. It affects 5 to 10 patients per million population each year and is 2 to 3 times more common than an acutely ruptured abdominal aortic aneurysm. Untreated, this is a lethal entity. The mortality rate is 28 percent at 24 h, 50 percent at 48 h, and 70 percent at the end of 1 week. Within 3 months, 90 percent of these patients are dead. Males are much more commonly affected than females. The vast majority of patients are hypertensive.

Etiology

The final common pathway leading to this entity is necrosis of the medial layer of the aortic wall, usually due to atherosclerosis. However, approximately 10 percent of these patients have cystic medial necrosis associated with Marfan's syndrome. Medial necrosis also occurs during pregnancy, with coarctation, with congenital abnormalities of the great vessels, and with various hormonal abnormalities. Half of the dissections occurring in young females occur during pregnancy.

Classifications

Dissecting thoracic aortic aneurysms are classified according to the location of the dissecting process and not the site of origin of the tear. In Debakey's classification, type I involves the ascending aorta as well as varying lengths of the distal aorta; type II is limited to the ascending aorta only and does not involve the arch or the more distal portions of the aorta; and type III is a dissection of the descending aorta, usually starts just distal to the origin of the left subclavian artery, and most commonly involves the entire descending aorta down to the iliac arteries. Many authors group types I and II together because the principles of treatment and the prognosis are the same. In the Debakey experience 36 percent of the patients presented with ascending aortic dissections and 63 percent with descending aortic dissections.

Presentation

Of these patients, 70 to 90 percent present with severe pain that is more intense than they have ever experienced. Chest pain radiating to the abdomen or legs, although classically associated with this condition, is in fact an uncommon presentation. The pain may be located in the back, the epigastrum, and/or the extremities. The most important characteristic of the pain is its severity and short duration of onset.

Patients may present with an acute stroke due to occlusion of a cerebral vessel or with paraplegia because of spinal ischemia. Congestive heart failure and pulmonary edema are present in 22 percent of patients. Less commonly, the initial presentation is acute ischemia of one of the lower extremities.

The blood pressure may be elevated, normal, or low. It should be measured in both upper extremities and one of the lower extremities. Significant differences in extremity blood pressures should suggest the diagnosis. Likewise, the patient who presents with both acute chest pain and an acute neurologic deficit (uncommon in acute myocardial infarction) should be suspected of having an acute dissecting aneurysm.

Diagnosis

The most important differential diagnosis is acute myocardial infarction. Less commonly, stroke, acute surgical abdomen, pulmonary embolism, or an acutely ischemic extremity due to thrombosis or embolus may be confused with an acute aortic dissection.

In addition to extremity blood pressure differences, physical examination may reveal the murmur of aortic insufficiency, signs of cardiac tamponade, or murmurs at the base of the neck, in the abdomen, or over the femoral arteries that have not been previously present.

The electrocardiogram is abnormal in 90 percent of these patients; however, changes compatible with acute myocardial infarction are rare.

A chest x-ray should be obtained immediately. A normal chest x-ray is rare. Roentgenographic findings suggestive of an acute aortic dissection are: (1) mediastinal widening; (2) a change in the configuration of the thoracic aorta as compared with old films; (3) extension of the aortic shadow beyond a calcified aortic wall; (4) a localized hump on the aortic arch; and (5) pleural effusion, most commonly on the left.

All patients with a suspected diagnosis of acute dissecting aneurysm should undergo aortography to establish the diagnosis. More recently, computed tomography (CT) with contrast enhancement has been used to evaluate these patients. The false lumen and its hematoma can usually be visualized and the extent of the aneurysm defined. However, this does not supplant arteriography and its usefulness in the acute setting is probably limited.

Management

The most important contribution of the emergency physician is to suspect the diagnosis and initiate proper diagnostic maneuvers. In institutions not equipped to definitively diagnose and/or treat this problem, arrangements should be made for transfer to such an institution as soon as possible. Hypertensive patients are treated by continuous intravenous infusion of nitroprusside using a pump. Frequent monitoring of blood pressure (preferably by an indwelling arterial line) is necessary. The patient may be given α-methyldopa and propranolol parenterally to establish long-term control of the blood pressure. Hypotensive patients can usually be resuscitated with small quantities of a crystalloid solution or blood.

Although some groups feel that all acute dissecting aortic aneurysms should be treated by emergency surgery most feel that the patient should be placed in an intensive care setting; that the blood pressure should be controlled to the lowest level compatible with good peripheral, visceral, and central nervous system perfusion; and that the patient should be carefully monitored. However, surgery should be performed on patients with aortic valvular insufficiency secondary to the aneurysm, cardiac tamponade, pending rupture or rupture, or continuing pain despite medical measures and on those whose blood pressure cannot be controlled. Of the patients stabilized on medical therapy, those with ascending aneurysms should undergo surgical treatment after a 10- to 14-day period of stabilization. The appropriate long-term therapy for those with descending aortic aneurysms is more controversial. Long-term results for surgical therapy as compared with medical therapy are approximately the same. However, surgical treatment of all aneurysms is favored by the recent observation of Debakey et al. that the most common cause of late death in their series of 467 patients was the later formation and rupture of an aortic aneurysm.

THORACIC AORTIC ANEURYSMS

Thoracic aortic aneurysms are most commonly located in the descending aorta but may occur in the ascending aorta.

Etiology

Formerly, syphilis was the most common cause of thoracic aortic aneurysms, but with control of this disease atherosclerosis has now replaced it. These aneurysms can occur in patients with Marfan's syndrome and cystic medial necrosis. Trauma is also a common cause of thoracic aortic aneurysms, but strictly speaking these are pseudoaneurysms and will not be discussed here.

Presentation

In approximately half the patients the diagnosis is an incidental finding on chest x-ray. It has been reported that 42 percent of patients had back or chest pain when first seen. Symptoms are usually due to compression or erosion of surrounding structures or to frank rupture. Large aneurysms (uncommon nowadays) may erode into the vertebral column or ribs. Dysphagia from compression of the esophagus, hoarseness from traction on the larnygeal nerve, cough because of bronchial compression, or hemoptysis because of compression of the left lung can occur. Hemoptysis from erosion into the esophagus or a bronchus also occurs.

Prognosis

The prognosis of this condition if left untreated is poor. Exact data are difficult to come by because most series are old and contain large percentages of syphilitic aneurysms. Nonetheless, a mean survival time of 2.4 years for untreated descending thoracic aneurysms and a 20 percent 5-year survival has been established. In most series the average survival time after onset of symptoms is less than 1 year.

Diagnosis

Diagnosis is accomplished by chest x-ray and aortography. The widened mediastinal or aortic silhouette is suggestive. Serial chest x-rays showing enlargement of the thoracic aorta indicate aneurysm formation. A CT scan is also useful in the nonemergent situation. Ultimately an aortogram must be performed to diagnose the size and extent of the aneurysm.

Management

The asymptomatic patient is not a problem for the emergency physician. Nonetheless, the patient suspected of having this diagnosis should be assured of adequate follow-up. Patients with symptomatic aneurysms that have not ruptured should be admitted for close observation and an expedient work-up.

The treatment of this entity is surgical. All patients with a symptomatic aneurysm or documented enlargement of their aneurysm should undergo surgery. Patients with asymptomatic aneurysms should undergo surgery if their overall condition permits.

EXPANDING AND RUPTURED ABDOMINAL AORTIC ANEURYSMS

Abdominal aortic aneurysms affect approximately 2 percent of the population. Of these cases 98 percent are infrarenal, which facilitates both diagnosis and surgical management. Approximately 90 percent of abdominal aortic aneurysms are atherosclerotic in nature, a small percentage being syphilitic or myotic in origin.

Over 80 percent of abdominal aortic aneurysms are asymptomatic when first diagnosed and are not emergency management problems. However, a symptomatic or ruptured aneurysm presents both diagnostic and management dilemmas. This entity is uncommon and a diagnosis may not be thought of unless one consciously searches for it and is aware of the many ways in which it may present. Treatment must be initiated on the basis of only clinical suspicion if inordinate delays are to be avoided and a reasonable salvage rate achieved.

An expanding aneurysm is one in which the aneurysmal wall is intact but symptoms are caused by compression of surrounding structures. Rupture is imminent in such cases. The ruptured aneurysm has lost continuity of the aneurysm wall at some point. If the rupture is contained, the patient will be temporarily normotensive. If it is open, shock or cardiac arrest will ensue.

Presentation

Patients with these entities present with the sudden onset of pain. Pain is severe and constant and cannot be relieved by changing position. It may be located in the low back, flanks, periumbilical area, or pelvis. It may radiate into the thigh, testicle, or perineum. There is no pattern that is clearly characteristic and the diagnosis should be considered in any patient over the age of 50 with a sudden onset of abdominal pain. In Szilagyi's experience the pain is usually somatic rather than visceral in nature. This is due to compression of the somatic sensory nerves in the retroperitoneum by the expanding aneurysmal sac or hematoma. Thus, the patient may present with a neurologic deficit caused by compression of the femoral or sciatic nerve.

A pulsatile abdominal mass is usually present on abdominal examination. However, this may be obscured by the presence of a retroperitoneal hematoma or low blood and pulse pressure. Seventy percent of patients are normotensive when first seen so that the hemodynamic stability of a patient should not dissuade the physician from making this diagnosis.

Any older patient presenting with the sudden onset of abdominal pain associated with an abdominal mass (whether pulsatile or not) or who is hypotensive with an abdominal mass (whether pulsatile or not) is presumed to have an expanding or ruptured abdominal aortic aneurysm. There are no laboratory studies that are of value in making this diagnosis. There is no place in the acute situation for ultrasonography, CT scanning of the aorta, or arteriography. The patient may well die during the delay caused by these studies.

Management

The definitive treatment of an expanding or ruptured abdominal aortic aneurysm is surgical. The goal of the emergency physician is to get the patient into an operating room as soon as possible.

If transfer is necessary, two large-bore intravenous catheters and a Foley catheter should be placed. Transfer should not await the availability of laboratory test results, blood products, or x-rays. If the patient is stable when first seen, intravenous fluid should be given at a rate adequate to maintain urine output but not to elevate the patient's blood pressure. Patients who become unstable or who are hypotensive on arrival in the emergency room should be resuscitated with fluids up to a systolic pressure of 90 to 100 mmHg. Mast trousers may be applied to the hypotensive patient in whom transfer is necessary. There is no wide experience with this particular mode of therapy but it seems a rational adjunctive measure to support the patient's blood pressure. Patients who become profoundly hypotensive or who do not respond to fluid resuscitation can only be saved by obtaining control of the aorta. This is most conveniently done by anterolateral thoracotomy at the left fourth intercostal space and cross clamping of the aorta just above the diaphragm. If this maneuver is necessary, the patient's survival is dependent upon restoring flow to the lower extremities within 30 to 45 min.

At an institution equipped to handle the problem definitively, the stable patient should be taken immediately to the operating room. The remainder of the work-up and preparation of the patient for surgery can be performed there. Two large-bore intravenous lines should be placed in the unstable patient upon arrival in the emergency room and the patient should then be transferred directly to the operating room. The patient without an obtainable blood pressure or who does not respond to fluid resuscitation will need immediate control of the aorta.

Prognosis

The overall mortality rate for this disease is approximately 45 percent in most centers. The patient who is stable upon admission has a better prognosis, with some centers achieving mortality rates as low as 15 percent but more commonly 30 to 35 percent. The patient who is unstable upon presentation has a poor prognosis, with mortality rates ranging from 60 to 80 percent. Salvage in this particular group of patients is dependent upon quick diagnosis and treatment.

BIBLIOGRAPHY

Debakey M, McCollum CH, Crawford ES, et al.: Dissection and dissecting aneurysms of the aortic: Twenty-year followup of five hundred twenty-seven patients treated surgically. *Surgery* 92:1118–1134, 1982.

Lawrie GM, Morris GC, Crawford EJ, et al.: Improved results of operation for ruptured abdominal aortic aneurysms. *Surgery* 85:483, 1979.

Miller DC, Stinson EB, Shumway NE: Realistic expectations of surgical treatment of aortic dissection: the Stanford experience, *World J Surg* 4:571–581, 1980.

Szilagyi DE: Clinical diagnosis of intact and ruptured abdominal aortic aneurysms, in Bergan JJ, Yao JST (eds): *Aneurysms: Diagnosis and treatment,* New York, Grune & Stratton, 1982, p. 205.

CHAPTER 19
PERIPHERAL VASCULAR DISEASE AND THROMBOPHLEBITIS

A. Joel Feldman

PERIPHERAL VASCULAR DISEASE

The emergency physician is increasingly becoming the first contact person for patients with acute vascular emergencies. In order to intelligently assess and initiate treatment in these patients it is important to have an understanding of the several etiologies of acute vascular disease and their underlying pathophysiology.

Acute Ischemia of the Extremities

Acute extremity ischemia is most commonly due to embolism, thrombosis in situ of a preexisting atherosclerotic lesion, or trauma. The latter diagnosis is obvious from the history and physical examination. The lower extremities are more frequently involved by both embolism and thrombosis in situ. Ninety percent of emboli originate in the heart, although infrequently the source is a proximally located arterial lesion (arterioarterial embolus). Thrombosis occurs at a site of a severe stenosis of the vessel (usually due to severe atherosclerosis) because of low flow through the stenotic area and abnormal intima. Because atherosclerosis is a systemic disease, the patient will frequently have evidence of chronic arterial occlusive disease on both history and physical examination. Both lower extremities may show diminished pulses, absent hair on the toes, thinning of the skin, and thickening of the nails.

There are a number of other conditions that may present with acute ischemia of the extremities. The false lumen of an acute dissecting thoracic aortic aneurysm involving the abdominal aorta may occlude the flow to one or both legs.

Patients with low cardiac output (either cardiogenic or hypovolemic) may present with acutely ischemic limbs not due to acute mechanical obstruction of a major artery but rather to decreased delivery of blood to the periphery. These patients are usually easily diagnosed because of the clinical setting of an acute myocardial infarction, blood loss, intravascular volume depletion (e.g., sepsis, dehydration), or treatment with intravenous vasopressors. Patients with severe atherosclerotic occlusive disease are at a much higher risk to develop ischemia or frank tissue loss in situations of low flow.

Intraarterial injection of illegal drug substances is an increasingly common problem. In our experience intraarterial injection into the femoral arteries rarely results in acute ischemia and tissue loss. Injection into the arteries of the wrist, hand, or fingers results in intense burning pain, frequently followed over a period of days by extensive swelling of the hand and digital gangrene of varying degree. Vasospasm, the presence of particulate matter used to cut the drug, crystallization of the injected substance upon injection, and arterial necrosis have all been implicated as causes of this injury.

Rarely, massive iliofemoral thrombosis may be confused with acute ischemia. This is discussed elsewhere.

Emboli most commonly lodge at the bifurcation of arteries and are more common in the lower extremities. In a recent series 46 percent of emboli lodged at the bifurcation of the femoral artery, 18 percent at the iliac arteries, 13 percent in the terminal aorta, and 10 percent in the popliteal arteries. The most common site of an upper extremity embolus was the distal brachial artery. Approximately 8 percent of emboli lodged in the visceral circulation, either in the renal or superior mesenteric arteries. Emboli may be multiple and the patient should be carefully examined for evidence of embolization to other extremities or to visceral arteries.

Pathophysiology

The severity of the ischemic episode depends upon the site of occlusion and the quality of collateral circulation around this point. Progressive thrombosis occurs in the stagnant column of blood both proximal and distal to the acutely occluded site. As thrombosis progresses, sources of collateral blood supply are occluded, causing progression of ischemia. Anticoagulation prevents this propagation and helps limit the ischemic insult.

Pain is the most common symptom of an acutely ischemic extremity. Loss of sensory nerve function (resulting in hypesthesia-anesthesia) and of motor nerve function (resulting in paresis or paralysis) occurs within minutes of severe ischemia. If the severe ischemic insult persists, muscle necrosis occurs. Much later, necrosis of skin, bone, and fat intervenes. The time sequence in which these events occur is dependent on the severity of ischemia. In general, patients presenting with sensorimotor deficits have a severe ischemic insult and if flow cannot be restored within 3 to 4 h permanent loss of function and possible gangrene may ensue.

Initial Evaluation

The history and physical examination are the most important parts of the initial evaluation of the acutely ischemic extremity. Both the normal and the symptomatic extremity are carefully examined because the former provides evidence of the patient's baseline condition. A careful sensorimotor examination is performed. The temperature and color of the skin of both extremities are noted. The presence of frank gangrene is important. The consistency of the limb musculature to palpation is evaluated. Of course, pulses are examined.

This initial assessment not only determines the severity of the ischemic insult but also provides a reference point for evaluating progression of ischemia and response to treatment.

Differential Diagnosis

The most common problem in acute ischemia of the lower extremities is differentiating embolus from thrombosis. The signs and symptoms of ischemia are the same regardless of the etiology. Nonetheless, various aspects of the history and physical examination tend to favor one diagnosis or the other. A history of cardiac disease (arrhythmia, myocardial infarction, valvular heart disease, etc.), an asymptomatic opposite extremity with normal pulses, and the absence of the skin changes of chronic arterial insufficiency favor embolism. Conversely, if the patient's history reveals no source for an embolus (no clinically significant heart disease), if the opposite extremity shows evidence of chronic arterial occlusive disease, and if there is a history of symptoms compatible with chronic peripheral vascular disease (claudication or rest pain), then thrombosis in situ is favored. Unfortunately, the patient with underlying chronic occlusive disease as well as cardiac disease who has thrown an embolus is quite common. Patients with emboli almost always have a known history of cardiac disease. Examination of the involved extremity may reveal an absent pulse when one is palpable at that level on the opposite extremity. An arteriogram is usually needed to differentiate the two entities.

Management

The management of these patients is outlined in Figure 19-1. After the history and physical examination, patients with salvageable

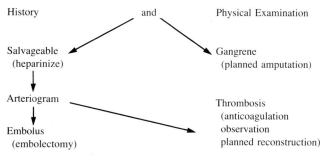

Figure 19-1. Management of acute ischemia of the extremities.

limbs are anticoagulated with 10,000 units of heparin intravenously. Patients suspected of having an acute aortic dissecting aneurysm are not anticoagulated. Patients whose history and physical examination clearly indicate an embolus undergo embolectomy. All others undergo emergent arteriography with visualization of both lower limbs. The radiographic appearance of the uninvolved limb will provide a clue as to the cause of ischemia in the symptomatic limb. A patient with a sharp cutoff on arteriogram most likely has had an embolic episode. On the other hand, thrombosis in situ frequently presents in the setting of diffuse atherosclerotic disease and commonly shows a tapering lumen. Patients thought to have emboli undergo immediate embolectomy if their condition permits. Those who have thrombosis are treated with anticoagulation and observation. A number of these patients will experience some improvement in their symptoms and may not require reconstruction as collateral flow improves with time. Those whose ischemia persists or worsens will need arterial reconstruction.

Arterial Trauma

Arterial injury is due to either blunt or penetrating trauma. Although penetrating trauma is more common, blunt trauma is potentially more dangerous since it is not so obviously associated with vascular injury. Severe soft tissue and bone injuries may obscure a vascular injury. The blunt trauma may appear so mild that an accompanying arterial injury may be missed unless it is searched for.

Diagnosis

The signs and symptoms of acute ischemia (''five Ps'') should be sought in patients suspected of having an arterial injury. Patients with severe ischemia frequently complain of pain. The patient may note paresthesias or paralysis due to direct nerve injury, ischemia distal to the injury, or nerve compression due to hematoma within the neurovascular sheath. Of course, a pulseless extremity and/or one with pallor distal to an injury indicates an arterial injury. Patients with any of these signs or symptoms should undergo arteriography. A biplane arteriogram obtained via transfemoral or transaxillary catheterization is preferred. If this is not possible, then the emergency room physician may elect to obtain an arteriogram of the involved extremity by placing a small intravenous catheter in the artery proximally and injecting the dye by hand. This provides less accurate information.

If the trajectory of a penetrating injury is thought to have passed in proximity to a neurovascular bundle, arteriography is indicated. This is true even in the absence of any obvious physical signs or symptoms of arterial injury. Under these circumstances, if good-quality biplane angiography is normal, then surgical exploration is not needed.

Patients with knee dislocations have a high incidence of accompanying popliteal arterial and venous injuries and arteriography should be performed in these patients.

A venogram of the injured extremity should be obtained, and popliteal venous injuries should be repaired if found. Injuries of more proximally located major veins are repaired if the patient's condition is stable and the repair does not unduly prolong surgery.

Emergency arteriography is contraindicated in any unstable

patient. Obviously, the patient's life takes priority over salvage of an extremity. Bleeding injuries are controlled by direct pressure and taken to the operating room, where the injury is explored and repaired. Other potentially life-threatening injuries take precedence over peripheral vascular injuries.

Symptomatic Popliteal Aneurysms

Any patient with acute ischemia of the lower leg may have a symptomatic popliteal aneurysm. Such aneurysms are among the most common of peripheral arterial aneurysms and present with either thrombosis of the aneurysmal sac or embolization of an intramural thrombus into the distal vasculature. Rupture is uncommon. These aneurysms are generally due to atherosclerosis and are more common in older males; 47 percent are bilateral and there is a high incidence (78 percent) of associated aortic, iliac, or femoral artery aneurysms.

A popliteal mass (whether pulsatile or not) in the symptomatic leg or a pulsatile mass in the asymptomatic extremity indicates a possible symptomatic aneurysm. An arteriogram is obtained to document the diagnosis and to plan operative treatment.

THROMBOPHLEBITIS

In patients with acute venous disease, thrombosis occurs because of mechanical injury to the vein, a hypercoagulable state, and/or venous stasis. The signs and symptoms of acute venous disease are quite variable and are related to the patient's underlying disease entity, and the location and extent of the thrombosis.

Superficial Thrombophlebitis

In the lower extremity superficial thrombophlebitis involves the greater or lesser saphenous veins or varicosities. Redness, tenderness, and induration are present along the course of the involved vein. If the greater saphenous vein is involved, it is clinically not possible to distinguish phlebitis from lymphangitis, as the major lymphatic drainage of the leg runs along the vein.

The diagnosis is confirmed by Doppler examination (with a reported 94 percent accuracy rate) or by obtaining a venogram. The Doppler examination, although easy to do, requires an experienced examiner. Superficial thrombophlebitis of varicosities or the lesser saphenous system is treated conservatively with bed rest, elevation, local heat, and analgesics as needed. Involvement of the greater saphenous vein below the knee is treated similarly. Thrombophlebitis of the saphenous vein in the thigh may also be treated conservatively unless there is some question of the involvement of the saphenofemoral junction. A venogram is then obtained. If the thrombotic process involves the iliofemoral system, anticoagulation as for deep vein thrombosis is performed.

Acute Deep Vein Thrombosis

The signs and symptoms of acute deep vein thrombosis are quite unreliable and confirmatory testing is necessary. Again, the lower extremity is most commonly involved. The classical findings of edema, warmth, erythema, pain, and tenderness are present in 23

to 50 percent of patients. Unfortunately, massive iliofemoral thrombosis can be present with minimal physical findings. Homan's sign is unreliable. The common femoral vein and popliteal vein are superficially located in the groin and popliteal fossa; tenderness, induration, or erythema in these areas is highly suggestive of acute thrombosis of the underlying vein.

A previous history of thrombotic disease, recent lower extremity trauma, treatment with estrogen, recent surgery (especially orthopedic or gynecologic surgery), advanced age, recent myocardial infarction, congestive heart failure, carcinoma, and obesity are all associated with an increased risk of deep vein thrombosis. Patients with one or more of these factors in their history should be evaluated by additional testing even if the physical examination is benign.

A large number of tests are available to diagnose deep vein thrombosis. The venogram remains the accepted standard. Venograms of both lower extremities should be performed to provide a comparison with the symptomatic side and also because occasionally a patient will have clinically silent deep vein thrombosis in the asymptomatic extremity.

The *phleborheogram* measures volume changes with respiration and with certain compressive maneuvers of the lower leg and foot. The overall accuracy in experienced hands in comparison with venography is approximately 90 percent. We find this procedure an acceptable alternative to venography. Iodine 125 fibrinogen uptake and Doppler examination of venous flow also may serve to diagnose deep vein thrombosis.

Management of Acute Deep Vein Thrombosis of the Lower Extremities

Patients who are at high risk for deep vein thrombosis based on history and/or physical examination should be heparinized immediately pending the results of confirmatory tests. Those not at high risk may await the results of these tests. We prefer the phleborheogram or venogram to establish the diagnosis. The patient is then treated with continuous intravenous infusion of heparin for 10 days. The patient is kept in bed with strict elevation of the legs for the first 4 days after the diagnosis is established. Local heat and analgesia are used as needed. Long-term anticoagulation with oral anticoagulants may be begun soon after the patient's admission.

Massive Deep Vein Thrombosis

Phlegmasia alba dolens (milk leg) is caused by extensive iliofemoral thrombosis with swelling of the entire leg to the groin. The leg frequently has a doughy consistency but is not tensely swollen. Arterial inflow is not compromised. The leg is treated as above.

Phlegmasia cerulea dolens is due to extensive iliofemoral thrombosis involving most of the venous collateral circulation as well. The leg is tensely swollen and cyanotic. Skin bullae may be present. Swelling within the muscular compartments of the leg may cause arterial insufficiency. If all venous outflow is occluded, stasis occurs in the capillary and arteriolar beds, and retrograde thrombosis of the arterial system will occur. Venous gangrene occurs in this setting.

The treatment consists of strict bed rest with maximum elevation of the affected extremity. Anticoagulation with heparin is instituted immediately. These patients may have intravascular volume depletion because of fluid sequestration within the affected extremity. Fasciotomy should be performed if indicated. Finally, amputation of gangrenous tissue may be necessary.

Deep Vein Thrombosis of the Upper Extremity

This most commonly involves the axillary and subclavian veins and is usually iatrogenic following catheterization. Effort thrombosis of the axillary or subclavian vein is seen in young persons following strenuous activity and may be more common in people who have some narrowing of the thoracic outlet.

The patient with axillary or subclavian vein thrombosis usually presents with mild swelling involving the forearm or occasionally the entire extremity. Edema is pitting and not tense. The color of the extremity is normal. Arterial flow is well preserved and pulses are present.

The risk of pulmonary embolism in this setting is between 12 and 15 percent. Accordingly, the patient should be treated with elevation of the extremity, application of local heat, analgesia as needed, and anticoagulation if not contraindicated by the patient's overall condition. Postphlebitic sequelae are common in these patients.

Streptokinase Therapy

Recently a number of centers have been using thrombolytic therapy in the treatment of patients with acute deep venous thrombosis. Streptokinase combines with plasminogen to form a plasminogen-streptokinase activator complex. This in turn can combine with a plasminogen-fibrin complex in the thrombus to cause lysis. The activator complex may also combine with circulating plasminogen, forming plasmin and causing fibrinolysis.

This is a useful treatment in experienced hands for appropriately selecting patients. It should be considered in patients with proven venous thrombosis of the iliofemoral or above-knee venous segments of less than 4 days duration. There are a number of contraindications to its use. Patients with a history of peptic ulcer disease, severe hypertension, recent stroke, liver disease, blood dyscrasia, recent surgery, recent arterial punctures, or intracranial neoplasms are not candidates for this treatment.

This method of treatment requires shorter hospitalization and may result in a lower incidence of postphlebitic sequelae.

BIBLIOGRAPHY

Adams JT, DeWees JA: Effort thrombosis of the axillary and subclavian veins. *Trauma* 11:923, 1971.

Astedt B, Robertson B, Haeger K: Experience with standardized streptokinase therapy of deep venous thrombosis, *Surg Gynecol Obstet* 139:387, 1974.

Dale, WA: The swollen leg. *Curr Concepts Surg* Sept 1973.

Elliott JP, Hageman JH, Belanger AC, et al.: Phleborheography: A correlative study with venography. *Henry Ford Hosp Med J* 28:189, 1980.

Salzman EW, Dykin D, Shapiro RM, et al.: Management of heparin therapy. *N Eng J Med* 292:1046, 1975.

SECTION 3
PULMONARY
EMERGENCIES

CHAPTER 20
PULMONARY
INFECTIONS

Introduction

Georges C. Benjamin

This section includes the pulmonary disorders that are of most significance in emergency medicine.

Bacterial pneumonia, an entity the emergency physician sees almost daily, is discussed. Less common causes of pneumonia such as the atypical pneumonias, mycobacterial infection, and Legionnaires' disease are also described.

The pathophysiology, prevention, and management of aspiration pneumonia are important for the emergency physician, because many factors associated with aspiration are likely to be present in emergency patients. Lung abscess, pleural effusion, and empyema generally involve prolonged hospitalization or extensive investigational procedures or both. Diagnosis, however, begins in the emergency department. Hemoptysis is a frequent emergency department complaint. Serious disorders may first reveal themselves in this manner and may, rarely, present with life-threatening bleeding.

The causes of acute respiratory failure are numerous but early recognition of the process and aggressive respiratory care in the emergency department can stabilize the patient before reaching the intensive care unit.

Asthma and chronic obstructive pulmonary disease and their complications probably form the largest group of disorders seen in emergency patients with lower respiratory tract problems. Many of these patients can be treated in the emergency department and discharged with follow-up care.

Finally, a group of disorders that are pathophysiologically unrelated except that they are caused or induced by environmental or therapeutic agents is discussed. This group includes near drowning, smoke inhalation, carbon monoxide poisoning, toxic gas inhalation, hypersensitivity pneumonitis, and radiation pneumonitis.

A. Bacterial Pneumonia

Georges C. Benjamin

Bacterial pneumonia is a disease frequently treated by emergency physicians. It remains a leading cause of death and is responsible for as many as 10 percent of hospital admissions in the United States. The pneumococcus accounts for up to 90 percent of all bacterial pneumonias, with *Escherichia coli, Pseudomonas aeruginosa, Klebsiella pneumoniae, Staphylococcus aureus, Hemo-philus influenzae,* and group A *streptococci* accounting for most of the rest. Other bacteria, such as *Legionella pneumophila* and the anaerobes, will be discussed in later sections. The frequency with which each of these organisms causes disease varies from study to study.

Patients with chronic diseases such as congestive heart failure,

Table 20A-1 Factors Predisposing to Bacterial Pneumonia

Debilitation
   Alcoholism
   The extremes of life
   Neoplasia
   Immunosuppression
Chronic diseases
   Diabetes
   COPD
   Valvular heart disease
   Congestive heart failure
   Leukemia
   Lymphoma
   Hemoglobinopathies
Viral infections
Chest wall disorders
   Myopathies and neuropathies
   Chest wall trauma
   Postoperative pain
Syncope
Seizures
Bronchial obstruction (tumor or foreign body aspiration)
Pulmonary embolism
Iatrogenic invasion
   Bronchoscopy
   Intubation, respiratory support
   Transthoracic procedures

diabetes, cancer, bronchiectasis, sickle-cell anemia, and hypogammaglobulinemia are at greater risk for pneumonia, as are smokers and postsplenectomy patients. Essentially all bacterial pneumonia is the result of aspiration of oropharyngeal contents. Therefore patients with seizures, obtundation, suppressed cough reflex, and increased secretions are also predisposed to it. These and other predisposing factors are shown in Table 20A-1.

HOST DEFENSES

Sterility of the lower airways and alveoli is due to a very effective system utilizing the cough reflex, mucociliary clearance, phagocytosis, and in situ bacterial killing. Cilia located in the tracheal bronchial tree are responsible for removing most infected particles greater than 5.0 μm.

Particles smaller than this are removed by alveolar macrophages and local factors (surfactant, complement, IgG, IgA) which limit bacterial growth. Because of a variance in the susceptibilities of different bacterial species to these clearance mechanisms, most pneumonias are ultimately the result of a single species. This is of interest in light of the multiplicity of organisms in oropharyngeal secretions.

LABORATORY TESTS

Laboratory tests useful in the emergency department diagnosis of bacterial pneumonia include the white cell count, chest x-ray, arterial blood gas, sputum examination, blood cultures, and pleural fluid examination.

White Cell Count

The white cell count remains a useful way to document the presence of the inflammatory response from pneumonia. In healthy young patients, marked elevation usually occurs. This elevation is not diagnostic, however, and the presence of a normal count does not rule out pneumonia or suggest a viral etiology. Also, in the elderly or debilitated patient, a normal or low white cell count may represent overwhelming sepsis. In these cases the presence of a left shift may be the only clue to bacterial infection.

Chest Radiograph

Radiographically, bacterial pneumonias are frequently characterized as in Table 20A-2. Note that these classic patterns frequently are the exception and serve only as a guide in radiographic diagnosis. Another reason to obtain a chest x-ray is to look for evidence of effusion, abscess formation, or pneumothorax. Special views such as the lateral decubitus and apical lordotic are frequently of value to further define the nature of pulmonary abnormalities. Patients with marked leukopenia or dehydration may not initially demonstrate an infiltrate. A diagnosis of pneumonia in these patients rests with a strong clinical suspicion on serial chest x-rays.

Pulmonary infarction, atelectasis, neoplasia, pulmonary edema, parenchymal scarring, and pleural thickening may all simulate pneumonitis radiographically. In these patients, clinical examination, history, and comparison with prior radiographs may aid in proper diagnosis.

Arterial Blood Gas

Ventilation-perfusion abnormality is the most common functional disorder in acute pneumonias. This is the result of sustained perfusion of poorly ventilated areas of the lung. Measurement of the oxygen content of arterial blood in patients with respiratory compromise is useful to document hypoxia and to ensure adequate oxygenation in patients on oxygen therapy. Arterial blood gases are especially important in patients with chronic lung disease because the acute hypoxia will be superimposed on an underlying ventilation-perfusion mismatch.

Sputum Examination

Sputum examination and culture remain the most important guides to proper antibiotic therapy. Frequently the patient is unable to generate an adequate specimen because of dehydration, obtundation, or a weak cough. Occasionally postural drainage or heated saline nebulization may be helpful to induce sputum.

Although not usually an emergency department procedure, transtracheal aspiration is frequently of value in patients who are unable to produce adequate sputum. Complications from this procedure include subcutaneous or mediastinal emphysema, cardiac arrhythmias, esophageal perforation, bleeding and infection. This procedure should be done by physicians thoroughly familiar with

Table 20A-2 Characteristics of Bacterial Pneumonia

Organism	Sputum	Chest X-ray	Therapy
Streptococcus pneumoniae	Rusty, gram-positive encapsulated diplocci (type III, thick)	Usually lobar in LLL, RLL, RML. Occasionally patchy, small pleural effusion, 10%	Phenoxymethyl penicillin 500 mg PO q 6 h for 10 days; erythromycin 500 mg PO q 6 h for 10 days or Aqueous penicillin G 20 million units/day q 4–6 h or procaine penicillin G 1.2 million units IM followed by phenoxymethyl penicillin 500 mg PO q 6 h for 10 days
Group A streptococci	Purulent, bloody, gram-positive cocci in chains, pairs	Often lower lobes. Patchy, multilobar large pleural effusion	See above
Hemophilus influenzae	Short, tiny, gram-negative, encapsulated cocci-bacilli	Patchy, frequently basilar, occasional pleural effusion	Ampicillin 500 mg PO q 6 h for 10 days or Tetracycline 500 mg q 6 h for 10 days or Chloramphenicol 50–100 mg/(kg·day) IV q 6 h and ampicillin 9–12 g/day IV q 6 h
Klebsiella pneumoniae	Brown jelly, thick; short plump, gram-negative, encapsulated paired cocci-bacilli	Upper lobes, lobular bulging fissure sign, abscess formation	Cephalosporin 6–12 g/day IV divided q 4 h or Aminoglycoside (gentamicin, tobramycin, or amikacin)
Staphylococcus aureus	Purulent; gram-positive cocci in pairs and clumps	Patchy, multicenter with early abscess formation, empyema, pneumothorax	Oxacillin 8–12 g/day IV or Nafcillin 40 mg/(kg·day) IV 10–14 days or Vancomycin 500 mg q 6 h IV
E. coli	Gram-negative cocci-bacilli	Patchy, bilateral, lower lobes	Ampicillin 6–8 g/day IV q 6 h or Cephalosporin 9–12 g/day plus gentamicin 3–5 mg/(kg·day) IV q 8 h (tobramycin or amikacin as needed)
Pseudomonas	Gram-negative cocci-bacilli	Patchy, mid- and lower lung, with abscesses	Gentamicin 3–5 mg/(kg·day) IV q 8 h plus carbenicillin 5–6 g q 4 h IV

the technique and its complications. It is contraindicated in the patient who requires restraint, has uncorrected hypoxia, or has a coagulopathy.

Gross examination of the sputum is done first and may reveal the bloody or rusty sputum of pneumococcal pneumonia (not diagnostic, as other bacterial pneumonias may involve rusty sputum); the thick "currant jelly" sputum produced by both type 3 pneumococcus and *K. pneumoniae;* the green sputum caused by *P. aeruginosa, H. influenzae,* and *Streptococcus pneumoniae;* or the foul-smelling sputum of an anaerobic infection. The sputum is then Gram-stained and viewed under the low-power objective (100×) to determine if the sputum is suitable for examination and culture. If more than 10 squamous epithelial cells are present per low-power field, the specimen is contaminated and of low diagnostic value. An adequate specimen should demonstrate more than 25 polymorphonuclear leukocytes and less than 10 squamous epithelial cells per low-power field. In addition, a predominant bacterial form should be evident, as a mixture of morphological forms suggests oropharyngeal contamination. Such contamination frequently makes interpretation difficult. Enteric organisms are uncommon habitants in the pharynx of healthy people. However, recent viral infections, chronic obstructive pulmonary disease (COPD), chronic bronchitis, recent hospitalizations, and debilitating diseases favor colonization with gram-negative bacteria.

Blood Cultures

Blood cultures are frequently of diagnostic value in patients who have presumed bacteremia, immunosuppression, rigors, or who are seriously ill. Two to three cultures from separate sites are done when indicated.

Pleural Fluid

Examination of the pleural fluid by thoracentesis, although generally not an emergency department procedure, is useful in ruling out empyema. Patients who may require a pleural biopsy should have only a diagnostic tap (10 to 20 mL) done by the emergency physician. Patients with respiratory compromise may require more extensive therapeutic drainage. The pleural fluid examination is further covered in Section 20E.

STREPTOCOCCUS PNEUMONIAE

Pneumococcal pneumonia is caused by *S. pneumoniae,* a gram-positive, lancet-shaped, encapsulated bacterium. Based on its capsular antigens it has been divided into at least 83 serotypes. Disease is usually caused by types 1, 3, 4, 6, 7, 8, 12, 14, 18, and 19 in adults and types 1, 6, 14, and 19 in children.

The frequency of this disease is 1 in 500 persons annually and the organism clearly is the most common cause of community-acquired bacterial pneumonia. Its peak incidence is winter and early spring, but it does occur year round. With the availability of antibiotic therapy the mortality from this disease has decreased dramatically from around 50 percent to less than 5 percent.

Clinical disease presents as an acute shaking chill, tachypnea, and tachycardia. A single rigor lasting several minutes is so common that recurrent rigors should suggest another etiology. Sharp chest pain which causes marked splinting on the affected side occurs in 70 percent of patients. Cough may be absent in the early phases but rapidly becomes a prominent symptom. In 75 percent of patients a rust-colored sputum develops. With type 3 pneumococcus a thick, jellylike sputum may be present and must be differentiated from that caused by *K. pneumoniae*. Additional symptoms include malaise, anorexia, myalgias, flank or back pain, and vomiting.

On physical examination, the classic signs of consolidation, including bronchial breath sounds, egophony, and increased tactile and vocal fremitus are present. Pleural friction rubs, cyanosis, and jaundice are occasionally found. Abdominal distention from acute gastric dilatation or paralytic ileus may also develop.

The white blood cell count generally ranges from 12,000 to 25,000 cells per cubic millimeter but may reach 40,000 per cubic millimeter. Normal or decreased white cell counts are seen and suggest overwhelming infection. The chest x-ray usually demonstrates a singular infiltrate in the right middle lobe, right lower lobe, or left lower lobe. The infiltrate frequently has a lobar or segmental pattern but patchy involvement is frequent in infants and the elderly. Occasionally bulging fissures similar to those seen with Klebsiella pneumoniae are noted. In 10 percent of patients a small, sterile pleural effusion is seen. Sputum culture is positive only in approximately 50 percent of cases and blood cultures only in 30 percent. This illustrates the difficulties in establishing a definitive diagnosis.

Untreated, this disease frequently resolves in 7 to 10 days by a clinical syndrome known as the crisis (prompt defervescence with diaphoresis and a rapid increase in well-being). Treated patients are often afebrile within 24 to 72 h, but in some the fever gradually decreases over 4 to 7 days. Physical signs take from 14 to 21 days to resolve, with radiographic signs resolving over another 21 days. Delayed resolution may be noted in some patients and is seen most frequently in the debilitated and the aged.

Complications include sepsis, lung abscess, congestive heart failure, meningitis, peritonitis, herpes labialis, septic arthritis, endocarditis, and pericarditis. In less than 20 percent of patients, empyema develops.

A poor prognosis is associated with type 2 and type 3 disease, multilobar involvement, leukopenia, bacteremia, jaundice, splenectomized states (including sickle hemoglobinopathies), congestive heart failure, chronic obstructive pulmonary disease (COPD), alcoholism, and diabetes.

Penicillin is still the drug of choice for pneumococcal pneumonia despite recently recognized resistant strains. The current recommendations for therapy are listed in Table 20A-2. In penicillin-allergic patients, erythromycin may be used. Tetracycline is not effective because of increased resistance.

HEMOPHILUS INFLUENZAE

H. influenzae is a gram-negative pleomorphic rod, which exists in both encapsulated and unencapsulated forms. The capsular forms are divided into six serotypes (a through f) based on their capsular antigens. Of these, type b is found to cause 95 percent of all human infections. Both forms are able to cause pneumonia but only the encapsulated form consistently causes bacteremia. The peak incidence of this disease occurs in winter to early spring and tends to occur in debilitated or immunocompromised patients.

The clinical presentation is one of fever, shortness of breath, and occasionally pleuritic chest pain. Lung examination may reveal rales without clear signs of consolidation. The white blood count is frequently normal but may be as high as 30,000. The chest x-ray usually demonstrates patchy alveolar infiltrates, generally without effusion. Lobar consolidation does occur but abscess formation is rare. This organism is frequently overlooked on Gram stains and diligence is required to find it and to recognize its small coccobacillary form.

Outpatient management consists of oral ampicillin or tetracycline (see Table 20A-2). For those patients requiring intravenous therapy, ampicillin and, if penicillin resistance is suspected, ampicillin or amoxicillin plus chloramphenicol is used.

Complications include septic arthritis, sepsis, meningitis, and, rarely, empyema. As with other serious pneumonias, the morbidity and mortality are highest in the young or compromised patient.

KLEBSIELLA PNEUMONIA

Klebsiella pneumonia is found most frequently in patients with alcoholism, diabetes, or COPD. It is a necrotizing lobar pneumonia, which is most frequently seen in the right upper lobe. In approximately 20 percent of cases empyema occurs within 24 to 48 h, along with intrapulmonary abscess formation in 4 to 5 days.

Klebsiella pneumonia presents as a sudden cough with rigors, shortness of breath, malaise, and often cyanosis; 80 percent of patients develop pleuritic chest pain. Pulmonary examination frequently reveals signs of consolidation and cyanosis. The white cell count is elevated in 75 percent of cases. Chest x-ray frequently reveals a necrotizing lobar pneumonia in the right upper lobe. In 35 percent of cases a bulging minor fissure is seen. Occasionally, perihilar and patchy infiltrates are also seen. Sputum examination reveals a dark brown tenacious sputum, occasionally blood-stained. Gram stain reveals short, plump, encapsulated gram-negative bacilli in pairs, which in poorly decolorized Gram stains, can be easily confused with pneumococci. Sepsis, empyema, and pneumothorax are complications of this disease.

Initial therapy usually consists of an aminoglycoside and a cephalosporin intravenously. Attention to airway management is a must, as frequently the sputum is so thick that clearance is difficult.

OTHER GRAM-NEGATIVE PNEUMONIAS

Other gram-negative organisms including *E. coli, Pseudomonas, Enterobacter,* and *Serratia,* are rare causes of pneumonia. Their presence should be considered in the recently hospitalized, debilitated, or immunosuppressed patient. Therapy usually consists of intravenous carbenicillin (or ticarcillin) and an aminoglycoside.

STAPHYLOCOCCAL PNEUMONIA

Staphylococci cause 1 percent of bacterial pneumonias. Although this pneumonia occurs sporadically, it has its peak incidence during influenza and measles epidemics. Patients presenting after a viral illness with the abrupt onset of productive cough, pleurisy, multiple chills, and hectic fever are suspect for this disease. Lung examination may show fine to coarse rhonchi and rales; however signs of consolidation are rare. The chest x-ray reveals a patchy infiltrate, which rapidly progresses to abscess formation and lobar consolidation. Empyema is common, white blood counts are usually above 15,000 per cubic millimeter; and blood cultures are usually negative unless the pulmonary involvement is metastatic. Gram stain of the sputum reveals large gram-positive cocci in pairs and clumps.

Patients at particular risk include intravenous drug abusers, hospitalized patients, and the debilitated. Therapy includes intravenous oxacillin or nafcillin unless penicillin resistance or allergy is suspected. In these patients vancomycin can be used.

STREPTOCOCCAL PNEUMONIA (GROUP A)

Although a rare cause of pulmonary infection, group A streptococci can cause rapidly progressive pneumonitis. The clinical syndrome is characterized by the sudden onset of fever, chills, and productive cough. In most patients pleuritic pain is a prominent symptom. Pulmonary examination usually reveals fine rales without signs of consolidation. The chest x-ray is usually consistent with a multilobar bronchopneumonia, often with a large pleural effusion. The sputum is frequently bloody and purulent. Gram stain reveals gram-positive cocci in pairs and chains. Penicillin is the drug of choice.

ADMISSION GUIDELINES

Pregnant patients and those with serious underlying diseases, volume depletion, toxicity, or severe hypoxia require hospital admission. Social admissions include all patients who cannot care for themselves at home. Patients who, after an appropriate evaluation, are felt to be well enough for outpatient therapy should be followed up in 3 to 5 days. A chest x-ray is frequently done after 1 month to document resolution of the infiltrate.

SUMMARY

Bacterial pneumonia is a problem commonly seen in emergency departments. Patients at risk for this disease include the chronically ill as well as those recovering from a viral respiratory tract infection. The chest radiograph and examination of the sputum remain the cornerstones of diagnosis for the emergency physician and complement the history and physical examination. Definitive diagnosis rests with a properly obtained and processed sputum culture. In patients who are unable to produce sputum and are not judged to be seriously ill, empiric therapy is frequently utilized with close clinical follow-up. Patients who are smokers or have been recently hospitalized should be especially considered at risk for gram-negative infection. Inpatient therapy is indicated for the toxic, markedly hypoxic, and debilitated, as well as those presumed to be infected by virulent organisms.

The opinions or assertions contained herein are the private views of the author and are not to be construed as official or reflecting the views of the Department of Defense or the Department of the Army.

BIBLIOGRAPHY

Austrian R, Gold J: Pneumococcal bacteremia with especial reference to bacteremic pneumococcal pneumonia. *Ann Intern Med* 60:759, 1964.

Barrett-Conner E: The nonvalue of sputum culture in the diagnosis of pneumococcal pneumonia. *Am Rev Respir Dis* 103:845, 1971.

Biggs DD: Pulmonary infections. *Med Clin North Am* 61(6):163, 1977.

Burmeister RW, Overholt EL: Pneumonia caused by hemolytic streptococcus. *Arch Intern Med* 111:367, 1963.

Chodosh S: Examination of sputum cells. *N Engl J Med* 282:854, 1970.

Everett D, Rahn A, Adaniya R, et al: *Hemophilus influenzae* pneumonia in adults. *JAMA* 238:319, 1977.

Finland, M: Pneumonia and pneumococcal infections. *Am Rev Respir Dis* 120:481, 1979.

George LW, Finegold SM: Bacterial infections of the lung. *Chest* 81:501–507, 1982.

Green GM, Jakab GJ, Low RB, et al: Defense mechanisms of the respiratory membrane. *Am Rev Respir Dis* 115:479–514, 1977.

Jacobs MR, Kournhof JH, Robins-Browne RM, et al: Emergence of multiply resistant pneumococci. *N Engl J Med* 299:735, 1978.

Jay SJ, Johanson WG, Pierce AK: The radiographic resolution of *Streptococcus pneumoniae* pneumonia. *N Engl J Med* 293:798–801, 1975.

Johanson WG, Gould KG: Lung defense mechanisms. *Basics Respir Dis* 6(2):66, 1977.

Johanson WG, Pierce AK, Sanford JP: Changing pharyngeal bacterial flora of hospital patients. *N Engl J Med* 281:1137–1140, 1969.

Kalinske RW, Parker RH, Brandt D, et al: Diagnostic usefulness and safety of transtracheal aspiration. *N Engl J Med* 276:604, 1967.

Manfredi F, Daly WJ, Beinke RH: Clinical observation of acute Friedländer pneumonia. *Ann Intern Med* 58:642, 1963.

Musher DM, McKenzie SO: Infections due to *Staphylococcus aureus*. *Medicine* 56:383, 1977.

Norden CW: *Hemophilus influenzae* infections in adults. *Med Clin North Am* 62(5):1037, 1978.

Quintliani R, Hymans P: The association of bacteremic *Hemophilus influenzae* pneumonia in adults with typable strains. *Am J Med* 50:781, 1971.

Ramirez-Ronda CH, Fuxeuch-Lopez Z, Nevarez M: Increased pharyngeal bacterial colonization during viral illness. *Arch Intern Med* 141:1599, 1981.

Reyes MP: The aerobic gram-negative bacillary pneumonias. *Med Clin North Am* 64(3): 363–383, 1980.

Scanlon GT, Unger JD: The radiology of bacterial and viral pneumonias. *Radiol Clin North Am* 11:317, 1973.

Smith JK, Wiener SL: The pneumonias. *Drug Ther Bull* 3:19, 1978.

Spencer CD, Beaty HN: Complications of transtracheal aspiration. *N Engl J Med* 286:304, 1972.

Tillotson JR, Lerner AM: Pneumonias caused by gram-negative bacilli. *Medicine* 45:65, 1966.

Tillotson JR, Lerner AM: Characteristics of pneumonia caused by *E. coli*. *N Engl J Med* 277:15, 1967.

Tuazon CU: Gram-positive pneumonias. *Med Clin North Am* 64(3):343–361.

Ziskind MM: The acute bacterial pneumonia in the adult. *Basics Respir Dis* 2(3), 1974.

B. Atypical Pneumonia

Kenneth Frumkin

INTRODUCTION

Since the late 1930s, a significant number of patients have been identified as having pulmonary infections "atypical" of the usual bacterial pneumonias. These illnesses are characterized by: a more prolonged clinical course; a longer incubation period; frequent absence of preceding upper respiratory infection; patchy, nonsegmental infiltrates; negative sputum Gram stain; normal to slightly increased white blood cell count; and failure to respond to the usual antibiotics. This group of "primary atypical pneumonias" has since been found to encompass respiratory infections caused by the wide variety of organisms discussed in this chapter.

MYCOPLASMA PNEUMONIA

Mycoplasma pneumoniae is responsible for 10 to 20 percent of all pneumonias and is the most common cause of nonbacterial pneumonia in adults. Occurrence is year-round, peaking in late fall and early winter. Worldwide epidemics occur every 2 to 6 years. Transmission is via respiratory secretions, and the disease is most often brought into the household by school-age children.

The usual age of patients with *mycoplasma* pneumonia is 5 to 30. The incidence is increased in closed populations and in persons with chronic bronchitis and chronic obstructive pulmonary disease.

Clinical Features

Most *mycoplasma* infections are inapparent, and most clinically evident disease involves only the upper respiratory tract, being manifested as a pharyngitis or tracheobronchitis. Only 3 to 10 percent of those infected are diagnosed as having pneumonia.

The incubation period is 2 to 3 weeks. Headache, fever, chilliness, malaise, and anorexia begin insidiously, followed by a sore throat and a dry cough with mucoid, nonpurulent sputum. Up to 50 percent of patients will have symptoms of an upper respiratory tract infection. Earache occurs in one-third. Anorexia, nausea, vomiting, and transient diarrhea are present in the first week of illness in 12 to 44 percent of patients. Hemoptysis, rigors, and pleurisy are rare.

Rhonchi and rales are commonly found on physical examination, but signs of consolidation are infrequent. Pharyngeal edema, tender cervical lymphadenopathy, skin rashes, and conjunctivitis occur occasionally, but *mycoplasma pneumoniae* does not cause rhinorrhea. Bullous myringitis is infrequent (3 to 10 percent). Exanthems are frequent, highly variable, and include Stevens-Johnson syndrome and erythema multiforme.

A less common clinical syndrome, associated with up to 25 percent of cases is lethargy and dyspnea. Symptoms increase over 1 to 4 weeks without fever, cough, myalgia, or chest pain. Chest radiographs show diffuse reticulonodular infiltrates.

The white blood cell count is less than 15,000 in 96 percent of patients, while the erythrocyte sedimentation rate is usually elevated. Infiltrates begin unilaterally in the lower lobes. Small pleural effusions and hilar adenopathy can be found in 20 to 25 percent (more frequently in children).

Fever, headache, and malaise resolve without treatment in 3 to 10 days, but the cough, rales, and radiographic abnormalities may persist for 3 to 4 weeks. Even with antibiotic therapy, symptoms and infiltrates occasionally reappear 7 to 10 days after the initial response.

Diagnosis

A fourfold rise in complement fixation (CF) titers from acute- to convalescent-phase specimens is diagnostic, while a single titer of 1:64 or greater is highly suggestive of infection. One-third to three-quarters of patients will develop cold agglutinin titers greater than 1:64 or a fourfold rise in this titer, but this is nonspecific. Cold agglutinins may also be positive in infectious mononucleosis, psittacosis, influenza, adenovirus infections, and a number of other disorders.

The differential diagnosis includes the other atypical pneumonias. In military recruits adenovirus pneumonia is a strong consideration, while viral pneumonias are the major differential concern in children.

Complications

Pulmonary complications [adult respiratory distress syndrome (ARDS), abscess, secondary bacterial infection, pulmonary function study abnormalities] are uncommon. Among hematologic complications, transient autoimmune hemolytic anemia is fairly common and is sometimes severe. Raynaud's syndrome, disseminated intravascular coagulation (DIC), and thrombocytopenic purpura have occurred. Cardiac complications have included myopericarditis, hemopericardium, congestive heart failure, and varying degrees of heart block.

CNS complications occur in 0.1 percent of patients and include acute psychosis, ataxia, aseptic meningitis, ascending paralysis, transverse myelitis, and cranial nerve palsies. As many as 20 percent will have no preceding respiratory symptoms.

Mild transaminase elevations, frank hepatitis, or pancreatitis can occur. Myalgias and arthralgias occur in 15 to 45 percent of patients but true arthritis is uncommon.

Treatment and Prophylaxis

Erythromycin (2 g/day) is the drug of choice, particularly if the diagnosis is in doubt and pneumococcal pneumonia is a possibility. Tetracycline also shortens the duration of the disease. A vaccine exists but is not yet believed useful for mass use.

VIRAL PNEUMONIA

Viral pneumonias are very common in early childhood, uncommon in adults, and difficult to distinguish from the other atypical pneumonias. The ''viral'' pneumonias of older children and young adults are usually mycoplasmal.

Etiology and Clinical Features

Respiratory syncytial virus is the predominant cause of viral pneumonia and bronchiolitis in children less than 6 months of age and of pneumonia in the 3- to 5-year age group. Annual 6- to 8-week epidemics occur in the winter and spring. A prodrome of fever, cough, and coryza precedes respiratory distress, a patchy bronchopneumonia, and pulmonary hyperexpansion.

Parainfluenza virus, the second most common cause of viral pneumonia in children, is also responsible for many cases of croup and bronchitis.

While adenovirus pneumonia is next in frequency in the pediatric age group, the only adults it strikes are military recruits. Fever and cough are associated with rhinitis, conjunctivitis, pharyngitis, and patchy lower lobe infiltrates.

Varicella is a serious cause of viral pneumonia. Of patients who develop varicella pneumonia, 90 percent are adults. Conversely, 15 percent of adults with varicella will develop primary varicella pneumonia. The disease is notoriously severe, particularly in women, and is aggravated by pregnancy. Generally, tachypnea, cough, dyspnea, and fever appear 1 to 6 days after the characteristic rash. Cyanosis, pleuritic chest pain, and hemoptysis each occur in 20 to 40 percent of cases. There are few clinical signs of pneumonia, but the chest radiograph shows widespread nodular densities, more concentrated in the perihilar region. Sputum specimens may reveal multinucleated giant cells.

Influenza is the only viral pneumonia of significance in adults, mimicking the other atypical pneumonias. Usually an acute, self-limited disease, influenza occurs every winter and is transmitted by droplet particle inhalation. The 2- to 4-day incubation period is followed by fever, frontal headache, myalgias, and a (generally) nonproductive cough. Pleuritic chest pain occurs with coughing but not with deep breathing. Of patients with uncomplicated influenza, 5 to 40 percent will have rhonchi, wheezes, or rales without pneumonia. The vast majority of patients with influenza who develop pneumonia (80 percent) will have a bacterial infection. More deadly than the associated bacterial pneumonias are the pure influenza pneumonias themselves. Influenza pneumonia follows the typical influenza prodrome, with sudden prostration, dyspnea, cyanosis, and diffuse, patchy infiltrates with dense air space consolidation. ARDS and death can occur in otherwise healthy adults, although older patients, those with preexisting cardiopulmonary disease, or patients in late pregnancy are at the greatest risk.

Diagnosis

The diagnosis of viral pneumonia is seldom confirmed by specific viral diagnostic techniques but rather by serologic evidence of infection in the presence of a compatible illness. Epidemiologic considerations may provide the only clues to the diagnosis (unless the pneumonia is associated with a recognizable viral illness such as varicella or measles).

Treatment and Prophylaxis

Adenine arabinoside may be used for the treatment of varicella in immunocompromised patients. Amantidine may be helpful in uncomplicated influenza.

Vaccination against influenza has been very successful. An adenovirus vaccine is available and is in use in the military. The measles vaccine successfully prevents measles and measles pneumonia, and immune serum globulin can prevent or modify measles in susceptible patients. Varicella-zoster immune globulin may protect immunocompromised children from this virus. When given prophylactically to household contacts, amantadine reduces the incidence of influenza by 60 to 75 percent.

PSITTACOSIS

Psittacosis is an infectious disease of birds, caused by *Chlamydia psittaci,* a gram-negative obligate intracellular parasite.

Although the disease is named for the psittacine order (parrots, parakeets, budgerigars, and cockatoos), any avian species can harbor it. The birds often appear perfectly healthy. Humans at risk for psittacosis include pet-shop owners, poultry raisers, pigeon fanciers, taxidermists, and zoo attendants. The organism is transmitted by inhalation of infected dust or droplets, only rarely by a bite. Person-to-person transmission may occur.

The infecting organism enters via the respiratory tract, travels to the reticuloendothelial system, where it replicates, and then travels via the blood to the lungs.

Clinical Features

Infection is most commonly asymptomatic. Clinically psittacosis most often resembles a systemic viral illness or a pneumonia with a viral prodrome. After an incubation period of 1 to 2 weeks or more, shaking chills, weakness, fatigue, and fevers to 105°F occur. Headache is almost always severe and is often the chief complaint. Photophobia, myalgias, and neck muscle stiffness may lead to the diagnosis of meningitis. Cough is usually nonproductive, but small amounts of mucoid or bloody sputum may occur. Only two-thirds of patients develop pneumonia. Upper respiratory tract infection symptoms are not prominent, although mild sore throat, pharyngeal injection, and cervical adenopathy are often present. Chest pain, pleural effusion, or friction rub are rare. Abdominal pain, nausea, vomiting, or diarrhea are present in 15 percent of cases. Epistaxis occurs in 25 percent.

As in most atypical pneumonias, physical signs are less prominent than the symptoms and radiographic findings. Signs of consolidation are usually absent, but some cases may mimic bacterial pneumonia both clinically and radiographically. Changes in mental status have been prominent in some epidemics. The liver is often enlarged and nontender, but jaundice is a rare and ominous sign. A number of features commonly described in early series have been only rarely documented in more recent large reviews: included are a faint macular rash (Horder's spots), splenomegaly, and relative bradycardia.

Radiographic and laboratory findings are unremarkable except for leukopenia (present in as many as 25 percent of cases) and the transient proteinuria and abnormal liver function tests found in 40 to 75 percent of a small series.

Diagnosis

A fourfold rise of CF antibody titer to at least 1:32 is diagnostic of psittacosis. Antibodies appear as early as the end of the first week, so even a low titer (1:16) during a compatible illness may be presumptive evidence. False positives may occur with brucellosis and Q fever.

The history of exposure to birds may be the only way to distinguish psittacosis from a large number of febrile disorders with or without pneumonia.

Complications

Unlike the majority of the atypical pneumonias, mortality without antibiotic therapy is considerable (20 to 40 percent). Reported complications have included encephalitis, pericarditis, endocarditis, myocarditis, hepatitis with jaundice, arthritis, anemia, DIC, thyroiditis, hemolysis with negative cold agglutinins, pancreatitis, proteinuria, oliguria, acute renal failure, exudative tonsillitis, and thrombophlebitis with pulmonary embolus. Relapses or secondary bacterial infection have been uncommon.

Treatment and Prophylaxis

Tetracycline (500 mg qid or 1 g/day IV) produces clinical improvement in 24 to 48 h and should be continued for at least 10 to 14 days after defervescence. Fever is usually gone in 2 to 3 days but may recur. Alternative therapy is chloramphenicol 2 to 4 g/day [30 to 50 mg/(kg·day)] PO or IV or penicillin 1 million units IM tid.

Doxycycline (100 mg/day for 10 days PO) has been used for prophylaxis in nonpregnant patients. Public health measures include quarantine for imported psittacine birds, tetracycline-impregnated feed, and serologic surveillance and treatment of turkey flocks. Patients are still susceptible to reinfection with another strain.

Q FEVER PNEUMONIA

When Q fever was first described in Australian abbattoir workers in 1935, the Q stood for "query," since the etiology was un-known. The disease is now known to be caused by *Coxiella burnetii*, an obligate intracellular rickettsial organism. Worldwide in distribution but rare in the United States, the organism is extremely resistant to antiseptics and harsh environments. It can live in dried soil or excreta for up to 18 months and in tap water or milk for 30 to 42 months.

The organism infects a wide variety of insects, rodents, and large domestic and wild animals. Transmission to humans is usually via inhalation of dust heavily contaminated by the excreta, placentas, and uterine discharges of infected sheep, goats, and cattle. Other less common sources that have been postulated include consumption of infected milk, entrance through skin abrasions or conjunctival innoculation, tick bites, or contact with infected hides or contaminated clothing or straw. Person-to-person transmission is rare but has been reported and attributed to droplet spray. Attack rates are high, and the infecting dose is believed to be as small as one organism.

After inhalation, the organism multiplies in the lungs and then spreads hematogenously to numerous other organs. Later, it is excreted in the urine.

Clinical Features

Infection may be asymptomatic. After an incubation period of 2 to 4 weeks, Q fever begins suddenly and is 10 times more likely to present as a febrile systemic illness than it is to present as an atypical pneumonia. Headache, chills, fluctuating fever, and myalgias occur in 60 to 85 percent of cases. As in psittacosis, headache and neck stiffness may be severe enough to suggest meningitis. Diaphoresis may be marked. Nausea, vomiting, cough, and arthralgias occur in 20 to 40 percent of cases, with pleuritic chest pain and diarrhea occurring less often. Cough develops late, after about 5 days, when rales are usually audible. The entire course usually lasts only 3 to 6 days and rarely exceeds 2 weeks. Pulmonary involvement is highly variable but is commonly about 50 percent.

Patients appear acutely ill. Fever is usually intermittent, with chills, sweats, and a relative bradycardia. Pulmonary examination may reveal only fine rales; consolidation is rare. Hepatomegaly may be present in as many as 51 percent and splenomegaly in 30 percent of patients. A mild erythema or a transient discrete trunkal maculopapular rash may be evident.

The chest radiograph is abnormal in half of the patients with Q fever, the abnormality usually appearing after the third or fourth day of illness. Infiltrates persist well beyond the period of fever and may take up to 10 weeks to resolve.

Laboratory findings include liver function abnormalities in as many as 85 percent of patients. Urinalysis revealed proteinuria in 62 percent in one series and sterile pyuria in 12 percent.

Diagnosis

A history of direct or indirect exposure to livestock or ticks in a patient with an atypical pneumonia should arouse suspicion of Q fever.

Definitive diagnosis is made by isolation of the organism, by an increase in specific antibody titer, or by direct fluorescent antibody staining demonstrating *C. burnetii* in tissue.

Complications

Even without treatment, mortality is low. The vast majority of cases are self-limited, commonly resolving in 1 to 2 weeks with or without therapy. Common complications include a prolonged course, which occurs in as many as 20 percent of patients. Persistent fevers, weight loss, and weakness can linger from 1 to 3 months. Relapse can occur in spite of antibiotic therapy. Chronic Q fever develops occasionally, even years after the primary infection, and is manifested as a subacute endocarditis.

Hepatitis has developed in as many as one-third of patients with the protracted form of the disease. Other complications have included thrombophlebitis with pulmonary embolus, hemolytic anemia, arteritis, thromboangiitis obliterans, pleuropericarditis, pericardial effusion, and myocarditis.

Treatment and Prophylaxis

Early treatment with 2 g/day of tetracycline or with chloramphenicol usually leads to a prompt clinical response and is believed to prevent relapse or chronic Q fever. Doxycycline (100 mg bid) is also being used with success.

Vaccines are available to protect slaughterhouse and dairy workers as well as livestock. Boiling or pasteurizing milk will prevent transmission.

TULAREMIA PNEUMONIA

Tularemia is an infectious disease of animals transmitted to humans by direct contact with infected animals or by insects. The causative organism is *Francisella (Pasteurella) tularensis,* a pleomorphic, nonsporulating, gram-negative bacillus, which, like other gram-negative organisms, produces an endotoxin.

The principal reservoirs for this organism in nature are ticks and wild rabbits, although up to 100 different species can be carriers. Infection occurs most commonly from contact with tissues or body fluids of infected animals and next most commonly from the bite of an infected arthropod. Infection occurs less commonly via animal bite, inhalation, or ingestion. Humans are very susceptible to infection and as few as 10 to 50 organisms can cause disease.

Cases peak in spring and summer in areas where ticks predominate but increase in winter in areas where rabbit-associated cases are prevalent. Hunters, butchers, and homemakers are most affected.

Clinical Features

Tularemia has a number of different clinical expressions, all with a 3- to 7-day incubation period (range 1 to 14 days).

The most common form (75 to 85 percent of cases) is ulceroglandular tularemia. It begins with an occasionally pruritic reddened papule, which soon ulcerates. This primary lesion, often overlooked, is followed by enlargement and suppuration of the regional lymph nodes. Bacteremia ensues with entrapment of the organism in the reticuloendothelial system. The glandular form of the disease is clinically identical except for the absence of an apparent portal of entry (5 to 10 percent). The typhoidal form (5 to 15 percent) is manifested by fever, prostration, and weight loss without a primary lesion or localized lymphadenitis. The organism can occasionally enter the conjunctivae (in the oculoglandular form of the infection) or the gastrointestinal tract.

Pneumonia only accompanies tularemia in a fraction of cases (30 to 80 percent of typhoidal and 10 to 15 percent of ulceroglandular cases). Even though inhalation of the organism can result in fever, headache, malaise, substernal discomfort, and a nonproductive cough, this "pneumonic" form may or may not be associated with pneumonia. When it occurs, tularemia pneumonia is secondary to hematogenous dissemination. It is manifested by fever (104 to 106°F), rigors, a nonproductive cough, hemoptysis, pleuritic pain, dyspnea, cyanosis, patchy, ill-defined infiltrates on chest x-ray, and a paucity of findings on physical examination. A rash (variable in nature) occurs in up to 20 percent of cases, beginning several days after the onset of other symptoms. Splenomegaly is detectable in many patients.

Diagnosis

Nearly all cases of tularemia are diagnosed serologically by a fourfold rise in titer, although a skin test is available. A single convalescent titer of 1:160 may be considered diagnostic of infection in patients with a clinically compatible illness.

Complications

Like psittacosis, tularemia produces significant mortality, said to be in the 5 to 15 percent range, without antibiotic therapy. Mortality is well below 1 percent with treatment. As with Q fever, the course may be prolonged, with high fevers persisting for as long as 4 weeks and lassitude, fatiguability, myalgia, irritability, or anorexia persisting for several months. Rare complications include endocarditis, pericarditis, peritonitis, appendicitis, osteomyelitis, and meningitis.

Treatment and Prophylaxis

Streptomycin, 0.5 to 1 g q 12 h for 7 to 14 days, is the drug of choice. Pulmonary lesions regress rapidly, but skin lesions and lymph nodes may continue to evolve. Tetracycline, chloramphenicol, gentamicin, and kanamycin are also effective. Relapse may occur, particularly if antibiotics are administered for less than 14 days, and is not due to antibiotic resistance.

An attenuated live bacterial vaccine exists and is particularly effective against the typhoidal form. However, immunity is incomplete after infection or vaccination. Streptomycin given after exposure will protect against developing the disease, while chloramphenicol and tetracycline given prophylactically only prolong the incubation period.

The best prophylactic measures are to avoid skinning or eviscerating rabbits or other wild mammals, to wear gloves when this must be done, and to avoid ticks.

The opinions and assertions contained herein are the private views of the author and are not to be construed as official or reflecting the views of the Department of Defense or the Department of the Army.

BIBLIOGRAPHY

Cunha BA, Quintiliani R: The atypical pneumonias. *Postgrad Med* 66:95–102, 1979.
File TM Jr, Tan JS, Murphy DP: Atypical pneumonia syndrome. *Primary Care* 8:673–694, 1981.

Levine DP, Lerner AM: The clinical spectrum of *Mycoplasma pneumoniae* infections. *Med Clin North Am* 62:961–978, 1978.
Moxley GF: Grand rounds: Psittacosis. *Va Med* 108:248–252, 1981.
Reichman RC, Dolin R: Viral pneumonia. *Med Clin North Am* 64:491–506, 1980.
Spelman DW: Q fever. A study of 111 consecutive cases. *Med J Aust* 1:547–553, 1982.

C. Legionnaires' Disease

Kenneth Frumkin

Legionnaires' disease captured the world's attention in July of 1976 following an outbreak at an American Legion convention in Philadelphia. Five months later the causative agent, a fastidious gram-negative bacillus, *Legionella pneumophila,* was isolated. The hearty organism, widely distributed in nature, is spread via the airborne route from cooling towers, evaporative condensers, and construction sites.

While sporadic cases are more common, there have been at least 17 epidemics in the United States. Most are seasonal (summer and fall). At greatest risk are men (2.6:1) in their mid-fifties. Persons who are immunocompromised (particularly following renal transplantation) or who have significant underlying illnesses are at greatest risk. Cigarette smoking, travel during the incubation period, and living or working near construction sites are also risk factors. Subclinical infection occurs.

CLINICAL FEATURES

Onset is usually abrupt, after a 2- to 10-day incubation period. Over two-thirds of patients will have rapidly rising fevers, recurrent rigors, headache, cough, myalgias, arthralgias, weakness, and malaise. Cough is initially nonproductive. Minor hemoptysis, dyspnea, and pleuritic chest pain are present in about one-third of cases, while coryza, photophobia, sore throat, and rash rarely occur.

Pulmonary findings are minimal early in the disease, in spite of apparent toxicity. Later, localized or generalized rales may progress to signs of consolidation. Tachypnea and relative bradycardia are reported in over 40 to 50 percent of patients.

The chest radiograph was initially abnormal in 87 percent of the Philadelphia cases and is not specific. Infiltrates are initially patchy, nonsegmental, and unilateral in over half of cases but become bilateral in as many as two-thirds. Small effusions, usually unilateral, are present in 9 to 16 percent.

Extrapulmonary manifestations are prominent: watery diarrhea occurs in up to 50 percent of cases, while nausea, vomiting, and abdominal pain are less common (20 to 25 percent). Headache is often severe. Disorientation, confusion, and even obtundation are present in up to half the patients. Tender hepatomegaly and jaundice can occur.

Laboratory abnormalities, found in 40 to 60 percent of patients, include a white blood cell count over 10,000, transaminase or urea nitrogen elevations, increased erythrocyte sedimentation rate, hyponatremia [and SIADH (syndrome of inappropriate secretion of antidiuretic hormone)], hypophosphatemia, and proteinuria. Microhematuria is present in as many as 16 percent. The CSF is usually normal. A Gram stain of sputum or transtracheal aspirate shows only small numbers of polymorphonuclear neutrophil leukocytes or monocytes with no organisms.

A prolonged clinical course and convalescence are the rule. Mortality has averaged 15 percent (5 percent with early diagnosis and treatment) but has been as high as 80 percent in compromised hosts not receiving specific therapy.

DIAGNOSIS

The diagnosis is often suggested by the characteristic clinical picture combined with a failure to respond to penicillin or ampicillin. Although it is not readily available, the quickest definitive diagnosis is made by direct immunofluorescent antibody staining of tissues, pleural fluid, or sputum specimens. The most commonly used criterion for diagnosis is a fourfold rise in indirect fluorescent antibody titer from acute to convalescent phase sera to at least 1:128. This may take 3 to 6 weeks for confirmation. A single titer on the same test of greater than 1:256 may indicate recent infection. The organism is best cultured on special media.

TREATMENT

Erythromycin is the drug of choice. Tetracycline therapy has met with irregular results. Rifampin is reserved for combination use in cases poorly responsive to erythromycin. Doses are 750 to 1000 mg of erythromycin IV every 6 h. To avoid relapse, therapy should be continued with oral erythromycin for a total of 3 weeks. Because delay in starting treatment affects the morbidity and mortality of Legionnaires' disease, most sources recommend erythromycin (with or without other antibiotics) early in cases of acute pneumonia until a clear-cut etiologic diagnosis can be made.

The opinions and assertions contained herein are the private views of the author and are not to be construed as official or reflecting the views of the Department of Defense or the Department of the Army.

BIBLIOGRAPHY

Ackley AM: Legionnaires' disease: An update. *Am Fam Physician* 24:165–170, 1981.

Balows A, Fraser DW (eds): International Symposium on Legionnaires' Disease. *Ann Intern Med* 90:489–707, 1979.

Cordes LG, Fraser DW: Legionellosis. *Med Clin North Am* 64:395–416, 1980.

Davis GS, Winn WC Jr, Beaty HN: Legionnaires' disease. *Clin Chest Med* 2:145–166, 1981.

Kirby BD: Legionnaires' disease and legionellosis. *Comp Ther* 8:8–12, 1982.

Shands KN, Fraser DW: Legionnaires' disease. *DM:* 1–40, Dec. 1980.

D. Tuberculosis

Steven C. Dronen

INTRODUCTION

Tuberculosis has been a significant cause of morbidity and mortality throughout recorded history. Early in this century at least 80 percent of the U.S. population was infected with tuberculosis before reaching the age of 20. Only in recent years has this epidemic subsided. Since the early 1950s this country has seen a dramatic and steady decline in the number of new cases and of tuberculosis-related deaths recorded per annum. This is primarily due to intensive public health efforts, an improved standard of living, and the use of effective chemotherapeutic agents. In this 30-year period the peak prevalence of chronic tuberculosis has gradually shifted from young to older adults, reflecting the aging of a patient population infected during childhood and a sharp decline in the number of new cases in children. Currently it is estimated that only 2 to 5 percent of this country's children are infected; this figure may be higher in socioeconomically depressed urban areas and among American Indians. It is ironic that the low prevalence of tuberculosis has resulted in an increased proportion of children and young adults who lack the acquired immunity of earlier generations.

An unfortunate by-product of the decreased prevalence of tuberculosis is lack of physicians' familiarity with the disease. As the majority of patients with tuberculosis have aged, so have the physicians whom they helped train. Younger physicians have in general had little experience in recognizing the often subtle manifestations of tuberculosis. Thus, to acquire knowledge of the varying clinical presentations of tuberculosis remains important for the modern physician.

PATHOPHYSIOLOGY

Mycobacterium tuberculosis is an aerobic, weakly gram-positive rod with acid-fast staining characteristics. The organism is an obligate aerobe with an optimal P_{O_2} of 140. Transmission of the tubercle bacillus is almost exclusively via the airborne route. In-fected individuals, especially those with cavitary disease, produce an aerosol of organisms suspended in tiny droplets as they talk, cough, or sneeze. The larger droplets are filtered by the mucociliary defenses of the upper respiratory tract, but the smaller droplets may reach the alveoli and initiate an infective process in the susceptible host. The lower lobes of the lungs are affected more often as they receive a greater total percentage of the tidal volume.

Tubercle bacilli multiply slowly in the human host, at a rate of once every 24 h. Most organisms would be unable to establish infection at this rate of growth, but tubercle bacilli invoke no tissue reaction. They are phagocytized but not killed and hence are free to multiply, forming a primary focus of infection. Within 3 to 10 weeks of exposure, the infection is disseminated to regional hilar lymph nodes. Bacilli then enter the bloodstream either via the thoracic duct or by direct spread into the pulmonary vasculature. This hematogenous seeding produces metastatic foci throughout the body, which may become active later in life. Foci are established preferentially at sites of high oxygen tension, especially the apices of the lungs (Simon foci) and also the kidneys and the growing ends of bones.

In the early stages of infection, previously unexposed persons have virtually no defense against multiplication of the organism. Infection induces a rich antibody response, but the role of immunoglobulins in control of the infection is unclear. T lymphocytes genetically coded to react with the tubercle bacillus begin to proliferate in response to the infection but do not reach sufficient numbers to bring the infection under control for 2 to 10 weeks. A positive tuberculin skin test is the specific indicator that immunity has developed.

Hematogenous dissemination of the primary infection usually occurs before the development of macrophage responsiveness. In approximately 5 percent of patients, cellular defenses are inadequate to control the primary infection and miliary or disseminated tuberculosis develops within weeks to months. In another 5 percent the primary infection is controlled, but a metastatic focus becomes reactivated at some later time. Reactivation of a pulmonary focus will occur within the first year in 4 to 5 percent of patients; tuberculous meningitis in children characteristically occurs within 3 months of the primary infection; tuberculous pleurisy generally occurs within 3 to 7 months; and bone or joint tuberculosis occurs within 1 to 3 years. In the remainder of cases, the infection is contained, memory lymphocytes become immunologically committed, and patients retain both tuberculin reactivity and immunity from primary infection for life.

At the present time most active tuberculosis occurs in adult patients whose initial infection was acquired many years previously. Several conditions have been identified as associated with an increased risk of conversion from the latent to the active form of the disease. Patients with diabetes, silicosis or in the postgastrectomy state, those with renal failure undergoing hemodialysis, those with cancer or organ transplants who are immunosuppressed, chronic psychiatric patients, and patients who have had intestinal bypass surgery for obesity are at increased risk.

CLINICAL FEATURES

The clinical manifestations of tuberculosis are quite variable and depend upon the stage of the disease, the site of involvement, and the age and general condition of the patient.

Pulmonary Tuberculosis

The Primary Infection

The initial pulmonary infection consists of one or more parenchymal infiltrates, with hilar and mediastinal lymphadenitis. Often there is no clinically significant associated illness, although a mild cough, fever, and malaise may develop. Infants are more likely to exhibit symptoms at this stage, specifically fever, lassitude, irritability, cough, and signs of bronchial obstruction. In most patients the primary infection is suppressed after development of tuberculin hypersensitivity and the disease enters a latent or asymptomatic phase.

Reactivation Tuberculosis

The clinical picture of reactivation or postprimary tuberculosis is somewhat dependent upon the site of involvement. The lungs are most commonly affected, but reactivation may occur in the kidney, liver, meninges, bones, or joints in the absence of pulmonary involvement. The classic symptoms of pulmonary tuberculosis are fever, night sweats, malaise, weight loss, and cough with sputum production. Gastrointestinal symptoms such as abdominal pain and anorexia will occasionally predominate. With progressive pulmonary involvement, pleuritic chest pain, sputum production, and hemoptysis become more prominent symptoms. Sputum is generally produced in the morning and is green to yellow in color. Hemoptysis is caused by the sloughing of a caseous lesion or bronchial ulceration and is usually slight. Frank bleeding is indicative of advanced disease. Dyspnea and other signs of respiratory failure are uncommon. Pleuritic chest pain generally indicates extension of the inflammatory process to the parietal pleura but may or may not be accompanied by an effusion.

Physical examination of the chest commonly fails to reveal the extent of the disease and may in fact be negative even in the presence of advanced disease. Apical posttussive rales are commonly described as indicative of active disease, but rales may persist after resolution. Other abnormal findings, such as basilar dullness, tubular breath sounds, tracheal shift, and impaired mobility of a hemithorax are seen as the disease progresses. A chest roentgenogram is necessary if there is clinical suspicion of the disease regardless of findings on auscultation of the chest.

Acute Tuberculous Pneumonia

Tuberculosis occasionally presents as an acute pneumonic process with chest pain, cough, sputum production, chills, fever and tachypnea. This is more common in blacks and in diabetics. Lobular or lobar involvement will produce signs of consolidation on pulmonary examination and may be indistinguishable from other bacterial pneumonias on roentgenographic examination. Pathologically, consolidation is followed by caseous necrosis. A sputum specimen usually reveals acid-fast bacilli.

Extrapulmonary Tuberculosis

Tuberculosis has been reported to involve most of the major organs through either lymphohematogenous dissemination, direct contiguous invasion, or spread via the various visceral conduits (gastrointestinal tract, ureters, etc.). Signs and symptoms of extrapulmonary involvement may coexist with clinically apparent pulmonary tuberculosis or may occur as isolated clinical manifestations. In the latter case it may be particularly difficult to arrive at the correct diagnosis. Tuberculosis may affect the meninges, pleura, larynx, gastrointestinal tract, peritoneal cavity, pericardium, lymph nodes, genitourinary system, skeletal system, and joints. A description of the clinical findings associated with all the various extrapulmonary sites of involvement is beyond the scope of this review. However, miliary tuberculosis and tuberculous meningitis will be discussed, as they are most likely to present as acute, life-threatening illnesses.

Miliary Tuberculosis

Miliary tuberculosis is an acute febrile illness caused by the hematogenous dissemination of tubercle bacilli. It is most likely to follow the hematogenous phase of primary tuberculosis in children and was a significant cause of mortality in this age group in the prechemotherapeutic era. Miliary tuberculosis is now seen with increasing frequency in the adult population and is usually due to reactivation and hematogenous seeding of an old focus. Patients with impaired immune responses are at increased risk; this includes patients with diabetes, alcoholism, leukemia, or lymphoma and those receiving immunosuppressive agents. When normal immune responses are incompetent, tuberculous lesions are able to form throughout the body, even in organs with low P_{O_2}'s.

The typical clinical presentation of miliary tuberculosis is the abrupt onset of fever, chills, malaise, and prostration. Headache is a frequent complaint. Less often, the disease may present insidiously with weeks or months of nonspecific symptoms such as weight loss, weakness, and low-grade fever. Consequently this diagnosis should be considered in all cases of fever of unknown origin.

Laboratory data may be of little value in making the diagnosis of miliary tuberculosis. Anemia and leukopenia are common findings. The tuberculin reaction is negative as much as 25 percent of the time, especially in the elderly. Chest roentgenograms are frequently normal when the patients present and then rapidly evolve to the characteristic miliary pattern for which the disease is named.

The complications of miliary tuberculosis are meningitis, pericarditis, peritonitis, and pleural effusion. Meningitis develops in about two-thirds of patients, usually several weeks after the onset of constitutional symptoms. The mortality rate associated with miliary tuberculosis is high, especially if treatment is delayed. It is essential that the diagnosis be entertained in the patient who presents with a nonspecific febrile illness, even in the presence of a normal chest film.

Tuberculous Meningitis

Tuberculous meningitis occurs secondary to the hematogenous dissemination of the organism in miliary tuberculosis or to the silent preallergenic bacteremia of primary tuberculosis. The meninges may be seeded directly or bacilli may spread to the subarachnoid space from a focus in the brain or spine. Once almost exclusively a disease of children, tuberculous meningitis is now seen more often in adults.

Classically, tuberculous meningitis presents insidiously over a 1- to 6-week period, with a nonspecific febrile illness. This is followed by the development of cranial nerve palsies, nuchal rigidity, personality changes, and a gradual depression in level of consciousness. The onset may also be abrupt, with severe headache, nuchal rigidity, and delirium or stupor. Fever is common but is often irregular and generally does not exceed 104°F. Signs of extrameningeal tuberculosis are present in about half of the cases, and 75 percent have a positive tuberculin test.

The typical CSF findings are elevated pressure and protein, decreased sugar, and a cell count in the range of 50 to 200 with a predominance of mononuclear forms. Acid-fast bacilli are usually not seen on the stained smear.

The patient presenting with tuberculous meningitis is frequently misdiagnosed, even in the presence of meningeal signs. The correct diagnosis will be reached more often if tuberculosis and its complications are thought of in any patient presenting with a nonspecific febrile illness.

ROENTGENOGRAPHIC FEATURES

In contrast to the pulmonary examination, the chest roentgenogram is critical to the diagnosis of pulmonary tuberculosis and is invaluable in gauging the extent of involvement and the response to therapy. Roentgenographic manifestations closely parallel the pathogenic varieties of this disease.

The roentgenographic findings of primary tuberculosis include patchy lower lung infiltrates and hilar adenopathy (the primary complex), pleural effusions, and, less often, atelectasis. The hilar adenopathy is especially prominent in children. Pleural effusion is more common in adults and may hide evidence of parenchymal

disease. Serial films may show complete resolution of these changes over a period of 6 months to 1 year. More often, the original lesion contracts to a small nodule (the Ghon tubercle), which eventually becomes calcified, as do involved hilar nodes.

Reactivation tuberculosis is strongly suggested by multinodular posterior apical infiltrates seen on posteroanterior (PA) or apical lordotic views. The posterior segment of an upper lobe is most commonly involved; less often the superior segment of a lower lobe is involved. Infiltrates of the middle lobe, lingula, and basal segments of the lower lobes rarely occur unless contiguous with upper lobe disease, except in patients with acute tuberculous pneumonia. The lobular involvement in this instance may be indistinguishable from other causes of pneumonia. Cavitation is a common feature of reactivation tuberculosis and is usually detected on the standard PA chest roentgenogram. Laminograms are valuable adjuncts in questionable cases. Other findings seen in reactivation tuberculosis are bronchiectasis and tuberculomas, which are small, discrete inflammatory nodules commonly containing concentric rings of calcification.

The chest roentgenogram is essential in demonstrating progression or healing of the disease process. Chemotherapy halts the exudative process, shrinking areas of parenchymal involvement and the walls of cavity lesions. These physical changes have distinct radiographic manifestations, which can be followed on serial examinations: the cavity wall decreases in thickness; fibrosis and scar contracture shift mediastinal and hilar structures toward the affected lobe and produce volume loss in that lobe and hemithorax; and pulmonary nodules become more clearly defined, decrease in size, and may begin to calcify.

Serial chest roentgenograms also have a role in evaluating the progression or reactivation of pulmonary tuberculosis. The appearance of old fibrotic areas does not change appreciably with time, so any change from earlier films is evidence of reactivation of tuberculosis or of the development of a new pulmonic process.

TREATMENT

Fresh air, sunshine, and prolonged hospitalization, once the mainstays of tuberculosis treatment, are no longer held to be of any value. Assuming the patient is compliant, the only important determinant of outcome is the selection of appropriate chemotherapeutic agents. The emergency department physician will generally not be involved in this decision but should have some familiarity with the agents in common use and their potential complications. Hospitalization of uncomplicated cases of tuberculosis is not necessary, nor should patients be removed from their home environment. Once chemotherapy is begun, infectivity is quite low.

There are currently 10 drugs available in the United States which have been approved for the treatment of tuberculosis. Except in special circumstances, multiple drug therapy is the rule because of the frequent occurrence of resistant organisms. For example, it is estimated that 1 bacillus in 100,000 is resistant to isoniazid. Traditionally, the duration of therapy has been 18 to 24 months, but recent studies suggest that a 9-month course of chemotherapy may be adequate.

Isoniazid and rifampin are considered the primary antituberculous drugs because of their effectiveness and low toxicity. Secondary drugs are ethambutol, para-aminosalicylic acid (PAS), pyrazinamide, and streptomycin. Although less effective and more toxic, these are acceptable companion drugs and help prevent the emergence of resistant organisms. Tertiary drugs are capreomycin, cycloserine, ethionamide, and kanamycin. Because of their toxicity and low effectiveness, they are used only when other agents are unsuitable.

There are complications associated with the use of all the antituberculous drugs. Isoniazid has been reported to cause hepatitis, peripheral neuritis, a hypersentitivity reaction that includes fever, rash, and a lupuslike syndrome, and CNS symptoms such as dizziness, muscle twitching, ataxia, optic neuritis, encephalopathy, and convulsions. Isoniazid also interferes with the metabolism of phenytoin, prolonging its half-life. The isoniazid-induced liver disease usually occurs within the first 3 months of treatment and is indistinguishable from viral hepatitis. In most cases complete resolution occurs after discontinuation of the drug.

The most serious side effects of rifampin are renal failure, hemolysis, and thrombocytopenia. A rifampin-induced hepatitis similar to that caused by isoniazid is also seen. The drug should be stopped if any of these side effects occur. Rifampin interacts with several drugs, including warfarin, oral contraceptives, methadone, and aminosalicylic acid. Self-limited effects not requiring discontinuation of the drug are an influenza-like syndrome and the appearance of orange urine, tears, and saliva.

Streptomycin, like other drugs in its class, is nephrotoxic and causes eighth nerve damage. Neuromuscular blockade has been observed in patients with myasthenia gravis and in those receiving muscle relaxants concomitantly.

The most important toxic effect of ethambutol is retrobulbar neuritis, which may be of the central or peripheral type.

PAS commonly causes anorexia and nausea and is rarely used in adults for this reason. Children tolerate the drug better, but hypersensitivity reactions have been reported in this age group.

BIBLIOGRAPHY

Addington WW: The treatment of pulmonary tuberculosis: Current options. *Arch Intern Med* 139:1391–1395, 1979.

Banner AS: Tuberculosis. Clinical aspects and diagnosis. *Arch Intern Med* 139:1387–1390, 1979.

Barlow PB: Treatment of tuberculosis. *Ann Thorac Surg News* 5:18–23, 1976.

Felton CP, Jones JM: Acute forms of tuberculosis. *Med Clin North Am* 57:1395–1402, 1973.

Geppert EF, Leff A: The pathogenesis of pulmonary and miliary tuberculosis. *Arch Intern Med* 139:1381–1383, 1979.

Glassroth J, Robins AG, Snider DE: Tuberculosis in the 1980's. *N Engl J Med* 302:1441–1450, 1980.

Leff A, Geppert EF: Public health and preventive aspects of pulmonary tuberculosis. *Arch Intern Med* 139:1405–1410, 1979.

Leff A, Lester W, Addington WW: Tuberculosis? A chemotherapeutic triumph but a persistent socioeconomic problem. *Arch Intern Med* 139:1375–1377, 1979.

Sahn SA, Neff TA: Miliary tuberculosis. *Am J Med* 56:495–505, 1974.

Sbarbaro JA: Tuberculosis. *Med Clin North Am* 64:417–431, 1980.

Scully RE, Mark EJ, McNeely BU: Case Records of the Massachusetts General Hospital. *N Engl J Med* 306:91–97, 1982.

Stead WW, Kerby GR, Schlueter DP, et al: The clinical spectrum of primary tuberculosis in adults. *Ann Intern Med* 68:731–745, 1968.

E. Pleural Effusions

John F. Keighley

Under normal conditions, a few milliliters of fluid are present in the pleural space, acting as a lubricant. When the rate of formation of this fluid exceeds its removal, accumulation occurs within the pleural space. Pleural effusions occur in a broad variety of diseases and the characterization of pleural fluid is important for diagnosis. In general, the symptoms accompanying the development of a pleural effusion are due to the underlying disease or to pleuritic irritation. In addition, large effusions or effusions that have accumulated rapidly may cause respiratory distress. In most instances, the evaluation of a pleural effusion requires in-hospital study.

PATHOPHYSIOLOGY

Pleural effusions may be broadly divided into two categories; transudates and exudates. *Transudates* are low-protein plasma filtrates and develop as a result of excessive hydrostatic pressure as in cardiac failure or as a result of insufficient oncotic pressure as in hypoproteinemia. *Exudates*, on the other hand, contain large amounts of protein and occur following a disruption of the normal formation-reabsorption mechanism. This breakdown may be due to damage to the pleural capillaries that permits leakage of protein-rich fluid into the pleural space, as occurs in inflammatory disease. The lymphatics are responsible for the reabsorption of large protein molecules so that lymphatic blockage, as seen in malignant disease, is also associated with the formation of an exudate. Common causes of pleural effusion categorized according to type are listed in Table 20E-1.

CLINICAL FEATURES

Pleural effusions may be asymptomatic, although generally there are symptoms and signs attributable to pleuritic irritation, to the underlying disease, or to respiratory embarrassment.

Table 20E-1. Etiology of Pleural Effusion

Transudates
   Heart failure
   Hypoalbuminemia
   Nephrotic syndrome
   Cirrhosis
   Postperitoneal dialysis
Exudates
   Infection
      Tuberculosis
      Fungi
      Viruses
      Mycoplasma
      Empyema
      Bacterial pneumonia
   Neoplasm
      Primary or metastatic
      Lymphoma
      Mesothelioma
      Chest wall neoplasms
   Pulmonary infarction
   Connective tissue diseases
      Rheumatoid arthritis and SLE
   Intra-abdominal disease
      Subdiaphragmatic abscess
      Acute pancreatitis
      Meigs' syndrome
      Ruptured pancreatic pseudocyst
   Miscellaneous
      Esophageal rupture
      Lymphedema
      Myxedema
      Familial Mediterranean fever
      Idiopathic
Trauma
   Hemothorax
   Chylothorax
   Urinothorax

Pleuritic pain commonly occurs when pleural effusion is due to infection. Generally it lasts only a few days but may recur following removal of the pleural fluid by thoracentesis. Though it may be mild, generally it is severe and may be described as knife-like, sharp, or cutting. The severity increases with inspiration and usually causes a sudden cessation of the inspiratory effect. The pain is less severe on expiration and is not present with breath-holding. Sudden respiratory movement, as with coughing or sneezing, is associated with severe pain. Although generally localized to the chest, the pain may be referred to the abdomen or the ipsilateral shoulder. Other causes of chest wall pain exacerbated by respiratory movement, such as rib fractures and costochondritis, must be differentiated from pleuritic pain.

Additional symptoms associated with pleural effusion include cough, shortness of breath, and fever. Cough may be secondary to moderate-sized effusions and is generally nonproductive. Similarly, large effusions, particularly when they have accumulated rapidly, may be associated with dyspnea. The presence of underlying lung disease will increase the severity of these symptoms.

Physical findings associated with pleural effusion are those relating to pleurisy and the presence of fluid. Underlying lung disease will modify these findings. Pleurisy is associated with chest wall splinting and, on auscultation, a pleural rib. The signs associated with the presence of fluid in the pleural cavity range from none to stony dullness on percussion, loss of breath sounds, and decreased tactile and vocal fremitus on the affected side. Atelectasis may occur in the region of the effusion and may be detected by an area of bronchial breathing and egophony at the upper limits of the effusion. The chest wall may not have the normal outward movement on inspiration. There may be some outward bulging of the intercostal spaces and a lag of inspiratory movement on the affected side. Tachypnea may be present owing to the inability of the patient to take a deep breath.

The first roentgenographic change may be a hazy obliteration of the costophrenic angle in the standard upright posteroanterior (PA) view. This represents the collection of approximately 250 mL of pleural fluid. On the lateral view there is generally some loss of clarity of the posterior costophrenic angle and, as more fluid accumulates, an upward concave density develops at the angle. It should be remembered that the overall height of the fluid is at least to the lateral upper border of the concave density.

In very ill patients, small effusions may pass undetected when the film is taken in the supine position. With moderate effusions, the lung field is hazy or ground-glass in appearance. This generalized haziness is more apparent in the lower central position, where the fluid is deepest and contrasts with the contralateral side. In most instances, the presence of fluid may be differentiated from pneumonia by the lack of an air bronchogram in the former. With large pleural effusions, there is general opacification of the lung field (Fig 20E-1).

Lateral decubitus views may aid in detecting relatively small effusions. When the affected side is dependent, layering of the fluid may be visible. When the side contralateral to the effusion is dependent, clearing of the costophrenic angle on the affected side may occur suggesting the presence of fluid; furthermore, the presence of underlying lung disease may become apparent.

Small subpulmonic effusions may be mistaken for elevation of the hemidiaphragm, but the loss of vascular shadows below the diaphragm on the affected side is a clue to their presence. The presence of subpulmonic effusions can usually be confirmed by a lateral decubitus view. Layering of fluid in the fissures increases their visibility. In patients with congestive failure, localized collections of fluid may occur in the fissures and appear as "phantom" or "pseudo tumors" on the PA roentgenogram. These "tumors" may rapidly resolve with diuretic administration.

Finally, it should be remembered that the roentgenographic appearance of fluid may also occur with old healed pleural disease so that a history of previous chest wall injury, thoracic surgery, or pleuropulmonary disease should be sought. Generally the availability of chest roentgenograms taken in the past will assist in this differential diagnosis.

DIAGNOSIS

Thoracentesis

While an estimate of the amount of fluid present may be made clinically and radiologically, accurate diagnosis requires laboratory examination of fluid obtained by thoracentesis.

Generally, diagnostic thoracentesis is required whenever the etiology of an effusion has not been established or chest roentgenogram findings need clarification. Therapeutic thoracentesis

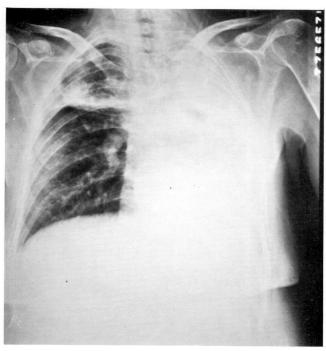

Figure 20E-1. Massive left pleural effusion and right upper lobe infiltrate. Tracheal and mediastinal deviation to the left indicates atelectasis of the left lung. Note the prominent, tortuous right pulmonary artery. (Courtesy Detroit General Hospital.)

may be used to alleviate respiratory distress secondary to a large pleural effusion or may be preparatory to the instillation of sclerosing or antineoplastic agents.

The categorization of pleural effusion is based upon fluid analysis after removal by thoracentesis. Generally, this procedure will be performed in an inpatient rather than emergency department setting.

Certain contraindications to, and common errors in the performance of, thoracentesis must be emphasized. Clinically significant coagulopathies are a temporary contraindication. Uncontrollable coughing or hiccups or an uncooperative patient may result in injury to the intercostal neurovascular bundle during needle entry or in laceration of the lung by the needle bevel, with a resultant pneumothorax and bronchopleural fistula. The liver or a subdiaphragmatic abscess may be entered during thoracentesis if inappropriate technique is used. The presence of cutaneous infection is a relative contraindication to thoracentesis.

Perhaps the most common error is performing a thoracentesis without a working diagnosis, for appropriate studies may be overlooked or an unnecessarily large number of studies performed. If in doubt, sufficient pleural fluid should be left behind so that thoracentesis and pleural biopsy may be repeated without hazard.

The difference in the anatomy of the intercostal space anteriorly and posteriorly is frequently not appreciated. To avoid damage to the neurovascular bundle anteriorly, the needle should be inserted midway between the ribs, whereas posteriorly it should be passed through the inferior portion of the intercostal space. In addition, the anatomy of small or loculated effusions should be clearly defined by roentgenography before proceeding with aspiration. In

difficult situations, ultrasound techniques may be required for accurate localization. The quantity of fluid removed should not exceed 1 to 1.5 L. The removal of quantities in excess of this limit can result in shock attributable to a variety of causes, development of unilateral pulmonary edema, hypoxemia, and severe chest pain. Postprocedure chest roentgenograms, observation of vital signs, repeated chest auscultation, and subsequent examination of the needle puncture site are necessary to detect development of complications.

Laboratory Studies

On gross examination, the fluid may appear clear and pale lemon-colored, suggesting a transudate, or dark amber with fibrin clots, suggesting an exudate. Between these extremes differentiation can only be made on the basis of detailed laboratory study. More important is the detection of bleeding into the pleural space. It is important to measure blood loss by the hemoglobin, hematocrit, or red cell count rather than to rely on descriptive terms that can be misleading. Frank pus may require a large-bore needle for aspiration. Chylous effusions have a characteristic milky appearance.

The minimum laboratory studies required for an undiagnosed pleural effusion should include red and white cell counts and differential, cytologic examination, and pleural fluid protein, lactic acid dehydrogenase (LDH), amylase, and glucose levels. In addition, cultures for aerobic, anaerobic, mycobacterial, and fungal organisms are generally obtained. At the same time, obtain serum protein, glucose, and LDH determinations to interpret the levels found in the pleural fluid. Approximately 60 percent of effusions can be differentiated into a transudate or exudate on the basis of these data and a specific diagnosis made. Of therapeutic importance is the separation of effusions that resolve spontaneously from those likely to require chest tube drainage. A pleural fluid pH greater than 7.3 suggests that spontaneous resolution will occur, whereas a pleural fluid pH less than 7.3 suggests an empyema or an effusion likely to loculate and require chest tube drainage.

To classify a sample of pleural fluid as an exudate, at least one of the following criteria of Light et al. should be present: (1) pleural fluid-serum protein ratio greater than 0.5; (2) pleural fluid LDH greater than 200 IU; and (3) pleural fluid-serum LDH ratio greater than 0.6. Reliance on the older method of differentiation by the pleural fluid protein level will lead to marked diagnostic error.

Depending on the clinical presentation, additional studies that may be required include total neutral fat, cholesterol level, complement, and rheumatoid factor. If inflammation or malignancy is suspected, it is preferable to perform a pleural biopsy at the time of the initial thoracentesis. A normal clotting profile should be present if pleural biopsy is to be done.

Specific Diagnoses

Certain symptom complexes occur frequently enough to suggest specific etiologies that will guide the clinician in ordering laboratory data.

Transudates due to congestive heart failure or cirrhosis occur commonly enough to present little difficulty in diagnosis. How-

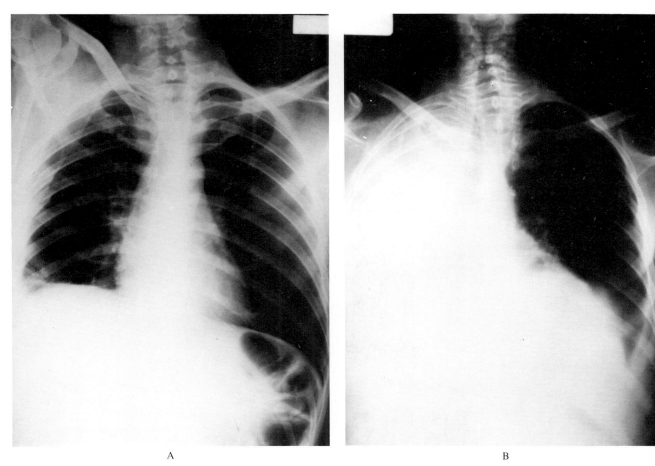

A

B

Figure 20E-2. A. This 40-year old man was treated for right lower lobe pneumonia on the basis of the chest film, which demonstrates elevation of the right hemidiaphragm, basilar infiltrate, and probably, a small right pleural effusion. (Courtesy Detroit General Hospital.) B. One week later he came to the emergency department because of the sudden onset of severe shortness of breath. Although carcinoma was the suspected diagnosis, the cause of the effusion was a ruptured pancreatic pseudocyst. (Courtesy Detroit General Hospital.)

ever, if the patient has cirrhosis or is an alcoholic, causes of pleural effusion may also include pancreatitis, rupture of a pancreatic pseudocyst into the pleural cavity (Fig. 20E-2A and B), empyema secondary to aspiration pneumonia, spontaneous esophageal rupture, tuberculosis, and trauma. Anasarca, particularly in a young person, suggests the nephrotic syndrome. In the patient with renal disease, pleural effusions may also occur following peritoneal dialysis.

Together, tuberculosis and malignancy comprise up to two-thirds of the causes of exudates in most published series. Precise proportions depend on the source of the series. Although the incidence of tuberculous pleural effusion is declining, malignant effusions associated with bronchogenic carcinoma continue to rise.

In children pneumonia is the most common cause of exudates, with malignancy the second most common. Tuberculous effusions tend to occur in adolescents and young adults but are by no means confined to this age group. Malignant effusions may be suspected in the older person, the heavy cigarette smoker, and patients with previous history of malignancy in other areas of the body. Clubbing and osteoarthropathy are also suggestive of malignant disease, although they are also found in cirrhosis, empyema, and

chronic obstructive pulmonary disease. Pleurisy with effusion may be secondary to inflammatory disease, pulmonary embolus, or, if there is a history of recent myocardial infarction, Dressler's syndrome. Rheumatoid arthritis is frequently associated with small pleural effusions that may, in fact, occur prior to the onset of arthritis. Arthritis and arthralgia associated with polyserositis suggest systemic lupus erythematosus. Carcinoma of the breast remains one of the most common causes of metastatic malignant pleural effusions in women.

SUMMARY

Pleural effusions occur in a wide variety of diseases and the characterization of pleural fluid is essential for diagnosis.

Radiologic signs of pleural effusion range from blunting of the costophrenic angle, to pseudotumors that resolve with diuresis, to opacification of the lung field. Lateral decubitus views may aid in detecting small effusions.

Pleural fluid is obtained by thoracentesis, and depending on the differential diagnosis, should be analyzed for cell count and differential; protein, LDH, amylase, and glucose levels; and cytology. Bacteriologic and fungal cultures should be obtained at this time.

In the United States most exudative pleural effusions are due to tuberculosis and malignancy.

BIBLIOGRAPHY

Berger HW: Tuberculous pleurisy—Critical review. *Chest* 63:88–92, 1973.
Black LF: The pleural space and pleural fluid. *Mayo Clin Proc* 47:493–506, 1972.
Gryminski J, Krakowka P, Lypacewicz G: The diagnosis of pleural effusion by ultrasonic and radiologic techniques. *Chest* 70:33–37, 1976.

Leuallen EC, Carr DT: Pleural effusion—A statistical study of 436 patients. *N Engl J Med* 252:79–83, 1955.
Light RW, MacGregor MI, Luchsinger PC, et al: Pleural effusions: The diagnostic separation of transudates and exudates. *Ann Intern Med* 77:507–513, 1972.
Potts DE, Levin DC, Sahn SA: Pleural fluid pH in parapneumonic effusions. *Chest* 70:328–331, 1976.
Sahebjami H, Loudon RG: Pleural effusion: Pathophysiology and clinical features. *Semin Roentgenol* 12:269–275, 1977.
Scerbo J, Keltz H, Stone DJ: A prospective study of closed pleural biopsies. *JAMA* 218:377–380, 1971.
Storey DD: Pleural effusion: A diagnostic dilemma. *JAMA* 236:2183–2186, 1976.
Vix VA: Roentgenographic manifestations of pleural disease. *Semin Roentgenol* 12:277–286, 1977.

F. Empyema

Judith E. Tintinalli

An *empyema* is the collection of purulent material in the pleural space or its loculation between fissures. It generally develops secondary to hematogenous or lymphatic spread from pneumonia, or by direct extension or rupture of a lung abscess into the pleural space. Other causes of empyema include esophageal perforation and mediastinitis; rupture of a mediastinal lymph node; direct extension from vertebral osteomyelitis, retropharyngeal or subdiaphragmatic abscesses; or infection as a complication of needle aspiration, thoracostomy tubes, or thoracotomy. The common causative organisms are *Staphylococcus,* gram-negative, and anaerobic organisms.

Presenting signs and symptoms are fever and chills, pleuritic chest pain, and shortness of breath. Weight loss, fatigue, and clubbing of the fingers may be present with chronic disease. On examination, dullness to percussion, decreased breath sounds, and diminished excursion of the affected hemothorax are evident.

The chest roentgenogram demonstrates an air-fluid level in the pleural space, or evidence of loculated fluid. The radiologic distinctions between empyema and lung abscess will be discussed in the section on lung abscess, Chapter 20G. Diagnosis is made by thoracentesis with aspiration of purulent material.

Complications of empyema include the development of an empyema necessitans or of a bronchopleural fistula or permanent loss of pulmonary parenchyma. *Empyema necessitans* is an encapsulated empyema that dissects into the subcutaneous tissues or through the chest wall.

An empyema may rupture into the bronchus, spreading infection throughout the tracheobronchial tree or causing airway obstruction. In chronic empyema or fibrothorax, restrictive lung disease may result.

Treatment is by tube thoracostomy with closed drainage or by open drainage and decortication.

SUMMARY

Empyema is the collection of purulent fluid in the pleural space, or its loculation in a fissure. It generally develops secondary to infection in the chest, thoracic spine, neck, or upper abdomen.

Diagnosis is by the radiologic demonstration of pleural fluid or an air-fluid level and by aspiration of purulent material on thoracentesis.

Major complications are the development of empyema necessitans, a bronchopleural fistula, or restrictive pulmonary disease.

Treatment is by tube thoracostomy with closed drainage, or open drainage and decortication.

BIBLIOGRAPHY

Bartlett JG, Gorbach SL, Thadepalli, H, et al: Bacteriology of empyema. *Lancet* 1:338–340, 1974.
Finland M, Barnes MW: Changing ecology of acute bacterial empyema: Occurrence and mortality at Boston City Hospital during 12 selected years from 1935 to 1972. *J Infect Dis* 137:274–291, 1978.
Marks MI, Eickhoff TC: Empyema necessitatis. *Am Rev Respir Dis* 101:759–761, 1970.
Ramilo J, Harris VJ, White H: Empyema as a complication of retropharyngeal and neck abscesses in children. *Radiology* 126:743–746, 1978.
Snider, GL, Saleh SS: Empyema of the thorax in adults: Review of 105 cases. *Dis Chest* 54:410–415, 1968.

G. Lung Abscess

Georges C. Benjamin, Judith E. Tintinalli

A lung abscess is a cavitation in the pulmonary parenchyma that develops as a result of local suppuration with central necrosis, usually after the aspiration of oropharyngeal secretions. As with other forms of pneumonitis, factors that suppress the cough or gag reflexes, such as anesthesia, tooth extraction, esophageal motility disorders, strictures, or carcinoma, predispose to aspiration. Other pulmonary disorders that may lead to lung abscess formation include pneumonia, pulmonary embolism with cystic infarction, carcinoma, septic emboli, vasculitis, and infected cysts. The presence of periodontal disease plays an important role in the formation of anaerobic lung abscesses by increasing the inoculum of organisms available for aspiration. Lung abscess is rare in edentulous people.

The flora in a lung abscess secondary to aspiration are usually polymicrobial, with as many as 60 percent exclusively anaerobes and the rest a mixture of both aerobes and anaerobes. The anaerobes include microaerophilic and anaerobic streptococci, *Fusobacterium*, and *Bacteroides*. Aerobic organisms such as *Staphylococcus aureus*, *Pseudomonas*, alpha streptococci, *Streptococcus pneumoniae*, *Proteus*, *Escherichia coli*, and *Klebsiella pneumoniae* can cause a severe necrotic pneumonitis with abscess formation. Mycobacterium, *Histoplasma*, *Coccidioides*, lung flukes, and *Entamoeba* can also present with abscess formation.

CLINICAL FEATURES

In patients with pulmonary aspiration, cavitation usually develops 1 to 2 weeks after the aspiration. Clinical illness is usually insidious but may present as an acute pneumonitis. Presenting signs and symptoms include a cough productive of a fetid and bloody sputum, fever, chest pain, shortness of breath, weakness, and weight loss. Oral examination usually reveals gingivitis and poor dentition. Signs of localized consolidation or cavitation may be present on pulmonary auscultation. Clubbing is rarely seen. Complete blood count usually reveals a leukocytosis with a left shift and anemia. Diagnosis is confirmed by chest roentgenograms that demonstrate the cavity (Fig. 20G-1). An air-fluid level is generally present. The most common sites for aspiration-induced abscesses are the posterior segment of the right upper lobe and the superior segments of the right and left lower lobes. A lung abscess that develops secondary to pulmonary parenchymal disease, carcinoma, opportunistic infection, or septicemia may occur anywhere in the lung.

Occasionally, it may be difficult to distinguish a lung abscess from empyema on the chest roentgenogram. Schachter et al. suggest several signs that favor the diagnosis of empyema over lung abscess. These include (1) the development of an air-fluid level at the site of a previous pleural effusion; (2) a cavity with an air-fluid level that tapers at the pleural border; (3) an air-fluid level that crosses a fissure; and (4) an air-fluid level that extends to the lateral chest wall.

Sputum Gram stains are of some value in the diagnosis of aerobic infection. However, only transtracheal or transthoracic aspiration are reliable for anaerobic culture since expectorated sputum is always contaminated with oral anaerobes. Pleural effusions are occasionally a source of positive cultures and should be cultured both aerobically and anaerobically. In patients with septic emboli, blood cultures are frequently positive.

COMPLICATIONS

Hemoptysis, although usually not life-threatening, may be of concern because of the risk of airway obstruction, which initially is more life-threatening than hemorrhagic shock. Mattox defines massive hemoptysis as the expectoration of 200 mL of blood per cough, 400 mL of blood per 24 hours, or hemoptysis requiring transfusion to maintain a stable hematocrit. Certain radiologic signs described by Thoms et al. are useful in identifying actual or

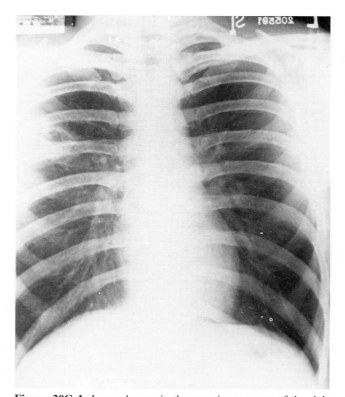

Figure 20G-1. Lung abscess in the superior segment of the right lower lobe.

Table 20G-1. Treatment of Lung Abscess

Aqueous penicillin G	6–12 million units/day
	Divided q 4 h IV then
	500 mg q 6 PO
Chloramphenicol	500 mg q 4 h IV, PO
Clindamycin	600 mg q 6–8 h IV then
	300 mg q 6 h PO

impending hemoptysis: (1) emptying and refilling of the abscess cavity on serial films; (2) variations in the lucency and height of the air-fluid level; and (3) variable parenchymal densities representing blood clots within the cavity. Other complications include chronic lung abscess, empyema, brain abscess, and bronchopleural fistula.

TREATMENT

Penicillin remains the drug of choice for uncomplicated lung abscess. Generally intravenous penicillin is given until clinical improvement occurs, followed by oral medications for up to 6 weeks. In patients with penicillin allergy, clindamycin or chloramphenicol are suitable alternatives (Table 20G-1). Elective bronchoscopy is valuable to evaluate the presence of a tumor or foreign body, to obtain material for culture, and to facilitate drainage. Surgery is indicated for life-threatening hemoptysis, tumor, and, rarely, a residual cavity.

Patients with life-threatening hemoptysis should be placed in Trendelenburg's position, vigorously suctioned, and oxygenated. If the side of the bleeding is known, the patient should be placed with that side down. Fluid and blood must be rapidly replaced as well and immediate consultation for bronchoscopy must be obtained, generally from a thoracic surgeon. Bronchoscopy can aid in localizing the bleeding site and can provide a route for suctioning, and the rigid bronchoscope can be used to maintain the airway. By use of a bronchoscope, the patient can be intubated with a double-lumen endobronchial tube (Carlens, Robert Shaw, or White), or selective endobronchial intubation can be done. The bleeding main-stem bronchus can then be occluded, which ensures a patent airway through the other mainstem bronchus. Both bronchoscopy and endobronchial intubation should be attempted only by trained, experienced individuals.

SUMMARY

Pyogenic lung abscess most commonly develops secondary to aspiration in patients with a suppressed cough reflex, depressed level of consciousness, or esophageal disorders.

The radiologic appearance of a lung abscess is generally characteristic, although carcinoma, pulmonary embolus with central cavitation, and occasionally empyema can be considered in the differential diagnosis.

The complications of lung abscess are rupture into the pleural cavity; failure of the abscess to heal; metastatic brain abscess; and massive hemoptysis. With massive hemoptysis, the immediate threat to life is generally airway obstruction. Adequate airway management and volume repletion are the cornerstones of management. Emergency thoracotomy may be necessary to control bleeding.

The opinions or assertions contained herein are the private views of the authors and are not to be considered as those of the Department of the Army or the Department of Defense.

BIBLIOGRAPHY

Bartlett JB, Finegold SM: Anaerobic infections of the lung and pleural space. *Am Rev Respir Dis* 110:56–77, 1974.

Crocco JA, Rooney JJ, Fankushen DS, et al: Massive hemoptysis. *Arch Intern Med* 121:495–498, 1968.

Johanson WG, Harris GD: Aspiration pneumonia, anaerobic infections, and lung abscess. *Med Clin North Am* 64(3):385–394, 1980.

Lorber B: ''Bad breath'': Presenting manifestation of anaerobic pulmonary infection. *Am Rev Respir Dis* 112:373–377, 1973.

Schachter EN, Kreisman H, Putman C: Diagnostic problems in suppurative lung disease. *Arch Intern Med* 136:167–171, 1976.

Takaro T, Scott SM, Bridgman AH, et al: Suppurative diseases of the lungs, pleurae, and pericardium. *Curr Probl Surg* 14:20–52, 57–62, 1977.

Thoms NW, Puro HE, Arbulu A: The significance of hemoptysis in lung abscess. *J Thorac Cardiovasc Surg* 59:617–629, 1970.

Weiss W, Cherniack NS: Acute nonspecific lung abscess: A controlled study comparing orally and parenterally administered penicillin G. *Chest* 66(4):348–351, 1974.

Zavala DC, Rhodes ML, Richardson RN, et al: Fiberoptic and rigid bronchoscopy. The state of the art. *Chest* 65:605–606, 1974.

CHAPTER 21
ASPIRATION
PNEUMONIA

Georges C. Benjamin, Judith E. Tintinalli

Aspiration pneumonia is an inflammation of the lung parenchyma resulting from the entrance of foreign material into the tracheobronchial tree. The clinical consequences of pulmonary aspiration of gastric contents were described in 1946 by Mendelson, who observed this complication in obstetrical patients undergoing anesthesia. Other situations predisposing to aspiration are shown in Table 21-1. The common factors in each of these risk categories are depression of the cough or gag reflex, alterations in the normal physiologic handling of secretions or gastric contents, and structural alterations of the normal physiologic protective mechanisms.

PATHOPHYSIOLOGY

The clinical and pathologic results of pulmonary aspiration depend on the pH of the aspirated material, the volume of the aspirate,

Table 21-1. Disorders Predisposing to Aspiration

1. Coma or depressed consciousness
   a. Drugs
   b. Anesthesia
   c. Alcohol
   d. Seizures
   e. Cerebral vascular accident
   f. Metabolic or infectious coma
2. Motility disorder
   a. Esophagus
   b. Incompetent swallowing mechanism
   c. Chronic debility
   d. Esophageal reflux (functional or surgical)
3. Iatrogenic
   a. Esophageal obturator airway
   b. Gastric lavage
   c. Feeding tubes
   d. Small volume–high pressure endotracheal tubes
4. Structural
   a. Tracheostomy
   b. Esophageal stricture
   c. Esophageal cancer
   d. Small bowel obstruction
5. Trauma
6. Childhood
   a. Force feeding
   b. Running with foreign body in mouth

the presence in the aspirate of particulate matter such as food, and bacterial contamination.

Aspiration of large particles of food or other objects that can cause upper airway obstruction is an important and easily reversible cause of mortality. This complication must be quickly recognized and treated.

Neutral Fluids

It is generally accepted that serious injury results if the pH of the aspirate is 2.5 or less. However, many of the early pathologic changes are nonspecific and occur regardless of the pH of the aspirate. These include collapse and expansion of individual alveoli, reflex airway closure, and interstitial edema. These changes occur within seconds, producing significant ventilation-perfusion mismatch and marked hypoxia. If material with a pH greater than 2.5 is aspirated, the severity of injury depends additionally on the composition of the aspirate and the volume. The aspiration of lipid materials results in a chronic granulomatous reaction resulting in lipoid pneumonia. The consequences of aspiration of neutral, clear liquids are more easily reversible with supportive therapy; however, large-volume aspiration results in high mortality and morbidity.

Neutral Fluids with Food Particles

Neutral fluids with food particles produce a persistent inflammatory reaction resulting in a hemorrhagic pneumonitis within 6 h after aspiration. As the pneumonitis progresses, a chronic granulomatous reaction develops which resembles the granuloma of pulmonary tuberculosis and may be visible on roentgenography.

Acid Aspiration

The aspiration of fluids with a pH of less than 2.5 results in severe pulmonary changes analogous to those produced by a chemical burn. Volumes as low as 1 mL/kg have been shown to result in pathologic changes throughout the pulmonary parenchyma within seconds. These changes include reflex airway closure, destruction of surfactant-producing alveoli, alveolar collapse, and pulmonary capillary destruction. In the first few hours after aspiration, intrapulmonary mucosal hemorrhage, bronchial epithelial degeneration, and pulmonary edema occur. Shunting may be massive and pulmonary compliance decreases. The loss of integrity of the alveolocapillary bed results in large fluid losses that can be severe enough to require volume repletion. Secondary bacterial infection results. In community-acquired aspiration, anaerobes comprise the most common bacterial isolates. In a patient who develops aspiration following hospitalization, gram-negative aerobes, including *Pseudomonas, Proteus,* and *Escherichia coli* in addition to anaerobes, are frequent isolates.

Foreign Body Aspiration

Foreign body aspiration remains a threat to life and is a leading cause of in-home accidental death in children under age 6. In patients in whom complete obstruction occurs, death from asphyxiation will occur in 4 to 6 min unless the condition is relieved. Peripheral aspiration results in lung abscess and pneumonitis distal to the point of obstruction. Pathologically, varying degrees of atelectasis and inflammation are present.

CLINICAL FEATURES

Aspiration of fluid and oropharyngeal bacteria can occur in healthy persons during sleep. Pathologic aspiration also can be silent and a high index of suspicion must be maintained in order to detect this problem. Signs of hypoxemia such as tachypnea, tachycardia, and cyanosis may develop immediately or may not be present for a number of hours. Auscultation of the chest may disclose wheezing, rales, or rhonchi, and the patient may produce large amounts of frothy, bloody sputum.

Blood gas abnormalities include marked hypoxia with respiratory alkalosis. Severe aspiration may result in respiratory failure with a combined respiratory and metabolic acidosis.

Hypotension and hypovolemic shock may develop rapidly owing to the outpouring of fluid into the alveolar spaces. Although the clinical picture may resemble pulmonary edema, left ventricular function remains normal and hemodynamic monitoring usually reveals a high cardiac index with normal to low right-sided pressures.

The chest roentgenogram may show a diffuse alveolar and interstitial infiltrate or a segmental or lobar infiltrate. The lower lobe of the right lung is most frequently involved because the right main-stem bronchus courses more directly toward the right lower lobe. If the patient is in the Trendelenburg position, the infiltrates tend to involve the axillary segment of the right upper lobe and the apical segment of the right lower lobe.

Patients with chronic aspiration may have repeated bouts of pneumonia, especially involving the right lower lobe or the axillary segment of the right upper lobe.

While acute respiratory failure is the most serious complication of acute pulmonary aspiration, chronic sequelae include pulmonary fibrosis, lung abscess, and empyema. The mortality due to this problem ranges from 40 to 70 percent for aspiration of fluids with a pH less than 2.5 and is higher for fluids with a pH less than 1.8.

TREATMENT

The prevention of aspiration pneumonia is the most important consideration in the management of patients at risk. This is accomplished by particular attention to airway management. Nasotracheal or orotracheal intubation should be considered in any patient with depressed or absent gag or cough reflexes. This is best done with a soft-cuffed endotracheal tube. Gastric lavage should be performed cautiously in a comatose or obtunded patient. Preventive measures include placing the patients in the Trendelenburg position on their left sides if possible, with endotracheal intubation before lavage. The presence of a nasogastric tube does not ensure that a patient's stomach is empty. The tube may not be positioned properly to completely evacuate the stomach, or large particles may be present that cannot be removed by the nasogastric tube.

The use of antacids to reduce gastric acidity does not appear to reduce the mortality from gastric aspiration, probably because of antacid-induced pulmonary toxicity. Recently H_2 receptor blockers such as cimetidine have been demonstrated to raise the pH of gastric secretions acutely in trauma patients requiring surgery. The long-term benefits of this approach remain to be demonstrated.

If pulmonary aspiration is observed, the trachea should be suctioned immediately and a sample of the aspirate checked for pH. Even in the best of circumstances, however, endotracheal suctioning cannot be expected to remove all the aspirate.

Bronchoscopy is indicated for removal of large aspirated particles and for further clearing of the large airways. Irrigation of the tracheobronchial tree with large volumes of neutral or alkaline solution appears to have no beneficial effect and may be harmful, since it may force the aspirate deeper into the terminal airways, increasing the extent of injury. Small amounts of saline may be used to clear the airway, but irrigation with large volumes of fluid should be avoided.

Oxygen should always be administered. Endotracheal intubation and mechanical ventilation are indicated for hypercarbia or in the management of severe hypoxemia that cannot be corrected with oxygen by nasal cannula or face mask. Continuous positive airway pressure or positive-end expiratory pressure (PEEP) is indicated if adequate oxygenation cannot be accomplished by the above means. Both increase functional residual capacity and diminish atelectasis and interstitial edema, resulting in a reduction of ventilation and perfusion inequality. In addition, Cameron and others have shown that PEEP decreases mortality if it is begun within 6 h after aspiration.

Fluid loss into the interstitium and alveoli should be compensated for by adequate volume replacement, generally with crystalloid solution. Despite the clinical finding of wet pulmonary rales, cardiogenic pulmonary edema is usually not present in uncomplicated aspiration pneumonia. Fluid replacement should be guided by changes in central venous pressure, by urine output, and by frequent monitoring of the pulse and blood pressure. If cardiac failure is suspected, it may be necessary to monitor the pulmonary capillary wedge pressure in order to administer fluids safely and effectively.

There are no data clearly indicating the therapeutic value of steroids in aspiration pneumonia. In a study of 43 patients with aspiration, Wolfe et al. found no significant difference in mortality between steroid-treated and nontreated groups. In patients who received steroids, however, the development of gram-negative pneumonia was more frequent. Some advocates favor an initial bolus of 30 mg/kg of methylprednisolone. Preparations with significant mineralocorticoid effects, such as hydrocortisone, are generally avoided.

The effectiveness of prophylactic antibiotic therapy on the eventual outcome of the disease is controversial. Some physicians believe that the patient should be monitored closely and antibiotics instituted when there is clinical evidence of infection. Those who administer steroids generally give antibiotics concurrently. If prophylactic treatment is selected, choose an antibiotic that is effective against the most likely infecting organisms, namely, selected aerobes and anaerobes.

Follow-up supportive care includes appropriate chest physical therapy; humidification and oxygenation; bronchodilators to treat bronchospasm; and serial blood gas determinations.

SUMMARY

Aspiration pneumonia is an inflammatory process caused by aspiration of gastric contents into the tracheobronchial tree. Injury is most severe if the pH of the aspirate is 2.5 or less. Severe injury is characterized by hypoxemia and pulmonary parenchymal destruction.

The hazard of aspiration exists in all patients with a depressed or absent gag reflex. Passage of a nasogastric tube can induce vomiting and aspiration, or it may facilitate aspiration because it renders the esophageal sphincters functionless.

Treatment consists of suctioning and lavage with small amounts of saline. Ventilatory support with the early use of PEEP may be beneficial. The efficacy of prophylactic antibiotics and steroids has not been established.

The opinions and assertions contained herein are the private views of the authors and are not to be construed as those of the Department of the Army or the Department of Defense.

BIBLIOGRAPHY

Arms RA, Dines DE, Tinstman TC: Aspiration pneumonia. *Chest* 65:136–139, 1974.

Bartlett JG, Gorbach SL, Finegold SM: The bacteriology of aspiration pneumonia. *Am J Med* 56:202–207, 1974.

Bynum LJ, Pierce AK: Pulmonary aspiration of gastric contents. *Am Rev Respir Dis* 114:1129–1136, 1976.

Cameron JL, Mitchell WH, Zuidema GD: Aspiration pneumonia: Clinical outcome following documented aspiration. *Arch Surg* 106:49–52, 1973.

Downs JB, Chapman RL Jr, Modell JH, et al: An evaluation of steroid therapy in aspiration pneumonitis. *Anesthesiology* 40:129–135, 1974.

Lorber B, Swenson RM: Bacteriology of aspiration pneumonia: A prospective study of community and hospital-acquired cases. *Ann Intern Med* 81:329–331, 1974.

Mendelson CL: The aspiration of stomach contents into the lungs during obstetric anesthesia. *Am J Obstet Gynecol* 25:191–205, 1946.

Ribaudo CA, Grace WJ: Pulmonary aspiration. *Am J Med* 50:510–520, 1971.

Roberts, RB: Pulmonary aspiration. *Int Anesthesiol Clin* 15:1–147, 1977.

Stewardson RH, Nyhus LM: Pulmonary aspiration. *Arch Surg* 112:1192–1197, 1977.

Wolfe JE, Bone RC, Ruth WE: Effects of corticosteroids in the treatment of patients with gastric aspiration. *Am J Med* 63:719–722, 1977.

Wynne JW, Modell JH: Respiratory aspiration of stomach contents. *Ann Intern Med* 87:466–474, 1977.

CHAPTER 22
ACUTE BRONCHIAL
ASTHMA

Richard M. Nowak

Asthma affects approximately 1 to 3 percent of the U.S. population and has an annual mortality rate of about 1 in 100,000 persons. It affects primarily younger people: one-half of asthma cases develop before age 10 and another one-third occur before age 40. Although asthma mortality is low (2000 per year), the morbidity is enormous.

Asthma is defined as a disease characterized by increased responsiveness of the tracheobronchial tree to various stimuli and manifested by widespread narrowing of the airways that changes in severity either spontaneously or as a result of therapy. This reversibility of airway obstruction must be objectively assessed by quantitating responses to different treatments at various times.

CLASSIFICATION

Asthmatic patients have been divided into those with extrinsic and those with intrinsic disease. Extrinsic asthma is characterized by a well-defined sensitivity to specific inhaled allergens, a personal or family history of multiple allergic diseases, higher levels of IgE in the serum, and positive immediate skin tests. It is usually seasonal in nature, has an onset usually in childhood or early adult life, and is intermittent in nature.

On the other hand, intrinsic asthmatics have no family or personal history of allergies and have normal serum IgE levels and negative immediate skin tests. This type of asthma tends to be perennial, begins in adulthood, and also tends to be more severe in nature than the extrinsic type. It may develop after a patient contracts an upper respiratory viral illness. Also, many different drugs including aspirin and other anti-inflammatory agents, analgesics, and yellow dyes (tartrazines, found in some medications used to treat asthma, such as theophylline compounds and steroid preparations, and in foods) may cause acute bronchospasm. Other causes of intrinsic asthma include the airborne irritants of industrial pollution, physical exercise, and/or simply breathing cold air. Emotional upset has long been known to exacerbate asthmatic attacks, presumably by altering the irritant receptor threshold to a wide variety of environmental stimuli.

The differentiation between the extrinsic or intrinsic variety of the disease does not affect assessment of severity nor response to treatment in the acute episode presenting to the emergency department.

PATHOLOGY

The lungs of patients suffering fatal asthma are uniformly over-distended and contain thick mucus plugs that occlude airway lumens to the level of the terminal bronchioles. On histologic section there is bronchial smooth muscle hypertrophy, edema of the mucosa and submucosa, marked thickening of bronchial basement membrane, and bronchial wall eosinophilic infiltrates. These pathologic features are present to a minor degree in asthmatics dying of nonrespiratory causes and also appear to be identical in both intrinsic and extrinsic asthma.

Pathophysiology of Asthmatic Bronchoconstriction

Traditionally, asthma has been regarded as an allergy-mediated phenomenon in which antigen-induced release of mediators from sensitized respiratory mast cells causes release and/or synthesis of the mediators of anaphylaxis. Histamine, the best studied of these, causes bronchoconstriction and increases vascular permeability. Other mediators include the bradykinins and the leukotrienes [formally referred to as slow-reacting substance of anaphylaxis (SRS-A)]. However, many asthmatics are not atopic and many atopic individuals do not have asthma.

Some investigators believe, however, that the primary problem in acute bronchial asthma is the stimulation of subepithelial tracheobronchial afferent vagal irritant receptors, resulting in a reflex, cholinergically mediated bronchoconstriction. The possible stimuli to these irritant receptors include histamine, viral infections, sulfur dioxide, ozone, and cigarette smoke.

There may be relationships between the mediators released and these abnormal neurogenic responses. For example, it is possible that antigen-antibody complexes may injure the epithelium and stimulate the irritant receptors with the vagal-induced bronchospasm or that the mediators were released by the antigen-antibody complexes and cause stimulation of the irritant receptors primarily. However, both mediator release and autonomic dysfunction probably play a varying integral role in the pathogenesis of both extrinsic and intrinsic asthma.

The influence of the nervous system on airway smooth muscle is becoming better understood (Fig. 22-1). The cholinergic system

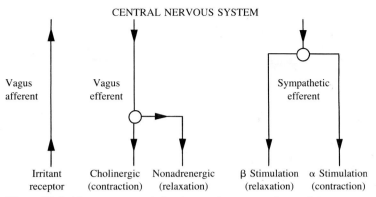

CENTRAL NERVOUS SYSTEM

Vagus afferent   Vagus efferent   Sympathetic efferent

Irritant receptor   Cholinergic (contraction)   Nonadrenergic (relaxation)   β Stimulation (relaxation)   α Stimulation (contraction)

Figure 22-1. Nervous system influence on airway smooth muscle.

constricts bronchial smooth muscle, and indeed normal patients who are taking anticholinesterases may develop some airflow obstruction. Sympathetic nerve stimulation causes little bronchodilatation in the proximal airways and it is most probable that the stimulation of the β_2-adrenergic airway receptors occurs as a result of systemic catecholamines from adrenal secretion. The nonadrenergic inhibitory nerves have been defined and cause airway relaxation, although there is little evidence that these serve a physiologic homeostatic function in antagonizing bronchoconstriction. α-Adrenergic stimulation promotes bronchoconstriction, but significant contractile effects are not observed except under conditions of β-adrenergic blockade.

The final common pathway in regulating bronchomotor tone is determined by the availability of intracellular calcium to the contractile apparatus of the respiratory smooth muscle cell, and hence both mediator and nervous system influence must affect a system or systems that modulate the availability of, or sequestering of, calcium.

Finally, Szentivanyi has developed a theory of β-*adrenergic blockade*. This suggests that the balance between the α- and β-receptor stimuli on bronchial smooth muscle and mast cells is upset by α-receptor-dominated increased bronchial tone and hyperreactivity secondary to a β-adrenergic defect. However, there does not appear to be significant evidence for the existence of a functional α-adrenergic airway control system.

The nonspecific inflammatory reaction seen in asthma is probably related to mucosal damage with resulting increased mucosal permeability. The plugging of the airways is probably secondary to both increased production and decreased clearance of mucus.

In summary, acute bronchial asthma may develop in a variety of different circumstances and is probably mediated to varying degrees by chemicals and/or nervous system influence. It is characterized by airway smooth muscle spasm, airway inflammation with edema, and mucus hypersecretion. The smooth muscle spasm probably accounts for the rapidly reversible types of acute asthma, while the inflammatory edema and mucus plugging of the airway may account for the nonresponsive forms of the disease.

CLINICAL PRESENTATION

The symptoms of an acute asthmatic attack consist of a triad of cough, dyspnea, and wheezing. These attacks often occur at night and are probably related to circadian variation in airway receptor threshold.

The cough is probably secondary to subepithelial vagal stimulation, often starts early, and may be associated with production of sputum and a sense of chest constriction.

Dyspnea is present, although the exact mechanism for its presence is unknown. The wheezing that develops is dependent on air movement velocity and turbulence, and its intensity will vary according to the radius of the bronchial tube. Thus, initially it is a low-pitched, coarse, discontinuous noise, which progresses with increasing airway obstruction to a high-pitched musical but low-intensity sound. Wheezing may disappear with severe airway obstruction because of insufficient velocity of airflow to produce sound. Also, some asthmatics only complain of intermittent episodes of cough and exertional dyspnea without wheeze, and they may represent variant aspects of asthmatic attacks.

ASSESSMENT OF ASTHMA SEVERITY

During an acute asthmatic episode it is important to objectively assess the severity of the airway obstruction in guiding treatment, utilizing either the forced expiratory volume in one second ($FEV_{1.0}$) or the peak expiratory flow rate (PEFR). The clinical modes of asthma assessment are more indirect measures of the problem, and thus are inherently less accurate and may lead to a serious underestimation of the severity of the attack.

History

Patients too dyspneic for speech have severe airway obstruction requiring aggressive therapy while a simultaneous attempt is made to obtain historical data from family and/or friends. The brief history should include the duration and onset of the attack, including recent therapy, the relative severity of this attack, and the previous need for corticosteroids, hospitalization, and the use of mechanical ventilatory support. The type and timing of asthmatic medications must be known in order to gauge current therapy.

Some suggest that the majority of life-threatening attacks evolve over days or weeks, others report progression in less than 24 h, and still others report no definite historical pattern.

Physical Examination

Alterations in consciousness and/or mentation are indicative of severe airway obstruction, but the restlessness and agitation seen are too nonspecific to consistently indicate hypercapnia. The leftward shift of the oxyhemoglobin dissociation curve causes difficulty in appreciating cyanosis. Wheezing is not an indicator of severity, as it does not correlate with any precision to the degree of functional derangement and may in fact be absent when maximal effort produces minimal airflow. Further, it may disappear on stethoscopic examination, with an $FEV_{1.0}$ of less than 60 percent of predicted normal.

A tachycardia of greater than 130 per minute indicates severe airway obstruction ($FEV_{1.0}$ less than or equal to 1 L) but many patients with severe asthma are not tachycardic. Despite treatment with large doses of sympathomimetic agents, the pulse rate drops as the airway obstruction decreases.

Because most patients with acute bronchial asthma are tachypneic and because the degree of tachypnea does not correlate with pulmonary function testing, the usefulness of tachypnea as a predictor of severity of obstruction is limited.

Although the presence of a significant pulsus paradoxus (a greater than 10 mmHg drop in systolic blood pressure during inspiration) signifies severe airway obstruction, its absence occurs in up to 48 percent of patients with an $FEV_{1.0}$ less than 1.0 L and it disappears rapidly with minimal improvement in airflow. Asthmatics who sit up and use their excessory muscles of respiration to lift the entire rib cage cephalad to facilitate breathing have severe asthma. However, the absence of these findings does not rule out severe obstruction ($FEV_{1.0}$ less than 1.0 L).

Laboratory Investigations

Complete Blood Count

The pretreatment white blood count (WBC) is elevated in one-half of cases, the range being 6100 to 28,000. The percentage of neutrophils is raised in one-third, and unless there is suspicion of pneumonia and/or sepsis, the WBC is of little value in the overall assessment. Eosinophilia (more than 350 eosinophils per cubic millimeter in non-steroid-treated patients) indicates probable reversible airway obstruction. However, routine pulmonary function testing is a more specific way to access asthma reversibility.

Sputum Analysis

Expectorated sputum may look purulent when eosinophils alone are present, while white blood cells are seen in up to 97 percent of cases. Examination of a Gram-stained sputum [with fewer than 10 squamous epithelial cells under low power (X100)] may contain Charcot-Leyden crystals (crystallized eosinophilic granules), Curschmann spirals (mucus and debris in the form of bronchiolar casts), and Creola bodies (columnar epithelial cells in clusters).

Chest Radiographs

Chest radiographs should be obtained when there is clinical suspicion of pneumonia or complications of asthma. They also should be obtained in patients who do not respond to optimal aggressive therapy because they are at risk of having unsuspected pulmonary collapse or consolidation.

Arterial Blood Gases

Many authors have demonstrated a poor correlation between arterial blood gases and asthma severity as measured by pulmonary function testing, which results in an inability to accurately predict the outcome. While it is true that more severe obstruction is manifest by normalization and eventual elevation of arterial P_{CO_2} with worsening of arterial hypoxemia, these situations can be identified by specific pulmonary function guidelines. Carbon dioxide retention and worsening hypoxemia develop when the $FEV_{1.0}$ drops to less than 1.0 L (less than 25 percent of predicted normal) or a PEFR to less than 200 L/min (less than 30 percent predicted normal). Blood gas analysis should be performed only on young asthmatics (age 16 to 40) who meet these criteria. For the very young or the older asthmatic, the decision to utilize arterial blood gases is a clinical one.

There are patients with severe airway obstruction who have relatively normal blood gases. These patients have severe airway obstruction not reflected in currently utilized severity scales. Further, repeat blood gas analysis after the identification of carbon dioxide retention and severe hypoxemia is unnecessary as long as the pulmonary function testing has improved to above the limits previously set.

Electrocardiogram

The electrocardiogram may show changes of right ventricular strain in 30 to 40 percent of patients; right axis deviation, clockwise rotation, and right-bundle branch block pattern being the most common findings. These reversible changes are seen in well-oxygenated hypocapnic patients, which suggests some etiology other than hypoxemia and/or hypocapnia. These changes should be thought of as an indicator of increased asthma severity but are not a contraindication to sympathomimetic therapy. All older patients, especially those with a history of heart disease, should have cardiac monitoring during therapy.

Pulmonary Function Testing

The PEFR and/or $FEV_{1.0}$ are the best tests for assessing asthma severity and responsiveness to treatment. The PEFR is a much easier study to carry out in a busy emergency department but it is effort- and volume-dependent.

The PEFR and/or $FEV_{1.0}$ are the key parameters for assessing severity of airway obstruction, β-adrenergic responsiveness and, thus, asthma resistance, and appropriate disposition after completion of therapy. Those patients with severe and nonresponsive asthma require admission or very closely monitored outpatient therapy (Table 22-1). Therapy should continue until the PEFR is greater than 300 L/min (60 percent of predicted normal) or the $FEV_{1.0}$ is greater than 2.1 L (60 percent of predicted normal) regardless of apparent clinical improvement. Resistant asthma can be identified by the responsiveness to initial sympathomimetic therapy. Thus, those patients with severe asthma and an initial PEFR less than or equal to 100 L/min ($FEV_{1.0}$ less than 0.7 L) who show improvement less than or equal to 60 L/min (0.3 L) 15 min after the initial sympathomimetic injection require early aggressive treatment, including corticosteroid administration, and will often require inpatient management (Table 22-1).

Table 22-1. Pulmonary Function Testing Criteria for Admission/Very Close Outpatient Follow-up (A) and for Early Aggressive Therapy (B).

A. ADMISSION/CLOSE OUTPATIENT FOLLOW-UP

	Pretreatment and posttreatment
PEFR (L/min)	< 100 and < 300
$FEV_{1.0}$ (L)	< 0.7 and < 2.1

B. EARLY AGGRESSIVE THERAPY

	Pretreatment and response to terbutaline (0.25 mg subcutaneous)
PEFR (L/min)	< 100 and < 60
$FEV_{1.0}$ (L)	< 0.7 and < 0.3

In older patients (over 40 years) or the young (less than 16 years) similar criteria are not available and clinical judgment and arterial blood gas analysis must be used.

Fischl et al. have developed an index scoring system to assess the severity of acute asthma. According to this index, a value of 1 is given for a pulse rate greater than or equal to 120, respiratory rate greater than or equal to 30, pulsus paradoxus greater than or equal to 18 mmHg, PEFR less than or equal to 120 L/min, dyspnea of moderate severity or greater, accessory muscle use of moderate degree or greater, and wheezing of moderate severity or worse. This results in a maximal score of 7, scores of 4 or higher being 95 percent accurate in predicting the risk of relapse within 10 days in patients discharged from the emergency department and 96 percent accurate in predicting the need for hospitalization after 12 h or less of emergency care. However, the weakness of the index lies in a reliance on subjective components; it does not allow for assessment of response to therapy, does not give directions for treatment, and has not been prospectively verified.

DIFFERENTIAL DIAGNOSIS

In treating patients who wheeze it is wise to remember that all that wheezes is not asthma. The following is a listing of problems that can mimic acute asthma.

1. Acute left ventricular failure (''cardiac asthma'')
2. Upper airway obstruction (laryngeal edema, neoplasm, foreign body inhalation)
3. Acute exacerbation of chronic obstructive pulmonary disease (COPD) or chronic bronchitis
4. Endobronchial disease (neoplasm, foreign body aspiration, bronchial stenosis)
5. Chemical irritants, insecticides, and cholinergic drugs
6. Pulmonary embolus (4 percent of cases)
7. Carcinoid tumors (20 to 30 percent of cases)
8. Allergic or anaphylactic reactions
9. Eosinophilic pneumonias
10. Invasive worm infestations

TREATMENT OF THE ACUTE ATTACK

Adrenergic Stimulants

Adrenergic agents bind to cell receptors leading to either α stimulation (vasoconstriction, uterine contraction, and bronchocon-

striction, especially under conditions of β-adrenergic blockade) and/or β excitation. While β_1 agonists produce a chronotropic and inotropic effect on the heart, β_2 agonists produce vasodilatation, bronchodilatation, and uterine smooth muscle relaxation. The effects on the bronchi are thought to be mediated through increased intracellular cyclic adenosine 3'5'-monophosphate (cAMP) secondary to the activation of the enzyme adenyl cyclase.

Subcutaneous Administration

Epinephrine

Epinephrine hydrochloride (adrenaline) has both α and β action but with β predominance. In the treatment of acute asthma, the usual subcutaneous adult dose is 0.2 to 0.5 mL of a 1:1000 aqueous solution repeated in 20 to 30 min for a total of three doses. The onset occurs in 5 to 10 min with a peak at 20 min and a duration of action of up to 3 h. Recent studies suggest that the bronchodilating effect steadily increases for up to 40 min after administration, and thus repeated doses prior to this time may be harmful, especially in the elderly. Tolerance or complete refraction may develop with repeated use in severe resistant asthma, especially if the patient is acidotic. Epinephrine should be used very cautiously in the cardiac or hypertensive patient.

A more sustained action is obtained by utilizing a 1:200 aqueous suspension of epinephrine in thioglycolate (Sus-Phrine) at a usual adult subcutaneous dose of 0.1 to 0.3 mL.

Terbutaline

Terbutaline hydrochloride is a β_2-specific, longer-acting (4 h) adrenergic drug given in a dose of 0.25 mg subcutaneously, which may be repeated in 30 to 60 min if necessary. Its bronchodilating effect equals that of epinephrine and its side effects include tremor and tachycardia.

Aerosolized Administration

Aerosols are becoming the mainstay of maintenance therapy and treatment for acute exacerbations of bronchial asthma, even if severe. Aerosolized adrenergic bronchodilators are as effective as those intravenously administered but have much less potential for side effects because of their topical administration.

The employment of intermittent positive pressure breathing for administration of these aerosolized agents has not been demonstrated to be superior to simple nebulization, and the positive inspiratory pressure delivered may act as an airway irritant to cause reflex bronchoconstriction or, worse yet, a tension pneumothorax.

Epinephrine

Epinephrine in pressurized aerosol form is currently available as a nonprescription medication (Primatene, Bronkaid). Its relatively short duration of action coupled with both α and β_1 stimulation make it a less than optimal agent for treatment of acute bronchial asthma. Also, there is potential for the development of serious resistance after repeated inhalation of epinephrine.

Table 22-2. Newer Sympathomimetic Agents for Use in Acute Bronchial Asthma

Agent	Availability*	α	Adrenergic Effects* β₁	β₂
			β_1	β_2
Catecholamines				
Isoetharine hydrochloride	N,M	0	+ +	+ + +
Resorcinols				
Terbutaline sulfate	S	0	+	+ + +
Metaproterenol sulfate	N,M	0	+	+ + +
Fenoterol	NA	0	+	+ + +
Saligenins				
Albuterol	M	0	+	+ + +

*N = nebulizer solution; M = metered-dose inhaler; S = solution for subcutaneous injection; NA = not available in the U.S.; 0 = none; + = slight; + + = moderate; + + + = notable.

Source: Adapted from George DB: Some recent advances in the management of asthma. *Arch Intern Med* 142: 933–935, 1982.

Isoproterenol

Isoproterenol hydrochloride (Isuprel) is the most potent of the sympathomimetic amines acting on β receptors and has the greatest therapeutic value as an aerosol. It is available as a Mistometer or as a solution (1:200 or 1:100) for inhalation therapy. The major problems associated with its use include: (1) β₁ cardiac stimulation, causing cardioacceleration and arrhythmias; (2) hypoxemia secondary to pulmonary vasculature dilatation and intrapulmonary shunting; (3) short duration of action (1 to 3 h); and (4) psychological dependency that may lead to significant abuse.

Because of these problems, the following newer longer-acting compounds, with more β₂ and less β₁ and α-stimulation, were developed (Table 22-2).

Isoetharine Hydrochloride

Although less potent than isoproterenol, isoetharine has more β₂ selectivity and lesser side effects. Maximal bronchodilatation is obtained in 5 to 15 min following inhalation, and subsequently the effect progressively declines to undetectable levels in 1 to 2 h.

Noncatecholamine β-Agonists

These agents are only slightly less rapid in onset of action than isoproterenol, with 75 percent of maximum effect obtained in 5 min. The peak bronchodilatation occurs between 30 and 90 min after inhalation, with little loss of effect until after 4 h. When these agents are given by inhalation in recommended doses, side effects are very uncommon. Recently metaproterenol, 5% solution, has been released in the United States for aerosolized administration in acute asthma (at a dose of 0.2 to 0.3 mL or 10 to 15 mg active ingredient, diluted with saline to 2.5 mL).

Although terbutaline sulfate is not approved for use in the United States, it has been extensively studied elsewhere at a dosage of 0.5 to 1.5 mg every 6 h by aerosol.

Albuterol (salbutamol), used extensively in other parts of the world, has recently become available in a metered-dose inhaler in the United States. The metered-dose device delivers 100 to 200 μg and is effective with minimal side effects. It appears that clinically important tolerance to inhaled albuterol does not develop unless overusage occurs.

Theophylline

Theophylline is a naturally occurring methylxanthine alkaloid. It is a competitive inhibitor of phosphodiesterase and prevents breakdown of the cAMP which mediates smooth muscle relaxation. Because it differs in action from the adrenergic agents, it would theoretically be expected to act synergistically with these drugs in causing bronchodilatation. However, the bronchodilating response in acute asthma to repeated doses of injected epinephrine or inhaled β agonists has been compared with the response to conventional loading and maintenance infusions of aminophylline, and there is general agreement that the response to the adrenergic agents by either route is superior to the response to aminophylline. Thus, some physicians recommend initial treatment with inhalation therapy utilizing the β₂-adrenergic agents. Further, those with severe asthma would be treated with intravenous aminophylline because of its additive bronchodilating effect, even though this may be quite small.

Since detailed pharmacokinetic studies of this drug and the resulting rational guidelines for loading and maintenance dosages in a variety of clinical situations have become available (Table 22-3), its use has markedly increased since 1973. Also, simple and reliable theophylline assays have been developed for monitoring serum levels in the therapeutic range of 10 to 20 μg/mL. If theophylline monitoring is unavailable and the patient has been taking oral theophylline preparations at home, some practitioners recommend decreasing the loading dose by 50 percent and others advise utilizing maintenance infusions alone. The maintenance infusions would depend on the clinical situation (Table 22-3). The only intravenous preparation available is aminophylline (theophylline ethylene diamine), which contains about 80% theophylline by weight.

The side effects of aminophylline include nausea, vomiting, abdominal cramps and diarrhea, cardiac arrhythmias, nervousness, headache, and grand mal seizures. The risk of these cardiac and neurologic toxic effects increases greatly with increasing levels above therapeutic. The presence of gastrointestinal upset correlates poorly with the serum level and should not be used to determine the presence or absence of toxicity.

Table 22-3. Guidelines for Intravenous Aminophylline Dosages for Treatment of Acute Bronchial Asthma

Loading dose (based on actual body weight)	5.6 mg/kg (over 20 min, peripheral IV)
Maintenance infusion (based on ideal body weight)	
Children to age 18	1.0 mg/kg/h
Adult smokers under 50	0.9 mg/kg/h
Adult nonsmokers under 50	0.5 mg/kg/h
Adults over 50	0.4 mg/kg/h
COPD, acute viral illness	0.6–0.7 mg/kg/h
Congestive heart failure	0.35–0.68 mg/kg/h
Liver dysfunction	0.25–0.45 mg/kg/h

Parasympathetic Antagonists

Recently, the development of ipratropium bromide, a quaternary isopropyl derivative of atropine, has brought about renewed interest in the anticholinergic therapy of asthma. The relative bronchoselectivity of this drug when given by the aerosol route is secondary to its poor lipid solubility and thus its minimal absorption across biologic membranes. This minimizes the undesirable side effects of atropine. Both inhalation ipratropium bromide (40 μg) and atropine methyl nitrate (1 to 2 mg) are effective, long-acting bronchodilators in acute asthma, alone or in combination with adrenergics, theophylline, and/or steroids. The effect of these parasympathetic antagonists occurs through a decrease in the concentration of cyclic guanosine monophosphate, resulting in bronchodilatation. This is exciting, as it is a completely separate physiologic pathway to bronchodilatation. However, the appropriate setting for routine use of anticholinergic medications in acute asthma needs to be defined before these agents replace currently effective treatment modalities.

Corticosteroids

Although there is ongoing debate concerning the usefulness of intravenous corticosteroids in acute asthma, it is still standard practice to administer intravenous steroids in resistant severe asthma and also to steroid-dependent asthmatics with an acute exacerbation. Because there is a lag time from administration to peak effect on pulmonary function, intravenous steroids should be administered as soon as the diagnosis of severe resistant asthma is made. This can be ascertained quickly by noting an initial $FEV_{1.0}$ less than or equal to 0.7 L (PEFR less than or equal to 100 L/min) and an improvement less than or equal to 0.3 L in $FEV_{1.0}$ (less than or equal to 60 L/min in PEFR) 15 min after initial subcutaneous β-agonist therapy. Recommended doses vary from 20 mg to more than 500 mg of methylprednisolone (or the equivalent) initially, to be repeated every 4 to 8 h with tapering off after the patient's pulmonary function shows improvement on testing. Such patients' problems consist of both smooth muscle contraction and mucosal edema with inflammation and thus require steroids as soon as possible.

There is no place in the treatment of acute bronchial asthma for inhaled steroids of high topical potency.

Other Treatments

Other Medications

Cromolyn sodium has no use in the treatment of an acute asthmatic attack. However, if the patient is receiving this medication and develops an acute exacerbation that does not subside quickly with therapy, the drug should be continued until airway obstruction is controlled.

Narcotics, sedatives, and tranquilizers are to be avoided in the acutely ill asthmatic as these patients are very vulnerable to depression of alveolar ventilation, with possible subsequent respiratory arrest. Anxiety should be treated with prompt reassurance by the physician, who should keep in mind that the etiologic agent may be hypoxemia and/or toxic levels of theophylline or β-adrenergic agents.

Expectorants add little to the therapy of acute asthma, and in fact acetylcysteine can produce bronchospasm in susceptible patients.

Viral infections are more common than bacterial infections and therefore routine use of antibiotics for all acute asthmatics seems excessive. However, the judicious use of antibiotics during winter months may decrease asthma accompanying respiratory infections in children.

While antihistamines are useful in allergic rhinitis they are relatively ineffective in asthma.

Hydration, Bicarbonate, and Oxygen

Most asthmatics are hypovolemic as a result of increased insensible water loss, diuretic drug effect, and poor oral intake. Consequently adequate hydration, taking into account the patient's cardiovascular status, will aid in sputum liquefaction with prevention of increased mucus plugging. Acidosis does depress the bronchodilating effect of β-adrenergic agents and this has resulted in recommendations to treat any pH below 7.25 with sodium bicarbonate. The best way to treat respiratory acidosis is by improving alveolar ventilation even if this necessitates tracheal intubation and assisted ventilation. However, with hypercarbia due to resistant disease, correcting the pH with bicarbonate while maintaining oxygenation may be preferable to barotrauma from high ventilator airway pressures. Adequate oxygenation must be maintained during therapy but supplemental oxygen appears to be only necessary in those patients with severe airway obstruction as defined by a PEFR less than 200 L/min or an $FEV_{1.0}$ less than 1.0 L.

Assisted Mechanical Ventilation

Although relatively uncommon, intubation and assisted mechanical ventilation may be life-saving maneuvers in the treatment of acute bronchial asthma. With the exception of apnea and/or coma there are no absolute criteria for the immediate institution of ventilatory support. Persistent hypercarbia or elevating arterial P_{CO_2} values, obviously exhausted patients, and continued poor or decreasing pulmonary function testing values aid decision-making concerning ventilatory support.

If intubation is necessary, stimulation of the mucus membrane nerve endings in the pharynx, larynx, or trachea by tube or laryngoscope may cause vagally mediated reflexes such as apnea, laryngospasm, further bronchospasm, and cardiac arrhythmias and/or bradycardia. These do occur more often in the awake, lightly anesthetized, and poorly oxygenated patient and can be treated with atropine.

Volume-cycled respirators with high pressure and flow capability are preferred to ensure adequate tidal volume (10 to 12 mL/kg, 10 to 12 respirations per minute) against changing resistance. Further, a relatively shorter inspiratory time, allowing a longer expiratory portion for lung emptying, meets the needs of most patients. Patients should be allowed to cycle the ventilator and if pain or restlessness is troublesome, analgesics such as meperidine or sedatives such as diazepam may be given. If there is continuing difficulty in ventilating the patient after these maneuvers, then muscle paralysis may be considered. Pancuronium bromide (Pavulon, 0.04 mg/kg intravenously) is preferred to d-tubocurarine in asthmatic patients as it does not cause histamine release.

Asthma and Pregnancy

Asthma affects approximately 1 percent of pregnant women, of whom one-third remain stable during pregnancy, one-third improve, and one-third have a worsening of their asthma. In practice, pregnant asthmatic patients are treated pharmacologically very much like nonpregnant asthmatics, with the exception that since some of the new β_2 specific agents lack clinical trials of any magnitude in the pregnant asthmatic, the ratio of benefit to potential risk must be weighed prior to their use. Also, the effects of the high intravenous corticosteroid dosages employed in severe resistant asthma have not as yet been fully evaluated in the pregnant patient.

Discharge Medications

Successfully discharged asthmatics have a relatively large reservoir of persistent peripheral airway obstruction. This requires continuous outpatient therapy over the next 4 to 5 days in spite of subjective improvements. This may include the longer-acting sustained-release anhydrous theophylline preparations, oral selective β_2 agonists, adrenergic aerosols, and in some cases corticosteroids. These drugs must be individualized for discharged patients in order to optimize patients' response once they leave the emergency department.

BIBLIOGRAPHY

American Thoracic Society: Definitions and classifications of chronic bronchitis, asthma and pulmonary emphysema. *Am Rev Respir Dis* 85:762–768, 1962.

Appel D, Shim C: Comparative effect of epinephrine and aminophylline in the treatment of asthma. *Lung* 159:243–254, 1981.

Arnaud A, Vervloet D, Dugue P, et al: Treatment of acute asthma. Effect of intravenous corticosteroids and beta 2 adrenergic agonists. *Lung* 156:43–48, 1979.

Arnold AG, Lane DJ, Zapata E: The speed of onset and severity of acute severe asthma. *Br J Dis Chest* 76:157–163, 1982.

Avery WG: Maximizing spirometry in reversible airways disease. *Ann Allergy* 47:410–414, 1981.

Bachus BF, Snider GL: The bronchodilator effects of aerosolized terbutaline. *JAMA* 238:2277–2281, 1977.

Banner AS, Shah RS, Addington WW: Rapid prediction of need for hospitalization in acute asthma. *JAMA* 235:1337–1338, 1976.

Barnes PJ, Wilson NM, Vickers H: Prazosin, an alpha₁-adrenoceptor antagonist, partially inhibits exercise-induced asthma. *J Allergy Clin Immunol* 68:411–415, 1981.

Beck GJ: Controlled clinical trial of a new dosage form of metaproterenol. *Ann Allergy* 44:19–22, 1980.

Bedell GN, Richardson RA: Safety and efficacy of albuterol aerosol in the relief of bronchospasm. *Ann Allergy* 47:392–393, 1981.

Ben-Zvi Z, Lam C, Hoffman J, et al: An evaluation of the initial treatment of acute asthma. *Pediatrics* 70:348–353, 1982.

Boggs PB, Stephens AL, Bhat KD, et al: A classification system for asthmatic patients. Clinical-physiological correlation. *Ann Allergy* 47:307–310, 1981.

Branscomb BV: Metaproterenol solution in the treatment of asthmatic patients by intermittent positive pressure breathing. *J Clin Pharmacol* 22:231–235, 1982.

Brenner BE: Bronchial asthma in adults: Pathogenesis, clinical manifestations, diagnostic evaluation and differential diagnosis. *Am J Emerg Med* 1:50–70, 1983.

Brenner BE: Bronchial asthma in adults: Treatment, acute respiratory failure, and recommendations. *Am J Emerg Med* 1 3:306–333, 1983.

Brown LA, Sly M: Comparison of Mini-Wright and Standard-Wright peak flow meters. *Ann Allergy* 45:72–74, 1980.

Cabezas GA, Graf PD, Nadel JA: Sympathetic versus parasympathetic nervous regulation of airways in dogs. *J Appl Physiol* 31:651–655, 1971.

Carden DL, Nowak RM, Sarkar D, et al: Vital signs including pulsus paradoxus in the assessment of acute bronchial asthma. *Ann Emerg Med* 12:80–83, 1983.

Cerrina J, Denjean A, Alexandre G, et al: Inhibition of exercise-induced asthma by a calcium antagonist, nifedipine. *Am Rev Respir Dis* 123:156–160, 1981.

Chervinsky P: Sixty day trial of a new inhalant dosage form of metaproterenol. *Ann Allergy* 38:107–111, 1977.

Chester EH, Racz L, Barlow PB, et al: Bronchodilator therapy: Comparison of acute response to three methods of administration. *Chest* 62:394–399, 1972.

Collins JV, Clark TJH, Harris PWR, et al: Intravenous corticosteroids in treatment of acute bronchial asthma. *Lancet* 2:1047–1049, 1970.

Cooke NJ, Crompton GK, Grant WB: Observations on the management of acute bronchial asthma. *Br J Dis Chest* 73:157–162, 1979.

Davis B, Gett PM, Sherwood JE: A service for adult asthmatics. *Thorax* 35:111–113, 1980.

Dolovich M, Ruffin RE, Roberts R, et al: Optimal delivery of aerosols from metered dose inhalers. *Chest* 80:911s–915s, 1981.

Dunnill MS: The pathology of asthma with special reference to changes in the bronchial mucosa. *J. Clin Pathol* 13:27–32, 1960.

Ellul-Micallef R, Fenech FF: Intravenous prednisone in chronic bronchial asthma. *Thorax* 30:312–315, 1975.

Elwood RK, Abboud RT: The short-term bronchodilator effects of fenoterol and iprotropium in asthma. *J Allergy Clin Immunol* 69:476–483, 1982.

Emermann CL, Nowak RM, Tomlanovich MC, et al: Theophylline concentrations in the emergency treatment of acute bronchial asthma: A lack of correlation with pulmonary function testing history of prior use and side effects. *Am J Emerg Med* 1:12–16, 1983.

Fairshter RD, Habib MP, Wilson AF: Inhaled atropine sulfate in acute asthma. *Respiration* 42:263–272, 1981.

Falliers CJ: Acute effects of albuterol aerosol in reversible obstructive airway disease. *Ann Allergy* 47:387–391, 1981.

Fanta CH, Rossing TH, McFadden ER: Emergency room treatment of asthma. Relationships among therapeutic combinations, severity of obstruction and time course of response. *Am J Med* 72:416–422, 1982.

Findley LJ, Sahn SA: The value of the chest roentgenogram in acute asthma in adults. *Chest* 80:535–536, 1981.

Fischl MA, Pitchenik A, Gardner LB: An index predicting relapse and need for hospitalization in patients with acute asthma. *N Engl J Med* 305:783–789, 1981.

Georg J: The treatment of status asthmaticus. *Allergy* 36:219–232, 1981.

George DB: Some recent advances in the management of asthma. *Arch Intern Med* 142:933–935, 1982.

George RB, Jenkinson SG, Light RW: Clinical effects of albuterol aerosol in the treatment of asthma. *Ann Allergy* 47:384–386, 1981.

Godfrey S: Worldwide experience with albuterol (salbutamol). *Ann Allergy* 47:423–426, 1981.

Gotz VP, Brandstetter RD, Mar DD: Bronchodilatory effect of subcutaneous epinephrine in acute asthma. *Ann Emerg Med* 10:518–520, 1981.

Gotz VP, Brandstetter RD, Mar DD: Subcutaneous epinephrine for acute asthma.

Hargreave FE, Dolovich J: Nonspecific bronchial responsiveness. *Chest* 82:23s–23s, 1982.

Hetzel MR, Clark TJ, Branthwaite MA: Asthma: Analysis of sudden deaths and ventilatory arrests in hospital. *Br Med J* 1:808–811, 1977.

Hiller FC, Wilson FJ: Evaluation and management of acute asthma. *Med Clin N Am* 67:669–684, 1983.

Hogg JC: The pathophysiology of asthma. *Chest* 82:8s–12s, 1982.

Hore PM: Asthma: The value of peak flow monitoring. *NZ Med J* 95:458–460, 1982.

Interactions between methylxanthines and beta adrenergic agonists. *FDA Drug Bull* 11:19–20, 1981.

Ishikawa S, Linzmayer I, Segal MS: Gas exchange and arterial blood gas tensions to terbutaline sulfate in older patients with reversible airway obstruction. *Ann Allergy* 39:303–305, 1977.

Isles AF, MacLeod SM, Levison H: Theophylline. New thoughts about an old drug. *Chest* 82:49s–54s, 1982.

I.V. dosage guidelines for theophylline products. *FDA Drug Bull* 10:4–6, 1980.

Jenne JW: A critique of dosing strategies for beta 2 adrenergic agents and theophylline. *Lung* 159:295–314, 1981.

Josephson GW, Mackenzie EJ, Lietman PS, et al: Emergency treatment of asthma: A comparison of two treatment regimes. *JAMA* 242:639–643, 1979.

Karentzky MS: Asthma mortality associated with pneumothorax and intermittent positive pressure breathing. *Lancet* 1:828–829, 1975.

Kelson SG, Kelson DF, Fleegler BF, et al: Emergency room assessment and treatment of patients with acute asthma. Adequacy of the conventional approach. *Am J Med* 64:622–628, 1978.

Kirkpatrick CH, Keller C: Impaired responsiveness to epinephrine in asthma. *Am Rev Respir Dis* 96:692–699, 1967.

Klaustermeyer WB, Hale FC: The physiologic effect of an intravenous glucocorticoid in bronchial asthma. *Ann Allergy* 37:80–86, 1976.

Knowles GK, Clark TJ: Pulsus paradoxus as a valuable sign indicating severity of asthma. *Lancet* 2:1356–1359, 1973.

Kreisman H, Frank H. Wolkove N: Synergism between ipratropium and theophylline in asthma. *Thorax* 36:387–391, 1981.

Larsson S, Svedmyr N: Bronchodilating effects and side effects of beta 2 adrenoreceptor stimulants by different modes of administration (tablets, metered aerosol and combination thereof). *Ann Respir Dis* 166:861–870, 1977.

Leff A: Pathophysiology of asthmatic bronchoconstriction. *Chest* 83:13s–21s, 1982.

Lilker ES: Asthma is a disease. A new theory of pathogenesis. *Chest* 82:263–265, 1982.

Martin TG, Elebaas RM, Pingleton SH: Use of peak expiratory flow rates to eliminate unnecessary arterial blood gases in acute asthma. *Ann Emerg Med* 11:70–73, 1982.

McCombs RP, Lowell FC, Ohman JL: Myths, morbidity and mortality in asthma. *JAMA* 242:1521–1524, 1979.

McFadden ER, Kiser R, DeGroot WJ: Acute bronchial asthma. Relationships between clinical and physiologic manifestations. *N Engl J Med* 288:221–225, 1973.

McFadden ER, Kiser R, DeGroot WJ, et al: A controlled study of the effects of single doses of hydrocortisone on the resolution of acute attacks of asthma. *Am J Med* 60:52–59, 1976.

McFadden ER, Lyons HA: Arterial blood gases in asthma. *N Engl J Med* 278:1027–1032, 1968.

Morrill CG, Dickey DW, Weiser PC, et al: Calibration and stability of standard and Mini-Wright peak flow meters. *Ann Allergy* 46:70–73, 1981.

Newhouse MT: Principles of aerosol therapy. *Chest* 82:39s–41s, 1982.

Nelson, HS: Beta adrenergic agonists. *Chest* 82:33s–38s, 1982.

Nicklas RA, Whitehurst VE, Donohoe RF: Combined use of beta-adrenergic agonists and methyl xanthines. *N Engl J Med* 307:557–558, 1982.

Nowak RM: Acute bronchial asthma. *Emerg Med Clin N Am* 1 1:279–293, 1983.

Nowak RM, Gordon KR, Wroblewski, DA, et al: Spirometric evaluation of acute bronchial asthma. *J Am Coll Emerg Phys* 8:9–12, 1979.

Nowak RM, Pensler MI, Sarkar DD, et al: Comparison of peak expiratory flow and FEV_1 admission criteria for acute bronchial asthma. *Ann Emerg Med* 11:64–69, 1982.

Nowak RM, Tomlanovich MC, Sarkar DD, et al: The usefulness of arterial blood gas analysis in acute bronchial asthma. The need for specific pulmonary function testing guidelines. *JAMA* 249:2043–2046, 1983.

Orehek J, Gayrard P, Grimaud CH, et al: Patient error in use of bronchodilator metered aerosols. *Br Med J* 1:76, 1976.

Ormerod LP, Stableforth DE: Asthma mortality in Birmingham 1975–1977: 53 deaths. *Br Med J* 1:687–690, 1980.

Patel KR: Calcium antagonists in exercise-induced asthma. *Br Med J* 28:932–933, 1981.

Patterson JC, Crompton GK: Use of pressurized aerosols by asthmatic patients. *Br Med J* 1:76–77, 1976.

Perks WH, Tams IP, Thompson DA, et al: An evaluation of the Mini-Wright peak flow meter. *Thorax* 34:79–81, 1979.

Petheram IS, Kerr IH, Collins JV: Value of chest radiographs in severe acute asthma. *Clin Radiol* 32:281–282, 1981.

Petty, TL: A critical look at IPPB. *Chest* 66:1–3, 1974.

Pierce RJ, Holmes PW, Campbell AH: Use of ipratropium bromide in patients with severe airways obstruction. *Aust N Z Med* 12:43–47, 1982.

Pierce RJ, Payne CR, Williams SJ: Comparison of intravenous and inhaled terbutaline in the treatment of asthma. *Chest* 79:506–511, 1981.

Pierson WE, Bierman CW, Kelley VC: A double-blind trial of corticosteroid therapy in status asthmaticus. *Pediatrics* 54:282–288, 1974.

Pliss LB, Gallagher EJ: Aerosol vs. injected epinephrine in acute asthma. *Ann Emerg Med* 10:353–355, 1981.

Pratt HF: Abuse of salbutamol inhalers in young people. *Clin Allergy* 12:203–208, 1982.

Rebuck AS, Chapman KR, Braude AC: Anticholinergic therapy of asthma. *Chest* 82:55s–57s, 1982.

Rebuck AS, Read J: Assessment and management of severe asthma. *Am J Med* 51:788–798, 1971.

Rossing TH, Fanta CH, Goldstein DH, et al: Emergency therapy of asthma: Comparisons of the acute effects of parenteral and inhaled sympathomimetics and infused aminophylline. *Am Rev Respir Dis* 122:365–371, 1980.

Rossing TH, Fanta CH, McFadden ER: A controlled trial of the use of single versus combined drug therapy in the treatment of acute episodes of asthma. *Am Rev Respir Dis* 123:190–194, 1981.

Roth NJ, Wilson AF, Havey HS: A comparative study of the aerosolized bronchodilators isoproterenol, metaproterenol and terbutaline in asthma. *Ann Allerg* 38:16–21, 1977.

Rothstein RJ: Intravenous theophylline therapy in asthma: A clinical update. *An Emerg Med* 9:327–330, 1980.

Sackner MA, Silva G: Effects of terbutaline aerosol in reversible airway obstruction. *Chest* 73:802–806, 1978.

Saunders NA, McFadden ER: Asthma—an update. *Disease-A-Month* 24:1–49, 1978.

Shenfield GM, Hodson ME, Clarke SW, et al: Interaction of corticosteroids and catecholamines in the treatment of asthma. *Thorax* 30:430–435, 1975.

Smith AP: Patterns of recovery from acute severe asthma. *Br J Dis Chest* 75:132–140, 1981.

Smith PR, Hevrich AE, Leffler CT, et al: A comparative study of subcutaneously administered terbutaline and epinephrine in the treatment of acute bronchial asthma. *Chest* 71:129–131, 1977.

Stellman JL, Spicer JE, Cayton RM: Morbidity from chronic asthma. *Thorax* 37:218–221, 1982.

Stewart CJ, Nunn AJ, Stableforth D, et al: Deaths in asthma: Disease of treatment. *Lancet* 2:747, 1981.

Strauss RH, McFadden ER, Ingram RH, et al: Enhancement of exercise induced asthma by cold air. *N Engl J Med* 297:743–746, 1977.

Szentivanyi A: The beta adrenergic therapy of the atopic abnormality in bronchial asthma. *J Allergy* 42:203–232, 1968.

Tai E, Read J: Blood-gas tensions in bronchial asthma. *Lancet* 1:644–646, 1967.

Van Arsdel PP, Glennon HP: Drug therapy in the management of asthma. *Ann Intern Med* 87:68–74, 1977.

Van As A: The accuracy of peak expiratory flow meters. *Chest* 82:263, 1982.

Webb-Johnson DC, Andrews JL: Bronchodilator therapy. *New Engl J Med* 297:476–482, 1977.

Weber RW, Petty WE, Nelson HS: Aerosolized terbutaline in asthmatics. *J Allergy Clin Immunol* 63:116–121, 1979.

Weinberger MW, Matthay RA, Ginchansky EJ, et al: Intravenous aminophylline dosage. *JAMA* 235:2110–2113, 1976.

Williams MH: Evaluation of asthma. *Chest* 76:3–4, 1979.

Williams SJ, Winner SJ, Clark TJH: Comparison of inhaled and intravenous terbutaline in acute severe asthma. *Thorax* 36:629–631, 1981.

CHAPTER 23
CHRONIC OBSTRUCTIVE
PULMONARY DISEASE

James Mathews

Chronic obstructive pulmonary disease (COPD) represents one of the major health problems in the United States. It accounts for more than 30,000 deaths annually and is responsible for a staggering amount of absenteeism. It represents the second highest cause of disability for male American workers, being preceded only by atherosclerotic heart disease. COPD frequently complicates the management and course of otherwise benign medical and surgical problems. Patients suffering from this disease complex frequently appear in the emergency department, often in severe distress, and represent a difficult management problem. The complications of both COPD and its therapy are life-threatening and must be dealt with rapidly and effectively.

CAUSES AND PREDISPOSING FACTORS

The majority of cases of COPD could be prevented by elimination of cigarette smoking. COPD in its full-blown state is seldom seen in nonsmokers. Even after the appearance of marked changes in the lungs, much can be reversed by cessation of smoking. Pipe and cigar smokers are also at a greater risk than nonsmokers, but their risk is less than that of cigarette users.

There are many other factors related to the development of COPD. Most common are environmental risks, particularly various types of industrial and vegetable dusts. Alone, their effect on the lungs seldom causes severe changes, but combined with cigarette smoking these agents produce serious lung disease, often at early ages.

Another cause of end-stage COPD is long-standing asthma with repeated respiratory infections. Even though most acute asthma is reversible between episodes, repeated attacks can result in the changes that gradually lead to COPD. Avoidance of causes of acute attacks, effective treatment, and strict avoidance of cigarettes by these patients are mandatory to prevent this entity.

Air pollution has not been proved to cause COPD. Long-term cigarette smokers who live in polluted environments have a higher incidence of COPD. Air pollution may induce acute exacerbations in patients suffering from COPD or chronic asthma, and in major metropolitan areas elevated ozone levels in the atmosphere may force patients with these problems to remain at home in an air-conditioned environment.

Mention should be made of two autosomal recessive genetic problems that lead to severe COPD. These are cystic fibrosis and α-1-antitrypsinase deficiency. More complete discussions of these are available in the bibliographic references.

Finally, even though many external findings of COPD may be present in an elderly patient, age in and of itself is not a cause of COPD.

PATHOPHYSIOLOGY

The earliest changes of COPD are completely silent. They are only demonstrable by highly sensitive measurements of pulmonary function, such as closing volume determination. These changes begin in the early twenties, are reversible with cessation of smoking, and have little or no clinical significance. As these changes progress, more symptoms and abnormalities begin to appear, until finally the full picture is present, usually at age 40 to 50. To understand the changes and effects of COPD, a brief review of basic pulmonary anatomy is necessary.

The respiratory tract has basically three divisions: the upper airway, which serves to warm, humidify, and filter air; the bronchial tree, which acts as a system of conduits; and finally, the actual area of gas exchange, comprised of respiratory bronchioles, alveolar ducts, and alveoli. Each terminal bronchiole, the last division of the bronchial tree not involved in gas exchange, divides into many respiratory bronchioles and alveoli. All the structures originating from a terminal bronchiole are collectively called the *acinus*. It is estimated there are over 300 million alveoli in the lung, with a surface area of over 70 m^2. A vast plexus of capillaries surrounds these alveoli, ensuring maximum diffusion transfer of oxygen between air in the alveoli and blood in the capillary. There is a tremendous functional reserve, and it is easy to see why marked changes in pulmonary anatomy may exist without obvious changes in arterial blood gases. By the time arterial blood gases deteriorate in COPD, very extensive irreversible changes in the lungs have occurred.

Several definitions are useful for clearer understanding of this disease process. Most of these are from the CIBA symposium on terminology, and are expanded upon in the references.

1. *Chronic bronchitis:* This term refers to the condition of subjects with chronic or recurrent excessive mucus secretion in

the bronchial tree. Infection of the bronchi is frequently but not necessarily present. (The words *chronic* or *recurrent* may be defined as occurring on most days for at least 3 months in the year in at least 2 years.)

2. *Emphysema (World Health Organization)* This term refers to enlargement of the air spaces distal to the terminal bronchioles, accompanied by destruction of the walls of these air spaces.

   a. Centilobular emphysema: This occurs with destruction of the respiratory bronchioles. These become confluent and produce enlarged spaces centrally, often with a surrounding rim of normal acinar tissue.

   b. Panlobular emphysema: In this entity, the entire acinus is involved, without sparing of particular structures. Respiratory bronchioles are much less involved. This type is particularly prevalent in α-1-antitrypsinase deficiency.

3. *Ventilation-perfusion imbalance:* Simply stated, this results whenever underventilated, normally perfused alveoli exist; it results in arterial hypoxemia. This situation results in a physiological shunt of blood through the lungs.

4. *Dead space:* This is the volume of air within the upper airway and bronchial tree that does not participate in gas exchange. The dead space is increased in diseases that destroy acinar structures.

The usual case of COPD secondary to chronic cigarette abuse is a combination of chronic bronchitis and emphysema. The earliest change in the lungs of smokers is enlargement of the mucus-secreting cells of the epithelium of the bronchial tree, resulting in increased secretions. As this progresses, chronic bronchitis results. In almost all such cases a certain amount of centrilobular emphysema occurs, secondary to repeated inflammation of the very sensitive respiratory bronchioles. More and more lung tissue is destroyed until either severe hypoxia or CO_2 retention or both occur as a result of these changes. These are followed closely by the development of pulmonary hypertension and cor pulmonale, conditions that have a poor prognosis. In these later stages, the patient has lost almost all functional reserve, and seemingly minor insults to the patient's health may quickly become life-threatening emergencies.

The course of this disease entity is very difficult to predict and is dependent upon multiple factors. At moderately advanced stages, cessation of cigarette smoking or removal from dust exposure may lead to virtually complete clearing of the pathology. Extensive bronchitis with large amounts of secretions may exist with little emphysematous changes and minimal abnormalities in pulmonary function. These patients may never develop emphysema but are at risk for progressive hypoventilation with partial collapse of acinar structures and resulting hypoxemia secondary to alveolar ventilation and perfusion imbalance. Other patients seem more likely to develop severe emphysema with increased dead space and CO_2 retention but little bronchitic change. The usual case of COPD is a combination of both forms of disease and in the end stage manifests both hypoxemia and CO_2 retention.

CLINICAL FEATURES

The diagnosis of COPD and the determination of its severity in a given patient are difficult at the bedside. There is poor correlation between the extent of disease and the symptoms related by the patient. Physical findings and x-ray data are extremely variable and also correlate poorly with the extent of disease. Pulmonary function testing and arterial blood gases will delineate the extent of impairment at a given point in time, but the axiom that patients are only as bad as their best result must be remembered. It is imperative that the emergency medicine physician know the signs, symptoms, and laboratory evaluation of the COPD patient.

The most common complaint of the COPD patient is shortness of breath or dyspnea, and frequently there is a chronic cough with sputum production (Fig. 23-1). A large percentage of patients may have small amounts of hemoptysis at some time in the course of their disease. Fatigue, weight loss, and general malaise often are present. A careful history of dust exposure may be revealing. Several physical findings may be present, although they correlate poorly with the severity of the disease. These include signs of hyperventilation with an increased anteroposterior (AP) diameter of the chest, tracheal deviation, and collapse of the lower lobes with expiration. A decrease in breath sounds throughout the lung fields is one of the most reliable signs. Scattered coarse rhonchi and expiratory wheezes are often found and heart sounds may be distant and heard best in the epigastrum. The pulmonary component of the second heart sound may be increased. The patient may be tachypneic and using accessory respiratory muscles and lip pursing. In certain cases, peripheral cyanosis and clubbing of the fingertips are present. It is not uncommon to find evidence of right-sided heart failure, with edema of the legs and distended neck veins.

Routine laboratory chemistries are of little diagnostic value in COPD. Determination of electrolytes is needed, especially in the later stages of the disease. The chest x-ray is seldom diagnostic; there is evidence of overinflation in about 60 percent of patients, including flattening of the diaphragm, increased AP diameter, a narrow and elongated heart shadow, and accentuation of thoracic kyphosis. If the diaphragm is concave downward, this is virtually diagnostic of emphysema. Increased lung markings are seen in patients with chronic bronchitic symptoms. ECG changes are nonspecific but may include arrhythmias, both supraventricular and ventricular in origin, and right axis shifts. Also P pulmonale and low voltage are frequent findings.

The most valuable diagnostic tools in COPD are bedside pulmonary functions and arterial blood gases. These studies are necessary to determine the present state of a given patient and to follow response to therapy. Bedside pulmonary functions include vital capacity (VC), forced expiratory volume in one second (FEV_1), and minute ventilation (MV).

The *vital capacity* represents the amount of gas expired from a full inspiratory effort without a time limit. As more and more obstruction occurs, vital capacity declines as dead space increases. This is usually of little clinical significance until a 50 percent reduction occurs. Any further impairment to vital capacity, such as that due to surgery or to chest injury, can produce acute ventilatory

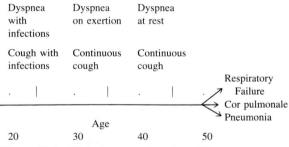

Figure 23-1. Clinical progression of COPD.

failure. Many techniques to measure this are available, but a simple spirometer will suffice and should be available in the emergency department.

The amount of air expired in the first second of a forced expiration from full inspiration is the FEV_1 and represents a measurement primarily of the degree of obstruction. At least 70 percent of the VC should be exhaled in the first second of a forceful expiration. This parameter is useful in following the course of a patient being treated for obstruction and bronchospasm. Like all pulmonary function tests, it is very dependent upon a good patient effort.

The *minute ventilation* measures the amount of air a patient is moving over 1 min. It is derived by measuring the tidal volume of each expiration for a period of 15 s, taking the average amount, and multiplying it by the number of breaths per minute. A more complete discussion of these parameters and their normal values is available in the bibliography.

The advent of arterial blood gas (ABG) determinations gives the clinician an invaluable tool for managing acutely ill patients. The basic parameters measured are blood pH, partial pressure of CO_2 (P_{CO_2}) and partial pressure of O_2 (P_{O_2}). These should be done on arterial specimens and should be available on a 24-h basis to the emergency department. Normal blood gases indicate respiratory and metabolic balance. Changes in these values correlate well with deterioration or improvement in the patient's condition. A brief discussion is indicated, and every emergency medicine physician must have a good understanding of this laboratory procedure.

The pH is a measurement of the acid-base balance in the body and is dependent upon both metabolic and respiratory components. It may remain near normal, even with severe abnormalities in metabolic or respiratory function, if the other system is able to compensate. The metabolic system takes time, and a rapid rise in P_{CO_2} leads to rapid decline in pH. As P_{CO_2} is the measurement of alveolar ventilation, a rapid increase in CO_2 must be corrected by improving this parameter. This will also correct the acidosis present. Chronic CO_2 retention is compensated for by a metabolic alkalosis achieved by retention of bicarbonate ion, so that the blood frequently has a near normal pH.

The level of oxygen in the blood is a result of complex interactions within the lungs. The most frequent cause of hypoxemia in COPD patients is ventilation-perfusion (V/Q) abnormality and resulting physiological shunting. Enrichment of inspired oxygen (FI_{O_2}) even with low flow rates of O_2 often markedly improves these values. In summary, the history, physical, and laboratory values of a patient with COPD are not diagnostic. A high degree of suspicion must be maintained. Definitive pulmonary function determinations will sustain the diagnosis and determine the degree of impairment. The arterial blood gas values are critical to the emergency medicine physician, as they demonstrate the ability of patients to ventilate their lungs, to maintain a normal pH, and to provide adequate amounts of O_2 to the tissues. Acute abnormalities in these parameters are life-threatening and must be corrected.

TREATMENT OF COPD AND ITS COMPLICATIONS

Therapy of COPD is aimed at avoiding the complications (see box) of the disease and also at maintaining and improving pulmonary function. Patients presenting to the emergency department

> **COMPLICATIONS OF COPD**
> - Depression
> - Disability
> - Infections
> - Pneumothorax
> - Pulmonary embolic disease
> - Peptic ulcer
> - Myocardial infarction
> - Congestive heart failure
> - Hypokalemia
> - Decreased phosphate
> - Oversedation

with COPD are often in acute distress. An outline of assessment and management of these patients follows.

A rapid but thorough history and physical are mandatory, along with a thorough review of medications. These patients have often taken an extensive array of bronchodilators, may be on digitalis and diuretics, and in certain cases are using steroids. These drugs may be responsible for their presenting complaints and may be complicating therapy. Certain tests and procedures need to be initiated early. An IV line should be established and basic laboratory studies made. These include electrolytes, complete blood count, ABG, and chest x-ray. Placing the patient on a monitor and obtaining an ECG is necessary.

Initial treatment is aimed at improving respiratory function and oxygenation. Marked bronchospasm often is present. The most useful drug for treatment of this problem is aminophylline given IV. A loading dose may not be needed, as these patients have frequently taken large amounts of theophylline before arriving. Aminophylline is potentially dangerous because of ventricular arrhythmias but if used judiciously is very safe. It also is a mild diuretic, has inotropic effects, and stimulates the respiratory center.

Oxygen therapy is needed, but O_2 must be considered a potentially dangerous drug. While waiting for blood gas results, an FI_{O_2} of 24 to 28 percent by a venturi mask system is a safe start. Injudicious use of O_2 may further depress respiratory function in patients with chronic CO_2 retention, as they are breathing on the O_2 drive and raising P_{O_2} rapidly shuts this off. Acute ventilatory failure may result. Administration of O_2 must be followed with serial blood gas determinations to avoid this complication of therapy.

Infection is often the cause of an exacerbation. The chest x-ray may not reveal an infiltrate, but cultures and antibiotics are indicated. Efforts to help mobilize secretions are important, and include hydration, IPPB, and ultrasonic nebulization. These last two modalities are more important after hospital admission than in the emergency department. Mucolytic agents and expectorants would seem to be of little use in the acute situation.

Electrolyte disturbances are frequent and should be corrected. Chronic CO_2 retention leads to a hypochloremic alkalosis and potassium wasting by the kidney. Diuretics may increase potassium losses and severe hypokalemia may result.

Cardiac disease is a frequent complication of COPD. There is a high incidence of myocardial infarction in these patients, and congestive heart failure is often present. Routine therapy and assessment of these conditions should be performed. Cardiac arrhythmias are common, especially those of supraventricular origin, and correlation of potential causes of the arrhythmias is mandatory. Specific drug therapy may be needed. The most frequent causes of arrhythmias in COPD patients are hypoxemia, hypokalemia, excessive use of sympathomimetic drugs, and digitalis toxicity.

Other common complications of COPD are peptic ulcer disease, pulmonary embolism, and spontaneous pneumothorax. The latter condition must be recognized early as it may prove rapidly fatal in these compromised patients. A chest x-ray is diagnostic, but immediate treatment may be critical. The usual physical findings of pneumothorax may be obscured as these COPD patients are often hyperresonant and have decreased breath sounds. A high level of suspicion must be maintained, and in any case in which a stable COPD patient has rapidly deteriorated without obvious cause, this problem must be considered.

Another complication is excessive sedation. This is an iatrogenic problem and is preventable. If sedatives are prescribed for a COPD patient, they must be used with extreme caution and should be given only if arterial blood gases are stable.

A certain number of patients do not respond to initial therapy and progress into acute ventilatory failure with severe acidosis. Respiratory efforts may need to be controlled by endotracheal intubation and assisted ventilation. On occasion this must be done immediately upon arrival of the patient. In most instances there is time for an attempt to improve the patient by the previously outlined therapeutic modalities. Careful observation of the patient and use of blood gas respiratory parameters will tell the physician when this is no longer safe and when ventilatory assistance needs to be initiated. Most of these patients will have to be sedated and paralyzed before intubation is attempted. Nasotracheal intubation is better tolerated by these patients but is not mandatory if the emergency medicine physician is not experienced in this technique.

Placing a COPD patient on a ventilator is not without management risks, particularly for those patients without reversible problems and who have reached end-stage disease. It is very difficult in most cases to determine this accurately, and the emergency medicine physician must always strive to maintain life and limb. If it is known that the patient is truly end-stage, intubation and mechanical ventilation should be avoided.

EMS CONSIDERATIONS

Two problems need reemphasis: the use of O_2 in patients with chronic CO_2 retention and avoidance of oversedation. Paramedics and other medical personnel must be aware of the danger of excessive O_2 in COPD and of its ability to cause increased ventilatory failure. They should be instructed on COPD in general and in the use of O_2 systems, particularly the Venturi type of mask. These patients must be observed carefully for signs of increasing ventilatory failure and acidosis. This means watching their respiratory efforts, maintaining vital signs, and observing any changes in their mental status. Sedation must be used very cautiously in COPD patients, as any depression in respiratory function may prove fatal. These patients are often very agitated, and the first reaction is to reduce their anxiety. Before this is done, the paramedic must make sure that one of the complications is not causing the restlessness. Paramedics may get involved in the treatment of

other complications in the field, including bronchospasm, spontaneous pneumothorax, and acute ventilatory failure. Techniques and drugs used should be well known to them.

SUMMARY

COPD is a commonly seen disease in most emergency departments, and its exacerbations and complications may be rapidly fatal to the patient. There are many pitfalls awaiting the physician who enters into treatment of these patients with COPD without adequate knowledge and information. Judicious use of potentially dangerous drugs and techniques will reverse the acute problems in most of these patients and will restore them to relative well-being. It is the responsibility of every physician to educate patients in the hazards of cigarette smoking and to encourage patients to give up the habit. If this can be achieved, this disease will eventually cease to exist.

BIBLIOGRAPHY

American Thoracic Society: Definitions and classifications of chronic bronchitis, asthma and pulmonary emphysema. *Am Rev Respir Dis* 85:762–768, 1962.

Ayers SM: Cigarette smoking and lung disease: An update. *Basics RD* 3(5):26–30, 1975.

Brummer DL (chairman): Chemoprophylaxis of chronic bronchitis, a statement by the committee on therapy. *Am Rev Respir Dis* 104:776, 1971.

Burrows B, Nevin W: Antibiotic management in patients with chronic bronchitis and emphysema. *Ann Intern Med* 77:993, 1972.

CIBA: Chronic respiratory disease. *Med Clin North Am* 57: May 1973.

Ebert RV, Pierce JA: Pathogenesis of pulmonary emphysema. *Arch Intern Med* 111:34, 1963.

Fletcher CM (ed): CIBA guest symposium report: Terminology, definitions, and classification of pulmonary emphysema and related conditions. *Thorax* 14:286, 1959.

Gilbert R, Ashutosh K, Auchincloss JR Jr: Clinical value of observations of chest and abdominal motion in patients with pulmonary emphysema. *Am Rev Respir Dis* 119(2,part 2):155–158, 1979.

Harless KW, Morris AH, Cengiz M, et al: Civilian ground and air transport of adults with acute respiratory failure. *JAMA* 240:361–365, 1978.

Hendeles L, Weinberger M: Guidelines for avoiding theophylline overdose. *N Engl J Med* 300:1217, 1979.

Hugh-Jones P, Whimster W: The etiology and management of disabling emphysema. *Am Rev Respir Dis* 117:343–378, 1978.

Medical Research Council: Definition and classification of chronic bronchitis for clinical and epidemiological purposes. Report by Committee on Aetiology of Chronic Bronchitis. *Lancet* 1:775–779, 1965.

Piafsky KM, Ogilvie RI: Dosage of theophylline in bronchial asthma. *N Engl J Med* 292:1218–1222, 1975.

Report of the Task Force on Chronic Bronchitis and Emphysema. *Natl Tuberculosis Assoc Bull* 53(5):1967.

Thurlbeck WM, Henderson JAM, Fraser RG, et al: Chronic obstructive lung disease: A comparison between clinical, roentgenologic, functional, and morphologic criteria in chronic bronchitis, emphysema, asthma, and bronchiectasis. *Medicine* 49:81–145, 1970.

U.S. Public Health Service: The health consequences of smoking: 1974. Publ. (CDC) 74-8704, Washington, 1974.

Wilson RW: Cigarette smoking, disability days and respiratory conditions. *JOM* 15:236, 1973.

CHAPTER 24
SPONTANEOUS AND
IATROGENIC
PNEUMOTHORAX

Judith E. Tintinalli

Spontaneous pneumothorax occurs without any obvious trauma. Iatrogenic pneumothorax is secondary to a diagnostic or therapeutic procedure.

SPONTANEOUS PNEUMOTHORAX

Spontaneous pneumothorax is more common in males than in females. It is generally due to the rupture of a pulmonary or subpleural bleb into the pleural space but may develop when excessive mechanical stress is placed upon a segment of weakened pleura. Leakage of air from the alveoli into the pleural space causes a rise in the intrapleural pressure, leading to pulmonary collapse. Spontaneous pneumothorax may occur in conjunction with pulmonary infection, such as tuberculosis, asthma or emphysema, pulmonary carcinoma, "honeycomb" lung disorders such as tuberous sclerosis or histiocytosis X, occupational pulmonary disease, sarcoidosis, postpulmonary irradiation, and Marfan's and Ehlers-Danlos syndromes. Rarely, cyclical pneumothorax may occur in young or middle-aged females. In such cases the development of pneumothorax is coincident with menstruation and may be related to the presence of pelvic, pleural, or diaphragmatic endometriosis. Some patients may have recurrent episodes of spontaneous pneumothorax. In some cases there is a history of deep inspiration or hyperventilation, followed by the generation of excessive intrathoracic pressures such as can be induced by screaming, coughing, or the Valsalva maneuver (when smoking marijuana).

Clinical Features

The most common symptom of spontaneous pneumothorax is sudden sharp chest pain, which is often pleuritic in character. The pain is generally anterior but it may radiate to the neck or back. Dyspnea, tachycardia, and tachypnea may be present if the degree of pneumothorax compromises pulmonary function. There may be a cough, occasionally productive of blood-streaked sputum. Subcutaneous emphysema involving the neck and chest wall may

be present if air has dissected through mediastinal structures (Fig. 24-1). On physical examination there may be decreased breath sounds and hyperresonance to percussion on the side of the pneumothorax. However in some patients, especially those with em-

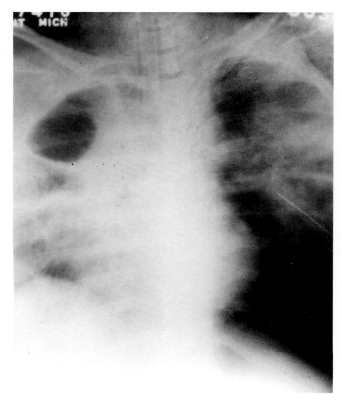

Figure 24-1. Spontaneous pneumothorax in a patient with COPD and active tuberculosis. The chest tube did not relieve the loculated pneumothorax, as is evident by persistent tracheal and mediastinal shift. The patient died of respiratory failure shortly after this film was taken. (Courtesy Detroit General Hospital.)

physema, the clinical findings may be subtle. In addition, the development of pneumothorax in this group is serious and can lead to respiratory failure. In every individual with chronic obstructive pulmonary disease pneumothorax should always be suspected as a cause for clinical deterioration.

A chest roentgenogram is necessary to confirm the diagnosis. Pneumothorax is characterized by hyperlucency and a lack of lung markings at the periphery of the lung and by the appearance of a fine line that represents the retraction of the visceral from the parietal pleura.

If a suspected pneumothorax is not visible on an inspiratory film, it may be seen on an expiratory film, since the constant volume of the pneumothorax is more evident when the size of the hemithorax decreases with expiration. A lateral decubitus film with the patient lying on the affected side may be helpful for the same reason.

A small amount of pleural fluid, usually represented by blunting of the costrophrenic angle, is generally present. Bullae or emphysematous blebs or pulmonary infiltration may be seen on the x-ray film.

Pneumothorax must be differentiated from skin folds, outlines of tubing, artifacts on the chest wall such as clothing, and bullae or cysts. Bullae and cysts have concave inner margins and rounded edges.

Hypotension, cyanosis, and marked respiratory distress may develop if the degree of pneumothorax is large, if underlying pulmonary function is poor, or if tension pneumothorax has developed (Fig. 24-2). Tension pneumothorax is characterized by severe dyspnea, cyanosis, and hypotension. The chest will be hyperresonant on the side of the pneumothorax and the trachea and mediastinal structures will deviate to the opposite side. Deviation of the mediastinal structures results in kinking of the inferior vena cava and a marked decrease in venous return. Uncorrected tension pneumothorax rapidly leads to cardiorespiratory collapse. Chest x-ray is generally not necessary to make this diagnosis. Procrastination in obtaining a confirmation chest x-ray can result in cardiac arrest in the patient.

IATROGENIC PNEUMOTHORAX

Iatrogenic pneumothorax can occur secondary to procedures such as cannulation of the subclavian vein, lung inflation at high pressures, intercostal nerve block, and thoracentesis. It is the most commonly described complication of subclavian vein catheterization and generally occurs if the angle of introduction of the needle is too sharp or if the tip of the needle is directed too deeply. It can also occur if catheterization is attempted while the patient is moving or during chest compression in CPR. It may be more common in apical procedures, as opposed to procedures generally performed at the lung bases such as thoracentesis, because airflow is greater in the apices than the bases. Consequently, subclavian vein catheterization should be approached cautiously in patients with hyperventilation or Kussmaul respirations. Simple pneumothorax can lead to tension pneumothorax rapidly in such circumstances. Chest x-ray is routinely performed immediately after subclavian vein catheterization to detect immediate pneumothorax, but delayed pneumothorax could also develop.

Lung inflation at high pressures can also lead to pneumothorax. Mouth-to-mouth or bag-mask ventilation in infants and children

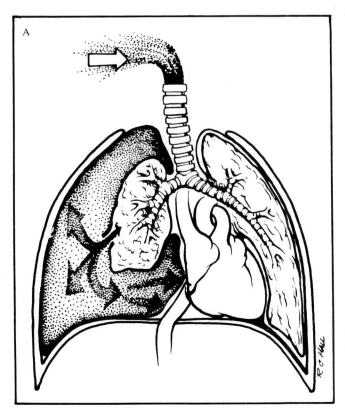
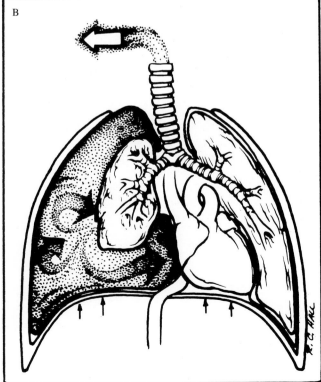

Figure 24-2. A. Tension pneumothorax (inspiration). B. Tension pneumothorax (expiration).

or even in adults can lead to pneumothorax or pneumomediastinum if excess airway pressures are generated. Pneumothorax has resulted when an oxygen cannula is inserted directly into an endotracheal tube. Oxygen is delivered at high flow rates through the cannula into the tube, but because the cannula itself nearly fills the tube lumen, adequate expiration is not possible. Lung pressures build up until pneumothorax results. The institution of mechanical ventilation or positive end-expiratory pressure can cause pneumothorax in patients with previous lung disease or can quickly lead to tension pneumothorax if there has been prior simple pneumothorax. In the latter case a thoracostomy tube is necessary before mechanical ventilation is begun.

In patients with recent subclavian vein catheterization or on mechanical ventilation, pneumothorax should be considered as a cause of cardiopulmonary deterioration. Intercostal nerve block for relief of pain from rib fractures or severe costochondritis should be followed by a chest x-ray to rule out iatrogenic pneumothorax.

TREATMENT

If the pneumothorax involves 20 percent or more of the hemithorax, tube thoracostomy, with water-seal or vacuum drainage, is generally performed. The technique of tube thoracostomy is discussed in the section on trauma.

If the pneumothorax is under 20 percent, the decision for tube thoracostomy varies with the clinical situation, the patient's pulmonary reserve, and the treatment philosophy of the institution. If tube thoracostomy is deferred, the patient must be frequently and carefully examined and serial chest x-ray films taken to detect the development of an increasing, or tension pneumothorax. If the pneumothorax is increasing, if the patient is on mechanical ventilation, or if general anesthesia is contemplated, tube thoracostomy should be performed. If tension pneumothorax is evident, the pressure should be immediately relieved by insertion of a large-bore needle into the pleural space, followed by tube thoracostomy.

On occasion, rapid expansion of pneumothorax with excessive negative pressure may result in the development of unilateral or even bilateral pulmonary edema. This is more likely to occur if there is bronchial obstruction. It is postulated that the increase in pulmonary blood flow with rapid lung reexpansion can cause transudation of capillary fluid into the alveoli. This condition is self-limited with judicious fluid management and respiratory care.

SUMMARY

Spontaneous pneumothorax can develop in healthy persons or in those with underlying pulmonary disease. Decreased breath sounds and hyperresonance of the affected side may be detected by physical examination, but a chest x-ray is often necessary to confirm the diagnosis. Iatrogenic pneumothorax can occur after subclavian vein catheterization, ventilation at high airway pressures, or intercostal block. Careful technique and close patient observation are necessary for the early detection and treatment of this complication.

Pneumothorax of 20 percent or more is generally treated by tube thoracostomy and vacuum drainage. The management of pneumothorax of less than 20 percent varies but tube thoracostomy is always necessary even with small pneumothorax if the patient is on mechanical ventilation. If tube thoracostomy is deferred, the patient should be carefully and frequently observed for an increase in pneumothorax or the development of tension pneumothorax. Tension pneumothorax should be recognized clinically and must be treated promptly by decompression.

BIBLIOGRAPHY

Childress ME, May G, Mottram, M: Unilateral pulmonary edema resulting from treatment of spontaneous pneumothorax. *Am Rev Respir Dis* 104:119–121, 1974.

Greene RG, McCloud TC, Stark P: Pneumothorax. *Semin Roentgenol* 12:313–325, 1977.

Knopp R, Dailey R: Central venous cannulation and pressure monitoring. *J Am Coll Emerg Physicians* 6:358–366, 1977.

Twiford TW, Fornoza J, Libshitz HI: Recurrent spontaneous pneumothorax after radiation therapy to the thorax. *Chest* 73:387–388, 1978.

Vestal B, Vestal R: Iatrogenic pneumothorax. An unusual cause. *JAMA* 235:1879–1880, 1976.

SECTION 4
TOXICOLOGY

CHAPTER 25
GENERAL APPROACH
TO POISONING

Lester Haddad

Poisoning or accidental ingestion occurs most commonly in the 1- to 5-year-old age group and in the elderly. Overdose or intentional ingestion, either from a suicide attempt, or for purposes of secondary gain or of abuse, is recognized in age groups from older childhood on. It is critical to determine if the cause of the toxic ingestion was not accidental so that proper psychologic intervention may be provided.

The general approach to the poisoning patient may be divided into nine phases:

- Emergency management
- History and physical examination
- Evaluation of major toxic signs
- Laboratory evaluation
- Elimination of the poison from the gastrointestinal tract, skin, and eyes
- Administration of a specific antidote if available
- Elimination of the absorbed substance
- Supportive therapy
- Observation and disposition

The presentation of the poisoning victim may be straightforward or subtle. Poisoning should always be suspected in the psychiatric patient; the trauma victim, especially the young victim; the patient exposed to a fire; the comatose patient where the etiology is unknown; the young patient with a life-threatening arrhythmia or arrhythmia of unknown etiology; or a patient with metabolic acidosis of unknown etiology. In addition, a patient may have two disorders simultaneously. For example, an accident victim may have had the accident because of an overdose. A psychiatric patient suffering from overdose may also have concomitant head trauma; or a patient with overdose may develop an acute episode of diabetic ketoacidosis.

EMERGENCY MANAGEMENT

Before specific evaluation, adequate ventilation and perfusion must be established, and the critical patient must be given appropriate emergency treatment.

An intravenous infusion of normal saline should be begun. All patients in coma should be given naloxone hydrochloride, at least 2 ampoules (0.8 mg) IV, followed by 50 g glucose IV bolus. Blood for glucose determination should be drawn before the IV is started or glucose is given.

A methemoglobin level of 15 mg/100 mL or greater is present if a drop of the patient's blood turns chocolate-brown when placed on filter paper.

HISTORY AND PHYSICAL EXAMINATION

History

Determine the type and amount of material ingested, inhaled, or splattered over the body. Nontoxic ingestions are listed in Table 25-1.

Prior medical history, current medications, and allergies should all be determined from family or friends if the patient is unable to relate the information. Determine whether the patient was on medication and whether empty bottles were found nearby. In the comatose patient, consider drug overdose until proved otherwise. Note what the patient was doing prior to the poisoning. Illness while fumigating a ship, for instance, suggests cyanide poisoning. A patient taken from a fire or found unconscious in a garage may have carbon monoxide poisoning. The patient should be asked if any self-treatment or home remedies have been administered—the cure may have been worse than the disease. The history from the patient is often inaccurate, however, owing to a number of factors such as fear, confusion, or disorientation. A patient who has ingested a street drug may be totally unaware of what actually has been taken.

For the patient with more obscure signs and symptoms, or those that suggest exposure to toxins, a detailed occupational and avocational history should be obtained.

Physical Examination

The physical examination can reveal the presence of a toxic syndrome and detect complications of the poisoning and underlying systemic disease. According to Done, the important toxic syndromes are anticholinergic, anticholinesterase, cholinergic, extrapyramidal, hemoglobinopathic, narcotic, sympathomimetic, and withdrawal syndromes (Table 25-2). An elevated temperature can

Table 25-1. Nontoxic Ingestions*

Abrasives	Elmer's glue	Petroleum jelly (Vaseline)
Adhesives	Etch-A-Sketch	Play-Doh
Antacids	Fabric softeners	Polaroid picture coating fluid
Antibiotics	Fish bowl additives	Porous tip marking pens
Baby product cosmetics	Glues and pastes	Prussian blue (ferricyanide)
Ballpoint pen inks	Hand lotions and creams	Putty (less than 2 oz)
Bathtub floating toys	3% Hydrogen peroxide, medicinal	Rubber cement
Bath oil (castor oil and perfume)	Incense	Sachets (essential oils, powder)
Birth control pills	Indelible markers	Shampoos (liquid)
Bleach (less than 5% sodium hypochlorite)	Ink (black, blue)	Shaving creams and lotions
Body conditioners	Iodophil disinfectant	Soap and soap products
Bubble bath soaps (detergents)	Laxatives	Spackles
Calamine lotion	Lipstick	Suntan preparations
Candles (beeswax or paraffin)	Lubricant	Sweetening agents (saccharin)
Chalk (calcium carbonate)	Magic markers	Teething rings (water sterility)
Cigarettes or cigars (nicotine)	Makeup (eye, liquid, facial)	Thermometers (mercury)
Colognes	Matches	Toothpaste with or without fluoride
Cosmetics	Mineral oil	Toy pistol caps (potassium chlorate)
Crayons marked AP, CP	Modeling clay	Vitamins with or without fluoride
Dehumidifying packets (silica or charcoal)	Newspaper	Watercolors
Deodorants	Pencil (graphite lead, coloring)	Zinc oxide
Deodorizers, spray and refrigerator	Perfumes	Zirconium oxide

*In the event of ingestion of large quantities, authoritative references should be consulted before final judgment is made.

occur with a great number of ingestions and a number of systemic disorders, but it is a hallmark of poisoning with salicylates, dinitrophenols, and anticholinergics. Hypothermia can be present because of exposure or hypoglycemia, or it can result from overdose with a number of agents. Bradycardia can be seen with digitalis or cholinergics, for example. Hypertension is characteristic of phencyclidine, amphetamines, and sympathomimetics.

Look at the skin. Are there needle tracks, burns, bruises, or lacerations? Are there pressure sores as seen in barbiturate or carbon monoxide poisoning? A "boiled lobster" appearance sug-

gests borate poisoning, particularly in a child who may have ingested Harris Famous Roach tablets or other boric acid derivatives.

Diaphoresis points to hypoglycemia and myocardial infarction, but it is also seen in organophosphate or salicylate poisoning. Jaundice and hepatic coma suggest causes other than poisoning, but if the patient has been transferred from a distant hospital, delayed hepatic failure could result from poisoning. Petechiae suggest meningitis or a coagulopathy. Myxedema or hypocalcemia should be suspected in a patient with a thyroidectomy scar.

Table 25-2. Toxic Syndromes (Multiple Etiology Symptom Complexes)

Syndrome	Causes			Manifestations
Anticholinergic	Belladonna alkaloids: 　Atropine (hyoscyamine) 　Belladonna alkaloids mixtures: belladonna leaf, fluid extract, tincture 　Stramonium 　Homatropine 　Methscopolamine 　Methylatropine nitrate 　Plants: *Atropa belladonna. Datura stramonium, Hyoscyamus niger, Amanita muscaria or pantherina* 　Scopolamine (l-hyoscine)			Parasympatholytic: 　Dry skin and mucuous membranes 　Thirst 　Dysphagia 　Vision blurred for near objects 　Fixed dilated pupils 　Tachycardia 　Sometimes hypertension 　Rash, scarlatiniform 　Hyperthermia, flushing 　Abd distension 　Urinary urgency and retention
	Synthetic anticholinergics:			Central:
	Adiphenine	Isopropamide	Pipenzolate	Lethargy
	Anisotropine	Mepenzolate	Piperiodolate	Confusion to restlessness, excitement, delirium
	Cyclopentolate	Methantheline	Poldine	Delirium, hallucinations
	Dicyclomine	Methixene	Propantheline	Delusions
	Diphemanil	Oxphenonium	Tiphenamil	Ataxia
	Eucatropine	Oxphencyclimine	Tridihexethyl	Respiratory failure
	Glycopyrrolate	Pentapiperide	Tropicamide	Cardiovascular collapse
	Hexocyclium			
	Incidental anticholinergics:			
	Antihistamines	Benactyzine	Tricyclic antidepressants	

Table 25-2. Toxic Syndromes (Multiple Etiology Symptom Complexes) (*Continued*)

Syndrome	Causes			Manifestations

Anticholinesterase	Organophosphates:
	  TEPP
	  OMPA
	  Dipterex
	  Chlorthion
	  Di-Syston
	  Co-Ral
	  Phosdrin
	  Parathion
	  Methylparathion
	  Malathion
	  Systox
	  EPN
	  Diazinon
	  Guthion
	  Trithion
				Muscarinic effects:
				  Sweating, constricted pupils, lacrimation, excessive salivation, wheezing, cramps, vomiting, diarrhea, tenesmus, bradycardia, fall in blood pressure, blurred vision, urinary incontinence
				Nicotinic effects:
				  Striated muscle: fasciculations, cramps, weakness, twitching, paralysis, respiratory embarassment, cyanosis, arrest
				  Sympathetic ganglia: tachycardia, elevated blood pressure
				CNS effects:
				  Anxiety, restlessness, ataxia, convulsions, insomnia, coma, absent reflexes, Cheyne-Stokes respirations, respiratory and circulation depression

Cholinergic	Acetylcholine *A. muscaria* *A. pantherina* *Areca catechu* Arecoline	Betel nut Bethanechol Carbachol *Clitocybe dealbata*	Methacholine Muscarine Pilocarpine *Pilocarpus* species	Same as Muscarinic under Anticholinesterases, also Nicotinic
Extrapyramidal	Acetophenazine Butaperazine Carphenazine Chlorpromazine Haloperidol	Mesoridazine Perphenazine Piperacetazine Promazine	Thioridazine Thiothixene Trifluoperazine Triflupromazine	Parkinsonian: Dysphonia, dysphagia, oculogyric crises, rigidity, tremor, torticollis, opisthotonos, shrieking, trismus, laryngospasm
Hemoglobinopathies	Carboxyhemoglobin Carbon monoxide Methemoglobin Sulfhemoglobin			Disorientation, headache to coma dyspnea, cyanosis with methemoglobinemia & sulfhemoglobinemia Cutaneous bullae, gastroenteritis Epidemic occurrence with carbon monoxide

Metal fume fever	Fumes of oxides of
	  Brass
	  Cadmium
	  Copper
		Iron
		Magnesium
		Mercury
			Nickel
			Titanium
			Tungsten
			Zinc
				Chills, fever, nausea, vomiting, muscular pain, throat dryness, headache, fatigue, weakness, leukocytosis, respiratory distress

Narcotic	Alphaprodine Anileridine Codeine Cyclazocine Dextromethorphan Dextromoramide Diacetylmorphine Dihydrocodeine Dihydrocodeinone Dipanone	Diphenoxylate (Lomotil) Ethoheptazine Ethylmorphine Fantanyl Heroin Hydromorphone Levorphanol Meperidine Methadone	Metopon Morphine Opium Oxycodone Oxymorphone Pentazocine Phenazocine Piminodine Propoxyphene Racemorphan	CNS depression Pinpoint pupils Slowed respirations Hypotension Response to naloxone Pupils may be dilated and excitement may predominate
Sympathomimetic	Aminophylline Amphetamines Caffeine Dopamine Ephedrine	Epinephrine Fenfluramine Levarterenol Metaraminol Methylphenidate (Ritalin)	Pemoline Phencyclidine Phenmetrazine Phentermine	CNS excitation Convulsions Hypertension Tachycardia
Withdrawal	Alcohol Barbiturates Benzodiazepines Chloral hydrate Cocaine	Ethchlorvynol Glutethimide Meprobamate Methaqualone	Methyprylon Narcotics Opioids Paraldehyde	Diarrhea, nydriasis, goose flesh, hypertension, tachycardia, insomnia, lacrimation, muscle cramps, restlessness, yawning, hallucinosis

Source: Adapted from Done AK: *Poisoning—A Systematic Approach for the Emergency Department Physician.* Presented Aug. 6–9. 1979 at Snowmass Village, Colo Symposium sponsored by Rocky Mountain Poison Center. Used by permission.

Smell the patient's breath. A fruity odor may be detectable with diabetic ketoacidosis. If the breath smells like silver polish, consider cyanide poisoning. Parathion smells like an insecticide. A cleaning fluid smell suggests carbon tetrachloride. Ether, turpentine, and gasoline all have a characteristic odor.

Listen to the lungs. In tricyclic antidepressant overdose or methaqualone ingestion, pulmonary edema may be a complication, and in all overdose patients, aspiration is a real possibility.

Listen to the heart. An arrhythmia in a young patient can result from overdose or electrolyte disturbance. Pancreatitis is common with methanol poisoning. Evaluate the extremities to detect thrombophlebitis, fracture or dislocation, or vascular insufficiency. Overdose patients who remain comatose and motionless for prolonged periods of time may develop rhabdomyolysis or the compartment syndrome.

EVALUATION OF MAJOR TOXIC SIGNS

The initial physical manifestations of poisoning and overdose are legion. One approach is to deal with five major acute toxic signs: cardiac arrhythmia, metabolic acidosis, coma, gastrointestinal disturbances, and seizures. Hepatic, renal, respiratory, and bone marrow failures are delayed complications.

Cardiac Arrhythmia

Obtain an ECG in all patients with significant poisoning. A patient may have no arrhythmia, but the ECG can provide important diagnostic clues, such as a prolonged QT interval in phenothiazine overdose or a widened QRS interval in tricyclic antidepressant, quinine, or quinidine poisoning. While many drugs cause a sinus tachycardia, sinus bradycardia is significant and suggests digitalis, cyanide, or physostigmine overdose. Table 25-3 lists the toxic causes of cardiac arrhythmias.

The patient with life-threatening ventricular arrhythmia or cardiac arrest should be managed using the basic principles of advanced cardiac life support. If tricyclic antidepressant overdose is suspected, sodium bicarbonate is indicated for ventricular arrhythmia or for conduction disturbances. In a referral patient with ventricular arrhythmia or cardiac arrest, the etiology of arrhythmia may be hyperkalemia, as renal failure may have already ensued,

Table 25-3. Common Toxic Causes of Cardiac Arrhythmia

Tricyclic antidepressants
Phenothiazines
Carbon monoxide
Cyanide
Cocaine
Digitalis
Propranolol
Physostigmine
Quinine
Chloroquine
Chloral hydrate
Phenol
Arsenic
Dinitrophenols
Fluoroacetate
Succinylcholine chloride

Table 25-4. Causes of a High-Anion-Gap Metabolic Acidosis

Uremia
Ketoacidosis
Lactic acidosis
Salicylate toxicity
Methanol poisoning
Ethylene glycol poisoning
Nondiabetic alcoholic ketoacidosis
Paraldehyde toxicity

and a trial of intravenous sodium bicarbonate or calcium chloride may be indicated in the event of cardiac arrest.

Metabolic Acidosis

Examples of agents that cause metabolic acidosis include cyanide, phenol, methyl alcohol, ethylene glycol, ethanol, salicylate, iron, and carbon tetrachloride. Metabolic acidosis must always be kept in mind from the beginning of evaluation and dealt with appropriately. While too involved to discuss here, the assessment of metabolic acidosis must include not only arterial blood gas analysis, but also serum sodium, potassium, chloride, carbon dioxide, BUN, glucose, acetone, and osmolality levels, and urine pH.

It can be helpful to determine the anion gap in the differential diagnosis of some toxic ingestions (Table 25-4). The serum osmolality can be measured either directly by determining the freezing point, or by calculation. The formula for calculating osmolality is:

$$\text{Serum osmolality} = (2 \times NA) + \frac{BUN}{3} + \frac{glucose}{18}$$

The normal serum osmolality is 280 to 295 mOsm. A measured osmolality that is elevated and more than 10 mOsm greater than the calculated osmolality, or an osmolal gap, suggests the presence in the serum of osmotically active substances measured by the osmometer that are not accounted for by the calculated osmolality. Substances such as ethyl alcohol, methanol, isopropyl alcohol, glycerol, or mannitol produce an increase in the measured osmolality over the calculated osmolality. A substance significantly contributes to osmolality only if it achieves relatively high blood levels and has a low molecular weight. Most drugs or intoxicants cannot be detected by using the osmolal gap. Drugs such as phenobarbital, amphetamines, diazepines, heroin, salicylates, phenothiazines, glutethimide, and methaqualone fall into this latter category.

Coma

One of the most common manifestations of acute poisoning is coma. The principles of managing the patient in coma are relatively straightforward. Draw blood and order appropriate studies. Save urine samples and initial gastric aspirate for laboratory studies.

Once blood is drawn, give all patients in coma 1 to 2 ampoules of 50% dextrose intravenously and up to 5 ampoules of Narcan (naloxone hydrochloride 0.01 mg/kg) IV push. These therapeutic measures should be repeated as necessary; the use of oxygen may be indicated.

It is important to determine the depth of the coma and the patient's neurological status. Special attention should be given to response to pain and verbal stimuli, presence or absence and type of reflexes, as well as disturbance of vital signs.

Rule out other causes of coma, such as trauma, diabetes, anoxia, meningitis, and others. Progression of localized signs suggests structural lesions. Extracranial signs such as jaundice, uremic frost, or thrombophlebitis may point to other causes. Pinpoint pupils are significant since they suggest opiates, phenothiazines, chloral hydrate, cholinergic agents (e.g., insecticides) or a brainstem (pontine) lesion. Dilated pupils are nonspecific.

Gastrointestinal Disturbances

Iron, lithium, mercury, phosphorus, arsenic, mushrooms, colchicine, and fluoride poisoning are some common toxic causes of severe vomiting, diarrhea, or both. The patient with iron poisoning will have severe, repeated episodes of vomiting, and may develop gastrointestinal hemorrhage., Lithium overdose may cause massive diarrhea. A patient with mercury poisoning usually has marked salivation and mucus-type diarrhea with later development of hemorrhagic colitis. One of the most striking presentations is from phosphorus poisoning, which produces luminescent vomitus and flatus.

The management of gastrointestinal disturbances is specific to each agent. As a general statement, one is often faced with hypovolemia and perhaps shock. Hypovolemia should be treated by fluid replacement with normal saline. In the event of hemorrhage, whole blood should be utilized.

Seizures

Common agents causing seizures are listed in Table 25-5. Seizures should be managed by establishing an airway and providing oxygenation. Simple isolated seizures may require observation and supportive care, while repetitive seizures or status epilepticus can be treated with intravenous diazepam. Keep in mind that seizures may be a sign of drug withdrawal.

LABORATORY EVALUATION

Blood samples should be drawn and several studies obtained. In every significant poisoning case, routinely obtain a CBC, serum electrolytes, BUN, glucose, arterial blood gases, and prothrombin time. For example, hyponatremia can cause coma; hypernatremia is seen in severe salicylate poisoning. Hyperkalemia can cause ventricular arrhythmias indistinguishable from those caused by several toxic agents. Carbon dioxide and arterial blood gases are necessary to diagnose metabolic acidosis. As previously mentioned serum acetone and serum osmolality, particularly in cases of alcohol, methanol, or ethylene glycol overdose, are important. A baseline prothrombin time is helpful in assessing delayed hepatorenal effects because the prothrombin time is often the earliest indication of hepatotoxicity.

It is important to maintain a proper perspective in the use of the toxicology screen. To delay treatment until the results of the toxicology screen are available can be disastrous. Poisoning must be recognized early if management is to be effective. In addition, most hospitals do not have the equipment required to perform

Table 25-5. Common Agents Causing Seizures

Tricyclic antidepressants
Phencyclidine
LSD
Phenol
Cocaine
Carbon monoxide
Propoxyphene hydrochloride
Lithium
Parathion
Ammonia
Camphor
Strychnine
Isoniazid
Phenothiazines
Chlorinated hydrocarbons

sophisticated emergency toxicology studies. Toxicology screens are too often misinterpreted. Treat the patient, not the laboratory. In proper perspective, however, the laboratory can help in the diagnosis and management of the poisoned patient.

In this author's opinion, any large emergency department should have access to the following toxicologic studies on a 24-h basis: serum acetaminophen, barbiturate, salicylate, iron, ethanol, methemoglobin, serum and red cell cholinesterase, carboxyhemoglobin, methanol, and lithium levels.

In a patient with poisoning of unknown etiology, save all urine for the first 24 h for diagnostic studies. Repeated daily urinalyses are important, as many agents, such as mercury and carbon tetrachloride, can cause delayed renal failure. Frequent monitoring of the urine pH is essential in the management of some poisonings, such as salicylate poisoning.

Since both phenothiazines and tricyclic antidepressants can produce coma and ventricular arrhythmias, a positive ferric chloride test indicating the presence of phenothiazines is of obvious diagnostic assistance. However, because the ferric chloride test can be misinterpreted, the physical examination is far more reliable than the laboratory in this instance. Dilated pupils suggest tricyclic antidepressant overdose, whereas pinpoint pupils suggest phenothiazine overdose.

The chest film is an aid for diagnosing aspiration or pulmonary edema. Iron, chloral hydrate, and phenothiazine tablets are radiopaque and can be demonstrated on a KUB film. Skull films should be obtained if the patient is comatose. A CT scan may be necessary if a structural CNS lesion may be present.

Finally, a spinal tap may be necessary to rule out meningitis in a patient with coma and fever.

ELIMINATION OF POISON FROM GI TRACT, SKIN, EYES

Aggressive removal of substances from the eyes, skin, and gastrointestinal tract is necessary to prevent toxic effects. For example, caustics and acids (such as battery acid and bleaches) should be removed from the eyes with copious irrigation for 15 to 30 min with either Dacriose solution or normal saline. Caustics should be removed immediately from the skin by copious irrigation. A patient exposed to insecticide poisoning should remove all clothes, and shower. Residual insecticide spray on the clothes will be continually absorbed.

The prognosis of the poisoning patient often depends on the aggressiveness with which poisons are eliminated from the gastrointestinal tract. A toxic substance can be neutralized or eliminated from the gastrointestinal tract by use of milk, ipecac, lavage, activated charcoal, demulcents, cathartics, and neutralizers administered over several phases.

Milk

Milk can be given to any conscious person who has ingested a poison except one who has ingested phosphorus. Milk can provide dilution; it is a demulcent; its high protein content can provide a substitute strata for agents such as caustics; and it is usually readily available.

Ipecac

If the patient is awake, give ipecac, 15 mL to a child and 30 mL to an adult, except in the following instances:

1. Following ingestion of a caustic
2. If the patient has seizures or is obtunded or comatose
3. If the patient has ingested a petroleum distillate, especially of low volatility and surface tension, such as charcoal lighter fluid

The one area of agreement among authorities with regard to the use of ipecac in petroleum distillate ingestion seems to be that when the petroleum distillate is a carrier for a more toxic substance, such as an insecticide or carbon tetrachloride, emesis should be induced.

Gastric Lavage

Gastric lavage is indicated in all significant cases of poisoning, with generally the same contraindications as listed above. Gastric lavage should not be utilized in petroleum distillate ingestion without prior endotracheal intubation. While gastric lavage is not indicated in alkali ingestion, it may have a role in the treatment of ingestion of an acid such as phenol, since acids tend to have a less severe corrosive effect upon the esophagus than alkalies.

Major points about gastric lavage include the following:

1. Use the largest-bore tube possible. In adults, pass a 36-Fr Ewald tube.
2. Protect the airway. Endotracheal intubation may be necessary in the comatose patient.
3. Tap water is sufficient for lavage in adults, but saline should be used in children since they are more susceptible to fluid and electrolyte imbalance.

There is some disagreement as to the comparative effectiveness of emesis induced by ipecac as opposed to gastric lavage. Some believe that gastric lavage, when properly done, is superior to emesis.

Activated Charcoal

Activated charcoal has an undisputed role in the management of the seriously poisoned patient. Prior to removal of the gastric tube,

give an adult 50 to 100 g of activated charcoal and 250 mL of water. The pediatric dose is 30 to 50 g. Ipecac and oral acetylcysteine given for acute acetaminophen overdose will be absorbed by activated charcoal.

Cathartics

There is much resistance to the use of cathartics in the treatment of poisoning patients, because changing of linen wastes valuable nursing time in a busy department. Nevertheless, cathartics are a legitimate means of eliminating poisons from the gastrointestinal tract and should be utilized. An effective cathartic for an adult is 30 g of magnesium sulfate (or 300 mL of a 10% solution). The pediatric dose is 250 mg/kg. Cathartics may not be of use in a patient who is deeply comatose and has an ileus. They should not be used in a patient who has or who may develop gastrointestinal hemorrhage, for example, in cases of iron ingestion. They are also contraindicated in caustic ingestion.

Demulcents

Examples of demulcents used in the management of poisoning include olive oil following electric dishwasher detergent ingestion, and Mylanta or other antacid to provide symptomatic relief for gastritis from salicylate ingestion.

Neutralizers

The following are specific instances in which a neutralizing agent instead of activated charcoal is indicated:

Mercury poisoning. Sodium formaldehyde sulfoxylate (20-g ampoule) is an effective neutralizing agent because it reduces mercuric chloride and other mercury salts to metallic mercury, which is considerably less soluble.

Iron poisoning. Sodium bicarbonate lavage is indicated in iron poisoning because sodium bicarbonate converts the ferrous ion to ferrous carbonate, which is poorly absorbed. After lavage, 200 to 300 mL of the bicarbonate solution should be left in the stomach.

Iodine ingestion. A solution of 75 g of starch in 1 L of water provides an effective lavage solution for neutralization following iodine ingestion. Lavage should be continued until the gastric aspirate is no longer blue.

Strychnine, nicotine, quinine, and physostigmine poisoning. In these instances, potassium permanganate is an effective neutralizing agent. A 1:10,000 solution is prepared by dissolving a 100-mg tablet in 1 L of water.

ANTIDOTES

Unfortunately, specific antidotes to poisons are uncommon. Table 25-6 lists the generally accepted antidotes.

Antidotes are divided into physiologic and specific. Atropine and 2-PAM chloride, used in organophosphate poisoning, are good examples of physiologic and specific antidotes, respectively. Organophosphates inhibit the enzyme cholinesterase, probably by phosphorylation. Toxic signs are considered to be an indirect con-

Table 25-6. Emergency Antidotes

Poison	Antidote	Adult Dosage*	Comments
Acetaminophen	*N*-Acetylcysteine	140 mg/kg initial dose	Most effective within 16 h
Arsenic	See mercury		
Atropine	Physostigmine	Initial dose 0.5–2 mg (IV)	Can produce convulsions, bradycardia
Carbon monoxide	Oxygen		
Cyanide	Amyl nitrite; *then*	Pearls every 2 min	Methemoglobin⁺ cyanide⁻ complex
	Sodium nitrite	10 mL of 3% solution over 3 min (IV)	Causes hypotension. Dosage assumes normal hemoglobin
		0.33 mL (10 mg 3% sol.)/kg initially for children	
	Sodium thiosulfate	25% solution—50 mL (IV) over 10 min; 1.65 mL/kg for children	Forms harmless sodium thiocyanate
Ethylene glycol	See Methyl alcohol		
Gold	See Mercury		
Iron	Deferoxamine	Initial dose: 40–90 mg/kg (IM) not to exceed 1 g	Deferoxamine mesylate—forms excretable ferrioxamine complex
Lead	Calcium disodium Edetate	1 ampoule/250 mL D₅W over 1 h	5-mL ampoule (IV) 20% solution. Dilute to less than 3% solution—Calcium displaced by lead
Mercury (arsenic, gold)	BAL (British antilewisite)	5 mg/kg (IM) as soon as possible	Each mL BAL in oil has dimercaprol, 100 mg, in 210 mg (21%) benzyl benzoate and 680 mg peanut oil—Forms stable nontoxic excretable cyclic compound
Methyl alcohol (ethylene glycol)	Ethyl alcohol in conjunction with dialysis	1 mL/kg of 100% ethanol initially in glucose solution; maintain blood level of 100 mg/100 mL	Competes for alcohol dehydrogenase; prevents formation of formic acid, oxalates
Nitrites	Methylene blue	0.2 mL/kg of 1% solution (IV) over 5 min	Often exchange transfusion is needed for severe methemoglobinemia
Opiates, Darvon, Lomotil	Naloxone	0.4–0.8 mg (IV) 0.01 mg/kg (IV)—children	Naloxone—no respiratory depression (0.4 mg/1 mL ampoule)
Organophosphates	Atropine	Initial dose: 0.5–2 mg (IV) 0.05 mg/kg (IV) initially for children	Physiologic: Blocks acetylcholine. Up to 5 mg (IV) every 15 min may be necessary in the critical adult patient
	Pralidoxime (2-PAM chloride) (Protopam)	Initial dose: 1 g (IV) Children: 25–50 mg/kg (IV)	Specific: Breaks aklyl phosphate–cholinesterase bond. Up to 500 mg every hour may be necessary in the critical adult patient

*Dosages listed may require modification according to specific clinical conditions.
Source: Adapted from the American College of Emergency Physicians poster on poisoning. Dallas, Tex, 1980.

sequence of this enzyme activation, for there is a local accumulation of acetylcholine. The clinical effects of organophosphate poisoning are thus, in effect, due to acetylcholine rather than the organophosphate directly. Atropine physiologically blocks acetylcholine, whereas 2-PAM chloride is a specific antidote for parathion. It cleaves the alkylphosphate parathion-cholinesterase bond, and thus liberates cholinesterase and allows cholinesterase to metabolize acetylcholine.

ELIMINATION OF ABSORBED SUBSTANCE

Aside from the gastrointestinal effects, the symptoms and signs of poisoning are caused by the absorbed poison. Elimination of the absorbed substance when an antidote is not available includes four modalities: forced diuresis, acidification or alkalinization of the urine, and dialysis and hemoperfusion.

Forced Diuresis

About 20 years ago, when barbiturates were one of the most common causes of overdose, fluid loading and forced diuresis

were accepted means of management for barbiturate poisoning; these means were extrapolated to all forms of poisoning. However, forced diuresis is now indicated less frequently since many overdose agents are metabolized in the liver while others can impair cardiopulmonary function. For example, methaqualone and the tricyclic antidepressants cause a susceptibility to drug-induced interstitial pulmonary edema, and fluid loading is contraindicated. In addition, the tricyclic antidepressants are markedly protein-bound and forced diuresis has no place in treatment. Thus, forced diuresis should be utilized only when specifically indicated such as in poisoning by phenobarbital, bromides, phencyclidine, lithium, salicylate, and amphetamines. Furosemide is usually the agent of choice, although osmotic diuresis with mannitol can be more useful in some instances, such as lithium overdose.

Acidification

Acidification of the urine is usually accomplished by ascorbic acid, 1 g every 6 h intravenously in an adult. Acidification is indicated in overdose with phencyclidine and amphetamines. If multiple drugs have been ingested, acidification may enhance the excretion of some and impair the excretion of others.

Table 25-7. Dialysis and Hemoperfusion of Common Drugs

Specific Emergency Indications	Dialysis Dependent on Clinical Condition	Dialysis never Specifically Indicated
Ethylene glycol	Boric acid	Chlordiazepoxide
Methyl alcohol	Chlorates	Cyanide
	Ethchlorvynol	Diazepam
	Lithium	Hallucinogens
	Salicylate	Iron
		Oxazepam
		Phenothiazines
		Tricyclic antidepressants

Alkalinization

Alkalinization of the blood is helpful in reducing arrhythmias secondary to tricyclic antidepressants. Alkalinization of the urine ionizes weak acids, such as salicylates and barbiturates, and prevents reabsorption by the renal tubule, thus increasing excretion.

Charcoal Hemoperfusion, Dialysis

Charcoal hemoperfusion, peritoneal dialysis, and hemodialysis can be valuable adjuncts to treatment. There are both specific and general indications for dialysis or hemoperfusion of drugs (Table 25-7). Examples of general indications for dialysis include (1) a patient with renal failure secondary to carbon tetrachloride or mercury poisoning who must be maintained until the kidneys recover; (2) a patient with cirrhosis who has ingested a lethal overdose of a dialyzable drug such as ethchlorvynol (which is metabolized by the liver); (3) a patient who has taken an overdose of an agent such as salicylate, methanol, or ethylene glycol, and who also has severe metabolic acidosis, electrolyte disturbance, or seizures.

A patient who only requires removal of the drug benefits most from charcoal hemoperfusion. Hemodialysis is obviously indicated in the patient who, in addition, has severe metabolic acidosis, electrolyte abnormality, or renal failure. Peritoneal dialysis can be useful if short-term dialysis is required, as in severe salicylate or lithium poisoning.

Immediate indications for dialysis include methyl alcohol, ethylene glycol, and perhaps *Amanita phalloides* ingestion.

Dialysis is not indicated in a patient who has ingested a substance that is markedly protein-bound, such as a tricyclic antidepressant; in a drug ingestion where the agent is rarely, if ever, lethal, such as diazepam; when the plasma concentration of the drug is not significant enough to ensure drug removal, such as gluthethimide; when the action of the agent is irreversible, such as cyanide; when the patient is in shock; or when the dangers of hemodialysis outweigh the benefits.

SUPPORTIVE THERAPY

Supportive therapy is the mainstay of treatment for the poisoned patient. All too often the agent is unknown, one is faced with a multiple drug overdose, or the patient is too critical to withstand anything other than supportive therapy.

- Intravenous fluids are indicated only to provide maintenance needs and replace losses, or to provide forced diuresis when indicated.
- Frequent arterial pH determinations should be monitored when using alkaline or acid therapy.
- Intensive nursing care is essential to avoid aspiration and the development of decubiti.
- Avoid the indiscriminate use of drugs or antidotes if they are not indicated or necessary.
- Treat hypothermia or hyperthermia.
- The management of hypotension may be difficult and must be individualized for each poison ingested.

OBSERVATION AND DISPOSITION

In-hospital observation of the patient with overdose may be necessary for several reasons.

First, some drugs, such as iron, acetaminophen, carbon tetrachloride, or mercury, have a latent phase in which the patient appears to recover from the initial insult, only to decompensate 48 to 72 h postingestion. Tricyclic antidepressant overdose has been reported to cause a fatal arrhythmia 6 days postingestion. Some drugs are associated with delayed effects, such as hypertension following phencyclidine ingestion, hemorrhagic colitis following mercury ingestion, and hepatic or renal failure following carbon tetrachloride ingestion.

Second, the patient may need observation because of an underlying disease that may be exacerbated during the overdose, for example, diabetic ketoacidosis.

Third, observation may be necessary both to evaluate and treat complications; for example, a skull fracture or other signs of trauma may not be evident until the overdose has been treated. Aspiration pneumonia or interstitial pulmonary edema may develop during the course of therapy.

The disposition of the poisoned patient may involve medical and psychiatric as well as social work follow-up. Overt or subtle suicide attempts or gestures indicate the need for psychiatric consultation. Some ingestions in the pediatric age group will require outpatient follow-up the next day, for example, a kerosene ingestion in a patient with a negative chest x-ray film and no respiratory distress. In addition, the question of child abuse should always be raised in the physician's mind when treating a pediatric poisoning or overdose.

BIBLIOGRAPHY

Haddad LM: General approach to the emergency management of poisoning, in Haddad LM, Winchester JF (eds): *Clinical Management of Poisoning and Drug Overdose.* Philadelphia, Saunders, 1983, pp 4–17.

CHAPTER 26
TRICYCLIC
ANTIDEPRESSANTS*

Lester Haddad

The tricyclics obtained their name originally from a three-ring structure—a central ring bounded by two benzene rings. The six tricyclics currently marketed differ by means of varying radicals attached to the central ring. The active agents responsible for both the antidepressant and the toxic effects of the tricyclic antidepressants (TCAs) are the parent compound, generally a tertiary amine, and its metabolite, a secondary amine. Laboratory values represent a combination of both the tertiary amine and its active metabolite. The tertiary amine imipramine is metabolized in vivo to its active desmethyl metabolite, which is the secondary amine desipramine. The tertiary amine amitriptyline is likewise metabolized to its secondary amine, nortriptyline. The tertiary amine doxepin is metabolized to desmethyldoxepin. The secondary amine protriptyline is also marketed as a tricyclic antidepressant.

The first tetracyclic antidepressant to be marketed in the United States is maprotiline (Ludiomil); this has been commercially available in England and Europe for some time. The tetracyclic antidepressants share the properties of the tricyclic antidepressants.

Indeed, if one considers the full gamut of agents in this category available in the United States and Europe, the term *tricyclics* is no longer *chemically* accurate, as there are now one- two-, and four-ring structured drugs with broadly similar properties. The term *tricyclic antidepressant* presently refers to a *pharmacologic* class of agents that have antidepressant properties.

In addition, the skeletal muscle relaxant cyclobenzaprine (Flexeril) and the anticonvulsant carbamazepine (Tegretol) are chemically related to the tricyclic antidepressants; the presentation and management of overdose are also similar.

How the TCAs produce their antidepressant effect is presently unknown and a subject of controversy. Hollister has extensively reviewed this subject.

Electrocardiographic changes, such as ST-T changes or widening of the QRS complex, may be seen at therapeutic levels. The lethal dose is quite variable, but it is generally given as 10 to 30 mg/kg. Tricyclic antidepressants have a narrow margin of safety. In a child, for example, a single dose of 75 mg imipramine may be therapeutic for enuresis, but a 200-mg dose may be lethal.

In lower toxic doses TCAs have a definite anticholinergic effect. In higher doses they prevent reuptake of norepinephrine into the adrenergic neurons, and this is believed to be the basis for their sympathomimetic effects. For this reason, TCAs should not be prescribed along with the monoamine oxidase inhibitors, methyldopa, the sympathomimetic amines, or agents such as atropine that have strong anticholinergic properties. The TCAs have a quinidine-like effect and can depress myocardial contraction, heart rate, and coronary blood flow. Drugs such as quinidine or procainamide, which may further depress myocardial function, should not be prescribed with the tricyclics.

Tricyclics are metabolized by the liver, excreted by the kidney, and are markedly protein-bound. The half-life of the TCAs varies from 24 to 76 h, but may be much longer, especially in overdose. Spiker and Biggs described a patient whose peak total tricyclic level was 1530 ng/mL; after 96 h, the patient's blood level had only fallen to 1280 ng/mL. Tricyclics are lipid-soluble, so that the tissue-to-blood ratio may be from 5:1 to 20:1. Myocardial levels may be from 10 to 100 times plasma levels. Because lipid stores are less in children, their blood levels may be higher.

CLINICAL FEATURES OF OVERDOSE

The first manifestations of TCA overdose are usually the anticholinergic effects. Flushing, dilated pupils, dry mouth, hyperpyrexia, confusion, hallucinations, hyperactive reflexes, clonus, choreoathetosis, and a positive Babinski sign have all been described. Confusion may rapidly lead to coma.

The myocardial effects are generally striking, and mortality is generally related to cardiotoxicity. The TCAs cause disturbances of both impulse formation and conduction. PR prolongation may be seen in the therapeutic range of the TCAs. *It has been demonstrated that a QRS duration greater than 100 ms is a sign of severe cardiotoxicity* (Fig. 26-1). Davies in Australia showed on His bundle electrocardiography that the HV interval was prolonged for *all* tricyclic agents studied except doxepin. In mild overdose, where anticholinergic effects are dominant, supraventricular tachycardia may be observed. When ingestions approach 20 mg/kg, the QRS complex widens, and PVCs, ventricular tachycardia, ventricular fibrillation, and first-degree, atrioventricular, or intraventricular heart block may develop. Hypotension and pulmonary edema may develop secondary to arrhythmias or depression of myocardial pump function.

*Portions of this chapter first appeared in Haddad, 1983, and are reprinted by permission of W.B. Saunders Company.

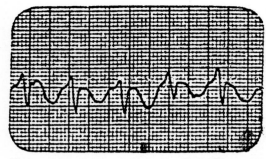

Figure 26-1. Widened QRS of amitryptyline overdose. On admission the ECG indicated a QRS interval of 0.12 s. The widened QRS, indicating serious toxicity, was confirmed by a tricyclic blood level of 126 (μg/100 mL) (1,260 ng/mL). (Courtesy Memorial Medical Center, Savannah.)

Pulmonary insufficiency may occur when the QRS duration is greater than 100 ms. The patient may then require respiratory support, and the mortality rate increases markedly.

TREATMENT

Alkalinization of blood with IV sodium bicarbonate has become the treatment of choice in the management of tricyclic antidepressant overdose.

Treatment must be aggressive from the start. All patients with known tricyclic antidepressant overdose in the prehospital phase are placed on electrocardiographic telemetry.

In the emergency department, the following steps are taken:

1. A catheter is inserted for immediate intravenous D₅W at a "keep open" rate. Maintenance intravenous fluids only are indicated throughout the hospital stay.
2. The patient is placed on cardiac monitor, and a 12-lead electrocardiogram is obtained.
3. Gastric lavage is performed with the usual precautions of airway maintenance, and 60 g of activated charcoal in 250 mL of water as a slurry is given to the patient after gastric lavage, followed by 30 g of sodium sulfate in 125 mL of water as a cathartic. Gastric lavage and activated charcoal are continued every 6 h throughout the hospital stay until the patient is stable, because the tricyclic antidepressants, as noted, are secreted into the stomach and hepatobiliary circulation.
4. To maintain a blood pH of 7.5 an intravenous drip of sodium bicarbonate is begun on all comatose patients, especially any patient who exhibits a QRS interval of 100 ms or more. This is usually begun with 2 ampoules of sodium bicarbonate in 1 L of D₅W. The resultant solution with 88 mEq of sodium will be roughly equivalent to one-half normal physiologic saline, plus 88 mEq of bicarbonate. When a patient is critical, this should be maintained until the patient has been stable for at least 24 h.
5. Proper oxygenation is necessary.
6. A general assessment of the patient is indicated. Has the patient aspirated? Is there evidence of concomitant trauma? Are there other underlying medical conditions requiring management? Are there indications of other drugs involved in overdose? In

short, a general approach to the poisoning patient must be utilized even when a specific agent is known.

These six steps in management are utilized initially for nearly all significant ingestions. Subsequent treatment depends upon observation of the clinical course of the patient. Patients generally remain asymptomatic except for slight drowsiness, develop manifestations of the anticholinergic syndrome, or become critical.

Management of Asymptomatic Patients

Patients who take insignificant amounts in an acute situational reaction or suicide gesture are generally asymptomatic except for slight drowsiness. They are managed with gastric lavage, instillation of activated charcoal, observation, and appropriate referral to either the family physician or a psychiatrist. Observation is critical even when minimal amounts are thought to be ingested, and, as the history is often unreliable, the patient may progress into the anticholinergic syndrome or develop critical signs. Even asymptomatic patients should be observed for about 4 h prior to transfer to the psychiatric unit.

Anticholinergic Effects

Patients who become comatose and flushed, have dilated pupils, and exhibit supraventricular tachycardia but no QRS widening on electrocardiogram manifest the anticholinergic effects of TCA overdose. These patients can usually be managed with gastric lavage, activated charcoal, physostigmine, cardiac monitoring, 12-h observation in the emergency department (or hospital, if there is no emergency department observation unit), and appropriate referral.

These patients are quite successfully managed with physostigmine, the reversible cholinesterase inhibitor that potentiates acetylcholine, thus reversing anticholinergic effects.

Generally, up to 2 mg IV of physostigmine given over 2 min in adults is the recommended initial dosage; this may need to be repeated every 15 to 30 min up to three or four doses, preferably on cardiac monitor, as physostigmine can produce a profound bradycardia; asystole has been described following its use. The initial intravenous dosage for children is 0.1 to 0.5 mg.

The use of physostigmine is most controversial in the face of concurrent intraventricular conduction defects, and its use in this setting should be avoided.

Seizures also have been treated with physostigmine, although both diazepam and alkalinization therapy are preferable, for physostigmine itself can cause seizures.

The use of physostigmine to reverse coma may be justified as a diagnostic trial on a one-time basis with tricyclic antidepressant overdose, but since awakening is only temporary and complications are common, repeated use of physostigmine for this indication probably is not warranted.

Slovis and associates, Rumack, and Burks and colleagues have reported on the use of physostigmine for the management of ventricular arrhythmias. There is no doubt that it can be effective, although there is risk of asystole. For those ventricular arrhythmias resistant to intravenous sodium bicarbonate, physostigmine perhaps should be the next agent of choice.

The Critical Patient

Patients who develop the following carry a significant risk of mortality and should be admitted to the coronary care unit (if resuscitation is successful in the emergency department): hypotension; intraventricular conduction defects of 100 ms or more; pulmonary edema, respiratory insufficiency, or respiratory arrest; ventricular arrhythmias, complete atrioventricular block, profound sinus bradycardia, or cardiac arrest, and exacerbation of preexisting conditions like diabetes mellitus, or other causes of significant metabolic acidosis such as concomitant salicylate overdose.

Management of these patients presents a significant challenge. Keynotes to success are aggressive, supportive therapy and prolonged observation for possible complications. For those patients who require ventilatory support, pulmonary consultation should be obtained if available.

Hypotension often responds dramatically to an intravenous bolus of sodium bicarbonate. Patients who are hypotensive from TCA overdose often also exhibit metabolic acidosis; these patients in particular respond to bicarbonate therapy.

The management of the patient with persistent hypotension unresponsive to bicarbonate is controversial. There are potential problems with both the use of fluid expansion and vasopressors, such as dopamine or dobutamine, but both may be required. If either fluid expansion or dopamine need be considered, Swan-Ganz catheterization may be necessary.

Ventricular arrhythmias secondary to tricyclic antidepressant overdose should first be managed with an intravenous bolus of sodium bicarbonate as described.

For those patients who do not respond to sodium bicarbonate, either phenytoin (Dilantin) or physostigmine is the next agent of choice.

Dilantin is a group II antiarrhythmic agent and is known to have application in arrhythmias of which the mechanism is associated with *unidirectional block with reentry,* such as postulated with the tricyclic antidepressants. The dosage in adults is 100 mg intravenously over 3 min. Its use has not been recommended in children.

Hagerman and Hanashiro recently recommended that phenytoin be initiated to reverse first-degree AV block and intraventricular conduction delay secondary to TCA overdose. Phenytoin was injected intravenously at a rate of 50 mg/min, not to exceed 500 mg in adults.

Propranolol is usually reserved for life-threatening ventricular arrhythmias in children with TCA overdose. The rationale for its use lies in its β-blocker effects, as the TCAs are sympathomimetic. The dose in children is usually 0.25 mg IV given as a bolus, or 0.1 mg/kg. Congestive heart failure, asthma, and heart block are contraindications to the use of propranolol.

Table 26-1 summarizes the use of agents in the management of TCA-induced ventricular arrhythmias.

While electric countershock usually converts ventricular tachycardia and ventricular fibrillation, it has been our experience that the patient's arrhythmia remains unstable and often reverts to a ventricular arrhythmia without drug therapy.

Finally, emergency pacemaker insertion may be indicated for severe bradyarrhythmia and heart block. A standby pacemaker should be inserted if these conditions appear progressive and are unresponsive to therapy.

Table 26-1. Therapy of TCA-Induced Tachyarrhythmias

Agent	Dosage
Agent of choice:	
Sodium bicarbonate	1 mEq/kg IV bolus followed by 44 mEq/250 mL D₅W IV drip
Physostigmine	Adult: Up to 2 mg IV push
	Child: 0.1–0.5 mg IV (Contraindicated if there is concurrent intraventricular conduction defect)
Phenytoin	Adult: 100 mg IV over 3 min
	Child: Not recommended
Propranolol	Adult: 0.50–1.0 mg IV bolus
	Child: 0.25 mg IV bolus
	Repeat q 5 min to maximum of three doses
Contraindicated:	
? Digitalis	
Quinidine	
Epinephrine	
Atropine	
Ineffective:	
Magnesium	
Calcium	
Potassium	
? Lidocaine	

BIBLIOGRAPHY

Arnsdorf MF: Electrophysiologic properties of antidysrhythmic drugs as a rational basis for therapy. *Med Clin North Am* 60:213–232, 1976.

Bigger JT, Giardina EGV, Perel JM, et al: Cardiac antiarrhythmic effect of imipramine hydrochloride. *N Engl J Med* 296:206–208, 1977.

Biggs JT, Spiker DG, Petit JM, et al: Tricyclic antidepressant overdose: Incidence of symptoms. *JAMA* 238:135–138, 1977.

Brown TC: Sodium bicarbonate treatment for tricyclic antidepressant arrhythmias in children. *Med J Aust* 2:380–382, 1976.

Brown TC: Tricyclic antidepressant overdosage: Experimental studies on the management of circulatory complications. *Clin Toxicol* 9:255–272, 1976.

Brown TC, Barker GA, Dunlop ME, et al: The use of sodium bicarbonate in the treatment of tricyclic antidepressant-induced arrhythmias. *Anaesth Intens Care* 1:203–210, 1973.

Burks JS, Walker JE, Rumack RH, et al: Tricyclic antidepressant poisoning: Reversal of coma, choreoathetosis, and myoclonus by physostigmine. *JAMA* 230:1405–1407, 1974.

Christensen KN, Andersen, HH: Deliberate poisoning with tricyclic antidepressants treated in an intensive care unit. *Acta Pharmacol Toxicol* 41(2): suppl:511–515, 1977.

Davies B, Burrows G, Dumovic P, et al: Effects on the heart of different tricyclic antidepressants, in Mendels J (ed): *Sinequan (doxepin HCL): A Monograph of Recent Clinical Studies.* Amsterdam, *Excerpta Med,* 1975, pp. 54–58.

Frejaville JP, Nicaise AM, Christoforov B, et al: Etude statistique d'une seconde centaine d'intoxications aigues par les dérives de l'iminodibenzyle (Tofranil, Pertofran, G 34, Surmontil) et ceux du dihydrobenzocyclohepadiene (Laroxyl, Elavil). *Bull Soc Med Hop,* 117:1151–1175, 1966.

Haddad LM: Tricyclic antidepressant overdose, in Haddad LM, Winchester JF (eds): *Clinical Management of Poisoning and Drug Overdose*. Philadelphia, Saunders, 1983, pp. 359–371.

Hagerman GA, Hanashiro PK: Reversal of tricyclic antidepressant—induced cardiac conduction abnormalities by phenytoin. *Am Emerg Med* 10:82, 1981.

Hollister LE: Tricyclic antidepressants. *N Engl J Med* 299:1106–1110, 1168–1172, 1978.

Moir DC: Tricyclic antidepressants and cardiac disease. *Am Heart J* 86:841–842, 1973.

Rumack BH: Anticholinergic poisoning: Treatment with physostigmine. *Pediatrics* 52:449–451, 1973.

Sesso AM, Snyder RC, Schott CE, et al: Propranolol in imipramine poisoning. *Am J Dis Child* 126:847–849, 1973.

Slovis TL, Oh JL, Teitelbaum DT, et al: Physostigmine therapy in acute tricyclic antidepressant poisoning. *Clin Toxicol* 4:451–459, 1971.

Spiker DG, Biggs JT: Tricyclic antidepressants: Prolonged plasma levels after overdose. *JAMA* 236:1711–1712, 1976.

Thorstrand C: Cardiovascular effects of poisoning with tricyclic antidepressants. *Acta Med Scand* 195:505–514, 1974.

Thorstrand C: Clinical features in poisonings by tricyclic antidepressants, with special reference to the ECG. *Acta Med Scand* 199:337–344, 1976.

Vohra J, Burrows GD, Sloman G: Assessment of cardiovascular side effects of therapeutic doses of tricyclic antidepressant drugs. *Aust NZ J Med* 5:7–11, 1975.

CHAPTER 27
LITHIUM

Lester Haddad

As lithium carbonate therapy is more widely used by psychiatrists in the management of their patients, the emergency physician is increasingly being called upon to manage lithium overdose. A review of therapeutic usage, physiology, and side effects will enhance an understanding of lithium intoxication. Commercial preparations of lithium include lithium carbonate, Eskalith, Lithane, and Lithonate.

Lithium carbonate is the drug of choice for the manic phase of manic depression. Patients with this type of illness usually make a dynamic presentation to the emergency department and characteristically display "stream of consciousness" talking, reduced need for sleep, marked hyperactivity, grandiosity, elation, impaired judgment, and aggressiveness to the point of hostility.

Lithium reverses manic symptoms within 1 to 3 weeks, and has been shown to increase the time period between attacks and shorten the duration of manic episodes.

A fascinating new role for lithium has been found in medical oncology. Since lithium has been shown to produce leukocytosis, it is now being tried in patients who develop leukopenia in the face of systemic chemotherapy. It has also been used in the management of inappropriate ADH syndrome and steroid psychosis in multiple sclerosis patients.

Other uses of lithium include the treatment of cyclothymic disorders, Huntington's chorea, and hyperactivity in children of lithium-responsive parents. It may have a role in management of treatment-resistant temporal lobe epilepsy.

The initial use of lithium may produce minor side effects that will usually resolve (Table 27-1).

PHARMACOLOGY

Lithium is a member of the same group of elements as sodium and potassium and shares physical and chemical properties of these two biological elements. It has a high ionization potential and is markedly water-soluble. Lithium salts are almost totally absorbed from the gastrointestinal tract, and 97 percent is excreted unchanged in the urine. Thus one does not speak of lithium metabolism, only lithium absorption, distribution, and excretion.

Lithium is evenly distributed through body water, and behaves as extracellular sodium ion and intracellular potassium ion. The mechanism of action in manic states is unknown.

The pharmacokinetics of lithium as described by Singer and Rotenberg are most easily related to partial ion substitution. Following administration, peak and plateau serum concentrations are achieved in 30 min. and 12 to 14 h, respectively. However, lithium crosses cell membranes at a relatively slow rate. This slow entry into and exit from the intracellular space accounts for the delay of 6 to 10 days in achieving therapeutic response to lithium, and also the difficulty in treating toxicity following long-term administration of the drug.

One-third to two-thirds of an oral dose is excreted in 6 to 12 h, followed by a slow excretion over 10 to 14 days. When lithium is discontinued after chronic administration, excretion occurs rapidly for the first 5 to 6 days, and more slowly for the next 10 to 14 days.

Desirable blood levels during therapy are 0.6 to 1.2 mEq/L (mmol/L) and are usually achieved with 900 to 1600 mg lithium carbonate daily, as reported by Hall and Schou. While toxicity is usually not observed under a serum level of 2 mEq/L, close observation and repeated studies are indicated in the 1.5- to 2-mEq/L range. Obviously, the toxic to therapeutic range is very narrow.

As lithium is excreted in breast milk, it should not be used by nursing mothers. Lithium may be teratogenic (Jefferson and Greist) and should not be used the first trimester of pregnancy.

Eighty percent of lithium is reabsorbed by the proximal tubule, but, unlike sodium resorption, none is reabsorbed by the distal tubule. Thus, 20 percent of the filtered load is excreted by the kidney. Sodium loading enhances excretion of lithium, whereas sodium depletion promotes lithium retention, according to Hall; Singer and Rotenberg; and Schou. Thus, loop diuretics such as furosemide, which do not affect excretion of lithium but increase sodium excretion, can precipitate lithium intoxication.

Lithium and Adenylate Cyclase

Hormones such as ADH bind to surface receptors localized on the plasma membrane. Their actions are actually mediated by "second messengers" located in the cell membrane, which in the case of ADH is cyclic AMP. When ADH couples to the receptor site, the complex activates *adenylate cyclase,* which produces cyclic AMP from ATP.

It is now known that lithium inhibits adenylate cyclase and thus inhibits the effect of ADH. Thus *polyuria* is often the first adverse effect seen with lithium administration. Loss of concentrated ability and nephrogenic diabetes inspidus have been described.

One can see that a ''vicious cycle'' develops with chronic lithium intoxication. Inhibiting adenylate cyclase and thus vasopressin, lithium leads to polyuria and thus salt and water loss, which in turn leads to further lithium retention, exacerbating the situation.

Lithium administration is also known to produce thyroid dysfunction.

CLINICAL FEATURES

Cardiac effects of lithium at therapeutic levels have been described by Tilkian et al. Reversible T wave abnormalities are most common, but disturbances of conduction, cardiac arrhythmias, and congestive heart failure have been described with toxic doses.

Table 27-1 lists the signs and symptoms of dose-related lithium intoxication, although these are highly variable depending on whether toxicity results from acute or chronic administration.

Lithium toxicity occurs in two fashions: from acute overdose and during chronic administration. While the emergency physician is usually faced with the overdose situation, the early signs of

Table 27-1. Signs and Symptoms of Dose-Related Lithium Intoxication

Initial response to therapy*:
  Fine tremor of hands
  Dry mouth
  Mildly increased thirst
  Mild polyuria
  Transient mild nausea
Blood level, mEq/L†:
  1.5: Nausea
       Vomiting
       Diarrhea
  2.0: Polyuria
       Blurred vision
       Muscular weakness
       Drowsiness
       Dizziness
       Vertigo
       Increasing confusion
       Slurred speech
       Transient scotomas
       Blackouts
       Fasciculations
       Increased deep tendon reflexes
  2.5: Myoclonic twitches
       Myoclonic movements of entire limb
       Choreoathetoid movements
       Urinary and fecal incontinence
       Increasing restlessness followed by stupor,
         followed by coma
  3.0: Epileptiform seizure
       Cardiac arrhythmias
  4.0: Hypotension
       Peripheral vascular collapse

*Not toxic signs

†May occur in different order or at lower serum levels in susceptible individuals.

Source: From Hall RC, Perl M, Pfefferbaum B: Lithium therapy and toxicity. *Am Fam Phys* 19:135, 1979. Used by permission.

chronic toxicity may be recognized and thus the sequelae of serious intoxication may be prevented.

Chronic Lithium Intoxication

Adverse renal effects. Lithium is known to cause nephrogenic diabetes insipidus (Hall et al.; Jefferson and Greist); impaired renal concentrating ability (urine is diluted with a constant specific gravity in the 1.010 to 1.012 range); reduced creatinine clearance, interstitial fibrosis, and frank renal failure. The presence of polyuria should indicate to the physician the possibility of such adverse effects, and the patient should be immediately worked up for assessment of renal status.

Lithium inhibits aldosterone effects on the distal tubule, reducing sodium reabsorption. With subclinical renal impairment, proximal tubular reabsorption is increased, thus increasing lithium reabsorption and causing lithium intoxication.

Sodium depletion. The most common cause of sodium depletion is the use of thiazide or other diuretics (Hall et al.; Schou; Oh). Sodium depletion increases lithium reabsorption as mentioned, thus producing lithium toxicity.

Hansen and Amdisen described 23 cases of lithium toxicity, 21 of whom developed intoxication during maintenance therapy. Toxic effects on the heart, brain, and kidneys were noted, and the severity of lithium intoxication related both to the lithium level and the duration of lithium intoxication. This has also been observed by other authors (Thomsen and Schou; Jefferson and Greist). Disorders of water and electrolyte metabolism preceded lithium toxicity in a majority of patients, with water loss due to impaired renal concentrating ability a major predisposing factor. Seventeen patients had apparent renal insufficiency. Treatment with sodium chloride in this group led to hypernatremia in some patients, and had no effect on lithium excretion. Hemodialysis in chronic lithium intoxication was the treatment of choice, although two patients expired, two developed persistent neurological sequelae, and five had residual renal impairment.

Acute Lithium Overdose

Acute overdose is usually manifested by neurologic changes varying from confusion, light coma, or seizures; coarse tremors, muscular twitching, or asymmetrical reflexes; and marked gastrointestinal disturbances. Diarrhea may be so severe that the flesh-colored lithium carbonate tablets may appear intact in the watery expulsion. Conduction disturbances, ventricular tachyarrhythmias, and congestive heart failure have been observed. *Shock* is common in the serious overdose.

EMERGENCY MANAGEMENT

Infusion therapy. An intravenous line with normal saline should be begun. In the event of hypotension, rapid infusion of 500 to 1000 mL may be necessary. Replacement of gastrointestinal losses is indicated. Normal saline infusion of from 3 to 6 L may be indicated as a trial to promote a lithium diuresis in the acute overdose situation, but this is dependent on the clinical situation. We usually place all patients on a normal saline infusion as a trial to promote lithium diuresis, at least until the serum lithium level is obtained. While the value of sodium diuresis is presently under question, a trial is certainly warranted in the emergency department especially in the face of hypotension and/or volume depletion.

Gastric lavage. No matter when the ingestion occurred, aggressive gastric lavage is indicated because lithium may be secreted into the stomach. Repeated gastric lavage every 6 h is indicated. Activated charcoal should be utilized following each dosage.

Blood, urine studies. In addition to serum lithium levels, blood and urine studies should include assessment of the patient's renal and electrolyte status; CBC; SMA-6; and serum magnesium, creatinine, calcium, and osmolality levels. Urine specific gravity and urinalysis should be done initially and repeated frequently, especially if an attempt to diurese the patient is undertaken.

Cardiac monitoring. The patient should be placed on cardiac monitor, and in the event of life-threatening ventricular arrhythmias, a trial of magnesium (in addition to the usual measures) may be indicated.

Diuresis. Administration of sodium chloride, sodium bicarbonate, aminophylline, and mannitol to promote an alkaline diuresis may be indicated for the patient who has a serum lithium level under 3 mEq/L and whose cardiac status and blood pressure are relatively stable. If the patient appears to be deteriorating in spite of this regimen, dialysis is indicated.

Hemodialysis. A patient with a serum lithium level of more than 3 mEq/L should be immediately admitted by a nephrologist for possible hemodialysis. Dialysis is effective in lithium overdose because lithium has a small molecular weight, is not protein-binding and does not have toxic metabolites, and has a high water solubility. Dialysis is dramatic and most usually successful in the acute overdose. In the chronic intoxication, however, dialysis may be fraught with difficulty and be associated with a significant degree of irritability, and neurologic, cardiac, and renal sequelae.

BIBLIOGRAPHY

Hall RC, Perl M, Pfefferbaum B: Lithium therapy and toxicity. *Am Fam Phys* 19:133–139, 1979.

Hansen H, Amdisen A: Lithium intoxication. *Q J Med* 47:123–144, 1978.

Jefferson JW, Greist JH: *Primer of Lithium Therapy*. Baltimore, Williams & Wilkins, 1977, pp 137–206.

Lyman GH, Williams CC, Preston D: The use of lithium carbonate to reduce infection and leukopenia during systemic chemotherapy. *New Engl J Med* 302:257–260, 1980.

Oh TE: Furosemide and lithium toxicity. *Anaesth Intens Care* 5:60–62, 1977.

Schou M: Pharmacology and toxicology of lithium. *Annu Rev Pharmacol* 16:231–243, 1976.

Singer I, Rotenberg D: Mechanisms of lithium action. *N Engl J Med* 289:254–260, 1973.

Thomsen K, Schou M: The treatment of lithium poisoning, in Johnson FN (ed): *Lithium Research and Therapy*. New York, Academic Press, 1975, pp 227–236.

Tilkian AG, Schroeder JS, Kao JJ, et al: The cardiovascular effects of lithium in man: A review of the literature. *Am J Med* 61:665–670, 1976.

Winchester JF: Lithium intoxication, in Haddad LM, Winchester JF (eds): *Clinical Management of Poisoning and Drug Overdose*. Philadelphia, Saunders, 1983, pp 372–379.

Worthley LIG: Lithium toxicity and refractory cardiac arrhythmia treated with intravenous magnesium. *Anaesth Intens Care* 2:357–360, 1974.

CHAPTER 28
BARBITURATES

Lester Haddad, Roscoe Robinson

Acute barbiturate intoxication is more often purposeful than accidental and more common in adults than children. A past history of one or more suicide attempts can often be elicited and follow-up psychiatric care is important.

PHARMACOLOGY

Barbiturates are chemical derivatives of barbituric acid (Fig. 28-1). The pharmacologic characteristics of each drug are largely determined by the side chains at R_1 and R_2. In general, agents with long side chains possess a short duration of action and a high degree of potency, and undergo hepatic degradation. Agents with short side chains have a longer duration of action and less potency, and are excreted primarily by the kidneys. Physiochemical properties of common barbiturates are listed in Table 28-1.

The pK is equivalent to the pH at which the ionized and non-ionized forms of an acid or base are equal in concentration. Barbiturates are weak organic acids whose pK values range between 7.2 and 8.0 (Table 28-1). A weak acid whose pK is close to the physiologic pH is less ionized in biologic fluids than one whose pK is considerably higher (Fig. 28-2). For example, about 5 percent of the total concentration of phenobarbital (pK 7.2) is non-ionized at pH 7.4, whereas 98 percent of secobarbital (pK 7.9) is nonionized at the same pH. Obviously, minor pH alterations can cause large changes in percent ionization if the pK of the drug is close to the physiologic pH. Phenobarbital is 50 percent nonionized at pH 7.2 but less than 4 percent nonionized at pH 7.5. Conversely, the degree of ionization is affected very little by pH changes of a similar nature when the pK is relatively high. For example, secobarbital is 99 percent nonionized at pH 7.2 and 98 percent nonionized at pH 7.5. Lipid-containing biologic membranes are freely permeable to the nonionized species but relatively impermeable to the ionized form. Although much less lipid-soluble throughout the usual range of blood pH, the tissue penetrance of agents such as phenobarbital can vary considerably because their degree of ionization is so responsive to minor changes of blood pH. Tissue solubility may thus be enhanced during systemic acidosis and diminished during systemic alkalosis.

Although all barbiturates undergo metabolic degradation by the liver to some degree, short-acting agents are principally metabolized in the liver and inactive metabolites are excreted in the urine.

Long- and intermediate-acting barbiturates are primarily excreted unaltered in the urine. Hepatic degradation is a relatively rapid process compared to renal excretion.

Renal Excretion

The unaltered drug is first filtered at the glomerulus, after which it undergoes renal tubular reabsorption by pH-dependent passive diffusion. The passive renal tubular reabsorption of these weak organic acids can be diminished by reducing the concentration of the nonionized form of the drug at the reabsorptive site by an increase in either the volume or pH of tubular fluid. Urinary alkalinization does not increase urinary excretion greatly except in the case of agents such as phenobarbital whose pK values are well below 8.0, which is the maximum urine pH. Variations in tubular fluid pH exert much less effect on the urinary excretion of drugs

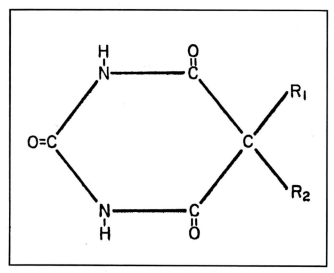

Figure 28-1. Chemical structure for derivatives of barbiturate acid. (From Robinson RR, Gunnells JC Jr, Clapp JR: Treatment of acute barbiturate intoxication. *Mod Treat* 8:563, 1971. Used by permission.)

Table 28-1. Physiochemical Properties of Common Barbiturates

Generic Name	Proprietary Name	pK	Plasma Protein Binding, %	Fatal Dose, g	Fatal Plasma Concentration, mg/100 mL
Long-acting (6 h):					
Barbital	Veronal	7.74	5	10	15
Phenobarbital	Luminal	7.24	20	5	8
Intermediate-acting (3–6 h):					
Amobarbital	Amytal	7.75			
Butabarbital	Butisol	7.74			
Short-acting (3 h):					
Pentobarbital	Nembutal	7.96	35	3	3.5
Secobarbital	Seconal	7.90	44	3	3.5

Source: Robinson RR, Gunnells JC Jr, Clapp JR: Treatment of acute barbiturate intoxication. *Mod Treat* 8:562, 1971. Used by permission.

such as pentobarbital or secobarbital whose pK values are close to 8.0. In general, long-acting barbiturates are much less bound to plasma proteins, and hence more dialyzable, than are short-acting compounds (Table 28-1).

CLINICAL FEATURES

The patient with barbiturate overdose represents the classic case of sedative overdose, and the chart showing stages of coma (Table 28-2) was originally developed to evaluate barbiturate overdose.

The patient usually presents in coma, and will often be hypothermic and cyanotic, have depressed respirations, and show clinical signs of shock. Persistence of the pupillary light reflex in spite of deep coma is a classic sign of barbiturate overdose. Corneal and deep tendon reflexes are often absent.

INITIAL EVALUATION

Acute barbiturate intoxication must be differentiated from other forms of coma or central nervous system injury. Information regarding occupation and possible trauma, and previous psychiatric illnesses, attempts at suicide, and drug usage should be obtained. Obtain an accurate history regarding the type, amount, and time of drug ingestion, the duration of coma, and the associated ingestion of alcohol. Alcohol is synergistic with barbiturates and will considerably increase the depth of coma.

Trauma, pressure sores, and bullous lesions on the skin suggest barbiturate overdose. Ascertain if the patient has jaundice, an enlarged liver, and a history of cirrhosis, as treatment will have to be modified in the presence of liver impairment.

After establishing an airway by endotracheal intubation and initiating an intravenous infusion of normal saline, obtain appropriate blood studies including serum barbiturate and alcohol levels.

Plasma barbiturate levels are notoriously unreliable. A plasma concentration of 3 to 5 mg/100 mL for short-acting drugs is often given as potentially fatal. However, because of synergism with alcohol, a short-acting level of 1.5 mg/100 mL may be potentially lethal. On the other hand, tolerance and chronic abuse may enable a patient with a blood level of 40 mg/100 mL to walk into the emergency department.

TREATMENT

Treatment of barbiturate overdose is directed to maintaining the patient's vital signs, avoiding complications, and eliminating the drug.

Ventilation

Respiratory arrest is often common in the severe barbiturate overdose, and endotracheal intubation and ventilatory assistance is often necessary.

Circulation

Hypotension can usually be corrected by fluid replacement with normal saline given in a bolus immediately in the emergency

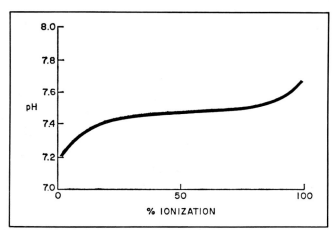

Figure 28-2. Titration curve for a weak organic acid (pK 7.5) against a base. Curve is similarly shaped for most barbiturates although its relationship to the vertical pH scale will vary according to specific pK value of each drug (pH = pK = 50 percent ionization). (From Robinson RR, Gunnells JC Jr, Clapp JR: Treatment of acute barbiturate intoxication. *Mod Treat* 8:562, 1971. Used by permission.)

Table 28-2. Stages of Coma

Group I: A patient who is comatose but will withdraw from painful stimuli such as venipunctures, slapping, pinching, etc. There is no circulatory embarrassment, and all reflexes are intact.

Group II: A patient who does not withdraw from painful stimuli but has no respiratory or circulatory depression. Most or all of the reflexes are intact.

Group III: A patient most or all of whose reflexes are absent, but who is without depression of respiration or circulation.

Group IV: A patient most or all of whose reflexes are absent, and who has respiratory depression with cyanosis, or circulatory failure and shock, or both.

It is important to emphasize that grouping of a patient should not be done until an adequate airway has been established because cyanosis and areflexia may be secondary to anoxia on an obstructive basis. When oxygenation is reestablished, the patient will be in a lighter group than at first.

In evaluating reflexes, primary emphasis should be given to the tendon reflexes. We have found that the pupillary and especially the corneal reflexes are often deceptive. Contrary to classic teaching, our experience has been that often the corneal reflex is the first to disappear and the last to return.

Source: Adapted from Reed CE, Driggs MF, Foote CC: Acute barbiturate intoxication: A study of 300 cases based on a physiologic system of classification of the severity of the intoxication. *Ann Intern Med* 37:291, 1952.

department. If hypotension does not respond to correction of hypoxia, dehydration, and rapid fluid replacement with normal saline, a vasopressor may be required. Dopamine is probably the agent of choice for correction of resistant hypotension.

Gastric Lavage

Aggressive gastric lavage with subsequent instillation of activated charcoal is indicated in all deeply sedated patients regardless of the time lapse since the ingestion. It is done following airway protection, usually with endotracheal intubation, and with a large-bore tube. The possible presence of ileus makes gastric lavage nearly always a worthwhile endeavor. The use of a cathartic such as magnesium sulfate is also indicated. Olive oil or castor oil may also be indicated, as it may dissolve concretions.

Alkalinization

Urinary alkalinization is a more effective form of therapy in patients with phenobarbital intoxication than in those who have ingested short-acting agents. For reasons outlined above, the urinary excretion of barbiturates with higher pK values is little affected by urinary alkalinization. However, if an alkalinizing agent such as sodium bicarbonate is used, a more favorable pH gradient between intracellular fluid and blood may be created, perhaps facilitating removal of barbiturate from peripheral tissues. Since phenobarbital excretion is enhanced tenfold by the use of sodium

bicarbonate, and since it is not contraindicated and may be helpful with short-acting barbiturates, the use of sodium bicarbonate is indicated, at least until definitive studies are available.

Forced Diuresis

The rate of urinary barbiturate excretion is directly related to increasing urine flow; this observation is consistent with the fact that filtered barbiturate is subsequently and partially reabsorbed via passive diffusion.

While the renal clearance of all barbiturates is increased at high rates of urine flow, forced diuresis is more effective for long-acting drugs such as phenobarbital than for short-acting drugs such as pentobarbital and secobarbital. Forced diuresis may excrete 20 percent of the filtered load of phenobarbital.

While some have recommended an average daily volume of 8 to 14 L to achieve maximum results, the danger of overhydration resulting in pulmonary edema, and electrolyte imbalance from intravenous infusion of fluids at the rate of 500 mL/h, indicate a more conservative approach, especially in a patient with underlying cardiac, hepatic, pulmonary, or renal disease.

The use of mannitol or furosemide or both to induce, and sustain diuresis is definitely indicated, especially for phenobarbital overdose. In adult patients, we have initiated diuresis with intravenous mannitol in the emergency department, and subsequently maintained diuresis with furosemide, 40 mg every 6 hours (in adult patients).

While hemodialysis or peritoneal dialysis has played a significant role in the management of barbiturate overdose in the 1950s and 1960s, conservative management with maintenance of vital signs, fluid and electrolyte balance, and alkalinization and forced diuresis are effective for the majority of these patients.

However, the patient with either hepatic or renal failure and other underlying illnesses may require dialysis, as well as patients with disturbance of vital signs. Charcoal hemoperfusion is also a useful modality in severe barbiturate overdose.

BIBLIOGRAPHY

Beveridge LW, Lawson AAH: Occurrence of bullous lesions in acute barbiturate intoxication. *Br Med J* 1:835–837, 1965.

Mann JB, Sandberg DH: Therapy of sedative overdosage. *Ped Clin North Am* 17:617–628, 1970.

Reed CE, Drigg MF, Foote CC: Acute barbiturate intoxication: A study of 300 cases based on a physiologic system of classification of the severity of the intoxication. *Ann Intern Med* 37:290–303, 1952.

Robinson RR, Gunnells JC Jr, Clapp JR: Treatment of acute barbiturate intoxication, in *Mod Treat* 8:561–579, 1971.

Spear PW, Protass LM: Barbiturate poisoning—An endemic disease: Five years' experience in a municipal hospital. *Med Clin North Am* 57:1471–1479, 1973.

Winchester JF: Barbiturates, in Haddad LM, Winchester JF (eds): *Clinical Management of Poisoning and Drug Overdose.* Philadelphia, Saunders, 1983.

Winchester JF, Gelfand MC, Knepshield JH, et al: Dialysis and hemoperfusion of poisons and drugs. *Trans Am Soc Artif Intern Organs* 23:770–773, 1977.

CHAPTER 29
NARCOTICS

George Sternbach

The number of narcotics addicts in the United States is estimated at 700,000, but the true incidence is probably much higher, and the mortality and morbidity associated with narcotic abuse is significant. This chapter will discuss these complications and their management.

Morphine is an opium alkaloid derived from the poppy, *Papaver somniferum*. Heroin is produced by the acetylation of morphine.

Street heroin is adulterated, usually in a 20 to 100:1 ratio, with a number of agents such as quinine, lactose, sucrose, mannitol, magnesium silicate (talc), procaine, or baking soda. Quinine is most commonly used, and in itself can produce auditory, ophthalmic, muscular, gastrointestinal, and renal toxicity.

CLINICAL FEATURES

Narcotic Intoxication

Acute narcotic intoxication is characterized by drowsiness, euphoria, miosis, conjunctival injection, and slowed respirations. Decreased sensitivity of the CNS respiratory center to carbon dioxide causes a decrease in minute and tidal volume. Nausea, vomiting, or pruritis can also occur.

Narcotic Withdrawal

The classic picture of narcotic withdrawal includes piloerection, lacrimation, yawning, rhinorrhea, sweating, nasal stuffiness, myalgia, vomiting, abdominal cramps, and diarrhea. The patient may be generally irritable, hyperactive, or confused.

Heroin withdrawal symptoms are generally seen about 12 to 14 h after the last dose, while symptoms of methadone withdrawal occur in 24 to 36 h. On occasion, the treatment of an overdose patient with naloxone may cause the patient to awaken with symptoms of withdrawal. Treatment of withdrawal is generally symptomatic.

The most common long-term treatment of narcotic withdrawal syndrome is through the substitution of methadone and the gradual withdrawal of that drug. Recently the antihypertensive agent clonidine has been utilized to effect narcotic detoxification. Clonidine has been shown to alleviate the symptoms of withdrawal, especially chills, lacrimation, rhinorrhea, abdominal cramping, sweating, myalgia, and arthralgia. Though the severity of symptoms is ameliorated, their presence is not entirely eliminated by clonidine. The mechanism by which the drug acts to reduce symptoms of opiate withdrawal appears to be by inhibiting adrenergic activity at α_2-adrenergic receptors. Side effects of clonidine treatment include hypotension, dizziness, drowsiness, and dry mouth. Dosage must be adjusted to individual reaction.

Narcotic Overdose

The cardinal physical findings of narcotic overdose are pinpoint pupils and hypoventilation. However, the pupils may be midrange or dilated if CNS hypoxia has occurred. Hypertension may be present secondary to hypoxia. An injection site may be visible or absent, depending on whether the patient injected the drug, inhaled it, or took it orally.

Street methods of overdose resuscitation include packing the victim in ice, pouring milk down the throat, and injecting milk or saline intramuscularly or intravenously. Complications of such resuscitation methods include hypothermia, aspiration pneumonia, and local cellulitis.

TREATMENT

The treatment of coma due to narcotic overdose is naloxone, at least 0.4 mg to 2 mg in an adult, and 0.01 mg/kg in a child or neonate. The drug may be given subcutaneously, intramuscularly, or intravenously. When administered intravenously, it is effective in 1 to 2 min. The dose may be repeated as needed. Naloxone can also be given as an IV infusion, with the dose titrated to clinical response; 2 mg of naloxone in 500 mL of normal saline or 5% dextrose produces a concentration of 0.004 mg/mL, or 0.4 mg/100 mL.

Through antagonism at opiate receptor sites in the CNS, naloxone rapidly reverses coma and respiratory depression caused by narcotics. Pentazocine has been shown to occupy receptor sites other than those of the opiates, and although naloxone can reverse the CNS depressant effects of this drug, larger doses are generally required. High-dose administration of naloxone has also been shown to reverse respiratory depression produced by propoxyphene and diazepam.

Many heroin addicts also use other drugs or alcohol so that overdose may be of a mixed type. Coma due to the action of other drugs will not be antagonized by naloxone.

The serum half-life of naloxone is about 1 h, with a duration of action of 2 to 3 h. Close observation and repeated injections or continuous intravenous administration may be necessary, since the action of the narcotic may be significantly longer than that of the antagonist. This is especially true with methadone, whose duration of action may be as long as 72 h.

Naloxone is virtually without adverse effect, even when given chronically and in large doses. Its action is purely narcotic-antagonistic, and the drug displays no intrinsic agonistic effects. In the truly addicted patient, however, its administration may precipitate a withdrawal syndrome of sudden and alarming proportions.

COMPLICATIONS OF NARCOTIC ABUSE

Skin

The appearance of the addict's skin is most characteristic. The tracks of repeated venous injections may be accompanied by the hallmark of subcutaneous use: small, oval, punctate, or depressed ulcers, or hyperpigmented atrophic lesions. Nonpitting edema of the upper or lower extremities is often seen in addicts of long standing. This results from occlusive thrombophlebitis, lymphatic obstruction, and lymphedema.

Infections

Among the most common sequelae of heroin addiction are infections. Narcotics cause inhibition of leukocyte motility and phagocytosis, and both humoral and cellular immune function abnormalities have been described in heroin addicts. In addition, the notorious lack of sterile technique among users contributes to the high incidence of infection. Recently, acquired immune deficiency syndrome (AIDS) has been reported in intravenous drug users.

Abscess, Cellulitis, Thrombophlebitis

Abscesses and cellulitis, especially of the hands and forearms, are common to subcutaneous injectors. These abscesses most often contain staphylococci, but may harbor other flora, including anaerobic bacteria. Small abscesses with no surrounding cellulitis can be treated with drainage and hexachlorophene soaks. More extensive lesions require antibiotic therapy, usually with an agent effective against penicillinase-producing staphylococci. Since septicemia or endocarditis cannot be ruled out with certainty in most patients with fever, hospitalization is often necessary, and blood cultures should be obtained before antibiotic therapy is begun.

Infections of the hand or fingers often require surgical drainage, for progression to gangrene can be rapid. Abscesses in the neck or groin are generally drained in the surgical suite because of their proximity to major vessels. Mycotic aneurysm should be considered in the differential diagnosis of abscesses in these areas.

Septic thrombophlebitis, most often involving the legs or thighs, is a common result of intravenous heroin use. It is characterized by painful swelling and warmth of the affected extremity. Unlike uncomplicated deep venous thrombosis, septic thrombophlebitis requires treatment with antibiotics, not heparin alone.

Mycotic aneurysm of the brain, neck, or groin can result in life-threatening hemorrhage. Masses in the neck or groin of a drug user should be carefully evaluated for pulsation or bruits, to rule out the presence of a mycotic aneurysm.

Endocarditis

Endocarditis is a serious complication. Louria reports mortality figures as high as 69 percent among addicts with endocarditis. Endocarditis may affect the left or right side of the heart, and the relative incidence varies widely in different reports.

Right-sided infections are the most common in addicts. These usually spare the pulmonic valve, attacking a previously normal tricuspid valve in almost all cases. Murmurs may be absent, faintly heard, or audible in atypical locations. Indeed, there may be no physical findings of tricuspid valvular disease per se, the diagnosis being made on the basis of multiple or repeated septic pulmonary emboli. The infecting organism is most often *Staphylococcus aureus*. The clinical picture of septic pulmonary emboli in these cases is often that of pneumonia with staphylococcal septicemia. The radiologic appearance may be one of pulmonary consolidation. Alternatively, round or wedged-shaped lesions may appear successively in the periphery of the lungs. On the other hand, initial chest roentgenograms may be unremarkable, or display only minor abnormality, with typical findings appearing only as the disease progresses. Pulmonary infarcts may progress to cavitation, abscess, or empyema formation. Following treatment, the chest film may revert to normal, or may display residual atelectasis or pleural thickening.

Left-sided cardiac valves may be affected in the presence or absence of previous aortic or mitral abnormality. The aortic valve in particular is susceptible even without preexisting disease. Classical physical findings of bacterial endocarditis are frequently present in left-sided disease. Organisms may be cultured from sites of extravascular embolization, such as Osler's nodes and Janeway lesions. *Escherichia coli, Streptococcus, Klebsiella,* and *Pseudomonas* species, as well as *Candida albicans,* are the most frequent pathogens involved in left-sided heroin-related endocarditis. It has been observed that of these, *C. albicans* never affects previously normal valves.

Complications of infective endocarditis include systemic embolization to the viscera, extremities, and brain; and acute valvular insufficiency. Focal CNS signs and progressive renal failure may develop. Embolization to a coronary vessel can result in acute myocardial infarction. Acute aortic insufficiency can lead to death within hours, and may be difficult to diagnose because the classic hallmarks of chronic aortic insufficiency, such as a widened pulse pressure and prominent diastolic murmur, are often absent. The clinical picture is most often one of unexplained dyspnea, tachycardia, and hypotension, followed by cardiovascular collapse. Acute mitral valve rupture is characterized by severe, sudden pulmonary edema. A loud mitral insufficiency murmur is usually present.

Malaria

Malaria was first described as a complication of narcotic abuse in Egypt in 1929. In the 1930s, the disease was considered endemic among addicts in New York City. A high mortality rate accompanied an epidemic of falciparum malaria that occurred in 1933. However, no further cases have been seen in this country. Some authors speculated that quinine adulterant in street heroin was acting to obliterate this complication. In 1971, however, a series of syringe-transmitted cases of vivax malaria were reported in California. Although it was postulated that the initial case originated in a serviceman returning from Vietnam, this could not be verified.

Any of the naturally occurring forms of malaria may be seen in the addict. Due to the rarity of the disease in this country, it is seldom considered in the differential diagnosis of the febrile addict. Indeed, many of the patients in the epidemic of 1933 were thought—on the basis of their chills, fever, and malaise—to be undergoing withdrawal. Though discomforting, acute narcotic withdrawal in the adult is, of itself, not life-threatening. Many of the symptoms, however, resemble those of a febrile illness, and the physician must be alert to the possibility of sepsis in a patient who appears to be undergoing withdrawal.

Tetanus

Tetanus was first described in addicts in 1876 and has been a relatively frequent observation among them ever since. An inordinately high mortality follows tetanus infection in the heroin user. It is a disease predominantly of the older, long-standing addict, especially the female. Some have speculated that adolescents and males are more likely to be protected by childhood or military immunization. Tetanus is more frequently seen in subcutaneous injectors, and many of these tend to be women, perhaps because the less prominent veins in many females preclude regular intravenous use. Emergency department patients should be routinely questioned on the status of their tetanus immunizations.

Pulmonary Complications

The occurrence of pulmonary complications in addicts is related to the duration of heroin use but not to the amount used or to overdose. Pneumonia is frequently seen. The bacterial agent is usually *Pneumococcus, Haemophilus, Klebsiella,* or *Staphylococcus aureus.* Factors predisposing the drug user to pneumonia include direct drug effects: slowing of the epiglottic, cough, and sighing reflexes; alveolar hypoventilation; aspiration of gastric contents; and alterations of humoral and cellular immunity.

Lung abscess may complicate bacterial pneumonia, aspiration pneumonitis, or pulmonary infarction. Pathogens may be either aerobic or anaerobic. Heroin addicts also contract tuberculosis more frequently than nonusers.

Pulmonary edema following use of heroin is a serious complication. Although the onset of symptoms usually immediately follows injection, it may also be delayed 24 to 48 h. The mechanism of onset is unclear, but it is characterized by an increase in capillary permeability with exudation of fluid into the alveoli. Whether the edema is due to hypoxia, an allergic reaction, or the direct toxic effects of heroin is unclear. Pulmonary edema is usually bilateral, though it may appear in one or only a part of one lung.

Physical signs include cyanosis, diffuse rales, tachypnea, tachycardia, and foamy sputum in the mouth. Extensive rales may be absent if pulmonary edema is perihilar or localized. Arterial blood gases reveal a profound hypoxemia, and there may or may not be hypercarbia as well.

The chest roentgenogram displays unilateral or bilateral, fluffy, ill-defined densities in an alveolar pattern, radiating centrally to peripherally. The heart size is usually normal but may be slightly enlarged. The differential diagnosis should include head trauma, subarachnoid hemorrhage, near-drowning, noxious gas inhalation, and allergic reaction.

The treatment of heroin-induced pulmonary edema consists of support of respirations, usually with a volume ventilator and the early use of positive-end expiratory pressure (PEEP), and the administration of naloxone. Other components of pulmonary edema therapy—digitalis, diuretics, or rotating tourniquets—are neither effective nor necessary. Response is usually dramatic, with physical findings clearing within 1 day and radiologic changes reverting to normal within 72 to 96 h.

Angiothrombotic pulmonary hypertension, a syndrome of pulmonary hypertension and cor pulmonale, results from recurrent embolization of injected material to the pulmonary vasculature. This is most frequently seen in those injecting oral preparations intravenously, but also affects heroin users, because of the talc and starch fillers in street heroin and the cotton through which the narcotic may be filtered prior to its use. Clinical presentation of the syndrome includes dyspnea, a pulmonic ejection murmur, and signs of right ventricular hypertrophy. Roentgenogram findings include a nodular, irregular shadow pattern that is symmetrical and perihilar in distribution.

Pulmonary function studies in chronic intravenous narcotic users have shown that diffusing capacity and vital capacity are decreased. It is uncertain whether these effects are due to a direct toxic action of heroin or represent sequelae of repeated episodes of the pulmonary diseases to which these patients are prone. Pulmonary infarction has been previously mentioned as a complication of right-sided endocarditis.

Hepatic Complications

The most common side effect of parenteral drug use is acute or chronic hepatic liver dysfunction. Liver function tests consistent with acute hepatitis were displayed in 10 to 15 percent of addicts tested, while approximately another 60 percent had less dramatic abnormalities. The latter are usually attributed to chronic hepatitis, and, indeed, in a study of addicts who died suddenly, 75 percent showed autopsy evidence of chronic hepatitis. This has commonly been assumed to be type B, or serum, hepatitis. It is being recognized, however, that hepatitis A—the infectious type—is also transmitted by needle, and is probably the disease seen in many younger addicts.

Experimental morphine addiction in animals has not been found to induce hepatitis or to exacerbate preexisting liver disease; so a toxic or allergic narcotic effect cannot be invoked to explain this extremely common association.

A large proportion of heroin addicts are heavy alcohol abusers as well, so liver disease in addicts may, in actuality, be alcohol-induced. Treatment of addicts with hepatitis is essentially the same as treatment for liver impairment of other origin. Progression from acute to chronic disease or a fatal outcome is best correlated with greatly elevated transaminase levels in the acute state.

Gastrointestinal Complications

Intestinal hypomotility, a direct narcotic effect, may give rise to ileus. The abdominal distension, obstructive bowel sounds, and dilated loops of bowel seen on radiologic examination can be associated with this condition and may mimic intestinal obstruction. Termed *intestinal pseudoobstruction,* this must be differentiated from the surgical abdomen.

Because of constipation due to hypomotility, there is a significantly increased incidence of symptomatic hemorrhoids and fecal impaction in narcotics addicts.

CNS Complications

The neurologic complications of heroin injection are many and varied. Some have clear etiologies and others are less readily explained. Traumatic mononeuritis is easily diagnosed because there is immediate postinjection pain and paresthesia in a definite nerve distribution. The loss of function sustained in this manner is usually permanent.

Heroin and merperidine overdose have been reported to cause seizures, although this is uncommon. These are usually grand mal and of short duration. The result may be a typical postictal stupor. Seizures induced by narcotics may also be focal, even in the absence of focal lesions. However, focal CNS lesions resulting in altered states of consciousness may have grave implications in view of the addict's increased propensity for meningitis and intracerebral abscess. Focal neurologic signs are not a feature of uncomplicated addiction per se. Subarachnoid hemorrhage is a less common, though well-recognized, complication of heroin addiction. This is thought to be due to vascular weakness caused by necrotizing angiitis or mycotic aneurysm.

The most frequent neurologic complication of narcotic abuse is nontraumatic mononeuropathy. This appears as a painless weakness 2 to 3 h after injection, with no history suggestive of pressure neuropathy. An entire brachial or lumbosacral plexitis may be seen, unrelated either to direct injection or to pressure effect. This often occurs in association with other neurologic complications.

Transverse myelitis involving thoracic segments of the spinal cord is seen particularly in patients reinstituting heroin injections after a 1- to 6-month abstinence. The cause is unclear, but it has been speculated to be toxic or hypersensitive mechanisms or vascular insufficiency to a portion of the thoracic cord. Horner's syndrome can occur as a result of neck injection.

Polyneuritis indistinguishable from Guillain-Barré syndrome has been reported. This may progress to respiratory failure.

The heroin user who has pain in the extremity may be the victim of a number of phenomena. Intraarterial injection, like neural trauma, results in immediate severe pain—in this instance along the distribution of the affected artery. Initial physical signs may be subtle and easily overlooked. The eventual outcome may include ischemic necrosis of the extremity. This end is more likely if the lower extremities are involved, less so if there is involvement of the arms.

The pathophysiology of this ischemic necrosis has been postulated to include several factors. Certainly, distal embolization of particulate matter poses a threat to the circulation via occlusion. Damage caused by the needle to the intimal layer of the vessel may also result in occlusion. Arteries may release catecholamines upon such insult, and although vasospasm has long been assumed to be a major factor in this process, recent work casts doubt upon this particular theory. Various therapeutic modalities have been employed, including sympathectomy and infusion of heparin or dextran, but the eventual outcome may not be greatly affected by such actions.

Muscular Complications

The drug user may be careless of the position of the limbs while in a deep drug-induced stupor, and arterial occlusion may result. A vicious cycle is established in which ischemic injury produces edema, which raises pressure in fascial compartments, which in turn aggravates ischemia. This "crush" syndrome creates a situation in which open fasciotomy may be necessary to save the involved extremity. The patient complains of increasing pain and progressive weakness as intrafascial pressure mounts, but external signs may be few. The physician may be forced to exercise clinical judgment upon hearing this history, with no more as a guide than a firm, wooden feeling to the extremity.

Signs of generalized sepsis along with raised pressure in the fascial compartment pose an even more ominous situation, these being the hallmarks of necrotizing fasciitis. This constitutes a spreading septic necrosis resulting from subfascial injection. The extremity is frequently dusky, edematous, and tender, and systemic signs of fever, tachycardia, chills, and leukocytosis are present. The bacterial agent is most likely to be streptococcal, staphylococcal, or a gram-negative organism. The entity produces a mortality rate as high as 30 percent. Treatment includes antibiotic therapy and surgical debridement.

Generalized necrosis of skeletal muscle sometimes occurs acutely in addicts. The rhabdomyolysis syndrome may occur in a variety of clinical situations, but if there is a mechanism peculiar to narcotic use of its intramuscular injection, this is unknown. Muscles over much of the body may be tender and edematous, and the extremities weak. The hallmark of this syndrome is myoglobin in the urine. Prompt treatment is in order to prevent renal damage.

A syndrome of fever, paraspinal myalgia, and periarthritis has been reported in association with the use of brown heroin. Although this clinical picture frequently mimics an acute febrile illness, no infectious organism has been implicated, and antibiotics do not affect the outcome of this self-limited illness.

Bone and Joint Pain

Bone or joint pain in the addict must call to mind at least two potential complications: septic arthritis and osteomyelitis. When injecting veins in the antecubital fossa or on the hand, the addict may inadvertently enter joint spaces at the elbow or wrist, thereby introducing foreign material and bacteria. Organisms may also spread hematogenously to infect sites distal to the site of their introduction. There is a curious predilection for the axial skeleton in such hematogenous metastases, particularly the sternoclavicular joint. Organisms infrequently seen in septic arthritis of nonaddicts, including *Pseudomonas aeruginosa* and *Serratia marcescens*, are frequently a cause.

Hematogenous osteomyelitis, though relatively rare, is a recognized complication of heroin addiction. There is a predilection for the spine, but other bones may be involved. *Pseudomonas* is a frequent pathogen. Osteomyelitis should come to mind whenever sudden back pain is a presenting symptom in a patient with evidence of self-injection. Indeed, the presentation of osteomyelitis may include little more than acute localized pain, as fever is rarely present, and the white blood count and x-ray films are normal early in the course. Spinal epidural abscess should also be considered in the differential diagnosis.

Amenorrhea

Secondary amenorrhea is common in female heroin users. In several studies, one-third to two-thirds of adolescent girls using narcotics ceased menstruating. An additional group displayed oligomenorrhea and hypomenorrhea. Normal menses resumed after discontinuation of the drug, but amenorrhea sometimes persisted for several months to a year. It has been thought that heroin produces amenorrhea by suppression of pituitary gonadotropin secretion.

Complications of pregnancy are frequent and include a high incidence of toxemia, as well as delivery of premature or growth-retarded babies. Up to 70 percent of babies born to drug-using mothers experience neonatal withdrawal, a potentially fatal condition.

BIBLIOGRAPHY

Armine ARC: Neurosurgical complications of heroin addiction: Brain abscess and mycotic aneurysm. *Surg Neurol* 7:385–386, 1977.

Bai J, Greenwald E, Caterini H, et al: drug-related menstrual aberrations. *Obstet Gynecol* 44:713–719, 1974.

Bakris GL, Cross PD, Hammarsten JE: The use of clonidine for management of opiate abstinence in a chronic pain patient. *Mayo Clin Proc* 57:657–660, 1982.

Bick RL, Anhalt JE: Malaria transmission among narcotic addicts. *Calif Med: The West J Med* 115:56–58, 1971.

Briggs JH, McKerron CG, Souhami RL, et al: Severe systemic infections complicating "mainline" heroin addiction. *Lancet* 2:1227–1231, 1967.

Brown SM, Stimmel B, Taub RN, et al: Immunologic dysfunction in heroin addicts. *Arch Intern Med* 134:1001–1006, 1974.

Brust JCM, Richter RW: Quinine amblyopia related to heroin addiction. *Ann Intern Med* 74:84–86, 1971.

Brust JCM, Richter RW: Tetanus in the inner city. *NY State J Med* 74:1735–1742, 1974.

Cherubin CE: Infectious disease problems of narcotic addicts. *Arch Intern Med* 128:309–313, 1971.

Cherubin CE: The medical sequelae of narcotic addiction. *Ann Intern Med* 67:23–33, 1967.

Citron BP, Halpern M, McCarron M, et al: Necrotizing angiitis associated with drug abuse. *N Engl J Med* 283:1003–1011, 1970.

Citron BP, Halpern M, Haverback BJ: Necrotizing angiitis associated with drug abuse: A new clinical entity. *Clin Res* 19:181, 1971.

Duberstein JL, Kaufman DM: A clinical study of an epidemic of heroin intoxication and heroin-induced pulmonary edema. *Am J Med* 51:704–714, 1971.

Eckenhoff JE, Oech SR: The effects of narcotics and antagonists upon respiration and circulation in man: A review. *Clin Pharmacol Ther* 1:483–524, 1960.

Feldberg W, Paton WDM: Release of histamine from skin and muscle in the cat by opium alkaloids and other histamine liberators. *J Physiol* 114:490–509, 1951.

Frand UI, Shim CS, Williams MH Jr: Heroin-induced pulmonary edema. *Ann Intern Med* 77:29–35, 1972.

Fultz JM, Senay EC: Guidelines for the management of hospitalized narcotic addicts. *Ann Intern Med* 82:815–818, 1975.

Gaulden EG, Littlefield DC, Putoff OE, et al: Menstrual abnormalities associated with heroin addiction. *Am J Obstet Gynecol* 90:155–160, 1964.

Geelhoed GW, Joseph WL: Surgical sequelae of drug abuse. *Surg Gynecol Obstet* 139:749–755, 1974.

Gelb AM, Mildovan D, Stenger RJ: The spectrum and causes of liver disease in narcotic addicts. *Am J Gastroenterol* 67:314–318, 1977.

Gifford DB, Patzakis M, Ivler D, et al: Septic arthritis due to pseudomonas in heroin addicts. *J Bone Joint Surg* 57A:631–635, 1975.

Gilroy J, Adaya L, Thomas VJ: Intracranial mycotic aneurysms and subacute bacterial endocarditis in heroin addiction. *Neurology* 23:1193–1198, 1973.

Goldin RJ, Chow AW, Edwards JE, et al: Sternoarticular septic arthritis in heroin users. *N Engl J Med* 289:616–618, 1973.

Gottlieb LS, Boylen TC: Pulmonary complications of drug abuse. *West J Med* 120:8–16, 1974.

Helpern M, Rho YM: Deaths from narcotism in New York City: Incidence, circumstances, and postmortem findings. *NY State J Med* 66:2391–2408, 1966.

Hunt LG: Prevalence of active heroin use in the US, in Rittenhouse JD (ed): *The Epidemiology of Heroin and Other Narcotics.* Monograph 16, National Institute of Drug Abuse, 1977, pp 61–86.

Husby G, Peirce PE, Williams RC Jr: Smooth muscle antibody in heroin addicts. *Ann Intern Med* 83:801–805, 1975.

Jaffe JH, Koschmann EG: Intravenous drug abuse: Pulmonary, cardiac, and vascular complications. *Am J Roentgenol Radium Ther Nucl Med* 109:107–120, 1970.

Jasinski DR, Martin WR, Haertzen CA: The human pharmacology and abuse potential of N-allynoroxymorphone (naloxone). *J Pharmacol Exp Ther* 157:420–426, 1967.

Johannesson T, Norn S: The effect of morphine on the histamine contents of brain and skin in the rat. *Acta Pharmacol Toxicol* (Kbh) 20:158–164, 1963.

Jones HR Jr, Siekert RG, Geraci JE: Neurologic manifestations of bacterial endocarditis. *Ann Intern Med* 71:21–28, 1969.

Jordan C, Lehane JR, Jones JG: Respiratory depression following diazepam. Reversal with high-dose naloxone. *Anesthesiology* 53:293–298, 1980.

Kaufer H, Spengler DM, Noye FR, et al: Orthopaedic implications of the drug subculture. *J Trauma* 14:853–867, 1974.

Kleber HD, Riordan CE: The treatment of narcotic withdrawal: A historical review. *J Clin Psych* 43:30–34, 1982.

Lamb D, Roberts G: Starch and talc emboli in drug addicts' lungs. *J Clin Pathol* 25:876–881, 1972.

Lewis R, Gorbach S, Altner P: Spinal pseudomonas chrondro-osteomyelitis in heroin users. *N Engl J Med* 286:1303, 1972.

Light RW, Dunham TR: Vertebral osteomyelitis due to pseudomonas in the occasional heroin user. *JAMA* 228:1272, 1974.

Litt IF, Cohen MI: The drug using adolescent as a pediatric patient. *J Pediatr* 77:195–202, 1970.

Litt IF, Schonberg SK: Medical complication of drug abuse in adolescents. *Med Clin North AM* 59:1445–1452, 1975.

Louria DB, Hensle T, Rose J: The major medical complications of heroin addiction. *Ann Intern Med* 67:1–22, 1967.

Martin WR: Naloxone. *Ann Intern Med* 85:765–768, 1976.

Martin WR, Fraser HF: A comparative study of physiological and subjective effects of heroin and morphine administered intravenously in post-addicts. *J Pharmacol Exp Ther* 133:388–399, 1961.

Maxwell TM, Olcott CO, Blaisdell FW: Vascular complications of drug abuse. *Arch Surg* 105:875–882, 1972.

Medical Staff Conference: Medical complications of heroin addiction. *Calif Med: The West J Med* 115:42–50, 1971.

Melluzzo PJ, Willscher M, Mason HDW, et al: Necrotizing fasciitis in narcotic addicts. *Am Surg* 42:251–253, 1976.

Moore RA, Rumack BH, Conner CS, et al: Naloxone underdosage after narcotic poisoning. *Am J Dis Child* 134:156–158, 1980.

Moser RJ: Heroin addiction. *JAMA* 230:728–731, 1974.

Most J: Falciparum malaria in drug addicts: Clinical aspects. *Am J Trop Med* 20:551–567, 1940.

Neufeld GK, Branson CG, Marshall LW, et al: Infective endocarditis as a complication of heroin use. *South Med J* 69:1148–1151, 1976.

Ngai SN, Berkowitz BA, Yang JC, et al: Pharmacokinetics of naloxone in rats and in man: Basis for its potency and short duration of action. *Anesthesiology* 44:398–401, 1976.

Oh I: *Serratia marcescens* arthritis in heroin addicts. *Clin Orthop* 122:228–230, 1977.

Pastan RS, Silverman SL, Goldenberg DL: A musculoskeletal syndrome in intravenous heroin users. *Ann Intern Med* 87:22–29, 1977.

Rea WJ, Wyrick WJ: Necrotizing fasciitis. *Ann Surg* 72:957–964, 1970.

Richter RW, Pearson J, Bruun B: Neurological complications of addiction to heroin. *Bull NY Acad Med* 49:3–21, 1973.

Rutherdale JA, Medline A, Sinclair JC, et al: Hepatitis in drug users. *Am J Gastroenterol* 58:275–287, 1972.

Sapira JD: The narcotic addict as a medical patient. *Am J Med* 45:555–588, 1968.

Schwartzfarb L, Singh G, Marcus D: Heroin-associated rhabdomyolysis with cardiac involvement. *Arch Intern Med* 137:1255–1257, 1977 (17 refs).

Shuster MM, Lewis MJ: Needle tracks in narcotic addicts. *NY State J Med* 68:3129–3134, 1968.

Smith WR, Wilson AF: Guillain-Barré syndrome in heroin addiction. *JAMA* 231:1367–1368, 1975.

Stern WZ: Roentgenographic aspects of narcotic addiction. *JAMA* 236:963–965, 1976.

Thadepalli N, Francis DK: Diagnostic clues in metastatic lesions of endocarditis in addicts. *West J Med* 128:1–5, 1978.

Thornton WE, Thornton BP: Narcotic poisoning: A review of the literature. *Am J Psychiatry* 131:867–869, 1974.

Washton AM, Resnick RB: Outpatient opiate detoxification with clonidine. J Clin Psych 43:39–41, 1982.

Wendt VE, Puro HE, Shapiro J, et al: Angiothrombotic pulmonary hypertension in addicts: ''Blue velvet'' addiction. *JAMA* 188:755–757, 1964.

White AG: Medical disorders in drug addicts: 200 consecutive admissions. *JAMA* 223:1469–1471, 1973.

Wright CB, Lamoy RE, Hobson RW: Hemodynamic effects of intra-arterial injection of drugs of abuse. *Surgery* 79:425–431, 1976.

Wynne JW, Goslen JB, Ballinger WE Jr: Rhabdomyolysis with cardiac and respiratory involvement. *South Med J* 70:1125–1127, 1977.

Young AW, Rosenberg FR: Cutaneous stigmas of heroin addiction. *Arch Dermatol* 104:80–86, 1971.

CHAPTER 30
COCAINE

Lester Haddad

Cocaine is the recreational drug of choice in the United States today. Unlike many drugs of abuse, cocaine has an extensive history. It has been called a status symbol, and its use has permeated the circles of the powerful and socially prominent.

"Of all drugs in the United States, cocaine is now considered the largest producer of illicit income; street sales of cocaine, the most expensive drug on the market, reached an estimated $30 billion in the United States alone." (*Time Magazine:* High on cocaine—A drug with status and menace, July 6, 1981.)

Cocaine is also lethal. In a recent National Institute of Drug Abuse report, over 111 deaths associated with cocaine were reported in a limited review. Cocaine can kill by the intranasal route, contrary to popular belief. In 1980, Dade County listed 135 murders committed during cocaine deals. The Medical Examiner's Office of Dade County also recently reported 68 deaths associated with the recreational use of illicit cocaine.

Cocaine ("coke" or "snow") usually costs $100 a gram. It is sold in grams or spoons (half grams) and is usually adulterated with mannitol, lactose, or sucrose. Caffeine, amphetamines, procaine, or lidocaine have all been substituted for cocaine. The user may get anywhere from 0 to 200 mg/dose. The cocaine is chopped with a razor blade into "lines," or columns, onto a piece of glass. The line is inhaled intranasally, usually through a rolled dollar bill.

The lethal oral dose is about 1,200 mg, while death has been reported to follow only 20 mg of parenterally administered cocaine.

PHARMACOLOGY

Cocaine is an alkaloid extracted from the leaves of *Erythroxylon coca,* a shrub that grows extensively in the valleys of the Andes Mountains. The alkaloid represents 1 to 2 percent of the coca leaf. Chemically, cocaine is benzoylmethylecgonine.

Javaid et al. report that the maximum high following intravenous injection occurs in 3 to 5 min and is over in 30 to 60 min. It takes about 60 min for effects to peak after nasal insufflation, and the effects gradually decrease over another 60-min period. Insufflation, or "snorting," is the most common route of administration among street users. The highest blood levels are achieved by intravenous injection; however, cocaine is absorbed in about 20 min when topically applied to the nasal mucous membranes, producing markedly elevated blood levels. It has been reported

that tracheal absorption is the greatest. Absorption of oral cocaine is markedly reduced by gastric hydrolysis.

Most cocaine is metabolized within 2 h in the liver to its principal metabolite, benzoylecgonine, which is promptly excreted unchanged in the urine. Stewart el al. point out that cocaine can also be metabolized by plasma cholinesterase.

PATHOPHYSIOLOGY

Cocaine is a powerful CNS stimulant causing an increase in heart rate, blood pressure, and temperature. It is also a powerful sympathomimetic.

Psychological effects in descending order of frequency are euphoria, stimulation, reduced fatigue, garrulousness, sexual stimulation, and increased mental ability, alertness, and sociality. When usage is intensified, negative effects occur, including perceptional changes such as seeing halo lights around objects or itching madly as if plagued by bugs.

Cocaine is not physically addicting as is heroin; however, it is psychologically addicting. Reportedly, the chronic user may have clinical syndromes manifested in an orderly progression from euphoria to paranoid psychosis. There may be a depressive aftermath and the user will often need cocaine to dispel the depression.

A kindling phenomenon or reverse tolerance to cocaine may occur. The kindling phenomenon has been defined as "a repetitive subthreshold electrical stimulation of the limbic system which produces increasing effects on electrical activity and behavior, eventually resulting in major convulsions or reaction to a stimulation that previously produced no effect."

Amphetamines produce effects similar to those produced by cocaine, and lithium is believed to antagonize the behavioral effects of cocaine, according to Caldwell and Fischman.

CLINICAL USE

Formerly cocaine was used for a variety of ailments. Freud, for instance, prescribed it as a stimulant; to relieve indigestion; as an aphrodisiac; as a local anesthetic; and in treating cachexia, alcohol and morphine addiction, and asthma.

Today, cocaine is used clinically only as a topical anesthetic intranasally prior to rhinoplasty or intranasal surgery, and prior to emergency nasotracheal intubation. It is no longer used in ophthalmic surgery.

Miller reports that cocaine blood levels during rhinoplasty have been recorded at less than 150 mg/mL. The usual topical therapeutic dose is 1 to 2 mL of a 10% cocaine solution (100 to 200 mg), but up to 200 mg intranasally may be necessary to prevent nasal hemorrhage during emergency nasotracheal intubation.

Gas or liquid chromatography is the preferred method of detecting cocaine and benzoylecgonine in the blood or urine; however, if this is not available, thin-layer chromatography is useful. The three-solution Scott field test is the method of choice for testing substances thought to be pure cocaine.

TREATMENT

Suspect cocaine poisoning in any young patient brought to the emergency department with generalized seizures or a ventricular arrhythmia of unknown cause that does not respond to lidocaine. The patient may or may not have hallucinations or be vomiting.

Initially, cocaine produces an excitable state, dilated pupils, rapid respirations, and tachycardia with elevated blood pressure.

With lethal doses, hyperthermia, status epilepticus, and ventricular arrhythmias or respiratory arrest or both may be presenting signs. It is important to document cocaine as the cause of intoxication since hyperthermia, seizures, and arrhythmias are constant concerns.

Ensure that the patient has a patent airway, obtain vital signs, and initiate cardiac monitoring. Insert an intravenous line.

In treating the cardiovascular effects of cocaine, propranolol has been effectively used. Since cocaine may potentiate the effects of epinephrine and norepinephrine, there is a clear rationale for propanolol use. However, Fennell et al. warn against its routine use, suggesting that the cardiovascular effects of cocaine are short-lasting and usually without rhythm disturbances other than tachycardia. This author's approach with propranolol has been conservative and reserved only for treating life-threatening arrhythmias. It is given in 1-mg increments IV push every 5 min, up to five doses.

Physostigmine is contraindicated in cocaine-induced arrhythmias because both cocaine and physistigmine can produce seizures.

Patients with seizures may be difficult to manage, as their seizures are often prolonged and recurrent. Status epilepticus is not unusual. Diazepam is the drug of choice for management of status elipepticus secondary to cocaine overdose. With seizures unresponsive to high doses of Valium, or those with associated opisthotonos, pancuronium bromide and mechanical ventilation may be necessary. Patients with recurrent seizures may develop a high-anion-gap metabolic acidosis, usually a lactic acidosis, which may require treatment. (Haddad, 1983.)

Dialysis has no role in treating cocaine poisoning because cocaine is rapidly metabolized and only small amounts produce symptoms.

The emergency physician may see cocaine intoxication following cocaine condom ingestion. Suarez recommends surgery rather than endoscopy for removal of intact condoms, as endoscopic manipulation may rupture the condoms.

BIBLIOGRAPHY

Caldwell J, Sever PS: The biochemical pharmacology of abused drugs. *Clin Pharmacol Ther* 16:625–638, 1974.

Catravas JD, Water IW, Walz MA, et al: Antidotes for cocaine poisoning, letter to the editor. *N Engl J Med* 297:1238, 1977.

Fennell WH, Fischman MW, Schuster CR, et al: Cardiovascular effects of cocaine. *N Engl J Med* 295:960–961, 1976.

Fischman MW: Physiological and behavioral effects of intravenous cocaine in man, in Ellinwood EH, Kilbey MD (eds): *Cocaine and Other Stimulants.* New York, Plenum Press, 1977, pp 647–664.

Flemenbaum A: Antagonism of behavioral effects of cocaine by lithium. *Pharmacol Biochem Behav* 7:83–85, 1977.

Gay GR, Inada DS, Sheppard CW, et al: Cocaine: History, epidemiology, human pharmacology, and treatment. A perspective on a new debut for an old girl. *Clin Toxicol* 8:149–178, 1975.

Gay GR, Sheppard CW, Inada DS, et al: An old girl: Flyin' low, dyin' slow, blinded by snow: Cocaine in perspective. *Int J Addict* 8:1027–1042, 1973.

Haddad LM: Cocaine, in Haddad LM, Winchester JF (eds): *Clinical Management of Poisoning and Drug Overdose.* Philadelphia, Saunders, 1983, pp 443–447.

Haddad LM: Cocaine in perspective. *JACEP* 8:374–376, 1979.

Javaid JI, Fischman MW, Schuster CR: Cocaine plasma concentration: Relation to physiological and subjective effects in humans. *Science* 202:227–228, 1978.

Kogan MJ, Verebey KG, DePace AC, et al: Quantitative determination of benzoylecgonine and cocaine in human biofluids by gas-liquid chromatography. *Anal Chem* 49:1965–1969, 1977.

Miller SH, Dvochik B, Davis TS: Cocaine concentrations in the blood during rhinoplasty. *Plast Reconstr Surg* 60:566–571, 1977.

Minutes, Ad Hoc Committee on Toxicology, American College of Emergency Physicians, Houston, Sept 19, 1978.

Minutes, Board of Director's Meeting, American College of Emergency Physicians, Houston, Sept 22, 1978.

Petersen RC, Stillman RE (eds): Cocaine. NIDA Research Monograph 13, May 1977.

Post RM: Cocaine, kindling, and reverse tolerance. *Lancet* 1:409–410, 1975*a*.

Post RM: Cocaine psychoses: A continuum model. *Am J Psychiatry* 132:225–231, 1975*b*.

Post RM, Kopanda RT: Cocaine, kindling and psychosis. *Am J Psychiatry* 133:627–634, 1976.

Price KR: Fatal cocaine poisoning. *J Forensic Sci Soc* 14:329–333, 1974.

Resnick RB, Schwartz LK: Acute systemic effects of cocaine in man: A controlled study by intranasal and intravenous routes. *Science* 195:696–698, 1977.

Stewart DJ, Inaba T, Tang BK, et al: Hydrolysis of cocaine in human plasma by cholinesterase. *Life Sciences* 20:1557–1563, 1977.

Suarez CA, Arango A, Lester JL: Cocaine-condom ingestion: Surgical treatment. *JAMA* 238:1391–1392, 1977.

Wallace JE, Hamilton HE, King DE, et al: Gas-liquid chromatographic determination of cocaine and benzoylecgonine in urine. *Anal Chem* 48:34–38, 1976.

Winek CL, Eastly T: Cocaine identification. *Clin Toxicol* 8:205–210, 1975.

CHAPTER 31
HALLUCINOGENS

Lester Haddad, Toby Litovitz

Hallucinogenic substances have been used for thousands of years in religious rites, but it was in the 1960s that abuse by the drug culture became evident. There are at least 12 different products taken by drug users to produce hallucinosis (Table 31-1). Over 90 percent contain either PCP [1-(1-phenylcyclohexyl)piperidine, or phencyclidine] or LSD (lysergic acid diethylamide), regardless of what the seller purports the particular drug to be. Thus, the medical management of hallucinogen abuse generally entails managing PCP or LSD ingestion.

PHENCYCLIDINE

Phencyclidine is presently the most commonly abused hallucinogen. It is excreted unchanged by the kidneys and as the glucuronides of its two known hydroxylated metabolites. It is a weak base with a pH of 9 and is ionized by acidification of the urine, which drastically reduces reabsorption at the renal tubule. If the urine is acidified to a pH of 5.5 or less, PCP excretion increases 100 times.

The acid media of the stomach also causes ion trapping because of the impenetrability of membranes to ions; however, upon passage to the alkaline small intestine, PCP is readily absorbed.

The half-life of 1 to 5 mg of phencyclidine is generally given as 30 to 60 min. This is the dose usually employed in street preparations to produce hallucinosis.

The clinical effects of phencyclidine overdose have been well described by Aronow and Done (Table 31-2). The most prominent signs are hallucinosis, hyperactivity (see Table 31-3 for classification), nystagmus, and marked sensory loss. The pupils are generally small and midpoint, and are often fixed. A person taking large doses (5 to 10 mg or greater) may have status epilepticus, and opisthotonos or decerebrate posturing, or respiratory arrest, or both. Hyperpyrexia or hypertension may also develop. Myoglobinuria from rhabdomyolysis, as described by Cohen et al., also occurs with subsequent renal failure. Frequently, a patient in coma exhibits rapid, unpredictable changes in the level of consciousness.

Phencyclidine has been reported to be associated with prolonged psychosis even after toxicologic studies show complete removal of the drug.

LSD

Until recently LSD was one of the most common hallucinogenic agents used. It was discovered by Albert Hoffman, a Swiss chemist working for a pharmaceutical company, who inadvertently discovered that LSD caused an "intense kaleidoscopic play of colors and fantasies." Further experiments established that as little as 100 μg could produce a full-scale LSD "trip."

LSD is an ergot derivative that somehow interferes with serotonin metabolism. It is not addicting but causes depersonalization, illusions, confusion, and reality distortion.

The hallucinogenic effects of LSD usually last from 2 to 4 h but can produce a permanent psychosis, particularly in someone of borderline stability. The phenomenon of LSD flashbacks has been well documented. Flashbacks can occur up to several months following the initial LSD ingestion but are generally more common in chronic abusers of LSD. Although LSD is not a depressant, there have been recent reports in the literature of massive doses (in milligrams) causing coma and respiratory arrest, as well as hyperthermia and bleeding. Systemic signs associated with LSD intoxication include hyperthermia (uncommon) and dilated pupils.

OTHER HALLUCINOGENIC AGENTS

Other agents with hallucinogenic properties include mescaline; psilocybin mushrooms; cannabinols; 3,4-methylene dioxamphetamine (MDA); dimethoxy-4-methyl amphetamine (DOM); dimethyltryptamine (DMT); diethyltryptamine (DET); wood rose; jimsonweed seeds; and nutmeg.

Mescaline is the active ingredient in peyote buttons, which are an intrinsic part of American Indian religious ceremonies. Usually 4 to 12 peyote buttons are consumed during each ceremony, and the effects are similar to those of LSD. The average hallucinogenic dose of mescaline is 5 mg/kg.

Psilocybin mushrooms are extremely scarce and found only in moist tropical climates, such as parts of Mexico, or in a southern climate such as that of Georgia, where they appear to grow overnight in cow pastures after a rainfall. Psilocybin is a mild hallucinogen but is treasured by the drug culture as providing the most vivid colors during hallucinosis.

Table 31-1. Agents, Drugs, and Chemicals Producing Hallucinosis

Agent	Street Name	Use	Route of Administration
Phencyclidine hydrochloride	Angel dust, angel mist, crystal, embalming fluid, hag, monkey tranquilizer, peace pill, PCP, lovely	Developed as human anesthetic, but too toxic. Marketed as Sernylan; used as veterinary anesthetic	Oral, parenteral
Lysergic acid diethylamide	Acid, LSD, psychedelic sunshine	Synthetic hallucinogen	Oral
3,4-Methylene dioxyamphetamine (MDA)	Love drug		Inhalation
2,5-Dimethoxy-4-methyl amphetamine	DOM, STP, serenity, tranquility, peace	Derived from amphetamine	
Dimethyltryptamine	Working person's LSD, DMT, Yurema	Basic to Brazilian Indian Kariri religion	Oral, subcutaneous, inhalation
Diethyltryptamine	DET		
Cannabinols: Marijuana, hashish, hash oil (THC)	Acapulco, bash, bhang, black Columbus, charas, dagga, frago, gold, gage, ganja, grass, hash, hashish, hay, jive, kef, leaves, LL, Mary Jane, MZZ, panatelle, pot, tea, weed	Natural hallucinogen derived from *C. sativa* (hemp plant)	Inhalation
Mescaline	Buttons, peyote, cactus, topi	Natural hallucinogen, poisonous alkaloid from flowering heads (mescal buttons) of *Lophophora williamsii*. Used by North American Indians (Native American church)	Oral
Psilocybin		Obtained from Mexican fungus *Psilocybe mexicana*. Used by Mexican aborigines to induce trances	Oral
Myristicin		Constituent of nutmeg; dried seed of *Myristica fragrans*	Oral
Morning glory, *Rivea corymbosa*	Mexican morning glory, heavenly blue, flower of the virgin, Mexican bindweed, ololiuqui, wood rose	Seeds contain lysergic acid amide, isolysergic acid, lysergic acid, and other indole alkaloids	Inhalation
Jimsonweed		Seeds of *Datura stramonium*	Oral

Cannabinols are marketed in three forms, all derived form the hemp plant *Cannabis sativa*. The first form, marijuana, is made from the flowering tops and leaves. Hashish is produced by drying the resin exuded by the plant. It is approximately five to eight times more potent than marijuana. The third form is a concentration of the active ingredient, Δ^9-tetrahydrocannabinol, which readily causes hallucinosis. It is usually marketed as hash oil (THC) but few street preparations actually contain THC.

Methylene dioxamphetamine and wood rose are also mild hallucinogens. Dimethoxy-4-methyl amphetamine was briefly used as a hallucinogen but was rapidly dropped because of its dangerous side effects. Death has resulted from the use of phenoghiazines to counteract the effects of this drug.

Dimethyltryptamine is referred to as the working person's LSD because it causes brief hallucinosis and can be taken during the lunch break. Diethyltryptamine has similar but longer-acting effects.

Ingestion of jimsonweed seeds produces anticholinergic or atropine-like hallucinosis. Anticholinergic hallucinosis can also be caused by abuse of tricyclic antidepressants such as amitriptyline, imipramine, perphenazine taken with amitriptyline, and nortriptyline.

CLINICAL FEATURES

The physician must determine whether the patient has ingested a hallucinogenic drug, is frankly psychotic, or has a toxic or organic psychosis induced by a condition such as hypoglycemia, hyper-

thermia, delirium tremens, or aspirin ingestion. A thorough history and physical examination are essential.

A straightforward case of hallucinogen overdose is that of a young patient aged 12 to 20 who has hallucinations and a history of ingesting an unknown substance approximately 2 to 3 h prior to admission. The most likely substance is LSD or PCP or, in certain areas of the country, jimsonweed seeds.

The patient is expected to be alert, and has a normal temperature and no evidence of bleeding or seizures.

The clinical picture can become complicated by the onset of prolonged hallucinosis, hypertension, hyperpyrexia, rhabdomyolysis, coma, or seizures.

TREATMENT

A patient with hallucinosis and hyperactivity but without organic systemic complications should be placed in a quiet, dim isolation room with a staff member who can reassure and calm the patient. Physical restraint should be used only if other measures fail. Intravenous diazepam is the drug of choice for sedation.

Suspect jimsonweed or TCA ingestion if the patient is hyperactive and has other signs of atropinism (flushed face, dry mouth, hyperpyrexia, dry skin). Obtain an ECG, and if it is normal, slowly give 1 to 2 mg physostigmine intravenously and monitor cardiac activity. If there is no improvement, and other causes of hyperactivity such as delirium tremens or thyroid storm have been ruled out, the patient has probably ingested LSD or PCP.

Since the prevalent hallucinogen is phencyclidine, treat the hallucinating patient as a phencyclidine overdose until proved other-

Table 31-2. Clinical Effects of Phencyclidine Overdose

Dose	Serum Level (est)	Symptoms	Psychological Changes
Low dose: <5 mg	20–30 ng/mL	Agitation and excitement Gross incoordination Blank stare appearance Catatonic rigidity Reactive pupils Horizontal or vertical nystagmus Loss of response to pinprick Flushing Diaphoresis Hyperacousis	Body image changes Estrangement Disorganization of thought Negativism and hostility Drowsiness and apathy Hypnagogic Feeling of inebriation Amnesia may or may not be present for the episode
Moderate dose: 5–10 mg (0.1–0.2 mg/kg)	30–100 ng/mL	Coma or stupor Pupils in midposition—reactive Nystagmus Vomiting Hypersalivation Myoclonus Muscle rigidity on stimulation Flushing Diaphoresis Fever Decreased peripheral sensation (pain, touch, position) Hyperacousis	Same as for low dose
High dose: >10 mg	100 ng/mL and up	Coma (unusually prolonged 12 h to days) Hypertension Opisthotonos Decerebrate positioning Repetitive motor movements Convulsions (0.5–1 mg/kg) Absent peripheral sensation Decreased or absent deep sensation Decreased or absent gag and corneal reflexes Diaphoresis Hypersalivation Flushing Fever Prolonged recovery phase marked by alternating periods of sleep and waking, misperception, disorientation, ''hallucinatory'' phenomena, and the clinical picture of the lower-dose states	No memory of episode

Source: Adapted from Aronow R, Done AK: Phencyclidine overdose: An emerging concept of management. *JACEP* 7:58, 1978. Used by permission.

wise. The management of PCP overdose has been adequately described by Aronow and Done and basically involves ion trapping or acidification of the urine to ionize PCP and thus prevent reabsorption by the renal tubule.

Utilizing the mechanism of ion trapping, urinary excretion of phencyclidine may be increased as much as 100-fold by acidification from pH 7.5 to pH less than 5.5. Forced diuresis with furosemide further increases

Table 31-3. Clinical Classification of Hyperactivity

Symptoms	Severity
Restlessness, irritability, insomnia, tremor, hyperreflexia, sweating, mydriasis, flushing	1+
Hyperactivity, confusion, hypertension, tachypnea, tachycardia, extrasystoles, fever (mild), sweating	2+
Delirium, mania, self-injury, marked hypertension, tachycardia, arrhythmias, hyperpyrexia	3+
Above symptoms, plus convulsions and coma, circulatory collapse, and death	4+

the clearance rate. As a result, many have recommended treatment with vigorous urinary acidification, either with 0.5 to 1.5 g of ascorbic acid IV or PO every 4 to 6 h, or with ammonium chloride in a dose of 1 to 2 g (IV or per nasogastric tube until the urinary pH is less than 5.5). Caution is advocated if ammonium chloride is chosen because of the attendant risks of severe acidosis, of aggravating underlying hepatic damage in chronic drug abusers, and of worsening potential myoglobinuric renal damage. Though the ion trapping and renal phencyclidine clearance data are quite impressive, clinicians should bear in mind that it is not yet clear whether phencyclidine is primarily inactivated by metabolism or by excretion in the urine. There have been no reported controlled clinical trials comparing treatment with and without acidification, and it is suggested that even the most rigorous urinary acidification may only increase the amount excreted by 10 to 13 percent. At this time, forced diuresis and acidification are indicated. Overall, the focus of treatment is intensive supportive care. (Litovitz, 1983.)

PCP ingestion has been associated with hypertensive crisis. For this reason, periodic blood pressure monitoring is necessary during the psychotic episode. If hypertensive crisis develops, give diazoxide or nitroprusside. Seizures may be treated with diazepam.

BIBLIOGRAPHY

Aronow R, Done AK: Phencyclidine overdose: An emerging concept of management. *JACEP* 7:56–59, 1978.

Burns RS, Lerner SE: Phencyclidine deaths. *JACEP* 7:135–141, 1978.

Cohen FC, Rigg G, Simmons JL: Phencyclidine-associated acute rhabdomyolysis. *Ann Intern Med* 88:210–212, 1978.

Eastman JW, Cohen S: Hypertensive crisis and death associated with phencyclidine poisoning. *JAMA* 231:1270–1271, 1975.

Fauman B, Baker F, Coppleson L: Psychosis induced by phencyclidine. *JACEP* 4:223–225, 1975.

Haddad LM: Management of hallucinogen abuse. *Am Fam Physician* 14:82–87, 1976.

Liden CB, Lovejoy FH, Costello C: Phencyclidine: Nine cases of poisoning. *JAMA* 234:513–516, 1975.

Litovitz TL: Phencyclidine, in Haddad LM, Winchester JF (eds): *Clinical Management of Poisoning and Drug Overdose*. Philadelphia, Saunders, 1983. pp 448–455.

Rappolt RT, Gay GR, Farris RD: Emergency management of acute phencyclidine intoxication. *JACEP* 8:68–76, 1979.

CHAPTER 32
SALICYLATES

Lester Haddad

Due to safety packaging, there has been a dramatic decrease in accidental poisoning from aspirin in the pediatric age group, but salicylate overdose is still common. Symptomatic adult salicylate overdose is more common than symptomatic pediatric poisoning in our experience. Salicylate is available in single or combination agents, as prescription or over-the-counter drugs. It is combined with other drugs in prescription items such as Fiorinal, Percodan, and Darvon Compound. Oil of wintergreen (methyl salicylate) contains the equivalent of 21 adult aspirin in 1 tsp (105 grains). Liquiprin is not salicylate but rather a suspension of acetaminophen. Salicylamide does not have the toxic effects of salicylates.

PATHOPHYSIOLOGY

Toxic effects of salicylate are encountered with a serum salicylate level of 30 mg/100 mL 2 h after a single ingestion. According to Done, a lethal dose is probably in the range of 8 grains per kilogram.

Salicylate stimulates the respiratory center, resulting in hyperventilation and respiratory alkalosis. The renal response is excretion of bicarbonate and potassium, resulting in a lowering of the plasma bicarbonate and hypokalemia. With very large doses, in the range of 80 to 100 mg/100 mL, the respiratory center is depressed.

Salicylates uncouple oxidative phosphorylation and inhibit dehydrogenases and aminotransferases, leading to the accumulation of organic anions such as acetoacetate and β-hydroxybutarate. While it was once thought that only children developed metabolic acidosis, Gabow et al. point out that metabolic acidosis can develop in both adults and children.

Toxic doses of salicylate usually cause fever. Dehydration is common in severe salicylate toxicity and is caused by hyperthermia, hyperventilation, and marked diaphoresis.

Hypernatremia can occur because of the increased loss of water in excess of salt from perspiration. Hypokalemia results from respiratory alkalosis and possibly from a direct effect on the renal tubule resulting in greater potassium excretion. Hyperglycemia and hypoglycemia have both been observed in salicylate poisoning; hyperglycemia seems to be more common in adults, whereas hypoglycemia is more common in children.

Salicylates cause hypoprothrombinemia with an increased tendency toward bleeding. Salicylate hepatitis has recently been described by Athreya et al. The occurrence of pulmonary edema in severe poisoning cases is not uncommon.

CLINICAL FEATURES

Symptoms of salicylate poisoning, as described by Hill and Done, include hyperpnea, confusion, lethargy, fever, tinnitus, and epigastric pain. Patients with normal hearing usually experience tinnitus with salicylate concentrations greater than 30 mg/dL. Altered consciousness is the most important indicator of severe salicylate concentration. Coma in the adult and convulsions in children are indicators of a poor prognosis. Often the diagnosis of salicylate poisoning is unsuspected and may be discovered after the patient has been admitted to other units of the hospital, such as the psychiatry ward. Suspect salicylate poisoning in a patient with fever of unclear etiology, especially in children; hyperventilation or diaphoresis; or coma or convulsions of unknown etiology. Once the diagnosis of salicylate poisoning is suspected proper laboratory evaluation of the patient is essential to appropriate therapy.

Serum salicylate, electrolyte, and acetone levels; arterial blood gases; CBC; prothrombin time; and urinalysis are all essential to the proper evaluation of salicylate toxicity. If available, a platelet count, prothrombin time, partial thromboplastin time, and a liver function screen are also helpful, as the patient may develop bleeding tendencies as well as salicylate hepatitis. Phenistix, reagent strips used to test for phenylketonuria, can also be used to detect salicylates in the urine, when present in moderate to large concentrations.

TREATMENT

One must first understand normal salicylate excretion to understand why urine alkalinization is the key to therapy of salicylate toxicity. Salicylate is normally absorbed, producing peak levels in approximately 2 h.

The Done nomogram can be a helpful tool in evaluating salicylate ingestion, but it should be combined with the clinical status (Fig. 32-1). If misinterpreted, the nomogram can lead a physician into complacency and mismanagement. Remember to treat the patient, not the nomogram. The nomogram should be used with the following cautions: (1) it is useful for acute ingestion only; (2) a patient with toxic levels in serum drawn 6 h previously should be treated; and (3) repeat blood levels are necessary to ensure that the value is not rising.

With a normal dose of salicylate, approximately 75 percent is bound to albumin as salicylate. Approximately 60 percent is excreted in the free form and up to 40 percent conjugated with

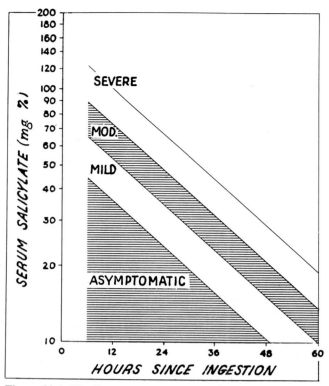

Figure 32-1. The Done nomogram correlates the serum salicylate level with the severity of ingestion at a given time after ingestion of a single dose of salicylate. (From Done AK: Salicylate intoxication: Significance of salicylate in blood in cases of acute ingestion. *Pediatrics* 26:805, 1960. Used by permission.)

glucuronide. However, only 10 percent of free salicylate will be excreted in acid urine, whereas up to 85 percent of free salicylate may be excreted in an alkaline urine. Only the *unionized* portion of salicylate is reabsorbed in the renal tubule, and since salicylate is a weak acid, it is ionized in an alkaline urine.

This is especially important, since the conjugation of aspirin with glycine proceeds at a constant rate—no matter how high the salicylate level. Thus, a substantial amount of aspirin excretion is unaltered, and in the face of an acid urine, up to 90 percent will be excreted in this fashion. Thus, at the normal pH of 5, the half-life of salicylate may be up to 200 h with toxic doses, as described by Hill.

On the other hand, when the urine is alkaline, the half-life of salicylate may be 4 h. Thus, in addition to lavage and activated charcoal, the keynote to therapy in salicylate poisoning is alkalinization of the urine. An outline of therapy is as follows.

Gastric Lavage

Gastric lavage with tap water is indicated for the adult patient with symptomatic salicylate toxicity. In a child, physiologic saline as a lavage solution is preferred to avoid electrolyte imbalance. Concretions of salicylate may develop in the stomach, and lavage with warm water or even gastroscopy may be indicated.

Charcoal

Activated charcoal reduces the absorption of salicylate to a marked degree. Continue lavage until the solution returns clear; then give 30 g of activated charcoal in 125 mL of water to a child, or 55 g of activated charcoal in 250 mL of water to an adult. Catharsis with magnesium sulfate is indicated, and antacids can be given to prevent or treat salicylate gastritis.

Urine Alkalinization

Intravenous bicarbonate therapy, 1 to 5 mEq/kg, and potassium replacement are necessary to correct metabolic acidosis and alkalinize the urine. Monitoring serum salicylate and electrolyte levels, as well as blood gases, every 4 to 6 h is essential to proper management. The most important test is probably hourly determination of the urine pH. If in spite of adequate bicarbonate therapy and potassium replacement, the urine pH is only 5 or 6 and the patient is not responding or is deteriorating, dialysis should be considered.

Tromethamine or THAM solution (tris-hydroxymethyl aminomethane) has been advocated for alkalinization but has never achieved wide popularity because it often causes profound respiratory and CNS depression. Tromethamine is contraindicated in patients with emphysema and renal compromise.

Acetazolamide is contraindicated in the management of salicylate poisoning, according to Done and to Gabow et al.

Dialysis

Dialysis is indicated if the patient does not respond to potassium replacement and bicarbonate therapy. Winchester et al. believe that dialysis is probably indicated for those patients with a salicylate level greater than 100 mg/100 mL. In this author's opinion, a brief trial of bicarbonate and potassium therapy, up to 6 h, is probably indicated when the salicylate level is 80 to 120 mg/100 mL. If no clinical or laboratory improvement is observed, or if the patient has pulmonary, renal, hepatic, or cardiac failure, dialysis should be promptly instituted.

Hemodialysis is four times more effective than peritoneal dialysis. However, peritoneal dialysis is simpler to perform and does not require the equipment and staff that hemodialysis requires. Because salicylate is avidly bound to serum proteins, it is not readily dialyzable unless protein is present in the dialysate to compete with serum proteins for binding of the drug. Peritoneal dialysis may be employed using a 5% solution of serum albumin. To prepare a 5% albumin solution, add 50 g (200 mL) of salt-poor albumin (a 25 g/100 mL vial supplies a 25% solution) to 800 mL of dialysate solution; use the 1.5% dialysate so the final osmolality is within the range of 280 to 350 mOsm/per liter. The final concentration of the dialysate should be albumin 5%, sodium 140 mEq/L, potassium 4 to 5 mEq/L (unless renal failure is present), and calcium 4 mEq/L.

Intravenous Fluids

In general, intravenous fluid therapy is necessary to correct dehydration, to provide adequate urine output, and to correct electrolyte deficit. If the patient is in shock and has an inadequate urine output, volume expansion with normal saline, up to 20 mL/kg over 45 min, may be necessary. After urine flow is established, half-normal saline is usually adequate unless the patient has developed hypernatremia. In that case, dextrose 5% in water may be indicated. The administration of intravenous fluids needs to be modified according to repeated clinical and laboratory assessment.

GENERAL MEASURES

Potassium replacement, up to 40 mEq/per liter of fluid, is essential to appropriate management of salicylate toxicity. Hypokalemia is a common problem and can cause arrhythmias, especially in the face of digitalis. Nephrogenic diabetes insipidus, rhabdomyolysis, ileus, and gastric dilatation are other possible complications.

Parenteral vitamin K is indicated to prevent the common complication of gastrointestinal bleeding secondary to salicylate gastritis.

Oliguria can be a serious complication. Measure the serum sodium, osmolality, BUN, and creatinine levels, and urine specific gravity. If necessary, obtain urine sodium and osmolality levels to distinguish between renal failure, inadequate fluid intake, and inappropriate ADH secretion. Inadequate fluid intake is suggested by an increase in the serum sodium and osmolality levels in the face of concentrated urine. Low serum sodium and low osmolality levels may indicate either hyponatremia or inappropriate ADH. In this instance hyponatremia is suggested by a low urine sodium level and a low specific gravity. Treatment is sodium replacement.

Inappropriate ADH secretion is indicated by a high urine osmolality, urine sodium greater than 40 mEq/L, and a specific gravity greater than 1.012. Treatment is fluid restriction.

BIBLIOGRAPHY

Anderson RJ, Potts DE, Gabow PA, et al: Unrecognized adult salicylate intoxication. *Ann Intern Med* 85:745–748, 1976.

Athreya BH, Gorske AL, Myers AR: Aspirin-induced abnormalities of liver function. *Am J Dis Child* 126:638–641, 1973.

Clarke A, Walton WW: Effect of safety packaging on aspirin ingestion by children. *Pediatrics* 63:687–693, 1979.

Done AK: Aspirin overdosage: Incidence, diagnosis, and management. *Pediatrics* 63(suppl):890–897, 1978.

Done AK, Temple AR: Treatment of salicylate poisoning. *Mod Treat* 8:528–551, 1971.

Gabow PA, Anderson RJ, Potts DE, et al: Acid-base disturbances in the salicylate-intoxicated adult. *Arch Intern Med* 138:1481–1484, 1978.

Hill JB: Salicylate intoxication. *N Engl J Med* 288:1110–1113, 1973.

Hrnicek G, Skelton J, Miller WC: Pulmonary edema and salicylate intoxication. *JAMA* 230:866–867, 1974.

Proudfoot AT: Salicylate poisoning, in Haddad LM, Winchester JF (eds): *Clinical Management of Poisoning and Drug Overdose.* Philadelphia, Saunders, 1983, pp 575–586.

Temple AR: Pathophysiology of aspirin overdosage toxicity, with implications for management. *Pediatrics* 62(suppl):873–876, 1978.

Winchester JF, Gelfand MC, Knepshield JH, et al: Dialysis and hemoperfusion of poisons and drugs. *Trans Am Soc Artif Intern Organs* 23:783–787, 1977.

CHAPTER 33
ACETAMINOPHEN

Christopher H. Linden, Barry H. Rumack

INTRODUCTION

Acetaminophen (N-acetyl-*para*-aminophenol, APAP) is marketed in liquid, tablet, capsule, and suppository formulations. APAP is present in hundreds of cough, cold, and pain-relief preparations which may also contain anticholinergics, antihistamines, muscle relaxants, narcotics, phenothiazines, and sympathomimetics. In cases of mixed overdosage, the more dramatic symptoms related to the ingestion of other drugs may mask the subtle, early symptoms of APAP toxicity. Unless a high index of suspicion is maintained, APAP poisoning may not be discovered until evidence of hepatotoxicity surfaces and it is too late for antidotal therapy to be effective.

PHARMACOLOGY

APAP is an effective antipyretic and mild analgesic and is equivalent and equipotent to aspirin in these actions. Its antipyretic activity appears to involve the inhibition of hypothalamic prostaglandin synthetase and be effected by cutaneous vasodilation. The inhibition of central nervous system, and perhaps peripheral, prostaglandin synthesis may also be responsible for APAP's analgesic activity.

The therapeutic dose of APAP is 15 mg/kg every 4 to 6 h in children and 325 to 1000 mg every 4 h in adults. The total daily dosage should not exceed 80 mg/kg in children and 4 g in adults. Most APAP preparations are well absorbed from the gastrointestinal tract. Peak serum concentrations of 5 to 20 μg/mL occur $\frac{1}{2}$ to 2 h following a therapeutic dose. Pharmacological effects are generally observed within 30 min and last about 4 h. In contrast to aspirin, cumulative effects have not been described following multiple doses of acetaminophen.

During absorption, some APAP may be metabolized to inactive products before it reaches the liver. Its apparent volume of distribution is 0.9 to 1.0 L/kg but tissue concentrations are variable. Rapid uptake by hepatocytes results in relatively high liver concentrations. Since plasma protein binding of APAP is low, it does not appear to significantly displace other drugs from such binding sites. In adults the plasma half-life is approximately 2 h after a therapeutic dose. It is slightly shorter in children, and perhaps with repeated administration, and is somewhat longer in neonates, the elderly, and those with underlying liver disease.

APAP is the active metabolite of phenacetin, another over-the-counter analgesic which it has largely replaced. An unidentified oxidizing derivative of the phenacetin metabolite, *p*-phenetidin, appears to be responsible for the methemoglobinemia, sulfhemoglobinemia, and hemolytic anemia that may occur following the ingestion of phenacetin. Since humans do not possess the metabolic machinery for converting APAP back to phenacetin, these toxicities do not develop after APAP ingestion. In contrast, other species such as dogs and cats are capable of this reverse synthesis, and APAP may be rapidly fatal if ingested by these common house pets.

APAP is metabolized primarily in the liver and to a limited extent in the kidney. About 90 percent of a therapeutic dose is converted to the inactive glucuronide and sulfate conjugates which are then excreted. The predominant metabolite in adults is APAP-glucuronide, whereas APAP-sulfate is the major metabolite in neonates. Paralleling maturation of the glucuronidation pathway, there appears to be a gradual transition of APAP metabolism with increasing age. The adult pattern is reached between ages 9 and 12 years. Less than 5 percent of a therapeutic dose is excreted as unchanged APAP, and a similar fraction is conjugated with glutathione by hepatic cytochrome P_{450}–dependent mixed-function oxidases (P_{450}-MFOs) and excreted as the mercapturic acid and cysteine conjugates.

MECHANISM OF TOXICITY

A highly reactive arylating metabolite of APAP is formed during its metabolism by the P_{450}-MFO pathway. This as yet unidentified compound is capable of causing hepatic necrosis by binding to hepatocyte protein macromolecules. While the amount of this intermediary formed by the metabolism of therapeutic doses of APAP can be rapidly detoxified by conjugation with glutathione, the increased production that results from the metabolism of toxic amounts eventually depletes glutathione. The metabolism of large quantities of APAP may also lead to saturation of the glucuronide and sulfate conjugations pathways and contribute to glutathione depletion by shunting more APAP into the P_{450}-MFO pathway. When glutathione is depleted by more than 70 percent, the capacity of the liver to detoxify the reactive intermediary is exceeded. Subsequent hepatic necrosis occurs in a centrilobular distribution corresponding to the region of greatest P_{450}-MFO activity.

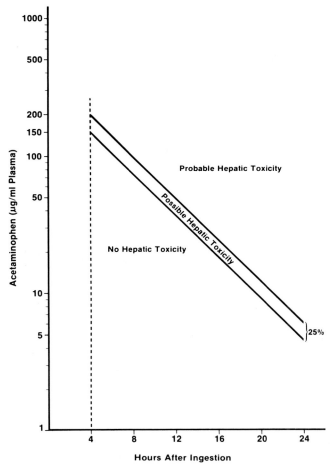

Figure 33-1. Semilogarithmic plot of plasma acetaminophen levels versus time. (Reprinted with permission from Poisindex.)

Although severe hepatic failure generally accounts for the CNS, cardiac, and renal toxicity that may be observed in APAP poisoning, there are rare instances where renal failure has developed in the presence of only mild hepatotoxicity. It is possible that highly reactive metabolic radicals are also generated during renal metabolism and cause direct nephrotoxicity.

CLINICAL FEATURES

Hepatic damage will develop when the rate of production of the reactive metabolite exceeds the supply and production of glutathione. These conditions may occur after a minimum acute ingestion of 140 mg/kg in children and 7.5 g in adults. However, because of individual variability in hepatic glutathione stores and P_{450}-MFO activity as well as historical inaccuracies, only a rough correlation exists between the amount of APAP ingested and the likelihood of toxicity. Prior use of drugs, such as antihistamines, phenytoin, barbiturates, and other sedatives which stimulate the P_{450}-MFO system, may enhance APAP toxicity. Conversely, the use of drugs, such as cimetidine, which inhibit this pathway may be protective. The effects of malnutrition and chronic ethanol consumption may also be protective. Spontaneous emesis may decrease the amount of APAP in the stomach and, hence, the amount absorbed. Children appear to be relatively resistant to

hepatotoxicity, perhaps because of early spontaneous vomiting as well as differences in APAP metabolism. Delayed treatment increases the likelihood of toxicity.

In contrast to the poor correlation between historical parameters and subsequent liver damage, the serum APAP concentration can be used to predict toxicity. The APAP nomogram (Fig. 33-1), derived from the evaluation of large numbers of overdose patients, describes this relationship. Hepatic damage is also likely when the serum APAP half-life is greater than 4 h, and hepatic coma is associated with a half-life exceeding 12 h. It should be noted that the nomogram applies only to acute ingestions and to the time period from 4 to 24 h following ingestion. APAP levels obtained sooner than 4 h after ingestion, during the absorption and distribution phases, will not reflect tissue levels and not be predictive of toxicity. Although levels obtained after 24 h will confirm the presence of APAP, treatment has not been shown to be effective after this point in time.

The clinical course of patients with toxic APAP levels can be divided into four stages (Table 33-1). During stage I, gastrointestinal symptoms are frequently present, particularly in children, although some patients may be entirely asymptomatic. These symptoms may be mild and are easily overlooked by parents, patients, and physicians. Since APAP does not cause direct CNS, cardiovascular, respiratory, or metabolic abnormalities, the ingestion of other drugs should be suspected if such findings are present.

Stage II begins with resolution of gastrointestinal symptoms and ends with the development of signs, symptoms, and laboratory evidence of hepatic, and occasionally renal, toxicity. The initial improvement is not indicative of the absence of subsequent toxicity, and treatment should continue if indicated by the nomogram. Hepatic enzymes, bilirubin, and the prothrombin time begin to rise about 36 h following ingestion. The patient may develop right upper quadrant abdominal pain, liver enlargement, and tenderness. Oliguria may also be observed and may be due to dehydration, direct APAP toxicity (acute tubular necrosis), or liver dysfunction (hepatorenal syndrome).

During stage III, the time of peak liver function abnormalities, gastrointestinal symptoms may reappear and mild jaundice may be evident. It is not uncommon for the SGOT (AST) to rise to over 10,000 IU/mL. The SGPT (ALT) may also rise to 100 times the normal level. If antidotal treatment is started within 16, and probably within 24, h of ingestion, complete recovery can be expected despite the striking elevation of hepatic enzymes.

Stage IV is characterized by the gradual return of liver function tests to normal. This usually occurs by the end of the first week but may take much longer, especially if the patient has not received antidotal treatment. Chronic hepatic dysfunction has not

Table 33-1. Stages of Acetaminophen Poisoning

Stage	Time Following Ingestion	Characteristics
I	$\frac{1}{2}$ to 24 h	Anorexia, nausea, vomiting, malaise, pallor, diaphoresis.
II	24 to 48 h	Resolution of above. RUQ abdominal pain and tenderness. Elevated bilirubin, prothrombin time, hepatic enzymes. Oliguria.
III	72 to 96 h	Peak liver function abnormalities. Anorexia, nausea, vomiting, malaise may reappear.
IV	4 days to 2 weeks	Resolution of hepatic dysfunction.

been reported. Following recovery, liver biopsies show normal histology unless underlying liver disease is present.

A small percentage of untreated patients develop confusion, stupor, coma, and finally death from fulminant hepatic failure. Hypoglycemia, renal failure, ECG changes suggestive of myocardial injury, jaundice, and hemorrhagic phenomena are associated findings. Pancreatitis has also been reported. In contrast to hepatic enzyme elevations, a bilirubin level of greater than 4 mg/dL and a prothrombin time of more than twice normal are associated with a poor prognosis.

TREATMENT

Children accidentally ingesting less than 140 mg/kg may be managed at home if the history is assuredly accurate. Ipecac-induced emesis is generally advisable, and close follow-up is necessary to confirm the absence of stage I symptoms.

Physician and laboratory evaluation are required for all children having ingested greater than 140 mg/kg and all adults having ingested more than 7.5 g. Inaccuracy of the history and the need for psychiatric assessment also make it mandatory that all intentionally overdosed patients be evaluated in person. Immediate gastric decontamination by emesis or lavage is recommended up to 12 h or longer following massive or mixed ingestions. Activated charcoal absorbs the antidote N-acetylcysteine (NAC) in addition to APAP and, hence, may interfere with the treatment of APAP overdosage. However, since activated charcoal absorbs most drugs, it is of potential benefit, especially when multiple drugs have been ingested. When charcoal is administered, it is advisable to allow 1 or 2 h for it to pass into the duodenum before giving NAC. If this will result in delaying the initiation of antidotal therapy longer than 16 h following ingestion, the charcoal may be lavaged from the stomach, and NAC may then be given immediately.

Blood for determination of the plasma APAP concentration should be drawn as soon as possible after 4 h following ingestion. Since the colorimetric assay may be unreliable, high-pressure liquid chromatography, gas chromatography, or enzymatic immunoassay (Emit) are the preferred methods of measuring APAP. A timed APAP level falling above the lower line on the nomogram (i.e., falling in either the possible or probable toxicity areas) indicates the need for NAC therapy. If an APAP level can not readily be obtained, antidotal treatment should be initiated on the basis of a history of ingestion of more than 140 mg/kg in children or 7.5 g in adults. Treatment can later be discontinued if the level is found by the nomogram to be nontoxic. Routine laboratory evaluation should include baseline SGOT (AST), SGPT (ALT), total bilirubin, prothrombin time, and urinalysis. If the patient is potentially toxic according to the nomogram, these laboratory tests should be repeated daily for at least 3 to 4 days or until they begin to return to normal if found to be elevated. Follow-up may be on an outpatient basis once antidotal therapy is complete and the patient is clinically well.

Following the observation that APAP-induced liver damage coincided with depletion of hepatic glutathione, various sulfhydryl donor compounds were administered in attempts to prevent hepatotoxicity. Although cysteamine and methionine were the first compounds to be used with success, NAC has emerged as the treatment of choice. After entering cells, NAC is metabolized to cysteine, a glutathione precursor. However, the exact mechanism by which NAC prevents hepatotoxicity is unclear. It may act by increasing the supply of glutathione, by combining directly with toxic intermediary, or by inhibiting the formation of this metabolite. It may also act as a sulfate precursor and prevent saturation of the sulfate conjugation pathway.

NAC is given orally using an initial dose of 140 mg/kg and maintenance doses of 70 mg/kg every 4 h for 17 more doses. NAC is widely available as the 20% respiratory mucolytic agent Mucomyst. Since Mucomyst smells and tastes like rotten eggs, it should be diluted to a 5% solution with three parts of a soft drink or fruit juice to increase its palatability. Nausea and vomiting are frequent side effects. The dose should be repeated if vomiting occurs within 1 h of administration. Diluting or chilling the solution, or administering it by nasogastric or duodenal tube, may be tried if repeated vomiting occurs.

NAC has been used intravenously in Europe and Canada by a treatment protocol limited to 20 h and using a lower total dose of NAC than the above oral protocol. The fact that oral NAC is absorbed into the portal venous system and then delivered directly to the liver may account for the slightly greater antidotal effectiveness of oral NAC when results of the two treatment protocols are compared retrospectively. The intravenous NAC protocol being studied by the Rocky Mountain Poison Center uses the same dosages as the oral protocol except that treatment is limited to 48 h.

It should be noted that although NAC has an FDA investigational new drug status, it is not officially approved for the treatment of APAP poisoning. Informed consent must, therefore, be obtained prior to initiation of treatment. Physicians needing assistance or wishing to enroll patients in either the oral or intravenous treatment study should call the Rocky Mountain Poison Center at the toll-free number, 1-800-525-6115.

BIBLIOGRAPHY

Clark R, Borirakchanyavat V, Davidson AR, et al: Hepatic damage and death from overdose of paracetamol. *Lancet* 1:66–70, 1973.

Cobden I, Record CO, Ward MK, et al: Paracetamol-induced acute renal failure in the absence of fulminant liver damage. *Br Med J* 284:21–22, 1982.

Donn KH, et al: Prevention of acetaminophen-induced hepatic injury by cimetidine. *Clin Pharmacol Ther* 31:218–219, 1982 (abstract).

Duffy JP, Byers J: Acetaminophen assay: The clinical consequences of a colorimetric vs. a high pressure liquid chromatography determination in the assessment of two potentially poisoned patients. *Clin Toxicol* 15:427–435, 1979.

Ferreira SH, Van JR: New aspects of the mode of action of nonsteroid anti-inflammatory drugs. *Annu Rev Pharmacol* 14:57–73, 1974.

Galinsky RE, Levy G: Dose and time-dependent elimination of acetaminophen in rats: Pharmacokinetic implications of cosubstrate depletion. *J Pharmacol Exp Ther* 219:14–20, 1981.

Gillette M Jr: An integrated approach to the study of chemically reactive metabolites of acetaminophen. *Arch Intern Med* 141:375–379, 1981.

Gilmore IT, Tourvas E: Paracetamol-induced acute pancreatitis. *Br Med J* 2:753–754, 1977.

James O, Roberts SH, Douglas AP, et al: Liver damage after paracetamol overdose: Comparison of liver-function tests, fasting serum bile acids and liver histology. *Lancet* 2:579–581, 1975.

Klein-Schwartz W, Oderda GM: Adsorption of oral antidotes for acetaminophen poisoning (methionione and N-acetylcysteine) by activated charcoal. *Clin Toxicol* 18:283–290, 1981.

Koch-Weser J: Acetaminophen. *N Engl J Med* 295:1297–1300, 1976.

Levy G: Comparative pharmacokinetics of aspirin and acetaminophen. *Arch Intern Med* 141:279–281, 1981.

Levy G, Houston JB: Effect of activated charcoal on acetaminophen absorption. *Pediatrics* 58:432–535, 1976.

Lovejoy FH Jr: Aspirin and acetaminophen: A comparative view of their antipyretic and analgesic activity. *Pediatrics* 62(suppl):904–909, 1978.

Miller RP, Roberts RJ, Fischer LJ: Acetaminophen elimination kinetics in neonates, children, and adults. *Clin Pharmacol Ther* 19:284–294, 1976.

Mitchell JR, Thorgeirsson SS, Potter WZ, et al: Acetaminophen-induced hepatic injury: Protective role of glutathione in man and rationale for therapy. *Clin Pharmacol Ther* 16:676, 1974.

Peterson RG, Rumack BH: Age as a variable in acetaminophen overdose. *Arch Intern Med* 141:380–385, 1981.

Peterson RG, Rumack BH: Pharmacokinetics of acetaminophen in children. *Pediatrics* 62(suppl):877–879, 1978.

Prescott LF, Illingworth RN, Critchley JAJH, et al: Intravenous *N*-acetylcysteine: The treatment of choice for paracetamol poisoning. *Br Med J* 2:1097–1100, 1979.

Prescott LF, Wright N, Roscoe P, et al: Plasma-paracetamol half-life and hepatic necrosis in patients with paracetamol overdosage. *Lancet* 1:519–522, 1971.

Rumack BH, Peterson RG, Koch GG, et al: Acetaminophen overdose: 662 cases with evaluation of oral acetylcysteine treatment. *Arch Intern Med* 141:380–385, 1981.

Sanerkin NG: Acute myocardial necrosis in paracetamol poisoning. *Br Med J* 3:478, 1971.

Wright N, Prescott LF: Potentiation by previous drug therapy of hepatotoxicity following paracetamol overdosage. *Scot Med J* 18:56–58, 1973.

CHAPTER 34
IRON

Lester Haddad

Iron poisoning was once the fourth most common poisoning in children. In Great Britain, it was second only to barbiturates as the most common cause of toxic death. With prompt recognition in the emergency department and greater awareness by the medical profession, the morbidity and mortality from iron poisoning have markedly decreased.

PATHOPHYSIOLOGY

The normal daily dietary intake of iron is about 15 mg. Approximately 10 percent is absorbed as ferrous iron. Most absorption takes place in the duodenum and upper small bowel. The absorbed iron is then transported in the plasma in the ferric state bound to a β-globulin, transferrin. The normal serum iron level is 50 to 150 μg/100 mL. Plasma transferrin is normally about one-third saturated. The total iron binding capacity ranges from 300 to 400 μg/100 mL.

Iron is transported to the reticuloendothelial cells of the bone marrow for hemoglobin synthesis, or for storage as ferritin and hemosiderin in the liver, bone marrow, or spleen.

There is no physiologic mechanism available for iron excretion. About 1.5 mg of iron is lost per day through sweat, bile, and desquamation of skin and mucosal surfaces. Menses in the female is, of course, the greatest normal cause of iron loss.

Ferrous sulfate ($FeSO_4$) and ferrous gluconate are the two most common preparations of iron. Ferrous sulfate tablets are usually 300 mg, of which 20 percent, or 60 mg, is elemental iron. Preparations of ferrous gluconate contain 36 mg elemental iron per 350-mg capsule, or approximately 12%. Ferrous fumarate preparations contain 33% elemental iron.

While the lethal dose of elemental iron is listed as 300 mg/kg of body weight, a potentially serious dose is 150 mg/kg and should be treated vigorously.

Iron intoxication results in necrosis of the mucosa of the gastrointestinal tract with hemorrhage and loss of fluid and electrolytes. Metabolic acidosis and shock are common: The etiology is unknown, but may result from dilatation of the splanchnic bed due to the direct effect of ferritin. Clotting mechanisms may be disturbed with subsequent increase in hemorrhage. The binding capacity of transferrin is rapidly exceeded so that free iron is present in the serum. Iron may then be sequestered in the liver and spleen.

CLINICAL PICTURE

The clinical picture may be divided into four stages. The first stage usually begins within 2 h after ingestion and is characterized by vomiting and diarrhea, which may be bloody.

The second stage is a latent period that may be present for up to 12 h and is characterized by a resolution of gastrointestinal symptoms. If vomiting and diarrhea have been severe, dehydration may be the most significant finding.

If a third stage develops, it usually occurs 48 to 96 h postingestion, and often begins abruptly with shock, and frequently metabolic acidosis (that may be resistant to bicarbonate therapy). This may progress to hepatic failure, coma, or convulsions. The prognosis for these patients is generally poor.

Finally, pyloric stenosis secondary to the early necrotic phase may occur in a delayed setting. There are no documented cases of patients who have recovered from hepatic failure secondary to hepatic cirrhosis.

TREATMENT

Generally, any child who has ingested over five iron tablets should be brought to the hospital for treatment. Milk, or ipecac if available, should be given at home. Treatment in the emergency department varies depending on the patient's condition. Most patients will have rather severe eructation if ingestion has been recent and is significant. If the patient is still asymptomatic, ipecac first is indicated. If the patient is already vomiting, proceed directly to lavage with a 5% solution of sodium bicarbonate. Sodium bicarbonate combines with iron to form ferrous carbamate, which is not absorbable. Following lavage, instill 100 mL 5% sodium bicarbonate into the stomach. After lavage, obtain a roentgenogram of the abdomen to show unabsorbed tablets, as iron is radiopaque.

Determine the serum iron level and total iron binding capacity (TIBC). A serum iron greater than the TIBC, usually 500 mg or more, is a definite indication for chelation therapy.

Baseline blood studies include a CBC, serum electrolytes, glucose, and BUN levels, as well as liver function studies, type and crossmatch, and blood gases. Metabolic acidosis, hypoglycemia, and liver failure usually occur later in the course of illness and are usually not seen in the emergency department unless the patient has been referred from another hospital without prior diagnosis and treatment.

Correlate the use of deferoxamine mesylate with the clinical setting. Some guides for use are described below.

Deferoxamine should not be used for patients with iron poisoning who have ingested relatively insignificant amounts. These patients can be managed successfully as outpatients following emergency treatment with ipecac and bicarbonate lavage.

Emergency use of deferoxamine is not indicated if the patient is asymptomatic, if the patient is experiencing minor symptoms such as abdominal pain, vomiting, or diarrhea without evidence of gastrointestinal bleeding, or if the serum iron level is less than the TIBC but the patient has ingested 150 to 300 mg/kg. In these cases, start an intravenous line and hospitalize the patient for observation.

If a lethal dose (300 mg/kg) of elemental iron has been taken, or if the patient is symptom-free or only mildly symptomatic but studies indicate free serum iron, initiate chelation therapy.

There may be hypovolemic shock secondary to blood, fluid, and electrolyte loss. If gastrointestinal bleeding is a presenting sign and shock ensues within 6 h of ingestion, volume replacement is indicated. At this point, Fischer and others recommend withholding chelation therapy, at least until serum iron studies indicate free serum iron. However, Robertson and others advocate the use of chelation therapy. If a lethal amount has been ingested or if there is free serum iron, we recommend chelation therapy along with volume replacement.

Coma following iron ingestion may be due to hypovolemic shock or, if it is 12 to 36 h postingestion, may be due to hypoglycemia or hepatic failure. Coma, shock, and convulsions are probable indications for chelation therapy. Deferoxamine can be given intramuscularly, or intravenously to the patient in serious condition with shock or coma. The recommended intravenous dosage is 10 to 15 mg/(kg · h) and should not be exceeded, as deferoxamine itself may produce hypotension. The intramuscular

dosage varies widely. For instance, Robertson suggests 20 to 40 mg/kg, whereas Chisholm mentions 90 mg/kg as an initial dose. Dosages should not exceed the adult dosage of 1 g intramuscularly initially, followed by 500 mg as needed at expanding time intervals. The total dose should not exceed 6 g in 24 h.

Unlike iron alone, the iron deferoxamine complex, ferrioxamine, is excreted in the urine. The urine is discolored by the complex from an orange-pink to a vin rosé color. A return to normal color indicates chelation is complete and deferoxamine can be stopped. This is confirmed when the serum iron concentration no longer exceeds the TIBC.

Dialysis is indicated only with renal shutdown. Chelation therapy is still necessary since only the ferrioxamine complex is dialyzable. Unfortunately, dialysis is not as effective as renal excretion.

BIBLIOGRAPHY

Aldrich RA, discussion, in Greengard J: Iron poisoning in children. *Clin Toxicol* 8:555–560, 1970.
Chisholm JJ: Poisoning due to heavy metals. *Pediatr Clin North Am* 17:591–615, 1970.
DeCastro FJ, Jaeger R, Gleason WA Jr: Liver damage and hypoglycemia in acute iron poisoning. *Clin Toxicol* 10:287–289, 1977.
Fischer DS, Parkman R, Finch SC: Acute iron poisoning in children. *JAMA* 218:1179–1184, 1971.
Greengard J: Iron poisoning in children. *Clin Toxicol* 8:575–597, 1975.
Haddad LM: Iron poisoning. *JACEP* 5:691–693, 1976.
Lacouture PG, Lovejoy FH: Iron Poisoning, in Haddad LM, Winchester JF (eds): *Clinical Management of Poisoning and Drug Overdose.* Philadelphia, Saunders, 1983, pp 644–648.
Murphy BI: Hazards of children's vitamin preparations containing iron, editorial. *JAMA* 229:324, 1974.
Robertson WO: Treatment of acute iron poisoning. *Mod Treat* 8:552–560, 1971.

CHAPTER 35
HYDROCARBONS

Regine Aronow

The term *hydrocarbon* has been used interchangeably and imprecisely with the term *petroleum distillate* in the medical literature. Petroleum distillates are hydrocarbons, but not all hydrocarbons are petroleum distillates. Hydrocarbons are derived principally from crude oil, coal, or plant sources. They represent compounds consisting of carbon and hydrogen in various configurations. They may be classified as aliphatic, or open-chain, compounds (e.g., methane, propane, naphtha, gasoline, kerosene, mineral spirits, mineral seal oil, motor oil, fuel oil, mineral oil, and lubricating oils); or cyclic, or closed-chain, compounds. Cyclic compounds are subclassified as alicyclic compounds—three or more carbons in a ring structure that act more like aliphatics (e.g., naphthenes, cyclohexane, cyclopentane, cyclopentadiene), aromatic compounds—unsaturated hexagonal rings (e.g., benzene, toluene, xylene, naphthalene), and cyclic terpenes (includes essential oils such as pine oil, turpentine). In addition, there is a large group of halogenated hydrocarbons (e.g., trichloroethane, trichloroethylene, tetrachloroethylene, carbon tetrachloride, methylene chloride).

These substances may be found in homes as ingredients in such products as cleaning and polishing agents, spot removers, charcoal lighter fluids, fuels, cosmetics, pesticides, adhesives, automobile maintenance products, paints, paint removers, paint and varnish solvents, and hobby and craft materials. Their toxic potential will depend on the unique characteristics of each, the concentration in the product involved, the other chemicals that may be present, and the total amount and the route of exposure.

LIQUID PETROLEUM DISTILLATES

In the past attention has been focused on the association of chemical pneumonitis with ingestion of various petroleum distillates and essential oils. This primarily involved small children ingesting kerosene, lighter fluids, or the red mineral seal oil furniture polishes. Approximately 1 out of every 200 children so exposed died from the resulting pulmonary complications.

Gerarde showed that the aspirational hazard associated with such substances depends on the combination of two physical properties: low viscosity and low surface tension. Viscosity is by far the most important factor, as it determines the likelihood of entry of the substance into the lung and the rate and extent of penetration into deeper structures via the bronchial tree. Viscosity is measured by the speed a substance goes through a calibrated orifice and is recorded in Saybolt Seconds Universal (SSU). The mortality in Gerarde's rat studies was inversely related to those petroleum products with SSUs under 60 (the lower the SSU, the higher the mortality rate). (Examples of the aspirational hazard of common hydrocarbons can be seen in Table 35-1.) Other important properties that influenced the results were the length of straight-chain substances and their boiling points. Small molecules were more irritating to the lung, and there was evidence of rapid absorption of the substance. Low boiling points resulted in the substance being in a vapor phase at body temperature and sometimes displacing air in the lungs.

The question of whether petroleum distillates were absorbed from the gastrointestinal tract and resecreted in the lung was unclear until the work of Bratton and Haddow in 1975 and Mann et al. in 1977 showed in test animals that naphtha and kerosene were only negligibly absorbed from the gastrointestinal tract and no pneumonitis occurred. Another question has been the etiology of the central nervous system depressant effects associated with exposure to petroleum distillates. Wolfsdorf in 1976 investigated the effect on the brains of primates of kerosene administered intrathecally, by intracardiac injection, into the carotid artery and into the portal vein, and came to the conclusion that the CNS manifestations following kerosene ingestion are due to the hypoxia secondary to aspiration pneumonia.

Most petroleum distillates represent mixtures, and, as technology has changed, so has the complex of what constitutes a given grade of a substance such as kerosene. There also may be differences among manufacturers which may account for variability in clinical manifestations. Additionally, even though there may be a high percentage of a hydrocarbon in a product, the physical properties of the total substance will influence its toxic and aspirational potential.

Generally, substances with SSUs under 60 spread on the saliva and can enter the lung just in the swallowing process; as little as 0.2 mL intrathecally can cause chemical pneumonitis. The patient who coughs, chokes, cries, or who has spontaneous emesis upon swallowing the petroleum distillate or essential oil should be assumed to have aspirated until proved otherwise. Many of these products cause a burning sensation in the mouth and act as gastric irritants. Belching for many hours after ingestion of gasoline is a frequent complaint. Loose stools often occur until the petroleum distillate is out of the gastrointestinal tract.

Respiratory distress and cyanosis may be evident within minutes of aspiration. This may be due to replacement of air in the lung

Table 35-1. Viscosity of Some Common Hydrocarbon Products

Less than 60 SSU:
   Mineral seal oil (furniture oil, signal oil)
   Gasoline
   Turpentine (pine oil, paint thinner)
   Kerosene (coal oil, jet fuel)
   Petroleum naphtha (lighter fluid)
   VM & P naphthas (varnish makers' and painters' naphtha)
   Petroleum ether (benzin)
   N-Hexane (solvent)
   Aromatic hydrocarbons (xylene, toluene, benzene)
   Halogenated hydrocarbons (trichloroethylene, tetrachloroethylene, tetrachloroethane, carbon tetrachloride)
   Mineral spirits (Stoddard solvent, Varasol)
   Petroleum naphtha (ligroin, racing fuel)

Greater than 100 SSU:
   Motor and lubrication oil (auto engine oil)
   Fuel oil and diesel oil (gas fuel)
   Mineral oil (liquid petrolatum)
   Plastic and rubber adhesives
   Petroleum jelly (Vaseline)
   Grease
   Tar

by the vaporized substance, bronchospasm, or an alteration of surfactant, causing atelectasis, pulmonary edema, and early distal airway closure.

On physical examination, the patient may exhibit CNS depression evidenced by lethargy, or stimulation, appearing inebriated or having seizures. There may be intercostal retractions, cough, increased pulse rate, tachypnea or dyspnea, and fever. On auscultation of the chest, there may be normal, coarse, or decreased breath sounds, and wheezing. X-ray findings do not correlate with physical findings. Patients with respiratory distress may not have early x-ray findings, and asymptomatic patients may have early findings or develop them several hours later. Typical distribution of the infiltrates may be bilateral basal, right basal, or perihilar with clear bases.

Rarely, intravascular hemolysis or cardiac arrhythmias have been associated with petroleum distillate ingestion. Pneumatoceles and pneumothorax may develop.

Industrial exposure to an aerosol mist of kerosene has been reported to cause pneumonitis in an adult.

Substances with an SSU of 100 or more are rarely aspirated. If they are, they cause a lipoid pneumonia which takes up to 6 weeks to resolve. These have a laxative effect on the gastrointestinal tract.

The first aid approach to the patient who has ingested a petroleum distillate or essential oil is based first upon determination of whether a toxic substance is contained in it. The toxic substance might be a pesticide such as an organophosphate (cholinergic poisoning), nitrobenzene (methemoglobinemia), triorthocresyl phosphate (peripheral neuropathy), or 2 to 5% benzene (myelotoxicity), among others. Then evaluate the condition of the patient and the type and amount of the substance ingested. Specific guidelines are as follows:

1. If there is severe breathing difficulty, coma, convulsions, or loss of the gag reflex, after endotracheal intubation and respiratory support are established, gastric lavage should be used to empty the stomach.

2. If significant symptoms are not yet present and a toxic substance is in the petroleum distillate, the stomach may be emptied by the administration of syrup of ipecac, preferably under medical supervision and with the patient in an upright position.

3. If excessive amounts (over 1 to 2 mL/kg) of a low-viscosity petroleum distillate have been ingested and the patient is asymptomatic, syrup of ipecac may be administered under medical supervision.

4. Do not empty the stomach if the ingested substance is 1 mL/kg or less of a low-viscosity petroleum distillate or any amount of a high-viscosity petroleum distillate not containing toxic additives.

5. Administer a demulcent to soothe gastric irritation. The use of olive oil or mineral oil to make the substance more viscous is not recommended. Milk is not recommended since it delays gastric emptying and may cause spontaneous emesis. The use of activated charcoal and saline cathartics has not been shown to be effective and may stimulate spontaneous emesis.

GENERAL MANAGEMENT

If patients are asymptomatic, they may be observed at home or in the health care facility for 6 h. If no symptoms develop, therapy will probably not be required. The x-ray does not determine therapy, but, if positive, it may be used to counsel the patient about general care. It is advisable to establish by telephone contact the condition of the patient in 24 h.

The symptomatic patient requires:

1. Stabilization of vital functions and administration of oxygen.
2. Monitoring of the electrocardiogram, blood gases, serum electrolytes, pulmonary function, and radiologic findings.
3. Treatment of bronchospasm with IV aminophylline; treatment of pulmonary edema with continuous airway expanding pressure and furosemide. Be cautious with IV fluids.
4. Evaluation of methemoglobinemia if cyanosis is persistent. If the level is over 30 percent treat the patient with 1% methylene blue, 0.1 mg/kg slowly IV.
5. Monitor for intravascular hemolysis and disseminated intravascular coagulation.

Warning. Do not use epinephrine, as petroleum distillates sensitize the myocardium and a serious arrhythmia may result.

Avoid. Steroids have not been shown to be beneficial, and they decrease mononuclear cell response, which in turn allows for increased bacterial growth in the lungs. They may, however, be used for shock-lung. Antibiotics are not indicated unless a specific organism has been isolated.

Comment. Pneumatoceles may be seen but do not require specific therapy. A few patients have been found to have chronic pulmonary disease or abnormal pulmonary function tests years later.

Petroleum distillate poisoning in small children does not seem to occur with the same frequency today as it did 20 years ago. Under the Poison Prevention Packaging Act of 1970, child-resistant packaging requirements were promulgated for the following products for home use:

Furniture polish in a nonemulsion liquid form, of low viscosity, and containing at least 10% mineral seal oil or petroleum distillates

Turpentine in a liquid form at least 10% by weight

Kindling and/or illuminating preparations as a prepackaged liquid, of low viscosity, containing at least 10% petroleum distillates

Paint solvents that contain 10 percent or more by weight of benzene, toluene, xylene

Dermal contact with or immersion in gasoline can cause second-degree burns. It is not established whether significant absorption of the gasoline can occur. If the burns are extensive and the gasoline contains lead, a blood lead level should be obtained. Chronic exposure to petroleum distillates has possibly been related to glomerulonephritis and distal tubule dysfunction.

GASES

Inhalation of the aliphatic gases methane, ethane (natural gas), butane, and propane (bottled LP gas) results in asphyxia. Symptoms are related to the degree of anoxia, and treatment should be directed to relieve it.

Intentional inhalation of gasoline fumes to achieve a pleasurable feeling is reported more commonly in children and teenagers. They are often in rural communities or on Indian reservations. The mental effects vary from inebriation to irritation and belligerence. Evidence of effects on the hematopoietic, hepatic, and renal systems should be sought. Documented physical effects relate to sudden death (without anatomically defined reason—due possibly to arrhythmias) or to tetraethyl lead poisoning. The latter may be manifest as polyneuropathy, cerebellar dysfunction, or the anorexia, pallor, nausea, vomiting, and encephalopathy that are also seen in inorganic lead poisoning. The lead toxicity should be evaluated and the case treated as inorganic lead poisoning with chelation if indicated. Gasoline has many other constituents, including benzene, which may influence the symptomatology. Intense psychotherapy may be necessary to interrupt the psychological addiction.

Alicyclic hydrocarbons are not apt to be found in household products. Many should be considered irritants and may cause narcosis on inhalation. Information about specific substances should be obtained from the regional Poison Control Center.

SOLVENTS

For the most part, aromatic hydrocarbons are solvents which evaporate readily at room temperature. The most commonly encountered ones are benzene, toluene, and xylene. Most exposures occur through inhalation. Table 35-2 shows the allowable threshold limit values and the metabolic products that may be tested for in the urine. In the event of aspiration, chemical pneumonitis may occur. Treatment is supportive and symptomatic. All these substances

may sensitize the myocardium, and so use of epinephrine is contraindicated.

Acute benzene exposure causes central nervous system depression. There may be euphoria, vertigo, headache, weakness, nausea, ataxia, drowsiness, tremors, and coma. Treatment is symptomatic and supportive after the patient has been removed from exposure. Chronic exposure to benzene has been associated with an initial stimulant effect on the bone marrow, followed by aplasia and fatty degeneration. A variety of symptoms may be associated with this. The National Institute for Occupational Safety and Health has characterized benzene as a leukemogen but this has not been proved. Most gasoline in the United States contains 2% benzene; in Europe, gasoline may contain up to 5% benzene.

There is little information available on the toxic oral dose of toluene or xylene. Either may cause a burning sensation on swallowing, nausea, vomiting, and central nervous system depression. Although a certain amount is metabolized in the body, most will be excreted by the lungs. Treatment is symptomatic and supportive. Hepatic or renal function should be monitored. A child who bites into a tube of adhesive containing one of these products needs only to have the mouth gently cleaned out.

On inhalation, xylene and toluene have similar effects. They may cause respiratory tract irritation and a state of inebriation which can progress to central nervous system depression. Death is usually due to respiratory arrest and asphyxia. Treatment is symptomatic and supportive. Liver and renal function should be monitored.

Intentional inhalation abuse of toluene either through huffing (liquid on a rag) or sniffing (poured into a container that one rebreathes into) has produced a variety of symptom complexes. Some of these are addictive behavior, acute brain syndrome, cerebellar dysfunction, encephalopathy, renal tubular acidosis, and hypokalemic periodic paralysis. Many patients may have hypokalemia, hypophosphatemia, hyperchloremia, and hypobicarbonatemia. Rhabdomyolysis has also been observed. As with all such exposures, there is seldom a single chemical involved. Treatment is symptomatic and supportive. Intensive psychotherapy may be required.

HALOGENATED HYDROCARBONS

Halogenated hydrocarbons represent a large class of diverse chemicals. A few aliphatic chlorinated ones that occur in readily available products which may be found in the home will be discussed (see Table 35-3). On ingestion, all these substances should be removed from the stomach (the method of removal depends on the patient's clinical status). Any of these substances may also be ingredients in products used for inhalation abuse. They all should

Table 35-2. Toxicity and Detection of Common Aromatic Hydrocarbons

Substance	TLV,* ppm	Fatal Amount, ppm	Urine Test
Benzene	10	20,000 at 5 min	Phenol
Toluene	100	10,000	Hippuric acid
Xylene	100	>10,000	Methyl hippuric acid

*TLV = threshold limit value.

Table 35-3. Toxicity of Common Halogenated Hydrocarbons

Substance	TLV,* ppm	Lethal Amount, ppm	Fatal Ingested Dose
1,1,1-Trichloroethane	350	14,000	500–5000 mg/kg
Trichloroethylene	50	15,000	3–5 mL/kg
Tetrachloroethylene	50	2,000	
Methylene chloride	100	15,000	0.5–5 mL/kg

*TLV = threshold limit value.

be considered to have the ability to sensitize the myocardium to epinephrine, and so its use is contraindicated.

1,1,1-Trichloroethane (methylchloroform) is used as a cleaning solvent and aerosol propellant. It has replaced carbon tetrachloride in many products. It volatizes at body temperature and can cause skin irritation. Moderate absorption occurs dermally. On inhalation, eye irritation, light-headedness, incoordination, impaired equilibrium, and central nervous system depression may occur. Death is usually due to respiratory failure or cardiac arrhythmias. Treatment is supportive and symptomatic. Hepatic and renal function should be monitored.

Trichloroethylene is used as a degreasing solvent and cleaning agent. It is absorbed through inhalation, ingestion, and the skin. It is an irritant to the respiratory and gastrointestinal tracts. Repeated skin contact may cause a vesicular dermatitis. Trichloroethylene is a central nervous system depressant. Euphoria, anesthesia, weakness, vomiting, abdominal cramps, loss of coordination, anosmia, changes in color perception, neuropathy, blindness, and cardiac arrhythmias may occur. Cutaneous vasodilation of the face, neck, shoulders, and back may occur with concomitant exposure to alcohol. This has been called ''degreasers' flush.'' Hepatic or renal necrosis may occur. Treatment is supportive and symptomatic.

Tetrachloroethylene (perchloroethylene) is used as a solvent and dry cleaning agent. It has been prescribed in 1- to 5-mL oral doses to treat hookworm. Information is not available on a lethal oral dose. It may cause central nervous system depression, liver damage, and peripheral neuropathy. Inebriation, dizziness, light-headedness, difficulty in walking, numbness, somnolence, coma, flushing, mild irritation of the eyes, nose, and throat, and impaired memory and vision may occur. Dermal exposure to the liquid for over 30 min has resulted in an extreme burning sensation and erythema. Treatment is symptomatic and supportive. Monitor for hepatic injury.

Methylene chloride (dichloromethane) is used as a paint remover, degreasing solvent, aerosol propellant, and refrigerant. It is an eye, skin, and respiratory tract irritant and moderate central nervous system depressant. It may cause bronchospasm or pulmonary edema. Methylene chloride is stored in fat and partially metabolized to carbon monoxide in the body. Elevation of carboxyhemoglobin levels may occur after exposure has ceased. Symptoms of excessive fatigue, weakness, light-headedness, somnolence, chills, nausea, incoordination, and pulmonary congestion may occur. Treatment is supportive and symptomatic. Carboxyhemoglobin levels and liver and pulmonary function should be monitored.

BIBLIOGRAPHY

Anas N, Namasonthi V, Ginsburg CM: Criteria for hospitalizing children who have ingested products containing hydrocarbons. *JAMA* 246:840–843, 1981.

Arena JM: Commentary. *J Pediatr* 87:637, 1975.

Askoy M, Erdem S, Dincol G: Types of leukemia in chronic benzene poisoning: A study of thirty-four patients. *Acta Hematol* 55:65, 1976.

Baker EL, Feldman RG: Paraoccupational exposure to mixed solvents. *J Toxicol Clin Toxicol* 19:27–34, 1982.

Barret L, Arsac Ph, Vincent M, et al: Evoked trigeminal nerve potential in chronic trichloroethylene intoxication. *J Toxicol Clin Toxicol* 19:419–423, 1982.

Bass M: Sudden sniffing death. *JAMA* 212:2075–2079, 1970.

Bauer M, Rabene SF: Cutaneous manifestations of trichloroethylene toxicity. *Arch Dermatol* 110:886–890, 1974.

Beamon RF, Siegel CJ, Landers G, et al: Hydrocarbon ingestion in children: A six year retrospective study. *JACEP* 5:771–775, 1976.

Beirne GJ: Goodpasture's syndrome and exposure to solvents. *JAMA* 222:1555, 1972.

Beirne GJ, Brennan JT: Glomerulonephritis associated with hydrocarbon solvents. *Arch Environ Health* 25:365–369, 1972.

Bennett RH, Forman HR: Hypokalemic periodic paralysis in chronic toluene exposure. *Arch Neurol* 37:673, 1980.

Benzon HT, Claybon L, Brunner EA: Elevated carbon monoxide levels from exposure to methylene chloride (letter). *JAMA* 239:2341, 1978.

Boeckx RL, Posti B, Coodin FJ: Gasoline sniffing and tetraethyl lead poisoning in children. *Pediatrics* 60:140–145, 1977.

Boor JW, Hurtig HI: Persistent cerebellar ataxia after exposure to toluene. *Ann Neurol* 2:440–442, 1977.

Bratton L, Haddow JE: Ingestion of charcoal lighter fluid. *J Pediatr* 87:633–636, 1975.

Brown J, Burke B, Dajani AS: Experimental kerosene pneumonia: Evaluation of some therapeutic regimes. *J Pediatr* 84:396–401, 1974.

Eade NR, Taussig LM, Marks MI: Hydrocarbon pneumonitis. *Pediatrics* 54:351–357, 1974.

Engstrom J, Bjurstrom R: Exposure to methylene chloride: Content in subcutaneous adipose tissue. *Scand J Work Environ Health* 3:215–224, 1977.

Feldman RG, Mayer RM, Traub A: Evidence for peripheral neurotoxic effect of trichloroethylene. *Neurology* 20:599–606, 1970.

Fischman CM, Oster JR: Toxic effects of toluene: A new cause of high anion gap metabolic acidosis. *JAMA* 241:1713–1715, 1979.

Forni AMA, Cappellini E, Pacifico E, et al: Chromosome changes and their evolution in subjects with past exposure to benzene. *Arch Environ Health* 23:385, 1971.

Gallassi R, Montajna P, Pazzaglia P, et al: Peripheral neuropathy due to gasoline sniffing. *Eur Neurol* 19:419–421, 1980.

Garriott J, Petty CS: Death from inhalant abuse: Toxicological and pathological evaluation of 34 cases. *Clin Toxicol* 16:305–315, 1980.

Garriott JC, Foerster E, Juarez L, et al: Measurement of toluene in blood and breath in cases of solvent abuse. *Clin Toxicol* 18:471–479, 1981.

Gerarde HW: Toxicological studies on hydrocarbons. *Arch Environ Health* 6:329–341, 1963.

Gold JH: Chronic perchloroethylene poisoning. *Can Psychiatr Assoc J* 14:627–630, 1969.

Greenberg LW, Coleman AB: A rare complication of hydrocarbon ingestion. *Clin Pro Child Hosp Nat Med Cent* 32:87–91, 1976.

Halevy J, Pitlir S, Rosenfeld J: 1,1,1-Trichloroethane intoxication: A case report with transient liver and renal damage. Review of the literature. *Clin Toxicol* 16:467–472, 1980.

Hansen KS, Sharp FR: Gasoline sniffing, lead poisoning and myoclonus. *JAMA* 240:1375–1376, 1978.

Harris, VJ, Brown R: Pneumatoceles as a complication of chemical pneumonia after hydrocarbon ingestion. *Am J Roentgenol* 125:531–537, 1975.

Hayden JW, Peterson RG, Bruckner JV: Toxicology of toluene (methylbenzene): Review of current literature. *Clin Toxicol* 11:549–559, 1977.

Herd PA, Lipsky M, Martin HF: Cardiovascular effects of 1,1,1-trichloroethane. *Arch Environ Health* 28:227–233, 1974.

Hydrocarbon exposure and proliferative glomerulonephritis. Editorial. *Lancet* 1:81–82, 1977.

Kaufman A: Gasoline sniffing among children in a Pueblo Indian village. *Pediatrics* 51:1060–1064, 1973.

King GD, Day RE, Oliver JS, et al: Solvent encephalopathy. *Br Med J* 283:663–664, 1981.

Kira S: Measurement by gas chromatography of urinary hippuric acid and methylhippuric acid as indices of toluene and xylene exposure. *Br J Ind Med* 34:305–309, 1977.

Kramer CG, Ott MG, Fulkerson JE, et al: Health of workers exposed to

1,1,1-trichloroethane: A matched-pair study. *Arch Environ Health* 33:331–342, 1978.

Law WR, Nelson ER: Gasoline-sniffing by an adult. *JAMA* 204:1002–1004, 1968.

Lewis JD, Mortiz D, Mellis LP: Long-term toluene abuse. *Am J Psychiatry* 138:368–370, 1981.

Longeley EO, Jones R: Acute trichloroethylene narcosis. *Arch Environ Health* 7:249–252, 1963.

Mann MD, Pirie DJ, Wolfsdorf J: Kerosene absorption in primates. *J Pediatr* 91:495–498, 1977.

Milby TH: Chronic trichloroethylene intoxication. *J Occup Med* 10:252–254, 1968.

Mofenson HC, Greensher J: The new correct answer to an old question on kerosene ingestion. *Pediatrics* 59:788, 1977.

Ng R, Darwish H, Stewart D: Emergency treatment of petroleum distillates and turpentine ingestion. *Can Med Assoc J* 3:537–538, 1974.

Perrone H, Passero MA: Hydrocarbon aerosol pneumonitis in an adult. *Arch Intern Med* 143:1607–1608, 1983.

Reinhardt CF, Mullin LS, Maxfield ME: Epinephrine-induced cardiac arrhythmia potential of some common industrial solvents. *J Occup Med* 15:953–955, 1973.

Robinson RO: Tetraethyl lead poisoning from gasoline sniffing. *JAMA* 240:1373–1374, 1978.

Savolainen H, Pfaffli P, Tengen M, et al: Biochemical and behavioral effects of inhalation exposure to tetrachloroethylene and dichloromethane. *J Neuropathol Exp Neurol* 36:941–949, 1977.

Sherwood RJ, Carter FWG: The measurement of occupational exposure to benzene vapor. *Ann Occup Hyg* 13:125, 1970.

Stewart RD: Acute tetrachloroethylene intoxication. *JAMA* 208:1490–1492, 1969.

Stewart RD, Rischer TN, Hoslso MJ, et al: Experimental human exposure to methylene chloride. *Arch Environ Health* 25:342–348, 1972.

Stewart RD, Hake CL, Peterson JE: Use of breath analysis to monitor trichloroethylene exposures. *Arch Environ Health* 29:6–13, 1974.

Stewart RD, Hake CL, Peterson JE: "Degreasers' flush": Dermal response to trichloroethylene and ethanol. *Arch Environ Health* 29:1–5, 1974.

Stockman JA: More on hydrocarbon-induced hemolysis. *J Pediatr* 90:848, 1977.

Strande CS: Carbon monoxide levels and methylene chloride exposure (letter). *JAMA* 240:1955, 1978.

Tahler SM, Anderson RJ, McCartney R, et al: Renal tubular acidosis associated with toluene sniffing. *N Engl J Med* 290:765–768, 1974.

Walkley JE, Pagnotto LD, Elkins HB: The measurement of phenol in urine as an index of benzene exposure. *Am Ind Hyg Assoc J* 22:362, 1961.

Wolfsdorf J: Kerosene intoxication: An experimental approach to the etiology of CNS manifestation in primates. *J Pediatr* 88:1037–1040, 1976.

Wyse DG: Deliberate inhalation of volatile hydrocarbons: A review. *Can Med Assoc J* 108:71–74, 1973.

Young RSK, Grzyle SE, Crismon L: Recurrent cerebellar dysfunction as related to chronic gasoline sniffing in an adolescent girl. *Clin Pediatr* 16:706–708, 1977.

CHAPTER 36
CAUSTIC INGESTIONS

Robert Knopp

Alkalies and acids are the most commonly ingested caustic substances. Devastating injuries to the gastrointestinal tract can result from ingestion of these substances.

The emergency physician plays an important role in the evaluation and management of patients who have ingested caustic substances. This discussion will be limited to emergency management of these patients.

INCIDENCE

It is estimated that 1.7 to 9.6 percent of accidental ingestions involve alkali or acid. Although many substances are involved, sodium hydroxide (lye) is the most frequent cause of severe injuries.

The frequency of caustic ingestions is highest in small children; 5000 to 8000 accidental lye ingestions occur yearly in children under the age of 5 years.

Adult ingestion of caustic substances often results in severe injury since the ingestion is usually intentional rather than accidental.

CLASSIFICATION OF CAUSTIC SUBSTANCES

A number of the commonly ingested acid and alkali substances are listed in Tables 36–1 and 36–2. There are two reasons why these substances are the most commonly ingested caustics:

1. Access: Most of these substances are household items located in the kitchen, bathroom, or garage. Easy access is the primary cause of caustic ingestion in small children.
2. Numerous cases exist where caustic substances have been placed in drinking containers (e.g., soda bottles). The patient inadvertently drinks from the container without realizing that the substance is a caustic.

PATHOPHYSIOLOGY

Most of the scientific studies on caustic ingestion have focused on the effects of lye on the gastrointestinal tract. There are very few studies of acid ingestion.

Solid lye ingestion produces deep tissue injury of the esophagus and less frequently the stomach. Ingestion of liquid lye, however, effects the esophagus and stomach with equal frequency. Several mechanisms have been proposed to explain the tissue injury that occurs after lye ingestion. Liquefaction necrosis occurs in tissues after exposure to lye. This is the result of the ability of lye to penetrate deeply into the tissues. The ingestion of liquid lye causes in seconds severe tissue injury which limits the effectiveness of virtually all nonsurgical treatment. Rumack has demonstrated that the reaction which occurs when lye comes into contact with the tissues involves the production of heat and resultant tissue injury. Saponification of fat also occurs from lye ingestion but is not a thermal injury.

Acid ingestion produces a different pathologic picture. Injury to the gastrointestinal tract occurs primarily in the stomach; 20 percent of these patients will have concomitant injury of the esophagus. Tissue contact with acid substances causes a coagulation necrosis.

The mechanism of injury in acid ingestion is purported to be dehydration and/or excessive heat generation.

Regardless of whether the substance ingested is an alkali or acid, tissue injury is dependent on a number of factors: (1) the nature, volume, and concentration of the substance; (2) contact time with the tissues; (3) presence or absence of stomach contents at the time of ingestion; and (4) tonicity of the pyloric sphincter.

COMPLICATIONS

The major complications from caustic ingestion can be divided into immediate (within 48 to 72 h) and delayed. The immediate complications occur as a result of hyperthermic injury to the tissues. Injury to the larynx, epiglottis, or vocal cords is an infrequent but potentially catastrophic problem which may cause soft tissue swelling and result in upper airway compromise.

The most frequent complication occurring during the first few days after ingestion of lye is perforation of the esophagus or stomach. Morbidity and mortality may occur from hemorrhage or infection. With acid ingestion the esophagus is less frequently involved; perforation is less frequent and usually involves the stomach.

Delayed complications can occur in both alkali and acid ingestions. Strictures of the gastrointestinal tract represent the most common delayed complication from caustic ingestion. Esophageal strictures occur most commonly after lye ingestion, whereas stricture of the pylorus is most common after acid ingestions.

Table 36-1. Common Alkali Substances

Sodium or potassium hydroxide (lye):
  Washing powders
  Paint removers
  Drain pipe and toilet bowl cleaners
  Detergents
  Clinitest tablets
Liquid:
  Liquid Plumber
  Drano
  Plunge
  Open-up drain cleaner
  Easy-off oven cleaner
Solid:
  Drano—granular
  Clinitest—tablets
Others:
  Sodium hypochloride (Clorox) bleach
  Nonphosphate detergents—sodium carbonate
  Sodium carbonate (Purex) bleach
  Potassium permanganate
  Ammonia—metal cleaners or polishers, hair dyes and tints, antirust
    products, jewelry cleaners
  Electric dishwashing agents

CLINICAL EVALUATION

Initial assessment of the patient involves the identification and treatment of life-threatening problems (airway obstruction, hemorrhage, etc.). In most instances, however, the patient will present in severe distress from pain, not shock or respiratory distress.

The diagnosis of gastrointestinal injury is usually confirmed by the history of ingestion and a brief examination of the mouth. The absence of oral lesions does not, however, preclude the possibility of esophageal burns. Reports in the literature document that from 2 to 15 percent of patients with esophageal burns have no oral lesions. Unfortunately, it has not been determined whether any of these patients developed strictures. The determination of the presence or absence of injury in patients whose histories are vague must often be left to the endoscopist.

The physician should attempt to elicit symptoms associated with ingestion of a caustic substance, such as difficulty in swallowing or pain in the mouth, chest, or abdomen.

Physical examination consists of attempting to determine whether signs of overt or impending perforation are present.

Table 36-2. Common Acid Substances

Hydrochloric acid:
  Metal
  Swimming pool cleaners
  Toilet bowl cleaners
Sulfuric acid:
  Battery acid
  Toilet bowl cleaners (sodium bisulfate)
Others [carbolic (phenol), nitric, oxalic, hydrofluoric, aqua regia
  (mixture of hydrochloric and nitric)]:
  Toilet bowl cleaners
  Slate cleaners
  Bleach disinfectants
  Soldering fluxes

MANAGEMENT

Stabilization (See Table 36-3)

Initial management of both acid and alkali ingestions is similar.

Respiratory distress is uncommon after caustic ingestion (Knopp, unpublished data). In 35 cases of caustic ingestion seen at Valley Medical Center in Fresno, California, during a 5-year period, only two developed respiratory distress. One required a tracheostomy.

The usual cause of respiratory distress in these patients is upper airway obstruction secondary to soft tissue swelling of the larynx, epiglottis, or vocal cords. Unless endotracheal intubation can be accomplished without additional trauma, a tracheostomy (or cricothyrotomy) may be necessary. With soft tissue swelling in the hypopharynx, there is a risk of perforation. Blind nasotracheal intubation in this situation is contraindicated. Although aspiration can occur with caustic ingestions, it has not been documented as a cause of acute respiratory distress.

Arterial blood gases should be obtained and oxygen started if the patient is in shock or respiratory distress. An intravenous line should be established. Central venous cannulation and pressure monitoring are necessary if signs of perforation or shock are present. Blood should be typed and crossmatched and baseline hemoglobin determined.

If the patient is complaining of severe pain due to oropharyngeal burns or perforation of the esophagus or stomach, meperidine or morphine may be given intravenously, once the diagnosis has been established. In cases of severe ingestion, after the patient has been stabilized, x-ray films of the chest and abdomen should be obtained for signs of esophageal or gastric perforation.

The patient is given nothing by mouth initially (except when diluents are indicated) because of the potential risk of vomiting or aspiration.

Diluents

The use of diluents in the treatment of caustic ingestions has provoked a great deal of controversy. Diluents are used for two reasons: (1) to move any solid alkali material adhering to the oropharynx and esophagus into the stomach where it can be neutralized, and (2) to dilute the caustic material and hopefully decrease the degree of tissue injury.

Table 36-3. General Management: Stabilization

1. ABCs and vital signs:
     Cricothyrotomy or tracheostomy
   Respiratory distress:
     Endotracheal intubation (may be contraindicated)
2. O$_2$ and ABGs if indicated
3. IV
4. CBC and T&C, four units
5. Physical exam
6. Analgesia—meperidine or morphine IV
7. X-ray of chest and abdomen
8. NPO

Alkalies

Recommendations in the older literature and on the labels of a number of alkali products advocate the use of acidic substances as antidotes. As recently as 1977, some medical literature still supported this idea. Although neutralizing a base with an acid seems logical, such a mixture actually produces an exothermic reaction releasing significant amounts of heat. This heat could produce a thermal injury and increase tissue damage. Therefore, the use of acidic substances such as lemon juice, acetic acid, or vinegar as an antidote is contraindicated.

Rumack and Burrington have demonstrated that milk or water is the preferred diluent in solid lye ingestion. They used water, milk, acetic acid, and lemon juice as diluents. Temperatures were recorded before and after each of the diluents was added. Milk was the most effective diluent in reducing the amount of heat generated. Water also appeared preferable to the acidic substances. Because of accessibility, milk and water are probably the best diluents. Unless there are contraindications, diluents are probably indicated in solid lye ingestions. There have, however, been no controlled studies demonstrating their benefit.

Diluents are of no value in liquid lye ingestion. By the time the patient reaches the emergency department, tissue injury is probably complete. The work of Ritter et al. shows that administering water to patients with gastric burns secondary to liquid lye ingestion may result in vomiting. Reexposure of the esophagus, larynx, and oral cavity to lye could increase tissue injury in these areas.

Acids

Although diluents have been recommended in acid ingestion, no studies have demonstrated their benefit. Rumack recommends milk or water for ingestion of concentrated acids. However, tissue injury may occur rapidly, and by the time the patient reaches the emergency department diluents may have no beneficial effect.

Contraindications to the use of diluents in the emergency department are listed in Table 36-4.

Emesis and Lavage

Gastric lavage or emesis is contraindicated in alkali ingestions. The potential hazards of such treatment are (1) reexposure of the esophagus to the alkali, (2) perforation of injured tissues, and (3) aspiration. Because tissue injury is often present by the time the patient reaches the emergency department, little benefit is gained by attempts to remove any remaining material.

Emesis is contraindicated in acid ingestions. Reexposure of the esophagus to the caustic and possible perforation of the stomach are the primary reasons for not inducing emesis.

Table 36-4. Contraindications to Diluent Use in the Emergency Department

1. Severe ingestions with signs of:
   a. Gastric or esophageal perforation
   b. Shock
   c. Upper airway obstruction
2. Ingestion of liquid lye

Controversy exists regarding the use of gastric aspiration and lavage in acid ingestions; although several authors recommend their use, no studies have been performed which demonstrate the advantages or disadvantages of such treatment. Those who recommend lavage specify that a soft rubber catheter be used and lavage considered only in patients seen soon after ingestion. Others advise against the use of gastric lavage regardless of the circumstances. Until further evidence is available demonstrating the benefit of gastric lavage, it probably should not be used in caustic ingestions.

Cathartics and Charcoal

Cathartics and activated charcoal are recommended in the early management of many overdoses; however, they are contraindicated in ingestions of alkali and acids for the following reasons: (1) alkalies and acids are poorly adsorbed by activated charcoal; (2) tissue injury occurs so rapidly that neither cathartics nor charcoal would be of any benefit when the patient reaches the emergency department; and (3) activated charcoal may limit the endoscopist's ability to identify tissue injury.

Steroids

Although opinions vary as to their efficacy, steroids are used in alkali ingestions to reduce the incidence of esophageal strictures. The use of steroids is based on studies by Spain. He observed that glucocorticoids inhibit fibroplasia and the formation of granulation tissue if given within 48 h of injury. Several studies have demonstrated a decreased incidence of esophageal stricture formation following lye ingestion in animals treated with steroids.

As a result of these studies, glucocorticoids have been given to patients with esophageal injury secondary to alkali ingestion. Unfortunately, no controlled studies exist to demonstrate that steroids decrease the incidence of esophageal stricture formation in humans. The side effects of long-term steroid administration are well documented, but in treating most caustic ingestions steroids are used only for a period of several weeks. The frequency of steroid-related complications in caustic ingestions has not been adequately studied. Steroids have been reported to cause an increased incidence of suppurative complications in animals as well as an increased risk of esophageal perforation in patients having ingested concentrated solutions of alkali. Moreover, steroids must be started within 48 h and probably are only effective in preventing strictures in circumferential esophageal burns.

Steroids may be useful in two specific circumstances: (1) patients with circumferential esophageal burns, and (2) patients with suspected esophageal burns (i.e., esophagoscopy cannot be used). In the emergency department, however, prior to endoscopy, the initial decision to use steroids will be based on a separate list of criteria.

Certain contraindications to steroid use must be considered. First, certain medical problems, such as an actively bleeding ulcer, would constitute a contraindication. Second, signs of gastric or esophageal perforation would contraindicate the use of steroids because severe irreversible tissue damage has occurred and steroids may tend to mask signs of perforation. Third, if more than

48 h has elapsed, the ability of steroids to prevent esophageal strictures is markedly reduced. Finally, noncircumferential esophageal burns probably do not cause esophageal stricture and do not require steroids.

Prednisone has been recommended for oral treatment in a dose of 1 to 2 mg/(kg·day). Most patients, however, will be unable to take oral steroid preparations, and methylprednisolone, 20 mg intravenously every 8 h for patients under the age of 2 and 40 mg every 8 h for patients over the age of 2 has been recommended.

Antibiotics

Antibiotics have been recommended for alkali ingestions in patients with signs of gastric or esophageal perforation and prophylactically in patients requiring steroid therapy for esophageal burns. There is some evidence that prophylactic antibiotics may be effective in reducing the frequency of suppurative complications associated with steroid therapy. Haller (1964) and Rosenberg (1953) demonstrated that cats and rabbits with esophageal burns from lye ingestion have a higher mortality from infections when treated with steroids alone than with a combination of steroids and antibiotics. Haller (1964) reported frequent mortality from aspiration pneumonia in cats treated with steroids alone.

Despite this experimental data, controversy exists over whether prophylactic antibiotics are beneficial, and no clinical studies have been published to resolve this controversy.

TREATMENT IN THE EMERGENCY DEPARTMENT

Treatment decisions regarding adults and older children involve three factors: (1) reliability of the patient, (2) presence or absence of specific symptoms (oropharyngeal, chest or abdominal pain, dysphagia, respiratory distress) or signs (drooling, shock, abdominal tenderness, etc.), and (3) presence or absence of oral burns. A small percentage of patients with no oral burns will have esophageal burns, but if these patients are reliable, the presence of signs or symptoms will alert the physician to the probability that gastrointestinal injury has occurred.

In patients with obvious signs or symptoms of alkali ingestion, endoscopy is required to determine the severity of the burn. Endoscopy is usually performed within 12 to 24 h of the time of injury. Recently the use of the pediatric endoscope has been advocated as a safer means of evaluating the gastrointestinal tract. In patients with signs of perforation, immediate operative intervention is required and endoscopy deferred.

Institution of steroid therapy is indicated in patients with signs or symptoms of caustic ingestion but no signs of esophageal or gastric perforation. Steroid therapy should be initiated as soon as possible, but withholding steroids until after endoscopy is an acceptable alternative if endoscopy is performed in less than 24 h.

Administration of prophylactic antibiotics remains controversial. Rumack and Becker (personal communication) do not recommend prophylactic treatment.

In small children or unreliable adults with a normal physical exam, the decision as to whether to perform endoscopy and initiate treatment is most difficult. Unless strong evidence exists that the ingestion did not occur or the substance was not caustic, endoscopy should probably be performed.

BIBLIOGRAPHY

Allen RE, Thoshinsky MJ, Stallone RJ: Corrosive injuries of the stomach. *Arch Surg* 100:409–413, 1970.

Ashcraft KW, Simon JL: Accidental caustic ingestion in childhood: A review. *Tex Med* 68:86–88, 1972.

Buntain WL, Cain WC: Caustic injuries to the esophagus. *South Med J* 74(5):590–593, 1981.

Cello JP, Fogel RP, Boland CR: Liquid caustic ingestion. *Arch Intern Med* 140:501–504, 1980.

Chodak GW, Passaro E: Acid ingestions. *JAMA* 239:225–226, 1978.

Chong GC, Beahrs OH, Payne WS: Management of corrosive gastritis due to ingested acid. *Mayo Clin Proc* 49:861–865, 1974.

Done A: Some caustic questions. *Emergency Medicine,* December 1975, pp 54–63.

Feldman M, Iben A, Hurley E: Corrosive injury to oropharynx and esophagus. *Calif Med* 118:6–9, 1973.

Genot A, Messier CA, Chicoine LUC: L'intoxication aux corrosifs. *Union Med Can* 97:279–282, 1968.

Goldfrank L, Kerstein R: The near-fatal mistake. *Hosp Phys,* December 1976, pp 20–25.

Haller JA, Andrews HG, White JJ: Pathophysiology and management of acute corrosive burns of the esophagus: Results and treatment in 285 children. *J Pediatr Surg* 6:578–584, 1971.

Haller JA, Bachman K: The comparative effect of current therapy on experimental caustic burns of the esophagus. *Pediatrics* 34:236, 1964.

Jelenko C: Acid trip to the stomach. *Emergency Medicine,* November 1972, pp 83–85.

Jelenko C: Chemicals that "burn." *J Trauma* 14:65–72, 1974.

Kirsh MM, Ritter F: Caustic ingestion and subsequent damage to the oropharyngeal and digestive passages. *Ann Thorac Surg* 21:74–82, 1976.

Knopp R: Caustic Ingestions. *JACEP* 8:329–336, 1979.

Krenzelok EP, Clinton JE: Caustic esophageal and gastric erosion without evidence of oral burns following detergent ingestions. *JACEP* 8:194–196, 1979.

Krey H: On the treatment of corrosive lesions in the esophagus: An experimental study. *Acta Otolaryngol* 102:1–45, 1952.

Middlekamp JN, Cone AJ, Ogura JH: Endoscopic diagnosis and steroid and antibiotic therapy of acute lye burns of the esophagus. *Laryngoscope* 71:1354–1362, 1961.

Middlekamp JN, Ferguson T, Roper C: The management of problems of caustic burns in children. *J Thorac Cardiovasc Surg* 57:341–347, 1969.

Picchioni AL: Activated charcoal—A neglected antidote. *Pediatr Clin North Am* 17:545–556, 1970.

Ray JF: Editorial. *Arch Intern Med* 140:471, 1980.

Ritter FN, Newman MJ, Newman DE: A clinical and experimental study of corrosive burns of the esophagus. *Ann Otolaryngol* 77:830–842, 1968.

Rosenberg N, Kundeman PH, Vroman L, et al: Prevention of experimental lye strictures of the esophagus by cortisone. *Arch Surg* 63:147–151, 1951.

Rosenberg N, Kunderman PH, Vroman L: Prevention of experimental lye stricture by cortisone II—Control of suppurative complications by penicillin. *Arch Surg* 66:593, 1953.

Rumack BH, Burrington JD: Caustic ingestions: A rational look at diluents. *Clin Toxicol* 11:27–34, 1977.

Scher L, Maull KI: Emergency management and sequelae of acid ingestions. *JACEP* 7:206–208, 1978.

Spain DM, Molomut N, Haber A: The effect of cortisone on the formation of granulation tissue in mice. *Am J Pathol* 26:710, 1950.

Webb W, Koutras P, Ecker R: An evaluation of steroids and antibiotics in caustic burns of the esophagus. *Ann Thorac Surg* 9:95–102, 1970.

Weisskopf A: Effects of cortisone on experimental lye burn of the esophagus. *Ann Otolaryngol* 61:81–691, 1952.

Wright JE, Hennessy EJ: Pyloric obstruction due to ingestion of corrosives. *Med J Aust* 2:761–767, 1972.

CHAPTER 37
ALCOHOLS

Judith E. Tintinalli

METHANOL

Methanol (wood or acetone alcohol) is obtained from distillation of wood, and is an important solvent in the manufacturing industry. It is a component of antifreeze, paint solvent, and canned fuels, and is used as a gasoline additive and home-heating fuel. Accidental poisoning can occur if it is substituted for ethyl alcohol in contraband liquor.

Pathophysiology

Methanol is converted in the liver, by the action of alcohol dehydrogenase, to formaldehyde, and, in minutes, to formic acid. The accumulation of formic acid in the blood is associated with the onset of clinical symptoms such as anorexia, photophobia, and hyperpnea, and can be correlated with the decrease in carbon dioxide content and the severity of metabolic acidosis. Formic acid accounts almost fully for the anion gap seen in methanol poisoning, while lactate, butyrate, and acetate account for only 2 to 3 percent. Formate metabolism in primates is implemented by a folate-dependent system. According to Noker et al., folate infusion of 2 mg/kg in monkeys decreased formate accumulation from methanol and reversed metabolic acidosis. This was true if folic acid was given before, during, or up to 18 h after methanol infusion. 4-Methylpyrazole (4-MP), alone or in combination with ethanol, may also be of value in methanol poisoning. 4-MP inhibits alcohol dehydrogenase and results in a dose-dependent inhibition of methanol elimination from plasma. In humans, pyrazole causes weight loss and hepatocellular toxicity, especially when given in conjunction with methanol. So far, toxic effects of 4-MP have not been demonstrated in primates, but it has not been used in humans. If 4-MP could be used with ethanol it would decrease the dose of ethanol needed, and 4-MP also has about a 24-h duration of action.

Formate concentrations are markedly greater in the vitreous humor than in the blood, and the structural changes in the eye may be caused by the interference of formate with enzymes critical to intermediary metabolism in the optic nerve itself. Optic disk edema can be produced in monkeys by formate infusion, even though a normal systemic pH is maintained.

Although most cases of methanol toxicity result from intentional or accidental oral ingestion, toxicity can also occur if methanol is absorbed through the skin or inhaled. Accidental inhalation has been reported when windshield solvent was applied to the interior of windows in a closed space, such as an automobile.

The toxic dose of methanol is variable. The smallest lethal dose reported is 15 mL, while doses as large as 500 mL have been reported without toxicity. Generally, a dose of 30 mL in an adult should be regarded as lethal. Toxicity is based upon the presence of folate deficiency and concomitant ethyl alcohol consumption, as well as the total dose of methanol absorbed. The volume of distribution of methanol is 0.64 L/kg. Animal experiments have demonstrated that pulmonary excretion can account for 14 to 75 percent of metabolism and renal excretion for 3 to 10 percent. Insignificant amounts are also excreted in sweat. Nevertheless, the respiratory tract is not felt to be a major route of excretion in humans, and forced diuresis does not significantly increase methanol clearance.

Clinical Features

The major toxic signs and symptoms of methanol ingestion are (1) visual symptoms; (2) CNS depression; (3) abdominal pain, nausea, and vomiting; and (4) metabolic acidosis (Table 37-1). A notable feature is the presence of a latent period of 8 to 72 h between the time of ingestion and the onset of symptoms. The onset of symptoms correlates with the appearance of metabolic acidosis. Visual complaints such as photophobia, blurred or indistinct vision, or descriptions of looking at a snowstorm are believed to occur universally in symptomatic cases of methanol poisoning. The pupils are frequently dilated and react sluggishly, if at all, to light. Hyperemia of the optic disk is evident at the onset of visual disturbances. Papilledema may develop within hours, and it is indistinguishable from that of elevated intracranial pressure. Microscopic findings include edema of the retina nerve fiber layer, and engorgement of the retinal veins. Optic atrophy and blindness can develop rapidly.

Methanol, like all alcohols, can produce confusion, lethargy, and obtundation. Generalized seizure activity may occur, and mental status may rapidly change from alertness to coma. Although cerebral edema has been described as a classic sign of methanol poisoning, only 10 percent of autopsied patients had evidence of cerebral edema in the series of 323 cases reviewed by Bennett et al.

Table 37-1. Clinical Features of Methanol Intoxication

8- to 72-h latent period
CNS depression
Severe metabolic acidosis
Blurred vision
Abdominal pain

Nausea, vomiting, and severe abdominal pain are frequent signs and symptoms and appear to be due to acute pancreatitis. In the study by Bennett et al., 80 percent of patients had evidence of hemorrhagic pancreatitis at postmortem examination.

Methanol poisoning is one of the instances in which a zero plasma bicarbonate can occur. A large-anion-gap metabolic acidosis and an osmolal gap (see below) are early laboratory clues to the diagnosis. The acidosis of methanol poisoning resembles lactic acidosis in that spectacular amounts of bicarbonate may be necessary to maintain the arterial pH and carbon dioxide content near reasonable limits.

The serum osmolality can be measured directly or determined by calculation:

$$\text{Serum osmolality} = (2 \times Na) + \frac{BUN}{3} + \frac{glucose}{18}$$

The normal serum osmolality is 280 to 295 mOsm. A measured osmolality (by freezing-point depression) that is elevated and more than 10 mOsm greater than the calculated osmolality is called an *osmolal gap*. An osmolal gap suggests the presence in the serum of osmotically active substances, such as ethyl alcohol, methanol, isopropyl alcohol, glycerol, or mannitol, measured by the osmometer, that are not accounted for by the calculated osmolality. A substance significantly contributes to osmolality only if it achieves relatively high blood levels and has a low molecular weight. Even if ethanol is present, an osmolal gap due to other substances can be detected by adding to the osmolality equation the contribution of ethanol, as [EtOH (mg/100 mL)]/4.6.

One can differentiate indirectly between alcohols by determining the presence of an osmolal gap or metabolic acidosis or both (Table 37-2). The alcohols do not cross-react on laboratory testing, and each substance must be qualitatively or quantitatively analyzed separately.

Treatment

The treatment of methanol poisoning consists of (1) general supportive measures, (2) correction of metabolic acidosis, (3) prevention of conversion of methanol to formic acid, and (4) elimination of methanol and formate.

Table 37-2. Clinical Differentiation of Unknown Alcohols

Alcohol	Osmolal Gap	Metabolic Acidosis
Ethylene glycol	Yes	Severe
Isopropyl alcohol	Yes	Variable pH, + ketones
Methanol	Yes	Severe
Ethanol	Yes	Variable serum pH Variable serum acetone Positive blood ethanol

Gastric lavage is indicated to remove any substance still present in the stomach. Adequate ventilation is essential to ensure maximum respiratory excretion. Adequate urine output should be maintained, but forced diuresis is not necessary. Fluid overload may exacerbate possible cerebral edema. Mannitol, glycerol, or corticosteroids can be given for cerebral edema, although their effectiveness in methanol poisoning has not been demonstrated.

For metabolic acidosis, administer bicarbonate and monitor the arterial pH as well as the serum bicarbonate level. Large doses are often necessary. The initial dose is usually 1 mEq/kg.

Ethanol is indicated whenever methanol poisoning is suspected because of a large-anion-gap acidosis and an osmolal gap. Ethanol and methanol are both substrates for the enzyme alcohol dehydrogenase, but ethanol has a nine-times-greater affinity for the enzyme than methanol and is preferentially metabolized, thus preventing the conversion of methanol to formic acid. McCoy et al. recommend an initial ethanol loading dose of 0.6 g/kg (given a volume of distribution of 0.6 L/kg) to produce a blood ethanol concentration of approximately 100 mg/100 mL, which can be maintained by an ethanol infusion of 66 mg/(kg·h) for nondrinkers or 154 mg/(kg·h) for chronic drinkers. One milliliter of absolute ethanol is equal to 790 mg of ethanol. The general agreement is that patients with a methanol level above 50 mg/100 mL should be treated by hemodialysis. Hemodialysis removes both methanol and formic acid. Peritoneal dialysis is not as effective, and should be utilized only if hemodialysis is not available. Sorbent-based hemodialysis has not proved effective in the removal of methanol. Gonda et al. recommend hemodialysis (1) if the blood methanol is greater than 50 mg/100 mL; (2) if more than 30 mL has been ingested; (3) if there is intractable acidosis; (4) if there is deterioration of vision or of CNS function.

During hemodialysis, the dose of ethanol should be increased since it, too, is removed by hemodialysis. McCoy et al. recommend increasing the ethanol infusion by an increment of 7.2 g/h during dialysis. Blood ethanol concentration should be monitored during both hemodialysis and during maintenance ethanol infusions, to remain at approximately 100 mg/100 mL.

ETHYLENE GLYCOL

Ethylene glycol is an aliphatic straight-chained polyalcohol. A colorless, odorless liquid, it is a component of various commercial products such as detergents, paints, pharmaceuticals, polishes, antifreeze, and coolants. Poisonings with ethylene glycol are uncommon but not rare.

Ethylene glycol is metabolized principally in the liver and kidney (Fig. 37-1), and toxicity is due primarily to the accumulation of the toxic intermediary metabolites—glycoaldehyde, glycolate, and glyoxylate. These compounds contain ketoaldehyde groups that inhibit oxidative phosphorylation, protein synthesis, and sulfhydryl-containing enzymes. Severe metabolic acidosis, due to accumulation of aldehyde, glycolate, and lactate, is a hallmark of ethylene glycol intoxication. Glycine production also consumes bicarbonate and contributes to acidosis. In addition, calcium oxalate precipitates in the kidneys, brain, liver, blood vessels, and pericardium, causing tissue destruction.

Ethylene glycol is converted to glycoaldehyde by the action of alcohol dehydrogenase. During this reaction the generation of large amounts of reduced nicotinamide adenine dinucleotide (NADH) can result in lactic acidosis if the NADH/NAD ratio is changed.

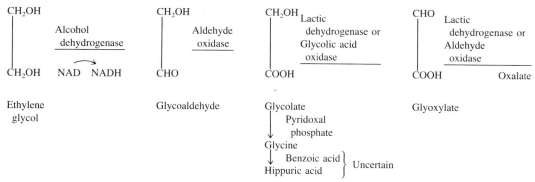

Figure 37-1. Pathway for metabolism of ethylene glycol.

Pyridoxal phosphate is a cofactor necessary for the conversion of the toxic glycolate to the nontoxic glycine. If all available pyridoxal phosphate is consumed, toxicity is enhanced, since more glycolate will be converted to glyoxylate and oxalate, and not to glycine.

The volume of distribution of ethylene glycol is 0.83 L/kg. The plasma half-life of ethylene glycol is about 3 h. However, metabolites are responsible for the toxicity, and these may have half-lives of up to 12 h. Ethanol administration prolongs the half-life of a metabolite to approximately 17 h.

Clinical Features

The lethal dose of ethylene glycol is about 2 mL/kg or about 100 mL in adults. The major signs and symptoms of ethylene glycol poisoning are those producing metabolic abnormalities and those affecting the central nervous system, cardiopulmonary system, and, finally, the renal system.

Central nervous system symptoms generally appear 1 to 12 h after ingestion, a time that correlates with peak glycoaldehyde production. Ataxia, nystagmus, ophthalmoplegia, papilledema, optic atrophy, myoclonus, focal or generalized convulsions, hallucinations, stupor, and coma may occur. Lumbar puncture may show elevation of the CSF pressure and protein, and polymorphonuclear pleocystosis. CSF cultures are sterile. At postmortem, calcium oxalate deposits can be demonstrated in the white and gray matter of the brain, blood vessels, and choroid plexus. There is a general cerebral edema and widespread petechiae.

Large-anion-gap metabolic acidosis usually accompanies the development of CNS symptoms. An osmolal gap is also present.

Hypocalcemia, on occasion severe enough to induce tetany, may develop because of precipitation of calcium as calcium oxalate. Myalgia and elevation of creatine phosphokinase levels have also been reported. Nausea, vomiting, and abdominal pain may develop in a great number of patients. Within 24 to 72 h, pneumonia, pulmonary edema, and fulminant cardiac failure may occur.

Renal failure may develop in 24 to 72 h. Both the aldehyde metabolites of ethylene glycol and oxalic acid have direct renal toxicity. The intratubular deposition of oxylate crystals is widespread.

Positive birefringent calcium oxalate and, possibly, hippurate crystals in the urine are pathognomonic of the diagnosis, although these crystals may be absent, especially in the early phase, even in severe poisoning. Microscopic hematuria, proteinuria, and renal epithelial cells are also commonly found on urinalysis. Azotemia and anuria may follow.

The diagnosis of ethylene glycol intoxication is based primarily on the clinical recognition of symptoms, since serum levels of ethylene glycol and oxalic acid are difficult to obtain, and treatment needs to be initiated quickly. In addition, there appears to be little correlation between the serum ethylene glycol level and the clinical condition of the patient.

Special aspects of laboratory evaluation include the determination of those studies important in the evaluation of an osmolal gap and a large-anion-gap metabolic acidosis: serum glucose, acetone, alcohol, BUN, creatinine, salicylate, and electrolyte levels; osmolality; and arterial blood gases. Methanol and paraldehyde poisoning, as well as alcoholic ketoacidosis, should also be considered in the differential diagnosis. Where available, specific toxicology studies, including methanol and ethylene glycol levels, should be obtained. Additionally, calcium, magnesium, and creatine phosphokinase levels should be obtained.

Treatment

Treatment must be initiated as soon as the diagnosis is suspected from an osmolal gap and large anion gap. Delay until toxicology results are received can result in serious or even irreversible deterioration.

Gastric lavage can be utilized to remove any product that has not yet been absorbed. Activated charcoal also decreases the gastrointestinal absorption by 50 percent.

Correct metabolic acidosis by the administration of sodium bicarbonate, while monitoring the pH and bicarbonate content. Treat hypocalcemia with calcium gluconate. Magnesium salts can also be administered concomitantly. Administer thiamine and pyridoxine, cofactors essential for the detoxificaton of ethylene glycol.

Maintain adequate urine output to enhance the renal clearance of ethylene glycol and oxalic acid. Loop diuretics such as furosemide or mannitol can be given. Fluid administration must be carefully monitored, however, to avoid the development of pulmonary edema.

Intravenous ethanol should be administered since it competes for alcohol dehydrogenase, and may inhibit the metabolism of ethylene glycol to toxic intermediaries. Ethanol must be given as soon as possible after ingestion since the half-life of ethylene glycol is about 3 h. To produce a level of 100 mg/100 mL a loading dose of 0.6 g/kg of absolute alcohol should be given.

Hemodialysis is indicated as soon as the diagnosis is made, before the development of renal failure. Both ethylene glycol and the intermediate aldehydes are dialyzable. Renal, CNS, and cardiopulmonary symptoms will be ameliorated, and severe metabolic acidosis will respond to dialysis as well.

ETHANOL

Although ethanol levels are widely used to evaluate the CNS status of intoxicated patients, there is marked individual variation as to the blood level and degree of intoxication. In many states, the legal limit of intoxication is 100 mg/100 mL. Although death from medullary failure is possible above 500 mg/100 mL, those with a high tolerance for alcohol can be ambulatory at even higher levels. At Detroit General Hospital, a patient with a blood alcohol of 999 mg/100 mL was treated in the emergency department and recovered within a few hours.

Alcohol is oxidized in the liver to carbon dioxide and water by alcohol dehydrogenase, a nicotinamide adenine dinucleotide (NAD) dependent enzyme. Another microsomal oxidase system, which is reduced nicotinamide adenine dinucleotide phosphate (NADPH) dependent, is thought to have a role in the oxidation of ethanol to acetaldehyde. A definite role has not been established for the microsomal ethanol oxidizing system (MEOS) in the metabolism of ethanol.

Although ethanol is generally metabolized at a constant rate, 20 mg/(100 mL·h), regardless of its concentration, the rate of metabolism may be increased in alcoholics.

Clinical Features

The clinical features of alcohol intoxication are similar to those induced by sedative-hypnotic agents. The signs of mild intoxication are colored by the individual's basic personality, and can range from euphoria, expansiveness, and loss of self-control, to general bad temper. Homicidal or extreme suicidal gestures or ideation while the patient is intoxicated indicate the need for psychiatric evaluation. Ataxia, slurred speech, nystagmus, and dullness or distortion of sensory perceptions are seen next. Tachycardia is common, as a result of peripheral vasodilation. An acute psychotic state, characterized by visual hallucinations and paranoid ideation, can be seen. With toxic levels, hypoventilation, hypothermia, and hypotension develop.

The patient with apparent alcohol intoxication must be carefully evaluated for a wide variety of coexisting abnormalities. Head and neck injury, hypoglycemia, electrolyte abnormalities, meningitis, sepsis, myopathy and neuropathy, bone marrow suppression, cardiac myopathy and arrhythmias, gastrointestinal bleeding, pancreatitis, liver disease and hepatic coma, polydrug abuse, or ethylene glycol or methanol ingestion are but a few of the complications that alcoholics can exhibit. The possibility of a number of alcohol-drug interactions should also be considered when evaluating the intoxicated patient and when prescribing agents for outpatient therapy (Table 37-3). The alcoholic patient, more often than not, has more than one disease, and meticulous emergency department evaluation should be the rule.

Motor vehicle accidents often occur while the driver is under the influence of alcohol. Physical examination of a trauma patient who is intoxicated is not reliable, as the sensory response to pain is dulled. Since the patient is unreliable as a historian, the mechanism of injury may be difficult to reconstruct. Repeat exam is always necessary, with chart documentation, when the patient is sober.

Chest pain in the intoxicated patient is difficult to evaluate, for patients are uncooperative and cannot describe symptoms well. Patients may go on a drinking binge to mask chest pain, or alcohol itself may precipitate angina. Common alcohol-related problems such as gastritis, esophagitis, and ulcer disease may be seen with noncardiac chest pain. Thus, complaints of chest pain in intoxicated patients should be evaluated carefully.

Treatment

For the patient with uncomplicated intoxication, observation until sober is generally all that is required. There have been isolated anecdotal reports of responses to naloxone, but there is no evidence to suggest that it should be administered routinely in alcohol intoxication unless concomitant opiate overdose is suspected.

Gastric lavage and the instillation of activated charcoal can be helpful if ingestion has been within 2 h, or if polydrug ingestion is suspected, and 50 g of glucose should be given intravenously for severe intoxication. Thiamine, 100 mg intramuscularly or intravenously, is often given to prevent the development of the Wernicke-Korsakoff syndrome.

Although fructose has been shown to increase the rate of disappearance of alcohol from the blood, clinical studies have not demonstrated its usefulness in speeding up sobriety. In the study of Levy et al., asymptomatic elevations of blood lactate and uric acid were noted with fructose therapy.

ALCOHOL WITHDRAWAL

The physiologic basis of the alcohol withdrawal syndromes remains undefined. A number of sleep disturbances, as demonstrated by the EEG, have been reported and appear to have a relationship to clinical symptoms. During alcohol intake, REM sleep decreases and delta sleep increases; during alcohol withdrawal, REM sleep increases and delta sleep decreases. Plasma and urine catecholamine levels are increased during withdrawal and may aggravate the symptoms.

The clinical features of alcohol withdrawal vary with the duration and intensity of drinking. Alcohol withdrawal can develop while the patient is drinking if there is a decrease in alcohol intake. Mild reactions include tremor, insomnia, and irritability. The full-blown syndrome of delirium tremens generally develops about 48 to 100 h after cessation of drinking, and consists of tachycardia, diaphoresis, hypertension, tremors, visual hallucinations, and paranoid ideation.

Alcohol withdrawal seizures, or ''rum fits,'' are major motor seizures that develop in patients with no underlying seizure focus and who show a normal EEG when abstinent. They generally develop before other signs of alcohol withdrawal, and consist of either a single, or a few, major motor seizures. Status epilepticus is rare and should suggest a mass intracranial lesion or barbiturate withdrawal. Focal seizures should always lead to evaluation for a mass lesion.

Table 37-3. Common Alcohol-Drug Interactions in the Alcoholic*

Drug	Effect
Aspirin and sodium salicylate	Gastritis
	Inhibit platelet aggregation
General anesthetics	Larger induction dose followed by increase in sleeping time
Phenytoin	Alcohol alters metabolism, leading to undertreatment or toxicity
Oral hypoglycemics	Large amounts increase half-life of alcohol
	Chronic alcoholism decreases half life; can produce a mild disulfiram reaction
	Hypoglycemia
Chloral hydrate	Tachycardia, palpitations, flushing, dysphoria
Disulfiram	Hypertension, tachycardia, headache, dizziness, nausea, vomiting, flushing
Antihypertensives, including ganglionic blockers and peripheral vasodilators	Additive effect on lowering of blood pressure
Anticoagulants	Additive effect with danger of hemorrhage
Tricyclic antidepressants	Can be synergistic or antagonistic; increased susceptibility to seizures
Antihistamines	Increased sedation
Antibiotics:	Mild disulfiram reaction
Chloramphenicol	
Izoniazid	
Metronidazole	
Quinacrine	
Griseofulvin	
Barbiturates and minor tranquilizers	Highest abuse potential; potent synergistic reaction
Major tranquilizers	Potentiate respiratory depression, hypotension, and hepatic dysfunction
	Increase susceptibility to seizures
Narcotics	Potentiates respiratory depression and sedation

*The effects of alcoholic liver disease in decreasing hepatic drug metabolism are not considered here.

Source: Adapted from Alcohol-drug interactions. *FDA Drug Bull* 9(2):10–12, June 1979.

Treatment

Hydration is necessary because of fluid loss from diaphoresis and decreased intake. Vomiting, diarrhea, and seizure activity may also contribute to fluid loss. Hypokalemia and hypomagnesemia are common and should be corrected.

Thiamine and multivitamins should also be given. Sixth-nerve palsy or oculomotor paralysis, ataxia, and dysarthria suggest the Wernicke-Korsakoff syndrome, and require the administration of 500 to 1000 mg thiamine intravenously.

Restraint is mandatory for patients with delirium tremens. In addition, those with impaired mentation or evidence of delirium tremens should not be considered competent to sign out of the emergency department against medical advice.

Sedative therapy is necessary to calm the patient, as well as to replace the withdrawn alcohol. The dose, route, and type of agent used is variable. Phenothiazines should be avoided because they increase mortality and enhance seizures and delirium. Paraldehyde, 10 mL rectally as needed, is absorbed slowly and erratically. Thompson et al. have shown it to be inferior to diazepam. Barbiturates and chloral hydrate have similarly been replaced by the benzodiazepines.

Although intramuscular chlordiazepoxide, 50 to 100 mg, as needed, is commonly used and clinically effective, absorption is erratic after intramuscular injection. Thompson recommends intravenous diazepam, 5 mg every 5 to 15 min, for sedation. The clinical dose response is variable, and Thompson has reported giving up to 215 mg IV diazepam for the initial calming dose, and a total of 2000 mg in the first 24 h. Such large doses require careful patient monitoring for respiratory depression and hypotension. In addition, the necessity for frequent IV bolus drug admin-

istration can be time-consuming in a busy emergency department. In severe cases, intravenous alcohol, to maintain a blood level of 100 to 150 mg/100 mL can be given. In summary, the ideal sedative agent for the management of delirium tremens has not yet been found.

The general management of alcohol withdrawal seizures is with the benzodiazepines. In a study by Sampliner, patients without an underlying seizure disorder were adequately treated with chlordiazepoxide alone. Those patients with an underlying seizure disorder, for whom anticonvulsants are indicated, should receive phenytoin. Barbiturates are cross-tolerant with alcohol and can be used to prevent and treat alcohol withdrawal seizures.

ISOPROPANOL

Isopropyl alcohol (isopropanol) is most commonly found in the home as rubbing alcohol. It is also used as a disinfectant, industrial solvent, and cleaning agent, and is a solvent in cosmetics. Isopropanol can cause toxicity by ingestion or by inhalation, as from alcohol sponging. It is more toxic than ethanol, its clinical effects last 2 to 4 times longer, and CNS depression is more significant. However, it is not as toxic as methanol or ethylene glycol. The lethal dose in adults is about 3 mL/kg. After oral ingestion, 80 percent is absorbed in 30 min and 99 percent by 2 h. However, once absorbed, it is secreted by the salivary glands and stomach.

The volume of distribution is approximately 0.7 L/kg. Metabolism follows first-order kinetics, with elimination at about 25 percent per hour. The major metabolic pathway of metabolism is probably oxidation via alcohol dehydrogenase to acetone. About 10 percent may be converted to glucuronide. Metabolism is much slower than that of ethanol. Despite the involvement of alcohol dehydrogenase in metabolism, ethanol has not been used clinically to inhibit isopropanol metabolism.

Because of the production of acetone, a major metabolic hallmark of isopropanol poisoning is the presence of ketones in the serum and urine. The half-life of acetone is approximately 28 h, and the prolonged clinical symptoms resulting from isopropanol poisoning may be related to the presence of acetone. Acetone is excreted primarily through the lungs, and with a small average ventilation per minute, it may take several days to eliminate a large amount. A portion of acetone can also be converted to glucose. Acetone produces severe CNS depression and can potentiate the depressant effects of isopropanol. Morbidity of isopropanol poisoning is determined by the serum level of both isopropanol and acetone. According to Alexander et al., a level of both isopropanol and acetone greater than 100 mg/100 mL is lethal.

Clinical Features

Signs and symptoms of isopropanol poisoning reflect involvement of a variety of body systems. CNS manifestations are similar to those associated with ethanol poisoning, although deep coma may develop rapidly. Severe hemorrhagic gastritis is a striking feature. Hypotension can result from vasodilation, direct myocardial depression, or hemorrhagic gastritis. Rhabdomyolysis and hepatocellular toxicity have also been reported.

The most characteristic and specific laboratory findings are an elevated anion gap, osmolal gap, acetonemia, and acetonuria. There is no acetoacetic acid or β-hydroxybutyric acid produced. Blood glucose is normal if the patient is not also diabetic. Therefore, the presence of acidosis and ketonemia concomitant with a normal blood sugar should suggest the possibility of isopropanol poisoning, in addition to the more familiar syndrome of alcoholic, nondiabetic ketoacidosis.

Treatment

Gastric lavage with continuous nasogastric suction should be performed. Intubation and ventilation may be necessary to ensure adequate respiratory elimination of acetone. Fluid and blood replacement is necessary to maintain adequate circulating volume and urine output in the face of hemorrhagic gastritis. For significant and persistent bleeding, endoscopy should be performed for definitive diagnosis. Acidosis is treated with sodium bicarbonate.

Hemodialysis is effective in removing both isopropanol and acetone. Fixed guidelines for its institution have not been published. However, it has been used in severe coma and for very high isopropanol levels, as long as a blood pressure can be maintained. Peritoneal dialysis can also be used. Controlled studies on such severely poisoned patients, comparing dialysis with supportive therapy, are not currently available.

BIBLIOGRAPHY

Methanol

Becker CE: Acute methanol poisoning—The blind drunk. *West J Med* 135:122–128, 1981.

Bennett I, Cary F, Mitchell G, et al: Acute methyl alcohol poisoning: A review based on experiences in an outbreak of 323 cases. *Medicine* 32:431–463, 1953.

Gonda A, Gault H, Churchill D, et al: Hemodialysis for methanol intoxication. *Am J Med* 64:749–758, 1978.

Hayreh MS, Hayreh SS, Baumbach GL, et al: Methyl alcohol poisoning. *Arch Ophthalmol* 95:1851–1858, 1977.

Jacobsen D, Jensen H, Wiik-Larsen E, et al: Studies on methanol poisoning. *Acta Med Scand* 212:5–10, 1982.

Keeney AH, Mellinkoff SM: Methyl alcohol poisoning. *Ann Intern Med* 34:331–338, 1951.

Keyvan-Larijarni H, Tannenberg AM: Methanol intoxication: Comparison of peritoneal dialysis and hemodialysis treatment. *Arch Intern Med* 134:293–296, 1974.

McCoy HG, Cipolle RJ, Ehlers SM, et al: Severe methanol poisoning: Application of a pharmacokinetic model for ethanol therapy and hemodialysis. *Am J Med* 67:804–807, 1979.

McMartin KE, Ambre JJ, Tephly TR: Methanol poisoning in human subjects: Role for formic acid accumulation in the metabolic acidosis. *Am J Med* 68:414–418, 1980.

McMartin KE, Ambre JJ, Tephly TR: Methanol poisoning in human subjects: Role for formic acid accumulation in the metabolic acidosis. *Am J Med* 68:414–418, 1980.

McMartin KE, Makar AB, Martin G, et al: Methanol poisoning: 1. The role of formic acid in the development of metabolic acidosis in the monkey and the reversal by 4-methylpyrazole. *Biochem Med* 13:319–333, 1975.

Noker PE, Eells JT, Tephly TR: Methanol toxicity: Treatment with folic acid and 5-formyl tetrahydrofolic acid. *Clin Exp Res* 4:378–383, 1980.

Ethylene Glycol

Ahmed MM: Ocular effects of antifreeze poisoning. *Br J Ophthalmol* 55:854–855, 1971.

Berger JR, Ayyar DR: Neurological complications of ethylene glycol intoxication: Report of a case. *Arch Neurol* 38(11):724–726, 1981.

Chadnapaphornchai P, Taher S, Bhathena D, et al: Ethylene glycol poisoning: Diagnosis based on high osmolal and anion gaps and crystalluria. *Ann Emerg Med* 10(2)94–97, 1983.

Moriarty RW, McDonald RH: The spectrum of ethylene glycol poisoning. *Clin Toxicol* 7:583–596, 1974.

Parry MF, Wallach R: Ethylene glycol poisoning. *Am J Med* 57:143–150, 1974.

Peterson CD, Collins AJ, Himes JM, et al: Ethylene glycol poisoning: Pharmacokinetics during therapy with ethanol and hemodialysis. *N Engl J Med* 304:21–23, 1981.

Stokes JB III, Aueron F: Prevention of organ damage in massive ethylene glycol ingestion. *JAMA* 243(20):2065–2066, 1980.

Winchester JF, Gelfand MC, Knepshield JH, et al: Dialysis and hemoperfusion of poisons and drugs. *Trans Am Soc Artif Intern Organs* 23:762–842, 1977.

Winek CL, Shingleton DP, Shanor SP: Ethylene and diethylene glycol toxicity. *Clin Toxicol* 13:297–423, 1978.

Ethanol

Alcohol-drug interactions. *FDA Drug Bull* 9(2):10–12, June 1979.

Gross MM, Goodenough DR, Hasty J, et al: Sleep disturbances in alcoholic intoxication and withdrawal, in Mellow NK, Mendelson JH (eds): *Recent Advances in Studies of Alcoholism*. US Government Printing Office, 1972, pp 317–397.

Levy R, Elo T, Hanenson IB: Intravenous fructose treatment of acute alcohol intoxication. *Arch Intern Med* 137:1175–1177, 1977.

Mellanby E: *Alcohol: Its Absorption into and Disappearance from the Blood under Different Conditions.* Med Res Comm, Spec Rep No 31. London, HM Stationery Office, 1919, pp 1–48.

Mendelson JH: Biologic concomitants of alcoholism. *N Engl J Med* 283:24–32, 71–81, 1970.

Sampliner R, Iber F: Diphenylhydantoin control of alcohol withdrawal seizures. *JAMA* 230:1430–1432, 1974.

Thompson WL: Mnagement of alcohol withdrawal syndromes. *Arch Intern Med* 138:278–283, 1978.

Thompson WL, Johnson AD, Maddrey WL, et al: Diazepam and paraldehyde for treatment of severe delirium tremens: A controlled trial. *Ann Intern Med* 82:175–180, 1975.

Victor WL, Adams RP: The effect of alcohol on the nervous system. *Res Publ Assoc Res Nerv Ment Dis* 32:526–673, 1953.

Isopropanol

Alexander CB, McBay AJ, Hudson RP: Isopropanol and Isopropanol deaths—Ten years' experience. *J Foren Sci* 27(3):1541–1548, 1982.

Mecikalski MB, Depner TA: Peritoneal dialysis for isopropanol poisoning. *West J Med* 137:322–325, 1982.

Winchester JF: Methanol, isopropyl alcohol, higher alcohol, ethylene glycol, cellosolves, acetone, and oxalate, in Haddad LM, Winchester J (eds): *Clinical Management of Poisoning and Drug Overdose.* Philadelphia, Saunders, 1983.

CHAPTER 38
ORGANOPHOSPHATES

Lester Haddad

Pesticides still account for a significant percentage of toxic deaths in the United States, especially in California, the farm belt, and the south.

In 1972, the Environmental Protection Agency estimated that 1230 children under 5 years of age were hospitalized, and 92 persons died from pesticide poisonings. Figures on chronic illness from pesticides are unknown and impossible to estimate.

Table 38-1 lists the common organophosphate insecticides. Table 38-2 lists other common insecticides. A discussion of herbicides, fungicides, and rodenticides is not included in this chapter. Because over 80 percent of all hospitalizations from pesticides are due to organophosphate insecticides, mostly involving children, farmers, and skilled and unskilled laborers, discussion here will be confined to recognition and management of organophosphate insecticides.

The organophosphates have achieved tremendous popularity because of their effectiveness as insecticides, and because they disintegrate into harmless radicals within days after application.

Organophosphate poisoning can be roughly divided into accidental poisoning of children by ingestion of pesticides present in garages or of dog tick and flea killers; accidental exposure among adult farm workers; and suicide attempts, the latter probably accounting for a slightly greater percentage. This parallels reports by the Environmental Protection Agency and by Namba et al.

Individual organophosphates differ widely in their ability to penetrate the skin, oral absorption, and toxicity. Tetraethylpyrophosphate, the first organophosphate synthesized in the mid-1800s, is probably the most dangerous by either the oral or dermal route. Malathion is at the other end of the spectrum because little is absorbed through the skin, and the oral toxicity is low. It is safe for home use.

PHARMACOLOGY

Acetylcholine is the chemical transmitter at synaptic junctions. Acetylcholinesterase hydrolyzes acetylcholine into its two primary fragments, acetic acid and choline. Both are essentially inert.

The two principal cholinesterases in humans are acetylcholinesterase and pseudocholinesterase. Acetylcholinesterase (true cholinesterase) is primarily found in nervous tissue and erythrocytes; pseudocholinesterase is found in the liver and serum. The organophosphates are powerful inhibitors of the cholinesterases and act by often irreversible binding of the phosphate radicals of the organophosphates to the active sites of the enzymes, forming phosphorylated enzymes, thus decreasing red cell and serum cholinesterase levels.

The toxicologic effects of the organophosphates are almost entirely due to the inhibition of acetylcholinesterase of the nervous system, resulting in accumulation of acetylcholine at synapses and myoneural junctions. The laboratory assessment of organophosphate poisoning is more accurately assessed by measurement of the red cell (true) cholinesterase rather than the serum (pseudo) cholinesterase. In addition, 3 percent of patients have a genetic variant causing low plasma cholinesterase levels.

The overabundance of acetylcholine initially excites and then paralyzes transmission in cholinergic synapses, which include (1) the CNS, (2) the parasympathetic nerve endings and a few sympathetic nerve endings such as the sweat glands (muscarinic effects), and (3) the somatic nerves and the ganglionic synapses of autonomic ganglia (nicotinic effects). The signs and symptoms of organophosphate poisoning are thus an expression of these three effects caused by excess acetylcholine (Table 38-3).

Parathion, an organic derivative of phosphoric acid, was recognized shortly after World War II as the most effective of the 50 or more organophosphates for insecticidal use. It is the most commonly used organophosphate and chemically is O,O-diethyl O-para-nitrophenyl phosphorothioate. It must be activated within humans by substitution of an oxygen atom for a sulfur atom to form paraoxon, which is the active cholinesterase inhibitor. When paraoxon combines with cholinesterase, a series of reactions ensue. These reactions are as follows:

1. The initial attachment occurs by electrostatic attraction.
2. The paranitrophenol, or "leaving," group separates from the parent molecule and is metabolized. The diethylphosphate that remains reacts chemically and becomes firmly attached. This "second stage" is still reversible by the specific antidote, pralidoxime (2-PAM) chloride.
3. If an antidote is not administered within 24 to 48 h, one of the ethyl groups leaves the phosphate moiety, and the cholinesterase molecule is irreversibly destroyed. Enzyme resynthesis, which takes weeks, must occur to restore cholinesterase. In the meantime, all that can be done for the critical patient is to provide complete pulmonary support until enzyme resynthesis occurs. Recovery has occurred after weeks of such therapy.

Table 38-1. Examples of Organophosphate Insecticides

Common Name	Product Example	Chemical Name	Estimated Fatal Oral Dose, g/70 kg
Agricultural insecticides (high toxicity):			
TEPP	Miller Kilmite 40	Tetraethyl pyrophosphate	0.05
Parathion	Niagara Phoskil Dust	O,O-Diethyl O-p-nitrophenyl phosphorothioate	0.1
Phosdrin	Mevinphos	Dimethyl-O-(1-methyl-2-carbomethoxyvinyl) phosphate	0.15
Disyston	Disulfoton	Diethyl-S-2-ethyl-2-mercaptoethyl phosphorodithioate	0.2
Guthion	Guthion	Dimethyl S-(4-oxo-1,2,3-benzotriazinyl-3-methyl phosphorodithioate)	0.2
Animal insecticides (intermediate toxicity):			
Ronnel	Korlan livestock spray (Dow)	O,O-Dimethyl O-(2,4,5-trichlorophenyl) phosphorothioate	10.0
Coumaphos	Co-Ral animal insecticide (Chemagro)	Diethyl-O-(3-chloro-4-methyl-7-coumarinyl) phosphorothioate	
Chlorpyrifos (Dursban)	Rid-A-Bug (Kenco)	O,O-Diethyl O-(3,5,6-trichloro-2-pyridyl) phosphorothioate	
Trichlorfon	Trichlorfon Pour On (Hess and Clark)	Dimethyl trichlorohydroxyethyl phosphonate	
Household use (low toxicity):			
Malathion	Ortho Malathion 50 insect spray	Dimethyl-S-(1,2-bis-carboethoxy) ethyl phosphorodithioate	60.0
Diazinon	Security Fire ant killer (Woolfolk)	Diethyl-O-(2-isoprophyl-6-methyl-4-pyrimidyl) phosphorothioate	25.0
Dichlorvos (Vapona, DDVP)	Shell No-Pest Strip	O,O-Dimethyl O-(2,2-dichlorovinyl) phosphate	

Source: Haddad LM: Organophosphate insecticides, in Haddad LM, Winchester JF (eds): *Clinical Management of Poisoning and Drug Overdose,* Philadelphia, Saunders, 1983, p. 705. Reprinted by permission.

CLINICAL FEATURES

The time interval between the exposure and onset of symptoms varies with the chemical, route of entry, and degree of exposure, but usually occurs up to 12 h postexposure and almost always prior to 24 h, as reported by Namba et al.

Symptoms may first suggest mild poisoning, but may rapidly progress to indicate severe poisoning. Initial symptoms usually include headache, intestinal cramping, vomiting, diarrhea, dizziness, weakness, excessive sweating, and salivation.

The development of coma, respiratory distress, ataxia, psychosis, convulsions, bradycardia, cyanosis, and paralysis indicates severe poisoning and aggressive emergency management must be instituted.

TREATMENT

A comatose patient who is diaphoretic with pinpoint pupils, who has the odor of an insecticide on the clothes or breath, and who

Table 38-2. Other Common Insecticides

Group	Chemical	Trade Name	Toxicity	Insecticide Use	Effects on Humans
Botanicals	Pyrethins	Hot Shot products	Low	Household	
Carbamates	Carbamates	Baygon Sevin	Moderate	Fruit, nuts, vegetables, forests, ranges	Reversible cholinesterase inhibitor
Organochlorine insecticides	Lindane	Isotox	Moderate	Cotton weevil	Interferes with axonal transmission of nerve impulses
	Toxaphene	Toxacil	Moderate	Tick mites	
	Chlordane	Chlordane	Moderate		
	Dieldrin	Dieldrite	Moderate	Field insects	
	Aldrin	Aldrite	Moderate		
	Endrin	Hexadrin	High		
Inorganic chemicals	Arsenic trioxide	Same	Extreme	Ants*	Inhibits sulfhydryl enzymes
	Arsine (gas) Paris green (copper acetoarsenite)	Same			Interferes with cellular oxidation

*Used now mainly as herbicide.

Table 38-3. Clinical Effects of Organophosphate Poisoning (Acetylcholine Excess)

Muscarinic effects:	
Sweat glands	Sweating
Pupils	Constricted
Lacriminal glands	Lacrimation
Salivary glands	Excessive salivation
Bronchial tree	Wheezing
Gastrointestinal	Cramps, vomiting, diarrhea, tenesmus
Cardiovascular	Bradycardia, fall in blood pressure
Ciliary body	Blurred vision
Bladder	Urinary incontinence
Nicotinic effects:	
Striated muscle	Fasciculations, cramps, weakness, twitching paralysis, respiratory embarrassment, cyanosis, arrest
Sympathetic ganglia	Tachycardia, elevated blood pressure
CNS	Anxiety, restlessness, ataxia, convulsions, insomnia, coma, absent reflexes, Cheyne-Stokes respirations, respiratory and circulation depression

Source: Adapted from Grob D, Harvey AM: The effect and treatment of nerve gas poisoning. *Am J Med* 14:52, 1953.

exhibits muscle fasciculations represents the classic presentation of organophosphate poisoning, and should be managed as such until proved otherwise. Specific steps in management include the following.

Remove clothing. Remove all contaminated clothing and wash skin and hair.

Establish an airway. Textbooks constantly suggest the importance of adequate oxygenation and ventilation prior to the use of atropine, as atropine is said to precipitate ventricular fibrillation in a poorly oxygenated patient.

Ipecac, charcoal, cathartic. Give ipecac if the patient is fully alert, even if a petroleum distillate is the carrier. If the patient is unconscious, intubate prior to use of gastric lavage. Both activated charcoal and then magnesium sulfate as a cathartic are indicated. Allow about 30 min for binding of the poison and charcoal before administering sodium sulfate.

Morphine, aminophylline, phenothiazines, and resperine are contraindicated. Vasopressors are considered only as a last resort.

Obtain blood studies. Specific blood tests include a serum, and preferably a red cell, cholinesterase. A depressed serum cholinesterase may be due to a genetic defect variant, but a depressed value of 25 percent or greater of the red cell cholinesterase is an indication of poisoning. Red cell cholinesterase levels may take up to 90 to 120 days to return to normal values, while serum cholinesterase recovers in days to weeks.

Physiologic Antidote

Do not wait for laboratory results before instituting treatment. If the patient presents the classic, full-blown picture, establish an airway, begin an intravenous infusion, provide oxygenation, and give atropine intravenously. Atropine should be used for 24 h as a physiologic antidote to competively block the effect of acetylcholine while the organophosphate is being metabolized. The ini-

tial dose is 2 mg for an adult and 0.05 mg/kg for a child. Up to 5 mg IV of atropine every 15 min may be necessary for the critical patient (i.e., patients with disturbances of vital signs—hypotensive, hypothermic, or in respiratory arrest). You may be hesitant to give such a "large" dose of atropine, but the patient severely poisoned by parathion may require hundreds of milligrams of atropine in the first 24 h. The early use of pralidoxime (2-PAM) chloride, the specific antidote, should obviate the need for such large doses of atropine.

Repeat atropine every 15 min until the patient exhibits reversal of cholinergic effects. Signs of atropinization include flushing, dry mouth, and dilated pupils. Remember that tachycardia is common, and that dilated and even unequal pupils are uncommon but have been described with organophosphate poisoning. However, dilated pupils which were once pinpoint, and a slow pulse which becomes rapid after administration of atropine, indicate the desired effects you wish to achieve. Signs of overatropinization include fever, delirium, and muscle twitching. The atropine dosage should be tapered after 24 h. Close patient observation is necessary, as delayed pulmonary edema has been described.

Specific Antidote

Remember, atropine has *no* effect on skeletal muscle and autonomic ganglia. The presence of muscle fasciculations, which is a striking clinical sign, and muscular weakness are a sine qua non indication for the use of the specific antidote, pralidoxime (2-PAM) chloride. Pralidoxime chloride is given intravenously, usually over a 30-min period. The dose is 1 g for adults, or up to 50 mg/kg for children. The effect is often dramatic, with disappearance of coma (usually temporary), fasciculations, and a return of strength and well-being. Up to $\frac{1}{2}$ g/h has been given to critical patients, but before the 24- to 48-h "critical" interval.

Pralidoxime chloride is of low toxicity and may prevent delayed complications of organophosphate poisoning, such as type II paralysis or late neuromuscular block, jake paralysis, and delayed peripheral neuropathy. There is a possibility of an insulating effect in preventing these delayed complications.

BIBLIOGRAPHY

Fisher JP: Guillain-Barré syndrome following organophosphate poisoning. *JAMA* 238:1950–1951, 1977.

Gadoth N, Fisher A: Late onset of neuromuscular block in organophosphorus poisoning. *Ann Intern Med* 88:654–655, 1978.

Ganendran A: Organophosphate insecticide poisoning and its management. *Anaesth Intensive Care* 2:361–368, 1974.

Haddad LM: Organophosphate poisoning, in Haddad LM, Winchester JF (eds): *Clinical Management of Poisoning and Drug Overdose.* Philadelphia, Saunders, 1983, pp 704–710.

Kass JB, Khamapirad T, Wagner ML: Pulmonary edema following skin absorption of organophosphate insecticide. *Pediatr Radiol* 7:113–114, 1978.

Namba T, Nolte CT, Jackrel J, et al: Poisoning due to organophosphate insecticides: Acute and chronic manifestations. *Am J Med* 50:475–492, 1971.

Peoples SA, Maddy KT: Organophosphate pesticide poisoning. *West J Med* 192:273–277, 1978.

Warriner RA III: Severe organophosphate poisoning complicated by alcohol and turpentine ingestion. *Arch Environ Health* 32:203–205, 1977.

CHAPTER 39
PHENOTHIAZINE
OVERDOSE

Michael Callaham

The phenothiazines are a group of drugs developed for their antipsychotic activities; the prototype is chlorpromazine, but more than 30 phenothiazines are on the market. The phenothiazines possess a three-ring structure of two benzene rings linked by a sulfur and nitrogen atom; this structure is similar to that of the thioxanthenes, dibenzodiazepines, and tricyclic antidepressant agents, among others. These drugs are erratically and unpredictably absorbed after oral administration; in overdose, undigested pills may remain in the bowel for long periods of time owing to their typical inhibition of peristalsis, and may be visualized on abdominal x-rays. Once absorbed they are highly membrane- or protein-bound and lipophilic, accumulating in the brain, lung, and other tissues. Their volume of distribution is 22 L/kg; thus the proportion of the total body dose in the bloodstream is small, and dialysis techniques are of limited usefulness. Typical half-life is 10 to 20 h, and effects may persist for days. They are largely metabolized in the liver and excreted as glucuronides. Less than 1 percent of excretion is renal. A few of the metabolites are also pharmacologically active.

Side effects of these drugs when used therapeutically, or abused, are common. Extrapyramidal effects are most common. Three types of reactions occur acutely: a parkinsonian syndrome with rigidity and rest tremor, akathisia (incessant movement and restlessness), and acute dystonic reactions, with facial grimacing, torticollis, oculogyric crisis, or other bizarre extrapyramidal movements which are often mistaken for malingering or hysteria. However, these dystonic reactions quickly resolve with intramuscular or intravenous diphenhydramine or benztropine. Tardive dyskinesia (stereotyped involuntary sucking and smacking of the lips) and perioral ("rabbit") syndrome appear late, after prolonged therapy. Also common during therapeutic use are orthostatic hypotension, due to the prominent α-blocking effect of phenothiazines on vascular receptors; this may cause syncope. Abnormalities of temperature regulation are also seen and may predispose to hyperthermia or even heat stroke.

FRANK OVERDOSE

The lethal dose of ingested phenothiazines ranges from 15 to 150 mg/kg, with a wide and unpredictable variability in individual susceptibility. The drugs have prominent anticholinergic effects which lead to tachycardia, flushed red skin, mydriasis, hyperthermia, and decreased peristalsis. The phenothiazines' α-adrenergic blocking properties produce vasodilation and hypotension. They possess the property of blocking norepinephrine uptake at the synapse, which causes adrenergic stimulation and possible arrhythmias. Phenothiazines also possess quinidine-like membrane-stabilizing and cardiodepressant properties which cause prolonged PR and QT intervals, and ST and T wave changes. Ventricular arrhythmias such as ventricular tachycardia have been reported, but are rare. Extrapyramidal reactions may occur with acute overdose. Coma is seen in large overdose, and although phenothiazines lower the seizure threshold, actual seizures seem to be a rare complication, at least in reported series. CNS depression caused by phenothiazines augments that of any analgesics, sedatives, antihistamines, and alcohol.

TREATMENT

Conservative supportive treatment is the foundation of therapy. Ingested pills should be removed by ipecac-induced vomiting, but since phenothiazines possess antiemetic properties, gastric lavage may be necessary. Remaining intact pills may be visualized on abdominal x-ray. Activated charcoal and cathartics should then be administered. Respiratory status should be monitored carefully and the patient intubated if needed. Tachycardia and most other anticholinergic signs do not need treatment. The ECG should be monitored, although serious ventricular arrhythmias are rare; they can be treated either with countershock or antiarrhythmic drugs which do *not* share the phenothiazines' membrane-stabilizing properties (e.g., quinidine, procainamide). Phenytoin is the drug of choice, followed by lidocaine. Because of the large volume of distribution of the phenothiazines, dialysis techniques are not useful in removing the drugs.

Hypotension is best treated with Trendelenburg's position and IV fluid loading. If this fails to produce adequate perfusion (as measured by urine output and other tests), then catecholamines with strong α-adrenergic properties (such as levarterenol or higher-dose dopamine) should be used. Agents with prominent vasodilatory effects, such as isoproterenol, should be avoided, particularly since catechols may increase cardiac irritability. Theoretically epinephrine may be hazardous, since its α-adrenergic properties are blocked by the phenothiazines, leaving the vasodilatory β-effects unopposed and exacerbating hypotension. However, there is no literature (either experimental studies or case reports) to lend support to this theory.

Seizures are rare, and can be treated with IV diazepam and phenytoin. Extrapyramidal effects are treated with oral, IV, or IM diphenhydramine or benztropine; the latter is just as efficacious and produces less sedative side effects.

Physostigmine, a cholinesterase inhibitor, has been used to reverse the anticholinergic effects of phenothiazines. Reversal of seizures, arrhythmia, hypotension, and CNS depression have been anecdotally reported; no controlled study has ever been done, however. Physostigmine has a short half-life (30 min) with a very narrow margin between therapeutic effect and toxicity, the major side effect being seizures. Since mortality from phenothiazine overdose is very low with good supportive care alone, this unpredictable and dangerous drug should be reserved for those cases in which it is the therapy of last resort.

BIBLIOGRAPHY

Barry D, Meyshens F, Becker C: Phenothiazine poisoning: A review of 48 cases. *Calif Med* 118:1–5, 1973.

Davis J, Bartlett E, Termini B: Overdosage of psychotropic drugs: A review. *Dis Nerv System* 29(3):160–164, 1968.

Lumpkin J, Watanabe A, Rumack B: Phenothiazine-induced ventricular tachycardia following acute overdose. *JACEP* 8:476–478, 1979.

Weisdorf D, Kramer J, Goldbert A, et al: Physostigmine for cardiac and neurologic manifestations of phenothiazine poisoning. *Clin Pharmacol Ther* 24(6):663–667, 1978.

CHAPTER 40
PHENYTOIN TOXICITY

Carl Sacks

Phenytoin (diphenylhydantoin, Dilantin), a much-used anticonvulsant and antiarrhythmic drug, can by corruption and exaggeration of its therapeutic qualities engender significant morbidity and mortality.

As an anticonvulsant, phenytoin works primarily by inhibiting the spread of seizures and to a much lesser degree by suppression of the focus itself. On a membrane level, stabilization is accomplished by stimulation of the sodium-potassium pump, blockade of passive sodium influx, and blockade of calcium influx. It also enhances the chloride ion–mediated inhibitory postsynaptic potential, and increases the concentration of γ-aminobutyric acid (GABA) in the brain. This unique substance is at the same time an inhibitory neurotransmitter for the cerebral cortex and a stimulatory neurotransmitter for the cerebellar cortex. It has been recently shown that cerebellar excitation can have a direct inhibitory effect on seizures, and electrical cerebellar stimulators have been used experimentally for this purpose. Conversely, when the cerebellum has been previously removed from an experimental animal, induced seizures are much more difficult to control.

Keeping in mind that efficacy and toxicity are clinical and not numerical manifestations, the following generalizations can be made: Phenytoin is therapeutic at blood levels of 10 μg/mL to 20 μg/mL. At 20 μg/mL, increasing cerebellar excitation and stimulation of the cerebellar vestibular pathways provoke an exaggeration of lateral gaze nystagmus. At 30 μg/mL the amplitude of lateral gaze nystagmus increases and there is spontaneous nystagmus, vertical nystagmus with upward gaze, and some degree of ataxia. At 40 μg/mL and beyond, the patient displays dysarthria, lethargy, confusion, and occasionally psychosis. Increased seizure activity is a well-documented complication of phenytoin toxicity. The mechanism is unknown. The danger is further increasing the phenytoin load to induce suppression. The lethal blood level of phenytoin is approximately 100 μg/mL. Death results uniquely from cardiac side effects.

A few dubious reports notwithstanding, the only well-documented examples of cardiac complications of phenytoin have been associated with the intravenous mode of administration.

The cardiac actions of phenytoin are the exact opposite of the digitalis glycosides. Phenytoin antagonizes digitalis-induced arrhythmias by decreasing the automaticity of the SA node, slowing the rate of conduction through the bundle of His, and reducing the automaticity and contractility of the myocardium. Exaggeration of these properties can lead to bradycardia, new heart block, aggravation of preexisting heart block, idioventricular rhythm, and cardiac standstill. Heart block may respond to 0.5 mg atropine intravenously, but resistant third-degree block should be treated by insertion of a temporary pacemaker. Hypotension is best treated by adjustment of fluids or in conjunction with positive inotropics. Not infrequently, intravenous administration of phenytoin is associated with hypotension and dizziness that is rapidly reversed by stopping the infusion or by decreasing the rate of administration.

Ten to fifty percent of phenytoin users exhibit bone demineralization and hypocalcemia, and, exceptionally, a ricketslike picture develops. The mechanism is postulated to be inactivation of vitamin D by phenytoin. The remedy is an increase in vitamin D intake.

Serum folate levels are 50 percent lower in patients taking phenytoin than in a comparable phenytoin-free control group. Approximately 1 percent of these patients will have a folate-dependent megaloblastic anemia. In addition, folate deficiency may be responsible for a myriad of birth defects found in children whose mothers took phenytoin during gestation, and lumped collectively under the name *fetal hydantoin syndrome*. Postulated mechanisms are impaired folate absorption and synthesis, accelerated metabolism, and increased use of folate in phenytoin metabolism. The anemia responds readily to increased folate. Some other hematological problems associated with phenytoin intake are thrombocytopenia, sometimes associated with phenytoin-dependent antibodies; a lymphomalike picture that responds readily to cessation of the anticonvulsant, and perinatal and, more rarely, infant bleeding, due to increased metabolism of vitamin K and inhibited production of the vitamin K–dependent clotting factors, especially factor VII. The symptoms respond readily to increased vitamin K intake.

Hypersensitivity skin rashes occur in up to 5 percent of people taking phenytoin. They range from the common and relatively innocuous morbilliform rash to the rare but lethal Stevens-Johnson syndrome. Lupus erythematosis has also been associated with phenytoin.

Approximately 50 percent of phenytoin users have gingival hypertrophy. Interestingly, this symptom correlates with increased concentration of the anticonvulsant in the saliva, not the blood. The salivary glands of those with gingival hypertrophy have an increased capacity to extract phenytoin from the blood and secrete it in saliva.

Additionally, the drug may be associated with hirsutism, coarse facial features, and hypoglycemia.

PHARMACOLOGY AND METABOLISM

Phenytoin is a weak acid with a pK_a of 8.3. It is only poorly soluble in water, but much more so in solutions of high ionic strength and alkalinity. Once in the bloodstream and in the steady state, it is 90 percent protein-bound, primarily to albumin. Only the free, non-protein-bound fraction is active. The volume of distribution is 0.64 L/kg for all of the drug and about seven times greater for the active, non-protein-bound fraction.

Phenytoin can be administered orally, intravenously, or intramuscularly. Oral phenytoin is administered as capsules or suspension. Peak blood levels are attained anywhere from 4 to 12 h after ingestion of the capsules, with prolonged absorption up to 48 h. Large amounts may cause an irritative gastritis which is best avoided by administering the drug with food or minimizing the dose. The oral solution of phenytoin gives peak blood levels in a mean time of 1.63 h postingestion.

Intravenous phenytoin is often associated with acute hypotension, often due to the diluent propylene glycol, and burning at the infusion site, due to its alkalinity. The probability of these complications is minimized if the infusion is given via piggyback IV and at a rate of 25 mg/min or less. The intravenous diluent should be normal saline. Hypotension or irritation that may occur in spite of the above precautions will rapidly terminate if the piggyback flow rate is reduced or stopped. In addition, the patient should be placed on a cardiac monitor to detect bradyarrhythmia or heart block during the infusion.

Some of the intravenously administered drug rushes across the blood-brain barrier before serum protein binding and steady-state equilibrium can be fully attained. Brain tissue levels are nearly maximal at the end of infusion, and maximal about 1 h postinfusion.

Intramuscular phenytoin crystallizes out at the injection site. There is considerable associated pain and local rhabdomyolysis. The absorption rate is slow and highly variable. Older studies reported that about 50 percent of the intramuscular dose was lost, while more recent studies indicate a bioavailability of 95 percent with a mean absorption of 5 days.

Only 2 percent of phenytoin is eliminated unchanged by the kidneys. The rest is conjugated and hydroxylated by the hepatic mitochondria. High blood levels are associated with both increased delivery and reduced metabolism. The latter is associated with hepatic damage of multiple etiology, or with other drugs that compete for the same enzyme system. Notable among the drugs that increase the half-life of phenytoin by direct competition are chloramphenicol, dicumarol, disulfiram, isoniazid, and some sulfonamides. Phenytoin intoxication, sometimes with normal serum concentrations, may occur if the amount of free, non-protein-bound drug increases. This may occur in any situation in which there is decreased production or increased loss of albumin, or if other substances are present and compete for binding sites. Phenylbutazone, sulfisoxazole, and possibly the salicylates have been implicated.

The elimination half-life of phenytoin can vary from 7 to 40 h, with an average of 24 h at therapeutic levels. The half-life is increased by hepatic disease or toxic blood levels, or if other agents are present that compete with the same metabolic enzyme system. The half-life may be decreased by products such as carbamazepine, alcohol, and phenobarbital, which enhance enzyme induction and biotransformation. When all the hepatic biotransformation sites are not occupied, there is a first-order, nonlinear relationship between time and the amount of phenytoin eliminated; that is, a constant fraction of the total dose is lost per unit of time. At high toxic doses, when all sites are saturated, the relationship is zero-order and linear, and a constant amount, approximately 3 g/day, may be metabolized.

Since phenytoin's pK_a is high, 8.3, attempts to augment renal elimination by alkalinization of the urine and forced diuresis are unproductive, and since phenytoin is highly protein-bound, hemodialysis and peritoneal dialysis are to little or no avail. Acute ingestion is best treated by induced emesis or gastric lavage with a large-bore tube, followed by oral administration of activated charcoal. Repeated oral doses of activated charcoal recently have been found to enhance the systemic elimination of related compounds and may be useful. Charcoal hemoperfusion has also been used for severe toxicity.

BIBLIOGRAPHY

Baehler RW, Work J: Charcoal hemoperfusion in the therapy for methpuxamide and phenytoin overdose. *Arch Intern Med* 140:1466, 1980.

Crompton M, Moser R: The interrelations between the transport of sodium and calcium in the mitochondria of various mammalian tissues. *Eur J Biochem* 82:25–31, 1978.

Delgado-Escueta AV, Wasterlain C: Management of status epilepticus. *N Engl J Med* 306:1337–1340, 1982.

DeLorenzo RJ: Role of calcium dependent regulator proteins in neurotransmitter release. *Trans Am Soc Neurochem* 10:100, 1979.

Diesz RA, Lux HD: Diphenylhydantoin prolongs post-synaptic inhibitions and GABA action in the crayfish stretch receptor. *Neurosci Let* 5:199–203.

Earnest MP, Marx JA: Complications of intravenous phenytoin for acute treatment of seizures. *JAMA* 249:762–765, 1983.

Fenton GW, Fenwick PBC: Chronic cerebellar stimulation in the treatment of epilepsy—A preliminary report, in Penoz J (ed): *Epilepsy, the Eighth International Symposium*, New York, Raven Press, 1977, p 333–340.

Goldschlarger AW, Karliner JS: Ventricular standstill after intravenous diphenylhydantoin. *Am Heart J* 74:410, 1967.

Haddad LM, Winchester JF (eds): *Clinical Management of Poisoning and Overdose*. Philadelphia, Saunders, 1983, pp 557–560.

Hansen JW, Mzrianthopoulous NC: Risks to the offspring of women treated with hydantoin anticonvulsants, with emphasis on the fetal hydantoin syndrome. *J Pediatr* 89:662–668, 1976.

Kutt H: Interactions of the Antiepileptic Drugs. *Epilepsia* 16:393–402, 1975.

Lipton RAM, Cooper AL: Some neurophysiological effects of cerebellar stimulation in man. *Can J Neurol Sci* 3:233–254, 1977.

Reynolds EH: Chronic antiepileptic toxicity. *Epilepsia* 16:319–3552, 1975.

Schwartz A, Lindenmayer GE: The Na^+K^+ adenosine transferase—Pharmacological, physiological, and biochemical aspects. *Pharma Rev* 27:3–134, 1975.

Voigt GC: Death following intravenous disodium phenylhydantoin. *Johns Hopkins Med J* 123:153, 1968.

Wasori M, Ionasescu V: Teratogenic effects of anticonvulsant drugs. *Am J Dis Child* 130:1022–1023, 1976.

Wilson JT, Juger B: High incidence of a concentration dependent skin reaction in children treated with phenytoin. *Br Med J* 1:1583, 1978.

Winnecker JL, Yeager H: Rickets in children receiving anticonvulsant drugs. *Am J Dis Child* 131:286–290, 1977.

Yaari Y, Pincus HJ: Inhibition of synaptic transmission of diphenylhydantoin. *Adv Neurol* 1:334–338, 1977.

Ziegler DK: Toxicity of diphenylhydantoin and the nervous system: A review. *Int J Neurol* 11:383, 1978.

CHAPTER 41
MUSHROOM POISONING

Christopher H. Linden, Barry H. Rumack

INTRODUCTION

The truism that "the most important step in making a diagnosis is to think of it" is particularly applicable to mushroom poisoning. A history of ingestion is often lacking and the nonspecific early symptoms of poisoning may be mistakenly attributed to other etiologies. Preschool children, the commonest victims of mushroom poisoning, may not volunteer a history of mushroom ingestion or they may be altogether incapable of giving a history. Unless they are seen eating the mushroom, the diagnosis may not be considered. Recreational users of hallucinogenic mushrooms are frequently reluctant to admit to mushroom ingestion. Although the opposite is true for amateur foragers and organic food enthusiasts who become ill after eating a mushroom meal, the interval between ingestion and onset of symptoms may be long enough that a cause-effect relationship is not realized and hence not mentioned to the physician.

Without a history of ingestion, the diagnosis of mushroom poisoning is virtually impossible to make on the basis of early symptoms. Regardless of the type of mushroom ingested, the initial symptoms of poisoning generally consist of nausea, vomiting, abdominal cramps, and diarrhea. From these symptoms alone, mushroom poisoning is indistinguishable from much more common illnesses such as viral gastroenteritis. The fact that mushroom poisoning occurs most frequently during the summer season is not particularly helpful since other forms of food poisoning are also more common during the warmer months. In the absence of a history, then, there is nothing to suggest that what appears to be a self-limited gastrointestinal process may progress to fatal hepatic necrosis. A high index of suspicion must be maintained to avoid missing the diagnosis of mushroom poisoning. Remembering to include this diagnosis in the etiologic differential of gastroenteritis may avoid subsequent morbidity, mortality, and litigation.

The identity of any available mushroom or spore specimen may be helpful in suggesting the offending species, but this information should be considered adjunctive and interpreted in light of the clinical findings. With few exceptions, the appropriate treatment is determined by symptoms and signs rather than the identification of the suspect mushroom. Since toxic and nontoxic mushrooms may be found growing side by side, they may be gathered together and eaten together. The mushroom available for identification may not be the one or the only one that was ingested and hence may not be responsible for observed toxicity. Symptoms may also be due to bacterial or chemical contamination of an edible mushroom. Alternatively, poisonous strains of reportedly edible mushrooms may exist. And finally, the treatment for poisoning due to one kind of mushroom may be detrimental if another kind is responsible for toxic symptoms.

Other reasons for treating the patient rather than the mushroom are based on variable individual response following the ingestion of a poisonous mushroom. Differing degrees of poisoning may be due to differences in metabolism, gastrointestinal absorption, and acquired or allergic sensitivity, as well as to the amount of toxin ingested. The amount of toxin in a given species of mushroom varies greatly and depends on such factors as mushroom maturity, geographic location, and growing conditions. The patient's age and method of preparation of the mushroom before consumption are also important variables. Both the very young and the elderly are more susceptible to fluid and electrolyte disturbances secondary to vomiting and diarrhea. Small children also appear to be more sensitive to the effects of ingested toxins. This may be related to the observation that children often pick and eat raw mushrooms, whereas adults generally cook them prior to ingestion and the fact that cooking renders some species of mushroom less toxic, although not necessarily safe.

Following the initial gastrointestinal phase, the clinical course of mushroom poisoning varies according to the type of mushroom ingested. On the basis of characteristic symptoms and signs, the physician should be able to arrive at a presumptive diagnosis of the responsible toxin. This situation is analogous to that encountered in diagnosing any type of poisoning due to an unknown toxin.

IDENTIFICATION

Although they do not contain chlorophyll, mushrooms (commonly called toadstools) are classified as plants because of their rigid cell walls. They are further characterized as fungi based on their spore-forming reproductive cycle and a filamentous or mycelial vegetative phase. What is commonly referred to as a mushroom is actually only the visible fruiting body of the plant. An extensive but invisible network of hyphae enables mushrooms to extract nourishment from either living or dead organic matter.

Contrary to popular belief, there are no easy rules of thumb for differentiating toxic from edible species of mushrooms. The fact that a mushroom did not turn a silver spoon black when the two were boiled in the same pot, that it was found growing on a wood substrate, or that an animal did not become ill after eating it does not make the mushroom edible. Similarly, the boiling, drying, or salting of a poisonous mushroom does not necessarily detoxify it.

Identification of a mushroom requires careful analysis of the shape, texture, and color of the pileus (cap), gills, stipe (stem), base, and spores. Its odor, food substrate (e.g., soil, wood, dung, or another mushroom), habitat, and geographic location, and the season of harvest are also helpful in identifying species. Since most physicians are not familiar with the complexities of mushroom identification, it is important to obtain the services of a competent mycologist. Prior arrangements will prevent confusion and costly or even fatal delays when an emergency arises. Mycologists may be located through university botany departments, botanical gardens, mycological societies and clubs, and poison centers. A listing of state mycological societies and color photographs of mushrooms and spores may be found in Poisindex.

When the suspect mushroom is available, it should be identified as quickly as possible. If a mycologist is not available in a particular area, the mushroom should be sent to one. The mushroom should first be dried in air, or by hot light or oven at 95° C (200° F) and then transported in a paper container to avoid decomposition. Alternatively, the physician may obtain telephone consultation with a mycologist or attempt to identify the mushroom utilizing one of the many available reference resources.

Spores are also very valuable for identification purposes, particularly when an intact mushroom of the variety thought to have been ingested is not available. Spores may be recovered from the patient's vomitus, gastric aspirate, or stool. They may also be found on the gills or in the pit of a partially eaten mushroom or remaining on the dish from which the mushroom was served. After suspending the specimen in a drop of water, microscopic examination using an oil immersion lens and a cover slip may reveal spores which have a fairly uniform appearance and can appear in an oval or popcorn-kernel-like shape. Spores are similar in size to red blood cells (8 to 20 μm). The parent mushroom may be identified by comparing observed spore features to those found in photographs and descriptions in reference texts. Features such as color, size, shape, surface texture, wall thickness, and the presence or absence of an apical pore are characteristics used in identification.

If no spores are seen on direct smear, the sample may be filtered through cheesecloth, using water as an emulsifier, and centrifuged for 10 min. The sediment may then be resuspended and examined. If spores are still not seen, the suspended sediment may be heat-fixed to the slide, stained with 1% acid fuchsin, dried, and examined again. This process will give spores a vivid red appearance. Spores may also be stained with Meltzer's solution, which can be made by dissolving 1.5 g potassium iodide, 0.5 g iodine, and 20 g chloral hydrate in 20 mL of water. The resulting spore wall color will be characteristic of the mushroom species. This feature may be quite helpful if the spore cannot be positively identified by its other characteristics.

GENERAL MANAGEMENT

As for all poisonings, good supportive care is the primary treatment for mushroom poisoning. Airway management, ventilatory support, oxygenation, and fluid and cardiac resuscitation should be the first priorities. Once vital functions have been stabilized, concern can then be focused on a detailed history, gastrointestinal decontamination, identification of the mushroom, and the use of antidotes.

Since most patients will have prominent vomiting and diarrhea, and some may develop hematemesis and hematochezia or melena, aggressive intravenous fluid resuscitation may be necessary and occasionally vasopressors may be required. The intravenous solution should contain glucose as well as electrolytes. Baseline CBC, electrolytes, BUN, and glucose should be determined. Serial measurements of these parameters may be helpful in guiding subsequent therapy. Further laboratory evaluation may be indicated depending on the clinical findings and the type of mushroom ingested.

With respect to the history it is important to determine the time of ingestion, how many varieties of mushrooms were consumed, who else ate them, the time of onset of symptoms, and the nature of the particular complaints. If gastrointestinal symptoms did not begin until 6 h or more after ingestion, it should be assumed that they are due to a mushroom containing a potentially lethal toxin (i.e., a cyclopeptide or monomethylhydrazine).

If the patient has not vomited spontaneously, gastric emptying procedures should be initiated. In the awake and alert patient, syrup of ipecac is recommended, whereas the comatose or convulsing patient should be lavaged using a large-bore (36F) orogastric tube. Activated charcoal may absorb any toxin remaining in the gut and is recommended in all cases. If the patient has not developed diarrhea, a saline cathartic should also be administered. The use of antispasmodics to treat gastrointestinal symptoms should be avoided unless specifically indicated (e.g., atropine for the cholinergic syndrome), since such therapy may delay spontaneous gastrointestinal evacuation and lead to increased toxin absorption.

All available mushrooms or parts thereof, as well as gastric contents and a stool sample, should be collected. Although untrained medical personnel may be able to make a preliminary identification by consulting standard reference sources, all specimens should be sent to a professional mycologist for positive identification.

SIGNS, SYMPTOMS, AND SPECIFIC TREATMENT

Of the thousands of species of mushrooms, less than 100 are capable of causing serious toxicity and only about 10 are normally associated with fatalities. As noted above, the initial stage of poisoning by nearly all toxic mushrooms begins with gastroenteritis. The subsequent toxic syndrome is characteristic of the particular toxin involved and determines the appropriate treatment. To simplify the symptomatic diagnosis and treatment, poisonous mushrooms can be divided into seven groups on the basis of the predominant toxin.

Group I mushrooms, those containing hepatotoxic cyclopeptides, include the deadly *Amanita* species (*A. phalloides, verna, virosc, bisporigia, ocreata, suballiacae,* and *tennifolia*), *Conocybe filaris,* some species of *Galerina* (e.g., *G. autumnalis, marginata, vererata*), and *Lepiota helveola.* The ingestion of one *A. phalloides* or 15 to 20 of the smaller *Galerina* may be lethal to an adult. The cyclopeptide molecules responsible for toxicity are eight-membered amino acid rings. These amanitotoxins cause the disintegration of nucleoli of liver cells due to their inhibition of

RNA polymerase II and hence interference with both DNA and RNA transcription.

The clinical presentation of patients poisoned by amanitotoxins can be divided into several stages, similar to those seen in poisoning by other hepatotoxins. Since disrupted protein synthesis is ultimately responsible for cell death, amanitotoxin poisoning begins with a latent or asymptomatic period usually lasting 6 to 12 h. However, symptoms may be delayed as long as 48 h, and the development of symptoms within several hours of ingestion does not rule out amanitotoxin poisoning since mushrooms causing early toxicity may have been coingested. Following the latent period, there is typically an abrupt onset of nausea, vomiting, thirst, colicky abdominal pain, profuse (''cholera-like'') diarrhea, and sometimes hematuria. Patients may develop severe dehydration, and the emesis and diarrhea may be bloody. Laboratory findings may include acidosis, hypoglycemia, leukocytosis, and abnormalities of serum sodium and potassium due to fluid and electrolyte losses. The hematocrit may decrease as a result of blood loss or occasionally increase due to hemoconcentration. The gastrointestinal phase, which lasts 12 to 24 h, may be terminated by a second latent period, during which liver enzymes, bilirubin, PT, PTT, BUN, and creatinine may begin to rise. Despite apparent clinical recovery, patients may then develop right upper quadrant pain, liver enlargement and tenderness, jaundice, coagulopathy, cardiomyopathy, asterixis, encephalopathy, seizure, coma, and other features of hepatic failure. Oliguria may indicate dehydration or true renal failure. Kidney dysfunction may occur without significant hepatotoxicity, but most often concomitant hepatic failure is present (hepatorenal syndrome). It is estimated that less than 5 percent of patients ingesting mushrooms containing cyclopeptides will develop fatal hepatic necrosis.

The mainstay of therapy for amanitotoxin poisoning consists of fluid, electrolyte, and metabolic support. A variety of antidotes and therapeutic interventions have been reported to be beneficial. Most regimens have only been studied using pretreatment experimental studies in animals but are of unproven effectiveness owing to lack of controlled postexposure studies in humans. However, these measures may be indicated because of the potentially fatal outcome. Thioctic acid (α-lipoic acid), a coenzyme in the Krebs cycle, has been used in a number of hepatic diseases, but its effectiveness is very questionable at this time. The usual dose is 25 to 150 mg IV every 6 h, and current sources are listed in Poisindex. Since this agent may cause hypoglycemia, supplemental dextrose should be given whenever it is used. High doses of corticosteroids have been recommended. The use of high-dose intravenous penicillin is theoretically attractive since it is thought to interfere with the binding of amanitotoxins to albumin, resulting in more free toxin available for renal clearance. Numerous other pharmacological interventions have been described but are not generally accepted. Charcoal hemoperfusion or exchange transfusion may be effective in removing toxin from the blood if performed early in the course of treatment. Both hemoperfusion and hemodialysis have supportive value in patients with hepatic and renal failure. In 1983 a liver transplant was performed in a child who developed massive hepatic failure after ingesting group I mushrooms.

Cyclopeptides are also present in *group IA* mushrooms such as *Cortinarius calisteus, cinnamomeus, gentilis, orellanus, rainierensis, semisanguineus,* and *speciosissimus.* In contrast to the amanitotoxins, the orellanine and orelline cyclopeptides are predominantly toxic to the kidneys.

Gastrointestinal symptoms develop during the first 24 h after ingestion but are usually mild and of short duration. Hence, patients poisoned by group IA mushrooms often do not seek medical attention until symptoms of renal failure appear. Such symptoms typically begin with the development of intense burning thirst, chills, night sweats, and flank pain several days to several weeks after ingestion. Examination may disclose flank tenderness, rising BUN and creatinine, hematuria, massive albuminuria, red cell casts, and oliguria. The pathologic lesion is described as a tubulointerstitial nephritis. Chronic renal failure may occasionally develop, but in many instances only temporary dialysis is necessary. As for the amanitotoxins, early hemodialysis or hemoperfusion may remove circulating orellanine and orelline cyclopeptides and prevent subsequent renal toxicity.

Species of *Amanita* (*A. muscaria, pantherina, gemmata, cokeri, cothurna*) also comprise the *group II* mushrooms, but are classified separately because they do not contain cyclopeptides. The predominant toxin is the hallucinogen muscimol. However, these mushrooms also contain the hallucinogenic insecticide ibotenic acid and the well-studied parasympathetic stimulant muscarine. Hallucinations produced by these mushrooms are often illusionary in nature and are characterized by visual misperceptions of color and shape with prominent religious overtones. Because of these properties, mushrooms of this group have been used in the rituals of Asian and African tribes for thousands of years, and drug cultists currently utilize them for recreational purposes. Unless the amount ingested is carefully titrated, severe toxicity may ensue.

Symptoms of muscimol poisoning usually begin within 20 to 90 min after ingestion, rarely last more than 8 h, and consist of an ethanol-like inebriation. An initial period of drowsiness may be followed by euphoria, confusion, ataxia, delirium, hallucinations, and manic behavior. There is often a fluctuating level of consciousness. In severe cases, patients may develop frank psychosis, seizures, and coma. These symptoms appear to be due to the central anticholinergic effect of muscimol. Peripheral anticholinergic findings such as dry mucosa, dilated pupils, warm and flushed skin, tachycardia, hypertension, absent bowel sounds, and urinary retention are frequently present.

In the presence of signs of both central and peripheral anticholinergic toxicity, specific indications for treatment with physostigmine include severe hypertension, hemodynamically compromising supraventricular tachyarrhythmias, seizures, and dangerously psychotic behavior. Physostigmine should be given as a slow intravenous bolus over several minutes in an initial dose of 1 to 2 mg in adults and 0.5 mg in children. Similar doses may be repeated if severe symptoms persist or recur.

Only occasionally do mushrooms of group II cause gastrointestinal symptoms, and such symptoms are usually mild if present. Similarly, marked cholinergic symptoms (see below) are infrequently present since these mushrooms usually contain very small amounts of muscarine. In general, mild sweating, salivation, and moderate gastrointestinal symptoms are the only ones observed.

The toxic mushrooms of *group III* contain monomethylhydrazine (MMH) and other hydrazones (''gyromitrins''). These chemicals are found in many species of *Gyromitra* (*G. esculenta, umbigna, infula, caroliniana, brunnea, fastigiate*), some *Paxina* species, and *Sarcosphaera coronaria.* MMH is also found as a by-product of many industrial processes and is used as rocket fuel. Its odor may be described as ammoniacal or fishy. MMH may cause methemoglobinemia, red blood cell hemolysis, and a syndrome resembling isoniazid (INH) poisoning. Methemoglobin levels above 15 to 20 percent of the total hemoglobin result in a blue-brown cyanosis unresponsive to oxygen. Arterial blood gases will reveal a normal P_{O_2} and calculated O_2 saturation. Direct measurement of the O_2 saturation, however, will show a value less than the calculated O_2 saturation by an amount equal to the percent of methemoglobin present. Such measurements can be used to estimate the methemoglobin level when it cannot be measured directly.

The similarity between MMH and INH intoxication is due to the fact that both agents are felt to interfere with the central nervous system neurotransmitter γ-aminobutyric acid (GABA). Since GABA is primarily found in inhibitory neurons, MMH poisoning results in central stimulation and is manifested by delirium, seizures, and coma in severe cases. Milder symptoms and signs consist of dizziness, vertigo, ataxia, weakness, muscle cramps, and hyperreflexia. There is a relatively long latent period from ingestion to onset of toxicity, with symptoms developing at 6 to 24 h and beginning with moderately severe gastroenteritis. In mild cases recovery may be complete in 24 h, whereas severe cases may end in death 5 to 7 days after ingestion.

Methemoglobinemia, hemolysis, seizures, and coma may be life-threatening. Specific treatment consists of intravenous methylene blue (1 to 2 mg/kg or 0.1 to 0.2 mL/kg of a 1% solution) for symptomatic patients with methemoglobin levels above 30 percent, blood transfusion for hemolytic anemia, and pyridoxine for CNS toxicity. Large doses of intravenous pyridoxine (vitamin B_6), beginning with 25 mg/kg and repeating as often as necessary, may be required to stop seizures. The rationale for the use of pyridoxine is that it provides substrate for the coenzyme pyridoxal phosphate, which catalyzes the synthesis of GABA. Supplemental pyridoxine appears to be able to compensate for the inhibition of this enzyme by MMH.

In contrast to the *Amanita* species of group II, mushrooms of *group IV* contain significant amounts of muscarine and predictably cause parasympathetic overstimulation. Such mushrooms include species of *Boletus* (*B. calopus, luridus, pulcherrimus,* and *satanas*), *Clitocybe* (*C. cerbissata, dealbata, illudesn,* and *riuulogg*), and *Inocybe* (*I. fastigata, geophylla, lilacina, patuoillardi, purica,* and *rimosus*).

Symptoms of muscarine poisoning are identical to those of the classic "cholinergic crisis" seen after organophosphate poisoning. In contrast to organophosphates, however, muscarine usually causes mild symptoms that are rarely life-threatening. Thirty minutes to 2 h after ingestion, patients may develop the "sludge" syndrome (*s*alivation, *l*acrimation, *u*rination, *d*efecation, or incontinence of urine and stool, *g*astrointestinal cramps, and *e*mesis), miosis, bradycardia, bronchospasm, excessive respiratory secretions, and, rarely, seizures.

Atropine is a specific antidote for cholinergic symptoms. The initial intravenous dose is 0.5 to 1.0 mg in adults and 0.01 mg/kg in children. Similar doses may be repeated as often as necessary to effect drying of pulmonary secretions.

Group V mushrooms contain coprine and include *Coprinus atramentarius* ("inky cap") and *Clitocybe calvipes*. Like disulfiram (Antabuse), a metabolite of coprine inhibits the enzyme aldehyde dehydrogenase. For up to 1 week following the ingestion of these edible species, the ingestion of ethanol may therefore precipitate a disulfiram-ethanol-like reaction. When the time between coprine and ethanol ingestion is longer than 24 h, patients unaware of this interaction are not likely to relate a history of mushroom ingestion. Hence, the cause of symptoms is often not appreciated.

Most symptoms of the coprine-ethanol reaction appear to be secondary to peripheral vasodilation and consist of flushing, diaphoresis, weakness, vertigo, confusion, hypotension, palpitations, chest tightness, and dyspnea. Other findings may include a metallic taste, nausea, vomiting, coma, and electrocardiographic changes suggestive of myocardial ischemia.

Symptoms are usually mild, last several hours, and resolve spontaneously. However, in severe cases, fluid resuscitation and antiarrhythmic agents may be required. Patients with persistent ECG abnormalities following an acute reaction should be admitted to rule out myocardial infarction.

The hallucinogenic indoles psilocin and psilocybin are the toxins that characterize *group VI* mushrooms. These mushrooms are popular with recreational drug users and have been used for centuries in the religious ceremonies of American Indians. Mushrooms containing the psychotropic indoles include numerous species of *Psilocybe* (*P. cubensis, caerulescens, cyanesceus, baeocystis, fimentaria, mexicana, pelluculosa, semilanceata, silvatica*), *Gymnopilus* (*G. aeruginosa, spetabilis, validipes*), and *Panaeolus* (*P. foenisecii, subbalteatus*), as well as *Conocybe cyanopus* and *Strophans coronilla*.

Thirty to sixty minutes (occasionally longer) after ingesting group VI mushrooms, patients develop a dysphoric state followed by hallucinations. The mood is usually elevated and the experience considered pleasant, but a "bad trip" may also occur. Findings may include mydriasis, vertigo, ataxia, tachycardia, paresthesia, weakness, and impairment of judgment and motor performance. The hallucinogenic-dysphoric episode generally lasts 4 to 6 h and may end in drowsiness progressing to sleep. Reassurance in a quiet atmosphere is usually the only treatment required. Diazepam is probably safer than an antipsychotic agent should pharmacological sedation be required.

Group VII mushrooms consist of those causing only gastrointestinal irritation. Most of the responsible toxins have not been identified. These mushrooms include such a great variety of species from diverse genera that a listing here is not feasible. Many of the "little brown mushrooms" found in backyards fall into this group. Not all people who ingest these mushrooms will develop symptoms.

Onset of nausea, vomiting, abdominal cramps, and diarrhea generally begins within $\frac{1}{2}$ to 2 h. Rarely, patients have developed paresthesia and tetany, probably as a result of hyperventilation. Symptoms usually last about 4 h, subside spontaneously, and do not require specific treatment.

CONCLUSION

Physicians must maintain a high index of suspicion in order to avoid missing the diagnosis of mushroom poisoning, particularly in patients presenting with gastrointestinal symptoms and without a history of mushroom ingestion. As for any drug overdose, the first priority in treatment is good supportive care. Although mushroom identification is important, specific therapy is dictated by the clinical presentation.

Dr. Linden is supported by a grant from the McNeil Consumer Products Division for research in clinical toxicology.

BIBLIOGRAPHY

Antkowiak WZ, Gessner WP: The structures of orellanine and orelline. *Tetrahedron Lett* 21:1931–1934, 1979.

Becker CE, Tong TG, Boerner U, et al: Diagnosis and treatment of *Amanita phalloides*–type mushroom poisoning: Use of thioctic acid. *West J Med* 125:100–109, 1976.

Chilton WS: Chemistry and mode of action of mushroom toxins, in Rumack BH, Salzman E (eds): *Mushroom Poisoning: Diagnosis and Treatment,* West Palm Beach, Fla, CRC Press, 1978.

Grzymala S: Étude clinique des intoxications par les champignons du genre *Cortinarins orellanus. Fr Bull Med Legale* 8:60–70, 1965.

Hatfield GM, Schaumbert JP: The disulfiram-like effects of *Coprinus atramantarius* and related mushrooms, in Rumack BH, Salzman E (eds): *Mushroom Poisoning: Diagnosis and Treatment,* West Palm Beach, Fla, CRC Press, 1978.

Lampe KF: Pharmacology and therapy of mushroom intoxication, in Rumack BH, Salzman E (eds): *Mushroom Poisoning: Diagnosis and Treatment,* West Palm Beach, Fla, CRC Press, 1978.

McDonald A: Mushrooms and madness: Hallucinogenic mushrooms and some psychopharmacological implications. *Can J Psychiatry* 25:586–594, 1980.

McDonald A: The present status of soma: The effects of California *Amanita muscaria* on normal human volunteers, in Rumack BH, Salzman E (eds): *Mushroom Poisoning: Diagnosis and Treatment,* West Palm Beach, Fla, CRC Press, 1978.

Mitchel DH: Amanita mushroom poisoning. *Annu Rev Med* 31:51–57, 1980.

Mitchel DH, Rumack BH: Symptomatic diagnosis and treatment of mushroom poisoning, in Rumack BH, Salzman E (eds): *Mushroom Poisoning: Diagnosis and Treatment,* West Palm Beach, Fla, CRC Press, 1978.

Rumack BH: Amanita poisoning: An examination of clinical symptoms. Presented at International Amanita Symposium, Heidelberg, Germany, 1978.

Rumack BH (ed): Poisindex, a computer generated microfiche poison information system (published quarterly). Micromex, Englewood, Colo, 1983.

Short AIK, Watling R, MacDonald WK: Poisoning by *Cortinarius speciosissimus. Lancet* 2:942–944, 1980.

Singer R: Hallucinogenic mushrooms, in Rumack BH, Salzman E (eds): *Mushroom Poisoning: Diagnosis and Treatment,* West Palm Beach, Fla, CRC Press, 1978.

SECTION 5
ENVIRONMENTAL
INJURIES

CHAPTER 42
FROSTBITE

Barry Heller

DEFINITIONS AND PATHOGENESIS

Injury due to cold may be generalized, as in hypothermia, or may occur locally, as in frostbite. Furthermore, local cold injury may occur at temperatures both above and below freezing. Nonfreezing cold injury can be divided into two groups on the basis of exposure to either dry or wet cold.

Trench foot, or immersion foot, occurs with exposure to wet cold for 1 to 2 days, with ambient temperatures above freezing. In this situation, the extremity often develops severe superficial damage resembling partial-thickness burns. Deep tissue destruction in this setting, however, is rare.

Pernio, or chilblain, refers to prolonged exposure of an extremity to dry cold at temperatures above freezing. This is seen most commonly in mountain climbers, and consists of small, superficial, painful ulcerations over chronically exposed areas. These lesions are often associated with hypersensitivity of the surrounding skin, pruritus, and erythema. On occasion, this process may be complicated by extensor tenosynovitis.

Freezing cold injury results in the clinical picture most often referred to as *frostbite*. The pathogenesis of frostbite remains controversial, however; there is evidence for both macrovascular and microvascular processes as well as direct cellular injury. When a body surface comes into contact with cold, there may be superficial tissue freezing to a depth dependent on the intensity and duration of cold exposure. Instantaneous, severe freezing can occur in tissue exposed to volatile hydrocarbons, such as gasoline, at low temperatures. Below this zone of freezing, capillary circulation slows and eventually halts secondary to cold-induced vasospasm and increased viscosity of blood. At this point, certain macrovascular responses have been shown to occur. Initially, the arterioles in the area constrict in an effort to decrease loss of heat at the site of the cold insult. Following this, capillary shunting occurs with arteriole-to-venule flow of blood. This is the body's physiologic effort to keep some blood circulating to the cold extremity while minimizing heat loss. However, chilled blood returning from the periphery to the heart may cause a drop in the core temperature as loss of body heat exceeds production capacity. To complicate matters further, the tissues once supplied by the capillaries, which are now being bypassed, remain devoid of oxygen and nutrients. With the inevitable drop in core temperature, shunting stops, allowing the extremity to freeze. This is the ulti-

mate physiologic mechanism of survival; sacrifice of an extremity in order to preserve the core of the organism. It is easy to see how this process can be worsened by shock, panic, and poor physical conditioning.

There is also evidence that ice crystals actually form in the extra- and intracellular spaces. The resulting shift of water leads to increased intracellular osmolality, intracellular dehydration, and ultimate denaturation of intracellular proteins. Intracellular ice crystals disrupt cellular architecture and function. Microvascular occlusion also has been shown to occur in the process of local cold injury. Low temperature leads to decreased flow of blood and sludging secondary to increased viscosity. Platelets aggregate, occluding venules, so that within 1 to 2 h capillary and arteriolar vascular beds are damaged. After thawing, protein-rich fluid leaks from the injured vasculature into the interstitial space (similar to burn injury). This leads to increased tissue pressure, further promoting venous stasis and occlusion, with eventual tissue damage and death.

The areas of the body most likely to suffer local cold injury are those farthest from the body's core, such as earlobes, cheeks, nose, hands, and feet. To prevent local cold injury, the body must be warm enough to supply warm blood to these areas. Adequate clothing and general physical condition of the body as a whole are therefore at least as important as warm covering for the hands and feet. However, local cold injury may occur in the presence or absence of generalized hypothermia.

There are several factors which influence the severity of cold injury. Obviously, the temperature and duration of exposure are of prime importance. Wet cold cools tissue much more quickly than dry cold, and the insulating effect of any piece of clothing is markedly diminished when the clothing is wet. Air movement accelerates heat loss so that the chilling effect of ambient temperature at $-7°C$ (20°F) combined with a 72.5-km/h (45-mi/h) wind is identical to that of $-40°C$ ($-40°F$) temperature on a windless day. Wind speed does not determine final tissue temperature because tissue cannot fall to temperatures below that of the ambient air, but it does greatly promote body and extremity heat loss.

High altitude also has a deleterious effect in terms of temperature regulation. Though blood has not been shown to be more viscous because of high altitude (in spite of increased packed red blood cell volume), water loss from increased respiratory rates can lead to relative dehydration and decreased blood flow. Furthermore, high altitude can lead to hypoxic conditions in the central nervous system, resulting in impaired behavioral responses and mechanisms of adaptation to cold and stress.

CLINICAL FEATURES

The initial clinical response to cold produces reversible skin changes known as "frostnip." The skin becomes blanched and numb, followed by a sudden cessation of cold and discomfort. This sudden loss of cold sensation at the injured location is a fairly reliable sign of incipient frostbite. If heeded instantly, frostnip will not progress to frostbite.

Frostbite has been divided on clinical grounds into as many as four different categories of severity ranging from hyperemia and edema to full-thickness necrosis. However, for purposes of recognition, treatment, and prognosis, two clinical classes of frostbite, *superficial* and *deep*, seem adequate. As frostnip progresses to frostbite, the frozen tissue remains cold to the touch, pale, gray, and bloodless. In superficial frostbite, the skin remains pliable and soft beneath the surface. In deep frostbite, the tissues feel woody and stony. Note, however, that this particular clinical distinction can be made only prior to thawing of the tissues.

In superficial frostbite, large, clear blisters appear in 24 to 48 h. Following this, the skin hardens, blister fluid is resorbed, and the skin blackens into a hard carapace. Within several weeks, a demarcation line occurs between blackened skin and healthy viable tissue. This carapace is in essence a dry gangrene of a very superficial nature (in contrast to that associated with arteriosclerotic-induced gangrene, which may include several tissue layers), peeling off bit by bit over several months and revealing a shiny, red skin beneath. This "new" skin will be abnormally tender and hypersensitive to heat and cold. Ultimately it will assume the characteristics of normal skin, but for unknown reasons will remain more susceptible to cold injury and frostbite compared with unaffected skin.

Deep frostbite involves deep structures including, in some cases, muscle, bone, and tendon, because nutritional capillary flow is never returned to these areas. The extremity appears deep purple or red and is cool to the touch. Although sensation and distal function are absent, the patient may be able to move distal parts because proximal muscles and tendons may be functional. In contrast to superficial frostbite, small, dark hemorrhagic blisters appear in 1 to 3 weeks. Edema is slow to form but may persist for months. Eventually, nonviable skin and deep structures demarcate, mummify, and slough.

It is important to remember that prediction of tissue loss is impossible for several months. However, the appearance of the tissue after initial thawing gives some clues to the severity of tissue damage. In mild or superficial frostbite, after thawing, the skin is sensitive to pinprick, has good color, and is warm to the touch. Furthermore, blisters of clear fluid occur early and extend to the tips of the digits. In deep or severe frostbite, after thawing, the distal portions remain cold and cyanotic. There is late appearance of small, dark vesicles, and failure of vesicles to extend to the volar pads of the distal digits. Once formed, if the blackened carapace corresponds to the original affected part, much tissue loss is unlikely. But if the contour of the pulp of the finger disappears, then the carapace will appear wrinkled, betraying the loss of tissue beneath it.

Laboratory tests are generally of little value in predicting severity of frostbite. However, technetium pyrophosphate scanning can identify nonviable bone with accuracy. Doppler and plethysmographic studies are of some assistance in the differentiation of mild from severe frostbite after thawing. Angiography is best reserved for evaluation of chronic vascular abnormalities of freeze-injured tissues.

The essential concept is that early prediction of actual ultimate tissue loss is impossible, in spite of the clues mentioned above. Therefore, early surgical intervention is contraindicated. Even an extremity with deep frostbite may return to almost normal, with minimal tissue loss, over several months.

TREATMENT

Frostnip is the only form of frostbite which should be treated at the scene. A site sheltered from the wind is used and the affected part is warmed by hand (without rubbing), by breathing through cupped hands, or by placing frostnipped fingers in the armpit. As the skin rewarms and color returns to normal, the patient will often experience a tingling sensation which heralds return of adequate circulation to the area. The patient may then continue working, but all members of the party must watch each other periodically for the signs described above.

For many years the common folk treatment of frostbite was rubbing the affected part with snow or another body part. This is to be discouraged as it causes skin breakage, increases chances of infection, and, in actuality, does not thaw tissues adequately. Wet or constrictive clothing should be removed. Alcohol is contraindicated until definitive warming can be accomplished and maintained, as alcohol causes increased heat loss on the basis of peripheral vasodilatation, while providing a false sense of security.

Rapid rewarming of the frozen part is the single most effective therapeutic measure for preserving viable tissue. This is best accomplished by immersion of the extremity in 42°C circulating water for 20 min or until a distal flush of the extremity is observed. Slow rewarming, in contrast, has been shown to be less effective and to increase tissue damage. Also dry heat, such as that from a campfire, is very dangerous as a thawing method. Because the frozen part is insensitive, there is a high chance of superficial burning and unnecessary tissue destruction.

Refreezing of thawed tissue drastically increases tissue damage and loss. If a patient develops frostbite on the trail, the extremity should not be thawed until definitive care can be given and maintained so that refreezing does not occur. This means that it would be more prudent to walk on a frozen foot to base camp or hospital rather than to thaw the foot first and then begin to hike to safety. Ideally, help should be brought to the victim.

As the definitive thawing is often quite painful, narcotic analgesics should be used liberally and tetanus prophylaxis administered appropriately. If the involved areas are large, intravenous fluid replacement should be considered. Antibiotics should be reserved for situations where infection is present or if there was an open wound on the extremity prior to freezing.

Local care of the extremity involves several basic principles. Unbroken vesicles should be left intact as they provide sterile covering. The injured extremity should be elevated to decrease further edema. With proper cradling of the extremity, it is best to leave it open to air during healing. The digits should be kept apart with soft, dry, absorbent dressings. These same dressings should be used to cover ruptured vesicle sites. Topical antibiotics, such as silver sulfadiazine, may be used, but should not substitute for definitive care of a clinically apparent infection. Weight bearing is proscribed on healing extremities. Whirlpool treatments with warm antibiotic solutions twice daily aid in gentle debridement, reduce the risk of infection, and soften the eschar for physiotherapy (which should include basic active range of motion exercises to prevent stiffness and contractures). Pressure dressings to decrease edema are discouraged as they tend to increase tissue destruction.

Again, early surgical intervention is not indicated for three reasons. First, it is impossible to assess the depth of frostbite in early stages. Second, the blackened, mummified carapace is protective to the underlying regenerating tissue. Third, premature surgery has been the most important cause of poor results and unnecessary tissue loss in this disease process. Keep in mind, however, that if wet gangrene and/or infection complicate the process, surgical intervention may be unavoidable.

Escharotomy and fasciotomy have been used in the past. However, since loss of circulation is due to primary vascular damage rather than occluding edema, these procedures are usually not indicated. If the eschar is preventing adequate range of motion, then escharotomy may be helpful.

Sympathectomy to increase blood flow has been advocated by several investigators with varying results. No rigorous study to date has demonstrated increased tissue salvage with this procedure and, thus, it remains controversial. Chemical sympathetic blockade also has been tried but found to be most useful in the chronic vasospastic sequelae of frostbite. Heparin and low-molecular-weight dextran have both been advocated in the treatment of frostbite, but clinical trials have not justified their routine use. Skin grafting procedures may be useful after final tissue loss is evident.

COMPLICATIONS AND SEQUELAE

There are several complications and sequelae of frostbite which should be kept in mind. Because of tissue and, more specifically, muscle damage, rhabdomyolysis and subsequent renal failure have been reported in several cases of frostbite. These complications should be anticipated and urinalysis and muscle enzyme determinations performed. It should be remembered that subsequent cold injury is more likely in a previously frostbitten extremity. Furthermore, healed frostbitten extremities demonstrate skin that is drier and more easily cracked with subsequent fissuring. This can be treated with moisturizing creams. Permanent depigmentation of the extremity may occur following recovery from frostbite.

Certain bony changes have been noted radiographically in extremities with a past history of frostbite. Three to six months following frostbite recovery, fine, irregular, punched-out lytic lesions appear at the MCP, MTP, PIP, and DIP joints of the extremities. These may be juxta- or subarticular and may extend into the joint. They are felt to be suggestive of chronic subperiosteal inflammation. Biopsy of the lesions reveals dense fibrous connective tissue. Clinical arthritis with fusiform soft tissue swelling and decreased range of motion may occur in these extremities and may be secondary to the above processes as well as to disuse, direct cold injury to bones and joints, and/or avascular necrosis as a result of thrombosis of digital arteries.

PREVENTION

Obviously, prevention is the best treatment for frostbite, and the above principles should be helpful in this regard. People working or traveling in cold weather and/or high altitude should be in good general health, assure themselves an adequate diet, dress appropriately, and avoid panic, fatigue, and alcohol consumption. Use of a buddy system to observe each other for frostnip and treat accordingly is very helpful. Frostbite should not be rewarmed on the trail and frozen feet, once thawed, should not be walked on. Cryotherapy (e.g., ice packs) for various disorders such as sprains or epididymitis, should be used with respect as there have been reports of iatrogenic frostbite to the scrotum, fingers, and toes.

SUMMARY

Local cold injury can occur in both freezing and nonfreezing conditions, usually affecting parts of the body distal to the central body mass. The pathogenesis of frostbite includes both disruption of cellular architecture by ice crystals as well as impaired vascular supply. The severity of frostbite is affected by the amount and duration of cold, wet versus dry conditions, wind chill, and altitude. Frostbite can be classified as superficial or deep by various clinical criteria, but eventual tissue loss cannot be predicted with accuracy until several months after the injury. The treatment of choice for local cold injury is rapid rewarming of the injured part in circulating water at 42°C, followed by meticulous local care to minimize tissue destruction. Surgical therapy is contraindicated early in the course unless the process is complicated by wet gangrene and/or infection. There are many sequelae and complications to frostbite injury, including hypersensitivity of skin, rhabdomyolysis, arthritis, radiographic bony abnormalities, and increased susceptibility to subsequent cold injury. A public and medical community well informed as to the dangers of cold, altitude, and wind, as well as protection from these and prompt action to combat developing cold injury, are of utmost importance in prevention of this injury.

BIBLIOGRAPHY

Boswick JA: Cold injuries. *Major Probl Clin Surg* 19:96–106, 1976.

Kyosola K: Clinical experience in the management of cold injuries: A study of 110 cases. *J Trauma* 14:32–36, 1974.

Mills WJ Jr: Frostbite and Hypothermia—Current concepts. *Alaska Med* 15:26, 1975.

Raifman M et al: Cold weather and rhabdomyolysis. *J Pediatr* 93:970, 1978.

Rosenthal L et al: Frostbite with rhabdomyolysis and renal failure: Radionuclide study. *Am J Roentgenol* 137:387, 1981.

Schumacker HB, Kilman JW: Sympathectomy in the treatment of frostbite. *Arch Surg* 89:575, 1964.

Snider RL, Rummell D, Merhoff GC, et al: Intra-arterial sympathetic blockade in the treatment of frostbite. *Surg Forum* 25:237, 1974.

Treatment of frostbite. *Med Lett Drug Ther* 18:105, 1976.

Ward M: Frostbite. *Br Med J* 1:67, 1974.

Washburn B: Frostbite, What it is—How to prevent it—Emergency treatment. *N Engl J Med* 266:974, 1962.

Weatherly-White RCA, et al: Pathogenesis of frostbite. *J Surg Res* 4:17, 1964.

CHAPTER 43
HYPOTHERMIA

Howard A. Bessen

Hypothermia is defined as a core temperature less than 35°C (95°F). While most commonly seen in cold climates, it may develop without exposure to extreme environmental conditions. Indeed, hypothermia is not uncommon in temperate regions, and may develop indoors during the summer. Failure to recognize and properly treat this condition leads to significant morbidity and mortality. This chapter reviews the etiology, physiology and pathophysiology, and management of hypothermia.

PHYSIOLOGY OF TEMPERATURE HOMEOSTASIS

Body temperature may fall as a result of heat loss by conduction, convection, radiation, or evaporation. Conduction is the transfer of heat by direct contact, down a temperature gradient, e.g., from a warm body to the cold environment. Since the thermal conductivity of water is approximately 30 times that of air, the body loses heat quite rapidly when immersed in water, leading to a rapid decline in body temperature.

Convection is the transfer of heat by the actual movement of heated material, for example, wind disrupting the layer of warm air surrounding the body. Convective heat loss increases markedly in windy conditions, a particular hazard for hikers and other outdoors enthusiasts.

Heat may also be lost by radiation to the environment (primarily from noninsulated body areas), and by evaporation of water. Evaporation of the water contained in exhaled, water-saturated air occurs over a wide range of ambient temperatures, and may be prevented by inhalation of warmed humidified air.

Opposing the loss of body heat are mechanisms of heat conservation and gain. In general, these mechanisms are controlled by the hypothalamus; thus, hypothalamic dysfunction may cause an impairment in temperature homeostasis. Heat is conserved by peripheral vasoconstriction and, importantly, by behavioral responses. If behavioral responses such as putting on clothing or coming indoors from a cold environment are impaired for any reason (e.g., drug intoxication or trauma), the risk of hypothermia is markedly increased.

Heat gain is effected by shivering, and by "nonshivering thermogenesis." The nonshivering component of heat production consists of an increase in metabolic rate brought about by increased output from the thyroid and adrenal glands.

HIGH-RISK PATIENTS

Individuals at the extremes of age, and those with an altered sensorium for any reason, are particularly susceptible to developing hypothermia.

The elderly often lose their ability to sense cold; neonates easily become hypothermic because of their large body surface area. Both groups have a limited ability to increase heat production and to conserve body heat. Individuals with an altered sensorium, if unable to carry out the appropriate behavioral responses to cold stress, may develop hypothermia despite otherwise intact thermoregulatory mechanisms.

ETIOLOGY OF HYPOTHERMIA;
CLINICAL SETTINGS

Table 43-1 lists the common causes of hypothermia. While there are other much less common causes, nearly all patients seen by the emergency physician will have hypothermia due to one or more of these causes.

"Accidental" hypothermia may be divided into immersion and nonimmersion cold exposure. Exposure to cold environmental conditions may lead to hypothermia even in healthy subjects, especially in wind and rain. Inadequate clothing and physical exhaustion contribute to the loss of body heat. As previously mentioned, the high thermal conductivity of water leads to the rapid development of immersion hypothermia. Though the rate of heat loss is determined by water temperature, immersion in any water less than 16 to 21°C (60 to 70°F) may lead to hypothermia.

Metabolic causes of hypothermia include various hypoendocrine states (hypothyroidism, hypoadrenalism, hypopituitarism), which lead to a decrease in metabolic rate. Hypoglycemia may also lead to hypothermia; the probable mechanism is hypothalamic dysfunction secondary to glucopenia.

Other causes of hypothalamic and CNS dysfunction (e.g., head trauma, tumor, stroke) may also interfere with mechanisms of temperature regulation. Wernicke's disease may involve the hypothalamus; this is a rare but important cause of hypothermia, since it is potentially reversible with parenteral thiamine.

In the United States, the vast majority of hypothermic patients are intoxicated with ethanol or other drugs. Ethanol is a vaso-

Table 43-1. Causes of Hypothermia: Clinical Settings

''Accidental'' (environmental) cause
Metabolic cause
Hypothalamic and CNS dysfunction
Drug-induced cause
Sepsis
Dermal disease
Acute incapacitating illness

dilator, and, because of its anesthetic and CNS-depressant effects, intoxicated subjects neither feel the cold nor respond to it appropriately. Other drugs commonly implicated in the development of hypothermia include barbiturates, phenothiazines, and occasionally insulin.

Sepsis may alter the hypothalamic temperature set point and is a well-known cause of hypothermia. Subnormal body temperature is a poor prognostic factor in patients with bacteremia.

Severe dermal disease may impair the skin's thermoregulatory functions. Significant burns or severe exfoliative dermatitis may prevent cutaneous vasoconstriction and increase transcutaneous water loss, predisposing to the development of hypothermia.

Finally, hypothermia may develop in anyone with an acute incapacitating illness. Thus, patients with severe infections, diabetic ketoacidosis, immobilizing injuries, and various other conditions may have impaired thermoregulatory function, including altered behavioral responses.

PATHOPHYSIOLOGY

Every organ system is affected by hypothermia. In general, body temperatures from 32 to 35°C (90 to 95°F) are considered to be ''mild'' hypothermia. In this temperature range, the patient is in an excitation (responsive) stage, in which physiologic adjustments attempt to retain and generate heat.

When temperature drops below 32°C, general excitation gives way to the slowing (adynamic) stage, in which there is a progressive slowdown of bodily functions. Metabolism slows, causing a decrease in both oxygen utilization and CO_2 production. Shivering ceases when body temperature falls below 30 to 32°C (86 to 90°F).

Hypothermia has a number of clinically important effects on the cardiovascular system. In the initial excitation phase, heart rate, cardiac output, and blood pressure all rise. With decreasing temperature, these parameters all decline. Cardiac output and blood

Table 43-2. ECG Changes in Hypothermia

T wave inversions
PR, QRS, QT prolongation
Muscle tremor artifact
Osborn (J) wave
Arrhythmias:
   Sinus bradycardia
   Atrial fibrillation or flutter
   Nodal rhythms
   AV block
   PVCs
   Ventricular fibrillation
   Asystole

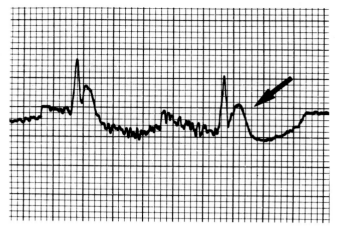

Figure 43-1. Rhythm strip from patient with temperature of 25°C (77°F), showing atrial fibrillation with a slow ventricular response, muscle tremor artifact, and Osborn (J) wave (arrow).

pressure may be markedly depressed by the negative inotropic and chronotropic effects of hypothermia, and further depressed by concomitant hypovolemia.

Hypothermia causes characteristic ECG changes, and may induce life-threatening arrhythmias (Table 43-2). The Osborn (J) wave, a slow positive deflection at the end of the QRS complex (Fig. 43-1), is characteristic, though not pathognomonic, of hypothermia.

Patients are at risk for arrhythmias at body temperatures below 30°C (86°F), and the risk of arrhythmias increases as body temperature falls. Although the various arrhythmias may arise at any time, the typical sequence is a progression from sinus bradycardia to atrial fibrillation with a slow ventricular response, to ventricular fibrillation, and, ultimately, to asystole. The hypothermic myocardium is extremely irritable, and ventricular fibrillation may be induced by a variety of manipulations and interventions which stimulate the heart, including rough handling of the patient.

Pulmonary effects of hypothermia include an initial tachypnea, followed by a progressive decrease in respiratory rate and tidal volume. Cold-induced bronchorrhea, along with a depression of cough and gag reflexes, makes aspiration pneumonia a common complication of hypothermia.

Much attention has been paid to the temperature correction of arterial blood gases in the hypothermic patient, yet the interpretation of blood gases remains problematic. Since the blood gas analyzer warms the blood to 37°C, thus increasing the partial pressure of dissolved gases, the machine will report a higher P_{O_2} and P_{CO_2}, and lower pH, than the actual values at the patient's body temperature. Correction factors and nomograms are available to determine the actual values in the patient's body; however, the ''normal'' values in hypothermia are not known. The simplest solution may be to use the uncorrected values as if the patient were normothermic. P_{CO_2} is often quite low secondary to depressed metabolism and decreased CO_2 production, and iatrogenic hyperventilation may lead to marked respiratory alkalosis.

Hypothermia causes a leftward shift of the oxyhemoglobin dissociation curve, potentially impairing oxygen release to tissues. These patients may have minimal oxygen reserve despite diminished oxygen requirements, warranting the administration of supplemental oxygen.

The central nervous system is affected by hypothermia, with a progressive depression of level of consciousness with decreasing temperature. Mild incoordination is followed by confusion, lethargy, and coma; pupils may be dilated and unreactive. These changes are associated with a decrease in cerebral blood flow. An even greater decrease in cerebral oxygen requirements may protect the brain against anoxic or ischemic damage.

Hypothermia impairs renal concentrating abilities and induces a "cold diuresis," leading to significant volume losses. Because of this concentrating defect, urine flow and specific gravity are unreliable indicators of intravascular volume and circulatory status. The immobile hypothermic patient is prone to rhabdomyolysis, and acute tubular necrosis may occur because of myoglobinuria and renal hypoperfusion.

Intravascular volume is also lost due to a plasma shift to the extravascular space. The combination of hemoconcentration, cold-induced increase in blood viscosity, and poor circulation may lead to intravascular thrombosis and subsequent embolic complications. Disseminated intravascular coagulation may occur because of release of tissue thromboplastins into the bloodstream, especially when circulation is restored during rewarming.

Endocrine function is fairly well preserved at low body temperatures. Plasma cortisol and thyroid hormone levels are usually normal or elevated unless the patient has a preexisting deficiency. Glucose levels may be normal, low, or elevated. Though hyperglycemia is common due to decreased insulin release as well as decreased glucose utilization, hypoglycemia may occur in up to 40 percent of patients.

Acid-base disturbances are common in hypothermia but follow no uniform pattern, and must be assessed individually. Acidosis may occur owing to severe respiratory depression and CO_2 retention, and to lactic acid production from shivering and poor tissue perfusion. Alkalosis may result from diminished CO_2 production with low metabolic rates, or from iatrogenic hyperventilation or sodium bicarbonate administration.

Pancreatitis (not only hyperamylasemia but true pancreatic necrosis) may occur in hypothermia. Hepatic function is depressed by cold, so that drugs which are normally metabolized, conjugated, or detoxified by the liver (e.g., lidocaine) may rapidly accumulate to toxic levels.

Finally, local cold injury and frostbite need special attention.

DIAGNOSIS

The diagnosis of hypothermia is often not obvious; exposure to profound cold is *not* necessary to produce hypothermia. Since standard clinical thermometers record only to 34.4°C (94°F), low-reading thermometers are required to accurately measure and monitor the temperature of hypothermic patients. Special low-reading glass and electronic thermometers are manufactured for this purpose, and should be available in every emergency department. Electronic thermometers with flexible rectal probes are often obtainable in a hospital's operating suite.

MANAGEMENT

The treatment of the hypothermic patient includes both general supportive measures and specific rewarming techniques. Therapy begins with careful, gentle handling; as mentioned above, almost any manipulation can precipitate ventricular fibrillation in the ir-

ritable hypothermic myocardium. Oxygen and intravenous fluids should be warmed, and patients should have constant monitoring of their core temperature, cardiac rhythm, urine output, and (in moderate to severe hypothermia) central venous pressure. In general, indications for endotracheal intubation are the same as in the normothermic patient. Concern has been raised regarding induction of arrhythmias during intubation; however, recent studies have shown a very low complication rate with gentle intubation after oxygenation.

Although arrhythmias in the hypothermic patient may represent an immediate threat to life, most rhythm disturbances (e.g., sinus bradycardia, atrial fibrillation or flutter) require no therapy and revert spontaneously with rewarming. In addition, the activity of antiarrhythmic and cardioactive drugs is unpredictable in hypothermia, and the hypothermic heart is relatively resistant to atropine, pacing, and countershock.

Ventricular fibrillation is often refractory to therapy until the patient is rewarmed. The patient in ventricular fibrillation should receive one or two attempts at electrical defibrillation. If this is unsuccessful, CPR should be instituted and rapid rewarming begun. As the myocardium warms, the rhythm may revert spontaneously or in response to electrical defibrillation.

Drug Therapy

Because a large proportion of hypothermic patients are thiamine-depleted alcoholics (and because Wernicke's disease may cause hypothermia), patients should be given supplemental intravenous thiamine, followed by 50 to 100 mL of 50% dextrose.

Administration of antibiotics, steroids, and thyroid hormone must be individualized. Serious, often occult, infections may either precipitate or complicate hypothermia. Though antibiotics are generally withheld until a definite infection is evident, a thorough search for infectious complications is clearly indicated.

As mentioned previously, serum cortisol is usually normal or elevated. Routine steroid therapy is generally not indicated, but hydrocortisone (100 mg) should be given to the patient with a history of adrenal suppression or insufficiency preceding the hypothermic episode, as well as to the patient with myxedema coma.

Hypothermia and hypothyroidism share many clinical features. While the majority of patients with myxedema coma are hypothermic, only a small minority of hypothermic patients are hypothyroid; thyroid hormone levels are most often normal or elevated. Thyroxine in large doses is necessary for the patient in myxedema coma, but may be quite harmful to other hypothermic patients. Therefore, thyroid hormone replacement is indicated only in patients with a known history of hypothyroidism, a thyroidectomy scar, or other strong clinical evidence of myxedema coma.

Rewarming Techniques

Modalities available for rewarming are listed in Table 43-3. The choice of rewarming method is a matter of great controversy. There are no prospective, controlled studies comparing the various rewarming methods in humans, and each method has its own advantages and disadvantages.

Passive rewarming allows patients to rewarm on their own, using endogenous heat produced by metabolism. Since patients often become hypothermic over a period of hours to days, slow

Table 43-3. Rewarming Techniques

Passive rewarming:
   Removal from cold environment
   Insulation
Active external rewarming:
   Warm water immersion
   Heating blankets
   Heated objects (water bottles, etc.)
Active core rewarming:
   Inhalation rewarming
   Heated IV fluids
   GI tract irrigation
   Peritoneal dialysis
   Hemodialysis
   Extracorporeal rewarming

passive rewarming is physiologically sound, avoiding rapid changes in cardiovascular status and the complications associated with active rewarming methods. However, temperature rises slowly with this method, and passive rewarming may be inappropriate for patients with cardiovascular compromise.

Active external rewarming (application of exogenous heat to the body) is often rapidly effective in raising body temperature, and has been used successfully in many patients. However, this method has several potential disadvantages. Application of external heat may cause peripheral vasodilation, returning stagnant, cold blood to the core. While warming the periphery, this may paradoxically cause central cooling (called *core temperature afterdrop*), potentially leading to arrhythmias. The peripheral vasodilation and venous pooling can lead to a relative hypovolemia and "rewarming shock." Washout of lactic acid from the peripheral tissues may lead to "rewarming acidosis," and an increase in metabolic demands of the periphery before the hypothermic heart can provide adequate tissue perfusion may lead to further tissue hypoxia and acidosis. Finally, resuscitation and monitoring of a patient immersed in warm water are technically difficult.

Active core rewarming has several theoretical advantages. Internal organs including the heart are preferentially rewarmed, decreasing myocardial irritability and returning cardiac function. Peripheral vasodilation is avoided, decreasing the incidence and magnitude of core temperature afterdrop, rewarming shock, and acidosis. However, some internal rewarming techniques are invasive and may be difficult to institute.

Inhalation rewarming—administration of warmed, humidified oxygen via mask or endotracheal tube—provides a fairly small heat gain, and is not effective for rapid rewarming. This is an important modality, however, as it minimizes heat loss from the lungs, a potential loss of up to 30 percent of the total metabolic heat production. Similarly, IV fluids should be warmed to avoid further cooling by the administration of fluids at room temperature.

GI tract (gastric or colonic) irrigation with warmed saline is technically simple, and patients can be lavaged with large volumes of fluid in a short time period. Care must be taken with the obtunded hypothermic patient, who may develop pulmonary aspiration if lavaged with an unprotected airway.

Peritoneal dialysis affords more rapid rewarming than any of the above internal modalities. It is widely available, and may be instituted rapidly and with little technical difficulty. It has been shown to be effective in both animal studies and human applications, and offers several potential benefits; in addition to allowing relatively rapid rewarming, peritoneal dialysis can remove toxic drugs and correct electrolyte abnormalities. Standard dialysis solution is warmed to 40 to 45°C (104 to 113°F), rapidly instilled, and then removed.

Rapid internal rewarming can also be accomplished through an extracorporeal circuit, employing heated hemodialysis or partial cardiopulmonary bypass. This consists of an arteriovenous shunt with an interposed heat exchanger; most commonly, blood is routed from the femoral artery to the rewarming apparatus, and back to the femoral vein. Profoundly hypothermic patients may be rewarmed in a very short time period with this method. Specialized equipment and personnel are required, however, and lack of immediate availability often precludes the use of this technique.

Finally, mediastinal irrigation via open thoracotomy should be mentioned, as it has been used as a rewarming technique in a few patients. This procedure has many serious complications, and offers virtually no advantages over the aforementioned modalities.

Choice of Rewarming Method

In deciding which rewarming modalities to use in any given patient, one must consider the duration, degree, causes, and consequences of the hypothermic state. Patients who become acutely hypothermic (e.g., cold water immersion) have little disturbance of volume, electrolyte, and acid-base status; in these patients, rapid external rewarming is usually safe and successful.

Patients with mild hypothermia, who are still in the "excitation" stage, generally improve on their own, regardless of rewarming method. At temperatures above 30°C (86°F), the incidence of arrhythmias is low, and rapid rewarming is rarely necessary. Hypothermia may be associated with drug toxicity; if the drug is dialyzable, peritoneal dialysis or hemodialysis should be considered for both rewarming and drug removal.

By far the most important consideration is the patient's cardiovascular status. Patients with a stable cardiac rhythm (including sinus bradycardia and atrial fibrillation) and stable vital signs do not need rapid rewarming. In these patients, passive rewarming and noninvasive internal modalities (e.g., warm moist oxygen and warm IV fluids) should be employed.

Patients with cardiovascular insufficiency or instability, including persistent hypotension and life-threatening arrhythmias, need to be rewarmed rapidly. As discussed above, the best method remains to be definitively determined. Though active core rewarming offers several theoretical and practical advantages, proponents of active external rewarming point out its ease of application and many examples of clinical success. It should be remembered that multiple rewarming modalities can be used simultaneously.

PROGNOSIS

Those providing care for hypothermic patients must recognize the crucial importance of associated disease processes. As previously discussed, many hypothermic patients have severe infections or other life-threatening illnesses. Studies have shown that patients with "uncomplicated" hypothermia (usually alcoholics with cold exposure) have a fairly low mortality rate; patients with significant associated diseases have a much worse prognosis. In terms of ultimate outcome, the underlying disease process is far more important than the initial temperature or the rewarming method chosen. Therefore, evaluation and treatment of these patients must include a search for associated diseases as well as treatment of the hypothermia itself.

The protective effect of hypothermia may have an important influence on prognosis; decreased oxygen requirements can protect the brain and other organs against anoxic and ischemic damage. This means that the usual criteria indicating death or irreversibility of disease are not valid in the hypothermic patient, who may even survive prolonged cardiac arrest without neurologic sequelae.

Hypothermic patients may recover completely after presenting in a rigid, apneic state with fixed and dilated pupils. Recovery has been documented with core temperatures as low 16°C (61°F), with cardiac arrest for over 3 h, and with cold water submersion for 40 min. Death in hypothermia must be defined as a failure to revive with rewarming; resuscitative efforts should be continued until core temperature is at least 30 to 32°C (86 to 90°F).

No one is dead until warm and dead!

BIBLIOGRAPHY

General Reviews

Carden D, Doan L, Sweeney PH, et al: Hypothermia. *Ann Emerg Med* 11:497–503, 1982.

Fitzgerald FT, Jessop C: Accidental hypothermia: A report of 22 cases and review of the literature; in Stollerman GH (ed): *Advances in Internal Medicine* Chicago, Year Book, vol 27, 1982, pp 127–150.

Reuler JB: Hypothermia: Pathophysiology, clinical settings and management. *Ann Intern Med* 89:519–527, 1978.

Stine RJ: Accidental hypothermia. *JACEP* 6:413–416, 1977.

Clinical Series

Fitzgerald FT: Hypoglycemia and accidental hypothermia in an alcoholic population. *West J Med* 133:105–107, 1980.

Hudson LD, Conn RD: Accidental hypothermia: Associated diagnoses and prognosis in a common problem. *JAMA* 227:37–40, 1974.

Miller JW, Danzl DF, Thomas DM: Urban accidental hypothermia: 135 cases. *Ann Emerg Med* 9:456–461, 1980.

O'Keeffe KM: Accidental hypothermia: A review of 62 cases. *JACEP* 6:491–496, 1977.

Weyman AE, Greenbaum DM, Grace WJ: Accidental hypothermia in an alcoholic population. *Am J Med* 56:13–21, 1974.

White JD: Hypothermia: The Bellevue experience. *Ann Emerg Med* 11:417–424, 1982.

Causes, Consequences, and Physiologic Effects of Hypothermia

Black PR, Van Devanter S, Cohn LH: Effects of hypothermia on systemic and organ system metabolism and function. *J Surg Res* 20:49–63, 1976.

Freinkel N, Metzger BE, Harris E, et al: The hypothermia of hypoglycemia. *N Engl J Med* 287:841–845, 1972.

Kearsley JH, Musso AF: Hypothermia and coma in the Wernicke-Korsakoff syndrome. *Med J Aust* 2:504–506, 1980.

Lewin S, Brettman LR, Holzman RS: Infections in hypothermic patients. *Arch Intern Med* 141:920–925, 1981.

Lloyd EL, Mitchell B: Factors affecting the onset of ventricular fibrillation in hypothermia. *Lancet* 2:1294–1295, 1974.

Ream AK, Reitz BA, Silverberg G: Temperature correction of P_{CO_2} and pH in estimating acid-base status: An example of the emperor's new clothes? *Anesthesiology* 56:41–44, 1982.

Tabaddor K, Gardner TJ, Walker AE: Cerebral circulation and metabolism at deep hypothermia. *Neurology* 22:1065–1070, 1972.

Wong KC: Physiology and pharmacology of hypothermia. *West J Med* 138:227–232, 1983.

ECG Changes

Clements SD, Hurst JW: Diagnostic value of electrocardiographic abnormalities observed in subjects accidentally exposed to cold. *Am J Cardiol* 29:729–734, 1972.

Thompson R, Rich J, Chmelik F, et al: Evolutionary changes in the electrocardiogram of severe progressive hypothermia. *J Electrocardiol* 10:67–70, 1977.

Trevino A, Razi B, Beller BM: The characteristic electrocardiogram of accidental hypothermia. *Arch Intern Med* 127:470–473, 1971.

Rewarming Modalities

Edwards RD: Accidental hypothermia. *JACEP* 6:426–427, 1977.

Frank DH, Robson MC: Accidental hypothermia treated without mortality. *Surg Gynecol Obstet* 151:379–381, 1980.

Gregory RT, Patton JF, McFadden TT: Cardiovascular effects of arterio-venous shunt rewarming following experimental hypothermia. *Surgery* 73:561–571, 1973.

Morrison JB, Conn ML, Hayward JS: Thermal increment provided by inhalation rewarming from hypothermia. *J Appl Physiol* 46:1061–1065, 1979.

Myers RAM, Britten JS, Cowley RA: Hypothermia: Quantitative aspects of therapy. *JACEP* 8:523–527, 1979.

Reuler JB, Parker RA: Peritoneal dialysis in the management of hypothermia. *JAMA* 240:2289–2290, 1978.

Welton DE, Mattox KL, Miller RR, et al: Treatment of profound hypothermia. *JAMA* 240:2291–2292, 1978.

Wickstrom P, Ruiz E, Lilja GP, et al: Accidental hypothermia: Core rewarming with partial bypass. *Am J Surg* 131:622–625, 1976.

Protective Effect of Hypothermia and Value of Prolonged CPR

Davee TS, Reineberg EJ: Extreme hypothermia and ventricular fibrillation. *Ann Emerg Med* 9:100–102, 1980.

Schissler P, Parker MA, Scott SJ: Profound hypothermia: Value of prolonged cardiopulmonary resuscitation. *South Med J* 74:474–477, 1981.

Sekar TS, MacDonnell KF, Namsirikul P, et al: Survival after prolonged submersion in cold water without neurologic sequelae. *Arch Intern Med* 140:775–779, 1980.

Southwick FS, Dalglish PH: Recovery after prolonged asystolic cardiac arrest in profound hypothermia. *JAMA* 243:1250–1253, 1980.

CHAPTER 44
HEAT EMERGENCIES

Michael Vance

It does not take long either to boil an egg or to cook neurones.

(D. Hamilton. *Anesthesia* 31:271, 1976.)

Body temperature is dependent on the balance between heat production and heat loss, and is maintained within narrow limits through a variety of mechanisms. Under normal circumstances, metabolic activity is the sole source of heat production. Therefore, increased metabolic activity (for example, during strenuous exercise) will result in increased body temperature. However, as ambient temperature approaches and exceeds normal body temperature, an additional source of body heat is provided by the surrounding atmosphere.

Heat loss is accomplished by radiation, convection, conduction, and evaporation. Responses to core temperature changes are directed by the anterior hypothalamus, and are mediated via the endocrine system, the autonomic nervous system, and neuromuscular activity. The primary response to increased core body temperature is cutaneous vasodilation, resulting in greater heat transfer from the skin to the atmosphere. However, as ambient temperature approaches body temperature, heat loss becomes increasingly dependent on evaporation of sweat produced by the activity of cholinergic sympathetic nerve fibers. The efficiency of evaporative heat loss is in turn influenced greatly by ambient humidity.

The body's temperature-regulating system generally functions well in the face of diverse metabolic and environmental conditions, and the human system is remarkably capable of adapting to dramatic changes through the process of acclimatization. Acclimatization occurs gradually over a period of days to weeks, and primarily involves alterations of sodium and water balance mediated by aldosterone. When a human being is initially exposed to a hot and humid environment, sodium and water are lost through sweating. In addition, blood is shunted to the skin to aid in heat dissipation. The net result is contraction of the extracellular fluid volume, decreased renal plasma flow, and consequently an increase in aldosterone secretion. The concentration of sodium in urine and sweat then decreases markedly (although potassium losses continue). Sodium retention results in expansion of extracellular fluid volume, and, at some point, acclimatization to the new environment is completed.

Heat cramps, heat exhaustion, and heatstroke develop from the inability to respond adequately to environmental conditions, inadequate correction of fluid and electrolyte deficiencies, and malfunction of the system through exogenous or endogenous causes. While one mechanism may predominate in one or the other heat disorders, multiple factors are most commonly responsible.

There is a great deal of overlap and interrelationship among all the heat disorders, and any particular patient may present a mixed picture. A number of predisposing factors are common to all forms of heat-related emergencies (Table 44-1). Obviously, anyone involved in physical exertion in a hot, humid environment, whether indoors or outdoors, is at risk for any of the heat disorders. As ambient temperature or humidity increases, and/or if the level of exercise is increased, the risk of a heat disorder increases proportionately, even among well-acclimatized persons. Other important factors are obesity, fatigue, alcoholism, and cardiovascular disease.

Certain drugs contribute to the development of heat disorders, particularly those such as the phenothiazines that alter the response of the hypothalamus (most likely through dopaminergic-blocking effects), and those such as the tricyclic antidepressants, whose anticholinergic properties may interfere with sweating (Table 44-2).

HEAT CRAMPS

Heat cramps are generally associated with strenuous physical activity. They are characterized by painful spasm of skeletal muscles, including muscles of the extremities and abdomen. The production of large amounts of sweat, which has a high sodium content, coupled with inadequate sodium replacement (typically through drinking tap water or other salt-poor fluid) results in hyponatremia leading to muscle cramps. Another factor which may contribute to the development of heat cramps is hyperventilation, which occurs commonly in association with the heat syndromes. Possibly due to the local accumulation of lactate, hyperventilation produces respiratory alkalosis, and an associated hypokalemia (due to

Table 44-1. Risk Factors Associated with Heat Emergencies

Age
  Infants (greater sweat losses, poorly developed compensatory
    mechanisms)
  Elderly (cardiovascular disease, multiple drug therapies)
Environment
  High ambient temperature
  High ambient humidity
Occupation
  Athletes:
    Professional, college, high school, "weekend" athletes
  Sports associated with strenuous exercise, brief bursts of high
    exertion, i.e., football, tennis; prolonged exertion, i.e., jogging,
    cross-country running
  Laborers:
    Construction workers
    Miners
  Military:
    New recruits
Pharmacologic factors
  Drugs with central effect on hypothalamus:
    Phenothiazine model
  Drugs with peripheral (anticholinergic) effects on sweat glands
  Tricyclic antidepressants
  Lithium intoxication
  Malignant hyperpyrexia following exposure to general anesthetics,
    i.e., halothane, succinylcholine; caffeine; potassium; and in patients
    with preexisting myopathies
Psychological factors
  Belief in the invulnerability of the young
  Peer pressure and competitive drive in real or imagined competition
  Voluntary restriction of fluid intake
Miscellaneous physical factors
  Alcoholism
  Illness, chronic or recent
  Inadequate electrolyte replacement
  Lack of acclimatization to heat stress
  Lack of exercise
  Lack of sleep
  Obesity
  Restrictive clothing
Sweat gland abnormalities:
  Congenital anhidrosis
  Cystic fibrosis
  Quadriplegia

intracellular potassium shifts) may contribute to the development of muscle cramps, paresthesias, and tetany.

Clinically, body temperature is normal, and there is generally no evidence of dehydration. Laboratory studies may show hyponatremia, hypokalemia, and respiratory alkalosis.

While painful, heat cramps are a benign entity and are effectively treated by oral or intravenous electrolyte replacement. However, episodes of muscular pain due to exertional rhabdomyolysis may be misdiagnosed as heat cramps. The serum creatine phosphokinase level is elevated, and there may be myoglobinuria if rhabdomyolysis is present.

HEAT EXHAUSTION

Heat exhaustion is characterized by volume depletion. Fluid and electrolyte losses due to sweating, coupled with inadequate re-

placement, may result in hypovolemia and tissue hypoperfusion.

The signs and symptoms of heat exhaustion are variable. Early complaints of fatigue may progress to light-headedness, nausea and vomiting, severe headache, and, finally, evidence of significant volume depletion with tachycardia, hyperventilation, and hypotension. The body temperature is normal or slightly elevated and there may be profuse sweating.

Laboratory studies will almost universally demonstrate hemoconcentration, although specific electrolyte abnormalities depend on the ratio of fluid and electrolyte losses to intake.

The definitive treatment of heat exhaustion is rest coupled with volume replacement. Rapid administration of moderate amounts of intravenous fluids may be necessary in occasional patients who demonstrate significant tissue hypoperfusion. The choice of solution is guided by laboratory determinations, but balanced salt solutions may be utilized until specific electrolyte abnormalities are determined to be present.

HEATSTROKE

Heatstroke is defined as the combination of hyperpyrexia [often to 41°C (106°F) or greater] and neurological symptoms. Lack of sweating is not an absolute diagnostic criterion. In contradistinction to heat cramps and heat exhaustion, heatstroke is a true medical emergency which may result in significant morbidity and mortality.

Risk factors associated with heat emergencies are summarized in Table 44-1. The central nervous system is particularly vulnerable to heatstroke. The clinical onset of heatstroke begins with an

Table 44-2. Drugs That Have Caused Heatstroke

Anticholinergic drugs:
  Atropine
  Scopolamine
  Benztropine mesylate (Cogentin)
Phenothiazine derivatives:
  Chlorpromazine (Thorazine)
  Mepazine (Pacatal)
Tricyclic antidepressants:
  Amitriptyline (Elavil)
  Desmethylimipramine (Norpramin)
  Imipramine (Tofranil)
  Nortriptyline (Aventyl)
  Protriptyline (Vivactil)
Monoamine oxidase inhibitors:
  Isocarboxazid (Marplan)
  Nialamide (Niamid)
  Phenelzine (Nardil)
  Tranylcypromine (Parnate)
Glutethimide (Doriden)
Lysergic acid diethylamide (LSD)
Amphetamine
Inhalation anesthetic:
  Ether
  Ethylchloride
  Halothane
  Nitrous oxide
Suxamethonium chloride (succinylcholine)

Source: From Shibolet S, Lancaster MC, Danon Y: Heat stroke: A review. *Aviat Space Environ Med* 47:281, 1976. Used by permission.

alteration of neurological function, frequently manifested by a sudden loss of consciousness with little or no prodrome. Irritability, bizarre behavior, combativeness, hallucinations, or coma may occur. Virtually any neurological abnormality may be present, including plantar responses, pupillary abnormalities, decorticate and decerebrate posturing, hemiplegia, and status epilepticus.

The mixed neurological picture associated with hyperpyrexia may present the clinician with a difficult "chicken-egg" problem, since cerebrovascular accidents may be accompanied by high fever. However, it cannot be overemphasized that a sudden alteration of consciousness in a setting of heat exposure must suggest the possibility of heatstroke, and prompt measurement of core temperature should follow. There are probably many episodes of early heatstroke that go unrecognized because mental status improves after cessation of exercise and removal of the patient from the hot environment. The patient may never seek medical care, or if the patient does consult a physician, the core temperature may not be measured or it may have declined by the time of evaluation. In addition, mild cases of heatstroke with cerebral dysfunction may occur at a much lower temperature than expected. In at least one study of volunteers undergoing heat stress, alteration of consciousness was produced when rectal temperature was 39.1°C (102.4°F).

The presence or absence of sweating has classically been one of the important distinctions between true heatstroke and the other heat emergencies. However, patients with early heatstroke may well demonstrate marked sweating, although many patients will at some point lose their ability to sweat and demonstrate the characteristic of hot, dry skin. The exact mechanism of the breakdown of the sweating mechanism is unclear, although direct thermal injury to the sweat glands is certainly an important factor. However, whatever the temporal relationship between the onset of clinical heatstroke and the failure of the sweating mechanism, there is no doubt that any abnormality of this organ system is an important contributing factor in the development of heatstroke. While an occasional patient with a rare problem such as congenital absence of sweat glands, cystic fibrosis, or quadriplegia will be encountered, the most common cause of impaired sweating is the administration of medications with anticholinergic properties.

Non-exercise-induced heatstroke may be encountered in the elderly or chronically debilitated patient whose cardiovascular system is unable to meet the metabolic demands of a hot environment. Exercise-induced heatstroke typically occurs in previously healthy persons under a wide variety of circumstances. In the greater Phoenix area, for example, roofers have the highest incidence of heatstroke, followed closely by tennis players. Regardless of the environmental setting or the presence or absence of predisposing or contributing factors, elevation of the core body temperature to critical levels results in widespread and disastrous effects on most body tissues. Temperatures in the range of 42°C (107.6°F) and above are associated with a poor prognosis, although clinical signs and symptoms may occur at much lower levels.

The status of the cardiovascular system is an important factor in the development of heatstroke. This is particularly true in the elderly and in other patient populations with preexistent cardiovascular disease. In the patient with a relatively intact cardiovascular response, heat stress will promote heat loss, with an increase in heart rate, cardiac index, and central venous pressure as a response to peripheral vasodilation. However, heart failure, pulmonary edema, and cardiovascular collapse can occur in young,

otherwise healthy persons suffering heatstroke. In any age group, the presence of hypotension, decreased cardiac output, and a falling cardiac index indicates a particularly poor prognosis.

Hepatic and renal abnormalities may also be found in patients with heatstroke. Centrilobular necrosis due to direct thermal injury results in abnormal liver function studies, although recovery is to be expected. Jaundice is unusual. Microscopic hematuria, proteinuria, and casts develop rapidly. Severe cases, especially those complicated by hypovolemia and a decreased renal blood flow, may progress to acute tubular necrosis (ATN) and renal failure. Exercise-induced heatstroke is often complicated by rhabdomyolysis, sometimes with massive myoglobinuria and renal failure.

Widespread hematologic disorders may be apparent both clinically and on laboratory evaluation. Purpura, conjunctival hemorrhages, petechiae, and pulmonary, gastrointestinal, and renal hemorrhages may be present. Coagulation studies may show decreased platelets, hypoprothrombinemia, and hypofibrinogenemia. Thermal injury to the vascular endothelium causes increased platelet aggregation, changes in capillary permeability, thermal deactivation of plasma proteins resulting in a decreased level of clotting factors, and, rarely, disseminated intravascular coagulation or fibrinolysis.

As expected, the fluid and electrolyte abnormalities vary with the onset and duration of the disorder, underlying disease (especially cardiovascular disease), and prior use of medications such as diuretics. The most important consideration with respect to fluid and electrolyte abnormalities in heatstroke is that dehydration and volume depletion may not occur in classic heatstroke, whereas they are common signs of heat exhaustion. Vigorous fluid administration may produce pulmonary edema, especially in the elderly. A myriad of blood gas abnormalities may be encountered, from respiratory alkalosis to severe metabolic acidosis.

Treatment

Once the diagnosis of heatstroke is made or suspected, rapid, aggressive therapy aimed at lowering the body temperature should be initiated immediately by whatever means available, whether in the prehospital or emergency department setting. In the field, remove the patient from external sources of heat; remove clothing; and promote evaporative cooling by applying cool or iced water to the entire skin surface by sponging or splashing, followed by fanning either by hand or mechanical means. This should be continued throughout transportation to an emergency receiving facility, and should be continued within the facility as well. There are a number of disadvantages to the use of an iced bath: it is more difficult to handle the patient; peripheral vasoconstriction may decrease heat transfer to the skin surface, although this may be overcome somewhat by vigorous skin massage; and intense shivering may actually increase endogenous heat production.

Intense shivering during any form of cooling therapy may be controlled with diazepam or chlorpromazine. While the latter is known to produce hyperpyrexia itself, this is believed to be due to effects on the hypothalamus, and is probably not a significant factor when external, artificial cooling methods are utilized. Hypothermia blankets and ice packs to the groin and axillae are also useful. Additional methods such as iced water gastric lavage and enemas, iced water peritoneal dialysis, and intratracheal administration of cold helium have also been suggested as methods of promoting heat transfer from the body, but are not widely used. Antipyretics such as salicylates have not proved useful in treating heatstroke.

While the rapid reduction of body temperature is the primary goal, additional supportive measures may be established early in the course of treatment, including oxygen therapy in conjunction with endotracheal intubation if necessary. An intravenous line, preferably a central venous pressure line, should be established, since most patients with true heatstroke do not have large fluid requirements. Early baseline determinations of clotting parameters and electrolyte levels, hepatic and renal studies, and a serum glucose level should be obtained. When blood gases are obtained, inform the laboratory of the patient's body temperature so that the appropriate corrections can be made (Table 44-3). Specific complications, such as heart failure, cardiovascular collapse, hepatic or renal failure, and myoglobinemia and myoglobinuria may be treated by standard approaches. Patients with depleted clotting factors must be carefully evaluated. Generally, they can be managed by administering platelets and fresh-frozen plasma.

Table 44-3. Temperature Correction Factors for pH, P_{O_2}, and P_{CO_2}*

Temperature				
°C	°F	pH	P_{O_2}	P_{CO_2}
28	82.4	1.0179	0.5333	0.6538
29	84.2	1.0165	0.5666	0.6923
30	86	1.0138	0.6083	0.7230
30.5	86.9	1.0131	0.6333	0.7384
31	87.8	1.0124	0.6583	0.7538
32	89.6	1.0096	0.7000	0.8000
33	91.4	1.0082	0.7500	0.8307
34	93.2	1.0055	0.8083	0.8769
35	95	1.0041	0.8666	0.9230
36	96.8	1.0027	0.9333	0.9538
37	98.6	1.0000	1.0000	1.0000
38	100.4	0.9986	1.0667	1.025
39	102.2	0.9972	1.1500	1.075
40	104	0.9945	1.2400	1.125
41	105.8	0.9932	1.3335	1.175
42	107.6	0.9905	1.4300	1.225

*To use: Multiply value determined at 37°C by corresponding body temperature (°C) to obtain corrected BTPS values. For example, as mentioned in the text concerning P_{O_2}, P_{CO_2}, and pH changes for temperature, an increase in temperature from 37°C (98.6°F) to 42°C (107.6°F) will produce only a 1 percent error in pH, but a 43 percent error in P_{O_2}, and a 23 percent error in P_{CO_2} unless corrected for temperature.

Source: Derived from Severinghaus JW: Blood gas calculator. *J Appl Physiol* 21:1108–1116, 1966.

OTHER CAUSES OF HYPERTHERMIA

In addition to heat syndromes resulting from heat exposure, there are a variety of other causes of hyperthermia. The first indication of many infectious diseases may be a markedly elevated temperature. A patient with severe dehydration may be hyperpyrexic because general hypoperfusion prevents effective dissipation of heat from the skin. Drugs producing an anticholinergic syndrome may cause hyperthermia through a combination of hypothalamic effects and decreased sweating. In fact, these patients, as well as those suffering from cerebrovascular accidents, including stroke and intracerebral or subarachnoid hemorrhage, may exhibit the classic signs of heatstroke: neurological dysfunction, hyperpyrexia, and hot, dry skin. When confronted with such a clinical picture, establishing a definitive diagnosis is difficult. It is most important to begin to aggressively lower the body temperature while awaiting resolution of the diagnostic problem.

Rarely, a person with a combination of underlying muscle disease and exposure to anesthetic agents may develop malignant hyperpyrexia, which is associated with an extremely high mortality.

BIBLIOGRAPHY

Barcenas C, Hoeffler HP, Lie JT: Obesity, football, dog days, and siriasis: A deadly combination. *Am Heart J* 92:237–244, 1976.

Boyd AE, Bellar GA: Heart exhaustion and respiratory alkalosis, letter to the editor. *Ann Intern Med* 83:835, 1975.

Clowes GH Jr, O'Donnell TF Jr: Heat stroke. *N Engl J Med* 291:564–567, 1974.

Conn JW: Aldosteronism in man. *JAMA* 183:775–781, 1963.

Denboroug MA: Malignant hyperpyrexia. *Frontiers in Medicine* (special issue) 51:56, 1976.

Ellis F: Heat wave deaths and drugs affecting temperature regulation. *Br Med J* 2(6033):474, 1976.

Forester D: Fatal drug-induced heat stroke. *JACEP* 7:243–344, 1978.

Hamilton D: The immediate treatment of heat stroke. *Anaesthesia* 31:270–272, 1976.

Knochel JP: Environmental heat illness. *Arch Intern Med* 133:841–864, 1974.

O'Donnell TF Jr: Acute heat stroke: Epidemiologic, biochemical, renal, and coagulation studies. *JAMA* 234:824–828, 1975.

Shibolet S, Lancaster MC, Danon Y: Heat stroke: A review. *Aviat Space Environ Med* 47:286–301, 1976.

Stine RJ: Heat illness. *JACEP* 8:154–160, 1979.

Tintinalli JE (ed): Heat stroke. *JACEP* 5:525–528, 1976.

Wadlington WB, Tucker A: Heat stroke in infancy. *Am J Dis Child* 130:1250–1251, 1976.

Wheeler M: Heat stroke in the elderly. *Med Clin North Am* 60:1289–1296, 1976.

CHAPTER 45
HUMAN AND
ANIMAL BITES

George Podgorny

HUMAN BITES

In addition to injury of the skin and soft tissues, infection must be considered as a complication in the treatment of a human bite. The human oral cavity is heavily populated with aerobic and anaerobic microorganisms, including fusospirochetes; as a result, infections of human bites are common.

The scalp and the dorsum of the hand are the most common locations of human bites. Scalp bites are frequent in children, while hand bites generally occur from contact between a closed fist of one individual and the open mouth of another. Other common locations of human bites include the penis, scrotum, vulva, breasts, ear, nose, and forearm.

Frequently, the injury is not reported as a human bite and is even vociferously denied to have been produced by the human mouth. Therefore, when treating cuts, scratches, and lacerations of the scalp, dorsum of the hand, or genitalia, consider the possibility that they were produced by a human bite.

A variety of organisms have been recovered from the human mouth and from cutaneous infections caused by human bites. These include aerobic and anaerobic streptococci, *Staphylococcus aureus*, other gram-positive cocci, gram-negative rods, and *bacteroides* species, among others.

Treatment

A wound due to a human bite should be meticulously cleaned and irrigated with copious amounts of sterile saline solution. Saline or other cleansing fluid should be poured perpendicularly or tangentially over the wound. Very small wounds can be irrigated with a syringe, directing the stream into the depth of the puncture wound. Devices are available that generate a steady or intermittent stream for irrigation. After copious irrigation, sterile gauze pads can be used to gently but firmly rub the area of the wound to remove any loosened debris, followed by additional irrigation. Inspect the wound for tooth fragments and, if they are present, remove them. Sharply debride any loose skin tags or loose underlying soft tissue. If the wound appears minor, antibiotics can be withheld, and the patient instructed to return if signs of infec-

tion develop. With more extensive wounds, antibiotics are given because it can be assumed that significant bacterial contamination has occurred.

The decision to perform primary closure of a laceration secondary to a human bite depends on the clinical circumstance. Some physicians prefer to leave all such wounds open. This methodology is certainly acceptable with small lacerations on extremities and genitalia, particularly in males. More extensive or gaping lacerations secondary to a human bite on the face, neck, and hands, particularly in females, present serious cosmetic problems. After adequate cleansing and debriding, loosely close such lacerations with synthetic sutures (silk should be avoided because a granulomatous reaction may result). Antibiotic coverage should include a penicillinase-resistant penicillin or cephalosporin.

If a portion of a finger, ear, or nose is bitten off, instruct emergency medical technicians and law enforcement personnel to bring all tissue to the hospital. Skin from some severed portions of the body can be removed and used for full-thickness grafts. The ear or a portion of it can be denuded and the cartilage buried in the subcutaneous tissue of the abdomen until the basic wound has been healed. The cartilage can then be reimplanted and a full-thickness graft applied. Tetanus prophylaxis is indicated for all bites.

ANIMAL BITES

Despite the wide variety of animal bites that may be encountered, the management consists of cleansing, debriding and repair of skin and soft tissue injury, and the prevention and treatment of rabies, tetanus, and other specific infections peculiar to the biting animal. Rabies prevention is discussed below, and tetanus is discussed in the section of the *Study Guide* on infections. Remember that with all animal bites adequate protection against tetanus must be assured.

Dog Bites

The most common animal bite is a dog bite. Large dogs can inflict serious injuries including crushing injuries of the face, head, and limbs, particularly in children. A canine bite, as do those of any carnivore, presents a danger of gross contamination from flora of the animal's mouth. Various organisms, such as streptococci, staphylococci, diphtheroids, clostridia, and even gram-negative organisms, have been cultured from animal bite wounds. *Pasteurella multocida* is also a common pathogen. Although not necessarily transmitted by bites, leptospirosis, a disease formerly thought to be limited to people with specific occupations, such as sewer, rice, sugar cane, farm, and abattoir workers, is now frequently demonstrated to be acquired from family pets. Even a healthy, immunized dog can shed the organisms.

An as yet unidentified gram-negative bacillus has been recognized as the cause of occasional fatal infection in individuals who have been bitten by dogs, and whose immunologic defenses are weakened by chronic illness or splenectomy. According to Butler et al., this organism is sensitive to penicillin, tetracycline, and carbenicillin, but resistant to gentamicin, colistin, and kanamycin.

Closure of a dog bite wound is frequently debated. Small puncture wounds or lacerations can be cleaned and left open. Most lacerations, except those of the hand with potential for joint or tendon involvement, should be closed primarily after meticulous irrigation and debridement. Hand wounds should be cleaned, debrided, and explored. If tendon or joint involvement is suspected, they should be left open, and antibiotics administered. Primary closure of simple hand wounds is still controversial. Following cleansing, debridement, and repair, treatment with a broad-spectrum antibiotic may be instituted. Penicillinase-resistant penicillin or cephalosporins should be used pending cultures.

Cat Bites and Scratches

Cats usually injure by scratching rather than by biting. The contaminating organisms are similar to those in dog bites, and treatment is as outlined for dog bites, although *P. multocida* is more commonly found in cat bite infections. Cat-scratch fever is an ill-understood disease, most likely caused by a virus related to the lymphogranuloma-psittacosis group. It is basically a nonbacterial, chronic, regional lymphadenitis which develops secondary to a primary cutaneous lesion. Biopsy may be necessary to distinguish it from lymphoma. Similar lesions are observed in patients who have scratches from sources such as thorns and fragments of animal bones. Occasionally, the wound may become suppurative, and incision and drainage may be necessary. The antibiotic of choice is tetracycline.

Miscellaneous Small Animal Bites

Bites by squirrels, rats, chipmunks, bats, raccoons, and mice usually result in puncture wounds. Meticulous cleansing and debridement are required.

Large Animal Bites

Bites of lions, tigers, and bears are rare and usually occur in a zoo or animal park setting. Such injuries can be extensive and life-threatening.

Monkey bites are not rare in the United States because of the number of monkeys used for scientific and educational purposes, as well as those that are kept in zoos or as personal pets. Since the flora of the mouth of the monkey is similar to that of the human, a monkey bite is treated just as a human bite is treated. In addition, herpes simplex virus may be transmitted from Rhesus monkeys.

Cows, horses, and camels occasionally inflict bites. The main consideration of these wounds is their magnitude. In a camel bite, the injured part is usually the victim's face and the cranium. In certain parts of the world, the most common cause of skull fracture is a camel bite.

Injuries caused by large animals are frequently massive and require resuscitation for hemorrhagic shock, followed by major surgical repair.

Rabies

Rabies is one of the most serious complications of animal bites. Rabies, or hydrophobia, is a viral disease transmitted by saliva of infected animals through a break in the victim's skin or mucous membrane. The virus is harbored in warm-blooded animals, more specifically, in carnivores.

About 50,000 animal bite exposures with potential for rabies occur in humans per year. In 1978, the Center for Disease Control (CDC) reported 3182 laboratory-confirmed cases of rabies, with 4 cases occurring in humans. Seven kinds of animals were implicated in 97 percent of the cases. These were skunks, 51 percent; bats, 20 percent; raccoons, 9 percent; cattle, 6 percent; foxes, 4 percent; dogs, 4 percent; and cats, 3 percent. Cases were reported of rabid swine, horses, mules, sheep, goats, bobcats, wolves, weasels, opossum, otter, mink, and in Puerto Rico, mongooses. Rabies is extremely rare in rodents such as rats and squirrels.

Pathophysiology

The virus is harbored mostly in the salivary glands, but it is also found in the intestine, pancreas, renal tubules, and occasionally in the adrenal medulla.

Spread of the virus begins from the point of inoculation along sensory nerves, into the posterior column of the spinal cord, and into the brain. If the point of inoculation is on the face, the spread is by cranial nerves.

Negri bodies, a pathognomonic autopsy finding of rabies, are located in the brain of the animal who has the disease. Negri bodies are $\frac{1}{2}$ to 10 μm in diameter, stain eosinophilic, and are present in the cytoplasm of the neuron. They are most abundant in the hippocampus. The entire nervous system is subject to invasion by the rabies virus. Perivascular infiltration by mononuclear cells results in demyelinization, and focal inflammation and hemorrhage. This is particularly marked in the basal ganglia and the spinal cord.

An animal may be a carrier several days prior to the appearance of the signs of rabies, and during that time, although the virus is present in the saliva, the animal's behavior is normal. Once the animal's behavior changes, and drooling, salivation, and aggressiveness occur, the rabid state is then obvious.

A rabid dog appears agitated, has a feeble bark, and may wander aimlessly. An indiscriminate attack on everything moving is characteristic of this condition. As the disease progresses, frothing at the mouth, dysphagia, and convulsions develop. Eventually paralysis and stupor lead to death of the animal.

Clinical Features of Rabies in Humans

In unvaccinated individuals, the incidence of rabies following a bite of a rabid animal has been estimated from 5 to 70 percent, the average being about 15 percent.

Incubation is 30 to 60 days with a range of approximately 10 days to 1 year. Prodromal symptoms include headache, malaise, sore throat, cough, and low-grade fever. Tingling, paresthesias, and sharp pain occur at the site of the bite. Following this the first phase of rabies is characterized by excitement, agitation, and restlessness. Pacing and painful contraction of pharyngeal muscles, fear of water, and drooling are common. Initially, hydrophobia develops during attempts to swallow liquid, but is later triggered by the sight, sound, or even mention of water. Cranial nerve paralysis, generalized autonomic hyperactivity, and hyperpyrexia may develop. Occasionally in this phase, general convulsions occur that may terminate in apnea and death. In the second phase, there may be a general flaccid paralysis, similar to the Guillain-Barré syndrome, or Landry's ascending paralysis. Unlike tetanus, there is no trismus present. There is usually an elevated white blood cell count. The cerebrospinal fluid shows elevation of protein and mononuclear pleocytosis.

Differential diagnosis of rabies includes hysteria secondary to dog bite, allergic encephalomyelitis secondary to rabies vaccine, poliomyelitis, Guillain-Barré syndrome, tetanus, and delirium tremens.

Treatment—Postexposure Prophylaxis

The decision to institute postexposure treatment must be made immediately, for the longer treatment is delayed, the less likely it is to be effective.

Postexposure prophylaxis consists of thorough cleansing and debridement of the wound, tetanus prophylaxis and infection control, and a combination of active and passive immunization (Table 45-1).

Physical and chemical cleansing is an effective means of eliminating the rabies virus at the site of infection. Scrub the area with soap and water and rinse thoroughly with water or saline to remove traces of soap. Then apply 40 to 70% alcohol, tincture or aqueous iodine solution, or 0.1% benzalkonium chloride.

The products currently indicated in rabies prophylaxis are human diploid cell vaccine (HDCV) for active immunity, and rabies immune globulin (RIG) for passive immunization.

Active immunization (vaccine) is used as a precautionary measure following a bite by an animal in the suspected group, or as preexposure prophylaxis for individuals such as animal handlers and veterinarians. Passive immunization with rabies immune globulin is advised when the animal responsible is or may be rabid. A combination of passive and active immunization is the best postexposure prophylaxis.

Rabies immune globulin is human antirabies γ-globulin concentrated by cold ethanol fractionation from the plasma of hyperimmunized human donors. It is supplied in 2-mL (300-IU) or

Table 45-1. Postexposure Antirabies Treatment Guide

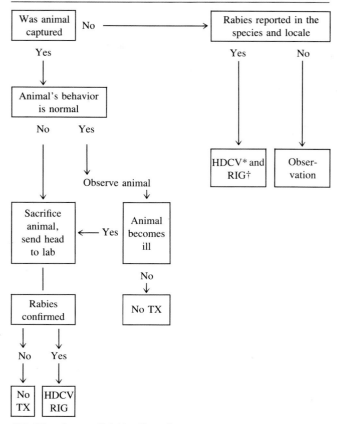

*HDCV = human diploid cell vaccine.
†RIG = rabies immune globulin.

10-mL (1500-IU) vials, and is available through the CDC and health departments of all the states and larger communities. The dose is 20 IU/kg. Half this dose is thoroughly infiltrated around the wound and the other half is given intramuscularly in the buttocks.

With the approval of human diploid cell vaccine by the FDA in 1980 we now have a safe, efficacious vaccine for the prophylaxis of rabies. Administration of HDCV is associated with protective antibody titers in a very high percentage of patients, while neuroparalytic and anaphylactic reactions are rare. Even local and systemic side effects are uncommon and mild with HDCV as opposed to previous vaccines. Postexposure prophylaxis consists of 5 intramuscular 1-mL vaccinations over a 28-day period. Following vaccination, antibody titers should be measured to assure protection; further immunizations are indicated if titers remain low. Preexposure protection may be indicated for those who are at risk of coming into contact with rabies.

Transmission may occur between humans as the virus can be isolated from the saliva of infected humans. Rabies has been transmitted via corneal transplant, and airborne transmission has been reported as well.

Rabies is a reportable disease. The physician should advise the patient and the public health department to secure the offending animal and observe it for approximately 2 weeks. Survival of the animal during this period indicates that the animal is not rabid. If the animal dies from any cause, postmortem examination of the animal's brain should be obtained. This can usually be arranged at laboratories of each state health department. If an offending wild animal can be captured or killed, its head should be sent to the proper laboratory for examination of the brain.

BIBLIOGRAPHY

Human Bite

Mann RJ, Hoffeld TA, Farmer CA: Human bites of the hand: Twenty years of experience. *J Hand Surg* 2:97–104, 1977.

Dog Bite

Butler T, Weaver RE, Ramani V, et al: Unidentified gram-negative rod infection: A new disease of man. *Ann Intern Med* 86:1–5, 1977.

Callaham ML: Treatment of common dog bites: Infection risk factors. *JACEP* 7:83–87, 1978.

Feigin RD, Lobes LA Jr, Anderson D, et al: Human leptospirosis from immunized dogs. *Ann Intern Med* 79:777–785, 1973.

Kizer KW: Epidemiologic and clinical aspects of animal bite injuries. *JACEP* 8:134–141, 1979.

Schultz RC, McMaster WC: The treatment of dog bite injuries, especially of the face. *Plast Reconstr Surg* 49:494–500, 1972.

Thompson HG, Svitek V: Small animal bite: The role of primary closure. *J Trauma* 13:20–23, 1973.

Cat-Scratch Disease

Margileth AM: Cat-scratch disease: Non-bacterial regional lymphadenitis: The study of 145 patients and a review of the literature. *Pediatrics* 42:803–818, 1968.

Lindsey D, Hirsch F: The infected cat bite. Type case of *Pasteurella multocida* infection. *Ariz Med* 38:623–625, 1976.

Veitch JM, Omer GE: Case report: Treatment of catbite injuries of the hand. *J Trauma* 19:201–202, 1979.

Rabies

Baer GM: Advances in postexposure rabies vaccination: A review. *Am J Clin Pathol* 70:(suppl):185–187, 1978.

Miller A, Nathanson N: Rabies: Recent advances in pathogenesis and control. *Ann Neurol* 2:511–519, 1977.

Plotkin SA, Wiktor T: Rabies vaccination. *Ann Rev Med* 29:583–591, 1978.

Rabies: Risk management, prophylaxis, and immunization. Public Health Service Advisory Committee on Immunization Practices. *Ann Intern Med* 86:452–455, 1977.

Recommendation of the Public Health Service Advisory Committee on Immunization Practices: *Rabies*. Atlanta, Center for Disease Control, April 1977.

Surveillance Summary Rabies—United States, 1977. *Morbid Mortal Weekly Rep* 27:499–501, 1978.

Warrell DA: The clinical picture of rabies in man. *Trans R Soc Trop Med Hyg* 70:188–195, 1976.

World Health Organization: *Sixth Report of the Expert Committee on Rabies*. Geneva, WHO Techn Rep No 523, 1973.

CHAPTER 46
INSECTS, TICKS,
AND SPIDERS

A. Insect Stings and Bites

Claude Frazier

Toxic reactions to multiple stings by members of the order of Hymenoptera and severe systemic reactions to one or two stings or to bites of some other insects such as deerflies, blackflies, horseflies, and kissing bugs can both present an emergency, life-threatening situation. (See Table 46A-1 for a listing of harmful arthropods of the United States.) However, fatalities due to biting insects are far rarer than those caused by the venom of Hymenoptera.

HYMENOPTERA STINGS

The normal response to Hymenoptera venom consists of pain, slight erythema, and some edema at the sting site, followed usually by pruritus.

Type of Reaction

Local reaction. A local reaction consists of marked and prolonged edema contiguous with the sting site. There are no systemic signs or symptoms, although a severe local reaction may involve one or more neighboring joints. The seriousness of a local reaction depends upon the sting location. For example, a local reaction occurring in the mouth or throat can produce airway obstruction. Stings around the eye or on the lid may result in the development of an anterior capsular cataract, atrophy of the iris, lens abscess, perforation of the globe, glaucoma, or refractive changes.

When subsequent local reactions become increasingly severe, the likelihood of future systemic reactions appears to increase and to be great enough, especially if skin tests are positive, to warrant immunotherapy.

Toxic reaction. A toxic reaction should be considered if there is a history of 10 or more stings. While symptoms resemble those of a systemic reaction, there is generally a greater frequency of gastrointestinal disturbance. Vomiting, diarrhea, light-headedness, and syncope are the principal features. There may also be headache, fever, drowsiness, involuntary muscle spasms, edema without urticaria, and occasionally convulsions. Urticaria and bronchospasm are not present. Symptoms usually subside within 48 h. Toxic reactions are believed to be a response to the non-antigenic properties of Hymenoptera venom.

Systemic or anaphylactic reaction. A generalized systemic reaction, whether in response to a single or to multiple stings, may range from the mild to the fatal, and death can occur within minutes. It is believed that the shorter the interval between the sting and the onset of symptoms, the more severe the reaction. Initial symptoms usually consist of itching eyes, facial flushing, generalized urticaria, and dry cough. Symptoms may intensify rapidly with chest and/or throat constriction, wheezing, dyspnea, cyanosis, abdominal cramps, diarrhea, nausea, vomiting, vertigo, chills and fever, laryngeal stridor, shock, loss of consciousness, involuntary bowel or bladder action, and bloody, frothy sputum. Such a reaction can be fatal within $\frac{1}{2}$ h, sometimes within 10 to 15 min, and, rarely, within 3 to 5 min. It is important to realize that initial mild symptoms can progress swiftly to anaphylactic shock. In addition, severe signs may overrun initial signs so that the physician is faced almost at once with respiratory failure and/or cardiovascular collapse.

Delayed reaction. A delayed reaction consists of serum-sickness-like symptoms of fever, malaise, headache, urticaria, lymphadenopathy, and polyarthritis that appear 10 to 14 days after a sting. Frequently, the patient has forgotten about the encounter and is puzzled by the sudden appearance of symptoms.

Table 46A-1. Harmful Arthropods of the United States

Class and Order	Common Name	Bite	Sting
Hexapoda (Insecta)			
Hymenoptera	Bees:		
	Bumblebees		×
	Sweat bees		×
	Honeybees		×
	Wasps:		
	Hornets		×
	Yellow jackets		×
	Ants:		
	Fire ants		×
	Harvester ants		×
Diptera	Mosquitoes	×	
	Deerflies	×	
	Horseflies	×	
	Stable flies	×	
	Blackflies	×	
	Biting midges	×	
Hemiptera	Bedbugs	×	
	Wheel bugs	×	
	Kissing bugs	×	
Coleoptera	Blister beetles		×
Lepidoptera	Puss caterpillars		×
	Browntail caterpillars		×
	Buck mouth caterpillars		×
Siphonaptera	Fleas (human, cat, dog)	×	
Anoplura	Lice (body, head, pubic)	×	
Arachnida			
Araneida	Black widow spiders	×	
	Brown recluse spiders	×	
Acarina	Mites	×	
	Ticks	×	
Scorpionida	Scorpions		×

Source: Frazier CA: *Insect Allergy.* St Louis, WH Green, 1969, p 469. Used by permission.

Unusual reactions. Infrequently neurological, cardiovascular, and urological symptoms are involved in a reaction to Hymenoptera venom, with signs of encephalopathy, neuritis, vasculitis, and nephrosis. A case of Guillain-Barré syndrome has been reported as a possible consequence of a Hymenoptera sting. Another unusual reaction is intense fear following a sting, with symptoms of faintness, excessive sweating, and an increased heart rate.

Pathophysiology of Systemic Reaction

A generalized systemic reaction to Hymenoptera venom is thought to be IgE-mediated. When, for example, an individual predisposed to allergy to bees is stung by one, there is usually an increase in the production of IgE antibodies, which become attached to the mast cells and basophils. This sensitizes the individual so that a subsequent sting by a bee may result in an antigen-antibody interaction that releases pharmacologically active mediators: histamine; the slow reacting substance of anaphylaxis (SRS-A), which is an acidic sulfate ester; and eosinophil chemotactic factors of anaphylaxis (ECF-A). It is these mediators which actually cause tissue damage and systemic symptoms.

The pharmacological effects of histamine are vasodilation, urticaria or angioedema, either an increased or decreased respiratory rate, fall in blood pressure, vomiting, and tenesmus. Histamine is believed responsible for symptoms of bronchoconstriction in a systemic reaction. SRS-A is also believed to be a constrictor of bronchial smooth muscle and may potentiate the effects of histamine. In addition to producing the eosinophil cell increase seen in an allergic reaction, ECF-A may serve to decrease the activity of SRS-A and histamine, and thus be responsible for decreasing the acuteness of the reaction. Platelet-activating factors may contribute to the reaction by platelet aggregation and degranulation.

Since there is still much to be learned about the precise mechanism of a systemic reaction to insect venom, explanations are often speculative. We do not know, for instance, the exact role of released bradykinin in the reaction, although we know the response can be contraction of bronchial smooth muscle and increased venular permeability.

Electrophoretic, chromatographic, and fractionating techniques have recently increased our knowledge of the chemical and immunological characteristics of Hymenoptera venoms. These venoms are similar in some substances but differ in others. For instance, honeybee venom contains histamine; wasp venom contains histamine and serotonin; hornet venom contains both histamine and serotonin, as well as acetylcholine. Pharmacologically active amines in the venoms have been identified as histamine, serotonin, acetylcholine, adrenaline, noradrenaline, and dopamine. Melittin and apamin are among the polypeptides, while phospholipase A and hyaluronidase are the major enzymes. The five important allergens in honeybee venom are phospholipase A, hyaluronidase, melittin, acid phosphatase, and diphenylpyraline (Allergen C). There is some controversy as to whether phospholipase A or hyaluronidase is the main allergen. The venom of other members of Hymenoptera differs from honeybee venom in several respects. Wasp venom contains histamine, 5-hydroxytryptamine, and kinins, while hornet venom contains these fractions plus acetylcholine. As Reisman (1979) points out, this allergenic specificity resides in the fact that bees belong to the superfamily Apoidea, while wasps, hornets, and yellow jackets belong to Vespoidea. It has been found that a common antigen occurs in the body of a wasp and a honeybee, but it is not common to their respective venoms. There is also a common antigen in the body of a bee and a yellow jacket. Cross-reactivity appears to be the greatest between the wasp and the yellow jacket, for they share a common body antigen as well as a common antigen in their venom sacs.

The venom of the imported fire ant is distinctive from that of other members of Hymenoptera in that it is mainly alkaloid and is the only venom that demonstrates necrotic activity. The venom is nonproteinaceous and, interestingly, is toxic to other insect species. It also exhibits antibiotic activity, which apparently explains why pustules that form at the sting sites are generally sterile.

Diagnosis

Identification of the offending insect can be difficult, except for the honeybee, which almost invariably leaves its stinger with venom sac attached in the lesion. A careful history is often necessary to distinguish members of Vespoidea from each other, and slides or pictures of the various species can aid the patient in recall. Some questions that can be asked in an effort to identify the offending insect are: Where did the encounter occur? Was a nest noted, and, if so, was it in the ground (yellow jackets), under eaves or windowsills (wasps), in bushes or low-hanging tree limbs (hornets)?

Skin tests are not always reliable in identification since most individuals allergic to insects are sensitive to two or three species. This high incidence of cross-reactivity underlines the importance of mixed species extracts in immunotherapy.

If edema persists at the sting site, secondary infection, such as cellulitis, must be considered. Severe local reactions on the foot or ankle can be misdiagnosed as gout if the insect bite is not visible.

Stings by the imported fire ant in the southern region of the United States are distinctive, both because of their groupings of three or four stings in the same general area and because of the typical pustules produced. In any case, few patients forget the painful nature of the event when they blunder into a fire ant mound or accidentally encounter these fierce ants going about their business.

Treatment

If a honeybee's stinger is present in the wound, scrape it out with a scalpel or even a fingernail. Never squeeze with fingers or tweezers since this will force more venom from the attached sac into the wound. It is especially important to remove stingers as quickly as possible in cases of multiple bee stings, for the venom sac of a honeybee continues to pulse even after the bee has torn free, thus pumping more venom into the lesion. Sting sites should be thoroughly washed with soap and water to minimize the possibility of infection. Analgesics may be administered if pain and discomfort are considerable, a likely contingency in the case of multiple stings and toxic reactions.

For local reactions ice packs at the sting site will help delay absorption of the venom and limit edema, while oral antihistamines and analgesics can relieve discomfort. If an extremity is involved and edema is significant, elevation and rest of the affected limb will help limit the reaction's duration, while prednisone 20 to 40 mg orally, daily for several mornings, will reduce swelling. Diphenhydramine hydrochloride, 25 to 50 mg orally, is effective in relieving pruritus. If secondary infection develops, antibiotics will be necessary.

While the initial symptoms of a systemic reaction may be mild and discounted by the patient, or even by the physician, it is important to remember that symptoms can intensify rapidly to become life-threatening in a matter of minutes. It is for this reason that it is vital to administer epinephrine hydrochloride; 1:1000, 0.3 to 0.5 mL for an adult, and 0.01 mL/kg for a child (never more than 0.3 mL). It should be injected subcutaneously and the injection site massaged to hasten absorption of the drug. The patient should then be observed for several hours to ensure that symptoms do not intensify.

More severe symptoms of a systemic reaction, such as chest constriction, nausea, faintness, and pronounced uneasiness, may require a second injection of epinephrine in 10 to 15 min. Antihistamines, such as diphenhydramine, 25 to 50 mg, should be administered intramuscularly.

If bronchospasm develops, a secure intravenous line should be established and an infusion of aminophylline administered IV over 20 to 30 min. The adult dose is 500 mg; a child's dose is 5 mg/kg. Blood pressure and heart rate should be monitored closely. Maintain an open airway and administer oxygen as needed. If laryngeal edema is severe and airway obstruction develops, insert an endotracheal tube or perform a tracheostomy. CVP monitoring to control IV administration to an optimum pressure (10 to 15 cmH_2O) is necessary. Persistent hypotension may call for an initial infusion of dopamine, 200 mg in 250 mL of normal saline, at 5 $\mu g/(kg \cdot min)$, which may be increased gradually to 20 to 50 $\mu g/(kg \cdot min)$. While steroids are of no help in combating the immediate problem, their administration tends to limit urticaria and edema and may prolong the effects of other measures. Hydrocortisone IV initially, then prednisone, 10 mg daily for 5 to 7 days, may help prevent delayed symptoms of nephrosis or central nervous system damage.

The patient who suffers a severe systemic reaction should be kept under observation for 24 to 48 h and examined for evidence of cardiac problems, bleeding, proteinuria, or neurological complications.

In treating a delayed reaction, it may be necessary to administer prednisone (8 mg for adults, half that dosage for children) at 8 a.m. for 3 days, then discontinue. Oral antihistamines, such as brompheniramine maleate 2 to 4 mg (four times a day for adults and half that for children), may also be of help.

While excessive fear may cause shocklike symptoms in a few patients, the physician must be sure that this is a psychological reaction rather than anaphylactic shock. Reassurance and relaxation generally resolve the stress symptoms of fright.

When ant stings or bites result in systemic reactions, especially if the bite is from the fire ant, treatment is the same as for other Hymenoptera stings, but since secondary infection is frequent, antibiotics may be necessary even if the reaction is nonallergic. On occasion, scarring is extensive enough to require skin grafts.

Long-Term Management

Once the acute systemic reaction to insect venom has been treated and resolved, attention should turn to the prevention of future problems, for there is always the possibility that an even severer systemic reaction will occur if the patient is restung. If skin tests are positive, immunotherapy should be initiated and the patient maintained thereafter on an optimum dose. While the question may become moot if the FDA revokes the license for whole-body extracts in favor of venom extracts, there is still controversy over the relative effectiveness and safety of both methods. Nor has the problem of which patients should undergo immunotherapy been totally resolved. Generally speaking, a rise in IgE levels indicates sensitivity and an increase in IgG levels may indicate protection, but unfortunately this is not always the case. Nor are skin tests and RAST 100 percent reliable in determining the need for patient protection, for patients who present negative results may have been sensitized by the skin tests themselves. It is therefore important that every patient who has had a systemic reaction be provided with an insect sting kit containing premeasured epinephrine and be carefully instructed in its use.

When immunotherapy with venom extracts is decided upon, the injection schedule may be rapid, with weekly visits until the optimum (for most patients) maintenance dose of 100 μg is reached. A slower schedule may also be used, with the advantage of fewer systemic reactions during the process, but the goal should remain 100 μg. It is believed that there are no contraindications to immunotherapy, although pregnancy may require extra caution against the possibility of systemic reactions during treatment.

Since we do not as yet have a foolproof method of determining when a protection level is reached, a patient deemed allergic to

Hymenoptera should be kept on maintenance injections indefinitely.

There are several insect sting kits available. Probably the simplest to use is the Ana-Kit, which contains a sterile syringe preloaded with two doses of epinephrine 1:1000, 0.5 mL in each dose with a stop between. The kit also contains a tourniquet, sterile alcohol pads, several antihistamine tablets, and instructions for self-injection. When prescribing this kit, the physician should stress that the patient must not rely on simply taking the antihistamine tablets, since these would not mitigate intensifying symptoms, but should inject the epinephrine subcutaneously at the first sign of a systemic reaction. Rather understandably some patients are loath to stick a needle into their own flesh (as are a good many bystanders offering help). Therefore, it is important to emphasize that the epinephrine is the only drug that can stave off intensifying anaphylactic symptoms long enough to obtain further medical aid.

A second kit, the Nelco kit, contains two doses of 1:1000 epinephrine in sealed ampoules of 0.5 mL each. However, breaking the ampoules and filling the sterile syringes provided may be exceedingly difficult for an inexperienced and probably badly frightened layperson. This decided disadvantage is balanced somewhat by the fact that there is less chance of contamination if a second injection proves necessary. In addition, the absence of antihistamine tablets leaves the patient no choice but to employ the epinephrine, which, in this author's opinion is a distinct advantage. The Nelco kit also contains a tourniquet, alcohol pads, simple instructions, and a list of recommended measures to avoid being stung, plus a salutary recommendation that the allergic individual wear a medical warning tag or bracelet.

A third kit, the Epi-Pen, differs from the other two in that it contains a single self-injecting syringe, spring-loaded, of epinephrine 1:1000. Its advantage is the ease of injection; its disadvantages are that to be on the safe side the patient should carry two kits and there is no way to measure a proper and lesser dosage for children.

Physicians should, as a matter of course, advise their patients who are allergic to insects to wear medic-alert tags, and they should provide those patients with a list of avoidance measures to prevent being stung (Table 46A-2).

Armed with these preventive measures—a medical warning tag and three insect sting kits, one for the home, one for the car, and one to carry in the field—the individual allergic to insects has taken every possible precautionary measure, as has the physician in recommending immunotherapy when deemed necessary.

MOSQUITO AND FLY BITES

From available evidence, it is apparent that a characteristic sequence of events takes place in all subjects exposed to mosquito bites over a period of time. Human reaction to bites of the mosquito may be classified as follows:

1. Immediate and delayed reactions, both negative
2. Immediate reaction negative; delayed reaction positive
3. Immediate and delayed reactions, both positive
4. Immediate reaction positive and delayed reaction negative

An immediate skin reaction to mosquito bites includes redness, wheal, and itching. A delayed reaction usually consists of edema and a burning pruritus. The immediate reaction tends to be of short duration, whereas a delayed reaction may persist for hours, days, and even weeks.

Table 46A-2. Prevention of Insect Stings

1. Seek and destroy Hymenoptera nests that may be in the vicinity of the home, outbuildings, and yard. Begin with the advent of warm weather and conduct the searches periodically until the first hard frost. This task, however, should not be undertaken by the insect allergic individual, but rather by a nonallergic person or by a professional exterminator.
2. Avoid going barefoot or wearing sandals outdoors.
3. When outdoors, wear light colors such as white, tan, khaki, or light green. Do not wear bright colors or flowery prints.
4. Do not use perfumed lotions, aftershaves, or shampoos during the warm months.
5. Cover up with long sleeves and long pants and wear gloves when working outdoors, and refrain from wearing floppy clothing that could entangle an irate stinging insect and from wearing bright jewelry that could attract one. Suede and leather articles may also not only attract but irritate Hymenoptera.
6. Anyone severely allergic to insects should not mow lawns, pick flowers, or clip hedges. Such an individual should be wary when eating outdoors, especially sugary food or drinks, and should avoid areas near garbage cans, littered picnic grounds, or fruit trees where fruit lies rotting on the ground.
7. If confronted by a member or members of Hymenoptera, remain calm, never swat or move hastily, but rather retreat as slowly and calmly as possible. If retreat seems impossible, lie on the ground and cover your head with your arms.

Hypersensitivity reactions are of three types: tuberculin, urticarial, and eczemoid. Arthus' phenomenon with skin necrosis occurs occasionally. The history of an allergy to mosquito saliva constituents consists of an increasing reaction to seasonal exposures with more and more pronounced edematous and pruritic lesions, accompanied sometimes by complications such as fever, malaise, generalized edema, severe nausea and vomiting, and necrosis with resulting scarring.

Fly Bites

Bloodsucking flies that stab and pierce the skin can cause some degree of pain and, commonly, subsequent pruritus. Several species, such as deerflies, blackflies, horseflies, and sand flies, can produce allergic reactions, although rarely as severe as those produced by Hymenoptera venom. There is also the possibility of myiasis with fly bites, but this, too, is rare in the United States.

The diagnosis of fly bites depends chiefly on the patient's history and a knowledge of the insects that frequent the area of the encounter.

Treatment

Treatment for the more severe normal reactions to insect bites is symptomatic, while treatment of systemic reactions is the same as it is for Hymenoptera venom. Prevention of secondary infection, especially in the case of fly bites, is important, although antibiotics should not be given prophylactically. Oral antihistamines and cyproheptadine or hydroxyzine hydrochloride are helpful in relieving pruritus; trimeprazine tartrate is particularly effective in relieving pruritus of mosquito bites. Use of topical antihistamines runs the risk of contact dermatitis. However, topical steroids are helpful when local reactions are severe or if scarring occurs.

Cold compresses may alleviate localized edema. For severe systemic reactions oral or parenteral steroids may be indicated. While immunotherapy has not proved as successful for mosquito or fly bite allergies as for Hymenoptera allergies, it is well worth the attempt for patients who suffer severe systemic reactions.

FLEA, LICE, AND SCABIES BITES

Flea Bites

Bites of fleas, lice, and scabies produce lesions so similar that diagnosis is often difficult. Flea bites are frequently found in zigzag lines, especially on the legs and in the waist area. The lesions have hemorrhagic puncta surrounded by erythematous and urticarial patches. Pruritus is intense, and often, even after the lesions clear, dull red spots persist. Children may develop impetigo as a complication.

The main concern in the treatment of flea bites is the possibility of secondary infection. The lesions should be washed thoroughly with soap and water. For children, it is important to keep the fingernails cut short to prevent scratching. To relieve discomfort and itching, starch baths at bedtime (about 1 kg starch to a tubful of water), local application of calamine, cool soaks, and an oral antihistamine such as trimeprazine may be helpful. For severe discomfort, application of a topical glucocorticoid cream or spray may be necessary.

If secondary infection develops, an antibiotic such as neomycin or polymyxin may be needed.

Lice

Body lice concentrate about the waist, shoulders, axillae, and neck. The lice and their eggs can often be found in the seams of clothing. The lesions begin as small, noninflammatory red spots that quickly become papular wheals. They are so intensely pruritic that their linear scratch marks are diagnostically suggestive of infestation.

The white ova of head lice can be mistaken for dandruff, but unlike dandruff, they cannot be brushed out, for they are glued to the hair itself.

Pubic lice leave bluish spots on the abdomen and thighs, and ova are evident on the shafts of pubic hairs. If sensitization to lice saliva and feces components takes place, delayed reactions may develop. Fever and malaise are possible, and secondary infection may produce enlarged lymph glands. Long periods of infestation may bring a decrease in pruritus and often impart a thick, dry, scaly appearance to the skin. A brownish pigmentation characteristic of vagabond's disease can occur on the neck, shoulders, and back, or can become generalized and include even the mucous membranes.

Treatment for body lice infestation consists of a thorough application of γ-benzene hexachloride (Kwell) or crotamiton (Eurax), plus sterilization of clothing, bedding, and personal articles. Kwell, however, must be employed with caution for infants and children since it can be absorbed more readily by their tender skin. It can be toxic to the central nervous system. Eurax should not be employed on raw or weeping areas. Head lice are treated with either of the above medications, daily shampoos, and fine combing of the hair. Personal articles should be sterilized.

Scabies

While scabies infestation resembles that of lice, scabies bites are generally concentrated around the hands and feet, especially in the webs between the fingers and toes. In children, however, the face and scalp may be infested as well. In adults, scabies frequently affects the nipples in females, the penis in males.

The scabies mite, an arachnid like the spider, is a universal pest that appears to follow a 30-year cycle of waxing and waning. During the last several years, there has been an epidemic of scabies infestation in the United States. In general, scabies infestation is more likely to occur by direct contact between the infested individual and the noninfested individual than by indirect contact with clothing and personal articles.

Diagnostically, pruritus is the dominant symptom, although it takes about a month for sensitization to develop and itching to begin. However, a patient who becomes reinfested, and who is already sensitized, develops inflammation and pruritus within a few hours of contact.

The distinctive features of scabies infestation is the burrow that the female mite digs into the skin to lay her eggs. Vesicles and papules form at the surface of these zigzag, whitish, threadlike channels that contain small gray spots at the closed ends where the parasite rests. Burrows tend to enlarge and be more visible in children. The burrows can be traced with a hand lens and the female mite scraped out with a needle or razor blade. A thin shaving of skin containing both burrow and mite can be examined under a microscope to establish diagnosis clearly. Unfortunately, the burrows are often disguised by the results of fierce scratching. These distinctive physical findings are then obscured by crusting, eczematization, and secondary infection.

Treatment

Treatment for scabies infestation consists of a thorough application of γ-benzene hexachloride (GBH; Kwell, cream or lotion) from the neck down, following a warm bath with liberal use of soap. The patient should be cautioned to keep the substance from eyes and mucous membranes and to avoid inhaling the vapors. Again, since GBH is toxic, it is questionable whether it should be employed for young children or pregnant women. A 5% sulfur ointment can be substituted if necessary, although it is apt to be somewhat odiferous and is definitely messy. It should be applied twice from the neck down, with a 24-h interval between applications, followed each time by a soap and water bath. A third application following the second by 12 h should be effective.

Crotamiton, which is also antipruritic in action, can be applied from the neck down in two applications 24 h apart and followed 24 to 48 h later by a bath. The safety of its use, too, is somewhat in doubt, and it should be employed with caution.

Patients should be warned that even after the scabies mites have been destroyed by the above methods, lesions and pruritus can persist. No further use of scabicide is needed, but calamine lotion, oral antipruritic agents, and analgesics will help alleviate discomfort. Antibiotics are only necessary where secondary infection is a problem.

KISSING BUG BITES

Triatoma species, commonly known as conenose or kissing bugs, are found mainly in the southeastern and Pacific coast regions of the United States. They feed on the blood of vertebrate animals, including humans. Their common name derives from their habit of feeding at night on any exposed surface of a sleeping victim, which commonly is the face. Since their bite is relatively painless, the victim is rarely aware of the attack.

Kissing bugs, like bedbugs, live in baseboards, between cracks in walls and floors, and in furniture.

Bites are usually multiple and consist of hemorrhagic papules or bullae if the bites occur on the hands or feet, and large wheals if they are on the trunk.

Diagnostically, kissing bug bites can be differentiated from bedbug bites in that they do not appear to form a linear formation nor do they leave the telltale brown or black patterns of excrement on the bed linen. They can be distinguished from spider bites, since the latter tend to be single lesions, and they usually can be distinguished from erythema multiforme by their unilateral, local distribution.

Treatment

Generally, treatment is symptomatic with cool local applications and mild analgesics to relieve pruritus. Some individuals become highly sensitive to the kissing bug and react with systemic symptoms, which should be treated as previously outlined for Hymenoptera venom. There are enough recorded cases of successful results with immunotherapy for allergy to kissing bugs to make it well worth the attempt for the hypersensitive individual.

CATERPILLAR STINGS

Some caterpillars possess hollow spines among their hairs which contain urticating poison that can cause symptoms ranging from local dermatitis to generalized systemic reactions. The puss caterpillar, larval stage of the flannel moth *Megalopyge opercularis*, is perhaps the most toxic in the United States and is especially hazardous for children who tend to find it intriguing and thus handle it.

Found primarily in the southeastern states and especially in Texas and Florida, the venom of the puss caterpillar has demonstrated hemolytic action in laboratory studies and an ability to increase vascular permeability. It is believed to be proteinaceous in nature.

The dominant feature of the puss caterpillar's sting is intense immediate pain, often rhythmic. Local edema and pruritus follow quickly, and a rash of red blotches and ridges develops. The lesions consist of white or red papules and vesicles, and frequently they form a perfect gridlike mark where the caterpillar made contact. The patient may be notably restless and frightened. In addition, generalized symptoms commonly occur with fever and muscle cramps. Shocklike symptoms have also been reported. Within several hours or days, local desquamation may develop. Lymphadenopathy has been described.

Treatment

Treatment should begin with immediate removal of broken-off spines by placing cellophane tape over the sting site. Calcium gluconate, 10 mL of a 10% solution, intravenously, is effective in relieving pain in severe cases, while tripelennamine usually brings relief in milder cases. Generalized symptoms are treated symptomatically.

BLISTER BEETLE STINGS

Blister beetles are found most frequently in the western section of the United States. When disturbed, they exude a vesicating agent, cantharidin, which can penetrate the epidermis to produce irritation and blistering within a few hours of contact. If ingested, cantharidin can produce intense gastrointestinal disturbances with symptoms of nausea, vomiting, diarrhea, and abdominal cramps. Initial contact with the beetle produces a burning, tingling sensation and a mild rash. Within a few hours, flaccid, elongated vesicles and bullae develop.

Treatment

Treatment consists of protecting the bullae from trauma by an occlusive dressing. Large bullae should be drained and an antibiotic ointment applied. If bullae occur on the feet, the patient should be advised to stay off the feet and wet dressings should be applied for 24 to 48 h.

INHALANT ALLERGY TO INSECTS

It should be noted that allergic respiratory disease can be caused by insect debris in the atmosphere, such as wing scales and chitin.

BIBLIOGRAPHY

Abbudn F: Myiasis in otolaryngology. *Ear, Nose Throat,* 59:32–46, 1980.

American Academy of Allergy: Monograph on Insect Allergy, 1981.

Baer H, Liu TY, Anderson MC, et al: Protein components of fire ant venom (*Solenopsis invicta*). *Toxicon* 17:397, 1979.

Feinstein RJ: Ticks. *Dermatologica* 1:13–15, 1978.

Frazier CA: Biting insect survey: A statistical report. *Ann Allergy* 32:200–204, 1974.

Frazier CA: Insect stings—A medical emergency. *JAMA* 235:2410–2411, 1976.

Frazier CA: A preventable emergency. *Mil Med* 141:222–223, 1977.

Geller RG, Yoshida H, Beaven MA, et al: Pharmacologically active substances in venoms of the bald-faced hornet, *Vespula (Dolichovespula) maculata,* and the yellow jacket, *Vespula (Vespula) maculifrons. Toxicon* 14:27–33, 1976.

Golden DBK, Valentine MD, Kagey-Sobotka A, et al: Regimens of Hymenoptera venom immunotherapy. *Ann Intern Med* 92:620–624, 1980.

Harves AD, Millikan LE: Current concepts of therapy and pathophysiology in arthropod bites and stings. *Int J Dermatol* 14:621–634, 1975.

Hatzel G, in Dworetzky M (ed): Insect sting allergy. Symposium and panel discussion. *NY State J Med* 62:3560–3572, 1962.

Hoffman DR: Honeybee venom allergy: Immunological studies of systemic and large local reactions. *Ann Allergy* 41:278–282, 1978.

Hoffman DR, Shipman WH: Allergens in bee venom. *J Allergy Clin Immunol* 58:551–562, 1976.

Hollman DR: Allergens in Hymenoptera venom. *Ann Allergy* 40:171–176, 1978.

Kern F, Sobotka AK, Valentine MD, et al: Allergy to insect stings, III: Allergenic cross-reactivity among vespid venoms. *J Allergy Clin Immunol* 57:554–559, 1976.

Lichtenstein LM, Valentine MD, Sobotka AK: Insect allergy: The state of the art. *J Allergy Clin Immunol* 64:5–12, 1979.

Lockey RF: Allergic and other adverse reactions caused by the imported fire ant, in Oehling A, et al (eds): *Advances in Allergology and Clinical Immunology.* New York, Pergamon Press, 1980, 441–448.

Mueller HL: Further experiences with severe allergic reactions to insect stings. *N Engl J Med* 261:374–377, 1959.

Nair BC, Nair C, Denne S, et al: Immunologic comparison of phospholipases A present in Hymenoptera insect venoms. *J Allergy Clin Immunol* 58:101–109, 1976.

Orkin M, Epstein F, Mailach HI: Treatment of today's scabies and pediculosis. *JAMA* 236(10):1136–1139, 1976.

Orange RP, Donsky GJ: Anaphylaxis, in Middleton E Jr, Reed CE, Ellis EF (eds): *Allergy—Principles and Practice.* St Louis, Mosby, 1978, 563–571.

Parish LC, Witkowski JA: Lice can happen to anyone. *Consultant,* September 1978, pp. 34–40.

Parrino J, Kandawalla N, Lockey RF: Treatment of the local skin response to imported fire ant sting. *J Allergy Clin Immunol* 63:135, 1979.

Paull BR, Yunginger JW, Gleich GJ: Melittin: An allergen of honeybee venom. *J Allergy Clin Immunol* 59:334–338, 1977.

Portnoy BL, Satterwaite TK, Dyckman JD: Rat bite fever misdiagnosed as Rocky Mountain spotted fever. *South Med J* 72:607–609, 1979.

Ramirez DA, Evans R: Adverse reactions to venom immunotherapy. *J Allergy Clin Immunol* 65:200, 1980.

Reisman RE, Arbesman CE, Lazell M: Observations on the aetiology and natural history of stinging insect sensitivity: Application of measurements of venom-specific IgE. *Clin Allergy* 9:303, 1979.

Reisman RE, Lazell M, Doerr J: Insect venom allergy: A prospective case study showing lack of correlation between immunologic reactivity and clinical sensitivity. *J Allergy Clin Immunol* 68:406, 1981.

Settipane GA, Chafee FH: Natural history of allergy to Hymenoptera. *Clin Allergy* 9:385, 1979.

Systemic reactions to Hymenoptera stings. *Med Lett Drug Ther* 20:54–55, 1978.

Yunginger JW, Paull BR, Jones RT, et al: Rush venom immunotherapy program for honeybee sting sensitivity. *J Allergy Clin Immunol* 63:340, 1979.

B. Tick-Borne Disease

George Podgorny

Ticks are small, oval or round in shape, and hard, and, along with mites and other insects, form the order of Acarina. These parasites are present, in one form or another, in most areas of the world. Ticks are particularly plentiful around congregations of warm-blooded animals, such as cattle, canines, or felines.

A tick uses its mouthparts to inflict a bite and, frequently, after a period of a few hours, manages to bury its head under or in the skin. In cases of infected ticks, the tick feces, body juices, and blood are all infective. Because of the above, ticks should not be crushed, either while attached to the patient or after being removed from the patient. Many substances, such as petrolatum, kerosene, oil, gasoline, and nail polish, if placed on the tick, will usually cause its retreat. When this is not possible, a 25-gauge hypodermic needle can be inserted gently between the mouthparts; with gentle traction the tick can be removed completely.

Ticks are vectors of such substantial and potentially fatal diseases as Rocky Mountain spotted fever, Q fever, tularemia, Lyme disease, tick paralysis, babesiosis, and boreliosis. The more common problems are discussed below.

ROCKY MOUNTAIN SPOTTED FEVER

Rocky Mountain spotted fever was first identified near the turn of the century in Idaho and Montana and is a misnomer, as the majority of cases are reported (in order of frequency) from the Carolinas, Virginia, Georgia, Tennessee, Maryland, and Oklahoma; cases have been diagnosed from Canada to Brazil. In 1982, almost 1000 cases were reported in the United States. Ninety-five percent of cases are seen in the spring and summer months.

The species of tick responsible for the spread of Rocky Mountain spotted fever are: In the west, the wood tick—*Dermacentor andersoni;* and in the southeast, the dog tick—*D. variabilis.* Only female ticks become infected, and they transmit the microorganisms transovarially to some of their offspring. Other ticks become infected by feeding on an infected mammal. As a result, the tick is not only the vector but also the reservoir of Rocky Mountain spotted fever. Two-thirds of patients give a history of exposure to ticks within 14 days of the disease, often with a history of travel to an endemic area.

The responsible microorganism is *Rickettsia rickettsii.* It is a gram-negative organism that stains red with Macchiavello's stain and purple with Giemsa's stain. Rickettsiae are obligate intracellular parasites, approaching the size of bacteria.

Rickettsiae enter the body through the respiratory tract or the skin. Lesions are widespread and primarily vascular with involvement of adjacent parenchymatous tissues. Destruction of endothelium with thrombosis is very common.

Fever is an almost universal finding, and headache occurs in 90 percent of patients. The classic nonfixed pink rash, with macules measuring from 2 to 6 mm in diameter, appears, in 90 percent of cases, typically between the second and sixth febrile days. The rash initially appears on wrists and ankles, and then spreads to palms and soles and eventually to the forearms. After about 6 to 12 h, the spread of rash becomes centripetal to the axillae, buttocks, trunk, neck, and face.

In 2 or 3 days, the rash becomes maculopapular, and additional petechiae can be provoked by the use of tourniquets or blood pressure cuff inflation (Rumpel-Leede phenomenon). Definitive diagnosis can be made through either the Weil-Felix reaction or through complement-fixation tests.

Prognosis

In mild cases, recovery occurs within 20 days. In general, the mortality rate for Rocky Mountain spotted fever, if untreated, is between 8 and 20 percent.

Treatment

The antibiotics of choice are chloramphenicol, a loading dose of 50 mg/kg of body weight, followed by the same dose divided daily thereafter; or tetracycline, 25 mg/kg loading dose, with the same dose divided daily thereafter. Treatment with antibiotics should be carried out for a minimum of 24 h after the patient becomes afebrile without taking antipyretics. Antibiotic therapy has reduced mortality to less than 4 percent.

LYME DISEASE

Lyme disease, named for the small Connecticut town where clusters of cases were first discovered and once thought to be an exotic form of arthritis, may become the second most important tick-borne disease in the United States. It may simply be an old problem becoming more virulent and recognized. Since 1982, about 500 cases have been confirmed in over 10 states in the northeast, the midwest, and as far south as North Carolina. The incidence of Lyme disease may approach that of Rocky Mountain spotted fever.

The insect vector for Lyme disease is the *Ixodes* tick. Various species, including *I. dammani, pacificus,* and *scapularis* have been incriminated in the United States. The potential wide vector indicates a growing need for the emergency physician to become familiar with the recognition and treatment of this disease. The causative organism discovered in ticks and victims of the disease is a serpentine spirochete which has been recovered from the blood, CSF, and skin lesions of patients with the disease. The organism must be cultured on a special medium used for culturing *Borrelia* organisms (Kelly's medium).

The course of the disease following a tick bite consists of three phases. The initial phase is characterized by large, distinctive circular skin lesions known as erythema chronicum migrans (ECM), seen in 85 percent of cases. Multiple smaller ringlike skin lesions are seen in 50 percent of those with ECM. Following the bite of an infected tick, patients may have malaise, fatigue, headache, fever, myalgia, lymphadenopathy, diffuse erythema, malar rash, conjunctivitis, and periorbital edema. Weeks or months later there may be temporary, transient cardiac abnormalities including AV block and myopericarditis, or neurologic abnormalities including meningoencephalitis and cranial or peripheral neuropathies. Still later, arthritis may develop. The arthritis is mono- or oligoarticular, affecting large joints, and may be chronic and recurrent.

The definitive diagnosis may be made by culturing the spirochete or by demonstrating a rise in antibody titer in the appropriate clinical setting. Therapy should be tetracycline, 250 mg, four times a day for 10 days in adults, or penicillin, 50 mg/(kg · day) in four divided doses, for 10 days in children. Erythromycin, 30 mg/(kg · day) should be used in penicillin allergic children. Early antibiotic administration appears to prevent the later stages of the disease.

TICK PARALYSIS

A tick bite, particularly in the neck, head, and spinal region, may cause an ascending flaccid paralysis, especially in children. Initial symptoms are extreme irritability, general malaise, and anorexia, followed by weakness and hyporeflexia, dysphagia, dysarthria, facial paralysis, nystagmus, and extraocular paralysis. Within 12 to 24 h, if the presence of the tick is not discovered and the tick removed, bulbar and respiratory paralysis may develop, and herein lies the danger. This paralysis is produced by a neurotoxin in the saliva of some tick species. According to Gormann and Snead, "the toxin produces a conduction block in the peripheral branches of motor fibers which results in a failure of liberation of acetylcholine at the neuromuscular junction." They also believe that the onset of truncal ataxia indicates cerebellar involvement.

Tick paralysis should be considered when there is a sudden onset of afebrile muscle weakness, early and symmetric loss of all deep reflexes, clear sensorium but marked apathy, ascending flaccid paralysis that may become bulbar, and ataxia.

Treatment consists chiefly of removing the tick and cleansing the lesion. However, severe symptoms of paralysis call for symptomatic treatment. Once the tick is gone, symptoms usually abate quickly.

TICK FEVER

Bites of various species of ticks can produce a nonspecific febrile illness. History of tick bite or the presence of the tick on the body are giveaways. Passage of a few days and particularly removal of the tick lead to the clearing of symptoms.

PROPHYLACTIC SUGGESTIONS

1. Use insect repellent and heavy clothing in tall grass or woods.
2. Conduct a careful self-examination after outdoor activity.
3. Keep grass short and remove overhanging shrubbery.
4. Examine pets for ticks.
5. Remove tick promptly and completely as soon as it is discovered.

BIBLIOGRAPHY

Rocky Mountain Spotted Fever

Feinstein RJ: Ticks. *Dermatology* 1:13–15, 1978.
Gorman RJ, Snead OC: Tick paralysis in three children, the diversity of neurologic presentations. *Clin Pediatr* 17:249–251, 1978.

Lyme Disease

Benach JL, Bosler EM, Hanrahan JP, et al: Spirochetes isolated from the blood of two patients with Lyme disease. *N Engl J Med* 308:740, 1983.
Burgdorfer W, Kierans JE: Ticks and Lyme disease in the United States. *Ann Intern Med* 99:121, 1983.
Steere AC, Bartenhagen NH, Craft JE, et al: The early clinical manifestations of Lyme disease. *Ann Intern Med* 99:76, 1983.
Steere AC, Grodzicki RL, Kornblatt AN, et al: The spirochetal etiology of Lyme disease. *N Engl J Med* 308:733, 1983.
Steere AC, Hutchinson GJ, Rahn DW, et al: Treatment of the early manifestations of Lyme disease. *Ann Intern Med* 99:22, 1983.

C. Venomous Spiders

George Podgorny

Spiders belong to the order Araneida within the class Arachnida. Most species of spiders produce some venom in order to paralyze and digest their prey. Occasionally the spider venom may be allergenic as well as toxic. Introduction of pathogenic microorganisms with a spider bite also presents a problem.

It is estimated that in the United States there are 15 or more species of spiders whose venom is capable of producing some neurotoxic symptoms. Only two of these species, however, are of any medical consequence because of an occasionally severe and very infrequently fatal outcome.

The minuscule size of the body and, therefore, of the available volume of venom are responsible for the fact that most spider bites hardly ever cause symptoms in humans. Most spider venoms contain neurotoxins and tissue lysins. This combination, when injected into the prey, paralyzes it while aiding in the digestion of the victim's body, the contents of which are sucked out later.

Two species of venomous spiders capable of producing some neurotoxic symptoms are usually present in the sunbelt during the warm period of the year.

Spider bites reported from unlikely locales are usually due to spiders brought into these areas along with fruits and vegetables or other produce.

BLACK WIDOW SPIDER

A native of this country, only the female black widow (*Latrodectus mactans* or *L. hesperous*) is of significance. She is glossy black with a body approximately 1 cm in diameter and a leg span approaching 5 cm. She frequently devours her mate; thus she is aptly named. She exhibits a very constant, discernible, hourglass-shaped, bright red marking on the ventral side of the abdomen. The male of the species is much smaller and displays only a small reddish dot on the abdomen. Occasionally, a younger female may lack the hourglass marking or may even appear to be a mottled brown. This spider is ubiquitous throughout most of the United States, particularly in the southeast. Its habitat is usually outdoors; the most common encounter occurs in an outhouse and involves genitalia of the human male. Despite various classic descriptions of how the black widow bite looks, it usually cannot be distinguished from a fleabite. Children, in particular, frequently report an initial sudden burning pain. Systemic symptoms develop usually anywhere from 2 to 12 h after the bite. The venom of the black widow produces diffuse central and peripheral nervous excitement with autonomic activity and muscle spasms. Symptoms include ascending paralysis involving muscular spasms, pain, and rigidity. Bites on lower extremities and genitalia usually produce abdominal symptoms, sometimes leading to the erroneous diagnosis of an acute abdomen. Abdominal guarding, rigidity, nausea, and vomiting can be extremely misleading. The sudden onset of symptoms and the usual lack of fever and leukocytosis, as well as the clinician's judgment and awareness, should help the physician avoid this diagnostic and therapeutic pitfall.

Bites on upper extremities cause chest symptoms, sometimes anginalike, pectoral spasm, and rigidity.

Treatment

In general, treatment should be supportive and should provide relief of pain. Slow intravenous administration of 10 mL of a 10% solution of calcium gluconate will serve as a diagnostic and therapeutic maneuver. The rapid relief of the pain and boardlike rigidity of the abdomen is comforting to the patient and welcome to the physician. Muscle relaxants such as methocarbamol and diazepam have been used with some success. A commercially prepared antivenom for black widow spider bite is available. It is an equine serum product and, therefore, should be used with caution and only after appropriate sensitivity testing.

The need for this antivenom is rare because most cases are self-limiting or respond well to treatment. Antivenom for *L. mactans* (made by Merck, Sharp, and Dohme) is available in vials of 6000 units. This lyophilized material is diluted in 2.5 ml of sterile water. A single vial constitutes a dose for intramuscular or intravenous injection.

A few recent reports indicate that in Florida *Latrodectus bishopi*, the so-called redleg spider, may produce symptoms in humans of poisoning resembling that of a black widow bite.

BROWN RECLUSE SPIDER

For the past 50 years, the range of the brown recluse spider (*Loxosceles reclusa*,) also known as the fiddleback spider, and the reports of bites from this spider have extended steadily from Louisiana toward Texas and Arkansas, as well as northeast and north, with cases reported as far east as Virginia and West Virginia. Despite the spider's reclusivity its frequent habitat is in abandoned buildings close to humans. This spider is somewhat nondescript: brownish to tan in color, small, and not unlike harmless spiders. A fiddle-shaped design is discernible on the dorsal thorax, but its outline may be vague and visible only with the aid of a magnifying glass. Most North American spiders have four pairs of eyes, while the brown recluse has only three pairs.

The venom of the brown recluse has a high content of lysins that cause vasculitis and necrosis. Bites of these spiders vary in severity from being almost asymptomatic to producing a major systemic reaction.

At the site of the local lesion, mild pain may be present initially, followed within hours to a day or two by an area of erythema; occasionally vesicles or ecchymoses appear, sometimes with a central blanched area. This blanched area becomes a vesicle which is eventually replaced by a necrotic crust. Removal of the crust shows a deep ulcer. The healing of such ulcers is variable, and occasionally excision and skin grafting become necessary.

Recent reports from Nashville indicate that at Vanderbilt University School of Medicine and Veterans Administration Hospital a project is underway to produce a brown recluse spider antivenom.

TARANTULA

Tarantulas (genus *Dugesiella*) are large, frequently hairy, jumping and running spiders. They are present particularly in the southwest United States. The tarantula's size, appearance, and undeserved reputation have created an aura of fatal danger. Tarantulas possess venoms which are quite mild and rarely problematic to humans; occasional allergic reactions may occur. Lately, tarantulas have become popular as pets. They are frequently seen in homes and occasionally utilized by jewelry stores to prevent unauthorized attempts to reach into the window displays.

BIBLIOGRAPHY

Hufford DC: The brown recluse and necrotic arachnidism, current review, *J Arkansas Med Soc* 74:126, 1977.

Podgorny G: Venomous reptiles and arthropods of the United States and Canada, in Haddad LM, Winchester JF (eds): *Clinical Management of Poisoning and Drug Overdose*. Philadelphia, Saunders, 1983, pp. 290–291.

Vorse M, et al: Disseminated intravascular coagulopathy following fatal brown spider bite. *J Pediatr* 80:1035, 1972.

CHAPTER 47
REPTILE BITES

George Podgorny

SNAKEBITE

Data concerning the incidence of snakebites in the United States are not available. Any figures cited represent educated guesswork, but a reasonable estimate is 8000 bites per year by venomous snakes and twice that number by harmless snakes. North Carolina shows the highest incidence of hospital admissions for venomous snakebites in the 48 contiguous states, followed by Arkansas, Texas, Georgia, West Virginia, Mississippi, and Louisiana, all with 10 or more admissions per year per 100,000 population. South Carolina, Oklahoma, New Mexico, and Florida follow.

A bite by a harmless snake is a minor nuisance, but its venomous counterparts can produce serious consequences. Although the annual mortality from venomous snakebites is unknown, it is believed to be somewhere between 50 and 100.

Most snakebites occur in the sunbelt. The peak months are July and August, followed by June and September, and then May and October. In general, snakes are poikilothermic and hibernate in cool temperatures. Abnormal and unexpected variations in temperature, however, can confuse snakes. Depending on the climate, snakes may be absent for a substantial portion of the year, or be present almost year-round. In geographical areas with four seasons, snakes emerge from hibernation late in spring and reenter it in mid-fall. Like all animals, the instinct of fight or flight is strongly present in snakes. Most snakes prefer to retreat rather than fight. Aggressive behavior usually represents an attempt to secure prey or is a defensive maneuver when the snake is unable to retreat. Snakes are more aggressive emerging from and immediately preceding hibernation. Because of relative dehydration during hibernation, venomous snakes possess more concentrated and, therefore, more potent venom immediately on emergence from hibernation. The snake's control over its venom-injection apparatus is poorly understood. However, a venomous snake, at the time of biting, may inject varying amounts of venom or none at all.

Although basically nocturnal, snakes more frequently encounter humans between 6 a.m. and 9 p.m. In the outdoors, human exposure to snakes occurs usually during agricultural activity, hunting, fishing, and professional or amateur study of nature. Exposure can also result during construction, surveying, camping, and military maneuvers, and during natural disasters such as earthquakes, floods, and brush or forest fires.

Indoor exposure to snakes takes place in locations such as zoos and animal research facilities, and bites often occur during amateur snake-keeping and -handling activities as a result of carelessness or daring. Resurgence of certain religious cults and their venomous snake–handling activities provides an additional setting for exposure.

Handling snakes that appear to be dead may result in a venomous snakebite secondary to postmortem reflex action of the snake's head.

Many venomous snakes, particularly pit vipers, possess fairly long and sharp fangs that can easily penetrate regular clothing. For this reason, humans should protect their extremities, the most common sites of exposure, when in snake-infested areas.

For those likely to encounter venomous snakes, additional protection is provided by pretesting for sensitivity to horse serum, so that horse serum antivenom can be given as quickly as possible if necessary.

Identification of Indigenous Venomous Snakes

Identification of the snake, either dead or alive, is important in order to determine whether it is harmless or venomous (Table 47-1). If the snake is not available, a reliable observer may have seen the snake well enough to identify it or describe it sufficiently. If the snake is venomous, it must be determined whether it is a pit viper or coral snake, and in the case of the former, whether it is a copperhead, cottonmouth, or rattlesnake.

Pit Vipers

Kin to vipers of the old world, pit vipers are more specific to the western hemisphere. The name is derived from the pit, a small indentation halfway between the snake's eye and nostril (Fig. 47-1). This represents a thermoreceptor organ that provides the snake with the ability to locate, track, and approach warm-blooded animals. In addition, all pit vipers possess anteriorly positioned, hollow, retractable fangs on the maxilla (Fig. 47-2). The anlage of the parotid glands produces the venom, and when the gland is squeezed by palatine muscles, the venom flows through a duct into the hollow fangs for injection.

Table 47-1. The More Common and Better-Known Indigenous Venomous Snakes of the United States

Family	Genus and Species	Common Name	Geographic Distribution
Crotalidae (pit vipers)	*Crotalus adamanteus* (rattlesnake)	Eastern diamondback	Eastern seaboard, tidal and adjoining areas from North Carolina to Florida and Gulf coast, Georgia, Alabama, and Mississippi
	C. horridus	Timber	North and northeast except Maine. West of Mississippi into central states and east Texas
	C. viridis	Prairie	Great plains, midwest, and prairie states
	C. atrox	Western diamondback	Texas, Oklahoma, and west into southeastern California
	C. cerastes	Mojave sidewinder	California, Arizona, Utah
	C. scutulatus	Mojave	Southwest Texas to California
	Sistrurus catenatus (rattlesnake)	Massasauga	Nebraska, Iowa, Colorado, Texas, Arizona
	S. milliarius	Pygmy	North Carolina to Florida, and west to Oklahoma and Texas
	Agkistrodon contortrix	Copperhead	Central Massachusetts to north Florida, west to Illinois and Texas
	A. piscivorous	Cottonmouth (water moccasin)	South Virginia to Florida; west to east Texas, Mississippi valley, Illinois and Indiana
Elapidae (coral snakes)	*Micrurus fulvius*	Eastern	Southeastern North Carolina to tip of Florida into Gulf coastal plain, Mississippi valley to central Arkansas, Texas, and adjacent Mexico
	Micruroides Euryxanthus	Western (Sonoran) (Arizona)	Southern Arizona, southwest New Mexico, and adjacent Mexico

There are three additional characteristics of pit vipers that aid in distinguishing them from harmless snakes. First, they have vertical pupils. Most harmless snakes have round pupils, although some venomous snakes also have round pupils. Obviously, identification of this characteristic should be undertaken carefully. Second, a pit viper's head is generally triangular in shape or, more precisely, is shaped like an arrowhead. Harmless snakes have oval or egg-shaped heads. Even in the hands of cognoscenti, this characteristic feature can be difficult to discern. A final distinction between pit vipers and harmless snakes lies in the pattern of plates on the snakes' undersides. On a snake's ventral side, somewhat caudad, are whitish, seemingly loose scales called the anal plates. In venomous snakes, scales are arranged in a single row from the anal plate to a point approximately a third of the distance away from the tip of the tail. In most harmless snakes, the scales are arranged in double rows from the anal plate to the tip of the tail.

Three genera of pit vipers need to be considered. The genus *Crotalus* includes almost all of the rattlesnakes, comprised of nearly 20 different species and variations. Two relatively well known rattlesnakes, the pygmy and the massasauga, belong to the genus *Sistrurus*. In addition to previously enumerated characteristics, all rattlesnakes, when intact and not suffering from congenital malformation, possess characteristic terminal rattles. The number and the size of the rattles do not denote the years of the snake's age; however, they reflect overall longevity. When all the rattles are missing, the tail's end is unexpectedly blunt. Rattlesnakes are

present over most of the continental United States (see Table 47-1). Except for the pygmy rattler, rattlesnakes usually grow to a large size, and their bites are potentially fatal.

The third genus of pit vipers, *Agkistrodon,* consists of two species. The water moccasin (*A. piscivorus*), also called cottonmouth because of its white buccal mucosa, is amphibious. It tends to be somewhat smaller than a rattlesnake, but is similar in terms of venom characteristics. The second species, the copperhead (*A. contortrix*), is so called because of the copperlike coloration of the mature adult. It is the most prevalent venomous snake in the United States but fortunately the least venomous of the pit vipers. It is responsible for a substantial number of venomous snakebites, particularly east of the Mississippi.

Coral Snake (Elapidae)

Two species of coral snakes are present in the United States. They are the only representatives of a totally different group of venomous snakes and are kin to cobras and kraits of the old world. The two species closely resemble each other. They are relatively small, shy snakes with a rather distinct pattern of red and black bands that are wider than the interspaced yellow rings. This has given rise to the following mnemonic rhyme: ''Red on yellow, kill a fellow—coral snake. Red on black, venom lack—harmless snake.'' The more plentiful of the species, the eastern coral snake

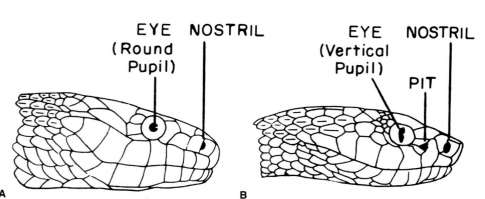

EYE NOSTRIL
(Round Pupil)

A

EYE NOSTRIL
(Vertical Pupil)

PIT

B

Figure 47-1. Lateral view of the head of a harmless snake (A), and of a pit viper (B). (Adapted from Blanchard.)

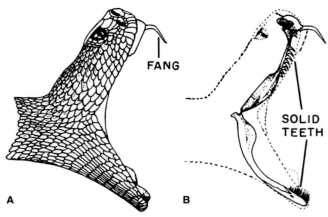

Figure 47-2. Lateral view of a head of a snake (rattlesnake) showing exposed fangs approximately in biting position. A. Tissues intact as in a live snake. B. Position of the tooth bearing bones. (Adapted from Pope.)

(*Micrurus fulvius*), has a black snout with the previously described coloration of the body.

Most of the head is black in the lesser of the species, the Arizona or Sonora coral snake (*Micruroides euryxanthus*), but the rest of its coloration is similar to the eastern coral snake (yellow rings may be narrower).

Variables Influencing Severity of Venomous Snakebite

In terms of pathophysiology and clinical approach, a venomous snakebite represents an undesirable and complex interaction between animal and human where usually the snake adversely influences the health of the victim depending on the variables related to the two organisms.

Snake Variables

The size and vitiation of the snake govern the type, quantity, and quality of venom available. The larger the snake (of the same species), the more venom it usually possesses and has available for injection. The condition of the snake is also important. A hungry, disturbed, and alert snake is deadlier. The angle of bite is significant, and so is its depth and the duration of the time of penetration of one or both fangs.

Snake venom is a highly complex biochemical compound. The following are some of the components that have been identified.

1. Blood coagulants, such as thrombin or prothrombin-like substances, anticoagulants, and agglutinins, which affect coagulation and red blood cells.
2. Cytolysins, proteolysins, and antibactericidin, which affect cellular blood components as well as the endothelium of the vessels. Antibactericidin contributes to suppuration, paralyzing the phagocytic activity of the white blood cells.
3. Neurotoxins A and B, which affect the nervous system, particularly the cardiorespiratory centers and higher central nervous system; neurotoxin B also affects the myoneural junction.
4. Cholinesterase and anticholinesterase, which affect the myoneural junction.

5. Cardiotoxin, which stimulates the heart.
6. Hyaluronidase, which facilitates the tissue spread of the venom.

The proportions vary depending on the type of snake. For instance, the venom of pit vipers is high in the hemopathic components, while venom from the coral snake is rich in neurotoxins.

Victim Variables

The size of the victim is important, children and infants being more vulnerable. The condition of the victim will seriously affect the outcome. Hypertension, diabetes, advanced age, debility, or coagulation disorders are aggravated by a venomous snakebite. Individuals with bleeding tendencies, such as hemophilia, or those on anticoagulant therapy, with active peptic ulcers, or with open wounds are susceptible to bleeding secondary to envenomation. Women who are menstruating will bleed excessively after a pit viper bite. Women who have endometriosis may bleed excessively and develop severe pain. Cases of abortion in pregnant women who have been bitten by pit vipers have been reported.

The location of the bite is of great importance. Venomous snakebites on the head and trunk are from two to three times more dangerous than those on the extremities. Venomous bites on the upper extremities are more serious than those on the lower extremities. Incidental penetration of fangs and injection of venom into a blood vessel is usually catastrophic.

Clinical Features

After identifying whether the snake is venomous or harmless, quickly examine the pattern of the snakebite on the victim. It is safe to assume that the bite is venomous if one or two fang marks are present. Rarely three or four marks may be present, according to the number of fangs. Absence of fang marks is presumptive evidence of a harmless snakebite or an unsuccessful attempt by the pit viper without penetration. Fang marks separated by 15 mm or more indicate a bite by a very large snake, while those separated by less than 8 mm point to a smaller snake. A coral snake bite may present an atypical pattern.

Signs and Symptoms

If the offending snake cannot be identified, the symptoms and signs are the only remaining criteria of severity. The signs and symptoms are divided into hemopathic, neurotoxic, and systemic manifestations.

Hemopathic Manifestations

Swelling, edema, ecchymoses, extravasation of blood, and bleeding from kidneys, lungs, peritoneum, rectum, and vagina may occur owing to endothelial damage of small vessels and lymphatic channels.

Changes in red blood cells and their ability to transport oxygen may result in bleeding, drop in hemoglobin, and tissue anoxia leading to necrosis. There may be local bleeding from areas such as the endometrium or urinary tract or bleeding from pathological foci, such as peptic ulcers, because of impaired coagulation mechanisms. Hypofibrinogenemia, with or without thrombocytopenia, disseminated intravascular coagulation, or fibrinolysis can occur.

While hemopathic and systemic signs, including swelling, edema, and pain predominate with pit viper bites, neurologic signs may also occur.

Neurotoxic Manifestations

The effects of neurotoxins A and B on the central nervous system are manifested by dysphagia, convulsions, and psychotic behavior. The myoneural junction is also affected by neurotoxin B, which results in locomotor disturbances, manifested by weakness of the muscles, fasciculation, paresthesias, and, in very extreme cases, paralysis. Neurologic signs predominate with coral and cobra bites.

Systemic Effects

General systemic signs and symptoms of venomous snakebite include elevation or depression of the temperature, nausea, vomiting, diarrhea, pain, and restlessness. Although tachycardia is common, severe bradycardia may develop. The pathogenesis of the bradycardia is obscure. Renal failure from acute tubular necrosis or bilateral cortical necrosis has been reported.

Coral Snakes

Coral snakes do not have retractable anterior fangs. Therefore, they need greater leverage to puncture the skin and a longer period to inject their venom. Coral snake venom has a blocking action on acetylcholine receptor sites, and is not responsive to treatment with neostigmine or edrophonium. The early signs of a coral snake bite are slurred speech, ptosis, dilated pupils, dysphagia, and myalgia. Frequently symptoms are not evident until a few hours after the bite. Death results from respiratory arrest secondary to CNS inhibition, as well as weakness and possible paralysis of respiratory muscles.

Absorption of coral snake venom is rapid, and fixation is at the myoneural junction. Mechanical measures of tourniquet, incision, and suction are not of value in retarding absorption.

Unless obvious signs and symptoms of venomous snakebite are present, the differential diagnosis may not be easy. Consideration should be given to bites of chiggers, occasionally of tarantulas, and some insects. Frequently, individuals with two chigger bites which are about 1 cm apart, seek medical treatment claiming that they have sustained a snakebite. Only in that context is the differential diagnosis necessary; certainly, the symptomatology is not related. Factitious "fang marks" are seen occasionally in supervised group environments such as summer camps, military installations, and correctional institutions.

Treatment

First Aid

Health professionals and laypersons who frequent areas where venomous snakes are known to be prevalent should know how to give rapid first aid and be equipped to do so. Knowledge of proper application of a venous tourniquet, indications and technique of adequate and safe incision, and proper suctioning are essential. These measures may be, to a limited extent, effective only if applied in the first 30 to 45 min after the bite.

The following first aid measures may be used in the field or in the emergency department. Have the victim lie down immediately, as rest decreases metabolism, spread, and absorption of venom. Immobilize the bitten limb in a dependent position and reassure the victim.

A tourniquet is used immediately after the bite only to occlude venous and lymphatic return. Do not occlude arterial circulation to an area that is already ischemic. Apply the tourniquet several centimeters proximal to the bite, and loosen it every 15 to 30 min. As swelling progresses, move the tourniquet proximal to the proximal margin of the edema.

Guidelines for the treatment of pit viper bites, including surgical, medical, and anticipatory measures, are listed in Table 47-2.

Table 47-2. Guidelines for Treatment of Pit Viper Bite

Grade of Envenomation	Symptoms and Signs within 2 to 4 Hours	Surgical Measures	Medical Measures	Anticipatory Measures
I. Minimal	Moderate pain, edema 2.5–15 cm, erythema, no systemic symptoms	Cleansing and debriding	Antibiotic, tetanus prophylaxis, antihistamine	Type and cross-match blood, CBC, urinalysis, clotting time
II. Moderate	Severe pain, tenderness, edema 25–40 cm, erythema, petechiae, vomiting, fever, weakness	If very early: tourniquet, incision, suction (if adequately trained)	As above, plus IV antivenin infusion in selected cases of bite of rattler and cottonmouth	As above; also be ready to treat hemorrhage
III. Severe	Widespread pain, tenderness, edema 40–50 cm, ecchymosis, systemic signs, vertigo	As above, tight tourniquet or cryotherapy (if antivenin not available and will not be available in 4–6 h)	As above; also IV electrolytes, follow coagulation parameters, and give calcium gluconate if indicated for seizures	As above; also be ready to intubate and support respiration if needed
IV. Very severe	Rapid swelling ecchymosis, CNS symptoms, visual disturbance, shock, convulsions	Tourniquet completely occluding limb (if antivenin not available)	IV antivenin in massive doses, blood transfusions	As above; also watch for cardiac arrest, renal failure, compartment syndrome in extremities

Surgical measures are not generally recommended but could be useful if carried out by a trained person within 30 min of the bite. Two incisions, 20 mm long and to the depth of subcutaneous fat and fascia, should be placed over and somewhat above the fang marks along the longitudinal axis of the limb. Place the incisions about 20 mm apart from each other. The complications of improper incisions include neurovascular or tendon injury, and infection. Cruciate incisions should be avoided because they will result in excessive scarring. There is no evidence that irrigation of the incision with saline alters the progression of symptoms.

Suction kits and devices are preferable to mouth suction. The mouth can be used if the aspirate is spit out periodically and the mouth washed out. Unless there are cuts or open sores in the buccal mucosa, there is no danger to the rescuer, except possible hypoesthesia of the mucous membrane. Snake venom is digested and destroyed by gastric juices.

Antivenom is available by prescription only and its use and storage by laypersons remains controversial. Therefore, the decision to issue antivenom to a nonphysician should be made on the basis of the circumstances of the environment, the logistics of communication with and transportation to a medical facility and personnel, and the ability of the individual to properly use and administer the antivenom. Proper information, training, and standing orders ought to be available to the EMS personnel. Physician supervision should be readily available particularly in situations where life or limb are endangered. Prior knowledge of the location of facilities that routinely store type-specific antivenom should be widely publicized to EMS and law enforcement personnel. In cases of severe envenomation, speedy transport and general resuscitative measures in transit should be implemented.

Medical Measures

Treatment should be directed toward general life support. Intravenous fluids should be administered. Blood samples should be sent immediately for typing and cross-matching, which may become impossible as envenomation progresses. In severe cases, intubation and ventilatory support are necessary.

Blood transfusions may be necessary if bleeding has been severe. Intravenous calcium gluconate, 10 mL of a 10% solution, has been recommended for the treatment of seizures, although the mode of action is obscure, and controlled studies of its effectiveness are not available. Cardiac arrhythmias are treated in the usual manner. Antihistamines are helpful for itching and urticaria.

Close evaluation of the symptoms, signs, and condition of the victim is necessary. The presence and extent of ecchymoses, discoloration, vesicle formation, and edema should be recorded. Marking progression of edema on the limbs is useful and can be done along with periodic measurement of the circumference of the limb at predetermined points.

Clinical laboratory determinations including CBC; platelet count; BUN, creatinine, and electrolyte levels; prothrombin time; blood type and cross-match; and urinalysis should be obtained.

Appropriate tetanus prophylaxis should be administered.

Snakebites are notorious for becoming infected. The microorganisms represent a mixed flora of both gram-positive and gram-negative. Broad-spectrum antibiotics are indicated pending culture and sensitivity.

Antivenom

Antivenom is given to neutralize the snake venom. There are two types of antivenom produced in the United States and approved by the FDA. Antivenin (Crotalidae) made by Wyeth Laboratories is polyvalent against the pit viper venoms of North and South America. It is supplied as a powder to be mixed with sterile water and comes in a self-contained kit with instructions. Crotalidae antivenin is prepared from hyperimmune equine serum of horses exposed to venoms of the eastern diamondback rattlesnake, western diamondback rattlesnake, tropical rattlesnake, and fer-de-lance. These venoms contain basic antigens common to most of the pit vipers of the Americas, including rattlesnakes and moccasins of the United States, Japan, and Korea, and of the fer-de-lance and bushmaster.

A second type of antivenom is specific against the eastern coral snake bite. There is no evidence that this antivenom is of any value in the treatment of Arizona coral snake bites, which are extremely rare.

All antivenoms are made from horse serum, so that the patient should be tested for sensitivity to horse serum as soon as there is a consideration of diagnosis of a venomous snakebite. Testing can be accomplished by the intradermal injection of 0.2 mL of horse serum diluted 1:10 or 1:100 depending on whether the patient has a possible history of sensitivity to equine serum. Appearance of a wheal with or without pseudopods, erythema, and severe itching within 15 to 30 min suggest a positive reaction. An alternative testing procedure is to place one or two drops of horse serum diluted 1:1000 into the conjunctival sac. Onset of edema, itching, and redness of the eye signify a positive reaction. In either instance, epinephrine for subcutaneous injection should be immediately available to counteract any untoward event. Instill epinephrine drops into the eye if allergic conjunctivitis results.

Horse Serum Sensitivity

The question of whether to give horse serum–based antivenom to individuals who show evidence or have a history of allergy to horse serum remains problematic. Clinical judgment should be used to weigh the advantages and disadvantages of administering antivenom in light of the severity of the venomous snake bite. Not only potential mortality, but morbidity and later complications should enter into clinical consideration. Guidelines for antivenom administration are listed in Table 47-3. Wingert and Wainschell have described a method for intravenous infusion in severely envenomated patients with sensitivity to horse serum, consisting of

Table 47-3. Guidelines for Antivenom Administration

Grade of Envenomation		Dose
I	None	None
II	Minimal	20–40 ml (2–4 vials)*
III	Moderate	50–90 ml (5–9 vials)
IV	Severe	100–150 ml or more (10–15 or more vials)

*Use of antivenom here controversial—use clinical judgment.

Source: Data from Antivenin (Crotalidae) Polyvalent package insert. Wyeth Laboratories, Philadelphia, Pa.

50 mg of diphenhydramine IV, followed by slow IV infusion of antivenom. Antivenom is necessary for severe envenomation, but for minimal envenomation, the risks of administration may outweigh the benefits. Complications of antivenom administration are serum sickness, which develops nearly universally in those receiving seven ampoules or more of antivenom; radiculitis or other neuropathies; and of course, anaphylaxis. Do not give antivenom if a patient is definitely sensitive to horse serum and the pit viper bite is within grades I or II. However, in grades III or IV, particularly in a child or infant, lack of antivenom will most likely be fatal.

Administration and Dose

Antivenom comes in vials of 10 mL each. Anywhere from 5 to 15 or more vials may be used depending on the severity of the bite and the type of snake involved. Compared with adults, in similar circumstances, children should be given proportionately more since the aim is to neutralize the venom, and they have received a greater amount of venom per kilogram of body weight. The amount of antivenom given to a child is based on grade and not on body weight. Antivenom should be given within 4 h of the bite; 12 h after the bite the use of antivenom is of uncertain value.

Antivenom should be administered as an intravenous infusion and regulated according to the advance or recess of the swelling and other symptoms. It should never be injected into a finger or toe, nor should it be injected into the area of the bite.

In most instances, bites of rattlesnakes and water moccasins should be treated with antivenom unless there is a contraindication or the bite is not considered to be severe enough to warrant antivenom administration. As a rule, the bite of the copperhead is self-limiting and will not require antivenom or treatment. Exceptions would be cases involving an unusually large snake, multiple bites, or a small or debilitated victim.

Helpful Hints

1. Absence of fang marks precludes envenomation.
2. In presence of venom injection, the fang marks will continue oozing nonclotting blood.
3. Marks without bleeding or with clotted blood probably represent insect bite or are factitious.
4. Very soon after a pit viper bite, mild ecchymoses appear around the fang marks.
5. Immediate severe burning pain is characteristic of pit viper bite.
6. Absence of microhematuria after a pit viper bite is a good prognostic sign indicating lack of severe envenomation.

Consultation Service

A national index is maintained by the Oklahoma Poison Control Center in Oklahoma City, Oklahoma (405-271-5454), for locating type-specific antivenins to use in exotic venomous snakebites. The international *Antivenin Index* lists medical consultants and inter-nationally available antivenins and the species against which they are effective.

Other Modalities

Cryotherapy or immersion of the limb in ice water (not saline) may further jeopardize the injured limb because of cold-mediated vasoconstriction, or frostbite, and has not been demonstrated to inhibit the destructive effects of venom. It is contraindicated in the management of snakebite.

Local injection of lidocaine or procaine may help relieve pain, but the local injection of epinephrine is contraindicated because it further potentiates tissue ischemia. Steroids are indicated for the management of serum sickness, but have no role in the management of acute envenomation.

In this author's opinion, excision of the local soft tissues should be undertaken only if envenomation is severe; if the bite is on the trunk; if no antivenom is available; if no more than 1 h has elapsed from the time of the bite; and if no anatomical contraindications exist. It should be carried out by, or in consultation with, a surgeon. The skin and subcutaneous tissue should be excised in a radius of 3 to 4 cm from the fang marks and deep to the fascia. In 72 h, apply a split-thickness skin graft unless the recipient site is infected. The skin of the excised specimen, if intact, can be removed and preserved as full- or split-thickness graft for later use. Huang et al. have reported good success with early excision, under 2 h, even with involvement of upper or lower extremities or digits; incision of lateral and nodal aspects of a bitten finger may relieve swelling and pain. Fasciotomy is useful only when indicated for anatomical considerations or compartment syndrome. Reports by Glass of definitive treatment of pit viper bites by fasciotomy and steroids in combination have not been duplicated.

Late Complications

Tissue necrosis and slough are frequently results of inadequate treatment of the pit viper bite. In the absence or delay of administration of specific antivenom, extensive vasculitis, necrosis, and sloughing of the skin and subcutaneous tissues may occur.

Fibrosis can result secondary to the bites of rattlesnakes and water moccasins. Bites of the hand, both on the dorsum and on the palm, are particularly susceptible to later fibrosis and contractures. Limitations of motion, both in flexion and extension, are frequently seen. Fibrosis is a component of healing and scarring.

Immunization

Periodic reports in quasiscientific and lay literature indicate that certain individuals who have been bitten frequently by venomous snakes develop active immunity and, in addition, their serum confirms passive immunity. Such reports are at best anecdotal and frequently charged with emotion. Several controlled attempts to produce immunity in humans have failed. At least two individuals known to the author who have sustained many venomous snakebites became just as ill with subsequent bites as they did with earlier ones.

Harmless Snakes

Bites of harmless snakes are significant only as contaminated puncture wounds. Harmless snakes have several rows of teeth, and frequently the imprints of the teeth are seen on the skin of the victim. Cleansing, debridement, and administration of tetanus prophylaxis, as indicated, usually suffice. The use of broad-spectrum antibiotics may be indicated because the mouth of the snake is a veritable collection of microorganisms. Infrequently, the bite of a harmless snake will produce swelling, itching, and erythema. This is an allergic reaction to the snake's saliva, and an antihistamine will quickly relieve the symptoms.

Recent reports indicate that a few types of snakes, so far considered harmless, may in fact be able, under certain circumstances, to produce small amounts of low-toxicity venom and cause a mildly symptomatic bite. The hog-nosed, corn, and lyre snakes have been implicated. Treatment of the local symptoms is sufficient.

GILA MONSTER BITE

The Gila monster (*Heloderma suspectum*) is a sluggish and shy lizard that lives in the southwest and, in undergoing evolutionary changes, has developed eight venomous glands in the floor of its mouth. The venom is secreted into the oral cavity and then flows along the teeth, which are grooved posteriorly. Because of this rather primitive and ineffective injection apparatus, lizards have to hang on tenaciously and chew on the soft tissues to introduce a sufficient amount of venom to immobilize the prey. To detach the monster from the victim, introduce a hemostat, stick, or spoon between the jaws posteriorly and pry them apart.

The venom of the Gila monster primarily contains neurotoxins, and produces pain, edema, and a mostly local reaction. Reports of death secondary to the bite are not substantiated. There is no antivenom available for a Gila monster bite. Use of a venous tourniquet soon after the bite, local measures, and tetanus protection are indicated treatments. There is some evidence that meperidine may be synergistic with the venom; thus it is contraindicated for pain.

SCORPION STING

The scorpion is a land cousin of the crustaceans. It has an elongated segmented body not unlike that of a shrimp and a pair of anterior appendages with grasping pincers. Its tail is medium to moderately long, and segmented. The last segment is equipped with a stinger or telson. The tail, particularly the terminal segment with the stinger, is extremely mobile, making it essentially impossible to pick up this animal with bare hands. In the United States, the scorpion's habitat and particularly its virulence are quite limited. Southern Arizona and portions of neighboring states are areas of prime distribution of the scorpion.

Clinical Features

Several species of scorpions of the genus *Vejovis* have a very mild venom that is more allergenic than venomous. The sting causes a sharp, burning sensation that lasts a few minutes. Other types of *Vejovis* are able to sting and produce marked local edema that resolves over a day or two. At times, the stings of the giant hairy scorpion (*Hadrurus arizonensis*) and other related scorpions produce edema, burning pain, and ecchymosis. Occasionally, with larger species, edema may progress a few inches up the limb.

Barring an anaphylactic reaction, no danger exists from stings of these scorpions. Adequate cleansing, tetanus prophylaxis, and administration of antihistamines are adequate.

The only significant group of Arizona scorpions are the *Centruroides*. Stings of some of the subspecies are immaterial. However, *C. sculpturatus* and *C. gertschi* cause primarily systemic rather than local effects. About three to four deaths are reported annually. At the time of the sting, there is an initial burning pain followed by cholinergic symptoms.

Treatment

Efforts to remove the venom locally are useless. Opiates are contraindicated, and the treatment consists of general life support in a hospital setting, antihistamines, and atropine to counteract the parasympathomimetic effects. Immersion of the limb in cold water is somewhat analgesic. Specific antivenom for *C. sculpturatus* is available in the scorpion-infested areas of the southwest.

BIBLIOGRAPHY

Snakebite

Arnold RE: Results of treatment of *Crotalus* envenomation. *Am Surg* 41:643–647, 1975.

Arnold RE: Treatment of snakebite, letter to the editor. *JAMA* 236:1843, 1976.

Clark RW: Cryotherapy and corticosteroids in the treatment of rattlesnake bite. *Mil Med* 136:42–44, 1971.

Gill KA: The evaluation of cryotherapy in the treatment of snake envenomization. *South Med J* 63:552–556, 1970.

Glass FG: Early debridement in pit viper bites. *JAMA* 235:2513–2516, 1976.

Huang TT, Lynch JB, Larson D, et al: The use of excisional therapy in the management of snakebite. *Ann Surg* 179:598–607, 1974.

Podgorny G: Ophidism: The snake bite. *N C Med J* 26:244–250, 1965.

Podgorny G: Treatment of snake bite, in Haddad LM, Winchester JF (eds): *Clinical Management of Poisoning and Drug Overdose*. Philadelphia, Saunders, 1983.

Rappolt RT, Quinn H, Curtis L, et al: Medical toxicologist's notebook: Snakebite treatment and international antivenin index. *Clin Toxicol* 13:409–438, 1978.

Sabback MS, Cunningham ER, Fitts CT: A study of pit viper envenomization in 45 patients. *J Trauma* 17:569–573, 1977.

Shastry JCM, Date A, Carman EH, et al: Renal failure following snake bite: A clinicopathological study of nineteen patients. *Am J Trop Med Hyg* 26:1032–1038, 1977.

Wingert WA, Wainschel J: Diagnosis and management of envenomation by poisonous snakes. *South Med J* 68:1015–1026, 1975.

CHAPTER 48
EMERGENCIES
RELATED TO
MARINE FAUNA

J. K. Sims

The primary considerations in human medical emergencies precipitated by marine animals include trauma (hemorrhage, tissue disruption, fractures, dislocations, shock), envenomation, infection, foreign bodies (foreign body granulomas), air embolism and decompression sickness in divers (from panic), near drowning, and underlying medical disorders which may complicate the immediate problem.

The marine milieu is not sterile. Over 20 separate species of human pathogenic bacteria have been cultured from seawater (e.g., *Acinetobacter, Aerobacter aerogenes, Aeromonas hydrophila, Alcaligenes faecalis, Bacillus subtilis, Bacteroides fragilis, Clostridium botulinum, Enterobacter aerogenes, Enterococcus* sp., *Escherichia coli, Klebsiella pneumoniae, Proteus mirabilis, Pseudomonas aeruginosa, Staphylococcus aureus, Streptococcus* sp., *Vibrio alginolyticus, V. parahaemolyticus*, lactose-positive vibrios). More than seven species of human pathogenic bacteria have been cultured from marine sediments (e.g., *Bacillus cereus, C. botulinum, C. perfringens, C. tetani, Salmonella* sp., *V. alginolyticus, V. parahaemolyticus*, lactose-positive vibrios, coliforms). Human tetanus has been proposed to have been contracted from marine sources (e.g., marine *C. tetani*). There is no single antibiotic which covers the full spectrum of human pathogenic bacteria which have been cultured from the marine milieu.

Open trauma caused by marine organisms is the rule, whereas closed marine trauma is extremely rare, except for electrical shocks from marine animals such as electric catfish, eels, stingrays, stargazer fish, and trauma due to tentacles of the octopus and the squid. Bites must be distinguished as either venomous or nonvenomous. The marine fauna responsible for the different types of bites are listed in Table 48-1.

Fish which produce trauma through impalement include the needlefish, although there is no known venom associated with this impalement. Marine organisms with grossly visible spines produce puncture wounds and are frequently venomous. Such organisms include crown of thorns starfish (*Acanthaster planci*), cone shells, sea worms, venomous sharks such as the dogfish shark (*Squalus acanthias*) with its dorsal fin spines, venomous catfish with dorsal fin spines, sea urchins, scorpionfish, stonefish, and stingrays. Marine wound contaminants include sand, silt, teeth (e.g., of sharks), fangs (e.g., of the sea snake), spines (e.g., of the stingray), spine integumentary sheath fragments, nematocysts (e.g., of jellyfish), shell fragments, rock fragments (e.g., lava rock, cochina), spicules (e.g., sponges), algae (e.g., seaweeds such as *Microcoleus lyngbyaceus*, the stinging seaweed formerly known as *Lyngbya majuscula*), oils (e.g., boat oil slicks), sticks, diatoms, and plankton.

Nematocyst envenomation by jellyfish, Portuguese man-of-war, anemones, stinging fire corals, stinging true corals, hydroids, and other coelenterates may produce tentacle marks with full-thickness dermonecrosis.

Coral cuts result from abrasive contact with stony corals. Local hemorrhage results and the wounds are at risk for the development of infection. Particulate matter such as sand, silt, and coral fragments may enter the wound, resulting in wound contamination by seawater and associated microorganisms. Soft tissue density roentgenographic techniques may be utilized for the localization of radiopaque foreign bodies such as sand and coral fragments. Trauma from underwater glass, metallic objects, lava rock, cochina rock, and other objects that cannot be seen by the victim may incorrectly be presumed to be a coral cut. Foreign body granulomas, abscesses, and draining infected cutaneous sinus tracts may complicate the chronic coral cut and give the appearance of a "growing" lesion, although at present there is no evidence for coral growth within the human body.

TREATMENT

Management of emergencies caused by marine fauna initially consists of providing for the ABCDs, as applicable:

A. Airway
B. Breathing
C. Circulation, including control of hemorrhage, restoration of circulating blood volume, and treatment of shock
D. Decontamination, including detoxification

Detoxification in cases of envenomation is often more important than the management of the traumatic lesion per se.

The treatment of open marine wounds consists of the following, as applicable:

- ABCD priorities—Rule out envenomation early

Table 48-1. Classification of Marine Fauna Bites

Venomous Bites	Nonvenomous Bites	Uncertain Status
Sea snake	Sharks	Pufferfish
Octopus (certain species)	Moray eels	Moray eels
Bloodworms	Barracuda	
	Grouper	
	Killer whale (Orcinus orca)	
	Dolphins (mammal form)	
	Scorpionfish and stonefish	
	Parrotfish	
	Seals	
	Sea lions	
	Sea turtles	
	Clams	
	Catfish	
	Needlefish	
	Most fish	

- Control of hemorrhage, treatment of shock, restoration of circulating blood volume, treatment of fractures, and surgical repair of wounds.

Soft tissue density x-rays may be utilized to detect foreign bodies such as shark teeth, stingray spines, sea urchin spines, shell fragments, sand, and other radiopaque materials, which should be removed during wound decontamination prior to closure. Wounds should be thoroughly cleaned out and the following measures used as appropriate:

- Primary closure should be used if the wound is thoroughly clean and not considered an infection risk. A number of coral cuts may not be in this category. Skin grafts may be performed if necessary.
- Secondary closure, or delayed closure, should be used for a thoroughly cleaned wound considered an infection risk and for a wound that cannot be thoroughly cleaned but which is not considered an infection risk.
- Tertiary closure, or closure by granulation, should be used for open wounds that cannot be thoroughly cleaned and which present risk of infection, as well as for wounds with high risk of infection, such as some coral cuts and shark bites.

Early operative intervention has been utilized successfully in primary closure and skin graft for contaminated wounds at high risk of infection, such as shark bites. Antitetanus immunization updating and antimicrobial therapy should be provided, as indicated, with consideration of the appropriate utilization of cefoxitin in penicillin-resistant clostridial infections such as those of *Clostridium tetani*. Gas gangrene and tetanus in particular should be sought for early and throughout the management of all open marine wounds, especially bites such as shark bites, large spine punctures such as stingray stings, and traumatic disruptions of the gastrointestinal tract by marine organisms. Physical examination, x-ray, and bacterial culture techniques should be used. Early hyperbaric oxygen treatment of clostridial infections and antimicrobial therapy, in particular, should be considered. Wounds should be evaluated at least 3 and 7 days after the injury, if possible, for assessment of wound healing progress and infection status. Whether or not to use prophylactic antibiotics with marine open wounds has not been resolved. However, with heavily contaminated acute wounds at risk for clostridial infections by organisms such as *C.*

tetani and *C. perfringens*, early utilization of septic shock dosages of antimicrobials such as the penicillins should be considered. Alternative medications of equivalent effect may be utilized in those persons for whom penicillins are contraindicated. Consideration should be given, in the event of potential or actual β-lactamase-producing *S. aureus* in a wound of clinical significance, to the utilization of oxacillin or other antimicrobials which are effective for these organisms. Moray eel bites and barracuda bites are associated with tendon, fascia, nerve, ligament, and blood vessel disruption. Because of the elongated teeth of these organisms, the resultant infections may be deep as well as superficial and may present serious complications for the patient since these bites are usually sustained on the hands or other extremities.

The treatment of closed marine wounds is usually similar to that of a nonmarine wound. However, electric marine animals generally only stun human beings (and initiate near-drowning or diving emergencies) and do not produce the superficial or deep burn trauma seen in the more severe electrical wounds from a nonmarine source. Thus specific treatment is not usually necessary.

Treatment of spine puncture wounds such as stingray stings; venomous fin puncture wounds by catfish, scorpion fish, and stonefish; venomous shark fin stings; crown of thorns starfish stings; surgeonfish stings; cone shell stings; and some sea urchin stings includes the following:

- ABCD priorities, with the envenomation frequently being more significant in terms of mortality than the actual tissue trauma.
- Injection of local anesthetic (appropriate to the patient), without epinephrine, at the puncture site.
- Injection of a naloxone-reversible analgesic, as needed, rarely for any of the sea urchin stings and not always for the very painful stingray stings in which venom is actually injected into the wound.
- Hot water treatment of the affected area; water should be as hot as can be tolerated without scalding (45 to 50°C), and treatment should continue for 7 min for sea urchin stings to 90 min or more for stingray and stonefish stings. Cone shell stings may not be relieved at all.
- Use of antivenom, if available (e.g., a stonefish antivenom is available).

Attention should be given to the patient's tetanus immunization status (see above); in particular, follow up for infection. Ice pack treatment locally of spine puncture wounds is usually not helpful, and pain may increase.

Coelenterate stings, for example, from jellyfish, Portuguese man-of-war, anemones, hydroids, stinging fire coral, and stinging true corals, may be treated locally, at either the tentacle mark sites or nematocyst contact sites, utilizing household vinegar and unseasoned papain meat tenderizers for those not allergic to papaya. If necessary, tentacles can be removed by using forceps or pliers, not hands, even those covered with surgical gloves. Other appropriate therapy, e.g., for anaphylactic reactions, asthma-like attacks, laryngospasm, and the like, should be used as necessary. Do not expose the sting sites, unless fully treated locally, to fresh water, or severe pain may occur.

Sponge poisoning may be treated with dilute vinegar soaks 3 to 4 times a day, with desquamation weeks after the initial insult heralding resolution of the problem in a number of cases. Anaphylactoid reactions may occur. Sponge poisoning may be confused with sponge fisherman's disease, a disorder attributed to anemone infestation of the sponge resulting in a coelenterate sting (see above).

Swimmer's itch is, in actuality, an extensive collection of aquatic disorders (freshwater and marine) manifested by itching, for which the primary etiologies are microbial, plant, and animal. Marine swimmer's itch includes marine fungal dermatitis, bacterial dermatitis from, e.g., *Pseudomonas* sp., schistosome dermatitis, sponge poisoning, coelenteratate stings of many varieties, stinging seaweed dermatitis, and others, for which the designation of *swimmer's itch* may be used either until the definitive etiologic agent has been identified or when the agent cannot be identified.

Many of the problems caused by marine fauna can lead to or complicate the management of serious medical emergencies, such as near drowning, and diving emergencies, such as air embolism and decompression sickness. Although emergencies precipitated by marine fauna are important, those caused by marine flora, such as stinging seaweed dermatitis due to the marine blue-green algae *M. lyngbyaceus,* and by marine microbes are also important both in themselves and in the differential diagnosis of problems caused by marine fauna.

BIBLIOGRAPHY

Arnold HL Jr: Portuguese man-of-war (''Bluebottle'') stings: Treatment with papain. *Straub Clin Proc* 37:30–33, 1971.

Davies DH, Campbell GD: The aetiology, clinical pathology and treatment of shark attack. *J R Nav Med Serv* 48:110–136, 1962.

Mullaney PJ: Treatment of stingray wounds. *Clin Toxicol* 3:613–615, 1970.

Sims JK: Environmental emergencies—Animal toxins. 1982 American College of Emergency Physicians Winter Symposium presentation syllabus, Kaanapali, Maui, Hawaii, April 22, 1982.

Sims JK, Enomoto PI, Frankel RI, et al: Marine bacteria complicating seawater near-drowning and marine wounds: a hypothesis. *Ann Emerg Med* 12:212–216, 1983.

Sims JK, Irei MY: Human Hawaiian marine sponge poisoning. *Hawaii Med J* 38:263–270, 1979.

Sims JK, Zandee van Rilland RD: Escarotic stomatitis caused by the ''stinging seaweed'' *Microcoleus lyngbyaceus* (formerly *Lyngbya majuscula*): Case report and literature review. *Hawaii Med J* 40:243–248, 1981.

Turner B, Sullivan P, Pennefather J: Disarming the bluebottle. *Med J Aust* 2:394–395, 1980.

CHAPTER 49
DYSBARISM

Kenneth W. Kizer

A. Dysbaric Diving Casualties

There are now about 3 million recreational scuba[1] divers in this country, and over 300,000 new sport divers are certified each year. In addition, diving has become an integral part of commercial, scientific, and military professions (Table 49A-1).

The health problems associated with diving are due to the hazards of the aquatic environment and the breathing of compressed gases at higher than normal atmospheric pressure. Table 49A-2 categorizes a number of diving-related medical problems. The intent of this chapter is to review the major problems of barotrauma of ascent and descent, nitrogen narcosis, and decompression sickness.

PHYSICAL PRINCIPLES

Pressure

Many adverse physical conditions are encountered in the underwater environment. These include cold, wetness, changes in light and sound conduction, increased density of the surrounding environment, and increased atmospheric pressure. Of these, the indirect or direct effects of pressure account for the majority of serious diving medical problems.

Pressure is force per unit area and is measured in a number of different units (Table 49A-3). The weight of air at sea level is equal to 14.7 pounds per square inch (psi) or 1 atmosphere absolute (ATA). Under water, pressure increases because of the weight of the water. Since water is much denser than air, large changes in pressure will accompany small fluctuations in depth. Thus, as shown in Figure 49A-1, at a depth of 33 feet of seawater (fsw) the pressure is 2 ATA and at 165 fsw it is 6 ATA.[2] The proportionate change in pressure per unit depth change is greatest near the surface and progressively diminishes with increasing depth.

[1]Scuba is an acronym for *s*elf-contained *u*nderwater *b*reathing *a*pparatus.

[2]In diving and hyperbaric medicine the most commonly used units of pressure and depth are ATA and fsw.

Since fresh water is slightly less dense than salt water, it takes a depth change of 34 feet of fresh water (ffw) to change the pressure 1 ATA. Scuba diving is generally done at pressures of less than 7 ATA, with the overwhelming majority in the 2- to 4-ATA range.

Since body tissues are composed mostly of water, which is not compressible, they are not directly affected by pressure changes. However, gases are compressible, and, consequently, the gas-filled organs of the body are directly affected by pressure changes.

Table 49A-1. Types of Commercial Diving

Recovery of natural resources:
  Oil and natural gas
  Minerals
  Fish and shellfish
  Pearls, corals, and shells
  Algae (e.g., kelp or limu)
  Wood (logging)
  Aquaculture
Salvage operations
Maintenance and repair work:
  Ship hulls
  Nuclear power plants
  Bridges and tunnels
  Piers and harbors
  Aquariums
Construction:
  Piers and harbors
  Bridges and tunnels
  Dams
Underwater photography and motion picture production
Marine studies:
  Biology
  Geology
  Archeology
  Other sciences
Rescue and recovery operations
Sport diving instructors and tour guides

Table 49A-2. Primary Problems in Diving Medicine

Environmental exposure problems:
  Motion sickness
  Near drowning and other immersion syndromes
  Hypothermia and heat illness
  Sunburn and other actinic radiation syndromes
  Irritant dermatitides
  Infectious diseases
  Physical trauma
Dysbarism:
  Barotrauma
  Dysbaric air embolism
  Decompression sickness
Breathing gas–related problems
  Nitrogen or other inert gas narcosis
  Hypoxia
  Oxygen toxicity
  Hypo- or hypercarbia
  Carbon monoxide poisoning
  Nitrogen oxide and other air contaminants
  High-pressure nervous syndrome
  Cutaneous isobaric counterdiffusion
Hazardous marine life
Miscellaneous:
  Dysbaric osteonecrosis
  Compression athralgia
  Hyperbaric cephalgia
  Hearing loss
  Carotogenic blackout
  Panic and other psychological problems

Source: Adapted from Kizer, 1983.

Gas Laws

Diving physiology is best explained by three gas laws.

The first is Boyle's law, which states that the volume of a gas is inversely proportional to its pressure at a constant temperature. This is expressed by the equation:

$$PV = K$$

where P is pressure, V is volume, and K is a constant. Thus, as shown in Figure 49A-1, when the pressure is doubled the volume of a unit of gas is halved, and conversely. Boyle's law explains the basic mechanism of all types of barotrauma.

The second is Dalton's law, which states that the pressure exerted by each gas in a mixture of gases is the same as it would exert if it alone occupied the same volume, or, alternatively, the total pressure of a mixture of gases is equal to the sum of the

Table 49A-3. Pressure Equivalents

1 atmosphere absolute (ATA)	= 33 ft salt water (fsw)*
	= 5.5 fathoms seawater
	= 34 ft fresh water (ffw)
	= 14.7 psi
	= 760 mmHg
	= 29.9 inHg
	= 1.033 kg/cm²
	= 1.013 bar
	= 10.06 m
	= 0 atm gauge

*1 fsw = 0.445 psi = 0.0303 atm.
Source: From Kizer, 1983.

partial pressures of the component gases. This is mathematically stated as:

$$P_t = P_{O_2} + P_{N_2} + P_x$$

where P_t is the total pressure, P_{O_2} is the partial pressure of oxygen, P_{N_2} is the partial pressure of nitrogen, and P_x is the partial pressure of the remaining gases in the mixture. This law explains why the partial pressures of component gases in a mixture change proportionately to changes in ambient pressure even though their absolute concentrations remain constant. This law is fundamental to the understanding of decompression sickness and other breathing gas–related problems.

Henry's law states that the amount of gas dissolved in a given volume of fluid is proportional to the pressure of the gas with which it is in equilibrium. The formula is:

$$\%X = \frac{P_X}{P_t} \times 100$$

where $\%X$ is the amount of gas dissolved in a liquid, P_X is the partial pressure of gas X, and P_t is the total atmospheric pressure. This law explains why more inert gas, e.g., nitrogen, dissolves in the diver's body as ambient pressure is increased with descent and, conversely, is released from tissue with ascent.

DIRECT EFFECTS OF PRESSURE

The pressure-related diving syndromes can be roughly divided into problems caused by the mechanical effects of pressure, i.e., barotrauma, and problems caused by breathing gases at elevated partial pressures, i.e., gas toxicities and decompression sickness.

Barotrauma is by far the most common affliction of divers. It can be defined as tissue damage resulting from contraction or expansion of gas spaces which occurs when the gas pressure in the body is not equal to ambient pressure. For purposes of discussion, barotrauma can be viewed according to whether it occurs during descent or ascent.

Barotrauma of Descent

Barotrauma of descent, or "squeeze," as it is known in common diving parlance, results from the compression of gas in enclosed

	Depth, fsw	Gauge Pressure, atm	Absolute Pressure, atm	Gas Volume, %	Bubble Diameter,* %
Air	0	0	1	100	100
Seawater	33	1	2	50	79
	66	2	3	33	69
	99	3	4	25	63
	⋮	⋮	⋮	⋮	⋮
	165	5	6	17	54

*Bubble diameter is probably more important than volume in consideration of the ability of recompression to restore circulation to a gas embolized blood vessel.

Figure 49A-1. Pressure-volume relationships according to Boyle's law. Gauge pressure is always 1 atm less than absolute pressure. (Adapted from Kizer, 1983.)

spaces as ambient pressure increases with underwater descent. Gas pressure in the various air-filled spaces of the body is normally in equilibrium with the environment; however, if something should obstruct the various portals of gas exchange, pressure equalization will be precluded. If the air-filled space is not collapsible, the resulting pressure imbalance will cause tissue distortion, vascular engorgement and mucosal edema, hemorrhage, and other tissue damage. Obviously, the ears and paranasal sinuses are most likely to be affected by such a process.

Aural barotrauma is the most common type of barotrauma and is a major cause of morbidity among divers, being experienced by essentially all divers at one time or another. There are three main types of aural barotrauma, depending on which part of the ear is affected, and they may occur singly or in combination.

The first type of aural barotrauma involves the external auditory canal and is generally referred to as *external ear squeeze*, or *barotitis externa*. The external ear canal normally communicates with the environment and, consequently, the air in the canal is replaced by water when a diver is submerged. However, if the external ear canal is occluded (e.g., by cerumen, foreign bodies, exostoses, earplugs, or a too-tight-fitting hood), water entry is prevented, and compression of the enclosed air with descent will have to be compensated for by tissue collapse, outward bulging of the tympanic membrane, or hemorrhage. This is typically manifested by pain and/or bloody otorrhea. Physical examination may reveal petechiae, blood-filled cutaneous blebs along the canal, erythema, or rupture of the tympanic membrane. As with other types of ear canal injury, treatment for this type of squeeze involves keeping the canal dry, prohibition of swimming or diving until healed, and, in special cases, antibiotics and analgesics.

The next and by far the most common type of aural barotrauma is middle ear squeeze, or *barotitis media*. This results from a failure to equalize the middle ear and environmental pressures because of occlusion or dysfunction of the eustachian tube.

The eustachian tubes normally open and allow equalization of middle ear pressure when the pressure differential between the middle ear and pharynx reaches about 20 mmHg. This can be facilitated by yawning, swallowing, or utilizing various autoinflation techniques (e.g., the Valsalva or Frenzel maneuver). If middle ear pressure equalization is not achieved, the diver will notice discomfort or pain when the pressure differential reaches 100 to 150 mmHg or, roughly, when there has been a 20 percent reduction in middle ear gas volume. As the pressure differential is further increased, there develops mucosal engorgement and edema, hemorrhage, and inward bulging of the tympanic membrane. Eventually, these will be inadequate to compensate for the gas volume contraction, and the tympanic membrane ruptures. Fortunately, this degree of injury is uncommon.

A number of factors may cause eustachian tube blockage or dysfunction, e.g., mucosal congestion secondary to upper respiratory infection, allergies, or smoking; mucosal polyps; excessively vigorous autoinflation maneuvers; and previous maxillofacial trauma. Persons with such conditions are at increased risk of aural barotrauma.

Divers having a middle ear squeeze usually complain of ear fullness or pain. As would be expected from the way that pressure changes with depth (Fig. 49A-1), most problems occur near the surface. The pain of a middle ear squeeze is substantial and usually causes the diver to abort the dive. If not, it will continue to worsen until the eardrum ruptures, at which time the diver may feel bubbles escaping from the ear and experience disorientation, nausea,

and vertigo secondary to the caloric stimulation of cold water entering the middle ear. This sequence of events has been responsible for many cases of panic and near drowning.

The otoscopic appearance of the tympanic membrane in cases of middle ear squeeze varies according to the severity of the injury and can be graded according to the amount of hemorrhage in the eardrum, with grades running from 0 (symptoms only) to 5 (gross hemorrhage and rupture). Utilizing this grading scheme facilitates communication when describing the injury but has little other function. Physical examination may also disclose blood around the nose or mouth and a mild conductive hearing loss, which is usually only temporary.

Treatment of middle ear squeeze involves abstinence from diving until the condition has resolved and use of decongestants, which may be combined with antihistamines if there is an allergic component to the eustachian tube dysfunction. A combination of oral and long-acting nasal spray decongestants is usually most efficacious. Antibiotics should be used when there is a tympanic membrane rupture or a preexisting infection, or after diving in polluted waters. Obviously, no diving should be done until a perforated eardrum has healed. Oral analgesics or topical aural anesthetics may be needed for a couple of days. In general, ear drops should not be used when there is a tympanic membrane perforation. Ideally, an audiogram should be obtained in anyone having more than a trivial squeeze, and serial audiograms should be obtained in patients having hearing loss. Most middle ear squeezes will resolve without complication in 3 to 7 days. Obviously, though, prevention is preferable; a diver should refrain from diving when unable to easily equalize pressure in the ears and should heed warning signs of ear pain.

The third type of aural barotrauma affects the inner ear and usually involves rupture of the round or oval windows, which results in the development of a perilymph fistula (PLF). The mechanism of injury in PLF is somewhat controversial, largely because there seems to be more than one set of circumstances under which it may occur. The basic requisite circumstance, though, is the sudden development of markedly different pressures between the middle and inner ears. This can occur after a rapid descent without adequately equilibrating the middle ear, resulting in excessive inward movement of the eardrum and stapes so that the oval window is imploded. Conversely, a forceful Valsalva maneuver may abruptly raise the cerebrospinal fluid pressure (which is transmitted to the perilymph) so much so that it causes an explosive outward rupture of either round or oval windows. Occasionally, PLF may develop during ascent. Whatever the case, the development of a labyrinthine fistula and consequent perilymph fluid leak will result in irreversible cochlear damage if not recognized and treated without delay. PLF almost always involves round window rupture in scuba divers.

Patients with inner ear barotrauma may complain of "blockage" in the affected ear, tinnitus, vertigo, disorientation, ataxia, or hearing loss, with the classic symptom triad being tinnitus, vertigo, and deafness. Examination will usually reveal findings of middle ear barotrauma, sensorineural hearing loss, and vestibular dysfunction. Management of PLF is also somewhat controversial, at least with regard to the indications for surgical exploration. Some experts prefer a trial of bed rest and symptomatic measures for vertigo before attempting surgical correction, while others advocate prompt exploration and, if present, repair of the fistula. Whichever route is taken, though, there is unanimity that no further diving should be done after a patient suffers a PLF.

Just as with the ears, any of the paranasal sinuses may fail to

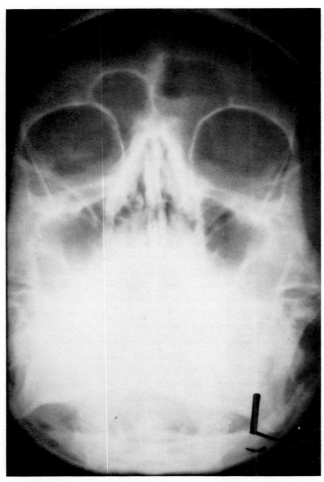

Figure 49A-2. Radiograph showing an air-fluid level in the left frontal sinus from a sinus squeeze. (Courtesy Castle Memorial Hospital, Hawaii; photo by K. W. Kizer.)

equalize pressure during descent. Manifestations of sinus squeeze include a sensation of fullness or pressure in the affected sinus, pain, or hemorrhage. Again, predisposing conditions for barosinusitis include upper respiratory infections, sinusitis, nasal polyps, or anything else that impairs the free flow of air from sinus cavity to nose. The maxillary and frontal sinuses are most often affected (Fig. 49A-2). Treatment for sinus squeeze is much the same as for middle ear squeeze, although antibiotics are usually indicated in cases involving the frontal sinuses.

Squeeze can also affect any other gas space that does not equilibrate with ambient pressure. For example, conjunctival and scleral hemorrhage may result from wearing goggles when diving. The same thing may happen if the diver fails to exhale into the mask during descent, resulting in telltale erythema, ecchymosis, and petechiae of the part of the face enclosed by the face mask— i.e., "face mask squeeze." Similarly, if an area of skin is tightly enclosed by a dry diving suit a "suit squeeze" may occur. Although the appearance of these injuries may be spectacular, no special treatment is required, and they usually resolve in a few days.

Another special kind of squeeze may occur in divers who, while holding their breath, descend below the depth at which their total lung volume is reduced to less than residual volume. As occurs in other types of barotrauma of descent, the underventilated lung

air spaces fill with tissue fluids and blood in an attempt to relieve the negative pressure. Clinical manifestations include chest pain, cough, hemoptysis, dyspnea, and pulmonary edema. Treatment includes administration of 100% oxygen, fluid replacement, and other supportive measures as clinically indicated. Because of the intrinsic lung injury and consequent potential for gas embolism, positive pressure breathing (e.g., PEEP or CPAP) should be avoided if at all possible. Overall, though, very few divers attempt to free-dive to depths likely to cause lung squeeze, and it is rarely seen.

Barotrauma of Ascent

If there has been adequate equilibration of the pressure in the body's air-filled spaces during descent, then the gas in those spaces will expand according to Boyle's law as ambient pressure decreases with ascent. The resulting excess gas is normally vented to the atmosphere. However, if this is prevented by obstruction of the air passages, the expanding gases will distend the tissues surrounding them; the resulting damage is known as *barotrauma of ascent* and is the reverse process of squeeze.

Although the ears and sinuses may be affected by barotrauma of ascent, this is unusual, since impediment of air egress is unlikely if pressure equalization can be achieved with descent. However, middle ear barotrauma of ascent, or *reverse squeeze,* as it is usually called, can occur, especially in divers having upper respiratory congestion treated with a short-acting nasal spray whose vasoconstrictive effect wears off while the diver is submerged. Similarly, *alternobaric vertigo* (ABV) resulting from unequal vestibular stimulation due to asymmetric middle ear pressure may occur during ascent. Although usually only transient, ABV may be severe enough to cause panic. Rarely, it may last for several hours after a dive.

Three other types of barotrauma of ascent should be discussed. The first of these may occur with either ascent or descent, although more commonly with ascent, and is known as *barodontalgia,* or, less accurately, "tooth squeeze." Several specific conditions are associated with this problem (e.g., pulp decay, peridontal infections, or recent extraction sockets or fillings), but it may be due to anything that causes a pressure disequilibrium in an air-filled space in or about a tooth. Although rare and usually self-limited, any diver presenting with a toothache after diving should be referred for dental evaluation after excluding maxillary sinus squeeze.

Another rather benign type of barotrauma of ascent is gastrointestinal barotrauma, which is also known as *aerogastralgia,* or "gas in the gut." This occurs most commonly in novice scuba divers, who are more prone to aerophagia, and is caused by expansion of intraluminal bowel gas as ambient pressure is decreased during ascent. Other predisposing conditions include repeated performance of the Valsalva maneuver in the head-down position (which forces air into the stomach), drinking carbonated beverages or eating a heavy meal before diving (especially one containing legumes or other flatogenic substances), or chewing gum while diving. Symptoms of gastrointestinal barotrauma include abdominal fullness, colicky abdominal pain, belching, and flatulence. It is rarely severe because most divers will readily vent any excess bowel gas during ascent; however, it has been known to cause syncopal and shocklike states. Only one case of actual gastric rupture from GI barotrauma is known to have occurred, and this was a very unusual case of a scuba diver who swallowed a large volume of water secondary to near drowning.

Table 49A-4. Manifestations of the Pulmonary
Overpressurization Syndrome

1. Pneumomediastinum
2. Subcutaneous emphysema
3. Pneumopericardium
4. Pneumothorax
5. Pulmonary interstitial emphysema
6. Pneumoperitoneum
7. Gas embolism
   a. Brain
   b. Heart
   c. Visceral

The last and most serious type of barotrauma of ascent is pulmonary barotrauma (PBT). Several different injuries can result from PBT of ascent, and these can be collectively referred to as the pulmonary overpressurization syndrome (POPS), or "burst lung" (Table 49A-4).

Diving equipment is designed to deliver compressed gas to the diver at the same pressure as the surrounding environment, e.g. at 33 fsw the diver breathes gas at 2 ATA. Consequently, the compressed gas will expand during ascent according to Boyle's law, and the diver must allow the expanding gas to escape from the lungs or it will rupture and dissect into the surrounding tissue. The resultant injury will depend on the location and amount of escaped gas. Overt symptoms may appear immediately upon surfacing or may be delayed for several hours. Mediastinal or sub-cutaneous emphysema are the most common forms of the POPS, and the patient usually presents with gradually increasing hoarseness, neck fullness, and substernal chest pain several hours after diving. Dyspnea, dysphagia, syncope, and other symptoms may be present as well. The history is usually diagnostic, although radiographs are indicated to verify the location of gas and exclude the presence of a pneumothorax (Fig. 49A-3).

The development of a pneumothorax while diving is serious, for intrapleural gas cannot be released to the environment and is likely to progress to tension pneumothorax during ascent, leading to syncope, shock, or unconsciousness upon surfacing.

Except for pneumothorax, which may require needle aspiration or tube thoracostomy, treatment of uncomplicated pulmonary overpressurization typically requires only observation, rest, and, sometimes, supplemental oxygen. Recompression is necessary only in extremely severe cases.

AIR EMBOLISM

The most feared complication of PBT is air embolism. Indeed, dysbaric air embolism (DAE) is one of the most dramatic and serious injuries associated with diving and is a major cause of death and disability among sport divers.

DAE results from the entry of gas bubbles into the systemic circulation via ruptured pulmonary veins. After passing through the heart, bubbles lodge in small arteries, occluding the more

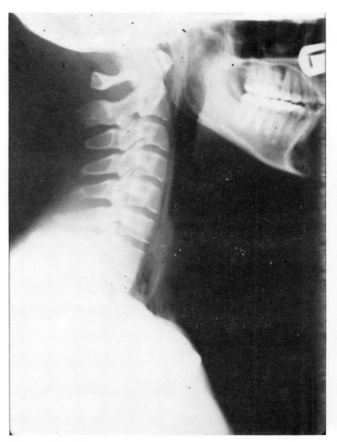
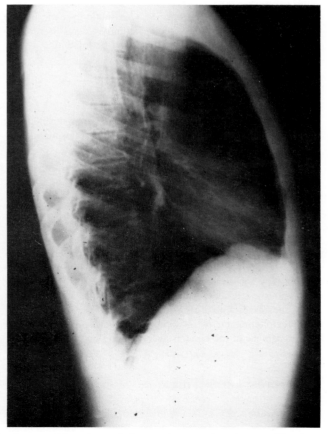

Figure 49A-3. Radiographs showing air dissecting through the mediastinum and into the neck from pulmonary barotrauma. (Courtesy Tripler Army Medical Center, Hawaii; photo by K. W. Kizer.)

distal circulation. The resulting manifestations will depend on the location of the occlusion, and, depending on the site, even minute quantities of gas can have disastrous consequences.

DAE usually presents immediately after a diver surfaces, at which time the high intrapulmonic pressure resulting from lung overexpansion is relieved, which allows bubble-laden blood to return to the heart. Although the classic history is that the diver ascends rapidly because of running out of air, panic, or some similar circumstance, this is not always the case, and localized overinflation may also result from focally increased elastic recoil of the lungs in some divers.

The presenting manifestations of DAE are usually dramatic. Coronary occlusion and cardiac arrest may occur, although the brain is by far the most often affected organ. The neurological manifestations are typical of an acute stroke, such as mono- or multiplegia, focal paralysis, sensory disturbance, blindness, deafness, vertigo, dizziness, confusion, convulsions, or aphasia. Asymmetric multiplegias are the most common presentation, and the differentiation of DAE from severe neurological decompression sickness is often impossible. Sudden loss of consciousness upon surfacing should always be assumed to be due to gas embolism until proved otherwise. Although hemoptysis is often mentioned in standard references as a presenting sign of DAE, this was noted in only 2 of 42 cases reviewed by the author. Other reported clinical findings such as visualization of bubbles in the retinal arteries or Libermeister's sign (a sharply circumscribed area of glossal pallor) are exceedingly rare.

Some patients with very severe initial neurological symptoms may quickly improve spontaneously. The mechanism of spontaneous recovery is not clear. Nonetheless, such patients should still be referred for recompression since even subtle dysbaric injuries may become irreversible without definitive care. Before recompression, pneumothorax should always be ruled out.

INDIRECT EFFECTS OF PRESSURE

Nitrogen narcosis and decompression sickness may develop as a result of breathing gases at higher-than-normal atmospheric pressure.

Nitrogen Narcosis

Nitrogen and other lipid-soluble inert gases have an anesthetic effect at elevated partial pressures. The narcotic effects are similar to those of alcohol and become evident in most divers between 70 and 100 fsw. Many divers are so markedly impaired at 200 fsw that they can do no useful work, and at depths over 300 fsw unconsciousness ensues. Although narcotic effects are reversed as the P_{N_2} decreases with ascent, nitrogen narcosis is not an uncommon precipitating factor in diving accidents and may impair a diver's memory of the circumstances leading up to the accident.

Decompression Sickness

Decompression sickness is a multisystem disorder resulting from the liberation of inert gas from solution with the formation of gas

bubbles in blood and body tissues when ambient pressure is decreased. The critical factor in its pathogenesis is increased tissue absorption of inert gas, which in most diving situations is nitrogen.

As an air-breathing diver descends underwater, the ambient pressure increases, and there develops a positive gradient of nitrogen from alveoli to blood to tissue. After a period of time at depth this gradient will diminish, eventually becoming zero as a new equilibrium is reached. The time that it takes for the new equilibrium to be achieved will depend on the alveolar-to-tissue inert gas gradient, the tissue blood flow, and the ratio of blood to tissue inert gas solubility. Consequently, the rate at which a diver reaches a new inert gas equilibrium will be an exponential function of the diffusion and perfusion characteristics of the different tissues.

The tissue absorption of increased gas is the first step to decompression sickness (DCS), but it is only when ambient pressure is decreased too rapidly to allow the diffusion of inert gas from tissues that DCS occurs.

The pathophysiology of decompression sickness consists of both mechanical and biophysical effects of bubbles (Fig. 49A-4). The major mechanical effect of bubbles in DCS is vascular occlusion; however, the bubbles in DCS form primarily in the venous circulation and thus impair venous return. However, the bubbles in DCS can form anywhere, such as in lymphatics, or intracellularly or extravascularly. Lymphedema, cellular distension and rupture, and intercellular dislocation can all compound the effects of vascular occlusion. Also, venous gas emboli may cause paradoxical arterial embolization via intrapulmonic and intracardiac shunts.

Bubbles also exert a variety of biophysical effects due to blood

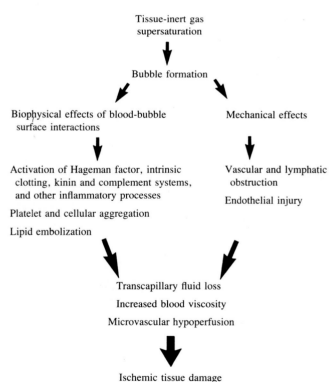

Figure 49A-4. Schematic representation of the pathogenesis of decompression sickness. (Adapted from Kizer, 1983.)

bubble surface interaction. In essence, bubbles are viewed by the immune system as foreign matter, and they incite an inflammatory reaction. The key step in the process is activation of Hageman factor, which, in turn, activates the intrinsic clotting mechanisms and kinin and complement systems, which results in platelet activation, cellular clumping, lipid embolization, increased vascular permeability, interstitial edema, and microvascular sludging. The net effect of all these processes is decreased tissue perfusion and ischemic injury.

The clinical manifestations of decompression sickness are protean (Table 49A-5), but the joints and spinal cord are most often affected. Technically, the term *bends* refers only to the musculo-skeletal form of DCS, but it is commonly used to mean any type of DCS. The various forms of DCS have also been arbitrarily categorized as either types I or II, with type I referring to the mild forms of DCS (skin, lymphatic, and musculoskeletal systems) and type II including the neurological and other serious types. Although this latter categorization is firmly entrenched in the literature, it is clinically more meaningful to refer to the systems affected when discussing patients with DCS.

Cutaneous manifestations of DCS include pruritus, subcutaneous emphysema, and scarlatiniform, erysipeloid, or mottled rashes. Localized swelling or peau d'orange may result from lymphatic obstruction.

Periarticular joint pain is typically described as a deep, dull ache, although it may be throbbing or sharp. There may be a vague area of numbness or dysesthesia around the affected joint. Movement of the affected extremity usually aggravates the pain, but inflation of a blood pressure cuff around the involved joint may relieve the pain for as long as the cuff is inflated. The shoulders and elbows are most often affected in scuba divers, although essentially any joint may be involved.

Neurological DCS may be manifested by a vast array of symptoms and signs, and even though specific types of diving characteristically produce certain neurological syndromes, the best rule is that essentially any symptom is compatible with neurological DCS. Classically, however, neurological DCS involves the lower thoracic and lumbar portions of the spinal cord and produces paraplegia or paraparesis, lower-extremity paresthesias, and bladder dysfunction. Historically, urinary retention was such a frequent manifestation of spinal cord DCS that a urethral catheter used to be part of the diver's standard equipment. Recently, Hallenbeck et al. have convincingly demonstrated that spinal cord DCS results from venous infarction of the cord due to obstruction of venous drainage in the epidural vertebral venous plexus.

Table 49A-5. Forms of Decompression Sickness

1. Cutaneous ("skin bends")
2. Lymphatic
3. Musculoskeletal (the "bends" or pain-only bends)
4. Neurological
   a. Spinal cord
   b. Cerebral
   c. Cerebellar (the "staggers")
   d. Inner ear
   e. Peripheral nerves
5. Pulmonary (the "chokes")
6. Cardiovascular (decompression shock)
7. Visceral

Pulmonary DCS results from massive venous air embolization and usually does not become symptomatic until at least 10 percent of the pulmonary vascular bed is obstructed. Signs and symptoms include chest pain, cough, dyspnea, shock, and pulmonary edema. The clinical course is often fulminant and downhill.

It has now been well demonstrated by ultrasonic techniques that many divers develop intravascular bubbles but no apparent illness; these have been called "silent bubbles."

A variety of laboratory abnormalities may be demonstrated in DCS, but most of them have little clinical relevance to acute care.

Dysbaric casualties should be rapidly referred for hyperbaric treatment. However, the patient should also be evaluated for life-threatening nondysbaric injuries and, if present, resuscitation commenced.

Since intravascular volume depletion and hemoconcentration are common in serious DCS, fluid replacement should be an integral part of therapy.

TREATMENT OF DIVING CASUALTIES

The Diving Accident History

Most diving problems can be properly diagnosed by history and physical examination alone. The specific diving accident history should encompass the following basic points.

1. The type of diving engaged in and the equipment used. Some kinds of diving or certain types of equipment are associated with specific problems, e.g., hypercarbia or oxygen toxicity with rebreathing apparatus. Make sure that the patient was actually breathing compressed air. For example, the author has responded more than once to the recompression chamber for an improperly evaluated snorkeler who was actually a near-drowning victim.
2. The number, depth, bottom time, and surface interval between repetitive dives for all dives in the 48 to 72 h preceding symptom onset. Even though this information may not be especially meaningful to you, having it available will facilitate communication with the diving medicine consultant, who will want to ascertain if required decompression steps were omitted.
3. In-water decompression. Again, this is relevant to the determination of the likelihood of the diver having DCS.
4. In-water recompression. Recompression with compressed air should never be attempted, for it almost always leaves the diver in a worse condition than originally and is fraught with other hazards.
5. Site of diving (e.g., ocean, lake, or quarry) and environmental conditions (e.g., water temperature, amount of surge) associated with the dive. Other things being equal, DCS is more likely to occur after diving in cold water.
6. Primary diving activity (e.g., spearfishing, photography). DCS is more likely after an arduous dive.
7. Presence of predisposing factors. A number of factors have been anecdotally related to the development of DCS. These include: advanced age (decreased tissue perfusion), obesity (increased absorption of inert gas), dehydration, recent alcohol intoxication, cold water (decreased peripheral perfusion), vigorous underwater exercise (increased gas uptake),

local physical injury (decreased local perfusion), and multiple repetitive dives in unacclimatized individuals (gradual buildup of inert gas).

8. Dive complications. These include running out of air, marine animal envenomation, trauma, or some other unexpected event. Musculoskeletal pain may be due to overexertion or muscle strain, and numbness in an extremity may be from a jellyfish sting rather than DCS.

9. Predive and postdive activities. Activities such as jogging, unpressurized airplane travel, etc., may precipitate DCS. Likewise, trivial dysbaric symptoms may become severe after similar activities.

10. Onset of symptoms. Certain conditions are more likely to occur at given times in the dive profile, and a differential diagnostic scheme can be derived on the basis of time of symptom onset.

Differential Diagnosis of Diving Accidents

In general, a scuba dive can be divided into five stages, each of which is associated with characteristic problems.

1. The predive surface phase. The predive surface phase includes all activities prior to going underwater and beginning to breathe compressed air. This often involves considerable surface swimming to the dive site. The most often encountered problems during this phase of the dive are motion sickness, hyperventilation, physical trauma, near drowning, and untoward marine animal encounters.

2. Descent phase. The primary problems associated with descent are the squeeze syndromes, especially aural barotrauma, although PLF and ABV may also occur. Similarly, carbon monoxide poisoning, hypoxia, or other breathing gas problems may develop early in the dive.

3. At-depth or bottom phase. Overall, few problems occur "on the bottom," and the most likely ones are physical trauma or encounters with dangerous marine life. Nitrogen narcosis may contribute to an underwater accident. PLF or gas mixture problems may first become symptomatic at this time.

4. Ascent phase. Again, barotrauma is the problem most often encountered with ascent, although much less frequently than during descent. The relationship of POPS, ABV, and PLF with ascent have already been discussed. Gas mixture problems may become manifest at this time, and hypercarbia can be experienced toward the end of a dive. Decompression sickness may occasionally occur while a diver is still submerged; if this happens it usually implies a serious problem.

5. Postdive surface phase. The postdive surface phase is divided into immediate (within 10 min of surfacing) and delayed (after 10 min). Any symptom occurring in the immediate postdive phase should be considered an air embolism until proved otherwise. Any symptom which begins more than 10 min after the dive should be viewed as decompression sickness until otherwise explained. More than half of all DCS patients will become symptomatic in the first hour after surfacing, with most of the rest experiencing symptoms within 6 h. A very few patients (1 to 2 percent) may note their first symptoms 24 to 48 h after diving. Other problems that may be first noted in the delayed postdive phase include mild forms of the POPS, sequelae of barotrauma, PLF, motion sickness, exhaustion, irritant or venomous dermatoses, and nondysbaric conditions related to physical activity.

Immediate Management

The victim should be rescued from the water and basic life support measures begun as needed. Hypothermia should be considered an aggravating factor in every aquatic accident victim.

If DAE is suspected the victim should be placed in the head-down position to prevent additional gas emboli from traveling to the brain. This position increases venous pressure, which should facilitate the passage of bubbles through to the venous circulation and, hence, back to the lung where they can be eliminated. Whether this truly happens or whether addition of the left lateral decubitus position is of any real benefit has never been demonstrated. In any case, unless transport to a hyperbaric chamber will take longer than 30 to 60 min these maneuvers should cause no harm. However, the head-down position does increase intracranial pressure, and may cause or worsen cerebral edema.

Supplemental 100% oxygen should always be given as soon as possible, being best administered by mask at 6 to 8 L/min. This facilitates offgassing of the nitrogen bubbles and improves oxygenation of damaged tissues.

Depending on local circumstances, patients with suspected DAE or DCS may be taken directly to the recompression chamber (Fig. 49A-5) or may need emergency department stabilization. Whichever the case, transportation should be as expeditious as possible. If air transportation is used, the patient should be subjected to the least possible pressure reduction so as not to cause any further gas expansion. Either a low-flying helicopter or light airplane, capable of flight at 1000 ft or less, should be used. Alternatively, aircraft that can be pressurized to 1 ATA (e.g., Lear jet or C-130 Hercules) can be used.

Advanced life support drugs should be administered according to the victim's condition and standard protocols. In general, most DCS victims will be at least mildly volume depleted, so parenteral

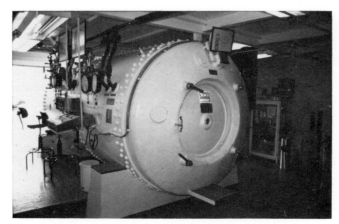

Figure 49A-5. Typical multiplace recompression chamber. The two compartments can be pressurized independently of each other up to 6 ATA, and as many as 12 persons can be seated in the chamber. (Photo by K. W. Kizer.)

and oral (if the patient is alert) fluids should be given at a brisk rate unless they are contraindicated for other reasons. High-dose parenteral corticosteroids are probably beneficial and should be given as soon as possible.

If the need for recompression or the location of the nearest hyperbaric treatment facility is uncertain, assistance is available 24 h/day through the National Diving Alert Network at Duke University (919-684-8111).

Hyperbaric Treatment

Space does not allow for a discussion of recompression treatment here. Suffice it to say that pressure and oxygen are the keystones of treatment for DCS and DAE and that they are administered according to well-established protocols. Various types of hyperbaric chambers may be utilized for treatment, and the relative merits of one type or another need not be recounted here.

The outcome of recompression treatment will, of course, depend on the severity of the disease, the delay in commencing hyperbaric treatment, and the victim's health prior to the accident. Overall, 80 to 90 percent success rates have been reported from a variety of sources, and even though recompression is more likely to be beneficial the sooner that it is commenced after the onset of symptoms, it should not be refused to someone who presents 2, 3, or more days after an accident, for dramatic recoveries have been reported after treatment delays of 7 to 9 days.

BIBLIOGRAPHY

Ah-See AK: Review of arterial air embolism in submarine escape, in Smith G (ed): *Proceedings of the Sixth International Congress on Hyperbaric Medicine*. Aberdeen, Wash, Aberdeen University Press, 1977, pp 349–351.

Behnke AR: Decompression sickness following exposure to high pressures, in Fulton JF (ed): *Decompression Sickness*. Philadelphia, Saunders, 1951, pp 53–89.

Blick G: Notes on diver's paralysis. *Br Med J* 4:1796–1798, 1909.

Bond GF: Arterial gas embolism, in Davis JC, Hunt TK (eds): *Hyperbaric Oxygen Therapy*. Bethesda, Md, Undersea Medical Society, 1977, pp 141–152.

Bove AA: The basis for drug therapy in decompression sickness. *Undersea Biomed Res* 9:91–111, 1982.

Brown FM: Vertigo due to increased middle ear pressure: Six year experience of the aeromedical consultation service. *Aerosp Med* 42:999–1001, 1971.

Cales RH, Humphreys N, Pilmanis AA, et al: Cardiac arrest from gas embolism in scuba diving. *Ann Emerg Med* 10:589–592, 1981.

Colebatch HJM, Smith MM, Ng CKY: Increased elastic recoil as a determinant of pulmonary barotrauma in divers. *Respir Physiol* 26:55–64, 1976.

Cramer FS, Heimbach RD: Stomach rupture as a result of gastrointestinal barotrauma in a scuba diver. *J Trauma* 22:238–240, 1982.

Elliott DH, Hallenbeck JM: The pathophysiology of decompression sickness, in Bennett PB, Elliott DH (eds): *The Physiology and Medicine of Diving and Compressed Air Work*, ed. 2. Baltimore, Williams & Wilkins, 1975, pp 435–455.

Elliott DH, Hallenbeck JM, Bove AA: Acute decompression sickness. *Lancet* 2:1193–1199, 1974.

Enders LJ, Rodriquez-Lopez E: Aeromedical consultation service case report: Alternobaric vertigo. *Aerosp Med* 41:200–202, 1970.

Farmer JC: Diving injuries to the inner ear. Candidate's thesis to Am Laryngol, Rhinol Otol Soc, 1978.

Ferjentsik E, Aker F: Barodontalgia: A system of classification. *Mil Med* 147:299–301, 1982.

Freeman P, Edmonds C: Inner ear barotrauma. *Arch Otolaryngol* 95:556–563, 1972.

Freeman P, Tonkins J, Edmonds C: Rupture of the round window membrane in inner ear barotrauma. *Arch Otolaryngol* 99:437–442, 1974.

Gillen HW: Symptomatology of cerebral gas embolism. *Neurology* 18:507–512, 1968.

Gillis MF, Peterson PL, Karagiones MT: In vivo detection of circulating gas emboli associated with decompression sickness using the Doppler flowmeter. *Nature* 217:965–967, 1968.

Golding FC, Griffiths P, Hempleman HV, et al: Decompression sickness during construction of the Dartford Tunnel. *Br J Ind Med* 17:167–180, 1960.

Goodhill V: Leaking labyrinth lesions, deafness, tinnitus and dizziness. *Ann Otol* 90:99–106, 1981.

Hallenbeck JM, Bove AA, Elliott DH: Mechanisms underlying spinal cord damage in decompression sickness. *Neurology* 25:308–316, 1975.

How J, West D, Edmonds C: Decompression sickness in diving. *Singapore Med J* 17:92–97, 1976.

Kizer KW: Corticosteroids in the treatment of serious decompression sickness. *Ann Emerg Med* 10:485–488, 1981.

Kizer KW: Delayed treatment of dysbarism; a retrospective review of 50 cases. *JAMA* 247:2555–2558, 1982.

Kizer KW: Dysbaric air embolism in Hawaii. Presented to the Seventh Annual Conference on the Clinical Application of Hyperbaric Oxygen. Long Beach, Calif, Memorial Hospital Medical Center, 9–11 June 1982.

Kizer KW: Dysbarism in paradise. *Hawaii Med J* 39:109–116, 1980.

Kizer KW: Epidemiologic and clinical aspects of dysbaric diving accidents in Hawaii. Presented to the Sixth Annual Conference on the Clinical Application of Hyperbaric Oxygen. Long Beach, Calif, Memorial Hospital Medical Center, 8–10 June 1981.

Kizer KW: Gastrointestinal barotrauma. *West J Med* 1981; 134:449–450, 1981.

Kizer KW: Management of dysbaric diving casualties. *Emerg Med Clin No Amer* 1:659–670, 1983.

Kizer KW, Goodman PG: Radiographic manifestations of venous air embolism. *Radiology* 144:35–39, 1982.

Lundgren CEG: Alternobaric vertigo—A diving hazard. *Br Med J* 2:511–513, 1965.

Lundgren CEG, Ornhagen H: Nausea and abdominal discomfort—Possible relation to aerophagia during diving: An epidemiologic study. *Undersea Biomed Res* 2:155–160, 1975.

Lundgren CEG, Tjernstrom O, Ornhagen H: Alternobaric vertigo and hearing disturbances in connection with diving: An epidemiologic study. *Undersea Biomed Res* 1:251–258, 1974.

McCormick JG, Holland WB, Brauer RW, et al: Sudden hearing loss due to diving and its prevention with heparin. *Otolaryngol Clin North Am* 8:417–430, 1975.

Menkin M, Schwartzmann RJ: Cerebral air embolism. *Arch Neurol* 34:168–170, 1977.

Miller J: Management of diving accidents—Author's response. *Emerg Med* 13:23–24, 1981.

Rivera JC: Decompression sickness among divers: An analysis of 935 cases. *Mil Med* 17:314–334, 1964.

Smith KH, Spencer MP: Doppler indices of decompression sickness; the evaluation and use. *Aerosp Med* 41:1396–1401, 1970.

Spencer MP, Campbell SD: Development of bubbles in venous and arterial blood during hyperbaric decompression. *Bull Mason Clin* 22:26–32, 1968.

Strauss RH: Diving medicine. *Am Rev Respir Dis* 119:1001–1023, 1979.

Waite CL, Mazzone WF, Greenwood ME, et al: Dysbaric cerebral air embolism, in Lambertson CJ (ed), *Proceedings of the Third Symposium on Underwater Physiology*. Baltimore, Williams & Wilkins, 1967, pp 205–215.

B. Blast Injury

The phenomenon of blast injury has been recognized for as long as humans have used explosives, although historically it has been mainly a wartime concern. However, in the past few decades there has been a dramatic increase in the incidence of peacetime civilian explosive blast injuries because of the popularity of the homemade bomb as a vehicle of social protest and the continued hazard of explosions in mining, grain storage, and other industries. In addition, blast injuries remain a prominent cause of fire-related morbidity, and they have become increasingly recognized as resulting from exploding automobile batteries and beverage bottles. Since emergency physicians are the ones most likely to supervise the prehospital management of such casualties, as well as provide the initial direct patient care, they need to be familiar with the pathophysiology and treatment of explosive blast injuries.

BLAST PHYSICS AND TERMINOLOGY

Explosives are materials which are rapidly converted into gases when detonated. *Blast* and *blast injury* are, respectively, general terms used to describe this gaseous decomposition and the damage occurring in an organism subjected to the pressure field produced by an explosion.

Blasts are characterized by the release of large quantities of energy in the form of pressure and heat, with the exact amount depending on the type and amount of explosive. If the explosion is confined within some sort of casing, i.e., a bomb, the pressure will rupture the housing and eject the resulting fragments at high velocity. The remaining energy is transmitted to the surrounding environment in the form of a blast wave, blast winds, ground shock, and fire.

The *blast wave* begins as a single pulse of increased pressure that rises to peak levels within a few milliseconds and then rapidly falls to a minimum pressure that is lower than the original atmospheric pressure (Fig. 49B-1). It is propagated radially outward from the explosion, with the sharply marginated periphery of the sphere becoming the blast, overpressure, or shock wave, as it has been variously called. The duration and level of the high pressure peak depends on the nature of the explosive, the conducting medium, and the distance from the detonation point. This blast wave pressure peak determines the *overpressure* that an object in its path is subjected to and is the main determinant of primary blast injury. Conversely, the negative pressure wave, or suction of the blast wave, lasts several times longer than the high-pressure wave but can never be greater than 70 mmHg (14.7 psi). Representative pressure effects are listed in Table 49B-1.

The rapidly expanding gases from an explosion also displace air, causing it to move away at very high velocity and produce transient *blast winds* that travel immediately behind the shock front of the blast wave. The blast wind may also accelerate loose objects (e.g., people) through the air, causing acceleration-deceleration injuries. In the immediate vicinity of an explosion this *windage* can cause atomization, or total disintegration, of a body, evisceration, or traumatic amputations, depending on the force of the explosion. Illustrative of the force of such winds, an overpressure of about 5200 mmHg (100 psi) produces a blast wind having a velocity of about 2400 km/h (1500 mi/h).

In addition to the amount and duration of overpressure caused by an explosion, the overall effect of the blast wave will also depend on the exact waveform of the overpressure (i.e., its rise time), the victim's body mass and orientation to the explosion, the presence of deflecting and reflecting surfaces in the environment, and the medium through which the shock wave is conducted. For example, because of the greater density of water and its relative incompressibility, blast waves produced by underwater explosions travel much faster and farther than those produced by above-ground explosions. Consequently, blast injuries in water occur at greater distances from the detonation point and tend to be more severe. Underwater blast injury has other peculiarities, too, but these are beyond the scope of this discussion.

CATEGORIES AND MANIFESTATIONS OF BLAST INJURY

Explosive blast injuries can be divided into four categories (Table 49B-2).

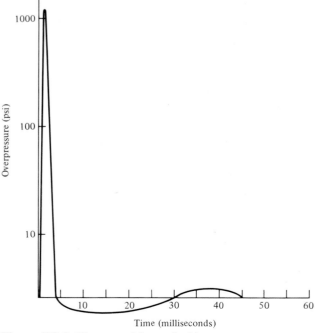

Figure 49B-1. The general form of a blast wave.

Table 49B-1. Selected Pressure Effects

Pressure, psi*	Effect
5	Possible tympanic membrane rupture
15	50% incidence of tympanic membrane rupture
30	Possible lung injury
75	50% incidence of lung injury
100	Possible fatal injuries
200	Death more likely than not

*1 psi = 51.7 mmHg

Table 49B-2. Categories of Blast Injury

Category	Injury by	Primary Target Organs
I. Primary blast injury	Blast Wave	Ears, lungs, GI tract, CNS
II. Secondary blast injury	Victim struck by flying debris	Integument, CNS, eyes, musculoskeletal system
III. Tertiary blast injury	Bodily displacement, i.e., victim impact with stationary objects	Abdominal viscera, CNS, lungs, integument, musculoskeletal system
IV. Miscellaneous	Inhalation of dust or toxic gases, thermal burns, radiation, other	Lungs, integument, eyes

Primary Blast Injury

Type I, or primary; blast injury, results directly from the sudden changes in environmental pressure caused by the blast wave. Tissues vary in their susceptibility to primary blast injury, with homogeneous or solid tissues being at least risk because they are essentially noncompressible and merely vibrate as a whole when subjected to a blast wave. Conversely, gas-filled organs are compressible and have tissue-gas interfaces, which means that displacement occurs wherever tissues of different densities interface, resulting in tissue distortion and tearing. Thus, primary blast injury mainly affects organs containing air and causes the most severe damage at the junctions between tissues, where loose, poorly supported tissue is displaced beyond its elastic limit.

There are three general mechanisms whereby a blast shock wave can damage living tissue. The first of these is known as *spalling* and occurs when a shock wave traveling through a medium of higher density (e.g., liquid) passes into a medium of lower density (e.g., gas), creating a negative reflection at the interface and, thus, fragmenting the surface of the heavier medium. This is analogous to hitting the outside of a rusty bucket with a hammer, which causes flakes to come off inside the bucket.

The second mechanism of injury is implosion of gas-filled spaces as the high pressure in the surrounding fluid or solid compresses these spaces. Similarly, because there is a pressure differential between the air-filled and vascular spaces, blood and fluid are forced into the air-filled spaces. This mechanism is of particular importance in the lungs, where it contributes to pulmonary hemorrhage. In addition, as the negative pressure wave follows the initial positive pressure, smaller internal secondary explosions occur as the compressed gas reexpands.

Third, tissues of different densities will be accelerated and decelerated at different rates relative to each other, producing shearing forces that can tear or otherwise damage the tissue.

The organs most vulnerable to primary blast injuries are the ears, lungs, central nervous system, and gastrointestinal tract. Abdominal visceral injury is relatively rare in air blast casualties but is of considerable concern in persons exposed to underwater blasts.

Otolaryngologic Manifestations

Overall, the ears are most often affected by explosive blasts, with hearing loss being the primary manifestation. Hearing can be damaged by one of three ways. First, the tympanic membranes may

rupture. This usually occurs in adults at a pressure differential between the middle and external ears of around 360 mmHg (7 psi), and most often presents as a linear perforation of the pars tensa. The second way is dislocation of the ossicles, which may accompany tympanic membrane rupture or occur as the sole injury. Lastly, deafness may result from blast effects on the inner ear, causing perilymph fistula formation and other damage. In addition to hearing loss, primary symptoms of inner ear damage include vertigo and tinnitus.

The paranasal sinuses are also susceptible to blast injury, usually manifesting barotraumatic damage similar to the squeeze syndromes that occur with compressed air diving.

Pulmonary Manifestations

Although less often affected than the ears, the lungs are generally the organs most severely affected by blast injury, and these injuries are likely to present a threat to life. (Of course, the severe injuries resulting from windage in the immediate vicinity of the explosion are also life-threatening.) The blast wave causes widespread alveolar damage because of its effects on tissue-gas interfaces, producing interstitial and intraalveolar hemorrhage and edema, parenchymal and pleural lacerations, and alveolar-venous fistulas. Because of the widespread nature of this damage a variety of specific injuries may be found, including pulmonary edema, pneumothorax and other extraalveolar air syndromes, and air embolism. Similarly, pulmonary contusions result from compression of the lung between the spine, thoracic wall, and rising diaphragm, as well as from being thrown against solid objects in the environment.

The actual symptoms experienced by victims of blast lung injury will vary with the severity and nature of their specific injuries, but, in general, they will present with dyspnea and other signs of pulmonary insufficiency, chest pain, hemoptysis, rales, rhonchi and other signs of pulmonary edema or hemorrhage, as well as symptoms of the pulmonary overpressurization syndrome.

Gastrointestinal Manifestations

As with the lungs, blast injuries to the stomach and bowels are due to damage at tissue-gas interfaces, producing hemorrhage into the wall and lumen along with perforations, which tend to be multifocal. Since the large bowel usually contains more gas than the small bowel, it tends to be most severely affected. Common clinical manifestations include abdominal pain, melena, signs of peritonitis, and free air in the abdomen. Evisceration and other gross damage may be found in victims who were very close to the detonation site, but these types of injuries are nearly always fatal.

Neurological Manifestations

Blast injuries of the central nervous system are of two main types. First are the direct shock wave effects, which produce a concussion syndrome and various types of intra- and extraaxial hemorrhage, and second are the effects of cerebral air embolism. As with dysbaric diving casualties, the actual neurological manifestations of air embolism are extremely varied.

Other Categories of Blast Injury

Type II, or secondary, blast injuries are largely due to the blast wind and result from the victim being struck by flying debris. Conversely, *type III, or tertiary, blast injuries* are those that result from the victim being displaced through space by the blast wind and impacting a stationary object; this sudden deceleration usually causes more harm than the acceleration through space. *Type IV blast injuries* include a wide variety of injuries resulting from inhalation of dust and toxic gases, exposure to radiation, thermal burns, and so on.

The myriad number of bodily insults that can result from these latter types of blast injury are far too numerous to list here. Of particular concern, though, are traumatic amputations, occurring in about 25 percent of severely wounded victims, and liver, spleen, or other visceral injury produced from the acceleration-deceleration forces of the blast wind. Likewise, bomb casing fragments or missiles such as nails, nuts and bolts, screws, ball bearings, etc., can cause high-velocity missile injuries.

MANAGEMENT OF BLAST CASUALTIES

Blast injury victims should be managed in the same manner as any multiple trauma victim, except that particular attention should be directed to the respiratory system. This includes giving special attention to maintenance of a patent airway (especially when maxillofacial, cervical spine, or other head and neck injuries are present), administering supplemental oxygen, judiciously using intravenous fluids and analgesics, evacuating pneumo- and hemothoraxes, and promptly implementing mechanical ventilation if signs of respiratory failure or inadequate oxygenation are present. Although positive pressure ventilation in one form or another may be necessary to maintain adequate oxygenation, its use is fraught with hazard, since the diffuse alveolar-capillary damage present in blast lung greatly increases the risk of causing extraalveolar extravasation of air, including air embolism.

Systemic air embolization presents particular problems in the management of blast casualties, since the effects on the brain, heart, and viscera caused by air emboli may be indistinguishable from other types of injury. Yet, the preferred therapy for air embolism is hyperbaric oxygen treatment (HBOT), which may not be readily available or may be impractical because of coexistent injuries or other logistical problems. Whenever possible, though, HBOT should be implemented as expeditiously as possible, being given in a manner similar to the treatment of dysbaric diving casualties, since it is usually very effective in reversing cerebral or coronary injuries.

Tympanic membrane rupture and other otolaryngologic trauma, as well as most other types of blast injury, should be treated essentially the same as they are treated when due to other causes. Closed abdominal injuries are always of particular concern and should be treated according to the patient's signs and symptoms, with prompt surgical exploration being undertaken whenever there are signs of peritonitis or peritoneal free air. Abdominal visceral injuries should be especially looked for in victims of underwater explosion. Lacerations, fractures, amputations, and missile wounds should be treated in the usual manner, except for delayed primary closure being the generally preferred method of wound management.

Explosions in confined spaces typically produce worse injuries than those occurring in the open because of the greater likelihood of inhalation injury from dust, smoke, and toxic gases. Again, though, the inhalation injury is treated essentially the same as that resulting from other circumstances.

Since primary blast injuries may not always be present when the victim is first evaluated, all blast-injured patients should be closely observed for at least 6 to 12 h after the accident. This is particularly true if there is perforation of the eardrums, which is generally an indication of significant exposure to high pressure.

BIBLIOGRAPHY

Benzinger T: Physiological effects of blast in air and water, in *German Aviation Medicine, World War II,* vol II. Washington, DC, U.S. Government Printing Office, 1950, pp 1225–1259.

Bergeson PS, Sehring, SA, Callison JR: Pop bottle explosions. *JAMA* 238:1048–1049, 1977.

Caseby NG, Porter MF: Blast injuries to the lungs: Clinical presentation, management and course. *Injury* 8:1–12, 1976.

Clemedson CJ: Blast injury. *Physiol Rev* 36:336–354, 1956.

Freund U, Kopolovic J, Durst AL: Compressed air emboli of the aorta and renal artery in blast injury. *Injury* 12:37–38, 1980.

Hadden WA, Rutherford WH, Merrett JD: The injuries of terrorist bombing: A study of 1532 consecutive patients. *Br J Surg* 65:525–531, 1978.

Hamit HF: Primary blast injuries. *Ind Med* 42:14–21, 1973.

Hirsch M, Bazini J: Blast injury of the chest. *Clin Radiol* 20:362–370, 1969.

Holekamp TLR: Ocular injuries from automobile batteries. *Trans Am Acad Ophthalmol Otolaryngol* 83:805–810, 1977.

Huller T, Bazini Y: Blast injuries of the chest and abdomen. *Arch Surg* 100:24–30, 1970.

Kerr AG: Blast injuries to the ear. *Practitioner* 221:677–682, 1978.

Kerr AG: Trauma and the temporal bone—The effects of blast on the ear. *J Laryngol Otol* 94:107–110, 1980.

Malpass CP, Martin LJ: Clinical aspects of ball-bearing bomb injuries. *Resuscitation* 6:53–58, 1978.

Marshall TK: Deaths from explosive devises. *Med Sci Law* 16:235–239, 1976.

Mondino BJ, Brown SI, Grand G: Ocular injuries from exploding beverage bottles. *Arch Ophthalmol* 96:2040–2041, 1978.

Murthy JMK, Chopra JS, Gulati DR: Subdural hematoma in an adult following a blast injury. *J Neurosurg* 50:260–261, 1979.

Nicholas EJH: Underground explosions in coal mines. *Med Sci Law* 16:240–243, 1976.

Pahor AL: Blast injuries to the ear: An historical and literary review. *J Laryngol Otol* 93:225–251, 1979.

Pahor AL: The ENT problems following the Birmingham bombings. *J Laryngol Otol* 95:399–406, 1981.

Rawlings JSP: Physical and pathophysiological effects of blast. *Injury* 9:313–320, 1977.

Roy D: Gunshot and bomb blast injuries: A review of experience in Belfast. *J R Soc Med* 75:542–545, 1982.

Russell RC, Baldwin JR, Law EJ: Burns due to grain dust explosions. *J Trauma* 20:767–771, 1980.

Siebert S: Ocular trauma from lead-acid vehicle battery explosions. *Aust J Ophthalmol* 10:53–61, 1982.

Stapczynski JS: Blast injuries. *Ann Emerg Med* 11:687–694, 1982.

Uretzky G, Cotev S: The use of continuous positive airway pressure in blast injury of the chest. *Crit Care Med* 8:486–489, 1980.

Weber FL, Babel J: Corneal trauma from protection of metallic mercury into the eyes. *Arch Ophthalmol* 97:1116–1120, 1979.

Williams RD, Ochsner RD, Morse PH: Explosion of automobile batteries as a cause of ocular trauma. *J L State Med Soc* 130:179–180, 1978.

C. Mountain Sickness and Other Acute High-Altitude Illnesses

INTRODUCTION

Once only the most hardy and extremely fit were brave enough to venture to the alpine reaches of the earth, but that is no longer the case. Since the early 1960s there has been a marked increase in the number of people participating in mountaineering and technical rock climbing. There are now estimated to be well over 100,000 active mountaineers in the United States and several times that many worldwide. Similarly, literally millions of hikers and skiers flock to high terrain in both winter and summer in search of adventure and wilderness escape. Unfortunately, many of these persons are middle-aged or older, relatively unconditioned, and/or poorly informed about the hazards of high altitude. These factors, combined with greater competition in recent years to go higher faster, has, not surprisingly, resulted in a dramatically increased incidence of mountain sickness and other high-altitude illnesses. Indeed, high-altitude illness is no longer a medical curiosity, but warrants the attention of all personnel involved in acute and preventive medicine.

Exposure to the reduced atmospheric pressure of high altitude can occur by climbing mountains; by flying in aircraft, spacecraft, balloons, or gliders; and by entering hypobaric (low-pressure or vacuum) chambers. The health hazards associated with such exposure will depend on both the type and degree of hypobaric exposure, but, overall, they can be grouped into two main categories. First are the problems due to the high altitude itself, i.e., the reduced barometric pressure, and second are problems due to the other hostile environmental conditions found at high altitude—cold, foul weather, avalanches, rough terrain, lightning, increased solar radiation, and so on. Since emergency physicians are much more likely to be involved with high-altitude problems associated with mountaineering than with aerospace accidents, this chapter will focus on mountain sickness and other similar acute high-altitude illnesses.

MOUNTAINEERING ACCIDENTS

Mountain climbing is among the most hazardous of sports. The risk of death for persons attempting to climb Mount McKinley and Mount Foraker in Alaska is between 1 and 2 percent, and 19 percent of all persons climbing these two peaks in 1976 suffered significant injury, illness, or death. Similarly, 10 percent of persons participating in expeditions to Nepal in 1975 perished, while nearly 20 percent of rock climbing accidents in Grand Teton National Park are fatal. Likewise, 8 percent of the mountaineering accidents on class V routes in the Sierra Nevada Mountains resulted in a fatal outcome between 1975 and 1980.

The chief contributing human factors in mountaineering accidents are poor judgment and lack of proper experience and preparation, including lack of knowledge about the effects of exposure to high altitude. Trauma, cold injuries (i.e., hypothermia and frostbite), and solar radiation syndromes (e.g., actinic keratitis

and sunburn) account for the majority of morbidity and mortality figures. Head injuries are the most frequent cause of death, and fractures of the lower extremities are the most common nonfatal serious injuries. Multiple injuries are common.

Management of traumatic and exposure problems in mountaineers is the same, at least in principle, as for similar conditions occurring in other situations, and will not be further discussed here. However, it should be noted that the vagaries of mountain rescue and resuscitation in a spartan wilderness setting typically require a high degree of improvisation and creative management skills.

In contrast to the traumatic and exposure problems associated with mountaineering, acute mountain sickness and the other maladies due to reduced barometric pressure at high altitude are distinct entities that require some special considerations in management, with regard to both specific treatment and prevention (especially insofar as prevention decreases the risk of other types of accidents).

HIGH-ALTITUDE ILLNESS

Despite the stories of Noah's landing on Mount Ararat, Empedocles' conquest of Mount Aetna, Hannibal's crossing of the Alps, and numerous other real or legendary historical accounts of mountain ascents, the earliest recorded case of altitude illness per se was described in 1590 by the Jesuit priest José de Acosta, who had sojourned to 5300 m (17,500 f) in the Peruvian Andes some 40 years earlier. Subsequently, other accounts appeared in the literature, with the first recorded fatalities from acute altitude illness occurring in 1875, when two French balloonists died at an altitude of 8500 m (28,000 f) above sea level. Since then it has become recognized that high-altitude illness includes a number of acute and chronic syndromes that typically occur at altitudes over 2400 m (8000 f) above sea level and that typically are caused by lack of oxygen.

The exact pathophysiologic effect of the hypoxia occurring at high altitude is not entirely clear, although it seems that the primary effect is impairment of the ATP-dependent sodium pump which normally maintains cellular osmolar equilibrium. Since ATP cannot be produced if there is insufficient oxygen to support oxidative cellular respiration, hypoxia prevents cells from being able to maintain their normal intracellular-to-extracellular sodium gradient. Consequently, they imbibe water, which results in cellular swelling and edema.

In addition to causing loss of the ability to maintain normal cellular osmotic gradients, hypoxia also induces changes in the secretion of antidiuretic hormone, somatotropin, and other hormones. Although these effects seem to be important, their exact significance is unclear at present. In any case, the net effect of the altered ability to handle water and electrolytes produces a spectrum of maladies that can occur either singly or in combination.

Acute High-Altitude Illness

Four different syndromes involving the brain, eyes, and lung constitute what is generally thought of as acute high-altitude illness.

Acute Mountain Sickness

Acute mountain sickness (AMS) is an acute, self-limiting illness resulting from the rapid exposure of unacclimatized persons to high altitude. This is the most common type of high-altitude illness, affecting about 20 to 30 percent of persons who travel to altitudes of 2400 to 2700 m (8000 to 9000 f) in less than 24 to 48 h, and nearly everyone ascending directly to altitudes above 3400 m (11,000 f). About 45 percent of the tourists who travel to the Khumbu valley in east Nepal to view Mount Everest develop AMS.

The most common symptoms of AMS are headache, nausea, vomiting, irritability, insomnia, dyspnea on exertion, and fatigue. The headache probably results from spasm or dilatation of cerebral blood vessels secondary to hypocapnia or hypoxia, respectively. Other reported symptoms include generalized weakness, lassitude, breathlessness, dizziness, impaired memory, reduced ability to concentrate, palpitations, and oliguria. Interference with sleep, resulting both from the headache and the development of Cheyne-Stokes breathing [which occurs in almost everyone at altitudes above 2700 m (9000 f)] may be especially bothersome.

In susceptible individuals, symptoms of AMS usually develop within 4 to 6 h of reaching altitude, attain maximum severity 24 to 48 h later, and then gradually abate after the third or fourth day. However, some affected individuals may not notice any ill effects for 18 to 24 h or may have prolonged symptoms.

Although causing considerable misery in those afflicted by it, AMS usually does not require any special treatment. While symptomatic, though, some relief can be achieved by minimizing activity, avoiding alcoholic beverages, forcing fluids, eating lightly, and not smoking. Symptoms are usually exacerbated by strenuous exercise. Aspirin or codeine may be taken for the headache, with supplemental oxygen being of value in patients with severe headache not relieved by mild analgesics. Continuous inhalation of oxygen during sleep may reduce sleep disturbances. Importantly, AMS may be a precursor to other much more serious forms of acute high-altitude illness.

The best way to prevent AMS is by acclimatization, i.e., by gradually ascending or staging one's ascent to altitude over a period of several days. However, when this is not possible (e.g., in rescue or recovery operations) or is intentionally omitted, administration of the carbonic anhydrase inhibitor acetazolamide (Diamox) is likely to ameliorate or completely prevent AMS. When used, acetazolamide should be given orally in doses of 250 mg every 8 to 12 h for 2 days before, during, and for 1 or 2 days after ascent. Higher doses may be needed on occasion. Although its use may not entirely prevent AMS, it certainly seems to shorten the time needed for acclimatization. It seems to be particularly effective in eliminating periodic breathing. Importantly, though, acetazolamide does not obviate the need for prompt descent in cases of more severe acute altitude illness.

High-Altitude Pulmonary Edema

High-altitude pulmonary edema (HAPE) was first reported in 1891 when a Dr. Jacottet died at an altitude of about 4300 m (14,140 ft) after ascending Mont Blanc [altitude 4760 m (15,623 ft)]. Although occasionally noted in the literature after this, it was not until Houston reported on it in 1960 that any detailed physiologic investigation was done. HAPE is now known to be a form of noncardiac pulmonary edema that affects unacclimatized persons who rapidly ascend to altitudes greater than 2300 m (7500 ft) above sea level, although rarely occurring at less than 3400 m (11,000 ft). Overall, HAPE has an incidence of between 0.15 and 0.6 percent in persons ascending above 2300 m (7500 ft).

The exact pathophysiology of HAPE still has not been precisely delineated, although it is probably related to the increased pulmonary artery pressure that develops in response to hypoxia. This may trigger the release of leukotrienes, which increase pulmonary arteriole permeability and, thus, leakage of fluid into extravascular locations. Consistent with this hypothesis is the interesting observation of severe HAPE developing at relatively low altitudes in a number of otherwise healthy individuals having congenital absence of one pulmonary artery. This very rare anomaly is associated with pulmonary hypertension, and the occurrence of HAPE in these persons at such modest altitudes is not likely due to chance alone.

Initial symptoms of HAPE usually begin between 24 to 72 h after arrival at altitude and are often preceded by strenuous exertion. Children and adolescents are particularly susceptible, as are long-time residents of high altitude who return to altitude after a transient descent to lower elevation. The duration of symptoms may be as short as 24 h in children. Shortness of breath, nonproductive cough, headache, weakness, and fatigue are typically the first symptoms. Concomitant symptoms of AMS may or may not be present, but are especially common in children. As HAPE worsens, so does the dyspnea and cough, which may produce frothy or bloody sputum. Generalized weakness, lethargy, disorientation, hallucinations, stupor, and coma may also develop, with the latter being very ominous. Death may follow if the victim is not promptly moved to a lower elevation.

Typical physical findings of HAPE include hyperpnea, rales and rhonchi, tachycardia, and cyanosis. Hypotension and low-grade fever may be present, but orthopnea is unusual. Laboratory studies may show signs of hemoconcentration, e.g., elevated hematocrit and high urine specific gravity, and chest radiographs, if obtained, may show patchy consolidation of the peripheral lung (which is in contrast to congestive heart failure, where the pulmonary edema is characteristically perihilar). The electrocardiogram may show ischemia or right ventricular strain. A four-point scale for clinically grading the severity of HAPE has been proposed (Table 49C-1), the use of which may be of value in communicating information about patients.

Proper management of HAPE is based on its prompt recognition, but this may be difficult in the field, where early symptoms may be attributed to pneumonia or ignored because of not wanting to abort a planned expedition. Once recognized, though, treatment should be initiated promptly, for this is a truly life-threatening condition.

The mainstays of treatment for HAPE are bed rest, administration of oxygen, and descent to a lower altitude, depending on the severity of symptoms. Mild cases may respond to bed rest only, but in more serious cases descent to lower altitude is mandatory. Indeed, descent is the only truly effective treatment for severe HAPE and should never be delayed in patients having serious symptoms. Fluid replacement and salt restriction may be helpful to some degree, but the value of furosemide and other diuretics is debatable. Other drugs commonly used in treating cardiogenic

Table 49C-1. Severity Classification of HAPE

Grade	Clinical	ECG	Chest Radiograph
1	Dyspnea on heavy exertion; minor symptoms	Tachycardia < 110	Consolidation of less than one-fourth of one lung
2	Dyspnea, weakness, fatigue with ordinary efforts; headache, cough	Tachycardia 110–120	Consolidation of at least half of one lung
3	Dyspnea, headache, weakness, and nausea at rest; productive cough	Tachycardia 120–140	Consolidation of at least half of each lung
4	Stupor, coma; severe ataxia and cyanosis; bubbling rales; sputum; hemoptysis	Tachycardia > 140; evidence of right ventricular strain	Consolidation of more than one-half of each lung

Source: Kizer KW: High altitude illness, in Edlich RF, Spyker D (eds): *Current Emergency Medical Therapy 1984*. Norwalk, Conn, Appleton-Century-Crofts, 1984, pp 231–234. (Adapted from Hultgren HC: High altitude medical problems. *West J Med* 131:8–23, 1979.)

pulmonary edema (morphine, digoxin, etc.) have not been found to be efficacious in treating HAPE, and use of acetazolamide has been associated with transient improvement followed by substantial worsening shortly thereafter.

Since the occurrence of HAPE is closely related to the speed of ascent, the altitude ascended, and the work expended in achieving altitude, it should be clear that the most effective way of preventing it is by acclimatization. Again, this may be achieved by either ascending gradually over several days or staging one's ascent so that one or more days are spent at intermediate altitudes, depending on the height of the final destination. Likewise, strenuous exertion should be avoided for 3 or 4 days after arrival at altitude.

High-Altitude Cerebral Edema

High-altitude cerebral edema (HACE) is the most severe form of acute high-altitude illness and was not really recognized until 1959. Fortunately, it is also the least frequent, almost always occurring above 3700 m (12,000 ft), although it, too, has been rarely reported at altitudes as low as 2400 m (8000 ft). Unlike AMS and HAPE, which typically result in no long-term sequelae, HACE may produce permanent neurological injury.

HACE may present with a wide array of neurological manifestations, although severe headache is the hallmark of the condition. Ataxia and clumsiness are also frequent, most likely being due to the particular sensitivity of the cerebellum to hypoxia. Of note, these symptoms are often initially attributed to the cold weather, rough terrain, or other environmental factors. However, as the condition progresses other symptoms develop. Typical among these are mental confusion, irritability, emotional lability, and hallucinations. The hallucinations may be visual or auditory. Importantly, affected individuals may become so paranoid and irrational that their behavior threatens both themselves and others, or judgment and dexterity may become so impaired that they are unable to perform necessary mental and physical tasks. If not promptly treated these physical aberrations quickly give way to lethargy, stupor, coma, and, eventually, death.

Other than the disturbed mental status, overt manifestations of HACE include papilledema, engorgement of retinal veins, and muscle weakness. The deep tendon reflexes usually remain until deep coma develops; spasticity or decerebrate posturing may develop in advanced cases. Despite the raised cerebrospinal fluid pressure, meningismus is rare. Urinary incontinence or retention may occur.

Management of HACE is largely expectant, with the only proven effective treatment being descent to a lower altitude. Although oxygen may relieve the headache, it is rarely available in sufficient quantities to be of more than transient benefit. Diuretics have not been found useful, and corticosteroids have been of equivocal benefit. Other pharmaceutical treatment modalities have been similarly disappointing.

High-Altitude Retinopathy

Spontaneous retinal hemorrhage and other vascular changes may occur at altitudes of 3700 m (12,000 ft), although they characteristically occur at higher elevations. This high-altitude retinopathy (HAR) occurs both as an isolated phenomenon and in association with other forms of acute high-altitude illness, especially HAPE and HACE, but rarely in simple AMS. The incidence of HAR is well over 40 percent according to some studies.

Although typically asymptomatic, HAR-affected individuals may complain of cloudy or blurry vision. Likewise, central scotomas may occur if there is hemorrhage into the macula. On ophthalmoscopy multiple and often bilateral hemorrhages may be present, along with hyperemia of the optic disk, cotton-wool spots, and dilatation and tortuosity of retinal vessels. Studies of retinal blood flow at higher altitude have shown it to be markedly increased compared with normobaric conditions.

The significance of HAR is unclear, since these hemorrhages tend to be self-limited and usually disappear without residua a few weeks after descent. However, macular hemorrhages may produce long-lasting central scotomas.

Acetazolamide does not prevent HAR, and the condition is usually not considered significant enough to necessitate descent, unless the hemorrhages involve the macula and interfere with central vision. At this time, there is no other specific treatment for HAR, and there are no good data on its prevention.

Miscellaneous Acute High-Altitude Problems

A variety of other medical problems are encountered at high altitude. For example, deep venous thrombosis and other thromboembolic phenomena are well-known complications of prolonged inactivity at altitude (such as might occur during a storm), dehydration (which is common at altitude), and hypoxia-induced polycythemia. Because of the obvious problems associated with anticoagulation, aspirin is the only useful drug in this setting. Another problem that may develop is edema of the face, hands, and feet. Diuretics have been used to treat this, but, overall, little has been written on the subject. Rarely, intravascular hemolysis may complicate the course of acute high-altitude illness.

A very rare problem that may develop with sudden exposure to the extremely low barometric pressure found at altitudes above 18,300 m (60,000 ft) is ebullism. This is the formation of water vapor bubbles in the body; that is, the body essentially boils. Obviously, ebullism is not relevant to mountaineers, but it is a concern in aerospace medicine and has been reported in industrial accidents involving vacuum chambers. Kolesari and Kindwall recently reported that they successfully recompressed a man accidentally decompressed in an industrial vacuum chamber to an altitude-equivalent of greater than 22,600 m (74,000 ft) for over 1 min. This case is the most severe nonfatal human altitude decompression ever reported.

Acute Aggravation of Preexisting Conditions

The reduced barometric pressure found at high altitude adversely affects a number of other medical problems, e.g., primary pulmonary hypertension, cyanotic congenital heart disease, chronic lung disease, ischemic heart disease, congestive heart failure, and sickle cell anemia. (Both S-S and S-C hemoglobinopathies are adversely affected at high altitude.) Obviously, persons having such conditions risk exacerbating their condition or developing complications at high altitudes and should avoid such exposures. Similarly, little is known about the high-altitude pharmacology of most of the commonly used drugs for these and other chronic medical conditions.

Chronic High-Altitude Illness

Although the acute forms of altitude illness are of prime interest here, it is worth noting that several forms of chronic high-altitude illness also occur. For example, subacute mountain sickness occurs when the symptoms of AMS do not disappear in 3 or 4 days as is usual, but, instead, persist for weeks or months, causing marked weight loss, insomnia, and mental and physical fatigue. This problem is rare, though, and can be cured just by descending to a lower altitude.

Long-term residents of high altitude may also develop a condition known as chronic mountain sickness, which is manifested by weakness, fatigue, somnolence, and confusion. Physical examination may reveal cyanosis, plethora, and clubbing of the digits, while polycythemia, hypoxemia, pulmonary hypertension, and right ventricular failure may be noted on more detailed evaluation. The underlying cause of these changes appears to be chronic alveolar hypoventilation due to a decreased respiratory response to hypoxia. Symptoms and signs disappear after the patient returns to lower altitude.

Distinct from chronic mountain sickness, polycythemia alone may develop as a result of the chronic hypoxemia associated with living at high altitude. Persons living at elevations above 3700 m (12,000 ft) typically have hematocrits in the mid- to high 50s.

Moderate degrees of pulmonary hypertension are also commonly found in persons living at high altitude. This most likely results from increased pulmonary vasoconstriction secondary to hypoxia, and, unlike the primary pulmonary hypertension occurring at sea level, pulmonary hypertension of high altitude is characteristically benign and reversible upon return to lower elevation.

SUMMARY

Heightened interest in mountain sports and increased access to previously remote mountain areas have produced a marked increase in the incidence of high-altitude illness in the last two decades. Since emergency physicians are the ones most likely to be called upon to care for these patients, they need to have an understanding of the protean manifestations and unique characteristics of these maladies. Above all, it should be understood that descent to a lower altitude is the definitive treatment for these conditions and that, in general, their occurrence can be completely prevented by proper acclimatization.

BIBLIOGRAPHY

Carson RP, Evans WO, Shields JL, et al: Symptomatology, pathophysiology, and treatment of acute mountain sickness. *Fed Proc* 28:1085–1091, 1969.

Claster S, Godwin MJ, Embury SH: Risk of altitude exposure in sickle cell disease. *West J Med* 135:364–367, 1981.

Cosio G: Mining work at high altitude. *Arch Environ Health* 19:540–547, 1969.

Cummings P, Lysgaard M: Cardiac arrhythmia at high altitude. *West J Med* 135:66–68, 1981.

Hackett PH, Creagh CE, Grover RF, et al: High-altitude pulmonary edema in persons without the right pulmonary artery. *N Engl J Med* 302:1070–1073, 1980.

Hackett PH, Rennie D: Rales, peripheral edema, retinal hemorrhage and acute mountain sickness. *Am J Med* 67:214–218, 1979.

Hackett PH, Rennie D, Levine HD: The incidence, importance, and prophylaxis of acute mountain sickness. *Lancet* 2:1149–1154, 1976.

Harber MJ, Williams JD, Morton JJ: Antidiuretic hormone secretion at high altitude. *Aviat Space Environ Med* 52:38–40, 1981.

Houston CS: High altitude illness—Disease with protean manifestations. *JAMA* 236:2193–2195, 1976.

Hultgren HN: High altitude medical problems. *West J Med* 131:8–23, 1979.

Hultgren HN: The risks of climbing. *West J Med* 128:536–537, 1978.

Hultgren HN, Marticorena EA: High altitude pulmonary edema—Epidemiologic observations in Peru. *Chest* 74:372–376, 1978.

Kolesari GL, Kindwall EP: Survival following accidental decompression to an altitude greater than 74,000 feet (22,555 m). *Aviat Space Environ Med* 53:1211–1214, 1982.

McFadden DM, Houston CS, Sutton JR, et al: High-altitude retinopathy. *JAMA* 245:581–586, 1981.

McLennan JG, Ungersma J: Mountaineering accidents in the Sierra Nevada. *Am J Sports Med* 11:160–163, 1983.

Reekie RJ: Tourism and acute mountain sickness in Nepal. *NZ Med J* 95:180–182, 1982.

Schussman LC, Lutz LJ: Mountaineering and rock-climbing accidents. *Phys Sportsmed* 10:53–61, 1982.

Scoggin CH, Hyers TM, Reeves JT, et al: High-altitude pulmonary edema in the children and young adults of Leadville, Colorado. *N Engl J Med* 297:1269–1287, 1977.

Singh I, Khanna PK, Cardiology DM, et al: Acute mountain sickness. *N Engl J Med* 280:175–184, 1969.

Sutton JR, Houston CS, Mansell AL, et al: Effect of acetazolamide on hypoxemia during sleep at high altitude. *N Engl J Med* 301:1329–1331, 1979.

Sutton JR, Lazarus L: Mountain sickness in the Australian Alps. *Med J Aust* 1:545–546, 1973.

Wilson R: Acute high-altitude illness in mountaineers and problems of rescue. *Ann Intern Med* 78:421–428, 1973.

Wilson R, Mills WJ, Rogers DR, et al: Death on Denali. *West J Med* 128:471–476, 1978.

CHAPTER 50
NEAR DROWNING

Bruce E. Haynes

Drowning is a special concern of the emergency physician because it, like other causes of accidental death, often strikes young, otherwise healthy individuals. The patient's prognosis after near drowning depends on the speed of rescue and resuscitation, emphasizing the importance of prehospital care and emergency department management.

DEFINITIONS

Almost as many definitions of drowning exist as authors in the field. One approach is to define drowning as death from suffocation after submersion in water, while those who suffer near drowning survive, at least temporarily, after suffocation by submersion in water. A few clinicians use the more generic term *immersion syndrome* to highlight the blurred margins between the two entities, although this term has also been used to refer to sudden death after immersion in cold water. Postimmersion syndrome, or secondary drowning, refers to the deterioration of a seemingly well patient after immersion.

EPIDEMIOLOGY

About 7000 persons die of immersion in the United States each year, making drowning the third leading cause of accidental death. Certainly many more—the exact number is uncertain—survive serious immersion accidents. Freshwater drowning, especially in pools, is more common than saltwater drowning, even in coastal areas. The peak incidence of death is in the teenage years, although children under the age of 4 are at increased risk and warrant special concern. Nonaccidental injury can be responsible for drowning in young children, and only a high degree of suspicion will protect a surviving victim or siblings.

Alcohol or drug use by victims or by supervising adults often plays a role in drowning; trauma, especially to the cervical spine, may result in some episodes. Overestimation of swimming skills, hypothermia, hyperventilation before underwater swimming, or seizure disorders may be factors in some near-drowning incidents.

CLINICAL COURSE

After the initiating event, panic frequently supervenes, followed by struggling in the water and desperate breath holding or hyperventilation. These soon lead to vomiting and aspiration of water and emesis. "Dry drowning" without aspiration results from laryngospasm and glottal closure and is thought to be responsible for 10 to 15 percent of deaths. Whatever the mechanism, the final common pathway is profound hypoxemia.

While both seawater and fresh water wash surfactant out of alveoli, fresh water also changes the surface tension properties of surfactant. Surfactant loss leads to atelectasis, ventilation-perfusion mismatch, and breakdown of the alveolar capillary membrane. Hypoxemia follows aspiration of small amounts of water and is seen experimentally with aspiration of 2.2 mL/kg of either fresh water or salt water. Contributing to hypoxemia may be aspiration of bacteria, algae, sand, particulate matter, emesis, and chemical irritants. Noncardiogenic pulmonary edema results from direct pulmonary injury, surfactant loss, inflammatory contaminants, and cerebral hypoxia.

Respiratory failure and ischemic neurologic injury are the threats to life after immersion, although associated injuries are occasionally severe. Modell et al. noted a mean arterial P_{O_2} of 67 mmHg among 40 near-drowning patients spontaneously breathing room air. More than one-third of their 91 patients were intubated, most requiring positive end-expiratory pressure (PEEP). Despite this high incidence of pulmonary dysfunction, only one patient with an arterial-P_{O_2}/FI_{O_2} ratio of more than 150 died, and that death resulted from neurologic injury.

Poor perfusion and hypoxemia lead to metabolic acidosis in a majority of patients; yet perhaps as a result of the young age of most drowning victims, the cardiovascular status is remarkably stable. Blood volume shifts depend on the nature and quantity of the fluid aspirated, although life-threatening changes are unusual, since most human drowning victims aspirate quantities of water far below those which produce significant disturbances. Electrolyte abnormalities in near-drowning patients brought to hospitals are seldom significant, and hematologic values are usually normal, although the clinician will occasionally see hemolysis resulting in anemia. Rarely, disseminated intravascular coagulation will occur.

Renal function is usually adequate, although proteinuria may occur and hemoglobinuria can follow hemolysis. Acute tubular necrosis can result from hypoxia or myoglobinuria.

THERAPY

Prehospital Care

Treatment of drowning begins at the scene with rapid, cautious removal of the victim from the water (Table 50-1). Cervical spine precautions should be observed if the mechanism of injury, such as diving or surfing, raises suspicion of such injury. The vast majority of spinal injuries are to the cervical spine after diving, and burst fractures predominate, especially at C5. Clues to spinal injury may be paradoxical respiration, flaccidity, priapism, unexplained hypotension, or bradycardia. Lifeguards and paramedics should scrupulously maintain spinal precautions during rescue if at all possible. Initial history may be unreliable and the physician should have a low threshold for obtaining cervical spine x-rays.

A patent airway must be maintained and ventilation assisted as needed, and all patients should receive supplemental oxygen. Cardiopulmonary resuscitation should be started on any arrested patient with even a remote possibility of success. Sodium bicarbonate should be administered to patients with moderately severe symptoms, and all patients, including those asymptomatic at the scene, should be transported to the hospital for evaluation.

In-water CPR is generally ineffective and dangerous for the rescuer, and should not be attempted unless a firm, stable surface is available. The efficacy of postural drainage is unproved. Experimental studies show little recovery of fresh water from the trachea but return of large amounts of salt water under study conditions. Human near-drowning victims aspirate much smaller quantities of water, and there is little evidence that aspirated water interferes with ventilation. Field limitations to postural drainage include lack of a controlled airway, interruption of ventilation or CPR, the danger of spinal injury, and the possibility of aggravating other undiagnosed injuries.

Hospital Care

Hospital evaluation and care of drowning victims emphasizes initial resuscitation, evaluation of associated injuries, treatment of respiratory failure, and, more recently, measures to protect the brain from hypoxic insult (Table 50-2).

The desirability of resuscitating patients, especially children, who arrive at emergency departments with CPR in progress has been debated since the 1970s. Peterson heightened the concern when he reported that all children requiring CPR on arrival at the hospital who survived were left with severe anoxic encephalop-

Table 50-1. Prehospital Care of Near-Drowning Victims

Rapid, cautious rescue
Cervical spine precautions
Cardiopulmonary resuscitation with administration of dextrose and naloxone
Supplemental oxygen on all patients
Sodium bicarbonate
Transport all patients

Table 50-2. Hospital Care of Near-Drowning Victims

Clear cervical spine
Laboratory studies:
  CBC, electrolytes, glucose, clotting studies, urinalysis
  Arterial blood gases
  Chest x-ray
  Electrocardiogram
Pulmonary support:
  Supplemental oxygen on all patients
  High-flow O_2 as needed
  Intubation and positive pressure (PEEP, CPAP)
Nasogastric tube
Foley catheter
Monitor:
  Oxygenation
  Acid-base balance
  Temperature
  Volume status
Evaluate and treat:
  Associated injuries
  Specific conditions: hypoglycemia, hypothermia, etc.

athy, while Pearn et al. in two similar studies reported almost no severe sequelae. More recent studies demonstrate that about 20 percent of patients who were comatose and flaccid with fixed, dilated pupils survived without significant neurologic deficit. Unfortunately the incidence of a persistent vegetative state was about the same (15 percent). It is the feeling of the author that all patients, including children, who are transported to the hospital deserve a resuscitation effort.

On arrival in the emergency department the integrity of the patient's cervical spine should be confirmed if clinically indicated, and associated injuries should be sought. Pulmonary insufficiency may be indicated by dyspnea, tachypnea, or use of accessory muscles of respiration. The physical examination may reveal wheezing, rales, or rhonchi, although the chest may be completely normal to auscultation after aspiration.

The patient's temperature is an important part of the evaluation, and those patients whose temperatures register at the low end of standard thermometers need further investigation. A hypothermia thermometer is best, but emergency departments seeing few hypothermia patients can usually obtain low-reading thermometers from their clinical laboratory or operating room. Hypothermia can immobilize a swimmer, resulting in drowning, may cause primary ventricular fibrillation, or may be responsible for a variety of adverse metabolic effects. Severe hypothermia often indicates prolonged immersion and is a bad prognostic sign after near drowning. Despite this, numerous persons have survived after prolonged immersion (up to 40 min) in cold water. These patients have body temperatures less than 30°C (86°F) after submersion in water less than 20°C (68°F). The nature of hypothermia's protective effect is unclear; it may be general slowing of metabolism or preferential shunting of blood to the brain, heart, and lungs (diving reflex). The similarity between severe hypothermia and death has led to the aphorism that no one is dead until warm and dead. Near-drowning victims who are hypothermic should be warmed to at least 30 to 32.5°C (86 to 90°F) before resuscitation efforts are abandoned.

A complete blood count; electrolytes including creatinine, BUN, and glucose; clotting studies; and urinalysis should be obtained. A baseline Gram's stain and culture of the trachea will be useful

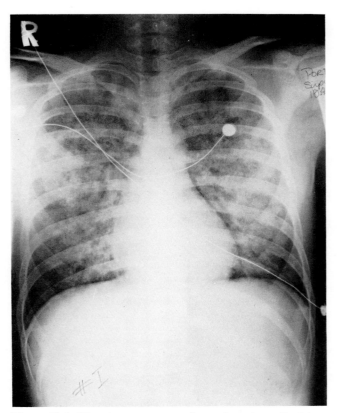

Figure 50-1. Chest roentgenogram of near-drowning patient demonstrating diffuse noncardiogenic pulmonary edema.

in intubated patients. Direct measurement of oxygenation and acid-base status by arterial blood gas analysis will guide pulmonary therapy and the need for sodium bicarbonate.

Roentgenograms of the chest do not necessarily correlate with arterial P_{O_2}, making direct measurement of arterial blood gases important. Despite this, the chest roentgenogram may have predictive value. Almost one-half of the patients with significantly abnormal films will require intubation, which is only occasionally required in patients with normal chest roentgenograms. The chest film may be completely normal after a significant near-drowning incident, or it may show generalized pulmonary edema (Fig. 50-1), perihilar infiltrates, or other patterns.

If not given in the field, an initial dose of 1 mEq/kg of $NaHCO_3$ should be administered while awaiting blood gas analysis if the patient has severe symptoms or is unstable. Standard treatment of bronchospasm, electrolyte imbalance (especially hypoglycemia), seizures, hypothermia, arrhythmias, and hypotension should be undertaken as needed. To avoid inducing arrhythmias, central venous catheters, if used, should not enter the heart in hypothermic patients. A nasogastric tube will empty the stomach and help prevent vomiting, and a Foley catheter will monitor urine output in unstable patients.

Attention must be focused on the patient's pulmonary status. All patients should receive supplemental oxygen during evaluation, and those with more than mild symptoms should be on 100% O_2 until adequate oxygenation is documented. If high-flow oxygen (40 to 50%) cannot maintain the arterial P_{O_2} greater than 60 mmHg in adults or 80 mmHg in children, the patient should be intubated and mechanical ventilation employed.

A few patients may require only increased oxygenation, and continuous positive airway pressure (CPAP) without mechanical ventilation will suffice. Only patients who are alert and unlikely to vomit are candidates for mask CPAP ventilation. The vast majority of intubated patients will require some form of mechanical ventilation such as intermittent mandatory ventilation (IMV) with CPAP or regular mechanical ventilation with PEEP. Intermittent positive-pressure breathing (IPPB) alone may benefit a few patients who are tiring without severe ventilation-perfusion mismatch, but in general has not been effective in severely ill patients.

Neither antibiotics nor steroids seem to alter the course of aspiration pneumonia or pulmonary edema in drowning, and they should not be given prophylactically in the emergency department.

POSTIMMERSION SYNDROME

The presence of a normal chest roentgenogram and normal blood gases does not protect against later deterioration in a few patients. Surfactant inactivation and loss during immersion, occasionally coupled with aspiration or bacterial pneumonia, lead to the occurrence of the *postimmersion syndrome*, or secondary drowning. Following a significant immersion the seemingly well patient will deteriorate after a latent period of 1 to 48 h. These patients may require no resuscitation at the scene and appear well in the emergency department, but later become dyspneic and require anything from supplemental oxygen to mechanical ventilation.

The syndrome is estimated to occur in 2 to 5 percent of patients after immersion in both fresh water and salt water. Many patients reported to have postimmersion syndrome in the past actually had mild near-drowning symptoms which could have alerted their physicians to the need for earlier treatment. Despite that, the syndrome may occur in asymptomatic patients and must be anticipated. There is no reliable way to predict who will suffer postimmersion syndrome; only admission and observation of all patients undergoing a significant episode will lead to early diagnosis and treatment. A "significant" episode is impossible to define exactly, but is generally one with some evidence of aspiration such as coughing, tachypnea, vomiting, or unconsciousness in the water.

PROGNOSIS AND CEREBRAL RESUSCITATION

Statistics on survival and the incidence of severe neurologic deficits after near drowning are difficult to interpret. Studies vary with regard to definitions, patient age, water temperature, treatment regimens, and many other variables. A number of recent studies show good-quality survival in about two-thirds of patients, while approximately 20 percent die and some 15 percent are left with severe neurologic deficits, including existence in a persistent vegetative state.

Conn et al. have attempted to treat severely ill children after near drowning with a regimen based on the principles of cerebral resuscitation. Their protocol includes moderate dehydration using fluid restriction and diuretics, mechanical ventilation to a $P_{O_2} >$ 150 and $P_{CO_2} = 30$, hypothermia to 30°C, muscular paralysis, use of corticosteroids, and barbiturate coma. They reported improved outcome among decorticate or decerebrate patients compared with retrospective control subjects at the same institution. Measures aimed at cerebral preservation have, in general, not benefited those who are flaccid with fixed, dilated pupils, although a few such patients survive with a good outcome.

Intracranial pressure monitoring may be able to predict survival fairly accurately, but has been little help in anticipating those who will be left with severe neurologic deficits. Not all flaccid patients with fixed, dilated pupils have elevated intracranial pressure (> 20 mmHg), but those who develop intracranial hypertension almost always die.

Routine measures such as muscular paralysis and hyperventilation are easily, and for the most part safely, accomplished in the emergency department. Techniques requiring close monitoring such as barbiturate coma, severe fluid restriction, or use of diuretics to control elevated intracranial pressure should be reserved for the intensive care unit. Cerebral resuscitative techniques are best employed at institutions experienced in their use. Only through prospective, randomized trials will the value of different therapeutic measures be established.

CONCLUSION

Near drowning is a common cause of accidental death, particularly in younger individuals. Prehospital care systems should be prepared to provide rapid, safe rescue, and field stabilization including advanced life support with adequate ventilation. All patients should be transported to a hospital for evaluation.

Hospital therapy is focused on treatment of noncardiogenic pulmonary edema and respiratory failure. The emergency physician's approach to the near-drowning patient will depend on the severity of the patient's symptoms and the degree of respiratory distress. Patients may be divided into four groups. One group will have no evidence of significant immersion and may be discharged from the emergency department after a short period of observation. Arterial blood gases and chest roentgenograms are not mandatory in the face of a benign history, but will lend weight to the decision to discharge the patient. Children should be placed in this group only with caution. A second group will be asymptomatic after a significant episode and need admission to observe for delayed symptoms. The third group will have mild to moderate hypoxemia corrected by oxygen therapy. They are admitted and then discharged when the hypoxia resolves if no complications ensue. The

final group will be composed of those patients suffering respiratory distress who require intubation. The prognosis in such patients usually depends more on their neurologic status than on their pulmonary condition.

Associated injuries, particularly to the cervical spine, must be sought and treated appropriately. Concurrent problems such as hypotension and hypothermia are treated in the usual manner.

Flaccid individuals with fixed, dilated pupils have survived without neurologic impairment, indicating that all patients deserve an attempt at resuscitation. The role of cerebral resuscitation is unclear and awaits prospective, randomized studies.

BIBLIOGRAPHY

Burke DC: Spinal cord injuries from water sports. *Med J Aust* 2:1190–1194, 1972.

Conn AW, Montes JE, Barker GA, et al: Cerebral salvage in near-drowning following neurological classification by triage. *Can Anaesth Soc J* 27:201–209, 1980.

Dean JM, McComb JG: Intracranial pressure monitoring in severe pediatric near-drowning. *Neurosurgery* 9:627–630, 1981.

Modell JH, Calderwood HW, Ruiz BC, et al: Effects of ventilatory patterns on arterial oxygenation after near-drowning in sea water. *Anesthesiology* 40:376–384, 1974.

Modell JH, Graves SA, Ketover A: Clinical course of 91 consecutive near-drowning victims. *Chest* 70:231–238, 1976.

Modell JH, Moya F, Newby EJ, et al: The effects of fluid volume in seawater drowning. *Ann Intern Med* 67:68–80, 1967.

Nussbaum E, Galant SP: Intracranial pressure monitoring as a guide to prognosis in the nearly drowned, severely comatose child. *J Pediatr* 102:215–218, 1983.

Pearn JH: Secondary drowning in children. *Br Med J* 281:1103–1105, 1980.

Pearn JH, Bart RD, Yamaoka R: Neurologic sequelae after childhood near-drowning: A total population study from Hawaii. *Pediatrics* 64:187–191, 1979.

Peterson B: Morbidity of childhood near-drowning. *Pediatrics* 59:364–370, 1977.

Ruiz BC, Calderwood HW, Modell JH, et al: Effect of ventilatory patterns on arterial oxygenation after near-drowning with fresh water: A comparative study in dogs. *Anesth Analg* 52:570–576, 1973.

Young RSK, Zalneraitis EL, Dooling EC: Neurological outcome in cold water drowning. *JAMA* 244:1233–1235, 1980.

CHAPTER 51
BURNS AND
ELECTRICAL INJURIES

Carl Jelenko III, Judith B. Matthews

In 1536, in Turin, Ambrose Paré discovered three burned soldiers in a stable. As he looked at them with pity, ''there came an old soldier who asked me if there were any way to cure them. I said no. And then he gently went up to them and cut their throats, gently and without ill will toward them. Seeing this great cruelty, I told him he was a villain: he answered he prayed God when he should be in such a plight, he might find someone to do the same for him, and that he should not linger in misery.''

There is none among us who at the present time and with the present ability to treat even the most seriously burned patient would consider acting as the old soldier did so gently. We have all experienced the pain of a small burn and so can empathize with any patient who is burned, but the advances in burn care from the early sixteenth century to the late twentieth century are frequently overlooked in their historical perspective.

BURNS

In the United States, an average of 2 million citizens per year will seek medical treatment for a burn injury. Of these, 100,000 will sustain a life-threatening injury requiring hospitalization, and 20,000 will die directly as a result of the burn or of complications resulting from the burn. Deaths due to postburn inhalation injuries resulting from the 750,000 annual residential fires, which in turn result in 57 percent of the deaths from fire, could be decreased by 50 percent by the installation of smoke detectors.

This discussion does not include burns due to cold, such as frostbite, which is discussed in Chapter 42.

Burns due to heat or flame are most frequently associated with concomitant clothing fire. Contributing to the increased incidence of residential fires and concomitant burn injury are the increased use of wood-burning fireplaces or stoves and/or the use of kerosene heaters to warm homes. In order to address these causes, some states, such as Maryland, have passed laws requiring all residences to have smoke detectors installed, and some local governments have made illegal the use of kerosene heaters.

A burn is the result of the impact of heat on the skin and underlying tissues.

Burns are classified as first-degree, second-degree, third-degree, and fourth-degree, or superficial, partial-thickness, deep partial-thickness, and full-thickness. Additionally, burns are classified as to cause, size, extent of body surface area damaged, age of patient, and other complicating trauma or chronic illness. Of all of these factors, the most important contributors to morbidity and mortality are age and extent of injury, particularly the extent of full-thickness body surface area (BSA) burned.

Prehospital Care

The patient should be evaluated with regard to airway, breathing, and circulation, followed by a 90-s survey for any hidden trauma. After this, the patient should be wrapped in a clean sterile dry sheet. *At no time* should burned clothing, dirt, or other materials be removed from the body surface. Ointments, unguents, or any other material *should not* be applied.

Ice should never be placed directly on the burn wound because of the potential for increasing the depth of the wound due to hypothermic effects. Small burns can be covered with cold (iced) water or saline, but *at no time* should ice come in contact with the wound. IV fluids and IV pain medication needs should be determined by EMS personnel in consultation via radio with a physician, and are frequently determined by the time required to transport the patient to the hospital.

All patients should be receiving O_2 at the highest concentrations possible during transport to minimize tissue damage. As in all cases where shock is of concern, the patient should be kept warm, with airway, vital signs, and level of consciousness continuously monitored during transport.

In many urban areas the patient will be transported to the designated burn trauma unit under local EMS protocols, if the magnitude of burn indicates the need for highly specialized care. In suburban and rural areas transport would be to the nearest emergency facility capable of stabilizing and/or treating the burned patient.

Evaluation

The extent of injury to an adult is most easily estimated using the rule of nines (Fig. 51-1). On a chart with the anterior and posterior outline of the body, the unclothed patient's burned areas are diagrammed, with partial- and full-thickness areas marked differ-

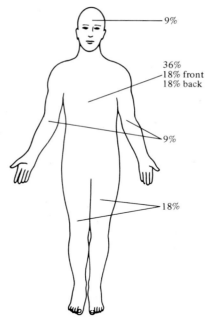

Figure 51-1. Rule of nines

Full-thickness (third-degree) burns present a charred surface or one that is pearly gray to white and, owing to destruction of nerve endings, is insensitive to pain or other sensation. The only definitive sign that a full-thickness burn has occurred is a translucent surface in the depths of which thrombosed veins are visible. Since complete destruction of all skin surface has occurred, full-thickness burns will heal only with skin grafting or scarring, which is a normal part of the healing of these lesions.

Of additional importance is where and how the burn occurred. Was it in an enclosed space such as a car or room? Were toxic products of combustion present? Does the patient have burns of the face? Singed nasal hairs? Sooty sputum? Any respiratory difficulties? If the answer to any of these questions is yes, the emergency physician should suspect a postburn pulmonary injury and give serious consideration to intubation of the patient. ABGs and chest x-rays are of no use in this setting; only fiberoptic bronchoscopy is of use in evaluation of postburn pulmonary injury.

Treatment

The emergency department health care team should take care in admission of the patient to the emergency facility to minimize contamination of the wound. This can range from wearing sterile gloves for the small injury to full gown, cap, mask, etc., for the

ently. The head is 9 percent of the BSA; the arm including the hand, the thigh, and the lower leg are each 9 percent of the BSA. The anterior trunk from the clavicles to the pubis, and the posterior trunk from the root of the neck to and including the buttocks, are each 18 percent of the BSA. The perineum comprises 1 percent of the BSA. Thus, a patient with the anterior trunk (18 percent BSA), perineum (1 percent BSA), and left thigh circumferentially burned (9 percent BSA) would have a total injury of 28 percent BSA.

In infants and young children it is preferable to use the Lund and Browder chart (Fig. 51-2), as this chart corrects for changes due to growth. For example, in the adult the head is approximately 9 percent of the BSA, but the head of the newborn is approximately 18 percent of the BSA. As with the rule of nines chart, the extent of injury is diagrammed on the chart, with areas of partial- and full-thickness burn marked differently.

On the same diagrams, it is also possible to note fractures, abrasions, lacerations, etc., that may have occurred at the time of burning. These charts should become a part of the patient's medical record, and, when transfer to a more highly skilled burn center is to occur, should accompany the patient.

The depth of a burn is dependent upon the tissue layers affected. A superficial partial-thickness (first-degree) burn involves minimal tissue destruction and is red and painful and possibly slightly edematous.

Partial-thickness burns and deep partial-thickness burns (second degree burns) occur when the tissue damage due to heat extends into the corium, or true skin, but leaves the hair follicles, sweat glands, and other adnexal structures present. From these structures metaplastic changes produce new skin. A partial-thickness burn is characterized by blistering and red to slightly whitish areas that are extremely painful to the touch. If the blisters have been abraded, ruptured, or stripped from the surface, they leave a bright red, moist or weeping area. Deep partial-thickness burns are characterized by areas that are very wet and painful as a presenting sign.

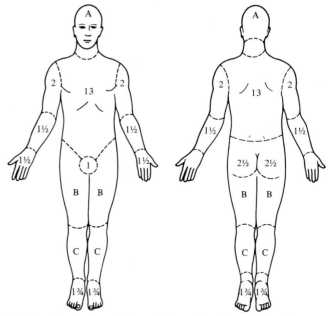

Relative Percentages of Areas Affected by Growth (Age in Years)

	0	1	5	10	15	Adult
A: half of head	$9\frac{1}{2}$	$8\frac{1}{2}$	$6\frac{1}{2}$	$5\frac{1}{2}$	$4\frac{1}{2}$	$3\frac{1}{2}$
B: half of thigh	$2\frac{3}{4}$	$3\frac{1}{4}$	4	$4\frac{1}{4}$	$4\frac{1}{2}$	$4\frac{3}{4}$
C: half of leg	$2\frac{1}{2}$	$2\frac{1}{2}$	$2\frac{3}{4}$	3	$3\frac{1}{4}$	$3\frac{1}{2}$

Second degree _____ and

Third degree _____ =

Total percent burned ____

Figure 51-2. Classic Lund and Browder chart

large burn. For psychological reasons one person should be assigned to talk to the patient on arrival, explaining what is going on and answering questions.

Immediately upon arrival, airway, breathing, and circulation should be assessed. Examination of the patient for hidden concomitant trauma should also be accomplished. Administration of O_2 by Ventimask at 38 percent augments tissue oxygenation.

If a high degree of suspicion exists that postburn pulmonary injury is present, after sedation an endotracheal or orotracheal tube should be placed, even though the patient may be alert, awake, and talking and has a P_{O_2} in the 100+-mmHg range. The mortality rate for the patient who requires a tracheostomy greatly exceeds the complications from tracheal intubation.

If the patient is to be admitted, or if there is question of a need for admission, an intravenous line should be established to prevent hypovolemic shock. It is preferable to establish this IV *above the waist* even if it is necessary to go through the wound itself.

During the development of the hypovolemic state, there will be vasoconstriction of the periphery and in the gastrointestinal tract. During this early period, there is extensive sloughing and micro-ulceration of the gastrointestinal tract from the stomach and duodenum down, and intestinal bacteria can invade the lymphatic and portal systems. In addition, a period of relative hypoimmunity occurs that includes ineffective phagocytosis. The burned tissue is less capable of retaining tissue fluids and probably has an increased likelihood of allowing transudation of plasmalike materials into the wound. Thus, early management includes the administration of adequate amounts of a balanced electrolyte solution such as lactated Ringer's Solution. Other fluid regimens are shown in Table 51-1.

The choice of which fluid regimen to use is up to the emergency physician and should always be modified as the patient's condition changes. If transfer to a burn center is planned, the fluid regimen of that center's choice should be used.

Keeping the patient warm while evaluating the extent of the injury is of great importance in the major burn patient, as hypothermia will rapidly develop. Ice applied directly to the burn will cause further damage and contribute to hypothermia.

Narcotics, used with caution, should be given intravenously unless contraindicated by other injuries such as head trauma or intraabdominal trauma. When not contraindicated, narcotics, specifically morphine sulfate, will help alleviate both anxiety and pain. IM injections should be avoided due to poor and irregular absorption from the muscle.

Tetanus toxoid, 0.5-mL booster, should be given IM in all burn patients. Where any doubt of previous immunization exists, 250 units of human immune globulin should be given IM in the opposite extremity. In the patient with small burns where *compliance* does not appear to be a problem, 0.5 mL tetanus toxoid may be given with a repeat dose in 2 weeks' time.

Since shock produces gastric distension with accompanying ileus, a nasogastric tube should be inserted in the major burn patient. At the same time an indwelling bladder catheter should be placed to monitor urine output.

Prophylactic antibiotics are no longer recommended by most burn centers, because of the development of resistant bacteria. However, in the child the high rate of positive cultures for streptococci in the oropharynx justifies the use of IV penicillin for 5 days prophylactically. Multiple cultures should be taken from various sites.

Baseline laboratory data should be obtained, such as complete blood count with differential, serum, and urine electrolytes, glucose, blood urea nitrogen, amylase, creatinine, clotting studies, LDH, CPK, SGOT, SGPT, blood type, blood and urine toxicology, arterial blood gases and carboxyhemoglobin, and urinalysis.

Table 51-1. Formulas for Treating Burn Shock

1. Parkland formula
    First 24 h:
        Give 4 mL lactated Ringer's Solution per kilogram body weight per % BSA burned
        Give one-half this amount in first 8 h and one-half in next 16 h postburn
    Second 24 h:
        Continue lactated Ringer's as needed
        Begin giving 2000 mL D_5W
        Add plasma or blood as needed
    Objectives:
        To maintain pulse rate below 110/min
        To maintain sensorium normal
        To maintain urine flow at 30–50 mL/h
2. Brooke formula
    First 24 h:
        Give 3 mL lactated Ringer's per kilogram body weight per % BSA burned
        Give one-half this amount in first 8 h and one-half in next 16 h after the burn
    Second 24 h:
        Give 2000 mL D_5W
        Give plasma as needed
    Objectives:
        To maintain pulse rate below 110/min
        To maintain clear sensorium
        To maintain urine flow between 30–50 mL/h
3. Monafo formula
    First 48 h:
        Give hypertonic lactated saline (300 mOsmol/L) at 2.7 mL/kg body weight per % BSA burned
        Add plasma after 24 h as needed
    Objectives:
        To maintain pulse rate below 110/min
        To maintain a clear sensorium
        To maintain urine flow between 30–50 mL/h
4. Jelenko formula
    First 48 h:
        Use HALFD solution containing per liter: 120 mEq sodium chloride, 120 mEq sodium lactate, 12.5 g human albumin
        Give 2.7 mL of this solution per kilogram body weight per % BSA burned
    Objectives:
        To maintain the mean arterial pressure (or the diastolic pressure) above 60 torr
        To maintain a urine flow of 30 mL/h
        To watch for an abrupt increase in serum sodium of 3–7 mEq/L and an abrupt drop in serum potassium of 0.3–0.7 mEq/L, which is considered the "endpoint"
    Therapy after the endpoint:
        Change solution to one containing per liter: 37.5 mEq sodium chloride (one-quarter normal), 20 mEq potassium chloride, 12.5 g albumin
        Maintain mean arterial pressure or diastolic pressure above 70 torr

Source: From Jelenko C III: Burn shock, in Frank HA, Wachtel TL (eds): Thermal Injuries, *Topics in Emergency Medicine* 3:3, Aspen, October 1981.

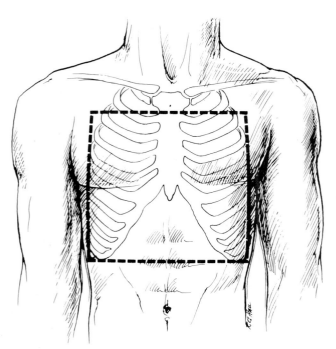

Figure 51-3. In escharotomy of the chest wall, the constricting eschar that may impair ventilation is cut and a floating square of tissue is defined.

If urine is positive for blood, urine should be tested for myoglobinuria. A 12-lead ECG should be obtained as well.

Debridement of the burn wound should be accomplished by gentle washing of the surface with an agent such as Ivory liquid or a similar detergent. Sharp debridement of loose tissue and any blisters that are already broken should follow. It is *inappropriate to rupture intact blisters*. A scrub brush or washcloth to "scrub" the surface will only serve to deepen the wound and increase trauma.

Following wound cleansing, a topical antibacterial agent such as silver sulfadiazine should be used. The agent should be smeared over the affected area in a $\frac{1}{16}$-in-deep layer. Occlusive dressings are a matter of individual choice, but should be applied if the patient is to be transferred to a burn center.

If the chest is burned circumferentially, particularly if the eighth to twelfth rib area is involved, mechanical restriction to respiration may occur. A circumferential burn of the arms, hands, fingers, legs, or toes may compromise vascular effectiveness due to edema. The Doppler flow probe is extremely useful in determining the presence or absence of pulses in the extremities. An escharotomy, or surgical excision in the eschar, may be necessary if pulses are diminished or absent or the developing edema restricts respiration. An incision through the skin so that fat bulges out of the wound is appropriate. Escharotomies should be performed on the lateral surfaces of the legs and arms, and the dorsum of the hand. If necessary, the fingers should be incised beginning at the medial surface distally, crossing the knuckle, and completing the incision on the lateral surface. Escharotomy of the chest wall requires an incision in the anterior axillary line commencing at the second rib and ending at the top of the twelfth rib (Fig. 51-3). The superior and inferior angles of these incisions should be joined by an incision that is perpendicular to the long axis of the body. Thus, a

floating square of tissue is defined that will move with respiration and alleviate restriction to ventilation.

Criteria for admission of patients to the hospital are listed in Table 51-2.

The outpatient management of the patient with burns over more than 20 percent of the BSA and/or full-thickness burns over more than 7 percent of the BSA (in children and adults over age 50, these figures should be 12 and 3 percent, respectively) begins with the diagramming of the size of the burn on either the rule of nines chart or the Lund and Browder chart. It is then advisable to medicate the patient for pain with modest doses of meperidene (25 to 50 mg) in combination with a mild tranquilizer (diazepam, 10 mg; promethazine, 25 to 50 mg). After approximately 20 min, during which the burns can be covered with gauze pads saturated with cool saline (ice should not touch burns) or 0.5 to 4% lidicaine can be administered, debridement can be accomplished with comfort. The burned area should be cleaned with a mild detergent such as Ivory liquid. All burned material clinging to the burn should be removed, as well as all broken blisters and abraded skin. Unbroken blisters should be allowed to remain whole.

Next the wound should be covered with silver sulfadiazine or gentamicin sulfate to a $\frac{1}{16}$-in thickness. Light, nonadherent dressings should be applied to prevent contamination. In the rare instance where a burned hand is managed on an outpatient basis, dressings should allow for the hand to be in the position of function and be loose and bulky to allow for movement under the dressing. Patients should receive a tetanus toxoid 0.5-mL booster if previously immunized, or should be started on a full immunization program.

It may be appropriate to institute an antibiotic such as penicillin, 250 mg qid PO, or cephaloxin, 250 mg tid PO, especially if the hands, feet, or perineum are involved. Pain management should be acetaminophen with 15 to 30 mg codeine. Some patients may require 2 to 3 days of meperidene, 25 to 50 mg PO.

All outpatient burns should be followed at frequent intervals beginning no later than 2 days after injury. If cleansing and dressing changes are required at home, the caregiver should be carefully instructed in how to apply dressings and topical agents. All patients should be encouraged to return immediately to the emergency physician if pain increases or if fever, chills, etc., occur.

Table 51-2. Criteria for Hospitalization of Burn Patient

Admit:
  Adults (5–50 years) with:
    Total burn ≥ 20%
    Full-thickness burn ≥ 7%
  Children (birth–5 years) or adults (≥ 50 years) with:
    Total burn ≥ 2%
    Full-thickness burn ≥ 3%
  Anyone with:
    Electrical injury
    Inhalation injury
    Burns of the hands, face, feet, or perineum
Admit to burn special care area any patient with:
  Electrical injury
  Inhalation injury
  Total burn of
    ≥ 30% in adults
    ≥ 20% in children and adults ≥ 50 yrs
  Full-thickness burn > 7%
  Arrhythmias, diabetes, liver disease, renal disease

Chemical Burns

In general, chemicals do not burn in the sense that they destroy tissue by hyperthermic activity, although selected ones can act in this manner.

Injurious chemicals can be classified as acids, alkalies, and vesicants. *Vesicants* include such entities as cantharides and mustard gas, and produce blistering and pandermic inflammation and vascular compromise.

Chemicals coagulate protein by reduction, oxidation, salt formation, corrosion, protoplasmic poisoning, metabolic competition, inhibition, desiccation, or ischemia. At times, although the original product may not be toxic, a toxic moiety is released during the chemical reaction.

Frequently, the area that appears to be involved may belie the true depth of the chemical involvement so that it is important to know the specific causative agent. Chemical agents that burn and emergency treatment measures are listed in Tables 51-3 and 51-4. The general supportive measures should be appropriate to the extent of the injury and the systemic effects of the individual chemical that has been contacted.

ELECTRICAL INJURIES

True electrical injuries are uncommon, affecting primarily skilled industrial workers and/or the curious infant or child who plays with an electric outlet or bites an electric cord. With the increased use of blow hair driers and electric curling irons, some increase in injuries sustained when these items plugged into household current are dropped into water is now being seen. Lightning injuries are discussed in Chapter 52.

In the curious infant or child and in patients injured in using electric appliances in the bathroom, alternating current in which the flow of electrons switches from positive to negative at 60 cycles per second is the cause of the injury. Alternating current produces entrance and exit wounds of approximately the same size.

In the industrial environment, direct current, in which the electrons flow in one direction with one positive lead and one negative lead, is the most common cause of injuries. Direct current produces a smaller entrance wound and a much larger exit wound.

These exit and entrance wounds are local lesions with a central area appearing whitened, coagulated, or charred, a middle zone of whitish to gray coagulation necrosis, and an outer area of bright red, edematous damaged tissue.

Electricity flows from the point of contact to the ground, producing heat proportional to the distance between these two points and the resistance of the tissues in between. The effects of electrical passage are generally worse with alternating current than with direct current. The current appears to follow the lines of least resistance. Skin has a resistance in the dry state of 40,000 Ω/cm^2. Nerve, blood vessel, muscle, and bone exhibit greater resistance and, therefore, incur greater damage in the reverse order of the listing. Electrical injury has been likened to crush injury in that the systemic effects are often similar. If muscle is injured, myoglobin is released systemically. The greatest threats to life are cardiac arrhythmias, renal failure secondary to myoglobinuria, and electrolyte abnormalities such as hyperkalemia and hypocalcemia due to massive muscle breakdown. Any or all of the major organs may be damaged, so that after first assuring oneself of the patient's airway, breathing, and adequate cardiac functioning (a 12-lead ECG is indicated in *all* electrical injuries with repeat ECGs at frequent intervals), a thorough review of all body systems is indicated. At this time it will not be possible to assess the full extent of tissue injury.

Of particular concern is the fact that electrical injury may induce progressive intravascular thrombosis. This process may occur over a period of several days and may account for extension and progression of the tissue damage. Muscle fibers in contraction are at a greater risk for damage than are relaxed muscle fibers. Often, one observes coagulation necrosis of slips of muscle fibers adjacent to totally unaffected muscle fibers even within the same muscle belly.

Treatment

After the safe extrication of the patient at the scene of injury, an immediate evaluation of airway, breathing, and circulation should be conducted. A monitor with defibrillator should be placed on the patient as soon as safely possible. If the patient is stable, a 90-s survey for indications of other injuries should be made. It is advisable to place a cervical collar on the patient and to place the patient on a wooden short or long backboard, especially where a history of a change in consciousness, pain, or a fall is present. The establishment of a large-bore IV line should be decided in consultation with medical control. Cardiopulmonary resuscitation, if initiated at the earliest possible time by advanced life support personnel and if successful, bodes well for survival. Transfer to an appropriate medical facility should be accomplished as expeditiously as possible.

If a large-bore IV line has not been established and arrhythmias are under control, then the IV is the priority of the emergency physician, with two lines preferable. A balanced electrolyte fluid should be infused. Fluid replacement should be determined by urine output per hour. It may be advisable to maintain an alkaline urine by the IV use of sodium bicarbonate, as myoglobin is less likely to precipitate in an alkaline solution.

Protection from and/or evaluation of cardiac arrhythmias with a 12-lead ECG should be accomplished. Blood studies should include a hemogram, plasma and urine myoglobin, blood and urine electrolytes, cardiac enzymes, arterial blood gases, and clotting studies.

Because of the potential extensive muscle necrosis that may attend electrical injury, particular attention should be paid to appropriate tetanus immunization, which should be given intramuscularly. *All* other medications should be given intravenously.

In addition to the management of the shock state discussed under thermal burns, which is equally appropriate in the electrically injured, careful attention to renal status is essential. Mannitol, 25 g/L, added to the IV infusion solution is often useful to enhance urine flow and minimize renal toxicity after initial fluid replacement has been completed.

Debridement should be extremely conservative, as the true extent of the injury is unknown at this time. In particular, debridement of lesions of the hands, fingers, and face should never be attempted in the emergency department.

Expeditious referral to a burn center should be accomplished for patients with electrical burns.

Table 51-3. Chemicals That Burn

Agent	Toxicity Tissue Action	Emergency Treatment
I. Oxidizing agents		
Chromic acid	5–10 g lethal. Coagulates protein, ulcerates, and blisters with perforation nasal septum; ulcerates skin and coagulates	Dilute Wash with dilute Na hyposulfite BAL for systemic toxicity
Chlorox (Na hypochlorite)	Releases free chlorine, coagulates protein	Milk, egg white, starch paste Lavage Na thiosulfate 1% solution
Potassium permanganate	Potent oxidizer producing thick, brownish-purple eschar of coagulated protein	Lavage Egg white
II. Reducing agents		
Alkyl mercury agents	5–50 mg/kg lethal; redness, bleb formation, partial-thickness lesions that deepen if blister fluid is not evacuated	Debride Remove blister fluid Lavage
HCL (see also muriatic acid below)	Rapid conversion of protein to coagulum salt of the acid; shallow ulcers form with coagulated eschar and base, prolonged action depending on exposure concentration	Avoid lavage Neutralize with soda lime, soap-magnesium hydroxide Demulcents
HNO$_3$		
III. Corrosives		
Phenol (cresol)	Soft, white coagulum caused by protein denaturization, absorption rapid	Dilute with water or cover with oil; avoid alcohol Demulcents May use activated charcoal PO
Phosphorous (white)	50–100 mg lethal; soluble in oils, fumes, and for burns, as it becomes P$_2$O$_3$	Lavage with KMnO$_4$ 1:5000 or 2% Cu(SO$_4$) or Cover with oil
Dichromate salts	10 g lethal; highly corrosive to skin and mucosa; soft yellow coagulum and indolent, deep ulceration; long action	Lavage with water 2% hyposulfite wash Lavage with buffer of 7% (w/w) KH$_2$PO$_4$; 18% (w/w) Na: HPO$_4$:H$_2$O) (70 g: 180 g: 850 mL)

Sodium metal; lye
Lyes:
  KOH
  NaOH
  NH$_4$OH
  LiOH
  Ba$_2$ (OH)$_3$
  CA (OH)$_3$
	(Also see salt formers)
	
	Liquefaction necrosis; soft, gelatinous, brown, friable tissue destruction; fulminant initial response; supporting structures often left intact; saponify fats, salt out collagen, dehydrate other cells
		Dilute
		Neutralize with weak acid
		Demulcents
		Appropriate systemic therapy

Na$_2$	Topical contamination: In presence of water forms NaOH and heat, and may explode	Cover with oil Avoid water Excise

IV. Protoplasmic poisons
Salt formers:
  Tungstic acid
  Picric acid
  Sulfosalicylic acid
  Tannic acid
  Trichloroacetic acid
  Cresylic acid
  Acetic acid
  Formic Acid
	5–50 mg/kg lethal; UC-F form the homologous proteinate when in contact with tissue; escharotic; firm to hard eschar with some sparing of underlying support structures occurs; may be absorbed and produce hepatotoxicity and/or nephrotoxicity; acetic is especially penetrating, formic especially long-lived	Liberal water lavage
		Demulcents
		Cover with oil

Metabolic competitor/inhibitor Oxalic acid	15–30 g lethal; affects mucous membrane; chalk white indolent ulcer; acts by binding Ca^{2+} and poisoning protoplasm	Immediate admin soluble Ca^{2+} salt solution in large volume Careful lavage IV calcium
Hydrofluoric acid	+ 1.5 g lethal; painful, indolent; deep ulcerations below tough coagulum	Boric acid wash NaHCO$_3$ wash Local infiltration of Ca gluconate Local MgSO$_4$ paste and/or hyamine 0.2% in iced alcohol or water

Source: Jelenko C III: Chemicals that burn. *J Trauma* 14:66–67, 1974. Used by permission.

Table 51-3. Chemicals That Burn (*Continued*)

Agent	Toxicity Tissue Action	Emergency Treatment
V. Desiccants		
H_2SO_4	Potent desiccant; produces hard eschar with indolent ulcer, deep destruction of all carbon-containing tissue; liberates considerable heat during reaction	Avoid water lavage Neutralize with magnesium oxide, lime water, soap Demulcents
Muriatic acid (conc. HCL commercial grade)	Slower coagulation process than H_2SO_4, but produces deeper, more severe ulcers and less heat; otherwise lesions similar	See H_2SO_4 and HCL above
VI. Vesicants		
Cantharides	5–50 mg/kg lethal; potent vesicant; severe partial-thickness lesions (Spanish fly)	Water lavage Avoid oils
DMSO	22 g lethal; causes hemolysis, histamine and serotonin release, edema, ischemia; water-soluble	Water lavage
Mustard gas	Severe blistering and partial-thickness necrosis of skin and mucosa; vesicles form, break down at 24–48 h, then ulcerate	Wash with oil, kerosene, or gasoline, then soap and water
Lewisite	0.1 mg/kg lethal; same actions as mustard gas, but slower action	BAL

Table 51-4. Treatment for Chemicals That Burn

I. Water lavage
  Chromic acid
  Potassium permanganate
  Cantharides
  DMSO
  Lyes:
    KOH
    NaOH
    NH_4O4
    LiOH
    $Ba_2(OH)_3$
    $Ca_2(OH)_3$
  Chlorox
  Phenol (cresol)
  Dichromate salts
  Tungstic acid
  Picric acid
  Tannic acid
  Sulfosalicylic acid
  Trichloracetic acid
  Cresylic acid
  Acetic acid
  Formic acid
II. Give calcium salts
  Oxalic acid
  Hydrofluoric acid
III. Cover with oil
  Na metal
  Phenol (cresol)
  White phosphorous
  Mustard gas
	IV. Special methods
	  Excision
	    Na metal
	  Weak acid lavage
	    Lyes
	  Boric acid or $NaHCO_2$ wash
	    Hydrofluoric acid
	  Dilute Na hyposulfite wash
	    Chromic acid
	  Milk, egg white, starch paste, or 1% Na thiosulfate
	    Chlorox
	  Avoid alcohol
	    Phenol (cresol)
	  1:5000 KMNO, or 2% Cu $(SO_4)_2$
	    White phosphorous
	  2% hyposulfite wash; monobasic/dibasic K–Na HPO_4 solution 7%/18% in water buffer wash
	    Dichromate salts
	  Debride and remove blister fluid
	    BAL
	    Alkyl mercury agents
	  Soda lime, soap as magnesium hydroxide washes
	    H_2SO_4, HCl, muriatic acid
	V. Avoid water lavage
	  Na metal
	  H_2SO_4
	  HCl
	  (Muriatic acid)
	VI. Avoid oils
	  Cantharides

Source: Adapted from Jelenko C III: Chemicals that burn. *J. Trauma* 14:67, 1974. Used by permission.

SUMMARY

The majority of patients with thermal burns seen by the emergency physician can be treated by managing pain, preventing tetanus, and treating the burn by gentle cleaning, debriding loose tissue and broken blisters, and applying a topical antibacterial cream and lightweight dressing. Criteria are listed for hospitalization and referral to a burn center. Early treatment includes intravenous infusions of the preferred electrolyte solution to maintain an appropriate urinary output and satisfactory cardiovascular status. An indwelling catheter is inserted to monitor urine output, a sump nasogastric tube is passed to prevent aspiration pneumonia, and oxygen by Ventimask at 38 percent or by endotracheal tube should be given to augment tissue oxygenation. With the exception of tetanus prophylaxis, all medications should be given intravenously. Where edema restricts blood flow or impedes respiration in circumferential burns, escharotomy may be necessary.

Causative agents and emergency treatment of a chemical burn are listed in Tables 51-3 and 51-4. It is important to know the specific causative agent because the depth of the injury is not apparent clinically and treatments vary. *The importance of poison control centers cannot be overemphasized.*

Electrical injury may precipitate cardiac arrhythmias, asystole, and ventricular fibrillation, which respond well to rapid initial management.

Initially, it is impossible to determine the full extent of electrical injury; therefore, lesions of the hands, fingers, and face should never be debrided in the emergency department. Treatment consists of initial resuscitation with a balanced electrolyte solution, management of shock, 12-lead ECG and blood and urine studies, mannitol to enhance urinary output and minimize renal toxicity, and antitetanus precautions.

Systemic effects of electrical injury are similar to those associated with crush injury and include renal failure secondary to myoglobinuria, and hyperkalemia and hypocalcemia due to massive muscle breakdown. Depending on the path of the electrical current, other problems may include coma, pancreatitis, necrosis, fractures, dislocations, and paralytic ileus.

BIBLIOGRAPHY

Thermal Burns

Braen GR, Jelenko C III: Thermal injuries, in Rosen P (ed): *Emergency Medicine*. St Louis, Mosby, 1983, pp 433–443.

Frank HA, Wachtel TL (eds): Thermal injuries, *Top Emerg Med* 3: 3, October 1981.

Garrison AF, Jelenko C III: Management of the acute burn patient. *Postgrad Med* 54:43–49, August 1973.

Jelenko C III, Garrison AF, McKinley JC: Respiratory problems complicating burn injury. *Postgrad Med* 58:95–102, October 1975.

Jelenko C III, Wheeler ML, Callaway BD, et al: Shock and resuscitation, II: Volume repletion with minimal edema using the "HALFD" method. *JACEP* 7:326–333, 1978.

Lloyd JR: Thermal trauma: Therapeutic achievements and investigative horizons. *Surg Clin North Am* 57:121–138, 1977.

Matthews JB, Jelenko C III: Psychosocial support of the burn patient, his family, and the burn team. *Life Support Nursing* 2:13–20, April 1979.

McKinley JC, Jelenko C III, Lasseter MC: Call for help: An algorithm for burn assessment, triage, and acute care. *JACEP* 5:13–16, 1976.

Moncrief JA: Topical antibacterial therapy of the burn wound. *Clin Plast Surg* 1:563–576, 1974.

Moncrief JA: Burns. *N Engl J Med* 288:444–454, 1973.

Paré A: "Journey in Divers Places," trans. The Harvard Classics, Vol 38, New York, Collier, 1910.

Pruitt BA, Erickson ER, Morris A: Progressive pulmonary insufficiency and other pulmonary complications of thermal injury. *J Trauma* 15:369–379, 1975.

Trunkey DD: Inhalation injuries, *Surg Clin North Am* 58:1139, 1900.

Chemical Injury

Berkhout PG, Paterson NJ, Ladd AC, et al: Treatment of skin burns due to alkyl mercury compounds. *Arch Environ Health* 3:592–593, 1961.

Cason JS: Report on three extensive industrial chemical burns. *Br Med J* 1:827–829, 1959.

Guzzardi LJ: Chemical injuries to skin, in Rosen P (ed): *Emergency Medicine*. St Louis, Mosby, 1983, pp 451–454.

Jelenko C III: Chemicals that burn. *J Trauma* 14:65–72, 1974.

Jelenko C III, Story J, Ellison RT: Ingestion of mineral acid. *South Med J* 65:868–871, 1972.

Rossway WH: Caustic skin burns following contact with solution from exhausted carbon dioxide absorption canister. *Anesthesiology* 27:100, 1966.

Tintinalli JE (ed): Hydrofluoric acid burns. *JACEP* 7:24–26, 1978.

Electrical Injury

Billings CE: Electric shock, in Beeson PB, McDermott W (eds): *Textbook of Medicine*, ed 14. Philadelphia, Saunders, 1975, pp 72–73.

Frank HA, Wachtel TL (eds): Thermal injuries, *Top Emerg Med* 3:3, October 1981.

Kay NRM, Boswick JA Jr: The management of electrical injuries of the extremities. *Surg Clin North Am* 53:1459–1468, 1973.

Kleiner JP, Wilkin JH: Cardiac effects of lightning stroke. *JAMA* 240:2757–2759, 1978.

Kunkle RF: Electrical injuries, in Rosen P (ed): *Emergency Medicine*. St Louis, Mosby, 1983, pp 455–461.

Luce E, Dowden WL, Su CT, et al: High tension electrical injury of the upper extremity. *Surg Gynecol Obstet* 147:38–42, 1978.

Rouse RG, Dimick AR: The treatment of electrical injury compared to burn injury: A review of pathophysiology and comparison of patient management protocols. *J Trauma* 18:43–47, 1978.

Solem L, Fischer RP, Strate RG: The natural history of electrical injury. *J Trauma* 17:487–492, 1977.

Strasser EJ, Davis RM, Menchey MJ: Lightning injuries. *J Trauma* 17:315–319, 1977.

Wallace JF: Electrical injuries, in Thorn GW, Adams RD, Braunwald E, et al (eds): *Harrison's Principles of Internal Medicine*, ed 10. New York, McGraw-Hill, 1983, pp 1305–1307.

Wray RC Jr: Electrical injuries, in Ballinger W, Rutherford RB, Zuidema GD (eds): *The Management of Trauma*, ed 2. Philadelphia, Saunders, 1973, pp 702–705.

Outpatient Management

Braen GR, Jelenko C III: Thermal injuries, in Rosen P (ed): *Emergency Medicine*. St Louis, Mosby, 1983, pp 433–443.

Haynes BW: Emergency department management of minor burns, in Frank HA, Wachter TL (eds): *Top Emerg Medi*, 3: 3, October 1981.

Shuck JM: Outpatient management of the burned patient. *Surg Clin North Am* 58:1107–1111, 1978.

CHAPTER 52
LIGHTNING INJURIES

Mary Ann Cooper

Lightning injuries have little relationship to injuries from high-voltage electricity. While lightning is an electrical phenomenon and follows the same laws of physics governing generated electricity, the substantial differences in the properties of a lightning strike account for the difference in the types and severity of injuries seen. Treating victims of natural electricity as though they were victims of human-generated electricity may well cause significant morbidity and mortality. Lightning kills 150 to 300 persons annually in the United States, more than any other natural disaster.

PATHOPHYSIOLOGY OF LIGHTNING INJURY

The voltage of lightning may vary from 10 million to 2 billion volts, the current from 2000 to 300,000 A, both much higher than technical electricity. Lightning is a direct current (dc) and acts as a massive dc countershock in its effects.

The factor that makes the greatest difference in the injury complex is the duration of the electrical exposure. With generated electricity the contact tends to be prolonged with resulting skin breakdown and sustained flow of the electric current internally causing extensive, deep internal damage to muscles, blood vessels, nerves, and other structures.

Lightning, on the other hand, has a duration of from 1 to 100 ms. The exposure is rarely long enough to cause breakdown of the skin, the primary insulator of the body to current flow. The current instead passes over the outside of the body, the so-called flashover phenomenon, similar to the current flow along the outside of a metal conductor. The majority of the current passes outside the body. Since the victim may be wet from sweat or rainwater, the flow of current may cause secondary first- and second-degree burns as the fluid in the sweat lines is turned to steam. The clothes may also be exploded off during this phase.

Thus, entry and exit burns and deep internal burns are rare with lightning injuries, although they are reported occasionally.

MECHANISMS OF INJURY

There are five main mechanisms of injury with lightning injury:

1. Direct strike
2. Side flash
3. Ground current
4. Thermal burns
5. Blunt injury

Direct strike is self-evident. Side flash occurs when lightning splashes from a tree, a structure, or another person to the victim. Ground current, or step voltage, injury occurs when the victim has one leg or some other portion of the body touching the ground closer to the strike point than another part of the body. This posture causes a potential difference between the parts. Thus, a current may flow between the body parts, usually with a lesser but still potentially significant voltage than a direct strike or flash. Thermal burns may occur as metal objects worn by the victim are heated up or as the clothes are ignited.

As lightning passes through the atmosphere it rapidly heats the air to 8000°C and then cools equally rapidly to 1500 to 2000°C. This rapid expansion and contraction accounts for the thunder and also an explosive effect on the victims. It is not uncommon for multiple victims to be injured by a single blast, possibly in a combination of explosive and ground current effects.

DIFFERENTIAL DIAGNOSIS

In the past lightning injuries have been confused with seizures, subrachnoid hemorrhages, and other intracranial vascular events, cardiac arrhythmias, assaults, and heavy metal poisoning. Points that may help with the diagnosis but are not essential include:

1. History of a storm
2. Outdoor occurrence of accident
3. Tympanic membrane rupture
4. Superficial linear or punctate burns or pathognomonic arborescent burns
5. Partial or complete clothing disintegration

INJURIES AND THEIR TREATMENT

Despite the flashover effect of the current there may still be a small internal leakage of current, depending on the body's resistance and the circumstances surrounding the strike. Less than 30 percent of lightning victims die of their injuries. However, 70 percent of survivors have some sequelae.

Cardiorespiratory Injuries

By far the most common cause of death is cardiac arrest. Lightning acts as a massive dc countershock, sending the heart into asystole.

While the rhythm may pick up again as a result of the heart's property of automaticity, the respiratory arrest that often accompanies it is more prolonged, often leading to secondary cardiac fibrillation and arrest due to hypoxia before appropriate resuscitative efforts can be mobilized. In the case of multiple victims, those who are breathing and moving can usually be left in favor of those who appear to be dead, since cardiopulmonary resuscitation may be their only chance of survival.

Treatment of arrhythmias is standard. All lightning victims should probably be monitored for 24 h, have an ECG and serial cardiac enzymes and isoenzymes. The use of prophylactic lidocaine may be efficacious but this has not been proved.

Burns

Burns are usually superficial and minor, generally requiring little treatment. Because they are superficial, myoglobinuria has been reported rarely but should be tested for. Fluid loading, the use of mannitol and other diuretics, and fasciotomies are rarely, if ever, needed. Fluid loading may further complicate cerebral edema in victims with neurological injury and is usually contraindicated unless the patient is in shock for some other reason. Tetanus prophylaxis should be instituted.

Neurological Complications

Almost two-thirds of severely injured patients present with lower extremity paralysis and one-third with upper extremity paralysis. The extremities appear cold, mottled, pulseless, and insensitive. This is usually due to vascular spasm and sympathetic instability and passes gradually in a few hours.

Seizures may occur as a presenting event, probably a result of hypoxia. They may be treated the same as other seizures.

A patient who presents to the emergency department unconscious and unresponsive has a grave prognosis. In the past, coma has often been a result of prolonged hypoxia prior to resuscitation, but it may also be a result of closed head injury. Fluid restriction should be the rule and computerized tomography is indicated to rule out a surgically correctable lesion.

A victim may have permanent neurological sequelae of paresis, trouble with fine calculations or other mental functions, insomnia, etc. It is not uncommon for the alert victim to be somewhat confused for a few days or have permanent amnesia for the events of the first few days after the shock, similar to a patient who has had electroconvulsive shock therapy.

Eyes

Cataracts are common and may occur at the time of injury or develop later. Optic nerve damage, retinal separation, and uveitis are common, so that dilated pupils cannot be relied on as criteria for brain death in lightning victims.

Ears

Over 50 percent of lightning victims have tympanic membrane rupture, either unilateral or bilateral, which may be from the concussive force or from basilar skull fracture. Treatment is usually conservative and expectant unless ossicular disruption has occurred or there is a CSF leak.

Table 52-1. Minimum Laboratory Examinations for Lightning Victims

CBC
UA, for myoglobin, if present; BUN, creatinine
Cardiac isoenzymes
ECG, monitor
Appropriate x-rays, including CT scan if decreasing LOC

Fractures

Fractures of scapulae, clavicles, skull, and long bones may occur but are much more unusual than in high-voltage electrical events.

Fetal Survival

Roughly half of the lightning strikes reported in pregnancy resulted in fetal wastage, one-fourth in neonatal death, and one-fourth in healthy living children.

Laboratory Examinations

Minimum laboratory examinations are listed in Table 52-1. More extensive laboratory analysis, x-rays, and monitoring may be indicated depending on the severity of injury.

SUMMARY

Lightning injury is not an uncommon occurrence and may affect multiple victims in a single event. While 150 to 300 persons are killed by lightning every year in the United States, this is only 30 percent of lightning victims, making it likely that the emergency physician may treat several victims of lightning strike in his or her lifetime. Cardiac arrest is the number one cause of death.

Nearly 70 percent of the victims will show some kind of usually temporary sequelae. Due to the almost instantaneous exposure to the current, though, there are seldom any deep internal burns as in high-voltage electrical injuries. Thus, deep muscle damage and myoglobinuria are rarely factors, so that fluid loading, fasciotomies, and diuretics are rarely needed. Particularly with comatose patients, fluid restriction should be the rule in order to minimize cerebral edema. An electrocardiogram and monitoring are essential since arrhythmias may occur for up to 24 to 36 h following injury. Treatment otherwise involves supportive care and common sense.

BIBLIOGRAPHY

Apfelberg DB, Masters FW, Robinson DW: Pathophysiology and treatment of lightning injuries. *J. Trauma* 14(6):453–460, 1974.

Bartholome CW, Jacoby WD, Ramehand SC: Cutaneous manifestations of lightning injury. *Arch Dermatol* 111:1466–1468, 1975.

Bergstrom LV, Neblett LM, Sando I, et al: The lightning damaged ear. *Arch Otolaryngol* 10:117–121, 1974.

Cooper MA: Prognostic signs for death in patients seriously injured by lightning. *Ann Emerg Med* 9:134–139, 1980.

Cooper MA: Lightning injuries, in Auerbach P, Geehr E (eds): *Management of Wilderness and Environmental Emergencies*. New York, Macmillan, 1983, pp 500–521.

Strasser EJ, Davis RM, Menchey MJ: Lightning injuries. *J Trauma* 17(4):315–319, 1977.

Taussig HB: Death from lightning and the possibility of living again. *Ann Intern Med* 68:1345–1353, 1968.

CHAPTER 53
TOXIC GASES
AND CHEMICALS

L. Scott Ulin

INTRODUCTION

The growth of our highly industrialized society, and the development and widespread use of plastics and other synthetic agents, increases the likelihood of exposure to toxic gases and chemicals. This threat is as close as products and furnishings in our own homes, the nearest highway or railroad track, or local supply stores and manufacturing plants.

There are over 35,000 chemical substances produced in the United States, and subsequently stored at sites located throughout the country. Several billion tons per year are shipped by air, sea, and land, or as many as 200,000 bulk shipments per day. Each year there are approximately 3000 trucking accidents and 100 major train derailments resulting in release of toxic agents. It is estimated that the total number of accidents involving hazardous materials is over 15,000 per year. Therefore, it is essential that all emergency medicine physicians be prepared to handle toxic exposures, whether as a single patient encounter or in a mass casualty situation.

GENERAL APPROACH

A prerequisite to successfully managing toxic exposures is a plan of action which has been established prior to the actual occurrence. When a hazardous material incident occurs, an initial assessment must be made and decontamination instituted. This includes identification, if possible, of the causative agent, the type and severity of injury, and the number of people affected. Often, the history will identify the offending substance. If the toxic source is unknown, certain key historical facts, physical examination findings, and laboratory data should be sought. If the toxic material is one for which an antidote exists, consideration should be given to its administration (see Table 53-1).

Table 53-1. Antidotes

100% oxygen
Methylene blue
Atropine and pralidoxime chloride
Cyanide Poison Kit (Lilly)
Calcium gluconate
Chelating agents

During the initial assessment, emergency medical care that can be rendered without further risk to the patient or staff should be provided. Once the patient is stabilized, a complete history and physical examination should be obtained, monitoring and close observation instituted, and good supportive care provided.

PREPLANNING

Every emergency department or acute care receiving facility should have a plan of action for handling toxic exposures, and make it a part of the policy and procedure manual. It must be readily available to medical team members in both triage and treatment areas. Components of such a plan are listed in Table 53-2.

The protocol should identify a separate receiving area for patients exposed to an agent capable of contaminating others and/or the environment, or when the toxic substance is unknown. This separate receiving site should have facilities for complete decontamination of the patient, including a collection system for wash water, and facilities for rendering emergency medical care once decontamination is complete. The location should be known to all police agencies, fire services, and emergency medical service providers.

Such a plan must delineate who has ultimate medical authority for all phases of operation, and who will be in charge at the triage, decontamination, and medical treatment areas. Responsibilities of all team members should be stated as well. A list of whom to notify, and in what order, as well as current phone or paging numbers should be available.

To protect the staff from inadvertent contamination, essential protective gear should be listed in the protocol and be immediately available for staff use. A minimum list would include hoods, face masks, gowns, double gloves, and shoe covers. Occasionally, this minimum protective gear will be inadequate and more extensive equipment will be needed, for example, self-contained breathing apparatus. In the receiving area, all unnecessary equipment and supplies should be covered by heavy plastic. Ventilation ducts should be sealed, unless a separate ventilation system exists.

Other information the plan should provide includes a resource list for obtaining different equipment and supplies at any hour, for example, extra oxygen tanks or specialized protective gear

Table 53-2. Essentials for a Toxic Exposure Plan

Notification list and in what order to call
Identification of receiving area
Specification of who will be in charge and of what
Minimal protective gear to be worn
A quick reference and resource list
Flexible enough to adjust for all situations
Reviewed yearly and tested through drills
Be readily available

such as acid suits. A reference directory listing books, outside agencies, and consultants should be present (see Table 53-3).

A plan of action is of no use if it is left sitting on the shelf. All emergency medical personnel should be familiar with it. Disaster drills should also include hazardous material scenarios. The plan should be reviewed and updated yearly.

DECONTAMINATION

Decontamination begins with ensuring adequate protection for medical team members, as alluded to previously.

When a patient arrives in the receiving area, his or her complete decontamination must be assured, since prehospital decontamination is often inadequate or nonexistent. Therefore, any clothing must be removed in the receiving area and the patient washed in a shower under a strong stream of water. The only medical care to be given prior to decontamination would be establishment of a stable airway, cervical spine immobilization, hemorrhage control, and treatment of major thoracic injuries, such as a sucking chest wound or tension pneumothorax. In general, rinsing should be continued for at least 15 min. If the toxic material is one that will react with water and the affected area of involvement is small, wiping with a dry, clean cloth can be done. However, if contamination is extensive, it is better to go ahead and quickly wash the patient with a rapidly flowing, strong stream of water.

Once decontamination is complete, the patient should be wrapped in a clean, dry blanket or sheet and passed to other medical staff members stationed outside the contaminated area. At this time, other emergency or urgent medical care required may be provided, as well as a more complete patient assessment. During decontamination, references should be consulted for any additional decontamination procedures needed, for example, washing with soap or application of special solutions.

Before leaving the contaminated area the staff should remove all protective gear and clothing except for the second pair of gloves. All equipment and supplies, as well as the patient's clothing and belongings, should be left behind. Once the staff member is in the safe area, protective gloves may be removed.

Table 53-3. Reference Sources

Clinical Approach to Poisoning and Drug Overdose, Haddad, L. M., and Winchester, J. F., W. B. Saunders Company, Philadelphia, Pa., 1983.
Clinical Toxicology of Commercial Products, Acute Poisoning, Gosselin, R. E., et al. The Williams & Wilkins Company, Baltimore, Md., 1976.
Hazardous Materials 1980 Emergency Response Guidebook, United States Department of Transportation, DOT-P 5800.2, 1980.
Chemical Hazards of the Workplace, Proctor, N. H., and Hughes, J. P. J. B. Lippincott Company, Philadelphia, Pa., 1978.
Recognized Regional Poison Control Center.

INITIAL MANAGEMENT

Once decontamination is completed attention should be directed toward the following priorities: assurance of adequate ventilation and circulation, consideration of possible cervical spine injury in unconscious patients, attempts to identify the toxic agent if not known, administration of an antidote if available and indicated, and good supportive care. As time permits, a thorough history and physical examination should be done.

Airway management and circulatory support are the most fundamental priorities and are rendered in the standard fashion, except in the following special situations. One-hundred percent oxygen should be administered to all patients suffering from exposure at a fire scene, or in the unknown situation when vague central nervous system complaints or altered mental status are found, until carbon monoxide poisoning is ruled out. If assisted ventilation is provided prior to transfer to the safe area, room air should not be used as it may be contaminated. Since many inhaled agents have the potential to produce upper airway obstruction, either by direct irritant injury with edema or by laryngospasm, early endotracheal intubation should be considered. Some toxic substances have the potential for such delayed pulmonary reactions as pulmonary edema or bronchiolitis obliterans. Therefore, even when the patient initially appears fine, close followup is necessary, whether the patient is discharged or admitted for observation. Specific therapeutic modalities will be discussed under inhalation injuries.

If the cause of toxic exposure is unknown, assessment should be directed toward identifying a toxic syndrome, which may aid in the diagnosis. A toxic syndrome is a constellation of signs and symptoms characteristic of poisoning by certain groups of toxins. Some examples of toxic syndromes follow.

Organophosphate or carbamate insecticide poisoning produces a cholinergic crisis. This syndrome is manifested by hypersalivation, lacrimation, diaphoresis, bronchospasm with pulmonary edema, bradycardia, miosis, muscular weakness, seizures, and coma.

Fumes from volatilized metals (i.e., zinc, aluminum, and copper oxide) produce a sudden-onset flulike syndrome with chills, fever, muscular pain, headache, fatigue, vomiting, and a dry throat. In the absence of pulmonary involvement, the disease usually subsides in 24 to 48 h and symptomatic therapy is all that is required. When there is pulmonary involvement, a severe and often fatal chemical pneumonitis with pulmonary edema may develop. Metal fume fever is an occupational hazard to workers in foundries, marinas, and shipyards.

The *hemoglobinopathy syndrome* results from exposure to a variety of agents which alter hemoglobin, making it incapable of oxygen transport. This syndrome includes carboxyhemoglobinemia, methemoglobinemia, and sulfhemoglobinemia. Signs and symptoms include headache, disorientation, dyspnea, coma, convulsions, tachycardia, nausea and vomiting, cutaneous bullae, and cardiovascular collapse. Cyanosis unresponsive to oxygen is seen in methemoglobinemia and sulfhemoglobinemia. Once the toxic agent is known or the toxic syndrome identified, emergency personnel can determine whether an antidote exists and use it. Of the many thousands of toxic substances in existence, antidotes or antagonists exist for only a few. However, when the appropriate antidote is used in specific situations, it can significantly reduce morbidity and mortality as well as be diagnostic of a specific toxin (see Table 53-1).

One-hundred percent oxygen is indicated in all cases of altered mental status or coma of unknown etiology, or exposure from a fire until carbon monoxide poisoning is ruled out. Administration may be accomplished by using a non-rebreathing oxygen mask with a reservoir applied tightly to the face or by insertion of an endotracheal tube. Methylene blue is used for methemoglobinemia with a level greater than 40 percent. Atropine is administered in organophosphate and carbamate insecticide poisoning, while pralidoxime chloride is used after atropine in organophosphate poisoning. The Cyanide Poison Kit (Lilly) contains amyl nitrite, sodium nitrite, and sodium thiosulfate, and is used for cyanide poisoning. Calcium gluconate counteracts the action of hydrofluoric acid on the skin. The chelating agents ethylenediaminetetraacetic acid (EDTA), British antilewisite (BAL), penicillamine, and deferoxamine are effective in heavy metal poisoning. Each antidote will be further discussed later in the chapter.

The key to the successful management of a patient suffering from toxic exposure is good supportive care, which includes close observation and hemodynamic monitoring for complications. Many toxic substances can cause progressive or delayed reactions. Others can be absorbed systemically, percutaneously or through inhalation, with secondary effects on distant organ systems. Specific complications to watch for are listed in Table 53-4.

HISTORY

Although the acuity of a toxic exposure may preclude a comprehensive history, certain facts should be ascertained to help assess the severity of the problem and identify the source. It is important to determine the circumstances surrounding the incident. Was there a fire or explosion? Did it occur inside or outside? Was there a sudden collapse of victims as seen with carbon monoxide or cyanide poisoning? What was involved? Was it, for example, the burning of tires with release of hydrogen sulfide? If it is of unknown etiology, what form was the toxin in? Was it a gas, vapor, fume suspension, or liquid?

Length of time of exposure and the interval since exposure are important. Prolonged skin contact with gasoline allows percutaneous systemic absorption. A gas of high water solubility normally affects only the upper airway, but with protracted exposure it can reach the lower airway as well.

At a fire scene, it is essential to determine if combustion was primarily complete (much fire and little smoke), which produces carbon dioxide; or incomplete (much smoke and little fire), which produces carbon monoxide. It is also important to ascertain what was burning. For example, burning upholstery degrades into hydrogen cyanide, and burning polyvinyl chloride (PVC) releases hydrogen chloride. The color of smoke also may give useful information; i.e., nitrogen dioxide imparts a red color. A history of strong irritant effects is significant in that most toxins produced

Table 53-4. Complications

Hypoxia
Arrhythmias
Hypotension
Seizures
Fluid and electrolyte disturbances
Pulmonary and cerebral edema
Hepatic, renal, and hemoproliferative failure
Aspiration

Table 53-5. Diagnostic Odors

Odor	Toxic Agent
Bitter almonds	Cyanide
Rotten eggs	Sulfides
Garlic	Arsenic, phosphorus, organophosphates
Shoe polish	Nitrobenzene
Disinfectants	Phenol, creosote
Violets	Turpentine

in a fire cause irritation except for cyanide. The presence or absence of unusual odors should be elicited. Hydrogen sulfide gives off a rotten egg smell and organophosphate insecticides give off a garlic-like odor (see Table 53-5).

Any patient complaining of vague or unusual central nervous system complaints may be suffering from a toxic exposure. Therefore, a detailed occupational and hobby activity history must be obtained.

PHYSICAL FINDINGS

Physical findings suggestive of a specific etiology are few; however, when found they may be diagnostic. As just mentioned, the odor on the breath, skin, and clothes should be checked. Fever in conjunction with a flulike syndrome is compatible with metal fume intoxication. Diaphoresis and hypersecretory activity are characteristic of organophosphate insecticide poisoning. The mouth and throat should be checked for burns. Conjunctivitis, rhinitis, and pharyngitis are seen in exposure to irritant gases that are highly soluble in water. Tachypnea, rhonchi, and rales will be seen in exposure to gases with low water solubility. Severe bronchospasm can be produced by pulmonary sensitizers such as grain dust. Pain out of proportion to a cutaneous injury is characteristic of hydrofluoric acid contamination.

Cyanosis unresponsive to oxygen therapy suggests methemoglobinemia. Violent hematemesis may be seen in heavy metal poisoning. Pressure bullae may be seen in carbon monoxide poisoning as well as flame-shaped retinal hemorrhages in normotensive people.

LABORATORY STUDIES

Laboratory studies needed include a complete blood count, electrolytes, blood urea nitrogen (BUN), blood sugar, hepatic and renal panels, arterial blood gases, and a urinalysis. As mentioned previously, a carboxyhemoglobin level should be obtained for all patients exposed to fire, smoke, fumes, or with central nervous system complaints of unknown etiology. A chest x-ray should be obtained for all patients with a history of toxic inhalation or pulmonary signs and symptoms. An ECG should be obtained for all patients exposed to agents of known cardiac toxicity or who have arrhythmias or chest pain.

Although most laboratory studies are nonspecific, some conclusions can be inferred. In patients exposed to smoke and fire, an elevated carboxyhemoglobin level is important even if it is not in the toxic range, for it may portend the inhalation of other more toxic gases as well. The finding of a normal arterial P_{O_2} and metabolic acidosis in a cyanotic patient is diagnostic of carbon monoxide poisoning or methemoglobinemia. Urine color can also help in diagnosis. Tetrahydronaphthalene gives urine a greenish color, methylene blue gives it a bluish color, and phenol and aniline dyes make urine dark. The appearance of chocolate-colored venous blood that does not change color on exposure to air can suggest methemoglobinemia, and arterial and venous blood specimens having the same color suggest carbon monoxide poisoning. In patients appearing in a cholinergic crisis, a decrease in the serum cholinesterase enzyme level points toward organophosphate poisoning.

ROUTES OF EXPOSURE

Primary modes of injury from exposure to toxic gases and chemicals are inhalation and cutaneous contact. Less common routes are ocular contact and ingestion. Inhalation is the most frequent route of injury, and the majority of cases are due to noxious gases, although occasionally metal fumes or direct chemical aspiration are the cause. Noxious gases are categorized into four classes (see Table 53-6).

Inhalation Injury

Simple asphyxiants are biologically inert and displace oxygen from the air. Signs and symptoms from these agents are due to the reduction of oxygen in the air. Symptoms first occur at a level of 12 to 15 percent, with loss of muscular coordination. Judgment becomes impaired when the oxygen level decreases to 10 to 12 percent. Collapse occurs when the level drops to 6 to 8 percent, and below 6 percent is fatal in 6 to 8 min.

Systemic toxins interfere with tissue oxygenation either by preventing the transport of oxygen, or inhibiting its use by the cell. Carbon monoxide has a much higher affinity for hemoglobin than oxygen and ties up the transport sites. Cyanide and hydrogen sulfide are gases which have an affinity for ferric iron present in the mitochondrial cytochrome oxidase system, and this binding prevents cellular respiration. The organ systems primarily affected by this class of noxious gases are the central nervous and cardiac systems.

Irritant gases produce direct mucosal damage to the respiratory tract. The primary location of injury depends on the water solubility of the substance. Agents with a high water solubility, such as ammonia, will be absorbed in the upper airways, producing rhinitis, pharyngitis, cough, and, if exposure is severe or pro-

Table 53-6. Noxious Gas Classification

SIMPLE ASPHYXIANTS

Carbon dioxide, hydrocarbons (butane, methane, propane)

SYSTEMIC TOXINS

Carbon monoxide, carbon disulfide, hydrogen cyanide, methylated halogens

IRRITANTS

Ammonia, halogens, hydrogen halides, nitric oxide, nitrogen dioxide, chloroacetophenone, phosgene, sulfur dioxide

COMBINED IRRITANTS AND SYSTEMIC TOXINS

Acetylene, aromatic hydrocarbons, hydrogen sulfide, metallic oxides (metal fumes), ozone

longed, laryngeal edema. Those agents with a low solubility in water, such as phosgene, will reach the lower airway, manifesting as pneumonitis, pulmonary edema, and bronchiolitis obliterans. Gases with an intermediate solubility in water will at first produce upper airway symptoms. However, if exposure is prolonged, lower airway damage can occur as well. Lower airway injury and subsequent findings may develop without any antecedent upper airway symptoms.

Combined systemic and irritant gases cause injury through both asphyxia and direct mucosal damage. Signs and symptoms are a combination of respiratory and central nervous system derangements. The patient with such an exposure may present with a wide variety of problems.

As previously stated, the cornerstone of treatment is supportive care. Mainstays of treatment include rest, hydration and humidification, supplemental oxygen, and close observation.

For patients exposed to simple asphyxiants, removal to fresh air may be all that is needed; however, any patient with an altered mental status or apparent hypoxia must be given 100 percent oxygen until carbon monoxide poisoning is ruled out. If hypoxia exists after the administration of oxygen, other toxic etiologies to consider include cyanide poisoning, exposure to hydrogen sulfide gas, and methemoglobinemia. If central nervous system excitation persists, judicious use of sedatives is appropriate.

Patients suffering from irritant gas inhalation are treated according to the signs and symptoms present. For rhinitis and pharyngitis without objective injury, reassurance and perhaps a decongestant are usually satisfactory. When tracheobronchitis is found, humidification with cooled steam should be started. If bronchospasm is present, bronchodilators should be utilized in the standard fashion: epinephrine or terbutaline subcutaneously along with nebulized β agonists. Aminophylline should be added to the regimen for nonresponders or those with severe bronchospasm. Parenteral corticosteroids should be given for intractable wheezing. If there is evidence of upper airway injury (burn, swelling, or stridorous respirations), impending upper airway obstruction must be considered and early endotracheal intubation or cricothyrotomy performed in a controlled environment. If pneumonitis develops with progressive respiratory insufficiency, positive end-expiratory pressure is added to maintain an arterial P_{O_2} greater than 60 torr. In this situation, steroids are controversial and antibiotics reserved for documented bacterial infection. When pulmonary edema develops, aggressive therapy with diuretics and vasodilators should be utilized. However, morphine sulfate is contraindicated in this situation. Because toxic gases have the capability of producing delayed pulmonary problems such as phosgene gas-induced pulmonary edema or upper airway obstruction from upper airway injury, repeat examinations and followup x-rays are advised during the first 72 h postexposure. Criteria justifying hospital admission include dypsnea on breathing room air, evidence of lower airway injury, severe upper airway inflammation, upper airway thermal injury, tracheobronchitis, or exposure to an agent known to cause severe lower airway injury.

Cutaneous Injury

Toxic gases and chemicals may produce several distinct patterns of injury upon dermal contact: burns, dermatitis, allergic reactions, and systemic effects. Treatment is dictated by the type of reaction present.

Thermal injury results from direct flame contact, contact with burning metals, or by an exothermic reaction. General burn care begins by halting the burning process, which includes removing smoldering clothing, smothering flames, decontamination, and, in the case of burning metals, covering with mineral oil. During evaluation adequate tetanus immunization must be assured.

Specific treatment depends upon the extent of burn injury. Minor burns are cleansed with a mild soap solution and any devitalized tissue is debrided. The burn is then dressed with a topical antibacterial cream and an occlusive dressing for comfort. All outpatient burns should be checked within 24 to 48 h after injury. Major burns are managed with an aseptic technique. Injured areas are covered with dry, sterile dressings or sheets, and large-bore intravenous catheters are inserted. Isotonic crystalloid and/or colloidal fluids should be given to correct underlying volume deficits and reduce further fluid loss. Small aliquots of intravenous analgesics should be administered to control pain, unless there are specific contraindications. Referral to a burn center should be considered in all these cases.

Dermatitis results from the direct contact of toxic substances on the skin. Therapy is determined by the extent of injury and the symptomatology present. When the affected area is small or localized, wet dressings may be applied for comfort and oral antihistamines prescribed for itching. When the reaction is severe or extensive, in addition to the wet dressings, dermatologic consultation should be obtained.

Allergic reactions may be of a contact type or due to prior sensitization. They are treated in the standard fashion with epinephrine and antihistamines. When anaphylaxis is severe or prolonged, parenteral steroids should also be administered and the patient admitted to the hospital.

Systemic toxicity from cutaneous injury may occur by two different mechanisms—either by percutaneous absorption or through denuded areas of skin that have lost their protective barrier. The ability of a drug to penetrate and attack skin is based upon lipid solubility. Agents with a high solubility, such as organophosphate insecticides or organic solvents, will be readily absorbed, while those of low solubility will not.

MANAGEMENT OF OCULAR EXPOSURE

If the patient arrives at the hospital suffering from ocular contact with toxic gases and chemicals, the adequacy of prehospital irrigation must be assured. If this is doubtful or if the patient still has symptoms, lavage should immediately be initiated using a physiologic solution such as normal saline. The goal of irrigation is to bring the pH of the lacrimal fluid back to normal, a pH of 7.0. If available, a topical anesthetic can be applied before lavage; however, delay in lavage should never be allowed. Flushing should be continued for a minimum of 15 min in each eye. If the substance is an alkali, lavage should be continued for a minimum of 30 min and may be necessary for up to 24 h or more. As just mentioned, the end point of irrigation is not a finite period of time but a return of the lacrimal pH back to normal.

After completion of the irrigation, visual acuity should be recorded for each eye. Unless contraindicated, fluorescein dye should be instilled and corneal abrasions searched for. Any eye injury found on examination should be treated in the standard fashion. Conjunctivitis is treated with cool compresses and perhaps vasoconstrictive eyedrops. Abrasions are treated with antibacterial drops, cycloplegics, and pressure patching. All eye injuries should receive ophthalmology referral for followup, and anything more serious than the above-mentioned problems should get an immediate ophthalmology consultation. Eyedrops containing steroids should not be used unless prescribed by the consulting ophthalmologist.

SPECIFIC AGENTS

Carbon Monoxide

Carbon monoxide is a systemic toxin which accounts for many thousands of deaths per year, and is a frequent cause of fire-related injuries in the United States. It is a tasteless, colorless, odorless, and nonirritating gas produced by the incomplete combustion of carbon-containing substances such as wood or cotton.

Carbon monoxide has an affinity for hemoglobin approximately 250 times greater than that of oxygen, which allows it to competitively combine with hemoglobin and form carboxyhemoglobin instead of oxyhemoglobin. The end result is functional hypoxemia. Its predominant effects are on the organ systems most sensitive to oxygen deprivation, the central nervous system and cardiac system. Clinical manifestations roughly correlate with the carboxyhemoglobin level. Symptoms begin as the level reaches 20 percent, with the person experiencing nausea, headache, and shortness of breath on exertion. As the level climbs to 40 percent, irritability, poor judgment, fatigability, visual disturbances, nausea, and vomiting will be seen. Between levels of 40 and 60 percent the patient develops tachycardia, tachypnea, syncope, ataxia, and confusion, which progress to convulsions and coma. At the level greater than 60 percent cardiovascular collapse and respiratory failure ensue.

Other organ systems affected include the skin and the musculoskeletal system, and neuropsychiatric manifestations may appear. Cutaneous manifestations may include erythema, edema, and bullae. Rhabdomyolysis may occur from pressure necrosis of muscle or as a direct toxic effect. An insidious and characteristic syndrome from carbon monoxide poisoning is the delayed development of psychiatric impairment 1 to 3 weeks after exposure. It is manifested by impaired judgment, difficulty with abstract thinking, poor concentration, and inappropriate euphoria. This phenomenon occurs in 10 to 30 percent of patients with carbon monoxide poisoning. An arterial blood pH below 7.4 portends a high chance of a patient suffering serious neurologic sequelae or death.

The goal of therapy with administration of 100 percent oxygen is to improve the oxygen content of the blood by maximizing the fraction dissolved in plasma (arterial P_{O_2}). This improves the availability of oxygen to the tissues and accelerates elimination of hemoglobin-bound carbon monoxide. The half-life of carboxyhemoglobin in room air is $4\frac{1}{2}$ to 6 h, but with 100 percent oxygen it is reduced to $1\frac{1}{2}$ h. Oxygen is continued until the level decreases to 10 percent. The definitive treatment of choice, if available, for severe carbon monoxide poisoning manifested by coma or a level greater than 40 percent is hyperbaric oxygen at 3 atm of pressure. This reduces the half-life to less than 60 min. The decision of whether or not to transfer a patient to a hyperbaric oxygen chamber should be based on proximity of the facility, the risk/benefit ratio of transferring a critically ill or unstable patient, and local medicolegal implications.

Additional management includes hemodynamic monitoring and close observation. Besides routine laboratory data and the carboxyhemoglobin level, creatine phosphokinase (CPK) and urine myoglobin must be measured to detect the development of rhabdomyolysis and renal failure.

Clinical recovery usually lags hours to days behind the blood level reduction. In addition, it must be remembered that the level of carboxyhemoglobin measured in the hospital may be considerably less than the original peak value, as prehospital and emergency department treatment will depress the value.

Cyanide Poisoning

Cyanide poisoning usually occurs from inhalation of toxic gases containing cyanide or ingestion of Laetrile. Hydrogen cyanide and its derivatives are widely used in industry for fumigation, ore extraction, electroplating, the production of synthetic rubber, and as fertilizer. Cyanides are also found in the home in silver polishes and rodenticides. The seeds of peach, plum, cherry, and almonds, and plants such as chokecherries and cassava beans contain amygdalin, which, when crushed and moistened (as by chewing and swallowing), produces cyanide. Laetrile is a synthetic amygdalin product which produces cyanide upon metabolism. Toxicity from Laetrile has become an increasing problem since its newfound popularity as a presumed anticancer drug.

Cyanide is a systemic toxin which has a strong affinity for iron in the ferric ($^{+3}$) state. The enzymes controlling oxidative processes of cellular function, especially the cytochrome oxidase system, contain iron in this ferric state. When cyanide is present, it reversibly binds to this iron form, inhibiting cellular respiration. Symptoms usually occur within seconds upon inhalation and within minutes following oral ingestion or skin contamination. They include giddiness, headache, palpitations, dyspnea, and unconsciousness. Historically, the diagnosis is suggested when there has been exposure to the products of combustion with sudden collapse, but without evidence of irritant gas effects; or by the presence of bitter almond odor, characteristic of cyanide poisoning. Physical findings include ataxia, coma, convulsions and death. Often the odor is present on the breath, skin, or clothing. Laboratory data helpful in the diagnosis include an arterial blood gas specimen with a normal oxygen tension, a decreased oxygen saturation, and a metabolic acidosis.

The rationale of therapy is to create a state of controlled methemoglobinemia which can compete for the cyanide ion forming of cyanmethemoglobin. This unbinds the more essential enzyme systems, and restores cellular respiration. The standard therapy available in the United States is the use of the Cyanide Poison Kit manufactured by Lilly. This kit contains amyl nitrite pearls, sodium nitrite solution, and sodium thiosulfate solution. The procedure for using this kit begins with breaking an amyl nitrite pearl and placing it on a gauze pad held under the patient's nose for 30 s out of each minute. This will create an initial methemoglobin level of approximately 5 percent and give the examiner time to prepare the other two components of the kit. Further amyl nitrite pearls should be used every 5 min.

The second step is administration of 10 mL of sodium nitrite. This dose should be administered at a rate of 2.5 to 5 mL per minute. It increases the methemoglobin level to nearly 40 percent, which is high enough to facilitate the competitive binding of cyanide to methemoglobin, yet low enough to protect against toxic methemoglobinemia. The side effects of intravenous sodium nitrite are hypotension, tachycardia, and vomiting. In children, the dose must be reduced and is calculated from the child's hemoglobin and total body weight. There is a chart in the kit giving the proper dose.

The third step is to administer sodium thiosulfate, which provides additional receptor sites for cyanide, forming thiocyanate, a relatively nontoxic product which is excreted by the kidneys. Sodium thiosulfate is given intravenously at a rate of 2.5 to 5 mL per minute also. The recommended dose of sodium thiosulfate for adults is 50 mL. The dosage for children is based upon the body surface area in square meters and should be available from a chart as well.

When poisoning has occurred by inhalation, removal to fresh air should allow the body to rapidly clear the cyanide that is already present. The need for use of the cyanide antidote kit in acute inhalational toxicity is not clear, since it does have the potential for toxicity itself. In a severe, life-threatening situation, sodium thiosulfate is indicated intravenously to help detoxify the cyanide present; however, the use of sodium nitrite in this situation is not validated and in fact may be harmful.

Methemoglobinemia

Methemoglobin is created by the oxidation of the iron in hemoglobin, from the reduced ferrous ($^{+2}$) form to the ferric ($^{+3}$) state, which is incapable of binding oxygen for transport to the tissues. Methemoglobin is normally present at 1 percent of the total circulating hemoglobin and maintained in equilibrium with the other 99 percent by a red cell enzyme called methemoglobin reductase. Nitrites, nitrates, aniline dyes, chlorates, and nitrobenzene increase the rate of oxidation of iron and upon toxic exposure overwhelm the capacity of this red cell enzyme. Sources of these agents are fertilizers, wax crayons, varnishes, solvents, shoe polishes, and laundry dyes.

Signs and symptoms of methemoglobinemia begin at a level of approximately 10 to 20 percent with the appearance of cyanosis, which will usually be asymptomatic. At a level of approximately 30 percent, nonspecific symptoms such as headache, fatigue, dyspnea, tachycardia, and dizziness develop. Obtundation will be found at a level greater than approximately 50 percent, and greater than 70 percent may be lethal. A diagnosis of methemoglobinemia should be considered when a patient presents with asymptomatic cyanosis or cyanosis which does not respond to oxygen therapy. The diagnosis can be made at the bedside by one of two tests. A drop of the patient's blood placed upon filter paper will appear chocolate-brown in color and not change its color upon exposure to air. This difference can be better appreciated if a drop of normal blood is placed next to the chocolate-colored blood. A few drops of 10 percent solution of potassium cyanide may be added to the patient's blood, and in the presence of methemoglobin will convert the chocolate-brown color to a bright red. Arterial blood gas measurements will show a normal oxygen concentration (arterial P_{O_2}) and a decreased oxygen saturation. The percent saturation must be measured directly however, because if it is derived from a nomogram, the value may indicate a normal oxygen saturation.

Besides the standard blood studies previously mentioned, renal and liver panels must be obtained as many of these agents can cause kidney and liver failure as well.

Methemoglobinemia must be differentiated from sulfhemoglobinemia, a pigment neither naturally occurring nor reversible. Sulfhemoglobinemia is felt to be due to oxidation by agents such as phenacetin and acetanilid. The blood color in these two hemoglobinopathies is similar; however, addition of potassium cyanide solution to the patient's blood in sulfhemoglobinemia will not convert the chocolate color to red as it does in methemoglobinemia.

Once the toxin is removed, methemoglobin reductase will spontaneously reduce the level of methemoglobin back to its usual low equilibrium state. Methemoglobin levels of 20 to 30 percent will revert to normal in 2 to 3 days without further therapy or causing any ill effects.

Methylene blue is the antidote for severe methemoglobinemia, manifested by symptoms of central nervous system derangement, or a methemoglobin level greater than 40 percent. Methylene blue enhances an alternate pathway for the reduction of methemoglobin, which involves the hexose monophosphate shunt, normally of little significance in physiologic hemoglobin metabolism. The dosage is 0.2 mL of a 1% solution (2 mg) per kilogram of body weight intravenously over 5 min. The dose may be repeated in 1 h and every 4 to 6 h thereafter should cyanosis persist. Total dosage should not exceed 7 mg/kg. Above this level methylene blue actually becomes toxic itself and can even act as an oxidant, further compounding the problem. Adverse reactions to methylene blue include nausea and vomiting, hypertension, confusion, diaphoresis and intravascular hemolysis.

Adjunctive therapy should include high oxygen flow to saturate the remaining normal hemoglobin and increase the physically dissolved oxygen in blood. Hyperbaric oxygen has also been shown to be useful, not only to saturate the blood, but also to decrease the rate of oxidation of hemoglobin. It should be considered for use in severe cases, especially those involving nitrite intoxication. As discussed under carbon monoxide poisoning the risk and/or benefits of transferring a critically ill patient to a hyperbaric oxygen chamber must be considered.

Organophosphate Insecticide Poisoning

Atropine and pralidoxime chloride are indicated for organophosphate insecticide poisoning, and atropine alone for carbamate insecticide poisoning. As mentioned previously, these toxins produce a cholinergic crisis by inhibiting the action of acetylcholinesterase which allows the accumulation of acetylcholine at synapses and myoneural junctions. Organophosphates cause irreversible inhibition, while carbamates produce reversible inhibition.

Atropine is the antagonist of choice and should be given in a test dose of 0.05 mg/kg up to a total of 2 mg whenever the diagnosis is suspected. This dose should be repeated in 15 min if there is no observable adverse effect. The goal of atropine therapy is to dry up all secretions, a state known as atropinization. There is no maximal total dose of atropine, and up to 5 mg intravenously may be needed every 15 min in a critically ill adult patient, i.e., one in respiratory arrest or with profound hypotension or hypothermia. Atropinization, once achieved, should be continued for at least 24 h. Prior to administration, adequate oxygenation must be ensured to reduce the risk of atropine-induced fibrillation in the hypoxic myocardium.

Atropine therapy has no effect on skeletal muscle or the autonomic ganglia; therefore, muscle fasciculations and weakness will persist. Pralidoxime (Protopam, 2-PAM) is given to reverse these effects and works by actually breaking the phosphate inhibition, allowing reactivation of the enzyme acetylcholinesterase. Prali-

doxime is not indicated in carbamate poisoning, as this inhibition will spontaneously reverse itself. The dose of pralidoxime is 20 to 40 mg per kilogram of body weight, up to a limit of 1 to 2 g intravenously over a 15- to 30-min period. This dose may be repeated up to 0.5 g per hour for critically ill patients. It should be given after atropine and within 24 h of exposure to be effective. Pralidoxime should never be withheld in an unknown toxic situation, when cholinergic findings are present.

Hydrofluoric Acid

Hydrofluoric acid is a powerful inorganic acid whose toxicity is due to its corrosiveness. The hallmark of toxicity is pain way out of proportion to the extent of injury present. Hydrofluoric acid readily penetrates intact dermis, whereupon it will dissociate, releasing the fluoride ion. This ion immobilizes intracellular calcium at the membrane level and subsequent increased potassium permeability occurs. The result is a spontaneous depolarization of nerve tissue, producing severe pain. Fluoride will continue to be active until medically deactivated. This can be achieved by injecting a 10% calcium gluconate solution subcutaneously, which precipitates fluoride as the insoluble salt, calcium fluoride. Treatment protocol is as follows:

1. If there is a history of contact but no evidence of significant injury, the area should first be flushed copiously with water and then covered with a dressing saturated in calcium gluconate solution.
2. If evidence of injury or pain is present, calcium gluconate infiltration subcutaneously is indicated.
   a. First administer a field or regional anesthesia to reduce pain.
   b. The solution is injected slowly through a 27-gauge needle and the area of infiltration is extended to at least $\frac{1}{2}$ cm beyond the margin of obviously burned skin.
   c. The lesion should then be covered with dressings soaked in the solution.
   d. If there is any possibility of exposure to the nail, the nail must be removed and calcium gluconate injected directly into the nail bed. If this is not performed, there is potential for the fluoride ion to erode into the phalanx, causing bony destruction.
   e. If pain recurs, the same procedure can be repeated in 24 h.
   f. Any patient who needs calcium gluconate infiltration, except for the most minimal of injuries, should be hospitalized for observation.

Phenol (Carbolic Acid)

Phenol and its derivatives, cresol, are used as disinfectants, deodorizers, and sanitizers. Upon exposure they cause a pattern of injury called coagulation necrosis, with formation of an eschar over the wound. The problem occurs because the phenol is trapped underneath the eschar, and cannot be removed by flushing the affected area with water. The treatment of choice is a special solution, usually available from industry, of polyethylene glycol and industrial methylated spirits in a 2:1 ratio. However, for emergency care, glycerol is an adequate substitute. The major hazard from phenol is systemic absorption with profound central nervous system depressant effects, leading to coma and death.

Metals

Metals have the ability to burn. Sodium and potassium may ignite spontaneously when exposed to air, and other metals such as magnesium, lithium, and aluminum will burn when ignited.

If burning metal fragments become embedded in the skin, they cannot be wiped off, and water is contraindicated as it causes a severe exothermic reaction. Therefore, to stop the burning process, the treatment of choice is to immerse in or cover the area with mineral oil which smothers the burning metal.

Lime (Calcium Oxide)

Lime reacts with moisture to form calcium hydroxide, an extremely caustic agent. Upon cutaneous exposure, it will draw water out of the skin, producing an exothermic reaction. In treating these cases, a strong stream and a large volume of water should be used for decontaminating the skin. If a small volume or a low flow is used, the ensuing exothermic reaction will be enhanced and can exacerbate any preexistent injury.

Heavy Metal Poisoning

Common poisons are various salts of lead, arsenic, thallium, mercury, and iron. Treatment of acute heavy metal intoxication involves a group of related chelating agents, EDTA, BAL, penicillamine, and deferoxamine.

Acute lead poisoning is relatively rare. Signs and symptoms of intoxication involve the gastrointestinal, neuromuscular, and central nervous systems. Suspected lead poisoning with acute symptoms must be confirmed with haste. Findings include leg cramps, muscle weakness, paresthesias, depression, and severe hematemesis. Tests the physician should obtain include a blood lead level and an erythrocyte protoporphyrin level.

Chelation therapy for lead poisoning involves the combined use of EDTA and BAL. Treatment protocol begins with administration of BAL in a dose of 4 mg/kg every 4 h. EDTA should be withheld until the second dose of BAL is given. EDTA is given intramuscularly in a child and intravenously in the adult. The dose is 50 mg/kg in 24 h in four divided doses. This is a painful compound, therefore the volume injected should be mixed with procaine to reduce the pain. If the patient is actively convulsing or in coma, the dose is increased to 75 mg/kg in 24 h. Up to 1 g in 24 h is the maximum for EDTA. In general, patients begun on this combined regimen are treated for at least 48 h, or until encephalopathy is resolved and serum levels are back to normal limits. Subsequently, EDTA is continued alone for a course of 7 days. Adverse effects of BAL include nausea, vomiting, and headache and are found in about half the patients. If BAL is not tolerated, adults can be given a slow IV drip of EDTA, 1 g in 250 mL of fluid twice daily.

Iron poisoning is relatively rare in the adult population. When acute iron poisoning occurs, the course is similar to the other heavy metal intoxications. Commonly there will be massive hematemesis and hematochezia, which continue to cardiovascular collapse and death. The decision to use the antagonist deferoxamine mesylate (Desferal), is based upon measurement of the total iron-binding capacity and free serum iron 4 to 5 h following exposure. If serum iron is greater than either 500 μg/100 mL or exceeds the total measured iron-binding capacity, deferoxamine therapy should be instituted. The dose is 90 mg per kilogram of body weight intramuscularly every 8 h for three doses. Otherwise, supportive therapy alone should suffice. If the patient is in shock or coma from acute iron poisoning, an hourly infusion of deferoxamine should be administered at 15 mg per kilogram of body weight and continued for 8 h. The main toxic effect associated with deferoxamine is hypotension. This is rarely seen unless the infusion rate exceeds the above doses. This agent will turn the urine a characteristic "vin rosé" color that marks excretion of the pigmented complex. Once the urine loses this characteristic color, chelation therapy can be stopped.

BIBLIOGRAPHY

Bayer MJ, Rumack BH: Topics in Emergency Medicine: Poisonings and Overdose, 1(3), 1979.

Caholane M, Demling RH: Early respiratory abnormalities from smoke inhalation. *JAMA* 251(6):771–773, 1984.

Cohen MA, Guzzardi LJ: Inhalation of products of combustion. *Ann Emerg Med* 12(10):628–632, 1983.

Garvin JM: Toxic and thermal Inhalations. Emergency Medical Services, May/June, 1980, pp. 10–15.

Gosselin RE, et al: *Clinical Toxicology of Commercial Products.* Baltimore, The Williams & Wilkins Company, 1976.

Haddad LM, Winchester JF: *Clinical Approach to Poisoning and Drug Overdose.* Philadelphia, Saunders, 1983.

Hedges JR: Acute noxious gas exposure. *Cur Top* Medical College of Pennsylvania. 2(10), 1978.

Jurkovich GJ, Moylan JA: Inhalation injury—a major burn complication. *Hosp Physician* Nov:92–98, 1983.

Kearney TE, et al: Chemically induced methemoglobinemia from airline poisoning. *West J Med* 140(2):282–286, 1984.

Litovitz TL, et al: Cyanide poisoning treated with hyperbaric oxygen. *Am J Emerg Med* 1:94–101, 1982.

Proctor NH, Hughes JP: *Chemical Hazards of the Workplace.* Philadelphia, J.B. Lippincott Company, 1978.

Tintinalli JE: Hydrofluoric acid burns. Emergency care conference. *Am Coll Emerg Phys* 7:24, 1978.

U.S. Department of Transportation: Hazardous Material—Emergency Response Guidebook. Washington, D.C., DOT-P 5800.2, 1980.

CHAPTER 54
Radiation Disasters

H. Arnold Muller

Emergency physicians are, of necessity, concerned with environmental hazards. One of those hazards is radiation. We cannot see, smell, feel, or hear it, yet it captured our attention during the Three Mile Island accident. We must learn about radiation and its hazards in order to be able to assume responsibility for leadership in the management of radiation accidents as well as radiation disasters. Thus, some elements of radiation physics, common sources of radiation (see Table 54-1), the tissue effects of radiation, the signs and symptoms of radiation injury, and the evaluation and therapy of radiation injuries and exposure will be briefly covered in this chapter.

PATHOPHYSIOLOGY

Radiation may be classified as *ionizing* and *nonionizing*. The former, ionizing, is produced by nuclear weapons and reactors, radioactive material, and x-ray machines. The term *ionizing* is derived from the effect that such radiation produces when it interacts with matter, i.e., it causes atoms to convert to ions as a result of the atoms' loss or gain of electrons. Biologic function may be affected if such ionized atoms are in the human body. On the other hand, light, radio, and microwaves are examples of nonionizing radiation.

Table 54-1. Common Sources of Radiation

Natural Sources of Radiation	Whole body, mrem/yr
Natural background radiation	35
Air	5
Building materials	34
Food	25
Ground	11
	Total 110

Technological Sources of Radiation	Dose rate
Coast-to-coast jet flight	5 mrem/round trip
Color television	1 mrem/year
One AP chest film	10 mrem

Source: Linneman RE: Background information on radiation. April 4, 1979 San Jose, Calif. General Electric Nuclear Energy Group. Used by permission.

Radiation is either *particulate* or *electromagnetic*. Electromagnetic radiation occurs in wave form. It belongs to a family of radiant energies that is described by wavelengths. Electromagnetic radiations, in order of decreasing energy content are: γ rays, x-rays, ultraviolet rays, visible rays, infrared rays, microwaves, and radio waves. γ Rays and x-rays are electromagnetic radiations that can cause ionization. They travel great distances and readily penetrate body cells. X-rays differ from gamma rays only in that they are produced outside of the nucleus of an atom. X-ray and γ rays can easily be detected by Geiger-Müller (GM) counters.

Although α and β particles are not electromagnetic they do cause ionization. α Particles consist of two protons and two neutrons (identical to a helium atom without electrons) that are emitted from the nucleus of radioactive atoms. α Particles travel only a few centimeters and may be stopped by paper or the keratin layer of the skin. β Particles are electrons emitted from the nucleus of radioactive atoms. They travel a few meters or more and barely penetrate the skin. Both α and β particles are harmful, however, if they contaminate wounds or are ingested or inhaled. Contamination of the body surfaces by α and β particles can be detected by appropriate counters.

Energy deposited by radiation is referred to as the dose. A rad, *r*adiation *a*bsorbed *d*ose, is 100 ergs of energy deposited in 1 g of material. A given rad dose from neutrons or α particles will produce three to twenty times as much biologic damage as the same dose in rads from x-rays or γ rays. The rem, *r*oentgen *e*quivalent *m*an, is a calculated radiation unit in which the absorbed dose in rads is multiplied by a quality factor to account for the biological effectiveness of the different types of radiation. For x-rays, γ rays, and β particles the rad and the rem are essentially equivalent. The dose of x- or γ radiation that will cause death to half who are exposed is 400 rem. At about 600 rad the mortality is near 100 percent. In pregnant women, there is generally little concern if fetal exposure is less than 1 rem. Indeed, the threshold for major malformation production is greater than 20 rem even between the eighteenth and thirty-fifth day, the most sensitive period of gestation. The human average annual "normal" exposure to radiation is 70 to 170 thousandths of a rem, 70 to 170 mrem. We generally use the term *rem* or *millirem* (mrem) when referring to biologic systems' exposure. It is important to remember that a person or object exposed to radiation does not become radioactive. It is only the presence of contamination, or radioactive dirt, that poses risk to personnel rendering treatment.

When considering the consequence of radiation exposure, we must take into account the time over which radiation was received. Equivalent doses received over a long time are less harmful than those received over a short period of time. For example, 100 rem delivered at 100 rem per year is much less harmful than 100 rem delivered at 100 rem per second. The radiation dose decreases inversely as the square of the distance from the source.

The biologic effects of radiation are a consequence of ionization. Free radicals are formed from water, and can cause DNA and RNA strands to be broken. Cell and chromosomal changes may be minor and not pose a hazard to the organism, or they may result in aberrations that are passed on to subsequent generations, or they may result in cell death or the inability to replicate.

Clinical Features

The most prominent systemic signs and symptoms of high (greater than 100 rem, i.e., 100,000 mrem) radiation exposure are malaise, nausea, vomiting, and diarrhea; seizures; erythema of the skin; and later, bleeding, anemia, and infection. Nausea and vomiting occur at about 100 rem exposure (see Table 54-2). If they develop within 2 h of exposure, it suggests a dose of more than 400 rem; after 2 h exposure, less than 200 rem; if none after 6 h exposure, less than 50 rem. Erythema indicates exposure greater than 300 rem to the skin; diarrhea indicates exposure greater than 400 rem; and seizures indicate exposure greater than 2000 rem to the head. Lymphocyte counts are useful prognostically. If after 48 h the lymphocyte count is 1200/mm³, the prognosis is good; 300 to 1200, fair; less than 300 mm³, poor. Bleeding, anemia, and infection may occur after a latent period of 20 to 30 days.

Erythema and brawniness of the skin develop in a few hours and progress over days, just as does a thermal burn. Loss of hair, vesiculation, and ulceration may eventually develop if the dose is high enough.

One can estimate the likelihood of significant systemic effects based on time of onset of nausea, vomiting, and diarrhea; changes in lymphocyte count, and by knowledge of the accident, the radiation source, the dose readings at the site of the accident, and the duration of exposure. Very often a health physicist at the scene of an industrial accident is able to provide one with such information. Severity of symptoms is variable and does not correlate with dose, but onset following exposure does. The quicker signs and/or symptoms develop, the higher the dose and the worse the prognosis. Initial symptoms (nausea, vomiting, and general malaise) generally subside within a few hours to several days and are followed by a latent period of 1 or more weeks. In general, if exposure is less than 125 rem, prognosis is good. For those with exposure to 200 to 1000 rem, observation is indicated and treatment need is probable to certain.

Following exposure to radiation, the exposed population would be concerned with delayed complications such as leukemia and thyroid carcinoma. Contraception should be practiced for several months to avoid congenital defects in offspring.

Table 54-2. Dose-Effect Relationships Following Acute Whole Body Irradiation (x- or γ ray)

Whole Body* Dose (rad)	Clinical and Laboratory Findings
5–25	Asymptomatic. Conventional blood studies are normal. Chromosome aberrations detectable.
50–75	Asymptomatic. Minor depressions of white cells and platelets detectable in a few persons, especially if baseline values established.
75–125	Minimal acute doses that produce prodromal symptoms (anorexia, nausea, vomiting, fatigue) in about 10–20% of persons within 2 days. Mild depressions of white cells and platelets in some persons.
125–200	Symptomatic course with transient disability and clear hematological changes in a majority of exposed persons. Lymphocyte depression of about 50% within 48 h.
240–340	Serious, disabling illness in most persons with about 50% mortality if untreated. Lymphocyte depression of about 75+% within 48 h.
500+	Accelerated version of acute radiation syndrome with GI complications within 2 weeks, bleeding, and death in most exposed persons.
5000+	Fulminating course with cardiovascular, GI, and CNS complications resulting in death within 24–72 h.

*Conversion of rad(midline) dose to radiation measurements in R can be made roughly by multiplying rad times 1.5. For example, 200 rad(midline) is equal to about 300 R (200 × 1.5).

Source: Mettler FD: Emergency management of radiation accidents. *JACEP* 7:302–305, 1978. Used by permission.

Treatment

Initial treatment of radiation-exposed patients must always first involve management of life-threatening injuries: airway impairment, bleeding, and circulation. Patients who have been irradiated, i.e., subjected to a high flux of γ rays or x-rays are not, as previously noted, radioactive. As such, no radiation will be detected on such a patient's body or clothes. Any tissue damage occurs instantaneously and will manifest itself in time. An irradiated person may sustain local or total body exposure. Following immediate management of life-threatening injuries, the patient should be checked with a Geiger-Müller counter for surface contamination and a determination made as to whether radioactive material has been ingested or inhaled. The Geiger-Müller counter is very useful for detecting β and γ radiation. If used to detect α radiation it must contain a special window because of the low penetrating power of α particles. The health physicist at the site should be contacted so that data regarding dose, nature of exposure, and duration of exposure can be obtained. A hotline to the regional decontamination area is most helpful for these and similar calls.

Treatment protocol is as follows: Cover open wounds, remove clothing, and deposit contaminated material in closed receptacles. Protect open wounds to avoid contamination while washing or disrobing the patient. Next, wash the patient with soap and water. If the patient is on a drainage table, contaminated water can be collected in containers. If radioactive material in the form of solid particles, liquid, or dust is inhaled or ingested or contaminates an open wound, then *incorporation* has occurred. Since such material will irradiate internal tissues and as such may well cause extensive cellular damage, and since some radioactive elements may become permanently incorporated in the body's molecules, immediate treatment (*decorporation*) is indicated. Radioactive actinide isotopes can be chelated effectively and subsequently excreted by the use of DPTA (diethylenetriaminepentaacetic acid). Such action should be taken within an hour of internal contamination! DTPA may be ordered from the Radiation Emergency Assistance Center/Training Site (REAC/TS) at Oak Ridge, TN. If one anticipates the possible future need for DTPA, then permission for current acquisition of it should be made with REAC/TS.

Potassium iodide will effectively block the uptake of radioactive iodine by the thyroid if it is given within a few hours of exposure. Many metals will be precipitated by antacids in the stomach in the form of insoluble hydroxides, and cathartics can shorten the internal transit time of such material. Aluminum phosphate gel reduces the intestinal absorption of radioactive strontium by 87 percent and barium sulfate will precipitate radium.

A baseline CBC, differential and platelet count should be taken during this initial treatment phase. For patients who have received 200 rem, protective isolation and blood transfusion may be necessary later. Bone marrow depression is usually evident 20 to 30 days after exposure.

Radiation burns are like electrical burns in that physical findings may be minimal initially. For β-particle burns, excision followed by full-thickness grafting may be necessary.

In addition to concern for adverse radiation effects one must also keep in mind the possibility that patients from a radiation accident scene may also have been exposed to chemical hazards. Thus, beryllium, which is present in many nuclear weapons, may be released as fumes and smoke, which in turn may cause respiratory distress, nervousness, and fever. Contamination of open wounds with beryllium results in greatly delayed wound healing. Treatment of the pulmonary problem includes, in addition to oxygen, EDTA, or another effective chelating agent.

Lead, used in nuclear weapon devices for shielding, will on burning release toxic fumes which can cause pneumonitis and dermatitis. Dermatitis and delayed-onset pneumonitis may also occur as a result of the inhalation of fumes secondary to the combustion of plastics, which are used in most nuclear devices.

Finally, one should keep in mind that if a U.S. nuclear weapon were to accidentally detonate, such detonation would in all probability be incomplete. It would, however, be associated with blast effects, fires, and the spread of radioactive material. Unexploded pieces of the explosive might be scattered around an accident site. Such pieces frequently look like natural rock and should not be touched or moved unless absolutely necessary for evacuation of casualties.

DECONTAMINATION IN THE EMERGENCY DEPARTMENT

Advance notice of the arrival of a radiation-injured patient is necessary so that the emergency department can be prepared. Given such notice, emergency department personnel can also advise on prior decontamination in the field.

Every nuclear facility must have identified primary and tertiary referral facilities. It is necessary to develop and maintain open channels of communication between the nuclear facility and the emergency department so that each will be prepared in times of individual injury or major accident. Do not rely on telephone communication being available within the hospital or between the hospital and other facilities in the event of a major nuclear accident or disaster. A predetermined plan involving backup radio communication is strongly advised. Periodic exercises in which the facility is suddenly faced with the hypothetical need to treat a few or hundreds of irradiated and/or radioactive-contaminated patients is the best means to ensure the capability of dealing with such problems.

In the emergency department, a designated area, the Radiation Emergency Area (REA), preferably with a separate entryway, should be available for the management of patients with radiation exposure and associated injuries. Contamination should be prevented by covering the floor with plastic or paper sheets and providing an isolated radiation area. Patients and personnel should be monitored for evidence of contamination. Personnel treating or attending the patient must be gowned and wear caps, masks, foot covers, double gloves, and personnel monitoring devices [i.e., film badge, thermoluminence dosimetry (TLD) badge and/or pocket dosimeters]. It may also be necessary to provide a lead shield to protect personnel. Exposure can also be minimized by decreasing exposure time (several people would share care of patient) and maintaining a distance from the patient whenever possible. Those providing care should not be exposed to more than 5000 mrem except to save a life. Individuals not involved in the treatment should be kept away from the roped-off area. All attendant personnel should be monitored and decontaminated and their garments appropriately disposed of following completion of their involvement in the treatment process. It is important to remember that everyone working in the REA must remain there and that traffic should never move in the reverse direction without first being appropriately monitored. Ambulance personnel and their vehicle(s) should also be checked for the presence of contamination before leaving the facility.

PREHOSPITAL DECONTAMINATION

Linnemann suggests an order of priority for treating a number of individuals involved in radiation accidents:

1. Injured and contaminated patients
2. Those with certain types of internal contamination
3. Patients exposed only to external total body radiation
4. Patients exposed only to external local body radiation

If treatment of great numbers of radiation-exposed and contaminated patients is necessary, different modes of treatment may be indicated. Home treatment with showers and garden hoses should be considered, as should treatment at nearby facilities such as schools. An alternative decontamination facility within the hospital should be such that ready access and shelter available from fallout may be provided for a large number of contaminated patients. Triage should be performed to identify those who may require decontamination. Those found to be contaminated should then pass through a disrobing area and a shower, and ultimately be garbed with hospital gowns and reassessed for residual contamination.

Under these circumstances all available Geiger-Müller counters and dosimeters would be commandeered. Provision should be made for initial and followup treatment of any injuries. One should also consider establishing a large holding area, with subsequent transfer, if necessary, to other institutions where there is no area-wide radiation risk.

HOSPITAL EVACUATION

It is conceivable that internal hospital evacuation may be necessary in the event of radiation threat. Emergency radiation disaster plans should include designation of preselected sites within the hospital which afford the most protection for patients and health care personnel. Such sites will usually be at ground level or below. As much "concrete" as possible should be placed between personnel and the environment. Provision should be made for ensuring appropriate medical equipment, food, medications, and electrical power and heat at the new care site (see Table 54-3). Consideration should be given to shutting off fans and air conditioning during the critical exposure period (plume phase). The duration of such an evacuation would be related to the type of radiation and its half-life, atmospheric conditions, availability of supplies, and the condition of the patients.

External evacuation in the event of a radiation threat can be even more chaotic if not properly planned. One central source must provide for the evacuation needs of the hospitals in the area, and determine the availability of off-site hospitals. Such an external evacuation would entail the need to categorize patients, effect discharge of ambulatory patients if possible, and provide clinical summaries plus radiographs and reports, a listing of medications and treatments needed, and a 24-h supply of food, water, and medications. Categorized patients would be taken to different and appropriate facility staging areas within the facility to await their external evacuation.

CERTAIN ASPECTS OF RADIATION ACCIDENTS AND DISASTERS DESERVE SPECIAL EMPHASIS

In the absence of nuclear war it is unlikely that most hospitals will receive any patients who have been involved in life-threatening radiation accidents. It is more likely that a given hospital's emergency department personnel would be called upon to handle a patient with routine injuries complicated by inadvertent radiation exposure and/or the presence of low-level radioactive contamination. Such a circumstance might result from an accident involving transportation of radioactive materials.

Linnemann reported in 1983 that radiation injuries are an infrequent medical event. Indeed, in the world's literature there are reported 131 accidents involving exposure of 356 people. Fifty-six required hospitalization for serious overexposure. There have been 19 deaths. In the United States we have had approximately 65 accidents resulting in 45 hospitalizations and 8 deaths. Reichter et al. report the majority of industrial radiation accidents involve personnel radiated from high activity sealed sources used in radiography. Nevertheless, as we plan for the more likely minor radiation accident, we must recognize that it is possible our country might sustain a terrorist attack with a nuclear weapon or suffer the accidental discharge and detonation of a nuclear weapon by another nation.

Whatever the basis for a radiation accident or disaster, prior communication, instruction, and staff exercise are the best preparation for any eventuality. And, as a corollary, ongoing communications with staff during an exercise or "real life" accident or disaster is a must. The role of the public relations department should not be forgotten, either. Such personnel are very important, for it is they who, under such circumstances, deal with the media and the public.

You are not alone. In addition to your own staff and others who are experienced and knowledgeable about radiation, there are other individuals and organizations, private, state, and federal, willing and able to promptly respond to your call for aid.

Remember, too, that nuclear facilities do not "blow up" like nuclear bombs. It is physically impossible. Rather, a nuclear plant accident is more apt to be associated with a potentially large number of people being slightly exposed, slightly contaminated, and very anxious.

Table 54-3. Emergency Supplies for Use in Radiation Emergencies

1. Radiation detection instruments including Geiger-Müller counter, spare batteries, film badges, ring badges, self-reading dosimeters
2. Surgical scrub suits
3. Surgical gowns
4. Surgical caps
5. Surgical masks
6. Surgical gloves
7. Plastic shoe covers
8. Adhesive tape
9. Plastic sheets and bags
10. Step-off pads
11. Plastic containers for collection of decontamination fluids
12. Decontamination stretcher
13. Roll of plastic floor covering for use in the hallway
14. Radiation "mark off" rope
15. Radioactive signs and labels
16. Filter paper for smears
17. Clipboard, paper, and pens
18. Assorted containers for sample collection

BIBLIOGRAPHY

Benson JM: Radiation safety. *J Fam Practice* 15:435–439, 1982.
DeMuth WE, Miller KL: A perspective on Three Mile Island. *Continuing Education for the Family Physician.* 17:18–24, 1982.
Jankowski CB: Radiation. *Am J Nurs* 1:90–97, 1982.
Leonard RB, Rucks RC: Emergency department radiation accident protocol. *Ann Emerg Med* 9:462–470, 1980.
Linneman RE: Initial management of radiation injuries. *J Radiation Protection* 5:1–16, 1980.
Linneman RE: Medical and public health consequences of the off-site release of radiation. Presented at the Medical Planning and Protocols for Nuclear Accidents Seminar at Lincolnshire, Ill., Sept. 1983.
Linneman RE: Radiation injuries. Presented at the Medical Planning and Protocols for Nuclear Accidents Seminar, Lincolnshire, Ill., Sept. 1983.
Miller KL, Demuth WE: Handling radiation emergencies. No need for fear. *J Emerg Nurs* 9:141–144, 1983.
Mobley JA: Nuclear accidents. *Am Fam Physician* 25:163–172, 1982.
Richter LL, et al: A systems approach to the management of radiation accidents. *Ann Emerg Med* 9:303–309, 1980.
Weidner WA, et al: The impact of a nuclear crisis on a radiology department. *Radiology* 135:717–723, 1980.

SECTION 6
THE DIGESTIVE SYSTEM

CHAPTER 55
ESOPHAGEAL
EMERGENCIES

James R. Mackenzie

INTRODUCTION

The esophagus is an enigma to most physicians. Benign esophageal disease masquerades as serious cardiac disease, serious cardiac disease masquerades as benign esophageal disease, and the signs and symptoms of serious esophageal disease are often at best occult. However, the emergency physician should realize that in spite of the sophisticated weapons used in our arsenal for the diagnosis of esophageal and cardiac disease, approximately 80 percent of esophageal problems can be diagnosed by history alone. It is the purpose of this chapter to explain the presenting symptoms of esophageal disease in terms of functional anatomy so that the emergency physician can use the symptoms to separate patients with diseases of esophageal origin from patients with diseases of nonesophageal origin. No attempt is made to discuss specific disease entities except as they relate to presenting problems. Resuscitative and diagnostic techniques are only discussed if they are specific to the emergency department management of esophageal problems.

GROSS AND FUNCTIONAL ANATOMY

Anatomical Relationships

The esophagus is defined by Jones and Shepard as "the portion of the digestive canal between the pharynx and the stomach." The esophagus begins at the hypopharynx opposite the sixth cervical vertebra and the lower border of the cricoid cartilage and ends at the cardia of the stomach opposite the body of the eleventh thoracic vertebra. It passes through three visceral compartments, the lower part of the neck (cervical portion), the superior and posterior mediastinum (the mediastinal portion), and the posterior epigastrium (the abdominal portion). The distance between the incisor teeth and the lower end of the esophagus is 40 cm ± 4 cm. The distance from the teeth to the esophagus is 12 to 15 cm, the cervical esophagus is 4 to 5 cm long, the mediastinal portion 15 to 20 cm, and the abdominal portion 2 to 3 cm (Fig. 55-1).

The esophagus is contiguous to numerous structures along its course, and pathology in any one of these structures may affect its function, usually by causing dysphagia or pain (Fig. 55-1). Diseased contiguous structures that may affect esophageal function include the spinal column (usually due to osteophytes) and descending aorta posteriorly; the larynx, trachea, and left main stem bronchus; the thyroid, carotid, and subclavian arteries; arch of the aorta, and the left atrium anteriorly; the lobes of the thyroid laterally (Fig. 55-2); and the stomach, diaphragm, and left lobe of the liver inferiorly. A detailed discussion of the anatomical relationship of the cervical, mediastinal, and abdominal esophagus can be found in several standard texts (e.g., Pope).

Conversely, esophageal pathology may cause symptoms to develop in contiguous structures, principally by invasion of esophageal cancer or liquid caustics into any of the above structures, which causes aspiration, coughing, or pneumonia; and the regurgitation of blood if vascular structures are invaded. Cancer of the esophagus is also a cause of hoarseness due to invasion of the recurrent laryngeal nerves, and chylothorax due to invasion of the thoracic duct which lies along the left border (Figs. 55-3 through 55-5). Benign or malignant perforation of the esophagus causes mediastinal emphysema and/or pyothorax (Fig. 55-5).

Functional Description of the Tube

The musculature of the pharynx forms a funnel of overlapping, flat, striated constrictor muscles which insert in front of the vertebrae at the median raphe posteriorly and sweep around to attach anteriorly. The superior constrictor arises from the pterygoid plate; the middle constrictor overlaps the superior constrictor and arises from the hyoid bone, and the inferior constrictor overlaps the middle constrictor and attaches to the thyroid and cricoid cartilages. The fibers of these muscles sweep downward and laterally as they approach their insertion. The uppermost striated muscle fibers of the esophagus sweep upward and laterally to insert into the cricoid cartilage.

The diamond-shaped defect between the downward lateral sweep of the inferior constrictor and the upward lateral sweep of the esophageal muscle is transversed by the fibers of the cricopharyngeal muscle (Fig. 55-6), dividing it into two triangles, the upper

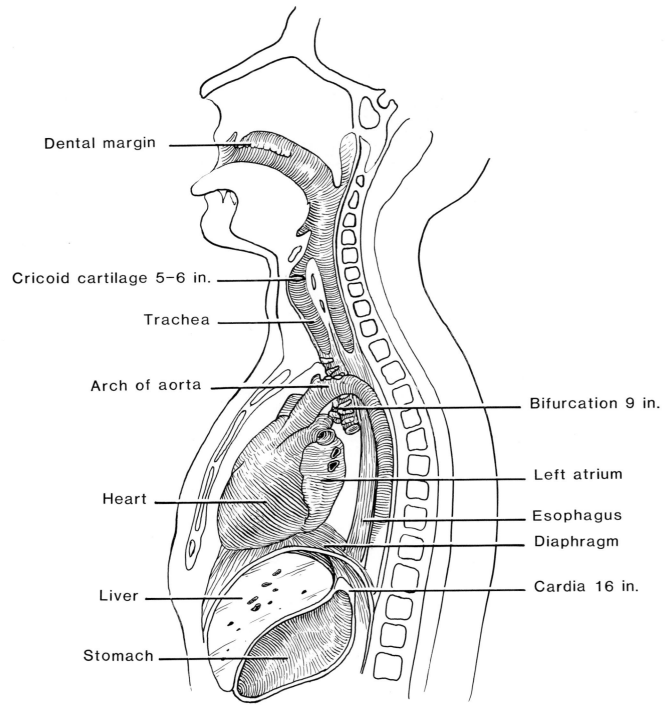

Figure 55-1. Anatomical relationships of the esophagus (seen from the left side). The esophagus is about 25 cm (10 in) long. The distance from the upper incisor teeth to the beginning of the esophagus (cricoid cartilage) is about 15 cm (6 in); from the upper incisors to the level of the bronchi, 22 to 23 cm (9 in); to the cardia, 40 cm (16 in). Structures contiguous to the esophagus that affect esophageal function are demonstrated (see text).

weak point and the lower weak point. Zenker's diverticula form at the upper weak point, presumably due to an incoordination of the contraction of the constrictor muscles and the relaxation of the cricopharyngeus during swallowing (Shackleford), but the pathogenesis is disputed.

The pharynx and esophagus lie immediately in front of the

prevertebral fascia and are surrounded by a layer of fascia which fuses with cellular tissue of the superior mediastinum. A layer of this tissue separates laterally in the neck to unite with the prevertebral fascia, forming the retropharyngeal space of Henke. The retropharyngeal and retroesophageal space are in direct communication with the superior mediastinum, and bleeding, perfora-

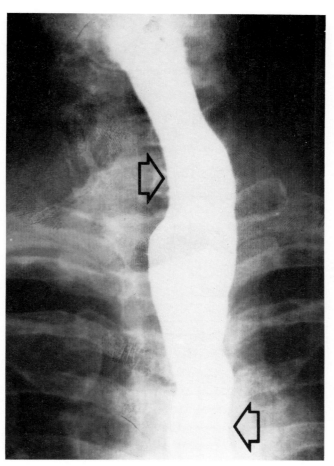

Figure 55-2. Anatomy—the relationship of the thyroid and aortic arch to the esophagus. Contiguous structures can cause esophageal dysphagia. An enlarged thyroid lobe (upper arrow) or an aneurysm of the aortic arch (lower arrow) are two of these causes.

tions, or abscesses in this space have a direct conduit to the superior mediastinum.

The esophagus is composed of an inner mucosal layer which covers a tough, fibrous submucosal layer. There are two muscle layers surrounding the mucosal and submucosal layers. The innermost is spiral to circular while the outer layer is longitudinal. There is no serosa and as a result, once the submucosa is perforated or destroyed the perforation tends to extend into the surrounding mediastinal structures, leading to a diffuse, malignant, and often rapidly progressive and fatal mediastinitis (Fig. 55-5) (Besson). The striated muscle of the upper esophagus gradually gives way to the smooth muscle which forms the rest of the esophagus and the gastrointestinal tract.

The mucosa and submucosa are the layers usually involved in peptic esophagitis, which in its extreme form results in scarring and stricture formation. However, it is only when the esophageal muscle layer is split beyond the submucosal scar in bougienage or by repeated dilatations that the muscle layer becomes involved in the scarring process. When the muscle becomes scarred, stricture formation continuously recurs after instrumentation. Elimination of the cause for esophagitis and one or two dilatations, on the other hand, eliminate the stricture (Maclean). Unfortunately,

ingestion of lye and some other corrosives involves and destroys the muscular layer to a greater or lesser degree, and dilatation of the scar formation in this layer tends to cause tearing and further scarring and stricture.

The Vessels

The Lymphatic System

Lymphatic supply of the esophagus is of principal interest to the surgeon, radiologist, and chemotherapist. However, cancer of the esophagus may cause cervical and paratracheal lymph node enlargement and pneumonitis on chest x-ray (Fig. 55-4), and scalene node enlargement on the physical examination. Invasion of the thoracic duct (usually by cancer) is a cause of pleural effusions seen on chest x-ray (Fig. 55-5). The chylothorax, which is the cause of the effusion, may be confirmed by thoracentesis.

The Venous System

The submucosal plexus of veins drains to an intercommunicating plexus which surrounds the esophagus. This network in turn anastomoses with the inferior thyroid vein in the neck, the azygous system in the thorax, and the coronary and short gastric veins (part of the portal system) in the abdomen. Obstruction of the portal system from such diseases as cirrhosis of the liver causes submucosal esophageal varices (Fig. 55-7).

The Arterial System

The anatomy of the arterial system is of principle interest to the surgeon. The arterial supply is segmental, gaining branches from the inferior thyroid artery in the neck, the aorta in the thorax, and the celiac plexus in the abdomen.

The Bleeding Esophagus

Bleeding from the esophagus, like bleeding from other parts of the gastrointestinal tract, may be classified according to the amount, severity (amount vs. time), source, periodicity of bleeding, and to symptoms produced by the bleeding at the time of presentation to the emergency department.

Amount

Bleeding from the esophagus can be classified according to the amount of blood replacement needed to restore blood volume while the patient is in the emergency department. There are four degrees of bleeding:

Mild Blood Loss

Mild blood loss (less than 10 percent loss of blood volume) is due to capillary bleeding or to sudden, nonrecurring arterial bleeding. Volume replacement for blood loss is unnecessary.

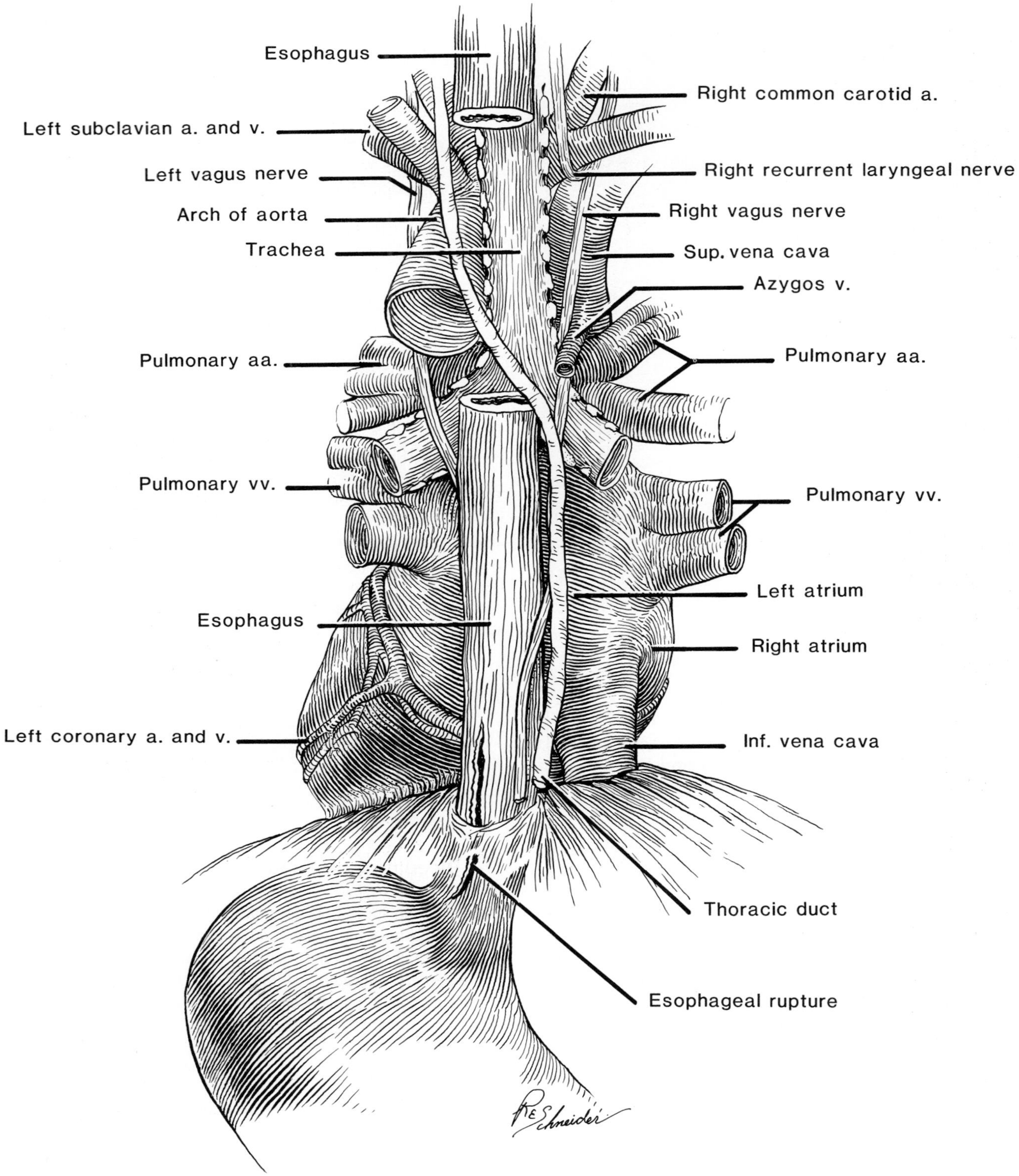

Esophagus

Right common carotid a.

Left subclavian a. and v.

Right recurrent laryngeal nerve

Left vagus nerve

Right vagus nerve

Arch of aorta

Sup. vena cava

Trachea

Azygos v.

Pulmonary aa.

Pulmonary aa.

Pulmonary vv.

Pulmonary vv.

Left atrium

Esophagus

Right atrium

Left coronary a. and v.

Inf. vena cava

Thoracic duct

Esophageal rupture

Figure 55-3. Anatomical relationships of the esophagus (as seen from behind). Structures contiguous to the esophagus that affect its function.

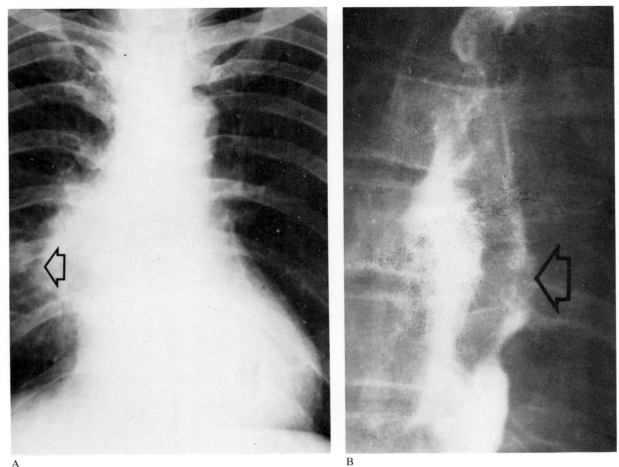

A   B

Figure 55-4. Anatomy of the structures contiguous to the esophagus. (A) This chest x-ray demonstrates how esophageal disease can masquerade as nonesophageal disease. A 56-year-old male with a 15-month history of dysphagia, recurrent pneumonia, chest and back pain, 20-lb weight loss, and anemia. Esophagoscopy and biopsy showed a poorly differentiated cancer of the esophagus. Chest x-ray shows infiltration of the cancer into the hilar lymph nodes (arrow). (B) The esophogram shows the cancer in the middle third of the esophagus.

Moderate Blood Loss

Moderate blood loss (10 to 20 percent loss of blood volume) is due to laceration of an artery or nondistended vein. Bleeding may or may not stop during treatment in the emergency department. Infusion of 1 L of crystalloid, and possibly 1 to 2 units of blood is needed to restore blood volume. The patient may be sent to a routine hospital bed if there is no need to continue intravenous replacement (signifying the bleeding source has stopped); or to a critical care unit if continued volume replacement in the emergency department indicates continued bleeding.

Major Blood Loss

Major blood loss (20 to 40 percent loss of blood volume) is due to a lacerated varix or an artery that has been eroded by a peptic ulcer but which cannot retract because it is bound down by scar tissue. The measure of major bleeding in the emergency department is that the patient needs at least 1 L of saline and 2 to 4 units of blood to restore blood volume. These patients must be sent to a critical care unit.

Life-Threatening or Massive Blood Loss

Massive blood loss (more than 40 percent loss of blood volume) can be due to a perforated artery at the base of a peptic ulcer, but is more likely due to a ruptured varix. The patient needs more than 4 units of blood in addition to the initial crystalloid replacement, and the source tends to continue bleeding. The source of gastrointestinal bleeding should be confirmed by endoscopy in the emergency department. If the esophageal varices are the cause of bleeding, then a Pitressin drip using 20 units in 200 mL of saline at 0.25 to 0.5 units per minute is given. If bleeding continues, sclerotherapy or Gelfoam embolization of the left gastric vein should be considered before use of a Blakemore or similar type tube. Other methods to control esophageal bleeding are inpatient unit decisions (Fiddian-Green; Dworken).

Comments

Classifying esophageal bleeding by the amount needed to restore blood volume in the emergency department is useful to the emergency physician for two reasons: First, the amount of blood

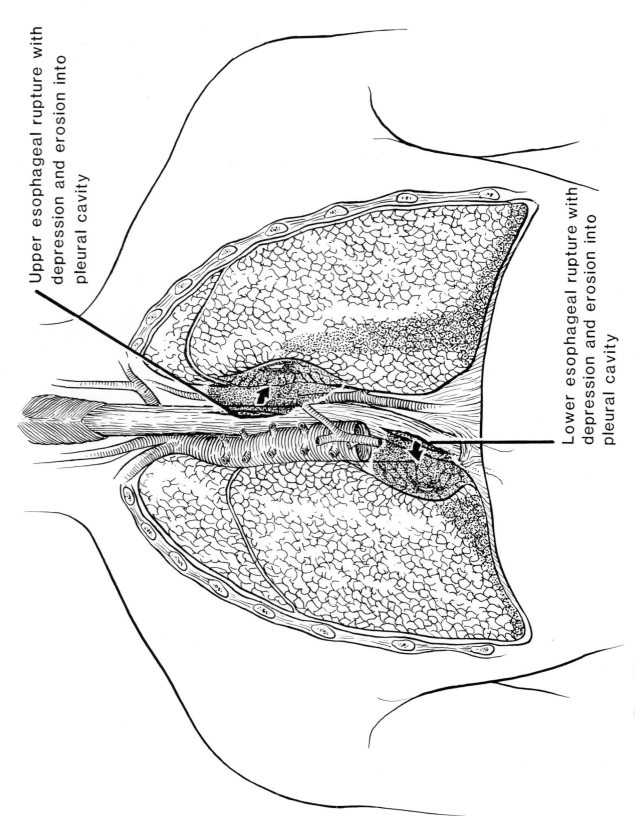

Upper esophageal rupture with depression and erosion into pleural cavity

Lower esophageal rupture with depression and erosion into pleural cavity

Figure 55-5. Anatomy—the relationship of the esophagus to the mediastinum and pleural cavities of the esophagus, seen from behind. It is clear that rupture of the lower esophagus is likely to extend to one of the pleural cavities (usually the left).

Unlike massive bleeding from other sites in the gastrointestinal tract, most esophageal bleeding, even when life-threatening, is treated nonoperatively (unless it is misdiagnosed as bleeding from a gastroduodenal site). It is, therefore, imperative for the emergency physician to establish the possible existence of a historical cause of bleeding—e.g., cirrhosis, heavy drinking—while the patient is able to give the history, or from friends and relatives while they are still in the emergency department, to avoid a misdiagnosis and a useless and possibly dangerous operation.

Severity

Severity of bleeding is a product of the amount vs. time. In the acute phase, massive bleeding within 10 to 30 min will kill the patient and is usually due to ruptured esophageal varices in a patient with portal hypertension (300 to 400 cmH$_2$O) (Fig. 55-7). Patients seldom bleed from their varices if the portal pressure is less than 180 cmH$_2$O. At the other end of the scale is the patient with very slow bleeding from peptic esophagitis, or who has intermittent arterial bleeding from an esophageal peptic ulcer, or an

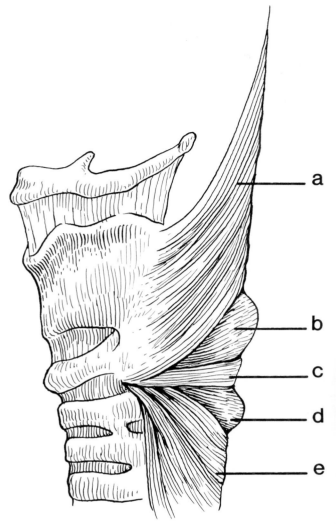

Figure 55-6. Anatomy of the esophagus. Diagram showing the weak points of the pharyngoesophageal segment: (a) oblique fibers of the inferior constrictor, (b) upper weak point, (c) cricopharyngeus muscle, (d) lower weak point (left lateral view), (e) muscular coat of the esophagus. (After a diagram by Terracol J, and Sweet RH: *Diseases of the Esophagus,* Philadelphia, W. B. Saunders, 1958, p 8, by permission.)

necessary to restore cardiovascular stability in the emergency department indicates the severity of bleeding and the urgency with which the patient must be brought to the unit providing definitive care. Second, once blood volume has been rapidly restored, continued drifting of the blood pressure and pulse, delay of capillary refill, or loss of urinary output indicates continued bleeding. Obviously, continued bleeding in the emergency department will shift the initial presenting bleeding classification to the next level of severity.

It must be emphasized that this classification can only be useful for emergency treatment of the patient if the emergency physician rapidly restores the blood volume so that observation of a subsequent drift of blood pressure and pulse will indicate continued bleeding. The infusion rate usually must be faster than 100 mL/min to accomplish this restoration in major or massive bleeding.

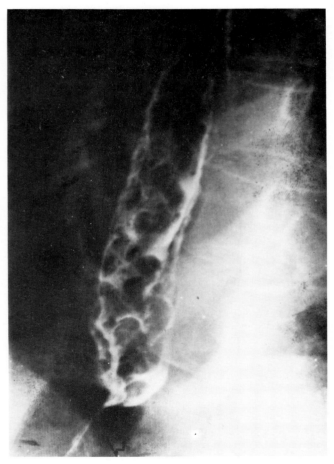

Figure 55-7. Esophageal varices. A 50-year-old male with cirrhosis and massive upper gastrointestinal bleeding which stopped with a Pitressin drip 24 h later shows esophageal varices reaching to the midesophagus. This patient would probably now have a Pitressin drip followed by esophagoscopy and an attempt at sclerotherapy to stop the bleeding.

ooze from an esophageal cancer (Fig. 55-4) who may appear with profound anemia, shortness of breath, or high-output heart failure.

Source

There are three sources of gastrointestinal bleeding:

Capillary bleeding is usually due to esophagitis. Capillary bleeding produces mild bleeding (from the emergency department definition) but it also tends to cause anemia, which may be profound because of its chronic and undetected nature. If bleeding from esophagitis produces emesis, it is a coffee-ground color rather than bright red because the blood drips into the stomach and is changed before regurgitation. Melena or vomiting of red blood in patients with capillary bleeding is rare because of the slowness of bleeding.

Arterial bleeding is usually due to an artery which has been perforated by a penetrating peptic esophageal ulcer or to a laceration of the esophagus due to instrumentation, foreign-body ingestion or to violent vomiting (Mallory-Weiss tear).

Arterial bleeding is usually mild or moderate, and presents with vomiting of bright red blood and/or melena. The bleeding is episodic and the bleeding episode has usually stopped by the time the patient reaches the emergency department, although he or she may be in hypovolemic shock from the event.

Venous bleeding from lacerations of the submucosal plexus of veins in a patient without portal hypertension may produce mild to moderate bleeding and is associated with arterial bleeding. However, the most common form of venous bleeding is from varices. It is usually massive and life-threatening, associated with portal pressure in excess of 180 cmH$_2$O, and usually with a liver-derived coagulopathy.

Periodicity

Esophageal lesions can produce a single bleeding episode, several episodes (episodic), or recurring episodes over a long time (chronic). Obviously, when patients arrive with a first bleeding episode they must be judged on criteria other than periodicity. However, if patients arrive with a history of episodic bleeding, it probably means that they have a lesion which will ultimately need operative correction. Finally, recurring and chronic bleeding lesions present with symptoms that are a consequence of their bleeding (see following discussion). These patients almost always need elective repair of their esophageal lesion.

Symptomatology

Patients with bleeding from the esophagus in addition to hypovolemia may present in one of three ways to the emergency department: (1) with anemia, which in its most severe, chronic form may be associated with a hemoglobin of 4 gms, shortness of breath, and high outpatient cardiac failure in the older patient; (2) with vomiting of blood or coffee-ground material (see above); or (3) with melena—the stool may be only guaiac-positive in slow bleeding, black in moderate bleeding, and wine-colored or even unchanged in massive bleeding from esophageal varices.

Neuromuscular Anatomy (Shackleford; Pope)

The esophagus is supplied by both an extrinsic and intrinsic nerve supply. The intrinsic nervous system includes Auerbach's and Meissner's plexuses. They are responsible for the contraction of both the longitudinal and circular muscles, and the coordination of deglutition, including relaxation of the upper esophageal sphincter (UES), the peristaltic wave, and relaxation of the lower esophageal sphincter (LES).

The intrinsic system is altered in motor disorders such as achalasia and diffuse spasm. It is also destroyed by ingestions of corrosives and by systemic diseases, principally the collagen vascular disorders such as scleroderma and others which are usually associated with Raynaud's syndrome.

The extrinsic nervous system can be divided into the parasympathetic and sympathetic system. The musculature of the upper esophagus is controlled by the spinal accessory nucleus, and the rest of the esophagus is under the control of the dorsal motor nucleus. The parasympathetic system consists of the vagus nerve which, in the neck, branches directly to the constrictors of the pharynx (superior laryngeal nerve) or to the pharyngeal esophagus by way of the recurrent laryngeal nerve, and to the thoracic esophagus by way of the vagal plexus surrounding it. The esophageal and bronchial plexuses of the vagus also supply the heart (Fig. 55-8). Presumably, reflex stimulation of the sensory ending in the esophagus by way of the dorsal motor nucleus and the vagus is the cause of bradycardia in esophageal intubation and endoscopy.

The sympathetic nerves arise from the cervical and thoracic ganglia and the superior and middle splanchnic nerves from both sides of the spinal cord. The branches from both sides mix together and supply sensation to the same area. Therefore, esophageal sensations such as dysphagia or pain are referred somatically to the midline. The segmental nature of esophageal innervation is evident at fluoroscopy. A patient with dysphagia can usually trace the passage of a barium-coated bolus of food down the esophagus with his or her finger while the progress of the bolus is observed by fluoroscopy (Pope). This would suggest that each level of the esophagus is segmentally represented by the afferent nerves in the cord instead of several segments being grouped together before innervation of the esophagus. In the abdomen, however, nerves from several segments are grouped together at the celiac ganglion before distribution to the foregut by way of branches of the left gastric and inferior phrenic arteries. As a result, abdominal esophageal pain cannot be differentiated from epigastric pain produced by the rest of the foregut (Fig. 55-8).

Nerves from the cervical and thoracic ganglia also supply the heart and other mediastinal structures (Figs. 55-1 and 55-8). For this reason pain or other sensations arising from the esophagus will be sensed by the patient in the same place as pain arising from these mediastinal structures (Fig. 55-8).

Deglutition and Propulsion of the Food Bolus: Physiology

Deglutition is initiated with the mouth opening to receive food and then closing, pursing of the lips to create an airtight seal, and mastication and mixing of the food with saliva so that it will slip easily down the pharynx and into the esophagus. The bolus is passed from the anterior part of the tongue backwards by a se-

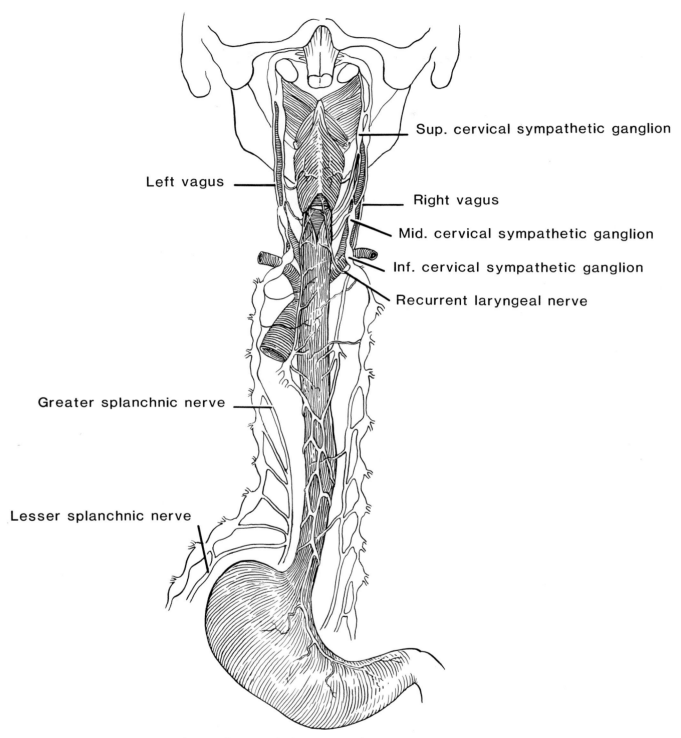

Figure 55-8. Anatomy of the esophagus—the sympathetic nervous system.

quential contraction of the tongue upward against the roof of the mouth backward against the hard and soft palate and posterior pharyngeal wall. At the same time there is a sequential contraction of the constrictor muscles from above downward. The pressure of the tongue and the contraction of the muscles of the soft palate and the superior constrictor cause an airtight closure of the nasal

pharynx to the food bolus. The resulting high-pressure wave which is created by the sequential contraction of the aforementioned muscles propels the food toward the esophagus. Any involvement of the muscles of the face, tongue, or pharynx, or their motor or sensory nerve supply may cause part of the bolus to drip out of the mouth, or to be propelled into the nose. This involvement may also weaken the propelling force, and the bolus may not be able to overcome the high-pressure area at the upper esophageal sphincter.

The laryngeal muscles contract involuntarily as the bolus is passed from the front of the tongue to the middle pharynx, causing the larynx to rise and be sealed from the pharynx by the epiglottis. The cricopharyngeal muscle forms the upper esophageal sphincter (UES) and is in tonic contraction at all times, except when it relaxes as the food bolus approaches. Dysfunction of laryngeal sensation or neuromuscular motor function, or failure of the UES to relax may cause the bolus to be aspirated, or impede its transfer to the upper esophagus.

The inability of the food bolus to be propelled directly into the esophagus from the mouth is called "transfer dysphagia." The causes are legion but essentially it results from interference in central nervous system coordination, and is seen in such diseases as stroke and multiple sclerosis, muscular disorders, or peripheral nerve destruction (e.g., as a complication of head and neck surgery). Incoordination of the forward propulsion of the bolus with the relaxation of the UES is thought to be the cause of a Zenker's propulsion diverticulum through the upper weak point (Fig. 55-6).

The bolus is then propelled caudad by a peristaltic wave which starts at the UES, and is controlled by the reflex arcs of Meissner and Auerbach's plexuses located between the inner and outer muscle layers. When the bolus reaches the distal 1 to 2 cm of the esophagus it meets another high-pressure area called the lower esophageal sphincter (LES), which relaxes to allow food to enter the stomach. A secondary peristaltic contraction wave will start at the level of the aortic arch, which is another area of raised pressure, and propel any leftover liquid caudad. Finally, a tertiary contraction wave may be initiated at the level of the lower one-third of the esophagus, usually by reflux of gastric contents. This may be an important mechanism for keeping the lower esophageal mucosa clear of gastric contents.

The LES appears to be under both intrinsic nervous and hormonal control. The practical use of these observations in treating reflux is yet to be discovered. Failure of the sphincter to relax causes achalasia of the more proximal esophagus, and is a cause of the motor disorders discussed later in the chapter.

PRESENTING SYMPTOMS

Patients present to the emergency department with clinical manifestation of their diseases (symptoms), not with esophageal dis-

ease. It is the job of the emergency physician to use these presenting complaints to separate those with life-threatening disease who need resuscitation from those with less urgent problems who need relief of their symptoms before being sent to the proper specialist for precise diagnosis and treatment. It is also the job of the emergency physician to separate those people with esophageal disease from those who may have similar symptoms arising from other diseased mediastinal structures, principally from the heart and tracheobronchial tree. The following discussions of these symptoms are designed to precisely define their meaning, to classify the more important causes of the symptom, and to discuss their importance to the emergency physician as a diagnostic tool.

Dysphagia (Pope)

Definition

Dysphagia is an awareness of something wrong with the smooth pattern of swallowing, i.e., the patient mentions that food sticks, hesitates, or pauses, or that it just won't go down right. The presence of dysphagia almost always signifies esophageal pathology. It is different from "globus hystericus"—the sensation of "something always stuck in the throat"—but is akin to transfer dysphagia, which is the inability to initiate the act of swallowing and is usually due to pharyngeal muscular weakness or central nervous system disease.

Cause

There are two basic causes for dysphagia, either mechanical narrowing of the lumen, or motor disorders (Table 55-1). Mechanical problems stem from pathology in the lumen (e.g., foreign body), in the wall (peptic stricture of the submucosa or esophageal cancer), or extrinsic to the esophagus from encroachment by surrounding structures (goiter, enlarged subcarinal lymph nodes). Motor disorders include those due to intrinsic muscular or nervous disorders of the esophagus or pharynx, and those due to central nervous lesions.

Characteristics (Table 55-2)

Dysphagia can be characterized by (1) the onset—the caliber, character, and temperature of food causing it; (2) the location of

Table 55-1. Causes of Dysphagia

Congenital	Obstructive	Neuromuscular
	Vascular abnormalities (dysphagia lusoria), webs	
Accquired inflammatory infections		Poliomyelitis, diphtheria, botulism, rabies, tetanus, chorea, herpes
Immunologic		Dermatomyositis, polymyosytis, myasthenia gravis, scleroderma, multiple sclerosis
Physical and chemical	Cervical spurs, Schatzki's ring, stricture, esophagitis (caustic, reflux)	
Traumatic	Foreign bodies, food, pills	
Vascular and heart	Aortic aneurysm, left atrial enlargement	CVA, Parkinson's, pseudobulbar palsy
Metabolic	Goiter	Lead, magnesium deficiency, thyrotoxic
Tumors	Benign and malignant tumors of esophagus, thyroid, larynx, tracheobronchial tree, lungs, pericardium, and esophagus	Brain tumors
Others	Achalasia, Zenker's diverticulum	Achalasia

Table 55-2. Characteristics of Dysphagia (Pope)

	Mechanical Narrowing (Tumors, Strictures)	Motor Disorder (Achalasia, Scleroderma)
Onset	Gradual or sudden	Usually gradual
Progression	Often	Usually not
Type of bolus	Solids (unless high-grade obstruction)	Solids and/or liquids
Temperature-dependent	No	Worse with cold liquids; may improve with warm liquids
Response to bolus impaction	Often must be regurgitated	Can usually be passed by repeated swallowing or by washing it down with fluids

the dysphagia, and (3) how it is relieved. Indeed, a correct diagnosis of the cause of dysphagia was made by the correct answers to 39 questions with a diagnostic accuracy of 80 percent (243 of 304 patients) (Edwards).

Mechanical problems cause solid foods to stick in the esophagus. The caliber of spongy-type foods which can be swallowed decreases relentlessly over a short period of time if dysphagia is due to esophageal cancer, and more slowly if it is due to benign stricture. Fluids can usually be swallowed until the stricture is far advanced, or the narrowing is suddenly blocked by a solid bolus of food or another foreign body (e.g., enteric coated pills). Peptic stricture can produce the same symptoms but usually the dysphagia is mild, and heartburn due to the esophagitis usually accompanies the dysphagia. Difficulty in swallowing liquids, especially if they are cold, is a symptom of a motor disorder.

The method of relief from dysphagia often helps in the diagnosis. Regurgitation of a bolus by self-induced vomiting suggests mechanical narrowing. In motor disorders the bolus usually passes after repeated swallowing, drinking water, or by throwing back the shoulders and performing a Valsalva maneuver.

Odynophagia (Pope; Wolff)

Definition

Odynophagia is defined as pain upon swallowing. It can be associated with bolus arrest (dysphagia) but may be experienced without arrest of the bolus. Odynophagia along with dysphagia are cardinal symptoms of esophageal disease.

Cause

Pain is associated with the lowering of the pain threshold of the esophageal nerve endings due to the mucosal surface being inflamed or congested. It is therefore seen most commonly in such conditions as reflux, radiation, or viral esophagitis.

Characteristics

Odynophagia appears at the time of bolus transmission and disappears when the material has left the esophagus. Therefore, unlike pain of cardiac origin, it comes with swallowing and disap-

pears within 10 s. It may be mild or so intense that the patient refuses to swallow solids, liquids, or saliva.

Esophageal Colic (Ach; Pope; Leriche)

Definition

Esophageal colic is an acute, agonizing, spasmodic, or crescendo-like pain.

Causes

Like all colic, it is due to an acute stretching or distension of a hollow muscular tube when the forward propulsion of the contents is blocked; or it is due to the acute vigorous contraction or spasm of the esophageal musculature secondary to stimulation. The spasm may be a direct consequence of odynophagia or heartburn but is not relieved by antacids. Colic is therefore found both in conditions that cause mechanical narrowing of the lumen with distension of the esophagus above the obstruction, and in motor disorders that cause esophageal spasm. Both distension and spasm may of course be caused by the same disease. The most common cause for colic is esophagitis.

Characteristics

The acute and crescendo-like pain is experienced substernally and radiates directly through to the back into the interscapular area. It may also radiate into the neck, jaw, or arms. It lasts from 5 to 10 s to hours and usually is indistinguishable from angina pectoris in terms of intensity, radiation, and relationship to exercise or relief with nitroglycerin, except that it usually takes 7 to 10 min for relief instead of 2 to 3 min. It is often an associated symptom in patients with dysphagia.

Heartburn (Pyrosis)

Definition

Heartburn is the most common symptom of esophageal disease. Unlike the first three symptoms, it is not associated with the swallowing of solids or fluids but rather with reflux of acid or alkali into the esophagus from the stomach.

Cause

Heartburn is due to acid or alkali refluxing onto a changed or inflamed esophageal mucosa. The inflammatory response depends upon the amount of acid or alkali refluxed and the rate at which it is cleared from the mucosal surface. Biopsy changes show thickening of the basal layer of the esophageal mucosa with extension of the dermal pegs to the free surface in the mildest cases of reflux esophagitis. In more severe cases the epithelial layer is obviously inflamed at esophagoscopy and microscopically the mucosa is covered with microulcers and the lamina propria has the classical pathological signs of inflammation.

In one-third of cases of heartburn the esophageal mucosa may look normal to the naked eye. In about one-third of patients with reflux but without heartburn, the mucosa will show inflammatory or wear-and-tear changes.

Characteristics

Heartburn is perceived as a burning felt over most of the substernal area. It appears after meals, especially large ones containing fat, is worse in recumbency or with lifting, and is relieved by antacids, if only temporarily. Symptoms are associated with a change in the pH of the lower esophagus and disappear when the pH returns to normal.

Regurgitation

Definition

Regurgitation is the retrograde propulsion of fluid into the mouth. It is different from rumination in which recently eaten food is propelled back into the mouth by a strong contraction of the abdominal wall musculature.

Cause

Regurgitation is usually due to the stomach or duodenal contents leaking through an incompetent lower esophageal sphincter (LES). It is, therefore, associated with reflux esophagitis and heartburn. It can also be associated with the emptying of a diverticulum or with regurgitation of the retained portion of fluid in achalasia.

Characteristics

Regurgitation is due to a weak LES, causes a bitter or acid taste in the mouth, and is associated with bending over, lying down, or lifting heavy objects.

Regurgitation of diverticular contents or from achalasia, on the other hand, usually produces undigested, foul-tasting food, with an odor from the mouth due to the presence of putrid food. Both types of regurgitation may produce aspiration, recurrent pneumonia, and failure to thrive (Wesley).

Water Brash

Water brash is the sudden appearance of a salty fluid in the mouth. It is probably due to the sudden outpouring of saliva and should not be confused with regurgitation.

Hematemesis and Melena (Dworken)

See discussion on the bleeding esophagus.

Definition

Hematemesis is the vomiting of blood, whether fresh and red or digested and black. ''Melena'' means black, and usually describes the passage of coal-black stools which have the clotted, gummy appearance of tar. However, melena is used in a wider clinical sense, although wrongly, to describe blood in the stool. In general, rapid bleeding from the esophagus tends to cause hematemesis and wine-colored stools, and slower bleeding coffee-ground emesis and melena, or even occult blood in the stool.

EXTRAESOPHAGEAL MANIFESTATION (EEM) OF ESOPHAGEAL DISEASE

It is important for the emergency physician to realize that many patients with esophageal disease will present to the emergency department with symptoms that do not directly relate to the esophagus but which are complications of their esophageal disease. These symptoms are referred to in this chapter as extraesophageal manifestations (EEM) of esophageal disease.

The common EEM of esophageal diseases in the adult include: pulmonary symptoms, weight loss due to starvation, and iron deficiency anemia. The EEM in infants and retarded children include pulmonary symptoms, failure to thrive, and hyperextension posturing (Wesley).

Pulmonary Manifestations

Material regurgitated or refluxed into the larynx and the tracheobronchial tree causes asthmatic-like symptoms in adults without a family history of asthma or a history of industrial exposure, nocturnal or early morning cough, nocturnal wheezing, hoarseness especially on arising, the need to repeatedly clear the throat, and a feeling of constant pressure deep in the neck. Patients may have recurrent bouts of pneumonia with radiographic changes in the right middle lobe and superior segments of both lower lobes. Infants, retarded children and adults, and debilitated people who have suffered strokes are especially prone to aspiration pneumonia.

Aspiration may be caused by transfer dysphagia while awake, reflux from an incompetent LES, or from retained food in achalasia or diverticula while asleep.

Starvation and Failure to Thrive (Wesley)

Starvation and failure to thrive is seen in infants, children, and adults. In adults it is seen with increasing obstruction of the esophagus due to stricture, achalasia, or cancer; or with reflux esophagitis, especially if esophageal colic is present or the patient is mentally retarded or debilitated by a stroke. It is important to recognize the cause of the starvation because many times the debilitation and/or mental retardation seen in these patients is due to caloric and essential vitamin and mineral deprivation in addition to the primary disease or to pulmonary complications.

Failure to thrive in retarded children can be partially reversed with correction of the reflux symptoms and the associated pulmonary complications. These patients will often show an improvement in the retarded state with better nutrition. A similar improvement is found in stroke victims whose caloric intake is improved. Totally dependent patients often return to self-feeding regimens with correction of pulmonary conditions caused by reflux, and with correction of starvation.

The diagnosis of reflux esophagitis as a cause of malnutrition in the child or the adult is complicated and necessitates hospitalization. It includes a barium swallow and the observation of radio-active nuclear materials in the lung after instillation of it into the stomach.

Hyperextension Posturing

Hyperextension posturing seen in some retarded children often improves with correction of reflux with aspiration and appears to be a complication of this symptom (Wesley).

Anemia

See discussion on the bleeding esophagus.

MANUAL SKILLS

Nasogastric Intubation (Fig. 55-9)

Indications

A nasogastric tube should be passed in all cases of gastrointestinal bleeding for diagnostic purposes, most cases of potential esophageal injuries due to ingestion, and intestinal obstruction. Exceptions include actual or suspected laceration or perforation of the esophagus (usual sites are at the upper weak point between the inferior constrictor and the crycothyroid muscle or at the level of LES), near-complete obstruction of the esophagus due to benign or malignant stricture, and in the presence of an esophageal foreign body. The nasogastric tube must be placed orally in patients with rhinorrhea associated with head trauma.

A relative contraindication for placement of a nasogastric tube is a lacerated posterior larynx from whatever cause. In this case the tube should be placed under the direct visualization of a laryngoscope (after the larynx has been anesthetized with a suitable local anesthesia).

Anatomical Considerations (Figs. 55-6, 55-9) (Hollingshead; Collins)

The following points should be recognized when passing a nasogastric tube:

1. Blocked nares: Use the other nares or the mouth.
2. The tip of the nose should be directed cephalad while the tip of the nasogastric tube is directed toward the floor of the posterior nares (rather than toward the roof of the anterior nares). This is the commonest cause for damage to the nasopharynx (Fig. 55-9).
3. The obstruction caused by the spasmodic closure of the soft palate pressing against the superior constrictor can be overcome by having the patient swallow. The conscious spasm will abate immediately after the swallow.
4. The next obstruction is at the level of the inferior constrictor approximately 15 to 20 cm from the ala of the nares. The tip of the nasogastric tube will catch, either on the lip formed by the cephalad surface of the cricothyroid muscle posteriorly, the pyriform fossa on either side of the larynx, or the vallecula anterior to the vocal cords or Killian's mouth (Fig. 55-9). These recesses disappear with a conscious swallow with or

without the use of water. However, the tube may continuously be directed into a Zenker's diverticulum if it is present (Fig. 55-6). In this situation, the tube may be guided past the opening of the Zenker's diverticulum by a Magill forceps under visualization of direct laryngoscopy.

The tip may be directed anteriorly by spasm of the constrictors through the vocal cords into the trachea. This problem can be alleviated by two maneuvers: first by advancing the tube past this area only during the swallowing motion when the larynx rises to and is covered by the epiglottis, thus making the curve from the posterior tongue continuous with the epiglottis and the anterior lip of the esophagus (Figs. 55-6, 55-9); and second by flexing the neck so that the chin is on the chest, thus directing the tip of the nasogastric tube posteriorly. Oral intubation with the patient sucking on the tube before swallowing will often overcome the problem when other maneuvers fail.

5. Insertion of the tube by way of the nasal or oral route directly into the esophagus using the Magill forceps and direct laryngoscopy may be used in the patient with an absent swallowing reflex or when it is dangerous to flex the neck as in the unconscious trauma patient.
6. Another method to overcome misdirection of the nasogastric tube is to place the second and third fingers over the tongue and direct the tips to touch the posterior pharyngeal wall. The tip of the tube is then directed over the dorsal groove formed by the approximation of the fingers.
7. The final obstruction to the passage of the tube is at the proximal end of the gastroesophageal junction. This hangup usually is overcome by gently injecting 15 to 20 mL of water to relax the lower esophageal sphincter. Occasionally the tip may fall into an epigastric hernia but this is rare.

Endotracheal Intubation

Indications

An endotracheal tube must be placed in all unconscious patients with gastrointestinal bleeding, or with a Levin tube in place; and in all patients who are to have a Blakemore tube placed for bleeding esophageal varices, whether they are conscious or unconscious.

Anatomical Consideration and Method (Collins; Dripps; Smith)

It is important to remember to intubate before placing a Blakemore tube in any patient and any type of esophageal tube in the unconscious patient. It is necessary to release the cuff pressure while passing the tip of the esophageal tube past the level of the balloon cuff of the endotracheal tube.

Endoscopy

Direct Laryngoscopy and Magill Forceps (Collins; Smith)

Indications

Endoscopy is indicated for removal of foreign bodies from the hypopharynx and those lodged in the constrictor muscle and to

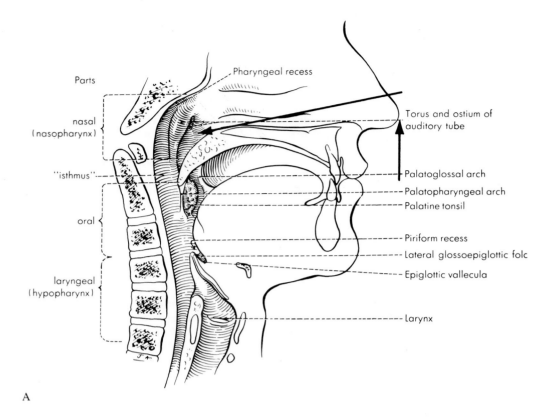

Parts

nasal
(nasopharynx)

"isthmus"

oral

laryngeal
(hypopharynx)

Pharyngeal recess

Torus and ostium of
auditory tube

Palatoglossal arch

Palatopharyngeal arch

Palatine tonsil

Piriform recess

Lateral glossoepiglottic folc

Epiglottic vallecula

Larynx

A

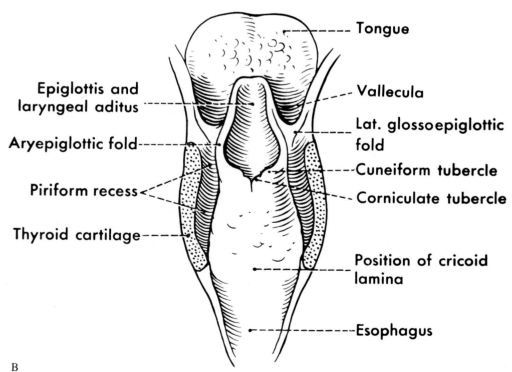

Tongue

Vallecula

Lat. glossoepiglottic
fold

Cuneiform tubercle

Corniculate tubercle

Position of cricoid
lamina

Esophagus

Epiglottis and
laryngeal aditus

Aryepiglottic fold

Piriform recess

Thyroid cartilage

B

Figure 55-9. Functional anatomy regarding the passage of tubes into the esophagus. (*A*) The arrows indicate that the tip of the nose needs to be elevated and the tip of the tube directed along the floor of the nares in order to make the curve at the isthmus. (*B*) and (*C*) The many recesses that impede the passage of esophageal tubes. Closure of the glottis eliminates them. (Hollingshed with permission by Hoeber)

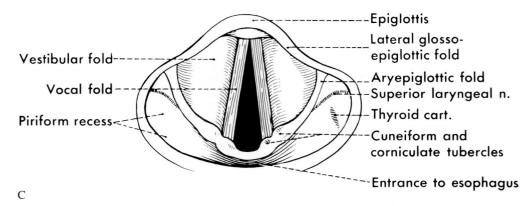

Vestibular fold

Vocal fold

Piriform recess

Epiglottis

Lateral glosso-epiglottic fold

Aryepiglottic fold

Superior laryngeal n.

Thyroid cart.

Cuneiform and corniculate tubercles

Entrance to esophagus

C

aid direction of the tips of esophageal tubes into the esophagus. Suffice it to say that local anesthesia must be used in the awake patient, the neck is not extended as in endotracheal intubation, the cervical vertebrae must be known to be intact, and a straight blade is more useful than a curved blade.

Esophagoscopy

Indications (Fiddian-Green)

Esophagoscopy should be used for removal of foreign bodies from the esophagus. It is also used in the emergency department to diagnose the site of gastrointestinal bleeding before introduction of a Blakemore tube or to confirm the absence of esophageal bleeding and varices in a patient going directly to surgery for massive bleeding from a suspected gastroduodenal site.

Anatomical Considerations and Procedure (Cotton)

Comments regarding nasogastric intubation apply to endoscopy. Obstructions can be visualized and the methods for overcoming them are the same.

Blakemore Intubation

Indications (Fiddian-Green)

Blakemore intubation is indicated for massive or uncontrolled bleeding suspected to arise from the lower 10 cm of the esophagus or from the cardia of the stomach, in which Pitressin (see discussion on the bleeding esophagus) and other measures fail to control the bleeding. Its best use is to stop bleeding from esophageal varices, but it has been used to temporarily stop bleeding from a bleeding esophageal peptic ulcer.

Contraindications include its use in patients bleeding from complete or incomplete lacerations of the esophagus (e.g., Mallory-Weiss); or peptic ulceration with stricture.

Anatomical Considerations and Procedure

A complete description of how to place the Blakemore tube can be found in the package with the tube. There are, however, some precautions:

1. The tube can be placed either through the nose or the mouth.
2. The same points of obstruction found in placing nasogastric tubes will obstruct passage of the Blakemore tube.
3. The oropharynx must be anesthetized prior to placement unless the patient is unconscious and without a gag reflex.
4. The site of bleeding must be identified by endoscopy prior to placement unless the rate of bleeding precludes it.
5. The airway must be protected by endotracheal intubation prior to placement.
6. The tip of the tube is best directed over a dorsal groove formed by the second and third fingers, which are in turn pressed loosely against the midposterior pharyngeal wall.

SYMPTOM COMPLEXES AND SPECIFIC DISEASES OF THE ESOPHAGUS WHICH ARE IMPORTANT TO THE EMERGENCY PHYSICIAN

Chest Pain of Esophageal Origin

Pain arising from the esophagus is the most alarming of the esophageal symptoms since it often mimics chest pain due to mediastinitis or heart pain. Indeed, patients with perforation of the esophagus may start out with pain from esophageal origin and then progress to pain due to mediastinitis such as in Boerhaave's syndrome (Fig. 55-14). However, the most common cause for alarm in emergency departments is the esophageal colicky pain that mimics myocardial infarction.

Pain due to esophageal pathology tends to be associated with dysphagia, odynophagia, pyrosis, epigastric bloating, belching, and reflux. If a careful search for these symptoms is made, then the vast majority of patients with esophageal causes for their chest pain will be separated from those who have myocardial infarction. Relief of chest pain by antacids; repeated swallowing, especially of warm liquids; and liberal use of a barium swallow will identify most of the leftover group.

Unfortunately, precipitation of pain by exercise and relief by rest is found in patients with atypical esophageal colic due to reflux esophagitis or diffuse spasm. Indeed, 55 percent of patients in Bennett and Henderson's studies had atypical esophageal chest pain precipitated by exercise. Nitroglycerin will produce pain relief in pain from both esophageal and cardiac origin, but pain relief in the esophageal group usually takes 5 to 10 min while pain from angina responds in 2 to 3 min, and not at all if it is a myocardial infarction. Both types of patients may also have ST elevations on an ECG.

The symptoms of chest pain due to mediastinitis are reviewed in the section on trauma, and in Figure 55-14.

Specific Types of Dysphagia (Pope)

Transfer Dysphagia

Transfer dysphagia is the inability to initiate the act of swallowing (deglutition). Inflammatory lesions which are painful and/or cause mechanical obstruction, and neuromuscular disorders are the usual causes for this disorder. Failure of the muscles of mastication and salivary lubrication also cause this problem, but less frequently.

Painful lesions of the tongue, oropharynx, and larynx can cause transfer dysphagia, along with odynophagia. Examples include pharyngitis of bacterial origin (streptococcal), viral origin (herpes), and fungus (*Monilia*); the latter two occurring especially in the immunocompromised patient. Parapharyngeal abscesses and tonsillitis may cause mechanical obstruction as well as odynophagia with dysphagia. Foreign bodies stuck in the throat especially in the young and the old (Fig. 55-10), and epiglottitis in the young also can lead to this symptom. Finally, cancers of the head and neck which invade the tongue and throat, and operations to cure the lesions are an increasing cause of transfer dysphagia.

Patients with mechanical causes of transfer dysphagia tend to drool because of mechanical obstruction and/or pain. They are often hoarse and have a bad cough because of the laryngeal involvement. The diagnosis is made by direct laryngoscopy, except in the child with possible epiglottitis, who must be intubated in the operating room under anesthesia.

Neuromuscular causes of transfer dysphagia include cerebrovascular accidents, polio and bulbar palsies, as well as dermatomyositis and polymyositis. The symptoms most associated with neuromuscular weakness are nasopharyngeal regurgitation or cough and hoarseness due to laryngeal aspirations. A Zenker's diverticulum may also be found associated with these diseases (Tables 55-1 and 55-2).

Three diseases, rare but curable, which cause transfer dysphagia in younger age groups, should be kept in mind: (1) myasthenia gravis, which improves immediately with a test dose of edrophonium (Tensilon) (2 mg, 3 mg, and 5 mg at 45-s intervals); (2) dysphagia from thyrotoxic myopathy, which has all the other manifestations of thyrotoxicosis; and (3) lead poisoning, which causes a gingival blue line in 60 percent of adults (although less frequently in children), basophilic stippling and clover-leaf morphology of the red blood cells on peripheral smear, and colicky and often intractable crampy pain.

Esophageal Body Dysphagia

Mechanical causes of esophageal body dysphagia in the young include congenital strictures, swallowing of foreign bodies, and vascular ring anomalies of the aortic arch. In the older patient the most common causes of dysphagia include reflux esophagitis, webs, rings, and cancer of the esophagus (Table 55-1). Increasingly, infections caused by herpesvirus and *Monilia* are the cause of dysphagia in the immunocompromised or suppressed patient, either secondary to systemic disease, or steroid or antibiotic suppression of the immune system. Aneurysms of the aortic arch and invading cancers of the lung and tracheobronchial tree are also less frequent but serious causes of dysphagia in the older patient.

The emergency physician should suspect mechanical causes of dysphagia, especially when they are related to the sticking of solid food and complete obstruction of the esophagus with regurgitation of undigested food or fluid (Table 55-2). Indirect evidence of an

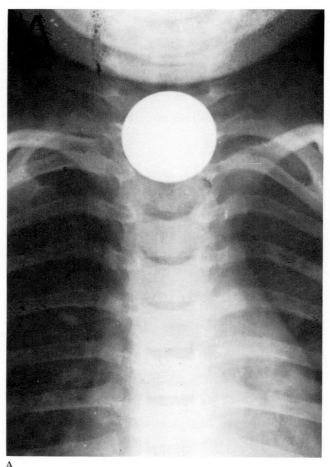

A

Figure 55-10. Foreign bodies in the esophagus. Swallowed foreign bodies lodged in the cervical esophagus at Killian's mouth (*A* and *B*) are a cause of dysphagia and drooling, especially in the infant and the mentally deficient or obtunded adult. Arrows point to the tracheal air shadow in *B*. Most of these foreign bodies can be removed by laryngoscopy and they can then be removed by esophagoscopy. If the foreign body passes Killian's mouth, the next two sites for lodging are at the aortic arch level and the LES. Usually, as was the case in *C*, the foreign body that passes Killian's mouth will pass into the stomach. The practice of using a Fogarty catheter to remove the foreign body is to be condemned since it may slip from the esophagus into the trachea.

inflammatory cause of dysphagia of the body of the esophagus is usually found in the mouth, e.g., herpes and monilias infections.

The most important neuromuscular causes of dysphagia include achalasia, diffuse spasm, and scleroderma; achalasia-caused dysphagia associated with esophageal retention; and regurgitation of retained food. X-rays show a dilated esophagus with a distal beak (Fig. 55-11). The diagnosis is confirmed by manometry of the LES, which remains high even during swallowing.

Diffuse spasm causes dysphagia associated with esophageal colic (see below). Segmental contractions are seen on barium swallow and some peristaltic waves interspersed with simultaneous, prolonged high-amplitude contractions on manometric studies. Many patients are admitted to the coronary care unit on several occasions before a barium swallow, esophageal manometry, and coronary

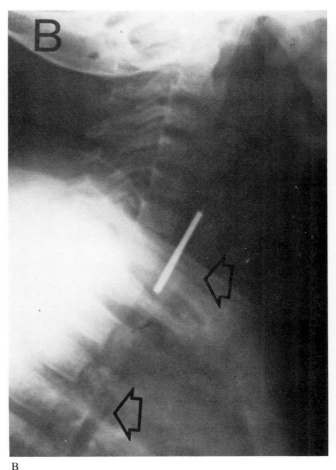

B

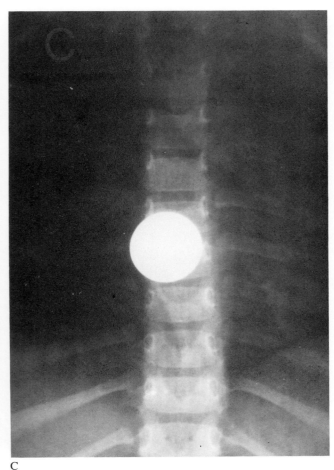

C

arteriography prove the esophageal rather than the myocardial origin of the pain. The emergency physician can minimize these coronary care unit admissions prior to diagnosis of spasm by searching for the history of dysphagia in these patients.

Dysphagia associated with scleroderma usually is associated with symptoms of reflux. If aperistalsis is seen on a simple barium swallow it is diagnostic, but often single or multiple contractions are seen, and therefore the barium swallow is not diagnostic.

It should be emphasized that if a patient has dysphagia, odynophagia, or esophageal colic, an emergency barium swallow, when positive, will lead to a diagnosis of mechanical or neuromuscular esophageal disease, and the emergency physician can then send the patient in the right direction for diagnosis. Unfortunately, motor diseases of the esophagus, except for achalasia, may not be evident at the time of the initial barium swallow, especially diffuse esophageal spasm.

Finally, patients may have primary muscle disease of the striated muscle of the upper one-third of the esophagus. Transfer dysphagia will also be present, which will lead to the diagnosis.

ESOPHAGEAL TRAUMA (Besson)

Etiology

There has been a 450 percent increase in esophageal injuries, both lacerations and perforations, in the past 30 years. In the 1950s foreign bodies were the most frequent cause of injury. However, while the incidence of foreign-body injuries remains stable, the incidence of instrumental perforation is three times higher, and perforation due to vomiting and cervicothoracic trauma with blunt and penetrating trauma is much higher. Increased recognition of injury is probably due to recognition by Gastrografin swallow and esophagoscopy (Fig. 55-12). The etiology of perforation at the various levels of the esophagus is seen in Figure 55-13. The cause of injuries to the cervicothoracic portion of the esophagus should be of special interest to the emergency physician, since the increased number of laryngoscopies and endotracheal and esophageal intubations performed by paramedics in the field under the most extreme emergency conditions is increasing; and since the number of these procedures plus the placement of nasogastric tubes by the emergency physician, again under extreme emergency conditions in the emergency department, is increasing. Also, the emergency physician in a large inner-city practice will see a number of penetrating stab and gunshot wounds to the cervical portion of the esophagus.

Pathogenesis and Clinical Presentation

The esophageal injury may be partial or full thickness. The partial thickness tears are usually innocuous and associated with dysphagia, odynophagia, esophogeal colic, and mild upper gastrointestinal bleeding. The full-thickness tears or perforations due to

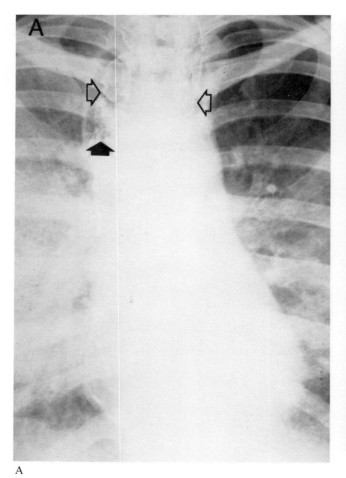
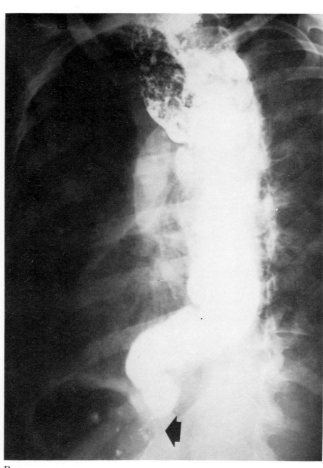

A   B

Figure 55-11. Achalasia. A 39-year-old female had a history of intermittent dysphagia, and sticking of the food bolus. The bolus could be propelled forward by a Valsalva maneuver. (*A*) The esophagus was barely outlined by barium to highlight the double shadow (between open arrows) and the fluid level (solid vertical arrow) seen on a plain chest film. The esophagus proximal to the LES which is closed is tremendously dilated (*B*). The solid arrow points to the beak-like deformity diagnostic of this disease.

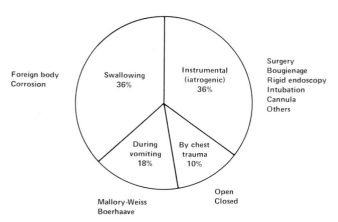

Figure 55-12. Pathogenesis of esophageal injuries. The diagram shows a detailed breakdown of the causes of injury. (After Besson A, Saegesser F: Trauma of the esophagus, in *Color Atlas of Chest Trauma, Vol II*. Oradell, NJ, Medical Economics Books, 1983, pp. 251–316.)

foreign bodies or instrumentation lead to mediastinitis. However, in one series the diagnosis was delayed for more than 24 h in one-half of cases, regardless of the level of perforation. If surgical repair of the perforation is made in less than 24 h, mortality is 5 percent, but if surgical treatment is delayed, mortality is 75 percent.

Laceration of the mucosa and submucosa (Mallory-Weiss syndrome) and perforation of the full thickness of the thoracic and abdominal esophageal wall (Boerhaave's syndrome) are associated with a sudden, violent, and usually repeated increase in the intraabdominal pressure against a weakened esophageal wall. The cause of the sudden increase in abdominal pressure is a Valsalva movement, which usually implies a closed glottis during hiccoughing, defecation, delivery, epileptic attack, or lifting a

Figure 55-13. Etiology of trauma by level of injury. (After Besson A, Saegesser F: Trauma of the esophagus, in *Color Atlas of Chest Trauma, Vol II*. Oradell, NJ, Medical Economics Books, 1983, pp. 251–316.)

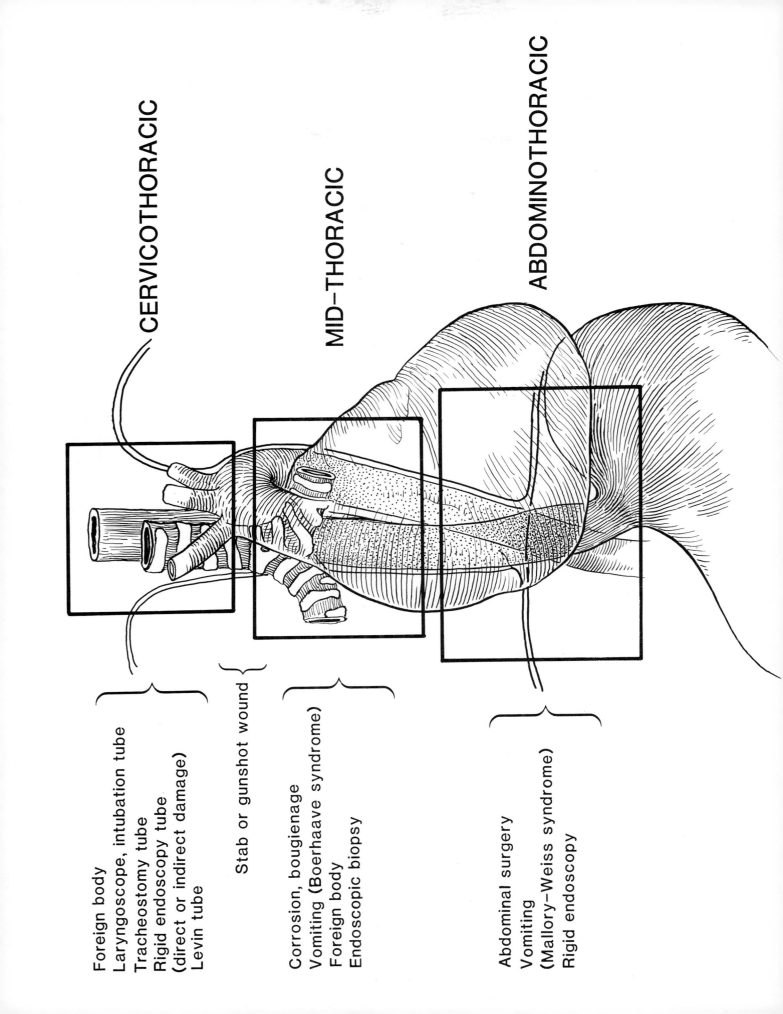

CERVICOTHORACIC

MID-THORACIC

ABDOMINOTHORACIC

Foreign body
Laryngoscope, intubation tube
Tracheostomy tube
Rigid endoscopy tube
(direct or indirect damage)
Levin tube

Stab or gunshot wound

Corrosion, bougienage
Vomiting (Boerhaave syndrome)
Foreign body
Endoscopic biopsy

Abdominal surgery
Vomiting
(Mallory-Weiss syndrome)
Rigid endoscopy

heavy weight; or external heart massage. The most common cause of increased intraabdominal pressure is violent and repeated emesis.

The predisposing causes for a weakened esophageal wall include emesis in which the mucosa at the gastroesophageal junction prolapses into the lumen through the gastroesophageal junction. The mucosa becomes edematous and even bruised and inflamed after such an event. The mucosa can also be weakened by the prolonged presence of a nasogastric tube, reflex esophagitis, epiphrenic hernias, or hemorrhage into the esophageal wall from rupture of a short gastric artery.

Mallory-Weiss lacerations are thought to occur in weakened mucosa, usually on the right posterolateral side, but Boerhaave's perforations tend to rupture on the left posterolateral side of the unsupported part of the abdominal esophageal wall. The lacerations or perforations tend to extend cephalad into the thoracic esophagus. The second most common site for both syndromes to occur is on the right side just below the level of the azygos vein.

Lacerations cause bleeding of the submucosal plexus of veins and arteries which is usually moderate and self-limiting. They may also produce dysphagia, odynophagia, and be associated with symptoms of reflux esophagitis (predisposing factor).

Perforations of the esophagus associated with Boerhaave's syndrome cause the most malignant type of mediastinitis. The force of expulsion of fluid through the perforation spreads it rapidly through the wispy and poorly perfused mediastinal tissue, causing an acid burn to the mediastinal blood vessels and rapid spread of very virulent bacteria. The patient complains of severe abdominal pain and chest pain which often radiates into the neck. Patients rapidly develop shock and septicemia, leading to death within 48 h. There is often an associated peritonitis with air under the diaphragm, as well as air fluid levels in the mediastinum (Fig. 55-14) and often pyopneumothorax (Fig. 55-5).

Symptoms of Laceration and Perforation

Bleeding and dysphagia following at least one episode of previous emesis are the common signs of laceration (see The Bleeding Esophagus). Severe and unrelenting chest and neck pain secondary to chemical and then bacterial mediastinitis, followed by shock and collapse, are the most outstanding symptoms related to perforation. The clinical and radiological signs of perforation are related to the level of the perforation and are reviewed in Figure 55-14.

Diagnosis

The most important clue to the diagnosis of esophageal injury is to suspect it from the history. All patients who swallow foreign bodies that stick in the esophagus are at risk for laceration and perforation. This is especially true of the infant and young child who swallow small alkaline batteries which lodge in the hypopharynx or at the level of the aortic arch. Patients who vomit blood and/or develop chest or abdominal pain after emesis are especially suspect. All unconscious patients who have had instrumentation of the pharynx, larynx, or esophagus, cardiopulmonary resuscitation in the field, or instrumentation or cardiopulmonary resuscitation in the emergency department (with the exception of very routine procedures) should be suspected of having a perforation.

Patients with penetrating wounds of the neck or chest and with crushing wounds to the chest must be suspected of having a ruptured esophagus. In addition, patients who have suspected splenic rupture treated nonoperatively should be observed for a late Boerhaave's rupture, since a predisposing factor to this syndrome is intramural rupture of a short gastric artery.

SPECIFIC DIAGNOSTIC MEASURES TO BE INITIATED IN THE EMERGENCY DEPARTMENT

All patients who come into the emergency department with chest pain or a history outlined in the previous paragraph must have a chest x-ray for evidence of foreign-body, perforation, mediastinal fluid, or cardiac and pleural effusions (Fig. 55-14).

If there is radiological evidence of perforation on posteroanterior and lateral chest x-ray, a water-soluble contrast study should be done to confirm the diagnosis. Esophagoscopy is only performed if a perforation is suspected but cannot be confirmed by contrast studies, or if there is upper gastrointestinal bleeding associated with a partial thickness laceration, or if the patient with chest trauma is unconscious and a contrast study cannot be done. In addition, all stuporous patients who have been instrumented in the field or who survive CPR should have endoscopy at the first appropriate moment after resuscitation to rule out an iatrogenic esophageal injury. Whenever esophagoscopy is performed, pharyngoscopy, laryngoscopy, and tracheobronchoscopy should also be performed to look for associated lesions.

Anyone suspected of having a perforation should be given intravenous antibiotics immediately (cephoxatin and clindamycin), since there will be a delay of at least 6 h between suspicion of perforation, diagnosis, and operative management. The time delay will be further aggravated if interhospital referral and transportation are involved in definitive care. On the other hand, an antibiotic is only effective if adequate tissue levels are reached within 6 h. It must be emphasized, however, that survival is inversely proportional to the length of time between perforation and operative repair.

Foreign-Body Ingestion

Most foreign bodies pass through the esophagus freely without incarceration or damage to the lining of the esophagus. Of those that have a difficult passage, some will damage the mucosa without incarceration, causing dysphagia, odynophagia, esophageal colic, or bleeding; some will be lodged without damage to the mucosa; some will be lodged with damage to the mucosa. Of those foreign bodies that become lodged, many will pass into the

Figure 55-14. Physical and radiological signs in chest pain due to perforation of the esophagus and to mediastinitis. (*A*) Cervicothoracic; (*B*) midthoracic; (*C*) abdominothoracic. Mediastinitis causes the most severe form of chest pain. The site and cause of the perforation can almost always be diagnosed by taking a careful history, physical examination, and by procurement of a chest x-ray. (After Besson A, Saegesser F: Trauma of the esophagus, in *Color Atlas of Chest Trauma, Vol II*. Oradell, NJ, Medical Economics Books, 1983, pp. 251–316.)

CERVICOTHORACIC

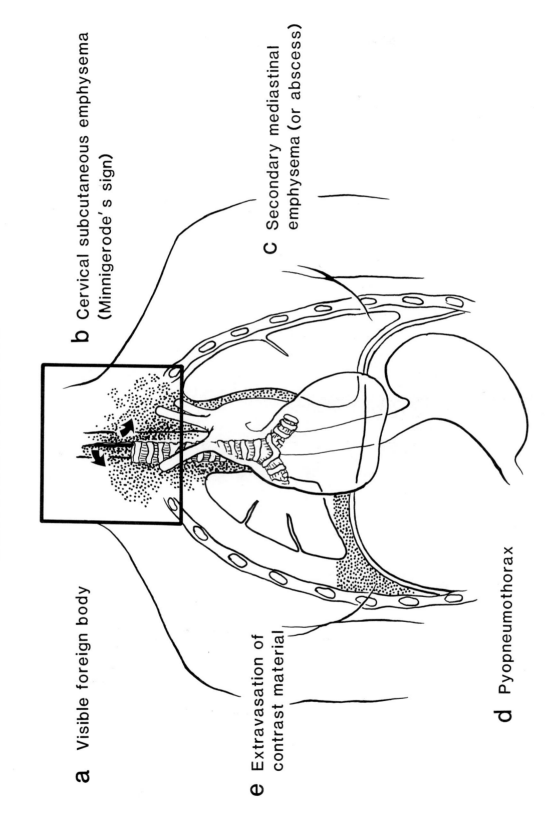

a Visible foreign body

b Cervical subcutaneous emphysema (Minnigerode's sign)

c Secondary mediastinal emphysema (or abscess)

d Pyopneumothorax

e Extravasation of contrast material

f Injury detectable by endoscopic means only

A

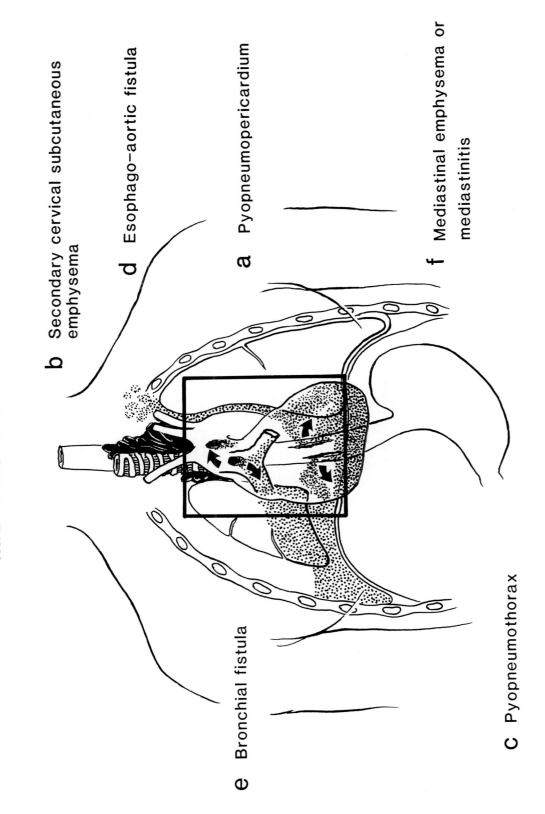

MID–THORACIC

b Secondary cervical subcutaneous
   emphysema

d Esophago–aortic fistula

a Pyopneumopericardium

f Mediastinal emphysema or
   mediastinitis

g Injury detectable by endoscopic or
   fibroscopic means only

e Bronchial fistula

c Pyopneumothorax

B (**Figure 55-14.** *Continued*)

ABDOMINOTHORACIC

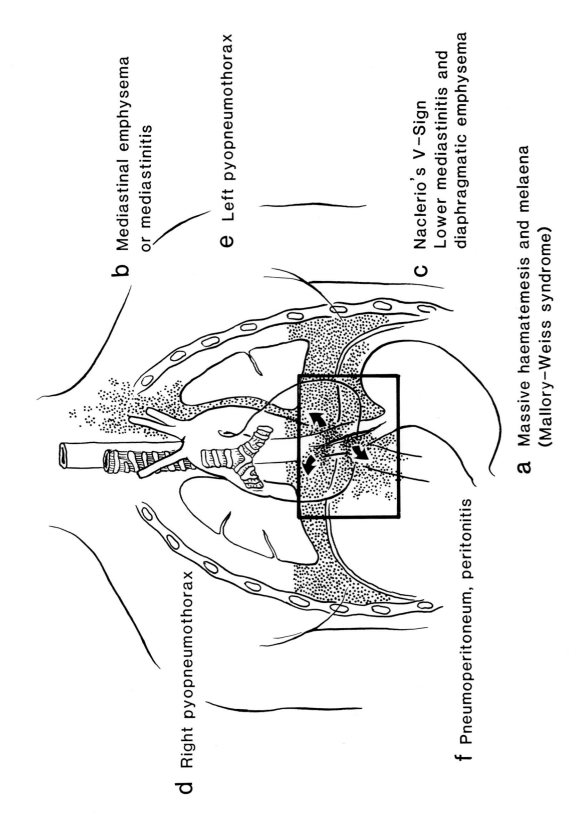

b Mediastinal emphysema or mediastinitis

e Left pyopneumothorax

c Naclerio's V–Sign Lower mediastinitis and diaphragmatic emphysema

a Massive haematemesis and melaena (Mallory–Weiss syndrome)

d Right pyopneumothorax

f Pneumoperitoneum, peritonitis

g Injury detectable by endoscopic or fibroscopic means only

C (**Figure 55-14.** *Continued*)

stomach after repeated swallowing (Fig. 55-10C) or will be re-gurgitated, especially a food bolus.

Foreign bodies lodge in the cervical esophagus, usually at Killian's mouth, in 82 percent of incarcerated foreign bodies in one series (Fig. 55-10A and B). Forty-five percent of these caused no injury; injury was superficial in 40 percent. Injury was deep or perforating in 12 percent of the cases lodged at Killian's mouth, in 11 percent of the foreign bodies lodged at the level of the aortic arch, and in 7 percent at the gastroesophageal junction.

The age distribution shows a peak in the first decade due to "inattentive swallowing" and a second peak at the sixth decade with a bell curve distribution between age 20 to 90. Most of the latter cases of ingestion are due to "insensitive swallowing" due to the presence of dentures or a stroke.

The types of foreign bodies are legion, but coins and pills predominate in the younger child and the mentally retarded. Lately, the small round alkaline batteries used in hearing aids, calculators, and cameras have become a common source of foreign bodies lodged in a child's esophagus. These batteries are very corrosive and cause ulcerations, scarring, or even perforations.

In adults the most common cause of foreign-body incarceration is a food bolus and the most common causes of injury are bone splinters, fish bones, and dentures. If a food bolus becomes lodged there is a high probability that there is underlying pathology in the esophagus, either due to webs, peptic stricture, achalasia, or cancer.

Diagnosis

Ingestion of foreign bodies is usually diagnosed because of the history of swallowing one, or because of dysphagia, odynophagia, or esophageal colic. Patients with foreign bodies lodged in their throats will have drooling or failure to eat. In both children and adults the history of having swallowed a foreign body or having one lodged elsewhere should cause a high index of suspicion of a new foreign-body ingestion.

Management (Besson; Cotton)

There are three principles in the management of ingested foreign bodies that cause damage or become lodged in the esophagus, or both.

1. The foreign body must be removed unless dislodgment is spontaneous. When it is not, most foreign objects can be removed with a laryngoscope and Magill forceps, or with a flexible pediatric endoscope and the foreign-body extraction tools designed for it. Sometimes the foreign body must be nursed into the stomach to better manipulate it for removal, e.g., to close a safety pin. Meat can often be removed by the ingestion of papain, a meat-tenderizing proteolytic enzyme. Some foreign bodies cannot be removed and must be extracted by surgery, but such cases are less than 5 percent of all foreign-body ingestions.

   A common recommendation in the pediatric age group is to pass a Fogarty catheter beyond the foreign body, inflate the balloon, and then remove the catheter, forcing the foreign body ahead of the balloon. This maneuver can be hazardous, car-rying the risk of the foreign body falling into the larynx and trachea, causing upper airway obstruction.

2. The esophagus must be inspected either directly by esophagoscope at the time of extraction or afterwards if perforation is not expected; or by water-soluble contrast to rule out perforation if it is expected.

3. It must be assumed that in all but the pediatric age group there is a reason for the lodgment of a foreign body and that reason must be actively sought.

BIBLIOGRAPHY

Ach RD: Adbominal pain, in Blacklow RS (ed): *MacBryde's Signs and Symptoms, Applied Pathologic Physiology and Clinical Interpretation,* ed 6. Philadelphia, JB Lippincott Co, 1983, pp 165–179.

Bennett JR, Atkinson M: The differentiation between oesophageal and cardiac pain. *Lancet* 2:1123, 1966.

Besson A, Saegesser F: Trauma of the esophagus, in *Color Atlas of Chest Trauma, II.* Oradell, NJ, Medical Economics Books, 1983, pp 251–316.

Blakemore AH: *Blakemore Esophageal-Nasogastric Tube—Instructions for Passing the Esophageal Balloon for the Control of Bleeding from Esophageal Varices,* Providence, RI, Davol Inc.

Collins VJ: Endotracheal anaesthesia II, technical considerations: *Principles of Anaesthesiology.* Philadelphia, Lea & Febiger, 1970, pp 322–354.

Cotton PB, Williams CB: *Practical Gastrointestinal Endoscopy,* ed 2. Oxford, Blackwell Scientific Publications, Ltd., 1982.

Dripps RD, Eckenhoff JE, Vandam LD: Intubation of the trachea: *Introduction to Anaesthesia—The Principles of Safe Practice.* ed 6. Philadelphia, WB Saunders Co, 1982, pp 180–195.

Dworken HJ: Gastrointestinal hemorrhage, in Shoemaker WC, Thompson WL, Holbrook PR (eds), *Textbook of Critical Care.* Philadelphia, WB Saunders Co, pp 591–597.

Edwards DAW: Flowcharts, diagnostic keys and algorithms in the diagnosis of dysphagia. *Scott Med J* 15:378, 1970.

Edwards DAW: Discriminating information in the diagnosis of dysphagia. *J R Coll Physicians Lond* 9:257, 1975.

Edwards DAW: Flowcharts, Diagnostic keys and algorithms in the diagnosis of dysphagia, *Scott Med J* 15:378, 1970.

Fiddian-Green RG, Turcotte JG: Evaluation of the bleeding patient, and variceal bleeding, in *Gastrointestinal Hemorrhage.* New York, Grune & Stratton, 1980, pp 3–80 and 233–328.

Henderson RD, et al: Atypical chest pain of cardiac and esophageal origin. *Chest* 73:24, 1978.

Hollingshead WH: The pharynx and larynx: *Anatomy for Surgery, I—The Head and Neck.* New York, Harper and Row, 1968, pp 440–446.

Jones T, Shepard WC: *Manual of Surgical Anatomy.* Philadelphia, WB Saunders Co, 1945.

Leriche R: *The Surgery of Pain.* Baltimore, Williams & Wilkins, 1939, p 434.

Maclean LD, Wagenstein OH: The surgical treatment of esophageal stricture. *Surg Gynecol Obstet* 103:5, 1956.

Pope CE: The esophagus, in Sleisinger MH, Fordtran JS: *Gastrointestinal Disease Pathophysiology Diagnosis Management,* ed 2. Philadelphia, WB Saunders Co, 1978, pp 196–199 and pp 495–610.

Shackelford RT: *Surgery of the Alimentary Tract,* ed 2. Philadelphia, WB Saunders Co, 1978.

Smith RM: Endotracheal intubation: *Anaesthesia for Infants and Children,* ed 4. St. Louis, The CV Mosby Co, 1980, pp 164–191.

Temple DM, McNeese MC: Hazards of battery ingestion. *Pediatrics* 71:100–103, 1983.

Wesley JR, Coran AG, Sarahan TM, Klein MD, White SJ: The need for evaluation of gastroesophageal reflux in brain-damaged children referred for feeding gastrostomy. *J Pediatr Surg* 16:866–871, 1981.

Wolff HG, Wolf SG: *Pain.* Springfield, Ill, Charles C Thomas Publisher, 1948.

CHAPTER 56

SWALLOWED

FOREIGN BODIES

Ronald L. Krome

Since young children, especially those aged 6 months to 3 years, have so much natural curiosity, they are peculiarly prone to swallow foreign bodies. High-risk factors in the pediatric age group include (1) curiosity and the proclivity to put foreign objects in the mouth, (2) the presence of social, developmental, or psychiatric factors, and (3) esophageal disease. The problem of ingested foreign bodies, however, is one that crosses age barriers. Especially in the elderly, a large bolus of ingested, incompletely chewed food can impact in the esophagus. Psychiatrically disturbed and prisoner patients are two adult populations who are also prone to ingest foreign bodies. In the latter group, the ingestion of razor blades or spoons seems to be favored. Overall, boluses of food and coins remain the most commonly ingested foreign bodies.

PATHOPHYSIOLOGY

Foreign bodies and boluses of food may lodge anywhere in the esophagus but are especially prone to lodge at points of pathologic or physiologic narrowing. Physiologic narrowing occurs at the cricopharyngeus muscle, the cardioesophageal junction, and at Schatzki's ring in the lower esophagus. Other points at which physiologic narrowing may occur are at the carina and behind the heart. In children, another common point for impaction is at the level of the aortic arch where the esophagus crosses the vertebral column.

The majority of ingested foreign bodies will spontaneously traverse the gastrointestinal (GI) tract without producing adverse results. Any object that passes the pylorus will most likely reach the rectum, assuming, of course, that the object has no sharp edges. Occasionally, an object will pass through the pylorus only to get hung up in the duodenum. Sharp or pointed objects, including bones, that lodge in the esophagus can produce perforation with the subsequent development of mediastinitis, cardiac tamponade, or an esophagoaortic fistula. These objects can also produce perforation anywhere along the GI tract. Alkaline disk batteries ingested and lodged in the esophagus have been known to break down and erode the esophageal wall, producing all the complications of esophageal perforation.

CLINICAL FEATURES

With an adult, the history of foreign-body ingestion or impaction of food is generally easy to obtain. Obstruction of the airway from a foreign body is discussed elsewhere. Objects lodged in the esophagus generally produce anxiety and discomfort. Substernal pain may also be present. There is a tendency for the patient to retch or attempt to vomit to dislodge the object. If an attempt is made to wash the object down, the patient may choke, cough, or aspirate.

Eventually, the patient may be unable to swallow his or her own secretions. The ingestion of a foreign body by a child is often not witnessed by an adult. In a child, coughing or choking occurs with acute aspiration. Wheezing and persistent coughing or respiratory distress can suggest a foreign body lodged at the bifurcation of the trachea, or in a bronchus. The child's inability to swallow and refusal to eat suggest a foreign body in the esophagus. The most common symptoms in the under-16 age group are as follows:

Vomiting
Gagging
Choking
Neck or throat pain
Inability to swallow
Foreign-body sensation in the chest

Physical examination should include the careful evaluation of the nasophrarynx, neck, and subcutaneous tissues for air resulting from perforation of a hollow viscus. Indirect or direct laryngoscopy should be done, especially when the patient complains of a sticking sensation, or when the patient has ingested a bone. There are times when the patient can localize the bone with a great degree of accuracy based on the sensation of sticking. The flexible laryngoscope is a valuable addition to the diagnostic tools available for this problem. Although most patients have no physical findings, the common ones in the 16-and-under age group are as follows:

Red throat
Palatal abrasion
Temperature elevation
Distress

Roentgenograms of the soft tissues of the neck, and posterioanterior and oblique views of the chest, should be obtained. The neck films, in addition to demonstrating the foreign body, may demonstrate air in the pretracheal space if perforation has occurred (Fig. 56-1). If bronchial obstruction is suspected, inspiratory-expiratory or lateral decubitus films may be helpful.

A flat object, such as a coin, will become lodged in the trachea in the sagittal plane. One lodged in the esophagus will become oriented in the frontal plane. The one lodged in the esophagus will show on routine chest films; the one in the trachea may not.

Pull tabs from aluminum beverage cans have been aspirated. These are difficult to detect on x-ray examination because they are relatively radiolucent and may overlie the more radiodense vertebral bodies.

TREATMENT

A nasogastric tube should be inserted to minimize aspiration of unswallowed fluids above the impaction. An esophagogram, using water-soluble contrast material can be done to visualize the obstruction. At times, having the patient swallow a barium-soaked cotton pledget is helpful in locating the obstruction, especially if the ingested material is not radiopaque.

Since the majority (80 percent) of ingested foreign bodies will traverse the entire GI tract without any problem, provided there are no sharp or jagged edges to the foreign body, treatment can be expectant once the object has passed through the pylorus. Virtually all symptomatic patients will require observation and esophagoscopy. Repeated abdominal films to monitor the contin-

uous movement of the foreign body should be made. The patient should have repeated abdominal examinations to detect the development of peritonitis that follows perforation. Any foreign body that becomes lodged in the esophagus or that does not pass through the pylorus should be removed using esophagogastroscopy. This is also true if the foreign body is lodged at the cricopharynx or upper esophagus. There are times when it is possible to pass a Foley catheter past the obstructing foreign body and then inflate the balloon and slowly extract the foreign body.

When meat is the offending foreign body, some have advocated the use of proteolytic enzymes such as an aqueous solution of papain (e.g., Adolph's meat tenderizer) to break up the food. Ritter has reported a 3 percent incidence of perforation following the use of such agents. If the meat contains bone, then perforation may occur because the bone is exposed as enzymatic dissolution of the meat occurs. Perforation may be secondary to focal ischemia that develops as a result of the distention of the esophageal wall by the impacted food bolus, enhancing the ability of papain to digest the wall. Papain given prior to esophagoscopy may increase the risk of perforation from the procedure, especially when the obstruction is not relieved and the papain and the bolus remain in place.

There have been reports of the use of intravenous glucagon in instances of food impaction in the esophagus. The postulate is that glucagon can dislodge an esophageal impaction because it relaxes the esophageal smooth muscle. For use in the emergency department, Glauser's group recommends intravenous glucagon, 1 mg, following a test dose to ensure that hypersensitivity does not exist. If the food bolus is not passed in 20 min, an additional 2 mg is given intravenously. If there is no relief, then esophagoscopy should be performed. Esophagograms should be made both before and after the administration of glucagon to confirm the obstruction and its relief. Ferrucci recommends the administration of a 2.5% suspension of papain if the food impaction is not relieved by glucagon. The dose is 10 mL in 240 mL of water administered in 20 mL sips.

Following the removal of a foreign body from the esophagus, the patient should have a complete evaluation of esophageal function, including motility studies, to ensure that there is no underlying pathology which led to the obstruction. Surgical removal of a foreign body is indicated for GI obstruction or perforation, for removal of a foreign body with toxic constituents, or if the length, size and shape of the foreign body suggest that it will not pass safely. Surgical removal may also be indicated if repeated films fail to demonstrate progress in motion of the foreign body over about 3 days. If GI bleeding develops, surgical intervention may also be indicated.

In one large, recent series, 12 percent of the patients required surgical intervention, virtually all for complications related to the ingested foreign body itself, although one patient had a complication related to instrumentation during an attempt at removal of the foreign body. In this same series, no patient under 12 years of age required surgery; most had the foreign body removed by endoscopy or passed the foreign body spontaneously.

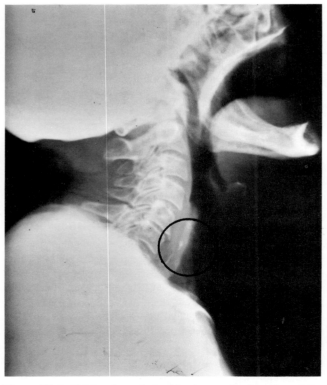

Figure 56-1. Chicken bone lodged in the proximal portion of the esophagus. (Courtesy of Detroit General Hospital.)

BIBLIOGRAPHY

Allen T: Suspected esophageal foreign body—Choosing appropriate management. *JACEP* 8:101–105, 1979.
Binder L, Anderson WA: Pediatric gastrointestinal foreign body ingestions. *Ann Emerg Med* 13:112–117, 1984.

Burrington JD: Aluminum ''pop tops.'' A hazard to child health. *JAMA* 235:2614-2617, 1976.

Dunlap LB: Removal of an esophageal foreign body using a Foley catheter. *Ann Emerg Med* 10:101–103, 1981.

Ferrucci LT, Long JA: Radiologic treatment of esophageal food impaction using intravenous glucagon. *Radiology* 125:25–28, 1977.

Glauser J, Lilja GP, Greenfield B, et al: Intravenous glucagon in the management of esophageal food obstruction. *JACEP* 8:228–231, 1979.

Gracia C, Frey CF, Bodai BI: Diagnosis and management of ingested foreign bodies: A ten-year experience. *Ann Emerg Med* 13:30–34, 1984.

Henry LN, Chamberlain JW: Removal of foreign bodies from the esophagus and nose with the use of a Foley catheter. *Surgery* 1:918–921, 1972.

Hoshmonal M, Kaufman T, Schramek A: Silent perforations of the stomach and duodenum by needles. *Arch Surg* 113:1406–1409, 1978.

Palmer ED: Backyard barbecue syndrome: Steak impaction in the esophagus. *JAMA* 235:2637–2638, 1976.

Selivanov V, Sheldon GF, Cello JP, et al: Management of foreign body ingestion. *Ann Surg* 199:187–191, 1984.

Spitz L: Management of ingested foreign bodies in childhood. *Br Med J* 4:469–472, 1971.

Tintinalli JE (ed): Respiratory stridor in a young child. *JACEP* 5:196–199, 1976.

Yee KF, Schild JA, Hollinger PH: Extraluminal foreign bodies (coins) in the food and air passages. *Ann Otol Rhinol Laryngol* 84:619–623, 1975.

CHAPTER 57
PEPTIC ULCER DISEASE

Ronald L. Krome

Although generally considered a chronic disease characterized by long asymptomatic periods interspersed with symptomatic episodes, peptic ulcer disease can run a rapidly fulminant course.

A peptic ulcer is a mucosal defect extending beyond the muscularis mucosae and occurring in acid-secreting epithelium. Regardless of the cause, the basic problem is that there is more acid than the mucosa can handle. Most peptic ulcers occur along the lesser curvature of the stomach or in the first portion of the duodenum. Less common sites include the distal esophagus, ectopic gastric mucosa in a Meckel's diverticulum, or on the margins of surgical anastomoses. Factors that predispose to ulcer formation include cigarette smoking, coffee, cola, or alcohol ingestion. Ulcer symptoms tend to become more severe in the spring and in the fall.

Duodenal ulcer is more common in emphysematous patients and in those with chronic pancreatitis. Gastric ulceration and erosive gastritis are associated with cirrhosis and/or heavy, chronic alcohol ingestion.

Endocrine abnormalities associated with an increased frequency of peptic ulceration are the Zollinger-Ellison syndrome and hyperparathyroidism. Ulcers associated with the Zollinger-Ellison syndrome tend to occur, or reoccur, in unusual locations and are very resistant to antacid therapy.

PATHOPHYSIOLOGY

Although clinically it may be difficult to distinguish gastric and duodenal ulcers, there are substantial differences in the development. Gastric ulcers are associated with prolonged gastric emptying times and low, or normal, gastric acid secretions. Duodenal ulcers are associated with hypersecretion, and there is no delay in gastric emptying. The development of gastric ulcers may be related to an impairment of the resistance of the gastric mucosa to hydrogen ions. The back diffusion of hydrogen ions into the gastric mucosa is thought to cause bleeding and ulceration. Some agents that alter the mucosal barrier in the stomach are bile salts, aspirin, alcohol, and indomethacin.

Several factors appear important in the development of duodenal ulcers, but not everyone with a duodenal ulcer demonstrates these characteristics. These factors include an increased number of parietal cells and an increased sensitivity of the parietal cells to stimulation, impaired inhibition of gastrin release when the antrum is acidified, and markedly increased gastric emptying with the rapid loss of the buffering capacity of food.

CLINICAL FEATURES

The primary manifestation of peptic ulcer disease is burning epigastric distress. The burning pain may extend across the upper abdomen, or, if the ulcer is located posteriorly and penetrates into the pancreas, the pain may go straight through to the back. The pain of a gastric ulcer tends to occur immediately after eating, while that of a duodenal ulcer tends to occur between meals. The burning pain also tends to wake the patient during the night.

Pain relief may result from a wide variety of over-the-counter medications, and the patient often will give a history of trying several different kinds before seeking medical attention. Even though almost one-third of patients with complications from their ulcer will give no history, the majority will describe the use, sometime in the past, of an over-the-counter medication for the relief of pain.

Characteristically, then, the pain is burning in nature, located in the epigastric region, occasionally radiating into the back (straight back), and may be worse at times when the stomach is empty— at night and between meals. Symptoms are usually periodic and recurrent. Definitive diagnosis is made with endoscopy and/or barium studies.

TREATMENT

Mild pain is generally treated with medical therapy: frequent feeding; avoidance of alcohol, coffee, tea, and smoking; antacids; perhaps mild sedatives or tranquilizers; and possibly anticholinergics, except when there is suspicion of pyloric obstruction or if bladder outlet obstruction may be present.

More severe pain requires more stringent treatment, which may include nasogastric suction, bed rest, sedation, and antacids. For a duodenal ulcer, 30 mL of antacid should be given 1 and 3 h after eating with an additional 30 mL at bedtime. If the patient is on nasogastric suction, no antacids are required, since the tube keeps the stomach empty and prevents the accumulation of acids. The buffering effect of antacids is prolonged if they are taken with food. Without food, the buffering effect lasts about 45 to 60 min.

The nasogastric tube serves not only to remove acid-containing gastric fluid but also decreases gastric retention, distention, and stasis. Gastric distention acts as a stimulus to the antrum, increasing gastrin secretion and then acid secretion.

Cimetidine, a member of a class of drugs that are histamine (H_2 receptor) antagonists and that inhibit gastric acid secretion, has been found useful in the treatment of duodenal ulcer disease. It has been shown to inhibit gastric acid secretion by about 70 percent.

The use of cimetidine has made a significant impact on the treatment of peptic ulcer disease. It appears as though the necessity for elective surgery for peptic ulcer problems has greatly diminished, although the incidence of perforation and rebleeding has not been significantly reduced. The use of cimetidine in bleeding has reduced the mortality from the initial bleeding episode.

When cimetidine has been used at a dosage of 400 mg twice a day, short-term healing of gastric and duodenal ulcers has been impressive, with a healing rate of 68 to 95 percent. Complications of therapy do occur, including interaction with other medications dependent on hepatic degradation.

COMPLICATIONS

In addition to intractable pain, i.e., pain that does not respond to conventional medical therapy, or pain that repeatedly incapacitates the patient for a prolonged period of time, the other major complications are bleeding, pyloric obstruction, and perforation.

Hemorrhage. Peptic ulcer disease, despite the advent of cimetidine, remains one of the major causes of massive upper gastrointestinal (GI) bleeding in the United States. Massive bleeding is generally defined as a loss of 1500 or 2000 mL of blood in an adult, or the need to replace 30 percent of a patient's blood volume over 12 h in order to maintain vital signs.

Initial management should consist of rapid fluid replacement using either Ringer's lactate or normal saline with transfusions of blood as indicated to maintain the patient's vital signs. Two large-bore intravenous lines should be inserted; one of them should be a central line to monitor central venous pressure (CVP). The rapidity of fluid replacement should be assessed by monitoring the patient's vital signs, CVP, and hourly urinary output. Transfusion of whole blood, or blood components, should be based on the patient's response to fluid administration. In addition, if the patient has angina or a past history of a myocardial infarction, transfusion may be indicated to maintain the patient's oxygen-carrying capacity. Oxygen should be administered at a flow rate of 6 to 8 L/min, depending on the presence of any intercurrent disease.

Nasogastric suction should be instituted to confirm the presence of acute and current bleeding and to begin lavage of the stomach. Constant nasogastric suction is indicated, with iced saline lavage to slow or stop the bleeding. Iced saline lavage is not universally successful, but it should be done in every patient. All clot should be removed. When transfusion becomes mandatory to maintain vital signs, some would consider surgical exploration.

Perforated ulcers are rarely the cause of massive upper GI bleeding, although they are often associated with some bleeding.

Definitive diagnosis should be established as quickly as feasible, since definitive therapy will depend on the cause of the bleeding. Endoscopic examination of the esophagus, stomach, and duodenum is becoming the new standard of diagnosis. Some believe that upper GI bleeding is an indication for emergency and immediate endoscopic examination. Other diagnostic tools include angiography and barium studies. To be diagnostic, angiography must be done while the patient is actively bleeding.

The chances of the patient's survival with minimum morbidity improve if the patient's bleeding can be controlled without emergency surgical intervention and surgery can be done on a more elective basis. Some people consider that one episode of massive bleeding from an ulcer is an indication for surgery, even if done on an elective basis. Cimetidine therapy may modify this position in time. However, if massive bleeding occurs, or active bleeding continues despite adequate fluid therapy and blood replacement, prolonged medical management is associated with a greater risk, and emergency surgical intervention is indicated.

Very little is known about the factors predisposing to recurrent hemorrhage from peptic ulcers. Patients with chronic ulcers seem to have an increased risk. According to Northfield, patients without any evidence of bleeding for 48 h are unlikely to rebleed in the near future. Patients with a large blood loss in the first episode are more likely to rebleed. Elderly patients, those with generalized arteriosclerosis, have a greater propensity to continue to bleed because the vessels are not soft enough to contract.

Obstruction. Since most ulcers heal by scar formation, when the ulcer is in the pyloric channel or in the antrum, there is a reasonable chance for pyloric obstruction to develop, or for antral narrowing to occur and produce gastric outlet obstruction. Obstruction can result in severe gastric distention with intractable vomiting, producing dehydration and metabolic alkalosis. Bile in the vomitus of a patient with peptic ulcer disease rules out, in essence, gastric outlet obstruction.

Treatment consists of constant nasogastric suction for a prolonged period of time. Fluid replacement and correction of electrolyte abnormalities is mandatory. Anticholinergic agents are contraindicated because they may aggravate the distention by decreasing gastric motility. Many surgeons consider that persistent gastric outlet obstruction after several days of nasogastric suction is an indication for surgical intervention.

Perforation. Despite the impact of cimetidine on the treatment of peptic ulcer disease and some complications, the incidence of perforation does not appear to have been significantly reduced. Perforation is characterized by the sudden onset of severe epigastric pain. If the gastric contents run down the colonic gutter, right lower quadrant pain may also occur. In this case, the picture may resemble that of acute appendicitis. The abdomen may be rigid. Percussion may reveal a lack of liver dullness in the right upper quadrant because of the presence of free air in the peritoneum. An upright view of the chest may show free air under the diaphragm, but this is not a universal finding. Free air under the diaphragm on an upright abdominal film is more difficult to detect. If free air is not demonstrated on the upright film of the chest, a lateral decubitus film of the abdomen may be helpful. If a further attempt to demonstrate free air is needed, the stomach can be filled with air using the nasogastric tube. Clamping the tube and allowing the patient to sit up for 5 to 15 min may make the air demonstrable. Shock results from primary chemical and secondary bacterial peritonitis; generalized sepsis will follow if aggressive treatment is not instituted. Posterior penetration may result in pancreatitis.

Treatment consists of constant nasogastric suction, fluid and electrolyte replacement, and appropriate antibiotic therapy. In the United States, surgery remains the definitive therapy for perforations.

STRESS EROSIONS AND HEMORRHAGIC GASTRITIS

The term *acute mucosal lesions* refers to a variety of lesions involving the gastric mucosa that include Curling's and Cushing's ulcers, stress ulcers, and acute erosive gastritis.

Stress erosions are superficial lesions that do not extend through the muscularis mucosae. They may be multiple and discrete, or diffuse and extensive, and most often they involve the body and fundus of the stomach. They are a very common cause of gastric bleeding. Multiple factors involved in the development of stress erosions include an increase in gastric secretion, an alteration in the mucosal barrier to hydrogen ions, and local ischemia.

Stress erosions or acute mucosal lesions can occur after a variety of systemic insults and can develop within hours in conditions such as CNS tumors, head trauma, fractures, burns, sepsis, or shock. Steroids, aspirin, and alcohol all predispose to the development of erosions. In a large series collected by Josen, acute hemorrhagic gastritis accounted for the bleeding in more than half of the patients.

The diagnosis is best made by endoscopic examination. Barium studies are of little help. Since surgery is rarely indicated in these patients, it is imperative that the diagnosis be established as quickly as possible in patients with upper GI bleeding.

Since the gastric mucosa will renew itself in 48 to 72 h, medical management is often effective. Cimetidine appears to be of some use in a preventative fashion. Nasogastric suction with iced saline lavage and the use of antacids may also be effective.

If bleeding is massive and cannot be controlled with the methods described, then surgery may be indicated. Because the lesions are generally extensive, the surgery will also need to be extensive.

BIBLIOGRAPHY

Barer D, Ogilvie A, Henry D, et al: Cimetidine and tranexamic acid in the treatment of acute upper gastrointestinal tract bleeding. *N Engl J Med* 308:1571–1575, 1983.

Bauman JH, Kimelblatt BJ, Caraccio TR, et. al.: Cimetidine-theophylline interaction: Report of four patients. *Ann Allergy* 48:100–102, 1982.

Brunner H: Pirenzepine and cimetidine in the treatment of peptic ulcer. *Scand J Gastroenterol* 17:207–209, 1982.

Chapman ML: Peptic ulcer: A medical perspective. *Med Clin North Am* 62:39–51, 1978.

Ching E, ReMine WH: Surgical management of emergency complications of duodenal ulcer. *Surg Clin North Am* 51:851–855, 1971.

Croker JR: Acute gastrointestinal bleeding in the critically ill patient. *Intensive Care Med* 5:1–4, 1979.

Dronfield, MW: Emergency situations: Acute gastrointestinal bleeding. *Br J Hosp Med* 19:97–108, 1978.

Eaves R, Korman MG: Twice-a-day dosage of cimetidine in the short-term treatment of peptic ulcer. *Med J Aust* 2:518–520, 1982.

Green PH, Gold RP, Marboe CC, et al: Chronic erosive gastritis: Clinical, diagnostic, and pathological features in nine patients. *Amer J Gastroenterol* 77:543–547, 1982.

Isenberg JI: H_2-Receptor antagonists in the treatment of peptic ulcer. *Ann Intern Med* 84:212–214, 1976.

Josen AS, Giuliani E, Voorhees AB, et al: Immediate endoscopic diagnosis of gastrointestinal bleeding. *Arch Surg* 111:980–986, 1976.

Lucas CE, Sugawa C, Riddle J, et al: Natural history and surgical dilemma of stress gastric bleeding. *Arch Surg* 102:266–273, 1971.

Midgley RC, Cantor D: Upper gastrointestinal hemorrhage—Diagnosis and management. *West J Med* 127:371–377, 1977.

Mouawad E, Deloof T, Genette F, et al: Open trial of cimetidine in the prevention of upper gastrointestinal haemorrhage in patients with severe intracranial injury. *Acta Neurochir* 67:239–244, 1983.

Northfield TC: Factors predisposing to recurrent hemorrhage after acute gastrointestinal bleeding. *Br Med J* 2:26–28, 1971.

Plamer ED: The vigorous diagnosis of upper gastrointestinal hemorrhage. *JAMA* 207:1477–1480, 1969.

Sedgwick CE, Reale VF: Upper gastrointestinal bleeding: Diagnosis and treatment. *Surg Clin North Am* 56:695–707, 1976.

Simonian SJ, Curtis LE: Treatment of hemorrhagic gastritis by antacid. *Ann Surg* 184:429–434, 1976.

CHAPTER 58
PERFORATED VISCUS

Ronald L. Krome

Nontraumatic perforation of the gastrointestinal (GI) tract is rare if the wall of the viscus is normal. Diligent search will reveal an etiologic factor either involving the wall or leading to rapid, marked increase in the intraluminal pressures. The underlying process may be inflammatory, neoplastic, or stone formation. The presence of an iatrogenic or self-ingested foreign body must be considered if no other obvious cause is present. Whatever organ is involved, the signs and symptoms of perforation are due first to chemical irritation of the peritoneum and then later to infection or sepsis. Therefore, the chemical composition of the contents of the viscus have a significant effect on the development of chemical peritonitis, including the onset and severity.

Sometimes the signs and symptoms of perforation precede those of the underlying disease or in fact may be the first presentation. At other times, there is a symptomatic period relating to the disease process before any signs or symptoms of perforation appear. Although most perforations of the GI tract are free into the peritoneum, they may be localized, walled off by the surrounding viscera or omentum, or they may occur into a limited or restricted space, e.g., the lesser sac. Perforations may also occur into the retroperitoneal space. Symptoms and signs, then, are generally determined by (1) the viscus involved, (2) the location of the perforation, (3) the volume and chemical composition of the leaking fluids, (4) the underlying disease, and (5) the host response mechanism.

Unless the patient has some significant contraindication, surgical intervention is indicated at the time of the diagnosis. One hopes that such intervention will occur before any significant contamination or sepsis has occurred.

PATHOPHYSIOLOGY

The combined surface area of the peritoneum (visceral and parietal) constitutes at least 50 percent of the area of the exterior body surface. Contact of intestinal contents with the peritoneum produces a sudden increase in capillary permeability with the subsequent exudation of large volumes of plasma into the peritoneal cavity, the bowel lumen, and the bowel wall and mesentery. As much as 4 to 12 L can be shifted into this "third space" within 24 h.

Inflammation of the visceral peritoneum produces a brief period of bowel irritability and hypermotility followed by bowel atony with paralytic (adynamic) ileus and distention. The inflamed bowel no longer absorbs fluid and secretes increased salt and water into the lumen. When distention becomes sufficient to compress capillaries and prevent, or compromise, circulation to the inflamed area, exudation ceases. The ultimate picture is one of severe hypovolemia and shock.

Hypovolemia, if severe enough, results in inadequate cardiac output, compensatory vasoconstriction, and inadequate tissue perfusion. Oliguria, severe metabolic acidosis, and respiratory insufficiency follow if the situation is not remedied rapidly. The peritonitis and resulting septicemia may evolve into septic shock. Because of the fluid loss into the third space, significant correction of the volume depletion is mandatory even in the presence of septic shock.

The local response to bacterial invasion from intestinal perforation is complex. Bacterial contamination is generally necessary to produce fatal peritonitis. Endotoxins and exotoxins increase cell permeability and compound the already significant fluid losses into the third space.

Distal obstruction, the amount of contamination, the elapsed time prior to the institution of treatment, and the host response to infection account for the variations in the clinical response to perforation.

PERFORATED ULCER

Gastric or duodenal perforations develop most commonly in benign rather than malignant ulcers, although malignant gastric ulcers may also perforate. Chemical peritonitis develops in the first 6 to 8 h and is due to the effect of the gastric acid and pepsin on the peritoneum.

In general, posterior duodenal ulcers penetrate into the pancreas rather than freely perforate into the peritoneum, and this produces pancreatitis. Free perforation is prevented because of the adherence of the pancreas to the posterior duodenum. Posterior gastric or duodenal ulcers may perforate into the lesser sac, resulting in abscess formation.

Anterior ulcers generally perforate into the peritoneal cavity, although the omentum may be adherent to the ulcer bed and limit the signs and symptoms. An antecedent history of ulcer disease is not always present, and perforation is not uncommonly the first manifestation of the disease. If carefully sought, though, a history of antacid use, mostly of over-the-counter preparations, will be found.

The pain of ulcer perforation is usually sudden and severe. The patient may even be able to give the exact time of onset. The pain is usually localized to the epigastric region, although if penetrating or posterior, it may radiate straight through to the back (not around to the back).

Upper GI bleeding of magnitude does not accompany perforation. Whatever bleeding occurs is minimal. Chronic blood loss may occur if the ulcer has been present for any length of time. Massive upper GI bleeding, as a rule of thumb, rules out the presence of a perforated ulcer.

GALLBLADDER PERFORATION

This is an uncommon problem. Perforation of the gallbladder, when it does occur, is associated with a high mortality. Peritonitis is the result of chemical irritation of the peritoneum as well as bacterial contamination. Of the two, bacterial contamination is more significant. Chemical irritation is due primarily to the cholate fraction of the bile.

Obstruction of the cystic or common bile duct by stones produces distention of the gallbladder with eventual compromise of the vascular supply and gangrene of the wall with perforation. The stones can erode through the wall of the gallbladder, cystic duct, or common duct. Such erosions more commonly produce fistulas between the gallbladder and another portion of the GI tract than free perforation into the peritoneal cavity. Large gallstones have been found to produce obstruction of the small bowel after such fistula formation, resulting in a syndrome known as *gallstone ileus.*

Gangrene can occur in the gallbladder free of stones, and perforations have been reported in acalculous cholecystitis, especially in diabetics.

Those most at risk are the elderly, the diabetic, those with atherosclerotic cardiovascular disease, and those with a history of stones and repeated cholecystitis. Perforations have also been reported in patients with sickle cell disease or hemolytic anemias. Infection is often associated with cystic or common bile duct obstruction and stone formation.

The diagnosis is often difficult. Although not always present, antecedent signs and symptoms of biliary disease should be actively sought. Gallbladder perforation should be suspected in an elderly patient with a tender right upper quadrant mass, fever, and leukocytosis who is deteriorating clinically or who develops signs of peritonitis. The bilirubin level may be elevated, and slight elevation of the amylase level is not unusual. Nonalcoholics may give a past history of episodes of jaundice or pancreatitis, which should suggest the possible presence of common duct stones. Subhepatic or subphrenic abscesses may form as a result of perforation of the gallbladder. The patient's temperature curve will demonstrate the typical pattern of an abscess if this occurs. Movement of the right leaf of the diaphragm may be restricted in the presence of either a subhepatic or a subphrenic abscess.

In this day and age, even in seriously ill patients, given the usual diagnostic accuracy of ultrasonography, this procedure should be performed in all patients suspected of having stones.

PERFORATION OF THE SMALL BOWEL

Nontraumatic perforations of the mid-GI tract are very uncommon. Jejunal rupture may result from certain drugs such as enteric-coated potassium tablets which produce ulcerations of the small bowel; infections, such as typhoid or tuberculosis; tumors; strangulated hernia, either internal or external; and rarely, regional enteritis.

In general, jejunal perforation produces a more severe chemical peritonitis than ileal rupture since the pancreatic juice that leaks out of the upper jejunum has a pH of about 8 and is rich in enzymes such as trypsin, lipase, and amylase. Fluid that leaks from lower jejunal and ileal perforations has less enzymatic activity, and the pH may also be lower. If, however, perforation is the result of obstruction, as in appendicitis followed by perforation, the clinical course is likely to be serious regardless of the level of perforation. This is because of the effect of the duration of the obstruction and the underlying inflammatory disease process.

Perforations of the jejunum and ileum, especially if due to regional enteritis, may become quickly walled off, and signs of generalized peritonitis may be delayed. Acute symptoms are limited in time. Free air may be detected on radiologic examination, or air may be seen in a retroperitoneal location, or in the wall of the bowel. There is a shift to the left and an elevated white blood cell count; the serum amylase level may also be elevated. Metabolic acidosis may be present. Tachycardia and fever elevation are common. The abdomen may be distended. Hypoactive bowel sounds are present. Tenderness, rebound, guarding, and rigidity, usually associated with peritonitis, may all be absent, especially in the elderly. Perforations of the appendix are more likely in the extremes of age and if symptoms are prolonged prior to exploration.

PERFORATION OF THE LARGE BOWEL

Nontraumatic perforations of the lower GI tract are most commonly the result of diverticulitis, carcinoma, colitis, and foreign bodies. Perforations of the colon produce signs and symptoms predominantly due to sepsis as opposed to chemical irritation.

Carcinoma of the large bowel detected by a perforation has a higher mortality than carcinoma detected because of obstruction, changes in bowel habits, or bleeding. If there is no obstruction, the more proximal the perforation, the more serious the clinical picture, probably because with more proximal rupture, the fecal stream is more liquid and disseminates rapidly. An antecedent history of partial or complete obstruction, change in bowel habits, and other findings consistent with carcinoma should be sought.

Perforation secondary to obstruction, as in carcinoma of the colon or acute diverticulitis with abscess formation, may be associated with a temporary amelioration of the abdominal pain because the local distention has been relieved, although this is not common. Perforation in diverticulitis is usually the result of abscess formation, so that signs and symptoms of the abscess, and a mass, may predominate. Perforation resulting from carcinoma is the result of erosion of the carcinoma and not rupture of a normal bowel wall. This is quickly followed, however, by evidence of peritonitis, hypovolemia, and sepsis.

Clinical Features

Usually vomiting is present. Bile in the vomitus indicates that the pylorus is open and that gastric outlet obstruction is not present. Coffee-ground vomitus may be present in patients with duodenal or gastric ulcer, or even in patients in whom common duct or cystic duct stones erode into the duodenum or stomach. A feculent smelling and looking drainage from the nasogastric tube, or vomiting of that sort of material, may indicate the presence of a long-standing small bowel obstruction or the presence of dead bowel. Abdominal distention, the inability to pass gas, and constipation are all signs and symptoms of the accompanying ileus or bowel obstruction.

Fever, tachycardia, a narrowed pulse pressure, oliguria, and tachypnea are signs of hypovolemia and sepsis. A fall in blood pressure usually indicates the presence of the full-blown shock state. Aggressive fluid therapy should occur before shock develops, while the patient's vital signs, including the urinary output, are monitored. Fluid correction and aggressive treatment of sepsis are a part of the resuscitation process in the emergency department, but often resuscitation cannot be completed until surgical intervention has occurred.

Marked tenderness is frequently detected on abdominal examination, usually accompanied with rebound tenderness over the area of inflammation. Rigidity is also present if generalized peritonitis has developed. Pain is aggravated by any motion of the patient, including sneezing and coughing. The patient frequently lies in the fetal position to reduce the pain by minimizing the tension on the peritoneum.

When rebound tenderness is present, it is usually referred to the area of perforation. Guarding is an unreliable sign. Bowel sounds are absent if adynamic ileus has developed as a result of the inflammation. If early obstruction is present, then the bowel sounds may be hyperactive. When the obstruction is long-standing, the bowel sounds disappear. If free air has accumulated, there may be a loss of liver dullness to percussion.

When a great deal of fluid is present in the peritoneum, then shifting dullness may be found. Rectal and pelvic examinations are essential to determine if any pelvic or lower abdominal masses are present, or if tenderness can be elicited.

Laboratory studies may be of little help. Leukocytosis with a

shift to the left is common. The blood urea nitrogen (BUN) level may be elevated if the degree of dehydration is significant. Electrolyte imbalance is frequent. Respiratory alkalosis is present early on in sepsis. Metabolic acidosis follows if the hypovolemia and sepsis are uncorrected. A mild elevation of the amylase level does not necessarily reflect pancreatitis since such elevations frequently accompany perforation, especially of the small bowel.

In cases in which the diagnosis of peritonitis is uncertain, peritoneal lavage may be useful. The fluid should be analyzed for blood, bacteria, bile, white blood cells, feces, and amylase. A Gram stain should be done, and a specimen should be sent for both aerobic and anaerobic culture. Of course, lavage may not be possible in the presence of surgical scars or marked abdominal distention.

Chest x-rays, upright if possible, should be made to rule out the presence of thoracic disease, and/or to detect free air under the diaphragm (Fig. 58-1). The leaves of the diaphragm are much more clearly demonstrated on this view. The left lateral decubitus film of the abdomen may also be helpful in detecting free air. In either case, the patient should be left in position for 10 min before obtaining the films.

The abdominal x-rays may show air-fluid levels in a stepladder pattern indicating the presence of mechanical obstruction, or simply dilated loops of bowel indicating adynamic ileus (Fig. 58-2). Air along the biliary tract may be present if a gallstone has eroded into the small or large bowel. Neighboring loops of bowel may be widely separated if the intestinal walls are edematous.

If free air is suspected but not detected, 200 mL of air can be instilled into the stomach through the nasogastric tube. The tube is then clamped. A sump tube cannot be used for this purpose unless both ports are clamped. The x-rays should then be repeated

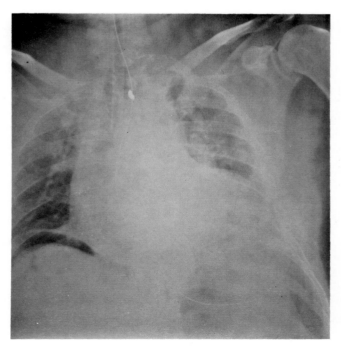

Figure 58-1. Perforated viscus as shown in upright chest film. (Courtesy of Detroit General Hospital.)

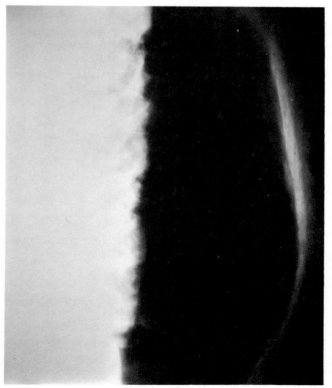

Figure 58-2. Perforated viscus as shown in cross-table lateral film of abdomen. (Courtesy of Detroit General Hospital.)

in about 10 to 15 min. The psoas shadows may be obscured by the presence of fluid in the abdomen or in the retroperitoneal space. If there is a distinct lack of gas in the intestine, dead bowel may be present.

Intravenous cholangiography or ultrasonography may be necessary to rule out the presence of cystic or common duct stones. The value of CT scanning in this area remains to be demonstrated. There is some suggestion that CT scanning may be helpful in detecting masses in the mesentery or adjacent to organs and that the procedure therefore can be used to indicate that perforation and abscess formation has occurred. Technetium-99m-labeled iminodiacetic acid hepatobiliary scans have been reported to show gallbladder perforations. These studies may not be universally available.

Treatment

Fluid resuscitation is mandatory as quickly as possible. It must be vigorous. In general, a balanced electrolyte solution should be used. Central venous pressure (CVP) and hourly urinary output should be monitored, in addition to the pulse and blood pressure, in continuous assessment of the patient's volume status. In the presence of blood loss, transfusions may be necessary. Nasogastric tube insertion should be done quickly, even if the diagnosis is suspected but not established. It can always be removed later. If left out until problems develop from distention or aspiration, there will be significant morbidity for the patient. Broad-spectrum antibiotics are indicated intravenously when the diagnosis of perforation is suspected. The particular antibiotics used should be discussed with the surgical consultant. Operative intervention is indicated as soon as possible, unless the risk of surgery exceeds the risk of death from the perforation.

BIBLIOGRAPHY

Ching EC, ReMine WH: Surgical management of emergency complications of duodenal ulcer. *Surg Clin North Am* 51:851–855, 1971.

Davis JH: Current concepts of peritonitis. *Am Surg* 33:673–681, 1967.

Donaldson GA, Welch JP: Management of cancer of the colon. *Surg Clin North Am* 54:713–731, 1974.

Donovan AJ, Vinson TL, Maulsby GO, et al: Selective treatment of duodenal ulcer with perforation. *Ann Surg* 189:627–636, 1979.

Emanuel B, Zlotnik P, Raffensperger JG: Perforation of the gastrointestinal tract in infancy and childhood. *Surg Gynecol Obstet* 146:926–928, 1978.

Giacobine JW, Silver, VE: Evaluation of diagnostic abdominal paracentesis with experimental and clinical studies. *Surg Gynecol Obstet* 110:676–686, 1960.

Haycock CE, Machtedo G: The use of peritoneal lavage as a diagnostic tool in emergencies. *JACEP* 3:397–400, 1974.

Hinchey EJ, Schaal PGH, Richards GK: Treatment of perforated diverticular disease of the colon. *Adv Surg* 12:85–109, 1978.

Howe HJ: Acute perforation of the sigmoid colon secondary to diverticulitis. *Am J Surg* 137:184–187, 1979.

Kay PH, Moore KTH, Clark, RG: The treatment of perforated duodenal ulcer. *Br J Surg* 65:801–803, 1978.

Koepsell TD, Inui TS, Farewell VT: Factors affecting perforation in acute appendicitis. *Surg Gynecol Obstet* 153:508–510, 1981.

Lee H, Vibhakar SD, Bellon EM: Gastrointestinal perforation: Early diagnosis by computed tomography. *J Comput Assist Tomogr* 7:226–229, 1983.

Marshak RH, Lidner AE, Maklansky D: Diverticulosis and diverticulitis of the colon. *Mt Sinai J Med (NY)* 46:261–276, 1979.

Massie JD, Austin HM, Kuvula M, et al: HIDA scanning and ultrasonography in expeditious diagnosis of acute cholecystitis. *South Med J* 75:164–168, 1982.

Schumer W, Burman SO: The perforated viscus: Diagnosis and treatment. *Surg Clin North Am* 52:231–237, 1972.

Schwesinger WH, Levine BA, Ramos R: Complications of colonoscopy. *Surg Gynecol Obstet* 148:270–281, 1979.

Stephen M, Loewenthal J: Generalized infective peritonitis. *Surg Gynecol Obstet* 147:231–234, 1978.

Taylor R, Weakley FL, Sullivan BH Jr: Nonoperative management of colonoscopic perforation with pneumoperitoneum. *Gastrointest Endosc* 24:124–125, 1978.

Weingart J: Obstruction of the duodenal bulb caused by gallstone perforation. *Endoscopy* 11:190–199, 1979.

Wilson DG, Lieberman LM: Perforation of the gallbladder diagnosed preoperatively. *Eur J Nucl Med* 8:145–147, 1983.

Yajko RD, Norton LW, Eiseman B: Current management of upper gastrointestinal bleeding. *Am Surg* 181:474–480, 1975.

CHAPTER 59
ACUTE APPENDICITIS

Ronald L. Krome

Appendicitis is the most common cause of emergency surgery of the abdomen in the United States and Great Britain, and it remains the most common surgical emergency in pregnancy. Although in the classic case the diagnosis may be straightforward, more often it is difficult. Most difficulty occurs in the very young, the very old, and the pregnant patient. In one study by Janik and Firor, 55 percent of the children under 6 years of age with only 2 days of symptoms had already perforated at the time of operation.

Obstruction of the appendiceal lumen is demonstrable in about 40 percent of cases and generally is caused by a fecalith. Other causes of obstruction include enlarged lymphoid follicles, inspissated barium, worms, tumors, and granulomatous inflammation due to Crohn's disease. Of the tumors, carcinoid is the most common. In the elderly, adenocarcinoma of the appendix has been reported. At least one author has recommended that carcinoma be considered in any patient over 55 years of age with more than 2 days of symptoms. Mucus secretion may produce progressive obstruction, leading to venous stasis, arterial compromise, and bacterial proliferation.

Although acute appendicitis may resolve with the use of intravenous antibiotics, more likely gangrene, perforation, and abscess formation will occur. Complications of abscess formation include septicemia and the development of fistulas between the appendix and the small bowel, large bowel, or bladder.

Despite the use of antibiotics and aggressive fluid resuscitation, perforation with subsequent abscess formation still occurs with alarming frequency. The essentials of successful management include early diagnosis, short preoperative resuscitation, and early surgical intervention.

CLINICAL FEATURES

The classic picture consists of (1) anorexia, (2) periumbilical or epigastric crampy pain, followed by nausea and vomiting, and (3) the development of severe, steady pain that eventually shifts to the right lower quadrant. The pain may radiate to the testicle or flank, especially if the appendix is in the retrocecal position. This picture is present in about 60 percent of patients. In general, the symptoms are present for less than a day, but in the very young and the very old they may last considerably longer. In patients who are over 40 years of age, the symptoms last longer in those who have perforated than in those who have not. Delay from admission to surgery tends to be longer in the elderly and is more often associated with perforation.

Anorexia is such a common symptom that its absence should lead one to question the diagnosis. Nausea and vomiting probably occur in one-half to two-thirds of patients. Symptoms in 53 patients over 40 with proven appendicitis are listed in Table 59-1.

At some time in the course of the process, pain is generally present in the area overlying the appendix. Careful history taking often extracts the information that the pain began in a more central location. Although left-sided appendicitis is exceedingly rare, it can occur if one of the following is present: situs inversus viscerum, malrotation of the gut, hypermobile cecum, or an extremely long appendix that crosses the midline.

Occasionally patients also have diarrhea or constipation. A prolonged history of intermittent episodes of diarrhea and constipation may be an indication that the patient has diverticulosis and the acute episode, in fact, represents an episode of acute diverticulitis. Regional enteritis may, of course, present exactly like acute appendicitis.

In women, a complete gynecologic history is mandatory. A number of gynecologic problems can present in a fashion similar to that of acute appendicitis, and their differentiation may be exceedingly difficult. Tubo-ovarian abscess, acute salpingitis, ruptured corpus luteal cyst, and ectopic pregnancy are among the more common gynecologic problems that must be considered. According to Lewis et al., the development of pain within 7 days of menses suggests the presence of pelvic inflammatory disease, while the development of pain 8 days or later suggests the diagnosis of appendicitis.

A urologic history should also be obtained since renal colic, pyelonephritis, and cystitis may mimic acute appendicitis. There

Table 59-1. Symptoms in Acute Appendicitis in Patients Over 40

Symptom	No.	%
RLQ pain	31	58
Nausea	26	49
Vomiting	24	45
Anorexia	19	36
Crampy abdominal pain	10	18
General pain—RLQ	9	17
Umbilical pain—RLQ	6	11
Diarrhea	6	11
Constipation	5	9
Fever	3	6

Source: Adapted from Stair T, Corlette MB: Appendicitis over forty. *Ann Emerg Med* 9:77, 1980.

are times when the inflamed appendix may overlie the ureter, further confusing the picture, because these patients may have red cells, white cells, and even bacteria in their urine specimens.

The temperature elevation is usually low-grade, i.e., a temperature of 37.7 to 38.3°C (100 to 101°F), unless localized or diffuse peritonitis is present. Fever may be present in fewer than half of the patients with rebound tenderness. In a large study of pediatric patients with acute appendicitis, the mean temperature was found to be 38.2°C (100.1°F). The temperature elevation does not appear to correlate with the presence or absence of perforation.

Right lower quadrant tenderness is most often present with appendicitis which has not yet perforated, or when only localized peritonitis exists. However, right lower quadrant tenderness may also occur with salpingitis, mesenteric adenitis, gastroenteritis, or even when nonspecific abdominal pain is present. The subsequent development of diffuse abdominal tenderness should suggest that perforation has occurred and that generalized peritonitis is present.

Rebound tenderness in the right lower quadrant, when present, is strongly suggestive of acute appendicitis. It is not, however, invariably present. In the series reported by Lewis et al., rebound tenderness was present in 48 percent of the patients who did not have acute appendicitis. The specific diagnoses in these cases were not listed, but pelvic inflammatory disease appeared to account for a large portion.

When the acute process has been present for some time, ileus may develop. Therefore, the bowel sounds may be diminished or absent. In general, however, the bowel sounds are of little help in establishing the diagnosis, except when entertaining the presence of an obstructing lesion.

Rectal examination must be done in all patients, and a pelvic examination in all women, except when there is no history of any sexual experiences. There may be little or no abdominal tenderness when the appendix is located in the retrocecal or pelvic positions. Tenderness, therefore, in the appropriate area on either rectal or pelvic examination can be helpful in establishing the diagnosis, although not pathognomonic of acute appendicitis. Lewis et al. noted rectal tenderness in 45 to 60 percent of their patients, regardless of the diagnosis. A rectal or pelvic mass may indicate the presence of a pelvic abscess.

Cervical tenderness on motion, the classic finding in acute pelvic inflammatory disease, may be present with acute appendicitis.

The white blood cell count is generally elevated, with the highest elevations occurring with perforation, usually in the area of 18,000. The white blood cell elevation is not of great help in establishing the diagnosis of acute appendicitis. The majority of patients do have a shift to the left, even when the count is not elevated.

Urinalysis should be done in all patients, since those with urinary tract infections, especially pyelonephritis, can present with a picture similar to that of acute appendicitis, including the finding of rebound tenderness in the right lower quadrant. If the appendix overlies the ureter, pyuria and hematuria can result even in the absence of a urinary tract infection, so that the laboratory results must be judged in light of the clinical picture.

Radiographs of the abdomen and chest, although frequently made, are not very helpful in establishing the diagnosis; they are more helpful in eliminating the presence of diseases that may mimic appendicitis. Such processes as small bowel obstruction or ureteral calculi may be eliminated by x-ray examination. Nonspecific findings in acute appendicitis include a sentinel loop in the right lower quadrant; dilatation of the cecum with air-fluid levels;

obliteration of the right psoas shadow, especially if perforation has occurred; scoliosis of the lumbar spine with curvature from the right; air in the appendix, or air bubbles in a right lower quadrant mass; and accumulation of fluid between the colon and the flank stripe. A calcified appendicolith has been reported in as many as 50 percent of children and 10 percent of adults with acute appendicitis (Fig. 59-1).

If the diagnosis is in doubt, a very cautious barium enema can be given. Nonfilling of the appendix is considered a presumptive sign of acute appendicitis, although exceptions can occur since not all cases of appendicitis are associated with luminal obstruction. Perforation may decompress the lumen and allow retrograde filling with barium; partial filling of a gangrenous or necrotic appendix can occur; or partial filling of a very long, inflamed appendix may be interpreted as complete and normal filling of the appendix.

Ultrasound has been used in some centers, generally to help make the differential diagnosis regarding the presence of a right lower quadrant mass, or a pelvic mass. It may also be helpful in women in distinguishing appendicitis from a tubo-ovarian abscess, or ectopic pregnancy.

Appendicitis in Pregnancy

Acute appendicitis during pregnancy presents a difficult and unique situation. As pregnancy progresses, the appendix moves to a more superior and lateral position. Consequently, the region of maximum tenderness, and the area of most pain, shifts from the right

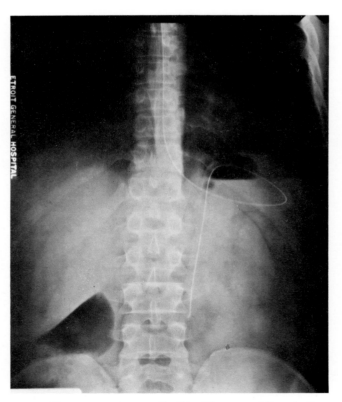

Figure 59-1. Calcified appendicolith. (Courtesy of Detroit General Hospital.)

lower quadrant to a more subcostal (right) position. Guarding may be absent or minimal. Gomez found that 88 percent of his patients had symptoms for less than 24 h. Nausea, vomiting, and anorexia were the most common. Most had right lower quadrant pain. Although he reported no fetal mortality in his study population, it has been reported in the 8 percent area, with a mortality as high as 30 percent when peritonitis was present. Acute appendicitis is most common during the second trimester of pregnancy.

Missed Diagnosis

When a normal appendix is found at the time of exploration, the most common diagnoses are probably mesenteric adenitis, gastroenteritis, nonspecific abdominal pain, or an acute gynecologic problem. In Lewis's series, one of these accounted for an erroneous diagnosis in one-third of the women and two-thirds of the men. The histories tended to be similar to that of acute appendicitis, but the tenderness was not as well localized to the right lower quadrant, and rebound was not as common.

Pelvic inflammatory disease is a very common missed diagnosis. The duration of symptoms is usually longer than in acute appendicitis, nausea and vomiting are not as common, and anorexia is often absent. Physical findings and laboratory studies are not usually helpful in distinguishing the two unless bilateral lower quadrant tenderness and/or cervical motion tenderness is present.

TREATMENT

In the United States, surgical intervention is the treatment of choice for all cases diagnosed as acute appendicitis. The patient suspected of having acute appendicitis must be given nothing orally. Intravenous fluids should be administered to maintain current needs and to correct any deficits that may be present. A nasogastric tube should be inserted. Antibiotics are indicated if perforation is suspected, but only after the commitment for surgical intervention is made. The incidence of wound infection, intraabdominal abscess, or perforation has not been shown to decrease with the prophylactic use of antibiotics. Any delay in operation increases the possibility of perforation and increases morbidity and mortality.

BIBLIOGRAPHY

Ackerman NB: The continuing problems of perforated appendicitis. *Surg Gynecol Obstet* 139:29–32, 1974.

Ackerman NB: Acute appendicitis in pregnancy. *Br Med J* 4:668–669, 1975.

Bonello JC, Abrams JS: The significance of a "positive" rectal examination in acute appendicitis. *Dis Colon Rectum* 22:97–101, 1979.

Brewer RJ, Golden GT, Hitch DC, et al: Abdominal pain: An analysis of 1000 consecutive cases in a university hospital emergency room. *Am J Surg* 133:219–223, 1976.

Fee HJ Jr, Jones PC, Kadell B, et al: Radiologic diagnosis of Appendicitis. *Arch Surg* 112:742–744, 1977.

Gilmore OJA, Browett JP, Griffin PH, et al: Appendicitis and mimicking conditions. *Lancet* 2:421–424, 1975.

Gomez A, Wood M: Acute appendicitis during pregnancy. *Am J Surg* 137:180–183, 1979.

Janik JS, Firor HV: Pediatric appendicitis: A 20-year study of 1,640 children at Cook County (Illinois) Hospital. *Arch Surg* 114:717–719, 1979.

Jordan FT, Mazzeo RJ, Hoshal VL Jr: Primary adenocarcinoma of the appendix. Can preoperative or intraoperative diagnosis be made? *Am Surg* 49:278–281, 1983

Law D, Law R, Eiseman B: The continuing challenge of acute and perforated appendicitis. *Am J Surg* 131:533–535, 1976.

Lewis FR, Holcroft JW, Boey J, et al: Appendicitis: A critical review of diagnosis and treatment in 1,000 cases. *Arch Surg* 110:677–684, 1975.

Marchildon MB, Dudgeon DL: Perforated appendicitis: Current experience in a children's hospital. *Ann Surg* 185:84–87, 1977.

Neuhauser EBD: Acute appendicitis: The x-ray examination. *Postgrad Med* 45:64–66, 1969.

Owens BJ, Hamit HF: Appendicitis in the elderly. *Am Surg* 187:392–396, 1978.

Parulekar SG: Ultrasonographic findings in diseases of the appendix. *J Ultrasound Med* 2:59–64, 1983.

Rajagopalan AE, Mason JH, Kennedy M, et al: The value of the barium enema in the diagnosis of acute appendicitis. *Arch Surg* 112:531–533, 1977.

Shimkin PM: Radiology of acute appendicitis. *Am J Roentgenol* 120:1001–1004, 1978.

Skoulas A, Steinhardt D, Chow CC: Appendicitis with symptoms in the left lower quadrant (letter to the editor). *JAMA* 225:638, 1973.

Smith DE, Jacquet JM, Virgilio RW: Left upper quadrant appendicitis. *Arch Surg* 109:443–447, 1974.

Stair T, Corlette MB: Appendicitis over forty. *Ann Emerg Med* 9:76–78, 1980.

Threatt BA, Appelman H: Crohn's disease of the appendix presenting as acute appendicitis. *Radiology* 110:313–317, 1974.

CHAPTER 60
INTESTINAL
OBSTRUCTION

Ronald L. Krome

Mechanical bowel obstruction occurs when there is a physical limitation to the bowel lumen and may result from either an extrinsic or an intrinsic lesion.

The overall mortality from mechanical bowel obstruction is estimated at 10 percent, with mortality determined by the development of complications, the duration of the obstruction, and the presence of concurrent disease in addition to the cause of the obstruction.

The most common cause of small bowel obstruction in the United States is adhesions resulting from surgery. Hernias, primarily inguinal, are the second leading cause. Although neoplasms, both benign and malignant, may cause small bowel obstruction, most often when neoplasms are the cause, they are extrinsic and the result of carcinomatosis. Intussusception, although rare in adults, may also occur.

Large bowel obstruction is most commonly, depending on the patient's age, caused by neoplasms. Mortalities are higher when tumors are the cause than when adhesions are the cause. Tumors that produce large bowel obstruction are generally located on the left side of the colon; blood loss is the most common sign of right-sided tumors.

Anything that produces abscesses can result in large bowel obstruction. When an abscess is present, it may be extremely difficult to differentiate it from a tumor.

Other causes of large bowel obstruction include cecal volvulus, sigmoid volvulus (more common), and Crohn's disease. Fecal impaction must be considered in the differential diagnosis in an elderly patient with bowel obstruction. The fecal impaction need not be in the rectum but can be higher in the colon. Consequently, rectal examination may not be helpful. To further complicate the diagnosis, these patients may have temperature elevation, vomiting, and watery diarrhea, all of which occur in patients whose bowel obstruction has other causes. Fecal impactions can also occur in patients who abuse narcotics, patients who are in nursing homes or psychiatric facilities, and those with neurologic diseases.

PATHOPHYSIOLOGY

Mechanical bowel obstruction occurs when the lumen of the bowel is compromised either completely or partially. Strangulation oc-

curs when either the arterial supply or the venous drainage of a segment of the bowel is compromised. Gangrene does not occur until vascular occlusion is complete.

A closed-loop obstruction occurs when the efferent and afferent loops of a segment of bowel are occluded. This can occur, for example, in the presence of a completely obstructing carcinoma of the colon if the ileocecal valve is competent. Pressure in the occluded loop rises quickly, compromising the venous drainage of the loop, resulting in gangrene and perforation. The signs of vascular collapse may be present before it is clinically evident that the patient has bowel obstruction. Volvulus is also associated with the closed-loop syndrome.

Perforation does not generally occur if the bowel is normal even if the obstruction is long-standing. Microscopic areas of gangrene develop as the distention progresses, and these are the areas that perforate. Perhaps one exception to this is in the cecum. Marked distention of the cecum can result in perforation even though gross gangrene is not present.

The local and systemic effects of bowel obstruction are generally the result of the accumulation of gas and fluids proximal to the obstruction. Bowel distention, disordered bowel motility, the absorption of systemic toxins, bacterial proliferation, and the diapedesis of bacteria across the distended bowel wall are all part of the picture of long-standing bowel obstruction. The distention develops because of the intestinal gas from swallowed air which cannot pass, and the presence of bacteria. Intestinal bacteria may seep across the bowel wall, even when the wall is intact, if the bowel is distended. The likelihood of bacterial seepage is increased when the vascular supply, venous or arterial, is impaired. Even in the absence of frank perforation, peritonitis and sepsis may result.

With early bowel obstruction, hyperperistalsis proximal to the level of obstruction may be intense enough that it contributes to bowel wall edema. The hyperperistalsis is responsible for the hyperactive bowel sounds heard on physical examination. Although peristalsis may also continue distal to the obstruction, it is not contiguous with the waves which begin proximal to the obstruction. This distal peristalsis may account for the continued propulsion of bowel contents, and the passage of flatus and stool may persist for a time following the development of the obstruction. The stool may be liquid.

In mechanical obstruction, peristalsis is normal until late in the course of the disease. Peristalsis continues even though the obstruction may not permit the passage of the bowel contents. In paralytic (adynamic) ileus, there is an abnormality of peristalsis as a result of either an inflammatory process or long-standing bowel obstruction. The inflammatory processes producing the ileus may involve the bowel directly or indirectly; in such cases peristalsis is diminished or absent. When bowel obstruction is long-standing, peristalsis is also diminished or absent, making differentiation between the two difficult at times. Early on, however, differentiation can be made based on the presence or absence of bowel sounds. X-rays are not diagnostic until differential air-fluid levels are seen, representing mechanical obstruction.

If the obstruction is uncorrected, venous compromise ensues, followed by arterial compromise, resulting in bowel wall infarction and perforation. Bacterial exotoxin or endotoxin and/or toxic breakdown products are absorbed, and this eventually leads to peritonitis and sepsis. Fluid accumulation in the obstructed and distended bowel may be significant enough to produce fluid and electrolyte losses of significant proportions.

Fluid and electrolyte losses can occur for other reasons as well. Fluid accumulation in the bowel wall related to edema may be significant. Intestinal fluid may exude across the bowel wall into the peritoneum, producing significant extracellular fluid accumulations. There is substantial fluid loss, with concomitant electrolyte depletion, as a result of vomiting and/or nasogastric suction. The hypovolemia resulting from these combined losses complicates the already compromised state of the patient in respect to the development of sepsis. Correction requires aggressive fluid replacement.

Colonic obstruction usually does not result in strangulation; this is more likely in small bowel obstruction. In addition, the large bowel is not as secretory or absorptive as the small bowel, so that large-volume fluid depletion is not as likely in cases of obstruction of the former as in cases of obstruction of the latter. From the therapeutic aspect, however, fluid replacement should be based on the patient's vital signs and urinary output, as well as on the central venous pressure monitoring which may be done. The most dangerous aspect of large bowel obstruction is perforation, with resulting soilage of the peritoneal cavity. Perforation may involve the cecum when solely on the basis of distention, provided the ileocecal valve is competent. The greatest tension on the wall occurs in the area of greatest diameter. Bowel wall infarction may act as a functional mechanical bowel obstruction since peristaltic waves are not transmitted through the infarcted segment.

CLINICAL FEATURES

Small bowel obstruction should be suspected in any patient with abdominal pain between the epigastrium and hypogastrium. In the presence of an abdominal surgical incision, the possibility becomes greater; the same is true if an inguinal hernia is present, although all external hernias should be suspected. Especially in the elderly, however, mesenteric ischemia or infarction should also be considered. Patients with lower abdominal pain, especially if elderly, should be considered to have colonic obstruction. Perineal pain may be a symptom of rectosigmoid obstruction. The pain of bowel obstruction is initially crampy and intermittent; as the obstruction persists and progresses, the pain becomes diffuse and generalized.

Vomiting frequently accompanies bowel obstruction; the higher the lesion, the sooner the vomiting develops and the greater its frequency. It is less common with large bowel obstruction and may not occur until the distention has extended to involve the small bowel. When bilious vomitus is present, whatever obstruction is present must be distal to the pylorus. The common duct enters the duodenum distal to the pylorus; for bile to be present in the vomitus, the pylorus must be open. Feculent vomitus may occur in the presence of lower small bowel obstruction, or in the presence of long-standing large bowel obstruction with incompetence of the ileocecal valve. If feculent vomitus is present, the obstruction should always be considered to be long-standing, or dead bowel should be considered to be already present.

The failure to pass flatus and stool is indicative of complete obstruction. In partial (incomplete) obstruction, both flatus and liquid stool can be passed. Even in the presence of complete obstruction, solid stool and flatus can be passed because of peristalsis distal to the obstruction.

In paralytic (adynamic) ileus, there is, by definition, an absence of peristalsis, and consequently stool and flatus are not passed. Bowel sounds are absent virtually from the beginning of the process. In mechanical obstruction, bowel sounds consist of high-pitched, tinkling rushes. Of course, in the late stages of mechanical obstruction, the bowel sounds disappear.

As time and the process proceed, abdominal distention becomes increasingly evident. If, however, the obstruction is a high-level small bowel or closed loop, the distention may be difficult to detect. Tenderness varies but is generally present. Guarding, a reflection of the pain felt by the patient, is not a reliable sign. Rebound tenderness and boardlike rigidity develop if peritonitis is present.

Rectal examination is a mandatory part of the evaluation of all patients with abdominal pain. It may establish the presence of fecal impaction, rectal tumors, or pelvic abscesses. Stool, if present, should be tested for blood, since even tumors that do not produce significant blood loss may be associated with sufficient bleeding to be detected on rectal examination. The absence of stool in the rectum is not an indication that complete obstruction is present. Following rectal examination, abdominal films may show air in the rectum or even in the sigmoid. Air in the rectum following rectal examination cannot be used to decide on the presence of an obstruction.

Pelvic examination is an integral part of the examination in women with significant abdominal pain. Pelvic abscesses may produce external mechanical obstruction by compressing the lumen of the bowel.

In thin patients, if hyperperistalsis is present, inspection may demonstrate the waves passing through the distended bowel. Cecal volvulus should be suspected when the bowel sounds are absent in the right lower quadrant and a sausage-shaped mass is found in the left upper quadrant. When there is a mass in the right upper quadrant, then a sigmoid volvulus may be present.

LABORATORY FINDINGS

Generally, laboratory findings reflect the degree of fluid loss with the associated electrolyte disturbances and acid-base imbalances. Leukocytosis ($>20,000/mm^3$) with a shift to the left is, of course, indicative of the presence of an inflammatory process and can occur with bowel gangrene, perforation, vascular occlusion, or an abscess. The serum amylase level is frequently mildly elevated in the presence of obstructed bowel. This elevation is primarily due to regurgitation from the pancreas or the systemic absorption of pancreatic enzymes from the ischemic bowel wall.

Elevation of the blood urea nitrogen (BUN) level correlates with the degree of dehydration or the presence of blood in the bowel lumen. The more complete and long-standing the obstruction, the more severe the dehydration is. Vomiting compounds the patient's dehydration, acid-base imbalance, and electrolyte disturbances. Dehydration and hypovolemia are reflected in the patient's vital signs and general physical appearance before any significant rise in the BUN.

Leukocytosis, elevation of the BUN, tachycardia, tachypnea, and elevated temperature, with or without a decrease in the blood pressure, are signs of toxicity and require vigorous fluid resuscitation. Decreased urinary output, monitored as part of the continuing evaluation of the patient, is an additional clue to the development of toxicity and sepsis. Broad-spectrum antibiotics, in keeping with local practice, are indicated.

Initial radiographic studies should include flat and upright views of the abdomen and radiographs of the chest. When possible, an upright radiograph of the chest should be obtained to rule out the presence of free air. The presence of air-fluid levels, with a stepladder pattern on the upright film, is considered fairly diagnostic of mechanical obstruction (Fig. 60-1). The presence of dilated loops of bowel without air-fluid levels is not diagnostic. Air in the rectum and/or sigmoid colon after a rectal examination does not help in deciding if a complete obstruction is present. There are times when dilated loops of bowel are present and ter-minate at the point of an obstruction, and this should be used as a clue to the diagnosis.

Sigmoidoscopic examination is a part of the diagnostic evaluation of patients with suspected obstruction, especially when the diagnosis is obscure. In general, sigmoidoscopic examination should be done before barium examination, so that the radiologist is aware of the results. If completely occluding lesions are seen, a barium enema examination may not even be necessary. Biopsy should not be done before barium enema examination because of the possibility of perforation.

During sigmoidoscopic examination, the examiner should not only look for masses, but should also look at the mucosa. Friable, erythematous mucosa, with or without a granular appearance, may be indicative of an underlying inflammatory disease. Dark blue, or frankly gangrenous mucosa is present when dead bowel, or bowel with compromised vascular supply, is entered with the sigmoidoscope.

If perforation of the bowel occurs during the sigmoidoscopic examination, the patient generally complains of the sudden onset of diffuse nonspecific abdominal pain. An upright chest x-ray may demonstrate free air under the diaphragm. A barium enema examination shows extravasation of the contrast material.

Barium enema examination is helpful in determining not only the presence of large bowel obstruction, but also its cause. Sooner or later every patient suspected of having a mechanical bowel obstruction needs to have such barium studies. The flexible colonoscope has not yet achieved widespread emergency use. The hazards of a barium enema examination include perforation, especially of already damaged bowel, or if a biopsy has been done; and the theoretical possibility of converting a partial bowel obstruction to a complete one with inspissated barium. A barium meal with small bowel follow-through may be useful if a mechanical small bowel obstruction is suspected. Once again, in theory, barium administered above a partial or a complete obstruction may increase morbidity and mortality. Miller and Brahme, however, studied 172 patients with mechanical small bowel obstruction in whom orally administered barium produced no untoward side effects.

Tachycardia, tachypnea, and a fever, even in the presence of a normal blood pressure, may be indicative of significant hypovolemia, with or without sepsis. In the elderly, the only signs of dead bowel may be the presence of deteriorating vital signs. Inflammatory lesions, of course, are commonly associated with tachycardia, tachypnea, and fever. Intraabdominal abscesses, like abscesses elsewhere, may be associated with spiking temperatures, so that the patient may be afebrile when initially seen. When the mechanical obstruction is of recent onset, vital signs may be within normal limits.

Mechanical obstruction and paralytic ileus are sometimes difficult to distinguish. Repeated radiographic examination, laboratory studies, and physical examinations, while correcting any electrolyte and fluid imbalances, may be the only way that the two can be differentiated. If possible, the same physician should repeat the examinations.

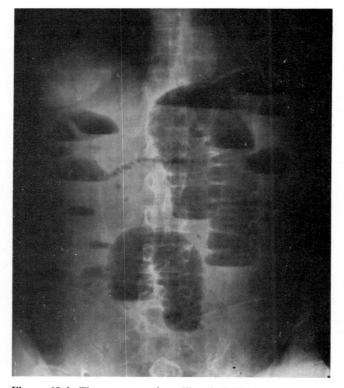

Figure 60-1. The presence of steplike air-fluid levels suggests a mechanical intestinal obstruction. (Courtesy of Detroit General Hospital.)

TREATMENT

The goals of successful treatment of patients with mechanical obstruction include (1) early initial recognition, (2) rapid correction of fluid and electrolyte imbalances without compromising the patient's cardiovascular status, and (3) early surgical intervention. Careful monitoring of the patient's vital signs, urinary output, and cardiovascular status is the key in managing fluid resuscitation. Central venous pressure monitoring, especially in the elderly, may be necessary, as well as use of a Foley catheter. Urinary output should be monitored. Nasogastric tube insertion is a vital part of the patient's management. Gastric contents are removed and the progression of intestinal distention minimized.

In the treatment of mechanical bowel obstruction, either large or small bowel, the use of a long tube remains almost a matter of philosophy. Some believe that these tubes should be inserted in all patients suspected of having a mechanical obstruction to minimize intestinal distention and to gain time before surgical intervention so that fluid and electrolyte disturbances can be corrected. Others feel that these tubes are difficult to pass, and therefore delays prior to surgery become unconscionably long. They also feel that these tubes, when passed, only compound fluid and electrolyte imbalances by removing large quantities of intestinal contents. In addition, when passed successfully the tubes may give a false sense of security by alleviating symptoms but not treating the primary problem.

If it is used, a long tube must not be connected to suction until there is x-ray confirmation of the tube's presence in the small bowel, beyond the pylorus. Therefore, the nasogastric tube must be left in the stomach, and it must remain connected to suction. The intestinal tube will not pass if peristalsis is not present, as for example in paralytic ileus. Once the long tube is beyond the pylorus and in the duodenum, peristalsis will propel it farther down the intestine.

Generally, unless the patient has a contraindication to surgical intervention, it is our recommendation that such tubes not be used. Surgical intervention is clearly indicated as soon as the diagnosis of mechanical bowel obstruction is made and the patient's condition permits.

Broad-spectrum antibiotics are indicated when a mechanical obstruction is confirmed before surgical intervention. The antibiotics used should be selected in consultation with the surgeon, but antibiotic protocols may need to be established even before a patient's arrival. In this circumstance the use of antibiotics is therapeutic and not prophylactic, since the presence of mechanical obstruction and intestinal distention go hand in hand, and these conditions ensure the development of sepsis, even if not clinically detected.

Since surgical intervention is necessary in virtually all patients with mechanical obstruction, evaluation, resuscitation, and treatment should proceed with all deliberate speed, but without compromising the patient.

VOLVULUS

Volvulus occurs whenever a freely movable loop of bowel twists on its mesenteric axis and fixation. It is usually related to incomplete fixation of a portion of the bowel during development. Sigmoid volvulus and cecal volvulus are the most common types. A history of chronic constipation and laxative abuse is present in nearly all patients. Persons predisposed to volvulus are the elderly, the psychiatrically disturbed, and those with certain neurologic diseases.

Symptoms of volvulus include obstipation and severe crampy, diffuse abdominal pain. This is usually intermittent, as the vol-

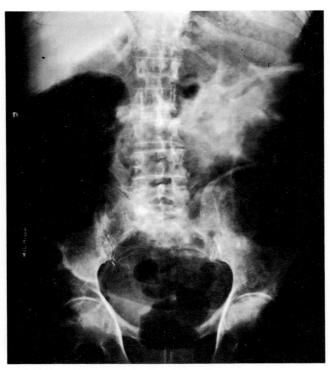

Figure 60-2. Sigmoid volvulus. (Courtesy of Detroit General Hospital.)

vulus twists and untwists. On physical examination, distention and tympany may be found. If gangrene has occurred, signs and symptoms of dead bowel are present. A sausage-shaped mass may be discovered on physical examination.

If a sigmoid volvulus is present, routine abdominal films may be diagnostic; a markedly distended loop of large bowel can be seen in the left side (Fig. 60-2). In cecal volvulus, the distended loop is present in the left upper quadrant, and there are few gas-filled loops of bowel in the right lower quadrant.

With sigmoid volvulus, sigmoidoscopic examination may be both diagnostic and therapeutic. Tapering closure of the sigmoid colon seen on this examination is the diagnostic clue. If a rectal tube is then gently passed, the volvulus can be reduced. There will be an explosive expulsion of gas and liquid feces as the tube is passed and the volvulus reduced. The examiner should be prepared. There is the danger of reducing a gangrenous loop of bowel when this is done, and the patient requires hospitalization, with careful monitoring, and further diagnostic studies. Definitive surgical intervention may be necessary to prevent recurrence.

Surgical intervention is indicated if the patient has had more than one episode of volvulus, or if gangrene is suspected.

BIBLIOGRAPHY

Anderson A, Bergdahl L, Van der Linden W: Volvulus of the cecum. *Ann Surg* 181:876–880, 1975.

Grodsinsky C, Ponka JL: Volvulus of the colon. *Dis Colon Rectum* 20:314–324, 1977.

Khoury GA, Pickard R, Knight M: Volvulus of the sigmoid colon. *Br J Surg* 64:587–589, 1977.

Laws HL, Aldrete JS: Small-bowel obstruction: A review of 465 cases. *South Med J* 69:733–734, 1976.

Miller RE, Brahme F: Large amounts of orally administered barium for obstruction of the small intestine. *Surg Gynecol Obstet* 129:1185–1188, 1969.

Sanner CJ, Saltzman DA: Detorsion of sigmoid volvulus by colonoscopy. *Gastrointest Endosc* 23:212–213, 1977.

Sharpton B, Cheek RC: Volvulus of the sigmoid colon. *Am Surg* 42:436–440, 1976.

Shatila AH, Chamberlain BE, Webb WR: Current status of diagnosis and management of strangulation obstruction of the small bowel. *Am J Surg* 132:229–303, 1976.

Stewardson RH, Bombeck CT, Nyhus LM: Critical operative management of small bowel obstruction. *Ann Surg* 197:189–193, 1978.

Sufian S, Matsumoto T: Intestinal obstruction. *Am J Surg* 130:9–14, 1975.

Valerio D, Jones PF: Immediate resection in the treatment of large bowel emergencies. *Br J Surg* 65:712–716, 1978.

CHAPTER 61
HERNIA

Ronald L. Krome

A hernia is classically defined as the protrusion of any viscus which is enclosed in a peritoneal sac from its normal position through a congenital or acquired opening into another area. This classic description does not include all hernias. It does not, for example, include internal hernias, herniation of omentum, herniation of preperitoneal fat, or traumatic herniation of a variety of organs.

An external hernia is one that protrudes through to the outside and can be seen or palpated. External hernias include femoral, inguinal, umbilical, and incisional hernias.

An internal hernia is one in which the herniated organ and the herniation itself occur within the confines of a body cavity. Examples of this are diaphragmatic hernias, both acquired and congenital, hernias through the foramen of Winslow into the lesser sac, or hernias through a tear in the omentum or mesentery.

An incisional hernia is one that results as a postoperative complication and occurs through a previous incision site. It is an acquired hernia.

A reducible hernia is any hernia in which the herniated organ can be returned to its normal anatomic position without surgical intervention, simply by manipulation.

An incarcerated hernia, or irreducible hernia, is one which cannot be returned to its normal anatomic position by manipulation, and therefore surgical intervention is necessary to replace the contents. Incarceration may be either acute or chronic. The incidence of incarceration is increased when the hernia occurs in association with a disease which causes increased intraabdominal pressure, for example, asthma, chronic obstructive pulmonary disease, benign prostatic hypertrophy, prostatism, and colon or rectal tumors producing obstruction and constipation. All these conditions may result in increased intraabdominal pressure because of the strain necessary to breathe, urinate, or defecate.

Incarceration is more likely to occur when the defect is small and the contents are large. This holds true wherever the hernia is; the incidence of incarceration decreases as the size of the defect increases. Once edema develops, and as it progresses, the hernia becomes increasingly difficult to reduce. Impingement of the vascular supply may result.

When the hernia is associated with vascular compromise, either venous or arterial, then it is said to be strangulated. As the vascular compromise progresses, or if it is not relieved, gangrene develops. Although all strangulated hernias are by definition incarcerated, not all incarcerated hernias are strangulated. Strangulated hernias require surgical intervention. Not all incarcerated hernias require intervention. Chronic incarcerations will most likely not stran-gulate, and therefore emergency surgery is not generally necessary.

Strangulation and incarceration may occur in both external and internal hernias.

PATHOPHYSIOLOGY

Inguinal hernia. A direct inguinal hernia is one that protrudes through Hesselbach's triangle, which is bounded by the inguinal ligament, the inferior epigastric vessels, and the lateral border of the rectus abdominis muscle. Direct hernias rarely, if ever, incarcerate (Fig. 61-1).

Indirect inguinal hernia. An indirect inguinal hernia is one that comes down the inguinal canal and occurs lateral to the inferior epigastric vessels. Incarceration of these hernias is not uncommon. Although indirect hernias are much more common in men because of the embryological descent of the testes, they do occur in women.

Femoral hernia. A femoral hernia is one that protrudes below the inguinal ligament into the femoral canal. They are much more common in women, most likely because of the different structure of the pelvis. Nevertheless, by far the most common hernia in the population as a whole is the inguinal hernia.

A hernia that occurs above the epigastric vessels, in the linea semilunaris, is called a spigelian hernia.

Bilateral inguinal hernias are referred to as a double hernia; a pantaloon hernia is an inguinal hernia with both direct and indirect components occurring on the same side. When one wall of the hernia sac is made up by the viscus involved, regardless of the anatomic location of the hernia, it is called a sliding hernia. There are therefore sliding inguinal hernias and sliding hiatal hernias. When an incarceration or a strangulation contains only one wall of a viscus, it is a Richter's hernia.

Although a number of factors play an etiologic role in the development of groin hernias, most often multiple factors are involved. Congenital developmental defects and heredity play roles in the indirect hernias present at birth. There is a failure to develop a portion of the abdominal wall. Persistence of the processus vaginalis peritonei in the inguinal canal, with an inguinal ring large enough to permit a hernia to occur, may be hereditary. Similarly, generalized connective tissue weakness may be hereditary.

Direct inguinal hernias have an increasing frequency as age increases and are uncommon in children. Indirect hernias, on the other hand, are more common in the younger age groups.

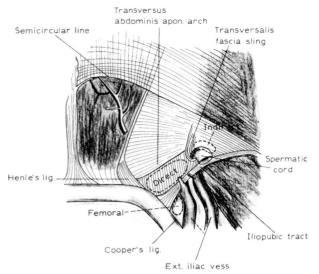

Figure 61-1. The posterior inguinal wall viewed from the preperitoneal side. The peritoneum and all preperitoneal fat and lymphoid tissue have been excised, exposing the transversalis fascia. The areas through which the three common groin hernias occur are indicated, as are the transversalis fascia analogues, which are utilized in the iliopubic tract repair. [From Nyhus LM: Preperitoneal approach in the repair of inguinal hernia in adults, in Ellison EH, Friesen SR, Mulholland JH (eds): *Current Surgical Management III*. Philadelphia, Saunders, 1965, p 465. Used with permission.]

A slow, chronic increase in intraabdominal pressure is a major factor in the development of acquired hernias and is the precipitating factor in indirect hernias, in spite of the existence of a congenital sac.

Umbilical hernias. Although an umbilical defect is common in the newborn, in the majority of cases the defect is closed by the second year of age. Obese patients, especially those in the older age groups, have an increased incidence of umbilical hernias, perhaps because of increasing intraabdominal pressure. Such hernias also develop with some frequency in persons with chronic and severe ascites. Pregnancy plays a significant role in their development. Umbilical hernias can incarcerate and strangulate, especially if the defect is small and the hernial contents are large.

CLINICAL FEATURES

The majority of hernias are asymptomatic and are detected either on routine physical examination or by the patient inadvertently. Mild symptoms, such as a sensation of "dragging" or a lump in the groin, may be the only manifestations. If incarceration is acute, pain may develop suddenly. When strangulation occurs, the patient may be toxic, with signs and symptoms of bowel obstruction or perforation. The most common complaint is a tender swelling or a sense of bulging.

Patients with incarceration frequently give a history of having a hernia. The patient can no longer return the hernia to its normal position and thus seeks help. Acute incarcerations are painful and tender; they may be accompanied by nausea and vomiting if partial or complete obstruction has occurred. The tenderness is due to inflammation of the bowel wall or omentum and the surrounding tissues. Incarcerated hernias are a leading cause of bowel obstruction in the United States, second only to postoperative adhesions.

Initial symptoms, produced by traction on a portion of the small bowel or omentum, may be located in the epigastrium. If only a portion of the bowel wall is caught in the defect (Richter's hernia), strangulation may occur without signs and symptoms of intestinal obstruction.

On physical examination, an abnormal swelling may be noted. If incarceration is present, the swelling is tender. The consistency of this mass varies depending on the contents of the hernia sac.

Tachycardia and mild temperature elevation frequently are present if incarceration is also present. Unrelieved incarceration or strangulation may result in bowel obstruction, perforation, abscess formation, or peritonitis and septic shock.

Groin hernias can be confused with tender lymph nodes and hydroceles. Lymph nodes are generally movable, firm, and multiple. Hydroceles will transilluminate and are not tender. Incarcerated hernias will not transilluminate and are tender. If bowel is contained in the hernia sac, bowel sounds may be heard and peristalsis may be seen. Testicular torsion may be confused with incarcerated hernias.

When incarceration is acute, the white blood cell count is slightly elevated with a shift to the left. Electrolyte abnormalities and elevation of the blood urea nitrogen (BUN) level occur as a reflection of both the patient's state of hydration and the toxic state. In the elderly, laboratory studies may not be reliable indicators of the patient's state.

Upright chest films should be obtained to rule out free air under the diaphragm, which may result from perforation or dead bowel. Flat and upright films of the abdomen, including the groin, should be obtained to assess the possible presence of bowel obstruction. Loops of bowel may be seen entering a hernial sac.

TREATMENT

If there is a good history that the incarceration is of very recent onset, an attempt can be made to reduce the hernia. If there is any question of the duration of the incarceration, no attempt should be made so that no dead bowel is reintroduced into the abdomen. Before an attempt is made to reduce the hernia, the patient should be placed in Trendelenburg's position and given some mild sedation. A warm compress over the area may make the task easier by reducing the swelling and relaxing the abdominal musculature. Only gentle compression of the hernia should be used, and nothing should be forced back. Attempts at reduction should be limited in time and force.

If the incarceration is tender, if it cannot be reduced, or if strangulation is suspected, the patient should not be fed by mouth, and a nasogastric tube should be inserted. Intravenous fluid should be started with the thought of correcting the patient's volume and electrolyte problems.

The treatment of choice for an incarceration which cannot be reduced, or for a strangulation, is surgical. Broad-spectrum antibiotics and vigorous fluid resuscitation may be necessary, but only as a prelude to operation.

BIBLIOGRAPHY

Berk JL, Weaver J, Siegler E: Delayed perforation of a strangulated hernia. *JAMA* 239:2781, 1978.

Conner WT, Peacock EE Jr: Some studies on the etiology of inguinal hernia. *Am J Surg* 126:732–735, 1973.

Dajee H: Traumatic abdominal hernia. *J Trauma* 19:710–711, 1979.

Ekwueme O: Strangulated external hernia associated with generalized peritonitis. *Br J Surg* 60:929–933, 1973.

Farrow GA, Thomson S: Incarcerated inguinal hernia in infants and children: A five-year review at the hospital for sick children, Toronto, 1955 to 1959, inclusive. *Can J Surg* 6:63–69, 1963.

James PM Jr: The problem of hernia in infants and adolescents. *Surg Clin North Am* 51:1361–1670, 1971.

Pfefferman R, Freund H: Symptomatic hernia: Strangulated hernia combined with acute abdominal disease. *Am J Surg* 124:60–62, 1972.

Read RC: Inguinal herniation 1777–1977. *Am J Surg* 136:651–654, 1978.

Rowe MI, Clatworthy WH: Incarcerated and strangulated hernias in children. *Arch Surg* 101:136–137, 1970.

CHAPTER 62
ILEITIS AND COLITIS

Howard A. Werman, Hagop S. Mekhjian
Douglas A. Rund

ILEITIS (CROHN'S DISEASE)

Crohn's disease is a chronic inflammatory disease of the gastrointestinal (GI) tract; its etiology is unknown. The disease was first described by Crohn, Ginzburg, and Oppenheimer in 1932 and was thought to involve only the distal ileum. Since then it has become clear that the disease can involve any part of the GI tract from the mouth to the anus. Characteristically, there is a segmental involvement of the intestinal tract by a nonspecific granulomatous inflammatory process. The ileum is involved in the majority of cases. In 10 to 15 percent of patients, the disease is confined to the colon, making differentiation from ulcerative colitis at times a difficult clinical problem. The terms *regional enteritis, terminal ileitis, granulomatous ileocolitis,* and *Crohn's disease* have been used synonymously to describe the same disease.

Etiology and Pathogenesis

Environmental as well as host factors have been incriminated as the cause for Crohn's disease. There is very little data to support the causative role of psychogenic factors. Cell-wall-defective pseudomonads and RNA-containing viruses have received some attention recently, but the evidence for their being a cause is inconclusive. Immunologic factors have received the greatest attention. There is considerable similarity between bacterial and gut mucosal cell antigens. It is postulated that T lymphocytes are sensitized by external antigens, and, in the presence of antibodies, the T lymphocytes produce cytotoxic changes in the gut mucosa. Some of the extraintestinal manifestations suggest a role for immune complexes at various involved sites.

Epidemiology

The peak incidence of Crohn's disease occurs between 15 and 25 years of age. There is a suggestion of a secondary peak at 55 to 60 years of age. The prevalence varies from 10 to 100 cases, and the incidence ranges from 1 to 7 cases per year per 100,000 population in the U.S. There is a strong suggestion that the incidence of the disease has been increasing over the past 20 years. The disease has a worldwide distribution but is more frequent in people of European extraction. It is four times more common in Jews than non–Jews and is more common in whites than blacks. Family history of inflammatory bowel disease is present in 10 to 15 percent of patients. Ulcerative colitis, as well as Crohn's disease, may be present in other family members, and siblings are more frequently affected with Crohn's disease.

Pathology

The most important feature of the pathology of Crohn's disease is the involvement of all the layers of the bowel as well as the mesenteric lymph nodes. In addition, the disease is discontinuous, with normal areas of bowel ("skip areas") intervening between one or more involved areas. On gross inspection the bowel wall is found to be thickened with a narrow lumen. The latter results in stenosis and obstruction of the intestine. The mesenteric fat often extends over the bowel wall ("creeping" fat). The appearance of the mucosa varies with the extent and severity of the disease. Longitudinal deep ulcerations are quite characteristic. These often penetrate the bowel wall, resulting in fissures, fistulas, and abscesses. Late in the disease a "cobblestone" appearance of the mucosa results from the crisscrossing of these ulcers with intervening normal mucosa.

Microscopically, there is an inflammatory reaction that extends through all layers of the intestine but is most marked in the submucosa. This inflammatory response consists of infiltration by mononuclear cells, lymphocytes, plasma cells, and histiocytes. Fissure ulcers frequently penetrate the muscle layer. Unlike the situation in ulcerative colitis, crypt abscesses are seen infrequently. Discrete granulomas consisting of epithelioid cells, giant cells, and lymphocytes are seen in 50 to 75 percent of the specimens. Although the finding of granulomas is helpful, it is not essential for the diagnosis of Crohn's disease.

Clinical Features and Course

The clinical course of Crohn's disease is variable and in the individual patient quite unpredictable. Diarrhea, abdominal pain, fever, and weight loss are present in 75 to 80 percent of patients. A patient with Crohn's disease may present with acute right lower quadrant abdominal pain and fever and on examination be found to have a mass in the right lower quadrant. The more common course is an insidious onset of recurrent abdominal pain, fever, and diarrhea for several years before the definitive diagnosis is made. Approximately 50 percent of patients develop perianal disease. In 10 to 20 percent of patients the extraintestinal manifestations of arthritis, uveitis, or liver disease could be the presenting symptoms. Crohn's disease should also be considered in the differential diagnosis of fever of unknown etiology.

The clinical manifestations as well as the course of the disease seem related in part to the anatomic distribution of the disease. This has been classified as disease involving only the small bowel, the colon only, or both as in ileocolitis. The latter is the most frequent pattern and is characterized by the highest recurrence rate following surgery. The incidence of hematochezia and perianal disease is higher when the colon is involved as in ileocolitis or Crohn's colitis. A slight increase in the incidence of arthritis may be associated with Crohn's colitis. With the exception of growth retardation, childhood-onset Crohn's disease seems to have a course similar to that of adult-onset disease.

Complications

The clinical complications of Crohn's disease can be classified as local and systemic. Perianal complications are seen in 50 to 80 percent of patients and include perianal or ischiorectal abscesses, fissures, fistulas, rectovaginal fistulas, and rectal prolapse. Other local intestinal complications include stricture formation, internal fistula formation, and, rarely, free perforation or massive hemorrhage of the bowel. Toxic megacolon is an infrequent complication associated with Crohn's colitis. The incidence of malignant neoplasms of the GI tract is three times higher than that of the general population but lower than the incidence associated with ulcerative colitis.

Systemic complications of inflammatory bowel disease often may precede bowel symptoms and thus may be the patient's presenting complaint. The incidence of these complications does not differ between patients with Crohn's disease and those with ulcerative colitis. Erythema nodosum, pyoderma gangrenosum, nongranulomatous anterior uveitis, and peripheral arthritis are seen. Ankylosing spondylitis can be detected in up to 20 percent of patients with inflammatory bowel disease, 80 percent of the latter with the antigen HLA-B27. Conversely, 18 percent with ankylosing spondylitis have inflammatory bowel disease. Hepatic disease is common in patients with inflammatory bowel disease and includes pericholangitis, chronic active hepatitis, primary sclerosing cholangitis, and cholangiocarcinoma. Growth retardation can be seen in children. Hyperoxaluria is a common and potentially treatable occurrence in patients with ileal disease and steatorrhea. This results from the colonic hyperabsorption of dietary oxalate and accounts for the occurrence of nephrolithiasis in 20 to 25 percent of patients with ileal disease.

When bowel symptoms are present, malnutrition, malabsorption, hypocalcemia, and vitamin deficiency can be severe. Added to the complications of the disease itself are complications associated with the treatment of the disease.

Diagnosis

In the majority of patients, the definitive diagnosis of Crohn's disease is made months or years after the initial symptoms. Oc-

casionally the initial presenting complaint is an extraintestinal manifestation such as arthritis or iritis. Not infrequently, these patients are operated upon for appendicitis or pelvic inflammatory disease only to have the diagnosis of Crohn's disease made at the time of surgery. A careful and detailed history for bowel symptoms before the onset of acute right lower quadrant pain usually provides clues to the correct diagnosis before surgery.

In addition to the clinical presentations, the major diagnostic tool remains x-rays of the GI tract. The classic findings in the small intestine include segmental narrowing, destruction of the normal mucosal pattern, and fistulas. The segmental involvement of the colon with rectal sparing is the most characteristic feature. Double-contrast barium enema examination can detect the mucosal abnormalities, but colonoscopy is by far the most sensitive technique for the detection of early aphthous ulcerations. Colonoscopy is also useful for delineating the extent of disease and for surveillance for the occurrence of colon cancer. Rigid sigmoidoscopy and biopsy are not helpful in the majority of instances because of the rectal sparing and the relatively low incidence of diagnostic biopsies.

Diseases that should be considered in the differential diagnosis of Crohn's disease include lymphoma, ileocecal amebiasis, tuberculosis and deep chronic mycotic infections involving the GI tract, and yersinial ileocolitis. Fortunately, most of these are relatively uncommon and can be differentiated by appropriate laboratory tests. Yersinial ileocolitis is a relatively acute problem that can be diagnosed by stool cultures. Acute ileitis should not be confused with Crohn's disease. Patients with acute ileitis usually recover without sequelae and should not be operated upon. When the disease is confined to the colon, ischemic bowel disease and pseudomembranous enterocolitis as well as ulcerative colitis have to be included in the differential diagnosis of Crohn's colitis.

Treatment

The aim of therapy in Crohn's disease includes relief of symptoms, suppression of the inflammatory disease, treatment of complications and maintenance of nutrition. In a disease that is virtually incurable, the emphasis should be on the relief of symptoms and the avoidance of complications.

Prednisone and sulfasalazine (Azulfidine) have both been demonstrated to be effective in inducing a remission in patients with active Crohn's disease. More recently, metronidazole (Flagyl) has been shown to be as effective as sulfasalazine. The presumed mechanism of action of sulfasalazine is the breakdown of the drug to 5-aminosalicylic acid, which appears to be the active component in suppression of the disease. Combination of 6-mercaptopurine or azathioprine with prednisone has been reported to increase the rate of remission and reduce the requirements for prednisone. The addition of sulfasalazine to prednisone does not improve the response rate and increases the risk of side effects. Broad-spectrum antibiotics have been used with improvement of radiographic appearance. There is no conclusive evidence that any drug is useful in maintaining remission in patients with Crohn's disease, unlike the situation with ulcerative colitis.

Diarrhea can be controlled by the use of loperamide (Imodium), diphenoxylate (Lomotil), and, in some cases, cholestyramine (Questran). The latter is particularly useful in patients who have limited ileal disease, no obstruction, and mild steatorrhea. Cholestyramine acts by binding bile acids and eliminating their cathartic action. The primary aim of dietary therapy is the maintenance of nutrition and the alleviation of diarrhea. Lactose intolerance is quite common in these patients and may be a major contributing factor to the diarrhea. This can be helped by the elimination of lactose from the diet. Reduction in dietary oxalate should be considered in every patient. In addition, supplementation of trace metals, fat-soluble vitamins, and medium-chain triglycerides should be considered in selected patients.

The indications for surgery are largely the complications of the disease. In addition, a patient may need surgery because of the failure of medical therapy. The recurrence rate after surgery approaches 100 percent. There has been some controversy about the recurrence rate following total colectomy for Crohn's colitis. The bulk of the evidence suggests, however, that if colectomy is done for carefully selected patients with Crohn's colitis, the recurrence rate is much lower than that of disease involving the small bowel.

ULCERATIVE COLITIS

Ulcerative colitis is a chronic inflammatory and ulcerative disease of the colon and rectum characterized most often clinically by bloody diarrhea. The etiology, like that of Crohn's disease, remains unknown even though extensive investigation into the cause continues to be carried out. Epidemiological considerations are similar to those of Crohn's disease: the disease is more prevalent in the United States and northern Europe, and peak incidence occurs in the second and the third decades of life. The incidence of ulcerative colitis in 1976 was about 10 per 100,000 and has not risen significantly in the last few years, even though the incidence of new cases of Crohn's disease has increased during this period.

Pathology

Ulcerative colitis is a process that involves primarily the mucosa and submucosa. Microscopically, the disease is characterized by mucosal inflammation with the formation of crypt abscesses, epithelial necrosis, and mucosal ulceration. The muscular layer and serosa are often spared. In the usual case the disease increases in severity more distally, the rectosigmoid being involved in 95 percent of cases. In the early stages of the disease, the mucous membranes appear finely granular and friable. In more severe cases, the mucosa appears as a red spongy surface dotted with small ulcerations oozing blood and purulent exudate. In very advanced disease, one sees large oozing ulcerations and pseudopolyps (areas of hyperplastic overgrowth surrounded by inflamed mucosa).

Clinical Features and Course

The clinical features and course of ulcerative colitis are very variable but somewhat dependent on the anatomic distribution of the disease in the colon. The disease can be classified as mild, moderate, or severe depending on the clinical manifestations. Patients with mild disease have fewer than four bowel movements per day, no systemic symptoms, and fewer extraintestinal manifestations. Of all patients, 60 percent present with mild disease, and in 80 percent of them the disease is limited to the rectum. Occasionally constipation and rectal bleeding is the presenting complaint. Progression to pancolitis occurs in 10 to 15 percent of patients. Patients with severe disease constitute 15 percent of those with ulcerative colitis. Severe disease is associated with more than six bowel movements per day, anemia, fever, weight loss, tachycardia, and more frequent extraintestinal manifestations. Severe disease accounts for 90 percent of the mortality from ulcerative colitis. Virtually all these patients have pancolitis. Moderate disease accounts for 25 percent of patients with ulcerative colitis. Their clinical manifestations are less severe and demonstrate a good response to therapy. These patients usually have colitis extending to the splenic flexure (left-sided colitis) but could have pancolitis.

The most frequent clinical course of ulcerative colitis is characterized by intermittent attacks with complete remission between attacks. This occurs in 75 percent of patients. In 15 percent of patients the disease is characterized by a chronically active course, and in another 10 percent the first acute attack is followed by a long period (10 to 15 years) of remission. The factors that are associated with an unfavorable prognosis and increased mortality include the severity and extent of disease, a short history before the first attack, and onset of the disease after 60 years of age.

Complications

Although blood loss from sustained hemorrhage may be the most common complication of the illness, toxic megacolon is a complication that must not be missed by the emergency physician.

Toxic megacolon develops in advanced colitis when the disease process begins to extend through all layers of the colon. The result is a loss of muscular tone within the colon and localized peritonitis. The colon begins to dilate as the muscular tone is lost. Plain radiography of the abdomen shows a long continuous segment of air-filled colon greater than 6 cm in diameter. If the colon continues to dilate without treatment, toxic megacolon develops. The distended portion of the atonic colon can perforate, causing peritonitis and septicemia. The mortality from this complication can be as high as 30 percent.

A patient with toxic megacolon appears severely ill; the abdomen is distended, tender, and tympanitic. Fever, tachycardia, and signs of hypovolemia are typically part of the portrait. Leukocytosis, anemia, electrolyte disturbances, and hypoalbuminemia are the supporting laboratory data.

Some of the more toxic aspects of the disease, like leukocytosis and peritonitis, can be masked in the patient taking corticosteroids. When such therapy is being administered, greater suspicion is required to make the diagnosis. Antidiarrheal agents, hypokalemia, narcotics, cathartics, and enemas have been implicated in precipitating toxic megacolon. Medical therapy with nasogastric suction, parenteral steroids, antibiotics, and intravenous fluids should be tried in preparation of the patient for possible surgery. However, prolonged medical treatment of these patients increases mortality; therefore, early surgical consultation must be sought for these patients with the aim of performing a colectomy on an elective basis.

Local complications like small rectovaginal fistulas occur infrequently in cases of ulcerative colitis. Perirectal fistulas and abscesses are much more common in patients with Crohn's disease than in those with ulcerative colitis.

Systemic complications of ulcerative colitis include peripheral arthritis, ankylosing spondylitis, episcleritis, posterior uveitis, and erythema nodosum.

Clincally apparent liver disease may occur in 1 to 5 percent of the patients. The liver disease may be any of the following: pericholangitis, chronic active hepatitis, fatty liver, or cirrhosis.

There is a 10- to 30-fold increase in the development of carcinoma of the colon in patients with ulcerative colitis. Carcinoma of the colon is the cause of 30 percent of the deaths attributed to ulcerative colitis. The major risk factors for the development of carcinoma of the colon are the extent and the duration of the disease. The cumulative risk of cancer after 15, 20, and 25 years is 8, 12, and 25 percent, respectively. Additional factors for increasing the risk of developing cancer include the onset of the disease in childhood and a family history of colon cancer. Carcinoma developing in patients with ulcerative colitis is more evenly distributed in the colon and is often multicentric and virulent in clinical behavior. The availability of fiberoptic colonoscopy allows us to perform periodic colonoscopies and biopsies to detect metaplastic changes that are thought to predict the development of colon cancer. In patients with pancolitis such surveillance should start 7 to 10 years after the onset of the disease.

Diagnosis

The diagnosis of ulcerative colitis rests on the following: a history of abdominal cramps and diarrhea, mucoid stools, stool examination negative for ova and parasites, stool cultures negative for enteric pathogens, and confirmation by sigmoidoscopic examination. The results of the latter examination are abnormal in 95 percent of the patients with ulcerative colitis. The changes vary depending on the severity and duration of the disease. Granularity, friability and ulcerations of the mucosa, and, in more advanced cases, pseudopolyposis are quite characteristic. Rectal biopsy is helpful in very early cases and in excluding amebiasis and metaplasia (see the section on pathology). Barium enema examination is useful in confirming the diagnosis and defining the extent of involvement of the colon. Colonoscopy is the most sensitive method for the diagnosis and definition of the extent and severity of the disease. In addition, in the evaluation of the patient for the development of metaplasia or colon cancer colonoscopy is extremely useful. Barium enema examination and colonoscopy should not be performed in moderately or severely sick patients. One should not shy away from performing a rigid or fiberoptic proctosigmoidoscopy, however, even in the severely ill patient, provided it is done gently and without the administration of any enemas or laxatives.

The major diseases that should be considered in the differential diagnosis of ulcerative colitis include infectious colitis, Crohn's colitis, ischemic colitis, irradiation colitis, and pseudomembranous colitis. When the disease is limited to the rectum, particular attention should be paid to sexually acquired diseases that are being seen with increasing frequency in the male homosexual population (''gay bowel disease''). Some of the more common diseases in this category include rectal syphilis, gonococcal proctitis, lymphogranuloma venerum, and inflammations caused by herpes simplex virus, *Entamoeba histolytica, Shigella*, and *Campylobacter*.

Treatment

The majority of patients with mild and moderate disease can be treated as outpatients. Corticosteroids are effective in inducing a remission in the majority of cases and constitute the mainstay of therapy in an acute attack. Daily dosages of 20 to 40 mg are usually sufficient and can be adjusted depending on the severity of the disease. The use of rectal steroids should be reserved for patients with ulcerative proctitis. Once clinical remission is achieved, steroids should be slowly tapered and discontinued. There is no evidence that maintenance dosages of steroids reduce the incidence of relapses. Sulfasalazine has been used in the treatment of acute attacks but is probably inferior to steroids, especially in the more severe cases. Its primary usefulness is in the form of adjunctive therapy and in the maintenance of a remission. Maintenance dosages of 1.5 to 2 mg/day significantly reduce the recurrence rate of the disease.

Supportive measures in the treatment of mild to moderately sick patients include the replenishment of iron stores, a nutritious diet with the elimination of lactose, and adequate physical and psychological rest. Hydrophilic bulk agents such as psyllium (Metamucil) can be used in some patients to improve stool consistency. The use of antidiarrheal agents should be minimized because of the risk of precipitating toxic megacolon and because the primary reason for the diarrhea is a diseased colon with impaired function which is unlikely to be improved by antimotility agents.

Patients with ulcerative colitis should be treated in the hospital. Intravenous steroids, replacement of fluids, correction of electrolyte abnormalities, antibiotics, and hyperalimentation may be considered for the individual patient. When toxic megacolon is suspected, nasogastric suction and a surgical consultation should be obtained, and the patient should be observed by frequent examinations and flat films of the abdomen. When the diagnosis of toxic megacolon is established and the patient fails to show dramatic clinical improvement within 48 to 72 h, emergency surgery should be considered. In addition to toxic megacolon, the indications for surgery are colonic perforation, massive lower GI bleeding, suspicion of colon cancer, and disease that is refractory to medical therapy (large doses of steroids required for the control of the disease). The surgical treatment of choice is total proctocolectomy with ileostomy. Selected patients could have a continent ileostomy. Unlike surgery in Crohn's disease, surgery in ulcerative colitis is curative.

PSEUDOMEMBRANOUS ENTEROCOLITIS

Pseudomembranous enterocolitis is an inflammatory bowel disorder in which membranelike yellowish plaques of exudate overlay and replace necrotic intestinal mucosa.

Three different syndromes have been described: neonatal pseudomembranous enterocolitis, postoperative pseudomembranous enterocolitis, and antibiotic-associated pseudomembranous colitis. In the latter, it is presumed that broad-spectrum antibiotics, most notably clindamycin, lincomycin, and ampicillin, alter the gut flora in such a way that toxin-producing clostridia can flourish in the colon. The result is a clinical picture of mucoid watery diarrhea that may progress to a full-blown ulcerative colitis. The disease typically begins 7 to 10 days after the institution of antibiotic therapy and in many cases begins up to 2 to 4 weeks after the antibiotic is discontinued.

The diagnosis is made by a history of antibiotic use and the observation of the characteristic yellowish plaques on sigmoidoscopy. Lesions may be limited to the right colon. For this reason colonoscopy may be needed in some cases. The diagnosis is definitively confirmed by the demonstration of the presence of *Clostridium difficile* toxin in stool filtrates.

The treatment of pseudomembranous colitis includes supportive measures such as the administration of fluids and the correction of electrolyte abnormalities. Severely sick patients may be hospitalized. Oral vancomycin, 125 mg four times a day, is effective in the majority of patients. The symptoms resolve in a few days. Relapses occur in 10 to 15 percent of patients, necessitating a second course of treatment with vancomycin. Other agents that are useful in the treatment of pseudomembranous colitis include bacitracin, 2 g/day; metronidazole, 250 mg four times per day; and cholestyramine (Questran) 8 to 12 g/day. The latter binds the toxin and presumably blocks its action. None of these latter agents are as good as vancomycin. Steroids and surgical intervention are rarely needed for patients with pseudomembranous colitis.

BIBLIOGRAPHY

Ileitis

Admans H, Whorwell PJ, Wright R: Diagnosis of Crohn's disease. *Dig Dis Sci* 25:911–915, 1980.

Block GE: Surgical management of Crohn's colitis. *New Engl J Med* 302:1068–1070, 1980.

Burham WR, Ansell ID, Langman MJS: Normal sigmoidoscopic findings in severe ulcerative colitis: An important and common occurrence. *Gut* 21:A460 (abstract), 1980.

Gebhard RL, Greenberg HB, Singh N, et al: Acute viral enteritis and exacerbations of inflammatory bowel disease. *Gastroenterology* 83:1207–1209, 1982.

Greenstein AJ, Sachar DB, Smith H, et al: Patterns of neoplasia in Crohn's disease and ulcerative colitis. *Cancer* 46:403–407, 1980.

Kirsner JB, Shorter RG: Recent developments in "nonspecific" inflammatory bowel disease (first of two parts). *New Engl J Med* 306:775–785, 1982.

Kirsner JB, Shorter RG: Recent developments in "nonspecific" inflammatory bowel disease (second of two parts). *New Engl J Med* 306:837–848, 1982.

Mekhjian HS, Switz DM, Melnyk CS, et al: Clinical features and natural history of Crohn's disease. *Gastroenterology* 77:898–906, 1979.

Mekhjian HS, Switz DM, Watts HD, et al: National cooperative Crohn's disease study: Factors determining recurrence of Crohn's disease after surgery. *Gastroenterology* 77:907–913, 1979.

Price AB: Overlap in the spectrum of non-specific inflammatory bowel disease—"colitis indeterminate." *J Clin Pathol* 31:567–577, 1978.

Rampton DS, McNeil NI, Sarner M: Analgesic ingestion and other factors preceding relapse in ulcerative colitis. *Gut* 24:187–189, 1983.

Sachar DB, Auslander MO, Walfish JS: Aetiological theories of inflammatory bowel disease. *Clin Gastroenterol* 9:231–249, 1980.

Shorter RG, Tomasi TB: Gut immune mechanisms. *Adv Intern Med* 27:247–280, 1982.

Singleton JW, Law DH, Kelley ML Jr, et al: National cooperative Crohn's disease study: Adverse reactions to study drugs. *Gastroenterology* 77:870–882, 1979.

Summers RW, Switz DM, Sessions JT Jr, et al: National cooperative Crohn's disease study: Results of drug treatment. *Gastroenterology* 77:847–869, 1979.

Surawicz CM, Meisel JL, Ylvisaker T: Rectal biopsy in the diagnosis of Crohn's disease: Value of multiple biopsies and serial sectioning. *Gastroenterology* 80:66–71, 1981.

Vesing B, Alm T, Barany F, et al: A comparative study of metronidazole and sulfadiazine for active Crohn's disease: The comparative Crohn's disease study in Sweden, II Result. *Gastroenterology* 83:550–562, 1982.

Winship DH, Summers RW, Singleton JW, et al: National cooperative Crohn's disease study: Study design and conduct of the study. *Gastroenterology* 77:829–842, 1979.

Colitis

Basler RD: Ulcerative colitis and the skin. *Med Clin North Am* 64:941–954, 1980.

Butt JH, et al: Dysplasia and cancer in inflammatory bowel disease. *Gastroenterology* 80:865–868, 1981.

Elson CO, et al: An evaluation of total parenteral nutrition in the management of inflammatory bowel disease. *Dig Dis Sci* 25:42–48, 1980.

Farmer RG: Colonoscopy in distal ulcerative colitis. *Clin Gastroenterol* 9:257–306, 1980.

Fonkalrud EW: Inflammatory bowel disease in childhood. *Surg Clin North Am* 61:1125–1135, 1981.

Glotzer, DJ: Operation in inflammatory bowel disease: Indications and type. *Clin Gastroenterol* 9:371–388, 1980.

Greenstein AJ, et al: Cancer in universal and left-sided ulcerative colitis: Factors determining risk. *Gastroenterology* 77:290–294, 1979.

Greenstein AJ, et al: The extra-intestinal complications of Crohn's disease and ulcerative colitis: A study of 700 patients. *Medicine* (Baltimore) 55:401–412, 1976.

Gueco MB, et al: Toxic megacolon complicating Crohn's colitis. *Ann Surg* 191:75–80, 1980.

Hamilton JR, et al: Inflammatory bowel disease in children and adolescents. *Adv Pediatr* 26:311–41, 1979.

Hodgson HJ: Assessment of drug therapy in inflammatory bowel disease. *Br J Clin Pharmacol* 14:159–170, 1982.

Janowitz HD: Inflammatory bowel disease. *Adolesc Med* 27:205–246, 1982.

Kirsner JB: Problems in the differentiation of ulcerative colitis and Crohn's disease of the colon: The need for repeated diagnostic evaluation. *Gastroenterology* 68:187–191, 1975.

Kirsner JB: Current medical and surgical opinions on important therapeutic issues in inflammatory bowel disease: A special 1979 survey. *Am J Surg* 140:391–395, 1980.

Klotz V, et al: Therapeutic efficacy of sulfasalzine and its metabolites in patients with ulcerative colitis and Crohn's disease. *N Engl J Med* 303:1499–1502, 1980.

Korelitz BI: Therapy of inflammatory bowel disease, including the use of immunosuppressive agents. *Clin Gastroenterol* 9:331–349, 1980.

Riddell RH, et al: Value of sigmoidoscopy and biopsy in detection of carcinoma and premalignant change in ulcerative colitis. *Gut* 20:575–580, 1979.

Ritchie JR: Prognosis of carcinoma in ulcerative colitis. *Gut* 22:752–755, 1981.

Smith JN: Complications and extraintestinal manifestations of inflammatory bowel disease. *Med Clin North Am* 64:1161–1171, 1980.

Stoke D, et al: Inflammatory bowel disease—relationship to carcinoma. *Curr Probl Cancer* 5:1–72, 1981.

Tedesco FJ: Differential diagnosis of ulcerative colitis and Crohn's disease and other specific inflammatory disease of the bowel. *Med Clin North Am* 64:1173–1183, 1980.

Telander RL: Surgical treatment of ulcerative colitis. *Surgery* 90:787–794, 1981.

Truelove SC, et al: Toxic megacolon part I: Pathogenesis, diagnosis and treatment. *Clin Gastroenterol* 10:107–117, 1981.

CHAPTER 63
COLONIC DIVERTICULAR DISEASE

Ronald L. Krome

The prevalence of colonic diverticular disease varies with geographic area and ethnicity. Most agree that a low-fiber diet is important in the development of diverticular disease, and the incidence is low in those populations that eat high-fiber foods such as whole grains, fruits, and vegetables.

PATHOPHYSIOLOGY

Although the pathogenesis of diverticula remains to be clearly established, their development appears to depend on two factors: the development of a pressure gradient between the colon lumen and the serosa, and a relative weakness of the muscles of the colonic wall. There appears to be no difference between the motility of the colon of those who develop diverticula and the motility of the colon of those who do not. Those with symptomatic disease, however, are more likely to have hypermotility. Diverticula appear to develop at the weakest point of the colonic wall, where the intramural vessels penetrate the circular muscular layer.

Diverticulosis of the colon can be preceded by muscular thickening and narrowing of the sigmoid lumen, but this is not universal. In about one-third of the cases, diverticula progress to the extent that they produce severe symptoms and signs. Medical treatment results in a clinical response in two-thirds of patients. Most recurrences are in the first 5 years of the onset of symptoms.

CLINICAL FEATURES

Clinical features generally depend on the progress of the disease and its complications (Table 63-1).

Early on, with relatively mild disease, the only symptoms may be related to the patient's bowel habits, with constipation and diarrhea alternating. Fever and leukocytosis may be absent at this time. Massive rectal bleeding may accompany diverticular disease and is not necessarily related to the number of diverticula present (see Chapter 64 on anorectal disorders).

In elderly patients with diffuse, nonspecific, lower abdominal pain, irregular bowel habits, and hypermotility, complete evaluation is necessary.

In elderly women with lower abdominal pain and a mass, fever, and leukocytosis, the distinction must be made between colonic and gynecologic disease. Walker et al. have described a series of women with diverticulitis who presented with lower abdominal masses but without fever, leukocytosis, or history compatible with colonic disease and were misdiagnosed as having a gynecologic mass.

Although diverticulitis of the cecum is rare, when it does occur it frequently mimics appendicitis. The diagnosis should be considered in the patient with an abdominal mass, fever, and leukocytosis when it is clear that the patient has had an appendectomy. When the diagnosis is in doubt, surgical intervention may be indicated.

Isolated rectal diverticula are very rare.

Generally considered a disease of the elderly, diverticular disease has been reported in those under 40 as well. In one series of patients under 40, the majority presented with acute diverticulitis and a few with rectal bleeding. Some patients required urgent surgical intervention because of the presence of significant acute complications. Of those treated medically, 45 percent subsequently required surgical intervention.

Colonic carcinoma should always be considered in the differential diagnosis, especially if signs and symptoms are present which are consistent with obstruction or perforation. The two can, of course, coexist.

Table 63-1. Clinical Features

Diverticulosis—multiple pseudodiverticula
  Asymptomatic
  Lower abdominal pain; bowel irregularity
  Hemorrhage—moderate to massive
Diverticulitis—necrotizing diverticular inflammation
  Local inflammation (microperforation)
  Abscess
  Fistula
  Peritonitis
  Obstruction
  Hemorrhage—minimal to moderate

Source: Adapted from Almy TP, Howell DA: Diverticular disease of the colon. *N Engl J Med* 302:324–331, 1980.

TREATMENT

Patients with uncomplicated, symptomatic diverticulosis generally experience relief of pain and improvement of bowel function when a high-fiber diet is instituted. Although anticholinergics are often prescribed, their effectiveness has not been clearly demonstrated.

Narcotics may compound the problem by increasing sigmoid pressure. Antibiotics are not indicated in uncomplicated disease, but should be used in the presence of bacteremia, fever, and leukocytosis; when there is a demonstrable, tender left lower quadrant mass; and for complications, such as peritonitis, abscess, fistula, or obstruction. The agent selected must be one that is effective against coliforms, streptococci, clostridia, and other bowel anaerobes.

For complicated diverticulitis, the patient should be given nothing orally, a nasogastric tube should be inserted, intravenous lines should be established, and surgical consultation should be obtained. Surgical intervention is still the treatment of choice, in general, for abscesses, perforation, fistula, and obstruction. Bleeding most often stops spontaneously. It is usually benign and at a slow, but steady rate. In the case of diverticulosis with bleeding that is massive or persistent, surgery may also be necessary. Parks found that 15 to 45 percent of patients hospitalized for diverticulitis required surgical intervention.

Nasogastric lavage should be done in the patient with rectal bleeding to ensure that the blood loss is not from the upper gastrointestinal tract. Colonoscopy and arteriography may be necessary to localize the bleeding site.

It appears that CT scanning is of little, if any, help in establishing the diagnosis. A mass may be detected, but it does not appear that the scan can yet differentiate the cause of the mass.

BIBLIOGRAPHY

Almy TP, Howell DA: Diverticular disease of the colon. *N Engl J Med* 302:324–331, 1980.

Bailey HR, Hernandez AJ Jr: Diverticulitis of the midrectum. *Dis Colon Rectum* 7:59–60, 1983.

Dawson JL, Hanon I, Roxburgh RA: Diverticulitis coli complicated by diffuse peritonitis. *Br J Surg* 52:354–357, 1965.

Eastwood MA: Medical and dietary management. *Clin Gastroenterol* 4:85–97, 1975.

Fisher JK: Abnormal colonic wall thickening on computed tomography. *J Comput Assist Tomogr* 7:90–97, 1983.

Gouge TH, Coppa GF, Eng K, et al: Management of diverticulitis of the ascending colon. 10 years experience. *Am J Surg* 145:387–391, 1983.

Kirwan WO, Smith AN, McConnell AA, et al: Action of different bran preparations on colonic function. *Br Med J* 4:187–189, 1974.

Ouriel K, Schwartz SI: Diverticular disease in the young patient. *Surg Gynecol Obstet* 156:1–5, 1983.

Parks TG: Natural history of diverticular disease of the colon. *Clin Gastroenterol* 4:53–69, 1975.

Painter NS, Truelove SC: The intraluminal pressure patterns in diverticulosis of the colon. *Gut* 5:201–213, 1964.

Schnyder P, Moss AA, Floeni FR, et al: Double-blind study of radiologic accuracy in diverticulitis, diverticulosis, and carcinomas of the sigmoid colon. *Clin J Gastroenterol* 1:55–66, 1979.

Schuler JG, Bayley J: Diverticulitis of the cecum. *Surg Gynecol Obstet* 156:743–748, 1983.

Sweatman CA Jr, Aldrete JS: The surgical management of diverticular disease of the colon complicated by perforation. *Surg Gynecol Obstet* 144:47–50, 1977.

Walker JD, Gray LA Sr, Polk HC Jr: Diverticulitis in women: An unappreciated clinical presentation. *Ann Surg* 185:402–405, 1977.

Welch CE, Malt RA: Abdominal surgery. *N Engl J Med* 300:648–653, 1979.

CHAPTER 64
ANORECTAL DISORDERS

Ronald L. Krome

There are a number of problems that involve the anorectal region; many of them occur because of disease within the intestine. In this chapter we deal only with those problems that are inherent to the anorectal region. The common symptoms of anorectal problems are as follows:

Bleeding
Constipation
Diarrhea
Discharge
Incomplete evacuation
Incontinence
Pain
Protrusion

HEMORRHOIDS

Hemorrhoids are one of the most common problems afflicting mankind. Internal hemorrhoids are dilatation of the venous plexus underlying the mucosa of the upper anal canal. They may be seen on sigmoidoscopy at the 4, 7, and 11 o'clock positions. External hemorrhoids are seen as dilatation of veins at the anal verge and can be seen with external inspection.

Although the cause is not always known, there is an association with constipation and straining at stool. They are very common during pregnancy and may be the result of increased pressure on the venous drainage of the rectum. One of the physiologic shunts of the portal system involves the hemorrhoidal veins. Consequently, increased portal pressure, as occurs as a result of chronic liver disease, may produce dilatation of the hemorrhoids and varix formation. The bleeding that results in this complex is extremely difficult to control. Tumors of the rectum and descending colon, often associated with constipation and tenesmus, may cause hemorrhoids.

Clinical Features

Uncomplicated hemorrhoids are usually painless, and the chief complaint is painless, bright red rectal bleeding with defecation. Bleeding is most often minimal, with blood being found on the surface of the stool or on the toilet tissue. Although the most common cause of rectal bleeding is hemorrhoids, other more serious causes should be sought in all patients who present with this as their chief complaint. Chronic, slow, blood loss may go unnoticed but may result in an anemia. Pain, when present, is most severe at the time of defecation and subsides with time.

As they increase in size, hemorrhoids may prolapse, requiring periodic reduction by the patient. The prolapse may persist. When prolapse occurs, the patient may develop a discharge and pruritus ani.

If the prolapse cannot be reduced, strangulation can result. Other complications include severe bleeding and thrombosis. Both strangulation and thrombosis are extremely painful and are accompanied by significant edema that must be treated before surgical intervention. Ulceration of the overlying mucosa may occur as well.

Treatment

Most treatment is local in nature and nonsurgical. Hot sitz baths, three to four times a day, will relieve pain and edema. Following the bath, the anus must be dried thoroughly. An analgesic cream or suppository should be used following the bath. The patient should be sure not to sit for a prolonged period on the commode. Stool softeners are helpful. Bulk laxatives can and should be used after the acute phase is adequately treated.

If symptoms are severe, thrombosed external hemorrhoids can be treated in the emergency department by making an incision directly over the palpated clot and extruding it. Bleeding may occur but will stop with the application of a compression dressing. Since there are often many clots, incision will relieve pain, but is not complete treatment. If pain is not severe, then the patient may be treated symptomatically. Complete treatment requires excision of the involved hemorrhoid.

Surgical intervention for hemorrhoids is indicated for intractable pain, severe unrelenting pruritus, continued bleeding, strangulation, and thrombosis. Surgical treatment can consist of sclerosing injections, the use of rubber band ligation, and excision.

FISSURE IN ANO

This common problem is a linear ulcer of the anal canal starting in the skin and sometimes extending into the area of the mucosa. It is often associated with swelling of the surrounding tissues, producing the characteristic sentinel pile, or hypertrophic papilla.

Most often it occurs in the midline posteriorly. In women, it may be in the midline anteriorly. A fissure not located in the midline should arouse suspicion that another cause is involved, e.g., an ulcerating neoplasm, syphilis, tuberculosis, Crohn's disease, etc. Most often a midline fissure is caused by the trauma produced by the passage of a particularly hard or large fecal mass and is associated with secondary infection. It is very painful, often associated with severe spasm of the anal sphincter and the retention of stool.

Clinical Features

On defecation there is severe pain which may last for hours. The pain diminishes with time, only to recur with each bowel movement. Sphincter spasm and pain may make the patient avoid defecation. Spasm may be so severe that the patient will not permit digital examination. Inspection of the anus will reveal the classic linear ulceration.

Treatment

Treatment is aimed at relieving the anal sphincter spasm. Hot sitz baths three to four times a day will relax the area and provide pain relief. The anus must be dried thoroughly after each bath. Local analgesic ointments, not containing hydrocortisone, are very helpful. A bulk laxative is used to ensure passage of a well-formed stool; this prevents scar formation from contracting the anus. Following defecation, the anus must be cleaned thoroughly. Healing is by the development of granulation tissue and reepithelization of the ulcerated area. If healing does not occur, the fissure may need to be excised.

ABSCESSES

Abscesses are common in the perirectal and perianal regions, as are fistulas, a common sequela. Abscesses may occur in any of the potential spaces near the anus or rectum.

Most abscesses point at the skin. There may be internal communication with the rectum or an anal crypt, and drainage, especially if spontaneous or inadequate, may lead to fistula development.

Ischiorectal abscesses are a different problem. The ischiorectal fossa forms a large potential space on either side of the rectum, communicating behind it, and with extensions anteriorly above the perineal membrane to the prostate in males. Infections in this area are insidious and can point in an area at some distance from the skin. The abscess can be quite large, and only a "mass" is detected on physical examination of the perineal area.

Most abscesses in this area are the result of obstruction of an anal gland which sits in the base of an anal crypt and normally drains into the anal canal. When obstruction occurs, the gland is blocked, resulting in infection and abscess formation. An element of cryptitis is frequently found if sought on anoscopic examination. There are a variety of diseases that are associated with the development of fistulous abscesses including gonococcal proctitis, Crohn's disease, and leukemia.

Clinical Features

Initially the patient notes a dull, aching pain or sensation in the rectal or anal area, becoming worse before defecation and better after defecation. The pain is increased by the increased pressure in the rectum that occurs just before defecation.

As the abscess spreads, increases in size, and comes nearer the surface, the associated pain becomes more intense. There is local tenderness that interferes with walking or sitting.

The patient appears markedly uncomfortable and may be febrile. A tender mass may be present, or there may be a tender, erythematous area with or without fluctuance. On rectal examination, a tender mass is detected. Leukocytosis may be present.

Treatment

Treatment is surgical. Drainage should be both early and extensive. All abscesses in this area should be drained in the operating room. It is only in the controlled circumstances of the operating room that adequate anesthesia can be obtained to allow the extensive incision and drainage that may be required. This is especially true when one is dealing with an ischiorectal abscess. Only the very small, subcutaneous abscess can be treated with soaks.

FISTULA IN ANO

An anal fistula is an abnormal tract which connects the anal canal with the skin and is lined with granulation tissue. A fistula in ano most commonly results from a perianal or ischiorectal abscess. It may, however, be associated with ulcerative colitis, regional enteritis, or tuberculosis. Although anterior-opening fistulas tend to follow a simple, direct course to the anal canal, posterior-opening fistulas follow a devious, curving path.

Clinical Features

As long as the tract remains open, there is a persistent, blood-stained discharge. More commonly the tract becomes blocked periodically. There are bouts of inflammation and even abscess formation that may be relieved by spontaneous rupture. An abscess may be the only sign of fistula in ano.

Treatment

The only definitive treatment is surgical excision of the fistula.

RECTAL PROLAPSE

There are three classes of rectal prolapse: (1) prolapse involving the rectal mucosa only, (2) prolapse involving all layers of the rectum, and (3) intussusception of the upper rectum into the lower rectum where the apex of the intussusception protrudes through the anus.

In the first group, the prolapse occurs because of the loose attachments of the mucosa to the submucosal layers, and there is an associated weakness of the anal sphincter. In the second and third groups, prolapse occurs because of the laxity of the pelvic fascia and muscles. Complete rectal prolapse occurs at the extremes of life. Mucosal prolapse is frequently associated with hemorrhoids.

Clinical Features

Most patients complain of prolapse because they are able to detect the presence of a mass, especially following defecation or when they stand or walk. A profuse mucosal discharge is present with some bleeding. The associated anal sphincter weakness leads to fecal incontinence.

Treatment

In young children, after appropriate analgesia and sedation, prolapse can be reduced and the precipitating problem treated. Surgical intervention is generally indicated in all other age groups, unless the prolapse is minimal. If vascular compromise appears to have occurred, reduction may be necessary on an emergency basis.

PILONIDAL SINUS

Pilonidal sinus or abscess occurs in the upper part of the natal cleft overlying the sacrum. The sinus is formed by the penetration of the skin by hair. The sinus is perpetuated by the presence of the hair and repeated bouts of infection. Although once thought to be congenital in nature, pilonidal sinus is now considered an acquired problem.

Clinical Features

The patient generally complains of a persistent discharge. When abscess formation occurs, the patient complains of a tender mass. A single opening, with hair protruding, is the most common finding, unless an abscess is present.

Treatment

Surgery is the treatment of choice. It is inappropriate to incise and drain these abscesses in the emergency department.

ANORECTAL TUMORS

Anorectal tumors are common and often malignant. The most common tumors are adenocarcinomas arising in the anal canal. Squamous cell carcinoma and malignant melanomas arise in the skin of the anus, but are uncommon. Inguinal adenopathy may be present in patients with epidermoid carcinomas of the anus. Generally, there is bleeding to a minor extent, with the bright red blood frequently admixed with the stool. Weight loss, anorexia, constipation, narrowing of the caliber of the stool, and tenesmus may all be symptoms of anorectal carcinoma. Complete obstruction may also occur.

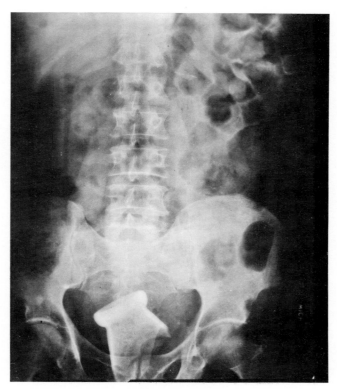

Figure 64-1. Milk bottle lodged in the rectum. Surgical consultation may be required for removal. (Courtesy of Detroit General Hospital.)

Anal canal tumors may produce rectal prolapse and tenesmus. Hemorrhoidal dilatation may also occur.

Villous adenomas frequently produce diarrhea and rectal discharge. The discharge may be copious and result in hypokalemia.

In most cases, rectal examination reveals a mass, and virtually all anorectal tumors can be detected by sigmoidoscopy.

RECTAL FOREIGN BODIES

The medical literature is replete with the variety of foreign bodies that have been reported to have been inserted into the rectum. Most foreign bodies are palpable, or detectable on sigmoidoscopic examination. Radiologic examination of the abdomen may reveal others (Fig. 64-1).

Perforation of the rectum or colon is the most frequent and serious complication. Perforation may be either extraperitoneal or intraperitoneal.

Treatment

Although most foreign bodies can be removed in the emergency department, some require surgical intervention. If the foreign body is removed in the emergency department and is of the size or shape to cause perforation, sigmoidoscopy and/or x-ray studies may be necessary to rule out iatrogenic perforation. Observation for 12 h, at least, should be done to ensure that perforation has not occurred.

Sphincter relaxation is mandatory for removal. Local infiltration anesthesia in the sphincter is frequently sufficient. Sedation is, of course, helpful. Suction created by a foreign body, such as a bottle, can be released by passing a catheter beyond the bottle and injecting air.

BIBLIOGRAPHY

Barone JE, Sohn NE, Nealon TF Jr: Perforations and foreign bodies of the rectum. *Ann Surg* 184:601–604, 1976.

Beahrs OH, Wilson SM: Carcinoma of the anus. *Ann Surg* 184:422–428, 1976.

Brenner BE, Simon RR: Anorectal emergencies. *Ann Emerg Med* 12:367–376, 1983.

Christiansen J, Kirkegaard P, Ibsen J: Prognosis after the treatment of villous adenomas of the colon and rectum. *Ann Surg* 189:404–408, 1979.

Eftaiha M, Hambrick E, Abcarian H: Principles of management of colorectal foreign bodies. *Arch Surg* 112:691–695, 1977.

Jahadi MR, Baldwin A: Villous adenomas of the colon and rectum. *Am J Surg* 130:729–732, 1975.

Sohn N, Weinstein MA, Robbins RD: Anorectal disorders. *Cur Probl Surg* vol 20, January 1983.

Trimpi HD, Khubchandani IT, Sheets JA, et al: Guide to the management of rectal abscesses. *Hosp Med* 12:79–88, 1976.

CHAPTER 65
DIARRHEA AND
FOOD POISONING

James Seidel

Vomiting, diarrhea, and gastrointestinal (GI) upset are common complaints in outpatient and emergency departments. The cause is most frequently food poisoning or an acute infectious illness. The majority of cases are mild, but systemic symptoms such as fever, rash, hypotension, and circulatory collapse may occur. Dehydration may be a prominent feature in the very young and old.

The causes of diarrheal illness include infection by viruses, bacteria, parasites, and fungi; antibiotic-induced enterocolitis; inflammatory bowel disease; cystic fibrosis; endocrinopathies; acrodermatitis enteropathica; lactose intolerance; milk allergy; or other extraintestinal infections such as otitis media or urinary tract infection.

Food poisoning may be caused by:

1. Toxic contaminants of food and water
   a. Heavy metals
   b. Organic chemicals: polyvinylchlorides
   c. Pesticides
   d. Radioactive substances
2. Bacterial, fungal, viral, and parasitic contaminants of food
   a. Invasive organisms
   b. Chemical metabolites of the microorganisms
3. Toxic substances naturally present in the food: akee fruit, mushrooms, thallophytes, fish (ciguatera, scombroid poisoning), dinoflagellates, shellfish.
4. Altered host response to a food substance, i.e., foods containing tyramine, monosodium glutamate, tryptamines, etc.
5. Food intolerance: shellfish, moray eel, chili pepper.

For the purpose of this brief review, we will only consider ciguatera fish poisoning and the infectious causes of food poisoning and diarrhea.

ETIOLOGY OF DIARRHEAL DISEASE

Viral Infections

The majority of cases of acute diarrheal disease, especially in children, are caused by viral infections and occur most often in the winter and the spring. Rotavirus has been studied most extensively and is responsible for endemic infantile gastroenteritis. Rotaviruses are most commonly seen in children under 1 year of age

but can occur in older children and adults. Typically the patient has fever, vomiting, and diarrhea, but may also have an upper respiratory infection or pneumonia. The diarrhea generally lasts for 3 to 10 days but may become protracted. Other viruses commonly associated with diarrhea are listed in Table 65-1 along with their clinical syndrome and typical clinical course.

Bacterial Infections

Bacterial infections are responsible for approximately 20 percent of acute infectious diarrheal illnesses. These agents may be divided into two classes; organisms that produce disease by direct invasion and those that produce enterotoxins that cause a secretory diarrhea, as depicted in Table 65-2.

Escherichia coli

Escherichia coli is the primary agent of traveler's diarrhea. Infection is acquired by ingestion of contaminated food and water. The ingested organism colonizes the intestine and elaborates an enterotoxin. Typically the patient experiences mild abdominal pain and watery diarrhea 2 to 4 days after infection. Infection may be fulminant and resemble clinical cholera but is usually self-limited and rarely associated with systemic symptoms. Thus only supportive therapy is required. *E. coli* may also produce invasive disease and a clinical picture similar to that described below for *Shigella*. Treatment with an antibiotic may be required in selective cases. The acquisition of enterotoxin production is plasmid-mediated; thus any serotype of *E. coli* may elaborate the toxin. Identification of enterotoxigenic organisms in the laboratory requires special techniques not widely available.

Shigella

Shigella infections are common in all parts of the world and are associated with food-borne, nosocomial transmission, and fecal and oral contamination. The organism is highly infectious, and ingestion of only 100 organisms may cause disease. The spectrum of illness may vary from mild—an asymptomatic carrier—to

Table 65-1. Viral Causes of Acute Diarrhea

Agent	Clinical Syndrome	Symptoms				
		Diarrhea	Vomiting	Fever	URI	Pneumonia
Rotavirus	Endemic infantile gastroenteritis	+ + +	+ +	+ +	+	±
Norwalk agent	Endemic gastroenteritis Family outbreaks	+ + +	+ +	+	−	−
Enteric type Adenovirus	Intestinal "flu"	+ +	+ +	+	+	±
Enterovirus	Variety of syndromes associated with mild GI upset	+	±	+ +	+	±

severe—a fulminant disease resulting in severe dehydration and death in the very young and old. The patient may become symptomatic 36 to 72 h after exposure. Infection is associated with abdominal pain and fever which may reach 40 or 41°C (104 or 105.8°F) in children. Bowel movements may be explosive and associated with blood and mucus in 50 to 75 percent of these patients. Young children may present with high fever and a febrile convulsion without a history of diarrhea; the diarrhea may begin in the emergency department, often when the child is being held for lumbar puncture.

A stool specimen should be transported to the microbiology lab in holding media as soon as possible. Even under the best circumstances, cultures may be negative in 30 percent of the cases and should be repeated. *Shigella*, like *E. coli*, generally causes a self-limited disease. The largest number of bowel movements are usually within the first 24 h, and dehydration may occur in young children. Deaths have been reported in infants within 8 h after the onset of symptoms. Although rare, bacteremia can occur with *Shigella* infections.

A complete blood cell count may be helpful in differentiating *Shigella* enteritis. The white blood cell count is generally elevated, and a marked left shift is observed. An absolute band count of greater than 800 is suggestive of *Shigella* infections.

Antibiotics promptly alter the course of *Shigella* infections but are only recommended in cases of *Shigella* dysentery or institutional outbreaks of *S. flexneri*. Although many strains are sensitive to ampicillin, trimethoprim with sulfamethoxazole is considered the treatment of choice by some authors. Without specific therapy the majority of patients have an uneventful recovery in 5 to 7 days. Complications of shigellosis include diarrhea and dehydration, Reiter's syndrome, arthralgias, and the hemolytic uremic syndrome.

Salmonella

This organism is ubiquitous in nature and is found in many animals as well as man. Most human infections occur as a result of contamination of food and water. Eggs, egg products, chicken, and turkey are often implicated as a source of infection. Pet turtles have also been known to carry the organism.

The clinical presentation is most often watery diarrhea associated with abdominal pain and cramping. Infection may produce septicemia with systemic symptoms including fever, cough, and meningismus (enteric fever). There may be a relative bradycardia associated with high fever; this is most often seen with infection of *Salmonella typhi*. Typhoid fever may present as an unremitting fever with abdominal pain, cramps, rose spots (10 to 20 percent), meningismus, and the absence of diarrhea. Drug addicts and persons with splenectomies or sickle cell disease are particularly susceptible to *Salmonella* infections. Uncomplicated *Salmonella* gastroenteritis should not be treated with antibiotics, but enteric fever should be treated in the hospital with antibiotics to which the organism is sensitive. Initial therapy should be with chloramphenicol or ampicillin.

Yersinia enterocolitis and Y. pseudotuberculosis

Domestic animals including household pets have been implicated in the transmission of *Yersinia* to humans. Food, water, and fecal-oral transmission have also been shown to occur. Infection is associated with gastroenteritis, colitis, dysentery, and fever. Mesenteric adenitis and pseudoappendicitis may also occur.

Yersinia is difficult to isolate in the laboratory, and when infection is suspected, one should specifically request the laboratory to isolate the organism. This may take days to accomplish, and often the symptoms have subsided when the report is returned from the lab. Symptomatic cases may be treated with ampicillin, chloramphenicol, or tetracycline, although experts do not agree about a precise treatment protocol.

Campylobacter fetus ssp. *jejuni*

Campylobacter fetus ssp. *jejuni* was first described in 1977 as a frequent cause of diarrhea. Isolation of the organism requires special laboratory techniques, and when such isolation has been per-

Table 65-2. Bacterial Causes of Acute Diarrhea

Invasive	Enterotoxin Producing	Unknown
Escherichia coli	*Clostridium perfringens*	*Vibrio parahemolyticus*
Salmonella	*Clostridium difficile*	
Shigella	*Staphylococcus aureus*	
Yersinia enterocolitica	*Vibrio cholerae*	
Campylobacter Fetus ssp. *jejuni*	*E. coli*	
	Bacillus cereus	
	Aeromonas hydrophila	

formed routinely, the organism has been shown to be as common as *Salmonella* and *Shigella* as a cause of bacterial diarrhea. The majority of patients present with fever and bloody diarrhea; two-thirds have abdominal pain, and one-third have vomiting. *Campylobacter* gastroenteritis is most frequently reported in children. Waterborne infections have been reported. Erythromycin is the treatment of choice in children, and tetracycline in adults. Parenteral treatment with gentamicin may be required to treat serious infections.

Clostridium perfringens

Clostridium perfringens is a common cause of food poisoning. The organism is a normal flora of the colon of humans and other animals, but only heat-resistant strains have been associated with enteritis. Human intestinal carriage of heat-resistant strains is in the range of 2 to 9 percent. The incubation period is 6 to 24 h, with an average of 12 h to the onset of symptoms. These include abdominal cramps and diarrhea. Constitutional symptoms such as headache, chills, and fever may occur, although they are not a prominent feature of clostridial food poisoning. Nausea and vomiting are usually not seen. Meat and meat products are usually implicated in the transmission of the bacteria. Clostridial food poisoning is generally self-limited and requires no therapy. Antitoxin to the beta toxin has been considered useful in the treatment of necrotizing enteritis of group C *C. perfringens*.

Clostridium difficile

An overgrowth of this organism has been associated with pseudomembranous enterocolitis, which may develop after the administration of antibiotics. The organism releases cytotoxins that produce a profuse diarrhea that may be indistinguishable from that of severe shigellosis. If untreated, the disease is associated with high mortality. Treatment includes the administration of vancomycin, the binding of the toxin with cholestyramine, and the administration of supportive fluids.

Staphylococcus aureus

Infections with *Staphylococcus* may occur after antibiotic therapy, with an overgrowth of the organism in the bowel and resultant enterocolitis. The enterotoxins may also contaminate food such as ham, poultry, meats, and dairy products. The organism and the enterotoxins it produces are the most common cause of food-borne disease. Vomiting and diarrhea are the most common symptoms, but abdominal cramps, headache, and prostration may occur when large amounts of toxin are ingested. The incubation period is 2 to 24 h with symptoms appearing most often 6 to 12 h after ingestion of the toxin. The disease is generally self-limited, and supportive therapy is all that is required.

Bacillus cereus

Recent work has shown that *Bacillus cereus* enterotoxins cause two clinical syndromes. *B. cereus* has been associated with a predominantly upper GI tract illness with vomiting that may develop 1 to 6 h after ingestion of contaminated food, particularly fried rice. A lower intestinal tract illness that resembles *C. perfringens* enteritis may also develop 6 to 24 h after ingesting a contaminated meal. *B. cereus* should be suspected if more than 10^5 organisms are isolated from the stool. Treatment is symptomatic.

Aeromonas hydrophila

Aeromonas hydrophila is a vibrio, found in soil and water, which can cause a choleralike GI disorder when contaminated food or water is ingested. The disease is mediated by an enterotoxin. Treatment is symptomatic, but serious infections can be treated with chloramphenicol or aminoglycosides.

Vibrio cholerae

Cholera is an acute infectious diarrhea caused by *Vibrio cholerae*. The disease is transmitted by contaminated water or food. A large innoculum of the organism is required to produce disease because of the acid sensitivity of the bacteria. The illness may begin with vomiting, but production of copious watery diarrhea is the hallmark of clinical cholera. Large volumes of "rice water" stool may lead to (1) severe dehydration due to loss of isotonic fluid from the bowel, (2) acidosis due to loss of bicarbonate in the stool, and (3) hypokalemia due to potassium loss in the stool. The disease may be complicated by renal failure and hypovolemic shock. Therapy is aimed at oral or parenteral replacement of fluids. Antibiotics may shorten the clinical course; tetracycline and trimethoprim with sulfamethoxazole are the drugs of choice.

Vibrio parahemolyticus

This organism has been associated with the ingestion of raw or improperly prepared seafood, particularly oysters, clams, and crabs. The spectrum of disease varies from mild gastroenteritis to explosive diarrhea associated with cramps, vomiting, and dysentery. The average incubation period is 12 h but may vary from 2 to 24 h. As is the case with cholera, symptomatic treatment is important. It is unclear if oral antibiotics are beneficial. In severe infections, however, tetracycline and chloramphenicol have been used.

Parasites

A variety of parasitic protozoa and helminths may produce diarrhea during the course of infection. Only two, however, are important in the United States as a cause of acute diarrheal disease.

Entamoeba histolytica

The prevalence of *E. histolytica* infection in the United States is probably between 1 and 5 percent. The majority of those infected are asymptomatic. These asymptomatic cyst passers may transmit the disease through the fecal-oral route as well as contaminate the environment with infected cysts. The disease may also be venereally transmitted through anal intercourse. Infection may cause colitis with abdominal cramps and diarrhea, or acute amebic dysentery with profuse bloody diarrhea. Vomiting is usually absent. Approximately 5 percent of the patients with dysentery develop extraintestinal amebiasis. The liver is the most common site of amebic abscesses, but they can also develop in the lung, heart, kidney, or brain. Treatment includes the use of metronidazole, tetracycline, or for severe infections, emetine hydrochloride or dehydroemetine plus chloroquine.

Giardia lamblia

Giardia is the most common intestinal parasite in the United States. Infection may be asymptomatic. Transmission is through fecal or oral contamination with infective cysts or through other contamination of water and food. Beavers have been shown to play a role in transmission through infection of mountain streams in Colorado and the northwest. Patients most often complain of abdominal pain and distention, postprandial urgency to defecate, and feeling bloated and gaseous. They may have profuse diarrhea that is foul-smelling. Classically the stools are floating, frothy, and foul-smelling. Diagnosis may be difficult as the cysts are only passed sporadically. At least three stools should be submitted for examination for ova and parasites. If these are negative and there is a high index of suspicion, an Enterotest (string test) or duodenal aspiration may be performed to look for trophozoites. Although metronidazole has been used effectively for the treatment of giardiasis, it is not approved for use in this infection. Quinacrine hydrochloride is the drug of choice.

Ciguatera Fish Poisoning

Although many exogenous toxins may cause GI upset, they are too numerous to discuss in this chapter. One, however, is worth mentioning briefly as it is becoming more prevalent in the southeastern United States: this is ciguatera fish poisoning. Fish whose ingestion can cause the disease are found in tropical and subtropical waters. These fish, particularly grouper, snapper, and kingfish, become sporadically poisonous when a particular dinoflagellate is present in the food chain in the late spring and summer months. The incubation period varies from 2 to 30 h after ingestion of the toxin (median 6 h). The illness may begin with vomiting and diarrhea, which are present in 78 percent of the patients. Neuromuscular and neurosensory manifestations may be particularly severe and lead to prolonged discomfort. These include myalgia of the legs and thighs, weakness, and dysesthesia and paresthesia of the perioral region and distal extremities. Occasionally patients describe a "burning" sensation of their feet or hands. Itching of various parts of the body is common and may be a late manifestation on day 2 or 3 of the illness. The disease is self-limited, and there is no specific therapy. Symptoms generally subside in several days, but some patients have reported having sensory problems for months after the ingestion of affected fish.

GENERAL MANAGEMENT

A complete history, including the time of onset of the symptoms, travel, and the relation of the symptoms to ingestion of a particular food, is important in determining the cause of the GI illness. The frequency, consistency, and odor of the stool and the presence of mucus or blood in the stool should also be determined. Physical examination should include all systems, as extraintestinal disease may cause GI upset and diarrhea.

Laboratory studies are not generally helpful in the acute management of food poisoning and infectious diarrhea. A high white blood cell count with a left shift may suggest a bacterial cause; however, this condition is not always present. In typhoid fever, one may see a relatively low white blood cell count and neutropenia. Electrolytes are indicated when dehydration is suspected, and urine specific gravity should be obtained. If a stool sample is available, a wet mount may be made by mixing a small amount of feces with normal saline on a slide. Microscopic examination of this preparation may show white and red blood cells, mucus strands, and trophozoites or cysts of parasitic protozoa. A Hemoccult test of the stool may also reveal the presence of blood. Cultures should be sent to the laboratory in transport media when *Salmonella, Shigella, Campylobacter,* or *Vibrio* infections are suspected because of the public health importance of these infections.

Many prescription and over-the-counter preparations are available for the treatment of diarrhea, vomiting, and GI upset. Few have been shown to be effective in altering the course of the illness. Most infectious and noninfectious GI illnesses are self-limited and do not require specific therapy. Antibiotics should be reserved for patients who are febrile and toxic, but antibiotics should be used only for diseases for which they have been shown to be effective. Contraindications to antibiotic therapy may exist in some uncomplicated infections, such as salmonellosis, as they prolong the carrier state. Other medications such as diphenoxylate hydrochloride with atropine (Lomotil) may provide temporary symptomatic relief and may be efficacious if the patient has uncontrollable diarrhea. These preparations and others that slow peristalsis and delay intestinal emptying may prolong the illness, as infective organisms and toxins have continued contact with the bowel. The mainstay of therapy is putting the intestinal tract at rest and maintaining hydration. Most patients can be managed with a clear liquid diet. Liquids may include clear fruit juices, sodas, gelatin dessert water, rice water, etc. The diet may be advanced to include rice, applesauce, bananas, and toast when the diarrhea has subsided. Small sips of clear liquids should be recommended when vomiting is prominent. Using popsicles is also recommended. Phenothiazine preparations may be used with severe vomiting but are not recommended in children because of a higher incidence of dystonic reactions. Hospitalization should be considered in the very young and old when there is evidence of dehydration.

BIBLIOGRAPHY

Black RE, Jackson RJ, Tsai T, et al: Epidemic *Yersinia enterocolitica* infection due to contaminated chocolate milk. *N Engl J Med* 298:76–79, 1978.

Communicable Disease Surveillance Center, PHLS: Surveillance of food poisoning and *Salmonella* infections in England and Wales 1170-9. *Br Med J* 281:817–818, 1980.

Harris JC, Dupont HL, Hornck RB: Fecal leukocytes in diarrheal illness. *Ann Intern Med* 76:697–703, 1972.

Lawrence DN, Enriquez MB, Lumish RM, et al: Ciguatera fish poisoning in Miami. *JAMA* 244:254–258, 1980.

Lowenstein MS: Epidemiology of *Clostridium perfringens* food poisoning. *N Engl J Med* 286:1026–1028, 1972.

Markell EK, Voge M: *Medical Parasitology,* ed 5. Philadelphia, WB Saunders Co, 1981.

Nelson J, Kumiosz H, Jackson L, et al: Trimethoprim-sulfamethoxazole therapy for shigellosis. *JAMA* 235:1239–1243, 1976.

Rodriguez WJ, Kim HW, Arrobio JO, et al: Clinical features of acute gastroenteritis associated with human reovirus-like agent in infants and young children. *J Pediatr* 91:188–193, 1977.

CHAPTER 66
CHOLECYSTITIS

Ronald L. Krome

It is estimated that from 5000 to 8000 deaths each year in the United States can be attributed to gallstone disease. It is also believed that about 800,000 new cases of cholelithiasis appear each year in this country. Cholecystitis is an acute inflammatory process involving the gallbladder and is most often, but not always, associated with gallstones. It is manifested by signs and symptoms of an acutely inflamed or obstructed gallbladder.

Acute cholecystitis may occur as a complication of a terminal systemic disease or as a postoperative complication of non–biliary tract abdominal surgery as long as 2 weeks after surgery. It also occurs in association with a number of other systemic diseases.

Cholecystitis has been reported in children as young as 14 days of age. In children, the cause is unknown, but steroids, marked obesity, and generalized sepsis with dehydration have all been associated with this problem. Most report a 50 percent incidence of calculi in infant cholecystitis.

In the elderly, there has been a high association between cholecystitis and a number of other medical problems: cardiovascular disease, hypertension, and diabetes mellitus. Hemolytic anemias, such as sickle cell disease, have also been associated with acute cholecystitis and cholelithiasis.

PATHOGENESIS

Gallstones are found in almost 30 percent of all persons over 40. The incidence increases with increasing age, with the highest incidence in those in their eighties.

In most, if not all, cases of cholecystitis, gallstones are present with some element of obstruction of the cystic duct. Most stones in the United States are composed of cholesterol; of these, 15 to 25 percent are radiopaque and their contents are mostly pigment.

Obstruction of the cystic duct leads to overconcentration of the bile trapped in the gallbladder. Inflammation of the gallbladder mucosa with increased secretion of fluid produces distention of the gallbladder, and this leads to increased intraluminal pressure. Most often, the bile is sterile. However, the blood supply of the gallbladder may be compromised by the distention, resulting in infection, gangrene, empyema, necrosis, or perforation.

Gangrene of the gallbladder and perforation occur in about 10 to 15 percent of cases. The perforation may be walled off in the right upper quadrant by the omentum and surrounding small bowel. In this case, an intraabdominal abscess (subhepatic abscess) develops. The abscess may subsequently erode into the small bowel, producing a biliary enteric fistula, although most often such fistulas are the result of erosion by a stone. Gallstones that erode through may be so large that they produce obstruction of the small bowel (gallstone ileus).

Emphysematous cholecystitis is an uncommon presentaton of acute cholecystitis resulting from gas-forming organisms. Although acute cholecystitis is more common in women, emphysematous cholecystitis is more common in men. Gangrene is more frequent and stones less frequent in emphysematous cholecystitis.

Acute cholecystitis may occur without gallstones. In about 6 to 8 percent of patients, there is a predisposing factor such as non–biliary tract surgery, trauma, burns, the postpartum state, hypertension, atherosclerosis, diabetes, myocardial failure, or phlebitis. In children there is an antecedent illness in 60 percent of the cases, and the disease tends to occur twice as often in boys.

CLINICAL FEATURES

In general, acalculous and calculous cholecystitis present with the same picture.

The most prominent symptom is severe upper abdominal pain, initially colicky in nature, but rapidly becoming continuous. The pain may be located in the right upper quadrant and may become worse with coughing or deep breathing if the inflamed gallbladder touches the diaphragm. Often there is a past history of fatty food intolerance, with pain, vomiting, frequent eructation, and flatulence. Although the pain may remain diffuse, it generally localizes in the right upper quadrant.

Nausea is frequent, but vomiting is neither frequent nor voluminous. If biliary obstruction is complete, there should be no bile in the vomitus. Fever and chills are additional complaints. Jaundice, if present, may be detected by the patient. When present, jaundice is the most serious complication of ductal obstruction. It may occur in the absence of obstruction and in the presence of acute cholangitis.

A temperature elevation may be present in the range of 38.3 to 38.8°C (101 to 102°F). There may be associated tachycardia and tachypnea. Tenderness and guarding may be present on palpation of the right upper quadrant. If perforation and generalized peritonitis have occurred, rigidity will be present. In about 25 percent of cases, a tender palpable mass is found in the right upper quadrant. There may be some abdominal distention. Ileus is common, and therefore the bowel sounds are diminished.

Sepsis may occur as a complication of biliary obstruction, perforation, or acute cholangitis. The incidence of acute cholangitis is highest in patients with choledocholithiasis. When sepsis occurs, it is presaged by the development of fever, chills, and severe pain.

Generally, there is some elevation of the white blood cell count with a shift to the left. Often there is mild elevation of the bilirubin and the alkaline phosphatase levels. The amylase level may also be elevated, but only to a mild degree.

In patients over 60 years of age, the temperature may not be elevated, peritoneal signs may be absent, and the white cell count, serum bilirubin, and alkaline phosphatase levels all may be normal. Because of the high incidence of concomitant disease, the mortality rate is higher in those over 60 years.

Plain films of the abdomen may reveal the presence of calculi. If emphysematous cholecystitis is present, air bubbles may be seen in the wall of the gallbladder or along the biliary tract. If perforation and abscess formation have occurred, extraluminal air-fluid levels may be seen in the right upper quadrant.

If a biliary enteric fistula has developed, air may be seen in the biliary tract, or a radiopaque stone may be seen in the small bowel.

In acute cholecystitis, if oral cholecystography is done, the gallbladder will not visualize. Infusion cholecystography with tomography may be useful but is generally not available on an emergency basis. Ultrasonography is useful in detecting gallstones and dilatation of biliary ducts, but it will not establish the diagnosis of cholecystitis. Although CT scanning is useful in detecting dilatation of ducts and the gallbladder, it is no more reliable than ultrasonography in detecting stones.

Endoscopic retrograde cholangiopancreatography (ERCP) is being more widely used to study both the biliary and the pancreatic duct systems to detect obstruction. Its added advantage is that the duodenum and stomach can be studied.

TREATMENT

Most authors agree that surgery is indicated when the diagnosis is established and the patient is stable. Emergency treatment includes the use of a nasogastric tube and intravenous fluids. Patients with acute cholecystitis should be hospitalized and treated with suction, fluids, and antibiotics. If the patient is unstable or has a complication of acute cholecystitis, surgery is most likely indicated.

Mortality rates are highest in those over 60 years of age and in those with acalculous cholecystitis.

BIBLIOGRAPHY

Adams TW, Foxley EG Jr: A diagnostic technique for acalculous cholecystitis. *Surg Gynecol Obstet* 142:168–170, 1976.

Ariyan S, Shessel FS, Pickett LK: Cholecystitis and cholelithiasis masking as abdominal crisis in sickle cell disease. *Pediatrics* 58:252–258, 1976.

Chenung LY, Maxwell JG: Jaundice in patients with acute cholecystitis: Its validity as an indication for common bile duct exploration. *Am J Surg* 130:746–748, 1975.

Glenn F: Acute acalculous cholecystitis. *Ann Surg* 189:458–465, 1979.

Glenn F: Acute cholecystitis. *Surg Gynecol Obstet* 143:56–60, 1976.

Jordan LJ Jr: Choledocholithiasis. *Curr Probl Surg* vol 19, December 1982.

Keddie NC, Gough AL, Galland RB: Acalculous gallbladder disease: A prospective study. *Br J Surg* 63:797–798, 1976.

McAvoy JM, Roth J, Rees WV, et al: Role of ultrasonography in the primary diagnosis of cholelithiasis: An analysis of fifty cases. *Am J Surg* 136:309–312, 1978.

McCluskey PL, Prinz RA, Guico R, et al: Use of ultrasound to demonstrate gallstones in symptomatic patients with normal oral cholecystograms. *Am J Surg* 138:655–657, 1979.

Mentzaer RM, Golden GT, Chandler JG, et al: A comparative appraisal of emphysematous cholecystitis. *Am J Surg* 129:10–15, 1975.

Pieretti R, Auldist AW, Stephens CA: Acute cholecystitis in children. *Surg Gynecol Obstet* 140:16–18, 1975.

Pinto DJ, Burke M, Wilkins A, et al: Infusion cholecystography in the diagnosis of acute cholecystitis. *Br J Surg* 66:173–176, 1979.

Pitluk HC, Beal JM: Choledocholithiasis associated with acute cholecystitis. *Arch Surg* 114:887–888, 1979.

Saharia PC, Cameron JL: Clinical management of acute cholangitis. *Surg Gynecol Obstet* 142:369–372, 1976.

Small DM: The etiology and pathogenesis of gallstones. *Adv Surg* 10:63, 1976.

Ternberg JL, Keating JP: Acute acalculous cholecystitis: Complication of other illnesses in childhood. *Arch Surg* 110:543–547, 1975.

Thompson J, Morrow DJ, Wilson SE: Acute cholecystitis in the elderly: A surgical emergency. *Arch Surg* 113:1149–1152, 1978.

Zwemer FL, Coffin-Kwart VE, Conway MJ: Biliary enteric fistulas: Management of 47 cases in native Americans. *Am J Surg* 138:301–304, 1979.

CHAPTER 67
ACUTE JAUNDICE

Richard Owen Shields Jr.

Jaundice is the yellowish discoloration of the scleras, skin, and mucous membranes by bilirubin. Long-standing hemochromatosis, the picrates, and carotene may also cause yellow-orange discoloration of the skin but do not discolor the sclerae.

Bilirubin, a breakdown product of hemoglobin from injured or senescent red blood cells, is produced in the reticuloendothelial system and transported on albumin to the liver. There it is conjugated as the diglucuronide and excreted via the bile channels into the small intestine. An increase in the production of bilirubin or a defect in the elimination pathway may produce clinical jaundice and hyperbilirubinemia.

Hyperbilirubinemia can be divided into two subtypes: conjugated and unconjugated. Unconjugated hyperbilirubinemia results from an increased bilirubin load or a defect in the hepatocytes' ability to take up and conjugate bilirubin. Conjugated hyperbilirubinemia may be either intrahepatic or extrahepatic in origin. Intrahepatic cholestasis is caused by decreased excretion of conjugated bilirubin, hepatocellular damage, and damage to the biliary epithelium. Obstruction of biliary outflow by a congenital defect, inflammation, a mass lesion, or gallstones produces extrahepatic cholestasis (see Table 67-1).

Emergency Department Evaluation

In the emergency department (ED), a patient with a new onset of jaundice poses a diagnostic challenge. Jaundice is present in a variety of diseases, some of which are benign and some of which are life-threatening. A careful history and physical examination coupled with judicious use of the laboratory frequently enable the emergency physician to make a reasonable diagnosis and decide if hospitalization is indicated. Often, however, more extensive diagnostic procedures (e.g., ultrasound, cholecystograms, CT scan, liver biopsy, etc.) are needed before the cause of the jaundice can be determined.

History

Jaundice without other complaints, and a family history of jaundice, suggest a hereditary cause. Viral hepatitis should be suspected in a young person with a history of intravenous drug abuse, contact with a jaundiced person, raw seafood ingestion, recent blood transfusion, ear piercing, tattoos, needle puncture, or foreign travel. Toxic hepatitis should be considered if there is a history of exposure to toxic chemicals or use of hepatotoxic drugs.

Older patients with right upper quadrant abdominal pain, vomiting, and fever probably have extrahepatic biliary obstruction. Heavy alcohol abusers with fever and abdominal pain are likely to have either alcoholic hepatitis or cirrhosis. Pruritus and dark stools imply cholestasis.

Physical Examination

Jaundice can most easily be detected in the mucous membranes of the mouth and the conjunctivas under natural light. The presence

Table 67-1. Causes of Jaundice

I. Unconjugated
  A. Hemolytic anemia
  B. Hemoglobinopathy
  C. Transfusion reaction
  D. Gilbert's disease
  E. Crigler-Najjar syndrome
  F. Prematurity in neonates
  G. Congestive heart failure
II. Conjugated
  A. Intrahepatic
    1. Infections
      a. Viral hepatitis
      b. Leptospirosis
      c. Infectious mononucleosis
    2. Toxic
      a. Drugs
      b. Chemicals
    3. Familial
      a. Rotor syndrome
      b. Dubin-Johnson Syndrome
    4. Alcoholic liver disease
    5. Other
      a. Sarcoidosis
      b. Lymphoma
      c. Liver metastases
      d. Amyloidosis
      e. Cirrhosis
      f. Biliary cirrhosis
  B. Extrahepatic
    1. Gallstones
    2. Pancreatic tumors or cysts
    3. Cholangiocarcinoma
    4. Bile duct stricture
    5. Sclerosing cholangitis

of ascites, edema, and spider angiomas suggests cirrhosis. Right upper quadrant tenderness, a positive Murphy's sign, or a palpable gallbladder might indicate biliary disease. Cachexia and an epigastric mass suggest a neoplastic process, while a hard, nodular liver may represent hepatic metastases. Hepatomegaly with pedal edema, jugular vein distension, and a gallop rhythm make congestive cardiac failure the likely cause of jaundice.

Laboratory

The total bilirubin level is elevated if clinical jaundice is present. With unconjugated hyperbilirubinemia, 85 percent or more of the total bilirubin is of the indirect fraction. A direct-reacting fraction of at least 30 percent and usually higher is present with conjugated hyperbilirubinemia. A bedside test to determine if bilirubin is conjugated or not is to test the urine for bilirubin. Conjugated bilirubin is water-soluble and appears in the urine at very low serum concentrations. Unconjugated bilirubin is bound to albumin and is not present in urine. Some degree of cholestasis is present if the alkaline phosphatase level is elevated to greater than three times normal. Anemia with reticulocytosis and an abnormal peripheral smear are characteristic of hemolysis. Markedly elevated transaminase levels are most compatible with a viral hepatitis. A prolonged prothrombin time, a low albumin level, anemia, and ethanol suggest alcoholic hepatitis or decompensated cirrhosis.

ACUTE HEPATITIS

Viral Hepatitis

Viral hepatitis produces inflammation of the liver and necrosis of hepatic parenchymal cells. The severity of illness ranges from inapparent, subclinical infections to fulminant hepatic failure and death. The initial prodromal symptoms are usually constitutional, may be quite variable, and may be abrupt or insidious in onset. Nausea, vomiting, fatigue, malaise, and alterations in taste are common. Low-grade fever with pharyngitis, coryza, and headache may lead to an early diagnosis of upper respiratory infection or "flulike" syndrome.

The majority of cases do not develop jaundice and recover uneventfully. In icteric cases, jaundice develops 1 to 2 weeks following the onset of the prodrome and may be preceded by a few days of pruritis and dark urine. Other prodromal symptoms usually diminish during the icteric phase, but malaise and gastrointestinal (GI) symptoms frequently persist. Right upper quadrant abdominal pain may develop because of hepatic enlargement. Physical examination during the icteric phase may reveal hepatomegaly, splenomegaly, and jaundice. In the recovery phase, the symptoms disappear, and complete clinical and biochemical recovery is the rule in 3 to 4 months.

The first biochemical abnormality is an elevation of the levels of serum transaminases (SGOT and SGPT) before the onset of the prodromal phase. The levels peak during the phase of clinical hepatitis and return to normal during recovery, the magnitude of the elevation not being a good indicator of the severity of the disease. A prothrombin time prolongation of more than a few seconds indicates extensive hepatic necrosis and a poorer prognosis, as does a persistent bilirubin level elevation of greater than 20 mg/100 mL. An early transient neutropenia is often followed

by a relative lymphocytosis with many atypical lymphocytes. Blood glucose levels may be depressed because of poor intake, depleted hepatic glycogen stores, and decreased hepatic gluconeogenesis.

Hepatitis A

Hepatitis A, formerly known as infectious hepatitis, is caused by a small RNA virus (HAV) (see Table 67-2) of the enterovirus group which is spread primarily by the oral-fecal route. Victims are usually children and adolescents with a seasonal peak of reported cases in fall and winter. About 30,000 cases are reported yearly in the United States, but this represents only a small minority of actual cases. Most cases of hepatitis A are mild, anicteric, and undiagnosed, as suggested by the fact that although more than 50 percent of the adults in the United States have serologic evidence of past hepatitis A infection, fewer than 10 percent of them can recall an episode of jaundice or hepatitis.

The incubation period for hepatitis A is 15 to 50 days with fecal shedding of virus in the final 1 to 2 weeks and during the first week of the prodrome. The onset of symptoms is more often abrupt than with hepatitis B or non-A, non-B. If jaundice develops, it appears several days to a week later and is usually mild. No carrier state or chronic liver disease has been described following hepatitis A infection. During the clinical phase of illness, IgM antibodies appear in the serum but are soon replaced by IgG antibodies which persist indefinitely.

Hepatitis B

Hepatitis B (formerly known as serum hepatitis) is caused by a double-stranded DNA virus with an inner core and an outer coat, both of which are antigenic. Hepatitis B is spread primarily by the percutaneous route, although in as many as 50 percent of acute cases no clear history of exposure can be obtained. Infective particles are present in blood, saliva, semen, and other body fluids and are responsible for at least some of the nonpercutaneous transmission of the disease. Hepatitis B virus (HBV) is maintained in humans in a large reservoir of chronic carriers, the carrier rate in the United States as a whole being 0.1 to 0.5 percent. Certain subpopulations such as intravenous drug abusers and patients on hemodialysis have a much higher rate.

The incubation period of hepatitis B is 70 to 160 days with a mean of 70 to 80 days. As is the case with hepatitis A, most cases are inapparent or anicteric. The onset of symptoms is usually insidious and is preceded in 5 to 10 percent of the cases by a "serum-sickness-like" illness with polyarthritis, proteinuria, and

Table 67-2. Distinguishing Features of the Hepatitis Viruses

Feature	Hepatitis A	Hepatitis B	Hepatitis NANB
Size	27 nm	42 nm	?
Nucleic acid	RNA	DNA	?
Incubation	15–49 days	70–160 days	15–160 days
Range (mean)	30 days	70–80 days	50 days
Oral-fecal	Yes	No	?
Percutaneous	Rare	Yes	Yes
Carrier state	No	Yes	Yes
Severity	Mild	Often severe	Moderate
Mortality	0.1–0.2%	1%	<1%

angioneurotic edema thought to be caused by circulating antigen-antibody complexes. With hepatitis B the symptoms tend to be more severe and prolonged than with hepatitis A, but complete recovery is expected in 90 percent of the cases.

Fulminant hepatitis develops in about 1 percent of the cases, characterized by encephalopathy, rapidly rising bilirubin levels, and a greatly prolonged prothrombin time. Complete recovery is possible, but 80 percent of those who develop coma die. About 10 percent of the cases develop either a chronic carrier state or chronic hepatitis.

The identification of three distinct hepatitis B antigens has provided serologic methods to diagnose and monitor patients with hepatitis B. Hepatitis B surface antigen (HB_sAg) represents the outer coat of the virus particle. It appears in the serum of more than 90 percent of the patients before the elevation of the transaminase level and clinical symptoms and persists until 1 to 2 months following the icteric phase, total antigenemia lasting about 6 months. Antibody to HB_sAg (anti-HB_s) appears in the serum from 2 weeks to 6 months following the disappearance of HB_sAg. The presence of anti-HB_s implies prior infection with HBV, and it is present in 5 to 10 percent of healthy, volunteer blood donors. Anti-HB_s is usually absent in chronic carriers.

The core of the HBV particle, called hepatitis B core antigen (HB_cAg), does not appear in the serum. Anti-HB_c does appear about 2 weeks after the appearance of HB_sAg, and during the time between the disappearance of HB_sAg and the appearance of anti-HB_s, it may be the only serologic evidence of recent infection. This is a period of active viral replication during which the patient is infectious. Anti-HB_c may persist for long periods after clinical recovery, but at low titers.

Hepatitis B e antigen (HB_eAg) is a soluble antigen found only in serum containing HB_sAg, and its presence implies higher infectivity. Antibody to HB_eAG (anti-HB_e) appears in the acute phase of illness and usually signifies reduced infectivity. The antibody persists for some months after HB_eAg is no longer detectable.

Hepatitis Non-A, Non-B

The term *hepatitis non-A, non-B* (HNANB) is used to denote typical viral hepatitis that is not caused by HAV, HBV, or other known viral agents. The etiologic agent is unknown, and there is substantial evidence favoring the existence of more than one agent. The terms *hepatitis C* and *hepatitis D* have been used by some authors but should be avoided until definite serologic identification is possible.

The incubation period of HNANB overlaps those of hepatitis A and hepatitis B, with a mean of about 50 days. Most cases are mild and anicteric. The clinical course resembles that of hepatitis B, although it is usually milder. The development of chronic hepatitis and a chronic carrier state appears to be more common with HNANB.

Some studies indicate that 3 to 7 percent of volunteer blood donors are asymptomatic carriers of HNANB, and HNANB now accounts for 90 percent of all cases of posttransfusion hepatitis. At this time, no screening method exists that can detect the carrier state.

Other modes of transmission of HNANB and its distribution in various populations are still poorly understood because of the lack of serologic markers.

Table 67-3. Indications for Admission with Viral Hepatitis

1. Encephalopathy
2. Prothrombin time prolonged >3 sec
3. Dehydration
4. Hypoglycemia
5. Bilirubin >20 mg/dL
6. Age > 45 years
7. Immunosuppression
8. Diagnosis uncertain

Emergency Department Management of Viral Hepatitis

No specific therapy is available for acute viral hepatitis. Strict bed rest, corticosteroids, antibiotics, and other therapies have been promoted, but none has been shown to be effective in shortening the course or lessening the severity of illness.

Outpatient management with emphasis on rest, adequate diet, good personal hygiene, and the avoidance of hepatotoxins (e.g., alcohol) is sufficient in the majority of cases. Patients in any of the categories listed in Table 67-3, however, should be admitted. Before the patient is discharged from the ED, blood should be sent for HB_sAg, anti-HB_c, and anti-HA analysis. The availability of follow-up care must be guaranteed. Documented cases of viral hepatitis should be reported to local public health agencies.

Use of Immune Globulins

Immune globulins are solutions of antibodies derived by cold ethanol extraction of pooled human plasma, and they contain both anti-HA and anti-HB_s. Hepatitis B immune globulin (HBIG) is derived from plasma known to contain high-titer anti-HB_s. Immune globulin (formerly called immune serum globulin or ISG) is 80 to 90 percent effective in preventing hepatitis A when given within 14 days of exposure. It also has some effect in preventing hepatitis B if given immediately after exposure. HBIG is much more expensive than immune globulin and should be reserved for use when there is known percutaneous or mucous membrane contact with blood known to contain HB_sAg. Serious adverse effects from the use of either globulin are rare.

The current recommendations of the immunization practices advisory committee of the Center for Disease Control regarding the use of immune globulins are summarized in Table 67-4. It must be noted that disagreements with the CDC guidelines exist with regard to dosages, indication for the use of HBIG, and the need for serologic evaluation of source and victim.

A highly effective vaccine for the prevention of hepatitis B is now available and is recommended for use in persons at high risk for contracting hepatitis B. This group includes intravenous drug abusers, homosexual men, the institutionalized retarded, immigrants from areas of highly endemic hepatitis B, hemodialysis patients, household and sexual contacts of chronic hepatitis B carriers, and selected health-care workers. The risk to health-care workers is proportional to their degree of exposure to blood products and cases of hepatitis B and to the number of preventive measures practiced. Emergency department personnel have been identified as being among those at high risk. The three-injection series induces protective levels of anti-HB_s in 85 to 95 percent of healthy adults and costs about $100. No serious immediate or long-term adverse effects of vaccination have yet been noted.

Table 67-4. Postexposure Immunoprophylaxis
for Viral Hepatitis

Source	Treatment
HEPATITIS A	
1. Household and sexual contacts of known cases	Immune globulin, 0.02 mL/kg IM
2. Day-care center, school, and custodial institution contacts of known cases if there is evidence of transmission	Same
3. Exposure to contaminated water or food before cases begin to occur	Same
HEPATITIS B WITH PERCUTANEOUS OR MUCOUS MEMBRANE EXPOSURE	
1. Known, HB$_s$Ag (+)	HBIG 0.06 mL/kg IM stat.; repeat in 1 month
2. Known, HB$_s$Ag (?)	
a. High-risk: drug abusers, hemodialysis or clinical hepatitis patients	IG 0.06 mL/kg IM stat.; get HB$_s$Ag; if (+) give HBIG 0.06 mL/kg IM ASAP; repeat in 1 month
b. Low-risk	Nothing, or IG 0.06 mL/kg IM
3. Unknown	Nothing, or IG 0.06 mL/kg IM
4. Newborns of HB$_s$Ag carriers	HBIG 0.5 mL/kg IM within 24 h; repeat at 3 and 5 months
HEPATITIS NON-A, NON-B	
	No specific recommendations

Note: IM = intramuscular; IG = immune globulin; HBIG = hepatitis B
immune globulin; and ASAP = as soon as possible.

Toxic Hepatitis

A large number of industrial chemicals and pharmacological agents are capable of producing hepatic injury. Some cause predictable, dose-dependent injury through a direct toxic effect of the agent or its metabolites. Others cause damage sporadically and unpredictably. These idiosyncratic reactions are not dose-related, may be delayed in onset, and may be accompanied by systemic signs and symptoms such as arthralgias, rash, fever, and eosinophilia.

Halothane, oxyphenisatin, methyldopa, isoniazid, and other drugs may produce morphological changes in the liver resembling those of an acute viral hepatitis. Other drugs such as anabolic steroids, oral contraceptives, chlorpropamide, chlorpromazine, and erythromycin estolate may produce cholestatic changes. Massive hepatic necrosis may be produced by carbon tetrachloride, phosphorus, acetaminophen, and mushroom poisoning (e.g., *Amanita phalloides*).

Some drugs and toxins including methyldopa, vinyl chloride, arsenic, and isoniazid have been implicated in the development of chronic active hepatitis and cirrhosis.

Halothane

Halothane hepatitis is an idiosyncratic reaction that may be immunologically mediated. It appears much more often in patients with multiple prior exposures to halothane and is more common in adults, especially women, and the obese. In about 25 percent of the cases, rash, fever, and eosinophilia are present. Severe icteric cases have a 20 to 40 percent mortality; thus it is imperative that even mild reactions to halothane be recognized so that susceptible patients are not reexposed.

Acetaminophen

Acetaminophen has become a very popular nonprescription analgesic and antipyretic, as well as an increasingly common cause of hepatic injury and death when taken in accidental or suicidal overdose. A toxic metabolite produces hepatic necrosis when the liver's capacity to conjugate (with glutathione) and excrete the metabolite is overwhelmed. Liver injury can be minimized or avoided when overdosage is recognized and treated as described in Chapter 33.

Methyldopa

Methyldopa causes minor, usually transient, elevations of transaminase levels in about 5 percent of those treated with this popular antihypertensive. In fewer than 1 percent of those treated, acute hepatitis, occasionally with cholestasis, develops, usually within the first 4 weeks of therapy. A prodrome of rash, arthralgias, and lymphadenopathy may precede the onset of jaundice. Clinical improvement occurs with discontinuation of the drug, but cases of chronic hepatitis and cirrhosis have been reported. The mechanism of hepatic injury is unclear but may be a combination of immunologic and direct toxic injury.

Chlorpromazine

Chlorpromazine induces intrahepatic cholestasis in 1 to 4 percent of those taking it, usually within 1 to 4 weeks of exposure. A prodrome of anorexia, nausea, vomiting, malaise, and pruritus may precede the onset of jaundice. Clinical recovery occurs within 4 to 6 weeks after withdrawal of the drug with only a rare fatality reported. Chlorpromazine-induced liver injury is not dose-related and appears to be immunologically mediated.

Treatment

During the evaluation of the patient with acute liver injury, it is important that the emergency physician obtain a detailed history of current and recent medications as well as possible occupational and recreational exposure to chemicals. Stopping the patient's exposure to the offending agent is vital, other treatment being nonspecific and supportive. Possible injury to other organs should be suspected as well with exposure to toxic chemicals.

ALCOHOLIC LIVER DISEASE

More than 10 million people in the United States are alcohol abusers, and alcohol-related injuries and illnesses are major causes of death and disability. Alcohol adversely affects all the organ systems of the body, but it is the liver that bears the brunt of alcohol's deleterious effects. Three syndromes of alcoholic liver injury—hepatic steatosis (fatty liver), alcoholic hepatitis, and alcoholic cirrhosis—have been described based on clinical and histologic criteria.

Hepatic Steatosis

Most people who regularly consume even moderate amounts of alcohol develop some degree of hepatic steatosis (also called fatty liver). It is usually a benign, asymptomatic condition in which fat is deposited in the hepatocytes. The most common clinical finding is nontender hepatomegaly with laboratory evidence of minimal hepatic dysfunction. Less commonly, patients with fatty liver develop a hepatic syndrome of jaundice, malaise, anorexia, and a tender, enlarged liver. Rarely, severe cholestasis or portal hypertension develops. When the patient abstains from alcohol and receives adequate nutrition, steatosis resolves in 4 to 6 weeks without residual scarring or necrosis.

Alcoholic Hepatitis

Alcoholic hepatitis is a syndrome characterized histologically by hepatocellular necrosis and intrahepatic inflammation. The clinical severity ranges from very mild illness to acute liver failure. More typically, the patient reports the gradual onset of anorexia, nausea, abdominal pain, weight loss, and weakness. Fever, dark urine, and jaundice are frequently reported.

On examination, tender hepatomegaly, low-grade fever, and jaundice are commonly noted. Laboratory evaluation usually shows elevation of the levels of serum transaminases in the range of 2 to 10 times normal, with SGOT levels characteristically greater than SGPT levels. Alkaline phosphatase and bilirubin levels are usually mildly elevated, although marked elevations may occur and imply more severe disease. Anemia, leukopenia, and thrombocytopenia are common and may be caused by the toxic effects of alcohol on bone marrow or by nutritional deficits. The prothrombin time is frequently prolonged a few seconds, but prolongation greater than 8 s is a poor prognostic sign. The presence of fever and leukocytosis in the alcoholic patient mandates a thorough search for concurrent pneumonia, peritonitis, urinary tract infection, sepsis, and meningitis.

Treatment

In-hospital treatment is mainly supportive with correction of electrolyte abnormalities, good nutrition with correction of specific deficits (e.g., folic acid, thiamine), rest, and abstinence from alcohol. Treatment is frequently complicated by the development of alcohol withdrawal symptoms. Symptoms of hepatic failure must be closely watched for and aggressively treated. A number of specific therapies have been advocated to speed recovery from alcoholic hepatitis or to halt the progression to cirrhosis, but at this time none is considered established. These include the use of corticosteroids, penicillamine, propylthiouracil, and insulin-glucagon combinations.

Unlike the situation with other types of toxic hepatitis, the histologic, biochemical, and clinical abnormalities of alcoholic hepatitis do not rapidly resolve with abstinence from the causative agent. Instead, from 15 to 50 percent of patients deteriorate during the first weeks of hospitalization despite abstinence and nutritional support. The overall mortality is 10 to 15 percent, and death results from hepatic failure with encephalopathy, GI bleeding, and infectious complications. Survivors face a convalescence lasting weeks to months, with a significant number going on to develop cirrhosis.

Emergency Department Management

Because of the difficulty of ruling out concurrent infection, the tendency toward clinical deterioration, and the significant mortality, all but the mildest cases of alcoholic hepatitis should be hospitalized. A complete blood count with differential and measurement of prothrombin time and levels of transaminases, alkaline phosphatase, bilirubin, albumin, blood urea nitrogen, creatinine, glucose, magnesium, and phosphorus, and urinalysis should be obtained. Intravenous hydration with correction of electrolyte abnormalities should be initiated as indicated. In the febrile patient, a chest radiograph and cultures of blood, urine, and ascitic fluid are needed. If the patient has an altered mental status, occult head injury, meningitis, hepatic encephalopathy, and hypoglycemia must be considered.

Alcoholic Cirrhosis

Alcoholic (or Laennec's) cirrhosis is the irreversible stage of alcoholic liver disease. The liver is usually a golden yellow and may be shrunken or enlarged. Nodules of regenerating hepatocytes are separated by bands of fibrous tissue which represent scarring from previous necrosis. The normal pattern of hepatic blood circulation is disrupted, with a resultant decrease in the total blood flow through the liver as well as the shunting of blood away from the remaining functioning hepatocytes and into the systemic circulation. This portosystemic shunting and concomitant portal hypertension result in many of the clinical findings of cirrhosis as well as the associated complications.

Cirrhosis develops in only about 10 percent of chronic alcoholics and may remain unrecognized in a significant number. Genetic, nutritional, and other factors probably are important, in addition to substantial alcohol consumption, in those who do develop cirrhosis.

Clinical Features

A characteristic clinical feature of symptomatic cirrhosis is a general, usually gradual, deterioration in health. Weight loss (sometimes masked by ascites and edema), weakness, peripheral muscle wasting, easy fatigability, and anorexia are the rule. Nausea, vomiting, and diarrhea are also commonly reported. Fever, usually low-grade and continuous, is much more common in alcoholic than in other types of cirrhosis and often develops in decompensated disease. Hypothermia may develop in the terminal stages, especially in the presence of sepsis or gram-negative infection. Jaundice, spider angiomas, palmer erythema, pedal edema, ascites, hepatosplenomegaly, and gynecomastia are frequently present.

Laboratory abnormalities include elevated bilirubin and alkaline phosphatase levels, a prolonged prothrombin time, a decreased albumin level, anemia (from chronic disease, GI losses, and nutritional factors), leukopenia, and thrombocytopenia.

Hyponatremia may be dilutional secondary to increased antidiuretic hormone activity or the result of total body sodium deficit, frequently aggravated by the injudicious use of diuretics. Hypokalemia is almost always present as a result of GI losses, secondary hyperaldosteronism, and diuretic use. Arterial hypoxemia is common in decompensated cirrhosis and may be caused by abnormal alveolar-capillary diffusion.

Management

The clinical course of cirrhosis is marked by periods of relative stability interspersed with episodes of decompensation. No therapy has been shown effective in reversing the histologic changes of cirrhosis. The mainstay of outpatient management is total abstinence from alcohol, which has been shown to significantly improve 5-year survival. Other measures include salt and water restriction, the cautious use of diuretics, and a nutritious diet with protein restriction as needed. Emergency department treatment may involve making alterations in diuretic dosage, correcting symptomatic anemia or fluid and electrolyte abnormalities, and recognizing and initiating treatment of the life-threatening emergencies seen in decompensated cirrhosis.

Complications of Alcoholic Liver Disease

Bleeding Esophageal Varices

Bleeding esophageal varices are the most dramatic, and, in terms of mortality, the most significant, complication of alcoholic liver disease with which emergency physicians are faced. The mortality from an episode of acute variceal bleeding averages 60 to 70 percent, with as many as 30 percent of all cirrhotics dying from this complication. The patient usually arrives in the ED hypotensive with massive hematemesis complicated by underlying coagulation and electrolyte disorders. A significant number of patients with documented esophageal varices who develop hematemesis, however, are bleeding from other lesions, including gastric or duodenal ulcers, gastric erosions, or a diffuse gastritis. Since definitive therapy for these conditions varies, emergency endoscopy may be needed to confirm the diagnosis.

Management

Initial management includes securing a stable airway and establishing at least two large-bore intravenous (IV) lines. Central venous pressure monitoring may be helpful in preventing fluid overload. Fresh whole blood or packed red cells augmented with fresh frozen plasma are rapidly infused to maintain perfusion and replace depleted clotting factors. Transfusion of platelet concentrates may be necessary if thrombocytopenia is severe (see Table 67-5).

Control of bleeding can be attempted using IV vasopressin, endoscopic sclerotherapy, tamponade with a Sengstaken-Blakemore or Linton-Nachlas tube, or emergency portal decompression. All these methods have significant morbidity even in experienced hands. The most technically easy and readily available method is IV vasopressin to constrict the splanchic arterial system and thus decrease portal venous pressure and bleeding. There appears to be no advantage to administering vasopressin via selective arterial

Table 67-5. Management of Variceal Bleeding

1. Secure the airway
2. Large-bore IV Lines
3. Volume replacement
4. IV Vasopressin
5. Esophageal tamponade
6. Endoscopic sclerotherapy
7. Portal decompression
8. Evacuate blood from GI Tract

catheterization. A continuous IV infusion should be given starting at 0.3 units/min and titrated up to 1.0 unit/min as needed. Complications include decreased cardiac output and prolonged antidiuretic hormone activity.

Emergency surgical portal decompression has a very high operative mortality and should be reserved for patients in whom less invasive methods have failed.

Particular attention must be paid during emergency treatment to the evacuation of blood from the GI tract with gastric lavage, vigorous catharsis, and enemas. Otherwise some patients in whom bleeding is controlled will die in hepatic coma.

Portosystemic Encephalopathy

Portosystemic encephalopathy (PSE, also referred to as hepatic encephalopathy and hepatic coma) is a neuropsychiatric syndrome of altered consciousness, impaired intellectual functioning, and elevated blood ammonia level seen in cirrhotics with extensive spontaneous or surgical portosystemic shunting. It results from an accumulation in the blood of substances which the damaged liver is no longer able to detoxify. The severity ranges from subtle changes in personality and performance to coma. Elevated blood ammonia clearly plays a role in the pathogenesis of PSE, but elevated levels of some amino acids (e.g., glutamine, tryptophan, tyrosine, and phenylalanine), short-chain fatty acids, biogenic amines, mercaptans, and putative false neurotransmitters have also been implicated.

PSE can be precipitated or exacerbated in susceptible patients by a variety of causes, some related to increased levels of ammonia and some to other mechanisms. Azotemia, either renal or prerenal, provides more urea to urease-producing intestinal bacteria, thereby increasing ammonia production in the gut. Gastrointestinal bleeding and high-protein diets also provide a large amount of nitogenous substrates. The careless use of analgesics, sedatives, and tranquilizers is a common cause of PSE in hospitalized patients. Hypokalemic metabolic alkalosis results in an increased pH gradient favoring the passage of ammonia into cells. Other metabolic derangements such as hypoglycemia, anemia, and hypoxia, as well as infection and hypotension, may also contribute.

Clinical Features

The patient arriving in the ED with PSE has the stigmata of chronic liver disease including edema, ascites, spider angiomas, and hepatosplenomegaly. Fetor hepaticus, a musty, sweetish odor on the breath attributed to elevated levels of mercaptans in the blood, is often noted. Asterixis (commonly called liver flap) is characteristic of, but not specific for, PSE. It is demonstrated most readily in the dorsiflexed wrist, but may be noted in other muscles as well. Neurologic examination may reveal a state of consciousness ranging from lethargy to coma with variable appearance of hyperreflexia, generalized seizures, and spasticity. Occult head injury should be suspected if focal or lateralizing signs are present.

Laboratory studies reflect the underlying liver failure with jaundice, prolonged prothrombin time, and decreased albumin levels. The acid-base status and the serum electrolytes must be followed closely. Arterial ammonia levels correlate more closely with the severity of PSE than venous levels, but there is a 24- to 72-h lag between the rise in ammonia levels and the onset of symptoms. Serial changes in arterial ammonia levels are more useful in evaluating the effectiveness of the treatment.

Treatment

The initial treatment of the comatose patient is to maintain oxygenation and perfusion. Precipitating factors such as GI bleeding should be treated aggressively. Specific treatment to lower ammonia levels is directed at cleansing the colon with cathartics and enemas, neomycin to suppress colonic flora, and lactulose. Lactulose is a nondigestible disaccharide which is degraded by bacterial action in the colon and produces an acidic diarrhea that traps ammonia in the intestinal lumen and eliminates it with the stool. Lactulose may be given orally, through a nasogastric tube, or via an enema. Many other therapies have been suggested and tried but not established. With meticulous supportive care and the aggressive treatment of complications, PSE is potentially reversible (see Table 67-6).

Hepatorenal Syndrome

Hepatorenal syndrome is a syndrome of acquired renal failure in patients with decompensated cirrhosis. The mortality of HRS approaches 100 percent. It probably represents a functional disturbance in the control of renal vascular tone with a decreased glomerular filtration rate due to intense vasoconstriction and shunting of blood away from the renal cortex. This results in the production of small volumes of concentrated urine with a very low sodium content, usually less than 10 mEq/L and a progressive azotemia unresponsive to attempts to expand intravascular volume. No significant histologic changes are evident in the kidneys of patients

Table 67-6. Precipitating Factors in PSE

1. Gastrointestinal Bleeding
2. Azotemia
3. Dietary Protein
4. Sedatives, Tranquilizers
5. Hypokalemic metabolic alkalosis
6. Severe anemia

dying with HRS. In fact, kidneys from HRS donors function normally if transplanted into recipients with normal hepatic function.

BIBLIOGRAPHY

American College of Physicians: Position Paper: Hepatitis B vaccine. *Ann Intern Med* 100:149, 1984.

Borowsky SA, Strome S, Lott E: Continued heavy drinking and survival in alcoholic cirrhotics. *Gastroenterology* 80:1405, 1981.

Boyer JL: The diagnosis and pathogenesis of clinical variants in viral hepatitis. *Am J Clin Pathol* 65:898, 1976.

Centers for Disease Control: Inactivated hepatitis B vaccine. *Morb Mortal Weekly Rep* 31:317, 1982.

Centers for Disease Control: Immune globulins for protection against viral hepatitis. *Morb Mortal Weekly Rep* 30:423, 1981.

Chojkier M, Groszmann RJ, Atterbury CE, et al: A controlled comparison of continuous intraarterial and intravenous infusions of vasopressin in hemorrhage from esophageal varices. *Gastroenterology* 77:540, 1979.

Dienstag JL: Non-A, non-B hepatitis. I. Recognition, epidemiology, and clinical features. *Gastroenterology* 85:439, 1983.

Dienstag JL: Non-A, non-B hepatitis. II. Experimental transmission, putative virus agents and markers, and prevention. *Gastroenterology* 85:743, 1983.

Gordon EK, Geiderman JM, Brill JC: Immunoprophylaxis of viral hepatitis. *Ann Emerg Med* 10:216, 1981.

Hoyumpa AM, Desmond PV, Avant GR, et al: Hepatic encephalopathy (clinical conference). *Gastroenterology* 76:184, 1979.

Johnson WC, Widrich WC, Ansell JE, et al: Control of bleeding varices by vasopressin. *Ann Surg* 186:369, 1977.

Jovanovich JF, Saravolatz LD, Arking LM: The risk of hepatitis B among select employee groups in an urban hospital. *JAMA* 250:1893, 1983.

Kiernan TW, Ramgopal M: Viral hepatitis: Progress and problems. *Med Clin North Am* 63:611, 1979.

Leevy CM, Kanagasundaram N: Alcoholic hepatitis. *Hosp Pract* October:115, 1987.

Lieber CS: Hepatic and metabolic effects of alcohol. *Gastroenterology* 65:821, 1973.

Mezey E: Medical problems associated with alcoholism. *Primary Care* 1:293, 1974.

Nielson JO: Clinical course and prognosis of acute hepatitis. *Ann Clin Res* 8:151, 1976.

Ostrow JD: Jaundice in older children and adults. *JAMA* 234:522, 1975.

Primstone NR, French SW: Alcoholic liver disease. *Med Clin North Am* 68:39, 1984.

Schenker S, Breen KJ, Hoyumpa AM: Hepatic encephalopathy: Current status. *Gastroenterology* 66:121, 1974.

Seeff LB, Hoofnagle JH: Immunoprophylaxis of viral hepatitis. *Gastroenterology* 77:161, 1979.

Tamburro CT: Chemical hepatitis. *Med Clin North Am* 63:545, 1979.

Weinstein MP, Iannini PB, Stratton CW, et al: Spontaneous bacterial peritonitis. *Am J Med* 64:592, 1978.

Zimmerman HJ: Jaundice due to bacterial infection (clinical conference). *Gastroenterology* 77:362, 1979.

Zimmerman HJ: Drug-induced chronic hepatic disease. *Med Clin North Am* 63:567, 1979.

CHAPTER 68
ACUTE PANCREATITIS

Donald Weaver

The diagnosis of acute pancreatitis rests primarily on clinical grounds. The severity of the disease may range from mild pancreatic edema to frank necrosis and hemorrhage. No clinical findings are pathognomonic, and the symptoms depend largely on the amount of glandular destruction. In the mildest form of pancreatitis, patients present with epigastric pain, abdominal distention, nausea, vomiting, and hyperamylasemia. Refractory hypotensive shock, blood loss, and respiratory failure may accompany the most severe forms. In 1977 Ranson and Posterbach proposed a schema to grade the severity of acute pancreatitis (Table 68-1). The use of such criteria has been helpful in projecting the outcome and in comparing clinical studies of different treatments.

Etiology

Acute pancreatitis is most often due to alcohol abuse or gallstones (Table 68-2). The incidence with which each is associated with pancreatitis depends largely on the age of the population and the type of reporting institution. Patients over the age of 50 who present in a community hospital setting most often have "biliary pancreatitis," while younger patients presenting to large inner-city emergency rooms almost always suffer from alcoholic pancreatitis.

Pathophysiology

A complete understanding of the pathophysiology of acute pancreatitis is lacking. The common-channel concept of Opie dominated the literature on pancreatitis for years, but anatomic studies of cadavers have shown that only a fraction of patients with pancreatitis have a true common channel. Moreover, in fatal cases,

Table 68-2. Etiologic or Contributing Factors in Acute Pancreatitis

Ethanol ingestion
Biliary tract disease
Trauma, penetrating or blunt
Penetrating peptic ulcer
Postoperative
Obstruction secondary to neoplasms, diverticula, roundworms, benign
  polyps
Perisphincteric fibrosis
Metabolic disturbances
   Hyperlipemia (Frederickson types I, IV, and V)
   Hypercalcemia
   Diabetes mellitus, diabetic ketoacidosis
   Uremia
   Hemochromatosis
   Hereditary pancreatitis
Viral infections
  Mumps
  Viral hepatitis
  Infectious mononucleosis
  Coxsackie group B
  Pregnancy—any trimester, postpartum
Collagen vascular disease
  Systemic lupus erythematosus
  Polyarteritis nodosa
Liver disease
Generalized infections
  Typhoid fever
  Salmonella typhimurium infection
  Scarlet fever
  Streptococcal food poisoning
  Dysentery
  Scorpion sting
  Other causes

Source: Adapted from Kowlessar OD: Pathogenesis of pancreatitis, in Clearfield HR, Dinoso VP (eds): *Gastrointestinal Emergencies.* New York, Grune & Stratton, 1976, p 226.

Table 68-1. Criteria for Projecting the Outcome from Acute Pancreatitis

On Admission	48 h Later
Age	Change in HCT (falling)
Blood sugar	Rise in BUN
White blood cell count	↓ Ca²⁺
SGOT	↓ Arterial P_{O_2}
Amylase	Rapid fluid sequestration
LDH	

careful dissection at postmortem examinations rarely discloses an impacted stone in the ampulla of Vater. In animal experiments, neither the anastomosis of bile ducts to the pancreatic duct nor the injection of bile into the pancreatic duct without pressure produces pancreatitis. Only when trypsin or bacteria are added to bile and the mixture is injected under pressure can consistent experimental pancreatitis be produced.

Table 68-3. Drugs Reported to be Associated with the Occurrence of Acute Pancreatitis

Oral contraceptives	Clonidine
Estrogens	Salicylates
Phenformin	Indomethacin
Azathioprine	Dextropropoxyphene
Corticosteroids	Calcium
Rifampin	Warfarin
Tetracyclines	L-Asparaginase
Isoniazid	Paracetamol
Thiazides	Ethacrynic acid
Furosemide	

It appears that a vascular insult is important either as a cause or perpetuator of acute pancreatitis. The hyperlipemic serum sometimes seen in patients following a drinking binge may be responsible for peripancreatic vascular sludging and relative pancreatic ischemia. Small-microsphere injections (8 to 20U) result in profound pancreatitis because of plugging of the terminal arterioles. The acinar and ductal injury which then results leads to extravasation of proteolytic enzymes, and this may be responsible for the progression of the inflammatory state. Alcohol increases pancreatic ductal permeability, and this may result in a similar escape of proteolytic enzymes.

Alcoholic pancreatitis may result from duodenal inflammation that produces some degree of pancreatic duct obstruction, with increased ductal pressure. The latter may occur secondary to sphincter of Oddi spasm or pancreatic hypersecretion.

Hyperparathyroidism has been associated with an increased incidence of pancreatitis, but the mechanism by which this occurs is unknown.

Patients with primary hyperlipemias (Frederickson types I, IV, and V) are susceptible to acute pancreatitis, but patients with pancreatitis may develop transient secondary hyperlipemia because of the release of an inhibitor of lipoprotein lipase during the attack of pancreatitis.

Various drugs, such as methyl alcohol, thiazide diuretics, and phenformin, can produce pancreatitis (Table 68-3). Inflammation and infection, such as mumps or hepatitis, can also result in pancreatitis. Penetrating posterior duodenal and gastric ulcers may involve the head of the pancreas, producing a local pancreatitis. Once the pancreas becomes edematous and swollen, especially if there is significant involvement of the head, partial obstruction of the common bile duct or even gastric outlet may occur. For these reasons elevation of the bilirubin level, and even clinical jaundice, may occur. Pancreatitis may also produce adynamic ileus secondary to the peritoneal irritation.

DIAGNOSIS

Laboratory

Since no clinical features are pathognomonic for acute pancreatitis, the diagnosis must often rest on the presence of abnormal results from laboratory tests, most often the serum amylase level. Amylase is a product of two genes located on chromosome 1. These genes are known as AMY_1 and AMY_2. Each organ that makes amylase expresses either one or the other, and no organ has been found that expresses both genes. The only known site to express the AMY_2 gene is the pancreas. All other organs such

as the fallopian tubes, ovaries, lungs, salivary glands, lacrimal glands, and endocrine glands express the AMY_1 locus. Pancreatic (AMY_2) amylase can be separated from nonpancreatic (AMY_1) amylase by a variety of electrophoretic techniques. Normally there is a nearly even distribution in the serum between AMY_1 and AMY_2 amylase. Multiple other isoamylases can occur but result from posttranslational modifications of the major isoenzymes.

During the last decade, recognition of the multiple organ sources of amylase has resulted in less reliance on the simple measurement of the serum amylase level as an indicator of pancreatic disease. In a recent study, 32 percent of the patients admitted with the clinical diagnosis of acute pancreatitis made on the basis of upper abdominal pain, nausea, vomiting, and an elevated amylase level, were found to have nonpancreatic hyperamylasemia. This suggests that the clinical criteria used to make the diagnosis of acute pancreatitis may be too variable.

Since the electrophoresis of serum to differentiate isoamylases is time-consuming (approximately 2.5 h), other laboratory tests have been proposed to improve the accuracy of pancreatitis diagnosis. Observations that the amylase-creatinine clearance ratio is high in patients with acute pancreatitis suggested that this might be a valuable diagnostic test. The ratio is determined using the following formula:

$$\frac{amylase\ clearance}{creatinine\ clearance}\% = \frac{urine\ amylase}{serum\ amylase} \times \frac{serum\ creatinine}{urine\ creatinine} \times 100$$

The normal clearance ratio is about 3 percent, and levels of 5 percent or greater are believed to be consistent with the diagnosis of acute pancreatitis. The mechanism for the increased renal clearance of amylase may be a tubular defect in the reabsorption of amylase. Unfortunately, elevated ratios have been found with other diseases, and not every patient with acute pancreatitis has an elevated ratio.

The level of lipase, another enzyme liberated by pancreatic disease, is nearly always elevated in acute pancreatitis. Although the lipase level is a more sensitive sign of acute pancreatitis than the serum amylase level, it too lacks specificity and immediate availability. Reports that the lipase level rises later and remains elevated longer than the serum amylase level have not been confirmed, but the course of the lipase level elevation more closely follows the clinical course than does the serum amylase level.

When pancreatic hemorrhage occurs, hemoglobin may be split by the action of pancreatic enzymes and methemalbumin be formed. The presence of this pigment in patients with acute pancreatitis indicates hemorrhagic pancreatitis. Unfortunately the finding of methemalbumin in the serum is not a pathognomonic sign since it may be elevated in any condition in which there is intraabdominal or retroperitoneal bleeding.

The finding of a wheat germ protein that inhibits the activity of salivary amylase nearly 100 times more than the activity of pancreatic amylase has led to a rapid test for approximating the levels of the serum isoamylases. Analysis of serum amylase levels before and after reaction with the inhibitor allows an estimation of what portion of the amylase comes from pancreatic sources. This test holds promise as a simple way to improve the accuracy of serum amylase interpretations. Patients with severe edema of the pancreatic head from pancreatitis may have elevation of the bilirubin and alkaline phosphatase levels.

As with most inflammatory conditions, leukocytosis is usually present but rarely exceeds 20,000/mL in uncomplicated pancreatitis.

Low calcium levels may be detected on laboratory analysis. Persistent hypocalcemia, less than 7 mg/100 mL, is associated with a poor prognosis. Hypocalcemia may result when calcium reacts with free fatty acids and precipitates as calcium soap, but a complete explanation for this phenomenon is lacking.

Radiographic

Plain radiographs of the abdomen have little role in the diagnosis of acute pancreatitis, although calcification (Fig. 68-1), when present, suggests preexisting pancreatic disease. More often their importance is to exclude other diseases which may be confused with pancreatitis. Patients with acute pancreatitis who show evidence of ileus, and air trapped in the small bowel near the inflamed pancreas, have been described as having a sentinel loop. Gaseous distention of the colon with a distally collapsed colon suggests colonic ileus (colon-cutoff sign). None of these signs is truly diagnostic of acute pancreatitis. Contrast studies of the upper gastrointestinal tract occasionally show narrowing or edema of the duodenum, but the routine use of this procedure or barium enema examination to confirm the diagnosis is not helpful.

Recently interest in ultrasonography or CT scanning of these patients has been shown. Evidence of pancreatic edema or lesser sac fluid may be indicative of acute pancreatic inflammation. The routine use of these tests is unnecessary and expensive and probably should be reserved to monitor late complications.

The injection of contrast material under pressure into the duct of an inflamed pancreas seems unwise. Although cases of severe pancreatitis following endoscopic retrograde cholangiopancreatography (ERCP) have been reported, these are rare, most likely

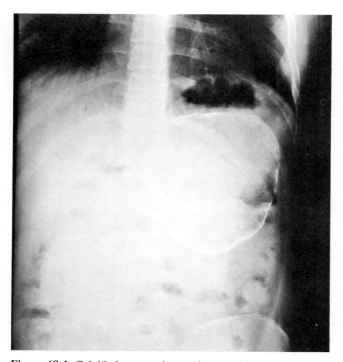

Figure 68-1. Calcified pancreatic pseudocyst. (Courtesy of Detroit General Hospital.)

because of prudence on the part of endoscopists. Isoamylase studies show that nearly all patients undergoing ERCP have a mild elevation of pancreatic amylase levels following the procedure.

TREATMENT

The mainstay of treatment for acute pancreatitis is fluid resuscitation. Recognition that profound shock may result from high-volume fluid sequestration in the retroperitoneum has lowered morbidity as resuscitation efforts have improved. Although some controversy exists about the optimum regimen of fluid replacement, most agree that the use of a balanced electrolyte solution is essential. The observation that albumin reduces the amount of pancreatic edema in a whole perfused pancreatitis model has suggested to some that colloid solution may be of benefit. Although an uncontrolled clinical trial of fresh frozen plasma given in large amounts to patients with acute pancreatitis seemed beneficial, most surgeons believe that these measures add little if anything to standard fluid regimens except cost. Fluids should be given in volumes adequate to ensure renal perfusion. When the pancreatitis is severe, admission to an intensive care unit with maximum hemodynamic monitoring is needed. A falling hematocrit should suggest hemorrhagic pancreatitis, and in this case blood replacement is mandatory.

Although the use of the nasogastric tube is widely accepted, no controlled clinical trial has shown its value in altering the course of the disease. The theoretical advantage of reducing pancreatic stimulation and its established value in preventing vomiting, however, make the nasogastric tube a standard part of therapy at most centers. Since acute pancreatitis is a self-limiting disease under most circumstances, attention to fluid needs, treatment of pain, and the prevention of vomiting is often sufficient treatment. A small number of patients may develop a severe systemic illness, complicated by acidosis, renal failure, severe hypocalcemia, and respiratory failure.

Acute pancreatitis is not a bacterial disease in its early stages, and the initial use of antibiotics is unwarranted. Sepsis when it occurs results from secondary infections and is usually encountered late in the course of the disease. The exception to this is when pancreatitis is complicated by biliary tract infection in the presence of choledocholithiasis.

The use of a variety of medications such as anticholinergic drugs, apoprotein, and cimetidine has been proposed to hasten the usual recovery from pancreatitis; however, none has been shown in controlled clinical trials to alter the course of the disease.

Peritoneal lavage should be considered for patients who fail to respond to initial supportive measures. The rationale for this approach is that the dilution or removal of "toxic" shock factors released by pancreatic necrosis may be beneficial to the patient. Although the precise mechanism by which peritoneal lavage benefits patients with acute pancreatitis is speculative, more than anecdotal observations by a number of clinicians have validated its usefulness in severe cases.

The role of surgery in the treatment of acute pancreatitis is limited. Patients whose clinical course deteriorates despite maximum supportive efforts should undergo laparotomy to ensure that another more treatable condition has not been missed and to debride and drain devitalized pancreatic tissue. Patients with gallstone pancreatitis and choledocholithiasis may benefit from early biliary tract decompression.

Acute pancreatitis can be considered to be a disease of limited duration. Failure to show significant improvement by the end of a week should lead the physician to suspect a complication such as pancreatic abscess, pseudocyst, or pancreatic ascites.

Pancreatic abscess or pseudocyst should be considered in any patient with an abdominal mass, an elevated serum amylase level, an elevated serum bilirubin level, and leukocytosis.

Pseudocysts may rupture spontaneously while the patient is under observation in the emergency department with catastrophic results. Erosion into the upper gastrointestinal tract or an adjacent vessel with massive bleeding has occurred.

Pancreatitis may be a difficult diagnosis to establish. It presents as an acute surgical abdomen, and repeated observation and surgical consultation are often necessary to determine the indicated treatment.

BIBLIOGRAPHY

Anderson WJ, Skinner DB, Zuidema GD, et al: Chronic pancreatic pleural effusions. *Surg Gynecol Obstet* 137:827–830, 1973.

Call T, Malarkey WB, Thomas FB: Acute pancreatitis secondary to furosemide with associated hyperlipidemia. *Dig Dis Sci* 22:835–838, 1977.

Cameron JL: Chronic pancreatic ascites and pancreatic pleural effusions. *Gastroenterology* 74:134–140, 1978.

Carey LC: Extra-abdominal manifestations of acute pancreatitis. *Surgery* 86:337–342, 1979.

Condon JR, Knight M, Day JL: Glucagon therapy in acute pancreatitis. *Br J Surg* 60:509–511, 1973.

Geokas MC, Van Lancker JL, Kadell BM, et al: Acute pancreatitis. *Ann Intern Med* 76:105–117, 1972.

Gilsanz V, Oteyza CP, Rebollar JL: Glucagon vs. anticholinergics in the treatment of acute pancreatitis. *Arch Intern Med* 138:535–538, 1978.

Glucagon therapy in acute pancreatitis. *Br Med J* 4:503, 1973.

Goldstein DA, Llach F, Massry SG: Acute renal failure in patients with acute pancreatitis. *Arch Intern Med* 136:1363–1365, 1976.

Hayes MF, Rosenbaum RW, Zibelman M, et al: Adult respiratory distress syndrome in association with acute pancreatitis—Evaluation of positive end expiratory pressure ventilation and pharmacologic doses of steroids. *Am J Surg* 127:314–319, 1974.

Interiano B, Stuard ID, Hyde RW: Acute respiratory distress syndrome in pancreatitis. *Ann Intern Med* 77:923–926, 1972.

Johnson SG, Ellis CJ, Levitt MD: Mechanism of increased renal clearance of amylase/creatinine in acute pancreatitis. *N Engl J Med* 295:1214–1217, 1976.

Kaplan MH, Dreiling DD: Steroids revisited. II. Was cortisone responsible for the pancreatitis? *Am J Gastroenterol* 67:141–147, 1977.

Kaye MD: Pleuropulmonary complications of pancreatitis. *Thorax* 23:297–306, 1968.

Kellum JM, DeMeester TR, Elkins RC, et al: Respiratory insufficiency secondary to acute pancreatitis. *Ann Surg* 175:657–662, 1972.

Levine RI, Glauser FL, Berk JE: Enchancement of the amylase-creatinine clearance ratio in disorders other than acute pancreatitis. *N Engl J Med* 292:329–332, 1975.

Lifton LJ, Slickers KA, Pragay DA, et al: Pancreatitis and lipase. *JAMA* 229:47–50, 1974.

Nakashima Y, Howard JM: Drug-induced acute pancreatitis. *Surg Gynecol Obstet* 145:105–109, 1977.

Paloyan D, Levin M, Simonowitz D: Azathioprine-associated acute pancreatitis. *Dig Dis* 22:839–840, 1977.

Ranson JHC, Turner JW, Roses DF, et al: Respiratory complications in acute pancreatitis. *Ann Surg* 179:557–566, 1974.

Robertson GM Jr, Moore EW, Switz DM, et al: Inadequate parathyroid response in acute pancreatitis. *N Engl J Med* 294:512–516, 1976.

Rovner AJ, Westcott JL: Pulmonary edema and respiratory insufficiency in acute pancreatitis. *Radiology* 118:513–520, 1976.

Salt WB, Schenker S: Amylase—Its clinical significance: A review of the literature. *Medicine* 55:269–283, 1976.

Sankaran S, Walt AJ: Pancreatic ascites: Recognition and management. *Arch Surg* 111:430–434, 1976.

Stanley JC, Frey CF, Miller TA: Major arterial hemorrhage: A complication of pancreatic pseudocysts and chronic pancreatitis. *Arch Surg* 111:435–440, 1976.

Warshaw AL, Fuller AF Jr: Specificity of increased renal clearance of amylase in diagnosis of acute pancreatitis. *N Engl J Med* 92:325–328, 1975.

Weaver DW, Bouwman DL, Walt AJ, et al: A correlation between clinical pancreatitis and isoenzyme patterns of amylase. *Surgery* 92:576–580, 1982.

SECTION 7
RENAL AND
GENITOURINARY
DISORDERS

CHAPTER 69
EMERGENCY
RENAL PROBLEMS

Dale Sillix

In caring for the patient with renal disease, the emergency physician is frequently handicapped in unique ways. The need to rapidly assess and treat potentially life threatening conditions, the frequent lack of historical information on the patient, and the unique health problems of this patient population all complicate the emergency physician's job. This chapter covers the emergency department diagnosis and treatment of acute renal failure and renal stones, and emergency care aspects of chronic renal insufficiency, dialysis, and renal transplants.

ACUTE RENAL FAILURE

Because of the burden of time, the assessment of the patient with an elevated serum creatinine level and oliguria or anuria must be swift but accurate. The diagnosis of acute renal failure (ARF) is one of exclusion. Obtaining any history of underlying renal disease is of major importance, as not only does chronic renal disease confound other diagnostic tests (i.e., urinary indices), but other mechanisms of determining chronicity such as kidney size, x-ray evidence of hyperparathyroid disease, and the absence of anemia are time-consuming and inaccurate. Once an underlying problem is excluded, the oliguric or azotemic patient falls into one of three categories of ARF: prerenal, renal, or postrenal azotemia.

Prerenal azotemia is caused by an intact kidney's responding to hypoperfusion from any cause (Table 69-1). Removing the extrarenal insult corrects the azotemia. Because of efficient autoregulation, the kidney is able to maintain a relatively constant blood flow at mean arterial pressures above 80 mmHg. Below this, renal perfusion and the glomerular filtration rate (GFR) fall, but tubular function and concentrating ability are generally spared. Prerenal azotemia may not be oliguric, however, if other factors inhibiting renal concentration are present such as impaired antidiuretic hormone (ADH) secretion (diabetes insipidus), impaired ADH responsiveness (lithium, demeclocycline, hypokalemia, hypercalcemia), diuretics, or a solute diuresis. The widespread use of nonsteroidal anti-inflammatory drugs has led to the increased recognition of the importance of prostaglandins in maintaining renal blood flow, particularly in those with sodium depletion, hypotension, heart failure, or underlying renal disease. The use of prostaglandin inhibitors in these patients carries a higher than normal risk of renal impairment (prerenal azotemia or frank renal failure).

Postrenal azotemia is caused by obstruction to urine flow anywhere from the tubule lumens to the end of the urethra (Table 69-2). Although complete obstruction usually presents as anuria, partial obstruction often presents as polyuria or wide fluctuations in urine output. With normal underlying renal parenchyma, obstruction must be bilateral before azotemia or oliguria can occur. Percussion or palpation of a distended bladder, a rectal or pelvic examination to evaluate prostatic or gynecological disease (especially cervical or endometrial carcinoma or endometriosis), and bladder catheterization to measure the postvoid residual volume in those with autonomic insufficiency (diabetics, or those with spinal disease or using anticholinergic drugs) excludes most cases of bladder obstruction. A kidneys, ureters, and bladder (KUB) study is helpful in evaluating renal stones, as 90 percent are radiopaque, and also indicates underlying chronic disease if the kidneys are small. A high-dose intravenous pyelogram (IVP) with a nephrotomogram is usually enough to exclude obstruction but should be used with extreme caution in diabetics, those with multiple myeloma, or those with chronic renal insufficiency because of the increased risk of dye-contrast ARF. Ultrasound examination is quick, involves no dye, and is usually quite adequate to rule out obstruction. Retrograde pyelography is limited by the risks of infection or ureteral edema but is usually definitive.

Urinalysis is helpful in cases of intraureteral or luminal obstruction such as acute crystalluria, necrotizing papillitis, blood clots,

Table 69-1. Causes of Prerenal Azotemia

Altered cardiac function	Congestive heart failure
	Pericardial tamponade
	Myocardial infarction
	Acute arrythmias
Decreased circulating volume	Hemorrhage
	Gastrointestinal losses
	Third spacing (burns, trauma, pancreatitis, etc.)
	Diuretics
	Sepsis
	Decreased oncotic pressure (nephrotic syndrome, liver disease)
	Hepatorenal syndrome
	Excessive antihypertension medications
	Prostaglandin inhibitors

Table 69-2. Causes of Postrenal Azotemia

Bladder obstruction	Urethral obstruction
	Prostatic disease (BPH, cancer)
	Functional (neuropathy, drugs)
	Bladder infection or carcinoma
Ureteral obstruction (bilateral)	Stones
	Blood clots
	Crystals (uric acid, oxalate)
	Papillary necrosis
	Tumors

Note: BPH = benign prostatic hyperplasia

or severe acute pyelonephritis. Hyperuricemia ARF occurs in patients with leukemias and lymphomas starting chemotherapy. In such case, the level of serum uric acid is usually over 20 mg/100 mL, hyperphosphatemia is present, and uric acid crystals are found in an acid urine. The treatment is diuresis, alkalinization of the urine, acetazolamide, and hemodialysis if the other treatments fail and the uric acid level is greater than 25 mg/100 mL. Acute oxalate nephropathy is seen in those who have ingested ethylene glycol or massive amounts of vitamin C. Blood clots are most common in those with coagulopathies, sickle cell disease or trait, or trauma. Papillary necrosis can cause significant obstruction in patients with a history of analgesic abuse, sickle cell disease, diabetes, or acute, severe pyelonephritis.

In adults, 10 to 20 percent of the cases of ARF are caused by primary parenchymal disease (Table 69-3). The rest are categorized as acute tubular necrosis (ATN), although not all cases have histologic confirmation of overt cellular damage. Glomerulonephritis (GN) can present as acute, rapid deterioration of renal function in cases of postinfectious (especially poststreptococcal) GN with ''smoky'' urine, edema, and oliguria, or as a more subacute deterioration in cases of crescentic or rapidly progressive GN (RPGN). RPGN is especially associated with Goodpasture's syndrome, systemic lupus erythematosus (SLE), disseminated vasculitis, endocarditis, or occult abdominal sepsis. Lupus nephritis has multiple forms of presentation; acute GN, nephrotic syndrome, and RPGN are the most dramatic. ARF caused by GN is usually obvious on urinalysis, with proteinuria (nephrotic and nonnephrotic range), hematuria (gross or microscopic), and red blood cell casts present. With acute inflammatory changes of the glomerular tuft, the urinary indices may be prerenal because of de-

Table 69-3. Causes of Acute Renal Failure

Renal parenchymal disease	Glomerulonephritis
	Hypertension (malignant or accelerated)
	Acute interstitial nephritis (drugs, hypercalcemia)
	Vasculitis (amphetamine abuse, hypersensitivity angiitis)
Acute tubular necrosis	
Ischemia	Prolonged, severe prerenal azotemia
	Dissecting aortic aneurysm
Nephrotoxins	Dye-contrast media
	Aminoglycosides, antibiotics
	Heavy metals (mercury, arsenic, platinum)
	Obstructive jaundice
Pigments	Rhabdomyolysis (myoglobinuria)
	Hemoglobinuria

creased glomerular perfusion. Acute oliguric interstitial nephritis frequently presents acutely with hematuria, eosinophiluria, fever, transient eosinophilia, and occasionally a rash. Penicillins (methicillin, ampicillin, penicillin G), rifampin, and sulfonamides are the common culprits, while phenytoin, thiazides, furosemide, allopurinol, and nonsteroidal anti-inflammatory drugs are less common causes. Polyarteritis has been reported with the use of penicillins and sulfonamides but is more characteristic of amphetamine abuse. Hypertension occurs in over half the cases of amphetamine-induced polyarteritis; multisystemic involvement is prominent, and hepatitis B surface antigenemia may be part of the cause.

Malignant hypertension is characterized by necrotizing vasculitis, a high diastolic blood pressure, progressive loss of renal function, hematuria, cardiac and CNS symptoms, and papilledema. Renin and aldosterone levels are high, and a hypokalemic metabolic alkalosis can be seen despite renal failure. Malignant hypertension is especially difficult to control in scleroderma and leads to rapid renal deterioration and death but may respond to angiotensin-converting enzyme blockade. Although earlier therapy of malignant hypertension included bilateral nephrectomy, good control of blood pressure can stabilize renal deterioration and even improve function. Blood pressure normalization should be swift and aggressive with care given to keep mean arterial pressure above 80 to 90 mmHg to prevent cerebral complications.

ATN accounts for the majority of the cases of ARF in adults, but an increasing number of these are nonoliguric. Nonoliguric failure appears to have much less morbidity and mortality compared with oliguric forms. Multiple studies have assessed the value of various agents in converting oliguric to nonoliguric forms. Mannitol has been used since the 1940s in experimental ARF models and consistently prevents ischemic damage if given prophylactically but is less useful when given after an insult. Loop diuretics (furosemide) work less consistently but have the advantage of not increasing extracellular volume. Several studies have demonstrated that furosemide can increase urine flow in oliguric ARF, but no difference is seen in the length of the oliguric period, the number of dialyses, or the mortality between those who respond to furosemide and those who don't. Although dopamine alone does not appear useful, a synergistic effect between dopamine and furosemide has been seen experimentally.

Ischemia is the most common cause or predisposing factor in ATN. In experimental studies there is a correlation between the degree of injury, the morphological findings, and the resultant functional impairment. The importance of plasma renin and angiotensin, of loss of autoregulation, and of prostaglandin synthesis has been receiving increased attention. The degree of oliguria is related to the severity of the ischemia.

Nephrotoxin-induced ATN has continued to increase in importance over the past decade. Antibiotics (aminoglycosides, amphotericin B) and radiographic contrast media are now major causes of ATN in hospitalized patients. Heavy metals are still important causes of ATN in suicides and industrial exposures. Inorganic mercury salts are highly toxic, and as little as 400 mg can cause significant damage. If the patient survives the major corrosive gastrointestinal (GI) complications after oral ingestion, proximal tubular necrosis is seen within 24 h. The prognosis for renal recovery is excellent if the nonrenal complications are managed. Arsenic is found in many herbicides and insecticides. Massive hemolysis and a direct toxic effect on the tubular epithelium contribute to the ATN. Treatment consists of gastric lavage, dimercaprol, and early hemodialysis. In oncology, platinum is a popular chemotherapeutic agent now used in outpatient settings; it can cause either ATN or severe hypomagnesemic hypocalcemia. Bismuth, silver, copper, and organic solvents (carbon tetrachloride, chloroform, and tetrachloroethylene) have all been reported as causes of ATN. Although organic solvents and acetaminophen usually produce primarily hepatic injury, the latter can cause ATN without severe hepatic injury.

Obstructive jaundice and acute pancreatitis are associated with an increased risk of ATN (spontaneous or postoperative), but the exact mechanisms are not clear.

Myoglobinuria can be traumatic (crush injuries, compartment syndromes, ischemia) and nontraumatic. Hypokalemia, alcohol, amphetamines, phencyclidine, and heroin as well as heat stress, enzyme deficiencies (McArdle's disease), and infections are associated with rhabdomyolysis and ATN. Hemolytic transfusion reactions as well as drug- or toxin-induced hemolysis are the causes of hemoglobinuric ATN.

The differentiation between prerenal azotemia and ARF can be difficult. If chronic renal failure is not present, if the urine sodium level is not being elevated by diuretics or by osmotic diuresis, and if obstruction is not present, urinary indices can be useful in diagnosing prerenal azotemia or ARF (Table 69-4). Urinary osmolality (Uosm) is more reliable than specific gravity in determining urinary concentrating ability. In ATN the majority of the patients have a Uosm below 350 mOsm/kg of H_2O, but up to 10 percent may have a Uosm above 500 mOsm/kg of H_2O. Urinary concentration may be lowered by large osmotic loads (glucose, x-ray dyes, mannitol), increased medullary blood flow, or severe malnutrition or liver disease. Ratios of the levels of urine to plasma creatinine, or urinary sodium levels, are useful, but there are large areas of overlap. The fractional excretion of sodium (FE_{Na}) and the renal failure index (RFI) discriminate better between the two groups and can be done on the very small amounts of urine seen in severely oliguric patient. They are compiled as follows:

$$FE_{Na} = \frac{U_{Na}/P_{Na}}{U_{cr}/P_{cr}} \times 100$$

$$RFI = \frac{U_{Na}}{U_{cr}/P_{cr}}$$

where U_{Na} = urinary sodium level
$\quad\quad P_{Na}$ = plasma sodium level
$\quad\quad U_{cr}$ = urinary creatinine level
$\quad\quad P_{cr}$ = plasma creatinine level

NEPHROLITHIASIS

The paradox of the emergency physician's role in dealing with patients with kidney stones is that although a large number of stone patients seek emergency care for acute symptoms, the emergency department is not well-suited for complete diagnosis or determination of long-term therapy. The emergency physician does, however, provide a pivotal role in first determining if renal calculi actually exist; second, uncovering any severe metabolic disorders needing immediate treatment; and third, convincing patients to seek follow up medical care if hospitalization is not needed at that time. The third point is as important as the others, for these patients are often younger (early thirties) and without other medical problems that would lead them to seek ongoing medical care, and renal stones often reoccur. Renal calculi are relatively common,

Table 69-4. Urinary Indices

Laboratory Test	Prerenal Azotemia	Acute Renal Failure
Urine osmolality (mOsm/kg of H_2O)	>500	<350
Urine sodium (mEq/L)	<20	>40
Urine/plasma creatinine	>40	<20
Fractional excretion of sodium	<1	>1
Renal failure index	<1	>1

accounting for 1 per 1000 hospitalizations, and their incidence may be increasing.

Renal colic from the passage of a stone through the ureter has a dramatic presentation. Pain begins insidiously, usually in the flank, radiating into the groin. The pain worsens over the next several hours, becoming excruciating and constant, until the stone is passed out of the ureter and the pain slowly regresses. During this period, management consists of hydration and analgesics. Stones less than 6 mm usually pass, but those over 6 mm may need surgical removal. Although the patient must always be given the benefit of the doubt, the severe pain and need for strong analgesics has led a few narcotic abusers to fake this disorder with a good story and a fingerprick-doctored urine sample. If there is any question, a second urine sample obtained under supervision will determine if the hematuria is of urinary tract origin.

The evaluation of the patient should start with a fresh void urine sample for immediate examination by the laboratory or physician, as cooling precipitates crystals even in normal urine. An abdominal x-ray (KUB) is next, as over 90 percent of renal stones are radiodense. The absence of a stone on KUB x-ray in the presence of renal colic and hematuria indicates a uric acid stone, a passed stone, a rare xanthine stone, or renal colic from blood clots, a tumor, or papillary necrosis. An IVP further defines the problem. Any stone passed should be sent for chemical analysis even though this takes weeks, as this not only provides the definitive diagnosis but may be the only opportunity short of surgery to obtain a stone.

More than 70 percent of the stones are calcium oxalate or phosphate. In the absence of definitive crystals on urinalysis, further diagnostic workup is not usually possible in the emergency department, as it involves serial collections of 24-h urine samples for calcium, oxalate, phosphorus, and uric acid analysis. The serum calcium level should be checked, as hyperparathyroidism, sarcoidosis, neoplasia, multiple myeloma, and rarely hyperthyroidism can present as stones. The serum electrolytes should also be determined, as distal renal tubular acidosis is a rare but very treatable cause of nephrolithiasis. This diagnosis is established by finding a urine pH greater than 6.0 in a noninfected urine in the presence of a nonanion-gap metabolic acidosis. Treatment consists of oral bicarbonate and potassium supplements if needed. Nephrocalcinosis on KUB x-ray should lead to an active search for any chronic hypercalcemic states (primary hyperparathyroidism, sarcoidosis, neoplasia, etc.) or distal renal tabular acidosis.

Struvite (magnesium ammonium phosphate) stones constitute 20 percent of the stones seen and are the most difficult to treat, as they occur in the presence of chronic urinary infection with urea-splitting organisms (*Proteus, Providencia, Staphylococcus aureas*, etc.) and some predisposition to chronic infection such as chronic urinary drainage catheters, bladder dysfunction or obstruction, congenital abnormalities, or ureteral diversions. Urinalysis shows a high pH (7.5 or greater) and pyuria. When large enough the stones are characteristically ''staghorn'', although cystine and uric acid stones may be staghorn on rare occasions. As bacteria are incorporated into the stones during stone growth, antibiotics alone are not enough to eradicate the infection. Management must consist of some combination of stone removal, antibiotics, and correction of the drainage problem.

Uric acid stones account for 5 percent of the stones seen, are radiolucent, and are found in patients with conditions that result in increased uric acid excretion such as gout, myeloproliferative disorders, or high-purine diets. Patients with persistent acid (pH less than 5.5) or concentrated urine may also be at risk. Treatment is hydration and urinary alkalinization. If the diagnosis is sure or the serum uric acid very high, allopurional may be needed. Cystine is a rare cause of stones (3 to 4 percent), but this condition is often easily diagnosed by family history (an autosomal recessive disorder) or urinalysis (''benzene ring'' hexagonal crystals in acid urine or positive cyanide nitroprusside test). Cystine stones are radiodense but less so than calcium-containing ones, so they may mimic uric acid stones. Treatment is consistent day and night hydration and urinary alkalinization, although rare cases may be put on D-penicillamine.

CHRONIC RENAL DISEASE AND DIALYSIS

More than 60,000 people in the United States are on maintenance hemodialysis, a smaller number are on some form of maintenance peritoneal dialysis, and uncounted numbers live with some form of chronic renal insufficiency. Chronic renal disease may be divided into four categories. In the first stage, renal reserve is lost,

Table 69-5. Complications of Chronic Renal Disease

Cardiovascular	Hypertension
	Myocardial infarctions
	Arrythmias
	Strokes
	Congestive heart failure
	Pericarditis
Hematologic	Anemia
	Splenomegaly
	Clotting abnormalities
	Lymphopenia
	Granulocyte dysfunction
Metabolic	Hyperparathyroidism
	Osteomalacia
	Glucose intolerance
	Hyperlipidemia
	Goiter
	Gonadal dysfunction
Neurologic	Uremic encephalopathy
	Peripheral neuropathy
	Subdural hematomas
Infections	Bacterial
	Viral
	Tuberculosis
	Fungal
Gastrointestinal	Bleeding
	Ascites
	Pancreatitis
	Hepatitis
Pulmonary	Pleural effusions
	Pulmonary edema

and at least half the normal function may be lost before the level of plasma creatinine rises above the normal level. Excretory and regulatory functions are intact. The second stage has some manifestations in insufficiency such as mild azotemia, loss of concentrating ability, and mild anemia. Mild insults such as fluid restrictions, diarrhea, vomiting, or prostaglandin inhibitors may lead to severe azotemia and acidosis. Outright renal failure marks the third stage. Anemia is more severe, urinary concentration is lost, hypocalcemia and hyperphosphatemia are present, and metabolic acidosis is seen. Hyperkalemia is not usually a problem until the fourth stage, uremia, which is the most symptomatic. All major organ systems are affected (Table 69-5). Because of the insidious nature of renal failure, a patient may present in the emergency department markedly uremic with no previous knowledge of renal disease, or renal insufficiency may be found on investigation of another problem. In the following sections, the major complications of severe chronic renal failure and dialysis are discussed.

Cardiovascular. Arterial hypertension is found in most patients nearing end-stage renal failure. Cardiac output is increased secondary to anemia, and total peripheral resistance is high. Correction of the anemia decreases the elevated cardiac index but does not decrease the blood pressure and may even increase it. Increased extracellular fluid volume and elevated renin-angiotensin levels both have varying degrees of importance in the cause and maintenance of hypertension. The majority of the patients on dialysis have volume-dependent hypertension, and a smaller number (10 percent) have volume-independent hypertension. Hemodialysis patients with severe hypertension seen in an emergency setting should be treated with short-acting antihypertensives if it is obvious that immediate hemodialysis is necessary, as longer-acting agents complicate hemodialysis with hypotensive episodes and hinder fluid removal. The majority of antihypertensive medications need little dose adjustment in renal patients.

Accelerated atherosclerosis is common in patients with severe renal insufficiency and on dialysis. In this population, deaths from myocardial or cerebral infarctions are increased fivefold over age-matched hypertensive controls. The majority of the patients have multiple risk factors: hypertension, smoking, hyperlipidemias, diabetes or glucose intolerance, hyperuricemia, and hyperparathyroidism with metastic calcifications. It is possible that uremia itself is a risk factor. There is a near universal finding of anemia, and thus oxygen-carrying capacity is decreased and myocardial metabolic demands are higher, leading to a greater chance of coronary insufficiency with additional insults (hypoxic episodes, acidosis) or demand (fever, increased blood loss). Heart failure can result from fluid overload, myocardial disease (infarction, arrhythmias), metabolic abnormalities (acidosis, electrolytes), high-output failure (arteriovenous shunts in accesses, blood loss), pericardial disease (acute, chronic restrictive pericarditis) or valvular damage (endocarditis). Therapy should be directed to the cause of the failure. Volume can be removed by diuresis, sodium restriction, or dialysis. Short-term ionotropic agents (dopamine, dobutamine) may be helpful, but long-term digitalis preparations must be used with caution to prevent overdosage. The smaller muscle mass seen in renal patients and the nondialyzability of these drugs make major dose adjustments necessary. Digoxin should be started at 0.125 mg every day or every other day, with changes based on blood levels.

Pericardial disease can present as uremic pericarditis, dialysis pericarditis, or constrictive pericarditis. Uremic pericarditis occurs in those not yet on dialysis or who have dropped out. It is readily responsive to treatment with dialysis: Dialysis pericarditis is seen in those already on maintenance hemodialysis. It ranges from a subclinical effusion seen on echocardiography to symptomatic forms. Constrictive pericarditis may result from either of the above. It is important to remember that pericarditis can also be caused by viral infections, tuberculosis, myocardial infarctions, and drugs. Because of the frequency of murmurs in renal patients, pericardial rubs may be difficult to evaluate in noisy settings. Elevated jugular venous pulses, hepatojugular reflux, and pulsus alternans are often present from congestive failure common in this setting, and pulsus paradoxus is a variable finding. Although the majority of the patients have some electrocardiographic changes, classic changes occur in less than a third. Over 95 percent have cardiomegaly and changes in the cardiac silhouette, while half have pleural effusions on chest x-rays. Fever and leukocytosis are common. The major complications are cardiac tamponade, constrictive pericarditis, and death. Mortality is 20 percent, and tamponade occurs in 10 percent of uremic and over 20 percent of dialysis pericarditis patients. The fluid is serosanguinous to bloody. The treatment of tamponade is surgical (pericardial window, pericardectomy), and pericardiocentesis should be used only in true emergencies when surgery is not possible, as it has a high morbidity and mortality, and recurrence of the effusion is high. Dialysis resolves the pericarditis in 90 percent of those with uremic pericarditis but in only 40 percent of those with dialysis forms. Anti-inflammatory agents (indomethacin) are not beneficial and may lead to worsening renal function or GI bleeding.

Clinical assessment of the cardiovascular status can be difficult. On auscultation, systolic murmurs are the rule, most benign systolic murmurs from high-output states. Diastolic murmurs are also common; they may be of valvular (aortic or pulmonary incompetence) or pericardial origin. Fourth heart sounds are common because of the hypertension. Third heart sounds, pericardial knocks (in constrictive pericarditis), and pericardial function rubs should be searched for actively. ECGs are often abnormal from myocardial ischemia, ventricular hypertrophy, pericarditis, arrhythmias, digitalis effects, or electrolyte (calcium and potassium) abnormalities. Chest x-rays may be of limited use unless serial ones are available to compare changes in cardiac silhouettes. Echocardiograms are sensitive and specific for determining pericardial effusions.

Hematologic. Anemia is found in almost all patients with creatinine levels above 3.5 mg/100 mL and worsens as renal function worsens. The primary causes of the anemia are decreased erythropoietin production, other inhibitors of erythropoiesis, hemolysis, excessive blood loss, and nutritional deficiencies. The anemia is usually normochromic normocytic, with burr cells seen in proportion to the azotemia. Splenomegaly is not rare and may complicate the anemia. Transfusions should be limited to times of real need, as the patients are at risk for the complications of the frequently transfused: hepatitis, cytomegalovirus infections, and iron overload. Androgens are used in some dialysis patients to increase the red cell mass, but their use is complicated by risks of virilization in women, acne, peliosis hepatitis (blood-filled liver cysts), and hepatocellular carcinoma.

A wide range of hemostatic abnormalities is present, and renal patients have an increased incidence of hemorrhagic problems, particularly GI bleeding. The prothrombin time (PT) partial thromboplastic time (PTT), and platelet count are normal, but the bleeding time is increased. Alterations in platelet release, aggregation, and adhesiveness are consistently found. Effective dialysis improves the bleeding abnormalities, but deamino-8-D-arginine vasopressin (DDAVP) has been suggested for temporary correction.

Lymphopenia is not corrected by dialysis, and defects in cellular immunity have been documented by skin-test anergy and the prolonged survival of skin hemografts. The results of in vitro tests of immune responsiveness are not consistently changed, nor are T-lymphocyte subpopulations altered from normal in the majority of studies. Some abnormalities in immune surveillance are probable, as abnormalities of null cells and natural killer cells have been described. Neoplastic disease is also increased in renal patients. The humoral immunity is less affected. Marked disagreement exists as to the presence of granulocyte dysfunction, with some noting depressed chemotaxis and chemiluminescence while others find no changes.

Metabolic. Renal osteodystrophy is a frequent complication and may be severely symptomatic, with bone pain, myopathies, and fractures. The bone disease results from secondary hyperparathyroidism, defective mineralization, chronic acidosis, heparin use in hemodialysis, and trace-element abnormalities. As hyperphosphatemia is a major problem, hypocalcemia should not be treated unless symptomatic to reduce the risks of metastatic calcifications. Phosphate binders should be used in all patients with hyperphosphatemia, with calcium supplements added later if needed.

The glucose intolerance seen is probably related to peripheral insulin resistance. The patients rarely have fasting hyperglycemia or ketosis but have prolonged elevations of glucose levels after carbohydrate loads. Spontaneous hypoglycemia is rare but does occur. Hemodialysis usually improves glucose utilization. Many have noted that diabetics have decreased insulin requirements as renal insufficiency worsens. A common explanation has been decreased insulin degradation by the kidney, but decreased functional cellular mass, decreased appetite, and decreased metabolic rates are probably better reasons. Tolbutamide is the only oral hypoglycemic safe to use in renal failure. The hyperlipidemias seen in renal patients may be related to their problems with carbohydrate metabolism as well as resulting from an impairment of lipoprotein lipase synthesis. Triglycerides are high, and cholesterol is often normal. Type IV hyperlipidemia is more common than types IIa and IIb. The hypertriglyceridemias may worsen after starting hemodialysis. Very low density lipoproteins (VLDL) levels are elevated and high-density lipoproteins (HDL) levels are decreased, a pattern common in those at risk for accelerated atherosclerosis.

Uremia may sometimes mimic myxedema coma, with pallor, hypothermia, edema, anemia, and stupor seen in both, but although goiters of unknown cause are seen in hemodialysis patients, no overt disturbances of thyroid function are caused by renal insufficiency. Hypothermia may be as severe as 35°C in advanced uremia, but most patients are started on dialysis before becoming severely uremic. Gynecomastia can be seen transiently after starting hemodialysis. Major abnormalities in levels of sex hormones lead to impotence and loss of libido in men, and infertility, amenorrhea, or menorrhagia in women. Conception is rare and is usually followed by spontaneous abortion.

Neurologic. Uremic encephalopathy is similar to other toxic and metabolic encephalopathies, as the signs fluctuate and include slurred speech, impaired sensorium, gait disturbance, asterixis, action tremors, multifocal clonus, and seizures. The development of these conditions seems to be related to the rate of renal failure rather than to an absolute level of serum creatinine. Uremic seizures are handled in an emergency as any other seizures until dialysis can be started. The peripheral neuropathy consists of a distal, symmetric, mixed sensorimotor polyneuropathy. Neurologic hemodialysis problems include subdural hematomas, Wernicke's encephalopathy, and dialysis dementia, a progressively fatal disorder of those on hemodialysis.

Miscellaneous. Infections are major complications in renal patients, and up to 60 percent of the patients suffer serious infections which contribute to death in many. The incidence of tuberculosis is 10 times greater than normal, and hepatitis B and cytomegalovirus infections can be a problem.

Ascites in patients on maintenance hemodialysis may develop without evidence of cirrhosis, heart failure, hypoalbuminemia, peritonitis, or carcinomatosis. The amylase levels are increased because of renal retention but are usually less than twice normal unless pancreatitis is present.

METHODS OF DIALYSIS

Hemodialysis (HD) is the most common method of maintenance dialysis, although there is increased interest in peritoneal dialysis (PD), especially continuous ambulatory peritoneal dialysis (CAPD). HD depends on an easily reached, high-flow, dependable angioaccess. Of the major types of angioaccesses, the oldest and least used is an external shunt (commonly a Scribner) connecting a peripheral (usually radial) artery and vein. These have major problems of infection, thrombosis, and accidental disconnection, risking large blood losses. They can be placed quickly and used immediately, however. Arteriovenous fistulas have lower complication rates with thrombosis and infection than the others but need several months to mature and occasionally develop steal syndromes or large, symptomatic shunting. In those with inadequate superficial veins, artificial arteriovenous conduits are made usually using Teflon polymers (GoreTex). They develop more rapidly (10 days to 2 weeks) than arteriovenous fistulas and are well-tolerated but can be complicated by infections or thrombosis. As blood flow rates are very high through these angioaccesses, exsanguination can occur if the angioaccess is disconnected or lacerated, major hematomas can occur if it is punctured, and thrombosis can occur after compression or trauma to the area. Blood drawing, the insertion of intravenous tubes, and blood pressure measurement should never be done in the arm with the hemoaccess. Rarely a patient may be seen with a temporary subclavian catheter for temporary hemodialysis. These catheters should be treated with the same asceptic technique as chemotherapy or parenteral nutrition catheters. A major cause of hospitalization in dialysis patients is vascular-access problems—usually infections or thrombosis.

Life expectancy is certainly not normal on HD, and patients die at an overall rate of 10 percent per year for the first 5 years. Diabetics, patients with other diseases, and older patients have a worse prognosis. Patients surviving 10 years show no evidence of progressive deterioration if hypertension and other problems are controlled.

Because of lower costs and increased personal freedom, CAPD is becoming more popular. This involves fluid exchanges through a permanent catheter (usually a Tenckhoff catheter) into the peritoneal space three to four times a day. Although many features (better fluid control, easier management of hypertension and the level of blood glucose) are superior to those of HD, the high rates of peritonitis and hyperlipidemias may be major problems.

Hemofiltration is a method of removing fluid, electrolytes, and small molecules over a period of hours or days by connection of a specially designed filter into an arteriovenous circuit which can be temporary (femoral vein and artery or Scribner) or permanent (arteriovenous fistula or graft). Fluid removal is readily titrated and may be more easily tolerated by a hypotensive hemodynamically unstable patient than HD or PD.

Dialysis can also be useful in drug overdosage. Indications for using dialysis include severe clinical intoxication, fatal blood levels, progressive deterioration while under medical management, and poisoning by agents known to produce prolonged toxicity. Phenobarbital, salicylates, methanol, ethylene glycol, and paraquat can be removed by HD, while other barbiturates, glutethimide, methaqualone, ethchlorvynol, meprobamate, trichloroethanol, and theophylline are better treated with hemoperfusion.

RENAL TRANSPLANTATION

More than 100,000 people have received a renal transplant in the 25 years of experience with them. In that time major strides have been made in the fields of histocompatibility and immunology, but much remains unsolved. The 1-year survival rate of those who received cadaver grafts is greater than 50 to 60 percent, and the 1-year survival rate of those who received grafts from living relatives is greater than 80 percent. These people are on permanent immunosuppression by drugs and suffer multiple complications from this and from unresolved uremic disorders. The causes of death after transplantation are infection (40 percent), cardiovascular disease (20 percent), suicide (15 percent), and GI problems (15 percent). Pneumococcal infections are particularly dangerous for those with splenectomies, but other agents include gram-negative infections, *Staphylococcus*, cytomegalovirus, toxoplasmosis, and fungi. Sites of infections include the lung (pneumonia), soft tissues, wounds, the CNS (meningitis and brain abscesses), and the heart (endocarditis). Perforations of the GI tract, peritonitis, and pancreatitis account for the GI deaths. Cardiovascular deaths result from conditions including myocardial infarctions, pulmonary emboli, and congestive failure.

Nonfatal complications after transplantation include hypertension (with or without renal artery stenosis), myelotoxicity from the drugs, hypercalcemia, RTA, steroid-induced diabetes mellitus, myopathies, cataracts, and osteoporosis. Hepatitis may be viral (hepatitis B or cytometalovirus) or drug-induced (azathioprine).

BIBLIOGRAPHY

Abrutyn E, Solomons NW, St. Clair L: Granulocyte function in patients with chronic renal failure. *J Infect Dis* 135:1, 1977.

Anderson RJ, Linas SL, Berns AS, et al: Non-oliguric acute renal failure. *N Engl J Med* 296:1134, 1977.

Andrews OT, Schoenfeld PY, Hopewell PC, et al: Tuberculosis in patients with end-stage renal disease. *Am J Med* 68:59, 1980.

Barratt LJ, Robinson MA, Whitford JA, et al: The diastolic murmur of renal failure. *N Engl J Med* 295:121, 1976.

Bismuth H, Kuntziger H, Corlette MB: Cholangitis with acute renal failure. *Ann Surg* 181:881, 1975.

Briggs WA, Pederson MM, Mahajan SK, et al: Lymphocyte and granulocyte function in zinc treated and zinc-deficient hemodialysis patients. *Kidney Int* 21:827, 1982.

Brown CB, Ogg CS, Cameron JS. High dose furosemide in acute renal failure: A controlled trial. *Clin Nephrol* 15:90, 1981.

Byrd L, Sherman RL: Radiocontrast-induced acute renal failure. A clinical and pathological review. *Medicine* 58:270, 1979.

Citron BP, Halpen M, McCarron M, et al: Necrotizing angiitis associated with drug abuse. *N Engl J Med* 283:1003, 1970.

Clarkson TW: The pharmacology of mercury compounds. *Annu Rev Pharmacol* 12:375, 1972.

Coburn JW: Renal osteodystrophy. *Kidney Int* 17:677, 1980.

Dunn MJ, Zambraski EJ: Renal effects of drugs that inhibit prostaglandin synthesis. *Kidney Int* 18:609, 1980.

Fine RN, Terasaki PI, Ettenger RB, et al: Renal transplant update. *Ann Intern Med* 100:246, 1984.

Goldstein DA, Llach F, Massry SG: Acute renal failure in patients with acute pancreatitis. *Arch Intern Med* 138:1363, 1976.

Gotloib L, Servadio C: Ascites in patient undergoing maintenance hemodialysis. *Am J Med* 61:465, 1976.

Kim KE, Onesti G, Swartz CD, et al: Hemodynamics of hypertension in chronic end stage renal disease. *Circulation* 46:456, 1972.

Kjellstrand CM, Campbell DC, von Hartitzsch, et al: Hyperuricemic acute renal failure. *Arch Intern Med* 133:349, 1974.

Kleinknecht D, Ganeval D, Gonzalez-Duque LA, et al: Furosemide in acute oliguric renal failure. A controlled trial. *Nephron* 17:51, 1976.

Lauer A, Saccaggi A, Ronco C, et al: Continuous arteriovenous hemofiltration in the critically ill patient. *Ann Intern Med* 99:455, 1983.

Ledingham RGG, Rajagopalan B: Cerebral complications in the treatment of accelerated hypertension. *Q J Med* 48:25, 1977.

Lee DB, Prompt CA, Upham AT, et al: Medical complications of renal transplantation. *Urology* 9:S7, S32, 1977.

Levitt MD, Ellis C: Serum iso-amylase measurements in pancreatitis complicating chronic renal failure. *J Lab Clin Med* 93:71, 1979.

Lifschitz, MD: Prostaglandins and renal blood flow: In vivo studies. *Kidney Int* 19:781, 1981.

Linder A, Cutler RE, Goodman WG, et al: Synergism of dopamine plus furosemide in preventing acute renal failure in the dog. *Kidney Int* 16:158, 1979.

Lopez-Ovejero JA, Saal SD, D'Angelo WA, et al: Reversal of vascular and renal crisis of scleroderma by oral angiotensin-converting enzyme blockage. *N Engl J Med* 300:1417, 1979.

Lundin AP, Adler AJ, Berlyne GM, et al: Tuberculosis in patients undergoing maintenance hemodialysis. *Am J Med* 67:597, 1979.

Madias NE, Harrington JT: Platinum nephrotoxicity. *Am J Med* 65:307, 1978.

Mamdani BH, Lim VS, Mahurkar SD, et al: Recovery from prolonged renal failure in patients with accelerated hypertension. *N Engl J Med* 291:1343, 1974.

Mannuccio PM, Remuzzi G, Pusineri F, et al: Deamino-8-D-arginine vasopressin shortens bleeding time in uremia. *N Engl J Med* 308:8, 1983.

Matas AJ, Simmons RL, Kjellstrand CM, et al: Increased incidence of malignancy during chronic renal failure. *Lancet* 1:883, 1975.

Miller TR, Anderson RJ, Linas SL, et al: Urinary diagnostic indices in acute renal failure. A prospective study. *Ann Intern Med* 89:47, 1978.

Mitchell JR, McMurty RJ, Statham CN, et al: Molecular basis for several drug-induced nephropathies. *Am J Med* 62:518, 1977.

Montgomerie JZ, Kalmanson GM, Guze LB: Renal failure and infection. *Medicine* 47:1, 1968.

Mroczek WJ: Malignant hypertension: Kidneys too good to be extirpated. *Ann Intern Med* 80:754, 1974.

Neff MS, Eiser AR, Slifkin RF, et al: Patients surviving 10 years of hemodialysis. *Am J Med* 74:996, 1983.

Neff MS, Goldberg J, Slifkin RF, et al: A comparison of androgens for anemia in patients on hemodialysis. *N Engl J Med* 304:871, 1981.

Raskin NH, Fishman RA: Neurological disorders in renal failure. *N Engl J Med* 294:143, 204, 1976.

Reaven GM, Swenson RS, Sanfelippo ML: An inquiry into the mechanism of hypertriglyceridemia in patients with chronic renal faiure. *Am J Clin Nutr* 33:1476, 1980.

Renfrew R, Buselmeier TJ, Kjellstand CM: Pericarditis and renal failure. *Ann Rev Med* 31:345, 1980.

Revillard JP: Immunological alterations in chronic renal insufficiency. *Adv Nephrol* 8:365, 1979.

Ritchey EE, Wallin JD, Shah SV: Chemiluminescence and superoxide anion production by leukocytes from chronic hemodialysis patients. *Kidney Int* 19:349, 1981.

Rowland LP, Penn AS: Myoglobinuria. *Med Clin North Am* 56:1233, 1972.

Rutsky EA, McDaniel HG, Thorpe DL, et al: Spontaneous hypoglycemia in chronic renal failure. *Arch Intern Med* 138:1364, 1978.

Schilsky RL, Anderson T: Hypomagnesemia and renal magnesium wasting in patients receiving cisplatin. *Ann Intern Med* 90:929, 1979.

Smolens P, Stein JH: Pathophysiology of acute renal failure. *Am J Med* 70:479, 1981.

Spector DA, Davis PJ, Helderman JH, et al: Thyroid function and metabolic state in chronic renal failure. *Ann Intern Med* 85:724, 1976.

Teitelbaum DT, Kier LC: Arsine poisoning report of five cases in the petroleum industry and a discussion of the indications for exchange transfusion and hemodialysis. *Arch Environ Health* 19:133, 1969.

Thurau K: Renal hemodynamics. *Am J Med* 36:698, 1964.

Tiller DJ, Mudge GH: Pharmacologic agents used in the management of acute renal failure. *Kidney Int* 18:700, 1980.

vanYpersele de Strihou, C: Acute oliguric interstitial nephritis. *Kidney Int* 16:751, 1979.

Vas SI: Microbiological aspects of chronic ambulatory peritoneal dialysis. *Kidney Int* 23:83, 1983.

Washer GF, Schroter GPJ, Starzl TE, et al: Causes of death after kidney transplantation. *JAMA* 250:49, 1983.

Winchester JF, Gelfand MC, Knepshield JH, et al: Dialysis and hemoperfusion of poisons and drugs—Update. *Trans Am Soc Artif Intern Organs* 23:762, 1977.

Woods, JW: Malignant hypertension: Clinical recognition and management. *Cardiovasc Clin* 9:311, 1978.

Woods JW, Blyte WB, Huffines WD: Management of malignant hypertension complicated by renal insufficiency. *N Engl J Med* 291:10, 1974.

CHAPTER 70
URINARY TRACT
INFECTIONS

Harold A. Jayne

Urinary tract infection is defined as significant bacteriuria in the presence of symptoms; it is one of the most common, most controversial, and least-appreciated problems in emergency medicine. About one in five women complain of dysuria each year. Urinary tract infection is a major cause of nosocomial gram-negative sepsis, and 1 percent to 3 percent of all patients with pyelonephritis die. Asymptomatic bacteriuria (ABU) is common, and its treatment (except in pregnancy) has not proved beneficial.

NATURAL HISTORY

The natural history of urinary tract infection varies with age and sex (Fig. 70-1). In neonates, a urinary tract infection is part of the syndrome of overwhelming gram-negative sepsis. The incidence of urinary tract infection in preschool children is about 2 percent, with the incidence in girls 10 to 20 times greater than that in boys; in school-age children, the incidence is about 5 percent, with a 50-times-greater incidence in girls. Asymptomatic bacteriuria has been studied extensively, but a detailed discussion is beyond the scope of this text.

Bacteriuria is rare in males under the age of 50 years unless there is a history of instrumentation or urethral stenosis. In men older than 50 years, the incidence increases because of prostatic obstruction and instrumentation.

Dysuria in females is a common clinical problem, and symptoms increase with age and sexual activity. Most urinary tract infections occur in otherwise normal females, probably secondary to sexual contact and local trauma. The infecting organisms are generally those found colonizing the perineum. A few patients appear to have a biological defect that allows bacteria from the gastrointestinal tract to colonize the vaginal vestibule. This group of women has a high incidence of calicectasis and renal cortical scarring, and there is often a history of childhood vesicoureteral reflux. About one-third of cases of dysuria are characterized by sterile urine; this is termed the urethral syndrome. Many of these patients have either low-grade or early *Escherichia coli, Chlamydia trachomatis,* or *Neisseria gonorrhoeae* infections. In fact, the definitions of urinary tract infection based on early studies that reported only upper tract disease may be inappropriate. Such studies established that colony counts of at least 10^5/mL are necessary to indicate the presence of bacteriuria. It may be that in lower urinary tract infection, significant bacteriuria may be present even when colony counts are less than 10^5/mL.

The majority of urinary tract infections in women recur because of either relapse or reinfection. Relapse is caused by the same organism and, when symptoms recur in less than 1 month, represents treatment failure. When symptoms recur in 1 to 6 months, the patient is most likely reinfected. Reinfection is from a different organism (usually enteric) or a different serotype of the same organism and often results from a defect in the defense mechanisms of the host. The recurrence of infection may indicate the presence of a tumor, tuberculosis, or renal calculi. Therefore, if recurrence develops more than three times in 1 year, a complete workup is warranted.

A urinary tract infection during pregnancy poses special problems. If it is untreated, ABU may develop into symptomatic bacteriuria. Symptomatic urinary tract infection and pyelonephritis have a high incidence in the third trimester and may lead to preeclampsia, sepsis, or miscarriage. This is the single case in which treatment of ABU is indicated.

BACTERIOLOGY

Urinary tract infections can be divided into complicated and uncomplicated. Complicated infections occur in patients with underlying renal or neurologic disease. Uncomplicated infections are those in which no defect can be demonstrated.

Most uncomplicated urinary tract infections are caused by gram-negative aerobic bacilli from the gut (Table 70-1). Anaerobic organisms do not grow well in urine. Complicated urinary tract infections are caused by unusual pathogens and should be managed by a urologist or nephrologist.

NORMAL HOST DEFENSE MECHANISMS

Urine is generally a good culture medium depending on the pH and the chemical constituents. Factors unfavorable to bacterial growth are a low pH (5.5 or less); a high concentration of urea; the presence of weak organic acids derived from a diet that includes hippuric acid (cranberry juice) and ascorbic acid (citrus fruits); and methionine (a sulfur-containing amino acid present in

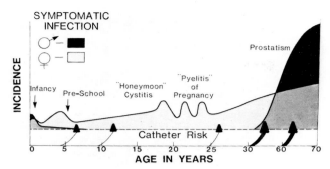

Figure 70-1. Natural history of urinary tract infections.

protein foods). Methionine is metabolized to inorganic sulfate, which is excreted with an obligatory increase in hydrogen ion movement, which acidifies the urine.

Bladder defense. A thin film of urine remains in the bladder after voiding. An intact bladder mucosa removes organisms from this film. This probably occurs by the production of organic acids by the mucosal cells and not by antibody formation or phagocytosis. The mechanism is ineffective if the bladder is incompletely emptied. Frequent and complete voiding has been associated with the reduction of recurrence of urinary tract infection.

Renal defense. Local antibodies are produced in the kidney and kill bacteria in the presence of complement. Local leukocytosis and phagocytosis also help eradicate bacteria.

Urinary hydrodynamics. Urinary hydrodynamics may be the most important host defense mechanism. Diuresis dilutes the bacterial inoculum, and frequent voiding tends to rid the bladder of bacteria.

DIAGNOSIS

If a urinary tract infection is suspected, the first step in establishing the diagnosis is the careful collection of urine for urinalysis and culture. The midstream voiding specimen is accurate if the patient is given and follows careful instructions. Instruct the woman to remove her underwear, face the back of the toilet, sit, spread the labia with one hand, cleanse from front to back with povidone-iodine swabs or liquid soap, pass a small amount of urine into the toilet, and then urinate into a sterile cup. Instruct the man to carefully cleanse the urethral meatus, retracting the foreskin if uncircumcised, and obtain a midstream specimen as described above.

If the sample is properly collected, it should contain no or few epithelial cells. Sources of contamination are material in the col-

Table 70-1. Bacterial Causes of Uncomplicated Urinary Tract Infection

Organism	Incidence
E. coli	80%
Klebsiella	
Proteus	
Enterobacter	
Pseudomonas	
Staphylococcus	Less than 5%
Group D streptococci	

lection bottle, menses, vaginal discharge, urethral or periurethral tissue, and organisms multiplying in the urine after collection. Bacteria in urine double each hour at room temperature. The use of a tampon enables a woman to obtain a clean-cup specimen if menstruation or a discharge is present.

Catheterization is indicated if the patient cannot void spontaneously, to relieve obstruction, if the patient is too ill or immobilized, if the patient is extremely obese, or when done as part of a urologic evaluation. However, routine catheterization should be avoided, as 1 to 2 percent of patients develop urinary tract infections after a single insertion of a catheter, according to Kunin. Women just prior to delivery are especially prone to develop infection from catheterization.

Suprapubic aspiration, described in the section on pediatrics, can be used to obtain a specimen in newborns and infants.

Blood or bile may be detected by gross examination of the urine. However, gross examination is never useful to determine whether urine is infected, as cloudiness is usually not due to white blood cells (WBC) or bacteria but to large amounts of protein or crystals.

Bacteriuria should be evaluated using a Gram stain of uncentrifuged urine, or an unstained drop preparation of centrifuged sediment. When the oil-immersion lens is used, the presence of any bacteria on a Gram stain of uncentrifuged urine is significant, and in 80 to 90 percent of the cases the culture correlates positively. When the dry high-power lens is used to examine a centrifuged urinary sediment, more than 15 bacteria per high-power field is significant. The problems with these methods of diagnosis are that (1) they fail to detect fewer than 10^4/mL colony counts, and gram-positive organisms can cause urinary tract infection at lower counts; (2) there is up to a 20 percent false negative rate; and (3) vaginal or fecal contamination can be falsely interpreted as positive. This may account for the finding that only 80 percent of women with colony counts of at least 10^5/mL are infected.

Pyuria can be present with many disorders such as trauma, irritation of the ureter by an overlying inflamed appendix, and gross contamination, as well as urinary tract infection. In women, pyuria is significant if there are more than 10 WBC per high-power field (HPF), but only if bacteria are present on microscopic examination. In men, more than 1 to 2 WBC/HPF can be significant in the presence of bacteria. Falsely negative pyuria is due to a number of factors. About one-half of women with symptomatic bacteriuria have fewer than 5 WBC/HPF. Ingestion of large amounts of fluids washes out the bladder and produces dilute urine. Partial treatment may clear pyuria when cultures are still positive. Pyuria can be intermittent, or absent, as in the case of an obstructed kidney.

The definitive diagnosis of urinary tract infection is made by a colony count greater than 10^5/mL from a midstream catch. If the patient is symptomatic, one culture is significant. For ABU, two to three positive cultures are necessary. There are qualifications to these statements that are beyond the scope of this chapter, but these are the standards with which more rapidly obtained diagnostic parameters are compared for use in the clinical setting.

CLINICAL FEATURES

The clinical signs of urinary tract infection in neonates and infants are anorexia, poor weight gain, irritability, and occasional vomiting. In preschool children, irritability, listlessness, and dysuria

Table 70-2. Oral Antimicrobial Agents Used in Treating Urinary Tract Infections

Drug	10–14 Day Dose	Comments
Sulfisoxazole (Gantrisin)	Children: Initially 75 mg/kg, then 150 mg/(kg·day) in divided doses 4–6 times per day Adults: Initially 2–4 g, then 2–4 g/day in 3–6 divided doses; single dose, 200 mg/kg PO	Low cost Broad-spectrum Resistance frequent because of high concentration of sulfas in stool Rash and bone marrow depression Causes hemolytic anemia in G6PD deficiency
Sulfamethoxazole (Gantanol)	Children: Initially 60 mg/kg, then 60 mg/kg in 2 divided doses Adults: Initially 2 g PO, then 1 g bid PO; single dose, 2 g PO	Displaces tolbutamide from serum protein binding site and may induce hypoglycemia Displaces warfarin from binding site and may increase anticoagulant activity Also inhibits intestinal bacterial synthesis of vitamin K, which may increase anticoagulant activity
Tetracycline	Children: 10–20 mg/(kg·day) in 4 divided doses Adults: 250–500 mg 2–4 times per day	Other tetracyclines do not achieve high urine concentrations Low cost Stains developing teeth; should not be used in patient under 8 years of age Causes negative nitrogen balance, aminoaciduria, and riboflavinemia May cause fulminant hepatitis in pregnant women Resistance frequent; causes stool bacteria
Ampicillin	Children: 100 mg/(kg·day) in 4 divided doses Adults: 250–500 mg qid; single dose, 2–3 g PO and 1 g probenecid (Benemid)	Reasonable cost, effectiveness overrated Diarrhea and morbilliform eruption 5–10% Leads to protoplast (L form) production *Proteus* particularly sensitive
Amoxicillin	Children: 20 mg/(kg·day) q 8 h PO Adults: 250–500 mg PO tid; single dose, 2–3 g PO and 1 g probenecid	Spectrum similar to that of ampicillin; slightly longer duration of action
Nalidixic Acid (NegGram)	Children: 55 mg/(kg·day) in 4 divided doses Adults: 1 g qid	Contraindicated in infants and children under 12 years old Useful for first few infections Resistance common GI complaints and allergy common Headache, visual disturbances, drowsiness, occasional toxic psychosis Hemolytic anemia seen in G6PD deficiency
Nitrofurantoin	Children: 5–7 mg/(kg·day) in 4 divided doses Adults: 100 mg tid or qid; single dose, 200 mg PO	Enteric bacteria develop less resistance Effective in upper and lower UTI Nausea, vomiting in 10–15% May cause interstitial pneumonia Contraindicated in azotemia, G6PD deficiency, and hemolytic anemia
Cephalexin	Children: 25–50 mg/(kg·day) in 4 divided doses Adults: 250–500 mg tid or qid	Expensive
Erythromycin	Children: 30–50 mg/(kg·day) in divided doses Adults: 500–1000 mg tid or qid	Relatively ineffective drug Kills L forms Usually effective against gram-positive organisms; in alkaline state, effective against enteric organisms

Note: G6PD = glucose-6-phosphate dehydrogenase

are common, but fever, chills, and flank pain are uncommon. Dysuria is a common complaint in school-age girls and is most often due to vulvovaginitis. Consequently, the physician should examine the vulva and make sure the method of urine collection is correct to prevent unnecessary treatment with antibiotics. Any female with a urinary tract infection must be followed since the recurrence rate is about 80 percent.

School-age boys less than 10 years old usually have fever with a urinary tract infection. The colony count may be less than 10^3/mL because infection with gram-positive cocci and *Proteus* is common. Boys aged 10 to 14 years are generally afebrile and have frequency and dysuria. The microbiology is variable.

The clinical symptoms of a urinary tract infection in adults are dysuria, frequency, and lower abdominal pain. In females, a vaginal examination is necessary to rule out vaginitis as the cause of dysuria. Fever, chills, and malaise may also be present.

Flank pain and costovertebral (CVA) tenderness can be associated with cystitis because of referred pain, but when these are found clinically, one should assume that pyelonephritis is present.

In the male, dysuria with discharge indicates urethritis, and a Gram stain of the discharge is necessary to establish the diagnosis. If gram-negative intracellular diplococci are present, the patient should be treated for gonococcal urethritis. If the Gram stain is negative, the diagnosis is most likely nonspecific urethritis, which is mainly chlamydial infection. A VDRL test and a culture for gonococcus should be obtained in both cases. Dysuria without a

Table 70-3. Guidelines to Management

Group	Ease of Management	Type of Patient	Clinical Characteristics	Organism	Probability of Tissue Invasion	Therapy
I	Excellent	Female, child or adult	Few previous episodes; reliable, with good follow-up available; less than 2 days between onset of symptoms and treatment	Usually *E. coli* sensitive to most agents	Low	One dose amoxicillin, sulfonamide, TMP/SMZ, kanamycin
II	Good	Female, child or adult	Few previous episodes; follow-up poor	Usually *E. coli* sensitive to most agents	High or low	3–10 days; prophylaxis for closely spaced recurrences
III	Fair	Female, child or adult	Many previous episodes; history of early recurrence, or diabetic, or renal transplantation	Variable; tends to have more resistant bacteria; susceptibility tests essential	High	4–6 weeks; prophylaxis for closely spaced recurrences
IV	Fair	Male, adult	Recurrent infections; some underlying anatomic abnormality	Variable; susceptibility tests needed	High; often prostatic colonization	4–12 weeks; prophylaxis for closely spaced recurrences
V	Poor	Male or female	Neurogenic bladder; large volume residual urine	Variable; susceptibility tests needed	High	Intermittent catheterization (treatment for symptomatic infections only)
VI	Very poor	Male or female	Continuous drainage required	Variable; susceptibility tests needed	Very High	Indwelling catheter closed drainage (treatment for sepsis only)

Note: TMP/SMZ = trimethoprim with sulfamethoxazole.

Source: Kunin CM: Duration of treatment of urinary tract infections. *Am J Med* 71:849–854, 1981.

discharge in the male should be evaluated with a clean-catch urine specimen. If bacteriuria is present, treatment followed by a complete urologic workup is indicated.

TREATMENT

Children

Antibiotic treatment for children, with the exception of treatment with tetracycline, is the same as that for adults. Urinary tract defects are common in children who have symptomatic urinary tract infection. All children who have demonstrated bacteriuria and significant culture results require urologic consultation, including diagnostic radiology. Care must be taken to ensure referral to a urologist who has knowledge of pediatric urinary tract infections.

Adults

Treat urinary tract infection if clinical symptoms are supported by a urinalysis demonstrating the presence of greater than 2 bacteria per HPF, 10 to 15 WBC/HPF and few epithelial cells. Obtain urine for culture from all patients except women with a first episode of urinary tract infection.

The selection of antibiotics depends on the bacteriology of the infection, patient sensitivity and compliance, drug toxicity, and cost. *E. coli* is susceptible to most oral agents: sulfonamides, tetracycline, ampicillin, nalidixic acid, nitrofurantoin, cephalexin, and penicillin G or V in high concentration. The dosage and com-

ments about some of these urinary antimicrobial agents are listed in Table 70-2.

Most antibiotics work in the general pH range of urine. However, *Proteus* and *Klebsiella* produce urease, which splits urea into ammonia and carbon dioxide, resulting in alkaline urine that decreases the effectiveness of nitrofurantoin and the tetracyclines. In these cases, oral agents to alter the pH of the urine are necessary.

Most authorities have, until recently, recommended treating the first episode with a soluble, short-acting sulfonamide for 10 to 14 days (Table 70-3). A sulfonamide can also be used to treat the next several episodes, but its effectiveness decreases as the bacteria develop resistance. Alternatively, tetracycline can be used in children aged 8 and over and in nonpregnant women. There is no evidence that ampicillin is any more effective than the sulfonamides. The cost of various antimicrobials is compared in Table 70-4. The urine should be bacteria-free in 24 to 48 h. If not, the antimicrobial agent must be changed according to the results of the culture and sensitivity. Therefore, arrangements must be made to have the patient seen in follow-up.

Recently, multiple investigational reports of shorter treatment regimens for uncomplicated infections have been published. Single-dose treatment appears to offer a number of advantages: cost and side effects are reduced, compliance is improved, and the development of resistant strains of bacteria is less likely. In addition, single-dose treatments may differentiate patients with more complicated infections, as relapse and failure to eradicate bacteriuria within 2 to 3 days is common in these patients.

Single-dose or three-day regimens have limitations. In a large series, those patients who demonstrated probable tissue invasion [those who were antibody-coated-bacteria (ACB) positive] had

Table 70-4. Cost Comparison of Urinary Antimicrobial agents

Generic Name	Brand Name	Cost of 10-Day Dose*
Sulfamethoxazole	Gantanol	$ 9.77
Sulfisoxazole	Gantrisin	6.28
Tetracycline, 250 mg		3.89
500 mg		5.13
Co-trimoxazole	Bactrim plain	13.45
	DS	19.93
Co-trimoxazole	Septra plain	13.45
	DS	19.93
Ampicillin, 500 mg		8.66

*Data source: Chicago-area pharmacies, 1983.

poor response to short-term therapy when compared with those who received traditional 10- to 14-day treatment. Since ACB testing is justifiable only in research settings, this raises questions about the efficacy of short-term therapy in episodic-care settings. Therefore, before an emergency physician decides to recommend a single-dose treatment, the patient's ability to obtain follow-up in 2 to 3 days must be ensured. If follow-up compliance is not expected, the patient should be placed on a 10- to 14-day regimen. A 3-day regimen may be as effective as a 10-day regimen, but only a few reports on this subject have been published, and such treatment is therefore not yet recommended.

For recurrent infection, culture and sensitivity tests are essential. The infection is often due to a new serotype of *E. coli,* or it may be due to newly resistant organisms, especially the L forms, which develop as a result of the antibiotics excreted into the gastrointestinal tract.

Agents recommended for recurrent infections include tetracycline, ampicillin, cephalexin, nalidixic acid, or nitrofurantoin. For frequently recurrent infections, sensitivity tests are essential. Nitrofurantoin can be used for several months in these cases, and it is especially good because it is not excreted in the stool, so the sensitivity of organisms to the agent remains high after repeated use in recurrent infections.

Adjunctive therapy consists of a high-protein diet to provide a more acidic urine, fluids to enhance diuresis, frequent voiding to diminish tissue contact with bacteria, and fruit juices such as cranberry juice and juices containing vitamin C to acidify the urine.

Once the infection is eradicated, management should be directed toward prevention of reinfection. This is designed to prevent ascending kidney infection. Approximately 80 percent of women who have demonstrated urinary tract infection develop recurrence. Since many factors are involved in reinfection and some of these are correctable, continuity of care is essential.

PYELONEPHRITIS

On occasion, it may be difficult to distinguish lower from upper urinary tract infection. Pyelonephritis is characterized by shaking chills and fever, flank pain, and CVA tenderness following several days of dysuria and frequency. The urine shows white blood cell casts and clumps, as well as bacteria.

Sophisticated differentiation consists of immunofluorescent antibody tests, and analysis for β-glucuronidase and lactate dehydrogenase isoenzymes. These are principally useful as research tools.

Factors that predispose to pyelonephritis are age, a short urethra, sexual trauma, pregnancy, congenital or acquired anatomic urinary tract abnormality, and neurogenic problems that result in incomplete bladder emptying. Young women of child-bearing age are more susceptible. Additional predisposing factors are diabetes mellitus, urinary tract instrumentation, renal calculi and nephrocalcinosis, vesicourethral reflux, and prostatic hypertrophy or prostatitis.

Complications of acute pyelonephritis are acute papillary necrosis with possible ureteric obstruction, septic shock, and perinephric abscesses. The latter condition is characterized by spiking fever, persistent pyuria, and CVA tenderness.

The decision to admit a patient with acute pyelonephritis is based on clinical judgment. Fluid replacement and parenteral antibiotics are necessary if the patient is vomiting or dehydrated. The probability of complications is not well established. Young, otherwise healthy, females have the least morbidity and mortality. However, 1 to 3 percent of patients with acute pyelonephritis die. Factors associated with an unfavorable prognosis are old age and general debility, renal calculi or obstruction, a past history of instrumentation, diabetes, analgesic abuse, sickle cell anemia or trait, underlying carcinoma, or cancer chemotherapy.

BIBLIOGRAPHY

Buckwold FJ, et al: Therapy for acute cystitis in adult women: Randomized comparison of single-dose sulfisoxazole vs trimethoprim-sulfamethoxazole. *JAMA* 247:1839–1842, 1982.

Freedman LR: Natural history of urinary infection in adults. *Kidney Int* 8:96–100, 1975.

Gillenwater JY, Harrison RB, Kunin CM: Natural history of bacteriuria in schoolgirls: A long-term case-control study. *N Engl J Med* 301:396–399, 1979.

Gleckman RA: Recurrent urinary tract infections. Therapeutic considerations. *Postgrad Med* 65:156–159, 1979.

Hodgson NB, Walsh JP: The management of urinary tract infections. *Surg Clin North Am* 55:1397–1401, 1975.

Komaroff AL, Pass TM, McCue JD, et al: Management strategies for urinary and vaginal infections. *Arch Intern Med* 138:1069–1073, 1978.

Kunin CM: Duration of treatment of urinary tract infections. *Am J Med* 71:849–854, 1981.

Kunin CM: Sexual intercourse and urinary tract infections. *N Engl J Med* 298:336–337, 1978.

Marshall JR, Judd GE: Guide for the management of women with symptoms arising in the lower urinary tract. *Clin Obstet Gynecol* 19:247–258, 1976.

McGuckin M, Cohen L, MacGregor RR, et al: Significance of pyuria in urinary sediment. *J Urol* 120:452–454, 1978.

Medical Research Council Bacteriuria Committee: Recommended terminology of urinary tract infection. *Br Med J* 717–719, September 1979.

Musher DM, Thorsteinsson SB, Airola VM II: Quantitative urinalysis. Diagnosing urinary tract infection in men. *JAMA* 236:2069–2072, 1976.

Rees DL: Urinary tract infections. *Clin Obstet Gynecol* 5:169–192, 1978.

Riff LJ: Evaluation and treatment of urinary infection. *Med Clin North Am* 62:1183–1199, 1978.

Rubenstein L, Mates S, Sidel VW: Quality of care assessment by process and outcome scoring. *Ann Intern Med* 86:617–625, 1977.

Seddon JM, Bruce AW: Cystourethritis. *Urology* 11:1–10, 1978.

Stamm WE, et al: Causes of the acute urethral syndrome in women. *N Engl J Med* 103:409–415, 1980.

Turck M: Therapeutic guidelines in the management of urinary tract infection. *Urol Clin North Am* 2:443–450, 1975.

CHAPTER 71
MALE GENITAL
PROBLEMS

Anthony J. Thomas Jr.

One of the most anxiety provoking medical problems presenting to an emergency department is the male with acute genital pain. The extensive sensory nerve supply to this area accounts for the severe symptoms even with relatively minor problems.

ANATOMY

Penis. The penis is composed of three cylindrical bodies: the two corpora cavernosa, which form the main bulk of the penis, and the corpus spongiosum, which surrounds the urethra (Fig. 71-1). The corpora cavernosa are the major erectile bodies, extending from the pubic rami and distally capped by the glans penis. These two cylindrical structures are encased in a thick tunic of dense connective tissue, the tunica albuginea. All three cylinders are collectively covered by a thinner Buck's fascia, which fuses with Colles' fascia at the level of the urogenital diaphragm.

The blood supply of the penis is primarily from the internal pudendal artery that branches to form the deep and superficial penile arteries. Lymphatic drainage is by the deep and superficial inguinal nodes.

Scrotum. The scrotal skin is thin, and the inner surface is lined with elastic and smooth muscles called the dartos tissue (Fig. 71-2). This layer is continuous with the superficial fascia of the abdomen and groin, while the areolar tissue deep to it continues as Colles' fascia.

The blood supply to the scrotum is primarily derived from branches of the femoral and internal pudendal arteries. Lymphatics from the scrotum drain into the inguinal and femoral nodes.

Testes. The testes usually lie in an upright manner with the superior portion tipped slightly forward and outward. The average size is between 4 and 5 cm in length and approximately 3 cm in width and depth. The overall volume is about 25 cm³. The testes are encased in a thick, fibrous tunica albuginea, and each rests within a separate tunica vaginalis. Between the tunica albuginea and the tunica vaginalis there is usually a small amount of fluid which acts as a cushion or buffer for the testes. With trauma or inflammation the fluid content may increase, resulting in a hydro-

cele. The testes are usually anchored to the posterior wall of the tunica vaginalis by a thin fibrous tissue, or mesorchium. Attachment to the scrotum is by the scrotal ligament, or gubernaculum. A lack of proper development of the mesorchium may result in a horizontal lie of the testes, predisposing them to torsion.

The blood supply to the testicles is by the internal spermatic, deferential, and external spermatic arteries. Venous return is primarily by the internal spermatic, epigastric, internal circumflex, and scrotal veins. The lymphatics drain toward the external, common iliac, and finally periaortic nodes.

The epididymis is a single fine tubular structure approximately 4 to 5 m long compressed into an area of about 5 cm. It is primarily of wolffian duct origin, with the efferent ducts at the head of the epididymis formed from portions of the mesonephros. The function of the epididymis is to allow sperm to mature and gain the ability to move.

Vestigial embryonic structures are often associated with the testes and epididymis. The appendix epididymis, a remnant of the epigentalis, is found attached to the globus major, or head of the epididymis. The appendix testis, a pear-shaped structure, is usually situated on the uppermost portion of the testis at the junction of the testicle and the globus major. The appendix testis is of müllerian duct origin, and neither it nor the appendix epididymis serves any known function in man, although oftentimes excruciating pain is caused by the torsion of one of them.

The vas deferens, a prominent portion of the adnexa of the scrotal contents, is a distinct muscular tube which should be easily palpable within the scrotal sac. It is of wolffian duct origin and extends cephalad from the tail of the epididymis, traversing the inguinal canal and crossing medially behind the bladder over the ureters to form the ampullae of the vas, where it joins with the seminal vesicles. These extend through the prostate as the paired ejaculatory ducts.

Prostate. The prostate begins its development from the urogenital sinus at approximately the third month of embryonic life. It continues to grow and in the young adult is approximately 10 to 15 g. As a man ages, the prostate may enlarge dramatically, causing significant obstruction of urinary outflow. The gland is

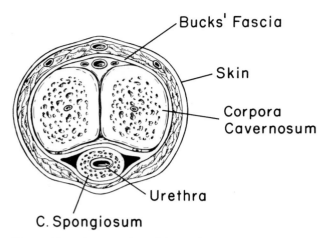

Figure 71-1. Cross section of the penis.

situated around the urethra between the bladder neck and the urogenital diaphragm. Positioned just anterior to the rectal ampulla, it offers itself to easy examination of its most posterior portion.

PHYSICAL EXAMINATION

The physical examination of the male genitalia should be carried out in a well-lighted and relatively warm room. If the patient is exposed to a colder atmosphere, the testes naturally draw up toward the perineum, making the examination more difficult. If the scrotum is drawn up tightly despite proper room temperature, a warm towel placed over the genitalia allows the scrotum and testes to descend and be comfortably examined.

Examination of the testes with the patient in an upright position determines if they are aligned along a vertical or a horizontal axis. Horizontally aligned testes may be more prone to torsion because of the lack of development of the mesorchium, the connective tissue which adheres the posterior portion of the testicle to the tunica vaginalis. Actual palpation of the testes should be performed with the patient in the supine position to prevent the occasional occurrence of a vasovagal response with hypotension, bradycardia and even syncope. A supine patient is more relaxed, and a careful bimanual examination of each testis, epididymis, and adnexa can be carried out.

The epididymis usually lies on the posterior aspect of the testis

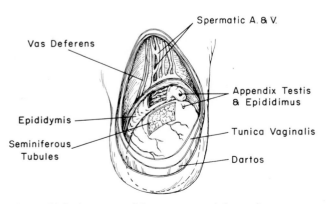

Figure 71-2. Anatomy of the scrotum and the testis.

and, if not inflamed or involved with other pathologic entities, has a soft fleshy feel similar to that of the earlobe.

The prostate can be properly examined with the patient in a number of positions. A modified knee-chest position or even the lithotomy position allows the examiner to more fully appreciate any abnormalities of the prostate and seminal vesicles.

When the prostate is palpated by rectal examination, it normally has a heart-shaped contour with its apex more distal, abutting the urogenital diaphragm. Normally the posterior lobe is quite small and thin, allowing palpation of the median raphe which distinguishes the two lateral lobes. The seminal vesicles, lying just superior to the prostate, cannot normally be distinguished unless there is inflammation, induration, or enlargement, which would suggest pathologic changes requiring further investigation.

A common analogy used to describe the consistency of a prostate is that normal tissue has the same resiliency as the cartilaginous tip of the nose, while areas in which one should suspect carcinoma feel more like the bony prominence of the chin.

It should be remembered that abdominal and genital examinations are closely linked in the male and some primarily abdominal problems may present as acute genital pain. Genital problems such as testicular torsion may present initially with lower abdominal discomfort.

EXAMINATION OF THE URINE

The accuracy of the information obtained from urinalysis is directly proportional to the technique used to collect the specimen. Although the first voided specimen in the morning is probably the best specimen to examine, as it relates to concentration and acidity as well as an overnight collection of urinary sediment, early-morning samples are often not practical and in an emergency room situation are usually irrelevant.

The uncircumcised male patient is advised to retract the foreskin and wash the glans with plain tap water. If hematuria or dysuria is reported, comparing the sediment and culture from a "three-cup specimen" may aid in detecting the location of the pathologic condition (Fig. 71-3).

The first 10 to 15 mL of voided urine represents the washout of the urethra and is voided into the first cup. Next, approximately 100 mL is voided and discarded, and a second container is used to collect the next 15 mL, representing urine from the bladder or kidneys. The patient is asked to retain some urine in the bladder just before the completion of voiding. The prostate is then massaged by rectal examination, with the examining finger moving from the lateral portion of the prostate to the medial aspect on both sides. A final 15 mL of urine is collected in a third cup, and this represents prostatic secretions. If urethritis exists, pyuria is present only in the first specimen. If prostatitis is present, the third cup shows pus cells, while if the bladder and/or kidneys are affected, all three cups contain white cells and bacteria.

COMMON PATHOLOGIC ENTITIES INVOLVING THE MALE GENITALIA

Scrotum. Because of the scrotal skin's loose, elastic capability, rather dramatic enlargement of the scrotum may occur secondary to either scrotal or testicular pathologic conditions.

Simple edema of the scrotal tissues may be present secondary to generalized anasarca, in severe cases of fluid overload, in hy-

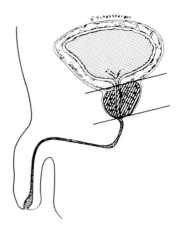

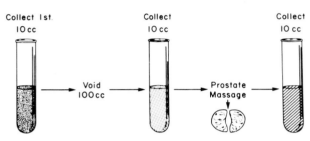

Figure 71-3. Three-cup urine collection used to establish the source of urinary tract infection.

poalbuminemia, or with congestive heart failure. Usually the lower extremities are also markedly edematous.

An acutely swollen, edematous scrotum with no demonstrable urinary problems is often a presenting sign of Fournier's gangrene, or idiopathic gangrene of the scrotum. This condition is usually acute in onset and is life-threatening if not cared for promptly. If the condition is seen in its later stages, the scrotal tissue may be obviously gangrenous (Fig. 71-4). The patient usually appears toxic, acutely ill. Subcutaneous emphysema may be present in the scrotum, thus making the scrotum crepitant to the touch. A roentgenogram of the scrotal area will confirm the presence of gas from gas-forming organisms in the tissue.

The cause may be a traumatic abrasion or scratch that allows the entrance of anaerobic streptococci beneath the skin, though a variety of other organisms have also been isolated from gangrenous scrotal tissue. This condition more commonly exists in men who are, for one reason or another, immunosuppressed, whether through self-induced immunosuppression such as chronic alcoholism or drug addiction, or from diabetes mellitus, or by iatrogenic immunosuppression due to steroid therapy.

Recognition and treatment should be rapid, and a combination of antibiotics such as penicillin, clindamycin, and an aminoglycoside are recommended along with immediate debridement of necrotic tissue once the patient is stabilized.

The physical findings of a urethral phlegmon are similar to those of Fournier's gangrene, but the patient also complains of marked urinary symptoms, usually retention or overflow incontinence. A phlegmon arises from the extravasation of urine through the urethra due to either stricture or trauma. The urine is usually infected and can cause acute necrosis of the skin; characteristically the necrosis does not go below the inguinal folds of the thigh but can extend upward even as far as the chest.

Again recognition and treatment must be prompt and consist of

the same broad-spectrum antibiotics, urinary diversion via cystotomy, and excision and drainage of the necrotic tissue.

Other acute problems of the scrotal skin may present themselves to the emergency room. Simple abscesses, particularly more common in diabetic men, should be dealt with as one would with an abscess in any other area of the body. Careful examination before definitive incision and drainage is necessary to be certain that the abscess involves only the skin and is not contiguous with the testes or epididymis, which may occur from chronic infections such as tuberculosis or bacterial epididymitis. This latter problem may require more extensive surgery, including orchiectomy.

Penis. Acute problems presenting to a busy emergency room regarding the penis are usually due to either trauma or inflammation. Infection and inflammation of the genitalia, especially sexually transmitted diseases, are discussed in Chapter 109. Balanitis, or balanoposthitis, is an inflammation of the foreskin. When the foreskin is retracted, the glans and inner prepuce appear purulent, excoriated, malodorous, and tender. This condition is common in the diabetic male and should suggest the diagnosis of diabetes in an otherwise asymptomatic patient. Treatment is aimed at cleansing the area with mild soap, application of antibiotic ointment, and circumcision when the inflammation has subsided.

Phimosis is a condition in which the foreskin cannot be retracted behind the glans. Infection, poor hygiene, or previous injury to the foreskin with subsequent scarring is often sufficient to cause this problem. If severe enough, scarring at the tip of the foreskin may result in total occlusion by the foreskin and the inability to void. Circumcision represents the definitive treatment for this problem. If urinary retention occurs, a rare problem, the tip of a hemostat can be gently inserted into the scarred end of the foreskin and gently opened, allowing the patient to void satisfactorily until elective circumcision can take place.

Paraphimosis is a condition which exists when the tight foreskin has retracted behind the glans and cannot be advanced over the glans to its natural position (Fig. 71-5). Edema of the glans occurs, and because of venous compression by the tight ring of skin, the glans may have a bluish appearance. Further progression without relief of this constricting band may lead to arterial compromise and gangrenous changes.

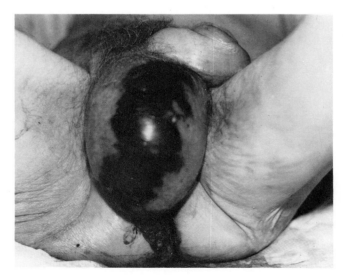

Figure 71-4. A patient with idiopathic gangrene of the scrotum. Note the sharp demarcation of gangrenous changes and the marked edema of the scrotum and the penis.

Phimosis

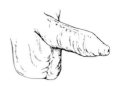

Paraphimosis

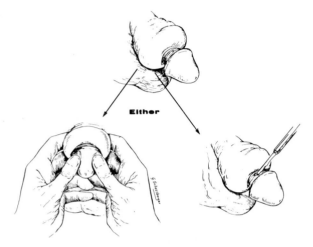

Either

Figure 71-5. Phimosis and paraphimosis. (The lower figure depicts the method of reduction.)

Paraphimosis represents a true urologic emergency, though certainly not life-threatening. If the edema in the surrounding tissue can be gently compressed, the foreskin may be pulled forward as demonstrated in Figure 71-5. If this condition is long-standing, present for a few days before being seen by a physician, the tight preputial ring should be gently washed with an antiseptic solution and infiltrated dorsally in the midline with approximately 1 mL of lidocaine (Xylocaine). The physician makes a superficial incision in this ring behind the glans, being careful not to cut below skin level. This immediately relaxes the foreskin and allows it to be drawn over the glans. Definitive circumcision can usually be done within 24 h after this maneuver.

Entrapment injuries. Various objects can be placed around the penis, causing occlusion of the venous and possibly the arterial blood supply. String, metal rings, and wire have been found wrapped around the penis for sexual, experimental, or accidental reasons. One of the most insidious objects found wrapped behind the coronal ridge is human hair (Fig. 71-6). This problematic condition is usually found in young circumcised boys aged 2 to 5 years. The child has marked swelling of the glans, and the offending hair may be all but invisible within a groove just behind the glans within the coronal sulcus. If the hair has been present long enough, the urethra may be partially or completely transected. The nerve supply on the dorsum of the penis may be interrupted as the partial amputation occurs. It is, therefore, vitally important to recognize this problem early before significant damage is done. Removal of the offending object often requires a certain degree of ingenuity and great care. The patient should not be sent home until the constricting object is removed and adequate delineation of the degree of injury is made.

Fracture of the penis. An acute tear or rupture of the tunica albuginea surrounding the corpora cavernosa is a rare but easily diagnosed lesion that should be immediately recognized so that appropriate therapy can be administered. The patient presents with an acutely swollen, tender penis, with blood discoloring the subcutaneous tissue. The history is usually one of trauma during intercourse or other sexual activity, and the patient describes a sudden "snapping sound" which heralds the fracture. Rarely, the urethra may also be injured along with the cavernous bodies. More commonly, only one of the cavernous bodies is injured, and treatment is aimed at evacuation of the hematoma and oversewing of the tunica albuginea.

Peyronie's disease. Peyronie's disease is not a urologic emergency, though the emergency physician should recognize the thickened plaque involving the tunica albuginea of the corporeal bodies and also the characteristic history of penile curvature with erection. If the condition is found on routine genital examination and the patient is concerned or bothered by the curvature, appropriate referral may be made.

Carcinoma. Carcinoma of the penis is a relatively rare disease estimated to occur in approximately 1 out of every 100,000 malignancies reported. It usually appears in the fifth or sixth decade of life in a man uncircumcised in infancy. There may be a nontender ulcer or warty growth beneath the foreskin on the glans penis. It is often hidden by an inflamed or tight foreskin and is therefore neglected. Thus in examining the uncircumcised male, it is important to retract the foreskin and examine the entire glans. Definitive diagnosis is made by biopsy.

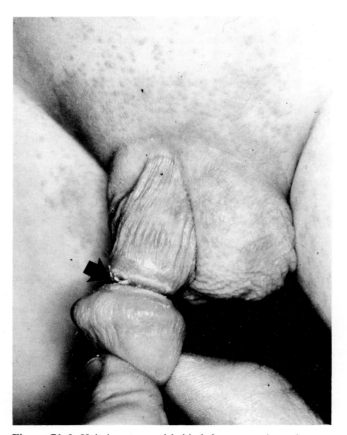

Figure 71-6. Hair is entrapped behind the corona (arrow), constricting and progressively amputating the glans.

Priapism. Priapism is a painful, pathologic erection in which the corpora cavernosa are engorged with stagnant blood. The glans penis and the remainder of the corpus spongiosum are soft and not involved in the erection.

The causes of this condition are multiple. It is often associated with sickle cell disease, sickle trait, high spinal cord injuries, leukemia, and drugs such as the phenothiazines. Much of the time, no specific cause is found. The diagnosis is easily made by observation and palpation of the hard, tender penile shaft and normal glans. Urinary retention may occur.

Treatment is directed at draining the stagnant blood by either irrigation with large-bore needles directed into the cavernous bodies or the creation of a shunt between the corpus spongiosum and the corpus cavernosum. This condition represents a true urologic emergency in that early treatment *may* prevent secondary fibrosis within the corpora that would result in impotence. If a patient with priapism presents to an emergency room, immediate treatment is primarily aimed at preparation for surgery.

Rarely do sedation or other medical treatments effectively alleviate the problem. Urgent urologic consultation should be sought.

Testes. Torsion of a testicle may occur at any age from before birth to and including the seventh decade of life. Most commonly, torsion occurs in the preadolescent, and unless the diagnosis is suspected and acted upon without delay, the salvage of a viable testis is unlikely.

Torsion of the spermatic cord results from a maldevelopment of the normal mesorchial attachments between the testicle and the tunica vaginalis. Characteristically, the testis prone to torsion tends to be aligned along a horizontal rather than a vertical axis (Fig. 71-7). This can only be determined with the patient in an upright position. It is not uncommon for the patient to give a history of engaging in strenuous physical activity or athletic events just before the torsion. It should also be noted that some young men experience intermittent torsion of the testis and are brought to the emergency room with a history of acute onset of testicular pain with sudden and dramatic spontaneous relief. Examination at that time reveals a relatively normal appearing testis, and in the absence of any inflammatory signs, the diagnosis of intermittent torsion and detorsion should be entertained, and the patient should be advised to seek urgent urologic consultation for possible orchiopexy.

It is imperative to think of testicular torsion as a true urologic emergency when a male has an acute onset of testicular pain and swelling. The pain may be sudden and severe and may initially be felt in the lower quadrant of the abdomen or in the testis itself. It takes only a few hours for rather startling swelling to occur. There is usually no associated fever, and the urinalysis is normal.

Emergency treatment is directed at preparing the patient for immediate testicular exploration, detorsion, and bilateral orchiopexy. It is not uncommon that younger boys present only after a delayed time because of embarrassment or other factors. If the testis can be detorsed within a period of 4 h from the onset of torsion, the chances of testicular viability are greatly improved. Certainly after 24 h, if the blood supply has been completely blocked because of a rotation of more than 360-degrees, it is unlikely that the testis can be salvaged. Regardless of the time factors, exploration should be performed without delay to confirm the diagnosis, and a contralateral orchiopexy should be performed, thereby saving the remaining testis from a similar fate. Recent evidence has shown that if the affected testis is significantly damaged, detorsed, and allowed to stay in the scrotal sac, there may be a significant impairment of fertility in the contralateral testicle.

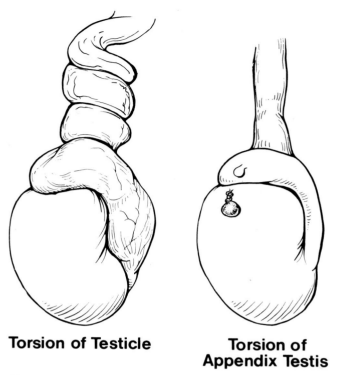

Torsion of Testicle   **Torsion of Appendix Testis**

Figure 71-7. Diagrams of testicular torsion and torsion of the appendix testis.

Differential diagnosis rests between testicular torsion, acute epididymitis, and torsion of the appendix testis or the epididymis. A Doppler stethoscope, if available, may be helpful in the differential diagnosis; the tip of the stethoscope is placed over the involved testis and the physician listens for the presence or absence of arterial pulsations. The contralateral side serves as the control. Hearing pulsations on the affected side is not an absolute indication that torsion has not occurred, as edema and erythema of the scrotal skin may produce sufficient increase in blood flow around the testis that this flow can be mistaken for testicular perfusion.

Another useful diagnostic procedure is the technetium testicular scan. Images of the scrotal sac area are obtained every 3 s for 60 s and then at 2-, 4-, and 6-min intervals. Decreased or absent uptake on the affected side, compared with the opposite side, is compatible with torsion (Fig. 71-8).

Though both Doppler examination and radioisotope scanning are useful, false positives and false negatives can occur, delaying the diagnosis and ultimate salvageability of the testis. Clinical judgment must be used in dealing with this problem, and if the diagnosis of testicular torsion cannot be absolutely ruled out, exploration is mandated.

Torsion of the appendices. The appendices of the epididymis and testis have no known physiologic function. The pedunculated structures are, however, capable of torsion and may cause pain and swelling similar to those of testicular torsion. If the patient is seen early in the acute event, the pain is most intense near the head of the epididymis or testes, and an isolated tender nodule can be palpated. When the testis is brought close to the skin, a blue reflection may be seen on the scrotal skin when light shines upon it. This ''blue dot sign'' is pathognomonic of torsion of the appendix testis or epididymis. If the diagnosis can be absolutely

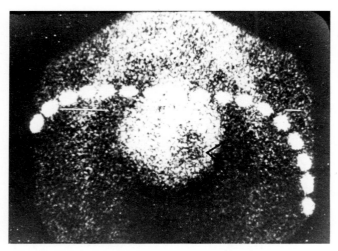

Figure 71-8. A testicular scan. The arrow points to the side of diminished activity indicating ischemia. In this case, testicular torsion was present.

ensured, immediate surgery is not necessary, as most of these appendices either calcify or degenerate and cause no harm to the patient. If the patient is seen later in the course of the acute episode, marked unilateral swelling may be present, and it may be impossible to differentiate the exact cause of the pain. Here again, experience dictates whether exploration needs to be carried out.

Epididymitis. Epididymitis or epididymal orchitis is most commonly due to a bacterial infection. The onset of pain is usually more gradual than that with torsion, and symptoms of urethritis, prostatitis, or cystitis may be present. This inflammation tends to occur in the young adult rather than in the adolescent. Fever may be present and the white blood cell count elevated. Urinalysis and careful examination of the prostate should disclose evidence of inflammation and/or infection.

Testicular scanning in the presence of epididymal orchitis usually reveals an increased uptake of the radioisotope in comparison with the nonaffected testicle.

Treatment of this condition is directed toward the specific bacterial infection. After adequate cultures are obtained, a broad-spectrum antibiotic such as tetracycline or ampicillin is given. Follow-up with medical and/or urologic consultation is imperative to ascertain whether all inflammatory changes have disappeared. Occasionally, a testicular tumor is present and an acute bleed into the tumor occurs, giving the patient some symptoms compatible with epididymitis. To simply treat this as an infection and disregard the follow-up may lead to a marked delay in the correct diagnosis and diminish the young man's chance of cure.

If epididymitis is present and the patient appears febrile and toxic, hospitalization and treatment of the infection with intravenous antibiotics is indicated. If the patient is not acutely ill and it is felt that he could do well at home, appropriate analgesics, antibiotics, and local treatment with ice pack and later sitz baths are quite effective in alleviating the symptoms. Dramatic improvement should occur within a couple of days.

Orchitis. Orchitis, or inflammation of the testicle, may occur in conjunction with other systemic diseases such as mumps or other viral illnesses. Orchitis usually presents as bilateral testicular tenderness and swelling over a few days' duration. A close examination of other systems often reveals the source of the orchitis.

Testicular malignancy. Any patient who presents with testicular swelling could possibly have a malignant tumor, and this diagnosis must always be borne in mind. A delay in diagnosis may allow the tumor to metastasize, lessening an otherwise relatively good outlook.

With the exception of a few rare tumors, most neoplastic growths of the testicle are malignant. They are uncommon, though not unheard of, in childhood and are relatively rare in the black population.

Pain is the presenting symptom in about 10 percent of these tumors. It is probably secondary to hemorrhage within the testis. Most tumors are painless, and the presenting sign is simply a large, often firm and irregular, testicle.

Some of these tumors produce large quantities of gonadotropins, and gynecomastia may be evident. If the periaortic lymph nodes are involved and enlarged, they may well be palpable in a thin patient. A chest roentgenogram may reveal the presence of metastatic disease.

In general, any testicular mass that cannot be specifically identified is a tumor until proved otherwise, and surgical exploration through an inguinal incision is indicated.

URETHRAL STRICTURE

Strictures, or narrowed areas, within the urethra may occur for a variety of reasons (Fig. 71-9). Postgonococcal strictures are more common in the older man, while younger men may develop strictures as a result of external trauma to the perineum or previous urethral instrumentation. The management of stricture disease is well beyond the scope of this chapter; however, patients with strictures and urinary retention may come to an emergency department, and if urologic consultation is not available within a reasonable period of time, some relief must be offered to them.

The passage of urethral sounds or filiforms and followers by a nonurologist should be discouraged, as untold damage to the genitalia may result from the injudicious use of these instruments by inexperienced persons.

If a male patient presents himself in urinary retention and a catheter cannot be easily placed through the urethra, then the possibility that a stricture is present must be considered. It is often important to diagnose the exact area of the stricture as well as its most proximal and most distal points. This information is easily obtained from a retrograde urethrogram.

The patient is placed on an x-ray table in a slightly oblique position with the lower leg in a flexed position and the upper leg straight. A plain film of the pelvis incorporating the urethra and scrotal area is then taken. The glans is washed with an antiseptic solution, and the tip of a sterile bulb syringe with approximately 20 to 30 mL of contrast material diluted with normal saline is placed just within the urethral meatus. With the physician's hand holding the penis on stretch, an x-ray exposure is taken while the contrast material is being *gently* injected into the meatus. This film delineates the exact area of the stricture and allows a more thorough understanding of the cause of the retention.

If a stricture is found, a 10 French or 12 French coudé catheter may be able to be maneuvered through the narrowed area into the bladder since this catheter has an angled bend near its beak. Occasionally there are false passages from previous attempts at dilatation or previous instrumentation, thus making the passage of a catheter almost impossible. Further manipulation of the urethra by catheter insertion may make these false passages worse and

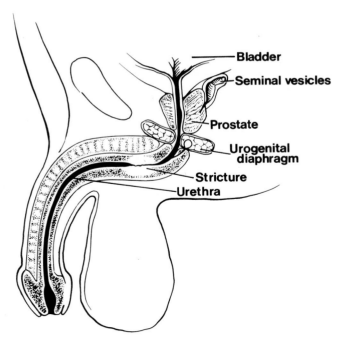

Figure 71-9. Stricture of the bulbous urethra.

could lead to unnecessary hemorrhage and possible sepsis, since many of these patients are infected. If two or three gentle attempts to pass a catheter fail, it is prudent to consult a urologist on an emergency basis before the urethra is severely traumatized. Suprapubic trocar cystotomy sets are available, but their use should be restricted to those specially trained in the procedure.

URETHRAL FOREIGN BODIES

Patients of any age, and especially young children, may present with a variety of foreign bodies lodged in the urethra and/or the bladder. These objects, ranging anywhere from bobby pins to ballpoint pens, usually require removal by cystoscopic manipulation or even open cystotomy. These patients require admission to a hospital, and antibiotic therapy, since most of them have infection caused by the foreign body. Bloody urine combined with infection and stranguria should alert the physician to the possible presence of a foreign body in the urinary tract. Often an x-ray of the bladder area discloses the source of these symptoms (Fig. 71-10).

URINARY RETENTION

Symptoms such as severe lower abdominal pain with an urgent need to void and a history of an inability to urinate for 6 to 8 h combined with a palpable lower abdominal mass most certainly suggest urinary outlet obstruction. The most common cause of outlet obstruction is benign prostatic hypertrophy. A past history of hesitancy, poor urinary stream, and nocturia can usually be elicited. A previous history of pelvic trauma or venereal disease suggests the possibility of a urethral stricture as the cause of retention.

Some drugs used commonly for symptomatic upper respiratory tract infections (ephedrine sulfate, phenylpropanolamine, antihis-

tamines, etc.) may cause urinary retention because of their sympathomimetic effect on the bladder neck. Discontinuing these drugs and alleviating the temporary problem of retention may return the patient to his normal voiding habits.

Most patients with bladder outlet obstruction are in distress. Some are not aware that the bladder is distended when there is a neurogenic component such as that found in some paraplegics, patients with diabetic neuropathies, and others with various neurologic disorders.

The passage of a urethral catheter alleviates the retention. If a patient is tense, the external sphincter may be contracted, giving the false impression that a stricture is present. Having the patient relax and breathe in and out through his mouth prevents this muscle from contracting and facilitates the passage of the catheter into the bladder.

The drainage of a distended bladder can be accomplished quickly without the need for repeated clamping of the catheter. Occasionally, when a bladder has been fully distended and rapidly drained, bladder mucosal edema develops and terminal hematuria occurs. This is usually self-limited.

The emergency room physician is often tempted to drain the distended bladder and then remove the catheter. However, the inability to void is likely to persist, and because of this, the catheter should be left in place. If retention has been chronic, a postobstructive diuresis may occur, demanding close attention to urine output and appropriate fluid replacement either by mouth or by an intravenous route. These patients require hospitalization, though it is prudent to observe the patient in the emergency department from the time the catheter is placed, accurately monitoring the intake and output. Occasionally, if not properly fluid-balanced, some patients tend to become hypovolemic and hypotensive with rather alarming speed. Replacement with appropriate electrolyte solutions matching intake with output plus insensible loss allows the kidneys to recompensate and the diuresis to dissipate within 24 to 48 h. If infection and retention are present, appropriate culture is necessary and immediate treatment with antibiotics recommended.

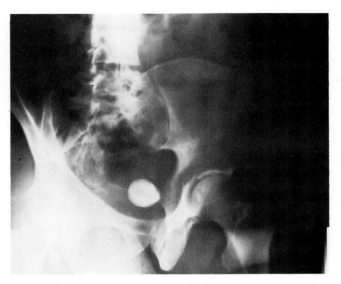

Figure 71-10. X-ray of the pelvis of a 32-year-old man who had passed a small lead pencil through the urethra into the bladder. Note the calcification around the pencil.

BIBLIOGRAPHY

Arya OP, Alergant CD, Annels EM, et al: Management of nonspecific urethritis in men. Evaluation of six treatment regimens and the effect of other factors including alcohol and sexual intercourse. *Br J Vener Dis* 54:414–420, 1978.

Birkhoff Wiederhorn AR, Hamilton ML, et al: Natural history of benign prostatic hypertrophy and acute urinary retention. *Urology* 7:48–52, 1976.

Blandy J: Emergency situations: Acute retention of urine. *Br J Hosp Med* 19:109–111, 1978.

Butler MR, Donnelly B, Komakanchat A: Intravenous urography in evaluation of acute retention. *Urology* 12:464–466, 1978.

Chambers RM, Baitera B: The anatomy of the urethral stricture. *Br J Urol* 49:545–551, 1977.

Doran J, Roberts M: Acute urinary retention in the female. *Br J Urol* 47:793–796, 1975.

Hahn LC, Nadel NS, Gittes H, et al: Testicular scanning: A new modality for the preoperative diagnosis of testicular torsion. *J Urol* 113:60–62, 1975.

Hinman F: Priapism: Reasons for failure of therapy. *J Urol* 83:420–424, 1960.

Hoffman LM, Suki WN: Obstructive uropathy mimicking volume depletion. *JAMA* 236:2096–2097, 1976.

Howe GE, Prentiss RJ, Cole JW, et al: Priapism: A surgical emergency. *J Urol* 101:576–579, 1969.

Jones P: Torsion of the testis and its appendages during childhood. *Arch Dis Child* 37:214–226, 1962.

Levy B: The diagnosis of torsion of the testicle using the Doppler ultrasonic stethoscope. *J Urol* 113:63–65, 1975.

Lewis-Jones DI, DeMarval MM, and Harrison RG: Impairment of rat spermatogenesis following unilateral experimental ischemia. *Fertil Steril* 38:482–490, 1982.

Mastrogiacomo I, Zanchetta R, Graziotti P, et al: Immunological and clinical study in patients after spermatic cord torsion. *Andrologia* 14:25–30, 1982.

Meares EM, Stamey TA: Bacteriologic localization patterns in bacterial prostatitis in urethritis. *Invest Urol* 5:492–518, 1968.

Skoglund RW, McRoberts JW, Ragde H: Torsion of the spermatic cord: A review of the literature and an analysis of 70 new cases. *J Urol* 104:604–607, 1970.

SECTION 8
GYNECOLOGY AND
OBSTETRICS

CHAPTER 72
GYNECOLOGIC
EMERGENCIES

Robert S. Hockberger

This section discusses the extremely common problem of vulvo-vaginitis, the increasingly important problems of pelvic inflammatory disease, the uncommon but serious problem of acute adnexal torsion, and an approach to evaluating the patient with abnormal vaginal bleeding. The goal is to enable the emergency physician to make a preliminary diagnosis, to provide adequate emergency care, and to either resolve the problem or ensure that the patient's well-being is maintained until a consultant can assume her care.

VULVOVAGINITIS

Vulvovaginitis is an inflammation of the external genitalia and/or vagina which is usually, but not always, secondary to infection with pathogenic microorganisms. The most common causes of vulvovaginitis are *Trichomonas, Candida albicans,* and *Gardnerella vaginalis.* Other important causes of inflammation include *Chlamydia trachomatis,* contact vulvovaginitis, and reaction to the presence of a foreign body.

Trichomonas Vaginitis

The incidence of *Trichomonas* vaginitis is approximately 2.5 million cases annually. The following points regarding *Trichomonas* infection are of clinical importance: (1) it causes cervical erosions which may predispose to malignant transformation, and it also causes cellular atypia which makes the cytologic findings difficult to interpret; (2) it is a sexually transmitted disease which causes prostatitis in approximately 40 percent of the males infected; (3) it inhibits spermatozoal motility and is therefore an occasional cause of male sterility; and (4) pregnant women who have *Trichomonas* infection at the time of delivery experience a twofold increase in the incidence of postpartum endometritis. Although transmission usually occurs during sexual intercourse, *Trichomonas* can survive for hours on wet sponges or towels, and for up to 24 h in urine (on toilet seats).

Patients complain of a gray to green malodorous discharge and mild pruritis, usually during or immediately following menses. Twenty percent of the patients have dysuria, and up to 10 percent of the patients complain of lower abdominal pain. On physical examination, only 20 percent of the patients are found to have a classic "strawberry" vagina secondary to diffuse punctate hemorrhages, but 80 percent exhibit diffuse erythema of the vaginal vault.

Diagnosis is made through use of the "hanging drop" slide test: a swab is taken from the vaginal vault (not the endocervix) and is placed within a drop of normal saline on a glass slide. Microscopic examination reveals motile, pear-shaped organisms slightly larger than white blood cells; the organisms contain flagella and undulating membranes.

Treatment in the nonpregnant patient is best accomplished by a single 2-g dose of metronidazole (Flagyl). Longer courses are more expensive, result in poor compliance, and are no more effective. Since metronidazole is an acetaldehyde dehydrogenase inhibitor, concomitant alcohol ingestion may precipitate an Antabuse-like reaction. Thus alcohol should be avoided within 24 h of metronidazole ingestion. Up to 80 percent of infected males are asymptomatic; thus all male consorts should be referred for therapy. Failure of the asymptomatic male partners to seek treatment is probably responsible for the high recurrence rate of this infection.

Metronidazole is also a folic acid inhibitor and therefore is not recommended for use in the first trimester of pregnancy. Clotrimazole vaginal suppositories (qhs for 7 days) is 70 percent effective in such instances and should be used when symptoms are severe.

Candida Vaginitis

Candida albicans is present as part of the normal vaginal flora in 25 to 50 percent of healthy asymptomatic women. Other normal vaginal flora such as lactobacilli and corynebacteria feed upon the glycogen in vaginal epithelial cells to produce the normally acidic (pH 3.5 to 4.1) vaginal milieu. Conditions which inhibit the growth of normal vaginal flora, diminish the glycogen stores in vaginal epithelial cells, or increase the pH of vaginal secretions cause colonization of candida and subsequent symptomatic infection. Precipitants of candida infection include the use of antibiotics or birth control pills, diabetes mellitus, pregnancy, the postmenopausal state, and the presence of menstrual blood or semen.

The primary complaint is vaginal pruritus. The discharge is

usually meager, thin, and watery, or may be absent. Patients occasionally complain of dysuria and/or dyspareunia. Physical examination reveals vulvar erythema, edema of the labia, vaginal erythema (20 percent), satellite lesions at hair follicles near the vaginal introitus, and an occasional "cottage cheese" discharge seen most often in pregnant patients.

Diagnosis is made by examining the discharge on a potassium hydroxide slide preparation. A drop of 10% potassium hydroxide is applied to dissolve the epithelial cells, leaving the yeast buds and pseudohyphae intact. The Gram stain, showing gram-positive oval bodies (spores) and gram-positive tubes (pseudohyphae), is a more sensitive test and should be done in all cases of recurrent infection.

Therapy is a vaginal cream or suppository with antifungal activity, e.g., nystatin bid for 14 days, or miconazole qd for 7 days.

Gardnerella Vaginitis

Also termed *Hemophilus* vaginitis, *Corynebacterium* vaginitis, and nonspecific vaginitis, *Gardnerella* vaginitis is caused by a gram-negative aerobic coccobacillus which is normally present in 10 to 40 percent of healthy asymptomatic women. No particular group of women seem to be at high risk for colonization, and it is not well-understood why from 20 to 90 percent of otherwise healthy "carriers" periodically become symptomatic.

Patients complain of mild pruritis and a slight vaginal discharge which has a disagreeable "fishy" odor. The results of the physical examination are usually normal except for mild vaginal erythema (20 percent) and the presence of a thin, frothy, gray-white vaginal discharge.

Pathognomonic clue cells (vaginal epithelial cells with adherent gram-negative rods) are seen in 50 percent of the wet mounts and 90 percent of the Gram stains performed on the vaginal discharge.

Treatment is moderately effective with metronidazole (500 mg bid for 7 days), ampicillin (500 mg qid for 5 days), or cephalexin (Keflex) (500 mg qid for 6 days). Sulfa creams are not effective for treating this type of vaginitis.

Gonococcal Vulvovaginitis

Gonococcal vulvovaginitis is seen only in prepubertal girls and postmenopausal women who possess thin vaginal walls and a higher vaginal pH, which promote gonococcal growth and invasion. The diagnosis is made by observing gram-negative intracellular diplococci on a Gram stain, or through positive culture results. When the condition is present in children, sexual abuse should be considered. Penicillin is the treatment of choice. The adult dosage is 4.8 million units of procaine penicillin intramuscularly accompanied by 1 g of probenecid orally. The pediatric dosage is 100,000 units/kg of aqueous penicillin G intramuscularly plus 25 mg/kg of probenecid orally, or, alternatively, 50 mg/kg of amoxicillin orally plus probenecid.

Cervicitis

Thirty percent of the women presenting with the complaint of vaginal discharge have cervicitis, not vaginitis, as the cause. The common causes of cervicitis are *Trichomonas,* gonococcus, and *Chlamydia trachomatis.* Diagnosis is made by observing normal vulvovaginal tissue and a purulent discharge from the endocervix.

If a Gram stain of the vaginal discharge reveals white blood cells but neither trichomonads nor gonococci, the tentative diagnosis of chlamydia cervicitis may be made. Cultures for gonococcus should be performed and treatment initiated with tetracycline (500 mg qid for 7 days) or doxycycline (100 mg bid for 7 days). Pregnant patients should be treated with a single dose of amoxicillin (3 g) plus probenecid (1 g PO). Treatment of trichomonas or gonococcus infections is as with vaginitis (see above).

Herpes Simplex

Herpes simplex type II vulvovaginitis is rapidly becoming one of the most common of all vulvar infections. Initial infections present with vulvovaginal pain, fever, and generalized malaise. Examination reveals tender inguinal adenopathy and 2- to 4-mm diameter clear fluid vesicles with erythematous bases which rupture to form small ulcers with pale yellow bases and an erythematous edge. The initial attack lasts approximately 3 to 6 weeks. Recurrent infections, which are very common, are less painful, usually have no systemic symptoms and no tender adenopathy, and are of shorter duration. Recurrent infections are probably not reinfections but, rather, reactivations of a virus which is never totally eradicated. Recurrences seem to be precipitated by a variety of physical or emotional stresses.

Diagnosis of herpes is made by seeing classic lesions as described, observing typical multinucleated giant cells with intranuclear inclusions on a Pap smear, or through viral culture results (which take approximately 72 h).

Treatment of herpetic vulvovaginitis is both symptomatic and specific. Symptomatic treatment includes Burrow's solution soaks, sitz baths, bed rest, and analgesics. Specific therapy with acyclovir (Zovirax) should be reserved for first infections in immunosuppressed patients to prevent dissemination of the herpetic infection. The ointment, which is applied every 3 h for 7 days, decreases the healing time, the pain, and the shedding of the virus. It does not, however, prevent recurrences and has negligible effect in the treatment of recurrences. Recent evidence suggests that IV acyclovir may be effective in decreasing the symptoms and viral shedding while shortening the clinical course of the primary infection.

The effects on infants born to women who have or contract herpes during pregnancy are covered in Chapter 74, "Obstetric Emergencies."

Contact Vulvovaginitis

Patients presenting with vulvovaginal pain, erythema, and edema without a vaginal discharge, who have a negative workup for possible causative organisms, may have contact vulvovaginitis. The usual causes include bubble bath, scented toilet tissue, vaginal deodorant sprays, and detergents used on undergarments. Treatment includes eliminating the cause, wet compresses or sitz baths, and topical application of steroid creams.

Foreign Body

Vaginal discharge, odor, and irritation may be caused by a foreign body in the vagina. In a child this may be any object that can be readily inserted into the vaginal orifice. In an adult this is often a forgotten tampon, diaphragm, or occasionally a condom. Treatment includes removal of the foreign body and application of a cleansing solution such as povidone-iodine to the vaginal vault and cervix. The patient is advised to douche daily with this solution and to seek follow-up consultation with a gynecologist to ensure that the local inflammation and irritation have resolved.

PELVIC INFLAMMATORY DISEASE (PID)

Pelvic inflammatory disease (endometritis, salpingitis or parametritis) is usually the result of an ascending bacterial infection following sexual intercourse but may arise de novo following delivery, abortion, or pelvic surgery and may in some instances be related to the presence of an intrauterine device (IUD). Approximately 60 percent of all acute PID is gonococcal-related. Up to 6 percent of the cultures from asymptomatic females show *Neisseria gonorrhoeae* in the endocervical canal, and 10 to 17 percent of these females develop acute PID. Nongonococcal PID, particularly secondary to *Chlamydia trachomatis* infection, is becoming increasingly more common.

It is estimated that approximately 1 million cases of PID were treated in the United States in 1980. The direct and indirect costs to society in that year were estimated at approximately $3 billion.

The classic patient is a sexually active female who presents with several days of progressive lower abdominal pain, often shortly following menses. Fever, chills, malaise, nausea, and vomiting are frequent accompanying symptoms. A history of previous episodes of PID, or the presence of an IUD, should heighten suspicion for this disease. Not all presentations are classic, however, and the possibility of ectopic pregnancy and adnexal torsion should be considered in all women with the complaint of lower abdominal pain.

On physical examination, fever, tachycardia, abdominal distension, and involuntary guarding are often but not universally found. Pelvic examination is often difficult because of patient discomfort. There may be extreme pain on palpation of the uterus, or movement of the cervix. The presence of only minimal pain on cervical motion, however, does not rule out the diagnosis of acute PID. Adnexal tenderness is usually intense bilaterally but may occasionally be greater on one side. The presence of an adnexal mass should raise the possibility of a tubo-ovarian abscess, ectopic pregnancy, or adnexal torsion. Culdocentesis may reveal purulent material.

The complete blood cell count may be normal or may show a marked leukocytosis with a left shift. The erythrocyte sedimentation rate (ESR) is usually elevated. A Gram stain of material from the cervix may reveal typical gram-negative intracellular diplococci. A Gram stain of purulent material obtained from culdocentesis may reveal the causative organism. Both aerobic and anaerobic cultures should be obtained. The yield of positive cultures increases if a sample from the anal canal is cultured at the same time as one from the cervix.

In a study by Jacobson, 905 cases of suspected PID were studied by laparoscopy. In all instances the clinical diagnosis of PID was made by gynecologic attending staff or senior residents. When compared with laparoscopy, their clinical diagnostic accuracy approached only 65 percent. Diseases commonly misdiagnosed as PID included surgical emergencies such as acute appendicitis and ectopic pregnancy. Approximately 20 percent of the patients diagnosed as having PID were found to have no pelvic pathology, were not treated, and in follow-up were found to have no recurrence of symptoms. Therefore, it is extremely important to make

every attempt to justify the diagnosis of PID before commencing antibiotic therapy. Routine culdocentesis and the more liberal use of laparoscopy should improve the diagnostic accuracy.

Outpatient Treatment

Asymptomatic gonorrhea should be treated with 4.8 million units of aqueous procaine penicillin intramuscularly plus 1 g of probenecid orally. An alternative approach consists of 3.5 g of ampicillin orally plus 1 g of probenecid. For patients allergic to penicillin, 500 mg of tetracycline qid for 5 days is recommended. In cases of penicillin-resistant gonococci, 2 g of spectinomycin intramuscularly should be used.

Treatment of *symptomatic* gonorrhea (acute PID) is as previously outlined but should be followed by 500 mg of ampicillin orally qid for 10 days. For patients allergic to penicillin, 500 mg of tetracycline orally qid for 10 days should be given.

If chlamydial infection is suspected, tetracycline, rather than ampicillin, should be given for 10 days in addition to IM penicillin.

Inpatient Treatment

Indications for hospitalizing patients with acute PID include the following: (1) clinical illness [fever over 38.6°C (101.5°F), the presence of peritoneal signs, and the inability to tolerate oral medications or fluids]; (2) pregnancy; (3) a palpable adnexal mass, i.e., suspected tubo-ovarian abscess; (4) uncertain diagnosis; and (5) failure to respond to outpatient management within 24 to 48 h.

Inpatient treatment for acute PID includes 20 million units of aqueous crystalline penicillin G daily until improvement is noted, followed by 500 mg of ampicillin orally to complete a 10-day course of therapy. For penicillin-allergic patients, 250 mg of tetracycline intravenously qid until clinical improvement occurs followed by 500 mg orally qid to complete a 10-day course of therapy is recommended. An aminoglycoside or clindamycin may be added as indicated by the results of a culture or Gram stain. Failure of the patient to respond to adequate antibiotic therapy within 24 to 48 h demands careful reevaluation of the initial diagnosis.

The possible sequelae of acute PID include chronic pelvic pain and the formation of adhesions, with an increased incidence of ectopic pregnancy and infertility.

ADNEXAL TORSION

Torsion of the ovary or fallopian tube is an uncommon but important cause of lower abdominal pain in females. It usually occurs in diseased adnexa (ectopic pregnancy, ovarian cyst or tumor, hydrosalpinx, pyosalpinx, etc.) at a point where a normal (thin) segment of fallopian tube acts as a pedicle about which a diseased (thick) segment twists, cutting off the blood supply to the distal segment, resulting in hemorrhagic necrosis. This disease can affect females from infancy to late adulthood.

The patients present with acute lower abdominal pain located from the flank to the groin, sometimes radiating to the thigh on the involved side. Nausea and vomiting are often present. Patients may have a history of previous episodes of similar symptoms probably caused by intermittent torsion and detorsion.

Physical examination reveals a palpable tender adnexal mass in approximately 80 percent of the patients. Most patients do not have a fever or an elevation in the white blood cell count until late in their disease. Culdocentesis may reveal blood or serosanguinous fluid.

If torsion is left untreated, necrosis of the involved organs can lead to peritonitis and shock. Diagnostic laparoscopy should be used liberally to help in early diagnosis. A strong case can be made that no patient should leave the emergency room with a diagnosis of pelvic inflammatory disease who has unilateral adnexal tenderness, and especially, who is afebrile. Further evaluation and observation including possible laparoscopy may be indicated.

ABNORMAL VAGINAL BLEEDING

The evaluation of abnormal vaginal bleeding may be an extremely complex problem. The endocrine physiology of the menstrual cycle is outlined in Figure 72-1. Conditions which cause abnormally high estrogen levels result in a prolonged proliferative phase and subsequent abnormal uterine bleeding secondary to irregular shedding of the endometrium. Such conditions include polycystic ovary disease, ovarian tumors, increased exogenous estrogen use, obesity, and thyroid or adrenal gland dysfunction. Abnormally low estrogen levels, as is seen with low-dose birth control pills, excessive exercise, and poor diet, can result in premature sloughing of the endometrium (spotting) or amenorrhea. Alterations in progesterone levels shortly after menarche and before menopause may also result in irregularity of the menstrual cycle.

Abnormal vaginal bleeding may also be seen as the result of neoplasms, infections, abnormal pregnancies, and trauma, as well as with metabolic and hematologic problems. Both benign and malignant neoplasms of the external and the internal genital organs may present as vaginal bleeding. Infections including acute ulcerative lesions of the vulva or vagina, acute and chronic cervicitis, venereal diseases, and endometritis may have vaginal bleeding as part of a symptom complex. Abnormalities of pregnancy including abortion, ectopic pregnancy, and trophoblastic disease should be considered. Bleeding may result from the presence of foreign bodies (particularly in children), lacerations from trauma (including sexual intercourse), and the presence of an IUD. Thyroid and adrenal disease, as well as the exogenous use of hormones, may result in abnormal bleeding. Finally, hematologic problems such as blood dyscrasias and anticoagulant use are additional possible causes.

The emergency physician cannot possibly evaluate a patient for all the potential causes of abnormal vaginal bleeding. In all instances, however, a search must be made for all easily identifiable and/or potentially life threatening causes of vaginal bleeding. The following points should be kept in mind:

1. Regardless of the cause of vaginal bleeding, an assessment of the patient's blood volume status should be made in all instances. The duration and magnitude of the bleeding; symptoms of weakness, lethargy, or syncope; and the patient's vital signs should be evaluated in all instances. The patient's hematocrit should be determined in any questionable case.
2. Careful physical examination should eliminate extragenital sources of bleeding such as urinary tract, perineal, and rectal bleeding, which may be misinterpreted by the patient as vaginal bleeding.
3. Examination for evidence of infections, trauma, or the presence of intravaginal foreign bodies should be performed.
4. All women of childbearing age presenting with abnormal vaginal bleeding of unclear cause should be considered to have an ectopic pregnancy until proved otherwise. The evaluation of this life-threatening disorder is discussed in Chapter 74, "Obstetric Emergencies."
5. If the emergency department evaluation of a patient with abnormal vaginal bleeding fails to reveal an easily identifiable and easily remediable cause for the bleeding, the patient should be referred to a gynecologist for evaluation of potential neoplastic, metabolic, or hematologic problems.

The term *dysfunctional uterine bleeding* (DUB) refers to abnormal endometrial bleeding with no apparent organic lesions. From the preceding discussion it is clear that this is a diagnosis which should be seldom, if ever, employed by the emergency physician. The treatment of abnormal vaginal bleeding should be directed at the identified cause of such bleeding. When no cause is found, and when blood loss is assessed as being insignificant, no therapy should be instituted. The patient should be referred to a gynecologist for further evaluation. Premature initiation of cyclic combination birth control pill therapy to "regulate" a patient's menstrual cycle may make further evaluation of the patient by the gynecologist more difficult.

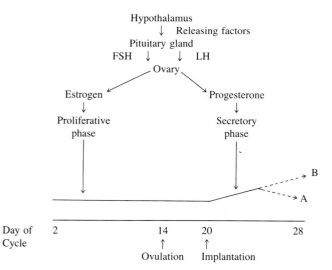

Day of Cycle 2   14   20   28

    ↑ Ovulation   ↑ Implantation

Figure 72-1. The endocrine physiology of the menstrual cycle. (*A*) In the absence of implantation, estrogen and progesterone levels fall, the endometrium sloughs, and the hypothalamus is stimulated to restart the cycle. (*B*) If implantation occurs, the fertilized ovum produces estrogen, progesterone, and HCG, and this causes development of the placenta and inhibits the hypothalamus from starting another cycle.

BIBLIOGRAPHY

Vulvovaginitis

Johannisson G: Genital *Chlamydia trachomatis* infection in women. *Obstet Gynecol* 56:671–675, 1980.

Lossick JG: Single dose metronidazole for treatment of vaginal trichomoneasis. *Obstet Gynecol* 56:508–510, 1980.

Pheifer TA: Nonspecific vaginitis. *N Engl J Med* 298:1429–1434, 1978.

Rein MF: Trichomoniasis, candidiasis, and the minor venereal diseases. *Clin Obstet Gynecol* 18:73–88, 1975.

Treatment of sexually transmitted diseases. *Med Lett* 24:29–34, 1982.

Vaginitis revisited (editorial). *Br Med J* 283:745–746, 1981.

Pelvic Inflammatory Disease (PID)

Jacobson L: Differential diagnosis of acute pelvic inflammatory disease. *Am J Obstet Gynecol* 138:1006–1011, 1980.

Jacobson L: Objectivized diagnosis of acute PID. *Am J Obstet Gynecol* 105:1088–1098, 1969.

Monif GR: Cul-de-sac isolates from patients with endometritis-salpingitis-peritonitis and gonococcal endocervicitis. *Am J Obstet Gynecol* 126:158–161, 1976.

Ory HW: Review of the association between IUD use and acute PID. *J Reprod Med* 20:200–204, 1978.

Sweet RL: Etiology of acute salpingitis: Influence of episode number and duration of symptoms. *Obstet Gynecol* 58:62–68, 1981.

Torsion of the Adnexa

Hockberger RS: Torsion of the fallopian tube. *JACEP* 7:315–317, 1978.

Skoglund RW: Torsion of the spermative cord: A review of the literature. *J Urol* 104:598–601, 1970.

Abnormal Vaginal Bleeding

Goldfarb JM, Little AB: Abnormal Vaginal Bleeding. *N Engl J Med* 302(12):666–669. March 20, 1980.

Reyniak JV: Dysfunctional uterine bleeding. *J Reprod Med* 17:293, 1976.

Shane JM, Haftolin F, Newark SR: Gynecologic endocrine emergencies. *JAMA* 231:393, 1975.

CHAPTER 73
SEXUAL ASSAULT

Vera Morkovin

This chapter covers emergency care of the female victim of sexual assault, but victims of homosexual assault (legally sodomy) should be treated with the same standards of care as other rape victims.

Caring for a victim of sexual assault requires the emergency department staff to perform two functions simultaneously. The patient's physical and emotional trauma must be diagnosed and treated, with concern for the delayed consequences. Also, evidence must be collected for the state to use in prosecuting an alleged perpetrator.

Old stereotypes about rape have changed in recent years. Rape is a crime of violence. Studies of rapists have shown that they are motivated by hostility, anger, and the drive for control, rather than by sexual desire. Victims feel helpless and fear death, since the assailant gains control by force or threats. Later, victims all develop some feelings of guilt and self-blame, even though they had to participate under duress. The victims' reactions appear to vary greatly depending on their age, prior sexual or other activities, cultural orientation, and expressive styles. Yet almost all have to cope with the aftereffects of these three traumatic emotions.

Awareness of these components dictates the emergency department management of the rape victim. She should be provided immediate privacy on arrival, and reassurance about her safety. She begins to regain control when the details of the procedure are explained and she is patiently asked to consent to all steps of the procedure. She should neither be pressured to talk nor left alone for long periods.

A nurse, physician, or counselor should obtain and document a detailed history of the actual assault, including force or threats used, which orifices were penetrated, and whether ejaculation occurred. Essential elements also include whether the victim bathed, voided, or changed clothes following the attack; any symptoms after the assault occurred; recent menstrual and contraceptive history; and recent sexual activity only if pertinent to the assault. Obtaining information about the past medical or sexual history is not necessary.

Documentation of the witnessed examination should include the condition of the clothing, any foreign material adhering to the body, any evidence of trauma even if minor, and a pelvic ex-

amination. Studies indicated for the patient's benefit include a Gram stain and culture of samples from the affected areas, serologic tests, a pregnancy test, and appropriate x-rays. The words *rape* and *sexual assault* refer to legal conclusions arrived at after a trial. The physician's diagnosis should avoid such terms and should be limited to the medical findings.

Evidential material to be collected may include plucked hair, fingernail scrapings, combings from the pubic area, clothing, fluid and swabs from the vaginal vault for sperm and acid phosphatase, saliva, and blood samples. These requirements vary in different jurisdictions, as do the instructions for packaging and labeling specimens and transferring them to authorities. It is always essential to maintain an unbroken chain of evidence. Even when collected, evidence may not be conveyed to law enforcement agencies without the patient's specific written consent. There is controversy about whether the physician should examine a wet mount for sperm. Those opposed point out that jurors might infer that motile sperm must be present for rape to have occurred.

Since the psychological sequelae of rape may be serious and prolonged, even in the absence of physical injury, the patient should receive counseling, as early as possible, from a trained volunteer, nurse, or social worker. It has been shown that this type of immediate intervention is effective in minimizing the severity of the rape-trauma syndrome; at the very least the patient should be told what feelings and reactions to expect and should be referred for counseling.

Before leaving she should be instructed as to the risks of infection and of pregnancy if applicable and offered treatment and/or referral relating to these. A follow-up visit in 6 weeks should be advised, and the patient should take home a written summary of what was done, as well as the above instructions.

BIBLIOGRAPHY

Burgess AW, Holmstrom LL: *Rape: Crisis and Recovery.* Bowie, MD, RJ Brady, 1979.

George, JE (ed): Rape and the emergency department physician, *Emerg Physic Legal Bull* 1 (2):1–8, 1975.

CHAPTER 74
OBSTETRIC
EMERGENCIES

Robert S. Hockberger

This chapter deals with the following topics: (1) the diagnosis of pregnancy; (2) the importance of caution in drug prescribing and x-ray utilization when treating a pregnant patient; (3) medical complications of pregnancy including nausea of pregnancy, pyelonephritis, thromboembolism, rubella, cholestatic jaundice, herpes simplex infections, hypertension, and Rh immunoprophylaxis; and (4) surgical complications including ectopic pregnancy, disorders causing bleeding during pregnancy, appendicitis in pregnancy, abdominal trauma in pregnancy, and emergency cesarean section.

DIAGNOSIS OF PREGNANCY

For the following reasons, the existence of pregnancy should be assumed in all women of childbearing age who present to the emergency department: (1) pregnancy may explain the presence of mild symptoms such as breast pain, nausea, urinary frequency, or general fatigue; (2) the complications of pregnancy must be considered in any woman of childbearing age with abdominal pain or vaginal bleeding; (3) the complications of pregnancy must be considered in the differential diagnosis of women of childbearing age with severe hypertension, seizures, thromboembolic disease, or jaundice; (4) radiation exposure and drug prescribing must take into account the potentially pregnant patient; and (5) the diagnosis and treatment of disorders such as herpes genitalis and rubella early in the course of pregnancy may hold grave consequences for the fetus and necessitate referral of the mother for genetic counseling.

Symptoms

The pregnant woman almost always has a history of a mistimed, light, or absent menses. During the first week of pregnancy, the woman usually notices mild breast tenderness and/or increased nipple sensitivity. During the second to third weeks the symptoms of fatigue, nausea, and urinary frequency usually occur. Often,

even in the absence of particular symptoms, multiparous women state that they "feel" pregnant.

Signs

At approximately 4 weeks of pregnancy, there may be a slight breast swelling and tenderness, and softening of the tip of the cervix may be found on physical examination. At 6 to 8 weeks of pregnancy, cervical softening extends to involve the isthmus, and a mild bluish discoloration of the cervix (Chadwick's sign) may be present. The abdomen may become slightly protuberant as the uterus displaces bowel from the pelvis. At 8 to 10 weeks, uterine enlargement and softening occurs. The uterus may be palpable abdominally after 12 weeks' gestation.

Pregnancy Test

All pregnancy tests are based on determination of the level of human chorionic gonadotropin (HCG), which is produced in small amounts by the fertilized ovum. After implantation of the ovum in the endometrium, trophoblastic cells initiate placental development with rapidly rising levels of HCG. HCG peaks at 50 to 60 days of pregnancy and decreases thereafter but is still detectable until 10 to 14 days postdelivery or after termination of the pregnancy.

A summary of available pregnancy tests is shown in Table 74-1. False negatives may occur when the urine is too dilute or has been stored at room temperature for too long, with ectopic pregnancy, and with missed abortions. False positive results occur with gross hematuria, proteinuria, tubo-ovarian abscess, thyrotoxicosis, persistent corpus luteal cyst, molar pregnancies, HCG-secreting tumors, and premature menopause. In addition, false positive results can occur with drugs: methyldopa (Aldomet), marijuana, methadone, aspirin (large doses), phenothiazines, anticonvulsants, antidepressants, and antiparkinsonian drugs.

Table 74-1. Available Pregnancy Tests

Test	Specimen	Test Time	Test Cost, $	Sensitivity, mIU/mL HCG	Days for a Positive	Error in Ectopic Pregnancy, %
Routine immunoassay (slide)	Urine	2 min	0.93–1.20	500–2000	25–28	20–50
Ultrasensitive immunoassay (tube or slide)	Urine or serum	1–2 h	1.75–1.84	200–250	7–14	6–10
Radioreceptor assay*	Urine	1 h	1.92	200	7–14	6–10
Radioimmunoassay†	Urine	1–48 h	0.72–1.35	1–25	2–7	0–1

*Measures β-human chorionic gonadatropin (β = HCG) and β-luteinizing hormone, which can give a false positive result with ovulation at midcycle and in postmenopausal women.

†Measures only β-HCG.

DRUG AND RADIATION EXPOSURE IN PREGNANCY

Drugs

Major congenital malformations occur in approximately 3 percent of all births in the United States, and another 9 percent have minor malformations. Perhaps only 2 percent of the malformations which occur in live births are attributable to a drug.

Antibiotics

The penicillins, cephalosporins, and erythromycin appear to be safe for use during pregnancy. Sulfonamides compete with bilirubin for albumin binding sites and can cause kernicterus when used in late pregnancy. Aminoglycosides should be avoided because of ototoxicity and nephrotoxicity. Tetracyclines may cause hepatocellular necrosis in the mother and hypoplasia of bones and teeth in the fetus. The gray syndrome observed in newborns following maternal chloramphenicol therapy provides a relative contraindication to the use of this drug during late pregnancy. Oxidant drugs such as the nitrofurantoins should be avoided in pregnant patients who are potentially deficient in glucose-6-phosphate dehydrogenase (G6PD). Metronidazole (Flagyl) and trimethoprim should be avoided.

Analgesics

Salicylates, with their potential adverse effects on platelet function, may be associated with an increased incidence of abortion and should be avoided. Nitrous oxide, which blocks vitamin B_{12} and folate metabolism, should not be used during the first trimester. Potent analgesics, such as morphine and meperidine (Demerol), may have CNS depressant effects on the newborn when used during late pregnancy or prior to delivery.

Anticoagulants

Warfarin (Coumadin) not only crosses the placenta, resulting in a warfarin embryopathy syndrome in as many as 50 percent of the infants exposed, but also is associated with an increased risk of hemorrhagic complications when used during the third trimester. Heparin, on the other hand, does not cross the placenta and has

not been associated with adverse fetal effects; its effects can be reversed readily by protamine sulfate. Heparin, therefore, is the anticoagulant of choice during pregnancy.

Anticonvulsants

Children born to mothers with epilepsy have a twofold to threefold increase in the frequency of malformations, especially facial clefts. It is difficult to separate the effects of phenytoin (Dilantin) from those of the maternal disease, other drugs, or the genetic liability of the offspring. Trimethadione (Tridione) has been linked to multiple malformations, as well as increased incidence of spontaneous abortions. Women in the reproductive years who are taking hydantoin or trimethadione should consider alternative therapy.

Psychotropic Drugs

Lithium may cause fetal cardiac defects and should be avoided during pregnancy. Conflicting reports concerning all other psychotropic medications (minor tranquilizers, phenothiazines, tricyclics, etc.) have led to the recommendation that they not be used, particularly in the first trimester, unless absolutely necessary for maternal health.

Asthma Medications

All medications currently employed for treating acute asthma appear to be safe during pregnancy. The inhalant route should be used if steroids are necessary. The reader should refer to current package inserts for the newer asthma drugs.

Antinauseants

Changes in eating patterns and dietary constituents may alleviate symptoms in many cases of nausea associated with pregnancy. If such is unsuccessful, the use of both prochlorperazine (Compazine) and trimethobenzamide (Tigan) is preferable to the development of dehydration and electrolyte imbalance.

Radiation Exposure

The incidence of birth defects may increase approximately 0.01 percent per rad of fetal radiation exposure. Studies such as skull series, cervical spine, chest, and extremity x-rays result in 1 to 10 millirads of fetal radiation exposure if the uterus is shielded during the procedure. Larger doses of radiation are delivered to the fetus with abdominal, pelvic, and lumbosacral spine x-rays.

When considering obtaining x-rays in potentially pregnant patients, (1) always take a menstrual history and consider pregnancy testing before obtaining any x-rays, unless the patient is using some form of contraception or has had ligation of the fallopian tubes, (2) never withhold necessary x-rays, (3) shield the uterus when possible, and (4) postpone ''elective'' x-rays in all women of childbearing age until the first 10 days following a normal menstrual period.

MEDICAL COMPLICATIONS

Nausea of Pregnancy and Hyperemesis Gravidarum

Approximately 50 percent of women experience nausea (morning sickness) during early pregnancy. The cause is probably HCG; the highest levels are found during the first trimester, when nausea is most prevalent. The nausea usually abates by the fourth month, and, as a general rule, the symptoms of nausea and vomiting in a patient pregnant more than 12 weeks should prompt consideration of another problem.

When the presence of other medical or surgical disease has been eliminated, the nausea of pregnancy may be treated with frequent small meals of dry food such as crackers, toast, and cereal during periods when the patient is symptomatic. Trimethobenzamide or prochlorperazine may be used if this fails to alleviate the symptoms. Starvation, dehydration, and acidosis may result from unremitting nausea and vomiting, a condition referred to as hyperemesis gravidarum. Hospitalization, intravenous rehydration, emotional support, and gradual reinstitution of oral nourishment have all but totally obviated the need for therapeutic abortion for this condition.

Urinary Tract Infection and Pyelonephritis

The pregnant woman is exposed to increased levels of progesterone, which decreases smooth muscle motility. This not only prevents the uterine musculature from contracting but also decreases both gastrointestinal (GI) and urinary tract motility and may cause or contribute to the 5 to 7 percent incidence of asymptomatic bacteriuria during pregnancy. An attempt should be made to eradicate the bacterial colonization of the urine in such cases. Before the third trimester, a sulfa drug is the drug of choice (except in G6PD-deficient patients), followed by ampicillin. When asymptomatic bacteriuria persists or is untreated, the likelihood that these patients will develop acute pyelonephritis approaches 30 to 40 percent.

Acute pyelonephritis complicates approximately 2 percent of all pregnancies. Because patients with acute pyelonephritis have decreased ureteral motility, an increased incidence of abnormal pathogens, an increased incidence of sepsis when compared with the nonpregnant population, and an increased incidence of premature labor, all such patients who present following the first trimester of pregnancy should probably be hospitalized for intravenous antibiotic therapy. Ampicillin is the drug of choice in such cases.

Thromboembolism

The risk of thromboembolism is increased five to six times in a pregnant woman, and this risk extends several weeks into the postpartum period. This is because of (1) increased levels of clotting factors (vitamin-K-dependent factors), (2) increased venous distensibility, and (3) increased uterine size, causing decreased venous flow below the vena cava.

Iodinated radiodiagnostic agents should not be used during pregnancy. These are concentrated 20 to 50 times more in the fetal thyroid than in the maternal thyroid. Therefore, even small doses may affect fetal thyroid development. Technetium-albumin combinations give excellent scans and should be used instead. If the scan is equivocal or fails to confirm a very strong suspicion of embolism, pulmonary angiography with shielding of the abdomen may be done.

The treatment of both deep venous thrombophlebitis and pulmonary embolism is with heparin. Low-dose subcutaneous heparin therapy is used instead of warfarin for up to 6 weeks postpartum.

Rubella

All women of childbearing age clinically diagnosed as having rubella (German measles) should have a pregnancy test. Up to 30 percent of women of reproductive age do not have adequate antibodies to protect against rubella infections. If a woman contracts rubella during the first month of pregnancy, the fetus has approximately a 50 percent chance of developing the classic rubella syndrome (cataracts, deafness, and patent ductus arteriosus). This drops to 25 percent in the second month and 10 percent in the third month. Treatment of the mother is symptomatic, but immediate referral for counseling is mandatory since if the infection occurs in the first 3 to 4 months of pregnancy, therapeutic abortion may be advisable.

Cholestatic Jaundice

Women of Scandinavian or Chilean descent seem to be particularly predisposed to developing cholestatic jaundice of pregnancy. This usually presents as mild jaundice, generalized itching, and GI upset during the third trimester of pregnancy. The conjugated bilirubin level is increased but is seldom above 5 mg/100 mL. The alkaline phosphatase level is elevated 7 to 10 times the normal pregnancy levels. Levels of other liver enzymes are less markedly elevated. Dramatic relief can be obtained with 10 to 12 g of cholestyramine resin (Questran) orally in three divided doses daily. Cholestatic jaundice may recur with subsequent pregnancies and has been associated with an increased incidence of fetal distress.

Herpes Simplex Infection

Herpes simplex type II vulvovaginitis is becoming a common venereal disease. Perhaps as many as 5 percent of the cultures of samples from the cervix are herpes positive in pregnant women. Infection diagnosed during the first trimester of pregnancy has been linked with an increased incidence of congenital malformations and spontaneous abortions. Hence referral of infected pregnant women for counseling and consideration of therapeutic abortion is advisable.

In addition, infants delivered through a cervical or vulvovaginal infestation of herpes stand a 30 to 40 percent chance of contracting neonatal herpes. In infected infants, manifestations may vary from a mild skin involvement to severe CNS impairment or death. Cesarean section should be considered in any patient in labor with active lesions or positive culture results whose membranes are intact or have been ruptured for less than 4 h.

Hypertensive Disorders of Pregnancy

Hypertension in pregnancy is classified into three categories: chronic hypertension without superimposed preeclampsia, preeclampsia, and eclampsia.

Chronic Hypertension

Women with chronic hypertension often experience exacerbations during pregnancy. Before 20 weeks' gestation, diuretics may be given if the diastolic blood pressure is consistently above 90 mmHg. During the second half of pregnancy, diuretics should be avoided because of the adverse effects they may exert on the uterine blood flow. Patients who cannot maintain a diastolic blood pressure below 90 mmHg in the absence of diuretic therapy should be hospitalized during the latter half of pregnancy. Bed rest alone is usually sufficient, but if not, methyldopa, hydralazine (Apresoline), and propanolol, in that order, have been used with some success.

Preeclampsia

Toxemia of pregnancy occurs in approximately 5 percent of pregnancies and is defined as the development of acute hypertension following the twenty-fourth week of gestation. It may occur in previously normotensive women or may complicate the pregnancy of a patient with chronic hypertension.

The cause is unclear, but decreased uteroplacental perfusion, a genetic defect, and an immunologic theory all have proponents. Regardless, the pathophysiology of this disease involves arteriolar

Table 74-2. Criteria for Diagnosing Preeclampsia

1. Mild preeclampsia
   a. SBP >140 mmHg or rise >30 mmHg above baseline or DBP >90 mmHg or rise >15 mmHg above baseline
   b. Proteinuria >300 mg and <2 g in 24 h
   c. Edema of hands and face
   d. Weight gain >2 lb/week
2. Severe preeclampsia
   a. BP >160/110
   b. Proteinuria >5 g/day (+4 dipstick)
   c. Generalized edema
   d. Weight gain >6 lb/week

Note: BP = blood pressure; SBP = systolic blood pressure; DBP = diastolic blood pressure.

Table 74-3. Protocol for Use of Magnesium Sulfate to Control Eclamptic Seizures or Other Seizure Activity

DOSAGE

Loading dose, 2–4 g IV. Push slowly over 5–10 min (20 mL of a 10% solution or 4 mL of a 50% solution = 4 g).
Maintenance dose, 1 g/h IV; continuous infusion.

PRECAUTIONS

Obstetrician should be notified immediately.
Respirations must be normal and greater than 16/min.
Follow deep tendon reflexes during administration.
Monitor urine output, generally with a Foley catheter, and ensure output of at least 30–40 mL/h, as magnesium is excreted solely through the kidneys.
Stop administration if the serum magnesium level is 10–12 mg/100 mL or when knee jerks disappear.

ANTIDOTE

1 g calcium gluconate IV slowly, if patient is not digitalis toxic

ADVERSE EFFECTS

Nausea, vomiting, and flushed feeling during loading dose
Depression of reflexes
Respiratory depression
Bradyarrhythmias, heart block, and cardiac standstill

LAB STUDIES

CBC; serum for BUN creatinine, glucose, sodium, potassium, chloride, bicarbonate, and magnesium levels; venous pH; and urinalysis.

Note: CBC = complete blood cell count; BUN = blood urea nitrogen; IV = intravenously.

vasospasm affecting the maternal brain, heart, lung, and kidney. Criteria for the diagnosis of preeclampsia are shown in Table 74-2.

Treatment. Patients with mild preeclampsia not exhibiting proteinuria should be instructed to decrease their activity at home or work, collect a 24-h urine specimen for protein quantification, and see their obstetrician in the next few days for follow-up. Any patient with mild preeclampsia exhibiting proteinuria should be hospitalized for bed rest, urine protein quantification, and consideration of medical therapy.

Patients with severe preeclampsia at fewer than 36 weeks of gestation should be hospitalized. The patient should rest in bed in the left recumbent position. Delivery should be induced in the following instances: (1) if there is evidence of a mature infant, (2) if the patient shows worsening blood pressure and renal function despite bed rest, and (3) if the patient requires drug therapy for the control of blood pressure.

Any patient with severe preeclampsia at greater than 36 weeks' gestation should be treated the same as a patient with eclampsia.

Eclampsia

Eclampsia is defined as the occurrence of grand mal seizures with severe preeclampsia. It occurs in approximately 1 in 1000 pregnancies, and in 1 in 75 twin births. Signs of impending eclampsia in a severely preeclamptic patient include (1) headache, (2) visual changes, (3) hyperreflexia or irritability, and (4) abdominal pain.

Treatment. The treatment of eclampsia is delivery. Magnesium sulfate (Table 74-3) should be administered before a pelvic examination of a patient with eclampsia or severe preeclampsia accompanied by any of the warning signs listed above as the stimulation of a pelvic examination can induce convulsions in such a patient. In addition, patients who must be transferred for definitive care should have magnesium sulfate before transportation. Both magnesium sulfate and hydralazine (Table 74-4) should be administered prophylactically approximately 20 min before delivery since the disease process inevitably worsens at the time of delivery.

The syndrome of disseminated intravascular coagulation (DIC) occasionally accompanies eclampsia. In such cases, coagulation studies (complete blood cell count, and assessment of platelets, fibrinogen, and prothrombin time) should be obtained. Heparin should not be administered. The treatment of DIC is delivery of the fetus. Abruptio placentae may occur in the preeclamptic or eclamptic patient and should be suspected in any such patient with abdominal pain or uterine tenderness.

Prognosis. Before the advent of magnesium sulfate and hydralazine therapy, fetal mortality was approximately 25 percent and maternal mortality varied from 5 to 10 percent. Since 1955, however, more than 170 women have been treated consecutively at Parkland Memorial Hospital in Dallas, Texas, with both magnesium sulfate and hydralazine. One maternal death and no fetal deaths have been reported to date.

Rh Immunoprophylaxis

The risk of isoimmunization of an Rh-negative mother against her Rh-positive fetus depends upon the number of Rh-positive red cells to which she has been exposed, and ranges from 3 to 65 percent. Exposure usually occurs during the third stage of labor when fetal blood cells enter the maternal circulation, although fetal-maternal hemorrhage has been noted as early as the second trimester.

The administration of Rh_0 (D) immune globulin (RhoGAM) within 72 h of delivery of a full-term infant reduces the incidence of Rh isoimmunization as the result of pregnancy from 12 to 1 percent. One vial of the immune globulin should be administered intramuscularly within 72 h of the presentation of an Rh-negative woman with a normal delivery, abortion, or ectopic pregnancy.

Postpartum Fever

Fever in the postpartum period is common, and evaluation is similar to that of any febrile patient. The process of delivery can result in trauma and devitalization of the structures of the pelvis and urinary tract, creating an environment conducive to infection. In any postpartum febrile patient, careful pelvic examination is necessary. Wound or episiotomy infections are uncommon, but when they occur they can be severe. Any patient who has been catheterized or has had a forceps delivery should be investigated for urinary tract infection.

Endoperimetritis is characterized by the development of a boggy, tender uterus and perimetrium 1 to 3 days postpartum. Uterine and cervical cultures are of little help in the diagnosis because vaginal and cervical flora are virtually the same in both uninfected and infected patients. Diagnosis is made on the basis of physical

Table 74-4. Treatment Protocol for Acute Hypertension Complicating Pregnancy, Primarily Pregnancy-Induced Hypertension

CRITERIA FOR TREATMENT

Diagnosis of toxemia or pregnancy-induced hypertension
SBP >180 mmHg
DBP >110 mmHg
Delivery anticipated in reasonable time period

GOALS OF THERAPY

Reduce SBP to about 150 mmHg
Reduce DBP to 90–100 mmHg
Prevent further compromise of blood flow to fetus and placenta by maintaining blood pressure at 150/90 to 150/100
Simultaneous preparation for delivery

TREATMENT*

1) 10–20 mg hydralazine IM, repeated as needed, or
2) Continuous hydralazine infusion 5 mg/h, with continuous blood pressure monitoring

*Drugs such as diazoxide and nitroprusside have little use in the treatment of obstetrically associated hypertension because of potential adverse effects on the mother or the fetus.

Note: SBP = systolic blood pressure; DBP = diastolic blood pressure; IM = intramuscularly.

examination and the finding of a foul lochia. Endoperimetritis is best treated with a broad-spectrum antibiotic such as ampicillin. Hospitalization for treatment with intravenous antibiotics should be considered.

Rarely, ovarian vein thrombophlebitis develops. The development of fever, malaise, or abdominal pain 4 to 5 days following delivery, with diffuse tenderness on pelvic examination, should suggest the possibility of thrombophlebitis. The presence of pulmonary embolism should heighten one's index of suspicion for this disease. The differentiation of pelvic thrombophlebitis from endoperimetritis is sometimes difficult, and thrombophlebitis should be suspected if the condition does not respond rapidly to antibiotics.

Premature Rupture of Membranes

Spontaneous premature rupture of membranes occurs in approximately 10 percent of all pregnancies. Although the exact cause is unknown, vaginal infections, coitus, and poor maternal health have been implicated. The time between premature rupture and spontaneous vaginal delivery is less than 12 h in 80 percent of the cases, between 12 and 24 h in 10 percent of the cases, and between 1 and 58 days in 10 percent.

Diagnosis. Patients usually present with a history of a trickle or a sudden gush of clear watery fluid from the vagina. The presence of urinary incontinence or a thin vaginal discharge must be ruled out by performing a sterile speculum exam of the vaginal vault to check for pooling of secretions. A positive nitrazine test (in the absence of vaginal bleeding) and the presence of ferning on microscopic glass slide examination confirm the presence of amniotic fluid. In no instance of suspected premature rupture of membranes should a bimanual examination be performed if the pregnancy is of less than 37 weeks' duration.

Treatment. Patients of more than 37 weeks' gestation with premature rupture of membranes should be hospitalized.

The treatment of premature rupture of membranes when gestational age is less than 37 weeks is controversial. Once the membranes rupture, the barrier to bacterial penetration is lost, and intrauterine infection may ensue. In such cases, both maternal and fetal mortality is high. The aggressive approach to treatment is delivery within 12 h of presentation, induced with intravenous oxytocin if necessary. Several centers, however, have been very successful with a more conservative approach. This approach includes (1) hospitalization in a facility which has a neonatal intensive care unit, (2) the administration of steroids to promote fetal lung development, and (3) induction of delivery once the infant reaches maturity, or, alternatively, if the mother develops a fever, an elevated white blood cell count, or any evidence of uterine tenderness.

SURGICAL COMPLICATIONS

Ectopic Pregnancy

Ectopic pregnancy is defined as the implantation of the fertilized ovum in any location other than the endometrium. The incidence in the United States is approximately 1 in 100 to 200 pregnancies. Approximately 1 in 20 cases results in fatal hemorrhage. Death in almost all instances is due to inadequate treatment. Ectopic pregnancy is the most common cause of maternal death among nonwhite women in the United States.

Associated factors include chronic salpingitis, the presence of an intrauterine device (IUD), and previous pelvic surgery. One to four percent of women become pregnant following tubal ligation. If this occurs, there is a 20 to 40 percent risk of an ectopic pregnancy.

Signs and symptoms. Classically, ectopic pregnancy presents as crampy, unilateral lower abdominal pain associated with abnormal vaginal bleeding following a period of amenorrhea (usually 5 to 7 weeks). Schwartz, however, found that less than 15 percent

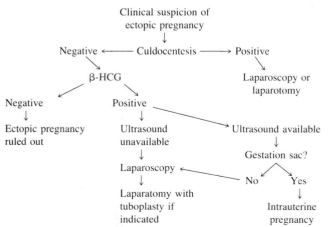

Figure 74-1. Differential diagnosis for ectopic pregnancy.

of the patients with ectopic pregnancies presented with this classic triad.

It is not the location, character, or duration of pain but the presence of lower abdominal pain in a pregnant patient which should lead to the suspicion of ectopic pregnancy. If rupture occurs, the pain may be severe and colicky and may be referred to the shoulders as the result of diaphragmatic irritation. Since the majority of ruptured ectopic pregnancies cause very slow leaks, the patient may tolerate larger amounts of free blood in the peritoneum with few signs. In addition, although an abnormal menstrual history is supportive of the diagnosis of ectopic pregnancy, a normal menstrual history is present in 10 to 15 percent of the cases.

Physical examination. Uterine enlargement may occur with ectopic pregnancy as a result of the action of placental hormones. The abnormally implanted placenta, however, produces lower levels of such hormones, and this results in a uterus which is larger than that of the nonpregnant woman but "small for dates." Ninety-five percent of ectopic pregnancies are located in the fallopian tube, and an actual "mass" is felt in 30 to 50 percent. In many instances, a vague and ill-defined sense of fullness rather than a mass may be detected on examination. Fullness in the cul-de-sac secondary to the accumulation of blood is felt in 50 to 80 percent. Guarding may preclude an accurate and diagnostic pelvic examination.

Culdocentesis. Culdocentesis should be performed in all instances of suspected ectopic pregnancy. The aspiration of free blood confirms the diagnosis of intraabdominal bleeding and is an indication for surgical intervention. Occasional false positive results are seen with ruptured corpus luteum cysts and torsion of the fallopian tube. Culdocentesis is approximately 90 to 95 percent accurate in instances of ruptured or leaking ectopic pregnancies, but may be negative if the ectopic pregnancy has not yet ruptured. A negative result from culdocentesis does not rule out ectopic pregnancy.

Pregnancy test. The routine immunoassay (slide test) may be negative in up to 50 percent of the cases. The radioreceptor assay is much more sensitive and is positive in up to 95 percent of the cases. False positive results are occasionally seen with ovulation at midcycle and in postmenopausal women. The radioimmunoassay for β-HCG is extremely sensitive and is positive in approximately 99 percent of the cases.

Pelvic ultrasound. The gray scale ultrasound detects a gestational sack at approximately 6 weeks following uterine implantation. Failure to visualize such a sack in a woman with lower abdominal pain and a positive pregnancy test is an indication for gynecologic consultation. The presence of an intrauterine pregnancy does not rule out a coexistent ectopic pregnancy. The presence of a small mass detected with ultrasound is compatible with a number of lesions including ectopic pregnancy, corpus luteum cyst, and hydrosalpinx. However, the absence of a definite mass does not rule out a ruptured ectopic pregnancy.

Differential diagnosis. The most commonly encountered misdiagnoses in ectopic pregnancy include pelvic inflammatory disease, ovarian cyst, dysfunctional uterine bleeding, incomplete or complete spontaneous abortion, and acute appendicitis. Adhering to a standardized approach similar to that shown in Figure 74-1 may decrease the incidence of misdiagnoses.

Treatment. Once the diagnosis is made or strongly suspected, treatment is surgical. In hypotensive patients, placement of a MAST suit, administration of crystalloid fluids through two large-bore intravenous lines, and early administration of whole blood are temporizing measures that may prove lifesaving.

A patient with an ectopic pregnancy who is Rh negative and unsensitized should be given RhoGAM to prevent Rh isoimmunization.

Vaginal Bleeding in Pregnancy

Abortion

First-Trimester Bleeding

The possibility of ectopic pregnancy must be eliminated in all patients with first-trimester vaginal bleeding. In addition, non-pregnancy-related causes of vaginal bleeding such as cervical polyps, acute or chronic cervicitis, vaginal trauma, and nonuterine bleeding from the urethra or rectum must be excluded. Once such possibilities are ruled out, only the diagnosis of abortion remains.

Threatened Abortion

Approximately 50 percent of all pregnant women have some vaginal bleeding in the first trimester. If there is no evidence of either cervical dilatation or expulsion of the products of conception, and if the pregnancy test remains positive, the diagnosis of threatened abortion is made. The patient should be advised to stay home and, after a 24-h rest period, resume normal activity as tolerated. Douching and intercourse should be avoided while the bleeding is present but are not otherwise contraindicated. The patient should be told to return if there is increased vaginal bleeding or abdominal cramping, or if the products of conception begin to pass. Any tissue passed should be brought in. Approximately 20 percent of these patients eventually completely abort.

Inevitable and Incomplete Abortion

If the cervix has begun to dilate or efface, or if the bag of waters has ruptured, the diagnosis of an inevitable abortion can be made. The nitrazine pH test differentiates vaginal secretions (acidic) from amniotic fluid (alkaline), but if there is any bleeding the test is unreliable. If the products of conception are through the endocervical canal and visible in the cervical os or in the vagina, the diagnosis of incomplete abortion is made. With both inevitable and incomplete abortions, admission is indicated, as the treatment is evacuation of the products of conception as quickly as possible.

Complete Abortion

In a complete abortion a patient has passed all the products of conception, the cervix is closed, the uterus is firm and nontender, and there is minimal, if any, bleeding. This is a difficult diagnosis to make unless the patient has brought in all the products of conception. If any doubt exists, or if bleeding continues, the patient should be hospitalized.

Missed Abortion

Missed abortion is the failure to expel the products of conception for 2 months after the pregnancy has terminated. Diagnosis is made by history, examination, and the conversion of a positive pregnancy test to negative. Treatment is uterine curettage.

Molar Pregnancy

Hydatidiform mole is a rare cause of late first trimester bleeding. Classically, there is excessive uterine growth, nausea, and vomiting, and/or the development of preeclampsia before 24 weeks of gestation. In addition, the patient has abdominal pain, is anemic, and has passed grape-like clusters of tissue characteristic of a mole.

Although a presumptive diagnosis may be made from the history and physical examination, the definitive diagnosis is made by ultrasound or by the identification of molar tissue in the vagina at the time of examination.

Treatment. Initially, intravenous oxytocin is given, and a careful suction dilatation and curettage is performed. Although the coexistence of a hydatidiform mole and a fetus is rare, it has been reported; consequently, an Rh-negative woman who is unsensitized should receive Rh immunoglobulin following the evacuation of a hydatidiform mole. Finally, all such patients should be entered in a trophoblastic disease register to ensure adequate follow-up of HCG titers. If the HCG titers plateau and do not fall, or fall and then rise again, chemotherapy for chorionic carcinoma is indicated.

Third-Trimester Bleeding

Third-trimester vaginal bleeding is bleeding that occurs after 28 weeks of gestation. In approximately 1 percent of all pregnancies, third-trimester bleeding results from placenta previa; in 1 to 2 percent, from abruption of the placenta. However, a placenta implanted low over the cervical os may bleed in the second trimester, and abruption may occur with or without bleeding. As with first-trimester bleeding, third-trimester bleeding may be secondary to cervical polyps, cervicitis, trauma to the cervix or vagina, or cervical cancer. A history should be taken and an examination should be performed to exclude the GI and urinary tracts as sources of bleeding. However, pelvic examination should be deferred (see below).

Placenta Previa

The ovum usually implants in the upper portion of the uterus near the entrance of the fallopian tubes. Ultrasound studies performed at 16 weeks of gestation, however, have shown that in approximately 5 percent of pregnancies, initial implantation occurs low in the uterus near the cervical os. In most instances, the low-implanted placenta migrates upward, away from the cervix, as pregnancy progresses. In approximately 1 percent of all pregnancies, migration does not occur, and when the lower uterine segment lengthens during late pregnancy, separation of the placenta from the uterine wall occurs, and bleeding ensues. The etiology of this "failure of migration" is unknown, but it is associated with advancing maternal age, multiparity, uterine anomalies, and twin gestations.

The clinical hallmark of placenta previa is *painless* bright red vaginal bleeding. In most instances, during a 1- to 2-week period the patient experiences intermittent episodes of bleeding which get progressively heavier. Exsanguinating hemorrhage is rare with initial bleeding episodes, unless the placenta is separated from the uterine wall during examination. Therefore, pelvic, vaginal, and rectal examinations are contraindicated in the initial evaluation of patients with painless bleeding late in pregnancy.

Stable patients with suspected placenta previa should be evaluated by pelvic ultrasound. If ultrasound fails to reveal placenta previa, further examination to identify other causes of vaginal bleeding can then be safely performed. If, on the other hand, ultrasound confirms the diagnosis, the patient is not in labor, and bleeding is slight or has subsided, the treatment is hospitalization and observation. The inhibition of labor, the following of serial hematocrits with the administration of blood transfusions when necessary, and the induction of delivery or cesarian section when the infant has reached maturity constitute the usual course of management.

If the patient with suspected placenta previa is in labor, or bleeding is severe or sustained, preparation for a double-setup examination in the operating room is necessary. The major maternal hazard is exsanguinating hemorrhage, and vigorous fluid resuscitation should ensue. Cesarean sections are usually performed since fetal anoxia may occur secondary to compression of placental vessels by the presenting part during vaginal delivery.

Abruptio Placentae

This is the premature separation of a normally implanted placenta. The incidence is less than 1 percent of all pregnancies in the United States. Although the cause is unknown, it has been associated with eclampsia, chronic hypertension, multiparity, megaloblastic anemia, and abdominal trauma.

The hallmark of abruption is *painful* uterine bleeding.

Bleeding begins at the point of separation between the placenta and the uterine wall. Significant blood loss may occur in the absence of overt vaginal bleeding. Under the force of maternal arterial pressure, bleeding continues with further dissection of the placenta. When vaginal bleeding occurs, the blood may be bright red, but most commonly it is dark or clotted because of the time delay. Physical examination may reveal a uterus that ranges from slightly tender to tetanic, depending upon the degree of hemorrhage into the myometrium. Fetal heart tones may be diminished, signifying fetal distress secondary to diminished fetal oxygenation from placental ischemia. In severe cases, DIC may occur. The resulting hemorrhage may produce maternal renal failure from acute tubular necrosis or bilateral cortical necrosis, and Sheehan's syndrome secondary to pituitary necrosis. Clinically, abruptio is divided into a mild syndrome, which occurs in approximately 90 percent of the cases, and severe abruptio.

Mild abruptio is characterized by separation of no more than 25 percent of the placenta. Abdominal pain is mild to moderate, vaginal bleeding is minimal or concealed, the uterus is slightly tender, the mother and infant appear well, and there is no evidence of DIC—hematocrit, platelet count, fibrinogen, fibrin split products, prothrombin time, partial thromboplastin time, blood urea nitrogen (BUN), and creatinine are normal.

If greater than 50 percent of the placenta is separated, the condition is called severe abruptio. Abdominal pain is moderate to severe, bleeding is variable, the uterus ranges from irritable to tetanic, there is evidence of maternal distress (significant pain, tachycardia, hypotension) and fetal distress (heart rate less than 120, greater than 160, or absent), and often there is evidence of DIC.

The mild form may progress to the severe form rapidly and, therefore, the treatment for all forms of abruptio placentae is immediate delivery. In the severe form, vigorous treatment of maternal hypotension with crystalloid fluid and whole blood transfusion is essential. The placement of central venous pressure lines should be withheld if there is clinical or laboratory evidence of DIC. A Foley catheter should be placed in hypotensive patients to allow accurate and timed recording of urinary output.

The only definitive treatment for DIC in the setting of abruptio placentae is delivery. Occasionally, cryoprecipitate or fresh frozen plasma and possibly even platelets may be necessary to stabilize the patient for the operative procedure itself. Unless labor is active and near termination, cesarean section is usually necessary. After delivery, patients improve rapidly, are usually stable within 6 to 8 h, and have normal coagulation profiles within 24 h.

Postpartum Hemorrhage

Postpartum hemorrhage, occurring in approximately 5 percent of all pregnancies, is the loss of greater than 250 mL of blood acutely following delivery, or the loss of greater than 500 mL of blood during the first 24 h following delivery. Patients who die from postpartum hemorrhage do so from a constant trickle of blood rather than from a sudden hemorrhagic event, at an average time of 5 h postdelivery.

The causes include (1) traumatic injury to the genital tract during delivery, (2) a retained placenta, and (3) uterine atony secondary to an overdistended uterus (large infants, twins, or hydramnios), general anesthesia, or prolonged labor.

The vaginal vault should be examined for evidence of lacerations. They should be sutured, or packed to await definitive closure. If the placenta is not normally delivered in the third stage of labor, an attempt should be made to manually express the placenta. If the placenta has been delivered, bleeding continues, and uterine atony is present, the uterus should be pushed up and out of the pelvis for bimanual massage. In addition, oxytocin should be administered as 5 mL in 1 L of 5% dextrose in water at a rate of approximately 20 to 30 drops per minute. If these procedures prove ineffective, surgical intervention may be necessary.

Occasionally, delayed postpartum hemorrhage from involution of the placental implantation site or retention of a placental fragment may occur 7 to 14 days following delivery. The treatment is dilatation and curettage.

Appendicitis in Pregnancy

Acute appendicitis complicates approximately 1 pregnancy in 1200. Diagnosis during the first trimester is usually not difficult, but as the pregnancy progresses and the uterus displaces the cecum cephalad and laterally, the clinical picture may become confusing. Rupture of the appendix in the third trimester is not uncommon and is associated with a 7 percent maternal mortality and a 36 percent fetal mortality.

Many women in the midst of a normal pregnancy suffer from anorexia, nausea, and vomiting. In addition, some studies have shown that up to 50 percent of pregnant women with acute appendicitis do not suffer from anorexia, nausea, or vomiting.

During late pregnancy, acute appendicitis is most commonly misdiagnosed as acute pyelonephritis. Patients with acute pyelonephritis usually complain of fever and *chills*. The temperature of patients with acute pyelonephritis is usually greater than 38.3°C (100.9°F), while the temperature of patients with unruptured acute appendicitis seldom exceeds 38°C (100.4°F). The diagnosis of acute pyelonephritis should never be considered in the absence of significant bacteriuria and pyuria. All pregnant patients in the third trimester who are diagnosed as having acute pyelonephritis should be admitted for intravenous antibiotics and observation. Patients should be clinically improved within 24 h and afebrile within 48 h. If such is not the case, a reconsideration of the initial diagnosis is in order.

Abdominal Trauma in Pregnancy

The incidence of abdominal trauma in pregnancy is approximately 6 percent. It is the most frequent nonobstetrical cause of death among pregnant women (14 percent of all maternal deaths). A number of factors make the evaluation of a traumatized pregnant patient difficult. The blood pressure in a pregnant woman is normally low (average 110/70), but a systolic blood pressure less than 80 mmHg should always be considered abnormal. Increased blood volume (approximately 35 percent) during pregnancy allows a loss of greater than 30 percent before vital signs change significantly. During trauma the maternal homeostasis is maintained at the expense of the uterus and fetus, with a disproportionately more severe fetal effect. The abdominal examination is altered by the presence of the uterus, particularly later in pregnancy. The hematocrit normally falls during pregnancy from an average of 41 to 37, while the white blood cell count rises from an average of 5000 to 15,000.

Except during the abdominal examination, pregnant patients should be allowed to lie on their sides. Prolonged supine positioning may compress the inferior vena cava, diminish right heart return, and result in tachycardia and syncope, which may erroneously be ascribed to the traumatic event. Culdocentesis is safely performed during the third trimester of pregnancy when the uterus has grown up out of the pelvic cavity. When physical examination and laboratory tests are equivocal and intraabdominal bleeding is suspected, culdocentesis may be performed to diagnose intraabdominal bleeding. Hospitalization for observation should be considered for all patients with ongoing abdominal pain, tenderness, or cramps; for all patients exhibiting vaginal bleeding or an amniotic fluid leak; when fetal heart tones are greater than 160 or less than 120; and for any questionable case.

Cesarean Section in the Emergency Department

Emergency cesarean section is justified if the mother is dead on arrival and the time lapse from her death until arrival is such that the fetus is potentially viable, that is to say, usually less than 15 min. The pregnancy should have proceeded far enough to allow fetal viability, that is, over 28 weeks of gestation. If an attempt at postmortem cesarean section is to be made, personnel must be immediately available for vigorous resuscitation of the infant after delivery.

This area is fraught with medical, legal, and ethical considerations, and extreme care must be taken in exercising this option.

BIBLIOGRAPHY

Diagnosis of Pregnancy

Hirsch HL: Routine pregnancy testing: Is it a standard of care? *Br Med J* 73:1365–1366, 1980.
Kosasa TS: Measurement of human chorionic gonadotropin. *J Reprod Med* 26:201–206, 1981.

Drugs and Radiation Exposure in Pregnancy

Beeley L: Adverse effects of drugs in the first trimester of pregnancy. *Clin Obstet Gynecol* 8:261–273, 1981.
Beeley L: Adverse effects of drugs in later pregnancy. *Clin Obstet Gynecol* 8:275–290, 1981.
Bracken MB: Exposure to prescribed drugs in pregnancy and association with congenital malformations. *Clin Obstet Gynecol* 58:336–344, 1981.
Hollengsworth M: Drugs and pregnancy. *Obstet Gynecol* 4:503–519, 1977.
Mole RH: Radiation effects on prenatal development and their radiological significance. *Br J Radiol* 52:89–101, 1979.

Medical Complications

Cunningham FG: Acute pyelonephritis of pregnancy: A clinical review. *Obstet Gynecol* 42:112–117, 1973.
Gilstrap MC: Acute pyelonephritis in pregnancy: An anterospective study. *Obstet Gynecol* 57:409–412, 1980.
Kappy KA: Premature rupture of the membranes: A conservative approach. *Am J Obstet Gynecol* 134:655–661, 1979.
Lindheimer MD: Pathophysiology of preeclampsia. *Annu Rev Med* 32:273–289, 1981.
Martin TR: The management of severe toxemia in patients at less than 36 weeks gestation. *Obstet Gynecol* 54:602–605, 1979.
Pritchard JA: Standardized treatment of 154 consecutive cases of eclampsia. *Am J Obstet Gynecol* 123:543–552, 1975.
Pritchard JA: The use of magnesium sulfate in preeclampsia-eclampsia. *J Reprod Med* 23:107–113, 1979.
Ries DL: Urinary tract infection in pregnancy. *Clin Obstet Gynecol* 5:169–191, 1981.
Roberts JM: Preeclampsia and eclampsia. *West J Med* 135:34–43, 1981.
Sibai BM: Late postpartum eclampsia controversy. *Obstet Gynecol* 55:74–78, 1980.
Sibai BM: Eclampsia. *Obstet Gynecol* 58:609–613, 1981.

Surgical Complications

Babaknia A: Appendicitis during pregnancy. *Obstet Gynecol* 50:40–44, 1977.
Booker D: Vaginal hemorrhage in pregnancy. *N Engl J Med* 290:611–613, 1979.
Brenner PF: Ectopic pregnancy: A study of 300 consecutive cases. *JAMA* 243:673–676, 1980.
Brown BJ: Uncontrollable postpartum bleeding. *Obstet Gynecol* 54:361–365, 1979.
Buchsbaum H: Accidental injury complicating pregnancy. *Am J Obstet Gynecol* 102:752, 1968.
Clark JM: Culdocentesis in the evaluation of blunt abdominal trauma. *Surg Gynecol Obstet* 129:809–810, 1969.
DeCherney AH: Contemporary management of ectopic pregnancy. *J Reprod Med* 26:519–523, 1981.

Espisito JM: Ectopic pregnancy: The laparoscope as a diagnostic aid. *J Reprod Med* 25:17–23, 1980.

Frisenda R: Acute appendicitis during pregnancy. *Am Surg* 45:503–506, 1979.

Gomez A: Acute appendicitis during pregnancy. *Am J Surg* 137:180–183, 1979.

Grimes DA: Fatal septic abortion in the United States (1975–1977). *Obstet Gynecol* 57:739–744, 1981

Hibbard BM: Abruptio placentae. *Obstet Gynecol* 27:155–167, 1967.

Jouppila P: Early pregnancy failure: A study by ultrasonic and hormonal methods. *Obstet Gynecol* 55:42–46, 1980.

Kelly MT: The value of sonography in suspected ectopic pregnancy. *Obstet Gynecol* 53(6):703–708, 1979.

Lowthian J: Appendicitis during pregnancy. *Ann Emerg Med,* 9:431–434, 1980.

Pelosi MA: Improved accuracy in the clinical diagnosis of ectopic pregnancy by the simultaneous use of pelvic ultrasound and radioreceptor assay of HCG. *Surg Gynecol Obstet* 149:539–544, 1979.

Rizos N: Natural history of placenta previa. *Am J Obstet Gynecol* 133(3):287–291, 1979.

Schwartz DO: BHCG as a diagnostic aid for suspected ectopic pregnancy. *Obstet Gynecol* 56:197–203, 1980.

Spirt BA: Abruptio placentae: Sonographic and pathologic correlation. *AJR* 133:877–881, 1979.

Webb MJ: Culdocentesis. *JACEP* 7:451–454, 1978.

SECTION 9
PEDIATRICS

CHAPTER 75
NEONATAL
RESUSCITATION
AND EMERGENCIES

Seetha Shankaran
Eugene E. Cepeda

NEONATAL RESUSCITATION

Resuscitation of the newborn infant in the delivery room or in the nursery must be performed as an emergency procedure. Any physician performing deliveries will find that 10 to 15 percent of the neonates he or she delivers require resuscitation.

Causes of Neonatal Asphyxia

It is important to anticipate the delivery of the high-risk neonate so that delivery room personnel may be alerted to the possible need for resuscitation.

Maternal Factors

Poor prenatal care
Age less than 16 or greater than 35 years
History of previous perinatal morbidity or mortality
Toxemia, hypertension
Diabetes
Chronic renal disease
Abruptio placentae, placenta previa, or antepartum hemorrhage
Drug abuse
Infection, prolonged rupture of membranes
Blood type or group isoimmunization

Intrapartum Factors

Abnormal presentation
Cesarean section
Prolonged labor or precipitous delivery
Cephalopelvic disproportion
Forceps delivery other than outlet or vacuum extraction
Prolapsed cord

Cord compression
Maternal hypotension
Analgesic or sedative drugs given within 2 h of delivery

Fetal Factors

Prematurity
Postmaturity
Multiple gestation
Acidosis (fetal scalp capillary monitoring)
Abnormal fetal heart rate monitoring
Meconium-stained amniotic fluid
Intrauterine growth retardation
Fetal malformation diagnosed by ultrasound

In the nursery similar physiologic mechanisms occur when an infant becomes apneic. The following is a list of conditions which should alert nursery personnel to the possibility of apnea:

Asphyxiation
Prematurity
Sepsis and/or meningitis
Congenital abnormalities
Respiratory distress
Seizures
Hypoglycemia, hypocalcemia

Principles of Resuscitation

The Apgar score (Table 75-1) is assessed at 1 and 5 min of age for every newly delivered infant. The 5-min Apgar score has been found to be the most sensitive indicator of morbidity following asphyxia. If the score is 2 or less at 1 min or 5 or less at 5 min of age, the neonate requires resuscitation. Although the scoring system has been useful in evaluating the amount of asphyxia the

Table 75-1. The Apgar Score

Sign	0	1	2
Heart rate	Absent	<100/min	>100/min
Respiratory effort	Absent	Weak cry	Strong cry
Muscle tone	Limp	Some flexion	Good flexion
Reflex irritability (when feet stimulated)	No response	Some motion	Cry
Color	blue:pale	Body pink; extremities blue	Pink

newborn has sustained, 1 min is too long to wait to make the decision to initiate resuscitation.

The following is a list of equipment needed for resuscitation:

Bag and mask with manometer attached, connected to a source of 100% oxygen. Oxygen should be heated and humidified.
Wall suction, sterile catheters, and bulb syringe
DeLee suction catheter with mucus trap
Laryngoscope with nos. 0 and 1 blade
Oral endotracheal tubes with stylet—size 1.5, 2, 2.5, and 3.0 mm diameter. The stylet should not extend beyond the orifice of the endotracheal tube.
Radiant heater with servomechanisms
Sterile umbilical vessel catheterization tray
Glucose oxidase test strips (Dextrostix)
ECG electrodes and heart rate monitor
Intravenous infusion equipment

Steps to Follow During Resuscitation

Maintain body temperature. When the cord is clamped, blot the infant dry with a sterile towel and place him or her under a radiant heater on a sterile table.

Clear the airway. Gently suction the nose and mouth with a bulb syringe. A 15-s examination should be performed to determine the need for resuscitation. This examination should include an assessment of heart rate, respiratory effort, color, and muscular activity.

Initiate breathing. If the infant is apneic or the respiratory rate is slow and irregular, administer positive pressure ventilation with a bag over the infant's face and 100% oxygen. The respiratory rate should be maintained at 40 breaths per minute with pressure applied to gently move the chest wall. In an infant who has not yet taken a breath, over 40 cm H_2O pressure may be necessary to expand the lungs. In mildly asphyxiated infants this will produce a prompt increase in heart rate and the onset of regular, spontaneous respirations. If both do not occur within 2 min, the trachea should be intubated under closely monitored conditions and assisted ventilation continued.

Cardiac massage. If the heart rate is below 50 beats per minute with assisted ventilation, cardiac massage should be initiated by placing both hands around the infant's chest with two thumbs over the mediasternum so that the sternum will be depressed two-thirds of the distance to the vertebral column at 120 compressions per minute. Cardiac massage may be stopped periodically to assess improvement. Ventilation and cardiac massage should be synchronized (1:3 ratio). The chest should expand, bilateral breath sounds should be heard in the axilla, and heart rate should increase

if resuscitation is effective. In most instances it is possible to obtain an adequate response with the use of external cardiac massage and assisted ventilation. If there is no response in 3 min, drug therapy should be considered. Any route of access to the circulatory system is acceptable, including a peripheral intravenous or umbilical vein or artery line.

Catheterize umbilical artery or vein. In an acidotic, hypoxic, and hypercarbic neonate it is often not possible to cannulate the artery because of vasoconstriction. The most expedient procedure is to insert the venous catheter through the ductus venosus into the inferior vena cava (10 to 12 cm) or avoid the portal system by anchoring it superficially (4 to 5 cm). The first blood sample aspirated should be analyzed for blood gases. Either capillary gases, in the absence of shock, or arterial gases should be monitored.

Drug Therapy in Resuscitation

Sodium bicarbonate. A base deficit of 14 mEq/L or more should be corrected by infusing 0.5M $NaHCO_3$ at the rate of 1 mEq/(kg·min) up to 5 mEq/kg total dose calculated by the formula:

$$mEq = 0.3 \times weight (kg) \times base deficit in mEq/L$$

The infusion should be slow and diluted 1:1 with sterile water. Bicarbonate should be used only if ventilation is being assisted effectively and P_{CO_2} is not elevated.

Tris-buffer. THAM (trimethamine) solution has the advantage of lowering P_{CO_2} and buffering metabolic acid, hence it is of benefit in severe mixed metabolic and respiratory acidosis. Tris-buffer may cause respiratory depression, hence it should be used only when ventilation is being assisted.

Dextrose. Ten percent dextrose in water ($D_{10}W$) at 100 mL/(kg·24 h) provides metabolic substrate and expansion of plasma volume. If the Dextrostix value is less than 45 mg/100 mL, 5 mL/kg of a 10 or a 15% glucose solution should be infused. Twenty-five percent dextrose infusions should be avoided because of occurrence of rebound hypoglycemia.

Epinephrine. 0.1 mL/kg of a 1:10,000 solution is given intravenously to stimulate the heart and cardiovascular system. Cardiac massage should continue following epinephrine administration.

Naloxone. 0.01 mL/kg is given to reverse narcotic depression. The time for peak concentration of transplacentally acquired narcotics in the fetus is 2 h, and delivery of a fetus at that time would predispose the infant to maximal depression on this basis.

Calcium gluconate. A 10% solution may be given intravenously (1 mL/kg) when severe bradycardia persists despite the previously outlined therapeutic measures.

Certain neonatal conditions require specific measures during resuscitation besides those outlined above.

Neonatal Shock

Risk factors for hypotension in the newborn infant are low birth weight, maternal sepsis, prolapsed cord, and acute onset of maternal vaginal bleeding. Clinical signs of hypovolemia in the neonate are pallor, tachycardia, mottling of skin, poor capillary filling, thready pulse, and hypotension (less than 45 mmHg in a

1000-g premature neonate or less than 60 mmHg in a term infant). A hematocrit should be obtained. Therapy consists of immediate plasma expansion in the form of whole blood, fresh frozen plasma, Plasmanate, or 5% salt-poor albumin, 10 to 20 mL/kg given intravenously over 10 min. Cord blood, obtained in a sterile manner in a heparinized syringe, may also be used for volume expansion.

Meconium Staining

Meconium staining of the amniotic fluid varies from 0.5 to 20 percent of all births. Meconium aspiration carries a 20 to 50 percent mortality rate; however, with proper management it is almost entirely preventable. When gross meconium is noted at the time of delivery, the following procedure should be followed: After delivery of the infant's head, but before delivery of the shoulders, the nose, mouth, and pharynx should be thoroughly suctioned with a DeLee suction catheter. Suctioning of the upper airway should be repeated as the infant is placed under a radiant warmer. The trachea should then be visualized with a laryngoscope and the meconium aspirated by direct suctioning through an endotracheal tube. Suctioning is repeated until no more meconium is present. The infant then may be ventilated with positive pressure as indicated. Failure to clear the trachea before assisted or spontaneous ventilation will disseminate meconium through the airways.

Complications of Asphyxia

Infants who were successfully resuscitated at birth should have continuous monitoring of vital signs, blood gases, fluid status, and clinical condition because of the possible complications of seizures, hypoxic-ischemic encephalopathy, intracranial hemorrhage, inappropriate antidiuretic hormone (ADH) secretion, persistent fetal circulation, ischemic cardiomyopathy, hypovolemia or shock, necrotizing enterocolitis, renal failure, or coagulopathy.

NEONATAL EMERGENCIES

Seizures

Seizures in neonates may represent primary central nervous system disease or a systemic or metabolic disorder. Experimental evidence suggests seizure activity itself may adversely affect the growing brain.

Types of Seizures

Subtle. These consist of ocular movements, facial, oral, and lingual movements, and respiratory manifestations such as apnea or stertorous breathing.

Tonic. These appear as decerebrate and decorticate posturing.

Multifocal clonic seizures. These are initially noted in one limb and migrate to another part of the body.

Focal seizures. These are well localized and accompanied by specific sharp activity on the EEG.

Myoclonic seizures. These seizures are expressed as jerking movements of the upper or lower extremities.

Tonic seizures are more common in premature infants. Multifocal and focal seizures are seen more commonly in full-term infants, while subtle seizures occur both in premature and full-term neonates. It is important to distinguish seizures from tremors or jitteriness, which may be seen in infants who have hypocalcemia, hypoglycemia, or drug withdrawal. Tremors are uniform fine movements which respond to sensory stimuli and do not occur spontaneously. They are not accompanied by eye, oral, or buccal movements.

Causes of Seizures

Hypoxic-ischemic encephalopathy. This is the most common cause of seizures. The seizures occur between 6 and 18 h of life. In full-term neonates there may be cerebral contusion, water-shed infarct, posterior fossa hematoma, or subarachnoid or subdural hemorrhage. In premature infants, hypoxic injury often results in periventricular-intraventricular hemorrhage. This type of seizure has the poorest prognosis of all seizures.

Metabolic disturbances. These are seen in premature infants and include hypoglycemia, hypocalcemia, hypomagnesemia, hypernatremia, and hyponatremia. Hypoglycemia, hypocalcemia, and hypomagnesemia are often associated with premature infants with perinatal asphyxia. Hypernatremia occurs in neonates with dehydration secondary to excessive fluid losses or treatment with large doses of sodium bicarbonate. Hyponatremia may be seen secondary to inappropriate ADH secretion or acute volume overload. Inborn errors of amino acid metabolism may present as seizures.

Meningitis or encephalitis. Seizures secondary to bacterial meningitis and encephalitis are associated with the TORCH complex (*to*xoplasmosis, *r*ubella, *c*ytomegalovirus infection and *h*erpes simplex infection) or Coxsackie B encephalitis.

Developmental abnormalities. Congenital hydrocephalus, microcephaly, and multiple congenital anomalies may cause seizures.

Drug withdrawal. Drug withdrawal rarely presents as seizures.

Pyridoxine deficiency or dependency. This condition occurs rarely but must be considered in neonatal seizures unresponsive to standard therapy.

Maternal anesthesia. A rare cause of seizures is inadvertent fetal scalp infiltration of maternal anesthetic agents.

Diagnosis of Seizures

A careful history, including intrapartum monitoring data and a physical examination, is essential when considering drug withdrawal, birth asphyxia, or metabolic disorders as a cause of seizures. A lumbar puncture with analysis of cell count and a Gram stain along with blood specimens for culture, sugar, calcium, and BUN should be obtained. The skull x-ray, echoencephalogram, and EEG can be obtained after seizures have been controlled. In a full-term infant a CT scan of the head may be necessary, as an echoencephalogram may not provide adequate visualization of the subarachnoid space or posterior fossa.

Treatment of Seizures

Treatment should be initiated while awaiting results of laboratory data. An intravenous access route should be established immediately and the airway maintained; assisted ventilation should be initiated if apnea persists. Hypoglycemia and hypocalcemia should be treated as stated earlier in the section under resuscitation. Hypomagnesemia is often associated with hypocalcemia and should be treated by intravenous administration of 2 to 4 mL of a 2% magnesium sulfate solution.

The anticonvulsant drugs used most frequently include phenobarbital and diphenylhydantoin. The loading dose of phenobarbital is 20 mg/kg intravenously, given slowly over 5 min, and the maintenance dose is 5 mg/(kg·day) IM or PO in two divided doses. In refractory cases, diphenylhydantoin may be administered as a loading dose of 20 mg/kg given slowly over 5 min followed by a maintenance dose of 3 to 5 mg/(kg·day) intravenously, in two divided doses. If seizures persist, paraldehyde (2 to 4 mL of a 4% solution) may be administered intravenously, using a glass syringe directly attached to the IV catheter, slowly over 10 min. Diazepam (Valium) is recommended for status epilepticus, as long as ventilation and blood pressure are supported. The dose is 0.01 mg/kg administered slowly and intravenously.

Diaphragmatic Hernia

A defect or failure of development through the posterolateral parts of the diaphragm at the foramen of Bochdalek or retrosternally at the foramen of Morgagni allows herniation of the gut into the chest cavity. Right-sided Bochdalek hernias are less common than those on the left. The defect occurs in 1 out of every 2200 births. It occurs equally in male and female full-term infants and rarely in prematures. Eighty percent of the hernias occur posterolaterally and do not have a peritoneal sac. Associated anomalies with diaphragmatic hernias include anencephaly, Arnold Chiari malformation, congenital heart disease, genitourinary anomalies, esophageal atresia, omphalocele, hydronephrosis, and cystic kidneys. Frequently the lungs are hypoplastic bilaterally.

Fifty percent of fetuses with diaphragmatic hernia will be unable to swallow or will have difficulty swallowing and the conditions will be associated with polyhydramnios. Ultrasound is able to detect the condition in utero and amniography confirms it.

Clinical and Radiographic Findings

Clinical findings are referrable to the respiratory and digestive tract. The chest is large while the abdomen is scaphoid. Bowel sounds are heard in the left chest and the heart is displaced to the right. Dyspnea, cyanosis, retractions, and vomiting are proportional to the amount of abdominal viscera herniated into the thorax. Radiologic study will reveal airfilled loops of bowel in the chest cavity and an absent diaphragmatic margin. The heart and lungs will be displaced.

Management

The infant should be intubated immediately and little or no attempt should be made to ventilate with a mask. High frequency and low pressures are used to ventilate and to prevent reactive respiratory acidosis and hypercapnia, which are potentially conducive to the development of pulmonary hypertension. A large-caliber (no. 10 French) tube should be placed in the stomach with low continuous

suction applied. An umbilical artery catheter is useful to monitor blood gases and pH. Any acidemia should be corrected and the pH should be maintained above 7.0; IV fluids should be given and the patient kept warm.

The outcome depends on the severity of lung hypoplasia and respiratory insufficiency present. One-fifth of all patients with this diagnosis die within the first hour of life. Mortality is 50 percent despite early diagnosis, transfer to a major medical center, and treatment. The outlook is better in those patients who survive after 24 h of age. Morgagni hernias, if they do not affect cardiac output, generally have a better prognosis than Bochdalek hernias. Common complications are pneumothorax, persistent fetal circulation, and overdistention of hypoplastic lungs and chylothorax.

Tracheoesophageal Fistula

A defect or absence of arrest in the separation of the trachea from the esophagus results in a persistent channel connecting the trachea and the esophagus. There are five types of tracheoesophageal fistulas (TEF) which are descriptive of the malformations possible: (1) esophageal atresia with a distal communication between the trachea and the esophagus, which occurs in 85 percent of all cases; (2) isolated esophageal atresia, occurring in 8 percent of all cases; (3) isolated TEF, occurring at a rate of 4 percent; (4) esophageal atresia with a proximal TEF, with an incidence of less than 1 percent of all cases; and (5) esophageal atresia with a double TEF, also occurring in less than 1 percent.

TEFs occur in 1 out of every 4500 births. One-third of the affected infants weigh less than 2500 g. The smaller the infant with TEF, the greater the number of other associated anomalies. Congenital heart malformations, vertebral anomalies, imperforate anus, and radial dysplasia are commonly associated with a TEF.

Signs and Symptoms

A history of polyhydramnios, early respiratory distress, bubbling mucus, coughing, and choking spells are noted. The neonate with a proximal blind pouch will be unable to handle his or her oral secretions so that there will be excessive drooling and regurgitation of feedings. The bowel becomes filled with air and the abdomen appears distended because of the communication between the trachea and esophagus. Rarely, the infant will present with pneumonia as a consequence of gastric secretion contaminating the lungs by way of the fistula.

Diagnosis

A catheter than cannot be passed more than 12 to 13 cm down the gastrointestinal tract is diagnostic of esophageal atresia. An x-ray may show the airfilled proximal pouch, and if the catheter is left in place it may coil in the proximal esophagus.

Management

It is important to provide respiratory support by assisted ventilation, if needed, and to correct acidosis, before any surgical repair can be undertaken. A plastic sump catheter should be left in the pouch and connected to constant, low-pressure suction. The patient should be maintained in the reverse Trendelenburg's or semi-Fowler's position to prevent further reflux of gastric secretions through the fistula into the trachea. Intravenous fluids and antibiotics are indicated. Other coexistent problems such as a heart defect should be palliated.

The majority (79 percent) of infants with TEF survive. A small number die prior to surgery (7 percent), as do some after surgery (6 percent). Late deaths (7 percent) occur as well. Complications of surgery are pneumonia, atelectasis, anastomotic leak, apnea, and tracheomalacia.

Pulmonary Air Leaks

Air leaks from the lung are a common occurrence in the neonatal intensive care unit. The air tends to collect in pockets and may present as a spectrum that includes pulmonary interstitial emphysema, pneumomediastinum, pneumopericardium, and pneumothorax.

According to Madansky, et al., asymptomatic pneumothorax was found in 1 to 2 percent of newborns studied consecutively with serial x-rays. The frequency of air leaks is related to the use of continuous positive airway pressure, positive end-expiratory pressure, mechanical ventilation, and cardiopulmonary resuscitation. Uneven ventilation caused by aspirated blood, mucus, meconium, and amniotic fluid debris can result in an air leak. Atelectasis, poor ventilation, and air trapping are common predisposing factors. The premature, low-birth-weight infant with surfactant deficiency has a high incidence of air leaks (27 percent), as does the newborn with meconium aspiration syndrome (41 percent).

Signs and Symptoms

The signs and symptoms of an air leak are those of respiratory distress. Grunting respirations, intercostal, sternal, and subcostal retractions may be seen. Cyanosis, an elevated respiratory rate, and elevated heart rate are common. Percussion and auscultation of the chest will reveal decreased breath sounds on the affected side of a pneumothorax, distant heart sounds, and a shift of the mediastinum. A high-intensity lamp may aid in the diagnosis. The light source is placed against the chest, causing the affected side to glow or transilluminate. A chest x-ray is diagnostic. Accuracy can be improved with a cross table lateral film of the chest taken along with anteroposterior and lateral views.

Treatment

A pneumothorax that is less than 20 percent of the volume of the affected side may be observed clinically and with serial radiographic studies every 4 h. Any pneumothorax with severe respiratory distress will need emergency treatment. When there is mediastinal shift and cardiovascular collapse, rapid decompression at the fourth intercostal space with a 21-gauge needle attached to a three-way stopcock and a large syringe can be lifesaving. A chest tube can be introduced by grasping the tube with a hemostat and passing it through a subcutaneous tunnel and hole in the intercostal space created by blunt surgical dissection. This technique will prevent the occurrence of lung perforation that may result

when the chest tube is introduced with a steel trocar. The chest tube should remain as long as the neonate receives positive pressure ventilation.

Gastroschisis and Omphalocele

An omphalocele is a defect in the umbilical ring which allows the intestines to protrude out of the abdominal cavity in a sac. A gastroschisis is a defect in the abdominal wall that allows the antenatal evisceration of abdominal structures. There is no sac present. There is some controversy as to the exact embryology of the two conditions.

Omphaloceles are found in 1 in 6000 to 10,000 births while gastroschisis occurs twice as frequently in the newborn population. Omphaloceles have double the rate (37 percent) of anomalies associated with it. Trisomy 13–15 and 16–18 and cardiac malformations are frequently found. Three specific syndromes are associated with omphalocele: the upper midline pentalogy of Cantrell, Haller, and Ravitch (sternal, ventral, diaphragmatic, pericardial, and cardiac defects); the lower midline syndrome (vesicointestinal fissure); and the Beckwith-Wiedemann syndrome (macroglossia, visceromegaly, and hypoglycemia).

The rate of other anomalies occurring with gastroschisis is about 18 percent, with intestinal atresias associated in 78 percent of the cases. Meckel's diverticulum, hydronephrosis, and patent ductus arteriosus are also reported.

Management

Emergency management of the two conditions is not different, especially when the sac in an omphalocele is ruptured. The eviscerated bowel should be wrapped in saline-soaked gauze and placed in a plastic bag to protect it from hypothermia and evaporative losses. A nasogastric tube should be secured to decompress the intestines. Rapid infusion of 20 mL/kg of 5% lactate may be necessary to restore vital signs, after which the infusion should be adjusted to maintain a urine output of at least 2 mL/(kg·h). Antibiotics, usually ampicillin, are routinely give intravenously.

Primary closure is the treatment of choice and is often accomplished within hours after birth. When the defect is large, a Silastic silo is used but survival nonetheless correlates with rapid closure and removal of the prosthesis.

Complications include gastroesophageal reflux, malabsorption, diarrhea, dehydration, and failure to thrive. The mortality of omphalocele is between 25 and 30 percent, due largely to congenital heart disease and sepsis, while death in patients with gastroschisis is associated with intestinal atresia.

Necrotizing Enterocolitis

Necrotizing enterocolitis (NEC) is a disease entity that affects the asphyxiated or stressed premature infant of less than 2000-g weight. Full-term newborns with congenital heart disease and dehydration have been reported to have this condition.

The exact cause of NEC remains unknown, and it is likely that there are multiple factors that can cause ischemia to the bowel wall and thus predispose it to infection. Recent papers have focused on hypertonic feeding solutions producing damage to mucosal epithelium of the intestine.

Signs and Symptoms

The signs and symptoms seen in decreasing frequency are as follows: abdominal distention, 90 percent; gastric distention, 81 percent; vomiting and regurgitation, 70 percent; apnea, 66 percent; gastrointestinal bleeding, 63 percent; and lethargy, 54 percent. Other signs are abdominal tenderness and redness and reducing substances in the stool.

Diagnosis

An anteroposterior, cross table lateral and upright view of the abdomen will aid in the radiographic diagnosis. Nonspecific findings are distention, air-fluid levels, and separation of intestinal loops suggesting mural edema. Pneumatosis intestinalis is the radiographic hallmark. Its presence indicates gas in the bowel wall and is present in 90 percent of cases. Portal venous gas is an ominous sign and pneumoperitoneum indicates perforation of the bowel.

Management

Medical management requires that the patient receive nothing by mouth, and gastric decompression. Cultures of blood, urine, and CSF should be obtained and systemic antibiotics started. Optimal vital signs should be maintained with liberal use of crystalloids and Plasmanate. Blood should be given when anemia is present. Respiratory support may be required, and any acidosis should be corrected. Patients with early NEC should have close clinical observation and serial x-rays to look for signs of gangrene or intestinal perforation, which will require surgical resection. Complications of NEC are bowel stricture fistula, abscess, malabsorption, and failure to thrive.

The Cyanotic Newborn

Cyanosis in the neonate may be central or peripheral. Central cyanosis is defined as cyanosis of the tongue, mucous membranes, and peripheral skin in the presence of 3 g or more of reduced hemoglobin. Peripheral cyanosis is defined as blue discoloration confined to the skin of the extremities; the arterial saturation will be greater than 94 percent. Peripheral cyanosis is common in the neonate and may persist for days. It is usually due to vasomotor instability secondary to a cold environment.

Causes of Central Cyanosis

Normal newborn infants have a P_{O_2} of around 50 mmHg by 5 to 10 min of age; hence it is pathologic for central cyanosis to persist longer than 20 min after birth.

Cyanotic heart disease. Congenital heart disease can present with cyanosis secondary to intracardiac right-to-left shunt including transposition of the great vessels, tricuspid atresia, truncus arteriosus, tetralogy of Fallot, and total anomalous venous return with obstruction (*Note:* all begin with ''t''), pulmonary atresia, and preductal coarctation.

Lung disease associated with cyanosis. These conditions include severe hyaline membrane disease, pneumonia, meconium aspiration syndrome, and persistent fetal circulation due to pneu-

monia or asphyxia. Mechanical interference with lung function by air leaks (pneumothorax), diaphragmatic hernia, lobar emphysema, or mucus plugs also cause cyanosis.

Central nervous system disorders. Intracerebral hemorrhage when severe may be associated with shock and cyanosis.

Polycythemia. The increased viscosity and stagnation of blood may produce apparent cyanosis.

Shock and sepsis. These lead to alveolar hypoventilation.

Methemoglobinemia. This is due to reduced oxygen-carrying capacity of the blood because of abnormal hemoglobin.

Diagnostic Approach to Central Cyanosis

Physical examination. Neonates with cyanosis secondary to cyanotic heart disease rarely have respiratory symptoms other than tachypnea. A murmur may be present. Neonates with lung disease producing cyanosis have respiratory distress, grunting, tachypnea, and sternal and intercostal retractions. The cyanotic infant with central nervous system disturbances or sepsis has apnea, bradycardia, lethargy, and seizures. Neonates with methemoglobinemia have minimal distress in spite of their cyanotic appearance.

Blood gas profile and response to 100% O₂ breathing. The ''hyperoxia test'' (the response in P_{O_2} to 100% oxygen breathing) may be of use to distinguish heart disease from other causes of cyanosis. The neonate with cyanotic heart disease will not increase the P_{O_2} because of the right-to-left shunting of the circulation. In the neonate with lung disease, there will be an increase in P_{O_2}. The neonate with persistent fetal circulation, central nervous system disorders, polycythemia, sepsis, and shock will increase the P_{O_2}. No response will also be elicited in the neonate with methemoglobinemia. When a specimen of blood is exposed to air it turns pink in all the conditions described above, except in methemoglobinemia, where it remains chocolate-colored.

Radiographic examination. The chest radiograph may demonstrate pulmonary oligemia with normal heart size in tetralogy of Fallot and pulmonary or tricuspid atresia, while pulmonary vascularity is increased in transposition of great vessels, truncus arteriosus, anomalous pulmonary venous return, and hypoplastic left heart. Neonates with lung disease have radiographs characteristic of the underlying disease.

Electrocardiogram and echocardiogram. These two studies will be useful in diagnosing cyanotic heart disease. Right ventricular hypertrophy may be seen in lung disease with associated pulmonary hypertension.

Management of Cyanotic Infants

Most of the cyanotic heart diseases are amenable to palliative or corrective surgery. Infants with severe or complete right ventricular outflow obstruction are dependent on the postnatal patency of the ductus arteriosus for maintenance of adequate pulmonary blood flow and systemic oxygenation. Short-term infusions of prostaglandin E_1(PGE₁) 0.05 to 0.1 µg/(kg·min) in these infants have allowed stabilization prior to surgery.

Congestive Cardiac Failure

Heart failure in the newborn infant is caused not only by structural heart disease but also by other systemic disorders.

Causes of Heart Failure

These include (1) structural heart disease (most common are transposition of the great vessels and hypoplastic left heart syndromes), (2) heart disease without structural abnormalities (myocarditis, cardiac arrhythmias, glycogen storage disease, and endocardial fibroelastosis), (3) respiratory disease with patent ductus arteriosus with left-to-right shunt, (4) anemia (hemoglobin less than 3.5 g/100 mL), (5) polycythemia, (6) cerebral arterial venous malformation, and (7) sepsis.

Signs and Symptoms

The most frequent symptoms of cardiac failure are feeding difficulties, tachypnea, increased sweating, tachycardia, rales and rhonchi, liver enlargement, and cardiomegaly. Less common signs and symptoms are ascites, gallop rhythm, pulsus alternans, or an increase in central venous pressure. Peripheral edema is exceedingly rare. A clear distinction between right heart failure (characterized by liver enlargement, tachycardia, dependent edema) and left heart failure (cardiomegaly, rales, tachypnea, and tachycardia) is not as obvious in the neonate as in the older child or adult.

Management

It is essential to closely monitor cardiac and respiratory rates and blood pressure. Blood gas levels should be monitored frequently for early detection of hypoxemia or acidosis.

Fluid intake. This should be restricted to 100 mL/(kg·day) and should be adjusted depending on the weight, liver size, and urine output. Electrolytes should be monitored closely. Anemia should be corrected with packed red cell transfusions.

Posture. The neonate should be on a 10 to 30° incline inside the incubator.

Digoxin. Infants with heart failure should receive digitalis unless the heart rate is below 100 beats per minute. The digitalizing dose of digoxin is 0.03 mg/kg PO for term neonates. For parenteral digitalization, two-thirds of the oral dose should be given. For digitalization, half the calculated digitalizing dose should be given initially, a fourth in 8 h, and another fourth in 8 h; start maintenance 12 h after the last digitalizing dose. The maintenance dose is one-fourth of the total digitalizing dose in two divided doses.

Diuretics. Furosemide (Lasix) is the drug with the most rapid response and should be used intravenously (1 to 3 mg/kg). Maintenance therapy with hydrochlorothiazide (Diuril) and spironolactone (Aldactone) to help conserve potassium may be necessary.

β-Adrenergic drugs. Neonates with severe heart failure from left-to-right shunts with cardiogenic shock and bradycardia may require β-adrenergic drugs for ionotropic action. Isoproterenol (Is-uprel) may be infused at 0.1 μg/(kg·min), increasing to 0.4 μg/(kg·min) until the heart rate is 140 beats per minute. Dopamine is useful in hypotensive shock and should be infused at 5 μg to 15 μg/(kg·min). Both medications should be discontinued slowly while monitoring heart rate and blood pressure.

BIBLIOGRAPHY

Apgar V: A proposal for new method of evaluation of the newborn infant. *Anesth Analg* 32:260, 1953.

Brown EG, Sweet AY: Neonatal necrotizing enterocolitis. *Pediatr Clin North Am* 29:1149, 1982.

Cockburn F, Brown JK, Belton NR, et al: Neonatal convulsions associated with primary disturbance of calcium, phosphorus and magnesium metabolism. *Arch Dis Child* 48:99, 1973.

Czerniak A, Dreznik Z, Neuman Y, et al: Chylothorax complicating repair of a left diaphragmatic hernia in a neonate. *Thorax* 36:701, 1981.

Gregory GA, Gooding CA, Phibbs RH, et al: Meconium aspiration in infants: A prospective study. *J Pediatr* 85:807, 1974.

Grosfeld JL, Dawes L, Weber TR: Congenital abdominal wall defects: Current management and survival. *Surg Clin North Am* 61:1037, 1981.

Harrison MR, De Lorimer AA: Congenital diaphragmatic hernia. *Surg Clin North Am* 61:1023, 1981.

Hertzlinger RA, Kandall SR, Vaughan HG, Jr.: Neonatal seizures associated with narcotic withdrawal. *J Pediatr* 91:638, 1977.

Heymann MA, Abraham MR: Ductus arteriosus dilatation by prostaglandin E$_1$ in infants with pulmonary atresia. *Pediatrics* 59:325, 1977.

Holder TM, Ashcraft KW: Developments in the care of patients with esophageal atresia and TEF. *Surg Clin North Am* 61:1051, 1981.

Lees MH, Jolly J: Severe congenital methemoglobinemia in an infant. *Lancet* 2:1147, 1957.

Lewis AB, Takahashi M, Lurie PR: Administration of prostaglandin E in neonates with critical congenital cardiac defect. *J Pediatr* 93:481, 1978.

Madansky DL, Lawson EE, Chernik V, et al: Pneumothorax and other forms of air leak in newborns. *Am Rev Resp Dis* 120:729, 1979.

O'Callaghan JD, Saunders NR, Chatrath RR, et al: The management of neonatal posterolateral diaphragmatic hernia. *Ann Thorac Surg* 33:174, 1981.

O'Neill JA: Neonatal necrotizing enterocolitis. *Surg Clin North Am* 61:1013, 1981.

Ostheimer GW: Resuscitation of the newborn infant. *Clin Perinatol* 9:177, 1982.

Pfenninger J, Bossi E, Biesold J, et al: Treatment of pneumothorax, pneumopericardium and pneumomediastinum. *Helv Paediatr Acta* 37:353, 1982.

Randolph J: Omphalocele and gastroschisis: Different entities, similar therapeutic goals. *South Med J* 75:1575, 1982.

Roberton NRC, Hallidie-Smith KA, Davis JA: Severe respiratory distress syndrome mimicking cyanotic heart disease in term babies. *Lancet* 2:1108, 1967.

Stevens DC, Fenton LJ, Wellman LR: Neonatal resuscitation. *South Med J* 34:15, 1981.

Volpe, JJ: Neonatal seizures. *Clin Perinatol* 4:43, 1977.

Wijesinha SS: Neonatal necrotizing enterocolitis: New thoughts for the eighties. *Ann R Coll Surg Engl* 64:406, 1982.

Williams R: Congenital diaphragmatic hernia: A review. *Heart Lung* 11:532, 1982.

CHAPTER 76
SUDDEN INFANT
DEATH SYNDROME

Carol D. Berkowitz

Sudden death may affect persons of any age, but it is especially devastating when it affects previously healthy individuals. Nearly 10,000 infants succumb yearly to sudden infant death syndrome (SIDS), also known as "crib death." An understanding of SIDS is essential for the emergency physician so that he or she can recognize the syndrome, initiate resuscitation, manage the "near-miss" SIDS, and counsel the family of the victim.

PATHOPHYSIOLOGY

Although over 70 different theories have been proposed, the main disturbance appears to be with the infant's ventilatory response. Death is due to respiratory rather than cardiac arrest, and some potential SIDS victims may be successfully resuscitated with ventilation alone. Arrhythmias probably occur only as a terminal event and prolonged QT syndrome is a very rare association.

Information implicating ventilation and hypoxemia has been obtained from two sources: autopsies of infants who succumbed to SIDS and studies of those who did not—so-called "near-miss" SIDS. This latter group represents infants who were found limp, cyanotic, pale and lifeless, without any respiratory effort, but who were successfully resuscitated.

Autopsies of SIDS victims reveal pathologic changes consistent with long-standing hypoxemia. Smooth muscle in small pulmonary arteries is thickened and extends into the periphery of the lung. Right ventricular hypertrophy may be noted. The brainstem shows astrogliosis. Intrathoracic petechiae and pulmonary edema indicate sustained perimortal hypoxemia.

Victims of near-miss SIDS are more prone to apnea. They experience cessation of breathing for 20 s or more, with cyanosis, pallor, or collapse. Newborns appear to have a unique response to hypoxemia, consisting of a brief increase in ventilation followed by respiratory depression. This is outgrown in most infants, but may persist in the SIDS victim. Additionally, studies of near-miss SIDS reveal that these infants demonstrate (1) hypoventilation and chronic hypoxemia; (2) a depressed ventilatory response to CO_2 breathing; (3) prolonged sleep apnea; (4) short frequent bouts of apnea; (5) increased periodic breathing (characterized by repeated cycles of 3-s pauses in breathing followed by normal breathing for less than 20 s); (6) a combination of the above and obstructive apnea. Obstructive apnea occurs in response to nasal occlusion,

and is an important contributor to SIDS in infants with upper respiratory infections. Infantile botulism may be responsible for the apnea in 5 to 10 percent of SIDS.

Young monkeys who receive a cold or wet stimulus to the area of the face supplied by the trigeminal nerve stop breathing and respiration fails to resume when the stimulus is removed. This "dive reflex" may be important in SIDS, as well.

Lastly, the young infant has few fatigue-resistant fibers in his or her respiratory muscles. The work of breathing increases during active sleep and with a respiratory infection. It is possible that this increased workload leads to respiratory muscle fatigue and subsequent apnea.

CLINICAL PICTURE

The diagnosis of SIDS is confirmed by autopsy, but there are many clinical and epidemiologic features which characterize the syndrome. Victims range in age from 1 month to 1 year, with peaks at $2\frac{1}{2}$ months and at 4 months. The infant frequently has been premature, or small-for-gestational age. The syndrome is rare in the first month of life, probably because the neonate has a better anaerobic capacity for survival, and with a gasp may be able to raise his or her arterial P_{O_2} over 20 torr and continue breathing. Thirty to fifty percent of the infants who are otherwise healthy have some infection, usually of the upper respiratory tract, at the time of the event. Otitis media and gastroenteritis have also been associated with SIDS. Infected infants tend to be older than non-infected infants, and males outnumber females in the infected group by 2:1. The sex ratio is equal in the noninfected group. There is a disproportionate number of babies from the lower socioeconomic group, though this is true for deaths in infancy from all causes. Mothers are frequently under 20 years, unwed, smoke, use drugs (particularly methadone), and have made few prenatal and postpartum visits. The event is more likely to occur during the winter months, and when the infant is asleep.

The sequence of events prior to the apnea may be a clue to the etiology. If the infant had stiffened or exhibited clonic movements the apnea may be postictal apnea following a seizure. With a seizure the infant is frequently awake prior to becoming apneic. Gastroesophageal reflux may lead to apnea, and also may occur in the awake infant following a feeding. A history of an upper respiratory infection followed by a paroxysmal cough with an apneic episode would be suggestive of pertussis. Hypoglycemia may also be associated with apnea, with or without a seizure.

Although it is an infrequent cause of SIDS, there are case reports of SIDS and near-miss SIDS attributed to child abuse. Child abuse is the diagnosed cause of death in 2000 cases a year. The presence of bruises, long bone fractures, internal hemorrhages, evidence of physical neglect, or trauma around the nares would be suggestive of abuse. A history of other unexplained infant deaths or a history inconsistent with the usual events surrounding a SIDS death may raise the suspicion of abuse.

MANAGEMENT

The usual scenario in the emergency department is the distraught mother who had fed her infant several hours earlier, went to check the sleeping infant, and found the baby blue and lifeless. Occasionally, resuscitation may be initiated by the parents; frequently the paramedics are summoned. The infant brought into the emergency department may have been revived or may need further CPR.

Resuscitatable Infant

The responsiveness of an infant to resuscitative efforts is probably most influenced by the duration of the arrest. Some infants present with evidence of livedo reticularis, blood pH of 6, and box-car venous pooling in the fundi. Attempts to resuscitate such an infant are usually unrewarding. Other infants will have been revived at home and one may be confronted by a completely well-appearing infant with a history of apnea. The physician may be uncertain of any serious preceding event. The finding of irregular respiration or poor muscle tone on physical examination would be evidence of a near-miss SIDS. Even in the absence of such findings, the child should be admitted for a minimum of 24 to 48 h of apnea monitoring. Occasionally parents may have misinterpreted acrocyanosis, postprandial regurgitation, or color changes with stooling as an episode of apnea. The burden of proof is, however, with the physician, and this infant too should be observed.

The child who is not fully revived in the field should receive the benefit of vigorous CPR, unless signs of irreversible death are apparent. Frequently the heart will resume beating even after prolonged arrest. The infant heart is a remarkably resistant organ, and may be revived after irreversible brain damage. If the resuscitation is successful, the infant should be admitted for further management and evaluation.

Near-Miss SIDS

The evaluation of the infant with near-miss SIDS is designed to rule out treatable causes of apnea and to determine if, in the absence of these other causes, the infant is at risk for recurrences of SIDS, an event reported in from 20 to 100 percent of near-miss SIDS.

The evaluation of the infant should include a complete history, particularly of the event itself, and take into account the perinatal and epidemiologic factors associated with SIDS. A history of other infant deaths should be obtained because of the familial incidence

of SIDS, or the possibility of child abuse. The physical examination should be complete with special emphasis on the neurological evaluation. The initial laboratory assessment should include a CBC, serum electrolytes, blood sugar, calcium, phosphate, magnesium, and a 12-lead ECG. A septic workup including blood cultures, cerebrospinal fluid analysis, urine culture, and chest x-ray is indicated in most cases. Stool should be sent for clostridial culture and botulinum toxin. Other studies should be obtained if suggested by the history and physical examination; these include serum and urine amino acids, sleep and awake EEGs, skull x-rays, barium swallow, and CT scan.

Apnea monitoring should be carried out in the hospital. Certain tertiary care centers are equipped to evaluate all near-miss SIDS for evidence of ventilatory abnormalities using responses to CO_2 breathing, nasal obstruction, diminished FI_{O_2}, and patterns of periodic breathing to determine which infant is at risk for further episodes of apnea.

Home Monitoring

Infants found to be at risk for recurrent apnea, and those with normal ventilatory responses but at epidemiologic risk may be sent home on theophylline preparations with monitoring devices. Theophylline is used frequently in treating apnea of prematurity, but its efficacy in the prevention of SIDS is unclear. The consensus of parents and physicians is that home apnea monitoring not only reduces parental anxiety but also reduces mortality to 0 to 10 percent.

Devices used for home monitoring usually measure chest wall movement. In infants with obstructive apnea, in whom the chest wall continues to move but the airway is occluded, the addition of a cardiac monitor to detect bradycardia is useful. Home monitoring does not mean simply supplying a family with a mechanical device. It involves the development of a medical team to support the family, interpret any episodes of apnea, and decide when home monitoring can be discontinued. Technicians who are available 24 h a day to maintain the equipment are also required.

THE SIDS VICTIM

The management of the nonresuscitatable SIDS infant and his or her family is equally challenging for the physician. Frequently, valiant though unsuccessful efforts are carried out in the emergency department, or the infant is revived briefly, only to succumb after several hours in the intensive care unit.

The major responsibility of the physician is then to notify, counsel, and educate the family. In most jurisdictions, victims of sudden and unexplained deaths must be referred to the coroner's office where autopsies are performed at the coroner's discretion. If the physician believes the infant is a victim of SIDS, the family should be so advised, but told that the final confirmation awaits the autopsy report. The emergency physician should reassure the family about their lack of responsibility for the infant's death and assuage their feelings of guilt. He or she should then serve as a facilitator maintaining contact with the family to advise them of the autopsy results. The hospital chaplain or social worker may provide additional support, but the physician's empathy is very supportive to the family. Most communities have organizations for parents of SIDS victims and information about these organizations can be obtained from the National Foundation for Sudden Infant Death, 1501 Broadway, New York, New York 10036. Parents should be referred to these organizations.

BIBLIOGRAPHY

Berger D: Child abuse simulating ''near-miss'' sudden infant death syndrome. *J Pediatr* 95:554, 1979.

Kelly DH, Shannon DC: Sudden infant death syndrome and near sudden infant death syndrome: A review of the literature, 1964–1982. *Pediatr Clin North Am* 29:1241, 1982.

Merritt TA, Bauer WI, Hasselmeyer EG: Sudden infant death syndrome: The role of the emergency room physician. *Clin Pediatr* 14:1095, 1975.

Shannon DC, Kelly DH: SIDS and Near-SIDS, Part 1. *N Engl J Med* 306:959, 1982.

Shannon DC, Kelly DH: SIDS and Near-SIDS, Part 2. *N Engl J Med* 306:1022, 1982.

CHAPTER 77
PEDIATRIC
CARDIOPULMONARY
RESUSCITATION

Robert C. Luten

The purpose of this chapter is to review the ABCs of cardiopulmonary resuscitation in children. Emphasis will be placed on pertinent differences between adults and children. Some subjects that are common to both groups have been reviewed elsewhere and will not be mentioned.

The most striking difference between adult and pediatric arrest is related to etiology. Adults, mainly because of coronary artery disease, tend to have a *primary* cardiac arrest. Adult advanced cardiac life support (ACLS) is based on this principle and heavily emphasizes recognition and management of cardiac disease. Children tend to have cardiac arrests *secondary* to other causes, mainly respiratory, and to a lesser extent shock syndromes. Attention to this basic difference can not only prevent cardiopulmonary arrest in sick children, but it also underlies many of the principles of successful pediatric resuscitation. Almost equally important for the emergency physician is that the similarities between the two groups be recognized, i.e., when the same principles of adult resuscitation apply to children. This actually holds true the majority of the time.

Besides these fundamental differences another type of difference distinguishes children from adults, and that is that children differ among themselves. What may be an appropriate drug dose for a 6-month-old is excessive for a 1-month-old and not enough for a 5-year-old. The same is true for many other aspects of resuscitation, e.g., endotracheal tube sizes, tidal volumes necessary for ventilation, cardiac compression rates, respiratory rates, etc. These are age-related differences which are not seen in adults. Many physicians perceive this type of difference as the major stumbling block to mastering successful resuscitation in children. In the section on Management Guidelines suggestions will be presented that can virtually eliminate age-related differences as problems.

In summary, pediatric cardiopulmonary resuscitation will be reviewed with emphasis on fundamental differences between children and adults, the similarities, and age-related differences. This chapter will follow the decision tree outlined in Figure 77-1.

AIRWAY

Obviously a child's airway is much smaller than an adult's and also varies in size, depending upon age. There are also some

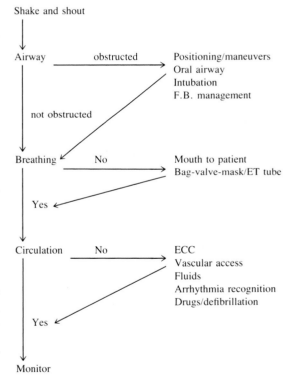

Figure 77-1. ABCs of cardiopulmonary resuscitation in children. (*Adapted from Fleisher G and Ludwig S (eds): Pediatric Emergency Medicine, Baltimore, Williams & Wilkins, 1983.*)

functional differences, more pronounced in the infant or young child, which must be addressed:

1. The airway lies higher and more anterior in the child's neck than in the adult. This is important when considering intubation.
2. The child has a prominent occiput and a hypotonic block of mandibular tissue. As will be demonstrated, unless these factors are considered when positioning a pediatric patient, airway obstruction may result.

Positioning/Maneuvers

The unconscious pediatric patient in a supine position is at risk for airway obstruction for the following anatomical reasons:

1. In the supine position the prominent occiput of the child causes flexion of the neck on the chest, occluding the airway. This can be corrected by *mild* extension of the head to the sniffing position. Overextension or hyperextension, as is recommended for adults, will cause obstruction. The sniffing position can be maintained by placing a towel or other object beneath the occiput (see Fig. 77-2).

2. Despite good head position the child's hypotonic mandibular

tissues may still occlude the airway posteriorly. This can be relieved by a chin lift or jaw thrust which elevates the mandible anteriorly and separates the tongue from the posterior pharyngeal wall. If these maneuvers are unsuccessful an oral airway or endotracheal tube should be considered (see Fig. 77-3).

Oral Airway

Oral airways are not universally accepted in pediatrics. However, they may be useful in the patient who does not respond to maneuvers to remove the mandibular tissues from the posterior pha-

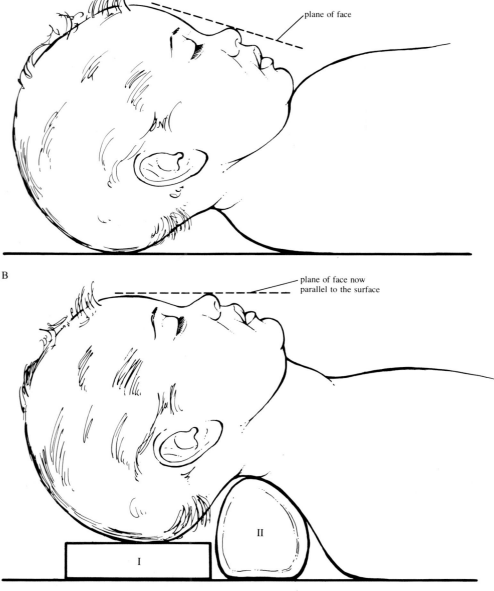

Figure 77-2. (*A*) Airway at high risk for occlusion. Flexion of the neck on the thorax is caused by a prominent occiput. (*B*) Sniffing position, which gives maximum possibility for a patent airway. Note the mild extension of the head. Flexion is now corrected by elevation of the head (I) and/or posterior neck support (II).

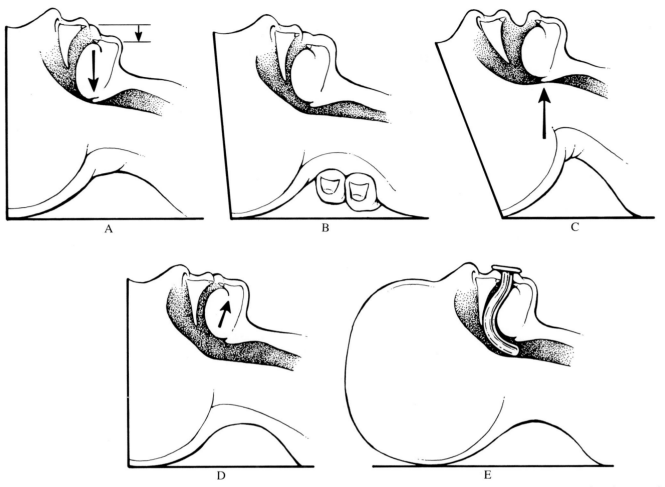

Figure 77-3. (*A*) Upper airway obstruction secondary to the hypotonic mandibular tissue collapsing against the posterior pharyngeal wall. The greater the flexion of the head secondary to the prominent occiput, the more pronounced the obstruction. (*B*) Partial relief of obstruction by means of head extension. (*C*) Extreme hyperextension causing obstruction at the level of the posterior pharynx. As the neck is hyperextended the strap muscles pull against the trachea, causing collapse anteriorly also. (*D*) The jaw thrust or chin lift elevates the mandibular tissue anteriorly, relieving the obstruction. (*E*) Oral airways may be used to maintain the tissue elevated from the posterior pharyngeal wall. (*Adapted from Fleisher G and Ludwig S (eds): Pediatric Emergency Medicine. Baltimore, Williams & Wilkins, 1983.*)

ryngeal wall. With the aid of a tongue blade they are inserted in much the same manner as is described for adults.

Intubation

Endotracheal intubation of infants and children is felt by many to be easier than the same procedure in adults. It requires much less effort and if done correctly is uniformly successful. It is beyond the scope of this chapter, and it would not be very helpful, to review the technique, which varies little with the adult procedure. There are, however, some differences related to patient anatomy and equipment which need to be understood.

As stated previously, hyperextension of the neck is not desirable. Not only does it cause airway obstruction by the hypotonic mandibular tissue as has been described, it can actually cause kinking of the trachea anteriorly because of the immature cartilaginous support. The sniffing position therefore should also be used for intubation.

Although there are many different variations, laryngoscope blades come in essentially two types: the curved (MacIntosh) and the straight (Miller), which has a curved tip. The curved type is rarely used in children less than 4 years old, except in controlled settings, for two reasons. First, because of the high anterior tracheal opening, the floppy mandibular mass of tissue may fill the field of vision when the blade is inserted in proper position. Second, one must have the exact size to fit the curvature of the tongue in order to perform the procedure. For these reasons a straight blade is preferred.

Tube sizes vary according to age. A general rule is that the correct tube size is approximately the same size as the end of the patient's little finger. Uncuffed tubes are used for children up to 7 or 8 years old, since the subglottic trachea usually narrows to form an adequate seal in this age group and cuffs are unnecessary. In emergency situations remember that *one can almost always intubate with a laryngyscope blade that is too large and ventilate with a tube that is too small, but not vice versa.*

Once the child has been intubated one person should be assigned to hold the endotracheal tube in place until it is securely fastened. This is done by grasping the tube at the level of the lips. In small infants minimum movements can easily displace the tube from the trachea into the esophagus.

Foreign-Body Management

Controversy exists as to the safest and most effective emergency maneuvers to use with the choking child. The American Academy of Pediatrics (AAP) specifically discourages two common maneuvers used with adult patients: (1) the Heimlich maneuver, because of the potential for injury to abdominal organs; and (2) blind finger sweeps, because of the possibility of pushing the foreign body further into the airway. Seriously differing opinion exists, but current AAP recommendations rely on the back blow and chest thrust to clear the child's airway.

The AAP recommends the following sequence for emergency treatment of the choking child who cannot cough, speak, or breathe: (1) With the infant's torso positioned prone and head down along the rescuer's arm or the older child draped prone and head down across the rescuer's knees, four blows are delivered to the interscapular area. (2) If the airway is still obstructed, the infant is repositioned supinely along the rescuer's arm or the older child is placed on the floor as for external cardiac compression, and four chest thrusts (cardiac compressions) are delivered. (3) Using the jaw thrust, the mouth is inspected, and a foreign body removed if seen. (4) If obstruction persists, mouth-to-mouth (or mouth-nose) ventilation is attempted. (5) If obstruction persists, the sequence is repeated. As mentioned, the back blow and chest thrust are controversial and thought by some to potentially worsen obstruction. Future investigation may well lead to revised recommendations.

It should be kept in mind that these recommendations are directed primarily at the first responder who has neither access to, nor the skills to use, airway management equipment. In the emergency department one would probably attempt direct laryngoscopy, visualization, and removal of the foreign body with McGill forceps before proceeding to the above maneuvers.

BREATHING

Mouth-to-Patient

Whether to employ mouth-to-mouth or mouth-to-mouth-and-nose ventilation depends solely upon the size of the patient. The rate of ventilation is shown in the following table.

Infants	20 breaths/min (every 3 s)
Children 1–8 years	15 breaths/min (every 4 s)
Children over 8 years and adults	12 breaths/min (every 5 s)

Bag-Valve-Mask

The self-inflating bag-valve-mask system is most commonly used. A pop-off valve set near 40 cmH$_2$O is a feature of many bags. There is a common misconception that children are more susceptible to pneumothoraces at high inspiratory pressure than adults. The fact is that pediatric lung compliance is very good and children can tolerate high pressures. The problem is that because of age-related differences children may receive three to four times

the required tidal volume necessary to ventilate, thereby producing excessive pressures and resultant leaks. The tidal volume necessary to ventilate children, whether it be mouth-to-mouth or bag-to-endotracheal-tube is the same as for adults, i.e., 10 to 15 mL/kg. It is impractical to calculate the tidal volume in the emergency situation. An easy shortcut is to start with minimal volumes and increase rapidly until adequate chest rise occurs. If a patient has poor compliance, requiring high pressures to ventilate, the pop-off valve may be occluded with a fingertip to produce adequate chest rise.

CIRCULATION

Adequacy of circulation is a clinical determination. In the absence of a pulse external cardiac compression must be initiated. If pulses are present, low cardiac output as determined by end organ perfusion (skin indications: cyanosis, mottling; central nervous system indications: coma, degree of alertness, renal indication: urine output) will determine whether further intervention is necessary.

External Cardiac Compression

Absence of pulses mandates external cardiac compression. The brachial pulse is recommended for monitoring purposes. The patient should be placed on a hard surface as with adults. An exception would be in smaller infants, when the wrap-around technique is used (see Fig. 77-4).

Compression should be over the midsternum and not the lower sternum as in adults. This usually corresponds to the transnipple line. Depending on the size of the child, one or two fingers should be used. In older children the heel of the hand is preferred. The depth of compression usually corresponds to one-fourth of the AP diameter of the chest. The rate of compressions is 100 per minute in infants, 80 per minute in children, and 60 per minute in adults. An easy way to remember this is to count aloud as shown in the following table. The ratio of ventilations to compressions is 1 to 5 for one- and two-person CPR.

Infants	One, two, three, four, etc.
Children	One and two and three and four, etc.
Adults	One thousand one, one thousand two, one thousand three, etc.

Vascular Access

Difficulty in obtaining rapid intravenous access is certainly one of the major differences between adult and pediatric resuscitative efforts. Whereas this is virtually never a problem with adult patients, it represents at least one of the most feared, though not necessarily always real, stumbling blocks in managing children. Vascular access must be viewed in perspective. Most traumatic arrests occur in older children and IV access is usually not a problem. Most medical arrests occur in infants less than 1 year old and it is in this subset of patients where difficulty may arise. Two important facts should be kept in mind. First, a significant portion of children will respond to airway management alone. This is not surprising since most cardiac arrests in children are secondary to a preceding respiratory arrest. Nowhere is it more important to follow the ABC's of resuscitation than in the management of pediatric patients. *Time spent securing vascular access at*

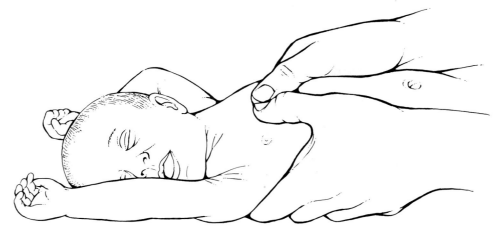

Figure 77-4. The wrap-around technique used in small infants.

the expense of adequate airway management is a common mistake in dealing with children, and nowhere is it more costly. Second, once a patient has been intubated, this route may be used to administer drugs, namely epinephrine, atropine, and lidocaine. The doses are the same as for IV administration.

Although central access is preferred over peripheral access for administration of drugs during CPR, this is rarely practical in the pediatric arrest situation. Most studies demonstrating the safety and efficacy of virtually all central venous approaches in children were done under controlled situations and mostly by experienced personnel. This is not the case in the emergency situation. The most frequently used peripheral sites are the scalp, the arm (hand or antecubital), the external jugular, femoral, or distal saphenous vein via cutdown. The distal saphenous vein offers the following advantages: the anatomy is constant; there is no artery, tendon, or major nerve in the incision area; it is easily extractable; and placement does not interfere with CPR.

A systematic approach according to each clinical situation is helpful to organize personnel and avoid confusion (see box).

PREARREST: (dehydration, early shock, etc.)

1. Percutaneous peripheral (i.e., antecubital vein)
2. Cutdown if unsuccessful (i.e., saphenous)

ARREST: (simultaneously)

1. Percutaneous peripheral
2. Saphenous cutdown
3. Percutaneous central—internal jugular (in experienced hands only)

Once an adequate IV line has been established using one of the above methods, efforts may be ceased in the other two areas. Modification of this approach will be determined by each physician's expertise and experience.

POSTSTABILIZATION:
Consider need for continuous cardiovascular monitoring using invasive procedures, i.e., CVP, arterial lines, Swan-Ganz catheters.

Fluids

There is an aura of mystery surrounding pediatric fluid and electrolyte therapy. Given the varying sizes of children, their changing metabolic needs with age and evolving renal function, it seems an impossible task for the nonpediatrician. However, in the arrest situation this becomes simplified. In the face of hypotension, isotonic fluid boluses of 20 mL/kg should be given as rapidly as possible and repeated depending upon response. If volumes of 40 mL/kg to 60 mL/kg are needed, a pressor agent should be strongly considered, preferably with the aid of a central venous pressure (CVP) catheter. In the normotensive patient or when the IV line is being used for drug administration only, it should be maintained at KVO. Fine fluid and electrolyte calculations and adjustments can be made after the emergency treatment has been completed. Overhydration, even when IV lines are set at KVO, is a common occurrence when adult equipment is used in pediatric resuscitations. *A pediatric microdrip should always be used when resuscitating children.*

Drugs

Specific to pediatric patients is the problem of dosage of respective drugs. Although a few minor differences exist between adult and pediatric drug therapy, the real differences are age-related. A drug may be given in many different doses because children come in many different sizes. Although this is perceived by many physicians as a major issue, with proper organization it should be no problem at all. However, a few basic concepts will be reviewed first.

Correct dosage of drugs for infants and children requires knowledge of three factors. First, body weight—actual or estimated. Estimated weight is acceptable (see Table 77-1). Most drugs are

Table 77-1. Body Weight Estimation Guidelines

Age	Weight, kg	
Term infant	3.5	Birth weight (BW)
6 months	7	$2 \times$ BW
1 year	10	$3 \times$ BW
4 years	16	$\frac{1}{4}$ adult weight of 70 kg
10 years	35	$\frac{1}{2}$ adult weight

given in a milligram per kilogram of body weight dose. Remember, recommended doses for drugs are given in ranges capable of yielding effective therapeutic effects. Therefore the fact that estimated weight varies slightly from true weight is not of great concern. In any event, clinical response will determine whether to increase or repeat the dose. The second factor is knowledge of the recommended dose. This is usually given in milligrams per kilograms of body weight or micrograms per kilogram. Finally, one must be familiar with calculations. It is in this area where many errors leading to overdosage or underdosage are made. Not only must the clinician be careful when multiplying the dose times the weight in kilograms (the most frequent error being the administration of one-tenth or ten times the correct dose because of a misplaced decimal point), but he or she must be familiar with serial dilution, percent solution, and microgram calculations (see box).

One way of avoiding these errors is to become familiar with the dosage and delivered quantity of the commonly used drugs for a 10-kg patient. Most cardiac arrests occur in patients less than 1 year of age. The 1-year-old infant weighs about 10 kg. Familiarity with the actual delivered amount of drug needed for a 10-kg infant allows the clinician to recognize gross under- or

---

CALCULATIONS

PERCENT SOLUTIONS

$$\text{Percentage} = \text{number of grams per 100 mL, \underline{regardless} of the substance.}$$

$$
\begin{aligned}
10\% \text{ solution} &= 10 \text{ g}/100 \text{ mL}\\
&= 0.1 \text{ g/mL}\\
&= 100 \text{ mg/mL}\\
D_{10}W &= 100 \text{ mg glucose/mL}\\
10\% \text{ CaCl}_2 &= 100 \text{ mg calcium chloride/mL}
\end{aligned}
$$

SERIAL DILUTION

$$
\begin{aligned}
1{:}100,\ 1{:}1000,\ 1{:}10{,}000 &= 1 \text{ g of \underline{any} substance per } 100/1000/10{,}000 \text{ mL}\\
1{:}10{,}000 \text{ Epinephrine} &= 1\text{g}/10{,}000 \text{ mL}\\
&= 1000 \text{ mg}/10{,}000 \text{ mL}\\
&= 1 \text{ mg}/10 \text{ ml}\\
&= 0.1 \text{ mg/mL}
\end{aligned}
$$

MICROGRAMS (μg)

$$
\begin{aligned}
1 \text{ μg} &= 1/1000 \text{ of a milligram or}\\
1 \text{ mg} &= 1000 \text{ μg}
\end{aligned}
$$

Example: How many μg/mL are in a 1:10,000 solution of epinephrine?

$$
\begin{aligned}
1{:}10{,}000 &= 1 \text{ g}/10{,}000 \text{ ml}\\
&= 1000 \text{ mg}/10{,}000 \text{ mL}\\
&= 1 \text{ mg}/10 \text{ mL}\\
&= 1000 \text{ μg}/10 \text{ mL}\\
&= 100 \text{ μg/mL}
\end{aligned}
$$

AIDS TO CORRECT DOSAGE

Knowledge of drug doses is not sufficient to assure that the patient receives the correct amount of drug. The physician must not only know the dose, but must avoid calculation errors by himself or herself and nursing personnel. Below are listed a few aids useful to ensure correct dosage.

1. Stock CRT carts, office, clinic, etc. with *one* preparation of each drug.
2. Post drug doses in clear view.
3. Obtain body weights on all patients in nonemergency situations and practice weight estimations.
4. Become familiar with actual delivered amount of drugs for the 10-kg patient.
5. Have dose per kilogram calculations for drugs (1–50 kg) on separate index cards kept in the CRT cart.

Example: 15 kg

Epinephrine	1:10,000	0.1 mg/mL	= 1.5 mL
Bicarbonate	8.4%	1 mEq/mL	= 15 mEq
Calcium chloride	10%	100 mg/mL	= 3 mL
Atropine	1:10,000	0.1 mg/mL	= 3 mL

6. Remember, dose-per-kilogram calculations should not exceed adult doses. This is usually reached at 50 kg.
7. Remember the "rule of 6" for IV drip medications.

overdosage, since most children who suffer arrest will require less than, or multiples of, this dose. Several aids to assure correct dosage are listed in the preceding box. *Use of index cards can eliminate drug dosage as a problem.* One does not have to remember dosages, calculate dosages, or worry whether the correct dose will be delivered to the patient.

Table 77-2 lists the doses of essential drugs or drugs used commonly in resuscitation.

The drugs delivered by constant infusion and the "rule of six" used to calculate their dosage are listed in the box below.

USEFUL DRUGS

RULE OF 6
FOR MEDICATIONS DELIVERED BY
CONSTANT INFUSION

Dopamine Dose = 5–20 μg/(kg·min)
Lidocaine Dose = 20–50 μg/(kg·min)
Isuprel Dose = 0.1–1.0 μg/(kg·min)

Dosage of medications delivered by constant infusions is calculated in terms of micrograms/(kg·min). Actual calculation can be confusing and a source of lethal decimal errors. The *"rule of 6"* can be used for *dopamine* and *lidocaine* to simplify dosage calculation:

6 mg × wt (kg), fill to 100 mL with D₅W

The medication is mixed in an intravenous set with a measured chamber and a microdrip (1 drop/min = 1 mL/h). Rate of administration is best set by an electric pump.

Example: A 10-kg infant requiring dopamine:

6 mg × 10 = 60 mg dopamine.

In a measured chamber *fill* to 100 mL with D₅W. Weight is now factored in so that:

1 mL/h = 1 μg/(kg·min)
5 mL/h = 5 μg/(kg·min)
10 mL/h = 10 mcg/(kg·min)

For *isoproterenol* the "rule of 6":

0.6 mg × wt (kg), *fill* to 100 mL with D₅W
1 ml/h = 0.1 μg/(kg·min)
5 mL/h = 0.5 μg/(kg·min)

The indications for the use of drugs are essentially the same for adults and children. Pharmacology of drugs has been well described in other sections and will not be addressed here. A few drug peculiarities pertaining to pediatric use are discussed in the following paragraphs.

Epinephrine. Symptomatic slow heart rates in adults are treated with atropine. This is true for infants and children also. However, in neonates epinephrine is used as the first-line drug. This is probably done more by convention than with basis in scientific study.

Atropine. As with adults, if atropine is given in too small a dose a paradoxical, centrally mediated bradycardia may be produced. This can be avoided by giving a *minimum* dose of 0.2 mg regardless of the size of the patient.

Sodium bicarbonate. Much has been written concerning the adverse effects of bicarbonate administration, especially in pre-

Table 77-2. Essential Medications

Drug	Concentration	Dose/kg	mL/kg
Epinephrine	1:10,000 (0.1 mg/mL)	0.01 mg	0.1 mL
Bicarbonate	8.4% (1 mEq/mL)	2 mEq	2 mL
Atropine	1:10,000 (0.1 mg/mL)	0.02 mg	0.2 mL
Calcium chloride	10% (100 mg/mL)	20 mg	0.2 mL

mature infants. Most of these complications are the result of rapid administration of this relatively hyperosmolar substance and the resultant rapid changes in osmolarity and pH. However, in the arrest situation there is no choice but to rapidly administer the drug initially. In the neonate or premature infant, sodium bicarbonate should be diluted 1:1 with *sterile water*, not saline, to reduce its concentration.

Calcium. Much has been written recently on the role of calcium in resuscitation. Traditionally it is indicated for electromechanical dissociation (EMD) and asystole although some investigators question its use. Calcium chloride is the preparation most used in cardiac arrests.

Arrhythmias

Another major difference is in the area of arrhythmia management. In contrast to adults, arrhythmias play only a small role in resuscitation of children. The principles of management, however, are the same for both groups *after* the underlying cause has been addressed, specifically, giving careful attention to correction of hypoxia and acidosis since rhythm disturbances are usually secondary to respiratory arrest and *not* primary cardiac events.

As is true in adult ACLS only unstable rhythms require immediate intervention (see box). Likewise, the classification of

---

DEFINITION—UNSTABLE OR SYMPTOMATIC RHYTHMS

The definition of unstable or symptomatic arrhythmias is determined by the clinical condition of the patient. This varies according to age.

ADULT: *Hypotension or collapse* (no rate)
Fulminant CHF—usually secondary to decreased diastolic filling during tachycardias
Ischemic chest pain—secondary to poor perfusion of coronary arteries

CHILD: *Hypotension or collapse* (no rate)
Fulminant CHF—rare

NEWBORN: *Heart rate not hypotension*

Blood pressure measurement is extremely difficult in the recently born infant.

SUMMARY: Infant or child—*blood pressure:*
Less than 60–70
Newborn—*heart rate:* Less than 80–100

These are only guidelines. Clinical evidence of end organ perfusion should always be correlated; i.e., mental status, cyanosis, mottling, etc.

unstable rhythms by heart rate is helpful in that many rhythms are treated in a similar fashion and need not be further differentiated to a specific diagnosis before intervention (see Table 77-3).

The most common rhythms seen in the pediatric arrest situation are the slow rates, specifically sinus bradycardia, which lead to asystole if untreated. It cannot be overemphasized that, in contrast to adults, arrhythmia recognition and management is probably the *least* important facet of successful pediatric resuscitation.

Defibrillation and Cardioversion

Electrical conversion is used on an emergency basis to treat ventricular fibrillation and symptomatic tachyarrhythmias. Ventricular fibrillation as a cause of cardiac arrest, as stated before, is a rare occurrence in children. The incidence of tachyarrhythmias is also much lower than in adults. Children can tolerate fast heart rates for long periods of time before terminal congestive heart failure or lethal arrhythmias develop. Most tachyarrhythmias can be cardioverted in a controlled situation or managed pharmacologically (see box).

DEFIBRILLATION AND CARDIOVERSION— ADULTS VS. CHILDREN

1. Blind defibrillation is not recommended. The incidence of ventricular fibrillation as a cause of arrest in children is very low.
2. Ventricular Fibrillation
   Adult—fixed doses
   Children—dose per kilogram
3. Tachyarrhythmias:
   Adults—dose varies according to the type of arrhythmia, i.e., atrial flutter, atrial fibrillation, and ventricular tachycardia
   Children—fixed doses regardless of the type of arrhythmia.

Defibrillators. Direct current (dc) defibrillators are recommended. It is preferable to use one that indicates both stored and delivered energy.

Paddle size. In general, the largest paddle that contacts in its entirety the chest wall should be used. This is usually 4.5 cm for infants and 8 cm for children.

Interface. Electrode cream, electrode paste, and saline-soaked gauze pads are all acceptable. Alcohol pads are to be discouraged as serious burns may be produced. Care must be taken so that the interface substance from one paddle does not come in contact with the substance from the other paddle. This creates a short-circuit and insufficient energy may be delivered to the heart.

Electrode position. The paddles should be placed so that the heart is between them. This can be difficult in small infants unless appropriate paddle sizes are used. One paddle is placed on the right of the sternum at the second intercostal space. The other is placed in the left midclavicular line at the level of the xyphoid. The AP approach can be used, but is less desirable.

Defibrillation dose. Initially, 2 Ws/kg should be used. The dose is doubled if unsuccessful. If the second attempt is unsuccessful,

Table 77-3. Summary of Treatment of Unstable Rhythms

Heart Rate	Most Common Diagnosis	Treatment
Slow	Sinus bradycardia	Atropine* (infant or child)
	Blocks: Second-degree	or → Isuprel
	Type I and type II	→ pacemaker
	Third-degree	Epinephrine (newborn)
Fast	Narrow QRS	Cardioversion
	PAT	
	Atrial fibrillation	
	Atrial flutter	
	Wide QRS	Cardioversion and
	Ventricular tachycardia	lidocaine
	Any supraventricular rhythm with aberrant conduction†	
Collapse (none)	Ventricular fibrillation	Bicarbonate, epinephrine, electrical defibrillation, lidocaine
	Asystole	Bicarbonate, epinephrine, atropine, calcium
	EMD	Bicarbonate, epinephrine, calcium, Isuprel

*By convention, epinephrine rather than atropine is given initially in newborns for slow rates. This is probably due to immature sympathetic innovation of the newborn heart, which requires extra adrenergic stimulation.

†Although wide SVT does not need lidocaine, in the unstable situation the differentiation between ventricular and supraventricular origin is often difficult. When in doubt, it should be treated as ventricular tachycardia.

epinephrine and bicarbonate should be given and the oxygen and acid-base status assessed before increasing the energy dose.

Cardioversion. Tachyarrhythmias are generally very sensitive to electrical conversion. There are no recent published standards for cardioversion. One can either use 1 to 2 Ws/kg and double this if unsuccessful, *or* place the defibrillator on the lowest possible energy setting and do the same. Of the two methods, the one that gives the lowest energy level is preferable.

SUMMARY AND MANAGEMENT GUIDELINES

In reviewing the ABC's of pediatric resuscitation the pertinent differences and similarities between adults and children have been presented. Once the clinician understands these differences it is relatively easy to apply general resuscitation principles to children. It is the age-related differences that are difficult to remember and which cause major problems in crisis situations. One should not have to memorize drug doses, tube sizes, cardiac compression ratios, etc. Through proper organization of equipment and the posting of pertinent information in an accessible area of the emergency department, any problem caused by difficulty in remem-

Table 77-4. CPR

	Infant	Child	Adolescent/Adult	
Compression/ventilation ratio	5:1	5:1	1. 15:2	2. 5:1
Cardiac compressions/minute	100	80	80	60
Respiratory rate	20	16	10	12

Table 77-5. Equipment

	Premature, 3 kg	Newborn, 3.5 kg	6 Months, 7 kg	1–2 Years, 10–12 kg	5 Years, 16–18 kg	8–10 Years, 24–30 kg
C-collars	-------	-------	Small	Small	Small	Medium
Chest tubes	10–14 F	12–18 F	14–20 F	14–24 F	20–32 F	28–38 F
NG tubes	5 feeding	5–8 feeding	8 F	10 F	10–12 F	14–18 F
Foley	5 feeding	5–8 feeding	8 F	10 F	10–12 F	12 F
O$_2$ masks	Premature Newborn	Newborn	Pediatric	Pediatric	Pediatric	Adult
BVM	Infant	Infant	Pediatric	Pediatric	Pediatric	Pediatric/Adult
Laryngo-scopes	0	1	1	1	2	2–3
ET Tubes	2.5–3.0	3.0–3.5	3.5–4.5	4.0–4.5	5.0–5.5	5.5–6.5
Suction catheters/stylets	6–8 F/6F	8F/6F	8–10F/6F	10F/6F	14F/14F	14F/14F
Oral airways	Infant	Infant/small	Small	Small	Medium	Medium/Large
IV equipment	22–24 angio 25 scalp	22–24 angio 23–25 scalp	22–24 angio 23–25 scalp	20–22 angio 23 scalp	20–22 angio 19 scalp	20–22 angio 19 scalp
Arm boards	6″	6″	6″–8″	8″	8″–15″	15″
BP cuffs	Newborn	Newborn	Infant/child	Child	Child	Child/Adult

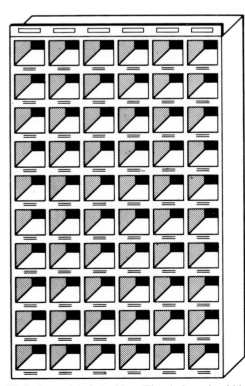

Figure 77-5. Age-related stocking. The shelves should be labeled horizontally with age and size and vertically with equipment corresponding to the equipment guidelines of Table 77-5. In a crisis situation all the correct size equipment is readily accessible if one knows the age *or* weight of the child.

bering the many age-related variables, or errors of calculation can be eliminated. Below are a few helpful suggestions.

1. Follow the Aids to Correct Dosage (see box on page 542), especially the use of index cards. This will eliminate the need to remember doses, will avoid calculation errors, and assure that the correct dose is delivered to the patient.
2. Post a chart containing the major age-related differences in an accessible area so that one can refer to it in the crisis situation (see Tables 77-4 and 77-5).
3. Age-related stocking: stock shelves following the equipment guidelines of Table 77-5 (see Figure 77-5).

Children *are* different from adults. This does not imply, however, that they cannot be managed appropriately in the crisis situation by the nonpediatrician. The key to successful resuscitation of children is in understanding fundamental differences and similarities between the two groups and reducing age-related problems to a minimum through proper organization.

BIBLIOGRAPHY

Chameides L: Guidelines for defibrillation in children. *Circulation* 56:502A–503A, 1977.

Courtney L, Crawford C, Morgan B: Management of cardiac and respiratory arrest in children. *Clin Pediatr* 8:(11)647–654, 1969.

Ehrlich R, Emmett S, Rodriguez-Torres R: Pediatric cardiac resuscitation team: A 6 year study. *J Pediatr* 84(1)152–155, 1974.

Eisenberg N: Epidemiology of cardiac arrest and resuscitation in children. *Ann Emerg Med* 12(11):672, 1983.

Friesen R, Duncan P, Tweet W, et al: Appraisal of pediatric CPR. *CMA Journal* 126:1055, 1982.

Greenberg H: Cardiac arrest in 20 infants and children and results of resuscitation. *Dis Chest*, 47:42, 1965.

Greensher J: Emergency treatment of the choking child. *J Pediatr* 70(1):110, 1982.

Guntheroth W: Neonatal and pediatric cardiovascular crisis. JAMA 232(2):168, 1975.

Kettrick L, Ludwig S: Resuscitation—Pediatric Basic and Advanced Life Support, in Fleisher G, Ludwig S (eds): *Pediatric Emergency Medicine*, Williams & Wilkins, 1983, pp. 1–29.

Melker R: CPR in neonates, infants and children. *Crit Care Quarterly* 1(1):49–65, 1978.

Orlowski JP: Pediatric cardiopulmonary resuscitation. *Emerg Med Clin North Am* 1:3–25, 1983.

Orlowski JP: Cardiopulmonary resuscitation in children. *Pediatr Clin North Am* 27(3):495–512, 1980.

Randolph J: Technique for insertion of plastic catheter into saphenous vein. *Pediatrics* 24:631–635, 1959.

Riemenschneider T: Cardiopulmonary resuscitation in infants and children. *J Fam Practice*, 8(3):597–603, 1979.

Riker W: Cardiac arrest in children. *Pediatr Clin North Am* 16(3):661–669, 1969.

Singer J: Cardiac arrests in children. *JACEP* 6(5):198–205, 1977.

Tahernia C: Managing cardiac arrest in infants and children. *Postgrad Med* 47:204, 1970.

CHAPTER 78
HEART DISEASE IN
INFANTS AND CHILDREN

James H. McCrory

The incidence of congenital heart disease is only 8 per 1000 live births. The incidence of acquired pediatric heart disease is also relatively rare. This low incidence rate contrasts sharply with the prevalence of cardiovascular disease in the adult population, in which the mortality from heart disease is almost 50 percent. Because of low incidence and age-related differences in presentation, recognition of heart disease in infants and children remains a challenge for the primary care physician.

Congenital heart disease is usually classified on the basis of presence or absence of cyanosis or on the nature of the anatomical defect (shunt, obstruction, transposition, or complex). The common acquired conditions include complications secondary to rheumatic fever and to severe chronic anemias, as well as myocarditis, pericarditis, endocarditis, and paroxysmal atrial tachycardia.

There are six common clinical presentations of pediatric heart disease: cyanosis, congestive heart failure, pathologic murmur in an asymptomatic patient, abnormal pulses, hypertension, and syncope. Table 78-1 lists the most common lesions in each category. Evaluation of a murmur is an elective diagnostic workup beyond the scope of this chapter, which will focus on those conditions presenting in the emergency department and requiring immediate recognition, therapeutic intervention, and prompt referral to a pediatric cardiologist.

TETRALOGY OF FALLOT

Most cyanotic lesions usually are recognized in the first few days of life before the infant is discharged from the newborn nursery. Failure of hypoxemia to resolve on Fi_{O_2} 1.00 distinguishes an intracardiac shunt from pulmonary disease.

Tetralogy of Fallot is a common cyanotic lesion that may escape detection in the nursery. It is therefore important for the emergency medicine physician to recognize this lesion, as well as to recognize and treat hypercyanotic spells. The degree of cyanosis is directly proportional to the severity of the pulmonary stenosis. In fact, cyanosis may be subtle or absent at rest, and clinically obvious only when the infant is active or crying.

The other cardinal features on physical examination are the holosystolic ventricular septal defect (VSD) murmur in the third intercostal space at the left sternal border and the diamond-shaped systolic murmur of pulmonary stenosis in the second intercostal

Table 78-1. Clinical Presentation of Pediatric Heart Disease

Cyanosis	TGA, TOF, TA, TAt, TAVR
Congestive heart failure	See Table 78-3
Murmur/asymptomatic pt.	Shunts: VSD, PDA, ASD
	Obstructions
	Valvular incompetence
Abnormal pulses	
Bounding	PDA, AI, AVM
Decreased	Coarctation, HPLV
Hypertension	Coarctation
Syncope	
Cyanotic	TOF
Acyanotic	Critical AS

Glossary:
AI = Aortic insufficiency
AS = Aortic stenosis
ASD = Atrial septal defect
AVM = Arteriovenous malformation
ECG = Electrocardiogram
HPLV = Hypoplastic left ventricle
PAT = Paroxysmal atrial tachycardia
PDA = Patent ductus arteriosus
TA = Truncus arteriosus
TAt = Tricuspid atresia
TAVR = Total anomalous venous return
TGA = Transposition of the great arteries
TOF = Tetralogy of Fallot
VSD = Ventricular septal defect

space at the left sternal border. The history may reveal exercise intolerance relieved by squatting. The main radiographic findings are a boot-shaped heart with decreased pulmonary vascular markings. A right-side aortic arch is present in 25 percent of tetralogies. Right ventricular hypertrophy with right axis deviation are the primary ECG abnormalities.

Dynamic obstruction below the pulmonary valve can lead to an acute increase in the right-to-left shunt and produce a *hypercyanotic spell* or *syncope with cyanosis*. Prolonged or recurrent syncope due to tetralogy of Fallot can be a life-threatening emergency, so that referral after initial stabilization is indicated for further diagnostic evaluation and possible urgent surgical intervention.

Initial medical management of a hypercyanotic spell includes placing the infant in the knee-chest position, maximizing the

Fi_{O_2}, and administering intravenous morphine. The infant should be made comfortable and kept quiet. The knee-chest position can be maintained while the infant is held upright in the mother's arms and the mother is seated. If the infant is aggravated by a face mask after consciousness has returned, then the mother can administer oxygen blown by the infant's face at a high flow rate. Direct manipulation of the infant is limited to establishing an intravenous line for medications. Morphine in the dosage of 0.1 mg/kg can relieve the hyperdynamic spell. If the syncope does not respond to this therapy, the dose of morphine can be repeated before considering usage of propranolol.

Because of the high mortality and CNS morbidity associated with hypercyanotic spells, surgical intervention is indicated. The two options are total repair, which requires heart-lung bypass, or a palliative shunt between the aorta and the pulmonary artery. Since many physicians consider that administration of propranolol is a contraindication to bypass surgery, initiation of this form of therapy should be done in coordination with the pediatric cardiologist and the cardiovascular surgeon.

CRITICAL AORTIC STENOSIS

Critical aortic stenosis is a noncyanotic lesion which can be life-threatening and may present at any age. In an older child, exercise intolerance with easy fatigability and chest pain can be present in the history. Prominent physical findings are a systolic ejection click and a diamond-shaped murmur which radiates to the neck and can be accompanied by a suprasternal thrill. Left ventricular hypertrophy with strain can be present on ECG and the chest x-ray may show poststenotic dilatation of the aorta, although neither of these signs is consistently present.

Syncope without cyanosis due to critical aortic stenosis can portend a sudden life-threatening arrhythmia. The patient should be kept strictly at rest, using sedation if necessary. Immediate referral for further diagnosis and possible urgent surgical repair is indicated.

CONGESTIVE HEART FAILURE

Recognition

The first task confronting the physician in the emergency department is to recognize congestive heart failure and to differentiate it from more common conditions, such as pneumonia or sepsis. The distinction between pneumonia and congestive heart failure in infants requires a high index of clinical suspicion and is a difficult one to make. Pneumonia can cause a previously stable cardiac condition to decompensate, so that both problems can present simultaneously. The common symptoms and signs of an infant presenting in congestive heart failure are outlined in Table 78-2.

Although hepatomegaly appears long before ascites, anasarca, or peripheral edema in right-sided failure in infants, it is usually a late sign. Hepatomegaly exists when the liver is more than 2 cm below the right costal margin in the absence of downward displacement by hyperexpanded lungs. In hepatomegaly, the liver border is rounded rather than sharp.

Both increased pulmonary blood flow in left-to-right shunts and pulmonary edema decrease lung compliance and thus result in tachypnea, which is the cardinal sign of left-sided failure in infants. Although the work of breathing is increased in congestive

Table 78-2. Recognition of Congestive Heart Failure in Infants

	Right-Sided Failure	Left-Sided Failure	Both
Cardinal signs	Hepatomegaly	Tachypnea Dyspnea and sweating on feeding	Cardiomegaly Failure to thrive Tachycardia
Unusual signs	Jugular venous distention Peripheral edema	Rales	

heart failure, the tachypnea is usually effortless because of the lack of airway obstruction. Since feeding is an infant's primary form of exertion, dyspnea and sweating during feeding can often be elicited in the history.

In addition to hepatomegaly and tachypnea, excessive fluid retention can be appreciated by weight changes in response to fluid restriction and diuresis, although such changes are not helpful for initial recognition. An important age-related difference is the fact that peripheral edema, jugular venous distention, and rales are unusual and late signs in infants.

Cardiomegaly evident on chest x-ray is universally present except in constrictive pericarditis. A cardiothoracic index greater than 0.6 is abnormal. Heart size can be difficult to judge on the posterior-anterior view because of the thymic shadow, but can be readily assessed on the lateral view. The primary radiographic signs of cardiomegaly on the lateral chest x-ray are an abnormal cardiothoracic index and lack of retrosternal airspace due to the heart's directly abutting against the sternum. On the posterior-anterior view, the thymic shadow can be distinguished from the cardiac silhouette by the "sail sign" if present, and by the scalloped border which is produced by compression of the thymus against the rib cage.

Differential Diagnosis

Once congestive heart failure is recognized, age-related categories simplify further differential diagnosis (Table 78-3). In the first few minutes of life, congestive failure occurs from a variety of noncardiac origins such as asphyxia, acidosis, hypoglycemia, hypocalcemia, anemia, and sepsis. In critically ill premature neonates, patent ductus arteriosus is the most common cause of

Table 78-3. Differential Diagnosis of Congestive Heart Failure Based on Age of Presentation

Age Spectrum	
1 min	Noncardiac origin: anemia, acidosis, hypoxia, hypoglycemia, hypocalcemia, sepsis
1 h	
1 day	
	PDA in premature infants
1 week	HPLV
2 weeks	Coarctation
1 month	
	VSD
	PAT
3 months	
1 year	Myocarditis
	Myocardiopathy
	Severe anemias
10 years	Rheumatic fever

congestive heart failure. Among full-term newborns, a hypoplastic left ventricle is the most common cause in the first week, and coarctation of the aorta in the second week of life. Transposition of the great arteries presents within the first 3 days of life, either with cyanosis or congestive heart failure.

Ventricular septal defects complicated by transposition of the great arteries, truncus arteriosus, aortic stenosis, or coarctation can present with failure at any time during the first few weeks. Large, uncomplicated ventricular septal defects can present with congestive heart failure. Onset of the failure is usually insidious between 1 and 3 months of age, when the left-to-right shunt increases as the pulmonary vascular resistance decreases to normal from high fetal values.

Onset of congestive heart failure after 3 months of age usually signifies acquired heart disease as opposed to congenital heart disease. The exception to this rule occurs when pneumonia, subacute bacterial endocarditis, or other complicating factors cause a previously stable congenital lesion to decompensate. Before 2 years of age, myocarditis, cardiomyopathies, and severe anemias are the most common diseases in the differential diagnosis. The peak incidence of rheumatic fever is between 8 and 12 years of age.

Assessment of Severity of Congestive Heart Failure

Clinical assessment also involves estimation of the degree of severity of the congestive heart failure. For example, depending on the size of the defect, a VSD may present in a variety of ways, ranging from mild tachypnea to chronic compensated congestive heart failure accompanied by growth failure. The onset of failure with a VSD is insidious because of the gradual increase in the amount of the left-to-right shunt produced by the gradual decrease in pulmonary vascular resistance during the first 2 months from high fetal values. Small ventricular septal defects present as a holosystolic murmur in an asymptomatic patient and can be hemodynamically insignificant even though the murmur may be louder than that of a large VSD.

In contrast to the gradual onset of failure with a VSD, coarctation of the aorta can present with abrupt onset of congestive heart failure precipitated by a delayed closure of the ductus arteriosus during the second week of life. The severity of the symptoms is directly proportional to the degree of obstruction and can vary from mild tachypnea to cardiogenic shock. Milder degrees of coarctation, on the other hand, present later in life with hypertension and diminished pulses in the lower extremities.

Initial Stabilization

The degree of severity of congestive heart failure outlined above dictates the types of therapeutic interventions necessary for the initial stabilization phase. The infant who presents with mild tachypnea, hepatomegaly, and cardiomegaly simply needs to be seated upright in a comfortable position and be kept in a neutral thermal environment to avoid the metabolic stresses imposed by either hypothermia or hyperthermia. If the work of breathing is appreciably increased by an increased pulmonary blood flow, 1 to 2 mg/kg of furosemide parenterally is indicated. If pulmonary edema is present, then the hypoxemia can usually be corrected by fluid restriction, diuresis, and an increased $F_{i_{O_2}}$, although continuous positive airway pressure is sometimes necessary.

Severe degrees of congestive heart failure can present with signs of low cardiac output or cardiogenic shock. Aggressive management is often necessary for secondary derangements, including respiratory insufficiency, acute renal failure, lactic acidosis, disseminated intravascular coagulation, hypoglycemia, and hypocalcemia.

For definitive diagnosis and treatment of congenital lesions, cardiac catheterization followed by surgical intervention is often necessary. Stabilization prior to definitive diagnosis with inotropic agents such as digoxin or dopamine are beyond the scope of this chapter and should be initiated in conjunction with the pediatric cardiologist.

PAROXYSMAL ATRIAL TACHYCARDIA

With the exception of paroxysmal atrial tachycardia (PAT), arrhythmias are uncommon in the pediatric age group. In infants, PAT presents with a 4- to 24-h history of poor feeding, tachypnea, pallor, and lethargy. In the older child, palpitations and chest pain can be prominent in the symptomatology. Physical examination reveals thready pulses and a tachycardia which can be too rapid to be counted accurately. Depending on the time since onset of PAT, other physical signs can vary from congestive heart failure to cardiogenic shock with pending arrest. Low cardiac output is secondary to inadequate ventricular diastolic filling time.

An ECG rhythm strip shows a ventricular rate of 220 to 360, as opposed to a range of 150 to 200 in adults with PAT. The QRS complexes are narrow and regular. P waves are absent or abnormal.

PAT must be distinguished from sinus tachycardia, which is the most common tachyarrhythmia in children. In sinus tachycardia, P waves are present. The normal range for heart rate in newborns is 120 to 200. Under age 5, it is not unusual to find a sinus tachycardia up to a rate of 200, due to fever, stress, or hypovolemia. The latter requires prompt recognition and adequate volume expansion.

Digoxin has been the time-honored standard of medical management of PAT in infants, but may take 4 to 6 h before the rhythm converts to a normal sinus rhythm. Intravenous verapamil is currently being utilized by many pediatric cardiologists for immediate conversion, followed by digoxin for chronic management. Since an error in administration of both of these medications can be lethal, initiation of digoxin or verapamil therapy should be done in conjunction with a physician familiar with their usage in infants.

Vagal maneuvers to convert PAT can be attempted, but are usually not successful until after the first dose of digoxin. The diver's reflex, which is elicited by submersing the face in ice water, usually produces the greatest vagal tone. An alternative to submersion is to place the ice water in a plastic bag which can be lowered briefly on the infant's face.

Cardioversion with 0.25 to 1 Ws per kilogram is indicated in infants and children presenting in profound cardiogenic shock with pending arrest.

BIBLIOGRAPHY

Artman M, Graham TP: Congestive heart failure in infancy: Recognition and management. *Am Heart J* 103(6):1040–1055, 1982.
Lees MH: Heart failure in the newborn. *J Pediatr* 75(1):139–152, 1969.
Talner NS: Congestive heart failure in the infant: A functional approach. *Pediatr Clin North Am* 18(4):1011–1029, 1971.

CHAPTER 79
THE FEBRILE CHILD

Carol D. Berkowitz

Fever is the most common chief complaint of children presenting to the emergency department and accounts for about 30 percent of pediatric outpatient visits. The physician evaluating the febrile child must differentiate the mildly ill from the seriously ill child, a challenge which may be compounded by the fact that no focus of infection is apparent. The extent of the diagnostic workup and the institution of appropriate management, including the use of antibiotics and/or the need for hospitalization, must be determined.

PHYSIOLOGY OF FEVER

Fever is defined as a rise in deep body temperature associated with a resetting of the body's thermostat. This thermostat is located in the preoptic region of the anterior hypothalamus near the floor of the third ventricle. Exogenous fever-producing substances (pyrogens) such as bacteria, bacterial endotoxin, antigen-antibody complexes, yeast, viruses, and etiocholanolone, may stimulate the formation and release of endogenous pyrogens. Endogenous pyrogens are produced by neutrophils, monocytes, hepatic Kupffer cells, splenic sinusoidal cells, alveolar macrophages, and peritoneal lining cells, and are felt to induce the synthesis of prostaglandins in the hypothalamus. The body's thermostat is then reset at a higher setting and the patient experiences a chill (because his or her own temperature is below that of his or her thermostat). Peripheral vasoconstriction, shivering, central pooling, and behavioral activity (putting on a sweater, drinking hot tea) lead to an increase in body temperature.

FEVER AS A SYMPTOM

The possible beneficial effects of fever have been debated for many years. Aside from these considerations, it is important to recognize that fever represents a symptom of some underlying disease, and one must determine what this disease is.

An initial question is "What degree of temperature elevation represents a fever?" The extent of the evaluation and the decision to hospitalize the patient is strongly influenced by the height of the fever and the age of the patient. Surveys suggest wide variability in the temperature considered a "fever" by various pediatric training programs. This figure has ranged from 38° to 39.4°C (100.4° to 103°F). It is important to recognize that oral temperatures are generally 0.6°C (1°F) lower than rectal temperatures and

axillary temperatures are 0.6°C (1°F) lower than oral temperatures. Additionally, body temperature normally varies from morning to evening with the circadian rhythm. The degree of variation is greatest in young women and small children, and is about 1.1°C (2°F).

The relationship between height of fever and incidence of bacteremia is discussed below. In general, higher temperatures are associated with a higher incidence of bacteremia.

AGE AS A FACTOR

The Infant Up to 3 Months

The age of the patient influences the extent of the workup. Early studies suggested that infants under the age of 3 months were at high risk for life-threatening infection. Recent studies based on outpatient data show that the incidence of bacterial infection, including bacteremia and meningitis, is about 3 to 4 percent, though serious nonbacterial infections (e.g., aseptic meningitis) are a frequent cause of fever in this age group.

The history and physical examination frequently provide clues to the diagnosis. A history of lethargy, irritability, and/or poor feeding suggests a serious infection. A history of viral illnesses in other family members suggests a similar diagnosis in the infant. The physical examination may reveal the focus of infection such as an inflamed eardrum. Inconsolable crying, or increased irritability when handled is frequently seen in infants with meningitis. Cough or tachypnea with a respiratory rate over 40 might suggest a lower respiratory infection and the need for a chest x-ray. The absence of any diagnostic abnormalities on history or physical examination suggests the need for extensive laboratory tests to detect occult infection. These tests would include a complete blood count and differential, blood culture, lumbar puncture, chest x-ray, urinalysis, and culture. Urinary tract infections may not produce symptoms other than fever, and so a urinalysis and culture should be included routinely in the workup. Antibiotic therapy and/or hospitalization should be instituted as suggested by the results of these studies.

There appears to be no "community standard of practice" regarding the need for hospitalization; some physicians hospitalize all febrile infants under 3 months and others hospitalize only those under 1 month. The ability of the physician to differentiate the well from the ill small infant has been questioned by some investigators who suggest that all such febrile infants need a septic workup and hospitalization. The decision not to hospitalize the small febrile infant must be made after careful clinical and appropriate laboratory assessment, and after assessing the reliability of followup.

Infants of 3 to 24 Months

Many of the considerations noted in the evaluation of the infant of less than 3 months are true for the older infant. Patients between 3 and 24 months have been the focus of considerable research because this group appears to be at higher risk for occult bacteremia. These studies have sought to identify clinical and laboratory characteristics of bacteremic patients.

Clinical judgment appears to be more reliable in the assessment of the older infant than it is in the younger infant. Characteristics that the evaluating physician should look for include willingness of the patient to make eye contact, playfulness and positive response to interactions, negative response to noxious stimuli, alertness, and consolability. The toxic infant will not respond appropriately.

Again, the history and physical examination will frequently reveal the source of infection. Viral illnesses, including respiratory infections and gastroenteritis, account for the majority of febrile illnesses, and usually have system-specific symptoms. Bacterial infections of the respiratory tract include most notably otitis media, pharyngitis, and pneumonia. Otitis media is generally caused by *Streptococcus pneumoniae* or *Hemophilus influenzae,* and antibiotic therapy should be directed at these organisms. Although pneumonia is commonly of viral etiology, it is appropriate to institute antibiotic therapy to ensure coverage of *H. influenzae.* The physical signs of meningitis, such as nuchal rigidity, Kernig's and/or Brudzinski's signs, may be inapparent in the child under the age of 2 years. A bulging fontanelle, vomiting, irritability which increases when the infant is held, inconsolability, or a febrile seizure may be the only signs suggestive of meningitis. Infants with aseptic meningitis should generally be hospitalized and assured adequate longterm followup because they are at higher risk for subsequent neurologic and learning disabilities.

The bacteremic infant may or may not have an obvious focus of bacterial infection. The height of the fever is a clue to which infants are bacteremic. Although bacteremia may be seen at lower temperatures, a temperature over 39.5°C (103.1°F) in infants 3 to 24 months is associated with a higher incidence of bacteremia. Certain laboratory tests have been recommended to assist in further identifying the bacteremic patient. White blood counts (WBC) over 15,000/mm^3, band counts $\geq$ 500/mm^3, total polymorphonuclear counts $\geq$ 10,000/mm^3, and band plus poly counts $\geq$ 10,500/mm^3 are associated with an increased incidence of bacteremia, although bacteremia also occurs in the absence of these findings. The incidence of bacteremia in children 3 to 24 months with a temperature $\geq$ 39.5°C (103.1°F) is about 5 to 6 percent. If one looks at patients with WBCs of $\geq$ 15,000/mm^3, the incidence increases to 12 to 15 percent. An erythrocyte sedimentation rate elevated to 30 mm/h or greater has the same significance as a WBC $\geq$ 15,000/mm^3. The organisms most commonly causing bacteremia in this age group are *S. pneumoniae* (65 percent) and *H. influenzae* (25 percent).

Is it important to do a blood culture and detect occult bacteremia? Opinions vary on the answer to this question. It is apparent that bacteremic patients do better if they receive antibiotics early on. Many of the bacteremic children have a focus of infection and so are treated anyway. Additionally, at least 25 percent of bacteremic patients with no focus of infection resolve their bacteremia without any antibiotics. Others develop soft tissue infections which are then appropriately managed. The ability of oral antibiotics to prevent development of bacterial meningitis in the bacteremic child is still unclear. The blood culture appears to be useful for keeping track of a patient who may not be returning for periodic evaluations. Therefore, from a medical and epidemiologic standpoint blood cultures are indicated in the suspicious or high-risk infant.

Once a blood culture is obtained, the physician has the additional dilemma of what to do with positive results. All patients with positive blood cultures should be recalled for repeat evaluation. If they are on the appropriate antibiotics, are clinically well, and have been afebrile, they should be instructed to complete their course of therapy. If they are afebrile, clinically well, but have never been treated with antibiotics, opinions differ about the need for additional blood cultures and/or antibiotic therapy. Generally, neither is necessary unless the child has developed a specific focus of infection. If, however, the patient continues to run a fever or does poorly even if on antibiotics, he or she should receive a complete septic workup (CBC, blood culture, lumbar puncture, chest film, urine culture), be admitted, and receive parenteral antibiotics.

Older Febrile Children

Children over the age of 2 are easier to evaluate. They can specify their complaints and have illnesses similar to younger children, particularly upper respiratory infections and gastroenteritis. The risk of bacteremia appears lower in this age group, but the incidence of streptococcal pharyngitis is higher, especially in children between the ages of 5 and 10. Infectious mononucleosis may present with fever, tonsillar hypertrophy, and exudate, like streptococcal pharyngitis. Marked lymphadenopathy and/or hepatosplenomegaly would be the clue to the diagnosis. Pneumonia in this age group may be caused by *Mycoplasma pneumoniae.* These children present with cough and fever. Rales may not be apparent early in the illness, though the chest film would show evidence of an infiltrate. Bedside cold agglutinins, if positive, provide a clue to the correct diagnosis. Children with pneumonia secondary to *Mycoplasma* should be treated with erythromycin, 30 to 40 mg/(kg·day) (maximum dose 1 g).

MANAGING THE FEVER

Once the issue of fever as a symptom has been addressed, it is appropriate to evaluate the role of fever-reducing measures.

Many parents are concerned about the harmful effects of the fever; many are aware of the risk of febrile seizures. Children who are prone to febrile seizures are generally not benefited by antipyretics alone. This is because the seizure frequently occurs early in the illness, often before the parents are aware the child is ill. Aside from febrile seizures, fever is not known to produce any harmful effects in children. Many children, however, feel uncomfortable during the fever, and so it is appropriate to institute measures directed at symptomatically reducing the fever.

The body loses heat in four ways: (1) radiation (60 percent), the heat that moves from the body to the air around us; (2)

evaporation (25 percent), heat lost through the evaporation of perspiration, water, or any liquid applied to the body surface; (3) convection (10 percent), heat lost when air currents blow over the skin; and (4) conduction (approximately 5 percent), heat lost by contact with a solid surface. Heat loss by convection is increased by the use of cooling blankets.

One can facilitate heat loss in a child using any combination of these measures. Unwrapping a bundled child increases heat loss through radiation, and rehydrating a dehydrated child will increase the heat loss through evaporation. Sponging also helps to reduce fever by evaporation. Sponging should be done slowly, using tepid water only. Very rapid cooling by sponging can result in peripheral vascular collapse, and death has been reported in the small critically ill infant. Sponging with ice water is uncomfortable and results in shivering; sponging with alcohol carries the risk of intoxication, hypoglycemia, and coma. Vigorous rubbing of the skin induces vasodilatation, and improves heat loss.

Studies have shown that sponging and antipyretics used together are more effective than either modality used alone. Acetaminophen and aspirin are equally effective and both drugs appear to work centrally to block prostaglandin synthesis. Heat is lost through peripheral vasodilatation and sweating.

Drug dosage is the same for either antipyretic and is 10 to 15 mg/kg per dose at 4-h intervals (maximum dose 600 mg). Increasing the dose does not result in a better or more sustained effect. Giving the drug by rectal suppository results in a slight delay in absorption. There are no studies to evaluate the efficacy of alternating the two drugs at 2-h intervals, in an effort to avoid the recrudescence of fever. Giving the drugs simultaneously at the usual dosage has been shown to produce a reduction in temperature that is sustained for 6 rather than 2 to 4 h.

The use of aspirin has been curtailed following reports linking aspirin and Reye's syndrome. Aspirin should not be used in children with chickenpox or with influenza-like illnesses. Aspirin's effects are cumulative, and more than half of the reported overdoses involve therapeutic misuse. Other side effects of aspirin include gastrointestinal upset and hemorrhage and coagulation disturbances. Acetaminophen is also toxic if taken in inappropriate doses, but there is no cumulative effect, and children are less prone than adults to hepatotoxicity.

SUMMARY

Fever is an elevation of the body's temperature caused by a resetting of the body's thermostat. It is a symptom of an underlying infection or inflammation. Infants under the age of 2 years with fever over 39.5°C are at increased risk for bacteremia. In addition to evaluating the patient for an underlying disease, the physician may treat the febrile child by unbundling, sponging, and with antipyretics to make him or her more comfortable (see Table 79-1).

Table 79-1. Management of the Bacteremic Child.

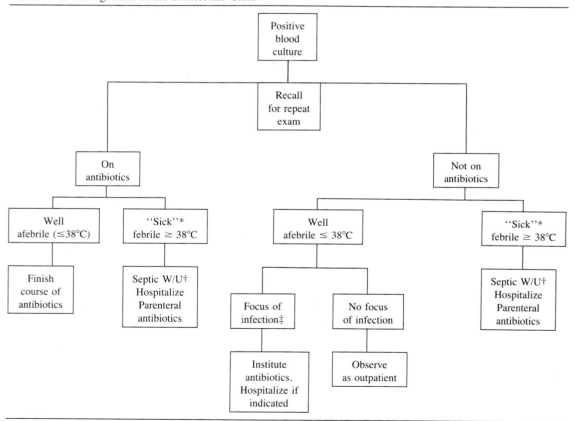

*"Sick" = irritable, lethargic, anorexic, vomiting.

†Septic W/U = blood culture, lumbar puncture, chest x-ray, CBC, differential, urinalysis, urine culture.

‡Focus of infection = otitis media, pneumonia, cellulitis.

BIBLIOGRAPHY

Baron MA, Fink HD: Bacteremia in private practice. *Pediatrics* 66:171, 1980.

Dinarello CA, Wolff SM: Pathogenesis of fever in man. *N Engl J Med* 293:607, 1978.

McCarthy PL, Jekel JF, Stashwick CA, et al: History and observation variables in assessing febrile children. *Pediatrics* 65:1090, 1980.

McCarthy PL, Dolan TF: The serious implications of high fever in infants during their first three months. *Clin Pediatr* 15:794, 1976.

Ringler DH, Anver MR: Fever and survival. *Science* 188:166, 1975.

Schwartz RH, Wientzen RL: Occult bacteremia in toxic-appearing, febrile infants. *Clin Pediatr* 21:659, 1982.

Soman M: Diagnostic work-up of febrile children under 24 months of age: A clinical review. *West J Med* 137:1, 1982.

Steele RW, Young FSH, Bass JW, et al: Oral antipyretic therapy. *Am J Dis Child* 123:204, 1972.

CHAPTER 80
PEDIATRIC UPPER RESPIRATORY EMERGENCIES

Nick Relich

The diseases which cause upper respiratory tract (URT) obstruction account for a significant percentage of pediatric emergency room visits. Some are very common and, ordinarily, quite benign, while others are much less common, yet are true pediatric emergencies. This chapter will deal with the causes of acute pediatric URT obstruction. Diseases of the lower respiratory tract, such as pneumonia, asthma, and bronchiolitis will be discussed elsewhere.

The physical examination sign common to all causes of URT obstruction is inspiratory stridor. This is a harsh, "raspy" noise produced by the flow of air through a partially obstructed airway. Stridor only on inspiration is indicative of obstruction at or above the larynx. Biphasic stridor, heard during expiration as well as inspiration, places the obstruction in the trachea, while expiratory stridor usually means obstruction below the carina. According to the American Thoracic Society's newly adopted definition of respiratory sounds, stridor is a type of "wheezing," i.e., a continuous sound originating from the airway. In common usage, though, only isolated expiratory stridor is referred to as "wheezing," while isolated inspiratory stridor is simply called "stridor." Throughout this chapter, "stridor" and "wheezing" will refer, respectively, to inspiratory and expiratory sounds, usually associated with prolongation of inspiratory or expiratory phases of respiration. Many other physical examination signs are present in patients with URT obstruction. The significance of these, especially in patients under 6 months of age, will be discussed before presenting specific disease entities.

PHYSICAL EXAMINATION

Cyanosis, while the most dramatic sign, has some inherent limitations. It depends to a great extent on the amount of hemoglobin in the blood and the status of the peripheral circulation. A child with severe anemia, for example, may have significant hypoxia without manifesting cyanosis. Conversely, a very young infant, whose hemoglobin has not yet fallen from the normally high levels found at birth, and whose peripheral circulation is normally somewhat sluggish, may show varying degrees of peripheral cyanosis in the face of a normal P_{O_2}. Detection of cyanosis is sometimes quite difficult in black children. And finally, even when present,

cyanosis is a late accompaniment of respiratory diseases. For all these reasons, cyanosis is of limited diagnostic value. However, when it is present, it is an extremely important and ominous sign.

Labored respirations consist of a triad of signs: tachypnea, chest retractions, and nasal flaring. Each of these signs has specific limitations that the physician must be aware of, especially in the infant less than 6 months old. However, as a group they are the most valuable signs of respiratory distress. They appear early in the course of the disease and worsen as the disease worsens, thereby serving as prognostic as well as diagnostic signs.

Tachypnea, an increased respiratory rate, is not specific for respiratory tract diseases. It is also seen in cardiac problems, as well as diseases that cause metabolic acidosis, e.g., diabetic ketoacidosis and salicylate intoxication. The physician must also be aware of the normal respiratory rate for the patient's age. Newborns *normally* breathe 40 to 50 times per minute. By 1 year of age, the respiratory rate is around 30 to 35, by 4 years 20 to 25, and by age 8 to 10 years it is the usual adult rate of 12 to 15. Even with these limitations, tachypnea is an early sign of respiratory distress, which correlates well with the severity of the disease.

Chest retractions and nasal flaring are much more specific for respiratory tract disorders than tachypnea. They are seen both in respiratory tract obstruction and parenchymal lung disease. Both appear early in the course of the disease. They also correlate well with the severity of the disease, although semantically it may be difficult to distinguish "mild" from "moderate" or "moderate" from "severe" retractions or nasal flaring. Both the increased airway resistance of parenchymal lung disease and URT obstruction cause a greater-than-normal negative inspiratory pressure to be generated. This increased negative pressure causes the soft parts of the infant's chest, which is compliant and poorly ossified, to retract inward. Most commonly, retractions are seen in the intercostal, subdiaphragmatic, and supraclavicular spaces. If severe disease is present, the entire sternum may retract on inspiration. Nasal flaring, an outward and upward flaring of the nares on inspiration, is thought to be a primitive reflex seen in young infants, who are obligate nose breathers for the first 2 to 3 months of life. It probably is an attempt to decrease the airway resistance at the nares, which is quite high in the young infant.

Coughing is uncommon in the infant less than 6 months old. This reflex is ordinarily not seen at this age, even in infants with large amounts of mucus in the airway. When a young infant does have a *persistent* cough, one should consider pertussis, *Chlamydia* pneumonia, or cystic fibrosis. Sneezing is much more common in this age group but is much less significant. Because of the importance of nose breathing to young infants, sneezing can occur quite often, usually in the absence of any respiratory disease.

Grunting is another important diagnostic sign. It occurs during expiration, when the glottis is partially closed, causing a delay and then a forceful, noisy expiration (the "grunt"). It seems to be the physiologic counterpart of end expiratory pressure in mechanically ventilated patients. In fact, it was through observations of neonates who grunted that continuous positive airway pressure (CPAP) and positive end-expiratory pressure (PEEP) first came to be used in the treatment of neonatal hyaline membrane disease. The importance of grunting is that it localizes the respiratory disease to the lower respiratory tract. That is, patients who grunt have pneumonia, asthma, or bronchiolitis. Patients with URT obstruction do not grunt. Therefore, not only is grunting specific to the airway, an early sign of disease which correlates with disease severity, but it also is specific to a particular location in the respiratory tract. A valuable sign, indeed.

Stridor is similar to grunting in its significance as a sign of respiratory distress. It appears early and correlates with disease severity. It is not only specific for the airway, but it is specific for the URT. That is, patients with stridor have URT obstruction. Patients with pneumonia, asthma, or bronchiolitis do not have stridor. These two signs, then, are the most important signs of respiratory distress in the pediatric patient. When seeing a child who has either stridor or grunting, the physician can be confident that the disease is not only localized to the respiratory tract but also to a specific part of the respiratory tract.

STRIDOR

The causes of stridor are listed in Table 80-1. These diseases are occasionally referred to collectively as "croup syndrome." This should not be confused with viral croup, which is one of the particular causes of stridor or "croup syndrome."

When confronted with a stridulous child, it is most helpful for the physician to ask two questions—the age of the patient and the duration of symptoms. The answers to these questions will narrow the differential diagnosis considerably. A child under 6 months old with a long duration of symptoms (weeks to months) characteristically has a *congenital* cause of stridor (see Table 80-1).

Table 80-1. Differential Diagnosis of Inspiratory Stridor

Congenital*	Laryngeal/tracheal webs, cysts, tumors, laryngomalacia,* vascular ring, ectopic thyroid, thyroglossal duct cyst, congenital vocal cord paralysis
Inflammatory	Viral croup,† epiglottitis,† retropharyngeal abscess, diphtheria, tetanus
Noninflammatory	Aspiration of a foreign body into the airway,† esophageal foreign body, gastroesophageal reflux, tetany, trauma, tumors

* = Most common causes under 6 months of age.

† = Most common causes over 6 months of age.

Most of these diseases present in the newborn nursery or in the pediatrician's office and are not emergency room problems.

Laryngomalacia, the most common congenital cause of stridor, is due to a developmentally weak larynx, which collapses with each inspiration. It is a self-limited disorder, resolving completely over 6 to 12 months, although there may be exacerbations with upper respiratory infections (URI). If asked, the mother will tell you, "He's breathed that way since he was born." It is usually an incidental finding and not the reason for the emergency room visit. It is a benign problem which requires no therapy.

The patient over 6 months with a relatively short duration of symptoms (hours to days) characteristically has an acquired cause of stridor. This may be inflammatory, such as viral croup or epiglottitis, or noninflammatory, such as foreign body aspiration. The remainder of the chapter will deal with the most common acquired causes of stridor: epiglottitis, viral croup, foreign body aspiration, and retropharyngeal abscess.

EPIGLOTTITIS

Clinical Findings

Epiglottitis is a life-threatening disease, a true pediatric emergency. The age of patients ranges from 2 to 7 years old; the etiology is almost always *Hemophilus influenzae*. Classically, there is an *abrupt* onset over several hours of high fever, sore throat, stridor, dysphagia, and drooling. The mother can often tell you the exact time of day the child became ill. Physical examination reveals a toxic-looking child with an ashen-gray color who is very apprehensive and anxious-looking, but with minimal movements. There is usually quiet breathing with little air exchange, no hoarseness but a whispering voice. The characteristic position is sitting up with chin forward and neck slightly extended—the so-called sniffing position.

Epiglottitis can also occur in teenagers and young adults, presenting with stridor, sore throat, fever, and drooling over several days, not hours. *Hemophilus influenzae* is still the most common organism, but gram-positive cocci are also common at this age. There are occasional reports of rapid-onset URT obstruction due to traumatic epiglottitis, secondary to blind vigorous attempts, usually by the parents at home, to remove a foreign body from the child's throat.

Diagnosis

The *ideal* approach is to take *all* patients with suspected epiglottitis to the operating room, administer anesthesia, and examine the airway with a laryngoscope while the patient is anesthetized. If the diagnosis of epiglottitis is made, the patient can be intubated. If it is ruled out, the patient can be returned to the emergency room or ward to continue the workup, secure in the knowledge that epiglottitis is *not* present. However, most hospitals do not have the luxury of a 24-hour-a-day in-house anesthesiologist available.

Therefore, a *less than ideal but perfectly acceptable approach* is the following: A portable lateral neck x-ray is done to establish the diagnosis. The physician *must* stay with the child at all times until the diagnosis is ruled out or the airway is secured. Do *not* send the patient to the x-ray department unattended. A portable

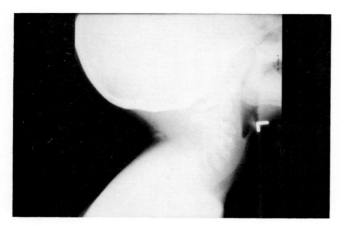

Figure 80-1. A normal lateral neck x-ray.

lateral neck x-ray is quite adequate for diagnosing epiglottitis. Once the diagnosis is made, the patient can be treated accordingly. Should total airway obstruction or apnea occur before the airway has been secured, children with epiglottitis can be bagged effectively. A bag and mask should stay with the physician at the bedside until the diagnosis is ruled out or the airway secured.

A few comments must be made on lateral neck x-rays. First, they must be taken with the neck extended or the anatomy will be impossible to see. Second, the x-ray should be taken during inspiration. The retropharyngeal space normally widens during expiration, and a film taken at that time may lead to a false diagnosis of retropharyngeal abscess. Fortunately, neither of these conditions is difficult to meet in the usual patient. The patient with epiglottitis is already in slight neck extension, and the audible stridor makes for easy timing of the film during inspiration.

A normal lateral neck x-ray is shown in Figure 80-1. There are four things to look for in any lateral neck x-ray done for airway

problems: the epiglottis, the retropharyngeal or prevertebral space, the tracheal air column, and the hypopharynx. The epiglottis is normally tall and thin, projecting up into the hypopharynx. In epiglottitis (Fig. 80-2), it is very swollen, and appears squat and flat, like a "thumbprint" at the base of the hypopharynx. The retropharyngeal space is normally 3 to 4 mm wide. The tracheal air column may need to be "bright-lighted" to be seen well. It should be of uniform width, without densities in the air column. Finally, the dimensions of the hypopharynx should be noted. Similarly to the gastrointestinal tract, although to a much lesser degree, the hypopharynx will distend proximal to a point of obstruction. This is illustrated by the different sizes of the hypopharynx in Figure 80-1 and those in Figure 80-2. While not specific for epiglottitis, this distension does indicate significant URT obstruction. To illustrate the dramatic increase in size in the infected epiglottis, Figures 80-3 and 80-4 show xerograms of a normal lateral neck and that of a patient with epiglottitis. The interested reader is referred to the literature for a more complete discussion of x-rays of the pediatric URT.

A *totally unacceptable approach* to the diagnosis is attempted visualization of the epiglottis with a tongue blade and flashlight in the emergency room. *Do not* attempt direct visualization of the epiglottis unless the patient is sedated *and* you are ready and able to do endotracheal intubation at that moment. The swollen, cherry-red epiglottis of the patient with epiglottitis is not as mobile as normal and does not pop up into view when gagging the patient with a tongue blade. Also, this forceful handling of the patient will cause increased anxiety and stridor, which may cause complete obstruction of the airway.

Airway Management

The airway must be secured either by immediate endotracheal intubation or immediate tracheostomy. The choice between these

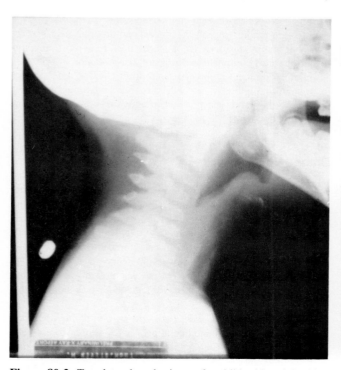
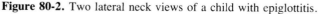

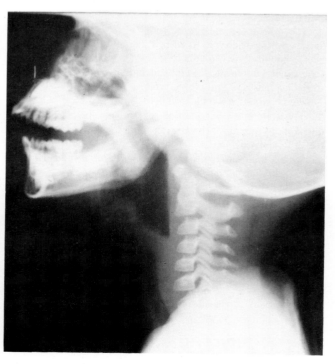

Figure 80-2. Two lateral neck views of a child with epiglottitis.

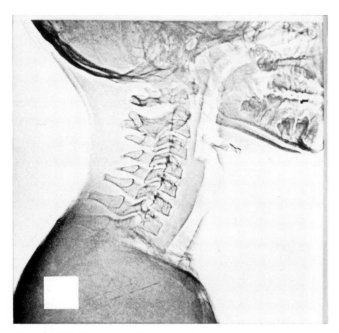

Figure 80-3. Xerogram of a normal lateral neck.

two depends on the particular institution and the 24-h availability of personnel trained in airway management. It is mandatory that each emergency department, along with the pediatric, anesthesia, and ENT departments, develop a protocol for managing the child with epiglottitis. Decisions concerning intubation or tracheostomy or transfer to a tertiary center must be made prior to the patient's arrival in the emergency room. It is totally unacceptable to "carefully observe the patient in an intensive care setting for signs of deterioration." What will surely be observed is the patient suddenly and totally obstructing his or her airway. The objective of airway management is to prevent this from occurring.

Most patients are treated with endotracheal intubation as soon

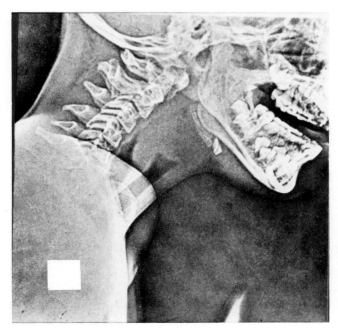

Figure 80-4. Xerogram of a child with epiglottitis.

as the diagnosis is made. This should be performed in the intensive care unit or operating room under controlled conditions on the sedated or anesthetized patient. We have had success using Valium and morphine for preintubation sedation, but some patients may require succinylcholine paralysis before intubation can be accomplished. If succinylcholine is used, the patient will have to be bagged via the endotracheal tube until the drug effect is over, usually several minutes. One should use an endotracheal tube that is one size smaller than ordinarily used for the patient's age, to reduce the incidence of postintubation sequelae. Nasotracheal intubation, following initial orotracheal intubation, is the preferred method in the literature; however, orotracheal intubation alone is also well tolerated. If an oral endotracheal tube is used, an oral airway must also be inserted to prevent the patient from biting down on the endotracheal tube.

Tracheostomy has a higher morbidity in the patient with epiglottitis than endotracheal intubation. However, in some hospitals without adequate availability of intubation personnel, tracheostomy may be the treatment of choice. Again, these decisions should be agreed upon ahead of time and made a part of the emergency room policy. Except for the patient who comes in in respiratory arrest and does not begin spontaneous ventilations after resuscitation (hypoxic brain damage), mechanical ventilation is not necessary. The duration of intubation is 24 to 48 h, after which time the patient can usually be extubated without visualizing the epiglottis. Once an endotracheal tube is in place, a lateral neck x-ray will not show the epiglottis. Occasionally, postextubation edema causes mild stridor which responds well to nebulized Vaponefrine.

Supportive Therapy

This includes IV hydration, humidification of the air to the endotracheal tube, and administration of oxygen as necessary. Because of the possibility of ampicillin-resistant *Hemophilus* infection, most physicians use ampicillin [200 mg/(kg·day)] and chloramphenicol [100 mg/(kg·day)] until sensitivities are available. Blood cultures are positive in 80 percent of the patients. It is recommended that oral antibiotics be continued after extubation for a total of 7 to 10 days. Steroids are not necessary. Sedation may be required for the duration of the intubation, either with IM Phenergan, Seconal, or rectal chloral hydrate, although verbal reassurance is often adequate, especially in the older child.

VIRAL CROUP

This is usually a benign, self-limited disease. The age range is 6 months—3 years; the etiology is almost always viral, usually parainfluenza virus. The disease occurs equally in boys and girls, although severe croup is more common in boys. The typical history is 2 to 3 days of a URI with a gradually worsening cough, especially at night. By the third or fourth day, there is a barking cough, stridor, and dyspnea, as well as varying degrees of anxiety. Examination shows marked stridor, retractions, tachypnea, hoarseness, and mild cyanosis in room air. The patient may be fairly calm with little distress until the physician begins the examination, at which time the patient's anxiety will increase markedly, causing a worsening of the stridor. Lateral neck x-ray will show a normal epiglottis, distended hypopharynx (in the moderate-to-severely afflicted patient), and a narrowed subglottic airway.

A PA chest x-ray shows a narrowed tracheal air column in the form of a "steeple" rather than the normal "square shoulder." X-rays in mild croup are usually normal.

Treatment is basically symptomatic, i.e. cool mist, oxygen PRN, and hydration either IV or PO. Antibiotics are not needed unless there is an associated bacterial illness (otitis media or tonsillitis). Steroids are probably not helpful, although controversy on this point continues in the literature. Mild sedation is often helpful, but codeine is contraindicated.

Spasmodic croup—recurrent episodes of croup, usually without a preceding URI or fever and almost always occurring at night—is thought to be due to allergy and is very sensitive to mist. Bacterial tracheitis, a more severe form of croup, has been reported with increasing frequency in the past few years. Also referred to as membranous laryngotracheobronchitis, it is usually caused by *Staphylococcus aureus*. The patient has significantly more respiratory distress because of the purulent secretions in the airway. The clinical presentation may be similar to epiglottitis. However, the x-ray shows either the typical findings of croup, or the purulent secretions in the trachea may mimic a foreign body. The patient may need intubation, as well as antibiotics.

In the severely ill patient, one must monitor blood gases and consider endotracheal intubation or tracheostomy. One can use Vaponefrine (racemic epinephrine) by nebulized aerosol via a face mask [intermittent positive pressure breathing (IPPB) is *not* necessary] for acute but sometimes temporary relief of obstructive symptoms. The dose is $\frac{1}{2}$ mL in 3 mL of normal saline. It can be repeated PRN, if a good response continues to occur and no cardiac toxicity, such as arrhythmia, is seen. Because of the possibility of rebound stridor, it is recommended that the patient severely ill enough to receive Vaponefrine should be admitted or watched in the emergency room for 6 to 12 h.

FOREIGN BODY ASPIRATION

Clinical Findings

Over 3000 people die from foreign body aspiration each year, and over half of these are children less than 4 years old. Foreign body aspiration is the most common cause of in-home accidental death in children under 6 years old. It usually occurs in the 1-to-4-year-old but may occur in children as young as 6 months. The most common foreign bodies are peanuts and sunflower seeds, but almost any conceivable type of object (metal, plastic, food, grass) may be aspirated. Under 1 year, eggshell aspiration during feeding is a common cause.

The patient may present with a variety of signs depending on the location of the foreign body and the degree of obstruction:—wheezing, persistent pneumonia, stridor, coughing, or apnea. Recurrent stridor and/or wheezing may indicate a foreign body which is changing position within the airway—stridor when it is proximal, and wheezing when it moves more distally. Stridor from a foreign body implies a location in the larynx, trachea, or mainstem bronchus. The usual location is in a mainstem bronchus, often the right, producing cough, unilateral wheezing, or stridor, and classical x-ray signs. Laryngeal and tracheal foreign bodies are less common but are not rare (10 to 15 percent of all foreign bodies). The patient with persistent stridor and "croup," who does not improve over 5 to 7 days, may have a foreign body in the trachea.

Classically, symptoms will occur acutely (choking, coughing, gagging) but usually subside with passage of the foreign body into the smaller airways. This, in turn, may lead to pneumonia, atelectasis, or wheezing. This triphasic course of symptoms (acute, latent asymptomatic period, delayed wheezing or stridor) is classic for mainstem bronchi foreign bodies. As many as one-third of the aspirations may not be witnessed or remembered by the parent. Often there is no history of aspiration, or it is obtained only in retrospect. The physician must have a high index of suspicion of a foreign body.

Upper esophageal foreign bodies can cause stridor. They may also cause dysphagia or failure to thrive, especially with a long-term radiolucent one such as an aluminum "pop top". However, even in the absence of dysphagia, one should keep in mind the possibility of an esophageal foreign body in the patient with stridor.

Diagnosis

If it is opaque, the foreign body can be seen easily on x-ray. However, most airway foreign bodies are radiolucent and must be diagnosed by a change in airway dynamics or appearance. Laryngeal foreign bodies can be outlined by air contrast on lateral neck x-rays. Tracheal foreign bodies can also be outlined on x-rays, although this may require special techniques such as xerograms or laminograms. Xerograms may also be useful in outlining small nonopaque foreign bodies in the lower airway.

A mainstem bronchi foreign body will cause air trapping in the involved lung on expiration, because the bronchus constricts around it during expiration and obstructive emphysema occurs. This leads to hyperinflation of the obstructed lung and a shift of the mediastinum, during expiration, away from the obstructed side (Fig. 80-5). This shift can be seen on inspiratory and expiratory PA chest x-rays or on fluoroscopy. If necessary, the x-ray technician can put pressure on the epigastrium during expiration, which leads to a maximal exhalation and allows for good timing of the films. In the young or uncooperative patient, it may be impossible to get accurately timed inspiratory and expiratory films.

This mediastinal shift may also be seen on bilateral decubitus x-rays of the chest. Normally, the "down" hemithorax is hypoinflated with an elevated hemidiaphragm and "splinted ribs". However, the reverse occurs on the side of the foreign body, where there is persistent hyperinflation and no loss of volume,

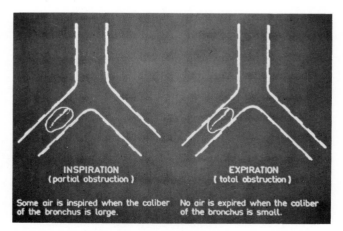

INSPIRATION
(partial obstruction)

EXPIRATION
(total obstruction)

Some air is inspired when the caliber of the bronchus is large.

No air is expired when the caliber of the bronchus is small.

Figure 80-5. Inspiratory and expiratory films in foreign body aspiration.

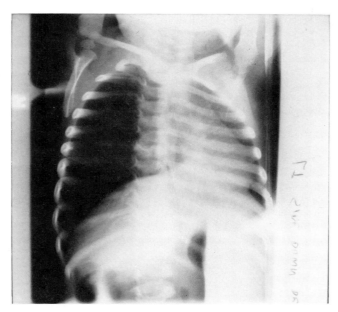

Figure 80-6. Normal decubitus film with left side down.

even when the affected lung is "down" (Figs. 80-6 and 80-7). These films can be done even in young, uncooperative patients.

Most importantly, it takes some time for these findings to occur. A single negative x-ray examination does not rule out the presence of a foreign body. A CT scan may be necessary for diagnosis in difficult cases. However, the most important rule is still to have a high index of suspicion. A preoperative diagnosis is made in only 60 percent of airway foreign bodies. If the physician still suspects the diagnosis, even though x-rays are not confirmatory, he or she should probably proceed to bronchoscopy anyway.

Esophageal foreign bodies are usually radiopaque and easy to

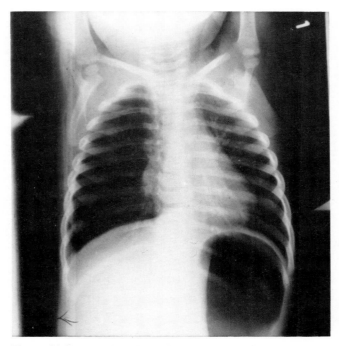

Figure 80-7. Decubitus film, right side down, in foreign body aspiration.

detect on x-rays. Flat esophageal foreign bodies, such as coins, are always oriented in the coronal plane, so that they are *en face* on a PA x-ray. Tracheal foreign bodies are almost always oriented in the sagittal plane because of absent cartilage in the posterior tracheal wall. However, these "rules" are not always obeyed. PA and lateral x-rays will place the opaque foreign body without a doubt. Radiolucent esophageal foreign bodies may require barium swallow, xerograms, or tomograms to make the diagnosis.

Management

Treatment of airway foreign bodies is by laryngoscopy of bronchoscopy with removal of the foreign body in the operating room under anesthesia. This may be a difficult procedure, especially in the young patient with very tiny airways. The foreign body may be too cumbersome to remove whole with the bronchoscope forceps, in which case a Fogarty catheter can be used for removal. Similarly, esophageal foreign bodies can be removed either by endoscopic forceps or with a Foley catheter. However, if the latter is used, the foreign body must be smooth, without sharp edges, in place for under 2 weeks, and there must be no underlying esophageal disease. It is almost never necessary to proceed immediately to bronchoscopy. One can usually wait and schedule it electively, especially if the patient has a full stomach.

Because of airway edema caused by the foreign body itself and the instrumentation necessary for removal, as well as chemical pneumonia in cases of food aspiration (especially peanuts), the patient with an airway foreign body will require respiratory care for 24 to 72 h after its removal. Antibiotics, steroids, oxygen, mist, and chest physiotherapy may all be necessary for 24 to 72 h after removal of the foreign body. The patient with a foreign body is not dramatically improved after bronchoscopic removal as the patient with epiglottitis is after intubation.

RETROPHARYNGEAL ABSCESS

The usual age of occurrence is 6 months to 3 years. Retropharyngeal abscess is rare in a child over 3 because of the normal regression in size of the retropharyngeal lymph nodes with age. It begins with a URI which localizes to the retropharyngeal lymph nodes over several days. Dysphagia and refusal to eat occur before significant respiratory distress. The child is usually toxic-looking, febrile, drooling, and has inspiratory stridor and dysphagia. Characteristically, these children assume an almost opisthotonic posture.

The diagnostic test is a lateral neck x-ray, which shows a widened retropharyngeal space (Fig. 80-8). The x-ray must be done in inspiration with the neck extended or a false-positive widening will be seen. Occasionally, lucencies or actual air-fluid levels can be seen within the widened retropharyngeal space. Physical examination of the pharynx shows a retropharyngeal mass which can often be seen with a tongue blade and flashlight. Palpation of the mass is dangerous for it may lead to rupture of the abscess.

Treatment is high-dose IV antibiotics, usually penicillin G, in doses of 100,000 units/(kg·day). The most common causative organism is β-hemolytic *Streptococcus*. If fluctuation or severe respiratory distress occurs, incision and drainage should be done in a controlled manner in the operating room by an experienced ENT physician. Complications include respiratory failure from obstruction; rupture of the abscess into the airway, causing either asphyxia

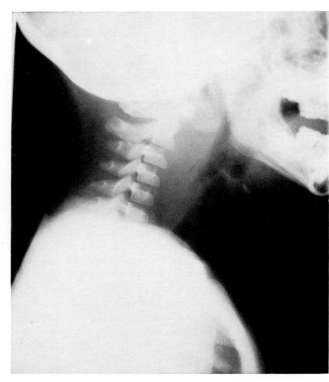

Figure 80-8. Lateral neck view in a child with retropharyngeal abscess.

or bronchopneumonia; and spread of the abscess into the adjacent soft tissues of the neck.

BIBLIOGRAPHY

American Academy of Pediatrics. Committee on Accident and Poison Prevention: First aid for the choking child. *Pediatrics* 67(5):744, 1981.

Bottenfield GW, Arcinue EL, Sarnaik A, et al: Diagnosis and management of acute epiglottitis—report of 90 consecutive cases. *Laryngoscope* 90(5):822–825, 1980.

Burrington JD: Aluminum "pop tops." A hazard to child health. *JAMA* 235(24):2614–2617, 1976.

Chernick V, Avery ME, Strieder DJ: Why intermittent positive pressure when normal inhalations will do? *J Pediatr* 91(2):361–362, 1977.

Denneny JC, III, Handler SD: Membranous laryngotracheobronchitis. *Pediatrics* 70(5):705–707, 1982.

Dunbar JS: Upper respiratory tract obstruction in infants and children. *Am J Roentgenol* 109(2):227–246, 1970.

Fogel JM, Berg IJ, Gerber MA, et al: Racemic epinephrine in the treatment of croup: Nebulization alone versus nebulization with intermittent positive pressure breathing. *J Pediatr* 101(6):1028–1031, 1982.

Hight DW, Philippart AI, Hertzler JH: The treatment of retained peripheral foreign bodies in the pediatric airway. *J Pediatr Surg* 16(5):694–699, 1981.

Liston SL, Gehrz RC, Jarvis CW: Bacterial tracheitis. *Arch Otolaryngol* 107(9):561–564, 1981.

Liston SL, Siegel LG, LaBeau RF: Epiglottitis. *Minn Med* 65(1):11–14, 1982.

Maze A, Bloch E: Stridor in pediatric patients. *Anesthesiology* 50(2):132–145, 1979.

Moskowitz D, Gardiner LJ, Sasaki CT: Foreign body aspiration: Potential misdiagnosis. *Arch Otolaryngol* 108(12):806–807, 1982.

Newman DE: The radiolucent esophageal foreign body: An often-forgotten cause of respiratory symptoms. *J Pediatr* 92(1):60–63, 1978.

O'Neill JA, Holcomb GW, Jr, Neblett WW: Management of tracheobronchial and esophageal foreign bodies in childhood. *J Pediatr Surg* 18(4):475–479, 1983.

Schloss MD, Gold JA, Rosales JK, et al: Acute epiglottitis: Current management. *Laryngoscope* 93(4):489–493, 1983.

Schuller DE, Birck HG: The safety of intubation in croup and epiglottitis. *Laryngoscope* 85(1):33–46, 1975.

Szold PD, Glicklich M: Children with epiglottitis can be bagged. *Clin Pediatr* 15(9):792–793, 1976.

Wesenburg RL, Blumhagen JD: Assisted expiratory chest radiography. An effective technique for the diagnosis of foreign body aspiration. *Radiology* 130(2):538–539, 1979.

CHAPTER 81
PEDIATRIC
BRONCHIOLITIS

Stanley H. Inkelis

Bronchiolitis is the term used to describe a clinical syndrome in infancy characterized by rapid respiration, chest retractions, and wheezing. It typically occurs during the winter and spring months, more often in male than female infants less than 2 years of age, with the greatest frequency between the ages of 2 and 6 months.

ETIOLOGY

The most common cause of bronchiolitis is the respiratory syncytial virus (RSV). It is the etiologic agent in approximately 75 percent of infants admitted to the hospital with this disorder. Other organisms which cause bronchiolitis are parainfluenza virus, influenza virus, mumps virus, adenovirus, echovirus, rhinovirus, *Mycoplasma pneumoniae, Chlamydia trachomatis,* and *Legionella pneumophilia* (suspected). Adenovirus, particularly types 3, 7, and 21, may cause a more destructive form of bronchiolitis, known as bronchiolitis obliterans, a chronic, obstructive lung disease. *Hemophilus influenzae* was at one time felt to be a cause of bronchiolitis, but this organism is not isolated more frequently in children with bronchiolitis than in controls.

PATHOPHYSIOLOGY

The most important pulmonary lesion associated with bronchiolitis is bronchiolar obstruction characterized by submucosal edema, peribronchiolar cellular infiltrate, mucous plugging, and intraluminal debris. These pathological changes lead to narrowing of the lumens of small bronchi and bronchioles, increasing airway resistance, and concomitant wheezing. The obstruction is not uniform throughout the lungs, so that some of the small bronchi and bronchioles are affected while others are not. However, normal exchange of gases in the lung is impaired. Hypoxemia is the major result of abnormal gas exchange in which alveoli are poorly ventilated but remain well perfused (ventilation-perfusion imbalance). Compensation for the hypoxemia results in hyperventilation, which is a more sensitive indicator of reduced oxygen tension than is cyanosis. Carbon dioxide retention does not occur in mild cases of bronchiolitis, but in more severe cases where larger numbers of alveoli are obstructed, hypercapnia and respiratory acidosis ensue. Carbon dioxide retention is associated with respiratory rates of greater than 60 and increases in proportion to the increasing rate.

CLINICAL FINDINGS

Bronchiolitis usually occurs in children in contact with family members who have an upper respiratory infection. The infant is first noted to have signs of upper respiratory infection, i.e., runny nose and sneezing, accompanied by a low-grade fever, 38° to 39°C (100° to 102°F), and decreased appetite. Lower respiratory symptoms develop over a few days and include dyspnea, tachypnea, intercostal retractions, wheezing, and cyanosis. In more severely affected patients, the symptoms may develop more rapidly, within a few hours.

On examination of the patient with bronchiolitis, one will typically see a tachypneic infant in mild to severe respiratory distress, with respirations ranging from 60 to 80 per minute, flaring of the alae nasi, and using the accessory muscles of respiration with intercostal and subcostal retractions. Cyanosis may not be present, but significant abnormalities of gas exchange may develop in the absence of cyanosis. Respirations are shallow because of the persistent distention of the lungs by trapped air. Diffuse, fine sibilant and/or musical rales are often present and the expiratory phase of breathing may be prolonged with audible wheezing. Barely audible breath sounds are a sign of impending respiratory failure. The liver and spleen may be palpated below the costal margins, suggesting hepatosplenomegaly; however, their position is secondary to downward displacement of the diaphragm from pulmonary hyperinflation. Signs of dehydration are often present, usually caused by inadequate oral fluid intake secondary to respiratory distress.

It is during the first 48 to 72 h after the onset of cough and dyspnea that the infant is most critically ill. Improvement occurs quickly after this time and the infant is usually fully recovered within a few days.

X-RAY AND LABORATORY FINDINGS

The chest x-ray shows hyperinflation of the lungs and an increased AP diameter on lateral view. There are sometimes small areas of atelectasis which may mimic pneumonitis. The white blood cell count and hemoglobin level are usually within the normal range. Viral cultures are positive in the majority of infants with bronchiolitis, with respiratory syncytial virus (RSV) being by far the most frequently identified. Blood gases almost always reveal hypoxemia, which correlates with the respiratory rate. Carbon dioxide retention occurs infrequently in children with bronchiolitis, but is present in those infants in severe respiratory distress.

DIFFERENTIAL DIAGNOSIS

Bronchiolitis and infantile asthma are very similar in their clinical presentation and their differentiation provides a challenge for even the best of clinicians. In fact, in some situations, it may be impossible to clinically differentiate between the two. The most important differential clue to infantile asthma is a history of recurrent episodes of wheezing and/or coughing in an infant, regardless of age. Other clinical features suggesting asthma are a positive family history of asthma or allergy, physical evidence of atopic disease in the patient, sudden onset of wheezing without preceding infection, markedly prolonged expiration, and rapid reversibility of bronchospasm with epinephrine or other sympathomimetic therapy.

The relationship between bronchiolitis and the subsequent development of asthma is very intriguing. Between 25 and 50 percent of children with bronchiolitis develop asthma later in life. It is not clear whether the airways of some children are initially hyperactive, thus predisposing them to bronchiolitis, or if the first viral infection and resultant epithelial damage sensitize irritant receptors and lead to hyperactive airways.

It is known that RSV and other viruses are potent stimulants of wheezing in the individual prone to asthma. This suggests that bronchiolitis may be the first attack of asthma in the atopic child and that these children may be more likely to wheeze if infected with RSV or other viruses. In most patients with RSV infection of any kind, IgE is bound to exfoliated nasopharyngeal epithelial cells. The persistence of cell-bound IgE in patients with RSV-induced bronchiolitis or asthma, in contrast to those patients with mild upper respiratory tract infection or pneumonia from RSV, may explain the recurrent episodes of wheezing that occur in infants after RSV-induced bronchiolitis. Other studies have demonstrated pulmonary function abnormalities in symptom-free children years after their episode of bronchiolitis, indicating that these children are left with residual parenchymal or airway lesions which may predispose them to chronic obstructive lung disease.

Other disease processes associated with wheezing which can be confused with bronchiolitis may be excluded by a careful history and physical and radiographic examination. Recurrent food aspiration from gastroesophageal reflux or tracheoesophageal fistula usually presents with a history of frequent vomiting after feeding and associated coughing and choking. Foreign bodies in the trachea, bronchus, or esophagus may be differentiated from bronchiolitis in that severe coughing, cyanosis, and respiratory distress usually develop suddenly in a well child who has recently been eating peanuts, popcorn, coins, seeds, etc. Often, the wheezing will be unilateral. A chest x-ray may identify the foreign body if it is radiopaque. If it is not, one may see hyperinflation on the affected side on an expiratory film. Since expiratory films are difficult to obtain in small children, bilateral, lateral decubitus films are very helpful. Normally, the dependent lung against the

table will have less volume than the other lung because of its immobility. However, if a foreign body is present on the side closest to the table, air trapping persists and hyperinflation is evident.

Bronchial stenosis is commonly manifested by wheezing and recurrent lower respiratory infection. This disorder can be diagnosed by bronchoscopy.

Children with cystic fibrosis on initial presentation may be difficult to differentiate from those with bronchiolitis. If there is a history of recurrent wheezing, pneumonitis, and respiratory distress in an infant who is failing to thrive, one must strongly consider this diagnosis.

Congestive heart failure from congenital heart disease or viral myocarditis may present in a fashion similar to bronchiolitis, especially with a palpable liver and spleen confusing the issue. A history of normal growth and development and the absence of a heart murmur makes the diagnoses of bronchiolitis more likely. The chest x-ray in congestive heart failure will usually demonstrate a large heart. An ECG is helpful if one remains unsure of the diagnosis. Infants with heart disease sometimes go into congestive heart failure with viral infections, and may present with both conditions at once.

Vascular rings, mediastinal cysts and tumors may compress the trachea or a bronchus. If one suspects a vascular ring but cannot see compression of the trachea on chest x-ray, a barium swallow may demonstrate constriction of the esophagus at the site of the ring. A mediastinal cyst or tumor will be apparent as a mass on chest x-ray.

Salicylate intoxication or other metabolic disorders may mimic bronchiolitis clinically because of the rapid respiratory rate. These disorders may be diagnosed by asking specifically about aspirin ingestion, obtaining measurements of arterial blood gas, salicylate levels, and serum electrolytes.

Bronchopulmonary dysplasia (BPD) presents with symptoms very similar to bronchiolitis. Infants with BPD, however, are usually premature and on a respirator for respiratory distress syndrome. Their chest x-rays show evidence of chronic lung disease not seen in the infant with bronchiolitis. Infants with BPD may develop bronchiolitis and present a confusing clinical picture.

Croup, epiglottitis, and other causes of upper airway obstruction usually present with inspiratory wheezing (stridor) but rarely with expiratory wheezing. If there is doubt about the diagnosis, chest and lateral neck x-rays may be helpful. If one is seriously considering the diagnosis of epiglottitis, however, one should follow the hospital protocol for this disease and, above all, never leave the patient unattended by a physician.

TREATMENT

Treatment for bronchiolitis is primarily supportive and should be based on the child's clinical condition. Almost all children with bronchiolitis are hypoxemic, especially when they are asleep. Consequently, the most important therapy for bronchiolitis is humidified oxygen at an Fi_{O_2} of 40%. This should be delivered by mask, hood, or tent, since nasal prongs may produce reflex bronchoconstriction. Arterial blood gases are useful in monitoring those patients in moderate to severe respiratory distress [respiratory rate (RR) > 60]. Mist has not proved helpful since almost no moisture reaches the lower respiratory tract to liquefy secretions.

Many children with bronchiolitis become dehydrated because of decreased fluid intake secondary to the excessive work of breathing and pulmonary insensible water loss. Intravenous fluids must be administered to these children, but should be given with some caution as pulmonary edema may occur with overaggressive fluid therapy. Hydration in excess of replacement and maintenance is unnecessary.

Routine administration of antibiotics has not proven beneficial in bronchiolitis. If the child is desperately ill, or if the infant's clinical condition suddenly deteriorates, one should consider bacterial infection superimposed on viral infection. In this case, a broad-spectrum antibiotic such as ampicillin may be useful. Prior to administering the antibiotic, tracheal secretions should be examined by Gram stain and by culture, and blood cultures should be obtained.

Corticosteroids have been studied extensively in bronchiolitis and have not been shown to alter the course of this disease.

Sedation should be avoided because of its effect on suppression of the respiratory drive. In very agitated infants, who are closely monitored, one may consider using chloral hydrate, 10 to 20 mg/kg per dose every 6 to 8 h.

Bronchodilator therapy in infants with bronchiolitis is controversial. Since many children with bronchiolitis go on to develop asthma, it is beneficial to give a trial of subcutaneous epinephrine, 1:1000, 0.01 mL/kg. If the child responds, it suggests that he or she has reversible bronchospasm and should be followed closely for future wheezing episodes. Although theophylline has never proved effective in children with bronchiolitis, theophylline preparations may be helpful at a starting dose of 3–5 mg/kg per dose in the child who has responded to epinephrine. Doses may have to be adjusted in order to obtain therapeutic levels of between 10 to 20 μg/mL. One must be careful in infants less than 6 months of age to monitor their theophylline levels closely since the half-life of theophylline is longer and the metabolism is more erratic than in older infants and children.

One may consider managing a child with bronchiolitis as an outpatient if the child is well hydrated, drinking fluids well, is not cyanotic, appears comfortable, and is not in visible respiratory distress (RR less than 60). Since hypoxemia is a common finding in bronchiolitic children, arterial blood gases should be obtained in most instances. Children who are not drinking fluids well and appear to be in respiratory distress should be admitted. Occasionally, children with severe bronchiolitis develop respiratory failure. These infants may need endotracheal or nasotracheal intubation for ventilatory support. Infants with a past history of respiratory distress syndrome resulting in bronchopulmonary dysplasia who develop bronchiolitis need close observation and should, in almost all cases, be hospitalized.

If the social situation is such that following instructions and giving adequate home care seem unlikely, or if parental anxiety is so great that the parents are having trouble coping with their child's illness, the child should be admitted. If one chooses to discharge a patient with mild bronchiolitis, parents should be given detailed instructions regarding hydration and increasing respiratory distress. All these children should be seen again 12 to 24 h after their presentation to the emergency department.

SUMMARY

Bronchiolitis is characterized by rapid respiration, chest retractions, and wheezing in the infant. It is most often caused by the respiratory syncytial virus and usually occurs in the winter and spring. Bronchiolitis is commonly confused with infantile asthma and attempts should be made to differentiate the two. Treatment is supportive. Bronchiolitis is usually a mild disease, but may cause significant respiratory distress and necessitate admission to the hospital.

BIBLIOGRAPHY

Brooks LJ, Cropp GJA: Theophylline therapy in bronchiolitis. *Am J Dis Child* 135:934–936, 1981.

Denny FW, Collier AM, Henderson FW, et al: The epidemiology of bronchiolitis. *Pediatr Res* 11:234–236, 1977.

Dunsky E: Bronchiolitis: Differentiation from infantile asthma. *Pediatr Ann* 6:45, 47–51, 55–56, July 1977.

Ellis EF: Therapy of acute bronchiolitis. *Pediatr Res* 11:263–264, 1977.

Gurwitz D, Mindorff C, Levison H: Increased incidence of bronchial reactivity in children with a history of bronchiolitis. *J Pediatr* 98:551–555, 1981.

Kattan M, Keens TG, Lapierre J, et al: Pulmonary function abnormalities in symptom free children after bronchiolitis. *Pediatrics* 59:683–688, 1977.

Mellins RB: Bronchiolitis—comments on pathogenesis and treatment. *Pediatr Res* 11:268–269, 1977.

McConnochie KM: Bronchiolitis: What's in the name. *Am J Dis Child* 137:11–13, 1983.

Simons ER, Friesen FR, Simons KJ: Theophylline toxicity in term infants. *Am J Dis Child* 134:39–41, 1980.

Tabachnik E, Levison H: Infantile bronchial asthma. *J Allergy Clin Immunol* 67:339–347, 1981.

Welliver RC, Kaul TN, Ogra PL: The appearance of cell-bound IgE in respiratory tract epithelium after respiratory syncitial virus infection. *N Engl J Med* 303:1198–1202, 1980.

Wohl MEB, Chernick V: Bronchiolitis: State of the art. *Am Rev Respir Dis* 118:759–781, 1978.

CHAPTER 82
PEDIATRIC ASTHMA

Stanley H. Inkelis

Asthma is a disorder of the tracheobronchial tree characterized by bronchial hyperirritability and subsequent obstruction to airflow after exposure to any one of many stimuli. Examples of these stimuli include extrinsic allergens, viral respiratory infections, vigorous exercise, cold air, cigarette smoke, and air pollutants. Narrowing of the airways is dynamic and either improves spontaneously or as a result of therapy. The symptom which is most characteristic of asthma is wheezing. However, the often-quoted statement, "all that wheezes is not asthma" is certainly true, and emphasizes the importance of the differential diagnosis which will be addressed later in this chapter. Asthma may occur, on the other hand, without evidence of overt wheezing and is often missed in children who are diagnosed as having recurrent pneumonia, recurrent or chronic bronchitis, or recurrent colds with chest congestion.

Asthma is one of the leading causes of chronic illness in children, with a prevalence rate of 5 to 7 percent. About 75 percent of children with asthma have their first symptoms before 4 to 5 years of age. One-fourth of the days lost from school because of chronic childhood illness can be attributed to this disorder. In addition, asthma ranks third among all chronic diseases for which physician visits are necessary. Consequently, it is important for all physicians caring for children to be aware of the different manifestations of asthma and to have a thorough understanding of its management. The prognosis for asthmatic children is very good. About half of these children will be free of symptoms by the time they are adults.

ETIOLOGY

The etiology of asthma is multifactorial. Immunologic, infectious, endocrine, and psychologic factors play a role in the development of asthma in different individuals. Rather than being one disease, asthma may, in fact, be a number of diseases that have in common the physiologic finding of reversible obstructive airway changes.

Asthma is usually divided into "extrinsic" and "intrinsic" forms. Environmental factors such as dust, pollens, dander, molds, and foods are the cause of asthma in children with extrinsic or allergic asthma. This is the most common type of asthma seen in children and represents type I immediate hypersensitivity in which IgE antibodies are produced in response to allergens. IgE antibodies bind to receptors of mast cells and basophils. Interaction with the antigens causes the release of mediators of inflammation such as histamine and leukotrienes [slow-reacting substance of anaphylaxis (SRS-A)].

In children with intrinsic asthma, no evidence of IgE involvement is found. There is little correlation with skin tests and known allergens. This type of asthma is seen most frequently in the first 2 years of life and in adults. The precipitant of asthma in these individuals is usually viral respiratory infection, most commonly caused by the respiratory syncytial and parainfluenza viruses.

Several theories have been proposed to explain, in more biochemical detail, the etiology of asthma. The β-adrenergic theory, proposed by Szentivanyi, suggests that asthma is due to abnormal β-adrenergic receptor–adenylate cyclase function, with decreased adrenergic responsiveness. Another theory proposes that increased cholinergic activity through increased irritant receptor sensitivity is the fundamental defect in asthma. Neither of these theories, nor others alone, fully explain the etiology of asthma but have helped physicians in their approach to the asthmatic child.

PATHOPHYSIOLOGY

Most of the information available regarding the pathology of asthma comes from postmortem examination. The lungs are hyperinflated and pale, and are difficult to collapse with pressure. Numerous tenacious mucous plugs exude from the larger and middle-sized bronchi. On microscopic examination, sloughing of mucosal cells, edema of the bronchial mucosa, and hyperplasia and hypertrophy of bronchial and bronchiolar smooth muscle are seen. Often, there is infiltration of the submucosa by eosinophils.

The combination of mucosal edema, bronchospasm, and mucous plugging results in airway obstruction which leads to increased airway resistance and gas trapping. Varying degrees of obstruction, atelectasis, and decreased compliance cause ventilation-perfusion mismatch. Hypoxemia occurs because of perfusion of inadequately ventilated portions of the lung. Early in severe asthma, carbon dioxide tensions are usually below normal because of compensatory hyperventilation. As the obstruction increases, the number of alveoli being adequately ventilated and perfused decreases, giving rise to CO_2 retention. A "normal" P_{CO_2} of 40 mmHg in the setting of asthma may be an indication of respiratory muscle fatigue and impending respiratory failure.

Acidosis results from both hypoxia and hypercapnea. Along with hypoxemia, acidosis leads to pulmonary vasoconstriction, pulmonary hypertension, right heart strain, and, occasionally, cardiac failure.

Infants with asthma have more severe respiratory symptoms and are more vulnerable to respiratory failure. The anatomic and physiologic reasons for this are (1) increased peripheral airway resistance, (2) decreased elastic recoil pressure and early airway closure, (3) deficient collateral channels of ventilation, and (4) an unstable ribcage and mechanically disadvantaged diaphragm.

Clinical Findings

Wheezing is the hallmark of asthma and is present in almost every child presenting to the emergency department with this disorder. The notable exceptions to this are (1) the child who is in extreme respiratory distress and is so "tight" that there is not enough movement of air to produce audible wheezing, and (2) the child who has a persistent nonproductive cough or who coughs and becomes short of breath with exercise. In the latter case, many of the patients will have findings characteristic of asthma on pulmonary function testing and will respond to bronchodilator therapy.

Attacks of asthma may be acute or may be of gradual onset. Exposure to allergens or bronchial irritants causes the acute attack of asthma which is most likely due to spasm of the large airways. Viral upper respiratory infections usually cause attacks of slower onset with a gradual increase in frequency and severity of cough and wheezing over a few days.

Other signs and symptoms in addition to wheezing and cough associated with asthma include tachypnea, shortness of breath with prolonged expiration and use of accessory muscles of respiration, cyanosis, hyperinflation of the chest, tachycardia, abdominal pain, a feeling of "tight chest," poor exercise tolerance, "recurrent chest colds," "recurrent" or "chronic" bronchitis, or "recurrent pneumonia."

On physical examination the chest is hyperinflated and hyperresonant to percussion. A barrel chest deformity suggests chronic, severe asthma. Expiratory wheezes are prominent; occasionally inspiratory wheezes will be heard as well. Musical rales may be present. The child usually is restless with tachypnea and tachycardia. If the child is in extreme respiratory distress, wheezing may be absent, as noted above. To make breathing easier, the child may assume a hunched-over, tripod-like sitting position. Cyanosis may be apparent. The liver and spleen may be palpable due to hyperinflation of the lungs and downward movement of the diaphragm. Successful treatment will produce color improvement and wheezing as air begins to move through the lungs.

Laboratory and X-ray Findings

Most asthmatic children have normal blood counts; however, an elevated white blood cell count does not necessarily indicate infection. Both the "stress" of an acute asthma attack and the injection of epinephrine may cause leukocytosis. Blood eosinophilia above 250 to 400 cells/mm^3 is common in asthmatic children with the total eosinophil count being preferred to estimation from differential white counts. Eosinophils in the sputum are usually present, as well. Sputum cultures are not very helpful in children.

A chest x-ray should be taken on every child with his or her first episode of wheezing or a history of persistent symptoms of asthma, i.e., "chronic cough," "chronic bronchitis," etc., (if no x-ray was taken previously) to rule out foreign body aspiration, heart disease, parenchymal disease, and congenital anomaly. One should obtain or strongly consider obtaining an x-ray on any child admitted to the hospital. Although the chest x-ray may be normal in an acute attack of asthma, the lungs are usually hyperinflated with flattening of the diaphragms, and increased bronchial markings. In addition, there may be patchy areas of infiltrate or atelectasis and, less commonly, pneumomediastinum and pneumothorax. Routine chest x-ray is not necessary, however, for the known asthmatic with an uncomplicated attack.

Pulmonary function tests are useful determinants of response to therapy in the asthmatic child. A spirometer or, for smaller children, a Wright pediatric peak flow meter are simple to use and are helpful in conjunction with clinical evaluation in identifying patients needing admission. A study by Wharton, et al., found that in children between 8 and 18 years of age, the peak flow rate taken prior to therapy was a poor predictor of the need for admission, but a peak flow rate of <150 L/min at 1 h after therapy was 89 percent predictive of later admission.

Arterial blood gases should be obtained from the radial or brachial artery in the moderate to severely ill asthmatic child to monitor for respiratory failure. Hypoxemia is commonly found because of ventilation and perfusion imbalance. The P_{CO_2}, which is usually low during the early part of an asthmatic attack, begins to rise as the obstruction increases. When the P_{CO_2} is >35, it is an indication for concern, and blood gases should be monitored frequently. The blood pH usually remains normal until the buffering capacity of the blood is superseded.

DIFFERENTIAL DIAGNOSIS

Some physicians are reluctant to diagnose asthma in a child less than 2 years of age, and label children who have recurrent episodes of coughing and wheezing with diagnoses such as asthmatic bronchitis, wheezy bronchitis, recurrent bronchiolitis, etc. There is good evidence, however, that approximately 5 to 10 percent of infants less than 2 years old have asthma.

The child with wheezing; a family history of atopic disease; past history of allergic disease, particularly atopic dermatitis; previous response to epinephrine; and an elevated IgE, is almost certainly an asthmatic. However, there are many variations on the theme of wheezing that do not always make the diagnosis of asthma as clear-cut as one might wish. Although, most often, wheezing is associated with asthma, the characteristic features of asthma may be found to some degree in a wide variety of chest and systemic diseases (see Table 82-1).

Table 82-1. Differential Diagnosis of Asthma

1. Bronchiolitis
2. Foreign body aspiration
3. Viral pneumonitis
4. Cystic fibrosis
5. Heart disease
6. Vascular rings
7. Gastroesophageal reflux
8. Stenosis: tracheal and bronchial
9. Alpha 1-antitrypsin deficiency
10. Neoplasms
    Adenomas
    Papillomas
11. Bronchopulmonary dysplasia
12. Bronchogenic cysts
13. Lymph gland enlargement
14. Hypersensitivity pneumonitis

The most common causes of wheezing in the infant are asthma and bronchiolitis. These are so similar in their clinical presentation that it may be impossible on first encounter with an infant to differentiate between the two. Acute bronchiolitis is primarily caused by the respiratory syncytial virus. It usually occurs in children between 2 and 6 months of age (but may occur until age 2 years) in the winter and spring months. There are often other family members with an upper respiratory infection (URI) and the infant's illness begins with signs of a URI. There is usually no history of associated atopic disease in the patient or family (see Chapter 81, "Bronchiolitis").

Considering that between 25 and 50 percent of children with bronchiolitis develop asthma later in life, it may be that bronchiolitis is the first attack of asthma in these children. A helpful way to differentiate between the two is by giving a trial of epinephrine. Those infants responding to epinephrine are more likely asthmatic. Since acute viral bronchiolitis is rarely a recurrent condition, infants with recurrent attacks (three or more episodes) of "bronchiolitis" should be considered asthmatic and treated as such.

Less common causes of wheezing in children are recurrent food aspiration from gastroesophageal reflux; a foreign body in the trachea, bronchus, or esophagus; cystic fibrosis; heart disease; vascular rings; mediastinal cysts and tumors; and bronchopulmonary dysplasia. More detailed signs and symptoms of these disorders may be found in the differential diagnosis section of Chapter 81, "Bronchiolitis."

TREATMENT

Theory

The treatment of asthma is aimed at decreasing smooth muscle spasm and reducing bronchial mucosal edema and mucus secretion. Treatment is based on the theory that cyclic AMP (cyclic adenosine 3′, 5′-monophosphate) and cyclic GMP (cyclic guanosine monophosphate) have opposing effects on bronchial smooth muscle and release of mediators from mast cells. Elevation of cyclic AMP causes smooth muscle relaxation and decreased synthesis and release from mast cells of mediators, while elevation of cyclic GMP causes constriction of bronchial smooth muscle and increased release of mediators from mast cells. Sympathomimetics and methylxanthines, the two types of bronchodilators most commonly used, increase levels of cyclic AMP. Sympathomimetics activate the enzyme adenyl cyclase which catalyzes ATP to cyclic AMP while methylxanthines inhibit the enzyme phosphodiesterase which degrades cyclic AMP.

Cyclic GMP appears to be controlled by the parasympathetic nervous system. The enzyme guanylate cyclase is increased by vagal stimulation or cholinergic drugs, thereby increasing the concentration of cyclic GMP. Atropine and other anticholinergic drugs have the reverse effect. The side effects associated with anticholinergic agents currently limit their use. However, these drugs may have significant potential for clinical use in the future if analogues of the present compounds can be found which produce fewer side effects.

Sympathomimetic (adrenergic) agents, which are often the first-line medication used in the treatment of asthma, exert their activity by combining with receptors on cell surfaces. The two types of

adrenergic receptors are α and β. Usually, drugs affecting α-adrenergic receptors are associated with excitatory functions while drugs affecting β-adrenergic receptors are associated with inhibitory functions (e.g., muscle relaxation). Stimulation of α-adrenergic receptors by agents such as norepinephrine decreases the amount of available cyclic AMP, and stimulation of β-adrenergic receptors increases the amount of available cyclic AMP. Consequently, adrenergic drugs which stimulate β receptors are useful in treating the asthmatic patient. The β-adrenergic system has two groups of receptors: the β_1 receptors, which control heart rate, myocardial contractility, and lipolysis; and the β_2 receptors, which control bronchiolar and arteriolar dilatation. Therefore, adrenergic drugs with more β_2-selective activity, such as metaproterenol, terbutaline, and salbutamol, affect bronchodilation without affecting an increase in heart rate and myocardial contractility that occur with epinephrine and isoproterenol, which stimulate both β_1 and β_2 receptors.

Treatment of Acute Attacks of Asthma

Most children presenting to the emergency room with asthma have an acute episode of airway obstruction that can be reversed relatively easily with bronchodilators. Epinephrine by injection has been the preferred treatment for acute asthma for many years, but bronchodilator aerosols, especially those with more selective β_2-activity, have been in favor more recently.

Aqueous epinephrine, 1:1000, may be administered subcutaneously at a dose of 0.01 mL/kg up to a maximum dose of 0.3 mL. This dose may be repeated twice at 20-min intervals. If there is no response, further administration of epinephrine is not indicated. If the patient improves, Sus-Phrine 1:200, a slowly absorbed epinephrine suspension that acts over 6 to 12 h, may be given to prolong the action of epinephrine. The dose is 0.005 mL/kg (half the dose of epinephrine) and should not be repeated any more often than every 6 to 8 h, since only 25 percent of the epinephrine is absorbed within minutes and the rest is released slowly over a period of hours. There is some evidence that Sus-Phrine alone, without previous administration of epinephrine, improves the clinical condition and pulmonary function as effectively as repeated doses of epinephrine.

Terbutaline (1 mg/mL), which is more β_2-specific, and appears to have greater potency and longer duration of action, may be given subcutaneously in place of epinephrine at a dose of 0.01 mL/kg (up to 0.3 mL). This dose may be repeated in 30 min if no adverse effects occur.

Isoproterenol (1:200) or isoetharine (1:100) can be given as a substitute for the repeated injections of epinephrine or terbutaline. Some physicians advocate using either of these agents as a one-time dose 20 min after the injections of epinephrine or terbutaline if the patient is not clinically improved enough for discharge from the emergency department. The dose is 0.25 mL for children under 10 years of age, and 0.5 mL for the older child diluted in 2 mL of saline, delivered nebulized with oxygen. The treatment may be given hourly if warranted by the clinical condition. Aerosolized metaproterenol (5%) may be used but is not approved for children less than 12 years of age. Aerosolized terbutaline and albuterol (salbutamol) have proved helpful in recent studies, but have not been approved by the Food and Drug Administration.

Close monitoring of the pulse, respiratory rate, auscultatory findings in the chest, and peak expiratory flow rate (PEFR) should be done before and after each treatment with adrenergic agents and should be recorded in the chart. The decision to repeat or withhold these agents should be based on the above clinical findings rather than rigidly following a protocol.

Patients who are partially responsive to sympathomimetic bronchodilators, i.e., there is improvement of wheezing and/or PEFR, deserve a trial of oral theophylline at a dose of 5 mg/kg in the emergency department if theophylline has not been given in the past 4 to 6 h. If there is a response to oral theophylline, the child may be discharged on oral theophylline at 5 mg/kg per dose every 6 h for a period of 5 to 7 days. Children less than 6 months and over 9 years of age should be started on doses of 4 mg/kg because of their slower clearance rate of theophylline. Infants less than 6 months of age have erratic clearance rates of theophylline and should have their serum theophylline levels monitored. Any child receiving theophylline should always be observed for signs of toxicity such as nausea, vomiting, restlessness, irritability, and seizures. If any of these signs appear, theophylline levels should be obtained and the medication stopped.

Patients who do not respond to sympathomimetic bronchodilators should be given intravenous aminophylline (85% theophylline) at 7 mg/kg diluted in 25 to 50 mL of saline over a period of about 20 min. If the child is a known asthmatic who has taken a dose of oral theophylline at home within 4 to 6 h prior to arriving at the hospital, or if oral theophylline has been given at the hospital, the loading dosage of aminophylline should be adjusted by deducting the amount given in the past 4 to 6 h from the ordinary bolus of 7 mg/kg of aminophylline. Canavan, et al., in a recent study have suggested that even if the child has taken theophylline within 6 h of arriving at the hospital, a loading dose of 6 mg/kg may be given with few side effects. In this study, time zero theophylline levels ranged from 0 to 24.0 μg/mL (mean 6.7 μg/mL) and peak theophylline levels ranged from 8.1 to 35.2 μg/mL (mean 15.2 μg/mL). There was no consistent relationship, in the immediate period after the bolus was given, between side effects and peak levels even if the peak level was > 20 μg/mL. If a recent theophylline level is known, one may calculate the loading dose with the knowledge that, as a general rule, 1 mg/kg of theophylline will raise the serum concentration by approximately 2 μg/mL. Another approach, advocated by some physicians, is to give 7 mg/kg of aminophylline to patients who have not taken a recent dose of theophylline and 5 mg/kg to patients who have taken a recent dose.

Corticosteroids should be considered in the outpatient management of an acute attack of asthma in the following cases: (1) a child who is well known to the treating physician or the hospital as one who responds for a short period of time to bronchodilators, but who subsequently develops wheezing again only to be admitted for status asthmaticus; (2) a child who has a second attack of asthma within a period of 1 week while on theophylline and/or metaproterenol, and who has responded on both occasions to sympathomimetic bronchodilators; or (3) a child who is chronically on corticosteroids or who has needed frequent short-term bursts in the past. Prednisone at 1 to 2 mg/kg per day, given as a single morning dose for a period of 5 days, is not associated with toxicity. If a child is receiving chronic steroid treatment he or she should be given high doses of prednisone for acute exacerbations and returned to a maintenance dose when the acute exacerbation is resolved.

Treatment of Status Asthmaticus

Status asthmaticus may be defined as severe, persistent wheezing and dyspnea that fail to respond to adequate doses of bronchodilators. Respiratory failure may occur in patients with status asthmaticus; this makes this disorder a true medical emergency. Hospitalization is mandatory for these patients.

All patients with status asthmaticus are hypoxemic and some are hypercapneic. Consequently, arterial blood gas levels should be obtained to determine baseline P_{O_2}, P_{CO_2}, and pH. These should be repeated frequently until the patient's clinical condition improves. Humidified oxygen should be administered to every child with status asthmaticus even before arterial blood gas results are reported. The P_{O_2} should be maintained between 70 and 90 mmHg. Mist tents are not indicated, both because water does not reach the lower airway in any significant way, and because mist irritates the airways of many asthmatics.

Many children with status asthmaticus become dehydrated. This is the result of several factors, including decreased fluid intake, excessive work of breathing, pulmonary insensible water loss, and the diuretic effect of theophylline. When hydrating children with status asthmaticus, it must be taken into account that they have increased secretion of antidiuretic hormone, and there is danger of overhydration and subsequent pulmonary edema. Consequently, fluid administration must be carefully monitored. Hydration in excess of replacement and maintenance is unnecessary and may be harmful.

In the patient who has metabolic acidosis, i.e., a pH of less than 7.3 and a base deficit greater than 5 mEq/L, intravenous sodium bicarbonate according to the following calculation may be helpful:

$$\text{Bicarbonate (mEq)} = 0.3 \times \text{body weight (kg)} \times \text{negative base excess (mEq)}$$

Give one-half of the calculated dose initially and the other half after repeating the blood gas measurements. The infusion rate should not exceed 10 mEq/min. Respiratory acidosis should be treated with appropriate medication and with assisted ventilation in those who fail to respond.

Aminophylline should be administered as a loading dose of 7 mg/kg diluted in 25 to 50 mL of saline given intravenously over a period of 20 min. This may be adjusted according to the recent intake of theophylline (see Treatment of Acute Attacks of Asthma). A theophylline level should be obtained prior to the administration of aminophylline if the child has been on an oral theophylline preparation. The loading dose should be followed by a constant maintenance infusion of aminophylline of 0.85 mg/(kg·h) for children 1 to 9 years old, 0.65 mg/(kg·h) for older children 9 to 16 years, and 0.45 mg/(kg·h) for adults. This will usually maintain serum concentrations of approximately 10 μg/mL. If there is significant fever, liver disease, or heart failure, the maintenance infusion should be reduced by 50 percent. Because infants, particularly those under 6 months of age, are erratic in their clearance rate of theophylline, a formula for infants less than 1 year of age is useful:

$$\text{Dose [mg/(kg·day)]} = 0.3 \times \text{age in weeks} + 8$$

It is extremely important to measure serum theophylline levels because of the variable clearance rates from one patient to the next. If, after the initial theophylline level is obtained, the patient continues to have significant wheezing, the dose of aminophylline can be increased until a theophylline level of 20 μg/mL is reached. Levels should also be measured whenever toxicity is suspected on the basis of symptoms such as gastrointestinal upset, central nervous system irritability, and headaches. Theophylline should be delivered by a constant infusion pump. If constant infusion cannot be delivered safely, boluses of aminophylline at 5 mg/kg every 6 h (or an amount which will give a serum concentration of 10 to 20 μg/mL) should be administered over a period of 30 min. Isoproterenol or isoetharine may be given every 4 h, or more frequently if needed, at the doses noted above.

Intravenous corticosteroids should be started in the child with status asthmaticus. The beneficial effects of corticosteroid therapy, i.e., decreasing inflammation, facilitating recovery from hypoxemia, increasing cyclic AMP, and possibly restoring β-adrenergic responsiveness to adrenergic drugs in patients who have become unresponsive to these drugs, outweigh the remote possibility of adverse effects from short-term corticosteroid use. Hydrocortisone (Solu-Cortef) or methylprednisolone (Solu-Medrol) may be administered. The dosage of hydrocortisone is 7 mg/kg initially and 7 mg/(kg·24h) by continuous infusion or in divided doses every 6 h. Methylprednisolone may be administered as 1 mg/kg initially and 4 mg/(kg·24h) by continuous infusion or in divided doses every 4 to 6 h. When the continuous infusion is discontinued, the patient should be maintained on oral prednisone at 1 to 2 mg/(kg·day) as a single morning dose for a total of 5 days.

Sedation is contraindicated in patients with status asthmaticus. Antibiotics should not be used routinely. If bacterial infection is suspected, attempts should be made to identify the causative organism; the patient should be started on a broad-spectrum antibiotic while the culture results are pending.

Occasionally, the patient with status asthmaticus develops respiratory failure. Clinical signs and symptoms of respiratory failure are decreased or absent breath sounds, severe retractions and use of accessory muscles, cyanosis on 40% oxygen, depressed level of consciousness, decreased response to pain, and poor skeletal muscle tone. Arterial blood gas levels are the final determinant of respiratory failure and must be monitored frequently in the distressed child. Respiratory failure may be defined as a $P_{O_2} < 50$ mmHg on 100% inhaled O_2, or $P_{CO_2} > 50$ mmHg. The child with a rapidly rising P_{CO_2} (e.g., from 35 to 40 mmHg in 1 h) who is receiving optimal therapy and is tiring, should be considered to be in respiratory failure and treated as such.

Although respiratory failure may be managed with intravenous isoproterenol in some children, the need for nasotracheal or endotracheal intubation and assisted ventilation is a likely possibility. Intravenous isoproterenol should not be used in children over 14 because of the increased frequency of cardiac arrhythmias in older adolescents. A second IV site should always be started because abrupt discontinuation of an isoproterenol drip can cause rapid rebound bronchospasm.

Intravenous isoproterenol by constant infusion should be started if the arterial P_{CO_2} is rising rapidly, but is < 55 mmHg, the arterial P_{O_2} is > 60 mmHg on oxygen, and there is no evidence of myocardial ischemia on ECG. The starting dose is 0.1 μg/(kg·min) by constant infusion pump and is raised by 0.1 μg/(kg·min) every 15 min until a good response is obtained or until the heart rate exceeds 200 (180 in large children), arrhythmia occurs, or other signs of toxicity such as chest pain or ischemic ECG changes occur. After a few hours, the drip is tapered slowly (over 24 to 30 h). Rebound bronchospasm is common after stopping the in-

fusion and is treated by resuming the previous rate. Isoproterenol can be mixed by adding 0.5 or 1.0 mg to 50 mL of D_5W to give 10 or 20 μg of isoproterenol/mL, respectively. Isoproterenol should be used only by those experienced with this drug in a properly equipped intensive care unit. If, for any reason, admission to the intensive care unit is delayed, initial therapy may be undertaken in the emergency department, but only with continuous cardiac monitoring and a constant infusion pump. An intraarterial catheter or someone skilled at obtaining arterial blood gases easily in children is essential for management of these patients.

Any child with a rising P_{CO_2} while on IV isoproterenol or a $P_{CO_2} > 55$ mmHg, or a $P_{O_2} < 50$ mmHg on 100% inspired oxygen, should be started on assisted ventilation. Although oral tracheal intubation can be used, nasotracheal intubation with 100% oxygen is preferred. This placement is both more secure and more comfortable for the patient. Rapidly changing lung compliances make the use of a volume respirator preferable. An initial tidal volume of 10 mL/kg should be used with a slower rate than the patient's preintubation rate to allow for sufficient expiratory time. A Swan-Ganz catheter should be placed if there is right heart strain, low pulse pressure, or low urine output. The patient may be given diazepam for sedation and pancuronium bromide for muscle relaxation. These medications will help with synchronization of respiration with the ventilator.

Management of Complications

Atelectasis occurs in 10 percent and pneumomediastinum occurs in 5 percent of children hospitalized with asthma. Treatment of atelectasis and pneumomediastinum should be conservative; they will usually resolve with drug therapy. Percussion and postural drainage are helpful for the resolution of atelectasis. Pneumomediastinal air is absorbed over 7 to 10 days.

Pneumothorax occurs rarely in children with asthma. When it does occur, a pneumothorax may be small and cause minimal respiratory compromise or it may be large or under tension, causing significant respiratory distress. A small pneumothorax may be managed conservatively and will often respond to the treatment of asthma. A large pneumothorax or tension pneumothorax will require placement of a chest tube.

Treatment of Chronic Asthma

An attempt should be made to determine the environmental factors which may trigger an attack of asthma. Some of these factors include allergens such as animal dander, pollens, house dust, molds, and foods; irritants such as smoke, perfumes, and aerosol spray products; and climate. If these environmental stimuli are identified, their removal may "cure" the child's asthma.

More often than not, the physician is unable to identify a precipitating environmental factor and must resort to medication to control a child's asthma. Theophylline is the first-line oral bronchodilator in the outpatient treatment of chronic asthma. Theophylline comes in many forms. Depending on the specific theophylline preparation chosen and individual patient clearance, it may be given every 6 h, every 8 h, or every 12 h. Sustained-release preparations, those given every 8 or 12 h, decrease fluctuations in serum concentrations and increase compliance. Some of these longer-acting preparations may be sprinkled on food, a method many children find more palatable than liquid preparations.

The initial dose for most children (see section "Treatment of Acute Attacks of Asthma") is 20 mg/(kg·day) (5 mg/kg per dose) given every 6 h. If one uses the longer-acting preparations, the daily dosage remains the same, but the amount per dose is calculated according to the frequency with which the medication is given. Depending on individual differences in metabolism, smaller or larger doses may be needed to maintain serum concentration between 10 and 20 µg/mL.

A β_2-adrenergic agent (metaproterenol, terbutaline, albuterol) is added if the response to theophylline is not satisfactory. Metaproterenol is the most commonly used of these medications in children. It is available as a liquid (10 mg/5 mL) or as a tablet (10 mg and 20 mg). The dose is 10 mg for children from 6 to 9 years of age or who weigh less than 27 kg (60 lb), and 20 mg in children who are over 9 years of age or over 27 kg (60 lb), given 3 to 4 times a day. The dose for children under 6 has not been clearly established, but dosages of 1.3 to 2.6 mg/(kg·day) are well tolerated. Terbutaline is available as 2.5- and 5-mg tablets. The dose for children from 12 to 15 years of age is 2.5 mg three times a day. For adolescents over age 15, the dose is 5 mg every 6 h, three times daily during waking hours. Terbutaline tablets are not currently recommended for children less than 12. Albuterol is available as 2-mg and 4-mg tablets. The starting dose for children over 12 is 2 mg or 4 mg three or four times a day. Albuterol is not recommended for children less than 12. If tachycardia, nervousness, tremors, palpitations, or nausea develop in patients taking β_2-adrenergic drugs, the dose should be reduced.

Metaproterenol and albuterol aerosols are very effective for exercise-induced bronchospasm. Two inhalations may provide more bronchodilation and fewer side effects than the oral preparations of these medications. However, patients and parents must be warned about the tendency to abuse these aerosolized agents.

Cromolyn sodium is another useful medication for the management of chronic asthma. It is administered as an inhaled powder preventing the release of mediators from mast cells and is a prophylactic drug when used on a regular basis; it has no bronchodilating effect once an attack of asthma has started.

Corticosteroids are rarely needed in the patient with chronic asthma. However, if the patient has chronic, intractable symptoms, continuous use of oral (prednisone) or aerosolized (beclomethasone) corticosteroids may be indicated. Treatment should begin with beclomethasone since fewer side effects are associated with it than with oral preparations. The latter should be reserved for the more intractable symptoms and should preferably be given as alternate-day doses. In any case of difficult-to-manage asthma, especially in a child in whom chronic steroids may be indicated, consultation with an allergist should be obtained.

SUMMARY

Pediatric asthma is characterized by tachypnea, wheezing, and cough. It is caused by multiple factors, the most common of which is exposure to environmental stimuli such as allergens, air pollutants, etc. Since there are many diseases which are associated with wheezing in children, it is important to differentiate them from asthma. Once the diagnosis of asthma has been established, control of the environment is an important adjunct to therapy. Pharmacologic therapy is aimed at decreasing smooth muscle spasm and reducing bronchial mucosal edema and mucous secretion. This is usually achieved with the use of sympathomimetics and methylxanthines. If a child is refractory to conventional outpatient management of asthma, he or she has status asthmaticus and must be admitted to the hospital for more intensive therapy. Once discharged from the hospital, the child must be followed closely and treated as necessary for long-term control of the asthma.

BIBLIOGRAPHY

Canavan JW, Ellerstein NS, Sullivan TD: Intravenous administration of aminophylline in asthmatic children taking theophylline orally. *J Pediatr* 97:301–303, 1980.

Dusdieker L, Green M, Smith GD, et al: Comparison of orally administered metaproterenol and theophylline in the control of chronic asthma. *J Pediatr* 101:281–287, 1982.

Easton J, Hilman B, Shapiro G, et al: Management of asthma. *Pediatrics* 68:874–879, 1981.

Francis WJ, Krastins IRB, Levison H: Oral and inhaled salbutamol in the prevention of exercised-induced bronchospasm. *Pediatrics* 66:103–108, 1980.

Leffert F: The management of acute severe asthma. *J Pediatr* 96:1–12, 1980.

Leffert F: The management of chronic asthma. *J Pediatr* 97:875–885, 1980.

Leffert F: Asthma: A modern perspective. *Pediatrics* 62:1061–1069, 1978.

Lulla S, Newcomb RW: Emergency management of asthma in children. *J Pediatr* 97:346–350, 1980.

Parry WH, Nortorano F, Cotton EK: Management of life threatening asthma with intravenous isoproterenol infusions. *Am J Dis Child* 130:39–42, 1976.

Richards W: Differential diagnosis of childhood asthma. *Curr Prob Pediatr* 4:1–36, 1974.

Siegel SC, Rachelefsky GS, Katz RM: Pharmacologic management of pediatric allergic disorders. *Curr Probl Pediatr* 9:1–66, 1979.

Simons FER, Pierson WE, Bierman CW: Respiratory failure in childhood status asthmaticus. *Am J Dis Child* 131:1097–1101, 1977.

Szentivanyi A: The beta adrenergic theory of the atopic abnormality in bronchial asthma. *J Allergy* 42:203–232, 1968.

Wharton R, McGloughlin J, Wise P: Serial peak flow rate is predictive of hospitalization in childhood asthma. Abstract. Ambulatory Pediatrics Association meetings. Washington, D.C., May 1983.

Wyatt R, Weinberger M, Hendeles L: Oral theophylline dosage for the management of chronic asthma. *J Pediatr* 92:125–130, 1978.

Zvi BZ, Lam C, Spohn WA, et al: An evaluation of repeated injections of epinephrine for the initial treatment of acute asthma. *Am Rev Respir Dis* 127:101–105, 1983.

CHAPTER 83
PEDIATRIC
BACTEREMIA, SEPSIS,
AND MENINGITIS

Joseph Zeccardi

Bacteremia, sepsis, and meningitis in children may be considered different points on a spectrum of bacterial invasion. Although all bacteremia does not progress through sepsis and meningitis, it is helpful to consider the three entities simultaneously.

BACTEREMIA

Much has been written on this condition in the past decade. Positive blood cultures with symptomatology confined to fever constitute the definition of bacteremia. Most bacteremias are caused by *Streptococcus pneumoniae* and *Haemophilus influenzae* with *Salmonella, Neisseria meningitidis,* and group A *Streptococcus* causing a significant minority. The incidence of various pathogens varies from study to study. However, the major cause is *Streptococcus pneumoniae,* which accounts for 60 to 80 percent, whereas *H. influenzae* accounts for anywhere from 10 to 30 percent. The preponderance of bacteremias are identified in the 6-to-24-months age population with many fewer occurring before or after that age. Bacteremia may progress to a focal infection such as meningitis, abscess, or sepsis, or the condition may spontaneously improve. Factors influencing susceptibility have not been well defined, so it is not possible to identify the child at risk for progression to sepsis or meningitis.

Diagnosis and Treatment

A number of studies have shown that the strongest evidence for bacteremia is in children under 24 months of age who have white blood cell (WBC) counts of 15,000 or more and a fever of 40°C (104°F) or higher. Therefore, a WBC count should be obtained in children in the following circumstances: (1) those 3 to 24 months old, with a temperature of 40°C or more without a demonstrable focus of infection; and (2) all patients 3 to 24 months old, who appear toxic and have a fever less than 40°C (104°F). Those children with a WBC count of 15,000 should have blood cultures done and antibiotic therapy administered on an ambulatory basis, on the presumption that therapy may reduce the incidence of progression to serious infection. Amoxicillin, 50 mg/(kg·day), is appropriate considering the likely bacterial causes. All discharged patients should be followed up within 48 h or less if the clinical condition warrants.

On reevaluation, the patient whose blood cultures are positive for *S. pneumoniae,* and who is asymptomatic and afebrile, may be treated with oral penicillin, 50,000 units/(kg·day), for the next 10 days. All children with blood cultures positive for *H. influenzae* should be admitted to the hospital. Children who continue to have symptoms or who develop a focus of infection should be admitted to the hospital for parenteral antibiotic therapy.

Children under 3 months of age with fever or who appear toxic should be admitted because of the possibility of sepsis, since neither the WBC count nor the physical assessment is reliable enough to distinguish those with sepsis from those with a more benign condition.

SEPSIS

Sepsis is bacteremia with focal findings in addition to fever. The commonest organisms causing sepsis in the neonate are group B *Streptococcus* and *Escherichia coli.* After the newborn period, *H. influenzae, Neisseria meningitidis,* and *S. pneumoniae* become the most frequently isolated pathogens with *Streptococcus* A, *Staphylococcus aureus,* and *Salmonella* reported much less commonly. Increased risk for sepsis includes exposure to communicable pathogens such as *Meningococcus;* suppressed immune competence from conditions such as primary immunodeficiency diseases or chemotherapy; hyposplenism due to surgical removal for hemoglobin disorders; and sickle cell disease or trait, which is associated with sepsis and bacteremia from *S. pneumoniae* and *Salmonella.*

Clinical Presentation

The patient's illness may range from hours, in the case of meningococcemia, to several days of mild to moderate symptoms, such as listlessness or poor feeding. Hypothermia rather than fever is more likely in those under the age of 3 months. Any child under the age of 3 months with hypothermia or fever should be admitted for treatment and evaluation of sepsis. Symptoms may progress through tachycardia, hypotension, cold and clammy skin, lethargy, or coma. Occasionally, hemorrhagic skin lesions may be noted.

Focal findings can be varied and include urinary tract infection or otitis, but the clinician should be alerted to sepsis when more than one focus is identified. Skin lesions indicative of embolic phenomena should also be sought.

Laboratory studies should include CBC with platelets, PT, PTT, fibrin split products, arterial blood gases, glucose, electrolytes, BUN, blood culture, SGOT and SGPT, and a spinal tap with cultures. Purpuric skin lesions should be opened with a lancet, smeared, and a Gram stain obtained. Laboratory studies will usually reveal a normal hemoglobin and hematocrit. The WBC count is almost always elevated, but neutropenia may accompany an overwhelming infection. The differential should show a shift to the left with immature forms. If there are hemorrhagic skin lesions, the platelets may be decreased on the smear and the platelet count will be lowered. Clotting studies may also be abnormal in the presence of disseminated intravascular coagulation. Measurement of blood gases will usually demonstrate a metabolic acidosis. Sodium may be lowered because of inappropriate antidiuretic hormone secretion. The BUN is usually normal. A lowered glucose may be noted in infants.

Treatment

If the patient is in shock, an infusion of 20 mL/(kg·h) of normal saline with 5% dextrose should be given following determination of the central venous pressure. Urinary output should be monitored with a catheter and maintained at 1 mL/(kg·h). Antibiotics of choice are ampicillin 200 mg/(kg·day) and gentamycin 7.5 mg/(kg·day). In the older child, because of the increased frequency of infection with *H. influenzae*, chloramphenicol at 100 mg/(kg·day) should be used instead of gentamycin. Chloramphenicol in the same doses is indicated in the infant with bloody diarrhea because of the possibility of *Salmonella* infection. Steroid therapy is still controversial, but pharmacologic doses in severely ill patients are commonly used by some physicians. Hypoglycemia should be treated with glucose in a dose of 1 g/kg utilizing a 25% solution and followed by 10% glucose infusion. Further stabilization may require infusion of packed red cells to correct blood loss or anemia, and platelet concentrates and fresh frozen plasma for bleeding disorders.

MENINGITIS

In children, *H. influenzae*, *S. pneumoniae*, *N. meningitidis*, *E. coli*, and group B *Streptococcus* are the commonest causes of meningitis. In the first month of life, group B *Streptococcus* and *E. coli* are usually the causative agents. After this period, *H. influenzae* becomes the most frequent cause of meningitis, with *S. pneumoniae* and *N. meningitidis* following in incidence. Unusual pathogens such as *Salmonella* should be considered in patients with sickle cell disease or those with a history of gastroenteritis. Bacterial invasion of the meninges occurs either directly from contiguous infection such as otitis, or seeding from sepsis. The mode of entry in the newborn can be from the maternal vaginal tract into the bowel or respiratory tract, whereas in the older child the nasopharynx is more frequently the site of entry for the organism. Splenectomized patients, patients with sickle cell disease or immune deficiency are at higher risk for meningitis following showers of bacteria. The clinician should look carefully for infections in the middle ear, sinuses, or associated fractures of these structures in addition to searching for midline defects such as meningomyelocele. Direct extension of infection from these sites may be associated with unusual organisms.

Clinical Presentation

The presentation varies significantly, depending on the age of the child. In the first 3 months of life, the degree of symptomatology is low, and the clinician needs to be especially alert to subtle findings. Increased or decreased activity level, vomiting, or decreased appetite as evidenced by poor sucking or rooting should alert the physician to infection in the infant. Increased irritability when held as opposed to being soothed is a useful symptom. The cuddling which normally would reduce crying may cause movement of the inflamed meninges and, therefore, more crying. A bulging fontanelle is a significantly late but important and reliable sign of increased intracranial pressure in meningitis.

Other late symptoms include a high-pitched cry and reduced consciousness. In the first few months of life, patients frequently do not have fever and may even be hypothermic. In the presence of fever over 38.5°C (101.3°F) or hypothermia below 36.8°C (98°F), meningitis must be ruled out by lumbar puncture.

Symptomatology becomes more reliable as the child develops beyond 3 months. Irritability and a significant change in sleep and wake patterns become much more noticeable. The child's level of activity is usually significantly decreased. As maturation continues, meningitis presents more frequently with nuchal rigidity and headache. Presenting complaints may also include back pain, petechial rash, and focal neurologic signs.

In a child older than 3 months, a febrile response is a more common finding. Seizures as an initial manifestation are rare in meningitis. However, in children under the age of 6 months with a fever, meningitis must be ruled out. Over the age of 6 months, controversy exists in management because the likelihood of a febrile seizure is greater. However, in general, a spinal tap is indicated in every case of a first febrile seizure or seizure with fever. If there is a definite history of febrile seizures, then a spinal tap need not be done unless there are other findings indicating the need for investigation. The patient with meningitis may also present in shock initially. The clinician presented with such a patient should search for skin lesions and nuchal rigidity in the febrile child with no history of blood or fluid losses. Signs of meningitis should be sought in febrile children with non-CNS problems such as vomiting, dehydration, or respiratory infections if the child appears to be more toxic than is usually expected from apparent primary problems.

Laboratory Findings

Accurate diagnosis is crucial and prompt therapy must be instituted in order to reduce mortality. The critical diagnostic procedure is the spinal tap. If the child appears stable, however, it is wise to obtain blood for CBC, electrolytes, glucose, osmolarity, clotting studies, blood culture, and type and crossmatch; then a spinal tap may be performed. The blood should be tested with a glucose oxidase tape. Immunoelectrophoresis may aid in the identification of the pathogen. Blood, urine, and cerebral spinal fluid may be submitted for this study. Cultures should be obtained from the most likely sites of entry including the throat, nasopharynx, stool, urine, and skin. The accuracy of cultures from the nasopharynx is low, but is higher from blood, urine, and skin. A spinal tap is necessary in all cases before antibiotic treatment is begun. Cerebrospinal fluid should be sent for cell count, differential, Gram stain, protein, and glucose. Culture of and sensitivity to aerobes should be done only if there is clinical indication that anaerobic and mycobacterial cultures should be added.

Rapid interpretation of cerebral spinal fluid results is important. A cloudy spinal fluid which is not blood-tinged indicates a need for immediate antibiotic treatment while awaiting the stat analysis. If (1) the WBC count is over 1000 cells per milliliter and is primarily polymorphonuclear, (2) the glucose is less than one-half of the blood sugar, and (3) the Gram stain demonstrates bacteria, the patient obviously has bacterial meningitis. Patients with less clear-cut findings should be admitted and retapped in 6 h. Antibiotics are generally withheld before retapping in order to avoid committing the patient to a prolonged and unnecessary course of parenteral antibiotic therapy. A completely clear tap in an infant with signs and symptoms of meningitis should be repeated within 6 to 8 h and the child admitted for close observation without antibiotics during this time. It is not unusual for symptoms to begin prior to the demonstration of bacteria in the cerebral spinal fluid. There is a lag period between the showers of bacteria and a positive Gram stain (especially in pneumococcal meningitis), and the onset of pleocytosis. Therefore, the Gram stain becomes an essential part of the evaluation despite the absence of any abnormal cells, protein, or glucose. Other tests that are helpful but not universally available are immunoelectrophoresis; cerebral spinal fluid, lactic acid dehydrogenase, and lactic acid concentrations; and the quellung reaction.

A urine sample should be sent for analysis, including osmolality measurement and culture. If immunoelectrophoresis is available, it should be obtained. Blood gas values should be obtained initially. Skin lesions may be incised with a lancet and a Gram stain obtained; the material should be cultured in an attempt to identify the pathogen. Additionally, Gram stains of the buffy coat may be useful in identifying the pathogen.

Treatment

After the spinal tap, an intravenous infusion should be started at a maintenance rate to avoid increasing intracranial pressure. A Foley catheter is appropriate in all cases. Seizures should be managed in the usual manner with Valium, 0.3 mg/kg, to terminate seizure activity, followed by loading with phenytoin or phenobarbital. Therapy for seizures should be specific and not prophylactic. Shock should be treated with volume infusion consisting of normal saline solution with 5% dextrose at 20 mL/kg. The patient's urinary output should be monitored and maintained at 1 mL/(kg·h). Methylprednisolone at 30 mg/kg is used by some, though its efficacy has never been documented. Positive inotropic or pressor agents may be necessary if the volume loading is unsuccessful. Cerebral edema or subdural effusions may lead to signs

of increased intracranial pressure. Treatment for signs of impending herniation should be instituted immediately using mannitol, 1 mg/kg, and dexamethasone, 0.15 mg/kg. Collections of fluid may be relieved by subdural taps. Fluid recovered should be treated as spinal fluid for laboratory purposes. The presence of cerebral edema is a significant risk and it should preclude a spinal tap. Cultures can be obtained from another site such as skin lesions or the pharynx, from urine and blood, and from any obviously infected site. A spinal tap may be attempted after a trial of therapy to reduce intracranial pressure. Then, a small needle, with the stylet held in the opening so that immediate control of leakage is possible, should be utilized, and the smallest amount of cerebral spinal fluid necessary for culture and Gram stains should be obtained.

Antibiotic Therapy

Although previously we divided decisions by 3 months of age because of the paucity of symptoms and increased risk, when considering antibiotic choice 2 months of age becomes a significant milestone, because during the second month *E. coli* and group B *Streptococcus* diminish in frequency while *H. influenzae* is isolated more frequently. *Haemophilus influenzae* becomes the major organism by the third month with *S. pneumoniae* and *N. meningitidis* following in incidence. Therefore, in the patient under 1 month, antibiotic therapy should include ampicillin and an aminoglycide. The choice of aminoglycide should be hospital-specific, depending on the sensitivity of the pathogens in the particular nursery. A common choice is gentamycin. The doses are: gentamycin, 5 mg/(kg·day) every 12 h for children under 7 days of age, and 7.5 mg/(kg·day) every 8 h for the patient over 7 days of age; ampicillin, 100 mg/(kg·day) every 12 h for patients under 7 days of age, and 200 mg/(kg·day) every 4 h for patients over 7 days of age.

In children in their second month and beyond, antibiotic choice changes to ampicillin and chloramphenicol because of the resistance of some strains of *H. influenzae*. Ampicillin is given in a dose of 300 mg/(kg·day), and chloramphenicol at 100 mg/(kg·day), given as a rapid IV infusion every 4 h. The patient must be monitored closely for signs of increasing intracranial pressure or focal neurologic signs.

Prehospital and hospital professionals and family who have had contact with the child will be concerned with prophylaxis. Family members should have cultures of the pharynx and one should consider prophylaxis with rifampin for meningococcemia. Rifampin is given in a dose of 600 mg twice a day, four doses in adults; and 10 mg/kg per dose for four doses for children between the ages of 1 and 12 years. Children 3 months to 1 year should be treated with 5 mg/kg every 12 h for 4 doses as prophylaxis. Prehospital and hospital professionals who transported and cared for the child do not need prophylaxis, but if mouth-to-mouth resuscitation has occurred, prophylaxis should be offered.

BIBLIOGRAPHY

Baltimore RS, Hammerschiag M: Meningococcal bacteremia. *Am J Dis Child* 131:1001–1004, 1977.

Bland RD, Lister RC, Ries JP: Cerebrospinal fluid lactic acid level and pH in meningitis. *Am J Dis Child* 128:151–156, 1974.

Dajani AS, Asmar BI, Thirumoorthi MC: Systemic *Haemophilus influenzae* disease: An overview. *J Pediatr* 94:355–364, 1979.

Dickerman JD: Splenectomy and sepsis: A warning. *Pediatrics* 63:938–940, 1979.

Gaudreau C, Delage G, Rousseau D, et al: Bacteremia caused by viridans streptococci in 71 children. *CMA Journal* 125:1246–1249, 1981.

Geiseler RJ, Nelson KE: Bacterial meningitis without clinical signs of meningeal irritation. *South Med J* 75:448–450, 1982.

Hierro FR, Palomeque A, Calvo M, et al: Septic shock in pediatrics. *Paediatrician* 8:93–108, 1979.

Laxer RM, Marks MI: Pneumococcal meningitis in children. *Am J Dis Child* 131:850–853, 1977.

Lerman, SJ: Systemic *Hemophilus influenzae* infection. *Clin Pediatr* 21:360–364, 1982.

Lewis JF, Alexander JJ: Blood cultures in bacteremia. *South Med J* 75:147–150, 1982.

McCracken GH, Eichenwald HF: Part II. Therapy of infectious conditions. *J Pediatr* 93:357–377, 1978.

Murray DL, Cocana J, Seidel JS, et al: Relative importance of bacteremia and viremia in the course of acute fevers of unknown origin in outpatient children. *Pediatrics* 68:157–160, 1981.

Onorato IM, Wormser GP, Nicholas P: ''Normal'' CSF in bacterial meningitis. *JAMA* 244:1469–1471, 1980.

Rosenberg N, Cohen SN: Pneumococcal bacteremia in pediatric patients. *Ann Emerg Med* 11:2–6, 1982.

Sullivan TD, Lascolea LJ, Neter E: Relationship between the magnitude of bacteremia in children and the clinical disease. *Pediatrics* 69:699–702, 1982.

Trigg ME: Immune function of the spleen. *South Med J* 72:593–599, 1979.

Wald EF, Minkowski JM: Bacteremia in childhood. *South Med J* 73:904–905, 1980.

CHAPTER 84
PEDIATRIC
SEIZURES AND
STATUS EPILEPTICUS

Michael A. Nigro

Approximately 4 million people in the United States (2 percent of the population) have some form of epilepsy. Many more experience seizures in association with febrile illnesses or other medical or surgical problems. The incidence of epilepsy varies; however, a study by Hauser and co-workers suggests 100,933 new cases per year. In children aged 0 to 9 years, the prevalence is 4.4 cases per 1000, and in those aged 10 to 19 years, the prevalence is 6.6 cases per 1000. A significant number of patients present themselves for emergency care of the initial or subsequent seizures. Simple febrile convulsions constitute a separate category, and there is an incidence of 3 to 4 percent in the pediatric population.

These numbers alone do not reveal the most important feature of the seizure phenomenon—the increased morbidity and mortality that are a direct result of seizures, their cause, or their treatment. Epidemiologic studies indicate a mortality two to three times higher in epileptic patients. The earlier the onset of seizures and the more deprived the social environment, the higher the morbidity and the mortality.

Typically a patient with seizures arrives at the emergency department with one of the following:

1. The initial or a recurrent seizure
2. Status epilepticus
3. Complications of medication
4. A history of seizures with an acute, underlying disease—e.g., sickle cell anemia, metabolic disease, or febrile illness—that needs treatment

Emergency care for seizures should include (1) safely stopping the seizure, (2) correcting and identifying immediately treatable or reversible causes, and (3) initiating appropriate diagnostic studies and arranging follow-up care. If management is difficult, the patient should be admitted. There are significant enough differences in the treatment of children that unless the physician is experienced in pediatric management or able to readily obtain pediatric consultation, the child should be transferred to a pediatric facility. When the treatment or the diagnostic studies promise to be complex, time is important in reducing morbidity.

DEFINITION

A *seizure* is an episodic, involuntary alteration in motor activity, behavior, sensation, or autonomic function. It represents an abrupt change in brain function. The term *epilepsy* indicates recurring seizures without a simple discernible or reversible cause. Physiologically, a seizure is an abnormal, sudden, and excessive electric discharge of neurons (gray matter) which propagates down the neuronal processes (white matter) to affect an end organ or end organs in a clinically measurable fashion.

The classification of seizures has been simplified. The International Classification of Epileptic Seizures, as described by Gastaut, is accepted as a standard (see Table 84-1).

THE FIRST SEIZURE

The first seizure in a child usually causes some degree of panic in the parents, and an accurate account of seizure and preseizure events may not be obtainable. If the seizure lasts seconds to minutes, and if others in the family have experienced seizures, an emergency visit may not be made. Unless the child is in status epilepticus, or seizures recur in the emergency room, the physician can defer immediate anticonvulsant treatment and concentrate on defining the cause and the risk of recurrence.

Hauser and co-workers categorized seizure recurrence for all ages according to the presumed cause. Of their patients, 73 percent were categorized as having idiopathic seizures, and 27 percent as having remote symptomatic seizures. Idiopathic seizures recurred in 17 percent of the patients by 20 months after the initial seizure, and in 26 percent of the patients by 36 months after the first seizure, but the recurrence rate was greater in patients with generalized spike-wave EEGs, and in patients with siblings who had had seizures. In patients with prior neurologic insult (cerebrovascular accident, meningitis, etc.) the recurrence rate was 34 percent by 20 months after the initial seizure.

Immediate diagnostic workup (see Table 84-2) can be initiated in the emergency situation, and if the seizure was brief and appears to be idiopathic, the decision to initiate anticonvulsant therapy can

Table 84-1. International Classification of Epileptic Seizures

I. Partial seizures (seizures beginning locally)
    A. Partial seizures with elementary symptomatology (generally without impairment of consciousness)
        1. With motor symptoms (includes jacksonian seizures)
        2. With special sensory or somatosensory symptoms
        3. With autonomic symptoms
        4. Compound forms
    B. Partial seizures with complex symptomatology (generally with impairment of consciousness)
        1. With impairment of consciousness only
        2. With cognitive symptomatology
        3. With affective symptomatology
        4. With ''psychosensory'' symptomatology
        5. With ''psychomotor'' symptomatology
        6. Compound forms
    C. Partial seizures secondarily generalized
II. Generalized seizures (bilaterally symmetric without local onset)
    A. Absences (petit mal)
    B. Bilateral massive epileptic myoclonus
    C. Infantile spasms
    D. Clonic seizures
    E. Tonic seizures
    F. Tonic-clonic seizures (grand mal)
    G. Atonic seizures
    H. Akinetic seizures
III. Unilateral seizures (predominantly)
IV. Unclassified epileptic seizures (due to incomplete data)

Source: Gastaut, 1970.

be deferred until the appropriate neurologic assessment is completed. The causes of the first seizure vary (see Table 84-3). Idiopathic seizures account for 26.3 to 47 percent of the children with seizures seen, depending on the study cited. Secondary seizures occur for a variety of reasons (e.g., inflammatory, structural, metabolic, or secondary to general illness).

In any group of seizure patients there is a subgroup in whom the seizure is a symptom of an underlying disorder, and in such cases correction of the primary problem makes seizure recurrence quite unlikely. Thus the primary goal must be to uncover disorders that are readily identifiable and reversible. Symptomatic seizures of hypoglycemia, hypocalcemia, and electrolyte imbalance can be treated immediately; there is little risk of recurrence, and they usually do not require anticonvulsant use. Seizures occurring as a result of intracranial infections and craniocerebral trauma may require only immediate or short-term anticonvulsant use. Symptomatic seizures of systemic lupus erythematosus (SLE), sickle cell anemia, leukemia, arteriovenous malformations, and neoplasms may be the heralding symptoms of a complex, yet treatable underlying disease.

If the initial seizure is prolonged and classified as status epilepticus, appropriate therapy and diagnostic workup must be initiated (Tables 84-2 and 84-6). If several seizures occur, or if the initial seizure is prolonged or occurs in a patient at higher risk for recurrence (such as one with prior neurologic insult), anticonvulsant therapy can be initiated. For tonic, tonic-clonic, clonic, or partial seizures, phenobarbital is used most often, and the initial doses need not be the higher, loading doses that are required in

Table 84-2. Diagnostic Studies in Seizure Patients*

Studies	Neonatal Seizure	First Seizure in Children	Status Epilepticus	Recurring Breakthrough (nonstable)
CBC with differential	X	X	X	—
Random blood sugar	X	X	X	X
Electrolytes	X	X	X	X
Creatinine	X	—	X	—
Magnesium	X	X	X	—
Calcium	—	X	X	X
BUN	—	X	X	—
Blood gases	X	—	X	—
Serum ammonia	X†	—	—	—
Urine and serum amino acid screen	X†	—	—	—
TORCH titers	X†	—	—	—
Lumbar puncture	X†	X†	X§	—
Anticonvulsant levels	—	—	X	X
EEG	X	X	X§	—
Echoencephalogram (real-time)	X†	—	—	—
CT scan	X†	X‡	X§	—
Chest x-ray	—	—	X§	X
Skeletal (x-ray) survey	X†	—	—	—
Cardiac/pulmonary evaluation	X†	—	X	—
Evaluation for superimposed medical problems	—	—	X§	X
Infectious disease workup	X	X	X§	X

*X = diagnostic studies to be performed; — = studies need not be performed.

†When history or physical examination warrant it.

‡If there is evidence of structural lesion or hereditary disorder.

§If indicated.

Table 84-3. Causes of Seizures in Children

I Infection
  A. Meningitis
  B. Encephalitis
    1. Acute—herpes, CMV, rubella
    2. Late—toxoplasmosis, CMV, rubella
  C. Intracranial abscess
    1. Epidural and subdural
    2. Parenchymal
II. Hypoxia
  A. Ischemic—hypoxic insults
  B. Hypoxemia
  C. Ischemia—maternal hypotension
  D. Intraventricular or cerebral hemorrhage (especially in premature)
III. Metabolic
  A. Hypoglycemia—less than 20 mg/100 mL in premature and 30 mg/100 mL in full-term infants
    1. Primary and transient
    2. Infant of diabetic mother
    3. Associated with hypoxia
  B. Hypocalcemia—less than 8 mg/100 mL
    1. Primary hypoparathyroidism
    2. Secondary with hypoxia
    3. Secondary with use of cow's milk formula (usually after 1 to 2 weeks of age)
  C. Hypomagnesemia—less than 1 mEq/L; usually associated with hypocalcemia
  D. Amino acidopathia, e.g., nonketotic hyperglycemia, urea cycle defect with hyperammonemia, maple syrup urine disease
  E. Organic acidemias
    1. Primary lactic acidemia
    2. Secondary lactic acidemia with hypoxia
    3. Methylmalonic acidemia
  F. Electrolyte imbalance
    1. SIADH with cerebral trauma or infection
    2. Iatrogenic—inappropriate IV fluids
    3. Inappropriate formula concentration by staff or parent
    4. Dehydration, compulsive water drinking, vomiting
  G. Other metabolic disorders
    1. Coenzyme dependency status (vitamin B_6)
    2. Kernicterus
    3. Galactosemia, fructose intolerance
  H. Renal disease, hepatic failure, hormonal disregulation (Addison's disease)
IV. Trauma
  A. Related to birth
    1. With forceps compression
    2. Precipitous delivery with vaginal compression
    3. Abdominal trauma, e.g., auto accident or abuse
  B. Neonatal period
    1. Abuse
    2. Unintentional doll shaking
  C. Postnatal—accidental and nonaccidental
    1. Open wound
    2. Closed head injuries or depressed fractures
V. Structural lesions
  A. Congenital anomalies, e.g., agenesis of the corpus callosum, porencephalic cyst, holoprosencephaly
  B. Acquired defects
    1. CVA from infection
    2. Trauma with late porencephaly and cerebral hemiatrophy
  C. Arteriovenous anomalies with or without hemorrhage
  D. Phakomatosis, e.g., neurofibromatosis, tuberous sclerosis, Sturge-Weber syndrome
  E. Congenital heart disease with cerebral ischemia or hypoxia
  F. Cerebral neoplasms
  G. Cerebrovascular disease—stroke associated with a variety of causes, e.g., SLE, sickle cell anemia
VI. Chromosomal aberrations, e.g., trisomies
VII. Drug withdrawal
  A. Neonatal
VIII. Illicit drug use
  A. PCP
  B. Alcohol
IX. Accidental ingestions, e.g., theophylline, heavy metals (thallium, lead, mercury, arsenic)
X. Idiosyncratic reactions to prescribed drugs
XI. Reye's syndrome
XII. Burn encephalopathy

Note: CMV = cytomegalovirus; SIADH = syndrome of inappropriate antidiuretic hormone; CVA = cerebrovascular accident; SLE = systemic lupus erythematosus; PCP = phencyclizine.

Table 84-4. Initial and Maintenance Doses in the First Seizure (Nonstatus Partial and Tonic, Clonic, and Tonic-Clonic Seizures of Childhood)

Drug	Initial Dose, mg/kg	Maintenance Dose, mg/(kg·24h)	Doses/Day	Therapeutic Level, µg/mL	Half-Life, h
Phenytoin (Dilantin)	8	4–8	1–2	10–20	24 ± 12
Phenobarbital	6	3–8	1–2	15–40	60 ± 20
Carbamazepine (Tegretol)	5	10–20	2–4	6–12	20 ± 5
Primidone (Mysoline)	5	10–20	2–4	5–12	12
Valproic acid (Depakene/Depakote)	10	20–60	2–4	50–100	6–12
Ethosuximide (Zarontin)	20	20–30	2–3	50–100	30
Clonazepam (Clonopin)	0.05	0.1–0.3	3–4	NA	18–50
Acetazolamide (Diamox)	10	10	1–2	NA	24–42

Note: NA = not applicable

status epilepticus. Phenytoin is the second most commonly used drug in this situation. Carbamazepine is considered equal to phenytoin in anticonvulsant properties but has a different spectrum of potential side effects.

Absence (petit mal) seizures rarely require emergency care, and an EEG should be obtained for confirmation before one starts drugs that are more specific, namely, ethosuximide, valproate, and acetazolamide.

FEBRILE SEIZURE

Febrile seizure is a unique and common form of seizure in childhood. Although various types occur (tonic, tonic-clonic, clonic), the characteristics of a febrile seizure separate it from other symptomatic and idiopathic seizure disorders. The National Institutes of Health Consensus Development Conference of Febrile Seizure defined it as "an event in infancy or childhood usually occurring between three months and five years of age, associated with fever but without evidence of intracranial infection or defined course." Typically, these seizures are generalized and last less than 10 min (some physicians say 15 to 20 min is more typical), and there is no postictal neurologic deficit. The EEG usually does not reveal paroxysmal (epileptic) activity, and there often is a family history of similar seizures. Typically a rapid rise in temperature, usually above 38.8°C (101.8°F), occurs at the onset of the illness and, on occasion, recurs several times in the course of the illness. Three to four percent of young children experience febrile seizures, and of these, 30 to 40 percent have recurrences, especially when the first seizure occurs under 1 year of age. The mortality from simple febrile seizures is extremely low.

Evaluation

The first febrile seizure warrants the most concern, because the benign nature of the illness has not been established; i.e., more concern regarding intracranial infection is justified with the febrile-seizuring child before the propensity for recurring simple febrile seizures has been established. The initial evaluation concentrates on serious causes, e.g., meningitis, encephalitis, and systemic illnesses. Lumbar puncture is warranted with the first febrile seizure or whenever intracranial sepsis appears likely. If a cause is not found and the child is ill, admission, workup, and therapy are warranted. Underlying diseases should be diagnosed. Toxic encephalopathy with fever as a symptom should be identified and treated. An EEG can be done electively, and, although its benefits are arguable, it can be helpful in identifying the child who is at greater risk of recurrent seizure.

Treatment

Therapy for the cause of the fever is the main goal. If a child appears well after experiencing a single febrile seizure, anticonvulsant therapy can be deferred, the child can be evaluated electively, and the family and attending physicians can decide whether anticonvulsants will be used. Phenobarbital at therapeutic levels (15 μg/mL) reduces febrile seizure frequency. If the child is ill, has had recurring seizures with this febrile illness, or has had several seizures with prior febrile illnesses, administration of

phenobarbital can be initiated and maintained until the child improves and a decision is reached regarding the use of long-term anticonvulsants. There are subgroups of febrile seizure patients who warrant long-term anticonvulsant (phenobarbital) use, including the child (1) with a preexisting neurologic deficit, e.g., mental retardation or cerebral palsy, (2) with repeated seizures in the same febrile illness, (3) under 1 year of age, (4) with prior nonfebrile seizures and siblings or parents with epilepsy, (5) with more than three febrile seizures in 6 months, or (6) whose parents request treatment, having been informed of the risks and benefits.

The protocol to follow when treating a child with febrile seizure is as follows:

1. Administer a loading dose of phenobarbital (10 mg/kg) orally, intravenously, or intramuscularly, followed by 4 to 6 mg/(kg·day) to attain therapeutic levels of 15 to 25 μg/mL.
2. Interrupt the fever gradually with tepid baths (use no alcohol) and give cautious doses of aspirin (controversy exists about use in Reye's syndrome) or acetaminophen.
3. Identify the source of infection and do a spinal tap if meningitis or encephalitis is suspected, or if unexplained febrile seizure occurs for the first time.
4. Arrange for follow-up studies with the child's family physician.
5. Admit the ill child without an easily treatable problem or one in whom recurrent seizures have occurred within several hours or 1 day.
6. Obtain an EEG when appropriate. An EEG may be helpful (if definitely abnormal) as a further indication of a convulsive disorder.

Phenobarbital is the most effective medication for febrile seizures. Phenytoin is less effective. Diazepam has been used rectally in Europe and Great Britain, but it is not in standard use in the United States. Valproic acid has been effective, but its relative toxicity increases its risk, which contraindicates its use in the prevention of febrile seizure.

NEONATAL SEIZURES

Seizures in the neonate are difficult to identify and often require aggressive therapy. All neonates experiencing seizures should be considered to be at serious risk from the underlying disorder and also to be at increased risk of epilepsy. Electroconvulsive activity should be of as much concern as the outward clinical signs of seizure. Prompt, effective anticonvulsant therapy and other specific therapies lessen the impact of short-term detrimental effects on long-term neurologic functioning. In many instances, the seizure itself is less important for its immediate effects than it is as an indicator of significant underlying disease (e.g., galactosemia, meningitis) that will ultimately have more effect on the morbidity and mortality.

The difference in seizure presentation is due to the predominantly inhibitory brain of newborns and the particular illnesses to which they are subject. Multifocal or fragmentary seizures occur more commonly at this age, and clonic or tonic movements independently affect the limbs simultaneously or fleetingly. Progressive migratory partial seizures (jacksonian) are rarely seen at this age. Autonomic seizures manifest as variable changes in respiration (tachypnea, depression, or apnea), temperature, and color (cyanosis), and also as cardiac arrhythmias and pupillary changes.

Table 84-5. Drug Regimen for Neonatal Seizures

1. Vitamin B$_6$ (pyridoxine), 50 mg IV—used in the absence of an obvious cause of seizures
2. Glucose 2 mL/kg (25% solution) bolus—given to infants stressed with proven hypoglycemia or when merely suspect
3. Calcium gluconate, 4 mL/kg IV
4. Magnesium—magnesium sulfate, 50%, 0.2 mL/kg IM—given to infants with a proven deficiency.
5. Phenobarbital loading
   Premature infant   10–20 mg/kg IV
   Full-term infant   10–15 mg/kg IV
6. Phenytoin (Dilantin), loading dose, 10–15 mg/kg IV
7. Diazepam (Valium) for continuous seizures, 0.2 mg/kg IV, repeat twice if necessary (see text)
8. Clonazepam (Clonopin), 0.1 mg/kg NG if high therapeutic levels of phenobarbital and phenytoin (Dilantin) are ineffective

Myoclonic seizures usually have hypoxic or metabolic causes and indicate a poor prognosis unless the cause is easily identifiable and readily reversible (e.g., hypocalcemia, hypoglycemia). They can, however, be refractory in metabolic disorders such as urea cycle defects and nonketotic hyperglycemia. Unilateral (partial or focal) seizures may be associated with structural lesions, and permanent neurologic deficit may be associated with them. The causes of neonatal seizures are diverse, but the majority of the seizures are attributable to a few well-defined causes (see Table 84-5).

Evaluation

Common neurologic nonepileptic problems encountered in the newborn are hyperexcitability in the tremulous infant, and non-epileptic cerebral manifestations of sepsis, cardiac disease, and hypoxia. Benign myoclonus is also seen. Respiratory immaturity with apnea is a particularly difficult problem at this age.

The workup includes early assessment for treatable causes. Sepsis and metabolic derangements are frequent causes of neonatal seizures. The highest incidence of neonatal seizures is in infants with hypoxia/ischemia, sepsis, or hypoglycemia.

Complex hereditary metabolic disorders—e.g., urea cycle defects with hyperammonemia; maple syrup urine disease; and methylmalonic acidemia—usually become evident days or weeks after feedings with protein are initiated. Others may appear symptomatic in utero or soon after delivery, e.g., nonketotic hyperglycemia, in which the mother reports fetal hiccoughs, and soon after birth the infant is flaccid, exhibiting myoclonic seizures.

Seizures in these metabolic disorders are a signal that significant CNS impairment may be present.

Some of these disorders may be completely controlled or the effects may be reversed with appropriate dietary manipulation (galactosemia) or coenzyme replacement (pyridoxine dependency, subtypes of methylmalonic acidemia).

In evaluating the infant, the cause of the seizures may be readily apparent. The dysmorphic newborn could have a chromosomal defect (trisomy, deletion) or be identifiable only by the combination of unusual features (Cornelia de Lange's syndrome). Neurocutaneous diseases infrequently cause seizures in the newborn but are readily identifiable by certain signs, e.g., encephalotrigeminal hemangiomatosis in Sturge-Weber syndrome, or achromic patches in tuberous sclerosis. Cutaneous herpes with seizures may be an indication that herpes simplex encephalitis is present. Chorioretinitis is a clear sign of an intrauterine infection which could

cause seizures (e.g., herpes, toxoplasmosis, cytomegalovirus, rubella). The laboratory assessment may require real-time ultrasound or a CT scan to diagnose cerebral hemorrhage or malformation.

Treatment

There are several factors influencing treatment in the neonate: (1) variations in the metabolic half-lives of drugs; (2) associated etiologic conditions, e.g., hypoxia prolongs the half-life of many drugs and may affect the renal or gastrointestinal clearance rate; and (3) the end point of seizure control may be harder to identify in neonates.

Effective seizure control is obtained by rapidly achieving therapeutic blood levels of the anticonvulsant chosen. Newborns have different rates of metabolism and excretion of anticonvulsants from older infants and children. In infants less than 7 days old, the half-life of phenobarbital, the drug of first choice, is 100 h, and after 28 days of continuous therapy, the half-life of the drug is reduced to 60 to 70 h.

In the presence of hypoxia with tissue acidosis and renal and hepatic compromise, anticonvulsant half-lives may be increased, with toxic levels reached more readily.

Blood levels of phenobarbital above 16 μg/mL are necessary to achieve seizure control, but levels above 40 μg/mL are of no proven benefit. Dosages of phenobarbital of 3 to 4 mg/(kg·day) maintain mid to high therapeutic levels and prevent toxicity.

Phenytoin is the second drug of choice in treating neonatal seizures and has the disadvantage of requiring intravenous use to obtain and maintain therapeutic levels. Loading doses vary from 10 to 20 mg/kg, and maintenance dosages of 3 to 4 mg/(kg·day) (similar to those of phenobarbital) are satisfactory and not likely to produce toxicity. Pyridoxine (vitamin B$_6$) is empirically used when no reasonable cause of the seizure is found. The only reasonable determinant of its effectiveness is a cessation of seizure activity. The electroencephalogram does not immediately improve with intravenous pyridoxine use.

In status epilepticus of the neonate, diazepam must be used with caution since its half-life may be prolonged, and respiratory depression superimposed on an immature and possibly compromised respiratory apparatus should be anticipated. Diazepam may exaggerate hyperbilirubinemia by uncoupling the bilirubin-albumin complex and should be used with caution in jaundiced babies.

Treatment principles in the management of neonatal seizures are as follows:

1. Identify and correct treatable causes (hypocalcemia, hypoglycemia, electrolyte imbalance).
2. Identify and treat associated problems such as sepsis, hyperbilirubinemia, acidosis, etc.
3. Initiate anticonvulsant therapy with appropriate loading doses, and carefully observe blood levels to adjust the maintenance dosage (see Table 84-5).

INFANTILE SPASMS

Infantile spasms are a unique form of seizures. The onset is typically between 3 and 9 months of age and may begin as late as 18 months. Concurrently, the child exhibits a regression in development. The spasms are very brief, lasting a split second, often with flexion or extension of the head and trunk. They occur singly or repeatedly in bursts of 5 to 20 spasms at a time, usually occurring several times per day and more often upon arousal from sleep or with sudden auditory or physical stimulation. The EEG is abnormal in most cases (hypsarrhythmic in 50 percent). Mental retardation is as high as 85 percent of patients with this disorder. Parents are often frustrated because medical professionals fail to diagnose these spasms as seizures.

There are many causes of infantile spasm (secondary type) including trauma, vitamin B_6 deficiency, infection, and metabolic disorders. The idiopathic type is the most alarming because it most often affects children with no prior neurologic disorder.

Recent studies indicate that early diagnosis and aggressive management with adrenocorticotropic hormone (ACTH) within a month of onset result in an optimum response. Since this is a neurologic emergency, hospitalization, neurologic referral, appropriate diagnostic workup, and initiation of treatment must be rapidly conducted. Aggressive management with steroids or anticonvulsants, careful monitoring of the EEG, and identification of side effects make this therapeutic problem beyond the scope of emergency care with one exception: identifying the problem.

HEAD TRAUMA AND SEIZURES

Head trauma can result in seizures of three types, classified according to the time of onset. Immediate seizures result from impact and presumably are due to traumatic depolarization of neurons. The risk of recurring seizures in these patients is remote unless there are more serious prognostic factors such as prolonged coma and penetrating head injury. Anticonvulsants are sometimes used because of the unknown potential for immediate recurring seizures. In the patient who recovers rapidly, chronic anticonvulsant use is usually not indicated. An exception would be a patient with a prior seizure history or a family history of epilepsy.

Early posttraumatic seizures occur within the first week of the trauma, and epilepsy results in 20 to 25 percent of these patients. These early seizures are presumed to result from the focal effects of contusions or lacerations and the associated hypoperfusion, which causes ischemia and related metabolic changes.

Treatment of immediate and early posttraumatic seizures requires the correction of neurologic problems (depressed fracture, hematoma), the reduction of cerebral edema, proper oxygenation (airway maintenance, correction of shock), and the careful administration of anticonvulsants. With immediate and early posttraumatic seizures when impaired consciousness already prevails, it is important to avoid the use of significant sedative medication (barbiturates or diazepam) if possible. Phenytoin may be used successfully with relative safety (see Table 84-4). The dosage is determined by the clinical presentation; rapid loading is warranted to obtain immediate therapeutic levels in the patient in whom repeated seizures are occurring or likely to recur, especially when a seizure may further aggravate associated medical or surgical conditions.

Immediate posttraumatic seizures warrant anticonvulsant therapy for initial control, while long-term management of immediate seizures remains controversial.

Late posttraumatic seizures occur after 1 week and may be seen as late as 10 years after the trauma. Structural changes such as atrophy with cicatrix and permanent local vascular changes, altered dendrite branching, and presumably modified neurotransmitter function account for the development and permanence of these seizures. Of these seizures, 40 percent are focal or partial seizures, and 50 percent are temporal lobe seizures, indicating the predilection for traumatic injury and known epileptogenic properties of this structure. The risk of recurring seizures in this group is reported to be as high as 70 percent.

Early and late posttraumatic seizures warrant long-term anticonvulsant therapy in view of the risk of immediate and later recurrence. Late-onset posttraumatic seizures are most likely to recur and long-term anticonvulsant therapy is necessary in these cases to prevent this risk. Patients at greater risk for chronic posttraumatic seizures include those with depressed skull fractures, posttraumatic amnesia more than 24 h after the trauma, dural penetration, acute intracranial hemorrhage, early posttraumatic epilepsy, and a foreign body in a cerebral wound. The more severe the seizure and the later the onset, the less likely remission will occur.

Emergency management of seizures related to trauma should emphasize neurosurgical assessment, the rapid, careful administration of nonsedative anticonvulsants, the interruption of the seizures, and the stabilization of the general medical condition.

BREAKTHROUGH SEIZURES IN THE KNOWN EPILEPTIC

When seizures recur in a known epileptic, something has occurred to alter the balance of the excitation-inhibition complex, and the seizure threshold has been lowered. Complete seizure control is not always possible. The child with mental retardation, cerebral palsy, and generalized (most often myoclonic) seizures is most likely to have recurring seizures. Tonic-clonic (grand mal) seizures are the most dramatic and often lead to emergency treatment. The usual causes of seizure breakthrough can be summarized as follows:

1. Lowered anticonvulsant blood levels.
   a. Due to noncompliance. This is a common cause, most often in the preteen or teen who has been given the responsibility for self-medication.
   b. Related to intercurrent infection. Anticonvulsant levels fall during acute infections (viral or bacterial) with or without fever. Quite often the child's seizure recurrence is an indication of the infection before the acute problem is evident, e.g., with varicella or otitis media.
   c. The interaction of different drugs. An example is the reduction of the phenytoin level by the induction of parahydroxylators when barbiturates are used concomitantly (see the section ''Problems of Anticonvulsant Use'').
2. Change in habits.
   a. Altered sleep patterns because of trips, holidays, or parties.
   b. A job, exams, or an emotional stress. In the active teen, this may lead to seizures. If a pattern develops, knowledge of the pattern is quite helpful in defining treatment.
   c. Alcohol use. This can lower the seizure threshold and can also increase noncompliance.
   d. The use of illicit drugs or prescription drugs that lower the threshold. Examples are phenothiazine, lindane (Kwell), and heavy metals.
3. Complicating factors of epilepsy management.
   a. Toxic levels of drugs. An example is phenytoin intoxication.
   b. The use of phenytoin in some myoclonic epilepsies.

c. Valproic acid. Its use in complex partial seizures with secondary generalization has been reported to increase the partial (focal) seizure.

d. Anticonvulsant-induced osteomalacia with hypocalcemia. This uncommon problem may increase the seizure frequency.

4. The progression of the underlying cause. Examples are subacute sclerosing panencephalitis, neoplasm, arteriovenous malformation, and degenerative disease (ceroid lipofuscinosis). Blume and co-workers reported that 16 of 38 children undergoing cerebral resection for intractable seizures were found unexpectedly to have a cerebral tumor.

5. The vagaries of epilepsy. An unprovoked episode of seizures may occur in a well child with adequate therapeutic levels of anticonvulsants.

6. Superimposed head trauma. This may precipitate seizures; however, this is an overrated factor.

When a child known to have epilepsy presents with recurring seizures, several steps may minimize the treatment time and disclose the reason for the breakthrough. The physician should first assess the obvious factors: the airway and the blood pressure. Next, if the patient is having seizures at the time, the physician should test for the levels of anticonvulsants, electrolytes, calcium, and glucose and should obtain a complete blood cell count with differential. An intravenous catheter should be inserted if the child is not alert, so that medication can be administered if necessary. If the patient is febrile, a source of infection should be sought.

Once these procedures have been completed, anticonvulsant management is initiated. Assume the anticonvulsant levels are low and give a partial loading dose. If the patient is compliant, give the daily dose of phenobarbital or phenytoin orally if the patient is able to swallow, or intravenously if not. If the patient is known to be noncompliant or if the levels of the anticonvulsant are found on testing to be significantly below the therapeutic range, give the daily dose twice, e.g., in the child on 60 mg of phenobarbital, give 60 mg initially and repeat the dose if the seizures recur despite levels in the low therapeutic range.

If the anticonvulsant levels are within a high therapeutic range and the child is well without an obvious source of infection or other cause of breakthrough, then one can decide if another anticonvulsant is necessary. One may decide to wait and see if there is a trend toward increased seizure frequency, warranting additional medication, or if this is a solitary episode, warranting observation, monitoring of drug levels, and follow-up. If the levels are within the high therapeutic range and seizures recur, additional anticonvulsants are warranted in appropriate loading doses (Table 84-4).

Recurring or frequent tonic, tonic-clonic, and clonic seizures warrant loading doses that produce therapeutic levels rapidly. Phenobarbital and phenytoin can be given orally or intravenously to achieve therapeutic levels. Primidone (Mysoline) and carbamazepine (Tegretol) are not typically used as emergency room drugs or given in large loading doses because of their side effects. Valproic acid (Depakene) or its enteric-coated form, divalproic acid (Depakote), is usually given orally; the enteric-coated form may be used with less likelihood of abdominal discomfort and nausea. Liquid valproate has been used rectally to achieve therapeutic levels rapidly (60 mg/kg with equal amounts of saline) in patients in status epilepticus. It can be given this way in patients temporarily unable to swallow.

Seizures which begin with focal features, partial or complex partial (temporal lobe, psychomotor) may appear less dramatic and typically warrant a slower modification of drug therapy unless the seizures are prolonged or postictal Todd's paralysis occurs. If the patient requires additional drugs, phenobarbital, phenytoin, and carbamazepine can be used interchangeably, although the last cannot be loaded rapidly without producing uncomfortable side effects. Patients with petit mal (generalized absence) epilepsy rarely are brought to the emergency room, since the seizures are not alarming to the parents. If some injury occurs because of the absence spells, or if the parent is unusually concerned and brings the child for emergency treatment, determining the blood levels of anticonvulsants is most useful. Addition of another anticonvulsant can be initiated, e.g., addition of ethosuximide (Zarontin), valproate, clonazepam (Clonopin), or acetazolamide (Diamox).

Most often the epileptic patient can be sent home, and modification of the drug regimen can be carried out by the attending physician. Following the initial evaluations, modification of drug therapy, and treatment for any superimposed problems, the emergency physician should (1) arrange for follow-up evaluations by the attending physician, (2) emphasize the need for compliance, and (3) provide continued treatment for infections.

STATUS EPILEPTICUS

Status epilepticus represents a state of "epileptic seizure that is so frequently repeated or so prolonged as to create a fixed and lasting epileptic condition." This definition applies to continuous seizures lasting at least 30 min. More specific classification is listed in Table 84-7.

Table 84-6. Doses for Status Epilepticus in Children

Drug	Recommended Loading Dose	Route	Repeat	Rate	Maximum Dose	
Diazepam (Valium)	0.2 mg/kg	IV	3 times	1 mg/min	5 mg	0–2 years
					10 mg	2 years and older
Phenobarbital	15 mg/kg	IV	0		400 mg	
Phenytoin (Dilantin)	15 mg/kg	IV	0	40 mg/min	1000 mg	
Paraldehyde*	0.3 mL/kg	Rectal	q 4 h		15 mL	
Clonazepam (Clonopin)	0.3 mg/kg	NG	q 6 h		10 mg	
Valproic acid (Depakene*)	60 mg/kg	Rectal	0			
Lidocaine	2 mg/kg	IV		5–10 mg/(kg·h)		

*See text

Table 84-7. Classification of Status Seizures

I. Primary generalized convulsive status grand mal (continuous and noncontinuous)
   A. Tonic-clonic status
   B. Myoclonic status
   C. Clonic-tonic status
II. Secondary generalized convulsive status (continuous and noncontinuous)
   A. Tonic-clonic status with partial onset
   B. Tonic status
III. Simple partial status
   A. Partial motor status including EPC
   B. Partial sensory status
   C. Partial status with vegatative or autonomic symptoms
   D. Partial status with cognitive symptoms
   E. Partial status with affective symptoms
IV. Complex partial status
V. Absence (petit mal) status

Note: EPC = epilepsy partialis continua
Source: Modified from Delgado-Escueta and Bajorek, 1982.

About 5 to 10 percent of chidren with epilepsy and 60,000 to 100,000 total epileptics experience one bout of status grand mal (SGM). This condition is a neurologic emergency which could be fatal. The longer the SGM persists, the greater the morbidity and the mortality and the more difficult it is to control the seizures. In patients with no neurologic sequelae, the mean duration of SGM is $1\frac{1}{2}$ h. Neurologic sequelae result when SGM lasts an average of 10 h. The mean duration of SGM in patients who die is 13 h.

Effects of SGM

Experimental models in animals provide evidence of the neurologic effects of SGM. Selective permanent cell damage in the hippocampus, amygdala, cerebellum, thalamus, and middle cerebral cortical layers develops after 60 min. of seizure activity. Even with artificial ventilation and correction of existing metabolic derangements, most changes still occur. This cell death results from the increased metabolic demands and the exhaustion of the continuously firing neurons. In addition, there are secondary effects which probably exaggerate the adverse effects of SGM. After unremitting SGM, the cerebral P_{O_2} and cytochrome A and cytochrome A_3 reductase decrease, enhancing the risk of cell damage. Calcium concentrations, arachidonic acid, arachidonal diglycerols, prostaglandins, and leukotriene increase in the neurons exaggerate or cause cerebral edema and cell death. Increased levels of cyclic AMP and increased release of prolactin, growth hormone, ACTH, cortisol, insulin, glycogen, epinephrine, and norepinephrine may contribute to the progression of cell damage with the loss of physiological responsiveness.

Late secondary effects include lactic acidosis, elevated cerebrospinal fluid pressure, hyperglycemia (followed later by hypoglycemia), dysautonomia with hyperthermia, diaphoresis, dehydration, hypertension followed by hypotension, and eventually shock. In addition, excessive muscle activity leads to myolysis, myoglobinuria, and renal failure. Neuropathologic studies indicate nucleovacuolation and ischemic nerve cell damage leading to neuronal dissolution.

Treatment

Treatment is best initiated when the type of seizure is identified. To obtain the most effective and rapid cessation of status epilepticus, the following specific therapeutic goals must be reached.

1. Specific delineation of the type and subtype of status epilepticus so that appropriate treatment can be chosen. For example, tonic-clonic generalized status is very responsive to diazepam or phenytoin; noncontinuous clonic or tonic-clonic seizures may be refractory to diazepam.
2. Identification and treatment of the reversible precipitating cause of status epilepticus, e.g., cerebral infection, trauma, electrolyte disturbance, brain abscess, hypoglycemia.
3. Rapid cessation of status epilepticus to prevent secondary effects that both prolong the seizures and cause irreversible neuronal damage.
4. Full support of medical systems to prevent unwarranted complications of the seizures or the treatment, e.g., respiratory depression, arrhythmia, aspiration pneumonia, shock, myoglobulinuria.

In treating the patient with continuous grand mal or tonic-clonic seizures, the end point is clear: the cessation of seizures. The amount of diazepam necessary to cause the seizures to cease has been derived from studies that confirm one significant point—complications usually occurred in markedly ill patients with complex disorders or with prior use of high dosages of other hypnotic drugs. The safety of diazepam to a maximum dose of 2.6 mg/kg over the course of treatment has been substantiated. Smith and co-workers described an effective dose of diazepam as 0.08 to 2.72 mg/kg in infants and young children with an average effective dose of 0.68 mg/kg. Many authors recommend initial doses of 1 mg/year of age with a maximum total dose of 5 mg in infants and 10 mg in children. Eckert reported maximum doses in adolescents as 35 mg in brief periods and 100 mg in 24 h.

A starting dose of diazepam of 0.2 to 0.5 mg/kg, given at a rate of 1 mg/min and repeated as needed to a maximum of 2.6 mg/kg, is recommended to stop continuous tonic-clonic and clonic seizures. This higher dose is rarely used since most patients stop seizing at lower doses and additional drugs such as phenytoin may be employed. Care must be taken to assure adequate ventilation.

The drug of choice in continuous SGM is diazepam, with 80 percent success within 5 min reported. To maintain the seizure-free state a long-term anticonvulsant is necessary. Therefore, after diazepam causes the seizures to cease, a phenytoin loading dose of 15 mg/kg is administered with maintenance dosages of 5 to 8 mg/(kg·day) to maintain therapeutic blood levels of 10 to 20 μg/mL. Phenobarbital may be necessary if phenytoin is ineffective.

The following 10 steps should be followed when treating continuous status grand mal (tonic-clonic status) (Table 84-6):

1. Assess basic functions immediately and maintain blood pressure, airway, and pulse.
2. Obtain blood to be tested for levels of anticonvulsants, electrolytes, BUN, calcium, glucose, and for a complete blood cell count with differential while inserting an IV catheter for fluid administration.
3. Administer IV a bolus of 25% glucose, 2 mL/kg.
4. Administer IV diazepam, 0.2 mg/kg, and repeat up to a total dose of 2.6 mg/kg or early signs of respiratory depression.

5. Administer IV phenytoin, 15 mg/kg, after diazepam is infused, at a rate less than 50 mg/min.
6. Administer IV phenobarbital, 10 to 15 mg/kg, if phenytoin is ineffective. When the patient requires step 6, transfer to ICU is warranted.
7. Administer rectally paraldehyde, 0.3 mL/kg, mixed with an equal amount of mineral oil, if step 6 is ineffective.
8. Administer IV a bolus of lidocaine, 2 mg/kg, if step 7 is ineffective.
9. In noncontinuous status grand mal, administer clonazepam (Clonopin) through nasogastric tube in a single dose of 0.2 to 0.6 mg/kg initially followed by 0.1 to 0.4 mg/(kg·day) maintenance.
10. General anesthesia.

Noncontinuous status epilepticus can be more difficult to treat since the end point is more elusive. Rapidly acting drugs such as diazepam are less effective, and a more sustained effect is necessary. Often noncontinuous status epilepticus is not responsive to appropriate therapeutic levels of phenytoin and phenobarbital. Large doses (0.2 to 0.6 mg/kg) of clonazepam via nasogastric tube may be used to produce the desired effect of rapid cessation of noncontinuous seizures, and the anticonvulsant effect maintained by additional drugs (phenytoin, phenobarbital) and clonazepam [0.1 to 0.3 mg/(kg·day)].

Paraldehyde can be very effective in noncontinuous status epilepticus. Although it is often given intramuscularly, rectal absorption can be quite effective and avoids the problem of sterile abscesses. Intravenous paraldehyde must be used cautiously because of its rapid pulmonary excretion and potential to produce pulmonary edema and metabolic acidosis. Paraldehyde should be administered only with glass syringes and rubber tubing in view of its degradation to toxic forms in the presence of certain plastics.

Absence (petit mal) status is a much simpler form of status epilepticus to deal with since it is exquisitely responsive to diazepam given intravenously. It rarely happens that a patient requires emergency care for this form of epilepsy.

Epilepsia partialis continua is a serious neurologic condition, although it does not appear threatening at first glance. The patient exhibits repeated continuous or minimally interrupted clonic jerking of one side of the body and usually one part of an extremity for days, weeks, or months. It is typically due to encephalitis or cerebrovascular accident and indicates a relatively poor prognosis. Its management is similar to that of noncontinuous SGM.

DIFFERENTIAL DIAGNOSIS OF SEIZURES

It is necessary to identify nonepileptic paroxysmal disorders to prevent confusion with epilepsy (see Table 84-8). Incorrectly diagnosing seizures instead of syncope, dyskinesia, or psychiatric disorders can be a problem in any circumstance, and in an emergency room one must avoid the pressure to make a diagnosis and treat too quickly.

The differential diagnosis of seizures must take into account many disorders that can produce loss of consciousness, unusual movements, impaired awareness, or bizarre behavior. Many of these disorders depend on age.

In the newborn, the problems partly reflect the intrauterine experience. Jitteriness or hyperexcitability appears as high-amplitude tremulousness easily brought out by passive movement of the extremities or jarring of the crib. The drug-withdrawn infant is

Table 84-8. Nonepileptic Paroxysmal Disorders

I. Loss of consciousness
  A. Syncope
    1. Vasovagal
    2. Valsalva maneuver
    3. Adams-Stokes
  B. Toxic
    1. Illicit drug use—narcotics, barbiturates
    2. Alcohol abuse
    3. Heavy metal poisoning
    4. Accidental ingestion of prescription medication
    5. Carbon monoxide intoxication
  C. Near miss sudden infant death syndrome (SIDS)
  D. Breatholding—cyanotic or pallid
  E. Metabolic
    1. Electrolyte imbalance—water intoxication
    2. Hypoglycemia
  F. Narcolepsy
II. Altered behavior
  A. Conversion reaction
  B. Effect of illicit drugs (PCP)
  C. Hyperkinetic due to theophylline intoxication
  D. Migraine with confusional states
  E. Drug interactions
III. Movement disorders
  A. Hyperexcitable infant
  B. Drug withdrawal
  C. Hyperexplexia—nonepileptic drop attacks
  D. Chorea
    1. Sydenham's poststreptococcal or idiopathic
    2. Paroxysmal, familial, nonfamilial
    3. Thyrotoxic
  E. Tourette's syndrome
  F. Sleep disturbance—myoclonus, night terrors, somnambulism

Note: PCP = phencyclizine.

irritable and tremulous, and may have diaphoresis, vomiting, and diarrhea; in addition, seizures may occur. Sepsis, hypoglycemia, and hypocalcemia may produce nonepileptic paroxysmal activity in addition to seizures. Near-miss sudden death syndrome (SIDS) remains a multifactorial condition in which seizures are part of the differential diagnosis and might be considered part of the cause.

In the older infant it is more common to see cyanotic and pallid breath-holding spells, which typically occur following an abrupt trauma (fall, minor spanking) or a verbal reprimand. The infant gives a sudden cry followed by prolonged inhalation or exhalation, resulting in no air exchange, and a Valsalva maneuver, often with bradycardia. A brief tonic nonepileptic seizure often occurs. Drug intoxication manifested by hyperkinesis, impaired awareness, or altered behavior (hallucinations) is usually accidental at this age. Later in childhood, phencyclidine (PCP) intoxication mimics complex partial seizures and may result in seizures with more severe overdoses.

Congenital heart disease can produce paroxysmal events at all ages. Abrupt mental status changes may occur in patients with pulmonary hypertension, aortic stenosis, tetralogy of Fallot, atresia of the ventricles, cardiac rhabdomyomas, etc. Acquired cardiomyopathy may result in decreased cardiac output (Adams-Stokes disease) or cerebrovascular accident.

Hyperkinetic movement disorders can be difficult to differentiate from complex partial seizures. Sydenham's chorea is infrequently seen today, and drug-induced chorea (ethosuximide, carbamazepine, diphenhydramine hydrochloride) and lupus-induced chorea are likewise very uncommon. Tourette's syndrome is more frequently seen, but rarely does the child appear acutely ill.

Immediate posttraumatic migraine may cause confusional states mimicking concussion or complex partial seizures. In the adolescent, syncope due to stretching and yawning or following hair combing (vasovagal) is more common.

Pseudoseizures represent a particular problem for the treating physician because the "seizures" appear to represent a significant threat to the patient's safety, and vigorous anticonvulsant therapy is often initiated. Unfortunately, pseudoseizures often occur in patients with documented epilepsy. Secondary gain should become evident in these cases. The "seizures" are atypical in that the patient may waken fully in the interictal phase and require repeated large doses of anticonvulsants even to the point of protracted drug-induced depression. Another form of pseudoseizures consists of those described by the parent and never observed by other witnesses.

To distinguish pseudoseizures from true epileptic spells, a bedside technique in the emergency room may be dramatic and diagnostic, and prevent overtreatment. One method is to gently insert a nasopharyngeal tube and observe the patient's response. The pseudoseizure patient will become responsive immediately. Experience dictates referral for patients with a diagnosis of pseudoseizure, or even hospitalization, to prevent recurrences, provide family education, and lessen the likelihood of inappropriate treatment.

Simple sleep myoclonus and night terrors are of concern to parents. They are, however, easily distinguished from nocturnal seizures.

Preventing misdiagnosis and mistreatment is an essential part of the emergency management of seizures and related disorders.

PROBLEMS OF ANTICONVULSANT USE

Unwanted features of anticonvulsants may be seen soon after the drug is initiated or may develop weeks, months, or years later. These problems may turn up during evaluation for other illnesses (e.g., macrocytic anemia) or be the basis for emergency treatment.

Immediate side effects often subside in time. Lethargy occurs more often with barbiturates, is usually dose-related, and subsides with chronic use and half-life stabilization. Irritability and changes in cognition can persist and be so significant that a nonbarbiturate anticonvulsant must be substituted. Rashes may occur within days or weeks of initiation of therapy but must be differentiated from concurrent viral exanthem. Pruritic and/or morbilliform rashes usually require cessation of medication. Stevens-Johnson syndrome, with bullous skin lesions affecting mucous membranes, is a serious potential reaction. There is a risk of serious sequelae—blindness, esophageal stenosis, or loss of life.

With valproic acid use, hepatic failure may occur within days or up to 2 years after first use. The drug reaction results in alteration of behavior, increasing lethargy, and vomiting. Levels of liver enzymes may be minimally to markedly elevated, and hyperammonemia with or without symptoms of hepatic failure may be found. Immediate cessation of valproate, hospitalization, and observation are necessary if symptomatic hepatic reaction is evident. In the asymptomatic patient with enzyme-level elevations, a reduction of the dosage and careful observation are warranted. Gastrointestinal side effects are common with initial use of valproic acid and may be so severe that more serious hepatic prob-

lems are considered. These side effects can be avoided by a more frequent dosage schedule, taken with meals, and by avoiding carbonated beverages and citric juices, or alternatively by using the enteric-coated form. Pancreatitis secondary to valproate use also has been reported.

Toxicity due to overdosage at any time can produce some readily identifiable symptoms and signs. Phenytoin toxicity occurs when serum levels exceed 25 μg/mL in most patients (above 20 μg/mL in some). Nausea, dysarthria, diplopia, and ataxia are seen early, with progression to impaired levels of consciousness and decerebrate posturing. Virtually all anticonvulsants produce ataxia and lethargy with significant overdosage. Cardiopulmonary monitoring during high-dose drug use in status epilepticus should be employed since cardiac collapse or respiratory depression can occur. Burning in the limb used for the infusion of phenytoin has also been reported. Using a free-flowing, well-positioned needle and a short tubing distance and infusing at a rate of 50 mg/min or less lessens the likelihood of phenytoin side effects. Chronic phenytoin use can result in folate deficiency with macrocytic anemia, acquired osteomalacia (increased vitamin D turnover), neutropenia (often transient), peripheral neuropathy, lupus-like syndromes, and myasthenic weakness.

Drug interactions may be quite dramatic. Valproate and aspirin can result in a bleeding diathesis. Antihistamines used in conjunction with barbiturates can be very sedating, warranting smaller doses of the antihistamine. When erythromycin is used, particular care must be exercised since the anticonvulsant levels may rise to toxic levels. The phenytoin levels are typically reduced by a change in protein binding when valproic acid is also used, but levels may still be therapeutic if free phenytoin is measured and found to be adequate. When barbiturates are used concomitantly, increased parahydroxylation can cause enhanced metabolism of phenytoin so that therapeutic levels fall, resulting in seizure breakthrough. Hyperbilirubinemia and hypoalbuminemia can affect anticonvulsant binding and blood levels.

Movement disorders (e.g., chorea) can result after several weeks' or months' use of ethosuximide and rarely with carbamazepine. The movements may be profound and usually respond promptly to the cessation of the drug and the use of diphenhydramine (Benadryl), 12.5 to 25 mg given intravenously. Clonazepam and diazepam can cause acute bladder dysfunction with urinary retention.

Many problems of dose-related toxicity can be avoided by maintaining therapeutic blood levels. There is, however, no set pattern or formula for the blood level, and it should depend upon seizure frequency, patient compliance, and careful observation for early clinical signs of toxicity. Idiosyncratic effects cannot be predicted, but families must be made aware that significant side effects can develop with little warning, and evaluation by a physician is recommended before a drug is dismissed. Obtaining the patient's history, consulting with the primary physician or consultant, and reviewing readily available drug information in the package insert or *Physician's Desk Reference* make emergency evaluation and treatment of anticonvulsant drug reactions simpler.

PITFALLS OF EMERGENCY MANAGEMENT OF SEIZURES

After the patient arrives for treatment, the initial assessment may be incomplete, resulting in inappropriate or inadequate therapy.

Not identifying treatable infections, electrolyte imbalance, child abuse, and accidental trauma can lead to rapidly progressive deterioration and demise, or may make seizure control difficult. By not ascertaining anticonvulsant levels in the patient with epilepsy, the physician loses an opportunity to determine if the anticonvulsant is ineffective or simply at too low a level.

If the emergency physician communicates with the primary physician, unnecessary studies, and drugs which either were ineffective or produced some side effects, can be avoided. Additionally, it is important to consult with the patient's physician when prescribing nonanticonvulsants which might interfere with anticonvulsants or produce unwanted side effects.

In the aggressive treatment of seizures (status epilepticus and recurring breakthrough seizures), inadequate loading doses or improper drug selection may prolong the seizures and worsen the prognosis. Excessive dosage can result in respiratory depression or hypotension and, in rare instances, can exacerbate the seizures. If nonepileptic paroxysmal disorders are not recognized, the patient is put at the additional risk of unnecessary medication and inadequate treatment of the real disorder.

The emergency physician cannot deal with all the problems facing the patient with epilepsy. Follow-up care by the primary physicians or appropriate consultants ensures better compliance and, one hopes, lessens emergency situations in the future.

BIBLIOGRAPHY

Berman PH: Management of seizure disorders with anticonvulsant drugs, in Prensky AL (ed): *Pediatric Neurology, Pediatric Clinics of North America*. Philadelphia, Saunders, 1976, pp. 443–459.

Blume BT, Gerven JP, Kaufmann JCE: Childhood brain tumors presenting as chronic uncontrolled focal seizures. *Ann Neurol* 12:538, 1982.

Commission on Classification and Terminology of the International League Against Epilepsy: Proposal for revised clinical and electroencephalographic classification of epileptic seizures. *Epilepsia* 22:489, 1981.

Craig WS: Convulsive movements occurring in the first ten days of life. *Arch Dis Child* 35:336, 1960.

Delgado-Escueta AV, Bajorek JG: Status epilepticus: Mechanisms of brain damage and rational management. *Epilepsia* 23(suppl 1):S29, 1982.

Delgado-Escueta AV, Treiman DM, Walsh GO: The treatable epilepsies (first of two parts). *N Engl J Med* 308:1508, 1983.

Delgado-Escueta AV, Treiman DM, Walsh GO: The treatable epilepsies (second of two parts). *N Engl J Med* 308:1576, 1983.

Desai BT, Porter RJ, Penry JK: Psychogenic seizures. *Arch Neurol* 39:202, 1982.

Dreyfuss FE, Sackellares JC: Treating epilepsy in children. *Curr Prescrib*:63, 1979.

Earnest MP, Marx JA, Drury LR: Complications of intravenous phenytoin for acute treatment of seizures. *JAMA* 219:762, 1983.

Eckert C: Neurologic Emergencies, in *Emergency-Room Care*, ed 4. Boston, Little, Brown, 1981, pp. 409–420.

Edwards R, Schmidly JW, Simon RP: How often does a CSF pleocytosis follow generalized convulsions. *Ann Neurol* 13:460, 1983.

Freeman JM: Neonatal seizures—Diagnosis and management. *J Pediatr* 77:701, 1970.

Gal P, Toback J, Boer HR, et al: Efficacy of phenobarbital monotherapy in treatment of neonatal seizures—Relationship to blood levels. *Neurology* 32:1301, 1982.

Gastaut H: Clinical and electroencephalographical classification of epileptic seizures. *Epilepsia* 11:102, 1970.

Gross M, Hureta E: Functional convulsions masked as epileptic disorders. *J Pediatr Psychol* 5:71, 1980.

Harrison RM, Taylor DC: Childhood seizures: A 25 year follow up—A social and medical prognosis. *Lancet*:948, 1976.

Hauser WA, Anderson VE, Levenson RB, et al: Seizure recurrence after a first unprovoked seizure. *N Engl J Med* 307:522, 1982.

Henderson BM, Levi JS: Febrile seizures in children. *Am Fam Physician* 11:114, 1975.

Holowach J, Thurston DL, O'Leary J: Prognosis in childhood epilepsy—Follow up study of 148 cases in which therapy had been suspended after prolonged anticonvulsant control. *N Engl J Med* 286:169, 1972.

Juul-Jensen P, Denny-Brown D: Epilepsia partialis continua. *Arch Neurol* 25:97, 1971.

Knauss TA, Marshall RE: Seizures in a neonatal intensive care unit. *Dev Med Child Neurol* 19:719, 1977.

Lombroso CT: A perspective study of infantile spasm: Clinical and therapeutic correlations. *Epilepsia* 24:135, 1983.

Lombroso CT: The treatment of status epilepticus. *Pediatrics* 53:536, 1974.

Lombroso CT, Lerman P: Breathholding spells (cyanotic and pallid infantile syncope). *Pediatrics* 39:563, 1967.

McInerny TK, Schubert WK: Prognosis of neonatal seizures. *Am J Dis Child* 117:701, 1970.

National Institutes of Health: Consensus Development Conference on Febrile Seizures, May 1980. *Epilepsia* 22:377, 1981.

Nelson KB, Eleenberg JH: Prognosis in children who have experienced febrile seizure. *Pediatrics* 61:720, 1978.

Niedermeyer E, Fineyre F, Riley T, et al: Myoclonus and the electroencephalogram—A review. *Clin Electroencephalogr* 10:75, 1979.

Painter MJ: General principles of treatment: Status epilepticus in neonates. *Adv Neurol* 34:385, 1983.

Pippenger CE: An overview of antiepileptic drug interactions. *Epilepsia* 23(suppl 1):581, 1982.

Riikonen R: A long term follow up study of 214 children with the syndrome of infantile spasms. *Neuropediatrics* 13:14, 1982.

Smith BT, Masotti RE: Intravenous diazepam in the treatment of prolonged seizure activity in neonates and infants. *Dev Med Child Neurol* 13:630, 1971.

Staudt F, Scholl ML, Coen RW, et al: Phenobarbital therapy in neonatal seizures and the prognostic value of the EEG. *Neuropediatrics* 13:24, 1982.

Tassinari CA, Daniele O, Michelucci R, et al: Benzodiazepines: Efficacy in status epilepticus. *Adv Neurol* 34:465, 1983.

Thurston JH, Thurston DL, Hixon BB, et al: Prognosis in childhood epilepsy—Additional follow up of 148 children 15–23 years after withdrawal of anticonvulsant therapy. *N Engl J Med* 306:831, 1982.

Wagman IH, DeJong RH, Prince DA: Effects of lidocaine on spontaneous cortical and subcortical activity. *Arch Neurol* 18:277, 1968.

CHAPTER 85
REYE'S
SYNDROME

Carol D. Berkowitz

Reye's syndrome is the most common neurologic complication of a viral illness in children. Early recognition and prompt management may be lifesaving and may significantly reduce the long-term morbidity.

The disorder was first reported by Reye, Morgan, and Basal in 1963. They described 21 children seen between 1951 and 1962 at the Royal Alexander Hospital for Children in Australia. These children had "encephalopathy and fatty degeneration of the viscera." Other authors in earlier reports had also noted encephalopathies of unknown cause associated with fatty accumulation in the liver, but it was only after the report by Reye and colleagues that the disorder became a recognized clinical entity. The incidence is now felt to be 1.3 to 2.7 cases per 100,000 per year in children under 17 years of age.

ETIOLOGY

The primary insult giving rise to Reye's syndrome appears to be a disruption of mitochondrial function in the brain and liver, as well as in other organs, such as the heart, kidneys, pancreas, and skeletal muscle. Electron microscopy demonstrates swelling and pleomorphism of the mitochondria, with disruption of the outer membrane and deformation of the cristae. Additionally, a heat-stable factor which affects mitochondrial function in vitro has been found in the serum of patients with Reye's syndrome. Cerebral edema occurs on a cytotoxic rather than a vasogenic basis and is the major pathologic complication.

It is uncertain what initiates the insult, but it may occur secondary to a virus, virus neutralization, genetic predisposition (e.g., heterozygotes for urea cycle disorders), exposure to toxins or drugs, or a synergistic interaction among these factors.

Influenza B and chickenpox are the viruses most frequently antedating Reye's syndrome. However, live virus immunization and other viruses have been associated with Reye's syndrome; the viruses include Coxsackie, influenza A, herpes (including simplex and zoster), reo, adeno, Epstein-Barr, echo, parainfluenza, polio 1, rubella, rubeola, and vaccinia.

Numerous toxins have also been implicated. Two disorders that clinically resemble Reye's syndrome are associated with the inges-

tion of specific toxins. Jamaican vomiting sickness follows the consumption of the unripe fruit of the akee tree, which contains hypoglycine A. Udorn encephalopathy, seen in southeast Asia, follows the ingestion of grains and nuts which contain aflatoxin B, a toxic metabolite of *Aspergillus flavus*.

The drug most recently implicated is aspirin. In 1980 a report from the Center for Disease Control showed a statistical correlation between the use of aspirin and the development of Reye's syndrome in a group of school-age children during an outbreak of influenza A. Children who developed Reye's syndrome had fever more often than controls, and among those who had fever, patients who developed Reye's syndrome used aspirin more frequently than those who did not. In addition, the group found increasing severity of Reye's syndrome with increasing aspirin dosage. Other investigators have corroborated these findings. The data are sufficiently convincing to make one recommend that children with chickenpox or influenza avoid aspirin.

Of interest is that salicylate diminishes mitochondrial function and uncouples oxidative phosphorylation, the phenomena seen in Reye's syndrome. Glycogen stores are diminished in the liver and muscle with both Reye's syndrome and salicylate ingestion.

Recent reports link pesticide exposure to Reye's syndrome.

CLINICAL PICTURE

The disorder presents in a biphasic manner. Initially, there is a viral illness. This is usually influenza B (most common in "epidemic" Reye's syndrome) or chickenpox (20 percent). Reye's syndrome occurs in 1 case per 1700 children afflicted with influenza B.

Clustering of cases of Reye's syndrome occurs in late winter and early spring, reflecting virus spurts. Following the initial phase of the acute viral illness, there is a recovery period. New symptoms, mainly vomiting, then develop. The vomiting may become pernicious; there is a subsequent alteration of mental status with either lethargy or *combative behavior which may progress to coma*, the encephalopathic phase. The mean duration between the two phases of the illness is 3 days but may range between 0.5 to 7 days, or may be as long as 2 to 3 weeks. Nonsurvivors have been noted to have a longer interval between the antecedent illness and the onset of Reye's syndrome.

The clinical features are influenced by the age of the patient. Reye's syndrome has been described in patients from early infancy to adulthood. Most children are between 6 and 11 years. The median age of children afflicted following chickenpox is 6 years as opposed to 11 years following influenza.

Infants under 1 year may present with seizures. These may be secondary to hypoglycemia or the cerebral insult. Respiratory disturbances, such as apnea or hyperventilation, are also noted, but the hallmark of Reye's syndrome, vomiting, may be minimal in the infant. Diarrhea, however, is more frequent. The child over the age of 1 may also have respiratory disturbances, particularly hyperventilation. Breathing may be shallow, irregular, or rapid, or may mimic that seen with ketoacidosis. Changes in mental status such as lethargy, irritability, disorientation, deliriums, hallucinations, and combativeness occur. Seizures are also seen in older children. Adults with Reye's syndrome resemble children with the disorder.

DIAGNOSIS

The diagnosis of Reye's syndrome should be suspected clinically in any one of the following circumstances:

1. A child showing an alteration of mental status, such as lethargy, irritability, or combativeness.
2. A child with right upper quadrant tenderness. Fifty percent of children with Reye's syndrome have hepatomegaly, and the liver may be either soft or firm.
3. A child with antecedent chickenpox, or during influenza season, who presents with new complaints.
4. A child with an abnormal neurologic examination. Fundal examination must be included because the finding of papilledema, although unusual, carries with it a higher mortality. More frequent neurologic findings include increased muscle tone and deep tendon reflexes, and dilated, sluggishly reactive pupils.
5. All infants with unexplained hypoglycemia and seizures.

It is crucial that the emergency physician maintain a high index of suspicion for this disorder, obtain the appropriate tests, and initiate early treatment.

LABORATORY

The detection of abnormalities is confirmatory evidence of Reye's syndrome. The following laboratory studies are suggested.

1. *Liver function tests*
   The liver panel should include tests for prothrombin time, partial thromboplastin time (prolonged), serum glutamic-oxaloacetic transaminase, serum glutamic-pyruvic transaminase (elevated 2 to 20 times normal), serum ammonia (elevated 2 to 20 times normal), and bilirubin (usually normal). It would be difficult to entertain the diagnosis of Reye's syndrome in the absence of abnormal liver function tests, or in the presence of an elevated bilirubin level (total greater than 5 mg/dL).

   Elevation of the blood ammonia level is the laboratory sine qua non of Reye's syndrome. The ultimate outcome does not completely correlate with the ammonia level, although levels greater than 350 μg/dL (venous) indicate a poor prognosis. The elevated ammonia level appears to be related to a disturbance of the urea cycle secondary to the mitochondrial dysfunction, since carbamoyl-phosphate synthetase and ornithine carbamoyltransferase, urea cycle enzymes, are located within the mitochondrial matrix.

   One may see a transient elevation of the liver function tests with chickenpox even in the absence of Reye's syndrome. Varicella hepatitis may also produce these laboratory abnormalities.

   Liver function studies return to normal in 3 to 5 days in Reye's syndrome. This rapid recovery is unlike that seen with acute yellow atrophy due to hepatitis or poisoning.

2. *Creatine kinase*
   Creatine kinase (CK) is also elevated. This includes MM (skeletal), MB (cardiac), but not BB (brain) fractions. The elevation of the CK level may correlate with the ultimate outcome; patients with the highest levels of CK have the highest mortality.

3. *Blood glucose*
   Hypoglycemia was initially considered a hallmark of Reye's syndrome. It is now felt to occur in about 40 percent of affected children, usually those less than 5 years old and especially those under 1 year. A low blood glucose level is correlated with a poor outcome. It is related to the diminished glycogen stores and the increased sugar utilization often seen with elevated ammonia levels.

4. *Serum electrolytes and blood urea nitrogen*
   These levels are either normal or reflect a degree of dehydration secondary to anorexia and vomiting. A baseline value of these tests is important in anticipation of diuretic therapy.

5. *Complete blood cell count and differential with platelet estimate*
   These values are usually normal. The white blood cell count may be elevated secondary to stress or metabolic acidosis. Platelet counts are rarely decreased.

6. *Amylase*
   The amylase may be elevated secondary to the pancreatic involvement noted in about 4 percent of children with Reye's syndrome.

7. *Urinalysis*
   This is a baseline examination in anticipation of fluid restriction and diuretic therapy.

8. *Lumbar puncture*
   Lumbar punctures may be performed, although there is some controversy about tapping a child with suspected elevation of intracranial pressure. The results of cerebrospinal fluid (CSF) examination are usually normal or may show a slightly low glucose level or mild monocytosis. The CSF examination is necessary to exclude a CNS infection.

9. *CT scan*
   The CT scan shows diffuse cerebral edema with slitlike ventricles.

10. *ECG*
    The ECG may show arrhythmia or evidence of myocarditis, although these are usually not severe enough to require treatment.

11. *Other laboratory studies*
    Other abnormal laboratory results include abnormal amino acid patterns, increased free fatty acid levels but diminished lipid levels, respiratory alkalosis and metabolic acidosis, and ketonuria.

PATHOLOGIC CONFIRMATION

The diagnosis of Reye's syndrome may be confirmed by liver biopsy. The biopsy is characteristic and shows microvesicular fat droplets in the hepatocytes without any inflammatory cell response. Electron microscopy reveals dilatation of the endoplasmic reticulum and the mitochondria. There is also an absence of glycogen stores.

The National Institutes of Health Consensus Development Conference on the Diagnosis and Treatment of Reye's Syndrome concluded that the clinical and laboratory findings are diagnostic in children over the age of 1 and liver biopsy is not necessary in all cases. Liver biopsy was recommended in infants under 1 year, children who have recurrences or atypical presentations (no prodromal illness, no vomiting), familial cases, or when unproven therapeutic interventions are planned.

DIFFERENTIAL DIAGNOSIS

The differential diagnosis must include those disorders producing hepatic and CNS dysfunction. The main disorders to be considered include the following:

1. *Fulminant hepatic failure*
   This may occur in association with infection (viral hepatitis), or drug or toxin ingestion. Salicylates, acetaminophen, isopropyl alcohol, and valproate may produce drug-induced hepatitis resembling Reye's syndrome. The absence of jaundice and the unique liver biopsy in Reye's syndrome help differentiate the two disorders.
2. *Pancreatic encephalopathy*
   This is a very rare disorder associated with a confusional state during a bout of acute pancreatitis.
3. *Infections of the CNS*
   Viral or bacterial meningitis or encephalitis may present with vomiting and lethargy. Varicella encephalitis is frequently confused with Reye's syndrome, but the absence of hepatic involvement leads to the diagnosis of encephalitis.
4. *Inborn errors of metabolism*
   These usually enter the differential diagnosis in young infants afflicted with Reye's syndrome, in familial cases, and in recurrent cases. These disorders include urea cycle defects (ornithine carbamoyltransferase and carbamoyl-phosphate synthetase deficiencies), organic acid disorders (glutaric aciduria and isovaleric acidemia), and systemic carnitine deficiency.

The liver biopsy usually helps to differentiate these disorders when differentiation on clinical or laboratory grounds is uncertain.

STAGING

Once the diagnosis is suspected and supported by the laboratory data, one should assign the patient to a stage. Lovejoy and co-workers have described five clinical stages helpful in determining the aggressiveness of the intervention.

Stage I
   Vomiting, *lethargy*, sleepiness, liver dysfunction. Mortality is less than 5 percent in this stage.
Stage II
   Disorientation, delirium, combativeness, hyperventilation, increased deep tendon reflexes, liver dysfunction.

Stage III
   Coma, increased respiratory rate, decorticate rigidity, intact pupils and oculovestibular reflexes, liver dysfunction. The mortality is 50 to 60 percent.
Stage IV
   Deepening coma, *decerebrate rigidity*, no oculovestibular reflexes, loss of corneal reflexes, minimal liver dysfunction.
Stage V
   Seizures, loss of deep tendon reflexes, *respiratory arrest*, flaccidity. *Liver dysfunction is absent.* The mortality is 95 percent in this group.

Staging based on the EEG is nonspecific and does not facilitate diagnosis but may have some predictive value. The neurologic symptoms as reflected in the staging move in a rostral to caudal manner, and seizures appear when there is brain stem dysfunction. Poor prognostic signs include the following:

1. Rapid passage through the first three clinical stages.
2. The onset of seizure while in stage III.
3. Initial ammonia levels greater than 300 μg/dL.

In addition, the following are associated with a poor outcome: a prothrombin time that is 13 to 14 sec greater than that of the control, an increased CSF pressure in stage III, and a type 3 EEG.

MANAGEMENT

The management of the noncomatose patient with Reye's syndrome is supportive, with intravenous fluids, including 10% dextrose, and observation in the hospital. The management of the comatose patient is directed toward preventing and reversing the potentially lethal complications. The focus is on managing the increased intracranial pressure, which is on a cytotoxic basis, secondary to mitochondrial dysfunction and impaired metabolism within the brain cell. This impairment results from the primary disruption compounded by the insult of metabolites resulting from deranged liver function. Few cases of herniation have been seen with Reye's syndrome in spite of massive swelling and flattening of gyri. Additionally, neuronal damage appears to be reversible, and neuronal necrosis is not extensive at the time of autopsy.

Elevated intracranial pressure is suggested by the presence of slitlike ventricles on CT scan and is documented with the use of an intracranial pressure monitor (subarachnoid or epidural bolt, or intraventricular catheter). The catheter transmits pressure via transducer to a recorder and also permits instant removal of CSF. It is preferred by many centers but is difficult to insert into the small ventricles and has an increased risk of bleeding and infection.

The main goal of management is to maintain the intracranial pressure at less than 15 torr. There is concern for the adequacy of cerebral blood flow when the cerebral perfusion pressure falls to less than 50 torr. The cerebral perfusion pressure equals the mean arterial pressure [diastolic + $\frac{1}{3}$ (systolic minus diastolic)] minus the intracranial pressure.

The following are measures to manage increased intracranial pressure and to ensure adequate cerebral perfusion.

1. The head should be elevated to 30° in a midline position. This ensures adequate cerebral venous return and helps reduce vasogenic swelling.
2. Intubation and controlled hyperventilation with a respirator may be used to maintain a P_{CO_2} of 20 to 25 torr. This achieves

optimum vasoconstriction and decreases the intracranial volume by decreasing the blood proportion. Further reduction of the P_{CO_2} to less than 20 torr may reduce flow so as to produce anoxia.

3. The patient may be paralyzed with pancuronium bromide, 0.1 to 0.2 mg/kg, to facilitate mechanical respiration and prevent an increase in intracranial pressure associated with movement.

4. *Furosemide* may be given orally in a dosage of 1 to 2 mg/(kg·day) divided every 6 to 8 h, or intramuscularly or intravenously 0.5 to 1.0 mg/(kg·day) in divided doses every 2 h; the maximum daily dose is 80 mg. The exact method by which furosemide works is unclear. It has been noted to produce an immediate effect with a reduction in pupillary size minutes after the dose is given. This occurs before the diuretic effect can occur.

5. *Mannitol* may be given as a bolus of 1 to 2 g/kg intravenously over 30 to 60 min. A continuous infusion may also be given using 1 to 2 g/(kg·h) or alternatively 13 g/(h·1.73 m²). The goal of continuous mannitol infusion is to maintain the serum osmolality at 310 mOsm. Glycerol is an alternative to mannitol and may be given at 1 to 2 g/(kg·dose) every 4 to 6 h orally. It has been noted to produce gastrointestinal irritation. Glycerol is a smaller molecule than mannitol and may recouple oxidative phosphorylation.

6. *Dexamethasone* is usually given as 0.25 to 0.5 mg/(kg·day) in divided doses every 4 to 6 h. The dosage may go up to 1 mg/(kg·day). Theoretically, the mechanism of action of dexamethasone is to stabilize vascular membranes and prevent leakage. Since the cerebral edema in Reye's syndrome does not have a vasogenic basis, it is unclear why dexamethasone should be effective. It is thought that intracellular membrane stabilization or decreased CSF production may be the mode of action.

7. *Pentobarbital coma* may be induced with an intravenous bolus, 3 to 5 mg/kg, followed by 2.5 mg/kg every 2 h. The serum should be monitored to achieve a level of 3.5 mg/dL. Pentobarbital is thought to decrease cerebral blood flow and the metabolic rate. Its use should be reserved for children whose elevated intracranial pressure is not responsive to other measures.

8. If positive end-expiratory pressure (PEEP) must be used, pressure should be kept at a minimum, so as not to impede cerebral venous return. Vigorous chest physiotherapy should not be given since this increases intracranial pressure. Gentle vibration and suctioning remove mucous plugs and facilitate ventilation.

In addition to the control of the elevated intracranial pressure, there are other considerations in the management of the child with Reye's syndrome.

1. *Fluid management*
   There is controversy about appropriate fluid management. Some maintain the child should be on full maintenance, while others state that the patient should receive between $\frac{2}{3}$ and $\frac{3}{4}$ maintenance fluids. Regardless of the regimen chosen, it is important to maintain urine output at a minimum of 0.5 mL/(kg·h) to avoid renal failure.

2. *Use of hypertonic glucose*
   Hypertonic glucose (10 to 15 percent) is recommended to provide a substrate for metabolism. Insulin may be given at 1 unit per 5 g of glucose, but patients seem to be in a hyperinsuli-

nemic state. Insulin may help reduce free fatty acids by stimulating lipoprotein lipase.

3. *Coagulation problems*
   Coagulopathy should be managed with the use of vitamin K, 5 mg given intravenously every 12 h. Fresh frozen plasma at a dose of 5 mL/(kg·dose) may be given, especially if one is contemplating any invasive procedures such as a liver biopsy or the placement of a subarachnoid bolt.

4. *CVP line*
   A central venous pressure (CVP) line is useful to monitor pressure in a patient who is being fluid-restricted. The CVP should be maintained at 4 to 6 cmH₂O to avoid renal complications secondary to dehydration.

5. *Ulcer prevention*
   There is a higher risk of ulcers and GI hemorrhage in patients with Reye's syndrome. The GI hemorrhage is exacerbated by the coagulopathy. Mylanta may be given via nasogastric tube, or patients may be managed with cimetidine.

6. *Neomycin*
   Neomycin, 500 mg by nasogastric tube every 6 h, is used in patients with hepatic failure.

Additional measures which have been tried with variable results include total body washout (removal of the blood and replacement with normal saline for a brief period of time), peritoneal dialysis (60 percent mortality), and exchange transfusion. Fresh heparinized blood must be used since banked blood has high ammonia levels. None of these measures offers any proven advantage.

COMPLICATIONS

Renal failure and pancreatitis are two additional complications which may occur with Reye's syndrome. Renal failure is an unusual complication, although the kidneys show pathologic changes affecting the tubules but not the glomeruli. These changes are reversible, and kidneys of children who have died with Reye's syndrome have been used for renal transplantation. In the three cases of renal failure with Reye's syndrome described in the literature, the children also exhibited a coagulopathy, and the renal failure was felt to resemble the hemolytic-uremic syndrome.

Pancreatitis occurs in about 1 out of every 25 cases of Reye's syndrome and may progress to acute hemorrhagic pancreatitis. Hypertension, hypercalcemia, and glucose lability may herald the onset of acute pancreatitis in these patients. The role of steroids in precipitating the pancreatitis is unclear. There may be an inherent predisposition to the development of pancreatitis in some patients with Reye's syndrome.

The lungs may also show some abnormalities with alveolar wall thickening and alveolar capillary block, but this does not appear to produce symptoms.

RECOVERY PHASE

The duration of coma is variable, but coma typically persists from 24 to 96 h. Some children, however, remain unconscious for several weeks.

The withdrawal of measures to regulate intracranial pressure may begin after the intracranial pressure has been maintained at

15 to 20 torr. If the intracranial pressure increases, the support must be reinstituted.

1. Ventilation may be decreased to allow the P_{CO_2} to increase by 5 mmHg every 4 to 6 h until it is in a normal range.
2. Once this has been achieved, pancuronium bromide may be discontinued.
3. The mannitol bolus may be decreased in frequency from every 8 h to every 12 h to every 24 h.
4. Steroids should be decreased by 50 percent per day.
5. Mechanical ventilation may be discontinued.
6. The bolt or the catheter may be discontinued.
7. Sedation may be discontinued.
8. Extra glucose and oxygen may be discontinued.

PROGNOSIS

The prognosis has improved significantly in recent years with the Center for Disease Control reporting a decline in overall mortality from 40 percent in 1973 to 25 percent in 1981. Infants under the age of 1 year and children admitted in stage V Reye's syndrome continue to do poorly. In others, the prognosis for survival and normal neurologic and cognitive functioning are excellent in spite of severe abnormalities at the time of the initial evaluation.

Early recognition of Reye's syndrome and the institution of appropriate management are the keys to a successful outcome for these children.

BIBLIOGRAPHY

Aprille JR: Reye's syndrome: Patient serum alters mitochondrial function and morphology in vitro. *Science* 197:908, 1977.

Baliga R, Fleischman LE, Chang CH, et al: Acute renal failure in Reye's syndrome. *Am J Dis Child* 133:1009, 1979.

Corey L, Rubin RJ, Hattwick MAW: Reye's syndrome: Clinical progression and evaluation of therapy. *Pediatrics* 60:708, 1977.

DeVivo DC, Keating JP: Reye's syndrome. *Adv Pediatr* 22:175, 1976.

DeVivo DC, Keating JP, Haymond MW: Acute encephalopathy with fatty infiltration of the viscera. *Pediatr Clin North Am* 23:527, 1976.

Ellis GH, Mirkin D, Mills MC: Pancreatitis and Reye's syndrome. *Am J Dis Child* 133:1014, 1979.

Haller J: Intracranial pressure monitoring in Reye's syndrome. *Hosp Pract* 15:101, 1980.

Huttenlocher PR: Reye's syndrome: Relation of outcome to therapy. *J Pediatr* 80:845, 1972.

Huttenlocher PR, Trauner DA: Reye's syndrome in infancy. *Pediatrics* 62:84, 1978.

Lovejoy FH, Smith AL, Bresnan MJ, et al: Clinical staging in Reye's syndrome. *Am J Dis Child* 128:36, 1974.

Mortimer EA, Lepow ML: Varicella with hypoglycemia possibly due to salicylates. *Am J Dis Child* 103:583, 1962.

Partin JC: Reye's syndrome (encephalopathy and fatty liver). *Gastroenterology* 69:511, 1975.

Reye RDK, Morgan G, Baral J: Encephalopathy and fatty degeneration of the viscera: A disease entity in childhood. *Lancet* 2:749, 1963.

Starko KM, Ray CG, Dominguez BS, et al: Reye's syndrome and salicylate use. *Pediatrics* 66:859, 1980.

Trauner DA: Treatment of Reye's syndrome. *Ann Neurol* 7:2, 1980.

Trauner DA: Reye's syndrome. *Curr Prob Pediatr* 12: 1982.

CHAPTER 86
PEDIATRIC GASTROINTESTINAL EMERGENCIES

Frederick A. Arcari

Implicit in the elucidation of the problem presented by a gastrointestinal (GI) emergency in childhood is the recognition of the import of age. A few years here or there in the adult have little bearing on the final diagnosis. On the other hand, the spectrum of the GI pathologic conditions of a 2-day-old infant is vastly different from that of a 2-week-old, and both are quite different from that of a 2-year-old.

Nevertheless, it should be recognized that many of the disease states classically considered to be "adult only" are found occasionally in infants and children: for example, cholecystitis, appendicitis, perforated duodenal ulcer, and ovarian torsion all may be found in children from the first year of life.

Obviously the successful management of GI emergencies depends on a thorough evaluation of symptoms and signs. Here again we are faced with a problem not present in most older patients, namely one of communication. The story is often secondhand, frequently and preferably provided by a parent, most often the mother. Most mothers are reliable in their recognition of changing states in their offspring. A mother who states, "My child is in pain" must be listened to and accorded credibility.

The important triad of symptoms referable to the GI tract consists of

1. Pain
2. Vomiting
3. Bleeding

These symptoms are so florid that little interrogation is necessary.

Unfortunately, because a child either is too young or too frightened to speak for him- or herself or has not been under continuous observation, trauma as a factor in the development of a GI emergency may be missed, particularly a form of trauma peculiar to children, the battered or abused child syndrome. In this situation there may be a purposeful attempt by the parent or caregiver to hide the background of the problem and confuse the physician by evasion and lies. Trauma must always be considered by the physician evaluating the pediatric patient presenting with what appears to be a GI emergency.

PAIN

Abdominal pain is a manifestation of a variety of disease states not necessarily related to the intestinal tract. This is particularly so in the 3- to 6-year-old, for example, with tonsilitis and pneumonia. Pain (subjective) as opposed to tenderness (objective) tends to be periumbilical in this age group. One ought to distinguish between two types of pain, peritonitic and obstructive.

1. Peritonitic pain tends to keep the patient relatively immobile, as for example in appendicitis.
2. Obstructive pain is usually spasmodic and associated with restlessness and motion, as for example with intussusception.

In the very young (up to 2 years of age), pain is described by the mother, the description being dependent on her familiarity with her own infant. She should be relied upon. Between 2 and 6 years of age, pain of GI origin is usually referred to the periumbilical region, and diagnosis requires correlation of the patient's observations and the physician's visual and tactile evaluation. The youngster with pain of peritonitic origin walks with obvious discomfort and prefers to lie quite still. In contrast, the youngster with obstructive pain may be unable to remain immobile on the couch.

VOMITING

Not all vomiting relates to GI disease. Intracranial hemorrhage, a space-occupying lesion of the skull, or pneumonia may initiate vomiting.

Vomiting or regurgitation may be a manifestation of a relatively minor problem, for example, a nervous mother, poor feeding habits, or gastroesophageal reflux. All of these diagnoses can be elucidated by careful questioning of the mother.

Bilious vomiting is always a serious manifestation in an infant or a child, and its cause must be defined before releasing a child from observation.

Vomiting (bilious or not) is a classic symptom of mechanical intestinal obstruction in the child. In the early phases of the condition, before the child has developed electrolyte abnormalities (as for example in the child with pyloric stenosis), or before the child has reached the stage of harboring gangrenous bowel (as with an internal volvulus), the child's general condition may appear to be good. In the early phases of such a process, it is not unusual that the youngster is hungry immediately after vomiting and even wants to feed vigorously. One must therefore not ignore the possibility of a serious underlying intraabdominal pathologic condition merely because the vomiting child appears to be systemically well.

BLEEDING

Apparent major GI bleeding in the newborn, whether vomited or evacuated per rectum, may be the result of the child's having swallowed maternal blood. Rarely do hemorrhagic states cause GI bleeding in the newborn. Small amounts of blood in the stool of an infant, if fresh, may be a manifestation of anal fissures, which are easily identified. In children 2 to 10 years of age, painless bleeding of small to moderate amounts of blood usually mixed through the stool might well be an indication of benign GI polyps.

Frequently the cause of minimal to moderate amounts of blood in the stool of an infant or a child may never be identified. Repeated episodes of bleeding require GI x-ray and endoscopic evaluation.

The presence of small to moderate amounts of blood in the stool of an infant (particularly if this is associated with vomiting) must lead the physician to consider the possibility of malrotation of the midgut. Once considered, the diagnosis becomes urgent and requires immediate investigation via either upper GI or barium enema examination. The urgency is because of the association of volvulus of the midgut with malrotation and the possibility of total midgut gangrene if the problem is not identified and corrected early in its course.

Major painless upper GI bleeding in the infant or child is most commonly the result of bleeding varices secondary to portal hypertension.

Major painless lower GI bleeding in the infant or child is frequently ascribable to a Meckel's diverticulum.

PHYSICAL EXAMINATION

It is essential that the physician examining the toddler or young child approach the youngster with an attitude of gentleness, concern, and warmth. The physician's voice should be conciliatory and relatively high pitched in order to allay the youngster's fears and suspicions. It is essential that another person with whom the child is comfortable and familiar be in the examining room at the time of the physician's examination. The child should be totally undressed at the time of examination, and the body should be observed for the presence of bruises, scars, petechiae, and particularly hernias.

GASTROINTESTINAL EMERGENCIES IN INFANTS IN THE FIRST YEAR OF LIFE

Malrotation

The complications of malrotation occur most commonly in the first year of life, although malrotation can give rise to symptoms at any time in a person's life. It is the most urgent of GI emergencies in infants and children because of the possible development of volvulus of the midgut with consequent gangrene of the bowel. The process from the first symptoms to the development of total midgut gangrene may occur within a few hours, and therefore the consideration of this diagnosis warrants immediate and urgent investigation. The presenting symptoms are usually vomiting (ultimately becoming bilious), with or without abdominal distention, and streaks of blood in the stool. This symptom complex usually occurs in a previously healthy child. However, there may have been past minor episodes of vomiting or abdominal discomfort that now become of import in the evaluation of the child's present state. Investigation of the child suspected of harboring a malrotation with possible midgut volvulus requires GI x-rays. Most commonly a barium enema is used in order to identify the anatomic position of the large intestine. However, the use of upper GI studies in order to identify the duodenal loop is becoming more popular.

Any child with vomiting and/or bloody stools who is identified as harboring an incompletely rotated bowel warrants urgent laparotomy in order to prevent the hazard of midgut volvulus and the consequent total midgut gangrene.

Incarcerated Hernia

An incarcerated hernia may be missed unless the infant or child is totally undressed at the time of examination. The symptoms stimulating the child's arrival in the emergency room may be irritability, discomfort, a scrotal mass, or vomiting. The differential diagnosis most frequently includes hydrocele of the cord or the testicle, undescended testicle, and torsion of the testicle. The incidence of incarceration of inguinal hernias is highest in the first year of life. In both boys and girls the incarcerated sac may contain small or large bowel. In girls there is a high incidence of cases in which ovary is present in the sac. In most instances, provided the child is examined gently and his or her confidence obtained, it is possible to achieve manual reduction of the incarcerated hernia (if it has been present for only a short period of time) without the use of sedation. When this maneuver is unsuccessful, most cases can be successfully reduced following the administration of intramuscular propoxyphene (up to 2 mg/kg of body weight in the first year of life). Following the administration of propoxyphene, the child should be left completely undisturbed in a dark room in the arms of the parent. Diapers should be left off, no urine cup should be applied over the external genitalia and there should be no interference with the child in order to obtain a blood sample. After an hour, only minimal disturbance is necessary to examine the child and observe the status of the incarcerated hernia. Quite often, as a result of the relaxation induced by propoxyphene, spontaneous reduction of the hernia is apparent. In the absence of spontaneous reduction, it is possible to attempt reduction without disturbing the child further, and in a large percentage of instances successful manual reduction can be achieved. The few patients that do not respond to these maneuvers must undergo surgical reduction.

It is not uncommon to read of a peculiar (to my mind) method aimed at achieving reduction of an incarcerated hernia. This involves suspending the child by the feet, over a crib, and applying crushed ice to the scrotum or the inguinal area! It must be obvious to the thinking physician that under no circumstances could a child subjected to this form of management relax!

Intestinal Obstruction

Intestinal obstruction presents in the infant and the young child in the classic manner, with symptoms of pain (manifested by irritability), vomiting (becoming bilious with the passage of time), abdominal distension, and later absence or diminution of bowel movements. The differential diagnosis of intestinal obstruction in the newborn includes the following:

1. Atresia
2. Incarcerated inguinal hernia
3. Malrotation
4. Malrotation with volvulus
5. Volvulus around a congenital intra-abdominal band
6. Duplication cysts of the intestinal tract
7. Postnecrotic stenosis of the colon
8. Hirschsprung's disease
9. Meconium ileus

Diagnosis necessitates immediate flat and upright films of the abdomen, which show, as depicted in Figures 86-1A and 86-1B, dilated loops of bowel with air-fluid levels. Such an appearance on the plain x-ray film warrants a barium enema examination, which helps to differentiate between Hirschsprung's disease, mal-

rotation, and colonic stenosis, and also separates lower large bowel obstruction from upper small bowel obstruction.

Once intestinal obstruction has been diagnosed, the patient should be prepared for surgical intervention.

Pyloric Stenosis

The child presenting in the emergency department with a history of nonbilious projectile vomiting must be considered to be harboring pyloric stenosis. It has become increasingly obvious that this is a familial disease, and if asked, the family may reveal that one parent (usually the father), aunts, uncles or siblings of the child have been treated for pyloric stenosis. The classic patient is a healthy 3- to 6-week-old infant with projectile nonbilious vomiting after feeding who is hungry enough after vomiting to take another feed. This of course is a description of the child early in the course of the disease, in the first 24 to 48 h. As time passes and vomiting becomes more prolonged, the systemic manifestations of dehydration and electrolyte imbalance are added to the picture. Examination of the patient may reveal the presence of gastric peristaltic waves traveling from the left quadrant to the midline across the abdominal wall. On palpation, with care and gentleness, the classic olivelike pyloric tumor may be identified. The differential diagnosis of pyloric stenosis includes gastroesophageal reflux, pylorospasm, and gastroenteritis. The diagnosis can be confirmed by obtaining an upper GI study. After rehydration and reestablishment of electrolyte balance, definitive treatment involves pyloromyotomy.

Intussusception

Intussusception presents with recurring attacks of cramping abdominal pain. The classic patient is an 8- to 18-month-old robust

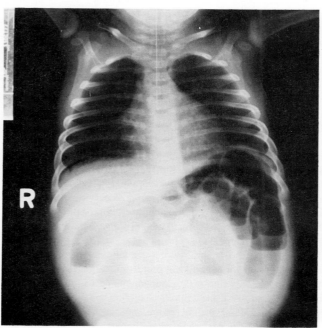

A

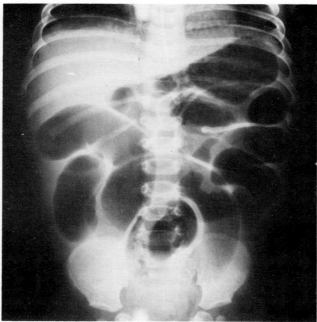

B

Figure 86-1. Mechanical intestinal obstruction (A) upright film; (B) flat film

infant without prior problems. Suddenly, out of the blue, the child appears to be in pain. The youngster may be playing quietly in the playpen and suddenly stop playing, begin to cry, and even roll around in discomfort. Just as suddenly, the pain ceases, and the child appears to be as happy and content as before the onset of the pain and returns to playing with toys. This process is repeated at decreasing intervals, with the duration of the painful attacks increasing. Vomiting is rare in the first few hours but usually develops after 6 to 12 h. The classic current-jelly stool associated with intussusception is a later manifestation of the disease complex, resulting from interference with mucosal circulation, and its absence should not delay investigation of the patient.

Examination between attacks may reveal the oft-described sausage-shaped tumor mass of intussuscepted bowel in the right abdomen. The absence of this finding, however, should not delay further investigation.

The presumptive diagnosis of intussusception is made on the basis of the history and may be seriously considered as a result of a telephone description of the child's problem by the mother. X-ray films of the abdomen may show, as in Figure 86-2A, a mass or filling defect in the right upper quadrant of the abdomen. Even in the presence of normal plain x-ray films, the history described demands a barium enema examination, which demonstrates the classic "coiled spring" shown in Figure 86-2B. The barium enema examination not only is a diagnostic tool in the management of this disease, but also is frequently curative. If it is obtained in the first 12 to 24 h of the disease, up to 80 percent of these cases can be corrected by barium enema alone. When barium enema does not resolve the intussusception, surgical intervention is indicated. If barium enema reduces the intussusception, the parents should be warned of the 5 to 10 percent chance of recurrence of the same process. Recurrence usually takes place within the first 24 to 48 h following the barium enema reduction.

GASTROINTESTINAL EMERGENCIES IN CHILDREN 2 YEARS AND OVER

Appendicitis

The classic progression of symptoms associated with appendicitis applies equally to children and adults. The events involve early anorexia followed by the development of mild to moderate periumbilical pain, then vomiting, and then the movement of the pain to the right lower quadrant of the abdomen. The youngster thought to be harboring an acutely inflamed appendix should be observed as the child walks into the examining room; in most instances the child appears to be in discomfort as he or she moves along. This discomfort associated with motion can be emphasized by asking the youngster to jump up and down before the child lies down on the examining table. On examination of the patient, the physician may find limited motion of the lower abdomen due to inflammation of the peritoneum, and, depending on the duration of the symptoms, there may be abdominal distention. Palpation reveals the presence of differential tenderness in the right lower abdominal quadrant; it is important to emphasize this differential tenderness and its localization in the right lower quadrant. Guarding and rebound tenderness may or may not be present in this same area.

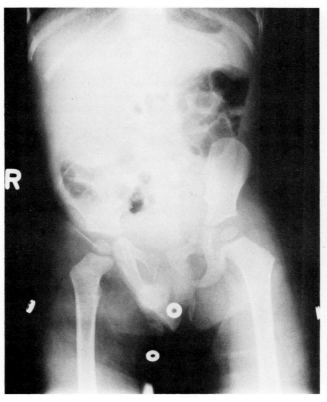

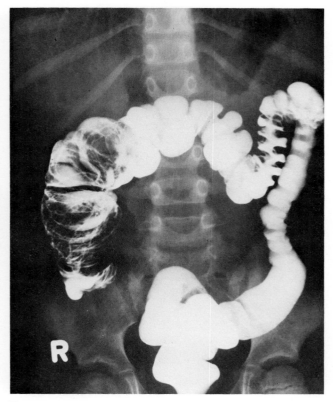

A   B

Figure 86-2. Intussusception. (A) plain film showing a filling defect in the right upper quadrant (B) with barium enema, showing a "coiled spring" in the ascending colon.

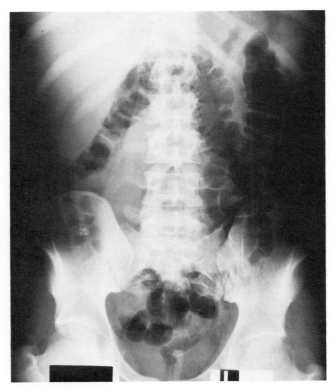

Figure 86-3. Appendicitis, appendicolith in the right lower quadrant.

The longer the duration of the symptoms, the greater the possibility of finding a mass in the right lower quadrant, representing localized perforation with the development of an appendiceal abscess. In the absence of definitive right lower quadrant tenderness, a rectal examination should be performed in order to detect the presence of a low-lying intrapelvic acutely inflamed appendix. The child may have a mild fever and an elevated white blood cell count in the range of 11,000 to 20,000. When there is doubt in the overall symptom complex, an x-ray may reveal the presence of an appendicolith (Fig. 86-3). Symptoms consistent with ap-

pendicitis together with the presence of an appendicolith warrant the clinical diagnosis of appendicitis, and laparotomy.

Red Herrings

The following may be misleading:

1. The temperature may be normal.
2. The white blood cell count may be normal.
3. The child may not be anorexic and may actually request food.
4. A heavily built child may manifest minimal right lower quadrant tenderness and minimal tenderness on rectal examination.
5. Gastroenteritis is not infrequently associated with appendicitis. Thus a child presenting with a several-day history of vomiting and diarrhea, perhaps even with siblings suffering from the same problem, should not have the diagnosis of appendicitis discounted on this basis. Intensification of pain in the presence of a history of gastroenteritis should suggest an acutely inflamed appendix secondary to gastroenteritis.
6. Appendicitis has been identified in children under 1 year of age and is not uncommon in the second year. The incidence of perforation in this age group is much higher because of the difficulty of making the diagnosis and the confusion with gastroenteritis.

Meckel's Diverticulum

A Meckel's diverticulum can cause a variety of signs and symptoms, such as bleeding, peritonitis, or obstruction. The presence of gastric mucosa in the diverticulum may give rise to an ulcer in the adjacent ileum, which may cause symptoms such as painless rectal bleeding or perforation with attendant peritonitis. Isotope scanning reveals the presence of a Meckel's diverticulum containing gastric mucosa in up to 50 percent of the cases. A negative scan does not eliminate the diagnosis.

Acute inflammation in a Meckel's diverticulum may simulate acute appendicitis or may initiate intussusception. Finally, the vitellointestinal remnant attaching the apex of a Meckel's diverticulum to the intraabdominal umbilical region may be the focus

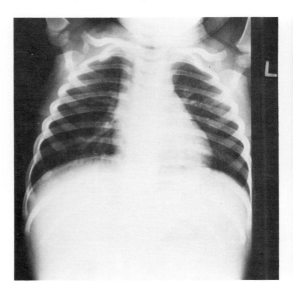

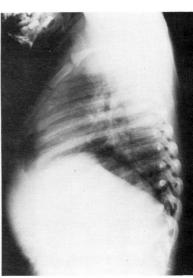

Figure 86-4. Foreign body—coin—in the stomach.

around which volvulus of the small bowel or an internal hernia develops, each of these giving rise to intestinal obstruction.

Colon Polyps

Single polyps or multiple or classic familial polyposis may give rise to painless bright-red lower intestinal bleeding. Most commonly the polyp is single, or perhaps there are two or three. These polyps are usually benign (juvenile) with no propensity for malignant degeneration. Frequently the parent describes what is obviously a prolapsed polyp, easily palpated on rectal examination. It is rare for bleeding originating in a polyp to be life-threatening.

Foreign Bodies in the GI Tract

It is safe to generalize that anything that reaches the stomach will eventually traverse the GI tract and be spontaneously evacuated per rectum (Fig. 86-4). Nails, open safety pins, pieces of glass, and coins are examples of objects that have traveled the complete journey. It may take months for a coin, for example, to complete the trip to the anus. Obviously a foreign body caught in the upper or mid esophagus and not moving on should be removed by esophagoscopy. (See Chapter 56, ''Swallowed Foreign Bodies.'') Very rarely is surgical removal of a foreign body in the stomach or distal to the stomach warranted.

Portal Hypertension

Portal hypertension is rare in children but is one of the common causes of major upper GI hemorrhage. Extrahepatic portal thrombosis, parenchymal liver disease associated with fibrocystic disease, and biliary cirrhosis in the youngster with congenital biliary atresia surviving as a result of portal enterostomy are examples of conditions which can result in portal hypertension and esophagogastric varices.

WARNING

All the problems and the associated manifestations described in this chapter may well be initiated by trauma, occult, abusive, or

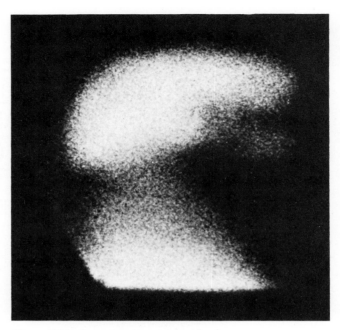

Figure 86-5. Scan showing a ruptured spleen.

florid (Fig. 86-5). Minimal trauma may shatter or rupture an abdominal organ that is diseased, as, for example, may occur in congenital obstructive hydronephrosis of the kidney.

BIBLIOGRAPHY

Benson CD: Infantile pyloric stenosis. *Prog Pediatr Surg* 1:63–88, 1970.

Ching E, Ching LT, Lynn HB, et al: Intussusception in children. *Mayo Clin Proc*, 45:724, 1970.

Grosfeld JL, Weinberger M, Gatsworthy HW: Acute appendicitis in the first two years of life. *J Pediatr Surg* 8:285, 1973.

Holter JC, Friedman S: Child abuse: Early case finding in the emergency department. *Pediatrics* 42:128–138, 1968.

McParland FA, Kieswetter WB: Meckel's diverticulum in childhood. *Surg Gynecol Obstet* 106:11–1L, 1958.

Stewart DR, Colodny AL, Dagget WC: Malrotation of the bowel in infants and children: A 15-year review. *Surgery,* 79:716, 1976.

CHAPTER 87
CHILD ABUSE: A
SPECTRUM OF DISEASE

Carol D. Berkowitz

Child abuse and neglect are problems which have been recognized with increasing frequency in recent years. In 1981, 845,330 cases of child abuse and neglect were reported in the United States. It is estimated that approximately 6 infants per 1000 live births are physically abused during childhood. The prevalence of physical abuse is about 500 cases per 1 million population per year. In spite of improved physician awareness and reporting, these figures are probably gross underestimates. The extent of sexual abuse is becoming recognized. It is estimated that one-fourth of all girls and one-sixth of all boys are sexually misused before adulthood.

The physician in the emergency department is often the first, and frequently the only, person to evaluate a child who is the victim of child abuse or neglect. Approximately 10 percent of all injuries in children under 5 years of age being evaluated in the emergency department result from inflicted, nonaccidental trauma. Failure to recognize this fact carries a high morbidity and mortality. Approximately 5 percent of these children will die from future trauma, and another 35 percent will be seriously injured again.

This chapter discusses the spectrum of the syndrome of child abuse and neglect, focuses on the features of the history and the physical examination which assist the physician with the diagnosis, and describes the legal obligations for reporting suspected cases.

SPECTRUM OF CHILD ABUSE AND NEGLECT

The concept of *maltreatment* of children, defined as harm to a child because of abnormal child-rearing practices, is a broadening of the initial description of the *battered child syndrome*. *Child maltreatment* is an all-inclusive term covering physical abuse; sexual misuse; emotional abuse; substance abuse; physical, nutritional, and emotional neglect; and supervisional neglect.

The ease with which the physician is able to recognize these disorders in part depends on his or her knowledge of normal children and normal development. The physical stigmata of maltreatment are characteristic, although the findings of neglect and sexual misuse are more subtle than those of gross physical trauma.

CHILD NEGLECT

Child neglect can result in an array of physical and emotional problems. Child neglect from early infancy results in the syndrome of failure to thrive (FTT). This syndrome usually affects children under the age of 3 years, although older children who remain in a nonnurturing environment show similar manifestations.

The patient is often brought to the emergency department because of other medical problems, such as intercurrent infections; skin rashes, particularly severe monilial diaper dermatitis; or acute gastroenteritis. The history of the acute illness may not alert the physician to the chronic nature of the underlying problem. The physical examination provides the clue to the diagnosis of long-standing malnutrition. Overall physical care and hygiene are frequently poor. The infant has very little subcutaneous tissue. The ribs protrude prominently through the skin, and the skin of the buttocks hangs in loose folds. There may be alopecia over a flattened occiput, reflecting the fact that the baby has been allowed to lie on his or her back all day. Muscle tone is usually increased (although sometimes these babies are hypotonic). This increased tone is most notable in the lower extremities, and infants may manifest scissoring, similar to infants with cerebral palsy.

FTT infants also show distinct behavioral characteristics. They are wide-eyed and wary. If brought in close proximity to the examiner's face, they may purposely turn away to avoid eye contact. They become irritable if interpersonal interaction is pursued. They are difficult to console and are not cuddly. They prefer inanimate over animate objects and spend much time with their hands in their mouths. When left alone, they assume a "straphanger's position" with their arms flexed at the elbows and extended over their shoulders.

Weights and lengths should be plotted on the appropriate growth curves. In general, weight is more adversely affected than length, although this depends on the duration of the neglect. Likewise, longstanding neglect results in a diminution in the rate of growth of the head.

In addition to observing for these physical signs, the physician should obtain certain historical information. This includes the birth weight (to assess the rate of growth); any maternal use of cigarettes, alcohol, and/or drugs during pregnancy; previous hospitalizations; and the parental stature. A full social service assessment should also be obtained, although this is usually done by a medical social worker.

Infants suspected of suffering from environmental FTT should be admitted to the hospital. Weight gain in the hospital is felt to be the sine qua non of environmental FTT. Many infants fail to gain weight until 2 to 3 weeks following admission; however, the hospitalization allows a more extensive social service assessment while the infant is in a protected environment. A skeletal survey of the long bones should be carried out to detect any evidence of physical abuse.

Children over the age of 2 to 3 years with environmental neglect are referred to as psychosocial dwarfs. Their short stature is a more prominent finding than their low weight. These children manifest a classic triad of short stature, a bizarre voracious appetite (eating from trash cans), and a disturbed home situation. They are frequently hyperactive and have delayed or unintelligible speech. Psychosocial dwarfs have been studied endocrinologically and have been found to have a low to normal level of growth hormone which fails to increase with stimulation with insulin or arginine. These children should also be admitted for evaluation and initiation of appropriate social intervention. The endocrinologic disturbances rapidly reverse following hospitalization or placement in a foster home.

SEXUAL MISUSE

Victims of sexual misuse are frequently difficult for the unexperienced physician to assess because of an unfamiliarity with the normal prepubertal genital exam. Children who have been sexually misused are brought to the emergency department because of symptoms referrable to the genitourinary tract, such as vaginal discharge; vaginal bleeding; dysuria; urinary tract infections; urethral discharge; behavior disturbances, such as excessive masturbation, genital fondling, or other sexually oriented or provocative behavior; encopresis; regression; nightmares; and so forth. In cases of sexual misuse, the assailant is known to the child 90 percent of the time. Usually 2 to 3 years of ongoing sexual misuse have occurred before the diagnosis is made.

The examining physician must maintain a high index of suspicion of sexual misuse when evaluating children presenting with the above complaints. The physical assessment should include an evaluation of the child's overall well-being. The skin should be examined for bruises. Common injuries in victims of sexual misuse include grip marks on the forearms and puncture wounds on the inner aspects of the lips resulting from a slap to the face. The age of the child and the degree of sexual development should be noted. Children of 8 to 11 years frequently disclose that they have been victims of sexual abuse for a significant period of time.

The genital examination should be confined to a careful inspection of the genitalia and perianal area. Generally, there is no need for a speculum examination. The normal prepubescent girl has full labia majora and small thin labia minora. The vaginal opening is covered by the hymen, a fine reddish-orange, thin-edged membrane. The hymenal orifice should be measured. Normally the orifice should be less than 3 to 4 mm in children under the age of 5 years and up to 5 to 6 mm in older, prepubertal girls. Chronic molestation results in multiple hymenal transections, giving the hymenal orifice an irregular appearance. These transections usually are located between 5 and 7 o'clock. Rounded hymenal remnants similar to hymenal tags are also seen. The hymenal orifice is larger than normal and frequently appears spacious or gaping, especially with the reflex relaxation of the pubococcygeal muscles. These children may show leukorrhea, and a fishy pungent genital odor may be present. Venereal warts, condyloma acuminatum, may be present. Synechiae may develop between the disrupted hymen and the posterior fourchette, and this appears as "tenting" of these structures on physical examination. Erythema, secondary to irritation and/or chronic manipulation, may be noted, along with small, fine blood vessels along the hymen or labia minora (neovascularization).

The genital examination in the sexually victimized young boy is less revealing. There may be a urethral discharge; the penis may become erect without tactile stimulation and remain erect. The perianal examination is often more revealing, even in the young female patient, because anal penetration is easier than vaginal penetration. Anal fissures may be noted. In addition, lateral traction on the buttocks results in relaxation of the external anal sphincter. Stroking the skin in the perianal area results in similar relaxation. Anoscopy using a 10 mL test tube may reveal extension of an anal fissure internally. Children who have been subjected to repeated oral copulation may show an equally relaxed gag reflex.

The laboratory evaluation of the sexually misused child should include cultures from the throat, vagina (or urethra), and rectum for gonorrhea, as well as a culture from the vagina (or urethra) for *Chlamydia*, and a serologic test for syphillis.

The child should be questioned directly about what happened. The child's name for the genitalia and other body parts should be recorded, and all statements that the child makes concerning the misuse should be recorded verbatim. A social service evaluation should be initiated at the time of the emergency department visit. Law enforcement and child protective services should be notified immediately, as outlined below.

PHYSICAL ABUSE

The spectrum of injuries in the child who has been intentionally traumatized is wide. Familiarity with this spectrum enables the physician in the emergency department to arrive at the correct diagnosis in a timely manner. Two-thirds of the victims of physical abuse are under the age of 3 years, and one-third are under 6 months. The physical vulnerability of such small children is easy to understand.

Historical data may raise suspicions of inflicted trauma. A history which is inconsistent with the nature or the extent of the injuries (e.g., a fractured femur in an infant from a fall off a bed), a history which keeps changing as to the circumstances surrounding the injury, a discrepancy between the story the child gives and the story the caretaker gives, a history of previous trauma in the patient or siblings, or a delay in seeking medical attention should raise one's index of suspicion of physical abuse. Knowledge of normal motor development assists the physician in determining the likelihood that the injury happened in the stated manner. Children under the age of 6 months are incapable of inducing accidents or accidently ingesting any drugs or poisons. The evaluating physician should record the developmental milestones the child has achieved, e.g., the age of sitting unsupported, walking, etc. Parental behavior in the emergency department should be observed, and it should be noted if the parents appear intoxicated or under the influence of drugs. The level of parental concern about the injury should also be noted.

Toddlers and older children should be questioned about the circumstances of the injury, and the comments should be recorded verbatim on the medical record.

The physical examination should note the child's overall hygiene and well-being. Normal children, especially toddlers who are just learning how to walk, may have multiple ecchymoses over the anterior shins, the forehead, and other bony prominences.

Most falls result in bruises on only one body surface. Bruises over multiple areas, especially the low back, buttocks, thighs, cheeks, ear pinnae, neck, ankles, wrists, corners of the mouth, and lips suggest physical abuse. Handprints may be observed, or there may be uniform but bizarre bruise marks caused by belts, buckles, cords, or blunt instruments. Bite marks produce bruising in a characteristic oval pattern, with teeth indentations along the periphery. Lacerations of the frenulum or oral mucosa may be present, especially in an infant who has been force-fed. Lacerations and abrasions in the genital area are seen in toddlers who are ''punished'' because of toilet-training accidents.

The duration of a bruise can be estimated by the color of the lesion. No discoloration is noted initially although the bruised area may be swollen and tender. Within a day or two the lesion becomes reddish-blue, and this lasts for about 5 days. This changes to green (days 5 to 7), then to yellow (days 7 to 10), and finally to brown (days 10 to 14) before resolving. For instance, reddish-blue lesions are inconsistent with a 2 week old injury.

Children with multiple bruises should be evaluated with a complete blood cell count, differential, and coagulation studies including a platelet count, a prothrombin time, and a partial thromboplastin time. Rarely, a child with leukemia, aplastic anemia, or thrombocytopenia is brought for evaluation because of multiple bruises.

Burns constitute another form of inflicted injuries. These may be scald burns caused by immersion in hot water. Such burns do not conform to a splash configuration; rather, an entire hand or foot (''glove stocking'' pattern) may be involved. There is sharp demarcation of the burn margin. The buttocks may be burned during toilet-training ''punishment'' by immersion in a bathtub filled with hot water. Knees, portions of the abdomen, anterior thighs, and feet are spared, and the buttocks and genitalia are scalded. Cigarette burns leave small (approximately 5 mm) circumferential scab-covered injuries. These lesions may resemble impetigo, as do scald injuries, which may resemble bullous impetigo. A culture of material from these lesions differentiates the burn from the infection. Other inflicted burns can result from forced contact with metal objects such as an iron, curling irons, or heater grids.

Skeletal injuries may be detected when a child presents with unexplained swelling of an extremity or refusal to walk or to use an extremity. These fractures may take any form, but spiral fractures caused by torsion (twisting) of a long bone, and metaphyseal chip fractures, suggest inflicted injury, especially when present in infants under 6 months of age. Skeletal surveys referred to as a trauma series (or trauma x) should be obtained. These include films of all long bones, the ribs, the clavicles, the fingers, the toes, the pelvis, and the skull. They may reveal periosteal elevation secondary to new bone formation at sites of previous microfractures or periosteal injury; multiple fractures at different stages of healing; fractures at unusual sites such as the ribs, the lateral clavicle, the sternum, or the scapula; or repeated fractures to the same site. Such x-ray findings are supportive of the diagnosis of child abuse.

Head injuries are a serious and potentially lethal form of child abuse. In addition to having bruises around the ears, eyes, and cheeks, these children may exhibit swelling of the scalp secondary to subgaleal hematomas or underlying skull fractures. Funduscopic examination may reveal retinal hemorrhages, which are usually associated with subdural hematomas. Such hemorrhages may result from direct trauma to the skull or severe shaking of the child. These children should be evaluated with a CT scan, and coagulation studies should be performed to rule out underlying coagulopathies. Additional eye injuries caused by trauma may include hyphema, lens dislocation, and retinal detachment.

Injuries to the abdomen are equally serious and are a common cause of death from child abuse. Symptoms include recurrent vomiting, abdominal pain and tenderness, diminished bowel sounds, and/or abdominal distension. A history of injury as well as bruising of the overlying skin may be absent. Abdominal x-ray films may reveal a distended stomach with a ''double-bubble sign'' secondary to a duodenal hematoma. Diffuse distention may also be noted. Laboratory studies may reveal anemia, an elevated amylase level from traumatic pancreatitis, or hematuria from kidney trauma. Other abdominal injuries caused by trauma may include hepatic or splenic rupture, intestinal perforation, or rupture of intraabdominal blood vessels.

Any serious injury in a child under the age of 5 years should be viewed with suspicion. Other injuries not specified above include those which the child states were inflicted by another, were self-inflicted, or were inflicted by an unknown assailant.

The behavioral interaction between the child, the parent, and the physician may provide supportive evidence of the diagnosis of abuse. These children are often very compliant and submissive. They do not resist the medical examiner and readily submit to painful procedures such as blood drawing. They are overly affectionate to the medical staff, frequently preferring the nurse or the physician over the parent. Sometimes they are protective of the abusing parent, try to foster to their needs, and lie to cover up the true nature of the injury.

Parental behavior is less uniform, but certain distinct characteristics may be noted. The parents may not interact with the child in a comforting or supportive manner during the examination. They may become angry at the physician early in the course of the evaluation and may refuse diagnostic studies. They may appear to be intoxicated or under the influence of drugs. They may have brought the child in for seemingly minor complaints and ignored the major injuries or lesions. They may insist on admission of the child for these minor problems and may readily confess they can no longer cope with the child. They may express fears of losing control.

The social service assessment may reveal an unstable home situation with frequent moves, poor parental support systems, low parental self-esteem (often caused by battering during their own childhood), and/or domestic violence. This adds further supportive evidence of a high-risk situation.

MANAGEMENT

Once the medical assessment has been completed, the physician must initiate the appropriate treatment. The medical management should be guided by the physical findings. Frequently these children require hospitalization.

Although the specifics of the laws surrounding child abuse and neglect vary from state to state, every state does require that suspected cases be reported. A verbal report is made initially to the police department and/or the child protection agency of the locality in which the child lives. Law enforcement officers often appear in the emergency department, especially if the child does not require hospitalization. The child may be removed from the home and placed in protective custody, taken to a juvenile facility, placed temporarily with other relatives, or placed in a foster shelter home. The final disposition is dependent on a court hearing. The physician is also required to complete an official report detailing the specifics of the evaluation and giving his or her diagnostic opinion as to why the injuries or neglect are nonaccidental. The report should use nontechnical terms, e.g. *bruise* instead of *ecchymosis*, so that law enforcement and social service workers can understand the extent of the injuries.

Physicians are sometimes hesitant to report suspected cases. They are not "100 percent" certain. They are fearful of the parental response to the report. They are concerned about removing a child from the natural home. It is important to remember that the physician is *required by law to report all suspected cases of abuse and neglect*. Failure to report *suspected* cases can result in misdemeanor charges and lead to a fine and/or imprisonment. Additionally, the physician is protected by the law from legal retaliation by the parents.

Parental anger is a natural response to the filing of a report of suspected child abuse. The physician should refrain from being accusatory. Instead, the physician should note his or her concern about the child's well-being and advise the family that a physician is required by law to report any suspicions. The physician should verbally acknowledge the anger but persist in the role of child advocate. This job is facilitated in hospitals which have child abuse teams available to assist the physician in the emergency department.

BIBLIOGRAPHY
Child Neglect

Cupoli JM, Hallock JA, Barness LA: Failure to thrive. *Curr Probl Pediatr* 10:5–43, 1980.

Money J: The syndrome of abuse dwarfism (psychosocial hyposomatotropism). *Am J Dis Child* 131:508, 1977.

Powell GF, Brasel JA, Raiti S, et al: Emotional deprivation and growth retardation simulating idiopathic hypopituitarism. II Endocrinologic evaluation of the syndrome. *N Engl J Med* 276:1279, 1967.

Sexual Abuse

Cantwell HB: Vaginal inspection as it relates to child sexual abuse in girls under thirteen. *Child Abuse Neglect* 7:171, 1983.

Orr DP: Limitations of emergency room evaluations of sexually abused child. *Am J Dis Child* 132:873, 1978.

Woodling BA and Kossoris PD: Sexual misuse; Rape, molestation, and incest. *Pediatric Clinics of North America* 28:481, May 1981.

Physical Abuse

Schmitt BD and Kempe CH: The pediatrician's role in child abuse and neglect. *Curr Prob Pediatr* 5:3–47, 1975.

Taylor L. Newburger E: Child abuse in the international year of the child. *N Engl J Med* 301:1205, 1979.

Wilson EF: Estimation of the age of cutaneous contusions in child abuse. *Pediatrics* 60:750, 1977.

SECTION 10
ENDOCRINE
EMERGENCIES

CHAPTER 88
HYPOGLYCEMIA

Gene Ragland

Hypoglycemia is a vast and complex subject with a wide variety of causes. Glucose is the main energy source of the brain, and prolonged, severe hypoglycemia has been reported to cause brain damage and death. The blood glucose level at which hypoglycemia occurs is variable but has been generally accepted as 35 to 55 mg/dL. Hypoglycemia occurs most often in insulin-dependent diabetics as a complication of insulin therapy. Treatment includes the administration of glucose, in most instances, and the outcome is usually favorable.

CNS GLUCOSE DEPRIVATION

The central nervous system (CNS) depends upon glucose as its sole source of energy, except under conditions of prolonged starvation, when it can utilize ketones to meet energy needs. Hypoglycemia can be defined as a fall in blood glucose concentration to a level that elicits symptoms due to glucose deprivation in the CNS. The symptoms of hypoglycemia are therefore due to CNS dysfunction. When hypoglycemia occurs suddenly, the symptoms are classified as adrenergic or sympathomimetic and include diaphoresis, pallor, tremulousness, tachycardia, palpitations, visual disturbances, mental confusion, weakness, and light-headedness. Hypoglycemia may also develop slowly so that the signs of acute hyperepinephrinemia are not seen. The usual clinical picture is that of more-prolonged CNS glucose deprivation. These symptoms are classified as neuroglycopenic and include fatigue, confusion, headache, memory loss, seizures, and coma.

The actual level of blood glucose that causes CNS deprivation and produces symptoms is highly individual. The glucose level may be influenced by factors such as age, sex, weight, dietary history, physical activity, emotion, and coexisting disease. Merimee, in a study of fasting hypoglycemia, found that more than half of the women had plasma glucose levels less than 50 mg/dL, while none of the men had levels that low. Other studies have reported that between 42 and 48 percent of normal asymptomatic subjects have random plasma glucose levels of less than 50 mg/dL. Additionally, many reports exist of asymptomatic individuals with plasma glucose levels of 35 mg/dL or lower and of individuals that are symptomatic with glucose levels in the "normal" range. The actual value of plasma glucose that defines hypoglycemia is somewhat arbitrary. The clinical state of the patient must be correlated with the glucose determination. In general, a reasonable lower limit of normal for the plasma glucose level in women is 35 mg/dL and in men is 55 mg/dL.

GLUCOSE HOMEOSTASIS

Glucose homeostasis in humans involves a complex, dynamic synchronized interaction of neural and hormonal factors. The primary glucoregulatory organs are the liver, the pancreas, the adrenal glands, and the pituitary gland, and glucose homeostasis is maintained by the interaction of insulin, glucagon, catecholamines, glucocorticoids, and growth hormone from these organs. This interaction is largely determined by glucose intake and varies in the fed and the fasting state. During the fed state, glucose intake stimulates the release of insulin, which initiates tissue uptake and storage of fuels. During fasting, low insulin levels initiate the mobilization of stored fuels from tissue sources.

The fed state begins with the ingestion of food and extends for 2 to 3 h. The fasting state begins 3 to 4 h after eating. Due to the human's continuous energy needs but intermittent food intake, fuel for use between feedings and during fasting must be stored. The major forms of stored fuel are glycogen in the liver, triglycerides in adipose tissue, and protein in muscle.

Following food intake and absorption from the gut, glucose stimulates the release of insulin from pancreatic β cells. Insulin promotes the uptake of glucose by the liver; the glucose is converted to glycogen and stored in that form. Insulin also acts on the liver to decrease glucose output by inhibiting glycogenolysis (breakdown of glycogen to glucose) and gluconeogenesis (formation of glucose from precursors). Insulin promotes the storage of other energy sources by restraining lipolysis and enhancing lipogenesis in adipose cells and by promoting the uptake of amino acids into muscle protein and inhibiting proteolysis.

In the fasting state, the most readily available source of glucose is hepatic glycogen, which is utilized first. Hepatic glycogenolysis is enzyme-mediated and is stimulated by glucagon and catecholamines. This glycogen reserve is depleted in 24 to 48 h, and other fuel stores must be mobilized if fasting is prolonged. As hepatic glycogen stores are exhausted, blood glucose and plasma insulin levels decrease. The inhibitory action of insulin on lipolysis and proteolysis is removed, and alternative fuel stores can be mobilized and utilized.

During fasting, after several hours' worth of liver glycogen has been utilized, gluconeogenesis becomes the primary source of blood glucose needed for brain metabolism. Gluconeogenesis occurs primarily in the liver. Amino acids, principally alanine, are mobilized from the muscles via proteolysis. This process is facilitated by low insulin levels and mediated by glucocorticoids from the adrenal glands. Glucagon aids the conversion of amino acids to glucose in the liver. Lactate, from recycled glucose, and glycerol, from fat breakdown, can also be transformed to glucose but are minor sources of energy. During nonprolonged fasting (e.g., overnight), 90 percent of gluconeogenesis occurs via proteolysis and conversion of amino acids to glucose. In starvation states, the kidneys play an important role in gluconeogenesis.

Fat stores are a major source of energy. Fat is stored as triglycerides (free fatty acids plus glycerol), and this process is promoted by insulin. Lipolysis can occur with low insulin levels and is enhanced by epinephrine and growth hormone. When triglycerides are broken down, free fatty acids (FFA) and glycerol are released. Most tissues, except brain and formed blood elements, can utilize FFA as a source of energy. This mechanism allows the body to conserve glucose for use in the CNS and to spare protein from breakdown for conversion to glucose. Additionally, the released glycerol can be converted to glucose in the liver. Growth hormone stimulates the preferential use of fat over glucose.

In brief summary, glucose homeostasis involves a complex interaction between insulin and the counterregulatory hormones glucagon, catecholamines, glucocorticoids, and growth hormone. The action of insulin depends upon its concentration, which is determined by the level of blood glucose through a sensitive feedback loop. In the fed state, insulin acts to convert glucose to stored energy and inhibits the release of other fuel stores. The glucose concentration during the transition from a fed to a fasting state depends upon the relative balance between glucose use and glucose production. The CNS is the primary consumer of glucose. The production of glucose during a brief fast occurs through glycogenolysis. When the fast is more than a few hours, such as overnight, gluconeogenesis is the primary mechanism responsible for glucose production. Hypoglycemia may result from disease of any of the glucoregulatory organs or as a perturbation of normal glucose homeostasis.

PATHOGENESIS

Hypoglycemia has been classified in a variety of ways. It has been divided into high-insulin states, low-insulin states, underproduction of glucose, underutilization of glucose, and the like. Table 88-1 lists the common causes of hypoglycemia seen in the emergency department and divides these into endogenous (or spontaneous) and exogenous (or induced) causes. Additionally, endogenous hypoglycemia is subdivided into that occurring in the fed and that occurring in the fasting state. This classification is arbitrary, and overlap between these divisions does occur.

ENDOGENOUS CAUSES

Fed Hypoglycemia

Hypoglycemia occurring during the fed state has also been termed *reactive* and *postprandial hypoglycemia*. Fed hypoglycemias are characterized by normal fasting serum glucose levels with a decline to hypoglycemic levels within 5 h of a glucose load. Most commonly fed hypoglycemia occurs several hours after eating, usually in the late morning or the late afternoon. The critical period in which hypoglycemia may develop is during the transition from the fed to the fasting state, between 2 and 4 h after the

Table 88-1. Causes of Hypoglycemia

ENDOGENOUS (SPONTANEOUS)

Fed—reactive—postprandial
  Alimentary
  Early diabetes mellitus
  Idiopathic or functional
Fasting
  Islet-cell tumor of pancreas (insulinoma)
  Extrapancreatic neoplasms
  Endocrine-related
    Pituitary insufficiency
    Adrenal insufficiency
    Glucagon deficiency
    Thyroid insufficiency
Hepatic disease
Miscellaneous
  Chronic renal failure
  Starvation
  Autoimmune
  Exercise
  Artifactual

EXOGENOUS (INDUCED)

Insulin
Factitious
Sulfonylureas
Alcohol
Miscellaneous drugs
Posthyperalimentation or hemodialysis

ingestion of glucose. The symptoms of postprandial hypoglycemia are of the sympathomimetic type. This entity may be suspected based upon the history. Diagnosis is supported by an abnormal 5-h glucose tolerance test (GTT) when the nadir of the plasma glucose level occurs concurrently with spontaneous symptoms.

Alimentary

The major causes of fed hypoglycemia are alimentary causes, early diabetes mellitus, and functional, or idiopathic. Following partial or total gastrectomy, gastrojejunostomy, or pyloroplasty, 5 to 10 percent of the patients may develop symptomatic hypoglycemia $1\frac{1}{2}$ to 3 h after a meal. The cause of this type of hypoglycemia appears to be rapid gastric emptying with a subsequent exaggerated insulin response. A close correlation of the hypoglycemia with peak insulin levels has been shown.

Postgastrectomy hypoglycemia is not the same as dumping syndrome, which is due to rapid dilution of a hyperosmolar load in the jejunum and produces symptoms of weakness, pallor, nausea, epigastric discomfort, palpitations, dizziness, and diarrhea. These symptoms occur within 10 min after a meal, subside within 1 h, and are not due to hypoglycemia. The symptoms of postgastrectomy hypoglycemia are usually of the sympathomimetic type but may also be neuroglycopenic. Alimentary hypoglycemia in the absence of gastrointestinal (GI) surgery has been described. Patients with this entity may have a gut defect with rapid glucose absorption, or release of gut factors that stimulate insulin secretion. Treatment of alimentary hypoglycemia is aimed at minimizing insulin release by decreasing the amount of ingested carbohydrate. Drug therapy with various agents has been largely unsuccessful to abort this type of reactive hypoglycemia.

Early Diabetes

Spontaneous hypoglycemia occurring 3 to 5 h after a meal may be seen as an early manifestation of maturity-onset (type II) diabetes. It is postulated that there is a delay in the early release of insulin with subsequent excessive insulin secretion in response to the initial hyperglycemia. The symptoms are usually brief and mild, lasting 15 to 20 min. A family history of diabetes is usual. In a study by Park and co-workers, 25 percent of genetic prediabetics (both parents diabetic) had glucose values of less than 50 mg/dL at some time during a 5-h GTT.

Functional

Functional, or idiopathic, hypoglycemia is a poorly understood, overdiagnosed, or misdiagnosed entity. It is usually described as occurring 2 to 4 h after meals or with minor deprivation of food such as a missed meal. The patient is often a healthy young adult with no known underlying cause of hypoglycemia. Symptoms of sweating, shakiness, weakness, light-headedness, numbness, confusion, and anxiety are commonly reported and may lead the physician to obtain a 5-h GTT. If the blood glucose level goes below 50 mg/dL, the patient is diagnosed as having hypoglycemia and placed on a high-protein, low-carbohydrate diet.

Many authors have expressed concern over this increasingly diagnosed entity. They have pointed out that a low blood glucose level during a 5-h GTT does not mean that the patient is hypoglycemic. One study found that 23 percent of the normal population had blood glucose levels below 50 mg/dL during a 5-h GTT. Another study of 650 subjects identified 10 percent of asymptomatic individuals with plasma glucose levels nadirs of 47 mg/dL or below during a GTT. Several investigations of patients diagnosed to have functional hypoglycemia have shown a poor correlation between the symptoms and the blood glucose levels during the GTT. Attempts to improve the accuracy of diagnosis have been made and include the simultaneous measurement of cortisol levels, the development of a hypoglycemic index in which the rate of fall of glucose is correlated with the glucose nadir, and the use of a mixed meal tolerance test rather than the standard oral glucose tolerance test. None of these approaches have met with universal acceptance as a means to diagnose functional hypoglycemia.

Yager and Young have termed this entity *nonhypoglycemia*. They believe this diagnosis has been popularized by the patient, the lay press, and the physician as a socially acceptable, quasiphysiologic explanation for a variety of somatic complaints. Many symptoms of hypoglycemia and chronic neurosis are similar. The relation of the diagnosis of hypoglycemia to psychiatric disturbance has been pointed out many times. Some studies have shown a correlation between a personality disorder evident by the Minnesota Multiphasic Personality Inventory (MMPI) and functional hypoglycemia. These studies show that diagnosed functional hypoglycemics have a conversion V pattern consistent with personality types who tend to somaticize emotional problems and are resistant to psychologic intervention or interpretation of their symptoms. Other studies have not substantiated the correlation between specific personality characteristics and functional hypoglycemia.

The true incidence of functional hypoglycemia is unknown. It is probably rare and may simply reflect the transition in inter-mediary metabolism between the fed and the fasting state. Certainly, functional hypoglycemia is diagnosed far more often than is justified. The American Diabetes Association in a recent statement identified the following criteria as necessary before the diagnosis of hypoglycemia is made: The occurrence of low blood sugar must be documented, the particular symptoms of which the patient complains must be shown to be due to low blood sugar, the symptoms must be relieved by the ingestion of food or sugar, and the particular kind of hypoglycemia that is producing the symptoms must be established.

It is important that the patient's symptoms be attributed to the correct underlying disorder. Accepting the diagnosis of functional hypoglycemia in an otherwise healthy person may lead to a delay in the evaluation of, or failure to evaluate, other possible causes, including psychiatric ones. It is the responsibility of the emergency physician not to perpetuate a false diagnosis but to educate the patient about the criteria for making this diagnosis. The use of the GTT to make the diagnosis of functional hypoglycemia may not be reliable. The documentation of a serum glucose level of less than 50 mg/dL concurrent with spontaneous symptoms that are absent at other times is a reasonable approach. Home blood glucose monitoring at periodic intervals and during all symptomatic episodes may be a simple method for assessing functional hypoglycemia.

Fasting Hypoglycemia

Fasting hypoglycemia is by far the most important hypoglycemic state for the emergency physician to recognize. Fasting hypoglycemia often reflects serious underlying organic disease. The hypoglycemia may develop slowly so that the signs of hyperepinephrinemia may not be seen. The patient may simply lapse into a coma that can be profound, prolonged, and life-threatening.

By definition, fasting hypoglycemia begins 5 to 6 h after a meal. Most patients with a disorder that causes fasting hypoglycemia develop low glucose levels during a 24-h fast. Occasionally a 72-h fast is required to establish or rule out this diagnosis. Not uncommonly, the patient is difficult to arouse in the morning following an overnight fast. Evaluation of the cause of this type of hypoglycemia requires hospitalization.

Islet-cell Tumor of the Pancreas

Islet-cell tumor of the pancreas, or insulinoma, is a rare cause of hypoglycemia. Hypoglycemia due to insulinoma may occur in the fasting or the fed state. In 80 percent of the cases, the tumor is small, single, and nonmalignant and is located anywhere within the pancreas. About 10 percent of the patients have multiple tumors and also a high association with multiple endocrine neoplasia (MEN), type I. The remaining 10 percent have metastatic malignant insulinoma.

Insulinoma occurs somewhat more often in women in the later decades of life (40 to 70 years). Most of the patients have symptoms consisting of various combinations of sweating, palpitations, weakness, diplopia, and blurred vision. Confusion or abnormal behavior is seen in 80 percent of the cases. Coma or amnesia for the hypoglycemic episode occurs in about half the patients and seizures in 12 percent. Symptoms occur at irregular intervals, more often in the late afternoon or early morning before breakfast and may be induced by exercise. The symptoms are of varying duration and are alleviated by food in the majority of instances. The interval between the appearance of the first hypoglycemic symptoms and the diagnosis of insulinoma is usually months (19 months) and may be years. Many of these patients are diagnosed to have a neurologic abnormality such as a convulsive disorder, a cerebrovascular accident, a brain tumor, or narcolepsy, or they may be thought to have a psychiatric problem such as psychosis or hysteria. Some patients have been diagnosed to have Adams-Stokes attacks.

The hypoglycemia of insulinoma is thought to be due to excess insulin secreted by the tumor. Most authors believe that hyperinsulinemia causes accelerated glucose utilization, but some evidence suggests that the hypoglycemia is due to the suppression of glucose production. The diagnosis of insulinoma is made by the demonstration of hypoglycemia and hyperinsulinemia at the time of spontaneous symptoms. A prolonged fast (72 h) may be required to provoke hypoglycemia, but most patients (75 to 90 percent) develop it before 24 h of fasting. A variety of provocative tests based upon the administration of insulin secretagogues, and several suppression tests utilizing insulin inhibitors, can be used as diagnostic aids. In most instances these are not needed, and inappropriate elevation of the concentration of plasma insulin in the presence of hypoglycemia remains the cornerstone of diagnosis. The ratio of immunoreactive insulin to glucose (IRI/G) can be determined to see if the insulin level is inappropriate to the concomitant level of blood glucose.

The differential diagnosis of insulinoma includes surreptitious self-administration of insulin. In an insulin-dependent diabetic, factitious hypoglycemia from excess insulin administration can be diagnosed by the determination of C-peptide levels. Proinsulin is converted to insulin and C peptide in the pancreatic β cells, and these two peptides are secreted in equimolar concentrations. If insulin is endogenously produced, the insulin and the C-peptide levels correspond. If insulin is exogenously administered, the insulin level is elevated but the C-peptide level is low. In patients who are not insulin-dependent diabetics, the presence of insulin antibodies in the serum points to the self-administration of insulin. These antibodies may not be detectable before 6 weeks to 2 months of exogenous insulin administration.

The treatment of insulinoma is surgical excision of the tumor, and this is curative in most cases. In those patients in whom surgical therapy is not feasible or curative or in whom surgery must be delayed, drug treatment and diet can be used. More frequent feedings using slowly absorbable forms of carbohydrate are indicated. Benign tumors can be treated with diazoxide and a natriuretic diuretic. Diazoxide acts to directly inhibit the release of insulin by the β cells and has an extrapancreatic hyperglycemic effect. The addition of a diuretic prevents edema caused by diazoxide-induced sodium retention. Diphenylhydantoin, propranolol, and chlorpromazine have also been used in the management of insulinoma. With malignant insulinoma, streptozotocin is the most effective antitumor agent to date. Several other chemotherapeutic agents have been tried with limited success.

Extrapancreatic neoplasms

Extrapancreatic neoplasms of widely divergent types and locations may cause hypoglycemia. Most evolve from mesoderm, but they may be epidermal or endodermal in origin. Hypoglycemia may be associated with, and caused by, neoplasms of virtually every histopathologic type. No histologic features serve to distinguish hypoglycemia-producing tumors from those that do not cause hypoglycemia.

The history in cases of tumor hypoglycemia is usually one of intermittent, severe episodes of neuroglycopenia developing over a few weeks or months. Whipple's triad of the features of tumor-induced hypoglycemia consists of hypoglycemia documented by laboratory analysis associated with physical symptoms of glucose deprivation which are relieved by glucose administration. Hypoglycemia-causing tumors may be unsuspected and discovered during systematic evaluation of a patient with fasting hypoglycemia; or hypoglycemia may occur as a late or preterminal event in a patient with known neoplasia.

Mesenchymal tumors are the most common tumors of nonpancreatic origin associated with tumor hypoglycemia. Approximately 30 percent of these tumors are located in the thoracic cavity, and 65 percent are in the abdominal cavity, especially retroperitoneally. These tumors include many histologic types, but fibrosarcomas and mesotheliomas are most common. Mesenchymal tumors are slow-growing and large and may be massive (20 kg or more). Other endocrinopathies may be present because of the ectopic production of a variety of hormones by these tumors. The presenting signs and symptoms may include profound hypoglycemia, depressed cerebral function, weight loss, and a large intrathoracic or intraabdominal mass. Approximately half these tumors are resectable, and this results in cure in the majority of cases.

Epithelial and endothelial tumors of various types such as lung, breast, renal, ovarian, and GI are capable of producing hypoglycemia. The epithelial tumors most often associated with hypoglycemia are hepatic carcinomas, adrenocortical neoplasms, and carcinoid tumors. Hepatic carcinomas are invariably large, occur more commonly in men than women (4 to 1), and usually have a rapid clinical course with a fatal outcome in 1 to 6 months. Hypoglycemia occurs as a terminal or a preterminal event. Adrenocortical neoplasms are usually malignant and large. Both sexes are equally affected at a younger age than that at which other hypoglycemia-causing tumors occur. Carcinoid tumors develop from cells of the amine precursor uptake and decarboxylation (APUD) series and may occur in a variety of locations. These tumors are slow-growing and elaborate a variety of biologically active substances. They are capable of producing hypoglycemia as well as the carcinoid syndrome. Diagnosis is made by the demonstration of increased 5-hydroxyindoleacetic acid (5-HIAA) in a 24-h urine collection.

Controversy exists about the mechanism by which extrapancreatic tumors cause hypoglycemia. Tumor hypoglycemia is a heterogenous disorder that no single mechanism can satisfactorily explain. Some researchers have identified tumor-secreted substances such as nonsuppressible insulinlike activity (NISLA) that may have insulinlike biological activity. Others attribute the hypoglycemia to increased utilization of glucose by the tumor, decreased gluconeogenesis from cachexia and depletion of substrates, or liver impairment due to metastasis or tumor products. Depression of glucagon secretion and activity has also been implicated as a cause of tumor hypoglycemia. Regardless of the mechanism of the hypoglycemia, the treatment is to maintain serum glucose levels by intravenous or oral therapy and to treat the tumor with surgical, radiologic, or chemotherapeutic measures as indicated.

Endocrine-Related

The crucial role of the counterregulatory hormones in the maintenance of glucose homeostasis has been reviewed. Deficiency of any of these hormones could result in hypoglycemia. Catecholamine deficiency has not been documented to cause hypoglycemia, but deficiency of glucagon, glucocorticoids, and growth hormone has. Glucagon and/or pancreatic α-cell deficiency is a rare cause of hypoglycemia. Glucocorticoid deficiency as a cause of fasting hypoglycemia is seen with primary or secondary adrenal insufficiency. Hypoglycemia is more pronounced with secondary adrenal insufficiency (hypopituitarism) because of concomitant growth hormone and glucocorticoid deficiencies. Patients with a growth hormone deficiency may have hypoglycemia in the fasting or the fed states even when the growth hormone deficiency is not accompanied by deficits in other pituitary hormones. Another endocrine-related cause of hypoglycemia is thyroid hormone deficiency, especially when severe enough to cause myxedema coma.

Hepatic Disease

Diffuse, severe liver disease, in which 80 to 85 percent of the liver is functionally impaired or destroyed, may result in hypoglycemia due to impaired glycogenolysis and gluconeogenesis. Diseases such as acute hepatic necrosis, acute viral hepatitis, Reye's syndrome, and severe passive congestion have been implicated. Metastatic or primary liver neoplasia may cause hypoglycemia if a large portion of the liver is involved, but liver metastases usually do not produce hypoglycemia. Chronic liver disease only rarely is a cause of hypoglycemia. Patients with hepatic failure severe enough to cause hypoglycemia are often in a coma. Hypoglycemia as a cause of the coma may be missed if it is assumed that the coma is due to hepatic encephalopathy.

Miscellaneous

Hypoglycemia has been described in a wide variety of other clinical situations. Spontaneous, fasting hypoglycemia with chronic renal failure has been well-documented since 1970. Diabetic and nondiabetic patients with chronic renal failure, who may be on long-term maintenance hemodialysis, have been reported to develop this complication. The pathogenesis of hypoglycemia under these circumstances is poorly understood. The hypoglycemia of chronic renal failure may be accompanied by a severe metabolic acidosis due to lactic acidemia. Hypoglycemia in this setting signals a poor prognosis since the majority of patients die within a few months after its onset.

Starvation-related hypoglycemia is occasionally seen. The majority of the case reports on starvation hypoglycemia involve children with kwashiorkor, but adult cases have also been described. Moderate hypoglycemia often occurs with protein-caloric malnutrition. With inanition, severe hypoglycemia that is refractory to therapy occurs rarely and is uniformly fatal. The mechanisms underlying this disorder are obscure, but the failure of gluconeogenesis due to the depletion of fat and protein stores is postulated. Abnormally increased glucose consumption by cells is another proposed mechanism. It has been recommended that an infusion of 20 percent dextrose and lactated Ringer's solution containing hydrocortisone be used to treat this condition.

Autoimmune hypoglycemia has been described. The presence of anti-insulin antibodies in patients not known to have received insulin injections has been confirmed in several reports. Fasting and fed hypoglycemia due to these autoantibodies has also been described. The mechanism responsible for the hypoglycemia is thought to be dissociation of the insulin-antibody complexes with the release of sufficient amounts of free insulin to cause hypoglycemia. Saturation of the insulin-binding capacity with the continued release of insulin from the pancreas has also been suggested. Additionally, hypoglycemia associated with antibodies to the insulin receptor has been identified. These autoantibodies may mimic the bioactivity of insulin on target tissues, causing hypoglycemia. Patients with other manifestations of autoimmune disease and severe fasting hypoglycemia should have this cause included in their differential diagnosis.

Two additional causes of hypoglycemia should be mentioned. Recognition of these conditions as a cause of hypoglycemia can save unnecessary evaluation and concern. Prolonged exercise may result in the development of frank hypoglycemia. With intense, continued exercise (longer than 90 min), liver glycogen stores are depleted, and the rate of glucose production may fail to keep pace with the rate of glucose use, resulting in a fall in the blood glucose concentration. Felig and co-workers studied 19 healthy men who exercised to exhaustion on a cycle ergometer. Hypoglycemia (< 45 mg/dL) occurred in seven subjects after 60 to 150 min of exercise. Despite the presence of hypoglycemia, each subject was able to continue intense exercise. With the current popularity of endurance training, a patient with exercise-induced hypoglycemia could present to the emergency department.

Artifactual hypoglycemia may occur in conditions in which the white blood cell count is markedly increased ($> 60,000$). Formed blood elements are avid consumers of glucose, and falsely low blood sugar levels may be reported in the presence of very high white blood cell counts. This apparent hypoglycemia is thought to be due to continued glycolysis by the large number of leukocytes between the time the blood is drawn and the time the glucose determination is made. Artifactual hypoglycemia has been reported in various leukemias, with nucleated red blood cells during a hemolytic crisis, and in polycythemia rubra vera. Polymorphonuclear leukocytes and lymphocytes are capable of producing this phenomenon, which seems related to extreme leukocytosis regardless of the underlying disease. True hypoglycemia has been reported in terminal leukemia and must be distinguished from artifactual hypoglycemia. The patient with a falsely low blood glucose level should be asymptomatic. The refrigeration of blood samples and the addition of an antiglycolytic agent, such as sodium fluoride, will decrease glucose consumption by the white blood cells.

EXOGENOUS HYPOGLYCEMIA

Exogenous, or induced, hypoglycemia is almost always due to drugs. The main drugs associated with hypoglycemia are insulin, sulfonylurea agents, alcohol, and salicylates. These drugs, alone or in combination, account for almost all cases of drug-induced hypoglycemia. All ages are subject to this complication. The total cases per decade are roughly equal after the age of 30. During the first 2 years of life, salicylates account for most cases of drug-induced hypoglycemia. During the next 4 years, alcohol is the most likely cause. Alcohol alone or in combination with insulin causes hypoglycemic coma in 7 out of 10 patients between 30 and 60 years of age who have drug-related hypoglycemia. Hypoglycemia caused by sulfonylurea agents is more likely after 50 years of age.

There are certain factors that predispose to all these types of drug-induced hypoglycemia. The most common denominator is restricted carbohydrate intake, ranging from a missed meal to chronic starvation. Other important contributing factors include abnormal liver or kidney function.

Insulin-Induced

Insulin reaction in the diabetic patient is by far the most common cause of hypoglycemia seen in the emergency department. A 1-year prospective study in a large emergency department identified 204 admissions of adults with severe hypoglycemia. Of these cases of hypoglycemia, 200 were due to insulin reactions in insulin-dependent diabetics and 3 were caused by chlorpropamide ingestion. Another study of 319 insulin-treated diabetics showed that severe hypoglycemia (coma or requiring treatment) occurred in 28 percent at least once during the period of 1 year. Over a 5-year period, 42 percent had a severe hypoglycemic reaction, and "mild" reactions occurred at least once a month in about half the patients. Hypoglycemia was the most common treatment complication, occurring in all but 2 of 73 patients with juvenile-type diabetes (type I) followed for 40 years or more. A follow-up study of 307 patients diagnosed to have diabetes mellitus before the age of 31 showed that death with or from hypoglycemia was more common than death in ketoacidotic coma (5 to 2 percent).

Multiple factors affect the severity and the frequency of insulin reactions. The severity of the diabetes is directly related to the incidence of insulin reactions. Those with the least endogenous insulin have the widest variation in blood glucose levels. It is well-documented that the counterregulatory hormones increase in response to insulin-induced hypoglycemia. A recent study of type I diabetics, several of whom had a history of repeated attacks of severe hypoglycemia, compared their counterregulatory metabolic and hormonal responses to those of controls to see if differences in the levels of the counterregulatory hormones were present. The peak levels of glucagon, catecholamines, glucocorticoids, and growth hormone were similar in the diabetics with and without clinical hypoglycemia. It was concluded that deficient counterregulatory hormone responses are important in the pathogenesis of insulin-induced hypoglycemic reactions, but that other factors in the daily lives of such patients also play a major part in determining whether reactions occur.

Some other factors that may precipitate hypoglycemia in an insulin-dependent diabetic include exercise, emotions, late meals, undereating of carbohydrates, alcohol ingestion, errors of insulin dosage, erratic absorption of insulin from subcutaneous sites, and overtreatment with insulin. Of these factors, overtreatment with insulin deserves further discussion. Excess insulin dosage may occur because of a physician error or when a patient attempts too-rigid control, especially when glucosuria is used as the principal indicator for the insulin dose. Following the classic report by Somogyi, excess insulin as a cause of both hypoglycemia and rebound hyperglycemia has been well-documented in adults and children. Travis found severe overcontrol in 22 of 135 children with unstable diabetes, and Rosenbloom and Giordano reported insulin overtreatment in 70 percent of 101 unselected diabetic children. Gale and co-workers found in overnight metabolic studies of 39 poorly controlled insulin-treated diabetic patients aged 9 to 66 years that 22 had nocturnal hypoglycemia (< 35 mg/dL).

Nocturnal hypoglycemia is often difficult to recognize clinically. It is most likely to be associated with the use of long-acting insulin preparations taken once daily. In Gale's series, hypoglycemia symptoms were mild or absent. Other features suggestive of insulin overtreatment were noted, however. These included lethargy, depression, night sweats, morning headaches, seizures, hepatomegaly due to gycogen accumulation, and acquired tolerance to high doses of insulin. Rosenbloom and Giordano also found polyuria, nocturia or enuresis despite increasing insulin dosage, excessive appetite, weight gain, mood swings, and frequent bouts of rapidly developing ketoacidosis as additional clues to the recognition of insulin overdosage (see Table 88-2). Fasting early-morning blood glucose levels may be normal in spite of nocturnal hypoglycemia. They may also be elevated and lead to an increase in the insulin dose and a worsening of the symptoms. When insulin-dependent diabetics are brought to the emergency department with symptoms of undetermined cause, the possibility of overtreatment with insulin should be considered. Follow-up arrangements should be made with their physicians through personal communication.

The question of rigid or tight control of diabetes is even more vital following a policy statement from the American Diabetes Association in 1976 calling for "a serious effort to achieve levels of blood glucose as close to those in the nondiabetic state as feasible." This therapeutic goal is based upon the belief that the long-term vascular complications of diabetes, particularly retinopathy and nephropathy, are decreased by reduction of the blood glucose concentration. To this end, newer methods for tight diabetic control have been introduced. These include home blood glucose monitoring with multiple insulin injections (2 or 3 times a day) based upon glucose levels, continuous subcutaneous insulin infusion using a portable pump, and the development of an artificial pancreas.

Several authors have cautioned against too-rigid control. In spite of the efficacy of home blood glucose monitoring and the apparent effectiveness of the infusion pump, complications have been reported. As of February 1982, 12 unexpected deaths had occurred in the estimated 4000 to 5000 patients receiving insulin by continuous subcutaneous infusion. Hypoglycemia was suspected as being a cause or a contributory factor in at least six of the deaths. An 18-month prospective study of 147 diabetic children and adolescents who received two daily injections of insulin showed 47 percent with at least one hypoglycemic reaction but only 4 percent with severe reactions. Interestingly, the episodes of frequent or severe symptomatic hypoglycemia occurred almost exclusively in

Table 88-2. Clinical Clues of Nocturnal Hypoglycemia

1. Lassitude, depression, difficulty with waking in morning
2. Early morning headaches or irritability
3. Night sweats, nightmares
4. Polyuria, nocturia, enuresis in children
5. Convulsions
6. Increased appetite and weight gain
7. Hepatomegaly
8. Morning ketonuria without glucosuria or disproportionate to glucosuria
9. Worsening of symptoms with increased insulin dose
10. Insulin dose greater than 1.0 unit/kg of body weight per day

the patients with well-controlled diabetes. No one would argue with the goal of better control of diabetes. Where the balance lies between the benefit of near-physiologic control and the risk of hypoglycemia is undetermined. The emergency physician, as one who is likely to see significant hypoglycemic reactions, is in a good position to help provide an answer to this question.

It is important to prevent hypoglycemic reactions in the insulin-dependent diabetic. Many diabetics accept mild reactions as a necessary nuisance and learn to recognize and abort them by the self-administration of glucose. Although most symptomatic insulin-induced hypoglycemia produces sympathomimetic reactions, neuroglycopenic symptoms may also occur and prevent recognition of the former by the patient. Relatives and close friends may be the first to notice confusion or subtle changes in behavior due to hypoglycemia. Additionally, studies with continuous blood glucose sampling in type I diabetics have suggested that less than a third of all hypoglycemic episodes are symptomatic. Recurrent, severe hypoglycemic reactions are demoralizing to the patient and the family. Such reactions interfere with work and are a hazard while driving. Hypoglycemic encephalopathy or death may occur with repeated, prolonged, and severe hypoglycemic episodes.

The best hope for the reduction of insulin-induced hypoglycemia depends upon the informed cooperation of the patient. Patient education is sadly lacking. One survey found that 40 percent of "trained" insulin-dependent patients could not demonstrate competence in a single area of diabetes management. The motivation of the patient is also important and often depends upon the doctor-patient relationship. A cooperative effort between the patient, the patient's primary physician, and the emergency physician is essential for the appropriate follow-up of a diabetic patient presenting to the emergency department.

When a diabetic patient is brought to the emergency department with depressed cerebral function or in coma, rapid differentiation between hypoglycemia and ketoacidosis must be made (see Table 88-3). Testing a drop of blood with a glucose reagent strip reliably allows differentiation between high and low blood glucose levels within minutes. If there is still uncertainty about the cause, 50 mL of a 50 percent glucose solution should be given intravenously after blood has been obtained for appropriate studies. The hypoglycemic patient benefits, and the patient in ketoacidosis is not unduly harmed.

Factitious Hypoglycemia

An occasional emotionally unstable patient surreptitiously administers insulin or an oral hypoglycemic drug to induce hypoglycemia and simulate organic disease. These patients may be medical personnel or diabetics, or they may be related to someone who is diabetic or in the medical profession. These patients often exhibit erratic patterns of hypoglycemia and usually deny drug misuse even when confronted directly. The use of insulin or oral hypoglycemia agents causes hyperinsulinemia, which may be mistaken for an insulinoma. Factitious hypoglycemia resulting from oral hypoglycemics can be diagnosed by detecting sulfonylurea agents in the blood. Insulin antibodies may be detected in the serum of patients who claim to have never used insulin if the insulin has been administered for 6 to 8 weeks. The measurement of C-peptide levels is indicated if insulin antibodies are not detected or if a diabetic patient is suspected of factitious hypoglycemia. The C-peptide levels are low if the source of the insulin is exogenous and high in cases of endogenous hyperinsulinemia. The correct diagnosis of factitious hypoglycemia can prevent needless surgery.

Sulfonylureas

The sulfonylureas are commonly used as oral hypoglycemic agents and include chlorpropamide, tolbutamide, acetohexamide, and tolazamide. They act to stimulate the release of insulin from the pancreas with a subsequent decrease in hepatic glucose output. These agents are commonly used to treat mild, type II diabetes. Approximately 5 percent of the patients on these hypoglycemic drugs have glucopenic reactions. These reactions may be profound, prolonged, and life-threatening. Sulfonylurea overdose and surreptitious self-administration may also produce hypoglycemia. Encephalopathy from recurrent hypoglycemic reactions induced by oral hypoglycemic drugs has been reported.

Other drugs may potentiate the hypoglycemic effect of sulfonylurea agents. In addition to those already mentioned, sulfonamides, bishydroxycoumarin, and phenylbutazone should be avoided in patients on sulfonylureas. All the sulfonylurea compounds have caused hypoglycemia, but chlorpropamide is responsible for the majority of the cases. Hypoglycemia due to chlorpropamide has

Table 88-3. Differential Diagnosis in Coma of a Known Diabetic

	Hypoglycemia	Ketoacidosis
History	Insufficient food, excess insulin, excess exercise	Insufficient insulin, infection, gastrointestinal upset
Onset	Following *short-acting insulin:* Sudden, a few hours after injection Following *long-acting insulin:* Relatively slower, many hours after injection	Gradual over many hours
Course	Anxiety, sweating, hunger, headache, diplopia, incoordination, twitching, convulsions, coma (headache, nausea, and haziness especially following long-acting insulin)	Polyuria, polydipsia, anorexia, nausea, vomiting, labored deep breathing, weakness, drowsiness, possible fever and abdominal pain, coma
Physical findings	Pale moist skin, full rapid pulse, dilated pupils, normal breathing, blood pressure normal or elevated, overactive reflexes, positive Babinski sign	Florid, dry skin, Kussmaul breathing with acetone odor, decreased blood pressure, weak rapid pulse, soft eyeballs
Laboratory findings	Second urine specimen sugar- and ketone-free, low blood sugar, normal serum CO_2	Urine contains sugar and ketone bodies; high blood sugar, low serum CO_2

Source: Ensinck JW, Williams RH: Disorders causing hypoglycemia, in Williams RH (ed): *Textbook of Endocrinology,* ed 6. Philadelphia, Saunders, 1981, p 873.

occurred during normal food intake, with intact renal function, and at ordinary dosages. Chlorpropamide causes the most prolonged hypoglycemia of all sulfonylurea drugs. Its half-life in the serum is 36 h, and 3 to 5 days are required for complete elimination from the body.

Sulfonylurea-induced hypoglycemia may be refractory to treatment by intravenous glucose alone. This is particularly true in nondiabetic patients in whom insulin-release mechanisms are intact. Infused glucose stimulates insulin release, which may further lower the blood glucose level. Diazoxide, 300 mg by slow intravenous infusion over a 30-min period, repeated every 4 h, has been successful in raising the blood glucose to supranormal levels without causing hypotension. All patients with sulfonylurea-induced hypoglycemia require hospitalization and prolonged treatment.

Alcohol

Alcohol-induced hypoglycemia is usually seen in malnourished chronic alcoholics. It may also occur in spree drinkers, in occasional drinkers who have missed a meal or two, and in children and adolescents exposed to alcohol for the first time. In Seltzer's series of 473 episodes of drug-induced hypoglycemic coma, alcohol accounted for 174 cases; 146 of these patients were adults and 28 were children. Severe alcoholic intoxication and hypoglycemic coma has also been reported from continuous sponging of a febrile child with rubbing alcohol. Rubbing alcohol may contain ethyl or isopropyl alcohol, both of which can be absorbed through the respiratory tract.

Patients with alcohol-induced hypoglycemia usually present in a comatose or a semiconscious state 2 to 10 h after alcohol ingestion. The presenting physical findings may include hypothermia, tachypnea, and the smell of alcohol on the breath. The absence of alcohol fetor does not rule out alcohol as a cause of hypoglycemia or coma. Most patients are unresponsive except to deep pain stimulation. Convulsions are a particularly frequent occurrence in children with alcoholic hypoglycemia. Laboratory findings, in addition to hypoglycemia, usually include an elevated blood alcohol level, ketonuria without glucosuria, and mild acidosis.

Alcohol-induced hypoglycemia is attributed primarily to the inhibition of gluconeogenesis during alcohol metabolism. Ethyl alcohol is metabolized primarily in the cytoplasm of the liver cells, utilizing nicotinamide adenine dinucleotide (NAD) as the hydrogen acceptor. During this process the rate of NAD reduction exceeds the rate of NADH oxidation, and the NADH/NAD ratio increases severalfold. The NAD available for those oxidation-reduction reactions necessary to sustain gluconeogenesis is thus decreased, and the level of plasma glucose subsequently falls. The chronic alcoholic with reduced caloric intake and depleted liver glycogen stores has no glucogenic reserve, and hypoglycemic coma results. The mechanism by which alcohol induces hypoglycemia in the well-fed person is less well defined.

Treatment with intravenous glucose is usually sufficient to correct alcohol-induced hypoglycemia. Thiamine should be given before glucose in chronic or suspected alcoholics. Glucagon is not recommended in the chronic alcoholic, as liver glycogen stores are usually exhausted. The mortality for alcohol-induced hypoglycemia is 11 percent in adults and 25 percent in children. This high rate is thought to be due to late recognition and inadequate treatment of this condition.

Miscellaneous Drugs

Several other drugs should be mentioned in relation to drug-induced hypoglycemia. Salicylate-induced hypoglycemic coma in children occurs most often because of parental overtreatment of febrile illnesses with aspirin rather than because of accidental ingestion. Salicylate toxicity and hypoglycemia should be considered in any child with coma, convulsions, or cardiovascular collapse. Salicylate-related hypoglycemia in adults most often occurs when aspirin is used in conjunction with other compounds that lower the levels of glucose. Propranolol has been reported to precipitate hypoglycemia, and several authors have expressed concern over the use of β-adrenergic blockers in diabetics. They believe that β-blockers may mask the adrenergic symptoms of hypoglycemia and increase the risk and the severity of hypoglycemic reactions. Experimental and clinical evidence is contradictory. Some researchers find that β-blockers potentiate insulin-induced hypoglycemia and delay the blood glucose recovery after hypoglycemic reactions, while others have disputed these findings. The β-blockers are widely used among diabetic patients for the treatment of angina and hypertension. Cardioselective β-blockers have been recommended when diabetics require β-blocking drugs. The possible induction, potentiation, or masking of hypoglycemia by β-blocking drugs in diabetics should be considered.

Drugs that have been found to cause hypoglycemia in isolated instances include *para*-aminobenzoic acid, haloperidol, propoxyphene, monoamine oxidase (MAO) inhibitors, and chlorpromazine. Disopyramide-induced hypoglycemia has been reported increasingly since 1978 and usually occurs in elderly patients who are poorly nourished and have mild abnormalities in glucose homeostasis.

A final cause of exogenous, or induced, hypoglycemia is the sudden cessation of a high-concentration glucose infusion. Hypoglycemia with this cause may occur in patients receiving hyperalimentation or hemodialysis. An occasional patient undergoing outpatient hemodialysis may be brought to the emergency department with hypoglycemia due to this cause.

Hypoglycemia of Infancy and Childhood

Hypoglycemia is relatively common in the pediatric age group. Many of the disorders already discussed cause hypoglycemia in neonates and children, but several metabolic and/or inherited abnormalities which can result in hypoglycemia occur exclusively in this age group. Only selected aspects of pediatric hypoglycemia will be mentioned.

Neonatal hypoglycemia occurs in approximately 4 infants per 1000 live births. The infant may be asymptomatic or have various symptoms consisting of limpness, tremors, irritability, convulsions, apnea, cyanosis, abnormal cry, and bradycardia. In the emergency setting, the infants at greatest risk of hypoglycemia are those born to diabetic mothers, especially if the mothers are on insulin or oral hypoglycemics, and infants born to mothers taking narcotics. Hypoglycemia also occurs in neonates in association with erythroblastosis fetalis, prematurity or postmaturity, hypoxia during delivery, and small size in relation to the gestational age. All neonates with plasma glucose levels less than 40 mg/dL, or infants suspected of hypoglycemia, should be treated with intravenous glucose infusion and referred to their pediatrician for hospitalization and evaluation.

The most common hypoglycemia in childhood is ketotic hypoglycemia, which accounts for more than half of all the cases. The precise mechanism of the hypoglycemia is unknown, but the underlying defect is probably present at birth. Manifestations of ketotic hypoglycemia do not occur until the child is stressed with caloric deprivation. Boys are affected twice as often as girls, and the onset is usually between 18 months and 5 years of age. The attacks are episodic, occurring in the morning or during periods of illness, vomiting, or deprivation of food. Ketonuria is frequently associated with the hypoglycemia. The hypoglycemic episodes respond promptly to the administration of glucose, and spontaneous remission of this disorder occurs by 8 to 10 years of age.

CLINICAL PRESENTATION

The clinical manifestations of hypoglycemia vary widely. Some patients are asymptomatic even though the hypoglycemia is significant. As glucose is the main source of energy for the brain, it is not surprising that most symptomatic hypoglycemia produces neurologic and mental dysfunction. The sympathomimetic symptoms of sudden hypoglycemia, and the neuroglycopenic symptoms, reflective of a gradual lowering of the blood glucose level, were described earlier in this chapter.

Hypoglycemia can cause other neurologic manifestations such as cranial nerve palsies, paresthesias, and transient hemiplegia. Hemiplegia may be due to endogenous or exogenous hypoglycemia. The paralysis is usually abrupt in onset, is associated with extensor plantar responses, and may last a few hours to a few days. This phenomenon is thought to be due to decreased glucose perfusion of a selected area of the brain because of arteriosclerotic narrowing of a blood vessel.

Moderate hypothermia may occur with hypoglycemia and can be a useful clue in cases of unsuspected hypoglycemia. Sweating, peripheral vasodilatation, hyperventilation, and reduced heat production contribute to hypoglycemic-induced hypothermia. When hypoglycemia is accompanied by elevated temperature, then infection, dehydration, or cerebral edema may be the cause.

Unsuspected hypoglycemia may masquerade as neurologic, psychiatric, or cardiovascular disorders. Hypoglycemia has been misdiagnosed as a cerebrovascular accident, a transient ischemic attack, a seizure disorder, a brain tumor, narcolepsy, multiple sclerosis, psychosis, hysteria, depression, and Adams-Stokes attacks. Particular care should be exercised when dealing with these entities so that hypoglycemia is not missed.

Evaluation of Hypoglycemia

The detection and the evaluation of hypoglycemia in the emergency department are limited. A history, a physical examination, selected x-rays, and laboratory studies, such as random glucose and urine chemistries, are the main investigative tools available to the emergency physician. One test that could assist in the diagnosis of suspected transient hypoglycemia is the cerebrospinal fluid glucose analysis. Gruber has reported that the CSF glucose level lags behind the blood glucose level during the return to the normal range. The delay in the return to a baseline level may be as much as 4 to 6 h. Transient hypoglycemia could be reflected in a low CSF glucose level at a time when the blood glucose concentration is normal. Other laboratory studies, such as a five-h glucose tolerance test, and measurement of the levels of insulin, insulin antibodies, and C peptides, should be obtained in conjunction with the patient's primary physician.

Fed hypoglycemic reactions are suspected based upon the proximity of the symptoms to eating, especially when a repetitive pattern is evident. A history of gastric surgery or relatives with diabetes may be obtained. A 5-h GTT may confirm this diagnosis. If functional hypoglycemia is suspected, home blood glucose monitoring or random blood glucose levels obtained at the time of the symptoms are indicated. Fasting hypoglycemia may occasionally be detected in the emergency department if the patient presents in a fasting state or if a random blood glucose level is low. Patients suspected of having fasting hypoglycemia should be admitted to the hospital for evaluation.

The plasma glucose levels should be determined in all patients who are comatose, have a seizure, have a disturbance of sensorium, have taken a drug overdose, smell of alcohol, or have "funny spells" that are undefined. Random glucose levels should be determined in all diabetic patients with clinically significant complaints.

TREATMENT

Many aspects of treating hypoglycemia have been discussed in conjunction with specific disorders. The armamentarium of the emergency physician in combating hypoglycemia consists of intravenous or oral glucose solutions, glucagon, and hydrocortisone.

Diabetic patients who present in coma, or other patients who have coma of uncertain cause, should be given 50 mL of a 50 percent glucose solution by intravenous bolus, after blood has been obtained for appropriate studies. In confirmed hypoglycemia, a follow-up infusion of a 5, 10, or 20 percent glucose solution should be started. Continuous intravenous glucose for 4 to 6 h is needed for most hypoglycemic reactions. Prolonged therapy may be indicated in some cases, and knowledge of the cause of the hypoglycemia should guide the duration of treatment. Care must be taken not to discontinue the glucose infusion too soon, as the hypoglycemia may recur.

The glucose level with the infusion running should be 100 mg/dL or greater. The blood glucose level should be monitored every 2 to 3 h. If the first liter of glucose solution fails to establish and maintain elevated glucose levels, 100 mg of hydrocortisone and 1 mg of glucagon should be added to each liter of infusate for as long as necessary. Persistent hyperglycemia, maintained by slow administration of 5 percent glucose, is a sign that the glucose infusion may be withdrawn. After intravenous therapy has been discontinued the blood glucose level should be determined in every patient discharged from the emergency department. These patients should be instructed to continue oral carbohydrate intake and to return if any symptoms of hypoglycemia recur.

The required duration of continuous glucose infusion is unpredictable. Most diabetics with insulin-reactions respond fairly rapidly to intravenous glucose. Similarly, alcohol-induced hypoglycemia usually responds quickly to glucose administration. Sulfonylurea-induced hypoglycemia can be prolonged and may not respond to intravenous glucose alone. Diazoxide as adjunctive therapy may be required. All patients with sulfonylurea hypoglycemia should be admitted to the hospital. One author has reported that greater and more prolonged increases in blood glucose concentrations occur when patients with sulfonylurea hypoglycemia are given glucagon intramuscularly rather than intravenously.

Glucagon is effective adjunctive therapy in selected cases. Glucagon acts to increase glucose production by the liver providing that glycogen stores are adequate. Glucagon can be administered intramuscularly, subcutaneously, or intravenously in 0.5- to 2.0-mg doses. It is effective in 10 to 20 min and may be repeated twice. If glucagon is given intravenously, continuous infusion should be used because of glucagon's short half-life in the circulation. Glucagon is not effective in the treatment of alcohol-induced hypoglycemia in chronic alcoholics because of the depletion of liver glycogen stores.

If a patient does not respond clinically to intravenous glucose, glucagon, or hydrocortisone, other causes of coma should be considered. Cerebral edema due to hypoglycemia has been reported. Osmotic diuretics, such as mannitol, may be indicated.

BIBLIOGRAPHY

Anderson JH, Blackard WG, Goldman J, et al: Diabetes and hypoglycemia due to insulin antibodies. *Am J Med* 64:868, 1978.

Anderson N, Lokich JJ: Mesenchymal tumors associated with hypoglycemia: Case report and review of the literature. *Cancer* 44:785, 1979.

Anthony D, Dippe S, Hofeldt FD, et al: Personality disorder and reactive hypoglycemia: A quantitative study. *Diabetes* 22:664, 1973.

Arem R, Jeang MK, Blevens TC, et al: Polycythemia rubra vera and artifactual hypoglycemia. *Arch Intern Med* 142:2199, 1982.

Arieff AI, Doerner T, Zelig H, et al: Mechanisms of seizures and coma in hypoglycemia: Evidence for a direct effect of insulin on electrolyte transport in brain. *J Clin Invest* 54:654, 1974.

Arky R: Pathophysiology and therapy of the fasting hypoglycemias. *DM*, February 1968, p 3.

Aynsley-Green A: Hypoglycemia in infants and children. *Clin Endocrinol Metab* 11:159, 1982.

Bale RN: Brain damage in diabetes mellitus. *Br J. Psychiatry* 122:337, 1973.

Bansal VK, Brooks MH, York JC, et al: Intractable hypoglycemia in a patient with renal failure. *Arch Intern Med* 139:100, 1979.

Barnett AH, Leslie D, Watkins PJ: Can insulin-treated diabetes be given beta-adrenergic blocking drugs? *Br Med J* 1:976, 1980.

Baruh S, Sherman L, Kolodny HD, et al: Fasting hypoglycemia. *Med Clin North Am* 57:1441, 1973.

Bleicher SJ, Levy LJ, Zarowitz H, et al: Glucagon-deficiency hypoglycemia: A new syndrome. *Clin Res* 18:355, 1970.

Blonde L, Riddick FA: Hypoglycemia: The "undisease." *South Med J* 69:1261, 1976.

Burns TW, Bregant R, Van Peenan HJ, et al: Observations on blood glucose concentration of human subjects during continuous sampling. *Diabetes* 14:186, 1965.

Cahill GF: Physiology of insulin in man. *Diabetes* 20:785, 1971.

Cahill GF: Starvation in man. *N Engl J Med* 282:668, 1970.

Cahill GF, Etzwiller DD, Freinkel N: "Control" and diabetes. *N Engl J Med* 294:1004, 1976.

Cahill GF, Soeldner JS: "A non-editorial on non-hypoglycemia." *N Engl J Med* 291:905, 1974.

Cameron AJ, Ellis JP, McGill JI, et al: Insulin response to carbohydrate ingestion after gastric surgery with special reference to hypoglycemia. *Gut* 10:825, 1969.

Charles MA, Hofeldt F, Shackelford A, et al: Comparison of oral glucose tolerance tests and mixed meals in patients with apparent idiopathic postabsorptive hypoglycemia: Absence of hypoglycemia after meals. *Diabetes* 30:465, 1981.

Cole RA, Benedict GW, Margolis S, et al: Blood glucose monitoring in symptomatic hypoglycemia. *Diabetes* 25:984, 1976.

Cotton EK, Fahlberg VI: Hypoglycemia with salicylate poisoning. *Am J Dis Child* 108:171, 1964.

Crofford OB, Spratt IL, Drash AL, et al: Statement on hypoglycemia. *Diabetes Care* 5:72, 1982.

Deckert T, Poulsen JE, Larsen M: Prognosis of diabetics with diabetes onset before the age of thirty one. I. Survival, causes of death, and complications. *Diabetologia* 14:363, 1978.

Eeg-Olofsson O: Hypoglycemia and neurological disturbances in children with diabetes mellitus. *Acta Pediatr Scand* 270(suppl):91, 1977.

Elias AN, Gwinup G: Glucose-resistant hypoglycemia in inanition. *Arch Intern Med* 142:743, 1982.

Exton JH: Gluconeogenesis. *Metabolism* 21:945, 1972.

Fajans SS, Floyd JC: Diagnosis and medical management of insulinomas. *Ann Rev Med* 30:313, 1979.

Fajans SS, Floyd JC: Fasting hypoglycemia in adults. *N Engl J Med* 294:766, 1976.

Fariss BL: Prevalence of post-load glycosuria and hypoglycemia in a group of healthy young men. *Diabetes* 23:189, 1974.

Felig P, Tamborlane WV: Insulin delivery devices. *Ann Intern Med* 93:627, 1980.

Felig P, Wahren J: Fuel homeostasis in exercise. *N Engl J Med* 293:1078, 1975.

Felig P, Brown WV, Levine RA, et al: Glucose homeostasis in viral hepatitis. *N Engl J Med* 283:1436, 1970.

Felig P, Cherif A, Minagawa A, et al: Hypoglycemia during prolonged exercise in normal men. *N Engl J Med* 306:895, 1982.

Field JB, Williams HE: Artifactual hypoglycemia associated with leukemia. *N Engl J Med* 265:946, 1961.

Field JB, Williams HE, Mortimore GE: Studies on the mechanism of ethanol-induced hypoglycemia. *J Clin Invest* 42:497, 1963.

Ford CV, Bray GA, Swerdloff RS: A psychiatric study of patients referred with a diagnosis of hypoglycemia. *Am J Psychiatry* 133:290, 1976.

Freinkel N, Arky RA, Singer DL, et al: Alcohol hypoglycemia, IV: Current concepts of its pathogenesis. *Diabetes* 14:350, 1965.

Frerichs H, Creutzfeldt W: Hypoglycaemia. I. Insulin secreting tumors. *Clin Endocrinol Metab* 5:747, 1976.

Gale E: Hypoglycemia. *Clin Endocrinol Metab* 9:461, 1980.

Gale E, Tattersall R: Brittle diabetes. *Br J Hosp Med* 22:589, 1979.

Gale EAM, Tattersall RB: Unrecognized nocturnal hypoglycaemia in insulin-treated diabetics. *Lancet* 1:1049, 1979.

Gerich J, Davis J, Lorenzi M, et al: Hormonal mechanisms of recovery from insulin-induced hypoglycemia in man. *Am J Physiol* 236:E380, 1979.

Goldberg IJ, Brown LK, Rayfield EJ: Disopyramide (Norpace)-induced hypoglycemia. *Am J Med* 69:463, 1980.

Goldstein DE, England JD, Hess R, et al: A prospective study of symptomatic hypoglycemia in young diabetic patients. *Diabetes Care* 4:601, 1981.

Gruber AB: Low CSF glucose level (hypoglycorrhachia) in symptomatic hypoglycemia. *JAMA* 247:1461, 1982.

Gutberlet RL, Cornblath M: Neonatal hypoglycemia revisited, 1975. *Pediatrics* 58:10, 1976.

Hadji-Georgopoulos A, Schmidt I, Margolis S, et al: Elevated hypoglycemic index and late hyperinsulinism in symptomatic postprandial hypoglycemia. *J Clin Endocrinol Metab* 50:371, 1980.

Hofeldt FD: Reactive hypoglycemia. *Metabolism* 24:1193, 1975.

Immerman SC, Sener SF, Khandekar JD: Causes and evaluation of tumor-induced hypoglycemia. *Arch Surg* 117:905, 1982.

Ingram TTS, Stark GD, Blackburn I: Ataxia and other neurological disorders as sequels of severe hypoglycaemia in childhood. *Brain* 90:851, 1967.

Järhult J, Farnebo LO, Hamberger B, et al: The relation between catecholamines, glucagon and pancreatic polypeptide during hypoglycaemia in man. *Acta Endocrinol* (Copenh) 98:402, 1981.

Johnson DD, Dorr KE, Swenson WM, et al: Reactive hypoglycemia. *JAMA* 243:1151, 1980.

Johnson SF, Schade DS, Peake GT: Chlorpropamide-induced hypoglycemia: Successful treatment with diazoxide. *Am J Med* 63:799, 1977.

Kahn CR: The riddle of tumor hypoglycemia revisited. *Clin Endocrinol Metab* 9:335, 1980.

Kedes LH, Field JB: Hypothermia: A clue to hypoglycemia. *N Engl J Med* 271:785, 1964.

Kennedy AL, Merimee TJ: The evaluation of hypoglycemia. *Compr Ther* 6:62, 1980.

Kennedy T: The management of the hypoglycemic patient. *World J Surg* 6:718, 1982.

Lager I, Blohmé G, Smith U: Effect of cardioselective and non-selective β-blockade on the hypoglycaemic response in insulin-dependent diabetics. *Lancet* 1:458, 1979.

Lang DA, Matthews DR, Phil D, et al: Cyclic oscillations of basal plasma glucose and insulin concentrations in human beings. *N Engl J Med* 301:1023, 1979.

Lev-Ran A, Anderson RW: The diagnosis of postprandial hypoglycemia. *Diabetes* 30:996, 1981.

Lock DR, Rigg LA: Hypoglycemic coma associated with subcutaneous insulin infusion by portable pump. *Diabetes Care* 4:389, 1981.

Maccuish AC, Munro JF, Duncan LJP: Treatment of hypoglycaemic coma with glucagon, intravenous dextrose, and mannitol infusion in a hundred diabetics. *Lancet* 2:946, 1970.

Marks V: Alcohol and carbohydrate metabolism. *Clin Endocrinol Metab* 7:333, 1978.

Marks V: Hypoglycaemia. 2. Other causes. *Clin Endocrinol Metab* 5:769, 1976.

Megyesi K, Kahn R, Roth J, et al: Hypoglycemia in association with extrapancreatic tumors: Demonstration of elevated plasma NSILA-s by a new radioreceptor assay. *J Clin Endocrinol Metab* 38:931, 1974.

Merimee TJ: Spontaneous hypoglycemia in man. *Adv Intern Med* 22:301, 1977.

Merimee TJ, Tyson JE: Hypoglycemia in man: Pathologic and physiologic variants. *Diabetes* 26:161, 1977.

Merimee TJ, Tyson JE: Stabilization of plasma glucose during fasting: Normal variations in two separate studies. *N Engl J Med* 291:1275, 1974.

Milner RDG: Neonatal hypoglycemia, 1979. *J Perinat Med* 7:185, 1979.

Molnar GW, Read RC: Hypoglycemia and body temperature. *JAMA* 227:916, 1974.

Montgomery BM, Pinner CA: Transient hypoglycemic hemiplegia. *Arch Intern Med* 114:680, 1964.

Moss MH: Alcohol-induced hypoglycemia and coma caused by alcohol sponging. *Pediatrics* 46:445, 1970.

Olson RL, Leichter S, Warram J, et al: Deaths among patients using continuous subcutaneous insulin infusion pumps—United States. *MMWR* 31:80, 1982.

Pagliara AS, Karl IE, Haymond M, et al: Hypoglycemia in infancy and childhood. Part I. *J Pediatr* 82:365, 1973.

Pagliara AS, Karl IE, Haymond M, et al: Hypoglycemia in infancy and childhood. Part II. *J Pediatr* 82:558, 1973.

Papaioannou AN: Tumors other than insulinomas associated with hypoglycemia. *Surg Gynecol Obstet* 123:1093, 1966.

Paz-Guevara A, Hsu TH, White P: Juvenile diabetes mellitus after forty years. *Diabetes* 24:559, 1975.

Peitzman SJ, Agarwal BN: Spontaneous hypoglycemia in end-stage renal failure. *Nephron* 19:131, 1977.

Pelligrino D, Yokoyama H, Ingvar M, et al: Moderate arterial hypotension reduces cerebral cortical blood flow and enhances cellular release of potassium in severe hypoglycemia. *Acta Physiol Scand* 115:511, 1982.

Permutt MA: Postprandial hypoglycemia. *Diabetes* 25:719, 1976.

Permutt MA, Kelly J, Bernstein R, et al: Alimentary hypoglycemia in the absence of gastrointestinal surgery. *N Engl J Med* 288:1206, 1973.

Polonsky K, Bergenstal R, Pons G, et al: Relation of counterregulatory responses to hypoglycemia in type I diabetics. *N Engl J Med* 307:1106, 1982.

Potter J, Clarke P, Gale EAM, et al: Insulin-induced hypoglycaemia in an accident and emergency department: The tip of an iceberg? *Br Med J* 285:1180, 1982.

Quevedo SF, Krauss DS, Chazan JA, et al: Fasting hypoglycemia secondary to disopyramide therapy: Report of two cases. *JAMA* 245:2424, 1981.

Ricci LR, Hoffman SA: Ethanol-induced hypoglycemic coma in a child. *Ann Emerg Med* 11:202, 1982.

Rizza RA, Cryer PE, Gerich JE: Role of glucagon, catecholamines, and growth hormone in human glucose counterregulation: Effects of somatostatin and combined α- and β-adrenergic blockade on plasma glucose recovery and glucose flux rates after insulin-induced hypoglycemia. *J Clin Invest* 64:62, 1979.

Rizza RA, Haymond MW, Verdonk CA, et al: Pathogenesis of hypoglycemia in insulinoma patients: Suppression of hepatic glucose production by insulin. *Diabetes* 30:377, 1981.

Rosenbloom AL, Giordano BP: Chronic overtreatment with insulin in children and adolescents. *Am J Dis Child* 131:881, 1977.

Rubenstein AH, Kuzuya H, Horwitz DL: Clinical significance of circulatory C-peptide in diabetes mellitus and hypoglycemic disorders. *Arch Intern Med* 137:625, 1977.

Rutsky EA, McDaniel HG, Tharpe DL, et al: Spontaneous hypoglycemia in chronic renal failure. *Arch Intern Med* 138:1364, 1978.

Santiago JV, Pereira MB, Avioli LV: Fasting hypoglycemia in adults. *Arch Intern Med* 142:465, 1982.

Scarlett JA, Mako ME, Rubenstein AH, et al: Factitious hypoglycemia: Diagnosis by measurement of serum C-peptide immunoreactivity and insulin-binding antibodies. *N Engl J Med* 297:1029, 1977.

Seltzer HS: Drug-induced hypoglycemia: A review based on 473 cases. *Diabetes* 21:955, 1972.

Senior B: Neonatal hypoglycemia. *N Engl J Med* 289:790, 1973.

Senior B, Wolfsdorf JI: Hypoglycemia in children. *Pediatr Clin North Am* 26:171, 1979.

Service FJ, Palumbo PJ: Factitial hypoglycemia: Three cases diagnosed on the basis of insulin antibodies. *Arch Intern Med* 134:336, 1974.

Service FJ, Dale AJD, Elveback LR, et al: Insulinoma: Clinical and diagnostic features of 60 consecutive cases. *Mayo Clin Proc* 51:417, 1976.

Silas JH, Grant DS, Maddocks JL: Transient hemiparetic attacks due to unrecognized nocturnal hypoglycaemia. *Br Med J* 282:132, 1981.

Skrabanek P, Powell D: Ectopic insulin and Occam's razor: Reappraisal of the riddle of tumour hypoglycaemia. *Clin Endocrinol* 9:141, 1978.

Skyler JS: Counterregulatory hormones, rebound hyperglycemia, and diabetic control. *Diabetes Care* 2:526, 1979.

Somogyi M: Exacerbation of diabetes by excess insulin action. *Am J Med* 26:169, 1959.

Siperstein MD, Foster DW, Knowles HC, et al: Control of blood glucose and diabetic vascular disease. *N Engl J Med* 296:1060, 1977.

Tattersall R: Brittle diabetes. *Clin Endocrinol Metab* 6:403, 1977.

Taylor JR, Sherratt HSA, Davies DM: Intramuscular or intravenous glucagon for sulphonylurea hypoglycaemia? *Eur J Clin Pharmacol* 14:125, 1978.

Taylor SI, Grunberger G, Marcus-Samuels B, et al: Hypoglycemia associated with antibodies to the insulin receptor. *N Engl J Med* 307:1422, 1982.

Tchobroutsky G, Goldgewicht C, Papoz L, et al: Hypoglycaemic reactions in 319 insulin treated diabetics. *Diabetologia* 21:335, 1981.

Travis LB: "Overcontrol" of juvenile diabetes mellitus. *South Med J* 68:767, 1975.

Turkington RW: Encephalopathy induced by oral hypoglycemic drugs. *Arch Intern Med* 137:1082, 1977.

Unger RH: The riddle of tumor hypoglycemia. *Am J Med* 40:325, 1966.

Unger RH: Meticulous control of diabetes: Benefits, risks, and precautions. *Diabetes* 31:479, 1982.

Viberti GC, Keen H, Bloom SR: Beta blockade and diabetes mellitus: Effect of oxprenolol and metoprolol on the metabolic, cardiovascular, and hormonal response to insulin-induced hypoglycemia in normal subjects. *Metabolism* 29:866, 1980.

Yager J, Young RT: Non-hypoglycemia is an epidemic condition. *N Engl J Med* 291:907, 1974.

CHAPTER 89
DIABETIC KETOACIDOSIS

Gene Ragland

Diabetic ketoacidosis is one of the most common and most studied endocrine emergencies. It occurs exclusively in the diabetic population and accounts for 14 percent of all diabetic hospital admissions in the United States. Diabetic ketoacidosis is characterized by hyperglycemia and ketonemia. A relative deficiency of insulin and a concurrent excess of stress hormones are responsible for the metabolic derangement. Therapy includes the replacement of insulin using low doses administered with various techniques.

Diabetic ketoacidosis may be the presenting manifestation of diabetes in an undiagnosed patient. It is seen more commonly in insulin-dependent diabetics. The greatest frequency of ketoacidosis is in the 0- to 19-year age group, which accounts for 65 percent of the estimated 40,000 patients admitted to U.S. hospitals for diabetic ketoacidosis each year.

PATHOGENESIS

The major metabolic abnormalities that occur during diabetic ketoacidosis are hyperglycemia and ketonemia. The metabolic derangements can be explained by relative insulin insufficiency and stress hormone excess. Insulin is the prime anabolic hormone and is responsible for the metabolism and storage of carbohydrates, fats, and proteins. The stress hormones, or counterregulatory hormones, are glucagon, catecholamines, cortisol, and growth hormone. Recent evidence implicates excess stress hormone secretion as a necessary event in the development of the severe metabolic decompensation seen in diabetic ketoacidosis.

Insulin

Ingested glucose is the primary stimulant of insulin release from the β cells of the pancreas. Insulin acts on the liver to facilitate the uptake of glucose and its conversion to glycogen. Insulin inhibits glycogen breakdown (glycogenolysis) and suppresses gluconeogenesis. The net effect of these actions is to promote the storage of glucose in the form of glycogen.

Insulin's effect on lipid metabolism is to increase lipogenesis in the liver and adipose cells and to simultaneously prevent lipolysis. Insulin promotes the production of triglycerides from free fatty acids and facilitates the storage of fat. The breakdown of triglycerides to free fatty acids and glycerol is inhibited by insulin. The overall result is the conversion of glucose to stored energy as triglycerides.

Insulin's action in protein metabolism is to stimulate the uptake of amino acids into muscle cells and to mediate the incorporation of amino acids into muscle protein. It prevents the release of amino acids from muscle protein and from hepatic protein sources.

Deficiency in the insulin-secretory mechanism of the β cells of the pancreas is the predominant lesion in diabetes mellitus. This defect results in insulin lack that may be partial or total.

Absolute insulin lack is rare but may be found in juvenile diabetics. In the typical maturity-onset diabetic patient, secretory failure involves primarily the initial rapid-release phase of insulin secretion. Minimal insulin inadequacy causes a decrease in the storage of body fuels, and β-cell failure is evident only by the abnormal response to a glucose load—abnormal glucose tolerance test (GTT). With more severe failure of insulin secretion, not only is fuel storage impaired, but fuel stores are mobilized during fasting, resulting in hyperglycemia. The increase in the blood glucose level is due to increased glycogenolysis and may elicit an increase in insulin secretion if β-cell reserve is present. The glucose metabolism and concentration may then return to normal.

When there is an absolute or relative failure of insulin secretion, hyperglycemia does not produce increased insulin activity. Loss of the normal physiologic effects of insulin results in catabolism, and hyperglycemia and ketonemia occur.

Stress Hormones

During insulin insufficiency, glucose transport into the cells is inhibited. The physiologic response to cellular starvation and other stresses is to increase the hormones glucagon, catecholamines, cortisol, and growth hormone. These hormones are grouped as counterregulatory hormones because of their antiinsulin effects. The relative roles of each and their mechanisms of action in diabetic ketoacidosis have not been completely elucidated. However, glucagon in excess has been implicated as the main hormone contributing to hyperglycemia and ketonemia. There is considerable evidence to support the hypothesis that excess counterregulatory hormone secretion, in conjunction with relative insulin deficiency, is an essential requisite to the development of diabetic ketoacidosis.

This evidence includes the failure of diabetic animals to develop ketoacidosis in the absence of counterregulatory hormones, the fact that at least one of these hormones has been found to be elevated in every case of diabetic ketoacidosis in which they were measured, a delay or reduction of ketoacidosis with pharmacologic blockade of individual stress hormones, and an increase in keto-genic activity when each of the counterregulatory hormones is infused in high physiologic concentrations. Additional evidence to support the role of these hormones in the genesis of diabetic ketoacidosis includes the fact that plasma insulin levels are not always below normal during diabetic ketoacidosis. In fact, no correlation has been reported between the plasma level of insulin during diabetic ketoacidosis and the severity of the ketoacidosis. Finally, the association between antecedent stress and diabetic ketoacidosis has long been recognized. Secretion of the counter-regulatory hormones characterizes all major forms of stress.

The counterregulatory hormones are catabolic and, in general, reverse the physiologic processes promoted by insulin. They affect carbohydrate metabolism by increasing glycogenolysis and gluconeogenesis, thereby raising the blood glucose level. Lipolysis is stimulated by glucagon and catecholamines, and this results in increased free fatty acids for conversion to ketones. Protein breakdown is accelerated and provides amino acids for gluconeogenesis. The net effect of relative insulin insufficiency and excess counterregulatory hormones is hyperglycemia and ketonemia (see Fig. 89-1).

Hyperglycemia occurs earlier than ketonemia during diabetic ketoacidosis. Glucose is underutilized because of insulin lack and overproduced because of enhanced glycogenolysis and gluconeogenesis. Gluconeogenesis is facilated by increased levels of glucogenic precursors such as glycerol and amino acids resulting from unopposed lipolysis and proteolysis.

Ketonemia occurs because of increased lipolysis and ketogenesis. Insulin deficiency and excess stress hormones lead to the breakdown of triglycerides and the release of large amounts of fatty acids into the circulation. These fatty acids are assimilated in the liver, where they are converted to ketone bodies. The peripheral utilization of ketones is decreased during insulin insufficiency, and they accumulate in the usual 3:1 ratio (β-hydroxy-butyrate to acetoacetate).

PRECIPITATING FACTORS

Factors known to precipitate diabetic ketoacidosis include omission of daily insulin injections and a variety of stressful events. Müller and co-workers in an investigation of the causes of human ketoacidosis identified some type of stress in 24 of 26 patients. Hockaday and Alberti found infection to be the cause of diabetic ketoacidosis in 56 percent of patients, and withdrawal of insulin to be the cause in 7 percent. Omission of insulin may be the primary factor causing diabetic ketoacidosis, or it may occur in response to other events and hasten the onset of diabetic ketoacidosis. In addition to infections, other stresses identified with the onset of diabetic ketoacidosis include cerebrovascular accidents, myocardial infarction, trauma, pregnancy, hyperthyroidism, pancreatitis, and emotional upset. An antecedent etiologic event may not be identified in some instances. Genuth reported that 35 percent of patients had no clear precipitating cause of diabetic ketoacidosis.

CLINICAL PRESENTATION

Most of the clinical manifestations of diabetic ketoacidosis can be related to the biochemical derangements. Hyperglycemia causes an increased osmotic load, and intracellular water is lost because cellular membranes are not freely permeable to glucose. In addition, osmotic diuresis produces total body fluid depletion. Dehydration, hypotension, and reflex tachycardia are the consequences. Osmotic diuresis also causes loss of sodium, chloride, potassium, phosphorus, calcium, and magnesium. The serum sodium level may be further decreased by a dilution effect in response to the hyperglycemia. The dilutional effect is a serum sodium decrease of about 5 mEq/L for every 180 mg/dL increase of blood glucose. Electrolyte loss may be worsened by repeated bouts of vomiting.

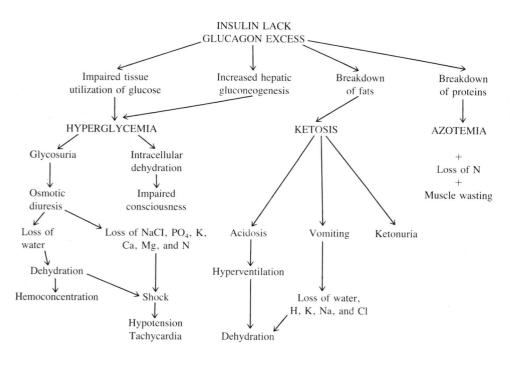

Figure 89-1. Metabolic consequences of insulin lack, accelerated by glucagon excess. (From Baruh S, Sherman L, Markowitz S: Diabetic ketoacidosis and coma. *Med Clin North Am* 65:117, 1981.

Ketonemia also produces clinical manifestations. Dissociation of hydrogen ions from circulating ketone bodies is responsible for the development of acidosis and the fall in the serum bicarbonate level. Some of the ketone bodies are oxidized to acetone, a neutral, soluble, volatile substance that causes the characteristic fruity odor on the breath of a patient with ketoacidosis. Hepatomegaly due to accumulation of fat within the liver may occur and should resolve with reversal of ketogenesis.

Acidosis produces other clinical consequences. Compensatory hyperventilation is commonly seen. Exchange of H^+ ions for K^+ ions across the intracellular membrane is partially responsible for the elevated serum potassium level seen in patients in diabetic ketoacidosis. Peripheral vasodilatation and vascular collapse can result from acidosis.

Some of the clinical manifestations seen during diabetic ketoacidosis have no clear explanation. There is no apparent correlation between the state of consciousness of the patient and the degree of ketonemia, hyperglycemia, electrolyte imbalance, or acidosis. The most direct correlation is with serum osmolality. Some degree of mental confusion or coma is more likely with serum osmolality levels above 340 mOsm/kg.

Nausea, vomiting, and abdominal pain are common presenting complaints. The cause of these disturbances is not clear. Gastric dilatation, paralytic ileus, and abdominal tenderness may be present. Although pancreatitis may develop as a result of ketoacidosis, the diagnosis is difficult since the serum amylase level and the amylase clearance can be elevated in both conditions. Of course, the reverse can occur, so that acute inflammatory or hemorrhagic pancreatitis can result in ketoacidosis. In general, abdominal signs and symptoms should disappear with the resolution of ketoacidosis, and carefully repeated evaluation is necessary to rule out a serious intrarabdominal disorder.

Finally, inappropriate normothermia is a clinical finding that is not well understood. Only 10 percent of patients have an elevated temperature in spite of the fact that infection is the most common precipitating factor of diabetic ketoacidosis. Absence of an elevated temperature may obscure the presence of an underlying infection. Therefore, infection must be actively searched for regardless of the patient's temperature.

Diabetic ketoacidosis may develop rapidly or over a few days. If the patient is able to maintain an adequate fluid and salt intake, a state of compensated ketosis may develop. During the early stages of ketoacidosis or when nausea and vomiting occur, the patient may decrease or omit insulin, thus hastening full-blown diabetic ketoacidosis. The typical patient has nausea, vomiting, abdominal pain, weight loss, dehydration, hypotension, tachycardia, hyperventilation or Kussmaul's respirations, and the odor of acetone on the breath.

LABORATORY

Laboratory abnormalities that are always present during diabetic ketoacidosis include elevated levels of blood glucose, β-hydroxybutyrate, and acetoacetate. Similarly, glucosuria and ketonuria are consistent findings. A decreased pH, low serum bicarbonate level, and decreased P_{CO_2} are present because of metabolic acidosis with respiratory compensation.

The serum sodium level is variable. More water is lost than solutes, and even if the serum sodium level is low, the patient is hypertonic. Initially, the serum potassium level is usually elevated

or normal, but it falls as the acidosis is corrected and potassium shifts intracellularly. The serum chloride level may be low if excessive vomiting has occurred. An increased anion gap acidosis is present because of ketonemia.

The diagnosis of diabetic ketoacidosis should be suspected based upon the clinical presentation previously described. Confirmatory laboratory findings include a blood glucose level greater than 300 mg/dL, a bicarbonate level less than 15 mEq/L, a serum acetone level greater than 2:1 dilution, and a pH less than 7.3. Venous blood should be drawn for a complete blood cell count and determinations of serum glucose, electrolytes, blood urea nitrogen (BUN), creatinine, phosphorus, and acetone. An arterial blood sample should be obtained for measurement of the pH and the carbon dioxide and oxygen tension levels. Urinalysis and a chest roentgenogram to search for infection, and an ECG to look for changes due to acute myocardial infarction and hyperkalemia, are necessary.

Differential Diagnosis

The differential diagnosis of the metabolic cause of coma in a diabetic patient includes hypoglycemic coma, nonketotic hyperosmolar coma, alcoholic ketoacidosis, and lactic acidosis. All these are life-threatening emergencies that require prompt recognition and treatment.

A rapid, reasonably accurate differentiation between these entities can be made in the emergency department (Fig. 89-2). The result of the analysis of blood gases should be available in a few minutes, and acidosis, if present, will be confirmed. While the physician is awaiting other laboratory results, a drop of blood can be tested for blood glucose and serum ketones.

Several reagent strips that measure blood glucose levels are currently available. The reacted strip can be interpreted visually by comparing it with a color chart, or can be read in a reflectance meter. Visual interpretation can only achieve a range rather than a precise number, but this method does reliably distinguish between hyperglycemic and hypoglycemic levels. Semiquantitative estimation of serum ketones can be made by testing a drop of blood with a nitroprusside-impregnated tablet. It should be remembered that the nitroprusside reaction measures acetoacetate but not β-hydroxybutyrate. This test can be misleading if most of the serum ketones are in the form of β-hydroxybutyrate. Additionally, lactic acidosis may occur simultaneously with diabetic ketoacidosis. Measurement of serum lactate levels may be indicated to determine the contribution of lactic acid to the metabolic

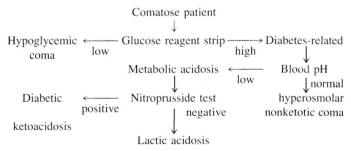

Figure 89-2. Differential diagnosis of metabolic causes of coma in a diabetic patient. (Adapted from Skillman TG: Diabetic ketoacidosis. *Heart Lung* 7:598, 1978).

acidosis. Finally, in mixed acid-base disturbance, the pH may not accurately reflect the degree of acidosis. The anion gap can assist in identifying unmeasured acids.

TREATMENT

Once the diagnosis of diabetic ketoacidosis has been established, thereapy must be started without delay. Specific therapeutic goals for diabetic ketoacidosis include rehydration and restoration of adequate intravascular volume, correction of electrolyte and acid-base imbalance, reversal of the metabolic consequences of insulin insufficiency, and avoidance of complications of therapy. Appropriate treatment of a precipitating cause of diabetic ketoacidosis must not be overlooked.

A variety of therapeutic approaches are advocated. Regardless of the approach used, frequent monitoring of the effects is essential. The levels of blood glucose, ketone bodies, potassium, and carbon dioxide should be determined every 1 to 2 h until recovery is well-established. A flow sheet to record vital signs, level of consciousness, intake and output, therapeutic measures, and blood chemistry determinations is recommended. Complete clearing of hyperglycemia and ketonemia usually requires 8 to 16 h.

Fluid Administration

Rapid fluid administration is the most important initial step in the treatment of diabetic ketoacidosis. The average patient in diabetic ketoacidosis has a water deficit of 5 to 10 L and a sodium deficit of 450 to 500 mEq. Normal saline is the most frequently recommended fluid for initial rehydration even though the extracellular fluid of the patient is hypertonic. The normal saline does not provide "free water" to correct intracellular dehydration, but it does prevent a too-rapid fall in extracellular osmolality and excessive transfer of water into the CNS. Some authors favor alternating the administration of normal saline with the administration of half-normal saline. Others recommend the use of half-normal saline plus enough bicarbonate to create a slightly hypotonic solution; this fluid combination is especially useful if the patient has severe acidosis.

The first liter of fluid should be administered rapidly, usually over half an hour. During the first 3 to 4 h, 3 to 5 L of fluid may be required. The blood glucose level and ketone body concentration fall after fluid administration and before implementation of any other therapeutic modality. With rehydration, tissue perfusion is restored, improving the effectiveness of insulin, and renal blood flow increases, allowing the excretion of ketone bodies.

The fluid should be changed to a hypotonic solution after the initial replacement of intravascular volume or if the serum sodium level is 155 mEq/L. Central venous pressure should be monitored during fluid replacement in elderly patients or in those with known heart disease.

Bicarbonate

Sodium bicarbonate is given to correct the negative effects of acidosis. At a pH of 7, peripheral vasodilatation, decreased cardiac output, and hypotension can occur. Respiratory and CNS depression can occur with severe acidosis (pH less than 6.8).

Caution must be used with the administration of sodium bicarbonate, since the attendant hazards of excessive alkali replacement can outweigh the potential benefits.

The hazards of bicarbonate administration include paradoxical spinal fluid acidosis, hypokalemia, impaired oxyhemoglobin dissociation, rebound alkalosis, and sodium overload.

It has been established that cerebrospinal fluid (CSF) acidosis is deleterious to brain function. Systemic acidosis per se does not cause mental aberration as long as the CSF is protected against large pH changes. When sodium bicarbonate is administered in large doses, the carbon dioxide loss is diminished, and extracellular fluid and levels of carbon dioxide and bicarbonate increase. Carbon dioxide diffuses freely across the blood-brain barrier, but bicarbonate difuses into the CSF much more slowly. The difference in the rates of movement into the spinal fluid results in an increase in CSF carbonic acid, a fall in CSF pH, and paradoxical spinal fluid acidosis.

Alkali administration causes a shift of potassium intracellularly. In a patient who already has total body potassium depletion, hazardous hypokalemia could result. During acidosis, the oxyhemoglobin dissociation curve shifts to the right, facilitating the offloading of oxygen at the tissue level. This beneficial effect of acidosis could be lost with sudden restoration of the pH toward normal. Final complications of excessive sodium bicarbonate administration include overcompensated rebound alkalosis and sodium overload.

Current recommendations are to administer sodium bicarbonate in modest amounts, i.e., 44 to 100 mEq, when the pH is less than 7. Remember that hydrogen ion production ceases when ketogenesis stops, that excessive hydrogen ions are eliminated through the urine and through the respiratory tract, and that ketone body metabolism results in the endogenous production of alkali.

Potassium

Virtually all patients with diabetic ketoacidosis have a deficiency of total body potassium. This deficit is created by acidosis, diuresis, and frequent vomiting. The deficient ranges from 400 to 1000 mEq, or an average of 5 to 10 mEq/kg. Potassium deficit is rarely evident in the initial determination of the serum potassium level. That value is usually normal or high because of a deficit of body fluid, diminished renal function, and intracellular exchange of potassium for hydrogen ions during acidosis. Hypokalemia in this clinical setting is an indicator of severe total body potassium depletion, and massive amounts of potassium for replacement are required during the next 24 h.

The goals of potassium replacement are to maintain a normal extracellular potassium concentration during the acute phases of therapy and to replace the intracellular deficit over a period of days or weeks. It is well known that with initiation of therapy for diabetic ketoacidosis, the serum potassium concentration falls. This is due to dilution of extracellular fluid, correction of acidosis, increased urinary loss of potassium, and the action of insulin in promoting reentry of potassium into the cells. If these changes occur too rapidly, precipitous hypokalemia may result in fatal cardiac arrhythmias, respiratory paralysis, and paralytic ileus. These complications are avoidable if the pathophysiology is understood and the effects of therapy are frequently monitored.

The ability of insulin to drive potassium into the cells is directly proportional to the insulin concentration. This factor has added support to the advocates of low-dose insulin techniques. Low-dose insulin therapy provides greater stabilization of the extracellular potassium concentration during the early stages of therapy.

Early potassium replacement is now a standard modality of care. Some authors recommend that small doses of potassium (20 mEq) be added to the intravenous fluid given initially. Others favor administering potassium within the first 2 to 3 h, when insulin therapy is initiated, or after volume expansion has been accomplished. If oliguria is present, renal function must be evaluated and potassium replacement must be decreased. Potassium determinations every 1 to 2 h and continuous ECG monitoring for changes reflecting the potassium concentration should be employed. From 100 to 200 mEq of potassium during the first 12 to 24 h is usually required. Occasionally, as much as 500 mEq of potassium may be necessary.

Insulin

The absence of the normal physiologic actions of insulin because of insulin deficiency results in the biochemical and clinical manifestations of diabetic ketoacidosis. Replacement of this deficient hormone is essential to reverse hyperglycemia and ketonemia and restore normal metabolic homeostasis. The amount of insulin required to achieve this therapeutic goal, the frequency of administration, and the route by which it should be administered have been widely debated for the last few years.

It should be emphasized that familiarity with a particular regimen, continuous monitoring, and attention to detail are the most important factors in successfully treating a patient in diabetic ketoacidosis. The amount and route of insulin administration are of secondary importance.

The traditional approach to insulin therapy recommends large doses of a rapidly acting insulin based upon the patient's state of consciousness and the degree of ketonemia. As much as 50 to 300 units are administered every 2 to 4 h. It is now clear that large doses of insulin are not required to reverse the metabolic derangements of diabetic ketoacidosis and that complications such as hypoglycemia and hypokalemia occur more frequently with large-dose insulin therapy.

Low-dose insulin techniques for treatment of diabetic ketoacidosis are generally simple, safe, and effective. Techniques for continuous intravenous infusion and intramuscular, subcutaneous, and intravenous bolus therapy have been developed. This approach has been used successfully in both adults and children.

The main arguments against the use of large doses of insulin are that they are not needed, they are less physiologic, and they produce more complications than low doses. It has been established that blood insulin concentrations of 20 to 200 microunits/mL inhibit gluconeogenesis and lipogenesis, stimulate the uptake of potassium by peripheral tissues, and achieve maximum rates of fall of blood glucose concentrations. Large-dose insulin regimens produce insulin levels of 250 to 3000 microunits/mL, far in excess of the concentration required for maximum therapeutic benefit. A continuous insulin infusion of 1 unit/h raises the plasma insulin concentration by 20 microunits/mL. Similarly, 5 units/h produces a therapeutic level of 100 microunits/mL. This level is generally sufficient to achieve normal metabolic homeostasis.

The half-life of insulin given intravenously is 4 to 5 min, with an effective biological half-life at the tissue level of approximately

20 to 30 min. Traditional intravenous bolus therapy every 2 to 4 h produces an uneven, intermittent insulin effect.

Finally, there is an increased incidence of complications associated with large doses of insulin. These include hypoglycemia, hypokalemia, and osmotic disequilibrium. The incidence of hypoglycemia with large-dose insulin therapy is 25 percent in most studies. Hypoglycemia using low-dose insulin techniques is almost nonexistent. A similar incidence of about 25 percent hypokalemia is reported with large-dose insulin therapy. With low-dose insulin therapies the occurrence of hypokalemia is less than 5 percent. Lastly, rapid shifts of glucose levels induced by large doses of insulin are more likely to produce osmotic disequilibrium and consequences such as cerebral edema. The more gradual, even insulin effect achieved by low-dose therapy avoids rapid fluid shifts and results in fewer complications.

All low-dose insulin techniques are effective in reversing the metabolic consequences of insulin insufficiency (see Fig. 89-3). All the various techniques have stated advantages, but continuous intravenous or intramuscular approaches have the most favorable outcome.

In continuous intravenous infusion of low doses of insulin, 5 to 10 units of regular insulin are administered per hour. [In children the dose of insulin is 0.1 unit/kg·h)]. The effect of insulin begins almost immediately after the initiation of the infusion, and a "priming" IV bolus is not required. Continuous insulin administration ensures that a steady blood concentration is maintained in an effective range, and this technique allows flexibility in adjusting the insulin dose. When the infusion is stopped, the insulin already in the blood is quickly degraded, providing greater control of the amount of insulin given in comparison to the intramuscular or subcutaneous routes.

Serious complications with continuous low-dose insulin infusion are minimal. The main disadvantage is that it requires an infusion pump and frequent monitoring to ensure that insulin is being administered in the desired amount. A separate intravenous site for the insulin infusion is desirable but not required.

The technique of low-dose intramuscular or subcutaneous in-

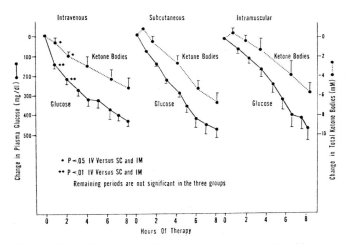

Figure 89-3. Change in levels of plasma glucose and total ketone bodies (β-hydroxybutyrate plus acetoacetate) after intravenous, subcutaneous, or intramuscular low-dose insulin therapy (15 patients in each group). (From Fisher JN, Shahshahani MN, Kitabchi AE: Diabetic ketoacidosis: Low-dose insulin therapy by various routes. *N Engl J Med* 297:238, 1977.)

sulin therapy is better suited to a hospital environment in which constant nursing supervision is not always possible. The main disadvantage to this approach, more marked with the subcutaneous route, is that insulin absorption may be erratic in a hypotensive, peripherally vasoconstricted patient. Erratic absorption may result in a delay in achieving adequate insulin levels. Further, delayed absorption can produce deposits of insulin that may later be absorbed, causing hypoglycemia. These problems can largely be eliminated by ensuring adequate hydration of the patient and by using small enough doses of insulin to preclude accumulation of large insulin deposits.

The onset of action of insulin given intramuscularly is delayed in comparison to that of insulin given intravenously. The most current protocols recommend an initial dose of 20 units of insulin intramuscularly, intravenously, or divided between these routes, followed by 5 to 10 units/h intramuscularly. The half-life of insulin given intramuscularly is 2 h. Hourly injections produce a continuous, effective blood concentration of insulin.

There are common problems with insulin therapy regardless of the technique used. The incidence of nonresponders to low-dose therapies is 1 to 2 percent. This low incidence suggests that the problem of insulin resistance has been exaggerated. If the patient fails to respond to low-dose insulin therapy in the first hour, most protocols recommend doubling the infusion rate or administering an intravenous bolus of insulin. The insulin dose is increased in a similar fashion each hour until a satisfactory response is achieved. The presence of infection is the main reason for failure to respond to low-dose insulin therapy.

Glucose should be added to the intravenous fluid when the blood glucose concentration falls to 250 mg/dL. Insulin therapy should not be stopped just because the blood glucose level declines but should be continued until the ketonemia and acidosis have cleared. Intravenous insulin should not be abruptly discontinued. An overlap period in which subcutaneous insulin is given should precede discontinuation of the insulin infusion.

Phosphate Replacement

The role of phosphate replacement during the treatment of diabetic ketoacidosis remains controversial. One author estimates that up to 90 percent of patients have acute hypophosphatemia within 6 to 12 h after initiation of therapy for diabetic ketoacidosis. The decrease is primarily due to a sudden shift of phosphate from the extracellular to the intracellular compartment following insulin administration and accelerated glucose storage. Phosphate is found in all body tissues, and this sudden shift deprives them of this essential constituent. Hypophosphatemia is usually most severe 24 to 48 h after the start of insulin therapy.

Phosphate plays an integral part in the conversion of energy from adenosine triphosphate (ATP) and in the delivery of oxygen at the tissue level through 2,3-diphosphoglyceric acid (2,3-DPG). In addition, many important enzymes, cofactors, and biochemical intermediates depend upon phosphate. Acute phosphate deficiency has been associated with a variety of clinical disorders including neuromuscular paralysis leading to respiratory failure and possibly myocardial dysfunction.

Acute hypophosphatemia can be corrected by intravenous or oral administration of phosphorus. Several oral forms are available but may cause diarrhea and be erratically absorbed. A commercial intravenous preparation (KH_2PO_4 plus K_2HPO_4) containing K^+ at a concentration of 4 mEq/mL and phosphorus at a concentration of 96 mg/mL can be used. Five milliliters of this commercial potassium phosphate preparation added to 1 L of intravenous fluid provides approximately 20 mEq of K^+ and 480 mg of PO_4^{2+}.

Hypophosphatemia is not associated with untoward consequences until a serum concentration of less than 1.0 mg/dL is reached. Phosphorus supplementation is not indicated and should not be given as long as the level remains above this concentration. Some authors have recommended the use of potassium phosphate salts instead of potassium chloride as a means of potassium replacement during therapy for diabetic ketoacidosis. Early routine use of potassium phosphate solutions to replace potassium should be discouraged. The need for phosphorus replacement, if at all, occurs several hours after therapy for diabetic ketoacidosis has begun, and potassium is usually required much sooner.

Several undesirable side effects from phosphate administration have been reported. These include hyperphosphatemia, hypocalcemia, hypomagnesemia, metastatic soft tissue calcifications, and hypernatremia and dehydration from osmotic diuresis. The serum phosphate level should be monitored during treatment of diabetic ketoacidosis, but the case for routine phosphate replacement has not been made.

COMPLICATIONS AND MORTALITY

Complications related to the disease state include aspiration of gastric contents by an unconscious patient, vascular stasis and deep vein thrombosis, and disseminated intravascular coagulation (DIC). Protection of the airway and evacuation of gastric contents are indicated in an unconscious patient. Prophylactic heparin therapy may help to prevent thrombotic complications.

Major complications related to the therapy of diabetic ketoacidosis include hypokalemia, paradoxical spinal fluid acidosis, and cerebral edema. These complications are usually due to excessive or too-vigorous therapeutic measures and are largely preventable. The goal of therapy of diabetic ketoacidosis is to produce a gradual, even return to normal metabolic balance. Rapid shifts of the levels of water, electrolytes, and other solutes can be avoided by using isotonic saline as the initial intravenous fluid, refraining from excessive bicarbonate administration, replacing potassium early in the course of treatment, and using low-dose insulin techniques. Above all, a basic understanding of the pathophysiology of diabetic ketoacidosis, constant monitoring of the patient, and attention to detail are essential to prevent complications of treatment of diabetic acidosis.

Diabetic ketoacidosis was invariably fatal prior to the introduction of insulin in 1922. Today in the best medical centers the mortality for patients in diabetic ketoacidosis is 5 to 15 percent. In less specialized centers the mortality may be as high as 20 to 30 percent, and in patients over 60 years of age, a 50 percent mortality from diabetic ketoacidosis is not uncommon.

In general, the greater the presenting serum osmolality, BUN, and blood glucose concentration, the greater the mortality. There is also increased mortality for patients presenting with a serum bicarbonate level of less than 10 mEq/L.

Of the factors responsible for precipitating diabetic ketoacidosis, infection and myocardial infarction are the main contributors to high mortality. Half the patients in diabetic ketoacidosis die when myocardial infarction is the precipitating event. Additional factors that reduce the chances of survival include old age, severe hypotension, prolonged and severe coma, and underlying medical problems, especially renal and cardiovascular disease.

PREVENTION

During the last few years, several developments in the outpatient management of insulin-dependent diabetics have occurred. These new approaches are directed toward a more even control of blood glucose levels in hopes of reducing the long-term complications of diabetes. These methods may also decrease the incidence of diabetic ketoacidosis and reduce the estimated 4000 deaths that occur in the United States each year because of diabetic ketoacidosis.

Conventional treatment of diabetes on an outpatient basis involves one or two injections of insulin per day and monitoring of urine glucose levels by the patient. Intensive management consists of self-monitoring of blood glucose levels and adjustment of insulin doses on the basis of the determinations. A drop of blood from a finger stick or earlobe prick is placed on a glucose reagent strip which can be read visually or in a reflectance meter. This method is more accurate than monitoring the urine glucose level and compares favorably with glucose determinations done in the laboratory. Insulin can be administered as two or more manual injections per day or as a continuous subcutaneous infusion via a portable pump.

Prevention of diabetic ketoacidosis also depends upon the reaction of the patient and the physician when the patient first detects metabolic decompensation (hyperglycemia, glucosuria, ketonuria) or comes under stress (infection, etc). Preventative measures under these circumstances include the substitution of regular insulin for intermediate-acting insulin and the monitoring of blood or urine glucose levels every 4 h. Patients should be instructed not to stop their insulin. Adequate caloric and fluid intake is important and can best be achieved with clear liquids supplemented with glucose as needed. Stress can be reduced by the use of antibiotics if infection is present and by controlling fever with antipyretics.

The outpatient can follow some parameters that may indicate the need for hospitalization. The patient's weight can be determined, and if the weight loss exceeds 5 percent of the usual body weight, severe dehydration is present. The inability to maintain hydration requires hospitalization. Other indicators include a basal respiratory rate exceeding 36/min, which would reflect compensatory hyperventilation in response to acidosis, and any change in the level of consciousness. The goal of prevention of diabetic ketoacidosis is worthy of aggressive pursuit. The emergency physician is in an ideal position to assist in this endeavor.

BIBLIOGRAPHY

Alberti KGMM: Low-dose insulin in the treatment of diabetic ketoacidosis. *Arch Intern Med* 137:1367, 1977.

Alberti KGMM, Hockaday TDR: Diabetic coma: A reappraisal after five years. *Clin Endocrinol Metab* 6:421, 1977.

Alberti KGMM, Hockaday TDR: Rapid blood ketone estimation in the diagnosis of diabetic ketoacidosis. *Br Med J* 2:565, 1972.

Alberti KGMM, Nattrass M: Severe diabetic ketoacidosis. *Med Clin North Am* 62:799, 1978.

Alberti KGMM, Hockaday TDR, Turner RC: Small doses of intramuscular insulin in the treatment of diabetic "coma." *Lancet* 2:515, 1973.

Alberti KGMM, Christensen NJ, Iversen J, et al: Role of glucagon and other hormones in development of diabetic ketoacidosis. *Lancet* 1:1307, 1975.

Ammon RA, May WS, Nightingale SD: Glucose-induced hyperkalemia with normal aldosterone levels. *Ann Intern Med* 89:349, 1978.

Asplin CM, Hartog M: Serum free insulin concentration during the treatment of diabetic coma and precoma with low dose intramuscular insulin. *Diabetologia* 13:475, 1977.

Assal JP, Aoki TT, Manzano FM, et al: Metabolic effects of sodium bicarbonate in management of diabetic ketoacidosis. *Diabetes* 23:405, 1974.

Barnes AJ, Kohner EM, Bloom SR, et al: Importance of pituitary hormones in aetiology of diabetic ketoacidosis. *Lancet* 1:1171, 1978.

Baruh S, Sherman L, Markowitz S: Diabetic ketoacidosis and coma. *Med Clin North Am* 65:117, 1981.

Beigelman PM: Potassium in severe diabetic ketoacidosis. *Am J Med* 54:419, 1973.

Beigelman PM: Severe diabetic ketoacidosis (diabetic "coma"): 482 episodes in 257 patients; experience of three years. *Diabetes* 20:490, 1971.

Bendezu R, Wieland RG, Furst BH, et al: Experience with low-dose insulin infusion in diabetic ketoacidosis and diabetic hyperosmolarity. *Arch Intern Med* 138:60, 1978.

Bureau MA, Bégin R, Berthiaume Y, et al: Cerebral hypoxia from bicarbonate infusion in diabetic ketoacidosis. *J Pediatr* 96:968, 1980.

Christensen NJ: Plasma norepinephrine and epinephrine in untreated diabetics, during fasting and after insulin administration. *Diabetes* 23:1, 1974.

Chupin M, Charbonnel B, Chupin F: C-peptide blood levels in ketoacidosis and in hyperosmolar non-ketotic diabetic coma. *Acta Diabetol Lat* 18:123, 1981.

Clements RS, Vourganti B: Fatal diabetic ketoacidosis: Major causes and approaches to their prevention. *Diabetes Care* 1:314, 1978.

Clumeck N, Detroyer A, Naeije R, et al: Treatment of diabetic coma with small intravenous insulin boluses. *Br Med J* 2:394, 1976.

Defronzo RA, Lang R: Hypophosphatemia and glucose intolerance: Evidence for tissue insensitivity to insulin. *N Engl J Med* 303:1259, 1980.

Defronzo RA, Sherwin RS, Felig P, et al: Nonuremic diabetic hyperkalemia: Possible role of insulin deficiency. *Arch Intern Med* 137:842, 1977.

Ditzel J, Standl E: The oxygen transport system of red blood cells during diabetic ketoacidosis and recovery. *Diabetologia* 11:255, 1975.

Drop SLS, Duval-Arnould BJM, Gober AE, et al: Low-dose intravenous insulin infusion versus subcutaneous insulin injection: A controlled comparative study of diabetic ketoacidosis. *Pediatrics* 59:733, 1977.

Duck SC, Weldon VV, Pagliara AS, et al: Cerebral edema complicating therapy for diabetic ketoacidosis. *Diabetes* 25:111, 1976.

Dupre J, Champion M, Rodger NW: Advances in insulin delivery in the management of diabetes mellitus. *Clin Endocrinol Metab* 11:525, 1982.

Edwards GA, Kohaut EC, Wehring B, et al: Effectiveness of low-dose continuous intravenous insulin infusion in diabetic ketoacidosis: A prospective comparative study. *J Pediatr* 91:701, 1977.

Fein IA, Rackow EC, Sprung CL, et al: Relation of colloid osmotic pressure to arterial hypoxemia and cerebral edema during crystalloid volume loading of patients with diabetic ketoacidosis. *Ann Intern Med* 96:570, 1982.

Felig P: Diabetic ketoacidosis. *N Engl J Med* 290:1360, 1974.

Felig P: Insulin: Rates and routes of delivery. *N Engl J Med* 291:1031, 1974.

Felig P: Pathophysiology of diabetes mellitus. *Med Clin North Am* 4:821, 1971.

Felig P, Bergman M: Intensive ambulatory treatment of insulin-dependent diabetes. *Ann Intern Med* 97:225, 1982.

Fisher JN, Shahshahani MN, Kitabachi AE: Diabetic ketoacidosis: Low-dose insulin therapy by various routes. *N Engl J Med* 297:238, 1977.

Fort P, Waters SM, Lifshitz F: Low-dose insulin infusion in the treatment of diabetic ketoacidosis: Bolus versus no bolus. *J Pediatr* 96:36, 1980.

Genuth SM: Constant intravenous insulin infusion in diabetic ketoacidosis. *JAMA* 223:1348, 1973.

Gerich JE, Lorenzi M, Bier DM, et al: Prevention of human diabetic ketoacidosis by somatostatin: Evidence for an essential role of glucagon. *N Engl J Med* 292:985, 1975.

Giammarco R, Goldstein MB, Halperin ML, et al: Renal tubular acidosis during therapy for diabetic ketoacidosis. *Can Med Assoc J* 112:463, 1975.

Gibby OM, Veale KEA, Hayes TM, et al: Oxygen availability from the blood and the effect of phosphate replacement on erythrocyte 2, 3-diphosphoglycerate and haemoglobin-oxygen affinity in diabetic ketoacidosis. *Diabetologia* 15:381, 1978.

Ginsberg HN: Investigation of insulin resistance during diabetic ketoacidosis: Role of counterregulatory substances and effect of insulin therapy. *Metabolism* 26:1135, 1977.

Gonzalez-Villalpando C, Blachley JD, Vaughan GM, et al: Low- and high-dose intravenous insulin therapy for diabetic ketoacidosis. *JAMA* 241:925, 1979.

Guerra SMO, Kitabchi AE: Comparison of the effectiveness of various routes of insulin injection: Insulin levels and glucose response in normal subjects. *J Clin Endocrinol Metab* 42:869, 1976.

Halperin ML, Bear RA, Hannaford MC, et al: Selected aspects of the pathophysiology of metabolic acidosis in diabetes mellitus. *Diabetes* 30:781, 1981.

Hamburger S: Diabetic ketoacidosis. *J Am Med Wom Assoc* 34:109, 1979.

Harrower ADB: Treatment of diabetic ketoacidosis by direct addition of insulin to intravenous infusion. A comparison of ''high dose'' and ''low dose'' techniques. *Br J Clin Pract* 33:85, 1979.

Heber D, Molitch ME, Sperling MA: Low-dose continuous insulin therapy for diabetic ketoacidosis. *Arch Intern Med* 137:1377, 1977.

Hockaday TDR, Alberti KGMM: Diabetic coma. *Clin Endocrinol Metab* 1:751, 1972.

James RC, Chase GR: Evaluation of some commonly used semiquantitative methods for urinary glucose and ketone determinations. *Diabetes* 23:474, 1974.

Johnston DG, Alberti KGMM: Hormonal control of ketone body metabolism in the normal and diabetic state. *Clin Endocrinol Metab* 11:329, 1982.

Johnston DG, Alberti KGMM: Diabetic emergencies: Practical aspects of the management of diabetic ketoacidosis and diabetes during surgery. *Clin Endocrinol Metab* 9:437, 1980.

Kanter Y, Gerson JR, Bessman AN: 2,3-Diphosphoglycerate, nucleotide phosphate, and organic and inorganic phosphate levels during the early phases of diabetic ketoacidosis. *Diabetes* 26:429, 1977.

Kappy MS, Lightner ES: Low-dose intravenous insulin in the treatment of diabetic ketoacidosis. *Am J Dis Child* 133:523, 1979.

Kaye R: Diabetic ketoacidosis—The bicarbonate controversy. *J Pediatr* 87:156, 1975.

Keller U, Berger W: Prevention of hypophosphatemia by phosphate infusion during treatment of diabetic ketoacidosis and hyperosmolar coma. *Diabetes* 29:87, 1980.

Keller U, Berger W, Ritz R, et al: Course and prognosis of 86 episodes of diabetic coma: A five year experience with a uniform schedule of treatment. *Diabetologia* 11:93, 1975.

Kitabchi AE, Ayyagari V, Guerra SMO: The efficacy of low-dose versus conventional therapy of insulin for treatment of diabetic ketoacidosis. *Ann Intern Med* 84:633, 1976.

Kitabchi AE, Young R, Sacks H, et al: Diabetic ketoacidosis: Reappraisal of therapeutic approach. *Ann Rev Med* 30:339, 1979.

Knochel JP: The pathophysiology and clinical characteristics of severe hypophosphatemia. *Arch Intern Med* 137:203, 1977.

Kohler E: On materials for testing glucose in the urine. *Diabetes Care* 1:64, 1978.

Kreisberg RA: Diabetic ketoacidosis: New concepts and trends in pathogenesis and treatment. *Ann Intern Med* 88:681, 1978.

Kreisberg RA: Phosphorus deficiency and hypophosphatemia. *Hosp Pract* 12(3):121, 1977.

Lavis VR: Treatment of diabetic ketoacidosis (letter). *Diabetes Care* 2:385, 1979.

Lentz RD, Brown DM, Kjellstrand CM: Treatment of severe hypophosphatemia. *Ann Intern Med* 89:941, 1978.

Levine SN, Lowenstein JE: Treatment of diabetic ketoacidosis. *Arch Intern Med* 141:713, 1981.

Liljenquist JE, Bomboy JD, Lewis SB, et al: Effects of glucagon on lipolysis and ketogenesis in normal and diabetic men. *J Clin Invest* 53:190, 1974.

Lundbaek K, Christensen SE, Hansen AP, et al: Failure of somatostatin to correct manifest diabetic ketoacidosis. *Lancet* 1:215, 1976.

Lutterman JA, Adriaansen AAJ, Laar AV: Treatment of severe diabetic ketoacidosis. *Diabetologia* 17:17, 1979.

Madison LL: Low-dose insulin: A plea for caution. *N Engl J Med* 294:393, 1976.

Malone JI, Brodsky SJ: The value of electrocardiogram monitoring in diabetic ketoacidosis. *Diabetes Care* 3:543, 1980.

Martin MM, Martin ALA: Continuous low-dose infusion of insulin in the treatment of diabetic ketoacidosis in children. *J Pediatr* 89:560, 1976.

Matz R: Diabetic acidosis: Rationale for not using bicarbonate. *NY State J Med* 76:1299, 1976.

McGarry JD: New perspectives in the regulation of ketogenesis. *Diabetes* 28:517, 1979.

McGarry JD, Foster DW: Hormonal control of ketogenesis: Biochemical considerations. *Arch Intern Med* 137:495, 1977.

McGarry JD, Foster DW: Ketogenesis and its regulation. *Am J Med* 61:9, 1976.

Miles JM, Rizza RA, Haymond MW, et al: Effects of acute insulin deficiency on glucose and ketone body turnover in man: Evidence for the primacy of overproduction of glucose and ketone bodies in the genesis of diabetic ketoacidosis. *Diabetes* 29:926, 1980.

Morris LR, Kitabchi AE: Efficacy of low-dose insulin therapy for severely obtunded patients in diabetic ketoacidosis. *Diabetes Care* 3:53, 1980.

Moseley J: Diabetic crises in children treated with small doses of intramuscular insulin. *Br Med J* 1:59, 1975.

Müller WA, Faloona GR, Unger RH: Hyperglucagonemia in diabetic ketoacidosis: Its prevalence and significance. *Am J Med* 54:52, 1973.

Munro JF, Campbell IW, McCuish AC, et al: Euglycaemic diabetic ketoacidosis. *Br Med J* 2:578, 1973.

Newman JH, Neff TA, Ziporin P: Acute respiratory failure associated with hypophosphatemia. *N Engl J Med* 296:1101, 1977.

O'Connor LR, Wheeler WS, Bethune JE: Effect of hypophosphatemia on myocardial performance in man. *N Engl J Med* 297:901, 1977.

O'Hearne J, Hamburger S: Phosphate therapy in the management of diabetic ketoacidosis. *Mo Med* 77:665, 1980.

Oh MS, Carroll HJ, Goldstein DA, et al: Hyperchloremic acidosis during the recovery phase of diabetic ketoacidosis. *Ann Intern Med* 89:925, 1978.

Ohman JL, Marliss EB, Aoki TT, et al: The cerebrospinal fluid in diabetic ketoacidosis. *N Engl J Med* 284:283, 1971.

Padilla AJ, Loeb JN: ''Low-dose'' versus ''high-dose'' insulin regimens in the management of uncontrolled diabetes. *Am J Med* 63:843, 1977.

Page MM, Alberti KGMM, Greenwood R, et al: Treatment of diabetic coma with continuous low-dose infusion of insulin. *Br Med J* 2:687, 1974.

Perkins RM, Marks JF: Low-dose continuous intravenous insulin infusion in childhood diabetic ketoacidosis. *Clin Pediatr* 18:540, 1979.

Pfeifer MA, Samols E, Wolter CF, et al: Low-dose versus high-dose insulin therapy for diabetic ketoacidosis. *South Med J* 72:149, 1979.

Piters KM, Kumar D, Pei E, et al: Comparison of continuous and intermittent intravenous insulin therapies for diabetic ketoacidosis. *Diabetologia* 13:317, 1977.

Posner JB, Plum F: Spinal-fluid pH and neurologic symptoms in systemic acidosis. *N Engl J Med* 277:605, 1967.

Raskin P, Fujita Y, Unger RH: Effect of insulin-glucose infusion on plasma glucagon levels in fasting diabetics and nondiabetics. *J Clin Invest* 56:1132, 1975.

Rosenbloom AL, Riley WJ, Weber FT, et al: Cerebral edema complicating diabetic ketoacidosis in childhood. *J Pediatr* 96:357, 1980.

Sacks HS, Shahshahani M, Kitabchi AE, et al: Similar responsiveness of diabetic ketoacidosis to low-dose insulin by intramuscular injection and albumin-free infusion. *Ann Intern Med* 90:36, 1979.

Sanders G, Boyle, G, Hunter S, et al: Mixed acid-base abnormalities in diabetes. *Diabetes Care* 1:362, 1978.

Schade DS, Eaton RP: Dose response to insulin in man: Differential effects on glucose and ketone body regulation. *J Clin Endocrinol Metab* 44:1038, 1977.

Schade DS, Eaton RP: Pathogenesis of diabetic ketoacidosis: A reappraisal. *Diabetes Care* 2:296, 1979.

Schade DS, Eaton RP: Prevention of diabetic ketoacidosis. *JAMA* 242:2455, 1979.

Schade DS, Eaton RP: The controversy concerning counterregulatory hormone secretion: A hypothesis for the prevention of diabetic ketoacidosis? *Diabetes* 26:596, 1977.

Sherwin RS, Hendler RG, Felig P: Effect of diabetes mellitus and insulin on the turnover and metabolic response to ketones in man. *Diabetes* 25:776, 1976.

Skillman TG: Diabetic ketoacidosis. *Heart Lung* 7:594, 1978.

Soler NG, Bennett MA, Fitzgerald MG, et al: Electrocardiogram as a guide to potassium replacement in diabetic ketoacidosis. *Diabetes* 23:610, 1974.

Soler NG, Bennett MA, Fitzgerald MG, et al: Intensive care in the management of diabetic ketoacidosis. *Lancet* 1:951, 1973.

Soler NG, Wright AD, Fitzgerald MG, et al: Comparative study of different insulin regimens in management of diabetic ketoacidosis. *Lancet* 2:1221, 1975.

Sönksen PH, Srivastava MC, Tompkins CV, et al: Growth-hormone and cortisol responses to insulin infusion in patients with diabetes mellitus. *Lancet* 2:155, 1972.

Standl E, Ditzel J: The effect of red cell 2,3-DPG changes induced by diabetic ketoacidosis on parameters of the oxygen dissociation curve in man. *Adv Exp Med Biol* 75:89, 1975.

Sullivan PA, Gonggrijp H, Crowley MJ, et al: Plasma angiotensin II concentrations in diabetic ketoacidosis and in hyperosmolar non-ketotic hyperglycemia. *Acta Diabetol Lat* 18:139, 1981.

Taylor AL: Diabetic ketoacidosis: Reassessment of therapeutic "truths." *Postgrad Med* 68(4):161, 1980.

Unger RH: Role of glucagon in the pathogenesis of diabetes: The status of the controversy. *Metabolism* 27:1691, 1978.

Unger RH, Orci L: The essential role of glucagon in the pathogenesis of diabetes mellitus. *Lancet* 1:14, 1975.

Vinicor F, Lehrner LM, Karn RC, et al: Hyperamylasemia in diabetic ketoacidosis: Sources and significance. *Ann Intern Med* 91:200, 1979.

Waldhäusl W, Kleinberger G, Korn A, et al: Severe hyperglycemia: Effects of rehydration on endocrine derangements and blood glucose concentration. *Diabetes* 28:577, 1979.

Wilson HK, Keuer SP, Lea AS, et al: Phosphate therapy in diabetic ketoacidosis. *Arch Intern Med* 142:517, 1982.

Winegrad AI, Clements RS: Diabetic ketoacidosis. *Med Clin North Am* 55:899, 1971.

Winter RJ, Harris CJ, Phillips LS, et al: Diabetic ketoacidosis: Induction of hypocalcemia and hypomagnesemia by phosphate therapy. *Am J Med* 67:897, 1979.

Young E, Bradley RF: Cerebral edema with irreversible coma in severe diabetic ketoacidosis. *N Engl J Med* 276:665, 1967.

Zack BG: Diabetic ketoacidosis in childhood. *Am Fam Physician* 26(7):107, 1982.

Zimmet PZ, Taft P, Ennis GC, et al: Acid production in diabetic acidosis; a more rational approach to alkali replacement. *Br Med J* 3:610, 1970.

Zipf WB, Bacon GE, Spencer ML, et al: Hypocalcemia, hypomagnesemia, and transient hypoparathyroidism during therapy with potassium phosphate in diabetic ketoacidosis. *Diabetes Care* 2:265, 1979.

CHAPTER 90
ALCOHOLIC
KETOACIDOSIS

Gene Ragland

Alcoholic ketoacidosis is a metabolically unique complication of alcoholism that frequently goes unrecognized. It is characterized by an anion gap acidosis due to high levels of ketoacids.

Alcoholic ketoacidosis was first described by Dillon and co-workers in 1940. It was not until the 1970s that it was further studied and defined. It occurs exclusively in relation to alcohol abuse but not just in chronic alcoholics. Thought to occur predominantly in middle-aged women, alcoholic ketoacidosis has now been reported with equal frequency in men, at a young age (23 years), and even in first-time drinkers whose food intake is minimal.

The true incidence is unknown. One report has postulated that approximately 20 percent of all ketoacidotic episodes may be of alcoholic origin. Another study, over a 2-year period, found alcoholic ketoacidosis to occur more frequently than diabetic ketoacidosis. The frequency is probably directly related to the incidence of alcoholism in a population. It undoubtedly occurs more often than it is diagnosed.

PATHOGENESIS

The precise pathogenesis of the ketosis of alcoholic ketoacidosis is not known. Several mechanisms have been postulated. McGarry has proposed a bihormonal concept to explain ketone body production. In his view, ketosis results from increased mobilization of free fatty acids from adipose tissue coupled with simultaneous enhancement of the liver's capacity to convert these substrates into acetoacetate and β-hydroxybutyrate.

It is known that during the metabolism of alcohol in the liver the rate of nicotinamide adenine dinucleotide (NAD) reduction exceeds the rate of mitochondrial NADH oxidation, causing a decrease in available NAD. This state persists for a few days in spite of no further alcohol consumption. An NAD-dependent step in the oxidation of fatty acids in the mitochondria of the hepatocyte is displaced in favor of ketone body formation.

It is also known that during alcoholic ketoacidosis insulin levels are low, whereas levels of cortisol, growth hormone, glucagon, and epinephrine are increased, possibly as a result of alcohol-induced hypoglycemia. This hormonal milieu promotes lipolysis, which increases the levels of free fatty acids available for conversion to ketones.

Additional mechanisms that may contribute to ketosis include the conversion of acetate, an alcohol breakdown product, to ketones; alcohol-induced mitochondrial structural changes which enhance the rate of ketosis; and mitochondrial phosphorus depletion, which inhibits the utilization of NADH and increases ketone body formation. Finally, vomiting and starvation superimposed on chronic malnutrition also contribute to ketoacidosis.

CLINICAL PRESENTATION

The usual history is one of heavy alcohol consumption or binge drinking with decreased or absent food intake for several days. Food and alcohol intake are usually terminated by nausea, protracted vomiting, and abdominal pain occurring 24 to 72 h before presentation. It is during this period that ketoacidosis develops.

Clinically the patient appears acutely ill with dehydration, tachypnea, tachycardia, and diffuse abdominal pain. Most patients are alert, but they may be mildly disoriented or occasionally comatose.

There are no specific physical findings. Diffuse or localized abdominal pain is the single most common physical abnormality. One patient underwent laparotomy before the correct diagnosis of alcoholic ketoacidosis was made. Evidence of dehydration such as hypotension, orthostatic changes in blood pressure, tachycardia, and decreased urine output may be present. The temperature varies from hypothermia to mildly elevated. Associated alcohol-induced disease such as gastritis, pancreatitis, hepatitis, infections, or delirium tremens may be found.

LABORATORY

A wide variety of laboratory abnormalities may occur. The alcohol levels are usually low or undetectable, as the alcohol intake is decreased or discontinued during the period of anorexia and vomiting. Essential to the diagnosis of alcoholic ketoacidosis is a large anion gap due to high levels of serum ketones. Most patients have a blood pH reflective of the underlying metabolic acidosis, but a significant number may present with normal or even alkalemic pH values.

Acid-Base Balance

In a letter to the *Annals of Internal Medicine*, Fulop and Hoberman compared typical laboratory data from patients with diabetic ketoacidosis to data from patients with alcoholic ketoacidosis (see Table 90-1). The alcoholic patients tended to have a higher blood pH, lower levels of serum K^+ and Cl^-, and a higher level of plasma HCO_3^- than the diabetic patients. This difference is attributed to the severe recurrent vomiting experienced by the alcoholic patients. Vomiting causes chloride depletion and metabolic alkalosis. In addition, respiratory alkalosis may occur secondary to fever, sepsis, or alcohol withdrawal and further increases the blood pH.

Ketones

The anion gap—$Na^+ - (Cl^- + HCO_3^-) = 12 \pm 4$ mEq/L— in the patient groups is very similar and is due primariy to high levels of β-hydroxybutyrate and to a lesser extent to lactic acid accumulation. The principal ketones are acetoacetate and β-hydroxybutyrate. These ketones are intermediates in the oxidation of fatty acids; they are normally produced in equal amounts and are not normally detectable in the serum. Acetoacetate and β-hydroxybutyrate are a redox pair and are interconverted by an oxidation-reduction reaction with NAD and NADH as cofactors. In alcoholic ketoacidosis, perhaps because of a lack of NAD, β-hydroxybutyrate accumulates to levels several times higher than the levels of acetoacetate. Acetone is a volatile, neutral ketone that is formed from acetoacetate by irreversible spontaneous decarboxylation. Its presence reflects the level and duration of acetoacetate elevation and is indicative of a sustained, severe acidosis.

Nitroprusside Test

The nitroprusside test is used to detect the presence of ketones in serum and urine. This is a semiquantitative test that gives a reaction with acetoacetate, is less sensitive to acetone, and does not detect β-hydroxybutyrate at all. There is no practical test that measures β-hydroxybutyrate levels. In most series on alcoholic ketoacidosis, the nitroprusside test has shown moderate or large ketonemia or ketonuria. But in a significant minority of patients, the reaction may be weakly positive or negative even though ketoacidosis, because of high levels of β-hydroxybutyrate, is pronounced. Reliance on this test alone as a measure of ketoacidosis may lead to failure to recognize the presence of ketoacidosis or to an underestimation of the severity of the ketoacidosis.

Glucose

The blood glucose level in alcoholic ketoacidosis varies from hypoglycemia to mild elevation. In most series it is normal or slightly increased. Glucosuria is usually mild or absent. A subset of alcoholic patients in whom hypoglycemia and ketoacidosis are coexistent has been described. The blood glucose levels ranged between 19 and 27 mg/dL, the pH averaged 7.19, and the mean anion gap was 25 mEq/L. This series consists of five men, but women with similar findings have been described by other authors.

The pathogenesis of alcohol-induced hypoglycemia includes acute starvation, depletion of liver glycogen stores because of chronic malnutrition, and inhibition of gluconeogenesis because of alcohol-induced alteration of the NAD/NADH ratio. Alcohol also causes decreased peripheral utilization of glucose, and this acts to balance the glucose-depleting processes. Devenyi asks if alcoholic hypoglycemia and alcoholic ketoacidosis are sequential events of the same process. He theorizes that alcohol-induced hypoglycemia occurs first, stimulating increased cortisol, growth hormone, glucagon, and epinephrine; this may correct the hypoglycemia and mobilize free fatty acids, which are converted to ketones. If this theory is correct, the diagnosis of alcoholic hypoglycemia or alcoholic ketoacidosis may depend upon the point in this process at which the disorder is detected.

Table 90-1. Comparison of Admission Laboratory Data* in Patients with Diabetic Ketoacidosis and Alcoholic Ketosis

Variable†	Diabetic Ketoacidosis		Alcoholic Ketoacidosis ($N = 18$)
	Oh and Co-workers ($N = 35$)	Our Series ($N = 27$)	
Blood pH	7.07 ± 0	7.17 ± 0.02	7.35 ± 0.05
Serum Na^+	135.5 ± 1.6	133.0 ± 1.2	135.2 ± 1.6
Serum K^+		4.9 ± 0.2	4.1 ± 0.3
Serum Cl^-	101.0 ± 1.4	97.3 ± 1.1	90.9 ± 3.9
Plasma HCO_3^-	9.4‡	6.7 ± 0.6	16.5 ± 2.4
$\Delta\ HCO_3^-$	14.6	17.3 ± 0.6	7.5 ± 2.4
Anion gap§	26.1	28.9 ± 1.1	27.8 ± 2.5
Plasma lactate	2.7 ± 0.3	2.1 ± 0.1	3.9 ± 1.2
Plasma 3-hydroxybutyrate	10.3 ± 0.3	10.8 ± 0.6	9.3 ± 1.1
Plasma lactate + 3-hydroxybutyrate	13.0	12.9 ± 0.6	13.2 ± 1.6
Excess anion gap¶	14.1	17.0 ± 1.1	15.8 ± 2.5

Source: Fulop M, Hoberman HD: Diabetic ketoacidosis and alcoholic ketoacidosis. *Ann Intern Med* 91:796, 1979.

*Data given as mean ± SEM.

†All units are in mEq/L except for blood pH.

‡This and all succeeding values in this column refer to 15 patients.

§Calculated as serum $Na^+ - (Cl^- + HCO_3^-)$.

¶Calculated as anion gap − 12 mEq/L.

DIAGNOSIS

The diagnosis of alcoholic ketoacidosis is easily established in those patients with an antecedent history of alcohol intake, decreased food intake, vomiting, and abdominal pain, and laboratory findings of metabolic acidosis, a positive nitroprusside test, and a low or mildly elevated glucose level.

Several factors may contribute to the faiure to recognize this metabolic disorder. The blood alcohol level may be zero, and, in the absence of a history of alcohol intake, this diagnosis may not be considered. The nitroprusside test may be weakly positive or negative in spite of significant ketoacidosis. The pH may be mildly acidotic, normal, or even alkalemic in the face of pronounced metabolic acidosis. There are no specific physical findings which suggest the diagnosis of alcoholic ketoacidosis. Alcoholic patients may have a variety of alcohol-induced associated illnesses which may obscure or distract from this diagnosis. Mental confusion or coma may be incorrectly attributed to alcoholic intoxication or other causes if the appropriate laboratory studies are not performed or if they are incorrectly interpreted.

Diagnostic Criteria

Soffer and Hamburger's criteria to define alcoholic ketoacidosis are a serum glucose level less than 300 mg/dL, a recent history of alcohol intake with a relative or absolute decline in ethanol consumption 24 to 72 h before hospitalization, a history of vomiting, and a metabolic acidosis for which other causes, such as diabetic ketoacidosis, lactic acidosis, renal failure, or drug ingestion, are excluded by clinical observations or laboratory studies. A positive serum nitroprusside test, because of its limitations, is not a criterion for diagnosis.

Differential Diagnosis

Cahill states that a positive nitroprusside test and a very low plasma bicarbonate concentration suggest ketosis with a high level of β-hydroxybutyrate. The combination of a barely positive nitroprusside test and a low plasma bicarbonate concentration signifies either a very reduced state with high concentrations of β-hydroxybutyrate or else a coincidental lactic acidosis. The measurement of serum lactate levels aids in this differential diagnosis.

The entity with which alcoholic ketoacidosis is most often confused is diabetic ketoacidosis. The magnitude of ketoacidosis is equal in these two disorders. It is important to make the proper distinction, as the treatment of each entity is different. In diabetic ketoacidosis, hyperglycemia and glycosuria are present. The serum glucose level in alcoholic ketoacidosis varies from hypoglycemia to mild elevation, and glucosuria is usually mild or absent. This differential diagnosis can be made in the emergency department.

TREATMENT

Therapy of alcoholic ketoacidosis is simple and effective and consists of the intravenous administration of a glucose and saline solution. Patients given only saline improve, but not as rapidly as those who are also given glucose. Thiamine, 50 to 100 mg intravenously, should be given before the glucose to prevent precipi-

tation of Wernicke's disease. Reversal of ketoacidosis usually occurs in 12 to 18 h.

Volume and Glucose

In one study, approximately 6 L of normal or half-normal saline during the first 48 h were required to restore and maintain intravascular volume. Cahill believes that volume repletion is necessary to correct insulin-release inhibition by adrenergic nerve endings in the islets of Langerhans as well as by circulating catecholamines. Glucose infusion stimulates insulin release, and insulin acts to inhibit lipolysis and terminate ketoacid production. Glucose may inhibit further ketoacid production by increasing oxidation of accumulated NADH via glucose-induced uptake of phosphorus by the hepatic mitochondria.

Insulin

Exogenous administration of insulin is not indicated in treatment of alcoholic ketoacidosis; this aspect of therapy differs from therapy of diabetic ketoacidosis. Inappropriate administration of insulin to a patient with a normal or low glucose level could be dangerous.

Bicarbonate

Administration of sodium bicarbonate is usually not required. As ketoacid levels fall, plasma bicarbonate levels increase, and the pH returns to normal. A small amount of bicarbonate may be indicated if the pH is less than 7.1 or if the patient is clinically deteriorating as evidenced by a weak, rapid pulse, hypotension, or inability to compensate by hyperventilation because of weakness. The role of phosphorus replenishment in therapy of alcoholic ketoacidosis is not clear.

Recovery

With recovery and reversal of the acidosis, β-hydroxybutyrate is converted to acetoacetate. As this process occurs, the nitroprusside test becomes more positive because of higher levels of acetoacetate. This factitious hyperketonemia may cause the uninformed clinician unnecessary concern, as it appears that the ketoacidosis is worsening. Clinical improvement of the patient and increasing blood pH values are more reliable parameters of recovery than the nitroprusside test.

Survival

The survival rates of patients with alcoholic ketoacidosis are good. Those patients that die usually do so because of other complications of chronic alcoholism. A thorough search for and treatment of associated alcoholic disorders is essential. Recurrent episodes of alcoholic ketoacidosis after subsequent alcoholic debauche are not uncommon. One patient was documented to have had 12 such episodes.

BIBLIOGRAPHY

Anwar A, Hamburger S: Alcoholic ketoacidosis. *Mo Med* 78:245, 1981.

Cahill GF: Ketosis. *Kidney Int.* 20:416, 1981.

Cooperman MT, Davidoff F, Spark R, et al: Clinical studies of alcoholic ketoacidosis. *Diabetes* 23:433, 1974.

Devenyi P: Alcoholic hypoglycemia and alcoholic ketoacidosis: Sequential events of the same process? *Can Med Assoc J* 127:513, 1982.

Dillon ES, Dyer WW, Smelo LS: Ketone acidosis of nondiabetic adults. *Med Clin North Am* 24:1813, 1940.

Fulop M, Hoberman HD: Alcoholic ketosis. *Diabetes* 24:785, 1975.

Fulop M, Hoberman HD: Diabetic ketoacidosis and alcoholic ketoacidosis. *Ann Intern Med Lett* 91:796, 1979.

Hasselbalch H, Selmer J, Kassis E: Alcoholic ketoacidosis presenting as an acute abdomen. *Dan Med Bull* 28:218, 1981.

Jenkins DW, Eckel RE, Craig JW: Alcoholic ketoacidosis. *JAMA* 217:177, 1971.

Kreisberg RA: Diabetic ketoacidosis: New concepts and trends in pathogenesis and treatment. *Ann Intern Med* 88:681, 1978.

Levy LJ, Duga J, Girgis M, et al: Ketoacidosis associated with alcoholism in nondiabetic subjects. *Ann Intern Med* 78:213, 1973.

Lumpkin JR, Baker FJ, Franaszek JB: Alcoholic ketoacidosis in a pregnant woman. *JACEP* 8:21, 1979.

McGarry JD, Foster DW: Hormonal control of ketogenesis. *Arch Intern Med* 137:495, 1977.

Miller PD, Heinig RE, Waterhouse C: Treatment of alcoholic acidosis—The role of dextrose and phosphorus. *Arch Intern Med* 138:67, 1978.

Platia EV, Hsu TH: Hypoglycemic coma with ketoacidosis in nondiabetic alcoholics. *West J Med* 131:270, 1979.

Schade DS, Eaton RP: Differential diagnosis and therapy of hyperketonemic state. *JAMA* 241:2064, 1979.

Soffer A, Hamburger S: Alcoholic ketoacidosis: A review of 30 cases. *J Am Med Wom Assoc* 37:106, 1982.

CHAPTER 91
LACTIC ACIDOSIS

Gene Ragland

Lactic acidosis is the most common metabolic acidosis. It occurs in association with a wide variety of underlying processes and may represent a well-tolerated, physiologic event or a life-threatening, pathologic condition. Lactic acidosis is classified based upon oxygen supply to the tissues. Type A is that clearly associated with clinically evident hypoperfusion or hypoxia, and type B includes all other forms, those in which there is no evidence of tissue anoxia. Lactic acidosis is often diagnosed during the evaluation of an anion gap acidosis. Treatment is directed toward identification and correction of the underlying disorder and restitution of normal acid-base equilibrium.

LACTATE HOMEOSTASIS

Lactate is a metabolic product of anaerobic glycolysis and under normal conditions is in equilibrium with its immediate precursor, pyruvate. The basal production of lactate in a 70-kg person is approximately 1300 mmol/day, and the normal lactate concentration in extracellular fluid is about 1 mEq/L. The maintenance of lactate homeostasis is a complex, dynamic process involving interorgan balance between lactate production and utilization. Virtually all body tissues are capable of producing lactate, but skeletal muscle, erythrocytes, brain, skin, and intestinal mucosa are the most active. The utilization of lactate takes place in the liver and kidneys and to a lesser extent in the heart and skeletal muscle. Lactate is primarily disposed of in the liver and kidneys via gluconeogenesis, a process that requires the conversion of lactate back to pyruvate.

LACTATE PRODUCTION

Lactate is formed from pyruvate as an end product of anaerobic glycolysis. This oxidation-reduction reaction requires reduced nicotinamide adenine dinucleotide (NADH) and hydrogen ion (H^+) and is catalyzed by lactate dehydrogenase (LDH). This reaction is expressed by the equation

$$\text{Pyruvate} + \text{NADH} + H^+ \xrightleftharpoons{\text{LDH}} \text{Lactate} + \text{NAD}$$

The equilibrium of this reaction strongly favors the formation of lactate. The normal ratio of lactate to pyruvate is 10:1. Lactate is a metabolic blind end; it cannot be utilized in any other intracellular reactions and must be converted back to pyruvate for gluconeogenesis or oxidation to CO_2 and H_2O via the Krebs cycle.

The result of this biochemical reaction is to produce energy in the form of adenosine triphosphate (ATP) and to oxidize NADH to NAD. A small amount of lactic acid is produced even at rest and under aerobic conditions. In the presence of oxygen and essential cofactors, lactate is converted back to pyruvate; it does not accumulate and maintains equilibrium with pyruvate.

A variety of factors may alter this normal process. The concentration of lactate in the cytosol depends primarily upon the concentration of pyruvate, the intracellular redox state (NADH/NAD), and the intracellular pH. The net effect of these multiple factors determines the intracellular concentration of lactate.

Pyruvate

Since lactate can be eliminated only by conversion back to pyruvate, lactate concentration is intimately interrelated to the fate of pyruvate. Pyruvate is a key intermediary at the junction of several important pathways. The major sources of pyruvate are glycolysis, in which pyruvate is formed from the oxidation of glucose, and transamination, a process by which pyruvate can be derived from amino acids, especially alanine. Pyruvate may be utilized via gluconeogenesis, in which pyruvate is a substrate in the formation of glucose, and mitochondrial oxidation, in which pyruvate enters the mitochondria for oxidation to CO_2 and H_2O. A variety of factors may alter these normal pathways. For example, rapid glycolysis can be induced by alkalosis, protein catabolic states may increase transamination, metabolic poisons may impair mitochondrial function, or key enzymes and cofactors may be inactivated or unavailable. The concentration of pyruvate, and thus the concentration of lactate, depends upon the net production and consumption of pyruvate by these various routes.

Redox State

The intracellular redox state is a critical factor in determining the concentration of lactate. The availability of oxygen at the tissue level is an important determinant of the cellular redox. During prolonged anaerobic conditions, lactate cannot be reoxidized back to pyruvate because of a lack of NAD. Normally, NADH can be reoxidized to NAD within the mitochondria via the electron transport chain coupled with oxidative phosphorylation. Electron transport abruptly ceases during anoxia, NAD is not available for lactate conversion, and lactate accumulates. This mechanism is thought to be operative during type A lactic acidosis. Other factors may alter the cellular redox, and consequently, alterations in the NADH/NAD ratio do not solely reflect tissue oxygenation.

Intracellular pH

A third major determinant of lactate concentration within the cytosol is the intracellular hydrogen ion concentration. Changes in the intracellular pH affect enzymatic reactions, lactate transport, and the lactate/pyruvate ratio. Some of these effects may counterbalance each other. In general, a fall in pH causes decreased lactate production, whereas an increase in pH causes increased lactate concentration. One important aspect of a change in intracellular pH is its effect on the liver. As the pH declines, lactate uptake by the liver decreases. Additionally, when the pH is 7.0 or less, the liver becomes an organ of lactate production instead of lactate clearance.

LACTATE UTILIZATION

The liver and kidneys are the major organs that consume lactate. Gluconeogenesis is the main pathway utilized by these organs in lactate removal. This process utilizes the hydrogen ions produced during the formation of lactic acid and thus acts to maintain acid-base balance. The liver normally clears more than half the total daily lactate load, and the kidneys remove approximately 30 percent. Some researchers believe that the kidneys have a negligible role in lactate clearance and that other extrahepatic sites are more important. Of the approximately 1300 mmol of lactate produced each day, 60 to 70 mEq of lactate is extracted by the liver every 2 h. The H^+ that is consumed by the liver during this period is roughly equivalent to the total amount of H^+ excreted daily by the kidneys. By virtue of the liver's ability to clear lactate, the role of the liver in the maintenance of the overall acid-base balance is very important. In addition, the liver has a large reserve capacity to extract lactate; this has been estimated to be as high as 3400 to 4000 mmol/day. Obviously, any situation which converts the liver from a lactate-consuming to a lactate-producing organ results in serious acid-base disturbance. Lactic acid clearance by the liver may be reduced with decreased hepatic blood flow or parenchymal hypoxia.

The kidneys carry out their role in lactate clearance primarily through gluconeogenesis, not excretion. The renal threshold for lactate is about 7 to 10 mEq/L, so the amount of lactate excreted by the kidneys at normal plasma levels is negligible. The kidneys may also dispose of lactate through oxidation, but this is not the preferred pathway. At a pH of less than 7.1, lactate uptake by the kidneys may be decreased, and at a pH of 7.0 or below, the kidneys—like the liver—may produce lactic acid.

Skeletal and cardiac muscle is capable of extracting some lactate from the circulation. The relative role of these sites of lactate clearance is not clear. Lactate utilization by skeletal muscle may depend on the concentration of lactate and whether the muscle is active or at rest.

LACTIC ACIDOSIS

Lactic acidosis can be thought of as an imbalance between the rate of production of lactate by tissues active in glycolysis and the rate of utilization by tissues active in gluconeogenesis. Disagree-

ment exists over whether the primary mechanism responsible for lactic acidosis is overproduction or underutilization.

Lactic acid is a strong organic acid that is almost completely dissociated at physiologic pH. The ratio of lactate ion to undissociated lactic acid at a pH of 7.4 is more than 3000:1. For each milliequivalent of lactic acid produced, equal amounts of hydrogen ion and lactate are liberated. Hydrogen ions are initially buffered by bicarbonate and other buffers and then consumed during the utilization of lactate via gluconeogenesis or oxidation. Acid-base balance is therefore maintained. Under circumstances of increased lactic acid production and/or decreased lactic acid utilization, body buffers are saturated by the excess hydrogen ions. When this is of sufficient magnitude, acidosis results. Whether the resultant lactic acidosis is clinically significant depends upon the underlying process responsible for the lactic acid accumulation and the preexistent acid-base status.

DIAGNOSIS

Lactic acidosis can be defined as a metabolic acidosis caused by the accumulation of lactate and hydrogen ion. It is accompanied by an elevated blood lactate concentration, but there is no consensus on what level of lactate defines lactic acidosis. The normal plasma lactate level is 0.5 to 1.5 mEq/L. In general, a lactate concentration of 4 to 5 mEq/L is considered indicative of significant acid-base disturbance. Some authors have included demonstration of a reduced arterial pH as a criterion for diagnosis. However, if there is a coexistent alkalosis, the pH could be normal or even alkalemic in the face of significant lactic acidosis.

The presence of hyperlactemia per se does not mean that the patient has clinically significant lactic acidosis. Many situations encountered clinically may result in elevation of blood lactate levels but not produce significant clinical consequences. Exercise; hyperventilation; infusions of glucose, saline, or bicarbonate, and injections of insulin or epinephrine may all cause elevation of lactate levels without clinical manifestations. Plasma lactate concentrations after vigorous exercise or maximum work have been reported to reach 14 to 30 mEq/L. In patients with grand mal seizures, levels of 12.7 mEq/L have been recorded. In spite of these high levels, the lactate production is self-limited, and the lactate is rapidly cleared from the circulation without untoward consequences. Persistent elevation of lactate levels may occur with chronic disorders such as severe congestive heart failure, pulmonary disease, liver disease, and diabetes mellitus. These levels are generally well-tolerated. To identify the patient in whom an increased lactate level is significant, the physician must assess the clinical state and correlate it with the extent to which increased lactate and hydrogen ion levels contribute to clinical abnormalities.

A presumptive diagnosis of lactic acidosis can be made in many instances. This diagnosis is based upon the recognition of an anion gap acidosis in a patient with a clinical disorder in which lactic acidosis is known to occur. For this impression to be confirmed, other causes of an increased anion gap metabolic acidosis must be excluded, and the plasma lactate concentration must be shown to be elevated.

Anion Gap Acidosis

The anion gap is generally determined by subtracting the concentration of chloride plus bicarbonate ions from the concentration

Table 91-1. Causes of Increased Anion Gap Metabolic Acidosis

Increased endogenous organic acids
   Diabetic ketoacidosis
   Alcoholic ketoacidosis
   Lactic acidosis
Decreased excretion of organic and inorganic acids
   Renal failure (uremia)
Ingestion of toxins
   Salicylates
   Methanol
   Ethylene glycol
   Paraldehyde
   Cyanide

of sodium ion: $Na^+ - (Cl^- + HCO_3^-)$. The normal value is 12 mEq/L $\pm$ 4. Any value greater than 16 mEq/L suggests the presence of an "unmeasured ion," usually an accumulation of organic anions. Most patients with lactic acisosis have an anion gap that averages 25 to 30 mEq/L. The major causes of anion gap acidosis in addition to lactic acidosis include diabetic ketoacidosis, uremic acidosis, alcoholic ketoacidosis, and ingestion of the toxins salicylate, methanol, ethylene glycol, paraldehyde, or cyanide (see Table 91-1). Laboratory determinations of the levels of arterial blood gases, electrolytes, glucose, blood urea nitrogen, creatinine, and lactate, and liver function studies and appropriate drug screens, should help establish the correct cause of acidosis.

Particular caution should be used with diabetic and alcoholic patients to ensure that the unmeasured anion is correctly identified. The major organic anion in diabetic and alcoholic ketoacidosis is β-hydroxybutyrate, which is not measured by the serum nitroprusside test. Lactic acidosis and ketoacidosis may occur simultaneously. If lactate levels do not account for the entire increase in the anion gap, ketoacidosis should be suspected, even with negative acetones. The bicarbonate level may provide additional help with this differential point. In uncomplicated diabetic ketoacidosis, the increase in the anion gap is identical to the decrease in the bicarbonate concentration, whereas in lactic acidosis, the increase in the anion gap is usually greater than the decrease in the bicarbonate concentration. In one prospective study of 57 hospitalized patients with an increased anion gap, 62 percent had increased lactate or keto anions. Anion gaps of 30 mEq/L or greater were virtually synonymous with lactic acidosis or ketoacidosis.

CLINICAL PRESENTATION

The clinical findings in lactic acidosis are nonspecific. No uniform signs and symptoms are indicative of this disorder. The onset may be abrupt, often occurring over several hours. Generally the patient appears ill. Hyperventilation or Kussmaul's respiration is the most constant feature. The level of consciousness may vary from lethargy to coma. Vomiting and abdominal pain sometimes occur. Hypotension and evidence of hypoxia occur with type A lactic acidosis but not with type B.

Laboratory abnormalities that occur during lactic acidosis include elevated lactate levels, increased anion gap, decreased bicarbonate levels, and decreased pH unless altered by compensatory alkalosis. Hyperkalemia has long been associated with metabolic acidosis. One review of a large series of patients with various

types of lactic acidosis showed that although many patients did have hyperkalemia, not all did. Organic acidosis may not elevate serum potassium levels. In this series, the serum potassium concentrations did not correlate well with the severity of the acidemia and were most likely to be elevated in those patients with underlying renal insufficiency or tissue destruction. Marked hyperphosphatemia and hyperuricemia may be seen. The white blood cell count is usually elevated and may reach leukemoid proportions. Hypoglycemia has also been reported in association with lactic acidosis, especially in conjunction with liver disease.

CLASSIFICATION OF LACTIC ACIDOSIS

Lactic acidosis is classified on clinical grounds and occurs in two principal clinical settings. According to Cohen and Woods' classification, type A lactic acidosis occurs with clinically evident tissue anoxia, such as during shock or severe hypoxia. Type B lactic acidosis includes all other forms, those in which there is no evidence of tissue anoxia (see Table 91-2). Spontaneous or idiopathic lactic acidosis has been described but is now felt to be nonexistent. Recognition of an increasing array of disorders in which lactic acidosis can occur without evident tissue anoxia has virtually eliminated this category. A new metabolic disorder, D-lactic acidosis, has been described. It occurs in patients with anatomically or functionally shortened small bowel. Bacterial fermentation produces D-lactic acid, which can be absorbed and cause an increased anion gap acidosis and stupor or coma. The plasma levels of L-lactate are normal. Treatment with neomycin or vancomycin results in correction of the metabolic abnormalities.

Type A Lactic Acidosis

This is the most common form of lactic acidosis seen in the emergency department and is most often due to shock. Hemorrhagic,

Table 91-2. Classification of Lactic Acidosis

Type A
  Clinically evident tissue anoxia (eg. shock, hypoxia)
Type B
  1. Various common disorders
    Diabetes mellitus
    Renal failure
    Liver disease
    Infection
    Leukemia and certain other malignant conditions
    Convulsions
  2. Drugs, toxins
    Biguanides (phenformin)
    Ethanol
    Fructose and other saccharides
    Methanol
    Various other drugs
  3. Hereditary forms
    Type I glycogen storage disease
    Fructose-biphosphatase deficiency
    Subacute necrotizing encephalomyelopathy (Leigh's syndrome)
    Methylmalonic aciduria
    Others

Source: Adapted from Cohen RD, Woods HF: *Clinical and Biochemical Aspects of Lactic Acidosis.* Oxford, Blackwell, 1976.

hypovolemic, cardiogenic, or septic shock have been shown to cause lactic acidosis. The pathogenesis of lactic acidosis during shock is inadequate tissue perfusion with subsequent anoxia and lactate and hydrogen ion accumulation. Clearance of lactate by the liver is reduced because of decreased splanchnic and hepatic artery perfusion, and hepatocellular ischemia. At a pH of around 7.0 or less, the liver and kidneys may become organs of lactate production.

The association between shock and lactic acidosis is so common that a presumptive diagnosis can be made in a critically ill patient in shock who suddenly develops severe hyperventilation and an increased anion gap acidosis. Treatment should be directed toward correction of the cause of shock. Some researchers have found a direct relation between mortality and the arterial lactate level in patients with shock. Others have found this relation to be obscure, and the clinical usefulness of the lactate concentration as a predictor of outcome to be unconvincing. In general, the higher the lactate level, the higher the mortality.

Hypoxia may also cause type A lactic acidosis. The hypoxia must be acute and severe. Adaptations such as polycythemia, diminished hemoglobin affinity for oxygen, and increased tissue extraction of oxygen protect patients with chronic, stable lung disease from developing lactic acidosis.

These patients may not develop significant lactic acidosis until an arterial P_{O_2} of 30 to 35 mmHg is reached. In patients with a diminished ability to compensate for a respiratory insult, lactic acidosis may arise at considerably higher arterial oxygen tensions. Acute asphyxiation, pulmonary edema, status asthmaticus, acute exacerbation of chronic obstructive pulmonary disease, and displacement of oxygen by carboxyhemoglobin, sulfhemoglobin, or methemoglobin have been associated with lactic acidosis.

Type B Lactic Acidosis

Type B lactic acidosis includes all forms in which there is no clinical evidence of tissue anoxia. This form may occur abruptly, over a few hours. The diagnosis may be missed or delayed because of no clear antecedent event, or because of lack of familiarity with the disorders associated with type B lactic acidosis. The mechanisms by which these disorders predispose to lactic acidosis are not well understood. By definition, the cardiovascular function is not impaired and the blood pressure is not decreased. Subclinical, regional underperfusion of tissue has been suggested as a possible cause. In many cases of severe type B lactic acidosis, circulatory insufficiency may occur after a few hours, making this condition clinically indistinguishable from type A lactic acidosis. Type B lactic acidosis is divided into three subgroups.

Type B₁

Type B_1 lactic acidosis comprises those cases that occur in association with other medical disorders such as diabetes, renal and hepatic disease, infection, neoplasia, and convulsions. There is no clear causal relation between diabetes and lactic acidosis, but the association between them has been noted by many authors. Cohen and Woods noted that 10 to 15 percent of diabetic patients who were in ketoacidosis had lactate levels of at least 5 mEq/L. Liver disease associated with lactic acidosis includes massive hepatic necrosis and cirrhosis. Decreased lactate clearance by the

liver because of insufficient liver tissue for gluconeogenesis may be the cause of lactic acidosis in this setting. Acute and chronic renal insufficiency is commonly associated with lactic acidosis but is probably not a cause in its own right. Some patients with severe infections, especially bacteremia, develop lactic acidosis for unknown reasons. Infection was present in 27 of 65 cases of type B lactic acidosis collected by Cohen and Woods. Myeloproliferative disorders such as leukemia, multiple myeloma, generalized lymphoma, and Hodgkin's disease are associated with lactic acidosis. Grand mal seizures may result in lactic acidosis because of muscular hyperactivity and probably hypoxia. Lactic acidosis in Reye's syndrome has been reported. A close correspondence between the stage of coma and lactate levels was noted.

Type B₂

This subgroup includes cases of lactic acidosis due to drugs, chemicals, and toxins. This category was formerly dominated by the oral hypoglycemic agent phenformin, which has been withdrawn from U.S. markets. Ethanol is currently the most common drug associated with lactic acidosis. During the oxidation of alcohol, NADH levels increase, causing utilization of the pyruvate-lactate pathway for the reoxidation of NADH. This reaction produces a moderate increase in the lactate level. In the presence of other causes of lactic acidosis, ethanol ingestion may cause increased acidosis. Other drugs associated with lactic acidosis include fructose; sorbitol; excess amounts of epinephrine and other catecholamines; methanol; and possibly salicylates. Many other drugs have also been implicated as causally related to lactic acidosis.

Type B₃

This form of lactic acidosis is rare and is due to inborn errors of metabolism such as type I glycogen storage disease (glucose-6-phosphatase deficiency) and hepatic fructose-biphosphatase deficiency. These congenital lactic acidoses include defects in gluconeogenesis, the pyruvate dehydrogenase complex, the Krebs cycle, and cellular respiratory mechanisms.

TREATMENT

The basic therapeutic goals in treatment of lactic acidosis are to identify and correct the underlying cause of the lactic acid accumulation and to counteract the deleterious effects of the acidosis. The presence of clinically significant lactic acidosis indicates a serious underlying disorder. The patient's survival primarily depends on whether the cause of the lactic acidosis can be recognized and treated effectively.

The specifics of therapy depend upon the cause of the lactic acidosis. Shock and hypoxia must be corrected as soon as possible. Adequate ventilation is imperative. Restoration of blood pressure, cardiac output, and tissue perfusion with well-oxygenated blood is essential. Volume replacement with fluids, plasma expanders, or blood, as indicated, should be instituted. Vasopressors should probably be avoided as they may decrease tissue perfusion and worsen the acidosis. Catecholamines are glycogenolytic and may enhance lactic acid production. In type B lactic acidosis, the underlying disorder may not be readily identifiable or amenable to therapy. Drugs known to be associated with lactic acidosis should be discontinued, and infection must be aggressively treated.

Sodium Bicarbonate

Treatment of acidosis with intravenous sodium bicarbonate ($NaHCO_3$) is a mainstay of therapy for lactic acidosis. The purpose of this therapy is to reverse the untoward effects of acidosis and allow time for other therapeutic modalities to correct the cause of the acidosis. If the cause of lactic acidosis can be quickly corrected, such as with respiratory failure or pulmonary edema, alkali therapy may not be needed. The undesirable effects of acidosis include depression of myocardial contractility and decreased cardiac output at a pH below 7.1. Arteriolar dilatation and hypotension may occur when the blood pH falls below 7.0. Additionally, a pH below 7.0 impairs hepatic utilization of lactate and may induce production of lactate by the liver and kidneys. These effects may be the cause of the cardiovascular collapse that occurs during the course of type B lactic acidosis.

In general, sodium bicarbonate should be given when the pH is 7.1 or less. Cohen and Woods believe it desirable to restore the pH to a normal range within 2 to 6 h and to maintain it there. Others recommend slower, cautious alkali administration because of its attendant hazards. Some undesirable effects include fluid and sodium overload, hyperosmolarity, alkaline overshoot which could increase lactate production, displacement of the oxyhemoglobin dissociation curve to the left, and paradoxical cerebrospinal fluid acidosis. Cardiovascular status and arterial pH should be continuously monitored during $NaHCO_3$ therapy.

The approximate dose of bicarbonate required to correct the acidosis can be calculated from the following formula:

$$HCO_3 \text{ deficit} = (25 \text{ mEq/L } HCO_3 - \text{measured } HCO_3)$$
$$\times 0.5(\text{body weight in kg})$$

This equation is based upon the assumption that bicarbonate distributes in a space equal to 50 percent of the body weight in kilograms.

Some patients may require massive amounts of sodium bicarbonate to correct acidemia. Those unable to tolerate fluid and sodium overload can be treated with a bicarbonate infusion, potent loop diuretic, or tris(hydroxymethyl)aminomethane (THAM). Hyperosmolarity can be reduced by adding 3 to 4 ampoules of $NaHCO_3$ (44 mEq/L) to a liter of 5 percent dextrose and water. This solution provides 132 to 176 mmol/L, respectively. Use of a potent loop diuretic creates intravascular space for fluid and sodium. A diuretic should be given in whatever dose is required to maintain a brisk diuresis (300 to 500 mL/h). Urinary sodium and potassium losses can be measured and replaced along with the urinary volume loss on an equal basis.

Oliguric patients require hemodialysis to permit administration of large amounts of sodium bicarbonate. Standard dialysis baths can be replaced by a bicarbonate bath so that the fluid and sodium chloride removed by the hypertonic solution can be replaced as the bicarbonate salt. Hemodialysis and peritoneal dialysis remove lactate. As there is no evidence that lactate ion per se is harmful, this approach is unnecessary. Removal of lactate, however, can minimize the rebound alkalosis that often occurs after correction of the acidosis.

There is often a delay of many hours between the return of the pH to the normal range and a fall in the blood lactate level. Cohen recommends patience during this period rather than the institution of more speculative forms of therapy. He recommends slowing the bicarbonate infusion after several hours of a normal pH. If the pH begins to drop, the bicarbonate infusion can be increased. When the pH stabilizes in an acceptable range, the infusion can be discontinued. As always, the clinical status of the patient is the best parameter to follow during recovery.

Additional Treatment

A variety of other therapies have been advocated in treatment of lactic acidosis. These include insulin, glucose, thiamine, methylene blue, vasodilator drugs such as sodium nitroprusside, and the experimental drug dichloroacetate. Most authors do not favor the use of insulin, or insulin in conjunction with glucose, in treatment of lactic acidosis. Insulin may be indicated in a diabetic patient with concomitant lactic acidosis or in a diabetic with an unexplained increased anion gap acidosis. Insulin therapy in these instances should be based upon individual need. Glucose infusion in the setting of hypoglycemia and lactic acidosis has been reported to correct the lactic acidosis.

Thiamine is a necessary cofactor for the enzyme that catalyzes the first step in the oxidation of pyruvate. This vitamin should be given to alcoholic patients with lactic acidosis, but a role for thiamine therapy in other patients has not been established. Methylene blue is a redox dye that is capable of accepting H^+ and thereby oxidizing $NADH_2$ to NAD^+ and theoretically limiting the conversion of pyruvate to lactate. Clinical trials have not supported the benefit of this drug. Vasodilator therapy is based upon the premise that tissue perfusion improves with reduced peripheral vascular resistance and increased cardiac output. The value of vasodilator agents in treatment of lactic acidosis remains to be proved.

Dichloroacetate (DCA) is an experimental drug that increases the activity of pyruvate dehydrogenase, and this promotes the oxidation of glucose, pyruvate, and lactate and thus reduces blood lactate levels. Since oxygen is required for this metabolic process, DCA has no role in treatment of type A lactic acidosis. Its role in therapy for type B lactic acidosis may be limited by the increased ketosis and neurologic complications that occur with its use.

The fact that so many experimental therapies have been tried in lactic acidosis reflects the poor outcome of this disorder with the use of current treatment. The mortality of patients with type A lactic acidosis is approximately 80 percent; with type B it is 50 to 80 percent. Earlier recognition and correction of the underlying disorder responsible for the lactic acidosis is the best hope for reduction of this high mortality.

BIBLIOGRAPHY

Aberman A, Hew E: Lactic acidosis presenting as acute respiratory failure. *Am Rev Respir Dis* 118:961, 1978.

Alberti KGMM, Nattrass M: Lactic acidosis. *Lancet* 2:25, 1977.

Arieff AI, Leach WJ, Lazarowitz VC: Effects of $NaHCO_3$ in therapy of experimental lactic acidosis. *Kidney Int* 14:645, 1978.

Arieff AI, Park R, Leach WJ, et al: Pathophysiology of experimental lactic acidosis in dogs. *Am J Physiol* 239:F135, 1980.

Bellingham AJ, Detter JC, Lenfant C: Regulatory mechanism of hemoglobin oxygen affinity in acidosis and alkalosis. *J Clin Invest* 50:700, 1971.

Berry MN, Scheuer J: Splanchnic lactic acid metabolism in hyperventilation, metabolic alkalosis and shock. *Metabolism* 16:537, 1967.

Breborowicz A, Szulc R: Removal of endogenous lactates via the peritoneum in experimental lactic acidosis. *Intensive Care Med* 7:297, 1981.

Cohen RD: Disorders of lactic acid metabolism. *Clin Endocrinol Metab* 5:613, 1976.

Cohen RD: The prevention and treatment of type B lactic acidosis. *Br J Hosp Med* 23:577, 1980.

Cohen RD, Iles RA: Lactic acidosis: Diagnosis and treatment. *Clin Endocrinol Metab* 9:513, 1980.

Cohen RD, Simpson R: Lactate metabolism. *Anesthesiology* 43:661, 1975.

Emmett M, Narins RG: Clinical use of the anion gap. *Medicine* 56:38, 1977.

Fields ALA, Wolman SL, Halperin ML: Chronic lactic acidosis in a patient with cancer: Therapy and metabolic consequences. *Cancer* 47:2026, 1981.

Fulop M: Lactic acidosis. *NY State J Med* 82:712, 1982.

Fulop M: Serum potassium in lactic acidosis and ketoacidosis. *N Engl J Med* 300:1087, 1979.

Fulop M: Ventilatory response in patients with acute lactic acidosis. *Crit Care Med* 10:173, 1982.

Fulop M, Hoberman HD, Rascoff JH, et al: Lactic acidosis in diabetic patients. *Arch Intern Med* 136:987, 1976.

Gabow PA, Kaehny WD, Fennessey PV, et al: Diagnostic importance of an increased serum anion gap. *N Engl J Med* 303:854, 1980.

Harken AH: Lactic acidosis. *Surg Gynecol Obstet* 142:593, 1976.

Hazard PB, Griffin JP: Sodium bicarbonate in the management of systemic acidosis. *South Med J* 73:1339, 1980.

Heinig RE, Clarke EF, Waterhouse C: Lactic acidosis and liver disease. *Arch Intern Med* 139:1229, 1979.

Herrera L, Kazemi H: CSF bicarbonate regulation in metabolic acidosis: Role of HCO_3^- formation in CNS. *J Appl Physiol* 49:778, 1980.

Huckabee WE: Abnormal resting blood lactate. I. The significance of hyperlactatemia in hospitalized patients. *Am J Med* 30:833, 1961.

Huckabee WE: Abnormal resting blood lactate. II. Lactic acidosis. *Am J Med* 30:840, 1961.

Huckabee WE: Lactic acidosis. *Am J Cardiol* 12:663, 1963.

Kapoor W, Carey P, Karpf M: Induction of lactic acidosis with intravenous diazepam in a patient with tetanus. *Arch Intern Med* 141:944, 1981.

Kreisberg RA: Glucose-lactate inter-relations in man. *N Engl J Med* 287:132, 1972.

Kreisberg RA: Lactate homeostasis and lactic acidosis. *Ann Intern Med* 92:227, 1980.

Kreisberg RA, Owen WC, Siegal AM: Ethanol-induced hyperlacticacidemia: Inhibition of lactate utilization. *J Clin Invest* 50:166, 1971.

Lloyd MH, Iles RA, Simpson BR, et al: The effect of simulated metabolic acidosis on intracellular pH and lactate metabolism in the isolated perfused rat liver. *Clin Sci Mol Med* 45:543, 1973.

Maguire LC, Sherman BM, Whalen JE: Glucose therapy of recurrent lactic acidosis. *Am J Med Sci* 276:305, 1978.

Murray BJ: Severe lactic acidosis and hypothermia. *West J Med* 134:162, 1981.

Naparstek Y, Friedlaender MM, Rubinger D, et al: Lactic acidosis and peritoneal dialysis. *Isr J Med Sci* 18:513, 1982.

Narins RG, Rudnick MR, Bastl CP: Lactic acidosis and the elevated anion gap (I). *Hosp Pract* 15(5):125, 1980.

Narins RG, Rudnick MR, Bastl CP: Lactic acidosis and the elevated anion gap (II). *Hosp Pract* 15(6):91, 1980.

O'Connor LR, Klein KL, Bethune JE: Hyperphosphatemia in lactic acidosis. *N Engl J Med* 297:707, 1977.

Oh MS, Phelps KR, Traube M, et al: D-Lactic acidosis in a man with the short-bowel syndrome. *N Engl J Med* 301:249, 1979.

Oliva PB: Lactic acidosis. *Am J Med* 48:209, 1970.

Orringer CE, Eustace JC, Wunsch CD, et al: Natural history of lactic acidosis after grand-mal seizures: A model for the study of an anion-gap acidosis not associated with hyperkalemia. *N Engl J Med* 297:796, 1977.

Oster JR, Perez GO, Vaamonde CA: Relationship between blood pH and potassium and phosphorus during acute metabolic acidosis. *Am J Physiol* 235:F345, 1978.

Park R: Lactic acidosis. *West J Med* 133:418, 1980.

Peretz DI, McGregor M, Dossetor JB: Lactic acidosis: A clinically significant aspect of shock. *Can Med Assoc J* 90:673, 1964.

Peretz DJ, Scott HM, Duff J, et al: The significance of lactic acidemia in the shock syndrome. *Ann NY Acad Sci* 119:1133, 1965.

Rehncrona S, Rosén I, Siesjö BK: Brain lactic acidosis and ischemic cell damage: 1. Biochemistry and neurophysiology. *J Cereb Blood Flow Metab* 1:297, 1981.

Relman AS: Lactic acidosis and a possible new treatment. *N Engl J Med* 298:564, 1978.

Rowell LB, Kraning KK, Evans TO, et al: Splanchnic removal of lactate and pyruvate during prolonged exercise in man. *J Appl Physiol* 21:1773, 1966.

Schwartz WB, Waters WC: Lactate versus bicarbonate: A reconsideration of the therapy of metabolic acidosis. *Am J Med* 32:831, 1962.

Stacpoole PW, Moore GW, Kornhauser DM: Metabolic effects of dichloroacetate in patients with diabetes mellitus and hyperlipoproteinemia. *N Engl J Med* 298:526, 1978.

Stacpoole PW, Moore GW, Kornhauser DM: Toxicity of chronic dichloroacetate (letter). *N Engl J Med* 300:372, 1979.

Stolberg L, Rolfe R, Gitlin N, et al: D-Lactic acidosis due to abnormal gut flora. *N Engl J Med* 306:1344, 1982.

Taradash MR, Jacobson LB: Vasodilator therapy of idiopathic lactic acidosis. *N Engl J Med* 293:468, 1975.

Tashkin DP, Goldstein PJ, Simmons DH: Hepatic lactate uptake during decreased liver perfusion and hypoxemia. *Am J Physiol* 223:968, 1972.

Tonsgard JH, Huttenlocher PR, Thisted RA: Lactic acidemia in Reye's syndrome. *Pediatrics* 69:64, 1982.

Tranquada RE, Bernstein S, Grant WJ: Intravenous methylene blue in the therapy of lactic acidosis. *Arch Intern Med* 114:13, 1964.

Tranquada RE, Grant WJ, Peterson CR: Lactic acidosis. *Arch Intern Med* 117:192, 1966.

Vaziri ND, Ness R, Wellikson L, et al: Bicarbonate-buffered peritoneal dialysis: An effective adjunct in the treatment of lactic acidosis. *Am J Med* 67:392, 1979.

Wainer RA, Wiernik PH, Thompson WL: Metabolic and therapeutic studies of a patient with acute leukemia and severe lactic acidosis of prolonged duration. *Am J Med* 55:255, 1973.

Warner A, Vaziri ND: Treatment of lactic acidosis. *South Med J* 74:841, 1981.

CHAPTER 92
NONKETOTIC
HYPEROSMOLAR COMA

Gene Ragland

Nonketotic hyperosmolar coma is a distinct medical syndrome characterized by severe hyperglycemia, hyperosmolality, and dehydration, but no ketoacidosis. This metabolic derangement occurs almost exclusively in the diabetic population but may occur in nondiabetics under certain circumstances. It was first described in 1886 but received little recognition until the modern description by Sament and Schwartz in 1957. Many names have been used to identify this entity, but the term *nonketotic hyperosmolar coma* is used in this chapter.

This syndrome shares many features with diabetic ketoacidosis, including hyperglycemia and hyperosmolality, but the lack of ketoacidosis is its main distinguishing feature. Nonketotic hyperosmolar coma occurs with one-sixth the frequency of diabetic ketoacidosis. Most authors believe that nonketotic hyperosmolar coma and diabetic ketoacidosis are part of a continuum, and that when present in pure form, they represent the opposite ends of a spectrum with regard to lipid mobilization. In general, a patient with nonketotic hyperosmolar coma has a blood glucose concentration greater than 800 mg/dL, usually 1000 mg/dL or more, a serum osmolality greater than 350 mOsm/kg, and a negative test for serum ketones. By comparison, the average blood glucose level of a patient in diabetic ketoacidosis is usually less than 600 mg/dL, the serum osmolality is rarely above 350 mOsm/kg, and the test for serum ketones is strongly positive.

Nonketotic hyperosmolar coma occurs most commonly as an acute complication of diabetes mellitus. The majority of patients have mild, maturity-onset diabetes that can be controlled by diet or oral hypoglycemic agents. Two-thirds of these patients have no previous history of diabetes, and nonketotic hyperosmolar coma is the initial manifestation of their disease. A small minority of insulin-dependent patients on parenteral therapy develop nonketotic hyperosmolar coma. Both extremes—nonketotic hyperosmolar coma and diabetic ketoacidosis—have been reported to occur in the same patient.

PATHOGENESIS

Any explanation of the pathogenesis of nonketotic hyperosmolar coma must explain why extreme hyperglycemia develops and why ketoacidosis does not. Neither of these questions has been answered with certainty. Simply put, extreme hyperglycemia develops because ketoacidosis does not. The failure of ketoacidosis to occur allows the underlying process to continue unrecognized and much higher levels of glucose to result.

Hyperglycemia

It has been theorized that when a patient with mild, maturity-onset diabetes is subjected to stress, the β cells of the pancreas respond to the increased glucose concentration by increasing the secretion of insulin. Continued diabetogenic stress eventually exhausts the insulinogenic reserve of the β cells, and plasma insulin levels fall. Because of the increased insulinogenic capacity of the patient with mild diabetes, higher levels of blood glucose occur before this reserve is depleted. If the patient is receiving insulin therapy, supplemental insulin allows additional time for β-cell recovery and further prolongs the time required for exhaustion of the insulin reserve. In addition, elevated levels of glucagon may promote gluconeogenesis in the liver, resulting in massive hyperglycemia.

Nonketosis

The reason ketoacidosis does not occur is not well understood. Experimental studies that have measured the levels of insulin, free fatty acids (FFA), glucagon, glucocorticoids, and growth hormone during nonketotic hyperosmolar coma have produced conflicting results. Some researchers found low levels of FFA, with normal insulin, glucocorticoid, and growth hormone levels. They believe that inhibition of lipolysis occurs because of relatively higher circulating insulin levels or lower lipolytic hormone levels than are present with diabetic ketoacidosis. When lipolysis is inhibited, the precursors required for ketone body formation are not released and ketoacidosis does not develop. It is known that the quantity of insulin required to inhibit lipolysis in adipose tissue is less than the quantity required to promote the utilization of glucose by peripheral tissues. Ketoacidosis may not develop because there is enough circulating insulin to inhibit lipolysis but an insufficient amount to protect against the development of hyperglycemia.

Other investigators have reported similar high FFA levels and low circulating insulin levels in both nonketotic hyperosmolar coma and diabetic ketoacidosis. Additionally, glucagon and glucocorticoids (cortisol) have been found to be increased to the same extent in both conditions. These authors conclude that in nonketotic hyperosmolar coma the FFA are mobilized to the same extent as in diabetic ketoacidosis, but that the intrahepatic oxidation of the incoming FFA is directed along nonketogenic metabolic pathways, such as triglyceride synthesis, because of an insulinated liver. Prehepatic and posthepatic insulin levels have been measured. In diabetic ketoacidosis, both pre- and posthepatic insulin levels are low, but in nonketotic hyperosmolar coma, prehepatic insulin levels twice the posthepatic ones have been found. Subscribers to this theory conclude that the liver is selectively bathed in insulin while the periphery is in a "diabetic" state. They conclude that the available insulin exerts its antiketogenic effect at the hepatic and not the adipocyte level.

Osmotic Diuresis

Regardless of the pathogenesis of nonketotic hyperosmolar coma, the effect of hyperglycemia in producing osmotic diuresis and fluid and electrolyte imbalance is understood. Total body water is normally distributed between the intracellular (two-thirds) and the extracellular (one-third) fluid compartments. The major osmotic solutes in the extracellular fluid are sodium and its anions. Potassium, magnesium, and phosphate are the major solutes in the intracellular compartment. Despite the difference in composition between these two compartments, the osmolality is equal because water is free to move across cell membranes and dissipate osmotic gradients.

When relative insulin insufficiency develops in the diabetic patient, hyperglycemia results from decreased peripheral utilization and increased hepatic production of glucose. Osmotically active glucose is located in the extracellular fluid compartment. During insulin insufficiency the cell membrane is not freely permeable to glucose, and water is drawn from the intracellular compartment into the extracellular compartment in an attempt to achieve equal osmolality. The presence of large amounts of glucose in the extracellular compartment tends to preserve that compartment at the expense of cellular volume. This relative expansion of the extracellular fluid volume may protect against hypotension until late in the course of nonketotic hyperosmolar coma.

In addition to the internal shifts in body fluids, an osmotic diuresis also occurs. Normally, antidiuretic hormone (ADH) from the posterior pituitary gland acts to maintain water balance. With severe hyperglycemia, glycosuria produces an increased volume and rate of urine flow through the kidneys. Despite maximum levels of ADH, water can no longer be maximally reabsorbed, and an increased volume of urine results. Total body water is decreased and serum osmolality is increased. Fluid losses during nonketotic hyperosmolar coma range from 8 to 12 L.

Sodium balance is also upset by osmotic diuresis. Sodium reabsorption normally occurs in the distal tubules, mediated by the renin-angiotensin system. The concentration gradient against which sodium must be actively transported into the distal tubules is increased as water reabsorption diminishes. Thus a large proportion of the filtered sodium remains unabsorbed and passes into the urine. Nevertheless, the water loss during osmotic diuresis is greater than the sodium loss, and the patient becomes hypertonic relative to sodium. Prolonged diuresis results in hypovolemia and hypertonic dehydration.

Total body potassium depletion is also a consequence of osmotic diuresis. The distal tubules are under maximal stimulation by aldosterone, and some sodium is reabsorbed in exchange for potassium. Because of the longer duration of osmotic diuresis with nonketotic hyperosmolar coma, potassium depletion is greater than that which occurs with diabetic ketoacidosis and may reach 400 to 1000 mEq. Potassium depletion may not become evident until the patient is rehydrated. Other solutes such as magnesium and phosphate are also lost during osmotic diuresis.

CLINICAL PRESENTATION

Nonketotic hyperosmolar coma can occur at any age, but it is rare in children and adolescents. It is most common in the middle-aged or elderly, with a mean age of 57 to 60 years, and occurs equally in men and women. It occurs most commonly in diabetics, although the majority are undiagnosed at the time of presentation.

Patients who depend upon others to meet their needs, such as infants, nursing home patients, and the mentally retarded, are particularly vulnerable to the insidious onset of nonketotic hyperosmolar coma. Inaccessibility to water coupled with an inability to communicate masks the early signs and symptoms. A substantial number of patients develop nonketotic hyperosmolar coma without any obvious cause, and most are found to have maturity-onset diabetes.

Precipitating Factors

Minor upper respiratory infections or gastroenteritis is capable of precipitating diabetic ketoacidosis, but an illness of greater magnitude is usually required before nonketotic hyperosmolar coma results. Infection is a common precipitating cause, especially gram-negative pneumonias. Other precipitating illnesses include myocardial infarction, cerebrovascular accidents, gastrointestinal (GI) hemorrhage, acute pyelonephritis, acute pancreatitis, uremia, subdural hematomas, and peripheral vascular occlusion. Chronic disease, especially renal and cardiovascular, is common among patients who develop nonketotic hyperosmolar coma.

A variety of drugs have been linked to the onset of nonketotic hyperosmolar coma. Most are dehydrating agents or have side effects of impairing insulin release from the pancreas or of interfering with the peripheral action of insulin. Thiazide diuretics and diazoxide possess both characteristics and are well-recognized causes of nonketotic hyperosmolar coma. Other drugs causally related to this syndrome include steroid compounds, diphenylhydantoin, mannitol, cimetidine, propranolol, and immunosuppressive agents. Diphenylhydantoin should not be used for treating seizures in nonketotic hyperosmolar coma.

Clinical situations that can result in severe dehydration or an excessive glucose load or both may produce this syndrome in nondiabetic patients. These include extensive burns, heatstroke, hypothermia, peritoneal or hemodialysis with a hypertonic glucose solution, and hyperalimentation; these causes are most commonly seen in hospitalized patients.

An occasional patient may have a history of ingesting enormous quantities of sugar-containing fluids. This patient is usually alert and has a lesser degree of dehydration than the usual patient with nonketotic hyperosmolar coma.

The prodromal period during the development of nonketotic hyperosmolar coma is longer than that for diabetic ketoacidosis. Metabolic changes occur over many days to several weeks. Symptoms of polyuria, polydipsia, and increasing lethargy are almost always present but may not be appreciated. Failure to develop ketoacidosis and its clinical manifestations may allow the underlying process to go unrecognized until stupor or coma develops. Decreased responsiveness is the main reason patients receive medical attention.

Physical Findings

There are no specific physical findings related to nonketotic hyperosmolar coma. Virtually all the patients are significantly dehydrated. The usual signs of dehydration including dry mucous membranes, shrunken tongue, absence of sweating, and soft, sunken eyeballs are common. Postural hypotension and reflex tachycardia may be present. One-third of the patients have vascular collapse and shock. Shock is especially common if gram-negative pneumonia is present. One-third of the patients also have fever. Respirations are variable. Kussmaul's breathing is not a feature of uncomplicated nonketotic hyperosmolar coma, but hyperventilation may be present if the patient is acidotic for other reasons. Shallow respirations with hyperpnea and tachypnea are usual. The smell of acetone on the breath is absent.

The most prominent physical findings are neurologic. Almost all patients exhibit some disturbance in mentation, ranging from inappropriate response to confusion, drowsiness, stupor, or coma. The higher the osmolality, the greater the obtundation. The average osmolality for a comatose patient with nonketotic hyperosmolar coma is 380 mOsm/kg. Depression of the sensorium does not correlate with the glucose concentration or with the pH of the plasma or cerebrospinal fluid. The absence of coma does not rule out the syndrome, and a high index of suspicion for this diagnosis must be maintained in a mentally alert patient.

The most common focal signs are hemisensory deficits or hemiparesis or both. Approximately 15 percent of the patients exhibit seizure activity, usually of the focal motor type (85 percent). Grand mal seizures can occur. Tremors, fasciculations, and a variety of other neurologic abnormalities including aphasia, hyperreflexia, flaccidity, depressed deep tendon reflexes, positive plantar response, and nuchal rigidity may be seen. In one series by Arieff and Carroll, 12 of 33 patients with nonketotic hyperosmolar coma were initially diagnosed as "probably acute stroke." This diagnosis was not confirmed in any of the patients.

Considering the age of the patient population and the frequency of neurologic findings, it is not surprising that the misdiagnosis of stroke or organic brain syndrome is common. Nonketotic hyperosmolar coma must be suspected in every elderly, dehydrated patient with glucosuria or hyperglycemia, especially if they are mild diabetics and on diuretic drugs or glucocorticoids.

LABORATORY

Confirmation of the diagnosis is with laboratory findings. The essential tests are blood glucose levels, serum osmolality, and serum ketone levels. A reasonable approximation of the blood glucose and serum ketone levels can be made promptly at the bedside by use of the nitroprusside test and glucose reagent strips. Additional tests should include a complete blood cell count and levels of electrolytes, blood urea nitrogen (BUN), creatinine, and arterial blood gases. The serum osmolality can be calculated using the following formula:

$$\frac{mOsm}{kg} = 2\ (Na\ +\ K)\ +\ \frac{glucose}{18}\ +\ \frac{BUN}{2.8}$$

The measured osmolality is usually higher than the calculated value and should be obtained when possible.

Serum electrolytes display a variable pattern. Serum sodium values usually range from 120 to 160 mEq/L, but because water is lost in excess of sodium through osmotic diuresis, the patient is almost always hypertonic. It should be remembered that there is a sodium decrement of 1.6 mEq/L for every 100 mg/dL increase in blood glucose. Total body potassium depletion is invariable and usually severe. Potassium loss in nonketotic hyperosmolar coma is greater than that with diabetic ketoacidosis because of the longer duration of osmotic diuresis, GI loss, and (sometimes) kaliuretic drugs.

The BUN level is almost always elevated because of extracellular volume depletion and underlying renal disease. The initial BUN level is usually 60 to 90 mg/dL and is elevated out of proportion to the creatinine level. Ratios of BUN to creatinine may be 30:1. Prerenal azotemia resolves with volume replacement, but 60 to 80 percent of the patients have continued elevation of renal function studies, reflecting chronic renal impairment.

Metabolic acidosis due to the accumulation of ketone bodies is not a feature of nonketotic hyperosmolar coma, but metabolic acidosis due to other causes can occur. In most series, 30 to 40 percent of the patients have a mild metabolic acidosis attributed to accumulation of lactic acid or due to uremia. However, in a significant number of these cases, no cause of the acidosis can be identified.

Because of the frequency of underlying chronic disease and precipitating illnesses, a search for a precipitating cause must be made. Urinalysis, chest roentgenogram, ECG, and cultures of the blood, urine, and sputum should be performed. Because of the frequency of fever and neurologic signs, including nuchal rigidity, a lumbar puncture may be required to rule out meningitis. Typical findings in the spinal fluid include a normal opening pressure, a markedly elevated glucose level (usually 50 percent of the serum value), a normal or slightly elevated protein level, and a serum osmolality essentially identical to that of the plasma.

TREATMENT

As with treatment of all life-threatening illnesses, attention to detail and constant monitoring are imperative in the treatment of nonketotic hyperosmolar coma. Serial measurements of glucose, electrolyte, and serum osmolality levels are essential. A flow sheet to record therapeutic measures and patient response is recommended. The specific goals of therapy of nonketotic hyperosmolar coma include correction of hypovolemia and dehydration, restoration of electrolyte balance, and reduction of serum glucose and hyperosmolality levels. Reasonable endpoints that can usually be achieved within 36 h are a blood glucose level of 250 mg/dL, a serum osmolality of 320 mOsm/kg, and a urine output of at least 50 mL/h.

Fluids

No agreement exists on the composition of the initial replacement fluid. Some authors advocate the use of isotonic saline (0.9 percent

NaCl), and others recommend the use of half-normal saline (0.45 percent NaCl). Those who advocate isotonic saline believe that the most immediate threat to life is hypovolemic shock. Even though the patient has lost water in excess of solute and is hypertonic, normal saline is still hypotonic to the patient with nonketotic hyperosmolar coma. Eighty percent of an isotonic fluid remains in the extracellular fluid compartment. Use of this type of fluid acts to correct the extracellular volume deficit, stabilize the blood pressure, and maintain adequate urinary flow. Once this has been achieved, hypotonic saline can be administered to provide free water for correction of intracellular volume deficits.

Those who recommend half-normal or hypotonic saline as initial fluid therapy argue that any osmotically active solute in the replacement fluid prolongs and enhances the hyperosmotic state. Further, since the patient has lost water in excess of solute, a hypotonic solution is the logical replacement.

All authors agree that if the patient is in hypovolemic shock, isotonic saline should be given until the circulatory volume has been restored. Most agree that if the patient has significant hypernatremia (155 mEq/L) or hypertension, hypotonic saline should be the initial fluid of choice.

Rarely a patient has hyperglycemia, hyponatremia, and a low or normal osmolality. This indicates a significant excess of water, probably due to the ingestion of enormous quantities. The ritualistic use of hypotonic saline in this setting can precipitate water intoxication.

There are no controlled studies that compare the advantages of isotonic solutions with those of hypotonic solutions in the initial management of nonketotic hyperosmolar coma. Regardless of the fluid used, there are guidelines to determine the rate and amount of fluid administration.

The average fluid deficit in nonketotic hyperosmolar coma is usually between 20 and 25 percent of total body water (TBW) or 8 to 12 L. In elderly subjects, it is assumed that 50 percent of the body weight is due to TBW. By using the patient's usual weight in kilograms, normal TBW and water deficit (20 to 25 percent of TBW) can be calculated. One-half of the estimated water deficit should be relaced during the first 12 h and the balance during the next 24 h. Ongoing insensible and urinary losses should also be replaced.

The fluid should be infused at a rate determined by the individual needs of the patient but in general it should be given rapidly until the blood pressure is stable and the urine output is adequate. Fluid administration is subject to the usual considerations of renal and cardiovascular status. Central venous pressure and urinary output should be constantly monitored.

Electrolytes

Electrolyte replacement is an essential part of therapy for nonketotic hyperosmolar coma. In the average patient, for every liter of body water lost, 70 mEq of monovalent ions is concomitantly lost. That translates into 300 to 800 mEq of sodium and potassium that usually needs to be replaced.

The sodium deficit is replenished by the administration of normal saline (154 mEq of Na per liter) or half-normal saline (77 mEq of Na per liter). Potassium replacement, as with diabetic ketoacidosis, should be started early in the course of treatment. Potassium supplement should be started within 2 h of the institution of fluid and insulin therapy or as soon as adequate renal function has been confirmed. Most authors recommend the infusion of KCl at a rate of 10 to 20 mEq/h during the acute phase of therapy (24 to 36 h). Potassium should be added to the initial intravenous fluid if the patient presents with hypokalemia.

Insulin

Traditionally it has been taught that the insulin requirement of a patient with nonketotic hyperosmolar coma is less than that of a patient with diabetic ketoacidosis. The difference in insulin requirement was attributed to decreased insulin resistance in the patient with nonketotic hyperosmolar coma because of the absence of acidosis.

Changing concepts pertaining to insulin resistance and to the amount of insulin required for successful treatment of diabetic ketoacidosis have led to a reappraisal of insulin therapy for nonketotic hyperosmolar coma. Recent reports in the medical literature have espoused the efficacy of low-dose insulin techniques in the treatment of nonketotic hyperosmolar coma. Continuous intravenous infusion of low doses of insulin and intermittent intramuscular injections of low doses of insulin have been reported to be effective in treating this medical emergency.

Five to ten units of regular insulin per hour should be given by continuous intravenous infusion or by intramuscular injection. If the intramuscular route is chosen, 20 units of regular insulin can initially be administered intramuscularly or by intravenous bolus. Often no additional insulin is required after the initial dose. No insulin should be given after the blood glucose level reaches approximately 300 mg/dL.

The reasons for not using large doses of insulin when treating nonketotic hyperosmolar coma are even more compelling than those stated for diabetic ketoacidosis. In addition to producing a more gradual reduction of the glucose concentration, thus avoiding hypoglycemia, hypokalemia, and cerebral edema, low-dose insulin techniques may help to avoid vascular collapse and renal shutdown in the patient with nonketotic hyperosmolar coma.

A high glucose concentration in the extracellular fluid compartment protects that compartment against hypovolemia at the expense of intracellular water. If the concentration of glucose is rapidly lowered by the administration of large doses of insulin, insufficient extracellular osmotic solute may result in a net intracellular shift of large volumes of water, producing hypovolemia and vascular collapse. Similarly, osmotic diuresis induced by hyperglycemia acts to protect the kidney against acute tubular necrosis (ATN) in the presence of reduced renal perfusion. If the blood glucose concentration is rapidly reduced, the osmotic diuresis decreases, and ATN may result. Acute tubular necrosis after institution of large-dose insulin therapy was reported in 5 of 30 patients in the series studied by Arieff and Carroll.

Glucose

Glucose should be added to the intravenous solution when the blood glucose level declines to 250 mg/dL. It is at this level that further rapid lowering of the blood glucose concentration may result in cerebral edema. Cerebral edema can be recognized clinically by the sudden onset of hyperpyrexia, hypotension, and deepening of coma in spite of biochemical improvement. Though cerebral edema during treatment of nonketotic hyperosmolar coma is rare, it is invariably fatal and can be prevented.

Additional Treatment

The role of phosphate replacement during treatment of nonketotic hyperosmolar coma is controversial. The plasma phosphorus level should be monitored during therapy, but a case for routine phosphate infusion has not been convincingly made.

Patients with nonketotic hyperosmolar coma are at risk for the development of arterial and venous thrombosis. Low-dose prophylactic heparin therapy should be considered.

MORTALITY

The overall mortality for patients with nonketotic hyperosmolar coma is 40 to 60 percent. This distressingly high figure is due in part to the older age of the patient population. One-half of the deaths can be attributed to preexisting disease or precipitating illness. The mortalities are higher for patients with significant renal impairment. There is no absolute correlation between survival and the degree of hyperglycemia or hyperosmolality, although patients with minimal alteration in consciousness do have increased survival rates.

Nonketotic hyperosmolar coma should be considered in every elderly dehydrated patient who presents to the emergency department especially with coma, altered sensorium, or neurologic abnormalities. Known mild diabetes mellitus; a family history of diabetes; drug therapy with diuretics, propranolol, or steroids; and social isolation increase the risk of development of this insidious disorder.

BIBLIOGRAPHY

Alberti KGMM, Hockaday TDR, Turner RC: Small doses of intramuscular insulin in the treatment of diabetic "coma." *Lancet* 2:515, 1973.

Arieff AI, Carroll HJ: Cerebral edema and depression of sensorium in nonketotic hyperosmolar coma. *Diabetes* 23:525, 1974.

Arieff AI, Carroll HJ: Nonketotic hyperosmolar coma with hyperglycemia: Clinical features, pathophysiology, renal function, acid-base balance, plasma-cerebrospinal fluid equilibria and the effects of therapy in 37 cases. *Medicine* 51:73, 1972.

Arieff AI, Kleeman CR: Cerebral edema in diabetic comas. II. Effects of hyperosmolality, hyperglycemia and insulin in diabetic rabbits. *J Clin Endocrinol Metab* 38:1057, 1974.

Arieff AI, Kleeman CR: Studies on mechanisms of cerebral edema in diabetic comas: Effects of hyperglycemia and rapid lowering of plasma glucose in normal rabbits. *J Clin Invest* 52:571, 1973.

Beigelman PM: Severe diabetic ketoacidosis (diabetic "coma"): 482 episodes in 257 patients; experience of three years. *Diabetes* 20:490, 1971.

Bendezu R, Wieland RG, Furst BH, et al: Experience with low-dose insulin infusion in diabetic ketoacidosis and diabetic hyperosmolarity. *Arch Intern Med* 138:60, 1978.

Bivins BA, Hyde GL, Sachatello CR, et al: Physiopathology and management of hyperglycemic hyperosmolar nonketotic dehydration. *Surg Gynecol Obstet* 154:534, 1982.

Blackwell SW, Burns-Cox CJ: Intravascular haemolysis complicating treated non-ketotic hyperglycaemic diabetic coma. *Postgrad Med J* 49:656, 1973.

Carroll HJ, Arieff AI: Osmotic equilibrium between extracellular fluid and cerebrospinal fluid during treatment of hyperglycemic, hyperosmolar, nonketotic coma. *Trans Assoc Am Physicians* 84:113, 1971.

Chupin M. Charbonnel B, Chupin F: C-Peptide blood levels in ketoacidosis and in hyperosmolar non-ketotic diabetic coma. *Acta Diabeto Lat* 18:123, 1981.

Danowski TS: Non-ketotic coma and diabetes mellitus. *Med Clin North Am* 55:913, 1971.

Ehrlich RM, Bain HW: Hyperglycemia and hyperosmolarity in an eighteen-month-old child. *N Engl J Med* 276:683, 1967.

Feig PU, McCurdy DK: The hypertonic state. *N Engl J Med* 297:1444, 1977.

Foster DW: Insulin deficiency and hyperosmolar coma. *Adv Intern Med* 19:159, 1974.

Fulop M, Rosenblatt A, Krietzer SM, et al: Hyperosmolar nature of diabetic coma. *Diabetes* 24:594, 1975.

Gennari FJ, Kassirer JP: Osmotitic diuresis. *N Engl J Med* 291:714, 1974.

Gerich JE, Martin MM, Recant L: Clinical and metabolic characteristics of hyperosmolar nonketotic coma. *Diabetes* 20:228, 1971.

Ginsberg-Fellner F, Primack WA: Recurrent hyperosmolar nonketotic episodes in a young diabetic. *Am J Dis Child* 129:240, 1975.

Goldman SL: Hyperglycemic hyperosmolar coma in a 9-month-old child. *Am J Dis Child* 133:181, 1979.

Gordon EE, Kabadi UM: The hyperglycemic hyperosmolar syndrome. *Am J Med Sci* 271:252, 1976.

Guisado R, Arieff AI: Neurologic manifestations of diabetic comas: Correlation with biochemical alterations in the brain. *Metabolism* 24:665, 1975.

Hare JW, Rossini AA: Diabetic comas: The overlap concept. *Hosp Pract* 14(5):95, 1979.

Joffe BI, Goldberg RB, Krut LH, et al: Pathogenesis of nonketotic hyperosmolar diabetic coma. *Lancet* 1:1069, 1975.

Johnson RD, Conn JW, Dykman CJ, et al: Mechanisms and management of hyperosmolar coma without ketoacidosis in the diabetic. *Diabetes* 18:111, 1969.

Joosten R, Frank M, Hörnchen H, et al: Hyperosmolar nonketotic diabetic coma. *Eur J Pediatr* 137:233, 1981.

Katz MA: Hyperglycemia-induced hyponatremia-calculation of expected serum sodium depression. *N Engl J Med* 289:843, 1973.

Keller U, Berger W: Prevention of hypophosphatemia by phosphate infusion during treatment of diabetic ketoacidosis and hyperosmolar coma. *Diabetes* 29:87, 1980.

Keller U, Berger W, Ritz R, et al: Course and prognosis of 86 episodes of diabetic coma: A five year experience with a uniform schedule of treatment. *Diabetologia* 11:93, 1975.

Knight G, Leatherdale BA: The role of race and environment in the development of hyperosmolar hyperglycaemic nonketotic coma. *Postgrad Med J* 58:351, 1982.

Lindsey CA, Faloona GR, Unger RH: Plasma glucagon in nonketotic hyperosmolar coma. *JAMA* 229:1771, 1974.

Mather HM: Management of hyperosmolar coma. *J R Soc Med* 73:134, 1980.

McCurdy DK: Hyperosmolar hyperglycemic nonketotic diabetic coma. *Med Clin North Am* 54:683, 1970.

Nardone DA, Bouma DJ: Hyperglycemia and diabetic coma: Possible relationship to diuretic-propranolol therapy. *South Med J* 72:1607, 1979.

Podolsky S: Hyperosmolar nonketotic coma: Death can be prevented. *Geriatrics* 34(3):29, 1979.

Podolsky S: Hyperosmolar nonketotic coma in the elderly diabetic. *Med Clin North Am* 62:815, 1978.

Podolsky S, Pattavina CG: Hyperosmolar nonketotic diabetic coma: A complication of propranolol therapy. *Metabolism* 22:685, 1973.

Rubin HM, Kramer R, Drash A: Hyperosmolality complicating diabetes mellitus in childhood. *J Pediatr* 74:117, 1969.

Sament S, Schwartz MB: Severe diabetic stupor without ketosis. *S Afr Med J* 31:893, 1957.

Shenfield GM, Bhalla IP, Elton RA, et al: Fatal coma in diabetes. *Diabete Metab* 6:151, 1980.

Stevenson RE, Bowyer FP: Hyperglycemia with hyperosmolal dehydration in nondiabetic infants. *J Pediatr* 77:818, 1970.

Vinik A, Seftel H, Joffe BI: Metabolic findings in hyperosmolar, nonketotic diabetic stupor. *Lancet* 2:797, 1970.

Whelton MJ, Walde D, Havard CWH: Hyperosmolar non-ketotic diabetic coma: With particular reference to vascular complications. *Br Med J* 1:85, 1971.

Wright AD, Walsh CH, Fitzgerald MG, et al: Low-dose insulin treatment of hyperosmolar diabetic coma. *Postgrad Med J* 57:556, 1981.

Yamashiro Y, Yamamoto T, Mayama H: Nonketotic hyperosmolar coma in two diabetic children. *Acta Paediatr Scand* 70:337, 1981.

CHAPTER 93
THYROID STORM

Gene Ragland

Thyroid storm is a rare, emergent complication of hyperthyroidism in which the manifestations of thyrotoxicosis are exaggerated to life-threatening proportions. Thyroid storm is most often seen in a patient with moderate to severe antecedent Graves' disease and is usually precipitated by a stressful event. It must be suspected and treated based upon a clinical impression, as there are no pathognomonic findings or confirmatory tests.

Thyroid storm used to occur most comonly with surgical treatment of hyperthyroidism. The use of antithyroid drugs and iodine in treatment and preoperative preparation of hyperthyroid patients has markedly reduced the incidence of surgically induced storm. Currently, thyroid storm is most often due to "medical" causes. It is reported to occur in 1 to 2 percent of patients hospitalized for hyperthyroidism.

Hyperthyroid patients who are undiagnosed or undertreated are at risk for this complication. Dobyns states that true storm occurs only in Graves' disease (toxic diffuse goiter), the most common cause of hyperthyroidism. Other authors have reported toxic multinodular goiter as an antecedent to thyroid storm. The sex incidence correlates with that for Graves' disease, occurring nine times more often in women than in men. The duration of uncomplicated thyrotoxicosis preceding the onset of storm varies from 2 months to 4 years. A majority of the patients have had symptoms of hyperthyroidism for fewer than 24 months. It is not possible to predict accurately which thyrotoxic patient will develop storm as there is no predisposition by age, sex, or race.

PRECIPITATING FACTORS

A wide variety of factors have been reported as precipitating events. Thyroid surgery for treatment of hyperthyroidism used to be the most common cause of storm. Current preoperative preparation has reduced this complication but not eliminated it. Other surgically related events known to precipitate thyroid storm include nonthyroidal surgery and ether anesthesia.

Medically identified causes of thyroid storm are numerous and now predominate over surgical ones. Infection is the most common precipitating event, and pulmonary infection is the most common of these infections. In diabetic patients, ketoacidosis, hyperosmolar coma, and insulin-induced hypoglycemia have provoked storm. Events known to increase the levels of circulating thyroid hormones and initiate storm in susceptible persons include premature withdrawal of antithyroid drugs, administration of radioactive iodide, use of an iodinated contrast medium during x-ray

study, poisoning with thyroid hormone, administration of a saturated solution of potassium iodide (SSKI) to patients with nontoxic goiters, and vigorous palpation of the thyroid gland in thyrotoxic patients. Additional events implicated as causes of storm include vascular accidents, pulmonary emboli, toxemia of pregnancy, and emotional stress. Finally, hospitalization may lead to storm because of the rigors of diagnostic procedures.

PATHOGENESIS

The exact pathogenesis of thyroid storm has not been defined. It is attractive to attribute storm to excess thyroid hormone production or secretion. The results of thyroid function studies are elevated in the vast majority of patients during storm, but the values are not significantly different from those found in uncomplicated thyrotoxicosis. An increase in free triiodothyronine (T_3) or free thyroxine (T_4) levels has been suggested as causative of storm. But storm has occurred in the absence of elevated free T_3 or T_4 levels. Something in addition to excess amounts or forms of thyroid hormones must occur during storm.

Adrenergic hyperreactivity due to either patient sensitization by thyroid hormones or altered interaction between thyroid hormones and catecholamines has been suggested. Plasma levels of epinephrine and norepinephrine are not increased during thyroid storm. One author has proposed two distinct adenyl cyclase systems in the heart, one responsive to epinephrine and the other to thyroid hormones. The exact role of catecholamines in storm awaits further study.

Altered peripheral response to thyroid hormone, causing increased lipolysis and overproduction of heat, is another theory. This theory maintains that excessive lipolysis due to catecholamine–thyroid hormone interaction results in excessive thermal energy and fever. Finally, exhaustion of the body's tolerance to the action of thyroid hormones, leading to "decompensated thyrotoxicosis," is a long-standing viewpoint. This implies an altered response to thyroid hormones rather than a sudden increase in their concentration.

CLINICAL PRESENTATION

Thyroid storm is a clinical diagnosis as there are no laboratory studies that distinguish it from thyrotoxicosis. Although the clinical presentation is extremely variable, there are some clues that may aid in making this diagnosis. A history of hyperthyroidism, eye signs of Graves' disease, widened pulse pressure, and a palpable goiter are present in most patients who develop thyroid storm. However, the history may be unobtainable and the usual features of Graves' disease absent, including no obvious goiter in up to 9 percent of patients with Graves' disease.

Diagnostic Criteria

The generally accepted diagnostic criteria for thyroid storm are a temperature higher than 37.8°C (100°F); marked tachycardia out of proportion to the fever; dysfunction of the CNS, cardiovascular system, or gastrointestinal (GI) system; and exaggerated peripheral manifestations of thyrotoxicosis. Some authors consider that the sine qua non of thyroid storm is fever accompanied by disproportionate tachycardia. It should be noted, however, that the diagnosis of thyroid storm requires more than fever in a hyperthyroid patient.

The signs and symptoms of storm usually occur suddenly, but there may be a prodromal period with subtle increases in the manifestations of thyrotoxicosis.

Signs and Symptoms

The earliest signs are fever, tachycardia, diaphoresis, increased CNS activity, and emotional lability. If the condition is untreated, a hyperkinetic toxic state ensues in which the symptoms are intensified. Progression to congestive heart failure, refractory pulmonary edema, circulatory collapse, coma, and death may occur within 72 h.

Fever ranges from 38°C (100.4°F) to 41°C (105.8°F). The pulse rate may range between 120 and 200 beats per minute but has been reported as high as 300 beats per minute. Sweating may be profuse, leading to dehydration from insensible fluid loss.

Central nervous system disturbance occurs in 90 percent of patients with thyroid storm. Symptoms vary from restlessness, anxiety and emotional lability to manic behavior, agitation, and psychosis to mental confusion, obtundation, and coma. Extreme muscle weakness can occur. Thyrotoxic myopathy can occur and usually involves the proximal muscles. In severe forms, muscles of the more distal extremities and muscles of the trunk and face may be involved. About 1 percent of patients with Graves' disease develop myasthenia gravis, producing an occasional confusing clinical situation. The response of thyrotoxic myopathy to edrophonium (Tensilon test) is incomplete, unlike the complete response that occurs with myasthenia gravis. Hypokalemic periodic paralysis may also occur in patients with thyrotoxicosis.

Cardiovascular abnormalities are present in 50 percent of the patients regardless of underlying heart disease. Sinus tachycardia is usual. Arrhythmias, especially atrial fibrillation, but also including premature ventricular contractions and other rhythm disturbances, may be present. In addition to increased heart rate, there is increased stroke volume, cardiac output, and myocardial oxygen consumption. Pulse pressure is characteristically widened. Congestive heart failure, pulmonary edema, and circulatory collapse may be terminal events.

Gastrointestinal symptoms develop in most patients in storm. Before the onset of storm, a history of weight loss of more than 20 lb is usual. Diarrhea and hyperdefecation seem to herald impending storm and can be severe, contributing to dehydration. During storm, anorexia, nausea, vomiting, and crampy abdominal pain may occur. Jaundice and tender hepatomegaly due to passive congestion of the liver, or even hepatic necrosis, have been reported. The occurrence of jaundice is a poor prognostic sign.

LABORATORY

There are no laboratory tests that confirm thyroid storm. Serum levels of T_3 and T_4 are usually elevated but do not distinguish uncomplicated hyperthyroidism from thyroid storm because of an overlap in values. Radioactive iodine (RAI) uptake during storm is frequently quite high but on occasion can be below the mean range found in patients with uncomplicated thyrotoxicosis. A rapid 1- to 2-h RAI uptake study, after β-blocking agents have been started but before treatment with antithyroid drugs and iodides, has been recommended. This test should not be performed in an acutely ill patient as it delays therapy. Others have recommended a 15-min dynamic flow study of the thyroid using Tc 99m pertechnetate. Although this test may demonstrate a hyperactive thyroid gland, it cannot resolve whether storm is present or not.

Routine laboratory data during thyroid storm show wide variation. Nonspecific abnormalities in the complete blood cell count, electrolyte levels, and liver function studies may be found. Hyperglycemia (>120 mg/dL) is common, and hypercalcemia is occasionally present. One series reported all patients to have low cholesterol levels with a mean value of 117 mg/dL. Plasma cortisol levels have been observed to be inappropriately low for the degree of stress, suggesting a lack of adrenal reserve.

APATHETIC THYROTOXICOSIS

Apathetic thyrotoxicosis is a rare, distinct form that usually occurs in the elderly and is frequently misdiagnosed. These patients may develop thyroid storm without the usual hyperkinetic manifestations and may quietly lapse into coma and die. There are some salient clinical characteristics which are helpful in establishing this diagnosis. The patient is generally in the seventh decade or older, with lethargy, slowed mentation, and placid apathetic facies. Goiter is usually present but may be small and multinodular. The usual eye signs of exophthalmos, stare, and lid lag are absent, but blepharoptosis (drooping upper eye lid) is common. Excessive weight loss and proximal muscle weakness are usual. These patients generally have had symptoms longer than nonapathetic thyrotoxic patients.

"Masked" thyrotoxicosis occurs when signs and symptoms referable to dysfunction of one organ system dominate and obscure the underlying thyrotoxicosis. Signs and symptoms referable to the cardiovascular system tend to mask thyrotoxicosis in apathetic patients. These patients frequently present with atrial fibrillation and congestive heart failure. In one series of nine patients, the diagnosis of hyperthyroidism was unsuspected in each case because of the predominance of cardiovascular symptoms. Congestive heart failure in this setting may be refractory to the usual therapy unless the underlying hyperthyroidism is diagnosed and treated.

The pathogenesis of an apathetic response to thyrotoxicosis is not understood. Age alone is not the determining factor, as apathetic thyrotoxicosis has been described in the pediatric age group.

A high index of suspicion must be maintained for this diagnosis. Every elderly patient with a small goiter and any of the described signs and symptoms may have apathetic thyrotoxicosis.

TREATMENT

The importance of early treatment of thyroid storm based upon the clinical impression cannot be overemphasized. Before therapy is begun, blood should be drawn for studies of thyroid function and cortisol levels, a complete blood cell count, and routine chemistries. Appropriate cultures in search of infection are indicated. An organized treatment protocol is desirable to avoid unnecessary delay in institution of therapy.

Specific therapeutic goals can be divided into five areas: general supportive care, inhibition of thyroid hormone synthesis, retardation of thyroid hormone release, blockade of peripheral thyroid hormone effects, and identification and treatment of precipitating events. Each of these goals must be pursued concurrently.

General Supportive Care

Adequate hydration with intravenous fluids and electrolytes to replace insensible and GI losses is indicated. Supplemental oxygen is needed because of increased oxygen consumption. Hyperglycemia and hypercalcemia can occur during storm; they usually improve with fluid administration but occasionally require specific therapy directed toward reduction of unacceptably high levels. Fever should be controlled through the use of antipyretics and a cooling blanket. Aspirin should be used with caution or not at all during storm because salicylates increase free T_3 and T_4 levels because of decreased protein binding. This objection to the use of aspirin is theoretical, as no untoward clinical effect from aspirin use has been demonstrated. Caution should also be exercised in the use of sedatives during thyroid storm. Sedation depresses the level of consciousness and reduces the value of this parameter as an indicator of clinical improvement. Sedation may also cause hypoventilation.

Congestive heart failure should be treated with digitalis and diuretics even though congestive failure due to hyperthyroidism may be refractory to digitalis. Cardiac arrhythmias are treated with the usual antiarrhythmic agents. Atropine should be avoided, as its parasympatholytic effect may accelerate the heart rate. Atropine also may counteract the effect of propranolol.

Intravenous glucocorticoids equivalent to 300 mg of hydrocortisone per day should be given. The role of the adrenal glands in the pathogenesis of thyroid storm is uncertain, but the use of hydrocortisone has been reported to increase the rate of survival. Dexamethasone offers an advantage over other glucocorticoids as it decreases the peripheral conversion of T_4 to T_3.

Inhibition of Thyroid Hormone Synthesis

The antithyroid drugs propylthiouracil (PTU) and methimazole act to block the synthesis of thyroid hormone by inhibiting the organification of tyrosine residues. This action begins within 1 h after administration, but a full therapeutic effect is not achieved for weeks. An initial loading dose of PTU, 900 to 1200 mg, should be given, followed by 300 to 600 mg daily for 3 to 6 weeks or until the thyrotoxicosis comes under control. Methimazole, 90 to 120 mg initially followed by 30 to 60 mg daily, is an acceptable alternative. Both these preparations must be given orally or via a nasogastric tube, as no parenteral form is available. The PTU has an advantage over methimazole because it inhibits the peripheral conversion of T_4 to T_3 and produces a more rapid clinical response. Although these drugs inhibit the synthesis of new thyroid hormone, they do not affect the release of stored hormone.

Retardation of Thyroid Hormone Release

Iodide administration promptly retards thyroidal release of stored hormones. Iodide can be given as strong iodine solution, 30 drops orally each day, or as sodium iodide, 1 g every 8 to 12 h by slow intravenous infusion. Iodide should be administered 1 h after the loading dose of antithyroid medication to prevent utilization of the iodide by the thyroid in the synthesis of new hormone.

Blockade of Peripheral Thyroid Hormone Effects

Adrenergic blockade is a mainstay of therapy for thyroid storm. In 1960 Waldstein and co-workers reported improved survival rates with the use of reserpine in a large series. Subsequently, guanethidine was shown to effectively ameliorate signs and symptoms of thyrotoxicosis due to sympathetic hyperactivity. Currently, the β-adrenergic blocking agent propranolol is the drug of choice. In addition to reducing sympathetic hyperactivity, propranolol also partially blocks the peripheral conversion of T_4 to T_3.

Propranolol can be given intravenously at a rate of 1 mg/min with cautious incremental increases of 1 mg every 10 to 15 min to a total dose of 10 mg. The effects of the drug in controlling cardiac and psychomotor manifestations of storm should be seen in 10 m. The lowest possible dose required to control thyrotoxic symptoms should be used, and this dose can be repeated every 3 to 4 h as needed. The oral dose of propranolol is 20 to 120 mg every 4 to 6 h. When given by mouth, propranolol is effective in about 1 h. Propranolol has been used successfully in treatment of thyroid storm in childhood. Younger patients may require a dosage as high as 240 to 320 mg/day orally.

The usual precaution of avoiding propranolol in patients with bronchospastic disease and heart block should be observed. In patients with congestive heart failure, the benefit of slowing the heart rate and controlling certain arrhythmias must be weighed against the risk of depressing myocardial contractility with β-adrenergic blockade. Urbanic believes the benefit outweighs the risk in this situation but recommends administration of digitalis before propranolol.

Propranolol should not be relied upon as the sole therapeutic agent in treatment of thyrotoxicosis or thyroid storm. One author has reported two cases in which thyroid storm developed in patients who were on seemingly adequate propranolol therapy for thyrotoxicosis. It is known that after single and repeated oral doses of propranolol, plasma propranolol levels are highly variable in normal controls and thyrotoxic patients. Treatment of thyroid storm must be comprehensive and individualized.

One author recommends gradual withdrawal of propranolol as storm is brought under control. He believes that the true status of the patient may be concealed, as propranolol masks the symptoms of hypermetabolism. Patients already on β-blockers may have their symptoms of thyroid storm masked and are at risk for delayed diagnosis.

Guanethidine and reserpine also provide effective autonomic blockade and are alternatives to propranolol. Guanethidine depletes catecholamine stores and blocks their release. When given 1 to 2 mg/(Kg·day) orally (50 to 150 mg), it is effective in 24 h, but it may not have its maximum effect for several days. Toxic reactions are cumulative and include postural hypotension, myocardial decompensation, and diarrhea. It has an advantage over reserpine because it does not cause the pronounced sedation observed with that drug.

Reserpine acts to deplete catecholamine stores. As the initial dose, 1 to 5 mg is given intramuscularly, followed by 1 to 2.5 mg every 4 to 6 h. Improvement may be seen within 4 to 8 h. Side effects include sedation; psychic depression, which can be severe; abdominal cramping; and diarrhea.

Identification and Treatment of Precipitating Events

A thorough evaluation for a precipitating cause of thyroid storm should be made. The treatment of thyroid storm should not be delayed by this evaluation, which may have to wait until the patient is at least partially stabilized. A precipitating event can be identified in 50 to 75 percent of cases.

Recovery

Following the initiation of therapy, symptomatic improvement should occur within a few hours, primarily due to adrenergic blockade. Resolution of thyroid storm requires degradation of the already-circulating thyroid hormones, whose biological half-life is 6 days for T_4 and 22 h for T_3. Storm may last from 1 to 8 days, with an average duration of 3 days. If conventional therapy is not successful in controlling storm, alternative therapeutic modalities include peritoneal dialysis, plasmapheresis, and charcoal hemoperfusion to remove circulating thyroid hormone. Following recovery from thyroid storm, radioactive iodine therapy is the treatment of choice for hyperthyroidism.

Mortality

The mortality in untreated thyroid storm approaches 100 percent. Decreased mortality has occurred with the use of antithyroid drugs. A 7 percent mortality for a 10-year period is the lowest ever reported, but 10 to 20 percent is still usual. Underlying illness is the cause of death in many cases. Prevention of thyroid storm is the ultimate solution to reduce mortality. In the interim, prompt recognition and treatment of this complication of hyperthyroidism offers the best hope for survival.

BIBLIOGRAPHY

Abuid J, Larsen PR: Triiodothyronine and thyroxine in hyperthyroidism: Comparison of the acute changes during therapy with antithyroid agents. *J Clin Invest* 54:201, 1974.

Ahmad N, Cohen MP: Thyroid storm with normal serum triiodothyronine level during diabetic ketoacidosis. *JAMA* 245:2516, 1981.

Ashkar FS, Katims RB, Smoak WM, et al: Thyroid storm treatment with blood exchange and plasmapheresis. *JAMA* 214:1275, 1970.

Ashkar FS, Miller R, Gilson AJ: Thyroid function and serum thyroxine in thyroid storm. *South Med J* 65:372, 1972.

Asper SP: The treatment of hyperthyroidism. *Arch Intern Med* 106:878, 1960.

Bayley RH: Thyroid crisis. *Surg Gynecol Obstet* 59:41, 1934.

Beahrs OH, Ryan RF, White RA: Complications of thyroid surgery. *J Clin Endocrinol* 16:1456, 1956.

Bernal J, Refetoff S: The action of thyroid hormone. *Clin Endocrinol* 6:277, 1977.

Blum M, Kranjac T, Park CM, et al: Thyroid storm after cardiac angiography with iodinated contrast medium: Occurrence in a patient with a previously euthyroid autonomous nodule of the thyroid. *JAMA* 235:2324, 1976.

Bridgman JF, Pett S: Simultaneous presentation of thyrotoxic crisis and diabetic ketoacidosis. *Postgrad Med J* 56:354, 1980.

Brooks MH, Waldstein SS: Free thyroxine concentration in thyroid storm: *Ann Intern Med* 93:694, 1980.

Brooks MH, Waldstein SS, Bronsky D, et al: Serum triiodothyronine concentration in thyroid storm. *J Clin Endocrinol Metab* 40:339, 1975.

Cerletty JM, Listwan WJ: Hyperthyroidism due to functioning metastatic thyroid carcinoma: Precipitation of thyroid storm with therapeutic radioactive iodine. *JAMA* 242:269, 1979.

Chandler PT, Chandler SA: Update on thyroid storm. *J Ky Med Assoc* 77:571, 1979.

Clute HM: The operative mortality in hyperthyroidism. *JAMA* 95:389, 1930.

Coulombe P, Dussault JH, Walker P: Catecholamine metabolism in thyroid disease: II. Norepinephrine secretion rate in hyperthyroidism and hypothyroidism. *J Clin Endocrinol Metab* 44:1185, 1977.

Das G, Krieger M: Treatment of thyrotoxic storm with intravenous administration of propranolol. *Ann Intern Med* 70:985, 1969.

Dillon PT, Babe J, Meloni CR, et al: Reserpine in thyrotoxic crisis. *N Engl J Med* 283:1020, 1970.

Dobyns BM: Prevention and management of hyperthyroid storm. *World J Surg* 2:293, 1978.

Dumlao JS: Thyroid storm. *Postgrad Med* 56(2):57, 1974.

Eriksson M, Rubenfeld S, Garber AJ, et al: Propranolol does not prevent thyroid storm. *N Engl J Med* 296, 263, 1977.

Freeman M, Giuliani M, Schwartz E, et al: Acute thyroiditis, thyroid crisis, and hypocalcemia following radioactive iodine therapy. *NY State J Med* 69:2036, 1969.

Galaburda M, Rosman NP, Haddow JE: Thyroid storm in an 11-year-old boy managed by propranolol. *Pediatrics* 53:920, 1974.

Goldfarb CR, Varma C, Roginsky MS: Diagnosis in delirium: Prompt confirmation of thyroid storm. *Clin Nucl Med* 5:66, 1980.

Goonewardena JN, Silva YJ: Thyroid storm in a decade of clinical practice. *W Va Med J* 75:124, 1979.

Grossman A, Waldstein SS: Apathetic thyroid storm in a 10-year-old child. *Pediatrics* 28:447, 1961.

Hanscom DH, Ryan RJ: Thyrotoxic crisis and diabetic ketoacidosis. *N Engl J Med* 257:697, 1957.

Herrmann J, Rudorff KH, Gockenjan G, et al: Charcoal haemoperfusion in thyroid storm (letter). *Lancet* 1:248, 1977.

Hoffenberg R: Thyroid emergencies. *Clin Endocrinol Metab* 9:503, 1980.

Jacobs HS, Mackie DB, Eastman CJ, et al: Total and free triiodothyronine and thyroxine levels in thyroid storm and recurrent hyperthyroidism. *Lancet* 2:236, 1973.

Jones DK, Solomon S: Thyrotoxic crisis masked by treatment with beta-blockers. *Br Med J* 283:659, 1981.

Lahey FH: The crisis of exophthalmic goiter. *N Engl J Med* 199:255, 1928.

Lahey FH: Non-activated (apathetic) type of hyperthyroidism. *N Engl J Med* 204:747, 1931.

Lamphier TA: Current status of diagnosis and treatment of thyroid storm. *Md State Med J* 29:67, 1980.

Larsen PR: Salicylate-induced increases in free triiodothyronine in human serum: Evidence of inhibition of triiodothyronine binding to thyroxine-binding globulin and thyroxine-binding prealbumin. *J Clin Invest* 51:1125, 1972.

Levey GS: Catecholamine sensitivity, thyroid hormone and the heart: A reevaluation. *Am J Med* 50:413, 1971.

McArthur JW, Rawson RW, Means JH, et al: Thyroid crisis: An analysis of the thirty-six cases seen at Massachusetts General Hospital during the past twenty-five years. *JAMA* 134:868, 1947.

McClintock JC, Gassner FX, Bigelow N, et al: Antithyroid drugs in the treatment of hyperthyroidism. *Surg Gynecol Obstet* 112:653, 1961.

McGee RR, Whittaker RL, Tullis IF: Apathetic thyroidism: Review of the literature and report of four cases. *Ann Intern Med* 50:1418, 1959.

Mackin JF, Canary JJ, Pittman CS: Thyroid storm and its management. *N Engl J Med* 291:1396, 1974.

Mazzaferri EL, Reynolds JC, Young RL, et al: Propranolol as primary therapy for thyrotoxicosis: Results of a long-term prospective study. *Arch Intern Med* 136:50, 1976.

Mazzaferri EL, Skillman TG: Thyroid storm: A review of 22 episodes with special emphasis on the use of guanethidine. *Arch Intern Med* 124:684, 1969.

Menon V, McDougall WW, Leatherdale BA: Thyrotoxic crisis following eclampsia and induction of labour. *Postgrad Med J* 58:286, 1982.

Nelson NC, Becker WF: Thyroid crisis: Diagnosis and treatment. *Ann Surg* 170:263, 1969.

Newmark SR, Shane JM: Hyperthyroid crisis (letter). *JAMA* 233:509, 1975.

Newmark SR, Himathongkam T, Shane JM: Hyperthyroid crisis. *JAMA* 230:592, 1974.

Oppenheimer JH, Schwartz HL, Surks MI: Propylthiouracil inhibits the conversion of L-thyroxine to L-triiodothyronine: An explanation of the antithyroxine effect of propylthiouracil and evidence supporting the concept that triiodothyronine is the active thyroid hormone. *J Clin Invest* 51:2493, 1972.

Ransom HK, Bayley RH: Thyroid crisis. *West J Surg* 42:464, 1934.

Roizen M, Becker C: Thyroid storm: A review of cases at University of California, San Francisco. *Calif Med* 115:5, 1971.

Rubenfeld S, Silverman VE, Welch KMA, et al: Variable plasma propranolol levels in thyrotoxicosis. *N Engl J Med* 300:353, 1979.

Serri O, Gagnon RM, Goulet Y, et al: Coma secondary to apathetic thyrotoxicosis. *Can Med Assoc J* 119:605, 1978.

Schottstaedt ES, Smoller M: "Thyroid storm" produced by acute thyroid hormone poisoning. *Ann Intern Med* 64:847, 1966.

Shafer RB, Nuttall FQ: Acute changes in thyroid function in patients treated with radioactive iodine. *Lancet* 2:635, 1975.

Shand DG: Individualization of propranolol therapy. *Med Clin North Am* 58:1063, 1974.

Shand DG: Propranolol. *N Eng J Med* 293:280, 1975.

Shanks RG, Hadden DR, Lowe DC, et al: Controlled trial of propranolol in thyrotoxicosis. *Lancet* 1:993, 1969.

Spaulding SW, Noth RH: Thyroid-catecholamine interactions. *Med Clin North Am* 59:1123, 1975.

Thomas FB, Mazzaferri EL, Skillman TG: Apathetic thyrotoxicosis: A distinctive clinical and laboratory entity. *Ann Intern Med* 72:679, 1970.

Urbanic RC, Mazzaferri EL: Thyrotoxic crisis and myxedema coma. *Heart Lung* 7:435, 1978.

Vagenakis AG, Wang C, Burger A, et al: Iodide-induced thyrotoxicosis in Boston. *N Engl J Med* 287:523, 1972.

Waldstein SS, Kaganiec I, et al: A clinical study of thyroid storm. *Ann Intern Med* 52:626, 1960.

Waldstein SS, West GH, Lee WY, et al: Guanethidine in hyperthyroidism. *JAMA* 189:609, 1964.

Wiersinga WM, Touber JL: The influence of β-adrenoceptor blocking agents on plasma thyroxine and triiodothyronine. *J Clin Endocrinol Metab* 45:293, 1977.

Williams DE, Chopra IJ, Orgiazzi J, et al: Acute effects of corticosteroids on thyroid activity in Graves' disease. *J Clin Endocrinol Metab* 41:354, 1975.

CHAPTER 94

MYXEDEMA COMA

Gene Ragland

Myxedema coma is a life-threatening expression of hypothyroidism in its most severe form. It occurs most often during the winter months in elderly women with long-standing, undiagnosed, or undertreated hypothyroidism. It may be precipitated by infection or other stresses, and the diagnosis must be suspected based upon the clinical presentation. Treatment should be prompt and requires the administration of thyroid hormone in large doses. The mortality is greater than 50 percent in spite of optimum therapy.

CAUSES OF HYPOTHYROIDISM

Hypothyroidism is a chronic systemic disorder characterized by progressive slowing of all bodily functions because of thyroid hormone deficiency. Thyroid hormone is secreted in response to stimulation of the thyroid gland by thyroid-stimulating hormone (TSH) from the anterior pituitary gland. The TSH release is promoted by thyrotropin releasing hormone (TRH) from the hypothalamus. Therefore, thyroid failure may be primary, due to intrinsic failure of the thyroid gland, or secondary, due to disease or destruction of the hypothalamus or pituitary gland (Table 94-1).

Primary Hypothyroidism

Primary thyroid failure is by far the most common, accounting for 95 percent of the cases of hypothyroidism. The most common cause of hypothyroidism in the adult is treatment of Graves' disease by radioactive iodine or subtotal thyroidectomy. The postoperative incidence of hypothyroidism is approximately 15 percent, and the condition is usually evident within 12 to 15 months after surgery. The incidence of hypothyroidism following destruction of thyroid tissue with radioiodine increases progressively with time, and at 10 years is 40 to 70 percent. The development of hypothyroidism as a consequence of effective surgical or radioiodine therapy may take years or decades; such patients must be followed indefinitely. If hypothyroidism develops, these patients are committed to replacement thyroid hormone therapy for life.

Autoimmune thyroid disorders are the next most common cause of hypothyroidism. These include primary hypothyroidism and Hashimoto's thyroiditis. Primary hypothyroidism is thought to be the end result of an autoimmune destruction of the thyroid gland and produces thyroid failure because of glandular atrophy. Hashimoto's thyroiditis is the most common cause of goitrous hypothyroidism in areas with adequate iodine and may cause hypothyroidism because of defective hormone synthesis. There is clinical and immunologic overlap of these entities. Other causes of primary thyroid failure are rare and include iodine deficiency, antithyroid drugs such as lithium and phenylbutazone, spontaneous hypothyroidism from Graves' disease, and congenital causes.

Secondary Hypothyroidism

Secondary thyroid failure accounts for 5 percent of the cases of hypothyroidism. Pituitary tumors, postpartum hemorrhage, or infiltrative disorders, such as sarcoidosis, may result in secondary thyroid failure. There are clinical and historical differences that distinguish primary thyroid insufficiency from pituitary failure (see Table 94-1). This differential diagnosis is difficult on clinical grounds and requires laboratory evaluation. In general, the TSH level is high in primary hypothyroidism and low or normal in secondary hypothyroidism. Disease of the hypothalamus may cause failure to secrete TRH and may result in thyroid failure. This condition has been termed *tertiary hypothyroidism*. A few hypothyroid patients have been identified who have presumed hypothalamic disease and respond to TRH administration by increasing TSH above baseline levels.

CLINICAL PRESENTATION

All patients who develop myxedema are hypothyroid, but not all hypothyroid patients have myxedema. Hypothyroidism is a graded phenomenon with various signs and symptoms along the clinical spectrum. With moderate to severe hypothyroidism, a nonpitting, dry, waxy swelling of the skin and subcutaneous tissue may occur, resulting in a puffy face and extremities. The term *myxedema* refers to this particular presentation of hypothyroidism.

The signs and symptoms of mild hypothyroidism may be subtle and the diagnosis difficult. With advanced hypothyroidism, the patients present with characteristic features. Typically, they complain of fatigue, weakness, cold intolerance, constipation, and weight gain without an increase in appetite. Muscle cramps, decreased hearing, mental disturbances, and menstrual irregularities are additional symptoms. Cutaneous features noted on physical examination include dry, scaly, yellow skin, puffy eyes, thinning of the eyebrows, and scant body hair. The voice may be deep and coarse and the tongue thickened. Paresthesias, ataxia, and

Table 94-1. Differentiation of Primary and Secondary Myxedema*

Primary (Thyroid)	Secondary (Pituitary)
Previous thyroid operation	No previous thyroid operation
Obese	Less obese
Goiter present	No goiter present
Hypothermia more common	Hypothermia less common
Increased serum cholesterol	Normal serum cholesterol
Voice coarse	Voice less coarse
Pubic hair present	Pubic hair absent
Sella turcica normal	Sella turcica may be increased in size
Plasma cortisol level normal	Plasma cortisol level decreased
Skin dry and coarse	Skin fine and soft
Heart increased in size	Heart usually small
Normal menses and lactation	Traumatic delivery, no lactation; amenorrhea
No response to TSH	Good response to TSH
Good response to levothyroxine without steroids	Poor response to levothyroxine without steroids
PBI <2μg/100 mL	PBI >2μg/100 mL
Serum TSH increased	Serum TSH decreased

*TSH signifies thyroid-stimulating hormone, PBI, protein-bound iodine.

Source: From Senior RM, Birge SJ: The recognition and management of myxedema coma. *JAMA* 217:61, 1971.

prolongation of the deep tendon reflexes are characteristic neurologic manifestations. Mild hypertension rather than hypotension is the rule. In advanced cases, delusions, hallucinations, and frank psychosis (myxedema madness) may occur. Abdominal distension and fecal impaction may be present. Cardiac findings include hypotension, bradycardia, enlarged heart, and low voltage on ECG. A surgical scar on the neck may be present, but a palpable goiter is uncommon.

Diagnosis of hypothyroidism in a patient with these signs and symptoms can be made essentially on clinical grounds. Abnormally low levels of thyroid hormones confirm the diagnosis. If the disease is not treated, death follows a progressive intensification of these signs and symptoms. The time from onset to death varies between 10 and 15 years. Appropriate therapy is L-thyroxine in an average maintenance dosage of 0.1 to 0.3 mg once daily. The dosage must be individualized and may be higher or lower. Other thyroid preparations are available and acceptable as replacement thyroid hormone therapy.

MYXEDEMA COMA

Myxedema coma is a rare complication of hypothyroidism, occurring in 0.1 percent of patients hospitalized with thyroid failure. The incidence is greater in women than men, with a ratio of 3.5:1. In one review, 60 of 77 patients were female. Myxedema coma is rare in a patient under the age of 50 years, and approximately half the patients are between 60 and 70 years old. A patient with undiagnosed hypothyroidism may present in coma, and this is the initial manifestation of the disease. More commonly, the disease progresses insidiously, and coma develops when the patient is subjected to stress.

Precipitating Factors

A precipitating factor can be found in most cases of myxedema coma. Exposure to a cold environment is a significant antecedent occurrence. In Forester's series, 73 of 77 patients developed myxedema coma during a cold season. In this setting, pulmonary infection and heart failure were identified as the most frequent precipitating events. Catz and co-workers found pneumonia as the precipitating cause of coma in 9 of 12 cases. Other stresses reported to initiate coma include hemorrhage, cerebrovascular accident, hypoxia, hypercapnia, hyponatremia, hypoglycemia, and trauma.

Significantly, it has been observed that greater than 50 percent of the patients whose cases were reported in the literature lapsed into coma after admission to the hospital. In this setting, the stress of diagnostic and therapeutic procedures, and acquisition of nosocomial infections, and the administration of certain drugs have been implicated as causative factors. Hypothyroid patients metabolize drugs more slowly than normal persons, and narcotics, anesthetics, phenothiazines, and other tranquilizers or sedatives have been reported to induce coma. One author noted that a prolonged (40 h) dystonic reaction to chlorpromazine occurred in a patient with myxedema coma, presumably because of the decreased rate of drug metabolism. Disastrous results may occur in a patient with advanced hypothyroidism and myxedema madness whose psychosis is treated with phenothiazines. The β-blocking drugs may cause myxedema coma by reducing thyroid hormone levels through peripheral conversion of thyroxine to triiodothyronine. Caution must be used when administering drugs, even in normal amounts, to hypothyroid patients. A final drug-related cause of myxedema coma is the failure of a patient who is dependent on it to take replacement thyroid hormone medication.

Clinical Presentation

The diagnosis of myxedema coma may easily be made in a patient who presents with the previously described general apearance and physical findings and with a history of previous thyroid hormone medication, radioactive iodine therapy, or subtotal thyroidectomy. Unfortunately, the diagnosis is not always that easy. A wide variety of clinical and laboratory abnormalities occur and may tend to occupy the physician's attention. Coma may be attributed to hypothermia, respiratory failure, and CO_2 narcosis; electrolyte imbalance and hyponatremia; hypoglycemia; congestive heart failure; stroke; drug overdose; and other causes. Indeed, any of these disorders may lead to or worsen coma in the hypothyroid patient, but unless the underlying thyroid failure is diagnosed and treated, therapeutic efforts are unsuccessful. The overall clinical picture must be correlated and the diagnosis of myxedema coma considered.

Hypothermia

Hypothermia, unaccompanied by sweating or shivering, is typical of patients in myxedema coma and occurs in 80 percent of the cases. Approximately 15 percent have a temperature of 29.5°C (85°F) or less; none of the patients in Forester's series survived a temperature at that level. One-fifth of his patients had a normal or elevated temperature, which is suggestive of underlying infection. It is not coincidental that most patients develop myxedema coma during the winter, as normal thermogenesis is impaired in hypothyroidism.

This important diagnostic sign may be missed if a low-reading thermometer is not used or if the mercury in the thermometer is not shaken down. A survey of emergency rooms found that only 20 percent had a low-reading thermometer; 30 percent did not have one in the emergency department but could obtain one elsewhere in the hospital, and the remaining 50 percent did not have access to one at all or were uncertain whether one was available! Hypothermia should be treated by gradual rewarming at room temperature. Too-rapid rewarming with hot baths, electric blankets, and the like may cause peripheral vasodilation and circulatory collapse.

Respiratory Failure

Hypoventilation, hypercapnia, and hypoxia are common in patients with myxedema coma and may be the cause of death in many instances. Multiple factors have been implicated as causes of respiratory failure. Impaired respiratory mechanics due to dysfunction of the muscles of the respiratory system may lead to alveolar hypoventilation, hypercapnia, and hypoxia, and loss of responsiveness of the respiratory center to these stimuli. Zwillich and co-workers have shown that with thyroid hormone replacement hypoxic ventilatory drive is increased but hypercapnic ventilatory drive is not.

Additional factors that may further impair pulmonary function include obesity, congestive heart failure, pleural effusions, ascites, parenchymal lung involvement by myxedematous infiltrate, enlarged tongue, and changes in the airway, which may occur over its entire length. Airway obstruction due to myxedematous infiltration of the laryngeal mucosa has been reported. These patients should be evaluated by chest roentgenography, determination of the arterial blood gas levels, and close monitoring. Drugs that may further depress respirations should be avoided. Mechanical ventilation may be required, and initial tracheostomy has been recommended because of the long recovery time for normal ventilatory function.

Hyponatremia

Water retention with electrolyte imbalance is another common finding in myxedema coma. Forester reported hyponatremia and hypochloremia in 46 percent of cases. The hyponatremia is dilutional and not the result of chronic sodium wasting. Extracellular volume expansion and impaired ability to excrete a water load occurs in hypothyroidism. Several mechanisms to account for the hyponatremia have been proposed. These range from deficiency of adrenal cortical hormones to decreased water delivery to the distal nephron to inappropriate secretion of antidiuretic hormone. Regardless of the etiology, hyponatremia is a potentially grave complication that can lead to water intoxication, brain edema, and death.

Conventional therapy of hyponatremia is fluid restriction unless the hyponatremia is profound. Hypertonic saline is recommended in patients whose serum sodium level is less than 115 mEq/L. A convincing case for a different therapeutic approach utilizing hypertonic saline, furosemide, and thyroid hormone has been pre-

sented. A review of the 24 hyponatremic-hypothyroid patients described in the literature since 1953 showed the serum sodium levels to range from 120 to 129 mEq/L in 8 patients, from 110 to 119 mEq/L in 10 patients, and to be less than 110 mEq/L in 6 others. All 6 patients treated with hypertonic saline survived, while 13 out of 18 who did not receive this treatment died. Intravenous furosemide induces negative water balance, while hypertonic saline replaces urinary sodium losses. Extreme caution must be used to avoid additional strain on the cardiovascular system during the administration of hypertonic saline.

Cardiovascular System

The cardiovascular system is altered in structure and function with advanced hypothyroidism. Hypotension, cardiac enlargement detectable on x-ray films, and bradycardia are the most significant abnormalities to occur during myxedema coma. In one series, 50 percent of patients who had blood pressures recorded had readings less than 100/60. Thyroid hormones and sympathomimetic amines act synergistically to maintain left ventricular performance and vascular tone. Hypotension may result from a decreased synergistic effect due to thyroid hormone deficiency. Left ventricular dysfunction and hypotension are usually corrected by thyroid hormone replacement. Vasopressors do not work well in the absence of thyroid hormone and should be used, with caution, only in cases of severe hypotension unresponsive to other therapy. Ventricular arrhythmia may occur because of the synergistic actions of simultaneously administered thyroid hormone and vasopressors on a myxedematous myocardium.

Cardiomegaly is seen on chest x-ray films in approximately 50 percent of myxedematous patients. Cardiac enlargement is thought to be due to either pericardial effusion or underlying heart disease and not to ventricular dilation induced by hypothyroidism. In one study, pericardial effusions were present in 30 percent of the patients, but only 70 percent with effusions were found to have cardiomegaly on x-ray films. Therefore, the presence or absence of cardiomegaly on x-ray films is not a reliable indicator of a pericardial effusion. Echocardiography may be required to determine if an effusion is present. In spite of the frequency of pericardial effusions, cardiac tamponade in myxedema coma is rare because of the slow formation of the effusion and the ability of the pericardium to distend. Most pericardial effusions resolve with thyroid hormone replacement, but some may require pericardiocentesis or pericardial fenestration.

Sinus bradycardia is the most common electrocardiographic abnormality during myxedema coma. Other findings include low voltage, flattening or inversion of the T waves, and prolongation of the PR interval. One-half of the patients studied by Aber and co-workers exhibited these typical changes. In spite of impaired cardiac contractility, pericardial effusions, and conduction disturbances, congestive heart failure is unusual in myxedema coma and probably is reflective of underlying heart disease.

Nervous System

Coma is the terminal expression of neurologic dysfunction in myxedema and may be directly due to a lack of thyroid hormone in the brain. A variety of neurologic symptoms premonitory of myxedema coma do occur. Psychiatric disorders were seen in 18 of 56 cases of myxedema and included slowed mentation, memory loss, personality changes, hallucinations, delusions, and frank psychosis. Cerebellar signs of ataxia, intention tremor, nystagmus, and difficulty with coordinated movements may occur. Twenty-five percent of those who develop myxedema coma initially present with grand mal seizure. Many of the neuropsychiatric abnormalities improve with thyroid hormone replacement, but permanent dementia may remain after treatment. The role of hypothermia, CO_2 narcosis, cerebral edema, and other metabolic disturbances in the genesis of coma must not be overlooked.

Gastrointestinal System

Patients with myxedema may have abdominal distension due to ascites, paralytic ileus, or fecal impaction. Acquired megacolon is almost uniformly observed and has been the cause of unnecessary abdominal surgery. Urinary retention may occur, causing lower abdominal discomfort from a distended bladder. The weight gain that occurs with hypothyroidism is due to accumulation of some adipose tissue and retention of fluid. Patients with myxedema coma may be emaciated because of long-standing illness and decreased food intake. The treatment of abdominal complications consists of thyroid replacement and conservative measures such as nasogastric aspiration and enemas.

Laboratory

A variety of laboratory abnormalities occur during myxedema coma. Although some laboratory findings are characteristic of myxedema coma, only thyroid function tests can confirm hypothyroidism. Serum thyroxine levels, triiodothyronine levels, triiodothyronine resin uptake, and TSH levels should be measured. The results of these tests will not be available for use in the emergent situation but can later be used to support the clinical impression.

Characteristic laboratory abnormalities of myxedema coma already mentioned include hypoxemia, hypercapnia, hyponatremia, and hypochloremia. Serum potassium levels are extremely variable from a low of 2 mEq/L in one study to more than 5 mEq/L in 10 of 19 cases in another study. Blood glucose levels are generally in the normal range, but severe hypoglycemia can occur. Hypoglycemia (less than 60 mEq/dL) was found in 4 of 23 cases and was implicated as the cause of death in 2 cases in a study by Forester. Hypercalcemia is a rare occurrence during myxedema coma. Hypocalcemia, especially in thyroidectomized patients in whom the parathyroids have been removed, has been described.

Elevated serum cholesterol levels occur in approximately two-thirds of myxedematous patients. One series reported a range from 160 to 680 mg/dL, while another author recommended the use of the serum cholesterol level as one of the "best confirmatory tests" of the presence of myxedema. Malnutrition may lower the serum cholesterol level in some cases. Carotenemia has also been reported and may be the cause of the yellowish skin discoloration. Occasionally, striking elevations of the levels of muscle enzymes such as creatine kinase (CPK), serum glutamic-oxaloacetic transaminase (SGOT), lactate dehydrogenase (LDH), and fructose-biphosphate aldolase may be present. The elevations are thought to be due to changes in membrane permeability in skeletal muscle rather than to muscle destruction. The concentrations of these enzymes fall quickly when thyroid hormone is replaced. Finally, in most hypothyroid patients the CSF protein level is elevated to 100 mg/dL or more. The CSF pressure may occasionally be increased to over 400 mmH$_2$O. The significance of these CSF abnormalities remains obscure.

TREATMENT

Patients with myxedema coma are critically ill with a multiplicity of precarious and complex management problems. Specific therapy requires the administration of large doses of thyroid hormone. This decision must be based upon clinical judgment and made with extreme caution. The recommended dose of thyroid hormone could be fatal to the euthyroid comatose patient and harmful to the patient with ordinary myxedema. Every attempt to rule out causes of coma unrelated to hypothyroidism must be made first.

Supportive Therapy

Coma in myxedema may be primary, from a cerebral lack of thyroid hormone, or secondary, due to complications or precipitating causes. Treatment of the secondary causes of coma already mentioned includes oxygen administration and ventilatory support for respiratory failure, avoidance of drugs that may further depress respiratory or metabolic function, gradual rewarming of hypothermic patients, correction of hyponatremia by fluid restriction or hypertonic saline and furosemide, correction of hypoglycemia by glucose infusion, and treatment of hypotension with thyroid hormone and vasopressors, as needed. A thorough search for precipitating causes of coma should be made. Antibiotics are indicated for underlying infection. Additional adjunctive therapy is hydrocortisone, 300 mg/day, to protect against adrenal insufficiency.

Thyroid Hormone

Thyroid hormone replacement is the most critical and specific aspect of therapy for myxedema coma. The treatment already mentioned is largely supportive and is not fully effective until adequate thyroid hormone is given. Disagreement exists over the type, dose, and route of thyroid hormone administration.

Intravenous thyroxine is the drug of choice of most authors. It has been shown to be fully effective within 24 h, with an onset of action in 6 h. The initial intravenous dose is 400 to 500 mg infused slowly; this is followed by the intravenous administration of 50 to 100 mg daily. Following the initial dose, some authors recommend no further thyroxine therapy until 3 to 7 days later. Once-daily therapy allows a smooth rise in hormone levels, as the turnover rate for L-thyroxine is about 10 percent per day. An oral dosage of thyroxine, 100 to 200 mg/day, can be started when possible. Cardiac arrest following the intravenous administration of L-thyroxine has been reported. The dose of thyroxine should be reduced in the face of cardiac ischemia or arrhythmias.

Triiodothyronine is an effective drug for treatment of myxedema coma. It has a more rapid onset of action than thyroxine but a shorter half-life. Repeated doses are required, which may cause abrupt cyclic changes in metabolic status. In addition, triiodothyronine must be administered orally or via nasogastric tube and has less predictable absorption by this route. In spite of these drawbacks, triiodothyronine, 12.5 mg every 6 to 8 h, can be used. Overall clinical improvement should be seen in 24 to 36 h.

BIBLIOGRAPHY

Aber CP, Thompson GS: Factors associated with cardiac enlargement in myxedema. *Br Heart J* 25:421, 1963.

Arieff AI, Llach F, Massry SG: Neurological manifestations and morbidity of hyponatremia: Correlation with brain water and electrolytes. *Medicine* 55:121, 1976.

Asher R: Myxedema madness. *Br Med J* 2:555, 1949.

Bacci V, Schussler GC, Bhogal RS, et al: Cardiac arrest after intravenous administration of levothyroxine (letter). *JAMA* 245:920, 1981.

Blum M: Myxedema coma. *Am J Med Sci* 264:432, 1972.

Brewster WR, Isaacs JP, Osgood PF, et al: The hemodynamic and metabolic interrelationships in the activity of epinephrine, norepinephrine and the thyroid hormones. *Circulation* 13:1, 1956.

Catz B, Russell S: Myxedema, shock and coma: Seven survival cases. *Arch Intern Med* 108:407, 1961.

Chiprut RO, Knudsen KB, Liebermann TR, et al: Myxedema ascites. *Am J Dig Dis* 21:807, 1976.

Crowley WF, Ridgway EC, Bough EW, et al: Noninvasive evaluation of cardiac function in hypothyroidism: Response to gradual thyroxine replacement. *N Engl J Med* 296:1, 1977.

Derubertis FR, Michelis MF, Bloom ME, et al: Impaired water excretion in myxedema. *Am J Med* 51:41, 1971.

Doniach D: Hashimoto's thyroiditis and primary myxedema viewed as separate entities. *Eur J Clin Invest* 11:245, 1981.

Doran GR, Wilkinson JH: The origin of the elevated activities of creatine kinase and other enzymes in the sera of patients with myxedema. *Clin Chim Acta* 62:203, 1975.

Dunn JT, Chapman EM: Rising incidence of hypothyroidism after radioactive-iodine therapy in thyrotoxicosis. *N Engl J Med* 271:1037, 1964.

Erwin L: Myxedema presenting with severe laryngeal obstruction. *Postgrad Med J* 58:169, 1982.

Evered D, Hall R: Hypothyroidism. *Br Med J* 1:290, 1972.

Forester CF: Coma in myxedema. *Arch Intern Med* 111:734, 1963.

Goldberg M, Reivich M: Studies on the mechanisms of hyponatremia and impaired water excretion in myxedema. *Ann Intern Med* 56:120, 1962.

Green WL: Hyperthyroid crisis (letter). *JAMA* 233:508, 1975.

Griffiths PD: Serum enzymes in diseases of the thyroid gland. *J Clin Pathol* 18:660, 1965.

Gupta OP, Bhatia PL, Agarwal MK, et al: Nasal, pharyngeal and laryngeal manifestations of hypothyroidism. *Ear Nose Throat J* 56:349, 1977.

Hamburger S, Collier RE: Myxedema coma. *Ann Emerg Med* 11:156, 1982.

Hoffenberg R: Thyroid emergencies. *Clin Endocrinol Metab* 9:503, 1980.

Holvy DN, Goodner CJ, Nicoloff JT, et al: Treatment of myxedema coma with intravenous thyroxine. *Arch Intern Med* 113:89, 1964.

Ivy HK: Myxedema precoma: Complications and therapy. *Mayo Clin Proc* 40:403, 1965.

Jellinek EH: Fits, faints, coma, and dementia in myxoedema. *Lancet* 2:1010, 1962.

Jones ER, Cook W, Lizarralde G: Myxedema crisis. *South Med J* 67:1481, 1974.

Kerber RE, Sherman B: Echocardiographic evaluation of pericardial effusion in myxedema: Incidence and biochemical and clinical correlations. *Circulation* 52:823, 1975.

Khaleeli AA: Myxedema coma: A report on five successfully treated cases. *Postgrad Med J* 54:825, 1978.

Khaleeli AA, Memon N: Factors affecting resolution of pericardial effusions in primary hypothyroidism: A clinical, biochemical and echocardiographic study. *Postgrad Med J* 58:473, 1982.

Lindberger K: Myxedema coma. *Acta Med Scand* 198:87, 1975.

Lowe CE, Bird ED, Thomas WC: Hypercalcemia in myxedema. *J Clin Endocrinol Metab* 22:261, 1962.

MacLean D, Griffiths PA, Browning MCK, et al: Metabolic aspects of spontaneous rewarming in accidental hypothermia and hypothermic myxedema. *Q J Med* 63:371, 1974.

McConahey WM: Diagnosing and treating myxedema and myxedema coma. *Geriatrics* 33(3):61, 1978.

Massumi RA, Winnacker JL: Severe depression of the respiratory center in myxedema. *Am J Med* 36:876, 1964.

Menendez CE, Rivlin RS: Thyrotoxic crisis and myxedema coma. *Med Clin North Am* 57:1463, 1973.

Michie MBE, Beck JS, Pollet JE: Prevention and management of hypothyroidism after thyroidectomy for thyrotoxicosis. *World J Surg* 2:307, 1978.

Mitchell JRA, Surridge DHC, Willison RG: Hypothermia after chlorpromazine in myxedematous psychosis. *Br Med J* 2:932, 1959.

Murakami K, Kasama T, Hayashi R, et al: Myxedema coma induced by beta-adrenoreceptor-blocking agent. *Br Med J* 285:543, 1982.

Newmark SR, Himathongkam T, Shane JM: Myxedema coma. *JAMA* 230:884, 1974.

Nichols AB, Hunt WB: Is myxedema coma respiratory failure? *South Med J* 69:945, 1976.

Nickerson JF, Hill SR, McNeil JH, et al: Fatal myxedema, with and without coma. *Ann Intern Med* 53:475, 1960.

Nicoloff JT: Treatment of hypothyroidism and myxedema coma. *Mod Treatm* 6:465, 1969.

Nofal MM, Beierwaltes WH: Treatment of hyperthyroidism with sodium iodide I[131]. *JAMA* 197:605, 1966.

Nordqvist P, Dhuner KG, Stenberg K, et al: Myxedema coma and CO_2-retention. *Acta Med Scand* 166:189, 1960.

Perlmutter M, Cohn H: Myxedema crisis of pituitary or thyroid origin. *Am J Med* 36:883, 1964.

Pittman JA, Haigler ED, Hershman JM: Hypothalamic hypothyroidism. *N Engl J Med* 285:844, 1971.

Ridgway EC, McCammon JA, Benotti J, et al: Acute metabolic responses in myxedema to large doses of intravenous L-thyroxine. *Ann Intern Med* 77:549, 1972.

Rosenberg IN: Hypothyroidism and coma. *Surg Clin North Am* 48:353, 1968.

Saberi M, Utiger RD: Serum thyroid hormone and thyrotropin concentrations during thyroxine and triiodothyronine therapy. *J Clin Endocrinol Metab* 39:923, 1974.

Sanders V: Neurologic manifestations of myxedema. *N Engl J Med* 266:547 and 599, 1962.

Senior RM, Birge SJ, Wessler S, et al: The recognition and management of myxedema coma. *JAMA* 217:61, 1971.

Shalev O, Naparstek Y, Brezis M, et al: Hyponatremia in myxedema: A suggested therapeutic approach. *Isr J Med Sci* 15:913, 1979.

Shenkman L, Mitsuma T, Suphavai A, et al: Hypothalamic hypothyroidism. *JAMA* 222:480, 1972.

Sherman FT, Daum M: Hypothermia detection: A survey of emergency room thermometry. Presented at 33rd annual scientific meeting of the Gerontological society, 1980.

Skowsky WR, Kikuchi TA: The role of vasopressin in the impaired water excretion of myxedema. *Am J Med* 64:613, 1978.

Smolar EN, Rubin JE, Avramides A, et al: Cardiac tamponade in primary myxedema and review of the literature. *Am J Med Sci* 272:345, 1976.

Toft AD, Irvine WJ, Sinclair I, et al: Thyroid function after surgical treatment of thyrotoxicosis. *N Engl J Med* 298:643, 1978.

Urbanic RC, Mazzaferri EL: Thyrotoxic crisis and myxedema coma. *Heart Lung* 7:435, 1978.

Utiger RD: Treatment of Graves' disease. *N Engl J Med* 298:681, 1978.

Wilson WR, Bedell GN: The pulmonary abnormalities in myxedema. *J Clin Invest* 39:42, 1960.

Wood GM, Waters AK: Prolonged dystonic reaction to chlorpromazine in myxedema coma. *Postgrad Med J* 56:192, 1980.

Zaenger P: Letter. *Br Med J* 285:888, 1982.

Zondek H: The electrocardiogram in myxedema. *Brit Heart J* 26:227, 1964.

Zwillich CW, Pierson DJ, Hofeldt FD, et al: Ventilatory control in myxedema and hypothyroidism. *N Engl J Med* 292:662, 1975.

CHAPTER 95
ADRENAL
INSUFFICIENCY AND
ADRENAL CRISIS

Gene Ragland

Adrenal insufficiency consists of decreased levels of or absent hormones produced by the adrenal glands and results from structural or functional lesions of the adrenal cortex or the anterior pituitary gland. Deficit of adrenal hormones may manifest clinically as a chronic, insidious disorder, or as an acute, life-threatening emergency. Therapy of adrenal insufficiency is specific and includes replacement of the deficient hormones.

Chronic adrenal insufficiency is due to a variety of causes. It may be primary (Addison's disease), due to failure of the adrenal glands. It may also occur secondarily because of failure of the hypothalamus or pituitary gland (hypopituitarism) or because of iatrogenic adrenal suppression from prolonged steroid use. Acute adrenal insufficiency (adrenal crisis) may result from certain acute events, or when a person with chronic adrenal insufficiency is subjected to stress and exhausts reserve adrenal hormones, or when replacement hormone medication is discontinued.

Adrenal Insufficiency

EPIDEMIOLOGY

The true prevalence of adrenal insufficiency is unknown. Addison's disease has been reported to occur with an incidence of 1 case per 100,000 population. In general, adrenal insufficiency is more common in the adult population but may occur at any age and in either sex.

ADRENAL HORMONES

The adrenal glands are divisible into the cortex and medulla. The adrenal cortex is essential for life and produces glucorticoid, mineralocorticoid, and androgenic steroid hormones. The medulla secretes the catecholamines epinephrine and norepinephrine, largely under neural control. No definite clinical condition has been ascribed to hypofunction of the adrenal medulla. Most of the manifestations of adrenal insufficiency occur when the physiologic requirement for glucocorticoid and mineralocorticoid hormones exceeds the capacity of the adrenal glands to produce them.

Cortisol

The major glucocorticoid is cortisol, which is secreted in response to direct stimulation by adrenocorticotropic hormone (ACTH) from the anterior pituitary gland. Secretion of ACTH is governed by the hormone corticotropin-releasing factor (CRF) from the hypothalamus. This normally occurs with a diurnal rhythm, with the highest levels in the morning and the lowest levels in the late evening. Upon stimulation by ACTH, the adrenal glands respond in minutes to secrete cortisol in direct proportion to the ACTH concentration. Cortisol is normally secreted at the rate of 20 to 25 mg/day. Through negative feedback inhibition, the plasma cortisol level acts to suppress ACTH release.

By an undefined mechanism, stress factors such as anoxia, trauma, infections, and hypoglycemia can also trigger CRF and ACTH release and produce cortisol levels several times normal. The release of CRF in response to stress is resistant to suppression through negative feedback inhibition.

Cortisol is a potent hormone and affects the metabolism of most body tissues. In general, cortisol acts to maintain blood glucose levels by decreasing glucose uptake at extrahepatic sites and by providing precursors for gluconeogenesis via protein and fat breakdown. Cortisol governs the distribution of water between extracellular and intracellular compartments and possesses a minor sodium-retaining effect. It also acts to enhance the pressor effects of catecholamines on heart muscle and arterioles. In supraphysiologic amounts, cortisol inhibits inflammatory and allergic reactions. Finally, through negative feedback inhibition, cortisol suppresses the secretion of ACTH and melanocyte-stimulating hormone (MSH) from the anterior pituitary gland.

Aldosterone

The major mineralocorticoid is aldosterone. The renin-angiotensin system and plasma potassium concentration regulate aldosterone through negative feedback loops. These mechanisms are probably of equal importance and far more important than the minor aldosterone-stimulating effect of ACTH.

Aldosterone acts to increase sodium reabsorption and potassium excretion, primarily in the distal tubules of the kidneys. Other tissue effects of aldosterone are minor in comparison with its regulation of sodium and potassium levels.

Androgens

Androgenic hormone production by the adrenal glands is regulated by ACTH and is trivial in comparison with the production of these hormones by the gonads.

PATHOGENESIS OF ADRENAL INSUFFICIENCY

Idiopathic

Primary adrenal insufficiency, or Addison's disease, is due to disease or destruction of the adrenal cortex and has a wide variety of causes (see Table 95-1). Approximately 90 percent of the ad-

Table 95-1. Pathogenesis of Primary Adrenal Insufficiency

1 Primary, chronic
 a Idiopathic (autoimmune)
 b Infiltrative or infectious
  (1) Tuberculosis
  (2) Fungal infections
  (3) Sarcoidosis
  (4) Amyloidosis
  (5) Hemochromatosis
  (6) Neoplastic (metastatic) disease
  (7) Adrenoleukodystrophy
 c Hemorrhage or infarction
 d Bilateral adrenalectomy
 e Chemotherapeutic agents (*o,p'*-DDD)
 f Congenital adrenal hyperplasia
 g Congenital unresponsiveness to ACTH
2 Primary, acute
 a Hemorrhage (adrenal apoplexy)
  (1) Fulminant septicemia
  (2) Newborn
  (3) Others
 b Discontinuation of replacement steroids

renal cortex must be involved before clinical manifestations of adrenal failure result. Idiopathic atrophy of the adrenal glands is the leading cause of chronic adrenal insufficiency. In one review of 108 cases of Addison's disease, 66 percent were classified as idiopathic. Idiopathic adrenal insufficiency has been further divided into autoimmune (70 to 75 percent) and truly idiopathic (25 to 30 percent). Another review of Addison's disease reported a 78 percent incidence between 1962 and 1972 of adrenal gland destruction due to autoimmune atropy.

There is an overwhelming association between idiopathic adrenal insufficiency and other diseases known to be autoimmune in origin. One review found a second disease of the pancreas, thyroid gland, gastric mucosa, or gonads in 53 percent of the patients with idiopathic adrenal insufficiency. Associated diseases include diabetes mellitus, Hashimoto's thyroiditis, pernicious anemia, primary ovarian failure. Other investigators have reported frequent association with hypoparathyroidism, chronic active hepatitis, malabsorption, chronic mucocutaneous candidiasis, alopecia, and vitiligo.

Infiltrative or Infectious

Adrenal tuberculosis has declined in frequency as a cause of Addison's disease but is still reported to be a cause in 17 to 21 percent of the cases. Fungal infections and other infiltrative processes are infrequent causes of adrenal insufficiency during active, disseminated disease. Metastatic carcinoma in the adrenal glands is a relatively frequent finding at autopsy in patients with certain carcinomas, but it only rarely causes adrenal insufficiency. In one review of 51 adrenal carcinomas identified by CT scan, 18 were primary and 33 were metastatic (13 from lung, 3 melanomas, and 17 from breast, kidney, ovary, prostate, and elsewhere).

Adrenal Apoplexy

Bilateral adrenal gland hemorrhage (adrenal apoplexy) is a rare occurrence that is seen in a variety of clinical settings and is seldom diagnosed during life. A review of 2000 consecutive autopsies, excluding newborns and patients with meningococcemia, yielded an incidence of bilateral adrenal hemorrhage (focal or diffuse) of 1.1 percent. The result of such hemorrhage varies from no apparent clinical consequences to primary adrenal failure to a cataclysmic clinical event.

In general, patients with a serious underlying condition whose adrenal glands are stressed are at risk for this complication. Stress-stimulated adrenal glands are hemorrhage prone. The association between adrenal hemorrhage and anticoagulant therapy with heparin and dicumarol is well-established. A classic example is the postmyocardial infarction patient who is on anticoagulant therapy. Adrenal hemorrhage in this setting is most likely to occur between the third and eighteenth day following institution of anticoagulation therapy. Sudden deterioration with hypotension and pain in the flank, costovertebral angle, or epigastrium should suggest this disastrous event. Associated findings may include fever, nausea and vomiting, and disturbed sensorium. Computed tomography and ultrasound can assist in establishing this diagnosis. Other stressful events that have been associated with adrenal hemorrhage include surgery, trauma, burns, convulsions, pregnancy, and adrenal vein thrombosis.

Adrenal crisis as a consequence of adrenal hemorrhage also occurs with overwhelming septicemia and in the newborn. Fulminant septicemia with meningococcus, pneumococcus, staphylococcus, streptococcus, *Hemophilus* influenza, and gram-negative organisms has been reported to cause adrenal hemorrhage. The Waterhouse-Friderichsen syndrome is a life-threatening disorder resulting from overwhelming septicemia due to meningococcemia. The patient is acutely ill and has shaking chills, severe headache, and a petechial rash that may progress to extensive purpura. Bilateral adrenal gland hemorrhage frequently occurs with this disorder. Vascular collapse and death may result unless the patient is promptly treated. Adrenal hemorrhage in the newborn may account for 1 percent of neonatal deaths but is rarely within the purview of the emergency physician.

Miscellaneous

Another cause of primary adrenal failure is bilateral adrenalectomy for metastatic breast or prostate cancer or for Cushing's syndrome. Following such a procedure the patient is totally dependent upon replacement corticosteroids for life. Chemotherapeutic agents such as mitotane (*o,p'*-DDD) used in treatment of Cushing's disease can produce adrenal failure. Finally, rare congenital and inherited disorders can cause adrenal insufficiency.

Secondary Causes

Secondary adrenal insufficiency may be due to disease or destruction of the hypothalamus or pituitary gland, resulting in impaired capacity of the pituitary to secrete ACTH. Those disorders responsible for secondary adrenal failure are listed in Table 95-2.

The most common cause of secondary adrenal insufficiency and adrenal crisis is iatrogenic adrenal suppression from prolonged steroid use. Rapid withdrawal of steroids from patients with adrenal atrophy secondary to chronic steroid use may result in collapse and death, especially under circumstances of increased stress. The first report of death presumed to be due to corticosteroid-induced adrenal suppression was in 1952. Confirmation of adrenal failure due to prednisone treatment was reported in 1961. Since that time numerous reports have supported the concept that ex-

Table 95-2. Pathogenesis of Secondary Adrenal Insufficiency

1 Secondary, chronic
  a Pituitary tumor (chromophobe adenoma, craniopharyngioma, hamartoma, meningioma, glioma)
  b Pituitary hemorrhage or vascular accident
  c Postpartum pituitary infarction (Sheehan's syndrome)
  d Infiltrative and granulomatous disease
     (1) Sarcoidosis
     (2) Hemochromatosis
     (3) Histiocytosis X
  e Internal carotid artery aneurysm
  f Head trauma (basilar skull fracture)
  g Infection (meningitis, cavernous sinus thrombosis)
  h Hypophysectomy
  i Pituitary gland irradiation
  j Isolated ACTH deficiency
2 Secondary, acute
  a Iatrogenic HPA suppression due to steroid therapy
  b Discontinuation of replacement steroids.

ogenous administration of glucocorticoids may cause hypothalamic-pituitary-adrenal (HPA) suppression and subsequent adrenal atrophy. This complication has been reported to occur not only with oral steroids but also with those given by the intrathecal, topical, and inhalant routes.

The mechanism of continued adrenal atrophy following discontinuation of exogenous steroids may be a failure of normal diurnal release of CRF. Stress-induced release of ACTH may remain intact, but the atrophic adrenal glands are unable to secrete sufficient cortisol to meet the physiologic requirements in response to stress. The shortest time interval or the smallest dose at which HPA suppression occurs is unknown. Any patient who has been on dosages of glucocorticoids equivalent to 20 to 30 mg of prednisone per day for more than a week should be suspected of having HPA suppression.

Following prolonged supraphysiologic dosages of steroids, it may take up to 6 to 12 months for recovery of HPA function when steroids are withdrawn completely. Until complete recovery has occurred, it is wise to assume the patient will need basal steroid therapy and supplementary therapy during intercurrent illness or stress. Adrenal suppression must be suspected based upon the history of prior steroid use. When in doubt about the HPA status of a seriously ill or deteriorating patient, steroids should be given!

CLINICAL PRESENTATION

Primary Insufficiency

The clinical manifestations of chronic adrenal insufficiency develop gradually with subtle signs and symptoms that provide a diagnostic challenge. The clinical presentation of Addison's disease can be explained on the basis of a deficiency of cortisol and aldosterone and a lack of feedback suppression of ACTH and MSH.

Cortisol deficiency manifests clinically with anorexia, nausea, vomiting, lethargy, hypoglycemia with fasting, and inability to withstand even minor stresses without shock. The ability to excrete a free water load with normal rapidity is also impaired and can lead to water intoxication. Lack of aldosterone results in impaired ability to conserve sodium and excrete potassium. The patient with aldosterone deficiency presents with sodium depletion, dehydration, hypotension, postural syncope, and decreased cardiac size and output. Renal blood flow is decreased, and azotemia may develop. Hyperkalemia is commonly seen but rarely is severe. Lack of suppression of ACTH and MSH secretion occurs because of deficient cortisol levels and results in increased pigmentation.

The overall clinical picture of a patient with Addison's disease is that of one who is weak and lethargic, with loss of vigor, and fatigue on exertion. The patient may have a feeble tachycardic pulse. Postural hypotension and syncope are common. In one series of 108 cases of Addison's disease, 88 percent had systolic blood pressure readings less than 110 mmHg. Another series of 86 patients with Addison's disease reported 91 percent with blood pressures below that level. In spite of the hypotension, the extremities usually remain warm. Heart sounds may be soft or almost inaudible on auscultation.

Gastrointestinal (GI) symptoms are a prominent feature of chronic adrenal insufficiency and include anorexia, nausea, vomiting, weight loss, abdominal pain, and sometimes diarrhea. In one series, anorexia and weight loss were present in 100 percent of the patients with Addison's disease, and other GI symptoms occurred in 87 percent.

Cutaneous manifestations of Addison's disease include increased brownish pigmentation over exposed body areas such as the face, neck, arms, and dorsum of the hands, and over friction or pressure points such as the elbows, knees, fingers, toes, and nipples. Hyperpigmentation has been noted in 92 to 97 percent of patients with Addison's disease. Pigmentation of mucous membranes, darkening of nevi and hair, and longitudinal pigmented bands in the nails may be seen. Vitiligo, mucocutaneous candidiasis, and alopecia may occur with Addison's disease that has an autoimmune cause. Women with Addison's disease may exhibit decreased growth of axillary and pubic hair because of adrenal androgen deficiency. This is not seen in men because of adequate testicular androgen.

Mentally these patients vary from alert to confused. Unconsciousness is rare unless the condition is preterminal. The sensory modalities of taste, olfaction, and hearing may be increased. Hyperkalemic paralysis is a rare, emergent complication of adrenal insufficiency; the patient presents with a rapidly ascending muscular weakness which leads to flaccid quadriplegia. Treatment of this complication consists of the intravenous administration of glucose and insulin or bicarbonate.

Laboratory

The usual laboratory findings in patients with primary adrenal insufficiency include hyponatremia, hyperkalemia, hypoglycemia, and azotemia. Hyponatremia is usually mild to moderate, and severe hyponatremia (<120 mEq/L) is rare. In one series, 88 percent of the patients with Addison's disease had a serum sodium level under 135 mEq/L. Hyperkalemia is usually mild, and the potassium level rarely exceeds 7 mEq/L. Initial potassium levels may be normal or low if protracted vomiting has occurred. Rarely, hyperkalemia may be severe and cause cardiac arrhythmia or paralysis.

Hypoglycemia, especially with fasting, is a characteristic finding in patients with primary adrenal insufficiency. One author noted that most of his untreated Addisonian patients were difficult to arouse in the morning because of hypoglycemia. Moderate elevation of the blood urea nitrogen (BUN) level may occur because of dehydration secondary to aldosterone deficiency. Azotemia is usually reversible with restoration of normal circulating blood volume.

Electrocardiographic changes may be seen in patients with Addison's disease. These changes include flat or inverted T waves, a prolonged QT interval, low voltage, a prolonged PR or QRS interval, and a depressed ST segment. The ECG changes reflective of hyperkalemia include tall peaked T waves, prolongation of the PR interval and QRS complex, and disappearance of P waves, and finally ventricular fibrillation may result. The chest x-ray film may show a small, narrow cardiac silhouette due to decreased intravascular volume. A flat plate film of the abdomen may show adrenal calcification, which is most commonly due to tuberculosis but may occur with infection or hemorrhage.

Primary versus Secondary

Significant clinical and laboratory differences exist between patients with primary and those with secondary adrenal insuffi-

ciency. With secondary adrenal failure, the capacity of the pituitary to secrete ACTH is impaired. The level of aldosterone is largely unaffected because of its regulation by the renin-angiotensin system and the plasma potassium concentration. The clinical manifestations of secondary adrenal failure are due to insufficiency of cortisol and adrenal androgens. In addition, insufficiency of other anterior pituitary hormones such as growth hormone, thyroid hormone, and gonadotropic hormone may cause clinical abnormalities.

Patients with secondary adrenal insufficiency are better able to tolerate sodium deprivation without developing shock. This is true because of intact aldosterone secretion. Hyponatremia, hyperkalemia, and azotemia are not prominent features of secondary failure. Hypoglycemia, however, may be more common in patients with hypopituitarism because of concomitant growth hormone deficiency. Hyperpigmentation does not occur with secondary failure because ACTH and MSH are eliminated at their source, the pituitary gland. Finally, with secondary failure, men as well as women may exhibit signs of androgen deficiency because of insufficient gonadotropic hormone from the pituitary.

DIAGNOSIS

Differentiation of primary from secondary adrenal failure on other than clinical grounds requires in-hospital evaluation. Primary adrenal insufficiency is diagnosed by demonstrating a low baseline plasma cortisol level and faiure to increase this level in response to exogenous administration of ACTH. Failure to respond to ACTH stimulation occurs because the adrenal cortex is damaged or destroyed and has no functional capacity to respond. Secondary adrenal insufficiency is diagnosed by demonstrating low plasma cortisol and urinary metabolite levels that increase in a stepwise fashion with repetitive ACTH stimulation over a period of days. A variety of tests to assess the integrity of the HPA axis are available.

There is a rapid screening test that can be performed in the emergency department and reliably distinguishes patients with normal adrenal function from those with adrenal insufficiency. This test is based on the fact that adrenal response to a single injection of ACTH is maximal within 1 h. Plasma for measurement of baseline cortisol level is drawn, and then 25 units of corticotropin (synthetic ACTH) is administered subcutaneously, intramuscularly, or intravenously. Another plasma cortisol level is obtained 30 to 60 min later. Normal persons should respond with a doubling of the baseline cortisol level. Patients with primary adrenal insufficiency show no increase in plasma cortisol levels, whereas those with secondary adrenal failure may show no, or a slight, response to corticotropin. A more prolonged period of ACTH stimulation is necessary to reliably distinguish primary from secondary adrenal insufficiency. This rapid screening test can be used to assess adrenal reserve in patients previously on steroid therapy.

TREATMENT

Glucocorticoid

Therapy of primary adrenal insufficiency consists of replacement of the insufficient hormones, cortisol and aldosterone, and, on

Table 95-3. Steroid Equivalents

Drug	Equivalent Dose, mg	Na + Retention
SHORT-ACTING		
Cortisone	25	2 +
Hydrocortisone (cortisol)	20	2 +
Prednisone	5	1 +
Prednisolone	5	1 +
Methylprednisolone	4	0
INTERMEDIATE-ACTING		
Triamcinolone	4	0
LONG-ACTING		
Dexamethasone	0.75	0
Betamethasone	0.6	0

occasion, supplemental androgen therapy in the female patient. The usual maintenance dosage for glucocorticoid replacement varies from 20 to 37.5 mg of cortisol per day. Various preparations may be used (see Table 95-3 for steroid equivalents). A generally accepted dosage schedule is 25 mg of cortisone acetate or 5 mg of prednisone in the morning, followed by 12.5 mg of cortisone or 2.5 mg of prednisone in the afternoon. This simulates the normal diurnal variation of cortisol secretion. A few patients, especially large active men, may require a total daily dose of 50 mg of cortisone or 10 mg of prednisone for optimum response.

Mineralocorticoid

Mineralocorticoid replacement in patients with primary adrenal insufficiency can be achieved by administration of the synthetic mineralocorticoid fludrocortisone acetate (Florinef), 0.05 to 0.2 mg/day. This dosage should be appropriately reduced in patients in whom hypertension develops. It is also important for the patient with Addison's disease to maintain an adequate dietary salt intake.

Androgen

The woman with primary adrenal insufficiency may show signs of androgen deficiency such as decreased growth of axillary and pubic hair. Supplemental androgen therapy can be achieved with 2 to 5 mg of fluoxymesterone (Halotestin) orally per day.

Secondary Insufficiency

Treatment of secondary adrenal insufficiency differs from that of primary adrenal insufficiency with regard to mineralocorticoid and androgen replacement. Patients with secondary adrenal failure usually do not require mineralocorticoid therapy and can maintain salt and fluid balance with a diet generous in sodium chloride. In the presence of hypotension, however, supplementary fludrocortisone acetate, 0.05 to 0.1 mg/day, is indicated. Evidence of androgen insufficiency may occur with male and female patients with hypopituitarism. Sufficient androgen in the female patient can be achieved with 2 to 5 mg of fluoxymesterone orally per day. Larger dosages of this preparation or long-acting testosterone (Depo-Testosterone) can be used in the male patient.

Various parameters to assess the adequacy of replacement steroids in treatment of chronic adrenal insufficiency have been used. Glucocorticoid replacement has been followed by measurement of the plasma cortisol level, the urinary free cortisol level, and the plasma ACTH and cortisol relation. The adequacy of mineralocorticoid replacement has been assessed by measuring the plasma potassium concentration and the plasma renin activity. In general, the patient's feeling of well-being indicates adequate therapy.

All patients with chronic adrenal insufficiency must be educated about the nature of their illness and the importance of maintaining their life-sustaining medication. They should wear a Medic Alert tag and carry a kit containing syringes of hydrocortisone or dexamethasone and cortisone acetate. Detailed instructions for emergent care and how to increase their medication during intercurrent illness and stress should be provided. Family members should also be familiar with the disease and know how to respond in an emergency. These patients must not be lost to medical follow-up.

Adrenal Crisis

Adrenal crisis is an acute, life-threatening emergency that must be suspected and treated based upon clinical impression. It is due primarily to cortisol insufficiency and to a lesser extent, aldosterone insufficiency, and occurs when the physiologic demand for these hormones exceeds the capacity of the adrenal glands to produce them.

Adrenal reserve may be exhausted in patients with chronic adrenal insufficiency when they are subjected to intercurrent illness or stress. A variety of conditions may precipitate crisis in this setting; these include major or minor infections, trauma, surgery, burns, pregnancy, hypermetabolic states such as hyperthyroidism, and drugs, especially hypnotics or general anesthetics. Adrenal crisis may also occur in patients with chronic adrenal failure if the patient fails or is unable to take replacement steroid medication. The most common cause of adrenal crisis is abrupt withdrawal of steroids from a patient with iatrogenic adrenal suppression due to prolonged steroid use. Finally, bilateral adrenal gland hemorrhage from fulminant septicemia or other causes can produce adrenal crisis.

CLINICAL PRESENTATION

The clinical manifestations of adrenal crisis are due primarily to insufficiency of cortisol and to a lesser extent, insufficiency of aldosterone. Patients appear acutely ill. They are profoundly weak and may be confused. Hypotension, especially postural hypotension, is usual. Circulatory collapse may be profound. The pulse is feeble and rapid, and heart sounds may be soft. Temperature elevation is common but may be due to underlying infection. Anorexia, nausea, vomiting, and abdominal pain are almost universal. The abdominal pain may be severe, simulating an acute abdomen. Patients in crisis may exhibit increased motor activity which can progress to delirium or seizures.

Laboratory findings in patients with adrenal crisis vary. The serum sodium level is usually moderately decreased but may be normal. Potassium levels may be normal or slightly increased. Rarely the potassium concentration may be markedly increased, and this can cause cardiac arrhythmias or hyperkalemic paralysis. Hypoglycemia is characteristic and on occasion can be profound.

TREATMENT

Treatment must be instituted promptly based upon clinical impression and should not be delayed for confirmatory testing of adrenal function. Therapeutic measures in treatment of adrenal crisis include replacement of fluids and sodium, administration of glucocorticoid, correction of hypotension and hypoglycemia, reduction of hyperkalemia, and identification and treatment of a precipitating cause of the crisis.

Fluids

A rapid infusion of 5 percent dextrose and physiologic saline should be started immediately. This acts to correct dehydration, hypotension, hyponatremia, and hypoglycemia. The extracellular volume deficit in the average adult in adrenal crisis is approximately 20 percent, or 3 L. The first liter should be given over 1 to 4 h, and 2 or 3 L may be required during the first 8 h of therapy. The functional capacity of the cardiovascular system is reduced with adrenal insufficiency, and the usual precautions with the rapid administration of saline should be observed.

Steroids

A water-soluble glucocorticoid should be administered promptly. As soon as the diagnosis of adrenal crisis is entertained, 100 mg of hydrocortisone sodium succinate (Solu-Cortef) or phosphate should be given in an intravenous bolus. In addition, 100 mg of hydrocortisone should be added to the intravenous solution. Usually, 200 to 400 mg of hydrocortisone is required during the first 24 h of therapy. One author recommends 100 mg of hydrocortisone every 8 h for 36 to 48 h. Cortisone acetate, 50 to 100 mg intramuscularly, can be given to provide a continuing source of hormone should the intravenous route be interrupted. Cortisone acetate should not be relied on as the sole source of replacement steroid as its absorption from an intramuscular site is unpredictable. Glucocorticoid therapy acts to correct hypotension, hyponatremia, hyperkalemia, and hypoglycemia.

Mineralocorticoid therapy is not required during the initial treatment of adrenal crisis. High dosages of hydrocortisone provide sufficient mineralocorticoid effect. As the total dosage of glucocorticoid is reduced below 100 mg/24 h, many patients need supplementary mineralocorticoid, which can be provided as desoxy-corticosterone acetate (Percorten), 2.5 to 5.0 mg intramuscularly once or twice daily.

Complications

Additional problems that may require therapeutic intervention during adrenal crisis are hyperkalemia and hypotension. Administration of fluids and glucocorticoid is usually sufficient to correct these disorders. If the serum potassium level is 6.5 to 7.0 mEq/L, especially if ECG changes reflective of hyperkalemia are present, one or two ampoules of sodium bicarbonate intravenously may be indicated. If hypotension persists following adequate volume replacement, supplement mineralocorticoid can be given. Vasopressors can be used to correct hypotension after intravascular volume has been replaced. Phenylephrine hydrochloride (Neo-Synephrine), 0.25 to 0.5 mg as an intravenous bolus, or 4 mg/L of physiologic saline as an intravenous infusion at a rate of 4 mg/min, can be used. Dopamine (Intropin) and metaraminol (Aramine) have also been used successfully to correct persistent hypotension in adrenal crisis.

The patient needs to be evaluated for a precipitating cause of adrenal crisis. Appropriate cultures and x-ray films should be obtained and the patient started on antibiotics if infection is present. Adrenal hemorrhage should be considered, especially if the patient is on anticoagulants. A detailed history pertaining to prior steroid therapy is essential.

Simultaneous Treatment and Testing

It is possible to treat adrenal crisis and to perform simultaneous, confirmatory diagnostic testing for adrenal insufficiency. Physiologic saline is administered, but instead of hydrocortisone, 4 mg of dexamethasone is added to the infusion. Additionally, 25 units of corticotropin is added to the solution and this liter infused in the first hour. Blood for plasma cortisol assay is obtained before and at the completion of the infusion. A 24-h urine collection for measurement of 17-hydroxycorticosteroid (17-OHCS) is collected. Additional corticotropin is added to subsequent intravenous solutions so that at least 3 units is infused each hour for 8 h. A third blood specimen for cortisol assay is obtained between the sixth and eighth hours of intravenous therapy.

If the patient has primary adrenal insufficiency, all plasma cortisol levels are low (<15 μg/dL), and the urinary 17-OHCS is also low, confirming the inability of the adrenals to respond to ACTH stimulation. An adequate rise in the plasma cortisol level excludes the diagnosis of adrenal insufficiency. A response indicative of partially intact adrenocortical reserve excludes the diagnosis of primary adrenal failure in favor of secondary adrenal insufficiency, but further testing is required to confirm this diagnosis. Other methods for simultaneous diagnosis and treatment have been described.

The adrenal crisis should begin to resolve favorably within a few hours after initiation of appropriate therapy. Intensive treatment and monitoring should continue for 24 to 48 h. Once the patient's condition has stabilized, the transition to the previously described oral maintenance program can begin. Usually, 7 to 10 days are required for this transition.

The main causes of death during adrenal crisis are circulatory collapse and hyperkalemia-induced arrhythmias. Hypoglycemia may contribute to demise in some cases. With prompt recognition and appropriate treatment, most patients in adrenal crisis should do well.

BIBLIOGRAPHY

Abrams HL, Siegelman SS, Adams DF, et al: Computed tomography versus ultrasound of the adrenal gland: A prospective study. *Radiology* 143:121, 1982.

Amador E: Adrenal hemorrhage during anticoagulant therapy, a clinical and pathological study of ten cases. *Ann Intern Med* 63:559, 1965.

Axelrod L: Glucocorticoid therapy. *Medicine* 55:39, 1976.

Baxter JD, Forsham PH: Tissue effects of glucocorticoids. *Am J Med* 53:573, 1972.

Burch WM: Urine free-cortisol determination; A useful tool in the management of chronic hypoadrenal states. *JAMA* 247:2002, 1982.

Cedermark BJ, Sjöberg HE: The clinical significance of metastasis to the adrenal glands. *Surg Gynecol Obstet* 152:607, 1981.

David DS, Grieco MH, Cushman P: Adrenal glucocorticoids after twenty years—A review of their clinically relevant consequences. *J Chronic Dis* 22:637, 1970.

Dunlop D: Eighty-six cases of Addison's disease. *Br Med J* 2:887, 1963.

Feek CM, Ratcliffe JG, Seth J, et al: Patterns of plasma cortisol and ACTH concentrations in patients with Addison's disease treated with conventional corticosteroid replacement. *Clin Endocrinol* 14:451, 1981.

Fraser CG, Preuss FS, Bigford WD: Adrenal atrophy and irreversible shock associated with cortisone therapy. *JAMA* 149:1542, 1952.

Glass AR, Smith CE: Stress-induced cortisol release in hypothalamic hypoadrenalism. *JAMA* 241:1612, 1979.

Gwinup G, Johnson B: Clinical testing of the hypothalamic-pituitary-adrenocortical system in states of hypo and hypercortisolism. *Metabolism* 24:777, 1975.

Himathongkam T, Newmark SR, Greenfield M, et al: Acute adrenal insufficiency. *JAMA* 230:1317, 1974.

Hughes IA: Congenital and acquired disorders of the adrenal cortex. *Clin Endocrinol Metab* 11:89, 1982.

Irvine WJ, Barnes EW: Adrenocortical insufficiency. *Clin Endocrinol Metab* 1:549, 1972.

Kehlet H, Binder C: Value of an ACTH test in assessing hypothalamic-pituitary-adrenocortical function in glucocorticoid-treated patients. *Br Med J* 2:147, 1973.

Kehlet H, Blichert-Toft M, Lindholm J, et al: Short ACTH test in assessing hypothalamic-pituitary-adrenocortical function. *Br Med J* 1:249, 1976.

Kozak GP: Primary adrenocortical insufficiency (Addison's disease). *Am Fam Physician* 15(5):124, 1977.

Leshin M: Acute adrenal insufficiency: Recognition, management, and prevention. *Urol Clin North Am* 9:229, 1982.

Levin J, Zumoff B, Kream J, et al: Cortisol measurement in patients receiving oral corticosteroid replacement treatment. *J Clin Pharmacol* 21:52, 1981.

Mason AS, Meade TW, Lee JAH, et al: Epidemiological and clinical picture of Addison's disease. *Lancet* 2:744, 1968.

Mulrow PJ, Forman BH: The tissue effects of mineralocorticoids. *Am J Med* 53:561, 1972.

Nelson DH: Regulation of glucocorticoid release. *Am J Med* 53:590, 1972.

Nerup J: Addison's disease—Clinical studies. A report of 108 cases. *Acta Endocrinol* 76:127, 1974.

Nerup J: Addison's disease—Serological studies. *Acta Endocrinol* 76:142, 1974.

Neufeld M, MacLaren NK, Blizzard RM: Two types of autoimmune Addison's disease associated with different polyglandular autoimmune (PGA) syndromes. *Medicine* 60:355, 1981.

Sampson PA, Winstone NE, Brooke BN: Biochemical confirmation of collapse due to adrenal failure. *Lancet* 1:1377, 1961.

Sheridan P, Mattingly D: Simultaneous investigation and treatment of suspected acute adrenal insufficiency. *Lancet* 2:676, 1975.

Speckart PF, Nicoloff JT, Bethune JE: Screening for adrenocortical insufficiency with cosyntropin (synthetic ACTH). *Arch Intern Med* 128:761, 1971.

Thompson DG, Mason AS, Goodwin FJ: Mineralocorticoid replacement in Addison's disease. *Clin Endocrinol* 10:499, 1979.

Thorn GW, Lauler DP: Clinical therapeutics of adrenal disorders. *Am J Med* 53:673, 1972.

Tyler FH, West CD: Laboratory evaluation of disorders of the adrenal cortex. *Am J Med* 53:664, 1972.

Tzagournis M: Acute adrenal insufficiency. *Heart Lung* 7:603, 1978.

Vesely DL: Hypoglycemic coma: Don't overlook acute adrenal crisis. *Geriatrics* 37(5):71, 1982.

Williams GH, Dluhy RG: Aldosterone biosynthesis—Interrelationship of regulatory factors. *Am J Med* 53:595, 1972.

Xarli VP, Steele AA, Davis PJ, et al: Adrenal hemorrhage in the adult. *Medicine* 57:211, 1978.

SECTION 11
HEMATOLOGIC
AND ONCOLOGIC
EMERGENCIES

CHAPTER 96
APPROACH TO THE BLEEDING PATIENT

Daniel Esposito

This section is intended both to provide a practical, clinical schema for identifying patients with abnormal bleeding and to provide insight into the interpretation of the common coagulation studies available to the emergency physician. Clinical and laboratory characteristics of specific hereditary and acquired bleeding disorders will be reviewed in the next two chapters.

SIGNS OF BLEEDING DIATHESIS

Trauma and tissue injury remain the most common causes of local bleeding and the clinician should always attempt to obtain historical or physical evidence of this. The following clinical findings should alert the physician to consider and evaluate the possibility of an underlying bleeding disorder:

- Inordinately profuse or prolonged bleeding after minor injury
- Spontaneous bleeding into joints (hemarthrosis) and deep subcutaneous tissues (hematomas)
- Concurrent multisystem or multisite bleeding
- Delayed bleeding several hours after trauma or surgery
- Diffuse petechiae, ecchymoses or both
- Spontaneous bleeding from mucous membranes, such as the conjunctivae, or oral, rectal, and vaginal mucosa, may indicate a severe bleeding diathesis that may ultimately be complicated by CNS hemorrhage

GENERAL CONSIDERATIONS OF HEMOSTASIS

Hemostasis involves the synergistic interaction of four essential systems: vascular integrity, platelets, coagulation factors, and fibrinolysis. The complexity of the clotting mechanism is often overexaggerated and the emergency physician may achieve a more lucid understanding by considering individual bleeding disorders as a lesion in one of these component systems. Table 96-1 outlines this concept and reviews clinical and laboratory features. The hybrid disorders—von Willebrand's disease and disseminated intravascular coagulation (DIC)—involve abnormalities in both platelets and clotting factors.

Vascular Bleeding

The primary defect leading to vascular bleeding is in either the blood vessel wall (inflammation) or the supportive connective tissue. Bleeding tends to be from smaller blood vessels. Increased vascular friability related to age (senile purpura) or steroid therapy has its genesis in diminished connective tissue support.

Platelets

Platelets participate at several levels of hemostasis by organizing at the site of vascular injury, by releasing adenosine 5′–diphosphate (ADP) that induces further aggregation; and by releasing platelet factor III and phospholipid which catalyze clotting. As in vascular bleeding, abnormal platelet number or function tends to cause small vessel bleeding (purpura).

Coagulation Factors and Clotting

Figure 96-1 outlines the intrinsic and extrinsic clotting cascades and schematizes the coagulation factors involved with the common coagulation screening tests. It should be reemphasized that tissue injury activates both pathways concurrently and that both systems may participate in producing an insoluble fibrin clot. With isolated (e.g., hemophilia) or combined (e.g., sodium warfarin) therapy with decreased factor (II, VII, IX, X) deficiencies, bleeding tends to be from larger blood vessels.

Fibrinolysis

The clotting process converts plasminogen to plasmin, a proteolytic enzyme that cleaves fibrin polymers into fibrin degradation (split) products and acts to lyse thrombi. Excessive fibrinolysis is the exaggeration of this homeostatic, thrombolytic mechanism and can produce bleeding by functionally altering other coagulation factors or by inducing excessive consumption of clotting factors as in DIC. The current use of streptokinase and urokinase (plasminogen activators) as thrombolytic agents in acute pulmonary

Table 96-1. Clinical and Laboratory Signs of Bleeding Disorders

Disorder	Clinical Stigmata	Laboratory Studies Abnormal	Laboratory Studies Normal	Miscellaneous Conditions
Vascular bleeding	Purpura (petechiae)	Prolonged bleeding time	Normal platelet count	Vasculitis Allergy to drugs, chemicals
	Telangiectasia of skin and mucous membranes (Osler-Weber-Rendu)	Positive tourniquet test may be present in vasculitis	Normal PT Normal PTT	Infections Immune diseases Hereditary telangiectasia Scurvy Abnormal connective tissue
	Perifollicular bleeding in scurvy Prolonged traumatic bleeding			

Platelet disorders	Purpura
	GI bleeding
	GU bleeding
	Epistaxis
		Prolonged bleeding time
		Low platelet count in thrombopenia
		Normal platelet count in thrombopathy
		  von Willebrand's
			Normal PT
			Normal PTT
				Thrombocytopenia
				Primary hemorrhage
				Thrombocythemia
				von Willebrand's disease
				Abnormal platelet function
				  Thrombocytopathy
				  Bernard-Soulier
				  Glanzmann's

Coagulation factor disorders	Hemarthrosis Delayed bleeding Prolonged traumatic bleeding Deep intramuscular bleeding Male predominance	PT PTT Specific factor assay	Normal platelet count Normal bleeding time Normal thrombin time except with heparin and fibrinogen disorders	Hemophilia Sodium warfarin therapy Heparin therapy Vitamin K deficiency Congenital hypo- + dysfibrinogenemia von Willebrand's disease (VIII)
DIC and fibrinolysis	Delayed bleeding in fibrinolysis Diffuse skin and mucous membrane bleeding Stigmata of chronic liver disease may be present	Variable prolongation in PT and PTT Low platelet count Low fibrinogen level Elevated fibrin degradation products		DIC–see Chapter 97 Primary fibrinolysis Liver disease Streptokinase and urokinase therapy

embolism can be complicated by generalized bleeding from hyperfibrinolysis and hypofibrinogenemia.

LABORATORY INTERPRETATION

Given a sufficient index of suspicion for abnormal bleeding, the emergency physician should attempt to identify the nature of the coagulopathy. The screening battery is outlined in Table 96-2. Interpretation of the platelet count, prothrombin time (PT), and partial thromboplastin time (PTT), are discussed below.

Platelet Count

Spontaneous bleeding generally does not occur if the platelet count exceeds 50,000 per cubic millimeter. Life-threatening CNS hem-

Table 96-2. Bleeding Screening Tests

Type of Bleeding	Screening Test	Adjunctive
Vascular	Platelet count	Tourniquet test
Platelet	Platelet count	Bleeding time
Clotting	Prothrombin time (PT)	Fibrinogen level
Fibrinolysis	Partial thromboplastin time (PTT)	Factor assays

orrhage may occur spontaneously with platelet counts below 10,000 per cubic millimeter. If a platelet count is not available, the physician can estimate the number of platelets by scanning the peripheral blood smear. In general, each platelet per oil immersion field represents 10,000 to 15,000 platelets per cubic millimeter. Platelet clumping on the smear may influence this and yield a factitiously low estimate.

Prothrombin Time Prolongation

The prothrombin time is the time required to induce clot formation in citrated plasma after the addition of tissue thromboplastin and calcium. Control values are in the 10- to 12-s range and are considered significantly prolonged when the patient's value is greater than three to four seconds above control. As illustrated in Figure 96-1 the PT can be affected by abnormalities in factors I, II, V, VII, or X and is normal in hemophilia. The PT is a valuable, reproducible study and an isolated prolongation (with a normal PTT) suggests sodium warfarin therapy, vitamin K deficiency, or liver disease.

Partial Thromboplastin Time Prolongation

The PTT measures the intrinsic pathway of coagulation. It is the time necessary to induce clot formation in citrated plasma after

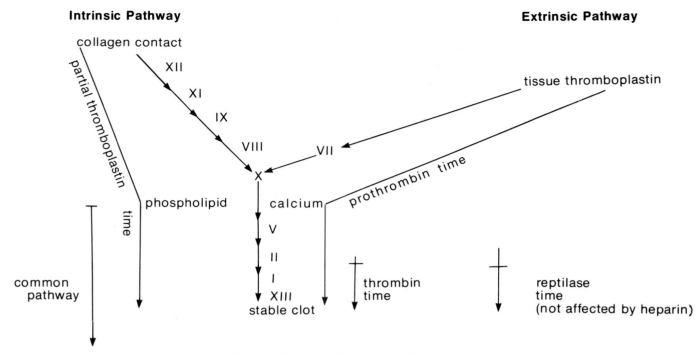

Figure 96-1. Schema of intrinsic and extrinsic mechanisms of blood coagulation.

the addition of calcium and contact with a surface (with kaolin activation it is called "activated" PTT). The control range is 25 to 35 s and varies widely depending on laboratory methodology. Significance is attributed to prolongations of 8 to 10 s above control. Isolated prolongation of the PTT suggests deficiency of factors VIII, IX, or XI or heparin effect.

Prolongation of PT and PTT–(Heparin and Sodium Warfarin Overdose, DIC, Hypofibrinogenemia)

Significant abnormalities in the common pathway (Fig. 96-1) may prolong both the PT and PTT. Since heparin acts primarily by inhibiting thrombin and factor X, heparin overdose can affect both studies. Similarly, sodium warfarin overdose may depress factors II, VII, IX, and X, affecting both pathways. In DIC, the rate of clotting factor consumption exceeds that of production (particularly fibrinogen, V, and VIII) and the additive antithrombin effect of fibrin-split products may prolong both the PT and PTT.

DIC Screen (See Chapter 97, "Acquired Bleeding Disorders.")

Because of the clinical importance of DIC, many laboratories are now establishing composite tests for defining the presence of intravascular coagulation:

Prolonged PT
Decreased fibrinogen level
Decreased platelet count
Increased fibrin degradation products

BIBLIOGRAPHY

Arkel YS: Evaluation of platelet aggregation in disorders of hemostasis. *Med Clin North Am* 60:881–911, 1976.

Ginsburg AD: Platelet function in patients with high platelet counts. *Ann Intern Med* 82:506–511, 1975.

Goulian M: A guide to disorders of hemostasis. *Ann Intern Med* 65:782–796, 1966.

Harker LA, Slichter SJ: The bleeding time as a screening test for evaluation of platelet function. *N Engl J Med* 287:155–159, 1972.

Lerner RG, Goldstein R: Tests of coagulation: Use and interpretation. *Med Clin North Am* 57:1609–1616, 1973.

Lewis JH, Spero JA, Hasiba U: Coagulopathies. *DM* 23:1–64, 1977.

Mason RG, Saba HI: Normal and abnormal hemostasis: An integrated view. *Am J Pathol* 92:775–811, 1978.

Stevens DJ: Vascular hemostasis: A review. *Am J Med Technol* 39:252–257, June 1973.

Zucker S, Mielke CH, Durocher JR: Oozing and bruising due to abnormal platelet function (thrombocytopathia). *Ann Intern Med* 76:725–731, 1972.

CHAPTER 97
ACQUIRED BLEEDING DISORDERS

Daniel Esposito

THROMBOCYTOPENIA

Acquired disorders that may underlie an abnormally low platelet count fall into two general categories: decreased platelet production and increased destruction. The list of etiologic agents is quite long and should be reviewed in a reference text. The more commonly encountered conditions include:

Decreased bone marrow production
  Aplastic anemia
  Malignant replacement of the bone marrow (leukemia, carcinoma, etc.)
  Drug suppression of the bone marrow (chemotherapy, radiation, alcohol, etc.)
  Infectious suppression (measles, tuberculosis)
  B_{12} and folic acid deficiency
Increased peripheral destruction
  Immune (idiopathic thrombocytopenic purpura, systemic lupus erythematosus, drug-induced, infectious mononucleosis, etc.)
  Disseminated intravascular coagulation (DIC)
  Hypersplenism
  Thrombotic thrombocytopenic purpura

The bleeding tendency is greatest when the platelet count is below 50,000 per cubic millimeter. Fatal, spontaneous bleeding may occur when the platelet count is below 10,000 to 20,000 per cubic millimeter. Large platelets (megathrombocytes) on the peripheral blood smear may reflect increased bone marrow production and imply a peripheral destructive process. Young, large platelets appear to be functionally hyperactive and may explain why patients with immune destruction tend to tolerate lower platelet counts than those with marrow failure. The demonstration of megakaryocytes and increased platelet destruction on bone marrow examination is important in excluding bone marrow failure as a cause of severe thrombocytopenia.

Management

Stabilization of intravascular volume status and maintenance of circulating hemoglobin should receive priority in any critically bleeding patient. Platelet transfusion is most effective when decreased platelet production is the underlying cause (i.e., normal peripheral survival). In general, one can assume an increment in the platelet count of 10,000 per cubic millimeter per unit of transfused platelets. Although platelet survival may be markedly shortened in peripheral destructive processes (particularly immune thrombocytopenia), and platelet transfusion as maintenance therapy is only slightly indicated, the patient with life-threatening bleeding should receive exogenous platelets as emergency therapy. Antibody suppressive therapy with corticosteroids and other immunosuppressive agents requires several days to improve platelet counts in the immune thrombocytopenias and are not commonly utilized in the emergency department.

HYPOPROTHROMBINEMIA

Sodium Warfarin Therapy and Vitamin K Deficiency

Prothrombin is a glycoprotein produced by the liver under the influence of vitamin K and is converted to thrombin in the common pathway of the coagulation sequence. Congenital prothrombin deficiency is exceedingly rare and bleeding due to abnormalities of prothrombin production is generally related to vitamin K deficiency, sodium warfarin therapy, or hepatic insufficiency. The multifactorial pathogenesis of bleeding in liver disease will be treated as a separate subject.

Fat-soluble vitamin K is necessary for the hepatic production of factors II, VII, IX, and X. Dietary and biliary insufficiency, as well as intestinal fat malabsorption, may lead to a bleeding diathesis characterized by a prolonged prothrombin time (PT) [variable prolongation of the partial thromboplastin time (PTT)] that reverses with parenteral vitamin K therapy.

Coumarin derivatives (warfarin or Coumadin, and dicumarol) are competitive inhibitors of vitamin K and are widely used oral anticoagulants in the treatment of thrombosis and thromboembolism. Their anticoagulant properties may be enhanced by a variety of drugs through protein displacement (phenylbutazone, clofibrate, idomethacin, etc.) or by metabolic inhibition (allopurinol, chloramphenicol, nortriptyline). With therapeutic doses, the PT is 2 to $2\frac{1}{2}$ times the control value and the PTT is generally normal. Otherwise, minor trauma may induce bleeding which, if uncontrollable by local compression, may require discontinuing the medication and reversal with vitamin K (oral or parenteral). Sodium warfarin overdose may produce fatal, spontaneous bleeding with prolongation of both the PT and PTT. Clinical judgment should dictate the need for volume-red cell replacement and emergency fresh frozen plasma infusion (see Chapter 100, ''Blood Transfusion—Components and Practices'').

LIVER DISEASE

Multiple factors may be responsible for abnormal (atraumatic) bleeding in acute and chronic liver disease. All four general categories of hemostasis may be individually or simultaneously affected as shown in the following outline:

Vascular
    Trauma
    Peptic ulcer disease and alcohol gastritis
    Variceal bleeding in portal hypertension
    Hemorrhoids
Platelets (thrombopenia)
    Alcoholic bone marrow suppression
    Hypersplenism
    Folic acid deficiency
    DIC
Clotting factors
    Vitamin K deficiency and malabsorption
    Insufficient production of factors I, II, V, VII, IX, X
    Chronic consumption coagulopathy (DIC)
Hyperfibrinolysis
    Hepatic inability to deactivate plasmin
    Inhibition of coagulation by circulating fibrin-split products
    Hypofibrinogenia

Bleeding in the presence of liver disease is, therefore, complex and requires diligent laboratory and clinical efforts to determine the nature and site of bleeding, degree of volume loss, and relative contribution of platelet and clotting factor abnormalities. The battery of laboratory studies should include: platelet count, PT, PTT, and fibrinogen level. Fibrin-split products may be obtained as a supportive test.

HYPOFIBRINOGENEMIA

Congenital hypofibrinogenemia and dysfibrinogenemia are rare, and clinical manifestations are quite variable (thrombosis, bleeding, wound dehiscence, or asymptomatic). Acquired hypofibrinogenemia is rarely an isolated phenomenon and is generally a composite feature of advanced liver disease, DIC, primary fibrinolysis, or increased fibrinolysis due to streptokinase/urokinase therapy. Prolongation of the PT, PTT, thrombin, and reptilase times may vary relative to the degree of fibrinogen level depression. Therapy is directed at the underlying etiology and replacement therapy with cryoprecipitate is utilized in the seriously bleeding patient. Pooled, fibrinogen concentrates have a high incidence of hepatitis transmission.

DISSEMINATED INTRAVASCULAR COAGULATION

DIC is a clinical syndrome characterized by diffuse bleeding from the skin, mucous membranes, and viscera. Widespread activation of the clotting mechanism results in consumption of the circulating clotting factors and platelets available for hemostatic homeostasis. When the rate of utilization exceeds production, diffuse bleeding ensues.

Any condition that is accompanied by significant tissue destruction can trigger and sustain unbridled intravascular clotting (e.g., burns, trauma, crush injury, malignancy, fetal death in utero, gangrene). In addition to tissue necrosis, DIC can be a sequela of drug reactions, amniotic fluid emboli, transfusion reactions, liver disease, and a host of infectious diseases. The clinical importance of DIC cannot be overemphasized and the reader is urged to read the review of the underlying causes and therapy by Gralnick.

The diagnosis of DIC may not always be achieved with absolute certainty (particularly in liver disease, TTP, etc.), however, the laboratory triad of prolonged prothrombin time, thrombocytopenia, and hypofibrinogenemia should signal its possible presence in the patient with multisite bleeding. Supportive laboratory evidence of DIC includes demonstration of elevated fibrin-split products and microangiopathic hemolytic anemia with fragmented red blood cells on peripheral blood smear.

Primary therapy should always be directed at the underlying cause when readily identifiable (sepsis, pregnancy, drug, or transfusion therapy), and early recognition and correction of hemodynamic instability through volume and red cell replacement are essential. Current consensus favors clotting factor (fresh frozen plasma), fibrinogen (cryoprecipitate or fresh frozen plasma), and platelet replacement in the uncontrollably bleeding patient, often in association with intravenous heparin therapy.

The continuous use of heparin to interrupt inappropriate coagulation activity may be effective prophylaxis in certain chronic DIC states such as carcinoma and acute progranulocytic leukemia.

BIBLIOGRAPHY

Thrombocytopenia

Amorosi EG, Ultmann JE: Thrombotic thrombocytopenic purpura: Report of 16 cases and a review of the literature. *Medicine* 45:139–159, 1966.
Baldini M: Idiopathic thrombocytopenic purpura. *N Engl J Med* 274:1245–1251, 1301–1306, 1360–1367, 1966.
Ellis LD, Dameshek HL: The dilemma of hypersplenism. *Surg Clin North Am* 55:277–285, 1975.

Garg SK, Lackner H, Karpatkin S: The increased percentage of mega-thrombocytes in various clinical disorders. *Ann Intern Med* 77:361–369, 1972.

Lacey JV, Penner JA: Management of idiopathic thrombocytopenia purpura in the adult. *Semin Thromb Homostas* 3:160–174, 1977.

Hypoprothrombinemia

Ansell JE, Kumar R, Deykin D: The spectrum of vitamin K deficiency. *JAMA* 238:40–42, 1977.

Koch-Weser J, Sellers EM: Drug interactions with coumarin anticoagulants. *N Engl J Med* 285:487–498, 547–558, 1971.

Liver Disease

Roberts HR, Cederbaum AI: The liver and blood coagulation: Physiology and pathology. *Gastroenterol* 63:297–320, 1972.

Hypofibrinogenemia

Colman RW, Robboy SJ, Minna JD: Disseminated intravascular coagulation (DIC): An approach. *Am J Med* 52:679–689, 1972.

Deykin D: The clinical challenge of disseminated intravascular coagulation. *N Engl J Med* 283:636–644, 1970.

Gralnick HR: Intravascular coagulation 2. Underlying conditions and therapy. *Postgrad Med* 62:81–87, Nov. 1977.

Mammen EF: Congenital abnormalities of the fibrinogen molecule. *Semin Thromb Hemostas* 1:184–201, 1974.

CHAPTER 98
HEMOPHILIA

Ronald Sacher

The hemophilias comprise a group of hereditary bleeding disorders that have in common a disturbance in intrinsic coagulation. These may be further subdivided into hemophilia A (classic hemophilia), hemophilia B (Christmas disease), and von Willebrand's disease.

GENERAL CONSIDERATIONS AND CLINICAL SYNDROMES

Classic hemophilia is a deficiency of normal functional factor VIII, Christmas disease is a deficiency of normal functional factor IX, and von Willebrand's disease is a deficiency of both antigenic and functional factor VIII and factor VIII von Willebrand's cofactor. The factors of the intrinsic coagulation pathway are measured by the partial thromboplastin time (PTT). Factors VIII and IX are important components of the intrinsic pathway and their deficiency is associated with prolongation of the PTT. The other factors unique to the intrinsic pathway, namely factors XII and XI, may also be genetically absent, but these constitute much less frequent and less severe clinical entities.

The prothrombin time (PT) measures the extrinsic coagulation pathway and factor VII is unique to this system. It is obvious that certain factors, such as X, V, II, and I, are common to both pathways. Thus a deficiency of factor VIII or IX would produce a prolonged PTT and a normal PT. This is a hallmark of the hemophilias. Obviously, identification of the deficient factor is essential to specifically define the type of hemophilia that is present. Identification will also affect specific treatment.

Genetic types

Classic Hemophilia (Hemophilia A)

Hemophilia A is a sex-linked genetic disorder resulting in deficiency of factor VIII coagulant activity. The deficiency is often defined as severe (less than 2 percent), moderate (2 to 5 percent), and mild (5 to 30 percent), depending on the level of factor VIII present. Only about 50 percent of severe hemophilias give a positive family history.

Hemophilia B

Hemophilia B is a sex-linked genetic disorder resulting in a deficiency of factor IX coagulant activity. Severe, moderate, and mild forms also exist. More than 75 percent of patients give a history of hemophilia. This disorder is clinically indistinguishable from hemophilia A.

von Willebrand's Disease

This disorder is an autosomal genetic disease resulting in a deficiency in factor VIII (VIII-C) coagulation activity, immunologic activity (VIII-ag), and the VIII von Willebrand's factor (VIII-vwf). The latter activity is the factor that corrects the platelet dysfunction found in von Willebrand's disease (see Table 98-1 for laboratory diagnosis of hemophilia).

This disorder is usually transmitted as an autosomal dominant inheritance with variation in expression of the disorder.

Clinical Syndromes of Hemophilia

Mild Disease

Mild disease may not be diagnosed until adult life, although very often the patients give a history of minor, but recurrent bleeding episodes in early life. Serious bleeding, however, rarely follows mild trauma but occurs following dental extractions, tonsillectomy, and other surgical challenges or severe trauma. Female carriers may easily bruise, producing cosmetically disturbing ecchymoses, and have excessive menstrual loss. Mild factor VIII or IX deficiency may occasionally have a normal PTT.

Moderate and Severe Disease

Moderate and severe disease usually presents in infancy or early childhood. The disease may become apparent following circumcision. In infants learning to walk, falling may produce recurrent

Table 98-1. Laboratory Diagnosis of Hemophilia

	PT*	PTT*	Factor* VIII-C	AG*	(Ristocetin Platelet Aggregation)	Bleeding Time	Factor IX
Hemophilia A	N	↑	↓	N	N	N	N
Hemophilia B	N	↑	N	N	N	N	↓
von Willebrand's (C)	N	↑	↓	↓	↓	↑	N

*See text for explanation of abbreviations.
Note: N = Normal; ↑ = prolonged; ↓ = decreased.

and severe muscle hematomas, lip lacerations, or tongue biting leading to severe bleeding episodes. Dental procedures may provoke severe bleeding. Hematuria may occur in adolescence and adulthood and may be spontaneous or associated with physical activity. The characteristic hemarthroses and muscle hematomas occur when the child is walking well, and the peak incidence is in schoolboys and adolescents.

Muscle hemorrhages are associated with stiffness and pain before the cardinal signs of swelling and warmth become apparent. Retroperitoneal hematomas may be difficult to diagnose and the patient may have groin pain at the insertion of the psoas muscle due to hemorrhage tracking down the fascial planes.

Joint hemorrhages are usually recognized by a sensation of joint fullness and limitation of range of movement. Pain and swelling become apparent. Knees, elbows, ankles, hips, and shoulders are affected in decreasing order of frequency. Chronic arthropathy may occur if treatment and consequently resolution of hemorrhage is delayed. Recurrent hemorrhages lead to synovial hypertrophy, chronic inflammation with fibrous adhesions, and joint ankylosis. Severe deformities can occur.

MANAGEMENT

Acute Medical Management

Replacement Therapy

Specific identification of the deficient factor is essential to proper management. All coagulation factors are present in fresh frozen plasma that can be given in a situation where the specific abnormality is unknown. However, the deficient individual usually requires a substantial amount of replacement therapy to achieve hemostasis and volume overload may be a problem. The average patient has approximately 40 mL of plasma per kilogram of body weight. Each 1 mL of normal plasma, then, has 1 unit of factor activity. The emergency physician should be able to calculate the amount of a given factor necessary to raise the patient's factor activity to the desired percent level of normal. Depending on whether bleeding is mild to severe, one may wish to raise the plasma level to 50 to 100 percent of predicted normal (see Table 98-2). Remember, since the half life of the antihemophilic factors

Table 98-2. Treatment Schedule for Severe Hemophilia (1% of Factor Present) without an Inhibitor

Disorders	Degree of Hemorrhage	Initial Dose of Concentrate in Units	Subsequent Doses	
Hemophilia A Classic hemophilia (factor VIII deficiency)	Minor Hemoarthrosis Muscle hematoma Mild hematuria	18 units/kg	10 units/kg q 8–12 h	Until objective bleeding and pain resolves; single dose may be sufficient.
	Moderate	26 units/kg	14 units/kg q 8–12 h	7–10 days to permit adequate healing
	Severe Life-threatening surgical procedure Major trauma Head injury	35 units/kg	18 units/kg q 8–12 h	7–10 days to permit adequate healing
Hemophilia B Christmas disease (factor IX deficiency)	Minor Hemarthrosis Muscle hematoma Mild hematuria	25 units/kg	5 units/kg q 12–24 h	Until objective bleeding and pain resolves; single dose may be sufficient.
	Moderate	35 units/kg	8 units/kg q 12–24 h	7–10 days to permit adequate healing
	Severe Life-threatening surgical procedure Major trauma Head injury	45 units/kg	10 units/kg q 12–24 h	7–10 days to permit adequate healing

is only 12 hours, the patient may need to be treated repeatedly, depending on the site, severity, and persistence of bleeding.

Fresh frozen plasma or cryoprecipitate may be used in the treatment of von Willebrand's disease. Since a unit of plasma is derived from a single donor, there is less risk of hepatitis than with pooled concentrates. Plasma may also be used to treat mild factor VIII or IX deficiency. Its use is limited by the volume needed since only 10 to 15 mL/kg is safely given in one dose with an expected rise of 20 to 30 percent in clotting factor activity.

The use of concentrates has made hemophilia management more practical. The dose of concentrate must be adjusted to the severity of the hemorrhage. Minor bleeding can be managed by a single infusion of several bags of cryoprecipitate in the emergency department. The patient is instructed to return if bleeding recurs. Cryoprecipitate is rich in factor VIII and contains approximately 5 to 10 units/mL of factor VIII activity. Single cryobags derived from a single donor contain about 10 mL total volume, i.e., 50 to 100 units of factor VIII activity per bag of cryoprecipitate.

Factor VIII concentrates are available in different total strengths. These concentrates are derived from pooled plasma, lyophilized, and then reconstituted with sterile water. The total activity is indicated on the container. The major advantage is that less volume is needed; however, since this product is derived from pooled plasma, it carries a greater risk of hepatitis and, more recently, of the acquired immune deficiency syndrome (AIDS). Furthermore, concentrates are more expensive. The approximate number of units per milliliter can vary considerably from preparation to preparation.

Lyophilized concentrates of factors II, VII, IX, and X (prothrombin complex) are used primarily for the treatment of factor IX deficiency. The complex is not separated for technical reasons and carries a higher risk of hepatitis as well as thromboplastin activity. Average factor IX activity is 20 units/mL concentrate.

Dosages and treatment schedules are outlined in Table 98-2.

Additional Features in Management

Local care, using ice packs and immobilization with an elastic bandage, can limit muscle hematomas and hemorrhage under the skin. Hemarthroses generally only occur in severe hemophilias and almost never in von Willebrand's disease. Temporary splinting is necessary to avoid further trauma, limit swelling, and help relieve pain.

Appropriate analgesia is important in the hemophilias. An increasing list of analgesics contain aspirin and should be avoided since they inhibit platelet aggregation and compound the hemostatic problem. Propoxyphene, acetaminophen, and codeine may be used as alternatives. Intramuscular injections must be avoided.

Anti-inflammatory agents, most specifically steroids, are used in hematuria, acute hemarthrosis, and chronic synovitis. The dosage is usually 1 mg/(kg·day).

Special Considerations

Occasionally a patient with severe hemophilia fails to respond to appropriate replacement therapy. These patients may constitute the small but therapeutically complicated group of patients with circulating anticoagulants (inhibitors). A hematology consultant should be called in to help in the management of this serious problem.

BIBLIOGRAPHY

Arnold WD, Hilgartner MW: Hemophilic arthropathy: Current concepts of pathogenesis and management. *J Bone Joint Surg* 59A:287–305, 1977.

Biggs R, Matthews JM: The treatment of haemorrhage in von Willebrand's disease and the blood level of factor VIII (AHG). *Br J Haematol* 9:203–214, 1963.

Gralnick HR, Coller BS, Shulman NR, et al: Factor VIII. *Ann Intern Med* 86:598–616, 1977.

Hoag MS, Johnson FF, Robinson JA: Treatment of hemophilia B with a new clotting-factor concentrate. *N Engl J Med* 280:581–586, 1969.

Hougie C: Disorders of hemostasis, in Williams WJ, Beutler E, Ersler AJ, Lichtman MA (eds): *Hematology*, ed 3. New York, McGraw-Hill, 1983, pp 1381–1397.

CHAPTER 99
SICKLE CELL ANEMIA

Daniel Esposito

Sickle cell anemia is a qualitative hemoglobinopathy inherited as an autosomal dominant trait with an approximate gene frequency in black Americans of 8 percent. Although a detailed account of the molecular mechanisms of the sickling phenomenon is beyond the scope of this volume the emergency physician's awareness of the pathophysiologic principles will greatly aid in approaching the extremely broad and often perplexing clinical manifestations of sickle cell anemia.

GENERAL

Pathogenesis

The biochemical abnormality of sickle hemoglobin is due to the substitution of B_6 valine for glutamic acid in the hemoglobin chain. This single substitution is responsible for the susceptibility of deoxygenated sickle hemoglobin to polymerize and aggregate which, in turn, induces red cell deformation.

By virtue of their shape change, sickled erythrocytes are unable to freely pass through the microvasculature and this ongoing process of thrombosis and hemolysis is largely responsible for the clinical expressions of ischemia, infarction, chronic hemolytic anemia, and multisystem compromise. *

Patients with sickle cell disease (homozygous-SS) have a clearly defined increased susceptibility to infection. Functional hyposplenism and autosplenectomy result from repeated erythrocyte stasis, thrombosis, and splenic infarction during childhood as a direct extension of the sickling process. Apart from diminished splenic and reticuloendothelial phagocytic function, deficient opsonin activity against pneumococci and *Salmonella,* as well as defective granulation and polymorphonuclear mobility, appear additive in predisposing to infectious complications.

Sickle Disease Variants

In populous urban settings the diagnosis of sickle cell anemia and related hemoglobinopathies is often first considered and evaluated in the emergency department. The following distinctions should be made.

Sickle Cell Anemia (Homozygosity) Hb SS

The most severe form of sickle syndromes occurs in the homozygous state, when 75 to 95 percent of circulating hemoglobin is of the sickle variety. Because of the likelihood of focal or disseminated microcirculatory thrombosis (crisis) with high sickle hemoglobin concentrations, the homozygous state should be considered in children who have unexplained bone pain, severe hemolytic anemia, jaundice, or recurrent left upper quadrant pain associated with splenic infarctions. The degree of severity is variable and the age at onset of symptoms may range from 6 months to 15 years.

Sickle Cell Trait (Heterozygosity) Hb AS

When the sickle gene is inherited from one parent and normal hemoglobin A from the other, one expects only partial expression of the abnormal gene. Erythrocytes will then contain both hemoglobin A and S in variable proportions depending on their synthetic rates. Since less than 50 percent of circulating hemoglobin is subject to sickling, the severe vasoocclusive and hemolytic manifestations do not occur. The reader is referred to the timely review by Sears on the morbidity of sickle trait.

Doubly Heterozygous (Heterozygous for S, Heterozygous for Another Abnormal Hemoglobin)

The most commonly encountered doubly heterozygous conditions are Hb SC, Hb SB thalassemia, Hb SD, and Hb S-fetal persistence. Patients may have severe systemic complications of sickle cell disease or may lead relatively asymptomatic lives. Distinction from sickle cell disease can only be accomplished with hemoglobin electrophoresis. Initial symptoms may manifest relatively late in life and the diagnosis often overlooked until the second to third decade. Recent attention to Hb SC disease and pregnancy complicated by bone marrow infarction and fat emboli further underscores the need to maintain an awareness of sickle disease variants.

DIAGNOSIS AND TREATMENT

Laboratory Diagnosis

Depression of the hematocrit and hemoglobin level due to sickle cell trait is uncommon; however, significant anemia, usually with a chronically elevated reticulocyte count, is invariably present in homozygous sickle cell disease. The hemolytic anemia serves as a constant bone marrow stimulus, and as a result elevated leukocyte and platelet counts are present in the "steady state" and serve little value in assessing the presence of infection. The diagnosis of sickle cell anemia is confirmed by the demonstration of sickle hemoglobin by electrophoretic separation.

The emergency physician can be relatively sure of the diagnosis if irreversibly sickled red cells are present on the peripheral blood smear. Since erythrocytes are exposed to oxygen during blood smear preparation, sickled red cells may revert to their normal shape. Irreversibly sickled cells on peripheral smear generally indicate homozygous disease or doubly heterozygous variants and are not seen in Hb AS patients. Most of the currently available screening tests for sickle hemoglobin (Sickledex, SickleScrene, Sik-L-Stat, SCAT) rely on the insolubility of sickle hemoglobin in a reduced environment. The turbidity thus produced constitutes a positive test, but does not distinguish between sickle trait or disease.

Clinical Manifestations and Management

Having considered the pathogenetic mechanisms of microcirculatory thrombosis, ischemia, and infarction, one can readily appreciate the panorama of systemic illness and organ dysfunction that befalls the homozygous sickler. The long-term deleterious effects of anemia and ischemia can produce a spectrum of chronic disorders, including progressive optic atrophy and blindness due to repeated vasoocclusion, hemorrhage, and neovascularization; chronic organic brain syndrome with epileptic foci; respiratory insufficiency with cor pulmonale; chronic congestive heart failure; progressive renal insufficiency and the nephrotic syndrome; and chronic, recurrent, ischemic leg ulceration. The reader is urged to review the sickle cell symposium in Lessin and Jensen, 1974, for added perspective and an overview.

Sickle cell crisis, acute respiratory insufficiency, arthropathy, and priapism are acute problems that are often encountered in the emergency department. They are discussed in detail below.

Sickle Cell Crises

Sickle cell crises include thrombotic crisis (vasoocclusive-infarctive); hemolytic crisis, exaggeration of the steady-state hemolytic process manifested as a dramatic fall in the hematocrit with concomitant jaundice; aplastic crisis, which is often induced by concurrent infectious suppression of the bone marrow or folic acid

deficiency with life-threatening depression of the hematocrit and reticulocyte count; and sequestration crisis, an uncommon feature of childhood sickle cell disease, clinically manifested as sudden painful enlargement of the liver and spleen with associated pancytopenia.

Thrombotic sickle crisis, which is universally more common than hemolytic or aplastic crisis, implies a sequential progression of pathological, symptomatic events that culminate in a clinical state of unremitting pain, prostration, and anxiety. Initially, gnawing pain may develop locally in the tibia, periarticular areas, back, abdomen, or chest. Paroxysmal pain may last only a few hours and subsequently recur with greater intensity and duration. "Impending" crisis seemingly refers to the sickle patient who has vague discomfort, a paucity of physical findings, and symptoms that initially appear easily manageable with fluid therapy and analgesics. The experienced emergency physician has no doubt seen this patient return several times in a 48- to 72-h period prior to the ultimate development of crescendo pain necessitating hospitalization. Thrombotic crisis is first and foremost a clinical diagnosis before it is a laboratory one and recent reports of elevated α-hydroxybutyrate dehydrogenase as a laboratory earmark of crisis have not, as yet, been substantiated. An element of increased hemolytic activity is commonly present and when baseline data are available, there may be an elevated reticulocyte count and a hematocrit below that of the patient's steady state. Laboratory studies should be further directed at identifying possible precipitating factors, including pneumonia, urinary tract infection, pharyngitis, acidosis, and dehydration.

Analgesics, rehydration, correction of acidosis, and treatment of infection remain as mainstay therapy for vasoocclusive crisis. Supplemental oxygen is advised but does little to improve oxygen tension in the stagnating microenvironment. Red cell transfusion should be reserved for significantly anemic patients (hematocrit less than 17 to 18 percent) as liberal transfusion to a hematocrit greater than 30 percent may increase whole blood viscosity and promote further sludging and vasoocclusion. Continued supplemental folic acid is indicated to meet the exaggerated red cell turnover rate. Antisickling agents (urea, sodium cyanate) have not proven clinically useful.

Acute Respiratory Insufficiency

Acute pulmonary manifestations include bacterial and mycoplasma pneumonias, thromboembolism, in situ pulmonary thrombosis, and acute pulmonary hypertension. Bone marrow infarction and pulmonic fat emboli have been described in Hb SS and Hb SC disease.

Central Nervous System

Acute neurological manifestations of sickle cell disease are primarily related to vascular occlusion, although narcotic overdose and withdrawal syndromes should also be considered in the individual with an altered sensorium. Subarachnoid hemorrhage, hemiplegia, and convulsions are the most common manifestations. Current therapeutic trends favor long-term transfusion programs in an effort to prevent irreversible cerebral damage. If stupor and coma are present, suspect severe anemia and aplastic crisis.

Arthropathy

It is convenient to consider an acutely tender and inflamed joint as another manifestation of thrombosis (synovial or periarticular); however, aseptic necrosis, septic arthritis, osteomyelitis, hemarthrosis, and gout are frequently responsible. When fever and monoarticular involvement coexist, diagnostic arthrocentesis may be necessary.

Priapism

Penile engorgement prolonged beyond several hours is uncommon but may occasionally occur in both sickle cell disease and sickle trait. Analgesia and ice compresses aid in relieving corpus cavernosal engorgement and urological consultation should be requested immediately.

Hematuria

Painless, gross hematuria is a common clinical feature of sickle cell trait and sickle disease. Relative hyperosmolarity of the renal medulla favors in situ sickling and subsequent papillary necrosis. Severe necrosis and substantial tissue sloughing may rarely obstruct the ureteropelvic junction, producing acute flank pain with hematuria.

BIBLIOGRAPHY

Baron M, Leiter E: The management of priapism in sickle cell anemia. *J Urol* 119:610–611, 1978.

Barrett-Connor E: Pneumonia and pulmonary infarction in sickle cell anemia. *JAMA* 224:997–1000, 1973.

Brewer GJ: A view of the current status of antisickling therapy. *Am J Hematol* 1:121–128, 1976.

Davey RJ, Esposito DJ, Jacobson RJ, et al: Partial exchange transfusion as treatment for hemoglobin SC disease in pregnancy. *Arch Intern Med* 138:937–939, 1978.

Finch CA: Pathophysiologic aspects of sickle cell anemia. *Am J Med* 53:1–6, 1972.

Gelpi AP, Perrine RP: Sickle cell disease and trait in white populations. *JAMA* 224:605–608, 1973.

Hand WL, King NL: Serum opsonization of Salmonella in sickle cell anemia. *Am J Med* 64:388–395, 1978.

Lessin LS, Jensen WN (eds): Sickle cell symposium. *Arch Intern Med* 133:529–705, April 1974.

Lusher JM, Haghighat H, Khalifa S, et al: A prophylactic transfusion program for children with sickle cell anemia complicated by CNS infarction. *Am J Hematol* 1:265–273, 1976.

Portnoy BA, Herion JC: Neurological manifestations in sickle cell disease. *Ann Intern Med* 76:643–652, 1972.

Schmidt RM, Wilson SM: Standardization in detection of abnormal hemoglobins: Solubility tests for hemoglobin S. *JAMA* 225:1225–1230, 1973.

Schumacher HR, Andrews R, McLaughlin G: Arthropathy in sickle cell disease. *Ann Intern Med* 78:203–211, 1973.

Sears DA: The morbidity of sickle cell trait: A review of the literature. *Am J Med* 64:1021–1036, 1978.

Seller RA, Jacobs NM: Pyogenic infections in children with sickle hemoglobinopathy, letter to the editor. *J Pediatr* 90:161–162, 1977.

Sennara H, Gorry F: Orthopedic aspects of sickle cell anemia and allied hemoglobinopathies. *Clin Orthop* 130:154–157, Jan.–Feb. 1978.

Sheehy TW, Plumb VJ: Therapy of sickle cell disease. *Arch Intern Med* 137:779–782, 1977.

Steinberg MH, Adams JG III: Laboratory diagnosis of sickling hemoglobinopathies. *South Med J* 71:413–416, 1978.

Steinberg, MH, Dreiling BJ, Morrison FS, et al: Mild sickle cell disease: Clinical and laboratory studies. *JAMA* 224:317–321, 1973.

White JM, Billimoria F, Muller MA: Serum α-hydroxybutyrate levels in sickle cell disease and sickle cell crisis, preliminary communication. *Lancet* 1:532–533, 1978.

CHAPTER 100

BLOOD TRANSFUSION— COMPONENTS AND PRACTICES

Steven J. Davidson

The cellular and noncellular elements of blood together serve multiple functions but rarely do patients require more than one of these components. Blood stored in preservatives and nutrient solutions in refrigerators is not the same substance removed from the donor or flowing in our patients' cardiovascular tree. Rather, as a living and metabolizing tissue, it inevitably undergoes change. Consideration of these changes as the physician orders blood for and subsequently initiates transfusion, the most frequent of all organ transplants, is the essence behind the rationales developed to assist safe and effective blood transfusion practice. Blood transfusion initiated in the emergency service in response to the usual indications is nonetheless frequently enough a prelude to special circumstances to warrant an awareness on the emergency physician's part of uncommonly employed but useful and life-saving modalities. Any transfusion carries with it certain risks to the recipient, most of which are not under the transfusing physician's control. Knowledge of these potential complications and awareness of the interventions that may ameliorate outcomes fulfills the transfusionist's ultimate responsibility of *primum non nocere*.

BLOOD COMPONENTS—DESCRIPTIONS AND INDICATIONS

Increasingly, physicians are provided with one or another of the various cellular (red blood cell, platelet, granulocyte) or noncellular [albumin, plasma protein fraction (PPF), fresh frozen plasma (FFP), cryoprecipitate, etc.] components of whole blood in response to requests for blood for transfusion. Particularly from the viewpoint of physiological rationale but admittedly with a view to maximal efficient use of a limited resource, component transfusion is usually preferred. The emergency physician most frequently will have cause to utilize red blood cell concentrates and will have secondary needs for fresh frozen plasma, cryoprecipitate and other coagulation factor concentrates, platelets, and human protein colloids including albumin and PPF. Rarely, and only under the circumstances of massive transfusion and infant transfusion, whole blood transfusion may be profitably employed.

However, even in this instance in which *freshness* is one of the most valuable charactistics, blood less than 72 h old can rarely be found. Regional blood banks are assured a supply of components, but the necessary interposition of transportation and processing time has severly curtailed the availability of fresh whole blood.

Transfusion of all but heat-treated components (albumin, PPF) carries with it the risk of hepatitis and, apparently, acquired immune deficiency syndrome (AIDS). Other infectious illnesses may be uncommonly transmitted. Incompatibility, isoimmunization, and allergic and toxic phenomena may be unwelcome sequelae in recipients. As with all therapeutic modalities, risk-benefit ratios should prevail; although in the emergency service thoughtful decision making may be rushed or incomplete.

Whole Blood

Fresh whole blood is a vanishingly rare commodity, whose primary value is probably to the patient suffering from massive exsanguination. Most of the country's blood supply is collected, quality-assured, and distributed by regional blood centers. Whether linked into the American Red Cross Blood Services (ARC) consortium or operating semi-independently under the American Association of Blood Banks (AABB) banner, these regional centers plan their activities on the basis of predictions and projections of previous years' utilization, and realistically emergency utilization is but a small fraction of most blood centers' work. Therefore, little whole blood is maintained in stock and most of what is available is anticipated for use in neonatal exchange transfusions.

The routine use of whole blood is inappropriate because in the majority of instances the blood is no longer "whole" at the time of administration. Within 24 h of initiating storage in citrate-phosphate-dextrose (CPD) or citrate-phosphate-dextrose-adenine (CDPA-1) solutions, blood stored at 4°C has no functioning granulocytes, and only 50 percent of the functional activity of platelets and coagulation factor VIII remains. Both platelet function and factor VIII levels reach negligible levels by 72 h. Since transportation and processing delays usually result in blood availability no sooner than 48 h after collection, unless special systems are implemented, fresh whole blood is rarely administered when whole blood is ordered.

Continued refrigerated storage of whole blood causes 50 percent reductions in factor V at 3 to 5 days and increased affinity of hemoglobin for oxygen at 4 to 6 days, with decreasing red blood cell (RBC) viability and deformability beginning at about the same time. At approximately the fifth day of refrigerated storage, hydrogen ion, ammonia, and potassium concentrations begin to rise and microaggregates of platelets, fibrin, and leukocytes collect rapidly. Viability of at least 70 percent of the administered RBCs at 24 h is the standard by which all storage of blood products is judged; CPD permits 21-day storage and CPDA-1 permits 35-day storage with the capability of meeting this standard. Decreased deformability limits the ability of red cells to travel through capillaries in tissues, while increased oxygen affinity by hemoglobin reduces tissue oxygenation. Fortunately these effects are reversed 24 to 48 h after the red cells are returned to their more ''natural'' environment of the vascular tree. Limited concentrations of labile clotting factors, excessive accumulations of metabolic by-products, volume overload, maximal risk of disease spread and exposure to immunizing stimuli, and lastly, overutilization of blood components not specifically indicated are all detriments to the use of whole blood. Usually, red cell concentrates and crystalloid infusions suffice when volume and red cell mass repletion are necessary; in massive transfusion, however, *fresh* whole blood transfusion when available is appropriate and may be helpful. Autotransfusion may be a helpful adjunct in these circumstances as well.

Cellular Concentrates

Packed Red Blood Cells (PRBCs)

Ideally PRBCs are transfused when red cell mass repletion is the primary aim. As with whole blood, typing and crossmatching are a necessity. They are prepared in closed systems to a hematocrit no greater than 80 and thus have a full 21- or 35-day refrigerated shelf life, depending on the storage medium. PRBCs and crystalloid solutions are ideal volume and red cell repletion fluids in the overwhelming majority of emergency transfusions. Objections based on rate of flow are easily overcome by dilution with warmed normal saline solution at time of infusion through Y set tubing providing that large-bore infusion catheters are being used. Warming the blood has the additional benefit of reducing the necessity for the patient to perform extra metabolic work, which would consume additional oxygen at a time when metabolic systems are maximally challenged.

Other objections lodged against the use of PRBCs include concerns about the volume of transfusion and provision of noncellular coagulation factors. PRBCs are *not* suited for volume repletion; rapid and continuing crystalloid solution infusions should be utilized for this purpose. The necessity for the additional provision of coagulation factors is vastly overstated. Of course, the reduced volume of plasma in each unit of PRBCs (approximately 10 percent of the original donor plasma remains in each unit) does not provide adequate levels of these factors, but except in instances of exchange transfusion or massive exsanguination with resulting ''resuscitation'' exchange transfusion, hepatic stores of the proteins involved in the coagulation cascades rapidly replenish intravascular stores.

The advantages to the use of PRBCs include the decreased burden of citrate, ammonia, and organic acids infused; the reduced risk of alloimmunization, since fewer antigens are infused; and the reduced risk of volume overload when multiple units are infused. Of course, the more appropriate use of other components harvested from the same donor unit most efficiently utilizes this scarce resource.

Washed Red Blood Cells

Washing of red cells stored in refrigerated liquid form or in frozen form is an expensive but growing practice. These products, most often utilized for patients with known allergic reactions to platelet, granulocyte, or plasma antigens, provide a pure PRBC unit with a 24-h shelf life; therefore they are only prepared on demand and infrequently used in the emergency service.

Platelets

Platelet ''packs,'' typically administered in multiples of 8 to 10 for bleeding resulting from thrombocytopenia or inadequate platelet function, are rarely necessary in the emergency service. ABO matching is not necessary although HLA matching may be performed in a few special circumstances. It is doubtful if it is ever done for emergency unit platelet transfusions. Surgery or injury may, in the face of symptomatic thrombocytopenia (range 40,000 to 100,000 platelets per cubic millimeter, assuming normal platelet function), result in bleeding correctable by platelet administration. However, spontaneous bleeding is uncommon at counts above 20,000 platelets per cubic millimeter although it is frequent and severe at platelet counts below 10,000 per cubic millimeter. Each platelet pack will typically increase platelet counts by 5,000 to 8,000 in a 70-kg patient. Platelets should be given rapidly, since their shelf life is brief (24 to 72 h based on method of preparation) and their effectiveness is diminished by refrigeration.

Noncellular Components

Fresh Frozen Plasma (FFP)

FFP, obtained by centrifugation from a single donor unit (pooled plasma is no longer available because of the heptatitis risk inherent in this product) and rapidly frozen, contains all noncellular coagulation factors in near normal levels. Units are thawed to order and ABO matched to the recipient prior to transfusion. Since hepatitis and other disease transmission risks are identical to those of whole blood and PRBCs, FFP should not be used for simple colloid volume replacement or expansion. In the emergency service it is most frequently administered as part of a ''resuscitation'' exchange transfusion in the treatment of the exsanguinating patient. One unit of FFP is customarily administered for every five to six units of whole blood or PRBCs given.

For the patient with an undiagnosed bleeding diathesis, FFP is the only source of all noncellular coagulation factors. At the risk of volume overload, FFP given in adequate volume will correct any deficiency and give normal coagulation mechanisms a chance to operate to the patient's benefit. However when a specific diagnosis is available, provision of the appropriate factor through the administration of lyophilized concentrates or cryoprecipitate is most appropriate.

Cryoprecipitate and Commercial Factor VIII Products

Classical hemophilia accounts for approximately 85 percent of patients with congenital abnormalities of coagulation factors. The majority of patients presenting to the emergency unit with this bleeding diathesis are aware of their diagnosis and usual therapeutic requirements. Cost differences between the commercial products and cryoprecipitate vary around the country but are of inconsequential concern in most areas. The use of paid pheresis donors and pooled plasma increases the risk of hepatitis transmission with the commercial products.

Dosage calculations may be facilitated by asking the patient, reading the package insert for the commercial products, or consulting the blood bank technician for assistance. The typical errors made by treating physicians do *not* relate to the estimate of dose but rather to the failure to start administration early and continue it long enough.

Fibrinogen is also present in large quantities in cryoprecipitate but not in the commercial products. The rare individual with congenital hypofibrinogenemia may be treated with cryoprecipitate.

Other Plasma Coagulation Factors

Factor IX deficiency (Christmas disease, hemophilia B) is a far less common congenital coagulopathy. Commerical products to treat episodes contain all the vitamin K–dependent coagulation factors, including factors II, VII, IX, and X. These products, prepared from pooled plasma collected from paid donors, involve a high risk of hepatitis transmission.

Albumin and Plasma Protein Fraction (PPF)

Colloid administration for maintenance or restoration of oncotic pressure has a hallowed history and a cloudy future. Since the colloid versus crystalloid resuscitation controversy rages on unsolved, the value of all these preparations remains unclear to this author. Both these products are chemically treated to eliminate the risk of hepatitis transmission. Albumin is available as a 25% "salt-poor" preparation (which in reality contains 160 mEq/L of sodium) hyperoncotic to plasma and as a 5% buffered solution isooncotic to plasma. The typical 25-mL ampoule (12.5 g) has an oncotic effect approximately equal to one unit of FFP.

PPF is a somewhat less expensive product containing 88% albumin, less than 1% globulins, and the remainder α and β globulins. It is isoosmotic with plasma containing 130 to 160 mEq/L of sodium. Its major risk is the presence of high levels of prekallikrein activator, which results in hypotension during rapid infusion in susceptible individuals.

Immune Globulins

The origin of immune globulins, best known as tetanus immune globulin, as blood products is often overlooked. Tetanus (Hypertet), hepatitis b (H-BIG), rabies (Hyperab) and a multiplicity of other hyperimmune globulins are prepared by hyperimmunizing donors who undergo plasmapheresis. Immune serum globulin produced at the same time as albumin or PPF is often used in an attempt to modify or prevent viral illnesses (rubella, poliomyelitis, rubeola) or treat hypogammaglobulinemia and agammaglobulinemia.

BLOOD TRANSFUSION PRACTICES

Transfusion of blood components in the emergency service commonly occurs at times of relative urgency. Such circumstances lead to incomplete communication, which can cause frustration for the clinician and anxiety for the blood bank personnel. *Absolute* identification of specimen and patient is an essential component of transfusion practice, and when "standard" inpatient systems are applied in the emergency service, time-consuming documentation may become a painful ordeal to the staff. However, specific and unique alternatives are often acceptable to the blood bank when such alternatives have been developed and approved in *advance* of need. The use of a uniquely coded bracelet with tear-off tabs for labeling specimen tubes and blood units is a quick and simple approach, readily acceptable to the majority of blood bank directors, which obviates the need for further identification beyond the usual identification of both phlebotomist and transfusionist.

Cross-Match Ordering

The emergency physician does not need to overorder the typing and cross matching of blood for transfusions on the premise that the patient has an unclear need. Determining the patient's type and the presence or absence of atypical antibodies ("type and screen" or "type and hold") is an adequate substitute for patients who fail to meet any of the following criteria:

1. Shock
2. Greater than 500 mL blood loss observed in the emergency unit
3. Grossly obvious gastrointestinal bleeding
4. Hemoglobin less than 10 mg/dL or hematocrit less than 30
5. Probability of a blood-losing operation (e.g., laparotomy for trauma, not appendectomy)

While these criteria aid in determining which patients might require cross matching for compatible donor units, they do not offer any guidelines for selection of the appropriate number to obtain for the given patient. This judgment must be made on clinical grounds while keeping in mind the likelihood of ongoing and future losses.

Cross-Matching Process

The properly labeled "clot tube" is centrifuged on arrival in the laboratory. Slide-typing techniques using modern potent reagents can be completed in 60 s. The immediate spin phase of the cross match can be completed in another 3 to 5 min. Within 5 min of arrival, incompletely cross-matched blood can be available in the majority of instances. These techniques are not necessarily those routinely employed for more leisurely or elective cross matches but are considered reliable, and when prearranged protocols are agreed to by both emergency service and blood bank, they are helpful in shortening the interval until blood for transfusion is available.

Full cross matching requires antibody screening in albumin and Coombs serum, both of which require time-consuming incubations at 37°C. These techniques, requiring an additional 30 min, can be completed after blood is released for transfusion in cases of extreme urgency. In all cases these steps will be completed so that the clinician can be apprised of any incompatibility potentially resulting in a delayed transfusion reaction.

Blood Administration Hardware

Patients who receive blood in the emergency service are likely to have multiple units transfused. The use of micropore filters and blood warming systems as well as pressure infusion pumps and special tubing can contribute positively to outcome.

Commonly, blood is "piggybacked" into running IV lines through the needle. Ideally, the use of IV extension tubing permits changing the running IV fluid to the blood without the decrease in flow rate caused by the needle. Alternatively, and perhaps optimally when PRBCs will be used, Y-type administration sets that have one inlet for the blood and another for the IV solution are useful. Warmed saline or Ringer's lactate solution can be run through the one arm of the Y, and when the blood becomes available, it may be warmed and diluted so as to flow faster. Only isoosmotic fluids not containing calcium or glucose should be used for this purpose.

Many vendors supply micropore ("millipore") filters for use in blood administration. Available in 20- to 40-μm pore sizes, they should be used for all homologous blood administered in the emergency service. They will contribute to slowing the rate of transfusion, and if unacceptable slowing occurs, pressure-infusion cuffs or three-way stopcocks with syringe pressure infusion may be utilized.

Warming baths and plates are becoming increasingly available at affordable cost. The energy and oxygen demand placed on a patient to warm a blood volume from 4 to 37°C is significant, and potentially life-threatening hypothermia occurs. All too often the patient is stripped naked during resuscitation, massively transfused, and subsequently subjected to a surgical procedure in the typical air-conditioned operating room. Warming of the blood and other fluids administered tends to be overlooked. Microwave warming systems, which were eagerly embraced in the past decade, have been shown to be unreliable and to contribute to the hemolysis of red cells. These should not be used.

SPECIAL SITUATIONS

Emergency Release

Typing and cross matching of blood for transfusion is one of the few laboratory studies for which no clinical correlates exist. For this reason the decision to abrogate full laboratory studies prior to initiating transfusion is fraught with risks, both in the acute situation and in ensuing days. Laboratory personnel, both physicians and technicians, are unable to accurately weigh the relative risks of delay of transfusion versus potentially fatal transfusion

reaction; therefore they tend to resist emergency release of both type-specific but incompletely cross-matched blood and type O blood. Only the emergency physician with the full clinical picture available can and should make the decision to proceed. Yet despite this caveat, the transfusion of type-specific but incompletely cross-matched blood or, rarely, type O (universal donor) blood may be lifesaving. Unfortunately, excessive anxiety about the appropriate indications may occasionally inhibit early emergency transfusion, resulting in an unfavorable outcome for the patient.

As with all crisis situations in medicine, clinical judgment remains the powerful arbiter by which decisions must be made. While indications overlap, when possible the additional 5 min necessary to secure type-specific rather than universal donor blood for emergency transfusion is generally preferred. However, when properly documented, the clinical decision to use incompletely cross-matched or universal donor blood is virtually always justifiable in the following circumstances:

1. Exsanguinating hemorrhage with no or insufficient initial response to the rapid infusion of crystalloid volume expanders
2. Profound shock resulting from exsanguination in previously compromised patients
3. Hemorrhagic shock in infants and small children (their smaller blood volume does not permit the luxury of delay in the repletion of red cell mass)
4. Any situation in which the typical delay of 20 to 30 min for cross-matched blood would further imperil the patient's eventual outcome

The use of O universal donor blood is still less widely sanctioned. Experience in wartime demonstrates the safety of its use in a young male population. Nearly $\frac{1}{4}$ million units were transfused in a 20-month period during the Vietnam conflict. Only 1 of the 24 hemolytic transfusion reactions resulting was a result of something other than misidentification. Smaller-scale civilian population studies have shown a small but anticipated increased risk in previously transfused individuals and in parous women.

All the military studies have used Rh-positive blood since only males were transfused and large quantities of Rh-negative blood are unavailable. The civilian studies and most civilian practice call for the use of Rh-negative blood since demand is far more episodic and local stores can be replenished more easily. In any case, whether one used Rh-positive type O in males, Rh-negative for females, or Rh-negative for all patients requiring critically urgent transfusions, only PRBCs should be transfused so as to limit the volume of antibody-containing plasma transfused. Unless more than 4 units of universal donor blood have already been transfused, reversion to the patient's hereditary (laboratory-determined) blood type is appropriate and usually decreases the strain on limited supplies of Rh-negative blood.

Autotransfusion

As practiced in the emergency unit, autotransfusion usually refers to the collection of blood from a traumatic hemothorax and its subsequent reinfusion into the same patient. Rarely, collection of intraperitoneal blood accumulating as the result of a presumed ruptured ectopic pregnancy may be reinfused prior to surgery.

Collection of hemothorax blood is facilitated by inexpensive, commercially available systems which provide simple filter-type processing of the collected blood. More elaborate (and expensive) systems which provide for cell washing are not necessary or appropriate in the emergency unit. Blood that drains through a chest tube placed by the usual technique is filtered through screen-type filters to remove gross clot and debris. CPD solution may be added, either by premeasurement or simultaneously with the collection of the blood, to inhibit coagulation in the system. When necessary the sterilely collected anticoagulated blood may be reinfused through a micropore filter.

Autotransfusion has the advantage of providing a rapidly available, warm, type-specific source of blood for the patient in urgent need. Its use is complementary to and not a substitute for homologous transfusion. Blood collected from the chest has functioning white cells and near normal levels of all noncellular coagulation factors with the exception of fibrinogen. Unfortunately, platelets are apparently altered in the process and those few which pass through the micropore filter do not function normally.

Complications directly attributable to autotransfusion are rare and mostly dose-related. Reinfusion of less than 4000 mL of autotransfused blood is rarely associated with any clinical manifestations of complications. Hemoglobinemia and hemoglobinuria are invariably present (to varying degrees) after autotransfusions. In most reported clinical series they have not been associated with renal failure. Disseminated intravascular coagulation (DIC) has been reported to occur in patients who had multiple other predisposing factors. Dilutional coagulopathy as a result of insufficient replacement of noncellular coagulation factors should theoretically be less common in patients receiving their own hemothorax blood.

Massive Transfusion

For clinical purposes *massive transfusion* can be defined as a transfusion of one-half of the patient's blood volume at one time or transfusion of one blood volume in a 24-h period. The first definition most commonly describes the emergency unit circumstances. Anticipation of the likelihood of massive transfusion allows for application of strategies designed to minimize if not eliminate its complications.

Hemostasis

Of most concern is the occurence of altered hemostasis. This condition, resulting both from dilution of humoral coagulation and from DIC subsequent to shock and tissue destruction, contributes to the hemorrhage for which the blood is being transfused. Since many clinicians are aware that the blood being transfused is to some extent contributing to the hemostatic defect (by dilution of humoral factors), they assume that the blood transfusion itself is the cause of the increased hemorrhage. By implication, the assumption that less blood is better if transfusion increases bleeding is an obvious and *wrong* conclusion. In reality the deficit of factors VIII and V present in all refrigerated blood is easily compensated for by use of FFP. Dilution of other factors as well occurs if only PRBCs and crystalloid are infused in large volume. The use of one unit of FFP for every five to six units of PRBCs or whole blood infused is good prophylaxis. Ordering one unit of FFP for every six to eight units of PRBCs crossmatched is an appropriate plan.

Dilutional thrombocytopenia is an often worrisome but rarely seen complication in exchanges of less than two blood volumes. At the time of ordering the second round of cross matches, 8 to 10 platelet packs may be appropriately ordered if continued transfusion is anticipated.

Hypothermia and Microaggregtes

Cold blood contributes to hypothermia, which increases the metabolic workload and depresses cardiac function. Patients in whom massive transfusion is anticipated must have blood warmed prior to infusion. Only systems that warm blood as it is infused are satisfactory from the viewpoint of both adequate warming and safety. These systems have been described in the section on "Blood Administration Hardware."

Similarly, microaggregates contained in all refrigerated blood have been implicated in the genesis of the adult respiratory distress syndrome. A dose-related effect has been postulated, and while other factors clearly contribute if they do not predominate, micropore filtration does relieve the lung of the burden of removing these microaggregates from the circulation.

Calcium and Citrate Toxicity

Citrate toxicity probably occurs in rare clinical situations. Citrated blood infusion to patients at rates greater than one mL/(kg·min) may be associated with the symptoms of perioral tingling and, rarely, carpal-pedal spasm in awake and alert patients. Potentially most at risk are infants and those with hepatic dysfunction either preexisting or secondary to continued shock or liver injury.

Citrate exerts its deleterious effect by chelating ionized calcium. Since citrate is always in excess in transfused blood, reduction of ionized calcium is likely until the citrate is metabolized. Of greatest concern is consequent depression of myocardial function; however, in the absence of shock myocardial depression has not been demonstrated at levels of ionized calcium one-third of normal. Total calcium levels may be elevated and are unreliable predictors of the need for calcium supplementation.

Calcium supplementation should not be routinely provided to massively transfused patients but rather to the individual who seems not to be responding to adequate replacement or is suffering from acute heart failure (while keeping in mind that the most common cause of these circumstances is hypovolemia). Electrocardiographic monitoring of the Q-T interval has been shown not to be useful in determining need for calcium. When used, calcium salts should be given by the intravenous route at a site distant from the blood transfusion, cautiously and in small doses. "Routine" calcium administration has been lethal in the past.

Summary

Collins has pointed out, "An intact circulation is a very good defense against the metabolic derangements of massive transfusion." The emergency physician can best preserve an intact circulation by anticipation of need and rapid, complete volume resuscitation.

CAVEATS AND COMPLICATIONS

Immediate Reactions

Febrile Reactions

Febrile reactions, which are probably the most common type of transfusion reaction, are characterized by the development of fever, chills, and malaise. They rarely progress to the development of hypotension or respiratory distress. Febrile reactions are thought to be the result of the infusion of platelets and leukocytes to which the recipient has antibodies. This thesis is somewhat complicated by the inevitability of protein denaturation that occurs in these cells during storage. In any case, the use of leukocyte-poor blood or washed PRBCs for patients known to have this type of reaction will prevent its occurrence.

Once a febrile reaction is recognized, the current transfusion should be terminated, since it is impossible to differentiate on clinical grounds between a simple febrile reaction and the more serious immediate intravascular hemolytic transfusion reaction. Anesthetized patients, infants incapable of shivering, and unconscious patients will not demonstrate and obviously will not report the symptoms of a febrile reaction. A search for red cell destruction (described below) should immediately ensue.

Allergic Reactions

True anaphylactic reactions to blood transfusion are comparatively rare, occurring approximately once in 20,000 transfusions. The genetically deficient IgA recipient is most at risk. Individuals with a history of multiple allergies should be carefully observed during transfusion. Individuals with a history of previous allergic reaction to transfusion who must be transfused should be premedicated with antihistamines administered intramuscularly or intravenously but not in the blood itself. Ideally, these individuals should be given washed PRBCs or blood from IgA-deficient donors.

The treatment of immediate hypersensitivity reaction to blood is the same as the treatment of any anaphylactic reaction: intravenous epinephrine in aliquots of 2 to 3 mL at a 1:10,000 concentration until symptoms are relieved and blood pressure maintained. Intravenous corticosteroids and antihistamines are useful but do not supplant the need for intravenous epinephrine. Obviously, the transfusion should be terminated.

Hemolytic Reactions

Intravascular hemolysis, the most serious immediate reaction, is, fortunately, a rare occurrence, which most often is the result of misidentification of patient, specimen, or blood unit. This antigen-antibody-mediated reaction results in the rapid destruction of transfused red cells by lysis occurring in minutes. The resulting release of free hemoglobin produces hemoglobinemia, hemoglobinuria, depletion of haptoglobin, and subsequent bilirubin elevation. Clinical manifestations include fever, chills, low back pain and other myalgias, and a burning sensation at the site of infusion and along the vein centrally. Later manifestations include a feeling of breathlessness or chest tightness, hypotension, and bleeding. Anesthetized and unconscious patients may manifest only hypotension, bleeding, and hemoglobinuria. The damaged red cells—

ghost cells—activate complement, which precipitates DIC and leads to renal and/or respiratory failure.

Laboratory evaluation includes determination of haptoglobin and free hemoglobin in blood serum and hemoglobin in urine, evaluation of the antigen-antibody reaction in the blood (Coombs test, both direct and indirect), and coagulation and renal function profiles. A quick, simple screen can be performed by saving a complete blood count tube and centrifuging it. A pale pink color suggests a free hemoglobin level of 50 to 100 mg/dL. A pale brown color may be evident at levels as low as 20 mg/dL. This "naked eye" screen does not supplant the need for full laboratory evaluation.

Treatment begins with discontinuing the current transfusion and instituting crystalloid infusion. Furosemide in 80 to 100 mg doses intravenously increases renal cortical blood flow and thus helps protect renal function. Mannitol, which increases urine flow by decreasing tubular absorption, does not have this salutory effect on renal blood flow and therefore should *not* be used. Large amounts of fluids must be administered to maintain intravascular volume. Careful monitoring of urinary output, maintaining a 0.5 to 1.0 mL/(kg·h) flow is essential. Following central venous pressures or pulmonary capillary wedge pressures will assure that volume depletion is not mistaken for renal failure subsequent to the hemolytic transfusion reaction.

Delayed Reactions

Extravascular Hemolysis

Unexplained decreases in hemoglobin levels days after transfusion are too infrequently recognized as a prime clinical manifestation of delayed extravascular hemolytic transfusion reactions. Coating by nonagglutinating antibodies of transfused red cells causes the removal of these red cells by tissue-bound macrophages, primarily in the spleen. Fever and chills do occur but may not be ascribed to the reaction. Confusion may occur because blood being administered at the time of the onset of symptoms rarely has anything to do with the reaction. Rather, a search through previously administered units must be processed in the laboratory.

Treatment includes fluid administration and redetermination of the compatibility for transfusion of all blood units destined for transfusion to the patient. Blood specimens for the determination of hemoglobin, bilirubin, and haptoglobin help to differentiate between extravascular and intravascular hemolysis. Repeat searches for atypical antibodies may now reveal the presence of a previously undetected antibody as a result of the anamnestic immunological response.

Infections

Viral hepatitis continues as the most common and severe infectious sequela to blood transfusion, occurring at a rate of 30,000 cases per year and resulting in 1500 to 3000 deaths annually. The non-A, non-B hepatitis virus is not dectectable by current screening methods and no specific proven therapy exists. Prophylactic administration of immune serum globulin may reduce the risk to patients destined to receive multiple unit transfusions, but extensive washing of red blood cells has not been shown to be efficacious.

Cytomegalovirus, Epstein-Barr virus, and a possible transmissible agent associated with AIDS are rarely transmitted by transfusion. Syphilis may be transmitted by fresh, untested blood units, but this is rare since all banked blood is tested for its presence and *Treponema pallidum* will not survive in citrated blood for more than 2 or 3 days. Malaria is rarely transmitted since strict rules preclude the collection of blood from donors who have traveled in endemic areas within 6 months prior to the intended donation or who have ever contracted the disease.

SUMMARY

Blood transfusion as practiced by the emergency physician requires first that the patient's true need for transfusion be determined and that this be followed by the selection of the appropriate component for transfusion, whether cellular, noncellular, or both. A knowledge of the cross-match process is useful to aid in decision making in those cases of extreme urgency in which the full process must of necessity be abrogated.

Proper technique for transfusion in the emergency service more typically follows the pattern of the operating room than the ward, with the use of micropore filtration, warming systems, and pressure infusors. The special procedures of massive transfusion, emergency release, and autotransfusion are more useful for emergency patients than most others. Complications of blood transfusion, the most common tissue transplant, are both immunologic and nonimmunologic. Differentiation and appropriate therapy of an already compromised patient are usually urgent. All these aspects of blood transfusion, while of less common concern to the emergency physician, must of necessity be part of that physician's knowledge base.

BIBLIOGRAPHY

Arens JF, Leonard GL: Danger of overwarming blood by microwave. *JAMA* 218:1045, 1971.

Barnes A: Status of the use of universal donor blood transfusion. *CRC Crit Rev Clin Lab Sci* 4:147, 1973.

Barnes A: Transfusion of universal donor and uncrossmatched blood: surgical hemotherapy. *Bibl Haematol* 46:132, 1980.

Clarke JR, Davidson SJ, Bergman GE, et al: Blood ordering for emergency department patients. *Ann Emerg Med* 9:2, 1980.

Collins JA: Problems associated with the massive transfusion of stored blood: Clinical review. *Surgery* 75:274, 1974.

Collins JA: Pulmonary dysfunction and massive transfusion. *Bibl Haematol* 46:220, 1980.

Davidson SJ: Emergency unit autotransfusion. *Surgery* 84:703, 1978.

Pineda AA, Brizica SM, Taswell HF: Hemolytic transfusion reaction: Recent experience in a large blood bank. *Mayo Clin Proc* 53:378, 1978.

Sinclair A, Jacobs LM: Emergency department autotransfusion. *Med Instr* 16:283, 1982.

Sohmer PR, Dawson RB: Transfusion therapy in trauma: A review of the principles and techniques used in the M.I.E.M.S program. *Am Surg* 45:109, 1979.

Walker AKY: Blood microfiltration: a review. *Anesthesia* 33:35, 1978.

Young GP, Purcell TB: Emergency autotransfusion. *Ann Emerg Med* 12:180, 1983.

CHAPTER 101
EMERGENCY
COMPLICATIONS
OF MALIGNANCY

Daniel Esposito

The increasing prevalence of malignant disease and the escalating frequency of complications resulting from local tumor effects, as well as from the adverse effects of medical treatments, demand that the emergency physician be educated to recognize potential life-threatening situations and initiate appropriate therapy. It is unlikely that complete evaluation and definition of malignant syndromes will be achieved in the emergency department. Therefore most of the clinical problems discussed in this chapter are in themselves sufficient grounds for immediate hospitalization.

The widespread use of a combination of chemotherapy and radiotherapy in both inpatient and outpatient arenas underlies the likelihood of emergency department exposure to the hemorrhagic and infectious complications of myelosuppression. It is apparent that many tumors produce similar syndromes by virtue of local compressive effects (spinal cord compression, upper airway obstruction, etc.). Other situations will be unique to certain tumors (e.g., the hyperviscosity syndrome of multiple myeloma-macroglobulinemia). The various situations that are considered imminently life-threatening are outlined in Table 101-1 with the intention of correlating pathogenic mechanisms with acute local or systemic compromise. A listing of the more frequent associated malignancies will be presented with each subtopic.

ACUTE SPINAL CORD COMPRESSION

Multiple myeloma
Non-Hodgkins and Hodgkins Lymphomas
Carcinoma of lung
Carcinoma of prostate
Carcinoma of breast

Ischemic dysfunction of the spinal cord due to extrinsic compression occurs most commonly with multiple myeloma and lymphoma. It is an uncommon presenting feature and is generally suspected in individuals with previously documented malignancy who develop paraparesis, paraplegia, sensory deficits, or urinary incontinence. Pain localized to involved vertebrae may be present and intensified by local percussion during the physical examina-

tion. However, as is often the case in lymphomas, if lytic bony lesions are not present, local pain is absent and the patient may have only a sensory-level or distal flaccid pralysis. Hypoesthesia and lower extremity weakness are early symptoms and should alert the emergency physician. Early treatment may avert progression to paraplegia.

The emergency physician's role includes not only suspicion and recognition of cord compression but also institution of measures to prepare the patient for potential emergency surgery. This would include assessment of fluid status, clotting parameters, anemia, and cardiorespiratory systems. CT scanning of the thoracolumbar spine may demonstrate the level of compression. Myelography is otherwise definitive. Emergency surgical decompression or emergency radiotherapy is necessary to prevent irreversible neural damage.

UPPER AIRWAY OBSTRUCTION

Carcinoma of larynx
Thyroid carcinoma
Lymphoma
Metastatic lung carcinoma

Acute upper airway obstruction is generally associated with aspiration of foreign bodies or food elements, with epiglottitis, or with other oropharyngeal infections. Malignancy-related obstruction to airflow is more insidious and often attended by voice change. This is generally a late manifestation of tumors arising in the oropharynx, neck, and superior mediastinum. Acute compromise is uncommon unless infection, hemorrhage, or inspissated secretions supervene. Rapidly growing tumors such as Burkitt's lymphoma and anaplastic carcinoma of the thyroid are capable of compromising airflow within weeks and should be suspected in afebrile individuals with laryngeal stridor and palpable anterior neck masses.

Fiberoptic or direct laryngoscopy is usually necessary to evaluate lumen size, as local anatomy is generally greatly distorted. Lateral soft-tissue x-rays are of great value in assessing laryngo-

Table 101-1. Emergency Complications of Malignancy

RELATED TO LOCAL TUMOR COMPRESSION

1. Acute spinal cord compression
2. Upper Airway obstruction
3. Malignant pericardial effusion with tamponade
4. Superior vena cava syndrome

RELATED TO BIOCHEMICAL DERANGEMENT AND SYSTEMIC COLLAPSE

1. Hypercalcemia of malignancy
2. Syndrome of inappropriate ADH (SIADH)
3. Hyperviscocity syndrome
4. Adrenocortical insufficiency with shock

RELATED TO MYELOSUPPRESSION AND INFECTION

1. Granulocytopenia and sepsis
2. Immunosuppression and opportunistic infections
3. Thrombocytopenia and hemorrage
4. Anaphylaxis and transfusion reactions

tracheal patency. Establishment of an effective airway is primary and surgical tracheostomy may be required prior to the initiation of radiotherapy.

MALIGNANT PERICARDIAL EFFUSION WITH TAMPONADE

Malignant melanoma
Hodgkins lymphoma
Acute leukemia
Carcinoma of lung
Carcinoma of breast
Carcinoma of ovary
Radiation pericarditis

Malignant involvement of the pericardium may give rise to chronic cardiac tamponade by inducing the formation of hemorrhagic malignant effusions. The hemodynamic consequences of such effusions are a function of the volume as well as the rapidity of accumulation. Large collections (greater than 500 mL) may be well tolerated if development is slow. If sudden intrapericardial bleeding occurs, the emergency physician may be confronted with acutely ill individuals with hypotension and dyspnea. Malignant involvement of the myocardium may also be present and contribute to reduced cardiac output. Significant fluid accumulations can occur from radiotherapy-induced pleuropericarditis, most commonly in patients treated with mediastinal irradiation for Hodgkins lymphoma.

The classical clinical features of cardiac tamponade include: (1) hypotension with narrow pulse pressure; (2) jugular venous distension; (3) diminished amplitude of heart sounds (quiet heart); (4) pulsus paradoxicus of greater than 10 mmHg; (5) low QRS voltage on EEG; and (6) cardiomegaly on chest radiograph with obscuration of the cardiophrenic angles. Neck vein distention and hypotension in acutely ill patients can also occur with massive pulmonary embolism or acute superior vena caval obstruction and should be considered in the differential diagnosis.

Confirmation of the diagnosis is most readily obtained by M-mode echocardiography, which can be performed in the emergency department. Emergency percutaneous pericardiocentesis may

be necessary and life-saving if profound vascular collapse is present. This may provide time for more definitive treatment, such as pericardectomy, pericardial window surgery, radiotherapy, or intrapericardial chemotherapy. The risks of aggressive mangement must be weighed against the benefits of such treatment modalities in patients otherwise terminally ill from widespread metastases.

SUPERIOR VENA CAVA SYNDROME

Small-cell (oat-cell) carcinoma of lung
Squamous cell carcinoma of lung
Lymphoma

The superior vena cava syndrome is frequently a de novo diagnosis first established in the emergency department. A history of previously documented malignancy is often lacking and patients may seek medical attention because of the insidious and progressive nature of their symptoms. Obstruction to blood flow in the superior vena cava elevates venous pressure in the arms, neck, face, and cerebrum. Patients with moderate obstruction complain of headache, edema of the face and arms, or a nondescript feeling of head congestion and fullness in the neck and face. As venous pressure rises, intracranial pressure also rises and frank syncope may ensue. Critical intracranial pressure elevations are a true medical emergency and are usually associated with bilateral papilledema.

On physical examination, neck vein and upper chest vein distention may be apparent. Facial plethora and telangiectasia often are prominent, but edema of the face and arms is generally subtle. Papilledema on fundoscopic examination indicates critical intracranial pressure and justifies early diuretic therapy. When tumefaction is located in the superior mediastinum, a palpable mass due to direct tumor extension can occasionally be appreciated in the supraclavicular space. Chest x-ray will demonstrate an enlarged mediastinum and possibly an isolated primary lesion in the lung parenchyma.

Prompt administration of diuretics and corticosteroids may help reduce venous pressure prior to initiation of mediastinal irradiation. In advanced disease radiotherapy to improve cardiodynamics is frequently necessary before tissue diagnosis can be obtained.

HYPERCALCEMIA OF MALIGNANCY

Multiple myeloma
Bony metastases from carcinoma of breast, prostate, or lung
Humoral-induced non-Hodgkins lymphoma and adult T-cell lymphoma-leukemia

Mild elevations of serum calcium are well tolerated and produce little in the way of symptoms. However, when serum calcium levels rise rapidly or exceed ionic thresholds, cardiac, neural, and muscular electrophysiology may be greatly altered and sudden death can occur. A number of mechanisms have been identified that promote release of bony calcium into the circulation. Bony involvement with myeloma or carcinoma of the breast, prostate, or lung will release calcium by local matrix destruction. Squamous cell carcinoma of the lung may produce a parathormone-like substance, and an osteoclast activating factor has been associated with non-Hodgkins lymphoma (diffuse histiocytic) and retrovirus adult T-cell lymphoma-leukemia.

Approximately 40 percent of patients with multiple myeloma will have hypercalcemia. An often encountered clinical triad includes back pain, constipation, and an insidious depression in the level of consciousness. Hypercalcemia from any cause may induce hypertension, constipation, and an altered sensorium. Elevated ionic (nonbound) calcium is responsible for neuromuscular dysfunction and therefore, serum calcium levels should be interpreted in concert with phosphorus, serum albumin, and blood pH determinations. The Q-T interval of the electrocardiogram will shorten as the serum calcium rises.

The majority of patients with malignancy-induced hypercalcemia will improve with saline infusion and intravenous furosemide (1 to 2 L saline load and 80 mg of IV furosemide). This will promote renal calcium excretion but depends upon adequate renal function and glomerular filtration. Because renal insufficiency is a common accompaniment in myeloma, assessment of blood urea nitrogen and creatinine levels is important to ensure both adequacy of response and avoidance of iatrogenic fluid overload. Hemoconcentration and dehydration may additionally aggravate elevating calcium. Short-term use of glucocorticoids may be life-saving in neoplastic hypercalcemia and should be used empirically in comatose or obtunded patients with serum calciums greater than 13. Mithramycin has been extremely effective in lowering serum calcium by reducing bone resorption. Doses of 15 to 25 mg/kg intravenously may rapidly reduce critical hypercalcemia.

SYNDROME OF INAPPROPRIATE ADH

> Malignancy of the brain, lung, pancreas, duodenum, thymus, prostate
> Lymphosarcoma

Ectopic secretion of antidiuretic hormone (ADH) may come from a variety of malignancies, but in any case the end result is the syndrome of inappropriate ADH (SIADH), which consists of serum hyponatremia, less than maximally dilute urine, excessive urine Na excretion (>30 mEq/L), and normal renal, adrenal, and thyroid functions. Treatment is aimed at removing the source of ADH secretion. Water restriction usually raises serum Na in the meantime, although hypertonic (3 percent) saline may be necessary in the face of seizures of arrhythmias.

HYPERVISCOSITY SYNDROME

> Multiple myeloma
> Waldenstrom's macroglobulinemia
> Chronic myelocytic leukemia

Viscosity is the flow-resisting characteristic of fluids. Marked elevations in certain serum proteins will produce sludging and a reduction in microcirculatory perfusion. IgA myeloma components and IgG subtype 3 proteins have a tendency to polymerize, leading to symptomatic hyperviscosity. Macroglobulinemia is the most common cause for hyperviscosity by virtue of the high molecular weight and high intrinsic viscosity of IgM proteins. Serum viscosity relative to water is normally 1.4 to 1.8 and symptoms develop at viscosities greater than 5 times that of water.

Fatigue, headache, anorexia, and somnolence are early nonspecific symptoms. As blood flow slows, microthromboses may occur, with the advent of local symptoms such as deafness, visual disturbances, and Jacksonian or generalized seizures. The diagnosis of hyperviscosity must be considered in the emergency department when patients with unexplained stupor or coma are found to have anemia, with rouleau formation on the peripheral blood smear. The most readily appreciated physical findings are in the ocular fundi and include "sausage-linked" retinal vessels, hemorrhages, and exudates. Laboratory evaluation should include coagulation, renal, and electrolyte profiles. Hypercalcemia can coincide, and when M-component protein concentrations are high, "factitious" hyponatremia due to the displacement phenomenon may also be present. A clue to the presence of hyperviscosity may be the laboratory's inability to perform chemical tests because of serum stasis in the analyzers, undoubtedly due to "too thick" blood. Serum viscosity and protein electrophoresis determinations are diagnostic.

The emergency physician's role is predominantly suspicion and recognition of the syndrome in patients with unexplained stupor and coma. Hyperviscosity is generally a presenting manifestation of certain plasma cell dyscrasias and a history of previously documented disease is often lacking. Initial therapy is rehydration followed by emergency plasmapheresis. When frank coma is present and the diagnosis rapidly established, a temporizing measure may be a two-unit phlebotomy with saline infusion and replacement of the patient's red cells.

The hyperviscosity syndrome associated with massive leukocytosis of chronic myelogenous leukemia is rheologically similar to the hyperviscosity syndrome of dysproteinemias. Altered mental status and vascular stasis occur because of white cell aggregation in the microcirculation. This is readily diagnosed from the complete blood count and white counts may be greater than several hundred thousand. The treatment consists of urgent leukopheresis and alkylating-agent chemotherapy.

ADRENAL INSUFFICIENCY AND SHOCK

> Carcinoma of the lung
> Carcinoma of the breast
> Malignant melanoma
> Retroperitoneal malignancies
> Withdrawal of chronic steroid therapy

Adrenal insufficiency may be related to adrenal gland replacement by metastatic tumors or to adrenocortical suppression by chronic therapeutic corticosteroid administration and its abrupt cessation. In either case, maximal adrenal function may be inadequate to support the individual when stressed by infection, dehydration, surgery, or trauma. Adrenal crisis and shock with vasomotor collapse may be sudden and fatal. The differential diagnosis of cancer patients with fever, dehydration, hypotension, and shock would more frequently include sepsis and hemorrhagic shock. Adrenal crisis is less common than bleeding and sepsis but empirically covered with intravenous corticosteroids.

Laboratory clues to the possible concomitant presence of adrenal insufficiency may be mild hypoglycemia, hyponatremia, hyperkalemia, and eosinophilia. Azotemia is, however, nonspecific and is often present in dehydration from any cause. In suspected cases, a serum cortisol should be drawn prior to steroid treatment.

Normal adrenal glands maximally produce approximately 300 mg/day of hydrocortisone when stressed. This has served as a guideline for replacement therapy. Adrenalectomized individuals are maintained on average doses of 35 to 40 mg of hydrocortisone per day and this is increased during potential stress. Appropriate emergency doses of hydrocortisone (Solucortef) would be 250 to 500 mg intravenously. Somewhat larger doses have been employed in septic shock.

GRANULOCYTOPENIA, IMMUNOSUPPRESSION, AND INFECTION

Overwhelming infection is a common cause of death in the immunocompromised host. A variety of factors may contribute to increased susceptibility to infection in cancer patients. Important factors include:

1. Malnutrition and cachexia
2. Granulocytopenia
3. Impaired humoral immunity and antibody production, as in chronic lymphocytic leukemia or multiple myeloma
4. Altered cellular immunity, as in Hodgkin's and other lymphomas
5. Postsplenectomy susceptibility to serious pneumococcal infections
6. Reactivation tuberculosis with concurrent corticosteroid therapy.
7. Polymicrobial enteric sepsis from bowel organism entry; carcinoma of colon or mucosal damage from chemotherapy.
8. Nosocomial infections transmitted through blood transfusion and blood products.
9. Immunosuppression and myelosuppression of chemotherapy

Both the frequency of infection and the mortality rate increase significantly when the circulating granulocyte pool is below 1000 to 1500 per cubic millimeter. Cancer patients are at risk for a variety of bacterial, viral, and fungal infections. Frequently encountered infections include pneumococcal sepsis and pneumonia; *Staphylococcus aureus* infection; enteric gram-negative pneumonia or sepsis, including *Pseudomonas* infections; and localized or disseminated varicella zoster viral and cytomegaloviral infections. Immunosuppression predisposes to invasion by organisms that are normally held at bay by host defenses and biocompetition from normal body flora. Such opportunistic infections include *Pneumocystis carinii* pneumonia (protozoal), disseminated candidiasis, aspergillosis, cryptococcal meningitis, pulmonary nocardiosis, and histoplasmosis.

Fever in the presence of malignancy is often difficult to define on clinical grounds alone. The emergency physician should assume an infectious etiology and initiate appropriate laboratory studies and cultures. Life-threatening gram-negative sepsis with hypotension should be aggressively treated after appropriate cultures. Fluids, antibiotics, and intravenous corticosteroids are advised. The choice of antibiotics has been a subject of debate and is indeed becoming a medical subspecialty in itself. However, few bacterial organisms would be missed with regimens containing a second- or third-generation cephalosporin (cefazolin, cefoxitin, cefotaxime) and an aminoglycoside (gentamicin, tobramycin, amikacin). Anaerobic coverage may be added (clindamycin) if peritonitis or abdominal symptomatology exists.

THROMBOCYTOPENIA AND HEMORRHAGE

Thrombocytopenia results from decreased bone marrow platelet production or increased peripheral destruction. Malignancy-associated thrombopenia is more commonly related to decreased production because of radiochemotherapeutic suppression (toxic myelophthisis), marrow replacement with tumor cells (malignant myelophthisis), or infectious suppression. Platelets may be rapidly destroyed in the peripheral blood when disseminated intravascular coagulation complicates malignancy. Autoimmune peripheral platelet destruction has commonly accompanied chronic lymphocytic leukemia and the lymphomas. Hypersplenism may also contribute to decreased platelet survival.

Spontaneous bleeding can occur when the platelet count is below 10,000 per cubic millimeter. The most frequent sites of hemorrhage are the gastrointestinal and genitourinary tracts; however, epistaxis may be a severe and significant management problem in the emergency department. Central nervous system hemorrhage may produce focal neural deficits or catastrophic decerebration. (See Chapters 96–99 on bleeding disorders.)

BIBLIOGRAPHY

Spinal Cord Compression

Bruckman JE, Bloomer WD: Management of spinal cord compression. *Semin Oncol* 5:135–140, June 1978.
Friedman M, Kim TH, Panahon AM: Spinal cord compression and malignant lymphoma. Treatment and results. *Cancer* 37:1485–1491, 1976.
Gilbert RW, Kim JH, Posner JB: Epidural spinal cord compression from metastatic tumor: Diagnosis and treatment. *Ann Neurol* 3:40, 1978.

Upper Airway Obstruction

Lockwood P: Airway obstruction in patients with carcinoma of the bronchus. *Respiration* 36 (1):50–56, 1978.

Malignant Pericardial Effusion with Tamponade

Biran S, Brufman G, Klein E: The management of pericardial effusions in cancer patients. *Chest* 71:182–186, 1977.
Memon A: Malignant effusions: Diagnostic evaluation and therapeutic strategy. *Curr Probl Cancer* 5 (8):1–30, Feb. 1981.
Spodick DH: Acute cardiac tamponade. Pathologic physiology, diagnosis, and management. *Prog Cardiovasc Dis* 10:64–96, 1967.

Superior Vena Cava Syndrome

Houser J: The Superior vena cava syndrome: A review of the literature. *IMJ* 156:459–462, 1979.
Lolich JJ, Codman R: Superior vena cava syndrome. Clinical management. *JAMA* 231:58–61, 1975.
Perez CA, Presant CA, Van Amburg AL III: Management of superior vena cava syndrome. *Semin Oncol* 5:123–134, June 1978.

Hypercalcemia of Malignancy

Burt ME et al: Incidence of hypercalcemia and malignant neoplasm. *Arch Surg* 115:704–707, 1980.

Delamore IW: Hypercalcemia and myeloma. *Br J Haemtol* 51:507–509, 1982.

Grossman B, Schechter GP, Horton JE, et al: Hypercalcemia associated with T-cell lymphoma-leukemia. *Am J Clin Pathol* 75:149–155, 1981.

Muggia FM, Heinemann HO: Hypercalcemia associated with neoplastic diseases. *Ann Intern Med* 73:281, 1970.

Sherwood LM: The Multiple causes of hypercalcemia in malignant disease (editorial). *N Engl J Med* 303 (24):1412–1413, Dec. 1980.

Zawada ET Jr et al.: Mangement of hypercalcemia. *Postgrad Med* 66(4):105–113, Oct. 1979.

Syndrome of Inappropriate Antidiuretic Hormone Secretion

Bartter FC, Schwartz WB: The syndrome of inappropriate secretion of antidiuretic hormone. *Am J Med* 42:790, 1967.

Cherrill DA, Stote RM, Birge JR, Singer I: Demeclocycline treatment in the syndrome of innappropriate hormone secretion. *Ann Intern Med* 83:654, 1975.

Harlow PJ, De Clerck YA, Shore NA, et al: A fatal case of inappropriate ADH secretion induced by cyclophosphamide therapy. *Cancer* 44:896, 1979.

Segaloff A: Managing endocrine and metabolic problems in the patient with advanced cancer. *JAMA* 245:177–179, 1981.

Hyperviscosity Syndrome

Cohen HJ, Rundles RW: Managing the complications of myeloma. *Arch Intern Med* 135:177–184, 1975.

Hild, DH: Hyperviscosity in chronic granulocytic leukemia. *Cancer* 46:1418–1421, 1980.

Kopp WL, Bierne GL, Burns RO: Hyperviscosity syndrome in multiple myeloma. *Am J Med* 43:141–146, 1967.

Granulocytopenia and Sepsis

Bodey GP, Buckley M, Sathe YS, et al: Quantitative relationships between circulating leukocytes and infection in patients with acute leukemia. *Ann Intern Med* 64:328–340, 1966.

Pizzo PA: Empiric antibiotic and antifungal therapy for cancer patients with prolonged fever and granulocytopenia. *Am J Med* 72:101–111, 1982.

Schimpff SC: Therapy of infection in patients with granulocytopenia. *Med Clin North Am* 61:1101–1118, 1977.

SECTION 12
DERMATOLOGIC
EMERGENCIES

CHAPTER 102
TOXICODENDRON
DERMATITIS (POISON
IVY, POISON OAK,
AND POISON SUMAC)

Thomas A. Chapel

Kligman states that the *Toxicondendrons*—poison ivy, poison oak, and poison sumac—are responsible for more cases of allergic contact dermatitis in the United States than are all other allergens combined. Fisher estimates that at least 70 percent of the population of the United States if casually exposed to the plants, would develop allergic contact sensitivity to the *Toxicodendrons,* and the percentage would be even greater if contact were more prolonged. Dark-skinned individuals seem less susceptible than others to *Toxicodendron* dermatitis and elderly persons are not as susceptible to poison ivy as are younger people.

CHARACTERISTICS OF *TOXICODENDRONS*

Poison ivy and poison oak are the principle causes of plant dermatitis in North America. Poison ivy occurs throughout the United States while poison oak is more common on the west coast. In the United States there are two species of poison oak, *Toxicodendron diversilobum* (western poison oak) and *T. toxicarium* (eastern poison oak). There also are two species of poison ivy, *T. rydbergii* a nonclimbing subshrub, and *T. radicans*, which may be either a shrub or a climbing vine. One species of poison sumac, *T. vernix*, occurs in the United States. It grows as a coarse, woody shrub or as a tree and it is found in wooded, swampy areas.

All species of poison oak and poison ivy have leaves with three leaflets, and poison sumac has 7 to 13 leaflets per leaf. The *Toxicodendrons* can also be recognized by their U- or V-shaped leaf scars, typical lenticels, and flowers and fruit that arise in the angle between the leaf and the branch. Off-white mature fruit is borne on a doubly branched structure called a *panicle.*

The leaves, stems, seeds, flowers, berries, and roots of the *Toxicodendrons* contain a milky sap, which darkens to the appearance of black lacquer on exposure to the air. The black deposit is present where plants have been injured and its presence proves that a suspicious plant is a *Toxicodendron*. This characteristic can be used by novices or persons working with unfamiliar vegetation to identify these plants. Guin suggests that several leafs from the

plant in question be crushed on a sheet of white paper. The sap stain from poison ivy, poison oak, and poison sumac darkens markedly within a few minutes. This black spot test is used only to augment classical methods of plant identification and care must be taken to avoid contamination of fingers and clothing with sap.

THE DERMATITIS-PRODUCING FACTORS OF THE *TOXICODENDRONS*

The antigenic oleoresin of *Toxicodendrons* is easily extracted from plant sap with alcohol and other solvents. The residue left after evaporation of the solvent is called *urushiol,* and its dermatitis-producing principle is pentadecylacatechol. The *Toxicodendrons* share similar antigens and therefore cross sensitivity exists between poison ivy, poison oak, and poison sumac.

Urushiol oxidizes and with complete oxidation is rendered non-allergenic. The speed of the breakdown is promoted by moisture and heat. The antigenic film on clothing or other objects may become inactive within 1 week in a hot, humid environment while the substance remains allergenic for much longer periods in a dry atmosphere. Washing with soap and water rapidly destroys the antigen. The allergenicity of the oleoresin is maximal in fresh plants and diminishes as the plant ages. However, sensitive individuals must avoid handling plants at any age, for even withered leaves produce contact dermatitis.

The persistence of the allergen permits its spread by contaminated fingers, clothing, tools, animals, and sports equipment. Smoke-carrying particles of the plant can, and often do, disseminate the disease. However, complete incineration of the plant destroys the allergen.

Toxicodendron antigen may remain under a person's fingernails for several days unless deliberately removed by thorough cleansing. Scratching with antigen-contaminated fingers disseminates the dermatitis to the face, genitals, and covered areas. The dermatitogenic effect of minute amounts of allergen in highly sensitized individuals is astonishing. Kligman contaminated the thumb of a nonsensitized subject with the juice from crushed leaves. The thumb was then pressed onto the back of a nonsensitized subject 99 times, then once onto the back of a highly sensitive individual. This sequence was repeated four more times. The fifth contact on the highly sensitive individual caused a slight dermatitis, even after 500 impressions.

PRESENTATION AND DIAGNOSIS

Clinical Features

Toxicodendron antigen enters the skin rapidly and in order to prevent a reaction the sap must be totally removed within 10 minutes after exposure. Under ordinary circumstances such prophylaxis is impossible. Contact dermatitis in susceptible people generally develops within 2 days following exposure. However, Fisher reports that in a few cases the eruption appears 8 h after exposure and, rarely, the interval may exceed 10 days.

The temporal difference in onset of the eruption and variations in the clinical expression of *Toxicodendron* dermatitis depends upon the patient's degree of sensitivity, the amount of contact with the allergen, and the regional variations in cutaneous reactivity. Mildly sensitive persons can probably withstand casual exposure to the plant without difficulty. Some individuals develop simple erythema, others erythema and papules, and yet others erythema, papules, vesicles, and bullae. The dermatitis usually begins with pruritus and redness. Streaks of erythema or papulovesicles in linear arrangement soon appear (Figs. 102-1 and 102-2). The linear configuration of some lesions is highly suggestive of *Toxicodendron* dermatitis; it is produced by portions of the plant rubbing across the skin or by dissemination of the allergen by scratching with contaminated fingernails. A common myth is that the disorder is spread by rupturing vesicles. However, blister fluid contains no antigen and therefore it cannot transmit the dermatitis.

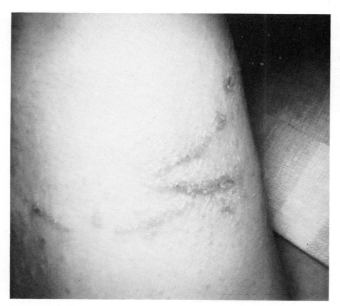

Figure 102-1. Erythematous, edematous papules and vesicles of poison ivy in typical linear arrangement.

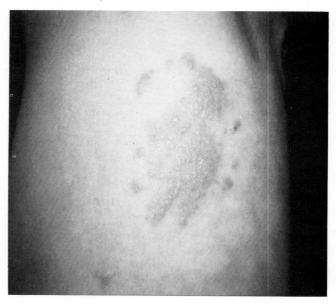

Figure 102-2. Plaque of poison ivy dermatitis with streaks of erythema and papulovesicles.

The eruption usually disappears without a trace but leukodermia or hyperpigmentation are occasional sequelae. Urticaria and erythema multiforme infrequently occur as a result of systemic absorption of *Toxicodendron* antigen.

Laboratory findings in patients with poison ivy dermatitis are minimal. Leukocytosis and eosinophilia of 5 to 10 percent occur in a small percentge of patients with severe dermatitis.

Differential Diagnosis

Toxicodendron dermatitis is quite distinctive but occasionally it may be confused with contact dermatitis of other origin. A mimic is phytophotodermatitis caused by lime, parsley, celery, figs, and buttercups. Juices from these plants contain psoralens, which are activated by long-wave ultraviolet light and produce a phototoxic eruption. The eruption consists of striate lesions and irregularly linear bullae in sun-exposed areas. The blisters usually heal with pigmentation that lasts for months. Poison ivy dermatitis is not photoactivated and it can be distinguished from phytophotodermatitis by lesions that occur on both covered and uncovered areas of the body.

TREATMENT

Treatment of *Toxicodendron* dermatitis is determined by the severity of the eruption. Mild dermatitis consisting of erythema, edema, and papules limited to a few anatomic regions can be managed with shake lotions such as calamine or steroid sprays, creams, or lotions. Compresses or soaks with cold or moderately hot water bring temporary relief from pruritus, and antihistaminics by mouth effectively control persistent itch.

More aggressive treatment is required for moderate and severe dermatitis with vesicles and bullae distributed over large areas of the body's surface. Compresses with cool aluminum sulfate diluted 1:10 (Domeboro) help dry lesions and minimize itch. Compresses are applied for 30 to 60 min two to three times each day until blisters dry. Large bullae can be aseptically aspirated with roofs left intact. Potassium permanganate baths aid in drying ruptured blisters. The patient dissolves one-half tablespoon of potassium permanganate crystals in a tub of lukewarm water and soaks for 15 to 20 min each day. Baths with colloidal oatmeal (Aveeno), mixed one cupful per tub of water, are also soothing. The pruritus accompanying severe dermatitis should be treated with antihistaminics in full therapeutic doses.

Systemic corticosteroids are effective in bringing relief and are often used if there are no contraindications. If corticosteroids are used, they should be initiated at a level equivalent to 40 to 60 mg of prednisone daily, gradually tapered over a 2- to 3-week period, and then discontinued. Shorter courses of corticosteroids should be avoided as they are frequently associated with a rebound exacerbation of the dermatitis.

The speed with which the eruption heals depends upon the severity and the extent of the cutaneous injury. Mild dermatitis often disappears within 7 to 10 days while severe eruptions often require 3 or more weeks for normalization.

PROPHYLAXIS

The salient points of *Toxicodendron* dermatitis must be explained carefully to patients and common myths should be dispelled. The best prophylaxis against recurrent dermatitis is avoidance of the *Toxicodendrons*. This requires that patients recognize poison ivy and related species. Display posters and illustrated pamphlets are helpful teaching aids in educating patients. Persons allergic to the *Toxicodendrons* may have cross reactions to Japanese lacquer and cashew nut trees, the mango, and the marking nut tree of India. Contact with these items also should be avoided.

Individuals exposed to *Toxicodendrons* should wash the entire body with soap and water and carefully clean their fingernails. Clean clothing should be worn and contaminated clothing laundered. Poison ivy, poison oak, and poison sumac growing in areas of unavoidable contact should be destroyed with herbicides or removed physically to prevent future reexposure.

Epstein and associates advise highly sensitive individuals at increased risk of reexposure because of work or hobbies to try hyposensitization. Hyposensitization requires oral administration of very large doses of urushiol over a 4- to 8- month interval. Unfortunately, hyposensitization lasts no more than several months after the last dose of oil.

BIBLIOGRAPHY

Epstein WL: Rhus dermatitis. *Pediatr Clin North Am* 6:843–852, 1959.

Epstein WL, Byers VS, Baer H: Induction of persistent tolerance to urushiol in humans. *J Allergy Clin Immunol* 68:20–25, 1981.

Fisher AA: The poison "rhus" plants. *Cutis* 1:230–236, 1965.

Kligman AM: Poison ivy (Rhus) dermatitis. An experimental study. *Arch Dermatol* 77:149–180, 1958.

Guin JD: The black spot test for recognizing poison ivy and related species. *J Am Acad Dermatol* 2:332–333, 1980.

Guin JD, Gillis WT, Beaman JH: Recognizing the *Toxicodendrons* (poison ivy, poison oak, poison sumac). *J Am Acad Dermatol* 4:99–114, 1981.

Maibach HI, Epstein WL: Plant dermatitis: Fact and fancy. *Postgrad Med* 35:571–574, 1964.

CHAPTER 103
EXFOLIATIVE
DERMATITIS

Thomas A. Chapel

Exfoliative dermatitis refers to a condition in which most or all of the skin surface is involved with a scaly erythematous dermatitis. Males are afflicted with the condition twice as often as females, and at least 75 percent of the patients are over the age of 40, as reported by Moschella. The widespread inflammatory exfoliation often is accompanied by immediate or delayed effects in other organ systems.

ETIOLOGY AND PATHOGENESIS

Exfoliative dermatitis is a cutaneous reaction produced in response to a drug or chemical agent or to an underlying cutaneous or systemic disease. The etiologic classification and relative incidence of the more common underlying conditions are listed in Table 103-1. Aside from acute exacerbation of a preexisting dermatosis or generalized exposure to a contact allergen, the mechanisms responsible for exfoliative dermatitis are not known. However, Lillie et al. postulate that drug-induced exfoliative dermatitis may be mediated by an excessive number of drug-sensitized suppressor-cytotoxic T lymphocytes and may represent a disorder of immunoregulatory T. cells.

Exfoliative dermatitis can have an abrupt onset when related to a drug or contact allergen or to malignancy. Outbreaks arising

Table 103-1 Causes of Dermatitis

Disease	Range of Reported Incidence (%)
Generalized flares of preexisting cutaneous disease	25–40
Psoriasis	
Atopic dermatitis	
Seborrheic dermatitis	
Lichen planus	
Pemphigus foliaceus	
Pityriasis rubra pilaris	
Contact dermatitis	
Drugs	3–10
Lymphoma, leukemia, solid tumors	10–40
Idiopathic	15–45

from an underlying cutaneous disorder usually evolve more slowly, and the identifiable features of the underlying disease may be lost. However, careful observation and a thorough physical examination can sometimes uncover changes characteristic of the primary disease.

In a study of 101 cases, Abrahams et al. found that exfoliative dermatitis tends to be a chronic condition, with a mean duration of 5 years and a median duration of 10 months. A shorter course often follows suppression of the underlying dermatosis, discontinuation of inciting drugs, or avoidance of the inciting allergen. Exfoliative dermatitis with no associated discernible cause can continue for 20 or more years. Death may occur and in general is attributable to hepatocellular damage from severe drug reactions or to underlying malignancies.

There is generalized erythema and warmth of the skin, accompanied by scaling or flaking of the epidermis. The patient usually has a low-grade fever and often complains of pruritus, a chilly sensation, and tightness of the skin. Chronic inflammatory exfoliation produces many changes, such as dystrophic nails, thinning of scalp and body hair, and patchy or diffuse postinflammatory hyperpigmentation or, less commonly, hypopigmentation. Gynecomastia and generalized lymphadenopathy are common in longstanding cases.

Active erythroderma is complicated by excessive heat loss, impairment of temperature regulation, and sometimes hypothermia. The widespread cutaneous vasodilation can cause increased cardiac output. In marginally compensated patients the hemodynamic changes may produce a high-output cardiac failure with dyspnea and dependent edema. Splenomegaly occurred in 3 to 14 percent of the 236 cases reported by Abrahams et al. and Nicolis and Helwig. When associated with exfoliative dermatitis, splenomegaly suggests an underlying leukemia or lymphoma.

The disruption of the epidermis results in increased transepidermal water loss, and continued exfoliation can result in significant protein loss and negative nitrogen balance. Steatorrhea sometimes results from the widespread inflammatory exfoliation, but the enteropathy resolves with improvement of the exfoliative dermatitis. The serum albumin level is lowered because of steatorrhea, cutaneous scaling, and plasma dilution arising from cardiovascular alterations.

DIAGNOSIS AND TREATMENT

Differential Diagnosis

The various ichthyoses may mimic exfoliative dermatitis; however, the presence of ichthyosis in other family members, the lifelong presence of disease, and the morphologic detail in scale and anatomic distribution make differentiation easy.

Clinical Evaluation and Treatment

A patient with a newly diagnosed case of exfoliative dermatitis or one who is experiencing an acute exacerbation should be hospitalized for dermatologic nursing care, supportive treatment, and investigative studies. Considerable effort must be made to determine the underlying etiology by a careful history of previous cutaneous disease and of recent drug use and laboratory tests to establish whether there is possible association with leukemia, lymphoma, or solid tumor. A cutaneous biopsy is indicated, and if there is significant lymphadenopathy, lymph nodes should likewise be biopsied. The patient should also be evaluated for cardiac failure and intestinal dysfunction.

Some patients respond to topical application of corticosteroid cream or ointment and oral antihistamines to control pruritus. However, many require systemic corticosteroids beginning with 40 to 60 mg of prednisone each day. If no response is observed, the dose may be increased by 20 mg. With a favorable response the dose is gradually tapered over weeks or months and eventually discontinued. When systemic steroids are used, the patient can apply bland lotions or creams rather than topical corticosteroid preparations. Tepid colloidal baths, such as cornstarch or oatmeal powder suspensions, are of some benefit.

SUMMARY

Exfoliative dermatitis is a cutaneous reaction produced in response to a drug or chemical agent or to an underlying cutaneous or systemic disease. It can be abrupt or insidious in onset. Clinically, it is characterized by generalized erythroderma and flaking or scaling of the epidermis.

Treatment includes control of the underlying cutaneous disorder, avoidance of the inciting drug or allergen, or treatment of the underlying malignancy. Topical steroids and antipruritic agents may provide relief in many cases, but for more serious disorders systemic corticosteroids may be necessary.

BIBLIOGRAPHY

Abrahams I, McCarthy J, Sanders S: 101 cases of exfoliative dermatitis. *Arch Dermatol* 87:96–101, 1963

Hasan T, Jansen CT: Erythroderma: a follow-up of 50 cases. *J Am Acad Dermatol* 8:836–840, 1983.

Nicolis GD, Helwig EB: Exfoliative dermatitis: A clinicopathologic study of 135 cases. *Arch Dermatol* 108:788–797, 1973.

CHAPTER 104
ERYTHEMA MULTIFORME

Thomas A. Chapel

PATHOLOGY AND CLINICAL CHARACTERISTICS

Erythema multiforme represents a spectrum of disease that ranges from trivial cutaneous lesions to severe, sometimes fatal, multisystem illness. Tissue reaction is of variable expression, yet the histologic features are sufficiently characteristic to differentiate this disorder from other erythematous and vesiculobullous eruptions. The histopathological spectrum of erythema multiforme has been described by Bedi and Pinkus. Bullae are subepidermal, and epidermal cell necrosis is often noted. The dermis is usually edematous and a lymphocytic infiltrate is often present about the capillaries and venules of the upper dermis. The disorder is a hypersensitivity reaction precipitated by many agents and conditions (Table 104-1).

Recent data suggest an important role for circulating immune complexes. Direct immunofluorescence studies of erythema mul-

Table 104-1 Common Etiologies of Erythema Multiforme

ASSOCIATED INFECTIOUS DISEASES

Herpes simplex infection, Types I and II
Mycoplasma pneumonia
Influenza
Mumps
Psittacosis
Cat-scratch disease
Typhoid fever
Diphtheria
Lymphogranuloma venereum
Histoplasmosis
Cholera

DRUGS COMMONLY IMPLICATED

Sulfonamides
Oral hypoglycemic agent: chlorpropamide
Phenytoin and related anticonvulsants
Pyrazolone derivatives: phenybutazone, oxyphenbutazone, phenazone
Barbiturates
Penicillins
Carbamazepine

MALIGNANCY WITH OR WITHOUT RADIATION THERAPY

Carcinoma
Lymphoma

tiforme skin lesions have shown deposits of complement components and immunoglobulin in the superficial dermal blood vessels or at the dermal-epidermal junction, and immune complexes have been detected in serum samples of patients with erythema multiforme.

It has been pointed out that infections are generally more important as the cause in children, while drugs (Fig. 104-1) and malignancies (Fig. 104-2) are more often implicated in adult cases. About half the cases lack an identifiable etiology. Many cases of erythema multiforme occur during epidemics of atypical pneumonia, adenovirus, and histoplasmosis.

The disorder occurs at any age, affects males twice as often as females, and is most common in the spring and the fall. The morphology of the cutaneous lesions is variable; they can be macular, urticarial, or vesiculobullous. The skin lesions typically begin as erythematous macules or urticarial-like plaques, and they often contain scattered petechiae. Unlike true hives, the urticarial lesions of erythema multiforme are not usually pruritic. Vesiculobullous lesions develop centrally within preexisting macules, papules, or wheals (Figs. 104-3 and 104-4). Blistering of the mucous membranes occurs in about a quarter of cases, and at times it represents the sole expression of the disease. The char-

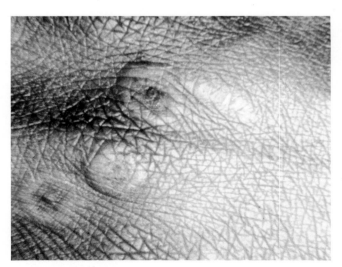

Figure 104-1. Erythema multiforme secondary to heroin snuff.

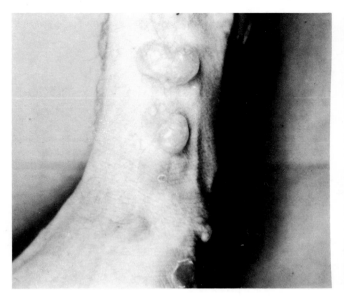

Figure 104-2. Erythema multiforme bullosum secondary to cancer of the stomach.

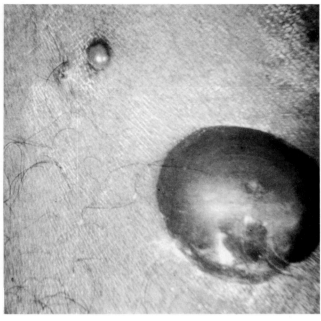

Figure 104-4. Erythema multiforme bullosum lesions are usually annular and sharply demarcated from normal skin.

acteristic iris lesions of erythema multiforme are erythematous plaques with dusky centers and bright red borders, resembling the bull's-eye of a target (Fig. 104-5).

The eruption has a predilection for dorsum of the hands, palms, soles, and extensor surfaces of the extremities. Lesions tend to appear in crops over a period of 2 to 4 weeks, and, rarely, over many months. The individual lesions heal in 7 to 10 days without scarring unless the site is secondarily infected. However, in dark-skinned patients postinflammatory hyperpigmentation or hypopigmentation is common. When associated with herpes simplex virus,

erythema multiforme can recur 5 to 7 days after each viral relapse and with drug incitant can recur upon repeat exposure.

The Stevens-Johnson eponym is reserved for the most severe bullous form of erythema mutiforme. It is frequently preceded by a prodrome of variable symptoms, such as fever, malaise, myalgias, and arthralgias, which probably stem from an underlying infectious disease. The mucocutaneous lesions have abrupt onset and are associated with marked constitutional symptoms and multisystem pathology. The mucosal surfaces of the lips, cheeks, palate, eyes, urethra, vagina, nose, and anus are involved (Figure 104-6). In severe cases the linings of the pharynx, tracheobronchial tree, and esophagus are also affected. The lesions begin as blisters, which rupture to leave shreds of necrotic grayish white

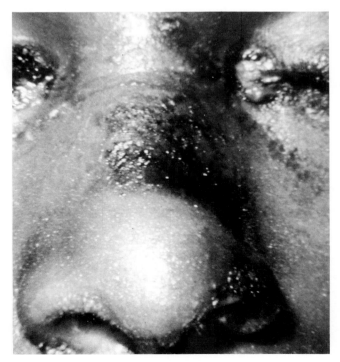

Figure 104-3. Bullous erythema multiforme of the face.

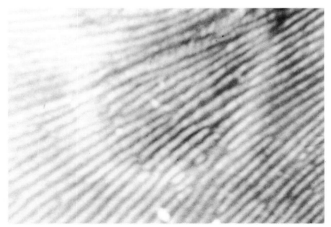

Figure 104-5. Erythema multiforme lesions tend to appear in crops over a period of 2 to 4 weeks.

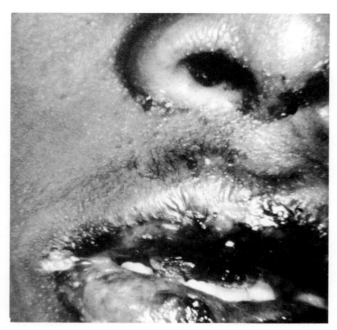

Figure 104-6. Bullous erythema multiforme of the mouth, a commonly involved orifice.

epithelium and blood-crusted denuded bases. Patients are often unable to eat because of the painful stomatitis. The eyes have a catarrhal or purulent conjunctivitis and vesicles are sometimes observed on the conjunctivae.

The Stevens-Johnson syndrome has substantial morbidity and a mortality rate of 5 to 10 percent. Denuded surfaces are susceptible to secondary bacterial infection and, when untreated, these can lead to scar formation. Nails may occasionally be shed, balanitis can lead to scarred attachment of the foreskin to the glans, and vulvovaginitis can lead to stenosis of the vagina. Hematuria, renal tubular necrosis, and progressive renal failure can occur but are rare. More common are significant ocular sequelae, including corneal ulceration, anterior uveitis, panophthalmitis, corneal opacities, and blindness.

Differential Diagnosis

Conditions to be differentiated include the migratory annular erythemas such as erythema annulare centrifugum; toxic erythemas of infectious or drug origin; blistering disorders such as bullous pemphigoid, pemphigus vulgaris, herpes gestationis; and the cutaneous and systemic vasculitides. Erythema multiforme has also been seen in association with erythema nodosum and topic epidermal necrolysis.

DIAGNOSIS AND TREATMENT

The clinical features are usually distinctive enough to permit a diagnosis, but a skin biopsy should be obtained in equivocal cases. Because erythema multiforme is a pattern reaction, appropriate investigative studies should be undertaken to determine the underlying etiology, and all drugs of potential etiologic significance must be stopped. Respiratory failure can develop secondary to mucosal sloughing. While renal complications are uncommon, kidney function should be monitored.

Patients with limited disease can be treated on an outpatient basis with topical corticosteroids. However, those with severe mucous membrane involvement require hospitalization and often several days of intravenous fluids. Relief from painful stomatitis can sometimes be achieved with diphenhydramine hydrochloride elixir or viscous lidocaine held in the mouth for 3 to 5 min before expectorating. Secondary infections require appropriate antibiotics, and ophthalmologic consultation is necessary if there is eye involvement. Secondary infection and oozing from denuded areas can be minimized by tub soaks in potassium permanganate (1:10,000) or by painting open areas with 0.25% gentian violet. Systemic corticosteroids give symptomatic relief but are of unproven value in influencing the duration and outcome of the disease. If corticosteroids are used, they should be initiated at a level equivalent to 80 to 100 mg of prednisone daily, gradually tapered off over a 3- to 4-week period, and then discontinued.

BIBLIOGRAPHY

Bedi TR, Pinkus H: Histopathological spectrum of erythema multiforme. *Br J Dermatol* 95:243–250, 1976.

Bianchine JR, Macaraeg P, Lasagna L, et al.: Drugs as etiologic factors in the Steven-Johnson syndrome. *Am J Med* 44:390–405, 1968.

Bluefarb SM, Szanto P: Erythema multiforme associated with acute renal tubular necrosis. *Arch Dermatol* 92:367–372, 1965.

Comaish JS, Kerr DNS: Erythema multiforme and nephritis. *Br Med J* 2:84–88, 1961.

Imamura S, Yanese K, Teniguchi S, et al.: Erythema multiforme: Demonstration of immune complexes in the sera and skin lesions. *Br J Dermatol* 102:161–166, 1980.

Kazmirowski JA, Peizner DS, Wuepper MD: Herpes simplex antigen in immune complexes of patients with erythema multiforme. *JAMA* 247:2547–2550, 1982.

Shelly WB: Herpes simplex virus as a cause of erythema multiforme. *JAMA* 201:153–156, 1967.

CHAPTER 105

TOXIC EPIDERMAL

NECROLYSIS

Thomas A. Chapel

Toxic epidermal necrolysis, also called the *scalded skin syndrome*, is composed of two distinct clinicopathologic entities: one associated with staphylococcal infection and the other due to a drug or chemical agent. Both forms are characterized by the sudden appearance of patches of intense, tender erythema that is followed by widespread loosening of skin and denudation to a glistening base.

The first form is called the *staphylococcal scalded skin syndrome* and usually afflicts children under the age of 5 years (Fig. 105-1). The disorder is associated with an underlying staphylococcal infection, and is due to the production of a toxin that cleaves the epidermis beneath the stratum granulosum. The exact mode of action of the toxin is unknown, although studies suggest an intercellular target or a specific receptor toxin interaction. Because the cleavage plane is intraepidermal, fluid loss may not be extreme, and despite widespread exfoliation the mortality rate is less than 5 percent.

CLINICAL FEATURES

Staphylococcal scalded skin syndrome comprises a spectrum of skin lesions ranging from localized bullous impetigo to generalized exfoliation. The disease begins as tender, erythematous patches of scarletiniform lesions that often follow an upper respiratory tract infection or purulent conjunctivitis. The initial lesions are characteristically distributed on the periorificial areas of the face, the neck, the axillae, and the groin. At this stage lateral pressure on the skin causes separation of the epidermis from the dermis (positive Nikolsky's sign). Large flaccid bullae sometimes develop and within 24 to 48 h the epidermis spontaneously separates in rumpled sheets revealing a moist, erythematous base. Despite widespread exfoliation of the skin the mucous membranes are not involved. The denuded bases dry rapidly leading to a postinflammatory desquamation that resolves in 5 to 7 days.

The form caused by a drug or chemical agent occurs chiefly in adults and is characterized by separation of the skin at the dermoepidermal junction (Fig. 105-2). The involved epidermis is necrotic but little infiltrate is seen in the dermis. The lesions of the scalded skin syndrome are widespread, and the mucous membranes are commonly involved (Fig. 105-3 and 105-4). At times, the skin lesions may resemble those of erythema multiforme. The complete loss of the epidermis is associated with slow healing, and reepithelialization takes one to three weeks. Drug related toxic epidermal necrolysis carries a 5 to 50 percent mortality due to fluid loss and secondary infection (Table 105-1).

Differential Diagnosis

Clinically, toxic epidermal necrolysis may be confused with pemphigus vulgaris, thermal or chemical burns, and severe erythema

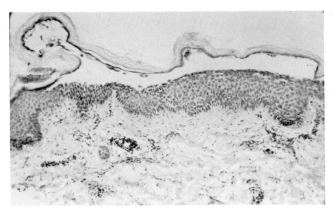

Figure 105-1. Staphylococcal scalded skin syndrome.

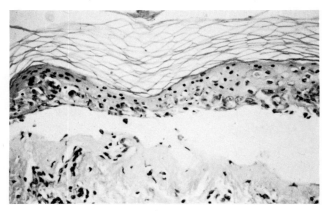

Figure 105-2. Drug-induced toxic epidermal necrolysis.

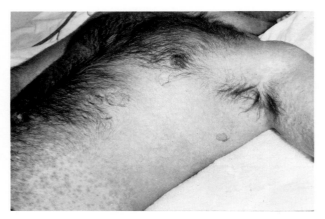

Figure 105-3. Toxic epidermal necrolysis secondary to a sulfone.

multiforme. Patients with a graft-versus-host reaction may have a reaction like the drug-induced form of toxic epidermal necrolysis.

DIAGNOSIS

The morphology of toxic epidermal necrolysis is sufficiently distinct to permit clinical diagnosis. However, the age of the patient is not an absolute indicator of the underlying etiology. A history of drug usage or chemical exposure and the results of bacterial culture and skin biopsy allow differentiation of the two forms. Amon and Dimond have suggested methods for more rapid differentiation. The level of separation in the cutaneum can be determined by examining the cells from denuded areas or by examining frozen sections of bullae roofs.

The first technique involves scraping the denuded bases with a no. 15 sterile surgical blade. The material collected is smeared on a clean glass slide and examined. In the staphylococcal scalded skin syndrome, a few acantholytic keratinocytes will be evident, while in the nonstaphylococcal type, inflammatory cells, cellular debris, and basal cell keratinocytes will be present.

The second technique involves histologic examination of a frozen section of skin peeled from a fresh lesion of toxic epidermal necrolysis. In the drug-induced form of the disorder the split is at

the dermal-epidermal junction and a full thickness of epidermis is present, while in the staphylococcal scalded skin syndrome only stratum corneum and a few granular cells are seen.

The growth of *S. aureus* on cultures obtained from the conjuctiva, nose, throat, perineum, and skin strongly suggests an infectious etiology. Definitive diagnosis is made by excisional or punch biopsy specimen of involved skin.

TREATMENT

A patient with toxic epidermal necrolysis has temporarily lost his skin barrier against percutaneous water loss. Adults with toxic necrolysis lose an average of 2 to 4 L/day by evaporation for the first 9 days. In general, greater losses of plasma occur within the first few days, whereas water loss predominates later in the course. At any rate, volume and electrolyte replacement should be done in the emergency department if there are signs of hypovolemia. The possibility of septic shock should also be considered in the differential diagnosis of hypotension.

Until barrier function is restored, the lesions of toxic epidermal necrolysis are treated as infected second-degree burns with tub baths of potassium permanganate and topical agents such as silver sulfadiazine.

Staphylococcal scalded skin syndrome should be treated with an oral or intravenous penicillinase-resistant penicillin, even though antibiotic therapy does not seem to alter the course of the cutaneous disease. Corticosteroids are contraindicated in staphylococcal scalded skin syndrome. Their value has not been proved in drug-related toxic epidermal necrolysis. If steroids are used in this form, large doses, equivalent to 200 mg prednisone daily, are recommended. If the drug has any beneficial effect, it should be obvious during the first week of therapy and the steroid can be abruptly discontinued thereafter. Antibiotics in drug-induced toxic necrolysis are reserved for treating disease caused by identified pathogens. If the eyes are involved, an ophthalmologist should be consulted.

SUMMARY

There are two forms of toxic epidermal necrolysis or scalded skin syndrome. The staphylococcal scalded skin syndrome generally occurs in children and, if appropriately treated, carries a favorable prognosis. The adult form is caused by a drug or chemical agent and carries a 5 to 50 percent mortality due to fluid loss and secondary infection.

The age of the patient is not an absolute indicator of the etiology. The two types are differentiated by a history of drug usage or chemical exposure and by the results of bacterial culture and skin biopsy.

Table 105-1. Drugs Most Commonly Implicated in Toxic Epidermal Necrolysis

Sulfonamides and sulfones
Pyrazolone derivatives: phenylbutazone, oxyphenbutazone, phenazone
Barbiturates
Antiepileptics
Antibiotics

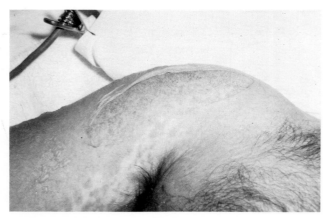

Figure 105-4. Closeup view of toxic epidermal necrolysis secondary to a sulfone.

The lesions are treated as infected second-degree burns with potassium permanganate tub baths and topical silver sulfadiazine. The form associated with staphylococcal infection is treated with antibiotics and steroids are contraindicated. In the drug-related form, steroids have not been shown to be of value.

BIBLIOGRAPHY

Amon RB, Dimond RL: Toxic epidermal necrolysis: Rapid differentiation between staphylococcal-induced disease and drug-induced disease. *Arch Dermatol* 111:1433–1437, 1975.

Birke G, Liljedahl S, Rajka G: Lyell's syndrome: Metabolic and clinical results of a new form of treatment. *Acta Derm Venereol (Stockh)* 51:199–209, 1971.

Elias PM, Fritsch P, Dahl MV, et al: Staphylococcal toxic epiderml necrolysis: Pathogenesis and studies on the subcellular site of action of exfoliation. *J Invest Dermatol* 65:501–512, 1975.

Elias PM, Fritsch P, Epstein EH Jr: Staphylococcal scalded skin syndrome: Clinical features, pathogenesis, and recent microbiological and biochemical developments. *Arch Dermatol* 113:207–219, 1977.

Koblenzer PJ: Acute epidermal necrolysis (Ritter von Rittershain-Lyell). *Arch Dermatol* 95:608–617, 1967.

Lillibridge CB, Melish ME, Glasgow LA: Site of action of exfoliative toxin in the staphylococcal scalded skin syndrome. *Pediatrics* 50:728–738, 1972.

Lowney ED, Baublis JV, Kreye GM, et al: The scalded skin syndrome in small children. *Arch Dermatol* 95:359–369, 1967.

Lyell A: Toxic epidermal necrolysis: The scalded skin syndrome. *J Contin Ed Dermatol* 16:15–31, 1978.

Peck GL, Herzig GP, Elias PM: Toxic epidermal necrolysis in a patient with graft-vs-host reaction. *Arch Dermatol* 105:561–569, 1972.

Rudolph RI, Schwartz W, Leyden JJ: Treatment of staphylococcal toxic epidermal necrolysis. *Arch Dermatol* 110:559–562, 1974.

Samuels ML, Howe CD, Frei E: Toxic epidermal necrolysis resembling erythema multiforme. *Tex Med* 64:44–50, 1968.

SECTION 13
INFECTIONS

CHAPTER 106
CUTANEOUS
ABSCESSES

Harvey W. Meislin

Skin infections and cutaneous abscesses are common emergency department problems, accounting for 2.5 to 5 percent of all visits. The time-honored treatment has been to surgically incise and drain the abscess.

BACTERIOLOGY

Anaerobic bacteria are known to be a part of the normal flora of the skin and all mucous membranes, including the mouth, vagina, urethra, and colon. Anaerobes outnumber aerobes in the oral cavity by 10 to 1. In the distal colon, this ratio is increased to greater than 1000 to 1. Twenty to thirty percent of the wet weight of stool is a solid mass of living bacteria, nearly all of which are anaerobic. Anaerobes are commonly seen in abscesses, usually in mixed cultures and primarily in the perineal areas. Their importance in infection of the CNS, the intraabdominal cavity, and the respiratory system is well documented.

Bacteroides fragilis (Table 106-1) is in general the only anaerobe resistant to penicillin and the most common gram-negative anaerobe in human feces. It is most common in abscesses involving the perineal region.

Staphylococcus aureus, the most prevalent aerobe in cutaneous abscesses, is found in all regions where abscesses originate in the skin. In several recent studies, *S. aureus* was found in about one-fourth of all abscesses, and almost always was isolated in pure culture. It was, however, isolated much less frequently than clinically expected (less than 50 percent of the time—Table 106-2). Two-thirds of all *S. aureus* infections were seen in abscesses from the upper torso (the head, neck, axilla, and trunk area). This organism has a well-recognized propensity for abscess formation and, in contrast to anaerobes, its potential for abscess formation is not as dependent on synergistic bacterial mixtures. It is significant that out-patient *S. aureus* showed a 97 percent resistance to penicillin G.

Proteus mirabilis, a normal inhabitant of feces, is the most common gram-negative aerobe found. It is seen mainly in cutaneous abscesses of the upper torso (Table 106-3). The reason for this is not clear, since *P. mirabilis* is not a normal inhabitant of the skin of the upper torso.

Escherichia coli, the most common aerobe seen in stool and intraabdominal abscesses, is cultured only rarely from any abscess and even more occasionally from perineal abscesses. It is a common misconception that foul-smelling pus is due to *E. coli* or other enteric aerobes; in fact, the pus of an *E. coli* abscess is odorless. The foul odor of abscesses in the perirectal area is due to the presence of anaerobic bacteria.

Neisseria gonorrhoeae, which may invade bartholin glands, is uncommon in vulvovaginal abscesses in which there is a predominance of anaerobes. One-third of abscesses seen will contain pure cultures, primarily of *S. aureus,* while anaerobes rarely exist in pure culture. Drug abuse–related abscesses often have more cellulitis, induration, and regional node involvement. Moreover, their course of development is often more rapid from the onset. This clinical picture is most likely due to the injection of necrotizing chemical irritants, not only from the drug itself but from other adulterants, resulting in sterile abscesses.

Table 106-1. Frequency of Isolation of *Bacteroides Fragilis*

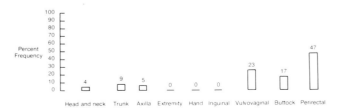

Percent chance of finding *Bacteroides fragilis* in each area

Table 106-2. Frequency of Isolation of *Staphylococcus aureus*

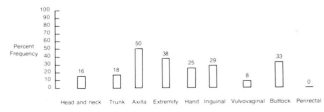

Percent chance of finding *Staphylococcus aureus* in each area

Table 106-3. Frequency of Isolation of *Proteus mirabilis*

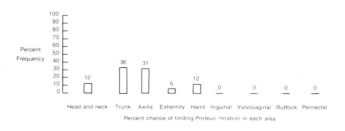

Percent chance of finding *Proteus mirabilis* in each area

Gram Stains

The Gram-stained smear is a reliable, quick, and readily available method of identifying offending pathogens from soft-tissue infections. With this method of presumptive identification, a rational choice of an appropriate antibiotic may be made before culture results are known. Unfortunately, the Gram-stained smear of an abscess will not differentiate aerobes from anaerobes. However, three specific patterns of Gram-stain morphology are consistently helpful:

1. If a Gram-stained smear of pus (carefully aspirated from an abscess cavity) shows only large gram-positive cocci in grape-like clusters, the abscess is almost certainly infected with *S. aureus*, which has been shown to exist most often in pure culture.
2. Gram-stained smears that show no bacteria at all are most likely from sterile abscesses.
3. A mixed Gram-stained pattern, with combinations of gram-positive and gram-negative cocci and rods, is indicative of a mixed aerobic and anaerobic infection.

CLINICAL PRESENTATION

Cutaneous abscesses occur in all areas of the body. Interruptions of the integrity of the protective epithelial layer of skin by minor traumas, such as cuts and abrasions, allow the normal flora of the skin and adjacent mucous membranes to invade the sterile subcutaneous spaces. Abscesses also originate within obstructed apocrine and sebaceous glands. These latter subcutaneous abscesses occur most often in the perirectal, axillary, and head and neck areas, which are richly endowed with these glands. The apocrine and sebaceous glands become active only after puberty, which probably accounts for the increased incidence of abscesses in adults.

Perirectal abscesses commonly arise from anal crypts, pilonidal abscesses often result from infection secondary to an ingrown hair and vulvovaginal abscesses usually begin in obstructed Bartholin's glands. In general, men present with head and neck, perirectal, and extremity abscesses while women present with axillary, vulvovaginal, and perirectal abscesses.

Patients most frequently complain of localized pain and swelling around the abscess site. Most date the onset of symptoms within the preceding week. Patients frequently attempt self-treatment by repeatedly squeezing or pinching the abscess soon after the onset is noted and may come to the physician with a traumatized, inadequately drained lesion.

Most normal patients who have cutaneous abscesses show little evidence of systemic toxicity. Although a slight tachycardia is common, it may be due to pain or anxiety as well as to the direct toxic effects of the infection. Induration, cellulitis, lymphedema, lymphangitis, and regional lymphadenopathy may be present. Fever is rare. In fact, fever in a patient with a cutaneous abscess may indicate an infection that is not localized. Similarly, fever may be evidence of compromise in the natural host defenses, which could predispose the patient to systemic infection. The physician should look for evidence of trauma, thermal injury, neoplasms (especially leukemia), diabetes mellitus, vascular insufficiency, collagen vascular disease, corticosteroid therapy, and chemotherapy, all of which lower the body's ability to combat infection.

Some patients, despite adequate treatment, may return with nonhealing or frequently recurring abscesses. Those in the perineal area may suggest the presence of an undiagnosed inflammatory bowel disease; 10 percent of patients with Crohn's disease have complications of perirectal abscesses and fistulas. Frequently recurring abscesses in the axillary and inguinal areas may be a sign of hidradenitis suppurativa. Likewise, nonhealing or recurring abscesses may be caused by any of the factors listed above that diminish natural host defenses.

TREATMENT

The primary treatment of the localized cutaneous abscess in the otherwise healthy nontoxic patient is incision and drainage alone. It has been shown that most patients, if treated properly, will not require antibiotics to heal. Taking cultures or preparing Gram-stained smears of the abscess, while providing definitive information about the infection's etiology, is not necessary for a successful outcome in these patients. Antibiotics are generally not indicated (Table 106-4).

Incision and Drainage

It is common to underestimate the extent of the abscess and the amount of pus that needs to be evacuated, especially in perineal and extremity abscesses, where tense induration alone, without fluctuance, may be the only clue to the presence of underlying pus. A physician who is uncertain about whether a subcutaneous infection is a simple cellulitis or an abscess should attempt a needle aspiration of the area. Any amount of aspirated pus is significant, since it indicates the presence of an abscess that usually demands surgical intervention. If no pus is aspirated, the infection is probably a cellulitis that has not yet loculated. These infections may be treated with frequent warm soaks and an anti-

Table 106-4. Treatment of the Cutaneous Abscess

Normal host defenses
  Incision and drainage
  No culture or Gram-stained smear
  No antibiotics
High-risk patient (septic, immunosuppressed, diabetic, special locations)
  Incision and drainage
  Culture and Gram-stained smear
  Antibiotics

biotic whose spectrum covers the common skin flora of the area involved. The efficacy of antibiotics in the treatment of cellulitis has not been documented. However, if antibiotics are used, a specimen for a Gram-stained smear and culture may be obtained by injecting 1 mL of sterile oxygen-free saline (nonbacteriostatic) into the cellulitic area, which is then reaspirated for examination. These patients must be followed until it is certain that the process is resolving, since some of these infections will proceed, despite antibiotics, to abscess formation, requiring incision and drainage.

Incision and drainage constitute an unavoidably painful procedure. Local anesthesia, properly used, anesthetizes only the dermal roof of the abscess. Large volumes of "local," infiltrated around the abscess in an attempt to achieve total anesthesia, only increase the swelling, ultimately causing more pain and further compromise to the blood supply. Regional blocks may provide anesthesia for the drainage of extremity abscesses. It is often comforting to the patient, as well as facilitating for the physician, to premedicate the patient with intramuscular opiates 30 to 40 min prior to the procedure. For a 70 kg patient, a dose of 50 to 100 mg of meperidine hydrochloride or 5 to 10 mg of morphine sulfate, with 25 mg of narcotic potentiator such as promethazine hydrochloride or hydroxyzine should be adequate. If the patient is especially anxious or pain-sensitive, intravenous diazepam, titrated to the level of hypnosis as indicated by slurred speech, may be necessary. Diazepam also has the advantage of being amnestic. In these patients, an intravenous line is indicated and the physician must be ready to intervene with appropriate airway management. Analgesia with 50 percent nitrous oxide is very useful and can be self-administered by the patient.

The patient should be positioned to allow complete visualization of the abscess site. Vulvovaginal abscesses are easily treated with the patient in the lithotomy position. Perirectal and pilonidal abscesses are best treated with the patient in a knee-chest, Sim's, or prone position. Wide adhesive tape extending from the buttock fold to the table edge may be used to retract the buttocks to ensure adequate exposure. The involved site is widely scrubbed with povidone-iodine and surgically draped. If no regional block is used, the skin through which the incision will be made should be anesthetized with 1% lidocaine or ethyl chloride spray to the extent of the fluctuance or, if no fluctuance is evident, over the central area of induration. If anaerobic cultures are needed, pus should be aspirated either percutaneously or immediately after the incision is made to prevent prolonged exposure to air.

An incision is made with a no. 11 scalpel blade into the abscess cavity, extending along the full length of the fluctuance in the plane of the natural skin folds. Bartholin's abscesses should be incised through the mucosal rather than the cutaneous surface. Pus should flow freely, providing adequate material for culture and Gram-stained smear. An abscess is not a simple sphere but includes fingerlike networks of loculated granulation tissue and pus, extending outward along planes of least resistance. Hence, the cavity should be probed radially to break up loculated pockets and thoroughly irrigated with saline until all pus and necrotic debris have been removed. Extreme caution should be used in areas such as the groin and neck, where large and important neurovascular bundle structures are in close proximity. The abscess may then be loosely packed from the skin to its depth with a plain gauze wick. Tight packing of an abscess does not allow drainage and may impede the healing process. It is not necessary to use iodoform gauze. Finally, a dry, absorbent dressing is applied. The perineal area is an especially difficult region in which to maintain an adequate dressing. A sanitary napkin seems to work well with both anterior and posterior abscesses in this area. If the gauze packing inadvertently becomes dislodged, the patient should be instructed not to replace it but rather to begin warm sitz baths for 20 to 30 min four times daily.

The abscess is rechecked in 48 h, except for facial abscesses, which are rechecked in 24 h, at which time the packing is removed. Patients who show minimal drainage, resolution of the surrounding cellulitis, and formation of healing granulation tissue should be instructed to begin warm soaks. Those patients who show continued drainage should have their abscesses repacked and then rechecked in 24 to 48 h. At the time that the infection shows clear signs of healing, no further follow-up is indicated.

Antibiotics

Antibiotics have a place in the treatment of a few specific patients. The use of antibiotics prior to and following incision and drainage has been considered in:

1. The clinically toxic patient with a significant fever
2. The patient with an abscess in the mastoid area or in the central triangle of the face, which is drained by the cavernous sinus
3. The patient at risk owing to systemic disease
4. The patient on immunosuppressive drugs or chemotherapy

For such patients a tentative identification of the invading bacteria may be made by:

1. Correlating the abscess site with the known bacteriologic data for similar sites to indicate the expected microflora of the abscess
2. Finding foul-smelling pus, which often indicates the presence of anaerobes
3. Preparing a Gram-stained smear of the pus, which will correctly identify sterile abscesses, mixed aerobic and anaerobic abscesses, and abscesses infected with S. aureus

Once tentative bacteriologic identification has been made, the most appropriate antibiotic can be chosen. If antibiotics are used for abscesses in the axilla, head, neck, and extremities, an oral antistaphylococcal drug such as dicloxacillin, erythromycin, or cephaloridine is required. Cephalosporins also are effective against P. mirabilis. Patients who are thought to be bacteremic should have blood cultures obtained and should be hospitalized.

Drug-related abscesses often contain penicillin-sensitive anaerobes, and S. aureus is seen less than one-fourth of the time. In patients treated with antibiotics, aerobic and anaerobic cultures should be obtained to identify the specific bacteriologic spectrum of the abscess so that the antibiotic choice can be modified when indicated. In general, B. fragilis is the only anaerobe resistant to penicillin and the aminoglycosides.

Tetracycline is a poor first choice, since many anaerobes are resistant to it. Clindamycin or newer-generation cephalosporin antibiotics are indicated in treating abscesses of the perineal area where anaerobes are suspected. Patients with nonlocalized or deep abscesses, abscesses near neurovascular bundles, or abscesses for which inadequate pain control prohibits complete drainage should be admitted to the hospital and have their abscesses drained in the operating room. Septic or immunosuppressed patients should likewise be admitted.

Cutaneous abscesses have been shown to contain a variety of both aerobic and anaerobic bacteria. Although anaerobes are found in abscesses in all areas of the body, they predominate in the perineal area. In the patient with normal host defenses, treatment of local cutaneous abscess consists of incision and drainage. Culture and antibiotics are generally not indicated.

BIBLIOGRAPHY

Anderson DK, Perry AW: Axillary hidradenitis. *Arch Surg* 110:69–71, 1975.

Brook I, Finegold SM: Aerobic and anaerobic bacteriology of cutaneous abscesses in children. *Pediatrics* 67:891–895, 1981.

Eisenhammer S: The anorectal fistulous abscess and fistula. *Dis Colon Rectum* 9:91–106, 1966.

Finegold SM, Bartlett JG, Chow AW, et al.: Management of anaerobic infections. *Ann Intern Med* 83:375–389, 1975.

Ghoneim ATM, McGoldrick J, Blick PWH, et al.: Aerobic and anaerobic bacteriology of subcutaneous abscesses. *Br J Surg* 68:498–500, 1981.

Gorbach SL, Bartlett JG: Anaerobic infections. *N Engl J Med* 290:1177–1184, 1237–1244, 1289–1294, 1974.

Meislin HW, Lerner SA, Graves MH, et al.: Cutaneous abscesses. Anaerobic and aerobic bacteriology and outpatient management. *Ann Intern Med* 87:145–149, 1977.

Meislin HW, McGehee MD, Rosen P: Management and microbiology of cutaneous abscesses. *J Am Coll Emerg Physicians* 75:5, 1978.

Simms MH, Curran F, Johnson RA, et al.: Treatment of acute abscesses in the casualty department. *Br Med J* 284:1827–1829, 1982.

J. Stephan Stapczynski

TETANUS

Tetanus is a potentially lethal neuroparalytic disease caused by tetanospasmin, an exotoxin elaborated by *Clostridium tetani*. In the United States 95 cases of tetanus were reported in 1980 and 60 cases in 1981. Despite modern medical therapy, tetanus still has a fatality rate over 40 percent. *C. tetani* is a gram-positive anaerobic rod, ubiquitous in nature, found primarily in the soil and feces of many animals, including humans. The organism cannot invade healthy tissue; it requires the proper anaerobic conditions for the spores to convert into toxin-producing vegetative forms.

Tetanospasmin is a protein of approximately 67,000 mol wt. The toxin enters the peripheral nerve endings and ascends the axons to reach the spinal cord and brain, where it irreversibly binds to and affects four areas of the nervous system. The major effect is at the level of the anterior horn cells of the spinal cord, where it causes a release of normal inhibition of muscular antagonists, leading to marked neuromuscular irritability and generalized spasms. The toxin stimulates the sympathetic nervous system, producing sweating, labile blood pressure, peripheral vasoconstriction, and tachycardia. Tetanospasmin inhibits release of acetylcholine at the myoneural junction. The toxin also binds to cerebral gangliosides, which is probably the cause of true seizures seen in some cases. There is no direct effect on the sensorium or sensory function.

Adults at highest risk for tetanus are the elderly, intravenous drug abusers, and those with decubiti or diabetic ulcers. Neonates and intravenous drug abusers have a higher case fatality rate than other patients with tetanus.

Clinical Features

In generalized tetanus, trismus is the presenting symptom in over 50 percent of cases. The severity of tetanus varies inversely with the incubation period. In mild cases the incubation period is longer than 10 days, stiffness is mild and may stay confined to an isolated muscle group (localized tetanus), true dysphagia or spasms never occur, and the case fatality rate is low. Patients with moderate cases experience a shorter incubation period, true dysphagia, and paroxysmal spasms but do not develop respiratory difficulty during attacks. Severe cases involve pronounced spasms with respiratory difficulty: glottal spasm may develop during these attacks, causing respiratory arrest.

Differential Diagnosis

The diagnosis of tetanus is based on the clinical picture—no specific ancillary test exists to make the diagnosis. Strychnine poisoning may mimic tetanus, with opisthotonus and seizures, but the signs resolve relatively quickly with supportive care and the poison is detectable in the urine. Other diseases may mimic parts of the clinical picture of tetanus: acute dystonic reaction to phenothiazines, hypocalcemic tetany, meningitis and encephalitis, early rabies, epileptic seizures, narcotic withdrawal, or localized head and neck infections.

Treatment

Emergency management should include the following:

1. Asphyxia is the most preventable cause of death. Maintaining the airway with endotracheal intubation and mechanical ventilation is necessary in severe cases.
2. Muscular spasms should be controlled with diazepam IV, titrated as needed. Very large doses may be required.
3. Neuromuscular blockade may be necessary to produce the full clinical benefit of mechanical ventilation. Pancuronium is recommended; the initial dose should be 0.06 mg/kg IV, with further doses as needed.
4. Further toxin production should be eliminated by wide surgical debridement of the causative wound.

5. Any remaining unbound toxin should be neutralized with 3000 to 10,000 units of human tetanus immune globulin [TIG (h), (Hyper-tet)] IM. There is no advantage to infiltrating the wound site with TIG. Studies in other countries where tetanus is still a common problem suggest that intrathecal administration of TIG is associated with a lower case fatality rate than intramuscular administration.

6. High doses of intravenous antibiotics are recommended: penicillin G 4 to 6 million units per day is the drug of choice, with tetracycline 2 g/day as the alternative in penicillin-allergic patients.

7. Patients should be in as quiet a room as possible; any stimulation, including noise, may precipitate generalized spasms.

8. Clinical tetanus does not produce immunity; the first dose of tetanus toxoid should be given in the emergency department.

9. If an acute dystonic reaction is a diagnostic possibility, a test dose of diphenhydramine 50 mg or benztropine mesylate 2 mg IV can be given to exclude this diagnosis.

Wound Management

Proper wound care includes cleaning, irrigation, debridement, and removal of foreign bodies from all wounds, even minor puncture wounds, abrasions, and burns. Since tetanus occasionally occurs after trivial wounds (conjunctival foreign body) or even without any detectable skin break, the concept of a clean wound without risk of tetanus is debatable. Current recommendations of the Public Health Service Advisory Committee on Immunization Practices for tetanus prophylaxis in wound management are given in Table 107-1. For children less than 7 years old, diphtheria-tetanus-pertussis vaccine (DTP)—DT if pertussis vaccine is contraindicated—is preferred to tetanus toxoid alone. For those over 7 years old, tetanus-diphtheria toxoid (Td) is preferred to tetanus toxoid alone.

The major hazard of too frequent tetanus toxoid adminstration is the development of an Arthus-type hypersensitivity reaction, generally beginning 2 to 8 h after injection. Systemic reactions such as urticaria or angioneurotic edema have been reported rarely. The only contraindiction to the use of tetanus toxoid is a history of neurologic or severe hypersensitivity reactions; local adverse effects alone do not preclude use. For unimmunized patients, complete protection includes Td at monthly intervals for three doses followed by a booster at 1 year.

Table 107-1. Summary Guide to Tetanus Prophylaxis in Routine Wound Management, 1981

History of Tetanus Immunization	Clean, Minor Wounds		All Other Wounds	
	Td	TIG	Td	TIG
Uncertain	Yes	No	Yes	Yes
0–1	Yes	No	Yes	Yes
2	Yes	No	Yes	No
3 or more and <5 years since last dose	No	No	No	No
3 or more and 5–10 years since last dose	No	No	Yes	No
3 or more and > 10 years since last dose	Yes	No	Yes	No

Source: Data from Immunization Practices Advisory Committee.

GAS GANGRENE

Clostridial myonecrosis, or *gas gangrene,* is a rapidly progressive soft tissue infection with muscle necrosis, gas production, and systemic toxicity. It is caused by one of six species of histotoxic *Clostridia,* with *C. perfringens* being the most common isolate. In the most common presentation of this disease, clostridial spores contaminate wounds when trauma produces an anaerobic environment appropriate for the development and growth of the toxin-producing vegetative forms. These forms elaborate exotoxins, which cause the tissue destruction, hemolysis, and "systemic toxicity" characteristic of gas gangrene. In the United States there are approximately 1000 civilian cases of gas gangrene per year, with a case fatality rate of about 30 percent.

Clinical Presentation

The incubation period is typically short, usually less than 3 days. The onset is acute, the first symptom being a sense of heaviness or weight in the muscle, followed rapidly by severe pain. Systemic toxicity is present, manifested by tachycardia, poor skin perfusion, and alterations in sensorium but usually only a slight elevation in temperature. At this early stage the primary wound is usually not pyogenic and crepitance is minimal. Within hours, a thin, brownish exudate develops and the skin becomes discolored. The discharge contains red cells and clostridia but very few white cells. Gas begins to develop within the muscle and is detected by palpable crepitance or by air visible on x-ray. Large cutaneous bullae filled with purple fluid may eventually appear. Bacteremia occurs in only 15 percent or less of the cases.

Differential Diagnosis

Other rapidly spreading, gas-forming soft tissue infections may be confused with gas gangrene: crepitant cellulitis, synergistic necrotizing cellulitis, necrotizing fasciitis, acute streptococcal hemolytic gangrene, and streptococcal myositis. While these syndromes may have a distinctive picture in their pure state, in practice it is often difficult to make a firm clinical diagnosis. Surgical exploration of the involved fascia and muscle is mandatory for correct diagnosis. In the early stage of gas gangrene the muscles are edematous and pale and still bleed when cut. Later, contractility is lost and dissection reveals beefy red, nonbleeding muscle tissue with gas bubbles between the fibers. Gram stain of the exudate or muscle tissue shows the gram-positive rods and very few leukocytes.

Treatment

Emergency management should include the following:

1. Immediate resuscitation requires volume expansion and blood to counteract shock and replenish red cells lost to hemolysis.

2. Antibiotics are recommended to suppress the spread of infection and treat bacteremia; they appear beneficial in animal models. Penicillin G 10 to 30 million units per day IV is the drug of choice, with chloramphenicol 4 g per day the alternative in penicillin-allergic patients. Some histotoxic clostridia

are resistant to tetracycline. Prior to surgery other gas-forming soft tissue infections may be a diagnostic possibility. Antibiotics to treat possible anaerobes (clindamycin or chloramphenicol), gram-negative rods (aminoglycosides), or staphylococci (semisynthetic penicillinase-resistant penicillin or vancomycin) should be given prior to surgery. The combination of cefoxitin 80 to 160 mg/(kg·day)and gentamicin 2 to 4 mg/(kg·day) IV in divided doses is a combination that provides adequate coverage in this situation.

3. Clearly, surgical debridement is the cornerstone of therapy, but the timing of surgery is less clear. Some authorities would delay definitive debridement until after 2 to 3 hyperbaric oxygen treatments in hope of limiting the eventual surgery required. Nevertheless complete removal of all infected tissue is the only therapeutic modality of proven effectiveness.

4. Hyperbaric oxygen is said to limit tissue necrosis, allow for better demarcation between viable and nonviable tissue at surgery, and reduce mortality from systemic toxicity. Partial pressures of oxygen (P_{O_2}) above 250 mmHg stop α-toxin production by the vegetative forms and P_{O_2}'s above 1520 mmHg are bactericidal to clostridia. Hyperbaric treatments are typically given with 100% oxygen at 3 atm pressure for 90 min, with two or three treatments in the first 24 h.

5. Polyvalent gas gangrene antitoxin should not be given. Antitoxin is theoretically of limited value, is unproven in animal or human studies, and has about a 10 percent incidence of allergic reactions.

6. Prevention of gas gangrene is best accomplished by care of the primary wound. There is evidence that prophylactic penicillin at the time of initial injury might reduce the incidence of clostridial infection, but the protection is not absolute.

7. The responsibility of the emergency physician is to recognize this very serious infection, initiate the resuscitation, and deliver the patient to wherever definitive care can be rendered.

CELLULITIS

Cellulitis is an inflammatory infection of the subcutaneous tissues, usually due to staphylococci and/or streptococci or, in young children, *Hemophilus*. In the preantibiotic era simple cellulitis had up to a 25 percent mortality.

Clinical Features

Simple cellulitis usually presents with local erythema and tenderness. Occasionally, spreading lymphangitis and regional lymphadenopathy are seen. If the condition is untreated, induration and suppuration develop. Fever, leukocytosis, or bacteremia is unusual in previously healthy individuals with simple cellulitis. Blood or wound cultures are usually not helpful in patients with simple cellulitis who can be treated as outpatients with oral antibiotics.

Treatment

1. Facial cellulitis in children is occasionally due to *Hemophilus influenzae* and may entail a high rate of bacteremia. Because of these risks admission to the hospital and treatment with intravenous antibiotics is advised. Coverage for possible pathogens include ampicillin 100 mg/(kg·day) or chloramphenicol 100 mg/(kg·day) to cover for *H. influenzae*, along with a penicillinase-resistant penicillin, [oxacillin 50 mg/(kg·day), or nafcillin 25 mg/(kg·day)] to cover for staphylococci or streptococci. Cefamandole 50 to 100 mg/(kg·day) can be used to cover for both *H. influenzae* and staphylococci.

2. Adults with cellulitis of the head or neck should probably be admitted for intravenous antibiotics. A penicillinase-resistant penicillin, cephalosporin, or vancomycin should be used.

3. Adults or children with cellulitis of either the trunk or extremity can usually be treated as outpatients with either an oral penicillinase-resistant penicillin, cephalosporin, or erythromycin.

4. Patients with high fever, systemic toxicity, poor host resistance (e.g., that due to diabetes, alcoholism, or immunosuppression), or underlying skin disease should have their cellulitis treated in the hospital with intravenous antibiotics.

ERYSIPELAS

Erysipelas is a distinctive variety of cellulitis caused by group A streptococci. This uncommon disease is found in infants, the elderly, and patients with predisposing skin ulcers. Usually it is found on the face, scalp, extremities, or genitalia, but it may occur anywhere.

Clinical Features

Erysipelas starts with the appearance of a small, raised, red, and painful plaque. The lesion expands slowly over several days to reach a maximal size around 10 to 15 cm. A sharp and distinct advancing edge is characteristic. Severe systemic toxicity, high fever, leukocytosis (around 20,000), and bacteremia are common. During convalescence, the rash desquamates. Untreated cases have about a 40 percent mortality.

Treatment

1. The patient should be admitted to the hospital. The affected part should be rested and elevated if possible, and wet dressings should be applied.

2. Penicillin G 4 to 6 million units per day IV should be given. Erythromycin or clindamycin can be used in penicillin-allergic patients. Clinical improvement is usually seen in 24 h.

BIBLIOGRAPHY

Tetanus

Armitage P, Clifford R: Prognosis in tetanus: Use of data from therapeutic trials. *J Infect Dis* 138:1, 1978.

Furste W: Editorial. The fifth international conference on tetanus, Ronneby, Sweden, 1978. *J Trauma* 20:101, 1980.

Furste W: Editorial. The sixth international conference on tetanus, Lyon, France, 1981. *J. Trauma* 22:1032, 1982.

Immunization Practices Advisory Committee: Diphtheria, tetanus, and pertussis: Guidelines for vaccine prophylaxis and other preventative measures. *MMWR* 30:392, 1981.

Jacobs RL, Lowe RS, Lanier BQ: Adverse reactions to tetanus toxoid. *JAMA* 247:40, 1982.

Rothstein RJ, Baker FJ: Tetanus. Prevention and management. *JAMA* 240:675, 1978.

Weinstein L: Current concepts. Tetanus. *N Engl J Med* 289:1293, 1973.

Leung FW, Serota AI, Mulligan ME, et al.: Nontraumatic clostridial myonecrosis: An infectious disease emergency. *Ann Emerg Med* 10:312, 1981.

Weinstein L, Barza MA: Current concepts. Gas gangrene. *N Engl J Med* 289:1129, 1973.

Gas Gangrene

Caplan ES, Kluge RM: Gas gangrene. Review of 34 cases. *Arch Intern Med* 136:788, 1976.

Darke SG, King AM, Slack WK: Gas gangrene and related infection: Classification, clinical features and aetiology, management and mortality. A report of 88 cases. *Br J Surg* 64:104, 1977.

Guidi ML, Proletti R, Carducci P, et al.: The combined use of hyperbaric oxygen, antibiotics and surgery in the treatment of gas gangrene. *Resuscitation* 9:267, 1981.

Kizer KW, Ogle LC: Occult clostridial myonecrosis. *Ann Emerg Med* 10:307, 1981.

Cellulitis and Erysipelas

Fleisher G, Ludwig S, Henretig F, et al.: Cellulitis: Initial management. *Ann Emerg Med* 10:356, 1981.

Ginsberg MB: Cellulitis: Analysis of 101 cases and review of the literature. *South Med J* 74:530, 1981.

Ho PWL, Pien FD, Hamburg D: Value of cultures in patients with acute cellulitis. *South Med J* 72:1402, 1979.

Uman SJ, Kunin CM: Needle aspiration in the diagnosis of soft tissue infections. *Arch Intern Med* 135:959, 1975.

CHAPTER 108
TOXIC SHOCK
SYNDROME

Ann L. Harwood

OVERVIEW

Toxic shock syndrome (TSS) was first described by Todd in seven children with Staphylococcus aureus infections. TSS is an acute febrile syndrome characterized by diffuse, desquamating erythroderma, mucous membrane hyperemia, vomiting, diarrhea, pharyngitis, and myalgias. It may progress rapidly to hypotension and multisystem dysfunction. There exists a convalescent peeling of digits, palms, and soles. Clinical recurrences seem to be the most common sequelae of TSS. In Table 108-1, a TSS case definition is given, and despite the general consensus of this case definition, there still is speculation regarding the existence and identification of less severe (subclinical) cases. This is in large part due to the fact that a definitive laboratory marker has not yet been confirmed.

Over the past 5 years the number of cases of TSS has increased dramatically, the disorder having been most evident in Minnesota and Wisconsin in late 1979 and early 1980. Epidemiological studies show that TSS can occur in men and children with focal staphylococcal infections, although the majority of cases occur among menstruating women. Continuous tampon use has been shown to be an important risk factor in these women.

PATHOGENESIS

In all reported cases of TSS, the association with coagulase-positive staphylococci has been consistent. The most impressive aspect of the pathogenesis of TSS appears to be the massive vasodilatation and rapid movement of serum proteins and fluids from the intravascular to the extravascular space. This is manifested by the rapid onset of oliguria, hypotension, edema, low central pressure, and the requirement for large amounts of fluid to restore and maintain blood pressure. The multisystem involvement seen in TSS may be a reflection of the rapid onset of hypotension and decreased perfusion, or there may be a direct effect of a toxin or toxins on the parenchymal cells of different organs. The precise pathogenesis of TSS remains unknown but current evidence suggests that pyrogenic exotoxin C, staphyloccocal enterotoxin F, or both, may play an important role. It is possible that these two toxins may enhance susceptibility to normal or sublethal amounts of endotoxin as well as directly damage cell membranes, thereby activating coagulation, kinin, and prostaglandin cascades.

The means by which S. aureus enters the host in TSS are probably numerous. Although an exogenous source of S. aureus has been suggested for nonmenstrual cases, no exogenous source has been identified for menstrual cases. It is presumed that women who develop menstrual TSS were colonized with S. aureus before the onset of menstruation.

CLINICAL FEATURES
AND LABORATORY FINDINGS

The most common form of TSS is that defined in Table 108-1. However, it is clear that this definition may exclude mild cases of TSS that present either as the first or as a recurrent episode. One must keep in mind the spectrum of the disease when evaluating such patients. A milder form of TSS may occur in any patient. It is generally characterized by fever and chills, myalgias, abdominal pain, sore throat, nausea, vomiting, and diarrhea. Hypotension does not occur and the illness is self-limited.

Severe TSS is an acute-onset, multisystem disease with symptoms, signs, and laboratory abnormalities reflecting multiple-organ involvement. Some patients may experience a prodrome consisting of malaise, myalgias, headache, and nausea. Most patients, however, will present with the sudden onset of fever and chills, headache, nausea, vomiting, and diarrhea. The patient may additionally complain of abdominal pain, cough, or sore throat. Patients may show edema of the face and extremities. Orthostatic lightheadedness or syncope may be present. In general, victims of TSS appear acutely ill upon admission. In the acute state, which usually lasts about 24 to 48 h, the patient may be obtunded, disoriented, oliguric, and hypotensive. Dermatologic manifestations include erythema of the skin and mucous membranes. Between the fifth and tenth hospital days a generalized pruritic maculopapular rash develops in about 25 percent of patients. In all cases, a fine generalized desquamation of the skin, with peeling over the soles, fingers, toes, and palms, occurs between 6 and 14 days after the onset of the illness. More than 50 percent of severely ill patients experience loss of hair and nails 2 to 3 months later. Other prominent signs and symptoms may include profound muscle

Table 108.1 Revised Case Definition of Toxic Shock Syndrome

Fever: temperature ≥ 38.9°C (102°F)

Rash: diffuse macular erythroderma

Desquamation 1 to 2 weeks after onset of illness, particularly of palms and soles

Hypotension: systolic blood pressure ≤ 90 mmHg for adults or below fifth percentile by age for children below 16 years of age; orthostatic drop in diastolic blood pressure ≥ 15 mmHg from lying to sitting; orthostatic syncope; or orthostatic dizziness

Multisystem involvement: three or more of the following:

  Gastrointestinal: vomiting or diarrhea at onset of illness

  Muscular: severe myalgia or creatine phosphokinase level at least twice the upper limit of normal for laboratory

  Mucous membrane: vaginal, oropharyngeal, or conjunctival hyperemia

  Renal: BUN or creatinine at least twice the upper limit of normal for laboratory or urinary sediment with pyuria (≥ 5 leukocytes per high-power field) in the absence of urinary tract infection

  Hepatic: total bilirubin, SGOT*, SGPT† at least twice the upper limit of normal for laboratory

  Hematologic: plateles ≥ 100,000/mm³

  Central nervous system: disorientation or alterations in consciousness without focal neurologic signs when fever and hypotension are absent

Negative results on the following tests, if obtained:

  Blood, throat, or cerebrospinal fluid cultures (blood culture may be positive for *Staphylococcus aureus*)

  Rise in titer to Rocky Mountain spotted fever, leptospirosis, or rubeola

*SGOT denotes serum aspartate (glutamic oxaloacetic) transaminase.

†SGPT denotes serum alanine (glutamic pyruvic) transaminase.

Source: Reingold et al.: *Ann Intern Med* 96:875, 1982.

weakness and tenderness and/or abdominal pain and tenderness; vomiting and diarrhea persist. The diarrhea is usually watery and profuse. Specific focal neurologic findings rarely occur but altered states of consciousness are common. Figure 108-1 illustrates the temporal relationships of the major manifestations.

Abnormal laboratory values have been remarkably consistent in the patient with severe TSS (Table 108-2). The majority of patients have leukocytosis, with increased and circulating immature granulocytes, prolonged prothrombin and partial thromboplastin times, hypocalcemia, low serum protein and albumin, and elevated blood urea nitrogen (BUN) alanine transaminase, bilirubin, and creatine kinase levels. Mild normochromic, normocytic, nonhemolytic anemia, thrombocytopenia, hypophosphatemia, and elevated serum creatinine are less common. If the patient's shock is severe, one will also note an acidotic pH.

Differential Diagnosis

There are other systemic illnesses characterized by fever, rash, and multisystem involvement that resemble TSS (Table 108-3). Kawasaki's disease (mucocutaneous lymph node syndrome) is characterized by fever, conjunctival hyperemia, and erythema of the mucous membranes with desquamation. The differentiation of Kawasaki's disease from TSS lies in the fact that more than 99 percent of those afflicted with Kawasaki's disease are under 7 years of age and it is not characterized by hypotension, renal failure, or thrombocytopenia. Septic shock must always be considered in the differential diagnosis of TSS. In general, the appearance of a rash and the characteristic laboratory abnormalities will aid in distinguishing these two entities. Scalded-skin syn-

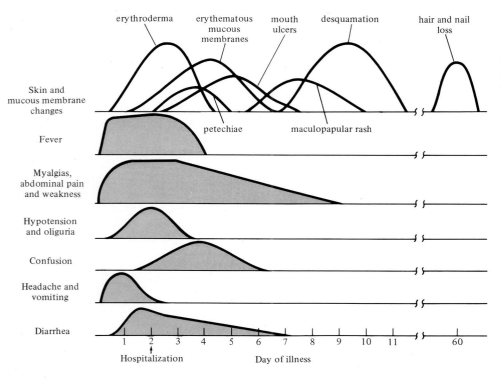

Figure 108-1. Composite drawing of major systemic, skin, and mucous membrane manifestations of toxic shock syndrome. (From Chesney et al: *JAMA* 246, 741–748, 1981.)

Table 108-2. Important Laboratory Abnormalities
(First Two Days of Hospitalization)

1. Present in > 85% of Patients*
   Coagulase-positive staphylococci in cervix or vagina
   Immature and mature polymorphonuclear cells > 90% of WBCs
   Total lymphocyte count < 650/mm³
   Total serum protein level < 5.6 g/dL
   Serum albumin level < 3.1 g/dL
   Serum calcium level < 7.8 mg/dL
   Serum creatinine clearance < 1.0 mg/dL
   Serum bilirubin value > 1.5 mg/dL
   Serum cholesterol level ≤ 120 mg/dL
   Prothrombin time > 12 s
2. Present in > 70% of Patients*
   Platelet count < 150,000/mm³
   Pyuria of > 5 WBCs per high-power field
   Proteinuria ≥ 2+
   BUN > 20 mg/dL
   SGOT > 41 units/L

*Results were available for at least 18 patients per category with the following exceptions: cervicovaginal cultures (12 patients), cholesterol level (15 patients), and prothrombin time (14 patients).

Source: Chesney et al.: *JAMA* 246:741–748, 1981

drome may be distinguished from TSS primarily by the lack of serious multisystem involvement.

MANAGEMENT

Management of TSS will vary depending on the severity of its presentation and the complications. Until an antitoxin is available, the most important aspect of acute management will be the use of fluids to restore intravascular volume. It is imperative to provide continuous monitoring of heart rate, respiratory rate, arterial blood pressure, urinary output, central venous pressure, and pulmonary capillary wedge pressure. During the first 24 h, patients with TSS may require 4 to 5 L of crystalloids and fresh frozen plasma. Pressor agents may be used if volume correction fails to restore normal arterial pressure. In addition to pulmonary wedge pressure,

Table 108-3. Differential Diagnosis of Toxic Shock Syndrome

Acute pyelonephritis
Septic shock
Acute rheumatic fever
Streptococcal scarlet fever
Staphylococcal scarlet fever
Legionnaires' disease
Pelvic inflammatory disease
Hemolytic uremic syndrome
Acute viral syndrome
Leptospirosis
Systemic lupus erythematosus
Rocky Mountain spotted fever
Tick typhus
Gastroenteritis
Kawasaki's disease

Source: Chesney et al.: *JAMA* 246, 741–748, 1981.

chest radiographic findings, blood gases, and serum electrolytes should be monitored. Close monitoring of these variables will lead to early recognition and management of complications.

If adult respiratory distress syndrome occurs, both mechanical ventilation and positive end-expiratory pressure will likely be necessary. Urinary output as well as renal function must be monitored hourly. Appropriate cultures should be obtained and the vaginal tampon, if present, should be removed. Some authors recommend irrigating the vagina with copious amounts of normal saline.

Although antimicrobial agents have not been shown to affect the outcome of the acute illness, they are recommended and have been given to most patients to eradicate the focus of toxin-producing staphylococci as well as to decrease the recurrence rate. Administration of intravenous methicillin or a cephalosporin in the highest recommended doses should be begun. The value of steroids is unproven in TSS. If the differential diagnosis of TSS includes septic shock, intravenous methylprednisolone may be beneficial. The majority of patients will become afebrile and normotensive within 48 h of hospitalization. The laboratory abnormalities seen initially will resolve within 1 to 2 weeks. Full anemia correction occurs in 4 to 6 weeks.

Sequelae

Potential sequelae of TSS include late onset rash, decreased renal function, prolonged neuromuscular abnormalities, and cyanotic extremities. The exact mechanism associated with the appearance of these is not yet clear. Possible explanations may include a delayed effect of the toxin, the presence of circulating immune complexes, or drug-mediated reaction.

Recurrences

TSS has a high tendency to recur. Up to 60 percent of patients who were not treated with β-lactamase-resistant antimicrobial drugs have had recurrences. Most recurrent episodes occur by the second month following the initial episode, although some have recurred in less than 1 month and some, more than 1 year later. In the majority of patients having a recurrence, it has been found that the initial episode has been the most severe, although deaths from severe recurrences have occurred from an initially mild case of TSS. As mentioned above, the usefulness of β-lactamase-resistant antimicrobials, as well as the discontinuation of tampon use have been substantiated in eradicating coagulase-positive staphylococci. Both these modalities have been shown to be instrumental in decreasing the incidence of recurrences.

NONMENSTRUAL TOXIC SHOCK SYNDROME

Although TSS has clearly been shown to predominantly affect previously healthy young women during their menstrual periods, the proportion of reported cases not associated with menstruation has been increasing. These cases either are associated with *S. aureus* infections or follow childbirth by vaginal delivery or cesarean section. Cases of TSS associated with subcutaneous and cutaneous lesions and with surgical wound infections show that life-threatening illness can result from innocuous or inapparent infections with *S. aureus* at these sites. Staphylococcal infections at virtually any site can be responsible for producing TSS.

Patients with TSS not associated with menstruation differ in age and racial distributions from those with menstruation-associated TSS, one-third of them being male. It is clear that TSS can occur in many clinical settings in patients of both sexes and of all ages and racial groups.

BIBLIOGRAPHY

Altemeir WA, Lewis SA, Schlievert PM, et al.: *Staphylococcus aureus* associated with toxic shock syndrome: Phage typing and toxin capability testing. *Ann Intern Med* 96:978–982, 1982.

Bergdoll MS, Crass BA, Reiser RF, et al.: A new staphylococcal enterotoxin, enterotozin F, associated with toxic-shock-syndrome *Staphylococcus aureus* isolates. *Lancet:* 1017–1021, May 9 1981.

Bergdoll MS, Crass BA, Reiser RF, et al.: An enterotoxin-like protein in *Staphylococcus aureus* strains from patients with toxic shock syndrome. *Ann Intern Med* 96:969–971, 1982.

Chesney PJ, Crass BA, Polyak MB, et al.: Toxic shock syndrome: Management and long-term sequelae. *Ann Intern Med* 96:847, 1982

Chesney PJ, Davis JP, Purdy WK, et al.: Clinical manifestations of toxic shock syndrome. *JAMA* 246:741–748, 1981.

Davis JP, Chesney PJ, Wand PJ, et al.: Toxic-shock syndrome. *N Engl J Med* 303:1429–1435, 1980.

Davis JP, Vergeront JM, Chesney PJ: Possible host-defense mechanisms in toxic shock syndrome. *Ann Intern Med* 96:986–991, 1982.

De Saxe JM, Wieneke AA, De Azevedo J, et al.: Staphylococci associated with toxic shock syndrome in the United Kingdom. *Ann Intern Med* 96:991–996, 1982.

Larkin SM, Williams DN, Osterholm MT, et al.: Toxic shock syndrome: Clinical, laboratory, and pathologic findings in nine fatal cases. *Ann Intern Med* 96:858–864, 1982.

Larsen B, Galask RP: Vaginal microbial flora: Composition and influences of host physiology. *Ann Intern Med* 96:926, 1982.

Maya M, Harwood AL: Toxic shock syndrome. *Ann Emerg Med* 11:75–79, 1982.

Reingold Al, Dan BB, Shands KN, et al.: Toxic-shock syndrome not associated with menstruation. *Lancet:* 1–4, Jan. 2, 1982.

Reingold AL, Hargrett NT, Dan BB, et al.: Nonmenstrual toxic-shock syndrome. *Ann Intern Med* 96:871–874, 1982.

Reingold AL, Hargrett NT, Shands KN, et al.: Toxic shock syndrome surveillance in the United States, 1980 to 1981. *Ann Intern Med* 96:875, 1982.

Schlievert PM, Kelly JA: Staphylococcal pyrogenic exotoxin type C: Further characterization. *Ann Intern Med* 96:982, 1982.

Schlievert PM, Osterholm MT, Kelly JA, et al.: Toxin and enzyme characterization of *Staphylococcus aureus* isolates from patients with and without toxic shock syndrome. *Ann Intern Med* 96:937–939, 1982.

Shands KN, Schlech WF, Hargrett NT, et al.: Toxic shock syndrome: Case-control studies at the Center for Disease Control. *Ann Intern Med* 96:895–898, 1982.

Shands KN, Schmid GP, Dan BB, et al.: Toxic-shock syndrome in menstruating women. *N Engl J Med* 303:1436–1442, 1980.

Stallones RA: A review of the epidemiologic studies of toxic shock syndrome. *Ann Intern Med* 96:917–920, 1982.

Todd J: Toxic Shock Syndrome: A perspective through the looking glass. *Ann Intern Med* 96:839–842, 1982.

Tofte RW, Williams DN: Toxic shock syndrome: Clinical and laboratory features in 15 patients. *Ann Intern Med* 94:149–156, 1981.

Tofte RW, Williams DN: Clinical and laboratory manifestations of toxic shock syndrome. *Ann Intern Med* 96:843–847, 1982.

Wannamaker LW: Toxic shock: Problems in definition and diagnosis of a new syndrome. *Ann Intern Med* 96:775–777, 1982.

CHAPTER 109
SEXUALLY
TRANSMITTED
DISEASES

David Nolan

Venereal or sexually transmitted diseases (STDs) have been regarded as including gonorrhea and syphilis (the major STDs) and chanchroid, lymphogranuloma venereum, and granuloma inguinale (the minor STDs). Other infections have also been known to be transmittable by genital contact: pubic lice, candidiasis, trichomoniases, herpes progenitalis. More recently, other conditions have been recognized as having venereal transmission potential, especially among homosexual and bisexual males. These include hepatitis B, numerous fecal-oral transmitted diseases, and acquired immune deficiency syndrome (AIDS).

These seldom present as true emergencies except for urinary obstructions or pelvic inflammatory disease (PID), but the patient may be having significant symptoms for which cure and amelioration is possible. The patient may also be aided by the discovery or prevention of another STD while the one that caused the visit is attended to. Further, the welfare of persons having sexual or other contacts with the patient, including children, may be served by the treatment of and advice to the patient. Lastly, in most states report of known or suspected STD is required of licensed practitioners.

The incidence and relative frequency of STDs are indicated by these recent (provisional) cases appearing in the California Department of Public Health's 1982 reports. Considerable underreporting is, of course, suspected:

Chancroid	323
Gonorrhea	112,032
Granuloma inguinale	4
Lymphogranuloma venereum	27
Syphilis	4,151

The basic information that follows can be augmented by most general texts, and updates on newer trends, cautions, and treatment revisions can be found in Morbidity and Mortality Weekly Reports and Medical letters, among other sources.

GONORRHEA

Gonorrhea (GC) is extremely common. It usually presents in the male as a purulent urethral discharge frequently associated with dysuria. The symptoms in the female are similar but more often overlooked. A considerable minority of cases are asymptomatic. In either sex, pharyngeal or anal infection may occur.

Complications more likely to come to emergency attention occur in the female as a result of invasion via the genital tract, producing PID, or in either sex after hematogenous spread to joints, heart, or meninges. All these can be destructive of tissue or life-threatening.

Diagnosis is made by smear of a discharge or lesion revealing gram-negative intracellular diplococci, together with culture of the organism *Neisseria gonorrhoeae*. Failure to obtain a positive smear or culture is common. Repeated cultures, including anal and pharyngeal, may be necessary to obtain a positive. Treatment is frequently started upon adequate suspicion or upon knowledge of exposure.

The disease is acquired by contact, usually genital, with an infected individual, but contamination of fingers or fomites can transmit the disease to another body site (e.g., the eyes) or another person. GC may also be acquired at birth in the vaginal canal. In young children it should be regarded as evidence of child abuse.

The incubation period is a few days to about a week and the communicable period is variable; if the case is untreated, it may be prolonged. The disease may be self-limiting. Communicability ceases promptly upon start of appropriate treatment. Treatment of adults usually employs one of the following:

Aqueous procaine penicillin G, 4.8 million units IM, half in each buttock at a single visit with 1 g probenecid PO (this should cure concurrent incubating syphilis)
Ampicillin, 3.5 g as a single oral dose, also with probenecid
Amoxicillin, 3.0 g as a single oral dose, also with probenecid

The above share antigenicity and can not be used if patient has significant penicillin allergy.
For penicillin-allergic individual, the drug of choice is either

Tetracycline HCl, 500 mg, PO qid for 5 days, total 10 g (not in pregnant females or children) or spectinomycin, 2 g as single IM dose.

Posttreatment cultures should be obtained 1 to 2 weeks after completion of treatment to rule out treatment failure. If the failure is due to a penicillinase-producing *N. gonorrhoeae* (PPNG), treatment should be repeated using spectinomycin. Failure may also be due to reinfection from an untreated sexual partner. Concurrent treatment of sexual partners is recommended.

SYPHILIS

Syphilis is a common STD transmitted by genital contact. It can be acquired congenitally and by blood transfusion (if the donor was in a very early stage of the disease). The infectious agent *Treponema pallidum* is a spirochete. It may be found in lesions, in infected mucous membranes, and in saliva, semen, and blood. It may enter via defects in skin or mucous membranes, even those too small to be easily noted.

The disease occurs in recognizable phases:

Primary: occurs with or without an ulcerated, usually genital, lesion approximately 3 weeks after exposure
Secondary: occurs with constitutional signs and/or symptoms and/or skin eruptions within weeks to months
Tertiary: involves cardiovascular and/or neurologic diseases; may take years

The presentation depends upon the stage of disease. All phases call for treatment.

Diagnosis in early phases may be made by examination of material from lesions by dark-field or phase-contrast microscopy. Serologic studies may reveal prior exposure to syphilis without indicating the time since exposure. Biologic false positives do occur. Treatment may be decided upon when prior effective treatment is not known to have been administered.

Treatment of known or suspected cases of primary syphilis through the first year after exposure is as follows:

For patients who can tolerate penicillin:
Benzathine penicillin G 2.4 million units IM, single dose, or
Aqueous procaine penicillin G 4.8 million units as 600,000 IM for 8 days
For those allergic to penicillin:
Tetracycline HC1 500 mg qid, PO for 15 days, or
Erythromycin 500 mg qid, PO for 15 days

Treatment in later stages is as follows:

For patients who can tolerate penicillin:
Benzathine penicillin G, 7.2 million units total as 2.4 million units, IM weekly for three consecutive weeks or
Aqueous procaine penicillin G 9.0 million units total as 600,000 units, IM daily for 15 days
For patients allergic to penicillin:
Tetracycline HC1 500 mg, qid, PO for 30 days or
Erythromycin 500 mg, qid, PO for 30 days

Treatment of the later stages should be followed by examination of serum or cerebrospinal fluid.

MINOR STDs

Chancroid

This disease is caused by *Hemophilus ducreyi,* which is acquired during sexual contact from discharges of ulcerations and/or sup-

purating lymphatic tissue. Lesions usually heal within weeks but are infectious during that time. The incubation period varies from 3 to 14 days.

Presentation is usually with one or more painful necrotic lesions or suppurating lymphadenopathy in the inguinal area. Lesions can also be located elsewhere, depending on the site of inoculation

The diagnosis is suspected on the basis of clinical presentation; a smear and subsequent culture are confirmatory. Histologic characteristics are also regarded as diagnositic.

Treatment is with sulfisoxazole, 4 g daily for 7 to 14 days. Tetracycline hydrochloride 2 g daily for 7 to 10 days may also be used. Drainage of fluctuant lesions hastens recovery.

Lymphogranuloma Venereum

This disease is caused by *Chlamydia trachomatis,* acquired by direct, usually genital, contact with open lesions of an infected individual. It is communicable while active lesions exist, and that may be for years. The incubation period is from 1 to 3 weeks if skin lesions appear first and longer if lymphadenopathy is the presenting sign.

The skin lesions are usually painless and may wax and wane, taking the forms of shallow ulcerations, papular or nodular lesions, or herpetiform vesicles. These are noted most often on genital tissue. Lymphadenopathy in the inguinal region follows. These latter lesions may become fluctuant, bind down overlying skin, and develop sinus tracts. In females sinus formation of greater extent involving the vagina and rectum may occur. Constitutional signs of chills, fever, headache, and general malaise may be present, and infection of the joints and meninges, while uncommon, has been noted. The course may be very prolonged but death is unusual.

Diagnosis is made by identification of leukocytes with intracellular inclusion bodies from aspirates of infected tissue. Culture is diagnostic if the laboratory is capable of *Chlamydia* culture. Biopsy may also reveal characteristic histology.

Treatment is with tetracycline hydrochloride, 500 mg qid PO for 10 days. Longer treatment may be necessary depending upon the extent of disease and the clinical response. Should tetracycline be prohibited by allergy or intolerance, the older therapy with sulfadiazine (4 g daily for 14 to 21 days) may be useful. Incision and drainage of fluctuant lesions may be indicated.

Late complications, including elephantiasis and rectal stricture, are not expected to respond to medications.

Granuloma Inguinale

This disease is caused by *Calymmatobacterium granulomatis*. It is thought to be an STD although heterosexual partners of patients rarely develop the disease. As indicated by the California reports listed above, it is uncommon in the United States. The incubation period may be as long as 3 months.

Presentation depends upon the stage of the disease, which begins as small lesions that are papular, nodular, or vesicular and develop slowly into extensive granulomatous and/or ulcerative lesions. These are found in skin and mucous membranes of the genital, inguinal, and anal areas. They may be quite painless. If they are untreated, great destruction of local tissues ensues. There may be subsequent squamous carcinoma. Healing should begin promptly with treatment. Diagnosis depends upon staining and histology of granulomatous lesions. Treatment is with tetracycline hydrochloride, 2 g, PO daily for 15 days. Streptomycin and chloramphenicol have also been used.

Trichomoniasis

Trichomoniasis is caused by the protozoon *Trichomonas vaginalis*. It is transmitted by contact, usually genital, with infected secretions of the genital and urinary tracts. It is communicable for the duration of the infection. The incubation period is from 4 to 20 days, but is usually about 1 week. Presentation is usually in the female, with vaginitis and copious, foamy yellow discharge, which has a foul odor. Diagnosis is made by identification of the motile parasite on a wet slide by microscopy. Treatment is with metronidazole, 250 mg, PO, tid for 7 days, or 2 g PO as a single dose, or 1 g PO twice for 1 day only. Sexual partners should be treated simultaneously.

Herpes Progenitalis

Herpes progenitalis is a very common disease caused by *Herpesvirus hominis*. Type 2 usually presents as recurring genital lesions of typical clustered vesicles, which can be very painful. Ulceration and crusting precede healing. In females, cervical and vulvar sites are the most common; in males, the glans and prepuce. Lesions may be seen at any site. Newborns who acquire the virus at birth may experience a devastating form of the disease. In females the primary infection may cause a self-limiting meningitis. A possible causal relationship with carcinoma of the cervix is being studied.

Type 1 virus can also cause genital lesions. Acquisition is usually by sexual contact. With or without visible lesions, the infected individual may be shedding virus and is contagious at such a time. The incubation period is 2 to 12 days.

The diagnosis is usually made by clinical findings but can be confirmed by paired sera if it is the primary infection, or more commonly by direct immunofluorescent tests, identification of intranuclear inclusion bodies, or virus isolation, depending upon the laboratory support available.

Treatment is still evolving. Currently it is focused upon various antiviral agents, including idoxuridine, adenine arabinoside, and acyclovir topically. Oral preparations are in trial states. Available evidence supports an improved rate of healing in some cases as well as a reduced time of virus shedding, but not cure.

Acquired Immune Deficiency Syndrome

Acquired immune deficiency syndrome (AIDS) is a newly recognized condition found primarily among male homosexuals and bisexuals and their consorts and, to a lesser extent, some other populations, including Haitians and hemophiliacs. AIDS is suspected to be caused by a communicable viral agent. Its epidemiologic similarity to the distribution of hepatitis B suggests transmission with blood products.

A prodrome of generalized lymphadenopathy is recognized. As the individual develops immune deficiency, any one (or more) of several infections and/or Kaposi's sarcoma may develop. Candidiasis, toxoplasmosis, cryptococcosis, histoplasmosis, mycobacteriosis, and the conditions caused by cytomegalovirus, herpesviruses, and *Pneumocystis carinii* are among the infections. The presentation depends upon which process is surfacing in this immune deficient person. Generally, there will be skin lesions, weight loss, lymphadenopathy, dyspnea, fever, and oral thrush.

The individual complicating processes should be treated as indicated. The underlying immune defect and its causative agent are as yet untreatable.

CHAPTER 110
MENINGITIS

Charles Rennie, III

The symptom complex of meningitis spans a wide spectrum, which ranges from the mild manifestations of some of the viral meningitides to the fulminant course of some of the bacterial variants. In 1978 approximately 17,500 cases of bacterial meningitis alone were estimated by Gold to have occurred in the United States. The diagnosis and treatment of meningitis is a great challenge to the emergency medicine specialist. Astute recognition of symptoms and aggressive management are keys to limiting morbidity and mortality. The mortality of untreated bacterial meningitis exceeds 90 percent; with early appropriate therapy it can be brought down to 10 to 20 percent. Sequelae, too, are significant (up to 70 percent in patients with bacterial meningitis) but can likewise be decreased with prompt therapy.

The primary etiologies of meningitis in the United States are bacterial and viral (with approximately 5000 cases per year being reported to the Center for Disease Control but the actual number being substantially higher). Less common etiologies include fungal, chemical, and neoplastic mechanisms. This discussion will focus primarily on the bacterial and viral diseases, although fungal meningitis will also be discussed. The subject will be approached from the clinician's viewpoint and will proceed from clinical presentation through laboratory work-up, diagnosis, treatment, and prophylaxis.

CLINCIAL PRESENTATION

Both viral and bacterial meningitis may present either acutely (symptoms appear in less than 24 h) or subacutely (symptoms may take as long as 107 days to appear). While bacterial meningitis more often presents acutely (25 percent versus 5 percent for viral), this cannot be used as an adjunct in distinguishing the two etiologies. One should suspect meningitis in any patient with an altered level of consciousness, unexplained seizures, severe unexplained headache, neck stiffness, unexplained fever, or new-onset focal neurological deficits. Although one cannot use these symptoms to distinguish between the two etiologies, they tend to occur more commonly with bacterial meningitis (see Table 110-1). Approximately 80 to 90 percent of patients with bacterial meningitis will have some alteration in level of consciousness, as opposed to only 25 to 50 percent of patients with viral meningitis. Seizures occur in approximately 30 percent of patients with bacterial and approximately 5 percent of patients with viral meningitis. Focal neurological deficits occur in up to 50 percent of patients with bac-

terial (30 percent cranial, 20 percent peripheral) but in less than 10 percent with viral meningitis. Headache, meningeal irritation, and fever are the most ubiquitous concomitants. Headache is usually a prominent symptom in both forms of the disease, although its absence does not exclude the diagnosis. Meningeal irritation is slightly more common in bacterial than in viral meningitis, (80 percent versus 60 to 70 percent) but again is common in both forms. Both forms usually present with fever, but that of the bacterial infection tends to be higher [approximately 80 percent over 38.9°C (102°F) versus 30 to 40 percent for the viral infection].

It must be emphasized that no group of the above symptoms is classic; many variations on the theme can occur. As with many other diseases, the very young and the elderly may present atypically and with considerably fewer symptoms. The very young patient may present with symptoms as ill-defined as irritability and poor feeding, with or without projectile vomiting. The elderly patient may present with nothing more than lethargy.

If the presentation is acute, the initial physical examination should be rapid and must be directed toward getting therapy underway within the first 30 min. Here, the focus is toward determining the presence of papilledema and/or a focal neurological deficit, either of which would be an indication for an emergent computerized tomographic (CT) scan prior to a lumbar puncture (LP). If neither is present, an LP should be performed and the patient started on antibiotics empirically by age and host factors. Only then should the Gram stain be looked at and the physical examination completed.

The complete physical examination, even though interrupted to begin therapy, should be thorough. Key aspects include not only those mentioned above but also a check for nuchal rigidity, Brudzinski's sign (flexion of hips and knees produced by passive neck flexion) and/or Kernig's sign (pain on passive extension of the knee past 120° with the hips flexed). A thorough neurological examination, including mental status, cranial nerve, and peripheral sensory and motor examinations, must be performed. In infants the status of the fontanelles must be assessed. A search for possible sources of infection, including ears, sinuses, posterior oropharynx, genitourinary tract, and chest is likewise important, since it may influence the choice of antibiotics.

The presence of a rash also should be noted. It is not uncommon for patients with viral meningitis (especially that due to the enteroviruses) to have a concomitant maculopapular eruption. A petechial, purpuric, or ecchymotic rash suggests meningococcemia,

Table 110-1. Clinical Findings in Meningitis

	Bacterial	Viral
Acute presentation (symptoms <24 h)	25%	5%
Headache	Prominent	Prominent
Meningeal signs	80%	60–70%
Fever	Common; 80% >38.9°C*	Common; 30–40% >38.9°C*
Alteration in mental status	80–90%	25–50%
Seizures	30%	5%
Focal neurological deficits	50%	<10%

*38.9°C = 102°F

although petechial reactions may also be produced by *Streptococcus pneumoniae*, *Hemophilus influenzae*, or *Staphylococcus aureus*. Even in the patient with a subacute presentation it is important that antibiotics be started within 2 h, so the work-up must be completed within this time frame.

LABORATORY STUDIES

Although other laboratory studies are useful or necessary, the most critical test is a detailed examination of the cerebral spinal fluid (CSF). A number of important considerations are involved in the LP and the examination of the CSF. These are detailed below and in Table 110-2.

Opening Pressure

The normal opening pressure (OP) is 150 ± 33 mmH$_2$O, with 95 percent between 94 and 216. It tends to be higher in patients with bacterial meningitis (the mean was 307 mmH$_2$O and the range 50 to 600 mmH$_2$O in a series of 106 patients), although papilledema is rare. Of patients with elevated pressures, one-third return to normal within 48 h and another third within 6 days. If papilledema or focal neurological deficits are present, the patient should be started on antibiotics empirically and receive an emergent CT scan prior to an LP. If papilledema is absent but the OP is >400 mmH$_2$O, several possible courses of action exist. The examiner can take a small amount of fluid and withdraw the needle (the damage has probably already been done); allow fluid to escape slowly (over minutes) until the pressure is below 200 mmH$_2$O; or initiate measures to decrease intracranial pressure (intubation, hyperventilation, mannitol) with the needle in place prior to removing any CSF. None of these methods has been conclusively demonstrated to be better than any of the others. Tentorial herniation may be manifested by fixed, dilated pupils, decerebrate or decorticate posturing, Cheyne-Stokes respirations, or cranial nerve def-

icits. Should this occur at any point during the LP, immediate measures must be undertaken to lower intracranial pressure.

Protein

Normal CSF protein is 38 ± 10 mg/dL (95 percent between 18 and 58). In viral meningitis protein is usually less than 100; in bacterial meningitis it is usually greater than 150, although there is considerable overlap. Protein also may be elevated in acute chemical meningitis. Normal values are somewhat higher (mean 90 mg/dL) in infants less than 6 months old owing to the immaturity of the blood-brain barrier. If blood is present in the CSF (traumatic LP or subarachnoid hemorrhage), the protein level may be elevated by 1 mg/dL for each 1000 red blood cells (RBCs).

Glucose

The normal steady-state CSF/serum glucose ratio is approximately 0.6. Both the entry and exit of glucose into and out of the CSF is determined by carrier-mediated diffusion. Infants less than 6 months of age have a mean ratio of 0.81, which is due to immaturity of this carrier system. If the serum glucose level changes abruptly, approximately 2 to 4 h is required for the CSF glucose level to equilibrate. Because of the saturation kinetics of the carrier exchange, the normal ratio decreases at higher serum glucose levels; at a serum glucose level of 700 mg/dL the ratio is about 0.4. Glucose levels are generally normal in aseptic meningitis, viral encephalitis, brain abscesses, and subdural empyemas. They are often less than 40 (CSF/serum ratio 0.4) in bacterial, fungal, and tubercular meningitis. Late in these entities, the glucose level may be profoundly depressed (less than 20). Hypoglycorrhachia also is seen in 15 to 20% of patients with subarachnoid hemorrhages, a low being reached 1 to 8 days posthemorrhage. The mechanism for this is unclear.

Cell Count

The normal cell count in the adult CSF is 0 to 5 mononucleated cells per cubic millimeter. In neonates it ranges up to 30 cells per mm^3 [60 percent polymorphonuclear leukocytes (PMNs) and 40 percent mononuclear cells]. In a traumatic tap or after a subarachnoid hemorrhage, one white blood cell (WBC) may be subtracted from the total WBC count in the CSF for each 1000 RBCs. Classically, bacterial meningitis patients have more than 500 WBCs per cubic millimeter, with a preponderance of PMNs, while patients with viral meningitis have less than 100 WBCs per cubic millimeter, with mononuclear leukocytes predominant; unfortunately, presentations often do not fit this picture. About 10 percent

Table 110-2. CSF Findings in Bacterial and Nonbacterial Meningitis

Parameter	Normal	Bacterial	Viral
Opening pressure (mmH$_2$O)	150 ± 33	Mean 307	Normal to sl ↑
Protein (mg/dL)	38 ± 10	>150	<100
CSF/serum glucose ratio	0.6 (Infants 0.81)	<0.4	0.6
Cell count (cells/mm^3)	<3 (mononuclear)	>500 (PMNs predominate)	<100 (mononuclear leukocytes predominate)
Gram stain	No organisms	Positive 70–90%	No organisms

of patients with bacterial meningitis will have less than 50 percent PMNs, while 10 percent of patients with viral meningitis will have more than 90 percent PMNs and 30 to 40 percent will have more than 50 percent PMNs. The initial LP examination in patients with viral meningitis may show a majority of PMNs but within 12 h approximately 90 percent of these patients will show a mononuclear leukocyte–predominant pleocytosis. One may see very low cell counts early in the course of meningitis, particularly with that caused by *Neisseria* or *H. influenzae* but also with overwhelming pneumococcal meningitis. In general, PMNs predominate not only in bacterial meningitis but also in subdural empyemas, ruptured brain abscesses, and chemical meningitis. Viral meningitis, tubercular meningitis, parameningeal osteomyelitis, collagen-vascular disease with CNS manifestations, syphilitic meningitis, viral encephalitis, meningeal neoplasms (and carcinomatosis), and cryptococcal and other fungal meningitides generally show a predominance of mononuclear leukocytes.

If RBCs are seen in the CSF, the most likely cause is either a traumatic LP or a subarachnoid hemorrhage. Cell counts should be done on the first and fourth tubes; approximately equal counts are strongly suggestive of hemorrhage.

On occasion the supernatant liquid of centrifuged CSF may be xanthochromic (a characteristic pink or yellow color). This is due to three pigments—oxyhemoglobin, bilirubin, and methemoglobin—which result from the breakdown of RBCs into their components. Therefore fresh CSF from a traumatic tap should not be xanthochromic. Oxyhemoglobin, which is pink and results from RBC lysis, appears within 4 h of hemorrhage and resolves after 8 to 10 days. Methemoglobin is brownish yellow and results from blood encapsulated in a subdural or intracerebral hematoma. Bilirubin is derived from both RBC lysis and hyperbilirubinemia. In the former it appears at about 10 h and resolves after 2 to 4 weeks. In premature infants xanthochromia due to bilirubin is normal and represents only immaturity of the blood-brain barrier. Xanthochromia may also be caused by hypercarotenemia or markedly elevated CSF protein (>150 mg/dL).

Search for Organisms

Stains and Cultures

The first test to be performed in a search for organisms is the Gram stain of the centrifuged specimen. This should generally yield organisms in 70 to 90 percent of cases, (87 percent as shown in one large series of meningitides caused by common bacterial pathogens—*H. influenzae*, meningococci, and pneumococci). The yield is somewhat lower (50 percent) for gram-negative enteric pathogens and lower still (30 percent) for *Listeria*. False negative results may also occur when the bacterial count in the CSF is less than 1000 per cubic millimeter. With select bacteria such as *H. influenzae* and *S. pneumoniae*, organisms can be identified via a quellung test with specific antisera that yield capsular swelling reactions.

If appropriate, an acid-fast stain also should be performed to search for mycobacteria. Specimens to be examined for the possible presence of fungi should be centrifuged and the sediment examined in India ink and/or 10 percent potassium hydroxide. However, several recent papers, most notably that of McGinnis, detail the low yield of this procedure; *Cryptococcus neoformans,* the most common of the fungal isolates, was detected on the first

LP in only 26.3 percent of 19 patients ultimately demonstrated to have cryptococcal meningitis. Repeat LPs raised this figure to only about 50 percent. Some recent papers emphasize the need for culturing large volumes of CSF (at least 5 mL), and there are numerous case reports of fungi being recovered only after 15- to 30-mL samples were cultured while downplaying the importance of ''wasting'' CSF on centrifugation and India ink stain.

Aerobic cultures should be sent routinely to the laboratory. Martin recommends using two blood agar plates, a chocolate agar plate, and a tube of tryptic soy broth. Anaerobic cultures need not be sent routinely (anaerobic isolates from positive CSF cultures run less than 10 percent) but should be sent in cases of antecedent trauma; previous CNS surgeries such as shunts, craniotomies, and laminectomies; head and/or neck infection or neoplasm; or concomitant or antecedent anaerobic infections or sepsis elsewhere in the body. Aerobic cultures should be held for 4 days before being discarded as negative; if the patient was on antibiotics before the cultures were made, they should be held for 1 week. If any suspicion of bacterial meningitis exists, multiple blood cultures and cultures of any underlying foci of infection should be obtained.

Over the past decade a number of additional diagnostic modalities have been proposed and utilized with varying success. CSF lactate levels have been utilized as a diagnostic adjunct but pose two problems. First, although CSF lactate is elevated to ≥ 35 mg/dL in 90 to 95 percent of cases of confirmed bacterial meningitis, it also is elevated in 20 to 30 percent of patients with presumed viral meningitis. Second, there is a high rate of false positives: craniotomies, CNS ischemia and/or anoxia, subarachnoid hemorrhages, intracranial neoplasms, and even closed head injury can all elevate CSF lactates.

Countercurrent immunoelectrophoresis (CIE) is the most widely used of the new diagnostic modalities. It can be performed rapidly (in substantially less than 1 h) and is effective in detecting antigens of *H. influenzae* group B, *S. pneumoniae*, *N. meningitidis* groups A and C, and group B streptococci. False positives are relatively infrequent. Unfortunately no antiserum is available for *N. meningitidis* group B, which accounts for approximately 50 percent of meningococcal meningitis in the United States. Also, the sensitivity of antisera varies both among species of bacteria and among manufacturers. CIE is useful in early or partially treated meningitis, where a Gram stain may be negative, and in confirming the results of a Gram stain in select bacterial meningitides.

Latex agglutination is another quick (less than 1 h in some cases) and effective method of confirming a bacterial etiology in meningitis. It has been well evaluated and is highly effective in detecting *H. influenzae* group B. Less data are available regarding detection of *S. pneumoniae* and *N. meningitidis* groups A and C, but commercial kits for the testing of both have recently become available. Early work with kits to detect group B streptococci is also promising.

Enzyme immunoassays also have been attempted with several bacteria. Although highly sensitive and requiring only dilute antisera, they are somewhat cumbersome and require 3 to 6 h to complete.

TREATMENT

Acute bacterial meningitis is a severe disease with a fulminant course and a significant mortality. For patients with acute presentations antibiotics should be instituted within 30 min. If the patient exhibits focal neurological deficits or papilledema, antibiotics should be initiated immediately according to age and host defense status (to be discussed below) and the patient should receive an emergent CT scan prior to LP. If the patient shows neither focal deficits nor papilledema, an LP should be performed and the patient started immediately on antibiotics appropriate for age and host defense status *without waiting for the Gram stain*. Antibiotics can be changed later according to the results of the Gram stain and culture.

Subacute presentations allow for a slightly greater work-up before initiating therapy. Here, therapy should be instituted within 2 h of presentation, which allows time to evaluate the Gram stain.

In initiating empirical therapy in patients with suspected bacterial meningitis, it is important that the emergency medicine specialist know which organisms predominate in which age groups and which organisms appear in patients with altered host defenses. A rough breakdown by age group in patients with normal host defenses is seen in Table 110-3.

Of those adults who are eventually diagnosed as having *S. pneumoniae* meningitis, 30 percent will give a history of otitis or mastoiditis and 25 percent will give a history of antecedent pneumonia. Other host factors are likewise (but by no means in all circumstances) linked with certain organisms. Alcoholics are prone to *S. pneumoniae* and *Listeria monocytogenes*. Patients with CNS shunts tend to develop staphylococcal infections. Patients with splenic dysfunction are prone to *S. pneumoniae*, and *H. influenzae* infections. Staphylococci, *S. pneumoniae*, and gram-negative rods predominate in patients with recent craniotomies. Hospital-acquired meningitis is often secondary to infection with gram-negative rods.

Recommended antibiotic regimens for suspected bacterial meningitis vary among authors to some extent, but there is broad general agreement. In infants under 2 months of age, the drugs of choice are ampicillin, 150 to 200 mg/(kg·day) IV in two to four divided doses, and gentamicin, 5 to 7.5 mg/(kg·day) IV or IM in three divided doses. Doses for patients less than 1 week of age should be at the lower end of this spectrum. Documented group B streptococcal meningitis may be treated with 300,000 to 400,000 units/(kg·day) of penicillin. In children from 2 months to 6 years of age, the antibiotics of choice are ampicillin, 300 to 400 mg/(kg·day) in six IV doses, and chloramphenicol, 100 mg/(kg·day) in four IV doses. In patients over 6 years of age penicillin [250,000 units/(kg·day) in four to six IV doses up to age 15, 15 to 20 million units/(kg·day) in six to eight divided doses IV for patients older than 15] or ampicillin [200 to 300 mg/(kg·day) in six divided doses up to age 15, 12 g/(kg·day) in six divided doses in adults] is used. Immune suppressed patients should be started on a regimen of penicillin (or ampicillin), gentamicin, and methicillin. The dosage should be adjusted to cover any organisms for which the patient may be at particular risk and it should also be adjusted in response to Gram stain and culture results.

None of the standard antibiotics used to treat meningitis penetrate the blood-brain barrier well. The penicillins penetrate the normal blood-brain barrier poorly, although their penetration is better under conditions of inflammation. Aminoglycosides penetrate poorly but are in part redeemed by small mean inhibitory concentrations. Chloramphenicol, which penetrates to a greater extent, is unfortunately bacteriostatic rather than bacteriocidal. First- and second-generation cephalosporins penetrate the CSF poorly also, but third-generation cephalosporins diffuse well across the inflamed blood-brain barrier and, in preliminary studies, have been

Table 110-3. Common Etiologies of Bacterial Meningitis

Age/Host Factors	Organism
0–4 weeks	*E. coli*
	Group B streptococci
4–12 weeks	Group B streptococci
	S. Pneumoniae
	L. monocytogenes
3 months–3 years	*H. influenzae* type B
	N. meningitidis
	S. pneumonia
3 years +	*S. pneumonia*
	N. meningitidis
Alcoholics	*S. pneumoniae*
	L. monocytogenes
CNS shunt	*S. aureus*
Splenic dysfunction	*S. pneumoniae*
	H. influenzae
Recent craniotomy	Staphylococci
	S. pneumoniae
	Gram-negative rods
Hospital-acquired meningitis	Gram-negative rods

highly effective in enteric gram-negative meningitis in adults. Moxalactam has been particularly successful in recent small trials. Not only are the concentrations in CSF 10 to 30 percent of those in blood (much better than with older cephalosporins) but mean inhibitory concentrations are approximately one-tenth those of previous cephalosporins. In one study, patients with bacterial meningitis treated with moxalactam showed a 25 percent greater response rate than those with other antibiotics.

OTHER CONSIDERATIONS

A number of vexing questions face the emergency medicine specialist in treating the meningitis patient. What if the LP is normal? Could the patient still have meningitis? The answer is yes, although such cases are rare. All such patients have shown clinical signs strongly suspicious of meningitis. A repeat LP in 8 to 36 h will generally show infection. Patients in whom the diagnosis is suspected should be admitted and observed and/or treated. A repeat LP should be performed in 8 to 12 h. If suspicion is high, antobiotic therapy should be initiated empirically prior to the second LP.

When is a repeat LP indicated? Several circumstances (other than that cited above) dictate a repeat LP: (1) a lapse of 24 to 48 h after initiating antibiotic therapy, at which time the culture and Gram stain should be negative (2) an initial LP in suspected viral meningitis (untreated) that shows a predominance of PMN leukocytes (90 percent will show lymphocyte predominance within 12 h) and (3) failure of any meningitis patient to improve or doubtfulness of the diagnosis.

What about patients who have received prior antibiotics (up to 50 percent in some series)? This has little effect on the overall WBC count but may decrease the number of PMNs to the "aseptic" meningitis range. The yield for the Gram stain and culture will decrease by 10 to 20 percent and that for blood cultures will decrease by 50 percent.

Under what circumstances can patients with presumed viral meningitis be sent home from the emergency department? The diagnosis of viral meningitis is usually made from both the LP and the clinical setting; generally the LP is typical and the patients are often young, present particularly in the early fall, and may have associated viral symptoms. Unfortunately, the symptoms overlap the clinical picture of bacterial meningitis, and 10 percent of patients with viral meningitis progress to severe symptoms. Only the most reliable of patients with clear-cut symptomatology should be managed as outpatients, and even these should be followed closely. If even slight doubt exists as to the diagnosis, the patient should be admitted and observed.

Finally, what should be done for those patients when it is necessary to transfer them to another facility? Any patients who show evidence of increased intracranial pressure or focal neurological deficits should not be transferred. Those who are transferred should have an LP performed and CSF and other appropriate cultures taken and should be on antibiotics. Cultures should either be sent with the patient (if practical) or incubated at the transferring institution. At least one spare tube of CSF should be sent with the patient.

SUMMARY

Meningitis represents a potentially high-morbidity, high-mortality group of diseases which challenges the emergency medicine specialist to provide rapid diagnosis and effective therapy. Patients who present with acute, fulminant symptoms should have antibiotics initiated within 30 min and prior to the LP; the choice and dosage of antibiotics should be determined by age and host factors and may require later adjustment based on CSF findings. Patients with more indolent symptoms should have antibiotics initiated within 2 h, which allows time for CSF examination prior to initiating therapy. Patients with neurological deficits or elevated intracranial pressure should receive an immediate CT scan after antibiotics are initiated empirically. No constellation of signs or symptoms is pathognomonic of either bacterial or viral meningitis; indeed, the symptoms overlap enormously. Perhaps the greatest aid in differentiating the forms of meningitis lies in thorough examination of the CSF. Newer laboratory methods hold promise for improving identification of specific bacterial agents.

BIBLIOGRAPHY

Bell WE: Treatment of bacterial infections of the central nervous system. *Ann Neurol* 9:313–327, 1981.

Berk SL, McCabe WR: Meningitis caused by gram-negative bacilli. *Ann Intern Med* 93:253–260, 1980.

Conly JM, Rould AR: Cerebrospinal fluid as a diagnostic body fluid. *Am J Med Infect Dis Symp,* 1983, pp 102–108.

Eng RHK, Seligman SJ: Lumbar puncture–induced meningitis. *JAMA* 245:1456–1459, 1981.

Feigin RD, Shackelford PG: Value of repeat lumbar puncture in the differential diagnosis of meningitis. *N Engl J Med* 289:571–573, 1973.

Gold, R: Bacterial meningitis—1982. *Am J Med Infect Dis Symp,* 1983, pp 98–101.

Kaiser AB, McGee ZA: Aminoglycoside therapy of gram-negative bacillary meningitis. *N Engl J Med* 293:1215–1220, 1975.

Kaplan SL: Antigen detection in cerebrospinal fluid—pros and cons. *Am J Med Infect Dis Symp,* 1983, pp 109–118.

Karandenis D, Shulman JA: Recent survey of infectious meningitis in adults: Review of laboratory findings in bacterial, tuberculous, and aseptic meningitis. *South Med J* 69:449–457, 1976.

Landesman SH, Corrado ML, Shat PM, et al.: Past and current roles for cephalosporin antibiotics in treatment of meningitis. *Am J Med* 71:693–703, 1981.

Martin WJ: Rapid and reliable techniques for the laboratory detection of bacterial meningitis. *Am J Med Infect Dis Symp,* 1983, pp 119–123.

McGinnis MP: Detection of fungi in cerebrospinal fluid. *Am J Med Infect Dis Symp,* 1983, pp 129–138.

Onomoto IM, Wormse GP, Nicholas P: Normal CSF in bacterial meningitis. *JAMA* 244:1469–1471, 1980.

Pickens SJ, Sangster G, Gray JA, et al.: The effects of preadmission antibiotics on the bacteriological diagnosis of pyogenic meningitis. *Scand J Infect Dis* 10:183–185, 1978.

Rahal JJ, Simberkoff MS: Host defense and antimicrobial therapy in adult gram-negative bacillary meningitis. *Ann Immunol (Paris)* 96:468–74, 1982.

Rubin SJ: Detection of viruses in spinal fluid. *Am J Med Infect Symp,* 1983, pp 124–128.

Sande ML: Editorial: Antibiotic therapy of bacterial meningitis with lessons we've learned. *Am J Med* 71:507–510, 1981.

SECTION 14
EYE, EAR, NOSE, THROAT—ORAL SURGERY

CHAPTER 111
OCULAR EMERGENCIES

Roland Clark

INTRODUCTION

Prompt recognition and management of ocular emergencies is mandatory for the preservation of visual function. Nonmedical staff should be prepared and trained to bring actual and potential ocular emergencies to the immediate attention of the clinical staff.

Whenever possible, physicians should be prepared to initiate early management. Many cases may be managed definitively in the emergency department. Firm referral patterns with the ophthalmology staff should be established so that emergency consultation will be available rapidly if the need should arise.

EYE EXAMINATION

Staff Preparation

In the emergency department setting, the physician and nursing staff are frequently isolated from the reception and secretarial staff. Non-medically trained personnel should be educated to be particularly alert for certain ocular complaints. At a minimum, these should include: (1) sudden onset of visual loss; (2) sudden onset of severe eye pain; (3) chemical eye injury; and (4) other severe injuries to the eye. Such patients should be escorted to the nurse-physician team for immediate evaluation.

History

In the acute situation, the taking of a history should be simultaneous with treatment. In any event, a history relative to the presenting complaint should be recorded. In addition, the examiner should search diligently for a past history of previous ocular problems and congenital ocular defects. In cases in which an intraocular foreign body may be present a close inquiry should be made into the history of activities involving striking metal on metal.

Physical Examination

A determination of the best visual acuity is the first step in any eye examination. If eyeglasses are normally worn, then the test should be conducted with eyeglasses in place. If the eyeglasses are not available, a pinhole occluder may be used to approximate the lens correction. While a Snellen eye chart is preferable, any printed material will do for testing as long as the examiner notes the testing material (i.e., newsprint, headlines, etc.)

Occasionally a patient with severe visual deficit may be unable to read any printed material. In this case, the patient may be able to count fingers or perceive hand motion, or may only be able to perceive light. This should be recorded.

The lids, cornea, anterior chamber, iris, and lens should be examined with the penlight. At the same time the direct and consensual pupillary response to light should be tested. The extraocular movements should be tested in the six cardinal positions of gaze and any nystagmus should be noted. Next, the disk, vessels, peripheral retina, and vitreous should be examined with a direct ophthalmoscope. The vitreous is evaluated by obtaining a well-focused view of the retinal vessels and then gradually increasing the diopter setting on the ophthalmoscope lens wheel. This brings the point of focus forward from the retina toward the lens and thus brings objects in the vitreous body into focus.

The optic disk should be examined to see that the outline is crisp and clear. The central optic cup normally accounts for less than one-third of the total diameter of the disk. To obtain a good view of the peripheral retina, it is necessary to dilate the pupil. Prior to instilling a mydriatic, the examiner should be certain that serial evaluation of pupillary function is not necessary for following a brain-injured patient.

The retinal venules are somewhat larger than the arterioles, the normal ratio being about 3:2. The examiner should be alert for either marked dilation of the veins or narrowing of the arterioles.

Visual fields should be evaluated when there is suspicion that a field defect may be present. Optic neuritis, branch retinal arterial occlusion, retinal detachment, and open-angle glaucoma all have associated visual field defects. Confrontation examination offers a simple screening test which will give a good estimate of the visual fields. Patient and examiner are seated opposite one another approximately 1 m apart. To test the right eye, the patient's left eye and examiner's right eye are occluded. The patient is instructed to look directly at the examiner's pupil. The examiner's hand is then moved through the visual field and defects are noted.

Examination of the cornea should be done with magnification, and the slit lamp is the preferred examining instrument. Following initial examination of the eye, a small quantity of fluorescein may be instilled into the eye and the area then examined with cobalt blue filtered light. Areas of damaged ephithelium will stain a brilliant yellow-green, whereas fluorescein is ordinarily orange in color. Fluorescein-coated strips of paper should be used rather than fluorescein solution, since the solution is an excellent culture medium for *Pseudomonas aeruginosa*.

Intraocular pressure should be measured with a Schiøtz tonometer after instilling a drop of topical anesthetic in each eye. The instructions enclosed with the tonometer should be followed carefully. The conversion table is used to translate the scale readings on the tonometer to millimeters of mercury. With the 5.5-g weight in place, a scale reading of 4 or more is equal to about 20 mmHg or less (i.e., normal). The scale readings are inversely related to the pressure, i.e., low scale readings indicate high pressure, and high scale readings indicate low pressure.

COMMON PRESENTING SYMPTOMS

Redness

Conjunctivitis

Bacterial Conjunctivitis

The most common presenting symptoms of bacterial conjunctivitis are redness and subjective sensation of multiple fine granular foreign bodies (''grittiness''). Bacterial conjunctivitis is rarely painful. It is characterized by a mucopurulent discharge of the lids and lashes which may be profuse enough to mat the lids together. Visual acuity is rarely affected. Pupillary reaction and fundoscopic examination are unremarkable. Determination of the intraocular pressure should be deferred until the infection has been cleared.

Staphylococcal allergic conjunctivitis. This is a special case of bacterial conjunctivitis. It is characterized by small white ulcers at the limbus (staphylococcal marginal ulcers). It is postulated that the disorder is due to an allergy to the staphylococcal toxin.

Treatment with topical 10% sulfacetamide drops or ointment is ordinarily effective for most cases of bacterial conjunctivitis. Drops should be instilled every 2 h while the patient is awake and every 4 h at night. Clearing can be expected in 3 to 5 days. Chloramphenicol and topical gentamicin are also very effective. However, the physician should defer the use of drugs which carry a greater risk potential, except when their use is specifically indicated. In the case of staphylococcal allergic conjunctivitis, a dilute corticosteroid is often added to abbreviate the treatment program. In any event, 3 to 5 days of treatment are usually sufficient. Patching should be avoided.

Chlamydial infections. Infections by *Chlamydia trachomatis* are another special case of bacterial infection. The organism is an obligate intracellular parasite which is the etiologic agent for eye infection and venereal infection in humans. Trachoma, the world's leading cause of preventable blindness, and inclusion conjunctivitis of the newborn are the most common ocular manifestations of this infection.

Trachoma is a chronic conjunctivitis which gradually produces scarring of the lids and cornea and ultimate blindness. It is usually heralded by the onset of a typical conjunctivitis characterized by lymphoid follicles in the conjunctiva. The treatment of choice is triple sulfa by mouth. Neonatal inclusion conjunctivitis is acquired from the female genital tract and produces an acute mucopurulent discharge. The usual recommended therapy is erythromycin.

Viral Conjunctivitis

Redness and subjective symptoms of itching and irritation usually fail to distinguish bacterial from viral conjunctivitis. Viral conjunctivitis is most frequently bilateral, while bacterial conjunctivitis may be unilateral. Moreover, the discharge of viral conjunctivitis is often watery, while that of bacterial conjunctivitis is purulent. However it is often difficult, if not impossible, to distinguish between the two on the basis of symptoms or clinical appearance alone. As a practical matter then, most conjunctivitis is treated with a topical antibiotic. The risks are few and the rewards may be great. Combination antibiotics are frequently used. One common formulation combines neomycin, polymyxin, and bacitracin. While the use of this combination is not contraindicated, the physician should recognize that neomycin may produce a hypersensitivity dermatitis in as many as 15 percent of patients.

Ordinarily the nonophthalmologist need not make a great effort to distinguish between the various kinds of viral conjunctivitis, although one should recognize that the adenoviruses are common offenders. However, there are certain viral entities that should be recognized clinically. They include the following:

Herpes zoster conjunctivitis. This conjunctivitis frequently has its onset as a typical viral conjunctivitis. Since this organism is the same one that causes common shingles, the condition is presumed to be an infection of the nerve root. Consequently, it is almost always uniocular. This infection usually progresses to a dermatitis in the distribution of the fifth cranial nerve, which leads to an extensive dermatitis very similar to shingles. Occasionally the cornea alone is involved. The nasociliary nerve supplies both the tip of the nose and the cornea. Thus, if the tip of the nose is involved the cornea will probably also be involved. With ocular involvement there is often a keratitis (inflammation and disruption of the cornea) and anterior uveitis (inflammation of the anterior segment of the eye). The keratitis can lead to catastrophic loss of vision. Therapy with some of the newer antiviral agents has shown promising results.

Vaccinia conjunctivitis. This form of conjunctivitis is preceded by exposure to a person who has received smallpox vaccine 1 to 4 days prior to the onset of symptoms. Typical lesions are found on the mating surfaces of the upper and lower lids (''kissing'' lesions). The lesions develop as a vaccination site on the lids and, as long as they remain confined to the lid, they resolve spontaneously. Topical antiviral medications may be helpful. Corneal involvement can represent a serious threat to vision. Hyperimmune globulin may be necessary, and ophthalmologic consultation is mandatory.

Epidemic keratoconjunctivitis. Epidemic keratoconjunctivitis is a highly contagious eye infection caused by an adenovirus (type 8). It is characterized by a diffuse conjunctivitis which produces marked discomfort. Tender ipsilateral preauricular lymph nodes appear a few days after the onset of symptoms. Approximately 1 week after the onset of symptoms a keratitis appears which is characterized by widely scattered subepithelial infiltrates. Epidemics are frequently traced to contaminated medical instruments. No specific therapy is indicated, but topical antibiotics may prevent secondary infection.

Allergic conjunctivitis. Pollens, high smog levels, and other environmental hazards frequently cause or aggravate allergic conjunctivitis. Vernal conjunctivitis, which usually occurs in the spring or fall, is a typical form of this problem. It is characterized by huge cobblestone papillae under the upper lid, itching, and tearing. A contact (allergic) conjunctivitis frequently occurs in postoperative cataract patients and other patients using eye drops. Common offenders are neomycin and atropine.

One particular subset of allergic conjunctivitis is due to reaction to insect protein. In the summer months it is common for small gnats and other flying insects to lodge as conjunctival foreign bodies. The reaction to them is frequently dramatic. Chemosis (swelling of the bulbar conjunctiva) may assume alarming proportions. The upper and lower lids may also swell dramatically. The conjunctiva is usually pale rather than red, and the eye may be very pruritic. The presentation is usually uniocular.

Treatment of allergic conjunctivitis consists of topical antihistamines, vasoconstrictors, and dilute corticosteroids when indicated. Cold compresses are very helpful. If no treatment is adminstered, the problem will usually resolve spontaneously in 24 to 48 h. Removal of the allergen, as in the case of an insect foreign body, is essential.

Chemical Conjunctivitis

Alkali burn. A burn produced by sodium hydroxide (lye) or other alkali is one of the few absolute ocular emergencies. The eye should be irrigated immediately at the scene with tap water for 15 to 20 min. Irrigation should continue in the emergency department with water or saline. Alkalis produce a liquefaction necrosis of the conjunctiva and cornea. Consequently, their corrosive action is unobstructed and they continue to dissolve soft tissue until removed. Hospital treatment may consist of irrigation for hours or days depending on the extent of the burn. Alkali burns of the eye should be seen immediately by an ophthalmologist.

Acid burns. Acid burns are extremely irritating and can be very serious. However, acids generally produce a coagulation necrosis of the cornea and their invasion is limited by the coagulum formed in the process. Immediate copious irrigation is still indicated, as is ophthalmologic consultation.

Foreign Bodies

Conjunctival Foreign Bodies

Foreign bodies that adhere to the conjunctiva should always be suspected as a cause of redness, pain, or tearing of the eye. An examination under magnification is indicated, and slit-lamp examination is preferred. Foreign bodies in the inferior cul-de-sac are usually quite apparent. Examination of the everted upper lid will reveal foreign bodies adherent to the conjunctival surface of the tarsal plate. After the foreign body has been identified, a drop of proparacaine hydrochloride should be instilled and the object removed with a cotton-tipped applicator.

Occasionally double eversion is indicated. To accomplish this, the lid is first singly everted. Using a lid elevator, the lid is everted once more to view the superior cul-de-sac. Alternatively, the conjunctiva of the superior cul-de-sac may be prolapsed into view by exerting firm pressure with cotton-tipped applicator after the upper lid has been singly everted.

Double patching of the eye will usually relieve a great deal of pain, but oral pain medication may be necessary.

Corneal Foreign Bodies

Corneal foreign bodies are a common problem and often cause a great deal of pain and redness. After completion of the examination, a drop of proparacaine hydrochloride should be instilled and the object removed with a corneal spud, burr or sterile hypodermic needle. This is best accomplished under slit-lamp magnification. After removal, antibiotics should be instilled and the eye doubly patched. Oral pain medication may be necessary, and the patient should be rechecked in 24 to 36 h.

Rust rings are usually present if a ferrous foreign body has been embedded for more than a few hours. The rust ring should be removed with the aid of the slit lamp. A battery-powered rust ring remover greatly facilitates this task. The rust ring should be removed completely, as persistence of the particles may cause recurrent ocular symptoms.

Eyelashes

Eyelashes are common ocular foreign bodies that usually settle in the inferior cul-de-sac. Occasionally the lash may lodge in the inferior punctum. In this case the patient usually has a medial conjunctivitis, with the temporal side clear. To avoid missing this common diagnosis, always check the puncta of the reddened eye.

Blepharitis

Blepharitis is a common condition characterized by chronic inflammation of the lid margins and occasionally the conjunctiva. Slit-lamp examination reveals scaling and a "greasy" appearance to the lid margins which is particularly prominent around the base of the lashes.

The condition is usually attributed to a staphylococcal infection of the skin and oil glands immediately adjacent to the lash follicles. Treatment consists of topical instillation of sulfacetamide drops and application of antibiotic ointment to the lid margins on retiring. This often can be facilitated by carefully scrubbing the lash margin with baby shampoo (nonirritating) to remove oil and scales.

Corneal Ulcer

With a corneal ulcer the eye is usually reddened and extremely painful. Slit-lamp examination will reveal a localized white flocculent infiltrate of the cornea. A hypopyon is a frequently associated finding which is characterized by the accumulation of a white inflammatory exudate in the anterior chamber. Corneal destruction and perforation are the major hazards. Immediate ophthalmic consultation and admission are mandatory.

Subconjunctival Hemorrhage

Subconjunctival hemorrhage is an extremely common condition characterized by objective findings of a very reddened eye with virtually no subjective complaints. The cause is the rupture of a small vessel beneath the bulbar conjunctiva. The objective appearance is characteristic. The bulbar conjunctiva is blood red and has a striking appearance. The condition is usually called to the attention of the patient by a concerned observer.

Rupture of these blood vessels is usually benign. Common causes include trivial trauma, foreign bodies, or violent valsalva maneuvers such as coughing or straining. Important differential considerations include hypertension and blood dyscrasias.

A patient who has not experienced this condition before is often terrified about impending blindness. After the other causes of subconjunctival hemorrhage have been eliminated, the patient may be reassured that the hemorrhage will resolve spontaneously in 10 to 14 days.

Ultraviolet Keratitis—Corneal Flash Burn

Virtually all ultraviolet radiation is absorbed by the cornea and the majority is absorbed by the corneal epithelium. Especially intense sources of ultraviolet radiation include arc welding and reflected sunlight. ''Welders' keratitis'' and ''snow blindness'' are both manifestations of excessive ultraviolet radiation to the corneal epithelium. Symptoms include intense pain, burning, blurred vision, and epiphora.

Slit-lamp examination reveals a diffuse punctate keratopathy, which is best seen by fluorescein staining and cobalt blue illumination under slit-lamp magnification. The examiner will note multiple pinpoint-sized areas of staining. These represent swollen and ruptured corneal epithelial cells. The experienced examiner will note diffuse corneal haziness under slit lamp, even without the use of fluorescein.

Management consists of topical anesthesia to facilitate examination, followed by snug double patching and systemic analgesia. The rapid healing properties of the cornea result in only slight irritation after 4 to 8 h of patching.

Indiscriminate use of topical anesthetics has led to grave consequences. Most of the topical anesthetics are cellular toxins in higher doses. Repeated administration will retard healing of the corneal epithelium. Furthermore, because anesthesia deprives the cornea of its normal protective reflexes, additional damage will almost surely follow. Permanent damage to the corneal stroma may then result from the increasingly frequent instillations of topical anesthetics that subsequently become necessary. Visual disability may ensue. Thus, firm double patching and adequate levels of systemic analgesia are the only rational modes of treatment.

Miscellaneous

Hordeolum (Stye)

A hordeolum is an acute inflammation of the meibomian glands, usually of the upper lid. Hordeola usually present as pustular vesicles at the lid margin.

Initial treatment consists of hot compresses and topical antibiotics. Surgical intervention is frequently necessary and consists either of drainage of the gland at the lid margin or eversion and incision with drainage of the gland from the posterior surface of the lid.

Chalazion

A chalazion is a chronic granulomatous inflammation of a meibomian gland, also most commonly of the upper lid. This condition usually presents as an uninflamed and nontender nodule of the lid several millimeters from the lid margin. The treatment for this is surgical and consists of curettage of the substance of the gland.

Acute Eye Pain

Acute Iritis

Acute inflammation of the anterior segment of the eye may be divided into two broad categories, traumatic and nontraumatic. Traumtic iritis will be discussed in a subsequent section. Nontraumatic iritis has a number of etiologies, and a complete discussion of the differential diagnosis is beyond the scope of this text. However, the emergency physician should be able to recognize the basic symptom complex and initiate management.

The onset of symptoms usually occurs over a period of hours. Symptoms include blurred vision, photophobia, and dull ocular pain, which is usually referred to the brow or temporal area.

Physical examination reveals a reddened and painful eye. The pupil is often constricted and direct and consensual photophobia is apparent on penlight examination. Close examination will reveal ciliary flush, a diffuse reddening of the sclera at the limbus. Visual acuity is usually decreased and intraocular pressure is decreased in the affected eye. Slit-lamp examination may reveal flare and cells in the anterior chamber. This is best seen with reduced room illumination and high magnification.

Management consists of mydriatics and topical steroids. Cycloplegia with cyclopentolate or homatropine markedly reduces ciliary spasm and pain, and steroids tend to reduce the inflammatory response of the anterior segment. Untreated inflammation of the anterior segment can lead to posterior synechiae (adhesions of the posterior leaf of the iris to the anterior lens capsule) or anterior synechiae (inflammatory attachment of the anterior iris leaf to the posterior corneal surface). These conditions produce a visual and cosmetic defect, and can lead to secondary glaucoma. Patients with iritis should be referred to an ophthalmologist for a detailed evaluation.

Acute Angle Closure Glaucoma

Congenital narrowing of the anterior chamber angle is the underlying etiology for acute angle closure glaucoma. Under a variety of circumstances the angle between the anterior iris leaf and posterior surface of the cornea may close completely, thus preventing the exit of the aqueous humor. Despite the elevated intraocular pressure, the ciliary body continues to produce aqueous humor and the intraocular pressure rises precipitously.

An acute angle closure may be precipitated in susceptible individuals by moving from daylight to a darkened environment, e.g., a movie theatre; or iatrogenically by the administration of mydriatics. The latter situation may be a beneficial diagnostic maneuver. The characteristic symptom is a unilateral dull, aching ocular pain, which is frequently accompanied by nausea and vomiting. Vision is blurred, with halos seen around lights. Physical examination will demonstrate a diffusely reddened and congested eye with reduced visual acuity. The cornea is often hazy and the pupil is mid-dilated and fixed to light. Intraocular pressures are extremely high, frequently 50 mmHg or greater.

Emergency management consists of frequent instillation of miotics such as pilocarpine, parenteral administration of carbonic anhydrase inhibitors (such as acetazolamide) to reduce aqueous humor production, and oral administration of hyperosmotic agents (such as glycerol). Miotics should also be instilled in the other eye, which is also susceptible to acute angle closure. In the clinical setting, prompt recognition and medical treatment will almost invariably control the attack. Definitive treatment is surgical. Peripheral iridectomy produces an open pathway for the exit of aqueous humor and will prevent subsequent attacks.

Open Angle Glaucoma

Open angle glaucoma is a chronic condition of elevated intraocular pressure. Constant elevation of intraocular pressure damages the optic nerve. Physical findings include elevation of the intraocular pressure, an increase in the optic cup/disk ratio, and arcuate scotomas emerging from the physiologic blind spot. Marked constriction of the peripheral visual fields with sparing of central vision is characteristic of late-stage chronic open angle glaucoma. Chronic glaucoma is not an ocular emergency; it is mentioned here to distinguish it from acute angle closure glaucoma.

Herpes Simplex Keratitis

The viral agent responsible for herpes simplex keratitis is herpes simplex virus. It produces an acute infection of the corneal epithelium, which is characterized by localized ocular pain frequently described as a foreign body sensation. Visual acuity is reduced if the lesion happens to fall on the visual axis. The eye is diffusely reddened and slit-lamp examination of the unstained cornea may reveal a localized area of haziness. Fluorescein staining will often demonstrate a dendrite figure, a branching pattern that resembles the outline of a forked lightning bolt.

Treatment consists of topical administration of antiviral agents and cycloplegics to reduce anterior chamber reaction. Dilute steroid drops are occasionally prescribed under ophthalmologic supervision. Ophthalmologic consultation is mandatory since progressive herpes simplex keratitis can lead to destruction of the cornea and grave visual disability.

Acute Visual Loss

Central Retinal Artery Occlusion

Acute occlusion of the central retinal artery is most commonly the result of atherosclerosis and its various manifestations: thrombosis, thromboemboli, and vasospasm. The patient experiences sudden monocular, painless loss of vision. Branch arterioles may be similarly affected, leading to sudden reduced vision and segmental visual field defects. Gross physical findings consist principally of a normal-appearing but sightless eye. Examination of the fundus reveals a very pale retina with a small pink dot in the vicinity of the fovea. Often no retinal arteries are visible.

Central retinal artery occlusion is an absolute ophthalmic emergency and the prognosis is extremely grave. Vigorous digital massage of the globe and/or anterior chamber paracentesis may reduce the intraocular pressure enough to allow atheromas to move peripherally. Immediate emergency ophthalmologic consultation is mandatory.

Central Retinal Vein Occlusion

A rigid atheromatous artery immediately adjacent to the central retinal vein may ultimately exert sufficient pressure to collapse the vein wall. This gradual process leads to occlusion of the vein. Symptoms are usually confined to uniocular painless decrease of vision, though some visual function may persist. Fundus examination will reveal a chaotically bloodstreaked retina with prominent dilated and congested veins. Management is beyond the scope of the nonophthalmologist and immediate consultation is mandatory.

Retrobulbar Neuritis

The usual presenting complaint in retrobulbar neuritis is loss of central vision in the affected eye. Peripheral vision is usually preserved, and visual field examination will define the degree of involvement. Other than loss of central vision, the physical examination findings are usually totally unremarkable.

The diagnosis of multiple sclerosis is associated with retrobulbar neuritis in approximately 25 percent of cases. Retrobulbar injections of steroids may be helpful, and ophthalmologic referral is necessary.

Eclipse Burn (Sun Gazer's Retinopathy)

Accidental or prolonged viewing of an eclipse, certain abnormal psychiatric states, and abuse of hallucinogenic or other mind-altering drugs (such as phencyclidine) predispose to so-called sun gazer's retinopathy. For uncertain reasons such patients may gaze directly at the sun with the unprotected eye for a prolonged period. Most ultraviolet light is absorbed by the ocular media. Lower-frequency radiation is transmitted to the retina, and direct viewing of luminous objects can produce photocoagulation of the macula. The result is often permanent complete loss of central retinal (macular) vision. The best visual acuity under these circumstances is ordinarily 20/200 or worse. Confrontation visual field examinations may not reveal this small defect. However, tangent-screen visual field testing will show a discrete ''gun barrel'' central visual field defect. Fundoscopic examination will demonstrate discrete disruption of the retina in the area of the macula.

Amarosis Fugax

Sudden temporary interruption of the blood supply to the retina will produce the fleeting uniocular visual loss termed *amarosis fugax*. The duration of visual loss may vary from only a few seconds to several minutes. By definition, complete visual function returns to the affected eye.

This phenomenon is usually attributed to vasospasm secondary to atherosclerosis. This alarming symptom should alert the physician and patient to the need for a diligent search for the treatable atherosclerotic disease.

Retinal Detachment

Spontaneous retinal detachment is painless. The patient experiences the gradual lowering or raising of a curtain over the visual field of the affected eye. A careful history will often reveal prodromal symptoms such as the perception of flashing lights in the peripheral visual field at night or the drifting of "spider webs" or "coal dust" across the visual field. The former symptom is due to mechanical trauma of the retina, while the latter two are a result of small vitreous hemorrhages drifting across the visual axis.

The retina detaches as the result of the seepage of the fluid portion of the posterior vitreous body through the retinal tear, causing separation of the loosely applied retina, much as water seeps behind wallpaper and strips it away from the wall.

Examination with a direct ophthalmoscope may reveal the undulating gray detached retina. Occasionally, vitreous hemorrhages resulting from rupture of retinal vessels bridging the tear will be noted as well. A diligent search with the indirect ophthalmoscope will usually demonstrate the retinal tear that is responsible for the detachment.

Initial management consists of preventing further retinal detachment when possible. As long as the macula remains attached, there is an excellent chance of preserving central retinal vision. If the detachment is inferior, the patient should rest in bed with the head elevated; if the detachment is superior, the patient should lie flat in bed. Prompt ophthalmologic consultation is indicated.

Hysterical Blindness

A variety of psychological factors may precipitate subjective complete loss of vision. The patient may be remarkably calm despite the gravity of this complaint, and the physician may note a variety of other clues that would suggest nonorganic visual loss. With the exception of the loss of subjective vision, the physical examination is unremarkable. Direct and consensual pupillary examination is normal, and the fundus has a normal appearance. Use of an optokinetic drum or strip will usually elicit optokinetic nystagmus, confirming an intact visual pathway. Management is by supportive referral for psychiatric evaluation.

TRAUMA

Lid Lacerations

Wounds that involve only the skin of the lid have an excellent prognosis. Closure may be accomplished with very fine (6-0 or 7-0) suture material. Ordinarily nonabsorbable material such as nylon should be used. However, suture removal may be very difficult with small children. Absorbable sutures may be used in these cases, although some skin reaction may occur. In 7 to 10 days any remaining sutures may be brushed away. Healing occurs rapidly due to the rich blood supply, and nonabsorbable sutures may be removed within 3 days.

There are at least five anatomical areas where more than the usual level of anatomical knowledge and suturing skill are necessary. These are discussed below.

Lacrimal canaliculi. The horizontal limb of the lacrimal canaliculi traverses the lid from the lacrimal puncta to the common canaliculus. The canaliculi lie about 1 mm beneath the lid margin. Any wound that affects the lid margin between the puncta and medial canthus has a high probability of damaging the canalicular apparatus.

Levator. Deep transverse lacerations of the upper lid threaten the levator mechanism. The presence of ptosis suggests involvement of the levator palpebrae tendon, and prompt ophthalmologic consultation is indicated. A careful search for any signs of ptosis must be made when the anatomy of the wound suggests this possibility.

Orbital Septum. Deep wounds of the upper lid may violate the orbital septum, which runs between the tarsus and the superior orbital rim. When this occurs, there is a high potential for: (1) prolapse of orbital fat, leading to a cosmetically unacceptable outcome; and (2) orbital cellulitis. The septum must be surgically closed, and prophylactic systemic antibiotics are indicated.

Canthal tendons. Penetrating wounds of the medial and lateral canthi may interrupt the canthal tendons. This will lead to a cosmetically unacceptable shortening of the palpebral fissure. Repair is technically difficult and should be performed by an ophthalmic surgeon.

Lid Margins. Through-and-through wounds of the lid margin and tarsal plate require meticulous realignment of the structures for a cosmetically acceptable result. If more than about 1 mm of the tarsal plate is lacerated, a complex three-layer closure is required.

Corneal Abrasions

Corneal abrasions are extremely common and the history will usually define the problem. The affected eye is painful and epiphora is common. Slit-lamp examination with fluorescein staining will reveal the abraded areas. Myriad extremely fine linear abrasions of the superior third of the cornea (the "ice rink sign") suggest the presence of a tarsal foreign body.

Removal of all foreign material and instillation of a topical antibiotic and firm double patching are indicated. If photophobia and signs of iritis are present, a short-acting mydriatic is indicated. Mydriasis and double patching will usually control pain, although occasionally systemic analgesics are required.

Corneal Lacerations

Recognition of small corneal lacerations may be difficult at times. Often slit-lamp examination may be required to identify even a full-thickness laceration. Clues include a "teardrop"-shaped pupil due to prolapse of the iris, and flattening of the anterior chamber resulting from loss of aqueous humor. Occasionally small fragments of black iris pigment may be present at the lips of the wound. They may be mistaken for foreign bodies. Repair should occur in the operating room under microscopic control.

Perforation of Globe

Penetrating wounds of lids should raise a suspicion of an occult perforation of the globe. The sclera is particularly thin under the rectus muscles and this is the area of highest risk.

Even though the perforation may not be visible, visual acuity is usually reduced, the globe is soft, and there may be vitreous hemorrhage visible on ophthalmoscopic examination. A rigid metal eye shield will protect the globe from inadvertent pressure with resulting extrusion of the contents of the globe. Immediate ophthalmologic consultation is indicated.

Hyphema

Small hyphemas (hemorrhages in the anterior chamber) may go unnoticed without slit-lamp examination. Larger hyphemas which do not resolve may lead to secondary glaucoma and blood staining of the corneal endothelium. Although initial hyphemas may be insignificant, recurrences are often more severe and the complication rate increases dramatically.

Management is directed toward enhancing absorption of blood and prevention of recurrence. Bed rest is necessary, while the use of patches, miotics, and topical steroids will vary with the preference of the individual ophthalmologist.

Traumatic Dislocated Lens

Blunt trauma to the globe may disrupt the zonules and result in dislocation of the lens. The lens usually falls backward into the vitreous cavity, although it may prolapse into the anterior chamber. In either case visual acuity is markedly reduced. Certain collagen disorders, such as Marfan's syndrome, predispose to spontaneous dislocation of the lens. With a high degree of suspicion on the part of the examiner, adequate slit-lamp and fundoscopic examination will confirm the diagnosis.

Blow-out Fracture of the Orbit

Blunt trauma to the globe transmits hydraulic forces throughout the entire orbital cavity. The floor and medial wall of the orbit are fragile particularly and subject to fracture. When the floor of the orbit is fractured under these circumstances, orbital contents such as the inferior rectus muscle and orbital fat may prolapse through the fracture and become trapped. The infraorbital nerve traverses the floor of the orbit and is also frequently involved. Symptoms include pain and diplopia on upward gaze. Physical examination may reveal enophthalmos and hypesthesia in the distribution of the infraorbital nerve. Paralysis of upward gaze will produce marked diplopia in the upper visual fields. Initial management is conservative and ophthalmologic referral is necessary.

Traumatic Retinal Detachment

A history of significant blunt ocular trauma should lead to a diligent examination of the entire retina for signs of retinal tears. Early recognition and therapy of the torn retina will prevent retinal detachment. Examination of the peripheral retina requires more skill in the use of the indirect ophthalmoscope and/or the Goldman contact lens. Findings of even a small amount of vitreous hemorrhage should raise suspicions of a traumatic retinal tear and lead to prompt ophthalmologic referral.

Intraocular Foreign Body

A history of work that involves pounding metal on metal should immediately raise the suspicion of an intraocular foreign body. The initial injury may be painless, and symptoms may not present for a day or more after the initial incident. Decreased visual acuity and dull, nonlocalizing ocular pain are usually the first complaints.

Small intraocular foreign bodies may leave only a minute wound on the lid or globe. The examiner should also search carefully for minute perforations of the iris leaf or early cataract formation resulting from violation of the lens capsule. A careful fundoscopic examination after dilation of the pupil may reveal the foreign body.

Metallic foreign bodies may be visible on plain x-ray films of the orbit, although specific localizing views may be necessary. Ultrasonic scanning of the globe and orbit are very helpful in the precise localization of foreign bodies, although this modality is not available in all institutions.

Virtually all intraocular foreign bodies must be removed. Innovations in the surgical approach to the vitreous body have greatly improved the prognosis for this injury.

Traumatic Iritis

Blunt ocular trauma followed by poorly localized, aching ocular pain, photophobia, and decreased visual acuity suggest a diagnosis of traumatic iritis. The pupil is constricted and a deep ciliary flush is usually present. Slit-lamp examination reveals cells and flare in the anterior chamber. Direct and consensual photophobia are due to iris and ciliary body irritability. Intraocular pressure is frequently lower than in the uninjured eye.

Initial treatment consists of topical short-acting mydriatics and dilute steroid drops. Mydriasis is a useful diagnostic tool as it will dramatically decrease ocular pain and photophobia secondary to iritis.

Traumatic Mydriasis

Blunt ocular trauma may selectively impair the function of parasympathetic innervation to the iris leaf and thereby result in mydriasis. This may be a local effect on the globe or may represent trauma to the ciliary ganglion located deep in the orbit. In either case the condition is usually temporary and managment consists of recognition and appropriate ophthalmologic referral.

DIAGNOSTIC DILEMMAS

Ophthalmic Migraine Manifestations

Migraine headache may present with ophthalmic symptoms manifested by visual phenomena. The patient may complain of objects taking on a "silvery" or "shimmering" appearance. This is frequently followed by the development of a scotoma, often described as a "fortification scotoma," in which the margin of the visual field defect is jagged or serrated in appearance. The scotoma may persist for several hours or even for a day or more. The usual course leads to complete resolution. Rarely, there may be a persistent peripheral scotoma after resolution of the migraine event.

Unilateral Dilated Fixed Pupil

The differential diagnosis of unilateral dilated fixed pupil is based on either a significant neurological event or the accidental (or intentional) instillation of a cycloplegic. To resolve this question, one drop of 1% pilocarpine is placed in the dilated eye and the instillation is repeated in 5 min. If at the end of 20 min the pupil is still fixed and dilated, the patient has instilled a cycloplegic.

Spasm of Accommodation

The hysterical or extremely anxious patient may occasionally present with what amounts to a full-blown manifestation of the near reflex. That is, the pupils are constricted, the eyes are convergent, and accommodation is at a maximum. The patient complains of blurred vision, particularly at a distance. Treatment should be directed at the underlying anxiety, although a drop of a short-acting cycloplegic in each eye may break the cycle.

Tunnel Vision

"Gun barrel" or tunnel vision is another manifestation of hysteria or anxiety. The patient complains of loss of all the visual field with the exception of the central area. A tangent-screen visual field examination will reveal a dense scotoma of all but the central visual field. If the scotoma is truly physiologic and not hysterical in origin, then doubling the distance between the examinee and the tangent screen will double the size of the central visual field. With hysterical tunnel vision the visual field size will remain unchanged.

OPHTHALMIC MEDICATIONS

Anesthetics

Proparacaine. Proparacaine has a rapid onset of action. Its duration of action is approximately 20 min, and the depth of anesthesia produced is adequate for most minor ocular procedures.

Tetracaine. This drug is somewhat more irritating than proparacaine and is less commonly used for ordinary office procedures. The onset of action is more delayed, the depth of anesthesia is greater, and the duration may be 1 h or more.

Cocaine. Topical cocaine is an excellent anesthetic and profound vasoconstrictor. Hence it is quite useful for minor surgical procedures. However, cocaine softens the corneal epithelium to the point where even minor corneal trauma may desquamate the entire surface.

Mydriatic Cyclopegics

Tropicamide. Tropicamide is a mydriatic cycloplegic with onset in 15 to 20 min. Its duration of action is fairly brief, and accommodation and pupillary reaction usually return within 1 to 2 h.

Cyclopentolate. Cyclopentolate is a somewhat more potent cycloplegic than tropicamide, with a longer duration of action.

Homatropine. Homatropine is a mydriatic cycloplegic, with a duration of action of 2 or 3 days.

Atropine. Atropine is a very long-lasting mydriatic, with a duration of action of up to 2 weeks.

Miotics

Miotics are used almost exclusively for the treatment of glaucoma. Pilocarpine is one of the most commonly used and is usually instilled four times a day in strengths varying from $\frac{1}{8}$ to 6 percent.

Antibiotics

Sulfacetamide. As the 10 percent solution or ointment, sulfacetamide is a relatively nonirritating and effective broad-spectrum antibiotic for the management of most external ocular infections.

Chloramphenicol. Chloramphenicol remains one of the most effective broad-spectrum antibiotics available for topical use. Most common gram-positive and gram-negative ocular pathogens are sensitive to chloramphenicol. Unfortunately, there is still some risk of bone marrow depression associated with its ocular use.

Gentamicin. This drug is particularly useful in the management of infections due to penicillin-resistant staphylococci and many of the gram-negative organisms. It is often used in conjunction with carbenicillin.

Neomycin. While neomycin is effective against many gram-negative organisms skin sensitivity, manifested by an erythematous, pruritic scaling dermatitis, may appear in as many as 10 to 15 percent of patients.

Steroids

Although reduction of the inflammatory response may be of great value from the standpoint both of comfort and of altering the pathophysiology of a disease process, steroid use should be limited to those cases which are seen in consultation with an ophthalmologist. A principal risk of topical steroid administration is acute exacerbation of ocular infections. In the case of herpes simplex keratitis, deep stromal scarring or corneal perforation may result from steroid use. Long-term administration for any reason may lead to glaucoma or cataract formation.

Miscellaneous

Acetazolamide. Acetazolamide, a carbonic anhydrase inhibitor, markedly reduces the output of aqueous humor by the ciliary body. Its principal use is in the management of acute angle closure glaucoma.

Glycerol. Orally administered glycerol acts as a hyperosmotic agent. Shortly after administration there is a notable reduction in intraocular pressure. Its ophthalmic use is ordinarily limited to the management of acute angle closure glaucoma.

TREATMENT TECHNIQUES

Eye Patch

A snugly fitting eye patch is appropriate treatment for minor abrasions of the cornea. The pressure of the patch reduces pain and, because the lid margin is immobilized, recurrent irritation of the damaged cornea by the lid margin is eliminated.

Double patching is the most common technique. The first patch is folded and applied against the closed eyelid. The second patch is then placed over the first. The bulk of this dressing fills the orbital recess so that when it is correctly taped in place moderate pressure is applied directly to the eye. The patch is commonly taped in place with three parallel strips of 1-in tape extending diagonally from the central forehead to the lateral cheek.

Eye Shield

Use of an eye shield is dictated by the fact that any pressure or contact with the globe must be avoided in cases where there is some question of interruption of the globe's integrity. If the globe is unprotected, accidental pressure may cause its contents to extrude through the wound. The eye shield provides this mechanical barrier of protection.

Foreign Body Removal

Conjunctival Foreign Bodies

Under ordinary circumstances conjunctival foreign bodies are easily removed with a cotton-tipped applicator after topical anesthesia. The examiner should search diligently for any remaining material after the first foreign body has been removed. The upper lid should be everted and the tarsal plate examined closely in every case.

Corneal Foreign Bodies

The slit lamp should be used when removing foreign bodies from the cornea whenever possible. After adequate topical anesthesia, an attempt should be made to sweep away the foreign body with a cotton-tipped applicator.

If the cotton-tipped applicator fails, the foreign body must be removed by sharp instrumentation. The most useful instrument is a sterile hypodermic needle used *bevel down* to prevent the tip from burying itself deeply in the corneal stroma. With magnification the foreign body can be meticulously dissected from the corneal surface.

Ferrous foreign bodies present a special problem. After the iron-containing particle has been present in the cornea for a few hours, a rust ring will develop. This should be removed along with the foreign body as it can produce recurrent irritation and permanent corneal staining. The rust ring can be removed with a sterile hypodermic needle. However, a small, electrically driven spherical corneal burr is particularly useful for quick and neat removal.

MISCELLANEOUS OPHTHALMIC PROBLEMS

Contact Lenses

Hard Corneal Contact Lenses

Occasionally, hard contact lenses will become "lost" somewhere in the conjunctival cul-de-sac. If the lens is not tinted, magnification and topical anesthesia may be necessary to find and retrieve it. Once visualized, the lens can easily be removed with a small rubber suction device designed for that purpose. All comatose patients should be examined for the presence of contact lenses, and they should be removed if present.

Soft Contact Lenses

These lenses may contain 60 percent or more water. They are comfortable, fragile, and expensive. If they become desiccated, they become brittle and are virtually impossible to remove intact. Repeated instillations of normal saline solution (without additives) will usually hydrate the lens sufficiently so that it can be removed. The removal technique consists of "pinching" the lens off the surface of the eye.

Intraocular Lens Implants

An increasing number of cataract patients have undergone lens implantation following cataract removal. These lenses have dramatically reduced the visual distortion previously associated with the use of heavy spectacle lenses for correction. The implanted lenses are held in place by a variety of methods, including loops, clips, sutures, and pins.

The most common complication seen in the emergency department is dislocation of the lens. This may result from pupillary dilation in a darkened environment or from minor direct trauma to the eye. Management consists of prescribing bed rest for the patient and contacting the ophthalmic surgeon. The surgeon will probably dilate the pupil, gingerly tap the front of the eye to pop the loop back under the iris, and then constrict the pupil with pilocarpine. Occasionally reoperation is necessary.

BIBLIOGRAPHY

Ballantyne AJ, Michaelson IC: *Textbook of the Fundus of the Eye*. London, Churchill Livingstone, 1970

Cogan DG: *Neurology of the Ocular Muscles*. Springfield, Ill., Charles C Thomas, 1970.

Duke-Elder S: *Neuro-ophthalmology*. St Louis, C.V. Mosby Co, 1971.

Duke-Elder S: *Ocular Adnexa* (Part 1), Volume XIII. St. Louis, C.V. Mosby Co, 1974.

Duke-Elder S: *System of Ophthalmology, Diseases of the Retina*, Volume X. St. Louis, C.V. Mosby Co, 1967.

Isselbacher KS, Adams RD: *Harrison's Principles of Internal Medicine*, 9. New York, McGraw-Hill Book Co, 1980.

Leopold IH: *Symposium on Ocular Therapy*, Volume 6. St. Louis, C.V. Mosby Co, 1973.

Moses RA: *Adlec's Physiology of the Eye-Clinical Application*, ed 5. St. Louis, C.V. Mosby Co, 1970.

Scheie A: *Textbook of Ophthalmology*, ed 9. Philadelphia, Saunders, 1979.

Walsh FB, Hoyt WF: *Clinical Neuro-Ophthalmology*, Volume II, Ed 3. Baltimore, Williams & Wilkins Co, 1969.

CHAPTER 112
OTOLARYNGOLOGIC
EMERGENCIES

Frank I. Marlowe, Ali Aghamohamadi

A. Otologic Emergencies

OTALGIA

Ear pain can usually be explained on the basis of the ear examination if there is evidence of otitis externa or media. When it cannot, sources of referred pain must be considered and sought to explain the pain. Cranial nerves V, VII, IX, and X and cervical nerves II and III supply sensation to the ear. The cervical nerve supply may be the source of referred pain in cervical arthritis and occipital neuralgia, but the cranial nerves are most likely to be associated with referred pain. Pain from the temporomandibular joint, mandibular teeth, or tongue may be referred to the ear by the trigeminal nerve. Herpes zoster oticus and Bell's palsy may cause otalgia by the facial nerve. The glossopharyngeal or vagus nerves may be the source of otalgia from tonsillitis, cancer of the tonsil, or foreign bodies of the hypopharynx, larynx, or cervical esophagus.

The management of otalgia is treatment of the underlying conditions, plus analgesics. If no cause for ear pain is found, treatment with analgesics and local heat is prescribed. An ear-nose-throat (ENT) consultation is necessary if pain is persistent.

INFECTIONS

Otitis Externa

The signs and symptoms of otitis externa are itching, pain, and discharge from the ear, with an intact drum. If the swelling is severe, hearing loss may be included. Pain may be severe and made worse by pressing on the tragus or by moving the auricle. Occasionally the entire auricle may be swollen and red, and tender enlarged lymph nodes can be palpated over the mastoid process, parotid area, and upper neck.

Treatment consists of cleaning the external ear canal by suctioning, or with a cotton-tipped applicator; an antibiotic-steroid

otic solution for 1 week; and, if desired, a $\frac{1}{4}$-in wide ribbon gauze moistened with an antibiotic solution can be inserted into the ear canal.

Systemic antibiotics are necessary if the auricle is enlarged and red or if there is lymphadenopathy. Drainage from the ear canal should always be cultured before initiating antibiotics. The patient should be told that symptoms will continue for 24 to 48 h before they improve, even though the treatment has been started. Malignant external otitis in the diabetic patient with external otitis that does not clear rapidly by routine measures should be suspected. These severe forms of otitis externa may lead to cartilage and bone destruction, and otologic consultation and hospitalization are necessary.

Furuncle

Furuncles of the ear canal cause pain until they spontaneously rupture and drain. Examination reveals a localized area of redness and tenderness at the external meatus.

The treatment is as for external otitis, along with incision and drainage.

The presenting sign of a preauricular sinus is usually a dimple in the preauricular area. Infection or abscess formation may occur if a cyst develops. Treatment is local heat application and 400,000 units of penicillin intramuscularly qid. Incision and drainage are necessary if the cyst is fluctuant, with delayed surgical removal of the cyst or sinus when the infection has resolved.

Bullous Myringitis

Bullous myringitis may be of viral or mycoplasmatic origin and causes persistent pain and, possibly, mild hearing loss. The tympanic membrane has blisters that may contain clear or hemorrhagic fluid. Bullous myringitis is treated by analgesics and application of local heat. If the pain is severe, the bullae may be ruptured by an otologist. If underlying otitis media is present, it should be treated.

Otitis Media

The symptoms of acute suppurative otitis media are fever, pain, and hearing loss. There will be a discharge if the tympanic membrane has ruptured. The tympanic membrane appears red with engorgement of the vessels, bulging, and thickened.

The treatment is ampicillin or amoxicillin for children up to adolescence and penicillin for older teens and adults for 10 days. Antibiotic-containing eardrops are indicated only when the tympanic membrane is ruptured and drainage is present in the ear canal. Topical heat and systemic analgesics are preferred to analgesic eardrops for the control of pain. Acute otitis media is discussed further in Chapter 80, ''Pediatric Upper Respiratory Emergencies.''

Myringotomy is indicated for severe pain, marked toxicity, and high fever, and complications such as facial nerve paralysis, meningitis, or brain abscess.

Chronic otitis media is treated by cleaning and suctioning of the ear, systemic antibiotics, and antibiotic-steroid eardrops. The patient should be referred to an otologist for further evaluation and treatment. A patient with chronic otitis and a cholesteatoma who has facial nerve paralysis, vertigo, or possible intracranial complications should have emergent referral to an otologist.

SUDDEN HEARING LOSS

Sudden hearing loss may occur as a result of lesions of the external ear (impacted cerumen), middle ear (fluid, blood, or pus in the middle ear), or inner ear (Ménière's disease, labyrinthitis, and syphilis). It can result from lesions of the internal auditory meatus, cerebellopontine angle, or from vascular spasm or occlusion. Most often, sudden deafness is idiopathic and is presumed to be of viral or vascular origin. The mechanism of sudden hearing loss associated with a viral etiology is unknown.

Vascular causes of sudden hearing loss are presumed to involve vasospasm or hypercoagulation states. The hearing loss may be mild or moderate in degree, but more frequently it is severe or total.

No specific therapy of proven value is available. A patient with sudden deafness should be evaluated on an emergency basis by an otologist.

VERTIGO

Vertigo is the hallucination of motion. In objective vertigo, the patient feels his environment is in motion; while in subjective vertigo, the patient feels he is moving. The sensation may be rotational; or the patient may experience undulating motions, feelings of unsteadiness, or rocking, without spatial disorientation.

Dizziness is a term used by both patients and physicians to express a variety of sensations, including vertigo. The sensations may have differential diagnostic significance, and a careful description of the sensation is essential.

Frequently, the patient may complain of dizziness when he actually has a sensation of unsteadiness of gait, a period of mental confusion, faintness, giddiness, or blurring of vision, all of which have little or no relationship to actual vertigo. Conversely, some patients use these latter terms when they have experienced vertigo.

Vertigo is divided into two forms, central and peripheral (Table 112-A1). Central vertigo can result from a variety of medical and neurologic conditions that affect the vestibular nuclei and their connections. Central vertigo does not usually have a severe rotational character. Nausea, vomiting, and other autonomic phenomena generally are absent. Usually there are physical findings that suggest a CNS lesion such as ocular palsy, unequal pupils, ptosis, facial palsy, sensory deficits, dysphagia, dysarthria, long tract signs, cerebellar ataxia, or papilledema. Hearing loss and tinnitus, which frequently accompany labyrinthine and eighth nerve disorders, are rarely seen with lesions confined to the brainstem or cerebellum. The presence of vertical nystagmus (upward and downward) indicates brainstem rather than labyrinthine disease. A careful history and physical examination and proper recording of findings is mandatory. A neurological consultation should be sought.

Peripheral vertigo is caused by diseases of the middle ear, inner ear, and eighth nerve. Peripheral vertigo is usually accompanied by decreased hearing that may be mild or severe.

The severe attack of peripheral vertigo can be controlled with parenteral antiemetics. Consultation with the otolaryngologist should be sought before treatment.

TRAUMA

Lacerations

Lacerations of the auricle can often be repaired in the emergency department using infiltration of field block anesthesia with 1% or 2% lidocaine without epinephrine. Avoid debridement of soft tissue and cartilage. Close the wound in layers: first the perichondrium or cartilage with 4-0 chromic catgut, and then the skin with 5-0 nylon interrupted sutures. Carefully approximate the natural ridges and folds. A mastoid dressing for 24 h is helpful.

Avulsion of all or part of the ear may often be replaced by the otolaryngologist as a free graft. If it is possible to completely restore the avulsed ear, the cartilage may be preserved by removing all the skin, and burying the cartilage in the abdominal wall. This will preserve it for future reconstruction.

Hematoma

Hematomas of the ear usually occur as a result of blunt trauma and are particularly common in wrestlers and boxers. Bleeding occurs between the cartilage and its covering perichondrium. Treatment of a hematoma is aseptic drainage by aspiration or by incision. A mastoid-conforming dressing should be applied after drainage. Complications include reaccumulation of the hematoma, deformity, and infection. Reaccumulation requires repeated aspiration or drainage. The cauliflower deformity results from the gradual replacement of the untreated hematoma by fibrous tissue, new cartilage formation, and calcification.

Perichondritis is characterized by a swollen, red, and tender

Table 112-A1. Differential Diagnosis of Vertigo

Disease or Condition	Vertigo	Nystagmus	Caloric Response	Cochlear Symptoms and Signs	Associated Symptoms and Signs	Comments
Endolymphatic hydrops (Ménière's disease)	Severe attacks with nausea & vomiting that lasts *hours* (not days or weeks)	Spontaneous during critical stage; postural in 25% of patients during first few weeks after an attack	Usually depressed in involved ear(s); progressive with recurrent episodes	Tinnitus (louder during attacks) Sensorineural hearing loss Recruitment and diplacusis usually present	Fullness in the ear during an attack; may also be noted before attack begins (as an aura)	Unilateral in 90% of patients Recurring attacks typical Interval is *variable* (days to years)
Benign positional vertigo	Always positional—provoked by certain head positions	Always positional—with latency, brief duration and fatigability	Normal	Absent	None	
Viral labyrinthitis or vestibular neuronitis	Severe 3–5 days, with nausea and vomiting Usually regresses over 3–6 weeks	Spontaneous during severe stage; may be postural during recovery phase	Usually depressed in the involved ear	Absent	Antecedent or concomitant acute febrile disease	Does not recur
Acoustic neuroma	Usually late; more often a progressive feeling of imbalance May be provoked by sudden head movements	Spontaneous type frequently present	Depressed or nonfunctioning labyrinth	Usually appear first Unilateral hightone sensorineural hearing loss and tinnitus Poor discrimination; rapid tone decay Recruitment usually absent	Decreased corneal sensitivity Facial weakness Diplopia Headache Positive radiologic findings Elevated CSF protein	Early diagnosis essential while lesion is small and may be removed with minimal sequelae
Vertebrobasilar insufficiency	Nearly always positional—provoked by certain head positions	Usually accompanies the vertigo	Normal	Absent	Arteriosclerosis; cervical arthritis; vascular malformations	Usually seen in older age group invariably with other symptoms of brainstem ischemia, visual symptoms being most common

Source: Wolfson RJ, Marlowe FI: Vertigo, in Schwartz GR, Safar P. Stone JH, et al (eds): *Principles and Practice of Emergency Medicine.* Philadelphia, Saunders, 1978, vol 1, p 584.

auricle. The causative organism is frequently *Pseudomonas* and the condition is best treated urgently by an otologist.

Foreign Body of the Ear

Children are particularly prone to acquire foreign bodies of the ear. Animate objects must be stupefied or killed before removal. Place a cotton tampon, well moistened with ether, at the external auditory meatus. After 5 min any insect will be stupefied. Then irrigate to flush the insect out.

Occasionally attempts to remove the object result in pushing it beyond the isthmus, the junction of the cartilaginous and bony canal. In patients in whom the object is lodged beyond the isthmus, removal may require general anesthesia. If the foreign body is distal to the isthmus, it may be grasped with a microforceps and removed. A larger object is removed by placing a hook or loop behind it and pulling it out. In some instances a stream of water may be directed superiorly to push the object out. However, vegetable foreign bodies should not be irrigated, as they will swell. Unless the child is calm during foreign body removal, it is best to use general anesthesia. Many instances of traumatic injury to

the tympanic membrane or the ossicles have been recorded because a child jumped during an attempt to remove a foreign body.

Thermal Injuries

With prolonged exposure to extreme cold, the upper and outer edge of the auricle becomes waxy and white; and may feel hard and cold. These signs, associated with loss of sensation, are diagnostic of frostbite. Frostbite is treated by rapid rewarming, with warm irrigations or application of warm compresses, at a temperature between 42°C (107.6°F) and 44°C (111.2°F), for not more than 20 min. Analgesics are necessary since the thawing process is usually painful. Avoid reexposure.

Contact with hot water bottles, hot liquids, or electrical currents may result in burns of varying degrees. Severe burns require cleansing of the wound by strict aseptic technique using detergent skin cleanser and saline solution. After thorough cleansing, excise all devitalized tissue and blisters. Apply silver sulfadiazine cream, and a thick mastoid dressing. Tetanus toxoid, antibiotics, and analgesics are indicated.

Chemical Injuries

Strong acids or alkalis produce a burn on immediate contact. Treatment consists of copious irrigation. Bathe the ear and the ear canal with saline or sterile water. Let the liquid remain for 2 or 3 min then aspirate and dry the auricle. Repeat this procedure three or four times, and thoroughly dry the ear and canal.

Traumatic Perforations

Perforations of the tympanic membrane may occur from a penetrating object such as a pencil or cotton-tipped applicator or after blunt trauma from an explosion.

In general, perforations heal spontaneously without specific treatment other than avoiding water in the ear. Careful follow-up is necessary. If the ear is contaminated, either from swimming pool water or by a penetrating object, administer a systemic antibiotic such as penicillin. Facial nerve palsy, hearing loss, or vertigo necessitate immediate ENT consultation. Otherwise, follow-up in a few days by an otologist for hearing assessment is sufficient.

Barotitis

Aerotitis may occur following barometric pressure changes such as those associated with flying or scuba diving. The sensation of a blocked ear and pain are the common complaints. Examination usually reveals a hemorrhagic or hyperemic tympanic membrane and fluid in the middle ear.

Barotitis is treated by analgesics, oral decongestants, topical nasal sprays, and middle ear inflation. Antibiotics should be given if secondary infection develops. Myringotomy is indicated if the pain is extremely severe and unrelenting, or if the fluid fails to resolve on medical therapy.

B. Acute Upper Airway Obstruction

Obstruction of the airway is one of the most demanding emergency problems the physician may encounter. Orderly and prompt evaluation followed by appropriate treatment can be lifesaving.

SIGNS AND SYMPTOMS

The most important signs and symptoms of upper respiratory obstruction are shortness of breath and stridor. Stridor may be either expiratory or inspiratory, and tends to be most marked in laryngeal disorders. In general, inspiratory stridor is associated with obstruction of the supraglottic or glottic larynx, while expiratory stridor is associated with subglottic obstruction. Other signs and symptoms that may be present are hoarseness or change in voice, difficulty in speaking, difficulty in swallowing either food or oral secretions, or loud wheezing.

History

A brief, but carefully obtained history is probably the most important single contribution towards an etiologic diagnosis of upper airway obstruction. It is of prime importance to establish the time of onset; the activities surrounding the onset, such as eating or holding something in one's mouth; and whether the obstruction is associated with systemic symptoms such as fever, cough, swollen glands in the neck, weakness, nausea, or vomiting.

Examination

Examination of the patient with acute upper airway obstruction may, of necessity, be brief, but this does not preclude its being thorough. The oral cavity must be examined with particular attention to the tongue, looking for inflammation or swelling. Similar examination of the area of the tonsils, uvula, and the hypopharynx must be employed. Examination of the hypopharynx and larynx requires facility with the use of the laryngeal mirror and headlight.

The neck must be examined for evidence of trauma such as abrasion, hematoma, ecchymosis, or crepitus, or for evidence of inflammation such as tenderness and lymphadenopathy. Auscultate the chest and neck to localize the source of stridor or wheezing, and to identify pulmonary disorders such as asthma or pneumothorax.

DIFFERENTIAL DIAGNOSIS

The causes of acute upper airway obstruction may be grouped into several categories: foreign bodies, trauma, irritants and corrosives, and inflammatory conditions including infections. Miscellaneous causes discussed are congenital anomalies, vocal cord paralysis, and cysts and neoplasms.

Foreign Bodies

Respiratory obstruction from a foreign body most often occurs in children, who are particularly prone to aspirating objects such as beans, buttons, beads, or parts from small toys that become lodged in the larynx. The problem most often occurs in children under 4. If a child is less than 1 year old, the foreign body is more likely to be lodged in the upper airway, that is, at or above the larynx. In the child that is older, the foreign body is more likely to involve the lower airway.

If the foreign body lodges in the upper airway at the larynx or above, the presenting symptoms are usually marked stridor and respiratory distress. Indeed, total airway obstruction may occur and profound asphyxia may be present. Wheezing is present if the aspirating foreign body passes past the epiglottis and lodges in one of the main bronchi. It may be unilateral, but because of the small chest size of the child, it may be readily heard in both lung fields. Aspiration of a foreign body should be considered in any child who has a rapid, sudden onset of wheezing or inspiratory stridor without prior upper respiratory tract infection and with no past history of wheezing events.

The diagnosis is made largely on the characteristic history of sudden onset of obstructive symptoms, associated with coughing or choking spells in a small child.

If the foreign body is suspected to be in the lower airway and the child is stable in regard to his respiratory status, both inspiratory and expiratory roentgenograms of the chest should be obtained. A plain film may demonstrate air trapping on the affected side. Inspiration and expiration views may demonstrate shift of the mediastinum away from the affected side. A better evaluation of the chest can be made under the fluoroscope if an esophageal foreign body is suspected. Both anteroposterior and lateral views of the chest should be obtained. The object ingested may be of sufficient radiodensity to be visualized. Even if the object is not radiopaque, air in the stomach may be regurgitated up the esophagus and thus outline the foreign object.

If the obstruction is of mild degree, it is important to refrain from doing anything that might convert a mild or partial obstruction to a total one. This caution refers particularly to the practice of turning very small children upside down and soundly smacking them on the back to expel a foreign body that perhaps has already entered the tracheobronchial tree. This is as likely to cause the foreign body to lodge in the subglottic area as it is to expel it. In the case of adults, the most commonly aspirated object is a bolus of meat. The use of back blows and abdominal or chest thrusts is discussed in Chapter 1A, "Basic Cardiopulmonary Resuscitation." If the foreign body is visible in the pharynx, it can be removed. Removal under direct visualization with a laryngoscope or bronchoscope may be necessary.

Recurrent or persistent pneumonia may develop distal to a foreign body obstruction in the lower airways.

Epiglottitis

Acute epiglottitis is characterized by the abrupt onset of rapidly progressive respiratory obstruction, usually in a child aged two to eight. In children the most common causative organism is *Hemophilus influenza*, type B. Acute epiglottitis is being reported with increasing frequency in adults also.

The clinical course is often characterized by the abrupt onset of severe sore throat, followed by pooling of pharyngeal secretions, drooling and dysphagia; fever that may reach 40.5°C (105°F); and rapid development of dyspnea and stridor. In most cases there is an upper respiratory tract infection prodrome. In over 50 percent of the cases, this may be present for as long as 12 to 24 h preceding the onset of recognizable symptoms. Restlessness, cyanosis, and exhaustion can rapidly develop. The face frequently reflects fear and apprehension, but oddly, there is little crying or struggling. Apparently, the entire effort is directed toward obtaining enough air, and quiet breathing provides more air than struggling. The chin is frequently thrust forward and the patient resists all efforts

to be placed on his or her back. Air hunger is usually marked, and suprasternal and infrasternal retractions are commonly present. The voice may be muffled or hoarse, but there is a striking absence of expiratory wheezing or the barking cough of croup.

Examination, which is best carried out with the patient in the sitting position, reveals a cherry-red, markedly swollen epiglottis. Complete respiratory arrest has been noted to occur suddenly, provoked by such seemingly innocuous events as attempting to visualize the laryngopharynx with a tongue blade or laryngeal mirror, or even the drawing of a blood sample. There is some evidence that inspection of the oral cavity is safe in the well oxygenated patient, and a short period of high-flow oxygenation by face mask seems to be a worthwhile precautionary measure. The diagnosis can often be made on the basis of a soft tissue lateral roentgenogram of the neck. The epiglottis will appear as a thumbshaped object on the lateral neck film (Fig. 112-B1). A normal epiglottis will appear slim, like the distal phalanx of the little finger (Fig. 112-B2). However, the best method for rapid diagnosis is direct visualization.

Instruments for immediate intubation, such as a laryngoscope and endotracheal tubes of the appropriate size, and/or a rigid bronchoscope should be readily at hand, and a physician skilled in their use readily available. With this preparation, a gentle attempt is made to visualize the epiglottis with a tongue blade that is directed inferiorly, and not placed near the base of the tongue or pushed posteriorly.

A similarly gentle visualization with a laryngeal mirror is also of value in making a rapid diagnosis. Some authors have suggested that once the presumptive diagnosis of acute epiglottitis is made, all examinations should be carried out in the operating room. The exact cause for respiratory arrest, which can occur with dramatic

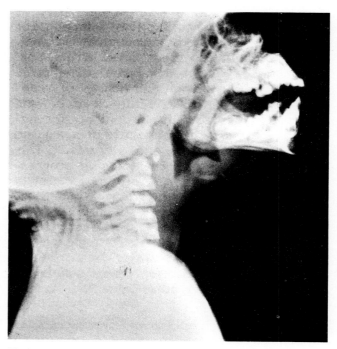

Figure 112-B1. The diagnosis of epiglottitis is confirmed by lateral neck film that shows an enlarged epiglottis encroaching the airway. (Courtesy of The Children's Hospital Medical Center of Akron.)

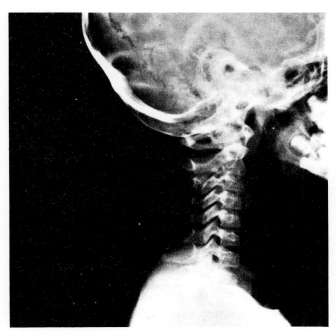

Figure 112-B2. Contrast the epiglottis in the previous film with the normal epiglottis shown in the film. (Courtesy of The Children's Hospital Medical Center of Akron.)

Table 112-B1. Advantages and Disadvantages of Tracheostomy and Endotracheal Intubation

Tracheostomy	Endotracheal Intubation
Necessitates surgery and its complications	Avoids surgery
Fewer laryngeal complications	More laryngeal complications (e.g., subglottic stenosis); decrease, however, with use of PVC tubes
More difficult and slower initially; reintubation easier	1 to 2 mm smaller than usual for age
Less likely displacement of tube; if displaced, more deaths	Quicker initially; however, reintubation more difficult
Higher mortality	More likely displacement of tube; if displaced, death less likely
Easier suction	Lower mortality
Less dead space; larger tube and therefore easier to ventilate	More difficult to suction
Probably takes less intensive care and sedation	More dead space; smaller tube and therefore more difficult to ventilate
Less uncomfortable to patient	Requires more intensive care and sedation
Often difficult to discontinue	Quite uncomfortable to patient
Larger tubes; therefore less easily obstructed	Easier to discontinue
	Smaller tubes and therefore easily obstructed

Source: Gross CW: Medical management, nasotracheal intubation, and tracheotomy in the treatment of upper airway obstruction in children. *Otolaryngol Clin North Am* 10:162, 1977. Used by permission.

suddenness, is uncertain, but some authors have suggested that the swollen epiglottis is drawn like a plug into the glottis, and the increased respiratory efforts serve only to impact the structure further. Other authors believe that the inflamed larynx is more prone to laryngospasm or that respiratory arrest results merely from rapidly progressing fatigue. Regardless of the exact mechanism, sudden arrest can and does occur, and if no artificial airway has been established, the patient dies.

Establishment and maintenance of an artificial airway is the primary and crucial part of the management of acute supraglottic laryngitis. With an experienced anesthesiologist available, immediate oral or nasal endotracheal intubation is carried out. An alternative, which is much less desirable, is positive-pressure oxygenation by mask as a temporizing measure. If the supraglottic structures are so swollen as to prevent passage of an endotracheal tube, a rigid bronchoscope is introduced with the aid of a laryngoscope to secure an airway and a tracheostomy may then be performed in an orderly fashion over the bronchoscope. This latter procedure requires the availability of an experienced otolaryngologist. Currently, there is considerable controversy surrounding the use of endotracheal intubation versus tracheostomy in the treatment of epiglottitis, and a detailed discussion of the pros and cons of each technique is beyond the scope of this paper, but Table 112-B1 delineates some of the pertinent points. In the final analysis, the method of treatment is largely determined by the facilities and the personnel available at the treatment center, and both methods are employed under appropriate circumstances with excellent results.

The medical treatment of acute epiglottitis includes broad-spectrum antibiotics, most commonly ampicillin (100 to 200 mg/kg) in divided doses, fluids, humidification and oxygenation, and possibly the use of steroids for their anti-inflammatory effect in reducing laryngeal edema.

Croup (Acute Subglottic Laryngitis)

Croup also parades under a host of other names such as inflammatory croup, spasmodic croup, and acute laryngotracheobronchitis. Croup is a common term used to denote a hoarse, barking cough associated with difficulty in breathing. Its occurrence in children in a nocturnal form is not uncommon, and it is secondary primarily to inflammatory change in the loose tissue of the subglottic area. Inflammation of this tissue causes a swelling that resembles the cherry red change noted in the epiglottis in acute epiglottitis, and indeed the loose tissues in both areas are quite similar. It is not uncommon to find that the vocal cords themselves appear normal or only slightly infected.

Laryngotracheobronchitis or croup generally occurs in the 1- to 5-year-old child. There is a history of one to three days of viral-like upper respiratory tract infection, with a slow and progressive onset of stridor. Symptoms are usually worse at night when the child is lying down. Croup may last for three to four days and may exhibit a cyclic pattern in terms of severity.

The patient with acute subglottic croup is in danger of asphyxiation but the danger is less imminent than in acute epiglottitis, as the course tends to be less fulminant or explosive. The treatment includes a cool, moist, humidified atmosphere, antibiotics, and steroids, along with supportive measures to prevent dehydration and drying of secretions. The patient is carefully observed, and the indication for intubation or tracheostomy is deterioration in spite of increased humidity, antibiotics, and steroids. This deterioration may be reflected in progressively worse blood gas determinations, or in a clinical change for the worse. In general, a respiratory rate over 40, a pulse rate greater than 160, or increasing restlessness with retraction of neck tissues indicate the need for an artificial airway. The symptoms and signs of supra-glottic versus subglottic laryngitis are compared in Table 112-B2.

Racemic epinephrine given by inhalation has proved to be of value in early croup, and according to some authors, it has reduced the need for intubation or tracheostomy.

When given, racemic epinephrine is mixed in a 1:8 dilution with normal saline solution in a sufficient quantity to provide 13 to 15 min of treatment. A typical dilution might be 0.5 mL of racemic epinephrine mixed with 4 mL of normal saline solution. When given, it should be regarded as a symptomatic and tem-porizing treatment. The effect of this treatment is variable, and if used repeatedly, it may be associated with a rebound phenomenon. If respiratory distress is moderate or severe, the child should be hospitalized regardless of the results with racemic epinephrine.

The controversy regarding the use of intubation versus trache-ostomy is similar to that in acute epiglottitis, with the most notable exception being that in acute laryngotracheobronchitis both the endotracheal tube and tracheostomy cannula traverse the in-flammed tissues, whereas in acute supraglottic laryngitis only the endotracheal tube actually traverses the inflamed tissues.

Spasmodic croup is a variant of croup that is essentially non-inflammatory in nature and occurs in infants and young children, often nocturnally. The child may awaken out of a sound sleep with a hollow, barking cough, and may shortly develop inspiratory stridor and dyspnea.

The symptoms are frightening for both the child and parents, and both cyanosis and air hunger can occur. The end of the attack is as abrupt as its onset, and the child worn out from exertion, commonly falls asleep. Treatment is conservative, and trache-ostomy is seldom, if ever, necessary.

Table 112-B2. Symptoms of Laryngotracheobronchitis and Acute Supraglottic Laryngitis

Laryngotracheobronchitis	Supraglottic Laryngitis
Mostly in children less than 2 to 3 years old	Mostly in children over 2 to 3 years old
More in winter	Occurs year round
Common	Uncommon
Viral, increased WBCs, lymphocytes	Bacterial, increased WBCs, PMNs
Does not extend above true vocal cords	Does not extend below true vocal cords
Prodrome of several days of "cold" and gradual onset of symptoms	No real prodrome or very short prodrome of sore throat and dysphagia; rapid onset and development of symptoms and course
Sick but not toxic	Toxic; high fever
Inspiratory and expiratory	Inspiratory obstruction and stridor, which occurs late
Hypoxia and cyanosis frequent	Hypoxia; no cyanosis
Not particularly affected by position	Frequently cannot lie down
Croupy cough	No cough
Hoarse voice	Clear voice but muffled
Larynx not tender	Larynx sometimes tender to movement
No drooling; able to swallow	Drooling; often cannot swallow
Recurrence not uncommon	Does not recur

Source: Gross CS: Medical management, nasotracheal intubation, and tracheotomy in the treatment of upper airway obstruction in children. *Otolaryngol Clin North Am* 10:159, 1977. Used by permission.

Trauma

Obstruction secondary to trauma may be due to direct trauma to the larynx or neck. Indirectly, obstruction may occur from bleed-ing in the pharynx or from a hematoma in the parapharyngeal structures, or from occlusion by the tongue. Relief of the obstruc-tion may involve a measure as simple as suctioning out the upper airway or altering the position of the patient's head so that ob-structing tissues resume a more normal position. Grasping and fixation of obstructing tissues is frequently an excellent means of counteracting the obstructive effect of injured tissues.

The possibility of an injury to the cervical spine should be considered at all times, since extension of the neck, in an attempt to place an airway or perform endotracheal intubation, can lead to paralysis.

In some forms of direct trauma to the larynx, such as may ocur in high speed vehicular accidents where the neck may strike the dashboard, marked respiratory distress may occur with little evi-dence of laryngeal injury. This most often is a result of bilateral vocal cord paralysis from a shearing injury to the recurrent lar-yngeal nerves in their position posterior to the cricothyroid joint articulation. There seems to be some misconception regarding unusual difficulty in intubating patients with vocal cord paralysis, but this is easily accomplished and is the initial treatment of choice. In some types of direct laryngotracheal injury, the extent of trauma may make nasal or endotracheal intubation impossible, and cri-cothyrotomy or tracheostomy may be necessary.

Irritants and Corrosives

Damage to the pharyngeal, laryngeal, and cervical tracheal mu-cous membranes can occur from steam, irritant gases (such as chlorine), corrosive liquids, burning gases, or hot air from a fire.

Examination may reveal burns of the oral mucous membranes, as seen in children with lye ingestions, and the assumption must be made that burns have occurred futher down in the aerodigestive tract until proven otherwise. Nasotracheal intubation is often done early, before the development of severe airway edema that can make intubation difficult or impossible. Otherwise, oxygenation and the use of steroids and antibiotics may be sufficient.

Angioneurotic Edema

The rapid and sudden onset of respiratory obstruction secondary to angioneurotic or allergic inflammatory edema may be quite striking and frightening for both the patient and physician. It is most likely to occur in an individual with a history of allergies and may follow the ingestion of foods such as shellfish, chocolate, peanuts, or strawberries, or it may be idiopathic. Examination may reveal massive edema of the tongue, or edema of the palate and uvula to such a degree that the uvula may resemble a large white grape (uvular hydrops). Edema may also involve the epi-glottis or larynx.

Treatment is administration of oxygen, epinephrine, and cor-ticosteroids, and the response is usually rapid and dramatic. Top-ical epinephrine may be helpful for uvular edema. Also, multiple scratches with a needle or knife blade on the uvula are almost always effective. In extreme or repetitive cases the tip of the uvula may be amputated by an otolaryngologist.

Peritonsillar, Retropharyngeal, and Parapharyngeal Abscess

These complications of pharyngitis, tonsillitis, or adenoiditis can cause airway obstruction. They are characterized by throat pain and swelling, fever and toxicity, and prior upper respiratory infection. Emergency otolaryngologic consultation is required, and treatment consists of antibiotics, and incision and drainage of the abscess.

Peritonsillar Abscess

Peritonsillar abscesses are rare in young children and most common in adolescents and young adults. The patient has a history of tonsillitis that was untreated or treated by a single injection of penicillin. The pain then localizes to one side and the patient begins to have drooling, alteration of voice, referred ear pain, and trismus. Fever and leukocytosis are present. On examination the tonsil is pushed down medially towards the midline or beyond, displacing the uvula.

Retropharyngeal Abscess

A retropharyngeal abscess usually occurs in a child less than 4 years of age. There is usually a history of upper respiratory tract infection. The signs and symptoms include fever, difficulty in breathing and swallowing, enlarged cervical nodes, and a stiff neck. Intraoral examination will show fullness or a mass in the posterior pharyngeal area. Palpation must be carefully done to avoid rupturing the abscess. A lateral soft tissue roentgenogram will help to confirm the diagnosis.

Parapharyngeal Abscess

The infection localizes in a space bounded by the pterygomandibular raphe, prevertebral fascia, hyoid bone, and base of the skull. The symptoms include marked trismus, fever, painful swallowing, altered voice, and stiff neck. On examination there will be pharyngeal swelling and displacement of the tonsil (but usually with little redness or other signs of tonsillar infection), and external swelling in the parotid regions. Trismus with an internal and external bulge, should suggest this diagnosis.

Miscellaneous Cases

Acute upper airway obstruction may also be noted secondary to the congenital anomalies. These may occur above the larynx, such as in choanal atresia (the newborn is usually an obligate nasal breather), or with malformations of the tongue. At the level of the larynx there may be webs, cysts, or atresia of the various cartilages. Below the level of the larynx there may be a tracheoesophagela fistula, vascular rings, or abnormalities of the greater vessels.

Bilateral vocal cord paralysis secondary to dysfunction of the recurrent laryngeal nerves may acutely impair the upper airway. This is most common following thyroid surgery, but it can occur following general anesthesia for any operative procedure, or it may be idiopathic. Inability to abduct the vocal cords may also occur in cricoarytenoid arthritis, or in conditions producing laryngeal tetany or spasm. The onset of the obstruction may be acute, or slow and insidious.

Cysts and neoplasms of the upper respiratory system can produce airway obstruction, and though usually slow-growing, the obstruction may appear acute at the time of presentation. Included in this group are benign neoplasms, such as subglottic hemangioma, and the more common malignant lesions of the larynx, as well as benign cysts such as dermoids and laryngoceles.

MANAGEMENT OF AIRWAY OBSTRUCTION

Endotracheal Intubation

The most rapid method for establishing an airway is endotracheal intubation. Properly executed, it is done without anesthesia, and often avoids the necessity for a traumatic, hurried tracheostomy. Following intubation, anesthesia may be administered while an orderly tracheostomy is performed. There are only rare instances, such as massive facial trauma or direct trauma to the larynx, in which intubation is not possible. This situation might also prevail in the case of impacted foreign body.

Cricothyrotomy (Laryngotomy)

Where endotracheal intubation is not possible, an obstructed airway is best relieved by an opening through the cricothyroid membrane. This may be done with a large-bore needle, or with a host of other devices designed for this purpose.

In the absence of these special devices, an incision is made into the cricothyroid membrane with a small surgical blade, and the opening maintained with any device at hand.

Emergency Tracheostomy

This procedure is carried out when the obstruction is too severe to allow time for an orderly tracheostomy, when facilities are unavailable for insertion of a bronchoscope or endotracheal tube, and when the surgeon believes that the patient cannot survive more than a few minutes without brain damage. The operation is fraught with difficulty, associated with high risk of complications, and is to be avoided at all costs by appropriate preplanning to avoid being placed in the position of having to do the procedure.

Orderly Tracheostomy

This procedure is the operation of choice for impending airway obstruction, and whenever possible it is performed with an endotracheal tube or bronchoscope in place, and an anesthetist in control of the airway. The techniques and selection of appropriate tracheostomy cannulas are beyond the scope of this discussion.

Otolaryngologic or surgical consultation should be obtained well in advance of the procedure as well as for the actual performance of the operative procedure, the day-to-day care of the tracheostomy, and the ultimate decannulation of the patient. Tracheostomy is *not* a minor surgical procedure to be carried out at the bedside.

BIBLIOGRAPHY

Otologic Emergencies

Ballenger JJ: *Deseases of the Nose, Throat and Ear,* ed 12. Philadelphia, Lea & Febiger, 1977.

DeWeese DD, Saunders WH: *Textbook of Otolaryngology,* ed 5. St. Louis, CV Mosby Co, 1977.

Fried MD, Baden E: Management of fractures in children. *Oral Surg* 12:129–139, 1954.

Newman MH, Olson NR, Singleton EF: *Handbook of Ear, Nose and Throat Emergencies.* Flushing, Medical Examination Publishing Co, Inc, 1973.

Snow JB Jr: *Introduction to Otorhinolaryngology.* Chicago, Year Book Medical Publishers, Inc, 1979.

Wolfson RJ, Marlow FI: Vertigo, in Schwartz GR, Safar P, Stone JH, et al (eds): *Principles and Practice of Emergency Medicine.* Philadelphia, Saunders, 1978, vol 1, pp 581–591.

Acute Upper Airway Obstruction

Allen T: Suspected esophageal foreign body: Choosing appropriate management. *J Am Coll Emerg Physicians* 8:101–105, 1979.

Aytac A, Yurdakul Y, Ikizler C, et al: Inhalation of foreign bodies in children. Report of 500 cases. *J Thorac Cardiovasc Surg* 74:145–151, 1977.

Cantrell RW, Bell RA, Morioka WT: Acute epiglottitis: Intubation versus tracheostomy. *Laryngoscope* 88:994–1005, 1978.

Daniidis J, Symeonidis B, Triaridis K, et al: Foreign body in the airways: A review of 90 cases. *Arch Otolaryngol* 103:570–573, 1977.

Gross CW: Medical management, nasotracheal intubation, and tracheotomy in the treatment of upper airway obstruction in children. *Otolaryngol Clin North Am* 10:157–166, 1977.

Hunsicker RC, Gartner WS: Fogarty catheter technique for removal of endobronchial foreign body. *Arch Otolaryngol* 103:103–104, 1977.

Katznelson D: On the diagnosis of foreign bodies in the respiratory tract in children: A point of view. *Clin Pediatr* (Phila) 17:107–108, 1978.

Liscott MS, Horton WC: Management of upper airway obstruction. *Otolaryngol Clin North Am* 12:351–373, 1979.

Majd NS, Mofenson HC, Greensher J: Lower airway foreign body aspiration in children. An analysis of 13 cases. *Clin Pediatr* (Phila) 16:13–16, 1977.

Steichen FM, Fellini A, Einhorn AH: Acute foreign body laryngotracheal obstruction: A cause for sudden and unexpected death in children. *Pediatrics* 48:281–284, 1971.

Strome M: Tracheobronchial foreign bodies: An updated approach. *Ann Otol Rhinol Laryngol* 86:649–654, 1977.

Tauscher JW: Esophageal foreign body: An uncommon cause of stridor. *Pediatrics* 61:657–658, 1978.

Tucker JA: Obstruction of the major pediatric airway. *Otolaryngol Clin North Am* 12:329–341, 1979.

CHAPTER 113
NASAL EMERGENCIES
AND SINUSITIS

Frank I. Marlowe, Ali Aghamohamadi

EPISTAXIS

The most frequent cause of epistaxis is spontaneous erosion of the superficial mucosal blood vessels situated near the anterior end of the nasal septum. Less commonly, bleeding originates from the branches of the ethmoidal arteries (resulting in bleeding from the roof of the nasal chamber or posterior septum), or sphenopalatine arteries (manifested by postnasal or lateral nasal wall bleeding). Local factors associated with nasal hemorrhage include ulcerations that result from excessive nasal dryness (nose picker's ulcer), nasal septal perforations, nasal trauma, nasal tumors, and hereditary hemorrhagic telangiectasia (Osler-Weber-Rendu disease).

Systemic diseases associated with epistaxis include hypertension, arteriosclerosis, blood dyscrasias, and coagulation disorders. Recognition and control of such associated conditions are important in successful mangement of the nosebleed.

General management of the severe nosebleed consists of maintaining the vital signs; obtaining a CBC, platelet count, prothrombin time, and PTT; and stopping the bleeding. Examine the patient in the sitting position to prevent swallowing and aspiration of blood. Instruct the patient to blow his nose of remaining blood. Using a headlight and nasal speculum, inspect the septum, floor, and lateral wall of both sides of the nose, to determine the site of bleeding. Topical vasoconstrictors can be applied in an effort to locate the bleeding point.

Anterior Epistaxis

Usually bleeding is from Kiesselbach's plexus (anterior inferior part of the nasal septum). Active bleeding can be controlled temporarily by pinching the nose for 4 to 5 min. After the active bleeding is controlled, the point may be cauterized with a silver nitrate bead or by electrocautery.

If bleeding cannot be controlled as above or if the source of bleeding is not accessible to cauterization, anesthetize the nasal chamber with a topical anesthetic such as 4% lidocaine or 2% cocaine and insert nasal packing. When packing is necessary, a properly sized Nasostat hemostatic nasal balloon or continuous strips of ½-in petrolatum gauze inserted under direct vision can be used to stop the bleeding.

The Nasostat hemostatic nasal balloon is a disposable rubber cuffed tube. First the cuff is inflated with 15 to 20 mL of air to make sure the bleeding stops. Then the air is removed and sterile saline is instilled. The Nasostat controls hemorrhage by exerting mechanical pressure on the site of the bleeding that may be in the anterior, middle, or posterior part of the nasal chamber.

The conventional nasal pack consists of petrolatum gauze strips that are placed in layers, starting either in the floor or roof of the nasal chamber, until the nasal chamber is tightly filled. To avoid displacement of the nasal septum to the opposite side, resulting in loosening of the pack, the other nostril may also be packed.

Whenever a nasal packing of any sort is used, the patient can be placed on a broad-spectrum antibiotic such as ampicillin until the packs are removed. A patient with anterior packing can be treated as an outpatient if the medical condition permits, and should be seen again in 24 h.

Posterior Epistaxis

If the bleeding site is in the nasopharynx or posterior end of the nasal chamber, it may be necessary to insert a posterior nasal pack. Posterior packs can be applied by using a gauze pack, Foley catheter, or Nasostat.

The patient with a posterior bleed should be admitted to the hospital for further care and evaluation. Humidified air, antibiotics and analgesics are generally necessary.

Posterior Gauze Pack

A satisfactory gauze pack can be fashioned by securing three strings of heavy suture material to a rolled 4 in × 4 in gauze sponge. The pack is inserted as follows:

- Anesthetize the nasal chambers.
- Spray the oropharynx with 4% lidocaine, or 5% cocaine.
- Insert the tips of two red rubber catheters, size Fr 8 or Fr 10, through the nostrils into the oropharynx.
- Grasp the tips of the catheters with a straight hemostat and pull them out of the mouth. (Now the tips of the catheters are out of the mouth and the ends are in the nostrils.)
- Fasten the ends of two of the strings to the tips of the catheters.

- Pull the ends of the catheters, which are in the nostrils, and make sure that you have fastened the strings to the proper tip on each side. By pulling of the catheters simultaneously the posterior pack is directed into the mouth and then into the oropharynx. The packing is placed in the nasopharynx by pushing with the second and third finger of the right hand, directing it behind the palate, while simultaneously pulling on the string from the bleeding nostril with the left hand.
- Strings from the right and left nostrils are tied on a gauze roll that is placed over the nasal columella. The third string of the posterior pack, which is in the mouth, is taped to the cheek. This string is to facilitate later removal of the packing from the nasopharynx and mouth.
- Anterior nasal packing should then be performed unilaterally or bilaterally.

Foley Catheter Balloon Tamponade

The insertion of a Foley catheter into the nasopharynx is as follows:

- Anesthetize the anterior nasal chambers as before.
- Insert a Foley catheter, Fr 10 to Fr 14 with a 20- to 30-mL bag, into the side that bleeds, advancing it along the floor of the nose until you see the catheter tip in the pharynx.
- Inflate the balloon with air or saline up to 20 mL and then pull to lodge it in the nasopharynx.
- Ask the patient or the nurse to pull moderately on the catheter while you pack strips of petrolatum gauze in both nostrils.
- Wrap one or two 4 in × 4 in gauze sponges around the stem of the catheter to close the anterior nasal opening. Pull moderately to make sure the bag has not slipped into the oropharynx.
- Keep the Foley in place by putting a Montgomery or Hoffman clamp around the stem of the catheter and on the 4 in × 4 in gauze sponges. Avoid excessive pull on the catheter and avoid pressure on the nasal skin.

NASAL TRAUMA

Fracture

The nasal bones make up the upper one-third of the nasal pyramid and the lower two thirds is made of cartilage. The midline dorsal support is provided by the cartilaginous septum and the lateral nasal vault is supported by paired upper and lower lateral cartilages. In severe trauma the septum may be fractured or displaced from its attachment to the nasal floor.

In evaluating nasal trauma, note any history of preexisting nasal deformity or surgery.

Frontal Nasal Trauma

Frontal nasal trauma displaces the nasal bones inward and downward, resulting in flattening and widening of the osseous dorsum. If the displacement is severe, the medial palpebral ligament may be displaced, leading to an increase in the intercanthal distance. Frontonasal fractures may also be associated with damage to the lacrimal duct, the ethmoid and frontal sinuses, obital margins, and the cribriform plate.

Lateral Nasal Trauma

Lateral nasal trauma displaces the nasal bones inwardly on the side of the applied force with outward displacement of the opposite nasal bone, resulting in step deformities between the nasal bone fragments or the nasal bone and the maxilla.

Unrecognized or untreated nasal fractures in children may lead to serious disturbances in nasal growth and contour, and are often overlooked. In small children, the external nasal structures are elastic and more resistant to fracture, but septal dislocation is common. If nasal fracture or dislocation is suspected, early treatment is necessary.

Edema, hemorrhage, and discoloration of tissues make it difficult to detect fractures and lacerations of the intranasal structures. To properly evaluate such injuries, carefully remove clots and debris and use a vasoconstrictor to shrink the mucous membrane. Mucosal lacerations commonly occur at the junctions of the cartilaginous and bony pyramid. Because of edema, accurate assessment of hematomas and lacerations may be especially difficult if the patient is seen hours after the injury. Edema of the lips, periorbital ecchymosis, and subconjunctival hemorrhage commonly accompany a nasal fracture. Subcutaneous emphysema is not uncommon. Movement of fragments with crepitation or pain may be prominent features, but it may be difficult to elicit fracture movement if the fragments are impacted. The most reliable guide in assessing nasal deformity is palpation of the nasal contour. Roentgenograms are obtained to confirm the diagnosis.

Early reduction of nasal fractures may be possible if swelling does not preclude an accurate assessment of nasal contour. Reduction of simple fractures should be done when the swelling subsides. Treatment of complex fractures, fractures associated with fractures of other facial bones, can be done in 7 to 10 days whenever the condition of the patient permits.

Complications are the development of a septal hematoma, CSF rhinorrhea, and hemorrhage. Bleeding may occur into the space between the septal cartilage and perichondrium. Such subperichondral hematomas appear as a soft unilateral or bilateral swelling of the nasal septum. Unless drained, the hematoma may result in aseptic necrosis of the septal cartilage or predispose to formation of a septal abscess. Drainage of nasal septal hematoma should be performed on an emergency basis by an otolaryngologist.

Cerebrospinal fluid rhinorrhea is characterized by clear nasal discharge. The rhinorrhea is usually unilateral and is increased by having the patient lean forward or by compression of the jugular vein. Neurosurgical consultation is required if CSF rhinorrhea is suspected, and nasal packing should be avoided if at all possible.

Nasal bleeding following trauma may be profuse, but it is generally of short duration. Hemorrhage that fails to cease spontaneously is best controlled by nasal packing.

Foreign Bodies

Nasal foreign bodies are the most common cause of unilateral nasal obstruction and rhinorrhea in children. The discharge is characteristically foul and may be temporarily controlled with antibiotics. There is always danger of aspiration of the foreign body into the lower respiratory tract.

Proper illumination and proper instruments are essential for safe removal. Suction secretions from the nostril, spray the nose with 1% phenylephrine, and visualize the object. Irregularly shaped foreign bodies may be gripped with a small alligator forceps, but round or smooth foreign bodies are best removed by a small hooked instrument that is used to engage the posterior end of the foreign body. Do not push the foreign body back into the nasopharynx because of the danger of aspiration. If the patient is uncooperative and cannot be restrained, general anesthesia may be required.

SINUSITIS

Acute paranasal sinusitis usually is precipitated by an acute viral respiratory tract infection. Swelling of the nasal mucous membrane produces obstruction of the ostium of the paranasal sinus; and the oxygen in the sinus is resorbed and relative negative pressure in the sinus develops and causes pain. This condition is spoken of as vacuum sinusitis. If the vacuum is maintained, a transudate of serum from the vessels of the mucous membrane occurs and fills the sinus. Bacteria may enter the sinus and cause a suppurative sinusitis. The causative organisms in acute sinusitis are generally gram-positive cocci, while in an acute exacerbation of chronic sinusitis, they are generally anaerobic or gram-negative organisms.

Acute maxillary sinusitis causes pain in the maxillary area, and toothache; frontal sinusitis produces frontal headache; ethmoid sinusitis causes pain in the retroorbital area and between the eyes, and frontal headache; and pain from sphenoid sinusitis is less well localized and may be referred to the frontal or occipital area. Fever and chills suggest extension of the infection beyond the sinus. Physical examination shows yellow or green purulent rhinorrhea and the mucous membrane of the nose is red and swollen, and there may be tenderness and swelling over the involved sinus.

Radiopacity of the paranasal sinuses due to a swollen mucous membrane or retained pus in the sinus usually is evident although sinus films may on occasion be normal.

Treatment includes antibiotics, drainage, and analgesics. The antibiotic of choice in acute sinusitis is penicillin with erythromycin as a second choice. In chronic sinusitis a broad-spectrum antibiotic such as ampicillin or a cephalosporin may be more effective.

Drainage can be improved by a topical vasoconstrictor such as $\frac{1}{4}$% phenylephrine. Systemic vasoconstrictors, e.g., ephedrine hydrochloride or pseudoephedrine, or phenylpropanolamine may be prescribed in conjunction with topical ones.

Complications of maxillary sinusitis are caused by uncontrolled spread of infection. Ethmoid sinusitis frequently is complicated by orbital cellulitis and abscess, especially in children. Redness and swelling of the eyelid, proptosis, and displacement of the globe laterally and inferiorly are signs of abscess formation. Orbital abscess and cellulitis are true emergencies, and require inpatient treatment, systemic antibiotics, and drainage where indicated.

Frontal sinusitis may cause osteomyelitis of the posterior table of the frontal bone leading to meningitis, epidural abscess, subdural empyema, and brain abscess; or destroy the anterior table and produce a large forehead abscess (Pott's puffy tumor). If frontal sinusitis fails to respond promptly to systemic antibiotics, the patient should be admitted to the hospital.

Barosinusitis

Barosinusitis results when a significant pressure differential develops between the atmosphere and the paranasal sinus cavity. Rapid descent in an aircraft or rapid ascent from underwater depths are common factors. Inflammatory, allergic, or neoplastic processes may obstruct air flow in and out of the sinus and gases within the sinus are slowly absorbed. Intense pressure differentials result in mucosal edema, intrasinus hemorrhage, or transudation, which are apparent on sinus roentgenograms. Relief of the pain may be dramatic as the sinus ostium opens. If spontaneous drainage does not occur, topical nasal vasoconstrictors are indicated.

BIBLIOGRAPHY

Goldstein E, Gottlieb MA: Roentgeno-oddities. *Oral Surg* 12:129–139, 1954.

Guthrie D: Foreign bodies in the nose. *J Laryngol* 41:454–457, 1926.

Hawkins DB, Kahlstrom EJ, MacLaughlin EF, et al: Foreign body of the right nostril and left bronchus. *Pediatrics* 59:303–304, 1977.

Hunter KM: Foreign body in the nasal fossa. *Oral Surg* 41:805, 1976.

Katz HP, Katz JR, Bernstein M, et al: Unusual presentation of nasal foreign bodies in children. *JAMA* 241:1496, 1979.

Malhotra C, Arora MML, Mehra YN: An unusual foreign body in the nose. *J Laryngol* 84:539–540, 1970.

Proctor DF, Anderson IB, Lundqvist G: Clearance of inhaled particles from the human nose. *Arch Intern Med* 131:132–139, 1973.

T'Ang CT: A large foreign body in the nasopharynx of an infant. *J Laryngol* 68:321–323, 1954.

Walike JW, Chinn J: Evaluation and treatment of acute bleeding from the head and neck. *Otolaryngol Clin North Am* 12:455–464, 1979.

Yarington CT: Sinusitis as an emergency. *Otolaryngol Clin North Am* 12:447–454, 1979.

CHAPTER 114
MAXILLOFACIAL
FRACTURES

Barry H. Hendler

GENERAL PRINCIPLES OF FRACTURE MANAGEMENT

The patient's general medical condition must always be the primary concern in the immediate posttraumatic phase of facial injury. It is rare for a patient to die as a direct result of maxillofacial injuries, yet because of the alarming nature, grotesqueness, and apparent severity of facial injuries, personnel may give these injuries priority over more critical problems.

In the absence of gross soft tissue injury, facial fractures are most often treated several days after initial assessment when an accurate plan for reduction can be developed through definitive radiologic evaluation and patient assessment, and the soft tissue swelling resolves. Three basic principles of treatment are (1) preservation of life; (2) maintenance of function, specifically the masticatory apparatus; and (3) restoration of appearance. The emergency physician functions to stabilize the patient and make the primary assessment of the patient's overall condition prior to consultation with the oral and maxillofacial surgeon.

Outlined below are orderly steps that should be taken for a patient with multiple trauma who also has incurred maxillofacial injuries.

Airway Obstruction

The adequacy of the airway is directly related to injuries of the face and jaw in three ways: (1) inhalation of blood clots, vomitus, saliva, tenacious mucus or portions of teeth, bone, and dentures; (2) inability to protrude the tongue because of posterior displacement or collapse of the bone at the symphysis of the mandible, with loss of anterior tongue support of the genioglossus and geniohyoid muscles (Fig. 114-1); and (3) occlusion of the oronasal pharynx by the soft palate after reposition of the maxilla.

Gross obstructions are usually easily noticed, but potential obstructions are often difficult to predict. Special care must be exercised whenever there is a wound involving the tongue, floor of the mouth, pharynx, or larynx.

In a patient with an associated head injury, deterioration in the level of consciousness can be associated either with CNS dysfunction, or with airway obstruction. Remove all loose foreign bodies, such as teeth or portions of fractured dentures, from the mouth and oropharynx. The conscious patient who has no other complicating injuries should be transported in an upright position, with the head forward, allowing him to maintain an open airway by coughing and expelling any blood or secretions that accumulate in the pharynx.

The unconscious patient or the patient with multiple injuries, should be positioned so that the tongue and contents of the floor of the mouth will be pressed forward or to the side, away from the pharynx, to minimize aspiration. Direct traction on the tongue with a suture can also be used. This suture must be passed through the dorsum of the tongue, as far back as possible in order to bring the tongue away from the posterior pharyngeal wall. Frequent suction of oral and nasal phryngeal secretions is extremely important.

Immediate restoration of the position of the soft palate is affected by forcibly disimpacting the maxilla. This is achieved by passing the index and middle fingers into the mouth with the tips hooked behind and above the soft palate in the posterior choanae, with the thumb placed on the alveolus in the incisor region. Counterpressure is then exerted by placing the other hand on the forehead and applying strong anterior traction to the jaw.

Emergency tracheostomy is seldom necessary, although occasionally it may be necessary to insert a naso- or endotracheal tube. It is far better to perform a tracheostomy on an elective basis, once tracheal intubation has been accomplished.

Hemorrhage

Control of hemorrhage and evaluation of thoracic, abdominal, pelvic, and extremity injuries are dicussed at length in Section 16, "Trauma." Control of hemorrhage in most facial wounds entails local pressure or packing of the wounds with sterile gauze, which suffices. Gross nasal bleeding may be controlled by pressure or by the placement of anterior nasal packs or a posterior nasal pack, as required.

Major facial and cervical vessels are anatomically associated with important cranial nerves (facial, trigeminal, and hypoglossal), and indiscriminate application of hemostats and ligatures may damage these structures.

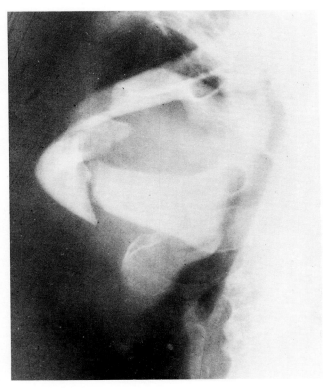

Figure 114-1. Bilateral edentulous mandibular fracture in the mental region. There is a loss of anterior tongue support with possible acute airway obstruction.

Spinal Cord Injury

In addition to intracranial injuries, dislocation or fracture of the cervical spine is frequently associated with severe maxillofacial trauma. When facial or skull x-ray films are ordered, films of the neck should also be obtained to verify the status of the cervical vertebrae. It is not uncommon to discover a cervical dislocation without any localizing neurologic defects, but excessive manipulation of the head may cause severe spinal injury. If it is necessary to establish an emergency airway before the status of the cervical spine is established, it is preferable to perform nasotracheal intubation or tracheostomy or cricothyrotomy with the neck stabilized in a neutral position rather than the hyperextended position generally recommended.

An arbitrary dividing line in fractures of the jaws is at the level of occlusal contact of the teeth. Fractures above this level involve the multiple bones comprising the framework of the middle third of the face, specifically the zygoma, zygomatic arch, maxilla, and nasal and orbital bones. Fractures below this level involve the mandible and its articulations, the bilateral temporomandibular joints (TMJ). In the middle third of the face, displacement is produced primarily by trauma itself, while in the mandible the pull of the attached muscles are a major cause of distraction of the fractured segment.

MANDIBULAR FRACTURES

The classic signs and symptoms of fracture of the mandible are (1) history of trauma; (2) malocclusion; (3) pain; (4) abnormal mobility or crepitus of the fracture segments; (5) interference with function and decreased range of motion; (6) deformity, either facial deformity or deformity of the dental arches; (7) deviation on opening; (8) swelling and ecchymosis; (9) mental nerve anesthesia; and (10) radiologic confirmation.

As with any facial fracture, the primary consideration in the treatment of fractures of the mandible is the assessment and treatment of the general condition of the patient. Mandibular fractures are rarely treated at the time of injury in the absence of gross soft tissue wounds.

There are several approaches to the examination of a patient to make the diagnosis of mandibular fracture. Extra- and intraoral examinations, as well as a radiologic survey, are required to complete the assessment of mandibular trauma.

Examination and Diagnosis

Extraoral Examination

This procedure will usually reveal unilateral or bilateral swelling, deformity, and ecchymosis associated with the ascending ramus or body of the mandible or both. The mandible should be palpated beginning at the mandibular condyle and proceeding along the entire length of the mandibular border, and any tenderness or break in contour of the posterior or inferior border should be noted. Point tenderness is pathognomonic of fracture and frequently a step deformity may be noted at the inferior border. Bilateral inferior alveolar nerves run through the inferior alveolar canal of the mandible and terminate as the mental nerves that supply sensation to the lower lip. Numbness of the lower lip on one or both sides is a strong indication of mandibular fracture.

Intraoral Examination

Bloodstained saliva will be evident in the mouth shortly after injury and if sufficient time has elapsed prior to examination, a marked fetor oris may be noted. The lower dental arch should be examined for disruption of arch continuity, gross malalignment of the teeth should be noted, and the teeth inspected for looseness. Malocclusion may indicate mandibular fracture. In cases where abnormal occlusion is suspected to have existed prior to the fracture, careful inspection of the wear facets on the teeth should be made in consultation with a dentist or oral and maxillofacial surgeon. More simply, patient should be asked to bite on the back teeth as if chewing, and tell the examiner if the bite has changed.

Movement of the mandible is also important. The patient should place the mouth through a full range of motion, with protrusion, lateral excursion, opening and closing, and any limitation of motion or associated pain should be noted. Unilateral subcondylar fractures will cause the mouth to deviate toward the side of fracture on maximum opening. The buccolingual sulcus of the mandible and the mucobuccal and labial gutters should be palpated and these areas examined for tenderness or alteration in contour, break in continuity of the mucosa, or existence of ecchymoses or a sublingual hematoma. A large sublingual hematoma can compromise the airway.

Roentgenographic Examination

A routine x-ray film series of the mandible involves three views: a posteroanterior (PA) view of the face and skull, and right and left lateral oblique views. The whole outline of the mandible is visible in the PA view, but owing to the superimposition of the zygomatic bone and the mastoid process, it may be impossible to accurately interpret the region of the condylar head. In the lateral oblique views, the outline of the mandible may be visualized from the first premolar to the condyle. In all cases, films of both sides of the mandible should be obtained to rule out bilateral or multiple fractures.

In the occlusal view, the x-ray tube is placed directly below the affected region of the mandible and directed at the film that rests upon the occlusal surface of the teeth. This view is particularly useful in evaluation of the mandibular symphysis, especially in those cases in which overshadowing of the cervical spine has somewhat obscured this region in the PA view. A reverse Towne projection view and a TMJ survey are additional roentgenograms to be obtained if fracture of the condyle is suspected. Dental films offer some information, especially in suspected alveolar fractures.

Perhaps the best roentgenogram for suspected fracture of the mandible is the panoramic view of the maxilla and mandible. This view is commonly utilized by oral and maxillofacial surgeons, for it is essentially a clear curved surface tomogram at the level of the facial bones taken by an x-ray beam moving around the head. The problem areas that frequently occur in interpretation with the PA and lateral oblique views are virtually eliminated.

Classification of Mandibular Fractures by Region

By site, the most common area of fracture is the angle of the mandible, followed closely by the condyle, molar, and mental regions. The symphysis is least frequently fractured due to the thickness of this area.

Alveolar Fractures

The most common type of mandibular fracture is a fracture of the alveolus, or tooth-bearing segment of the mandible. Alveolar fractures are most frequently observed in the anterior or incisor region, since this area is more directly exposed to trauma. Viable teeth should be preserved even if they have been avulsed, and no segments of alveolus should be removed if they are firmly attached to mucoperiosteum (Fig. 114-2). Injudicious debridement of the oral cavity will leave the patient with large defects in the alveolus that cannot be corrected prosthetically. Direct pressure should be applied with gauze sponges to the attached dental segments and they should then be covered with a saline-soaked sponge. Most alveolar fractures can then be stabilized with wires or arch bar fixation.

Condyle Fractures

Unilateral fractures of the condyle will cause the jaw to deviate toward the side of fracture on maximum opening. In a bilateral subcondylar fracture the patient usually has an anterior bite, oc-

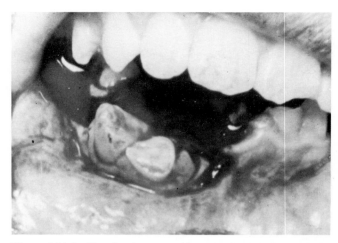

Figure 114-2. Alveolar fracture with avulsed teeth. Preservation of supporting bone and viable teeth is an important early consideration.

clusion on the posterior molars, and no contact of the incisor teeth (Fig. 114-3).

Symphysis Fractures

Fractures of the mandibular symphysis are easily noted by observation of displacement of the lower incisor teeth, disruption of arch continuity, and the ease with which segments can be moved on bimanual palpation (Figs. 114-4 and 114-5).

Angle and Body Fractures

Unfavorable angle fractures are usually acted upon by muscle pull of the pterygomasseteric sling causing the proximal fragment to ride superiorly. This is best observed by roentgenographic examination.

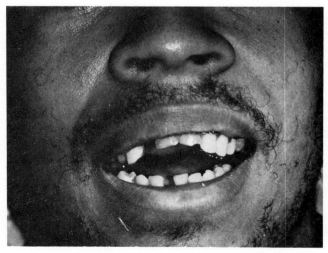

Figure 114-3. Anterior open bite secondary to bilateral subcondylar fractures.

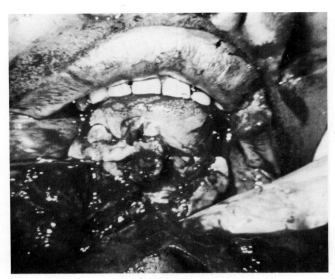

Figure 114-4. Through-and-through avulsive-type laceration of lower lip associated with compound-comminuted symphysis fracture. Intraosseous and intermaxillary fixation must be accomplished prior to soft tissue closure. Gross soft tissue trauma requires immediate surgical intervention.

Edentulous Fractures

Since many teeth may be missing in one or more of the fragments and the occlusion may be difficult to evaluate, the only way to accurately diagnose edentulous or partially edentulous mandibular fractures is by roentgenography.

Treatment

Most mandibular fractures can be reduced and fixed in position by wiring upper and lower teeth in occlusion. Nonviable, loose teeth in the fracture site should be removed unless essential for

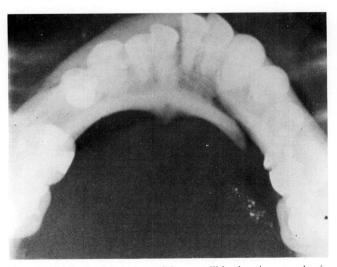

Figure 114-5. Occlusal view of the mandible showing symphysis fracture with telescoping of fragments.

splinting and alignment of the fractures. When many teeth are missing in any or all of the fragments, the problem is more complex, but still lends itself to surgical management.

It is essential for the emergency physician to preserve any dental appliances that may be utilized by the oral and maxillofacial surgeon in intraoral fixation of fractures.

When there are teeth on either side of the fracture site that can be brought into satisfactory occlusion with opposing maxillary teeth, a closed reduction is indicated. When the fracture line is unfavorable and posterior to the last tooth in the dental arch, or in a large edentulous segment, open reduction is most often required.

Tetanus prophylaxis must be instituted in any case of mandibular fracture where soft tissue injuries exist and there is a risk of contamination. Since most mandibular fractures are compounded intraorally, the risk of infection is always present. Antibiotic therapy is indicated with penicillin or a cephalosporin, the current drugs of choice. However, decision on antibiotic maintenance therapy should be made by the surgeon in charge.

MIDFACIAL FRACTURES

Since fractures of the midface can be divided into several categories by anatomic region, each type of fracture will be dicussed individually regarding diagnosis, roentgenographic examination, and treatment. Obviously these fractures can occur in any and all combinations depending on the multiplicity and direction of force.

Zygomatic Arch

Isolated fractures of the zygomatic arch are uncommon, because the force must be directly over the midlateral position of the arch to break it.

Clinical Features

A facial dimpling or depression over the affected region of the zygomatic arch may be evident. This depression may be palpated to elicit point tenderness. In addition, owing to mechanical impingement of the coronoid process of the mandible by the inwardly fractured arch, the patient may not be able to open the mouth or, rarely, may have a partially open mouth and be unable to close it or move it in lateral excursion.

Radiologic Examination

The zygomatic arches are best visualized by a modified basal view of the skull. Other names for this survey include submentaloccipital, submental-vertical, or jug-handle view of the skull (Fig. 114-6).

Treatment

Treatment of zygomatic arch fractures is usually delayed. Criteria for surgical intervention are residual cosmetic deformity or restriction

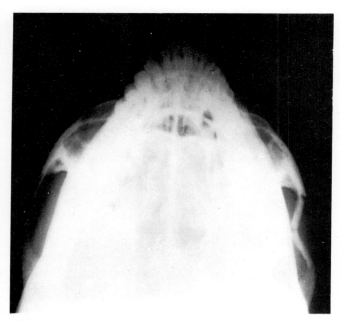

Figure 114-6. Basal view of skull demonstrating unilateral fracture of the zygomatic arch.

of mandibular motion. Frequently several days elapse for resolution of facial swelling before surgery is contemplated.

Zygoma or Zygomatic-Maxillary Complex

The zygoma has major articulations with the frontal bone, maxilla, zygomatic process of the temporal bone, and lateral wall of the sinus, and it is usually subjected to multiple fractures at or near these articulations. A blow to the zygomatic prominence is unlikely to shatter the bone, but probably will result in a line of fracture at the frontal zygomatic suture line; the zygomaticomaxillary suture line or infraorbital rim; the lateral wall of the maxillary sinus at the buttress of the zygoma; or at the zygomatic arch slightly behind the suture, between the short temporal process of the zygomatic bone and the longer zygomatic process of the temporal bone.

Frequently the central portion of the orbital floor will also fracture as part of the zygomaticomaxillary complex. A comminuted depressed fracture may lead to serious complications with entrapment of extraocular muscles. This type of orbital floor fracture should not be confused with the blowout type of orbital fracture.

A pure blowout is caused by direct intraocular trauma, forcing the eye posteriorly, at which time a plunger effect takes place upon the surrounding structures, particularly the relatively incompressible periorbital fat. The dense, strong, laterally angled outer wall of the orbit resists this force that is reflected downward on the thin bone of the floor of the orbit. The bone is forced into the underlying cavity of the maxillary antrum, thus the term orbital blowout. Extraocular muscle entrapment often occurs with this type of fracture.

Clinical Features

The major clinical signs of a fracture of the zygomatic bone or zygomaticomaxillary complex are: (1) edema of the cheek and periorbita; (2) facial flattening shortly after injury or after initial edema subsides; (3) circumorbital or subconjunctival ecchymosis; (4) unilateral epistaxis; (5) anesthesia of the cheek, upper lip, teeth, and gum; (6) step deformity and tenderness over the inferior orbital margin, the frontal zygomatic suture line area, the zygomatic arch, and the lateral wall of the maxillary sinus (intraorally in the region of the zygomatic buttress); (7) diplopia with possible asymmetry of the ocular levels; (8) limitation of mandibular movement; and (9) emphysema of the overlying tissues.

Within 2 or 3 h of injury, the underlying skeletal deformity will be masked by edema. Therefore a great number of these injuries remain undiagnosed until swelling subsides so that resultant disfigurement can be evaluated.

A characteristic flattening of the upper part of the cheek can be noted, either immediately following injury or after the acute phase of edema has subsided, usually in 3 to 5 days (Fig. 114-7).

Palpation, beginning at the medial aspect of the superior orbital margin, will often elicit step deformities at the infraorbital rim and at the frontal zygomatic suture area. The tip of the index finger should be carefully passed around the entire orbital rim. Owing to the thinness of the overlying tissue, step defects are usually easily palpated. Then palpation should proceed along the prominence of the zygoma and along the zygomatic arch. Point tenderness at the fracture sites is usually elicited.

Circumorbital ecchymosis and severe lateral subconjunctival hemorrhage are often present. Carefully examine the pupillary level on both sides to detect unilateral depression of the ocular level. Visual acuity and the range of ocular movements should be tested. Complaints of diplopia or blurring of vision should be noted.

Limitation of mandibular movement may be a result of mechanical obstruction by the depressed zygomatic bone or arch. Intraorally, ecchymosis of the upper buccal sulcus is often evident. Anesthesia of the teeth, gum, cheek, upper lip, and lateral ala nasi on the affected side is caused by injury to the infraorbital nerve at the zygomaticomaxillary fracture site. Subcutaneous em-

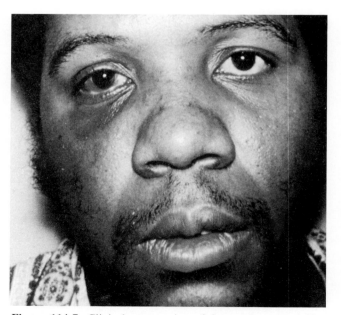

Figure 114-7. Clinical presentation of fractured zygoma. Note facial flattening and lateral subconjunctival hemorrhage.

physema may be caused by fracture of the lateral antral wall at the zygomatic buttress. Unilateral epistaxis may occur, but this usually ceases spontaneously.

Radiologic Examination

The Waters' projection and a basal view of the skull are most important in the initial evaluation of fractures of the zygomatic bone. The Waters' or occipitomental projection, commonly used to visualize the maxillary sinus, offers complete visualization of three of the four areas that commonly fracture and displace in zygomaticomaxillary complex injuries: the frontozygomatic suture area; the zygomaticomaxillary or infraorbital area; and the lateral wall of the maxillary sinus. The presence of opacity or an air-fluid level in the sinus may signify antral hemorrhage secondary to trauma.

A basal view of the skull demonstrates the fourth point of fracture at the zygomatic arch. This view can also demonstrate inward displacement of the prominence of the zygoma and confirm intrusion or rotation of that bone in relation to the undisplaced zygoma on the opposite side. Further evaluation can be obtained through orbital tomograms that confirm fractures at the aforementioned articulations, as well as suspected fractures of the floor of the orbit. Frequently, herniation of orbital contents through the roof of the maxillary antrum can be seen on tomography.

Treatment

The treatment is surgical, through a number of approaches. Detailed discussion is beyond the scope of this text.

Orbital Floor Fractures

Fracture of the orbital floor may occur as a component of a massive zygomaticomaxillary complex fracture, which usually causes comminution of the thin orbital floor, or as an isolated fracture—the less common orbital blowout fracture—caused by a very rapid increase in intraorbital pressure. The force producing a blowout fracture is usually delivered by a blunt object directed at the glove and lids (e.g., a fist or ball) that is slightly larger than the orbital inlet and penetrates the orbital space for only a short distance. The sudden increase in pressure fractures the bony orbit at areas of weakness, usually at the orbital floor or the medial wall.

Direct entrapment of extraocular muscles is a rare finding. In some instances a large volume of orbital soft tissue may protrude into the maxillary sinus, lowering the glove level, and if the soft tissue is not retrieved and the orbital floor reconstructed, occlusal motility will be impaired.

Clinical Features

The two most common presenting ocular problems from orbital floor injury are diplopia and lowering of the glove. Diplopia occurs particularly in zygomaticomaxillary fractures when the thin orbital floor is fractured and comminuted as the stronger zygomatic complex is depressed downward and medially.

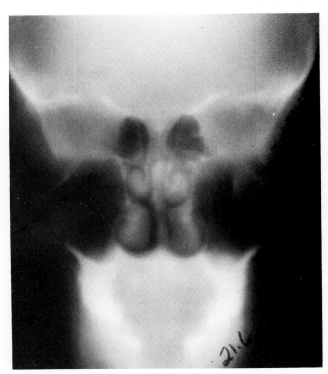

Figure 114-8. Orbital tomogram showing classical "teardrop" herniation of orbital tissue into the maxillary sinus.

X-ray Findings

Diagnostic studies should include Waters' view x-rays and tomograms. On x-ray, the orbital floor may appear fragmented and displaced bony fragments may be seen in the maxillary sinus. In orbital floor fractures, orbital soft tissue may be seen protruding into the upper portion of the maxillary sinus (Fig. 114-8). In either fracture there may be emphysema of the soft tissues of the orbit. The soft tissue shadow on the x-ray usually appears as a semilunar mass protruding into the upper half of the maxillary sinus.

Treatment

The goal of treatment of orbital floor fractures is to relieve restricted extraocular muscle function and elevate the lowered glove. This can be accomplished through an infraorbital approach, which permits direct inspection of the floor, removal of the small pieces of comminuted bone, and reconstruction of the orbital floor with an implant of alloplastic material. Some workers have suggested the use of autogenous bone as an alternative to alloplastic material; however, harvesting the bone requires another operation and actually the bone adds no advantage.

The alloplastic implant should be placed over the defect subperiosteally and rest passively in place. It should be as thin as will allow proper support of the soft tissues.

MAXILLA FRACTURES

Fractures of the alveolar process alone are, again, the most common form of maxillary fracture and have been previously discussed.

Le Fort Fractures

The characteristic of most maxillary fractures is a separation of attachments to the bony framework of the face or the skull. Studies by the French scientist, René Le Fort, at the turn of the century, produced the Le Fort classification of midfacial maxillary fractures (Fig. 114-9).

Le Fort I or Horizontal Maxillary Fracture

As in all the Le Fort-type fractures, a free-floating jaw is encountered. The horizontal fracture is one in which the body of the maxilla is separated from the base of the skull above the level of the palate, and below the attachment of the zygomatic process. The fracture line runs from the lateral nasal apertures, along the lateral wall of the maxillary sinuses bilaterally, and across the pterygomaxillary tissue to the lateral pterygoid plates.

Diagnosis of Le Fort I Fractures

Many horizontal maxillary fractures are not significantly displaced and their diagnosis may be missed at first examination. Displacement is dependent upon the force of the blow and the muscular pull. Diagnosis is most easily made by grasping the alveolar process and anterior teeth between the thumb and forefinger and causing a forward-backward motion. The visualization of movement of the entire upper dental arch is noted and the patient has, at the very least, a Le Fort I fracture. Roentgenographic survey often does not establish the diagnosis.

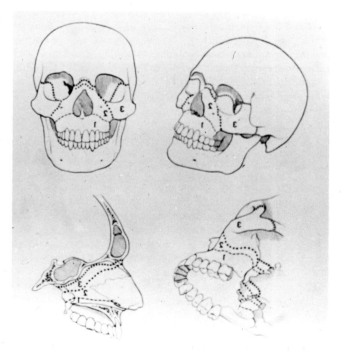

Figure 114-9. Schematic of midfacial fracture lines: Le Fort I, II, and III. (From Dingman RO, Natvig P: *Surgery of Facial Fractures.* Philadelphia, Saunders, 1964, p 248. Used by permission.)

Le Fort II or Pyramidal Fracture

The pyramidal fracture consists of vertical fractures through the facial aspects of the maxilla extending upwards to the nasal and ethmoid bones. The fractures extend through the maxillary sinuses and the infraorbital rims bilaterally across the bridge of the nose.

Clinical Features

The entire midface, nose, lips, and eyes are swollen. Bilateral subconjunctival hemorrhage is present and there is often blood in the nares. If clear fluid is seen in the nose, cerebrospinal rhinorrhea must be differentiated from mucus extravasation. A Dextrostix reagent strip can be applied to the fluid as a test for glucose, or a sample of fluid can be taken for glucose analysis. An empirical test consists of collecting some of the fluid on a cloth and if it stiffens on drying, it is mucus. Any patient with suspected cerebrospinal rhinorrhea should be evaluated by the neurosurgical service prior to obtaining a consultation with the oral and maxillofacial surgery service. Cerebrospinal rhinorrhea is a result of fracture of the cribriform plate of the ethmoid bone. It is for this reason that a clinical examination for suspected Le Fort II fracture must be done gently with as little movement as possible. However, the diagnosis of Le Fort II fracture can usually be confirmed by grasping the premaxilla, as with the Le Fort I fracture, in conjunction with palpation of the base of the nose (Fig. 114-10).

Radiologic Examination

The diagnosis of Le Fort II fracture is usually confirmed by a Waters' view of roentgenogram for evaluation of the infraorbital rims bilaterally, together with bilateral orbital tomograms. Films of the nasal bones should also be ordered.

Le Fort III Fracture or Craniofacial Dysjunction

The Le Fort III fracture extends through the frontozygomatic suture lines bilaterally, across the orbits, and through the base of

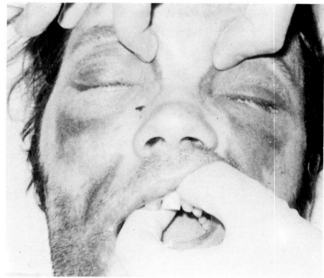

Figure 114-10. Method of examining for Le Fort II fractures of maxilla.

the nose and the ethmoid region (Fig. 114-11). The lateral rim of the orbit is separated and the infraorbital rim may be fractured, along with associated fractures of the zygoma. A pyramidal or horizontal fracture may also be present.

Clinical Features

A characteristic "dishface" may be evident because of retroposition of the entire midface at a 45° angle, along the base of the skull. On profile, the face appears spooned-out in the nasal area and the patient often has an anterior open bite. As the face is repositioned by the force of impact, the teeth in contact on occlusion are the posterior molars while there is no contact of the anterior or incisor teeth. Cerebrospinal rhinorrhea is more common than with the Le Fort II fracture. Palpation should be done gently (Fig. 114-12). If movement of the midface and zygoma occur concurrently, Le Fort III fracture can be confirmed clinically.

Radiologic Examination

A Waters' view roentgenogram and bilateral orbital tomograms confirm the diagnosis.

Treatment

The usual treatment of midfacial fractures is to support the sagging face and restore normal occlusion. The bones of the face must be mobilized and displacements of the zygoma, lacrimal, and other facial bones corrected. Fractures of the nasal bones are usually treated by closed reduction with intranasal reduction and manual molding. Tetanus toxoid and antibiotic prophylaxis should be administered.

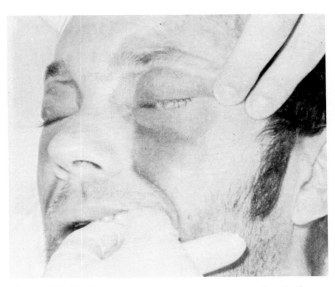

Figure 114-12. Movement of zygomas on examination indicates probable Le Fort III fracture.

COMPUTERIZED TOMOGRAPHY IN MAXILLOFACIAL TRAUMA

The use of computerized tomography (CT) in the evaluation of maxillofacial injuries has been an extremely helpful adjunct in assessing orbital fractures, midfacial trauma, and potential airway obstruction. This technique not only can be used when conventional techniques fail but actually offers some distinct advantages as a primary assessment tool.

These advantages may be listed as follows:

1. Soft tissues are clearly displayed and related to the bony framework so that exact margins of lesions can be defined.
2. Both axial and coronal views are available as well as sagittal reconstruction.
3. Blurring does not occur as with conventional tomograms.
4. There is approximately 40 percent less radiation exposure than with the latter.
5. Density determination and identification (e.g., blood, pus, muscle) of tissues are possible by measuring their absorption values.
6. It is the diagnostic modality of choice in the assessment of intracranial lesions.

Orbital and Midfacial Fractures

Fractures of this region are often complicated by edema, making initial clinical assessment of bony injury difficult. Since the bones are thin and lie in various planes, superimposition often occurs and may be further obscured by the dense cranial base.

Fractures of the cribriform plate of the ethmoid can be identified, which is especially important in the diagnosis of cerebrospinal fluid leakage. In addition, persistent leaks can be evaluated by the intrathecal placement of metrizamide (Fig. 114-13).

CT is the only technique that clearly shows the complete skeletal distortion often occurring in middle third fractures. The amount of comminution and degree of displacement, especially at the

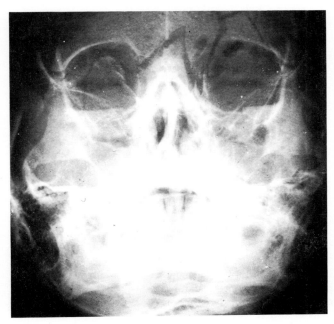

Figure 114-11. Waters' view roentgenogram of Le Fort III fracture. Note bilateral fracture at the frontozygomatic area and the craniofacial dysfunction.

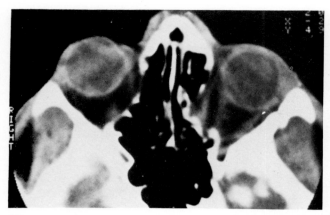

Figure 114-13. Orbital CT scan showing enophthalmos and fracture of the medial wall of the orbit. Note that the extraocular muscles can also be visualized.

posterior aspects of the maxilla, are often unobtainable by a routine radiographic study (Fig. 114-14).

Slices 5 mm in thickness are used routinely for maxillofacial and orbital evaluation, along with selective use of 1.5-mm slices. Slices are usually contiguous. Reconstruction of images in other planes can be extremely worthwhile. Axial scans of the oropharyngeal area may demonstrate gross soft tissue swelling as an aid to assessment of upper airway obstruction. Direct coronal CT is contraindicated in patients with suspected or unstable cervical spine fracture because of the manipulation required for proper positioning.

DISTURBANCES OF THE TEMPOROMANDIBULAR JOINT

Dislocation of the Mandibular

Acute dislocation causes considerable pain, discomfort, and swelling. The anatomic structure of the TMJ fossa and anterior articular eminence of that fossa may predispose to dislocation. The weakness of the connective tissue capsule forming the temporomandibular ligaments also may be a predisposing factor. The capsule may have loose attachments, may be excessively stretched, and more rarely, may be torn. Dislocation is generally caused by trauma to the chin while the mouth is in the open position, but it may occur while yawning, laughing excessively, or opening the mouth widely to chew food. Dislocation can also occur by overstretching the mouth while the patient is under general anesthesia. In addition, hysterical dislocations have been recorded.

Clinical Features

In an acute dislocation, the condyle becomes locked anterior to the articular eminence and is prevented from sliding back by muscular trismus. The external pterygoid, masseter, and internal pterygoid muscles then go into spasm. Characteristically the patient has the mouth open, and is unable to close the anterior teeth. Bilateral dislocation will thus present with an anterior open bite, but if the dislocation is unilateral, the jaw is displaced toward the unaffected side. The head of the condyle may produce swelling in front of the ear below the zygomatic arch. Since the jaw is

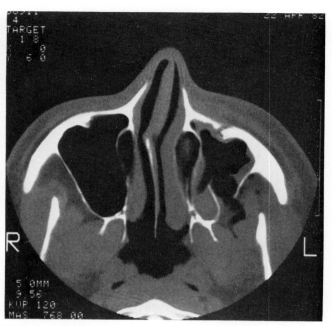

Figure 114-14. Zygomaticomaxillary complex fracture showing fractures at the medial and posterior lateral walls of the sinus.

locked in an open position, talking and swallowing are difficult. Examination of the TMJs will demonstrate the condyle in front of the anterior articular eminence of the joint fossa.

Radiologic Examination

The roentgenogram may be an important aid in differentiating dislocation from fracture of the condyle, since these conditions may produce similar occlusal disturbances.

Treatment

Temporomandibular joint dislocation can usually be successfully treated by manual manipulation. Occasionally, owing to the intensity of the muscle spasms, the oral and maxillofacial surgeon must inject the muscles of mastication with a local anesthetic solution to enable them to relax. More frequently, 10 mg of diazepam is injected slowly to aid in muscle relaxation and to allay some of the anxiety of the patient during the relocation procedure.

The emergency physician can easily master the manipulation, which consists of grasping the mandible with both hands, one on each side, with the physician facing the patient, thus reversing the process of dislocation. The patient should be in a sitting position with the physician straddling the patient's knees. The thumbs are then wrapped in gauze and placed on the occlusal surfaces of the posterior teeth with the fingertips placed around the inferior border of the mandible in the region of the mandibular angles. Downward pressure is then exerted while the jaw is opened wide to free the condyle from the stuck position anterior to the eminence. The chin is then pressed back after it has been forced down so that the mouth is closed while the condyle returns to the fossa. Since the jaw may snap back quickly, the gauze protects the physician's thumbs and avoids injury.

After reduction of an acute dislocation, the patient is cautioned against further wide excursions of the mandible, and placed on a soft diet for 1 week. Analgesics and muscle relaxants help override the acute phase of trauma.

In chronic dislocations, or in acute recurrences, a Barton bandage is applied for 2 weeks to prevent the patient from opening the jaw widely. In severe cases, intermaxillary wiring and fixation may be applied to restrict and control jaw motion during healing. Chronic dislocation may occasionally require surgical intervention, with most procedures aimed at recontour of the articular eminence to prevent dislocation or eliminate locking.

The Temporomandibular Joint (TMJ) Syndrome

Temporomandibular myofascial pain dysfunction syndrome, commonly called the TMJ syndrome, is a dysfunction of the normal mandibular articulation that produces complex clinical symptoms.

No clear etiology has been established. It is believed that the disease is a neuromuscular disturbance and that occlusal factors are contributory in nature. In addition to irregularities of the teeth and occlusion, factors such as trauma, psychic tension, and neuromuscular habits, such as bruxism and clenching of teeth, are all considered to play a major role in the development of this syndrome.

Clinical Features

Typically, the patient with the TMJ syndrome will have unilateral facial pain, mainly around the immediate region of the joint. The pain is of a dull, aching character that intensifies toward evening because of the use of the jaw during the day. Pain may be referred to the temporal, supraorbital, occipital, and cervical regions.

Commonly, the patient will have acute otalgia mimicking external otitis or otitis media, yet the otologic examination is negative. Inability to open the mouth widely is another complaint. The mouth may deviate on opening toward the side of the mandibular dysfunction or facial pain. Stiffness of the jaw generally worsens with use. Myofascial spasm or trismus may also be associated with clicking of the affected joint.

Clinical examination will usually reveal acute tenderness over the lateral capsular ligament of the TMJ, anterior to the external auditory canal. Placing the fingers on the joint and having the patient open and close the mouth will elicit this tenderness. The masseter and the internal pterygoid muscles may also be tender.

Radiologic Examination

Radiologic diagnosis is usually unrewarding. TMJ films are taken in the open and closed position. It is uncommon to find irregularities of the joint unless the patient has temporomandibular degenerative joint disease. In that case, osteophyte proliferation and flattening out or erosions of the head of the condyle are characteristic changes.

Treatment

The TMJ syndrome is treated by physiotherapy, dietary restrictions, analgesics, muscle relaxants, and occlusive therapy. Warm, moist compresses should be applied to the affected side of the face for 15 min four times a day for 7 to 10 days. A pureed diet should be followed for 1 to 2 weeks. Analgesics and muscle relaxants help disrupt the pain–muscle spasm–pain cycle.

It is surprising how often relief can be obtained by placing the upper and lower jaws in their proper occlusal relationship and maintaining the joint in its maximum rest position. When the acute phase has subsided, or as an adjunct to the treatment of the acute phase, the patient should be referred for a dental consultation for equilibration of occlusion, and for possible construction of bite splints to disarticulate the posterior teeth and help relieve muscle spasm.

Direct intraarticular injection of steroids is beneficial in many patients who do not respond to conservative therapy.

Arthritis of Temporomandibular Joint

Rheumatoid arthritis generally has a clear history with multiple joint involvement. In children, TMJ ankylosis is a common sequela, and the patient develops ankylosis, micrognathia, and a foreshortened mandible owing to the interference with the epiphyseal center of growth by the disease. In the adult, chronic rheumatoid arthritis is more common and the onset is more insidious, with slowly progressive changes causing limitation of motion. Active and passive motion becomes limited and aggravates the pain, and in the chronic stage the range of motion remains permanently limited.

Clinical Features

On palpation, both pain and crepitation may be noted. Periods of pain, exacerbation, and remission and morning stiffness that wears off during the day are common characteristics. Chronicity of adult rheumatoid arthritis again may cause TMJ ankylosis.

Roentgenographic Examination.

Roentgenograms show no bone changes in the early stages of the disease, but as rheumatoid arthritis progresses, radiolucent changes in the bone and eventually, evidence of resorption will be apparent.

Treatment

Treatment of the acute phases of TMJ arthritis does not vary significantly from the treatment of TMJ syndrome. Physiotherapy and anti-inflammatory drugs may be prescribed. Surgery may be indicated in cases of significant limitation of motion or fibrous and/or bony ankylosis of one or both joints.

Computed Tomography of the Temporomandibular Joint

CT has proved extremely useful in evaluating internal derangements of the TMJ. This joint is particularly difficult to examine with conventional radiographic means because of complex anatomic superimposition (Figs. 114-15 through 114-17).

While CT scanning can produce a clear representation of the

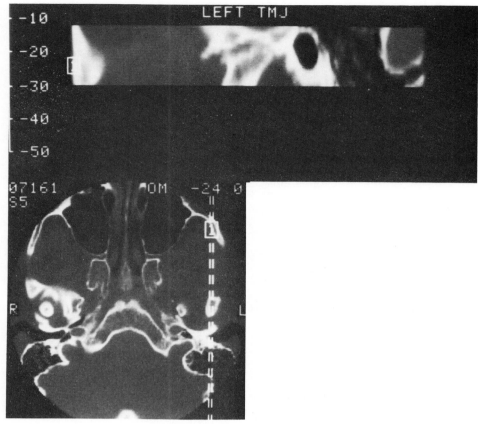

Figure 114-15. CT scan sagittal reconstruction of a patient with rheumatoid arthritis showing advanced degeneration of the condylar head.

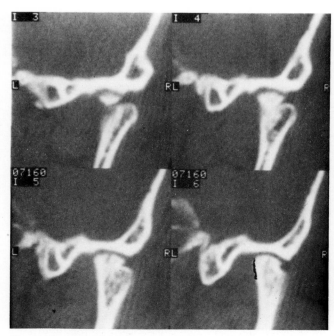

Figure 114-16. Multiple level view CT scan of the patient in Figure 114-15 showing erosion of the condylar head.

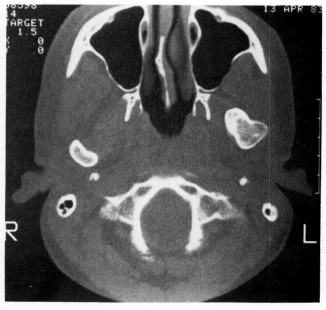

Figure 114-17. Posttraumatic CT scan of a patient with condylar hyperplasia (osteocondroma) with pseudoarthrosis and dislocation.

condylar head by magnification to permit study of intrabony defects, increasing use is being made of CT in the study of aberrations of the meniscus. Scans are routinely obtained by standard technique with use of 1.5-mm sections 1.5 mm apart and a third- or fourth-generation scanner. The "blink mode" highlighting technique is then used to show graduations in density between the meniscus and surrounding soft tissues. Studies show that CT in selected cases can replace arthrography, which is invasive, and is diagnostic in only the most skilled hands.

SPREAD OF ODONTOGENIC INFECTION—FASCIAL PLANES OF HEAD AND NECK

Periapical, Periodontal Infections

Acute infections of the oral cavity and jaws run the gamut from minor to life-threatening. The most common infection is the periapical abscess or the acute alveolar abscess that usually begins in the periapical region as a result of nonvitality or degeneration of the pulp of a tooth. These infections are usually easily treated with endodontics or extraction. Periodontal abscesses adjacent to the crowns of teeth can cause acute suppuration and swelling of the marginal gingiva.

Treatment

Superficial drainage of these abscesses, as well as ongoing periodontal therapy, is usually sufficient treatment.

Pericoronal Infection

Impacted third molar teeth commonly present with pericoronal infection, which can occur at any time throughout life. The most usual periods of pericoronal infection occur in early adulthood when food debris or microorganisms are trapped between the gingival or gum tissue and the crown of an impacted or partially erupted tooth, causing acute swelling of the adjacent tissues.

Treatment

Pericoronal infection is generally best treated by irrigation with sterile saline solution, warm salt rinses for 24 to 48 h, and antibiotics.

As in all minor dental-associated infections, oral phenoxymethyl penicillin in dosages of 250 to 500 mg four times a day is the drug of choice. In many instances, however, the progression of oral infection may cause acute fascial cellulitis.

Fascial Cellulitis

The severity of cellulitis depends upon the virulence of the organism, the resistance of the host, and the location and spread of infection through the fascial compartments.

The fascial spaces are formed by a deep cervical fascia that consists of the superficial and investing layer, the pretracheal layer, the prevertebral layer, and the carotid sheet. The superficial and investing layer surrounds the neck. Inferiorly, the fascia is at-

tached from the clavicle, sternum, and the spine of the scapula, to the inferior border of the mandible, zygomatic arch, mastoid process, and superior nuchal line of the occipital bone. Anteriorly, it blends to be attached to the symphysis menti and the hyoid bone. Posteriorly, it is attached to the ligamentum nuchi and the spine of the seventh cervical vertebra. The fascia splits as it attaches to the inferior border of the mandible. It thus encloses the parotid gland, and masseter and internal pterygoid muscles in the region of the ascending ramus. This split forms the masticator space.

Masticator Space Infection

Spread of infection, particularly in lower molar teeth, commonly invades the area between the internal pterygoid and masseter muscles. This space communicates superiorly above the level of the zygomatic arch into the superficial and deep temporal pouches. Since the mandibular periosteum is firmly attached inferiorly, infection tends to spread into the masticator space, and its extension inferiorly into the neck is prevented by the fascial reinforcement.

Clinical Features

Clinically, masticator space infection is dominated by trismus, pain, and swelling, usually within a few hours of acute onset (Fig. 114-18). The clinical signs increase rapidly to reach a peak in 3 to 5 days. Trismus is intense owing to severe irritation of both the masseter and internal pterygoid. As a result, visualization of the oral pharynx is often impossible, making intraoral evaluation of the source of infection extremely difficult.

Treatment

High-dose intravenous antibiotic therapy, generally 15 to 20 million units of penicillin daily, or 600 mg of clindamycin q 8 h if anaerobes are suspected, is the treatment of choice.

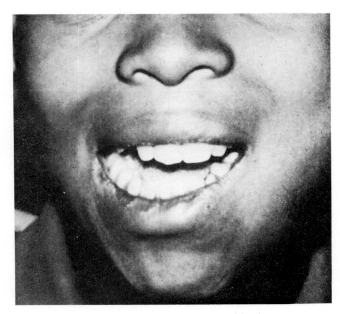

Figure 114-18. Masticator space infection with trismus.

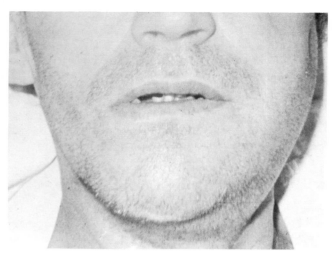

Figure 114-19. Combined fascial space infection involving the masticator, paraphyaryngeal, and temporal spaces.

Parapharyngeal Space Infection

The lateral pharyngeal space or parapharyngeal space is a deeply situated fascial space lying lateral to the pharynx and medial to the masticator space. It extends from the base of the skull to the level of the hyoid bone and is bound medially by the superior constrictor of the pharynx, laterally by the mandible and the internal pterygoid muscle, superiorly by the petrous portion of the temporal bone, and inferiorly by the submandibular gland and the posterior belly of the digastric muscle.

Infections of the parapharyngeal space are extremely serious (Fig. 114-19). This space is often involved by infections from the palatine tonsils, mastoid air cells, parotid gland, deep cervical lymph nodes, and teeth. Spread of dental infection directly from the masticator space is a common presentation.

Clinical Features

The clinical picture is marked by rapid onset, high fever, and marked swelling, usually obliterating the inferior border of the mandible and the lateral neck. There is severe pain due to the accumulation of pus and tissue fluid between the internal pterygoid and superior constrictor of the pharynx. The patient has marked trismus, difficulty swallowing, and there may be respiratory distress. Visualization of the posterior pharyngeal wall and soft palate is difficult or impossible. A further complication is mediastinal extension.

Treatment

Treatment of this condition is vigorous antibiotic therapy, careful observation of the airway, and incision and drainage. External incision is usually preferred because of the easy access to the submandibular, masticator, and parapharyngeal spaces through one incision. Tracheostomy may be necessary.

Ludwig's Angina

Ludwig's angina is a bilateral boardlike swelling involving the submandibular, submental, and sublingual spaces with elevation of the tongue. It is most often secondary to infection of the lower second and third molars. Brawny induration is characteristic and there is no fluctuance present.

Predominant organisms are hemolytic streptococci, *Staphylococcus,* or mixed aerobes and anaerobes. The presence of anaerobes accounts for gas in the tissues.

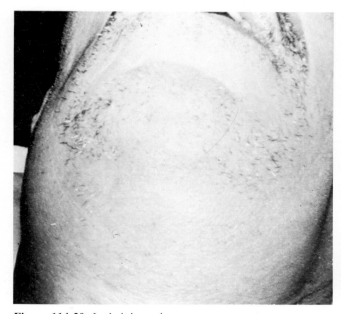

Figure 114-20. Ludwig's angina.

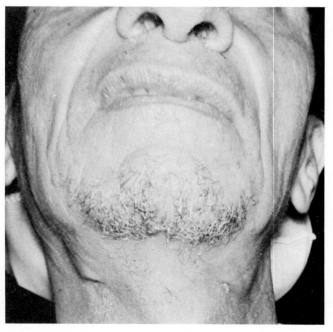

Figure 114-21. Postoperative view of Ludwig's angina in Figure 114-20.

Clinical Features

Chills, fever, difficulty in swallowing, stiffness of tongue movements, and trismus are common presenting signs (Fig. 114-20 and 114-21). Respiration becomes increasingly difficult as the tongue is elevated and the oral pharynx becomes occluded; the larynx may become edematous.

Treatment

Treatment consists of high-dose intravenous antibiotic therapy, and tracheostomy may be necessary. Incision and drainage superficial and deep to the mylohyoid muscle and medial to the mandible may be required if antibiotic therapy is not successful. As in parapharyngeal space infection, mediastinal extension can occur.

BIBLIOGRAPHY

Akamine RN: Diagnosis of traumatic injuries of the face and jaws *Oral Surg* 8:349–358, 1955.

Buzzard EM, Crampton-Smith H, Hayton-Williams DS: Symposium: Medical and surgical considerations in the treatment of maxillofacial injuries. *Br Dent J* 116:63–72, 1964.

Hagan EH, Huelke DF: An analysis of 319 case reports of mandibular fractures. *J Oral Surg* 19:93-104, 1961.

Helms CA, Katzberg RW, et al.: Computed tomography of the temporomandibular joint meniscus. *J Oral Maxillofacial Surg*, 41:512–517, 1983.

Hendler BH, Quinn PD: Fatal mediastinitis secondary to odontogenic infection. *J Oral Surg* 36:308–310, 1978.

Hendler BH, Wagner D: Problem—Blow to the jaw, trauma rounds. *Emerg Med* 5:60–62, 1973.

Hendler BH, Wagner D: Injury to the lip and oral mucosa, trauma rounds. *Emerg Med* 6:278–280, 1974.

Huelke DF, Harger JH: Maxillofacial injuries: Their nature and mechanisms of production. *J Oral Surg* 27:451–460, 1969.

Le Fort R: Etude experimentale sur les fractures de la machoire superieure. *Rev Chir* (Paris) 23:360–379, 479–507, 1901.

Noyek AM, Kassel EE, et al.: Sophisticated CT in complex maxillofacial trauma. *Laryngoscope* 96:1–17, 1982.

Sicher H: Structural and functional basis for disorders of the temporomandibular articulation. *J Oral Surg* 13:275–279, 1955.

Smith B, Converse JM: Early treatment of orbital floor fractures. *Trans Am Acad Ophthalmol Otolaryngol* 61:602–608, 1957.

Solinitzky O: The fascial compartments of the head and neck in relation to dental infections. *Bull Georgetown Univ Med Center* 7:86, 1954.

CHAPTER 115
GENERAL DENTAL EMERGENCIES

James T. Amsterdam

There are four categories of general dental emergencies of importance to the emergency physician: (1) oral-facial pain, primarily of odontogenic origin; (2) dentoalveolar trauma; (3) hemorrhage; and (4) oral medicine emergencies, including oral manifestations of systemic disease. An understanding of the anatomy of the stomatognathic system, especially the tooth and attachment apparatus, is essential for the recognition and managment of these emergencies.

STOMATOGNATHIC SYSTEM

Anatomy of the Teeth

A tooth is a homogenous body of dentin, a microporous structure that surrounds a central pulp—the neurovascular supply—from which it is nourished and was initially derived. The pulp continuously lays down additional dentin throughout life. The coronal portion of the tooth is that part that is normally seen in the mouth and is covered by enamel, the hardest substance in the body. The root portion serves to anchor the tooth and is covered with cementum, a substance much softer than enamel.

Thirty-two teeth are generally found in the permanent dentition, consisting of four types of teeth–incisors, canines, premolars, and molars. Generally, beginning from the midline and counting backward, the normal dental anatomy will consist of one central incisor, one lateral incisor, one canine, two premolars, and three permanent molars. The third molar is commonly referred to as the wisdom tooth. Agenesis of any of these teeth can occur or additional (supernumerary) teeth can be present. It is best for the emergency physician simply to describe the type of tooth and location involved in a particular emergency, e.g., an upper right second premolar or a lower left canine.

Useful dental nomenclature consists of the following terms:

Facial: referring to that part of a tooth that faces the oral vestibule
  Incisors to canines: *labial*
  Premolars to molars: *buccal*
Oral: referring to that part of a tooth that faces the tongue (lingual) or palate (palatal)
Approximal: referring to the contacting areas of adjacent teeth; those closest to the midline are mesial, those toward the posterior aspect of the mouth distal

Occlusal: referring to the biting surface of the premolars and molars
Incisal: referring to the biting surface of the incisors and canines
Apical: referring to the tip of the root
Coronal: toward the biting surface of the tooth

The Normal Periodontium

The normal periodontium can be divided into two major components, the gingival unit and the attachment apparatus.

The *gingival unit* is composed of the soft tissues investing the teeth and alveolar bone. The *gingiva* is covered by a keratinized stratified squamous epithelium, extending from the free gingival margin to the mucogingival junction. Apical to the mucogingival junction is the *alveolar mucosa,* which is covered by a nonkeratinized stratified squamous epithelium and is continuous with the mucosa of the lip and cheek.

In healthy individuals the gingiva is attached tightly to the tooth except for a 2 to 3 mm cuff of tissue surrounding the neck of the tooth (*gingival sulcus*) and bounded on one side by enamel and on the other by a continuation of the gingival epithelium. The *attachment apparatus* or anchoring mechanism consists of the cementum covering the root, the alveolar bone surrounding the root, and the periodontal ligament. The periodontal ligament is composed of collagen fibers of which one end inserts in the alveolar bone and the other end in the cementum, forming a fibrous attachment, not a calcific union. The anatomy of the dental unit (crown and root) and the periodontium is illustrated in cross section in Figure 115-1.

ORAL AND FACIAL PAIN

If pain is of odontogenic origin, patients usually will be able to localize the pain. The emergency physician should also recognize nonodontogenic causes for facial and oral pain, e.g., temporomandibular joint disturbances, which require therapeutic manipulations as well as palliative treatment (see Chapter 114, "Maxillofacial Fractures") and consider ischemic heart disease in the adult presenting with mandibular pain of unclear etiology.

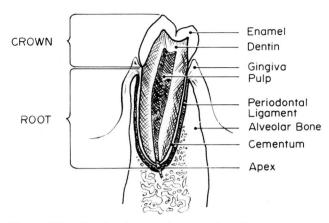

Figure 115-1. The dental anatomic unit and attachment apparatus.

Odontogenic Pain

Tooth Eruption

The earliest pain of odontogenic origin is associated with eruption of the primary teeth in the infant. Although there is some controversy about whether diarrhea and low-grade fever are associated with tooth eruption, an infant with dental pain may indeed refuse to eat or drink and become dehydrated. Management is directed toward: (1) pain control; (2) control of diarrhea if it is present; and (3) adequate hydration. Topical application every 15 to 30 min of a swab dampened with paregoric has been found to be a useful method of analgesia. Adult patients may suffer from pain associated with erupting teeth, most commonly third molars. The gingiva surrounding crowded, malerupted, or impacted third molars has a tendency for food impaction and subsequent inflammation, termed *pericoronitis.* Local therapy consists of saline irrigation and mouth rinses; if fluctuance and pus are present, incision and drainage may be useful. If local infection, fever, and/or generalized systemic involvement are evident, antibiotics of choice (phenoxymethyl penicillin or erythromycin 250 to 500 mg qid) are prescribed. Once local inflammation has resolved, definitive treatment involves surgical removal of these third molar teeth, requiring referral to an oral-maxillofacial surgeon in 48 h.

Dental Caries

The most common odontogenic pain, odontalgia or toothache, is associated with a carious tooth. A history of sudden or gradual onset of sharp to dull throbbing pain localized to a specific area of the mouth, which is aggravated by changes in temperature or possibly relieved by cool temperature, is consistent with caries. Moreover, such a history is consistent with significant pulpal involvement and may indicate that the tooth in question is abscessed (periapical abscess). The pain may be generalized or referred to other areas such as the ear, temple, eye, neck, or even opposite jaw. Physical examination frequently will reveal a grossly decayed tooth (or teeth), or there may be no apparent pathology. Localization is most easily accomplished by percussing individual teeth with a tongue blade; if abscessed, the individual tooth will elicit a sharp pain when tapped. Patients are treated with analgesics, such as codeine, acetaminophen-codeine combinations, or even

on occasion parenteral narcotic analgesics. Patients who have undergone endodontic treatment may experience exquisite pain, secondary to instrumentation during therapy and/or the buildup of gas in the tooth after it has been sealed (pericementitis), which may be unrelieved by an analgesic; a general dentist or endodontist should be notified.

It is important to rule out any associated oral or facial swelling secondary to abscessed teeth since the patient's pain may be from tense, swollen tissues. Swelling may range from a parulis (a small swelling in the gingiva opposite an abscessed tooth) to subperiosteal extension or facial cellulitis. Fluctuant swellings require incision and drainage, antibiotics, and warm saline rinses every 2 h until seen the following day for definitive treatment.

Postextraction Pain

Pain experienced immediately (24 h) after an extraction, termed *periosteitis,* responds well to analgesics. Severe pain 2 to 3 days after an extraction and associated with a foul odor and taste in the mouth is termed *alveolar osteitis* (dry socket). This pain is often excruciating and not relieved by oral analgesics. The pathophysiology is due to a combination of loss of the healing blood clot and a localized infection (localized osteomyelitis). Treatment consists of irrigation of the socket and application of a medicated dental packing or simply of a 1-in strip of iodoform gauze dipped in eugenol or camphophenique, which may be performed by the emergency physician. The patient should be seen by a dentist in 12 to 24 h.

Periodontal Emergencies

Peridontal Abscess

A swelling of the gingiva secondary to entrapment of plaque and debris in a so-called pocket (space between the tooth and the gingiva) is termed a periodontal abscess and may result in severe pain. Abscesses of this nature usually respond to local therapy consisting of warm saline irrigation and, when appropriate, antibiotics. Larger abscesses may require incision and drainage.

Acute Necrotizing Ulcerative Gingivitis

Acute necrotizing ulcerative gingivitis (ANUG) is an acute destructive disease of the periodontium found most often in adolescents and young adults. ANUG is the only periodontal lesion in which bacteria (fusobacteria, spirochetes) actually invade nonnecrotic tissue. Patients complain of generalized gingival pain associated with a foul taste and odor. Signs that may be present are fever, malaise, and regional lymphadenopathy. On physical examination the gingiva appears edematous and fiery red; the interdental papillae (tissues between the teeth) are edematous, ulcerated, and covered with a grayish pseudomembrane (Fig. 115-2).

ANUG is initially managed with antibiotics (tetracycline 250 mg qid, preferred or phenoxymethyl penicillin 250 mg qid) and warm saline rinses, as well as with the application of topical local anesthetic agents such as viscous lidocaine or 10% carbamide peroxide in specially prepared anhydrous glycerol. Symptomatic

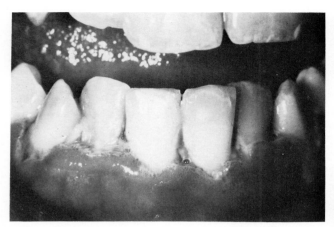

Figure 115-2. Acute necrotizing ulcerative gingivitis. (Courtesy of Dr. J. Giangrasso.)

improvement is impressive; however, underlying destruction of alveolar bone requires referral to a dentist for follow-up.

Oral Medicine Emergencies

Although it is beyond the scope of this chapter to discuss myriad oral medicine emergencies that may result in pain, there are several important classes that represent common problems.

Oral Lesions

Patients frequently present to the emergency department with a variety of oral lesions, not because of the oral lesions themselves but because of the pain that they produce. It is often difficult to distinguish a primary herpetic gingivostomatitis from a recurrent infection, herpangina, or herpes zoster. Such ulcerations when recognized are often best treated palliatively in the emergency department with topical anesthetic agents, e.g., viscous xylocaine, and warm saline rinses. These lesions are usually secondarily infected, and since much of the pain is due to the secondary infection itself, prescription of antibiotics is often appropriate (Fig. 115-3). In most circumstances the prescription of topical or systemic corticosteroid preparations should be avoided. Although steroids have been useful in treatment of erythema multiforme, their use with viral infection is not indicated. Owing to the complexity of the differential diagnosis of oral vesicular lesions, their definitive treatment is best managed by a dentist.

Paroxysmal Pain of Neuropathic Origin

Tic douloureux, or trigeminal neuralga, is the most common cause of paroxysmal pain of neuropathic origin involving the trigeminal (fifth) cranial nerve. The diagnosis is made primarily on history. Patients report a paroxysmal pain, i.e., episodes of sudden pain separated by pain-free periods, which are recurrent, excruciating, normally of short duration, and resemble the pain due to a severe electric shock. The key to the diagnosis is the fact that the pain follows the anatomical distribution of the cranial nerve involved. Often a similar pain can be initiated by minor sensory stimuli to

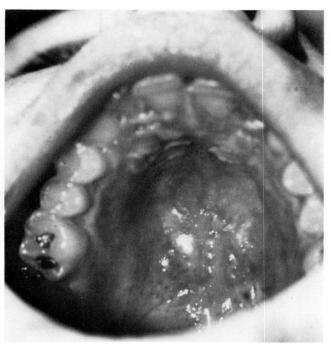

Figure 115-3. Systemic lupus erythematosus—characteristic ulcer with secondary infection.

areas called *trigger zones*, that consistently reproduce the pain. Tic douloureux may respond well to administration of carbamazepine. The pain of tic douloureux may not necessarily be idiopathic, as it may be the result of a tumor such as a cerebellopontine angle tumor (e.g., acoustic neuroma), a nasopharyngeal carcinoma, or a manifestation of multiple sclerosis. Any patient in whom the diagnosis of tic douloureux is made requires a careful neurologic examination, a referral to a dentist to rule out any oral pathology, and a referral to a neurologist for a full work-up to rule out any intracranial pathology.

Nonparoxysmal pain of neuropathic origin may develop (1) in patients who have suffered for a long time from tic douloureux, (2) secondary to surgical trauma along the distribution of the fifth cranial nerve, most frequently the mandibular branch, or (3) in association with viral infections, drugs, or heavy metal intoxication. Other neuropathies, such as alcoholic and diabetic sensory neuropathies, may be seen in the oral cavity.

Other

The differential diagnosis of oral facial pain includes a variety of other entities such as vascular problems, e.g., headache of cluster type, and rheumatologic disorders, e.g., giant-cell arteritis and polymyalgia rheumatica. In any differential diagnosis of jaw pain, referred pain from an ischemic myocardium must be considered.

Oral Manifestations of Systemic Disease

Several systemic diseases are associated with important oral manifestations. Patients may present with complaints related to the oral manifestation alone.

Diabetes Mellitus

Acute gingival abscesses and sessile or pedunculated gingival proliferations (granulation tissue that protrudes from under the gingiva, producing a red gingival hypertrophy) occur frequently in diabetics. Uncontrolled diabetes is associated with more severe manifestations. Dry burning mouth, gingival tenderness, lip dryness, spontaneous gingival bleeding, and tooth mobility may be seen. Chronic oral disease, particularly periodontal disease, may contribute to out-of-control diabetes.

Collagen Vascular Disease

Systemic lupus erythematosus (SLE) may be associated, in addition to characteristic facial lesions, with large intraoral necrotic ulcerations, which may be secondarily infected (Fig. 115-3).

Scleroderma may be present with a characteristic facies or thickening of the periodontal ligament on x-ray. Midline lethal granuloma or Wegener's granulomatosis may present with large intraoral ulcerations (primarily on the palate). All ulcerations of the oral cavity that do not respond to palliative treatment warrant biopsy within 7 to 14 days.

Granulomatous Disease

Rarely, tuberculosis may manifest itself orally as granulomatous ulcerations. Other infections, such as actinomycosis, must be ruled out. These lesions may frequently be confused with syphilitic ulcerations in the oral cavity (the tongue and tonsil area being common locations).

A more benign and common entity is a pedunculated or sessile mass, termed the *pyogenic granuloma*. This is a proliferation of highly vascularized connective tissue in response to nonspecific

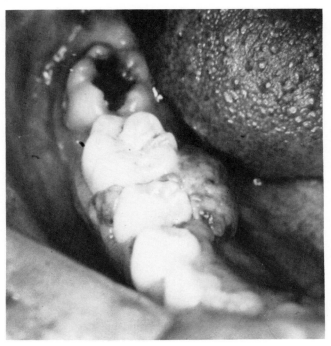

Figure 115-4. Pyogenic granuloma.

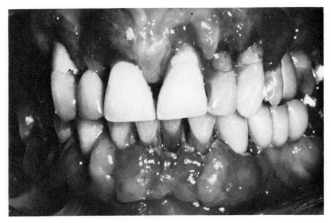

Figure 115-5. Oral manifestations of leukemia.

infection seen on the gingiva. A specific pyogenic granuloma occurring primarily during pregnancy is referred to as a *pregnancy tumor* (Fig. 115-4). The tumor is benign and frequently recurs if removed during the pregnancy. If the tumor does not regress by 2 to 3 months postpartum, definitive removal is indicted.

Blood Dyscrasias

Acute leukemia, particularly the acute granulocytic form, causes massive infiltration of leukemic cells into the gingival tissues, resulting in a hyperplastic gingivitis so marked as to almost cover the teeth; it is edematous and bluish in color. Chronic leukemia rarely causes oral disorders.

Complications that occur during the disease include toxemia, septicemia, gingival hemorrhage, marked discomfort, and loss of appetite. During the acute phase of the disease, only those procedures that are necessary to alleviate the discomfort and hemorrhaging should be performed (Fig. 115-5).

The interoral signs and symptoms of thrombocytopenia purpura consist of gingival bleeding, intramucosal hemorrhages, and prolonged bleeding from trauma. In addition, gingival hypertrophy has been reported.

Dilantin Hyperplasia

Dilantin hyperplasia of the gingiva occurs in approximately 40 percent of patients receiving the drug and is more prevalent in younger patients. Its severity is said to be unrelated to either dilantin dosage or blood levels. The initial appearance of dilantin hyperplasia is an enlargement of the interdental papillae, which encroaches on the crowns of the teeth, with the marginal gingival tissue lobulated, firm, and pale pink in color. Inflammation secondary to local irritants alters the appearance of the hyperplastic gingiva and responds to improved oral hygeine. Surgical removal of tissue is effective, but hyperplasia recurs if the drug is continued.

DENTOALVEOLAR TRAUMA

The simplest type of dental trauma involves the fracture of anterior teeth. The management of dental fractures is based on: (1) the extent of the fracture in relation to the pulp of the tooth, and (2) the age of the patient. A classification, the Ellis system, has been developed to describe the fracture anatomy of teeth. However, the emergency physician may also use a descriptive classification of traumatic injuries to teeth and supporting structures, as advocated by Johnson (Fig. 115-6).

Fractures

The Ellis class I fracture involves only the enamel portion of the tooth. This is generally a minor problem and requires immediate intervention only if a sharp piece of tooth is causing trauma to soft tissues. In such situations the rough edge may be smoothed with something as simple as an emery board and/or the patient may be referred to a general dentist for cosmetic restoration.

The Ellis class II fracture is a more complicated fracture in that it involves not only the breaking of the enamel but also exposure of dentin. The patient may complain of sensitivity to heat, cold, or even air. The immediate treatment of the Ellis class II fracture is dictated by the age of the patient, since less dentin is present in younger patients (under 12 years). Passage of microorganisms through the microtubules of exposed dentin can contaminate the pulp. Therefore management of Ellis class II fractures in younger patients requires immediate placement of a calcium hydroxide dressing on the exposed dentin, which is then covered with dry gauze or tinfoil. The patient requires dental referral within 24 h. Older patients (12 to 14 years), who have a greater dentin to pulp ratio, may be advised to avoid extremes in temperature and to seek dental care the following day. Patients with severe Ellis class II fractures (which may be recognized by a pinkish tinge to the dentin) should be treated in the same way as younger patients; analgesics may also be required. The correct management of Ellis class II fractures may obviate the need for root canal therapy. The emergency physician should warn any patient who has sustained trauma to the anterior teeth, no matter how minor, that disruption of the tooth's neurovascular supply may have occurred; long-term complications may be pulpal necrosis and/or resorption (dissolving) of the tooth.

Ellis class III fractures of the teeth involve, in addition to fracture of enamel and exposure to dentin, actual exposure of the pulp. The Ellis class III fracture may be differentiated from the Ellis class II fracture by gently wiping the tooth clean with a piece of gauze to eliminate the possibility of blood from soft tissue trauma. The tooth is then examined for any red blush of dentin or frank drop of blood. A patient may complain of exquisite pain or no pain if the neurovascular supply is disrupted. Ellis class III fractures are true dental emergencies and require immediate attention from a general dentist or an endodontist, since delay in treatment may result in significant pain and probably abscess formation. If a dentist is not immediately available, the tooth may be temporarily covered with tinfoil so as to minimize pulpal irritation and pain. Analgesics should be prescribed and the patient should be told to see a dentist as soon as possible. The emergency physician would be ill-advised to introduce any instrument into the tooth for removal of pulpal tissue since instrument breakage or tooth fracture may result, making endodontic treatment difficult or impossible. Over-the-counter topical dental analgesic preparations should be neither prescribed nor applied. Although these agents may give the patient temporary relief from pulpal pain, they often cause severe soft tissue irritation and sterile abscesses. In all cases of tooth fracture, the soft tissue should be palpated for tooth fragments and radiographed if swelling limits the examination.

Subluxated and Avulsed Teeth

The same force that may result in the fracture of an anterior tooth may also result in actual loosening of the tooth, termed *subluxation*. A traumatized tooth should always be examined for subluxation by use of finger pressure or by application of gentle rocking pressure with two tongue blades on each side of the tooth. A more subtle indication that a tooth has been traumatized is the appearance of blood in the gingival crevice of the tooth. Minimally mobile teeth heal well with soft diet for 1 to 2 weeks. Grossly mobile teeth require prompt stabilization. As a temporizing procedure for teeth that are very loose, it is often useful to have the patient bite gently on a piece of gauze to keep the tooth in place pending examination by a dentist or oral-maxillofacial surgeon.

A tooth that has been completely avulsed from the socket constitutes a true dental emergency. If the patient is unaware of the location of the missing tooth, a complete intrusion of the tooth below the level of the gingiva must be ruled out with a radiograph. Intruded primary ("baby" teeth) are allowed to erupt for 6 weeks. Permanent teeth are surgically repositioned with a forceps and stabilized. Failure to diagnose intruded teeth may result in cosmetic deformity and/or infection. The management of an avulsed tooth depends upon the age of the patient and the length of time that the tooth has been absent from the oral cavity. Avulsed primary anterior teeth in the pediatric patient (aged 6 months to 5 years) are not replaced in their sockets. Reimplanted primary teeth have a high tendency to ankylose or fuse to the bone itself, with resulting facial deformity.

A permanent tooth should be replaced in its socket as soon as possible if it has been avulsed for less than 2 to 3 h. A percentage point in the chance for successful reimplantation is lost for each minute that the tooth is absent from the oral cavity. When a call is received about an avulsed tooth, determine the age of the patient. If it appears that the tooth is permanent, the parent or patient should be instructed to quickly rinse the tooth under running tap

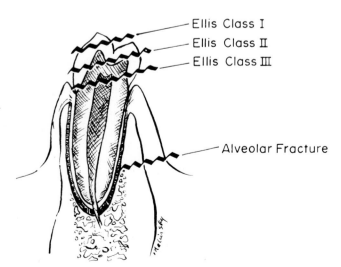

Ellis Class I
Ellis Class II
Ellis Class III

Alveolar Fracture

Figure 115-6. Ellis classification for fractures of anterior teeth.

water and to reimplant it immediately in its socket. If actual reimplantation is not possible, the patient should be advised to bring the tooth to the emergency department as quickly as possible in moist gauze, or preferably, in a glass of milk. Ideally, the patient may also be allowed to place the tooth in the mouth to bathe in saliva, being careful not to swallow the tooth.

If the tooth has not been reimplanted by the time the patient reaches the emergency department, it should be held by the crown at all times, rinsed under saline or running water, but *not* scrubbed (so as to conserve as much of the remaining periodontal ligament fibers as possible for reattachment) and reimplanted into the socket. If a blood clot prevents such reimplantation or in the case of a long time interval since avulsion, the clot should be quickly suctioned or debrided under local anesthesia and then the tooth should be reimplanted.

Avulsed teeth require immediate stabilization or they will exfoliate; biting on gauze is a temporizing measure. Although stabilization is normally performed by the general dentist or oral-maxillofacial surgeon, there are situations in which stabilization may be performed by the emergency physician. Indications would be a single avulsed tooth that has been placed back into the socket with satisfactory alignment, e.g., no prematurity of occlusion on jaw closure. Any tooth stabilized by the emergency physician should be evaluated by the general dentist or oral-maxillofacial surgeon within 24 h.

Several techniques are at the disposal of the emergency physician for stabilization of subluxated or avulsed teeth. A simple method described by Medford involves the application of a periodontal dressing (Coe-Pak), consisting of zinc oxide and a catalyst, that sets when mixed to a semi-hard consistency. When this is molded over the reimplanted tooth and adjacent teeth, 24 h of stabilization can be achieved.

Alveolar Fractures

Avulsed teeth are stabilized for approximately 10 days to 2 weeks and then placed back into function to avoid ankylosis. When there are concomitant alveolar fractures, the stabilization of avulsed or subluxated teeth also serves to stabilize the alveolar bone; stabilization is then left for a minimum of 6 weeks. Indiscriminate loss of alveolar bone will lead to much more difficult prosthetic restoration of this area than the removal of any ankylosed tooth. Generally, prophylactic antibiotics, e.g., phenoxymethyl penicillin, 250 to 500 mg qid, are used when avulsed teeth are reimplanted in the oral cavity, and appropriate tetanus prophylaxis should also be instituted.

Soft Tissue Injury

Closure of associated lacerations of the gingiva, mucosa, lips, and other facial soft tissues is performed after the teeth have been stabilized in the oral cavity. Stabilization of these teeth involves various methods of wiring, application of plastic materials, or both, all of which require stretching of soft tissues, especially the lips and oral mucosa. Thus, carefully placed sutures will simply be torn and this will increase the soft tissue injury.

The emergency physician should await final stabilization of the dentoalveolar component before instituting soft tissue closure and plastic repair. Dentists and oral-maxillofacial surgeons commonly close mucosa with 4-0 chromic or 3-0 black silk suture; gingival lacerations are sutured with 4-0 black silk. The patient should be advised to keep the intraoral area clean with warm saline irrigations and local application of hydrogen peroxide with swabs. Lip sutures should be covered with a thick coating of an antibiotic ointment or petrolatum jelly.

Intraoral lacerations, especially through-and-through lacerations resulting in communication between skin and oral cavity, are at increased risk for infection. Antibiotic coverage is advised. The patient should have the wound checked in 48 to 72 h.

HEMORRHAGE

Spontaneous Hemorrhage

Oral hemorrhage may be spontaneous from the gingiva. The history should include inquiry as to recent dental scaling or prophylaxis. If this history exists, bleeding usually responds to peroxide mouth rinse and local pressure with gauze compresses. Spontaneous gingival hemorrhage may also be the initial presentation of a systemic process such as leukemia or coagulopathy. The extent of the hemorrhage, age of the patient, and results of general examination determine the need for laboratory testing.

Hemorrhage Secondary to Extraction

Most commonly, the patient has bleeding secondary to dental extractions. Such bleeding is usually controlled by having the patient apply sustained pressure by biting gauze. Spitting, smoking cigarettes, and the use of straws create a negative pressure intraorally that exudes blood clots from sockets and aggravates postextraction bleeding.

If the bleeding fails to respond to gauze pressure and large clots are present, the clots should be wiped from the oral cavity, the socket suctioned, and gauze pressure attempted once again. If this is unsuccessful, local anesthesia consisting of 2% lidocaine with 1:100,000 or 1:50,000 epinephrine may be infiltrated in the area of the socket and gingiva and gauze pressure reapplied for 20 min. If oozing persists, a small piece of absorbable gelatin sponge can be placed in the socket and secured with one or two 3-0 black silk sutures.

If there is sustained, vigorous oozing after all the above procedures, a screening coagulation profile consisting of a complete blood count, platelet count, prothrombin time, and partial thromboplastin time should be drawn, since extraction is often the initial manifestation of a coagulopathy.

In some instances, postextraction bleeding is due to improper surgical technique or flap design and lack of a sufficient number of sutures for hemostasis. Flaps may be sutured together and gauze pressure applied.

Postoperative Hemorrhage

In case of bleeding after periodontal surgery, the emergency physician should contact the periodontist, for periodontal packs placed during surgery are extremely important to wound healing and incorrect placement can result in treatment failure.

BIBLIOGRAPHY

Amsterdam J, Hendler B: Approach to oral facial pain *Curr Top Emerg Med*, 2(10), 1981.

Amsterdam J, Rose L: Dental alveolar trauma. *Curr Top Emerg Med*, 2(9), 1981.

Amsterdam J, Strawitz J: Squamous cell carcinoma of the oral cavity in young adults, *J Sur Onco* (19)2, 1982.

Amsterdam J, Wagner D, Rose L: Interdisciplinary training: hospital dental general practice/emergency medicine. *Ann Emerg Med* 9:310–313, 1980.

Amsterdam J, Hendler B, Rose L: Dental emergencies, in Schwartz, Safer, Stone, et al, (eds): *Principles and Practice of Emergency Medicine*, ed 2. Philadelphia, Saunders, (in press).

Amsterdam J, Hendler B, Rose L: Dental emergencies, in Roberts J, Hedges J, (eds): *Emergency Department Procedures*. Philadelphia, Saunders, (in press).

Dice WH, Pryor GJ, Kilpatrick WR: Facial cellulitis following dental injury in a child. *Ann Emerg Med* 11:541, 1982.

Hendler B, Amsterdam J: Spread of infection of dental origin. *Curr Top Emerg Med* 2(8), 1982.

Hendler BH, Wagner D: Injury to the lip and oral mucosa, trauma rounds. *Emerg Med* 6:278, 1974.

Johnson R: Descriptive classification of trauma—the injuries to the teeth and supporting structures. *J Am Dent Assoc* 102:195, 1981.

Laskin D: The role of the dentist in the emergency room. *Dent Clin North Am* 19:675, 1975.

Lynch M, (ed): *Burket's Oral Medicine*, ed 7. Philadelphia, J.B. Lippincott, 1977.

Medford HM: Temporary stabilization of avulsed or luxated teeth. *Ann Emerg Med* 11:490, 1982.

Rose L, Hendler B, Amsterdam J: Spread of infection of dental origin. Part 1. *Consult Mag* 23(12):110–135, 1982.

Rose L, Hendler B, Amsterdam J: Spread of infection of dental origin. Part 1. *Consult Mag* 23(II):149–162, 1982.

Rose LF: General health affecting periodontal disease and therapeutic response, in Goldman HM, Cohen DW, (eds): *Periodontal Therapy*, ed 6. St. Louis, CV Mosby, 1979.

Weisgold A, Baumgarten H, Rose L, et al: Dental medicine, in Kaye D, Rose L, (eds): *Fundamentals of Internal Medicine*. St. Louis, CV Mosby, 1983, pp 1228–1251.

CHAPTER 116
ANESTHETIC
NERVE BLOCK

James T. Amsterdam

Intraoral and extraoral regional anesthesia is both simple and convenient for use by the emergency physician to induce anesthesia in areas of broad distribution in the face with a minimum amount of anesthetic and tissue distortion. Local anesthetic blocks are effective for closing facial lacerations, especially of the lips, forehead, and midface, where infiltration frequently swells and distorts the tissues.

The procedures and techniques described generally carry a low morbidity. The supraperiosteal and mental infiltrations can generally be learned through reading and experimentation; more sophisticated blocks are best performed after supervison by a more experienced physician, dentist, or oral-maxillofacial surgeon.

Anatomy of the Fifth (Trigeminal) Nerve

The fifth or trigeminal nerve takes its origin from the midbrain, enlarges into the Gasserian or semilunar ganglion, and divides into three branches.

The *first* or *ophthalmic division* is the smallest branch and leaves the cranium through the superior orbital fissure, supplying structures within the orbit, forehead, scalp, frontal sinuses, and upper eyelids. The *second* or *maxillary division* supplies the maxilla and associated structures such as the teeth, periostium, mucous membranes, maxillary sinus, soft palate, lower eyelids, upper lid, and side of the nose. After exiting from the cranium via the foramen rotundum, the nerve enters the interior orbital fissure, follows along the infraorbital groove, and enters the infraorbital canal, becoming the infraorbital nerve and terminating at the infraorbital foramen to give branches to the lower eyelids, side of the nose, and upper lip.

The second division consists of four major branches. The first branch consists of two short sphenopalatine nerves to Meckel's or the sphenopalatine ganglion, which give off the nasopalatine and anterior palatine branches, which innervate the palatal mucosa. The second branch consists of the posterior superior alveolar nerve, which courses down the posterior surface of the maxilla, supplying all the roots of the third and second molars and two roots of the first molar. A third branch consists of the middle superior alveolar nerve, which branches off about midway within the infraorbital canal, supplying the maxillary first and second bicuspid teeth and the mesiobuccal root of the first molar. Finally, the fourth branch consists of the anterior superior alveolar nerve, which branches

off from the infraorbital canal about 5 mm behind the infraorbital foramen, descending in the anterior wall of the maxilla to supply the maxillary central, lateral, and cuspid teeth, labial mucous membrane, periosteum, and alveoli on one side of the median line. There is an intercommunication between the anterior, middle, and posterior superior alveolar nerves.

The *third* or *mandibular division* exits from the cranium through the foramen ovale, dividing into three principle branches: (1) the long buccal nerve, which supplies branches to the buccal mucous membrane and the mucoperiostium over the maxillary and mandibular molar region; (2) the lingual nerve, which courses downward superficially to the internal pterygoid muscle, entering the base of the tongue to supply the anterior two-thirds of the tongue, lingual mucous membrane, and mucoperiosteum; and (3) the largest of the branches, the inferior alveolar nerve, which descends between the ramus of the mandible and the sphenomandibular ligament to enter the mandibular canal accompanied by the inferior alveolar artery and vein supplying the teeth. At the mental foramen the nerve bifurcates into an incisive branch, which continues forward to supply the anterior teeth, and the mental nerve, which exits from the mental foramen to supply the integument of the chin, the skin, and the mucous membrane of the lower lip. The mental foramen is located approximately between the apices of the lower first and second bicuspids or premolars.

EQUIPMENT AND ANESTHETICS

Intraoral local anesthesia is conveniently performed with a mono-jet aspiring dental syringe which employs Carpules of anesthetic and disposable needles, although a standard syringe may be used (Fig. 116-1). A needle no smaller than 27-gauge is recommended for deep block techniques; however 30-gauge needles are convenient and less painful for supraperiosteal infiltrations, especially in children. Generally, a long needle is used for block techniques and a short needle for infiltrations. Other adjuncts that are helpful include topical local anesthetic agents, such as gels or sprays.

Anesthetic agents most frequently employed are 2% lidocaine with a vasoconstrictor, such as 1:100,000 or 1:50,000 epinephrine. However, many other anesthetic agents, with or without vasoconstrictor agents, are readily available. Owing to the rich vascularity of the oral cavity, vasoconstrictors are important in sustaining the

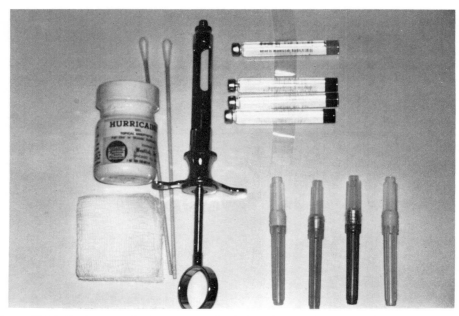

Figure 116-1. Basic set-up for intraoral anesthesia includes a topical anesthetic, a monojet aspirating dental syringe, Carpules of anesthetic, and a disposable needle.

duration of anesthesia and should be used wherever possible when no medical contraindications exist.

TECHNIQUES

Supraperiosteal Infiltration

The most common application for intraoral local anesthesia is the supraperiosteal infiltration for anesthetizing individual teeth. The area to be anesthetized is selected, dried with gauze, and wiped with a topical anesthetic. The mucous membrane of the area is grasped with a piece of gauze and pulled downward in the maxilla and upward in the mandible to fully extend the mucosa and delineate the mucobuccal fold. The fold is then punctured, with the bevel of the needle facing the bone, the area is aspirated, and

approximately 1 to 2 mL of local anesthetic is deposited at the apex (root tip) of the tooth involved. Infiltration of the area around the maxillary canine and the first premolars will anesthetize the middle and the anterior superior alveolar nerves; lacerations of the upper lip can be treated by bilateral injection in the canine fossa areas (Fig. 116-2). Similarly, infiltration between the apices of the mandibular first and second premolars provides sufficient anesthesia to block the mental nerves exiting from the mental foramen that supply the lower lip. This technique is referred to as a *mental infiltration* as opposed to a mental block (Fig. 116-3). A true

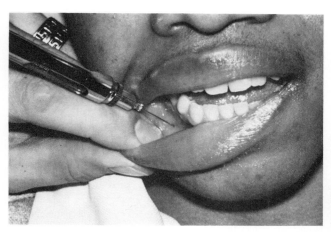

Figure 116-2. Supraperiosteal injection technique—mental infiltration.

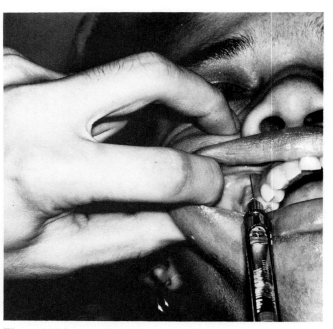

Figure 116-3. Infraorbital block—intraoral approach.

mental block would involve the introduction of the needle into the mental foramen, which can cause neurovascular damage. Lacerations of the midline of the lip require deposition of anesthetic to the side of the midline opposite to where the block was attempted in order to anesthetize crossing-over fibers.

Infraorbital Block

Intraoral Approach

The infraorbital block injection can be used to anesthetize the midface (Fig. 116.3). A solution of local anesthetic deposited at the infraorbital foramen not only will anesthetize the middle and anterior superior alveolar nerves but also will unilaterally anesthetize the main trunk of the infraorbital nerves, which supplies the skin of the upper lip, nose, and lower eyelid. The infraorbital foramen is found by palpation between the infraorbital ridge on a vertical line with the pupil as the patient stares straight ahead. While keeping the palpating finger in place, the cheek is retracted as in the supraperiosteal injection and puncture is made in the mucosa opposite the upper second bicuspid approximately 0.5 cm from the buccal surface. The needle should be directed parallel with the long axis of the second bicuspid until it is palpated at the foramen, a depth of approximately 2.5 cm. If the entry is too acute initially, the malar eminence will be encountered prior to approaching the infraorbital foramen. Also, if the needle is extended too far posteriorly and superiorly, the orbit may be entered. Therefore, the procedure should be halted if the physician is unsure of the location of the needle or if patient cooperation is unsatisfactory. When the location is assured and aspiration has been performed, approximately 1 to 2 mL of solution is injected.

The infraorbital foramen may also be approached from an extraoral route. In the extraoral approach, similar landmarks are used to locate the infraorbital foramen, and the needle can be felt to pass through the skin, subcutaneous tissue, and quadratus labii superioris muscle. Care must be taken not to anesthetize the facial artery and vein since they may lie on either side of the needle. Vasoconstrictors should not be used in this technique if possible. If vasoconstrictors are employed and severe blanching of the face occurs, warm compresses should be immediately applied to the face.

Inferior Alveolar Block

In some situations the emergency physician may find the inferior alveolar nerve block and lingual nerve block useful (Fig. 116-4). This injection is somewhat more difficult than the other techniques described and is best demonstrated prior to initial attempts. The inferior alveolar nerve block will provide anesthesia to all the teeth on that side of the mandible and to the lower lip and chin areas traversed by the mental nerve. It is primarily useful for anesthetizing patients with complaints of severe dentoalveolar trauma, postextraction pain, dry socket, pulpitis (toothache),or periapical abscess.

The technique involves palpation of the retromolar fossa with the index finger so that the convexity of the mandibular ramus can be palpated. The tissues are then retracted toward the buccal (cheek) side and the pterygomandibular triangle is visualized. The syringe should be held parallel to the occlusal surfaces of the teeth and angled so that the barrel of the syringe is lined between the

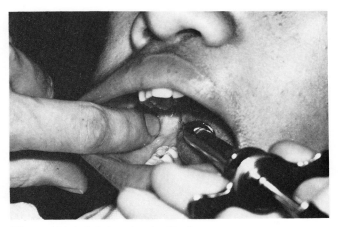

Figure 116-4. Inferior alveolar block.

first and second premolars on the opposite side of the mandible. Puncture is made in the triangle and the needle should be felt to pass through the ligaments and the muscles covering the internal surface of the mandible and to stop when it has reached the posterior wall of the mandibular sulcus. The needle should then be withdrawn slightly, the area aspirated, and approximately 1 to 2 mL of solution deposited. In children the angulation is not parallel to the occlusal surfaces of the teeth; the barrel of the syringe must be held slightly higher since the mandibular foramen is lower. The lingual nerve may be anesthetized by placing several drops of anesthetic solution in its path while withdrawing the syringe, thus anesthetizing half of the tongue.

Complications include inadvertent administration of anesthetic posteriorly in the region of the parotid gland, anesthetizing the facial nerve (Fig. 116.5). This will cause temporary facial paralysis, affecting the orbicularis oculi muscle and result in inability to close the eyelid. The eye must be protected until the local anesthetic has worn off (approximately 2 to 3 h) and the patient reassured.

Supraorbital Nerve Block

The injection technique is similar to that used for the infraorbital nerve, extraoral approach. The supraorbital notch should be palpated

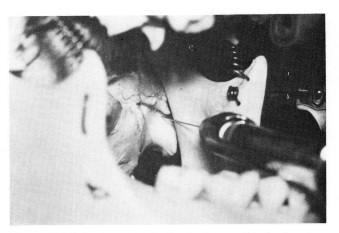

Figure 116-5. Inadvertent injection in the parotid gland region, resulting in anesthesia of the facial nerve.

and the anesthesia applied in this location. Occasionally local infiltration of the wound is required for complete anesthesia of the scalp and forehead.

General Precautions

Needles no smaller than 27 gauge should be employed for block techniques as the higher gauge makes aspiration difficult and may lead to inadvertent intravascular injection. When an intraoral block technique is employed, the needle should never be inserted to its full length at the hub to avoid inadvertent breakage.

A final precaution for intraoral local anesthesia is that the injection should not be made into or through an infected area. This is especially important in inferior alveolar nerve blocks, where tracking of an infection can be serious and difficult to treat and can result in trismus, lack of access, and direct extension to parapharyngeal spaces. Therefore, local anesthesia should be employed very superficially prior to incision and drainage, unless a block can be performed far proximal to the site of infection.

BIBLIOGRAPHY

Amsterdam J, Hendler B, Rose LF: Dental emergency procedures, in Roberts J, Hedges J (eds): *Emergency Department Procedures*. Philadelphia, Saunders (in press).

Bennett CR: *Monheim's Local Anesthesia and Pain Control in Dental Practice*, ed 6. St. Louis, C. V. Mosby Company, 1978.

Manual of Local Anesthesia and General Dentistry. New York, Cook-Waite Laboratories, Inc. 1947.

SECTION 15
NONTRAUMATIC
MUSCULOSKELETAL
DISORDERS

CHAPTER 117
MUSCULOSKELETAL
DISORDERS

Joseph J. Weiss

Musculoskeletal problems presenting in the emergency department are rarely life-threatening, and therefore the emergency physician usually does not have to concern himself with making a precise diagnosis. However, timely intervention when the patient is seen can provide significant relief, and the evaluation may yield valuable information in establishing the final diagnosis.

PHYSICAL EXAMINATION

The reader is referred to the monograph by Polley et al. for a complete description of joint examination. However several comments are in order.

In palpating the proximal interphalangeal (PIP) and distal interphalangeal (DIP) joints, a two-hand technique should be used, as it facilitates identifying minimal amounts of fluid. When checking the patient's hand strength, the examiner's two fingers should be placed in the palm from the lateral side to the medial side, as the last three fingers are the phalanges that grip.

The same two-hand technique is satisfactory for palpating wrist effusions. To detect early inflammation, the range of motion of the wrist is evaluated; a slight loss of 70° to 45° is often the first sign of carpal bone inflammation.

The examiner should not be concerned if a patient lacks a full range of motion in the elbows; limitation of extension to various degrees, by as much as 10 to 15°, is common in women. Asymptomatic enlargement of the olecranon bursa is also frequently seen, and its presence does not provide a diagnosis of olecranon bursitis.

Shoulder effusion is difficult to identify by either inspection or palpation; it is often revealed by comparing the affected with the nonaffected shoulder. In most instances of shoulder arthritis, the presence of inflammation is revealed by loss of range of motion. A simple way to test shoulder motion is to ask the patient to place both hands behind the head and look up to the ceiling. If the patient can do the maneuver, then external rotation is intact. Next the patient should place both hands behind the back as if about to scratch it. If the patient can reach from L5 to T10, internal rotation is unimpaired. Adduction from 0° to 90° is not helpful. Almost every patient with shoulder pain has some impairment of this motion, which is not diagnostic.

Hip motion is most rapidly evaluated by the Fabére maneuver. The patient should lie supine and bring the hip up in flexion, followed by abduction and external rotation, and should complete the test with extension by taking the heel down the contralateral tibia.

The presence of knee pathology is assessed by palpating from one side of the knee and looking for a "bulge" sign at the other side. This move can uncover as little as 3 mL of excess fluid. Medial or lateral laxity and the presence of recurvatum is important in evaluating trauma but does not provide useful information when looking for evidence of inflammation.

Ankle irritation is best tested for by flexion, extension, and rotation of the ankle. Assessment for the presence of fluid is done by palpating for the extensor hallucis longus tendon. If it is readily palpable, ankle joint swelling is not present. If palpation gives a sense that the tendon is boggy or difficult to identify, then fluid is present in the joint. The usefulness of this test is not diminished in patients with ankle edema.

REMOVAL AND EVALUATION OF SYNOVIAL FLUID

Aspiration

The ability to aspirate a joint is essential for the emergency physician. Removal of synovial fluid relieves pressure on the distended joint and often provides the patient immediate relief from pain. In many other cases synovial fluid holds the key to diagnosis and therapy.

The main potential complication in joint aspiration is the introduction of infection because of faulty aspiration technique. To prevent this problem, the area over the site of aspiration should be prepared as follows: Initially the area is scrubbed with surgical soap, then the physician, wearing sterile gloves, swabs the area with 2% iodine followed by 95% alcohol. The iodine must be washed off by the alcohol, as iodine is a potential irritant to the skin and joint. Next, a sterile drape is placed over the prepared site. A local anesthetic, 1% or 2% lidocaine, is then administered with a 25-gauge needle. A local anesthetic containing epinephrine is not necessary and is contraindicated for finger joints. A 20-gauge needle should be used for aspiration unless there is reason to believe the joint contains thickened material such as clotted blood, in which case an 18-gauge needle is preferable.

Figures 117-1 through 117-5 illustrate useful landmarks for aspiration of the wrist, elbow, shoulder, knee, and ankle.

Hip aspiration is not a procedure for the emergency physician. Surface landmarks are deceptive, and accurate introduction of an aspiration needle usually requires localization under fluoroscopy.

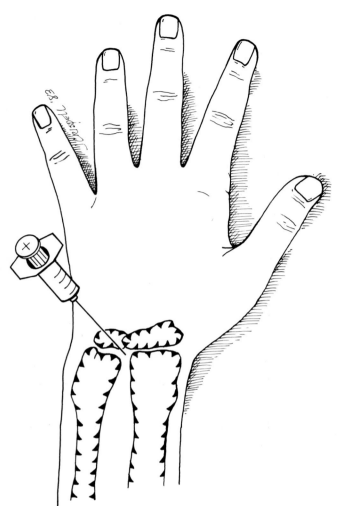

Figure 117-1. Wrist aspiration: Palpate the edge of the radial and ulnar styloid process and estimate the midpoint line. Next palpate anteriorly until the radial notch is felt. Insert the needle at this point.

If hip aspiration is necessary, obtain the assistance of an orthopedic surgeon or rheumatologist.

Two methods are presented for shoulder aspiration (Fig. 117-3). Most physicians use the anterior approach, but others believe the posterior approach has more usefulness as it provides identifiable landmarks in muscular or obese patients.

Synovial Fluid Evaluation

Once a synovial fluid specimen has been obtained, its proper handling is essential. The mnemonic below summarizes the essential laboratory examinations.

MNEMONIC FOR LABORATORY EXAMINATION OF SYNOVIAL FLUID

C—Culture, cell count, crystals
A—Appearance
P—Protein content
S—Sugar and stain (Gram stain)

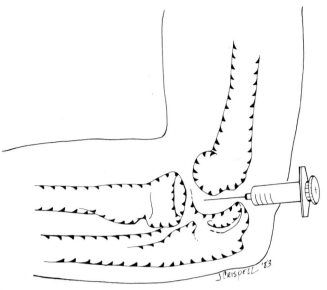

Figure 117-2. Elbow aspiration: Palpate the lateral epicondyle and the olecranon, place the needle between these landmarks and in the direction of the patient's thumb.

Gout or pseudogout are important considerations in the differential diagnosis of acute joint pain and swelling. Therefore it is helpful if the physician can evaluate synovial fluid for urate (gout) or calcium pyrophosphate (pseudogout) crystals. This is done by placing a drop of aspirated synovial fluid on a glass slide and covering the drop with a coverslip. Next a polarizer is placed over the microscope light source and another polarizer put over the coverslip. The polarizer is rotated over the light source until the microscopic field is absolutely dark. Any birefringent material will then shine brightly. Urate crystals are needle-shaped (Fig. 117-6) and calcium pyrophosphate crystals are rhomboid. The type of crystal present can be confirmed by using a red compensator. One can be made from two pieces of cellophane tape applied to a glass slide. This compensator is placed over the light-source polarizer. If the crystal turns yellow when parallel to the compensator and blue when at right angles to it, the crystal is said to be negatively birefringent. This pattern characterizes gout crystals. If the crystals are blue when parallel to the compensator and yellow when perpendicular, the crystal is called positively birefringent. This pattern is typical for pseudogout crystals.

If joint infection is in the differential diagnosis, then it is necessary to culture the joint fluid. In cases in which gonococcus is suspected, the laboratory should be alerted so that an aliquot of synovial fluid will be plated on chocolate agar with CO_2 incubation.

Culture for tuberculosis or fungal disease is not an emergency department responsibility; such causes for joint infection are rare and are sought during follow-up observation after other obvious infectious agents have been excluded.

A cell count plus differential leukocyte count of the synovial fluid, while a time-honored test, has its limits. Synovial fluid counts of under 1000 white cells represent noninflammatory fluid regardless of the differential count. Counts of over 10,000 white cells usually have 80 percent or more polymorphonuclear leukocytes (PMNs) and can be found in rheumatoid arthritis, gout, and infection. Cell counts of 1000 and 10,000 white cells are not

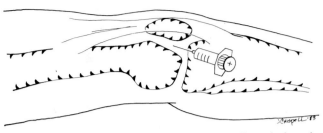

Figure 117-4. Knee aspiration: Palpate the patella and place the needle just medial or lateral to the mid third; aim the needle below the patella and in the cephalad direction.

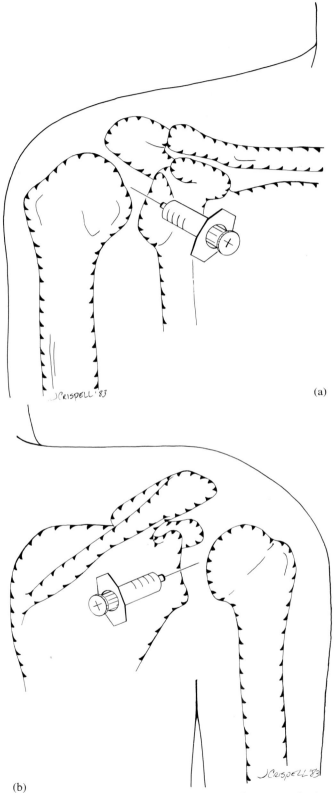

(a)

(b)

Figure 117-3. Shoulder aspiration. (*A*) Anterior approach: Approximate a point 1 to 2 cm below the acromial process and aim the needle in the posterior direction. (*B*) Posterior approach: Approximate a point ½ cm below the scapular spine and point the needle anteriorly in the direction of the acromial process.

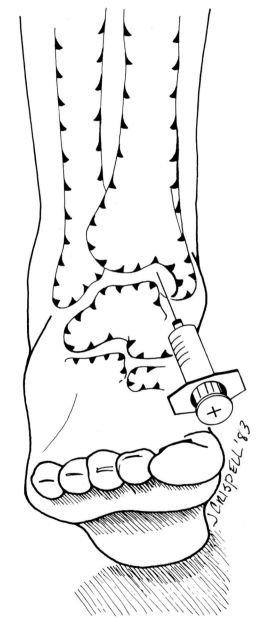

Figure 117-5. Ankle aspiration: Palpate the medial and lateral malleolus, draw an imaginary line between these landmarks. Next approximate the position of the extensor hallucis longus as it passes this imaginary line. Then place the needle just medial or lateral to the tendon, perpendicular to the skin surface, on the line.

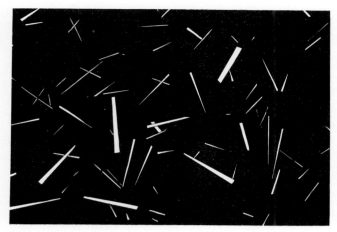

Figure 117-6. Gout crystals are needle-shaped.

helpful clinically, as such numbers are found both in osteoarthritis and in early inflammatory conditions. However, if the differential count is predominantly lymphocytic, then a viral etiology is most likely.

A Gram stain is indicated in any case of suspected joint infection. A positive smear is found in only 10 to 15 percent of cases of infectious arthritis, but the test is simple to perform and if positive, provides an immediate diagnosis. Therefore it is worth undertaking routinely.

The appearance of the fluid provides information. For example, hemorrhagic fluid on initial aspiration is a sign of recent joint trauma. If the aspiration itself was traumatic, the fluid's dark color quickly clears. A check as to whether the fluid aspirated is joint fluid is made by taking a drop between the first and second finger and observing whether the fluid stretches out into a thin band. Joint fluid will show such a "string sign," even if it has poor viscosity. Anesthetic fluid will not form such a string, and fibrin will form a short irregular line.

A protein content below 2.5 g/dL is characteristic of noninflammatory joint fluids; such a result is consistent with osteoarthritis or recent trauma. A protein content of at least 3g/dL is found in inflammatory conditions such as infection, gout, and rheumatoid arthritis.

Synovial fluid glucose concentration may provide a distinction between bacterial and noninfectious causes of joint swelling. In a bacterial infection the glucose concentration of the synovial fluid is less than two-thirds that of a concomitant serum sample; in some cases of infectious arthritis the synovial glucose concentration may be zero. In noninfectious conditions, even with high white counts, synovial glucose is two-thirds or more of concomitant serum glucose. There are two qualifications to this statement: first, if the synovial cell count is high and the fluid is not analyzed for hours, whole blood glycolysis may lower the synovial glucose concentration to levels compatible with infection. Second, if a patient with an infectious arthritis has taken any antibiotic within 12 h of the aspiration, it is possible that the infection was sufficiently suppressed so that synovial glucose levels will remain within expected limits.

If only a small amount of fluid is obtained, the following sequence of ordering tests is suggested:

1. Culture
2. Crystals/Gram stain
3. Glucose
4. Cell count and differential
5. Protein

ROENTGENOGRAPHIC STUDIES

The following mnemonic summarizes important features of bone and joint films.

> **MNEMONIC FOR EVALUATING X-RAY STUDIES OF THE JOINT**
>
> S—Soft tissue swelling
> E—Erosions
> C—Calcification (including periostitis)
> O—Osteoporosis
> N—Narrowing (joint space)
> D—Deformity
> S—Separations (i.e., fractures)

In practice, swelling about a joint is best noted on physical examination. Erosions are most often seen at the edges of the joint and are usually noted as breaks in the cortex at the synovial joint–cartilage junction. Such a finding is typical for rheumatoid arthritis. Larger erosions, called rat bite erosions, are seen in the first tarsal-metatarsal joint and are associated with gout.

Calcifications are ectopic, irregular spicules of bone, which are the hallmarks of calcific tendinitis. Often the x-ray film must be viewed under a bright light to see such calcifications. These spicules should be distinguished from sesamoid bones, which are regular and circular.

Juxtaarticular osteopenia is characteristic of early rheumatoid arthritis. Actual lysis or sequestration of bone is a late finding of joint infection and is not likely to be seen in the patient with acute joint pain. Evaluation of joint narrowing requires experience and is often subjective. Bone deformities are usually evident clinically, but roentgenographic studies are helpful in defining the extent of ulnar drift or of flexion abnormalities in the fingers and feet.

Pathologic or inapparent fracture is always a possibility in a person with joint complaints, and one reason for ordering an x-ray is to evaluate for the presence of metastatic or primary bone tumors. Finally, in the patient who has an underlying Charcot's joint, the x-ray will show a number of small fractures, giving a "bag of bones" appearance.

OTHER LABORATORY EXAMINATIONS

In patients with arthritis who are suspected of having infectious hepatitis, liver function studies are worth ordering. If rheumatoid arthritis or systemic lupus erythematosus is under consideration, then determinations of antinuclear antibodies (ANA), latex rheumatoid factor (latex RA), complete blood count (CBC), and Westergren sedimentation rate are in order. An antistreptolysin O (ASO) titer or a streptozyme assay is necessary to confirm a case of suspected rheumatic fever. In some instances, as will be explained later, the emergency physician will order a test whose results will not be available immediately. The purpose of such an order is to provide the physician responsible for ongoing care with necessary information.

DISPOSITION AND TREATMENT

Table 117-1 summarizes the indications for hospitalization. It may be appropriate to admit a patient with arthritis for rest and analgesic and/or anti-inflammatory medications only. The need for repeated aspiration is also a reason for admission. It could be argued that the patient can return to the emergency department for this procedure. However, in cases of suspected infection or Reiter's syndrome, daily and perhaps twice daily aspiration may be needed. In such instances responsibility for patient compliance is not appropriate for the emergency physician. In addition, multiple visits to the emergency area should be kept to a minimum.

While intraarticular steroids are efficacious in noninfectious arthritis, their use in the emergency department should be minimized. The reason is that precise diagnosis in the emergency department is often impossible, and physicians cannot be completely confident that they are not injecting steroid medication into an infected joint. Furthermore, patient cooperation for follow-up is uncertain. Finally, in many instances joint aspiration in itself is adequate therapy.

Polyarticular Pain and Swelling

Polyarticular involvement means pain and/or swelling affecting three or more joints. Usually joint involvement is symmetrical and includes the hands and shoulders, knees, or ankles.

Table 117-2 summarizes the main points of differential diagnosis as applicable to the emergency physician. It may take weeks to months to establish the exact diagnosis, and the responsibility of the emergency physician is not to do this but rather to start the patient on the appropriate pathway that will lead to the best and least expensive care while the diagnosis and long-term therapy are being established.

At present the most common viral cause of a symmetrical polyarthritis is serum hepatitis. Often the patient will have a concurrent urticarial rash. Rubella is another frequent viral cause of polyarthritis. The condition occurs most often in persons of the same age group as those who are most often afflicted with rheumatoid arthritis or systemic lupus erythematosus (ages 18 to 30). An inquiry about recent rubella vaccination can make the distinction between these choices.

The arthritis of adult rheumatic fever does not skip from joint to joint but is symmetrical and involves multiple joints, especially the knees and ankles, simultaneously. It occurs equally in men and women and is extremely rare as a first attack in any individual over age 30 to 35.

In evaluating an individual with symmetrical polyarthritis, a selective physical examination is in order. The skin is examined carefully for papulosquamous eruption in cases of suspected lupus, rubella, or rheumatic fever; urticarial lesions are searched for if infectious hepatitis is a consideration. If the patient is febrile, careful ausculation of the heart to detect a possible murmur is in order. Complete joint examination is necessary to establish the number and symmetry of the joints involved.

Emergency laboratory studies should include ANA, CBC, latex RA, and serum glutamic oxaloacetic transaminase determinations. The CBC is useful to uncover a leukopenia characteristic of systemic lupus or the lymphocytosis that accompanies viral infection. A baseline CBC is necessary before initiating aspirin administration with its risks of gastrointestinal bleeding.

Roentgenographic studies are of value in cases of suspected rheumatoid arthritis, as juxtaarticular osteopenia, a hallmark of the condition, may be present.

Whenever physical examination reveals a joint effusion, the physician should undertake aspiration if possible. Fluid in the small joints is not accessible to the aspiration needle, but fluid in the wrist, shoulder, knee, or ankle can be aspirated. Table 117-3 indicates what information analysis of synovial fluid can yield in instances of polyarticular joint swelling.

Table 117-4 summarizes emergency treatment for polyarticular pain and/or swelling. The best initial therapy for rheumatoid arthritis (RA) and its variants such as systemic lupus erythematosus (SLE) is aspirin and rest. If the patient cannot take aspirin, acetaminophen should be prescribed. The nonsteroidal anti-inflammatory medications have not yet been found to be of value in a consistent way. The physician with the responsibility of taking long-term care of the patient should make the arbitrary decision as to which, if any, of these newer agents to use.

Table 117-1. General Indications for Hospitalization of Patients Presenting with Musculoskeletal Problems

Incapacitated, i.e., unable to give self-care at home in bathing, dressing, feeding, toilet care, and ambulation.
Unable to obtain appropriate rest at home.
Specific therapy requires hospitalization.
Repeated aspirations in order.

Table 117-2. Differential Diagnosis of Multiple Joint Pain and Swelling

Condition	History	Physical Examination	Laboratory Studies
Rheumatoid arthritis, SLE, and variants	Previous attack with remission, multiple joint pain, A.M. stiffness	Symmetrical fusiform swelling of involved joints; in SLE a rash on sun-exposed areas	Latex +, ANA + (in SLE), CBC, elevated sedimentation rate, AP x-ray, hands and wrists
Viral arthritis, rubella	Skin rash, or recent vaccination	Macular rash	ANA, CBC, latex RA within normal limits
Infectious hepatitis	Contact with a person with hepatitis, recent hives	Urticaria, tender liver edge, hands and wrists with symmetrical swelling or pain on palpation	ANA, CBC, latex RA within normal limits; abnormal liver functions
Rheumatic fever	High fever, history of rheumatic fever, recent sore throat	Murmur of mitral insufficiency or stenosis, erythema marginatum, temperature 38.3°C (101°F) or greater, bilateral involvement of knees and ankles	Elevated ASO or streptozyme titer, positive strep throat culture; ANA, CBC, latex RA within normal limits; elevated sedimentation rate, elevated C-reactive protein

Table 117-3. Joint Aspiration Analysis in Polyarticular Joint Pain and Swelling

Procedure	Comments
Cell count	Cell count of 10,000 or more, 80–100% PMNs, is compatible with SLE, RA, or rheumatic fever. Counts of 1000–10,000 often present in SLE. Cell counts under 10,000 and predominantly lymphocytes are indicative of viral infection.
Culture and crystals	Negative
Appearance	Opaque, mucin clot variable
Protein	At least 3 g is indicative of an inflammatory response, a characteristic of all conditions mentioned in Table 117-2.
Glucose	Synovial glucose 60% or more of serum glucose indicates a nonbacterial inflammation.

The arthritis associated with viral conditions, including rubella, is usually short-lived. Flares can occur, and follow-up care is advisable.

The arthritis of infectious hepatitis is usually transient and disappears when jaundice occurs. However, some patients develop a polyarteritis syndrome, and the hepatitis itself can be severe. Thus, the emergency physician must make provision for follow-up.

Patients suspected of having rheumatic fever require admission. Precise diagnosis is not possible by multiple outpatient visits. Evaluation for bacterial endocarditis must be made to rule out that possibility for the patient with a heart murmur and fever. Also, as rheumatic fever is treated with large doses of aspirin, up to 90 to 120 grains per 24 h, hospitalization is essential to ensure patient compliance and to monitor possible salicylate toxicity.

Oligoarticular Pain and Swelling

Table 117-5 presents a summary of the salient features in the differential diagnosis of patients with oligoarticular (less than three joints) involvement.

Osteoarthritis and the closely related conditions, trauma, and aseptic necrosis are the most frequent causes for an emergency visit due to pain and/or swelling in a single joint. In such instances, joint pain often is related to the sudden distention of the joint capsule and may be extreme.

Table 117-4. Treatment of Polyarticular Pain and Swelling

Condition	Treatment	Comment
RA or SLE	Rest, aspirin, 9–12 tablets per day. Admit to hospital if unable to give self-care or obtain adequate rest	Follow-up medical care necessary
Viral rubella	Aspirin, 9–12 tablets per day	Follow-up medical care necessary
Infectious hepatitis	None	Follow-up medical care necessary
Rheumatic fever	Admit to hospital	Needs supervised aspirin administration; blood cultures to rule out bacterial endocarditis

In considering septic arthritis, the emergency physician should question the patient about a preceding episode of shaking chills or fever, as such an episode is typical of a transient bacteremia. In women a menstrual history should be obtained, since the bacteremia often begins concomitantly with menstruation. The patient's skin, especially the palms and oral cavity, should be inspected for pustulovesicular lesions. Such findings are characteristic of gonorrhea. Preparation of cultures from the cervix, pharynx, urethra, and rectum in Thayer-Martin media is recommended even if the physician plans to aspirate the involved joint. Gonococci are fastidious organisms and may grow out from one source and not the others.

In cases of gout and pseudogout, history is of particular value. The joint pain rapidly becomes intense and usually the patient will comment that "no matter how much it hurts now, it's not as bad as when I left home to come here." In all the other oligoarticular conditions, pain is usually minimal initially and gradually increases in intensity over time. When possible gout or pseudogout is being considered, the patient should be asked about previous episodes. Often there will be a history of similar pain that lasted for seconds or minutes and then disappeared as suddenly as it had come.

Radiologic studies are essential in evaluating for osteoarthritis and its variants. Occult fracture, metastatic carcinoma, or a bone tumor can present in a similar fashion.

To definitely diagnose gout or pseudogout, one must find crystals in a synovial fluid aspirate. Once the physician identifies crystals, the diagnosis is secure. While infection and gout do occur concomitantly, the association is rare. If crystals are seen in the fluid, culture of the fluid is not necessary.

Reiter's syndrome can present a diagnostic problem if the characteristic psoriasis-like skin lesions are absent and the patient has no conjunctivitis. The presence of both oligoarticular arthritis, especially in the lower extremities, and urethral discharge is compatible with Reiter's disease and gonorrhea. Synovial glucose levels are helpful if the patient has not received prior antibiotic therapy. In bacterial infection, glucose levels are depressed; in Reiter's syndrome, the synovial fluid glucose is within normal limits.

Table 117-6 summarizes therapy. In cases of gout, colchicine remains the treatment of choice. It is most effective if taken immediately when a gouty attack occurs. The dose is one tablet per hour until either the attack stops, 12 tablets have been taken, or diarrhea ensues. Intravenous colchicine, given as a single dose of 3 mg, is also useful. Strict precautions are necessary to avoid subcutaneous leakage of the solution, as a painful skin slough will result.

The more delay there is between the onset of the attack of gout and the initiation of therapy, the less effective is oral or intravenous colchicine. Unfortunately, when a patient with gout is seen by the emergency physician, a great deal of time, from 4 to 12 h, has usually elapsed since the onset of the attack. If such is the case, phenylbutazone, 300 mg/day in divided doses, is the treatment of choice. In this dosage, this medication is well tolerated, possible gastrointestinal upset is kept to a minimum, and bone marrow suppression is not a problem. Indomethacin can also be used but in the doses recommended, 200 mg/day for 2 to 3 days, gastrointestinal upset frequently occurs.

For therapy in osteoarthritis and trauma, aspirin is still the first choice. If the patient cannot or will not take aspirin, acetaminophen will provide relief.

Patients with joint infections require hospitalization. While it is

Table 117-5. Differential Diagnosis of Oligoarticular Joint Pain and Swelling

Condition	History	Physical Examination	Laboratory Findings
Osteoarthritis, trauma, aseptic necrosis	Occupational history, recent trauma	Swelling but little heat	Clear fluid on aspiration, low cell count; synovial glucose within normal limits; x-ray film may reveal loose body, fracture, or area of lucency.
Infection, especially staphylococcal or gonorrheal	Episode of fever or chills, recent IV drug use, urethral or cervical discharge, onset with menstruation	Hot swollen joint, urethral or cervical discharge; skin pustules (gonorrhea)	Positive Gram stain of culture of synovial fluid; aspiration yields cell count 20,000 or more, 90% PMNs; synovial glucose markedly decreased compared with serum glucose
Crystalline disease, gout, pseudogout and calcific tendinitis	Previous fleeting pain in affected joints, rapid onset of exquisite pain	Diffuse swelling over involved areas	Joint aspiration yields crystals, cell count 20,000 or more, 90–100% PMNs; synovial glucose two-thirds or more of serum glucose; x-ray film shows stippling in pseudogout, fleck of calcium in calcific tendinitis; serum uric acid elevated in gout
Reiter's syndrome	Male, history of urethral discharge, onset after sexual activity or diarrhea	Psoriasis-like lesions on palms or soles; conjunctivitis, urethritis	Joint aspiration yields 25,000 WBC or more, 90–100% PMNs; negative culture, synovial glucose within normal limits

possible to treat gonococcal arthritis on an outpatient regimen, such an approach is not practical for the emergency physician as it is difficult to judge the patient's capability of compliance. Furthermore, at times a joint infection is stubborn, seeming to resist antibiotic treatment, and frequent aspirations, even on a twice daily basis, are needed. Such a program of care is not possible on an outpatient basis.

Patients suspected of having Reiter's syndrome also need hospitalization. Repeated joint aspirations are required to confirm that no joint infection is present and to provide the patient with relief from the intense inflammation.

Table 117-6. Treatment of Oligoarticular Joint Pain and Swelling

Condition	Treatment	Comment
Gout	Colchicine 1 tablet/h until relief is obtained, 12 are taken, or diarrhea occurs	Needs medical follow-up
Gout, pseudogout, calcific tendinitis	Phenylbutazone, 300 mg/day in divided doses × 5 days	Needs medical follow-up
Osteoarthritis, trauma	Aspirin 12 tablets/day plus rest	Needs medical follow-up
Joint infection	Hospitalization	Requires frequent aspiration and IV antibiotic therapy
Reiter's syndrome	Hospitalization	Frequent aspiration and repeat joint culture to substantiate no bacterial growth; complete bed rest required for involved joints

Other Bone and Joint Conditions

Charcot's Joint

The most common presentation of a Charcot's joint is a painful swollen ankle. It should be kept in mind that above pain-insensitive areas is a plane in which pain fibers are at least partially intact. When the swelling associated with the ongoing trauma reaches this area of intact fibers, the patient seeks medical care.

Diagnosis is not difficult. The appearance of a swollen, boggy extremity brings up the possibility of trauma and makes radiologic study mandatory. Resulting films will show the classic bag of bones appearance. At present the usual cause is not syphilis but diabetic peripheral neuropathy. Patients usually need hospitalization for control of their diabetes and instruction on joint care.

Painful Shoulder

The emergency physician can assess the painful shoulder by using the approach discussed for oligoarticular complaints. However, Reiter's disease is an unlikely cause and calcific tendinitis a strong possibility. In addition, two other conditions, adhesive capsulitis and rotator cuff tear, need attention when assessing the painful shoulder. Bicipital tendinitis—inflammation of the biceps tendon as it passes in the groove between the greater and lesser tubercle—is often considered but rarely seen as an acute cause of shoulder pain.

Patients with a painful shoulder will require follow-up care, as treatment often requires prolonged physical therapy or repeated injection; at times, shoulder arthrography is needed to make the proper diagnosis. None of these responsibilities should fall to the emergency physician, whose first concern is diagnosis. X-rays are needed to rule-out unsuspected fracture or occult bone or metastatic carcinoma or to prove the presence of calcific tendinitis. In addition, an anterior-posterior chest film is necessary if Pancoast's tumor is a consideration.

If tendinitis is the most likely diagnosis, phenylbutazone provides an excellent treatment. The dosage is 300 mg/day in divided doses. In cases of calcific tendinitis, injection of steroid, 10 to 40 mg, into the area of tenderness is also reasonable therapy. The usual site of involvement in calcific tendinitis is near or at the insertion of the supraspinatus tendon at the greater tubercle. Injection into this area is safe, but accurate localization is difficult; for this reason injection therapy is a second choice after phenylbutazone. The technique for injection is similar to that described earlier in the section on shoulder aspiration.

If the etiology of the shoulder pain is uncertain, then the patient should receive analgesia in the form of aspirin or heat.

Irritable Hip

The usual causes for irritable hip in the adult are: (1) osteoarthritis, (2) aseptic necrosis, (3) metastatic carcinoma, and (4) infection.

Hip pain is characterized by a complaint of discomfort radiating down the groin. If the condition has been present for several days, the pain may radiate down the front of the knee or to the buttocks. This discomfort is secondary to muscle strain as the patient attempts a modification in gait to prevent the irritation.

Physical examination provides limited information, although usually the physician can establish loss of hip motion. Swelling of the hip capsule is difficult to assess because of the large amount of tissue between the hip joint and surface landmarks. X-ray films are essential, as they may reveal the presence of osteoarthritis, aseptic necrosis, or occult carcinoma. Often a single anterior-posterior view of the pelvis will serve as a screening x-ray examination. Women of child-bearing age should be asked about possible pregnancy before this view is ordered.

Evaluation for hip infection is done as discussed previously. The patient should be questioned regarding recent fever or chills or a history of intravenous drug use preceding the hip pain. If infection is a consideration, the emergency physician should obtain rheumatologic or orthopedic assistance for aspiration or should have fluoroscopy available.

Patients with aseptic necrosis or advanced osteoarthritis need referral to an orthopedic surgeon for possible arthroplasty or prosthetic replacement. Obviously, patients found to have their hip pain on the basis of malignancy will need hospitalization for evaluation and appropriate pain relief.

De Quervain's Tenosynovitis

Figure 117-7 illustrates the important anatomy involved in De Quervain's tenosynovitis. While the original description reported inflammation of the extensor pollicis brevis and abductor pollicis longus, the present definition has been expanded to include involvement of the extensor pollicis longus.

Usually De Quervain's tenosynovitis is related to a repetitive use of the hand in a motion connected with the patient's occupation or avocation. The emergency physician should ask the patient about work or hobbies with this relationship in mind. A positive Finkelstein's test confirms the diagnosis. In this test the patient makes a fist over the flexed and adducted thumb. In pa-

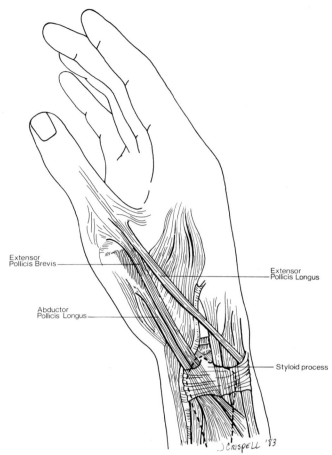

Figure 117-7. Anatomy of the wrist to illustrate the position of the abductor pollicus longus, extensor pollicis brevis, and extensor pollicis longus at the radial styloid process.

tients with De Quervain's tenosynovitis, this maneuver reproduces the patient's discomfort. X-rays are taken to rule out osteoarthritis of the first carpal-metacarpal joint or evaluate for a possible calcific tendinitis of the pollicis tendon.

Emergency department treatment consists of instructions to rest the joint and to use aspirin for analgesia. Additional rest can be provided by splinting the wrist. Such splinting can be done by placing the wrist in a position of 20° of dorsiflexion with a plaster or plastic half-cast. As with all other musculoskeletal problems, follow-up by a physician prepared to give ongoing care is necessary.

Tennis Elbow

Tennis elbow is a variant of De Quervain's tenosynovitis. In tennis elbow the cause is a repetitive motion with strain on the common extensor tendon, which originates at the lateral epicondyle. If the same problem occurs owing to strain on the common flexor tendon of the medial epicondyle, the condition is called bowler's elbow.

X-rays are necessary to exclude occult fracture or calcific tendinitis. Treatment is similar to that of De Quervain's tenosynovitis: rest of the involved tendon and aspirin. Splinting of the elbow has not proved practical to date.

Olecranon Bursitis

If enlargement of the bursa on the flexor surface of the olecranon is not causing the patient pain, no intervention is in order. In such cases the enlargement is secondary to a repetitive occupational motion or a nervous habit. The treatment is to remove the cause or pad the elbow.

If there is pain at the site of olecranon bursal enlargement, aspiration is necessary. The possibility of gout or infection arises. Rather than draining the bursa completely, as is done with other effusion, a 25-gauge needle should be used to aspirate from the top edge of the olecranon bursa. Only enough fluid for crystal examination, culture, cell count, and glucose concentration determination should be obtained. The reason for not draining the bursa is that the bursa has a predilection for infection. Minimizing the amount of fluid withdrawn and the size of the needle used will decrease the chance of this complication.

Gout in the olecranon bursa is treated as outlined previously. If there is a question of infection of the bursa, the patient should be admitted until the matter is settled and/or treatment is initiated.

Muscle Pain and Weakness

Most muscle pain seen in the emergency department is related to unusual use of the involved muscles; history will elicit this information. Treatment consists of heat, rest, and aspirin.

If muscle weakness is the patient's complaint, the physician must consider the possibility of polymyositis. If muscle weakness is the only problem, the patient should remain at rest and seek follow-up care. Any alteration in the ability to swallow, ambulate, or breathe demands admission. A creatine phosphokinase (CPK) determination should be made for a baseline assessment. At times patients with acute rhabdomyolysis may present with minimal complaints. If the patient's CPK level is 80 to 100 or more times normal levels, hospitalization is required. Under such conditions the patient is at risk for renal failure, and sustained and large amounts of intravenous fluids are needed to prevent this complication.

Fibrositis

Patients may come to the emergency department because of exquisite tenderness in soft tissue sites. Common areas of pain in fibrositis include the C7 spinous process, the midtrapezoid area bilaterally, the tip of the scapula, and the costochondral junctions (Tietze's syndrome).

In the emergency department the most efficacious way to care for these patients is to inject a local anesthetic into the sites of pain and refer the patient for follow-up care.

Carpal Tunnel Syndrome

Compression of the median nerve at the wrist is the usual reason for numbness of the hand. However, it is also necessary to rule out vascular insufficiency, which may produce evidence of skin atrophy, loss of hair, skin fold, or nail thinning. An Allen's test should be performed on physical examination. If there is good peripheral blood flow, the patient should be questioned specifically for possible carpal tunnel syndrome.

Patients with median nerve compression will be awakened at night by hand numbness and pain. The patient soon learns that vigorous shaking of the hand relieves the discomfort. This maneuver helps because the numbness results from nerve compression caused at least in part by soft tissue swelling. When the hand is shaken vigorously, the effect is to stimulate venous return and decrease tissue swelling about the median nerve.

The physician should not be surprised if the patient notes that the pain travels to areas other than the first to third fingers. It is possible to feel tingling up the arm as far as the shoulder. The mechanism is thought to involve antidromal transmission of nerve impulses from the hand up to the brachial plexus.

Physical examination in patients with median nerve compression may reveal thenar atrophy. The patient may have a positive Phalen's sign (flexion of the wrist produces discomfort) or Tinel's sign (tapping over the median nerve causes pain similar to the patient's complaint).

If the median nerve compression is the diagnosis, the patient should be referred to a surgeon experienced in performing carpal tunnel release operations.

Low Back Pain

The starting point in the evaluation of low back pain is to establish that the discomfort the patient reports as back pain does indeed involve the back.

The patient should show the emergency physician the area of discomfort. If the patient does point to the back, the physician can focus on the possibilities presented in Table 117-7. This list is not exhaustive but includes the most common and important causes of back pain. Unusual conditions such as lumbar stenosis are best diagnosed in the follow-up evaluation.

Referred pain as listed in the table means pain that is secondary to a more serious diagnosis, i.e., meningitis, dissecting aneurysm, or posterior penetrating duodenal ulcer. In such instances the underlying problem is apparent quickly. Back pain may also be part

Table 117-7. Differential Diagnosis of Back Pain

Referred—meningitis, aortic aneurysm, peptic ulcer, pyelonephritis, pancreatitis
Osteoarthritis
Vertebral disk compression
Osteoporosis
Primary or secondary carcinoma
Ankylosing spondylitis and variants
Infection—TB or psoas abscess, epidural abscess, or lumbar osteomyelitis
Pelvic inflammatory disease, ectopic or intrauterine pregnancy

of pyelonephritis, the diagnosis being recognized by the associated fever and dysuria. Patients with asymptomatic bacteriuria and low back pain will still have back discomfort after the bacteriuria is eliminated.

The causes of osteoporosis and associated vertebral collapse are numerous—hyperparathyroidism, malabsorption, and multiple myeloma, to name a few. For the emergency physician it is sufficient to have established that osteoporosis is present; it is the responsibility of the physician giving ongoing care to investigate the etiology.

A similar point can be made about ankylosing spondylitis and its variants. Spondylitis can be caused by inflammatory bowel disease, Reiter's syndrome, psoriasis, or *Yersinia* infection. It is the responsibility of those doctors involved in follow-up to evaluate such possibilities.

It is useful to ask the patient how long the back pain has been present. In the case of referred pain, the discomfort is sudden and of short duration, usually being present less than 3 to 4 h. It should be kept in mind that acute vertebral compression can be present in the same way. If pain has been present for days or weeks, it is likely to be of musculoskeletal origin. The physician should establish whether stress from work, acute injury, or strenuous activity has occurred and should then question the patient concerning radiation of the pain. Pain remaining in the back area or radiating into the buttocks or down to the knees is typical of nonneurogenic back pain. The radiation probably results from strain on the gluteus and quadriceps muscles as the patient unconsciously attempts to find a position of pelvic tilt that minimizes the back pain.

Anterior nerve root involvement characteristic of vertebral disk compression causes pain in a dermatome distribution. The patient will describe discomfort that begins in the buttocks area and runs down to the foot or heel in a linear fashion.

To evaluate the possibility of infection the physician should inquire if the patient is an intravenous drug user, has a history of tuberculosis, or has had a recent fever. These conditions precede seeding of the vertebral spine or psoas area.

Physical examination is summarized in Table 117-8. The main purpose of this examination is to confirm the presence of vertebral disk compression or uncover ankylosing spondylitis. An objective method of determining limitations of back mobility is Schober's test. With the patient standing erect the physician should mark the L5–S1 vertebral boundary. Then the physician should measure 5 in from this mark and make another mark on the lumbar spine at that point. The patient should then bend forward as far as possible. The physician should remeasure the distance between these two marks while the patient maintains the flexed position. Normal motion in forward flexion is an increase of 2 in.

Table 117-8. Physical Examination of Low Back Pain

CNS—knee jerk (L3,L4)
   Ankle jerk (S1)
   First toe dorsiflexion (L5)
   Walk on toes (plantar flexion strength)
   Walk on heels (dorsiflexion strength)
   Pinprick in dermatome distribution L3–S1
Bones and joints—Schober's maneuver
   Occiput-to-wall motion
   Chest expansion
   Hip flexion and rotation

The peripheral CNS examination focuses on the anterior root involvement occurring secondary to vertebral disk compression. The bone and joint examination emphasizes the areas of involvement in spondylitis: cervical extension, intercostal expansion, and lumbar flexion. Hip movement is evaluated to check that the patient's back pain is not hip or thigh discomfort and to see if hip joint involvement, a characteristic of spondylitis, is present.

The most important laboratory examination is radiologic evaluation of the back. Anterior-posterior views of the pelvis and a lumbosacral spine series suffice. Routine views of the sacroiliac joints are not in order; in most cases of spondylitis or infectious sacroiliitis, diagnosis can be made from the pelvic and lumbosacral roentgenologic studies.

Back films should be obtained if there is concern for osteoarthritis, osteoporosis, primary or secondary carcinoma, acute vertebral compression, Paget's disease, psoas abscess, or ankylosing spondylitis or if neurologic deficit is present.

Spondylolisthesis or spondylolysis may be detected on routine x-ray. Spondylolisthesis is the forward slippage of one vertebra upon another. It most commonly involves L5 on S1 and is usually associated with a defect in the vertebral arch. Spondylolysis is the presence of arch defects without slippage. Patients with these defects can present with low back pain or nerve root compression; initial management is symptomatic, with referral to a consultant.

Care of the painful back involves rest and patient education. There is a role for therapeutic exercises and, under appropriate circumstances, for back bracing. The mode of therapy most applicable depends on the duration of the patient's pain, the severity of nerve root involvement, and the level of the patient's usual and necessary activities. The presence of nerve root compression indicates the need for orthopedic or neurosurgical evaluation.

In the emergency department the physician's goal should be to provide symptomatic relief. No therapy accomplishes this aim better than bed rest. Complete bed rest, at home if possible and in the hospital if not, is the immediate treatment of choice. Equally important is a firm mattress. Such support is best achieved by having the patient place a $\frac{3}{4}$-in plywood board between the mattress and bed frame. Heat to the back has not proved useful in the acute attack, although in prolonged cases ultrasound may help.

The role of muscle relaxants is controversial. Many are available, but diazepam, 5 to 10 mg every 8 h, seems to provide the most consistent results. Probably the reason is its effect on tension and anxiety rather than any specific pharmacological action on spinal musculature.

BIBLIOGRAPHY

Barnert AL, Tery EE, Perselen RH: Acute rheumatic fever in adults. *JAMA* 232:925, 1975.

Begg RE: Epicondylitis or tennis elbow. *Ortho Rev* 9:33, 1980.

Bohan A, Peter JB, Bouner RC, et al: A computer assisted analysis of 153 patients with polymyositis and dermatomyositis. *Medicine* 56:255, 1977.

Butler MJ, Russell AS, Perry JS, et al: A follow-up study of 48 patients with Reiter's syndrome. *Am J Med* 67:808, 1979.

Duffy J, Lidsky MD, Sharp JT: Polyarthritis, polyarteritis, and hepatitis B. *Medicine* 55:19, 1976.

Horwitz CA: Laboratory diagnosis of rheumatoid disease. *Postgrad Med J* 67:93, 1980.

Howell DS, Moskowits RW: Symposium on osteoarthritis. *Arthritis Rheum* 20(suppl):596, 1977.

Lee CK, Hansen HT, Weiss AB: The "silent hip" of idiopathic ischemic necrosis of the femoral head in adults. *J Bone Joint Surg* [Am] 62:795, 1980.

Masi A, Eisenstein J: Disseminated gonococcal infections and gonococcal arthritis. *Semin Arthritis Rheum* 10:173, 1981.

Polley HF, Hunder GG: *Rheumatologic interviewing and physical examination of the joints,* ed 2. Philadelphia, Saunders, 1978.

Rodnan GP: Treatment of the gout and other forms of crystal-induced arthritis. *Bull Rheum Dis* 32:43, 1982.

Sharp JT, Lidsky MD, Duffy J, et al: Infectious arthritis *Arch Intern Med* 139:1125, 1979.

Simkin P: The pathogenesis of podagra. *Ann Intern Med* 86:230, 1977.

Sinhar S, Munichoodappa CS, Kozak GP: Neuropathy (Charcot joints) in diabetes mellitus. *Medicine* 51:91, 1972.

Weiss JJ: Rheumatologic conditions of the wrist. *Primary Care* 4:319, 1977.

Weiss JJ: Clarifying diagnosis and therapy of acute shoulder pain. *ER Reports* 2:147, 1981.

SECTION 16
TRAUMA

CHAPTER 118
INITIAL APPROACH TO
THE TRAUMA PATIENT

Ronald L. Krome

INTRODUCTION

Trauma is the leading cause of death in young people today, and has been for some time. In most patients, death is the result of respiratory or central nervous system failure or injury. Although we are breaking new ground in the arena of cerebral and cardiac resuscitation, most trauma deaths are best treated by simple, basic techniques and the application of knowledge already available. Perhaps the single hallmark of treatment and management is the attention to detail necessary in the patient with multiple injuries.

The care of the trauma patient is a continuum from the prehospital arena through the emergency department into the operating room. The level of care provided at each step depends upon the availability of appropriately trained personnel and equipment necessary for them to perform their tasks. Most patients who have sustained multiple-system injury will, sooner or later, require hospital attention. Some will require services which can be found only in the setting of a trauma center.

PREHOSPITAL CARE

Care rendered by the prehospital provider should be aimed at identifying and correcting those problems which will mitigate against safe transport of the patient. If paramedics are available, then IV fluids can be started, an airway established, the spine protected, and the patient transported. Fluids should be either normal saline or Ringer's lactate. Airway insertion should always be done while protecting the neck. Oxygen should be administered at 10 to 12 L/min. The rest should be left until the patient arrives at a hospital.

Although cardiac arrest is frequent in the field with these patients, external cardiac massage will not be effective until volume is replaced and those injuries which impinge upon ventilation corrected. What is needed is stabilization and quick transport.

Military Antishock Trousers (MAST)

These are discussed in greater detail in Chapter 1B. Some discussion is mandatory in this section, however. Although MAST are beneficial in patients with hypovolemic shock, their application should not delay definitive therapy.

The trousers consist of three compartments—one for each leg and one for the abdomen. Each compartment may be separately inflated, beginning with the legs and ending with the abdominal portion. Some trousers have an inflation valve so that the pressures can be measured as inflation progresses. Most physicians would recommend that the gauges not be used, but that inflation continue until the Velcro binders crinkle, or until there is a change in the patient's blood pressure and/or pulse.

In the past, it was felt that the trousers would provide an autotransfusion of 700 to 1400 mL of blood into the central circulation. Recent studies now dispute this. Although some controversy still continues concerning the exact mechanism of action of the trousers, it does appear that peripheral resistance increases, and this plays a role in the improvement of the blood pressure and pulse.

In any case, the application of MAST is not a substitute for adminstration of fluids. In reality, MAST should be looked upon as a method of gaining time until bleeding can be controlled and volume replaced. There may be some disadvantages to their use (Table 118-1).

Inflation of the abdominal portion is believed to limit the patient's ability to ventilate adequately. Some physicians suggest that use in patients with chest injuries is contraindicated, although there has not been any documentation of this in the literature. Prolonged high-pressure inflation has been shown to be associated with some complications—lactic acidosis and hypokalemia in the extremities—which, when the trousers are deflated, aggravate the already existing acidosis. Inflation longer than 24 h, especially when the pressure is elevated, has been associated with tissue necrosis in the legs. There are reports of patients who developed anterior tibial compartment syndromes when the trousers were left inflated 12 to 24 h. In these cases the abdominal portion was

Table 118-1. Potential Disadvantages of MAST

1. Examination of covered areas is limited.
2. Ventilation may be impaired by inflation of the abdominal portion.
3. Possibility of functional impairment of covered extremity.
4. Metabolic acidosis may result from decreased blood flow to extremities.
5. Pulmonary edema or pulmonary bleeding may be intensified.
6. Urination, defecation, vomiting may be triggered by abdominal inflation.

deflated while the leg compartments were left inflated. This may be more likely to occur when MAST are inflated in the presence of an already existing leg injury.

Regardless of the method by which MAST work or their limited complications, they have been a significant improvement in the treatment of hypovolemic shock and hypovolemia in both prehospital and hospital settings. However, it is imperative that rapid volume repletion occur while the trousers are in place and inflated, and that bleeding be stopped. MAST help in buying time, but are not definitive therapy. If surgery is indicated, they should be deflated in the operating room, after anesthesia has been induced, and with everything and everybody ready to proceed. MAST should be deflated, slowly, but as soon as possible.

Trauma and the Emergency Physician

The emergency physician who cares for the trauma victim has a vital role in the EMS system. In consultation with the prehospital care provider, using radio communication, he or she directs prehospital care and decides which facility the patient should be transported to as well as the method of transportation (helicopter vs. land ambulance). The prehospital providers can relay much vital information to the treating physician which only they can provide. This includes (1) the mechanism of injury, (2) exposure to noxious gases, (3) ambient weather conditions, and (4) the presence of drug paraphernalia or alcohol.

The trauma surgeon is an integral part of the care of the patient with multiple injuries. This necessitates that a community trauma plan include consideration of the utilization of trauma centers. Today there can be little doubt that mortality and morbidity rates are improved for the patient with multiple injuries when he or she is cared for in a trauma center. Community plans must include use of these centers as well as up-to-date transportation modes for the most economical utilization of all community resources.

MANAGEMENT OF THE PATIENT WITH MULTISYSTEM INJURY

Management of these patients requires a logical approach, the establishment of priorities, and close attention to detail. Steps in management are (1) initial stabilization, (2) multisystem evaluation, and (3) appropriately timed consultations.

Initial Stabilization

Cardiopulmonary Resuscitation

The first priority in management is the institution of cardiopulmonary resuscitation in the patient who has no vital signs. Although the first step, done almost simultaneously with institution of the airway and administration of fluids, is external cardiac compression, its use in the multisystem-injured patient may be limited.

Principal problems in resuscitating these patients are the marked fluid depletion (blood loss), flail chest, cardiac tamponade, hemo- and/or pneumothorax, and multiple rib fractures without flail. In addition, there are a number of other injuries which must be recognized and treated if resuscitation is to be successful.

All bleeding must be stopped or, at least, volume repletion must exceed volume depletion for successful resuscitation. In addition, anything which limits the ability of the patient to ventilate must be corrected. Evidence is accumulating, reconfirming older beliefs, that cardiac output with internal massage is much better than that obtained with external compression.

When traumatic cardiac tamponade is present, emergency thoracotomy, either in the operating room or in the emergency department, is generally indicated. Signs include: (1) shock, (2) narrowed pulse pressure, (3) muffled heart sounds, and (4) a markedly elevated central venous pressure. Not all these signs may be present in all patients, but clinical suspicion should be raised by the presence of neck vein distention. Pericardiocentesis is both diagnostic and therapeutic. If nonclotting blood is obtained, then the diagnosis is established; removal of blood from the pericardium will relieve the tamponade for a short time. Definitive surgical intervention is mandatory, however. Some institutes recommend emergency thoracotomy at the time of recognition of the tamponade. Others feel that less aggressive action is required in the patient who improves after tapping. It is our recommendation that emergency thoracotomy be done at the time of recognition of the tamponade.

There are those who believe that any penetrating chest wound in proximation to the heart, regardless of the patient's vital signs, is an indication for emergency thoracotomy. If the patient is stable, this should be done in the operating room. In any case, profuse bleeding from the chest after the insertion of a chest tube is considered an indication for thoracotomy. In general, this is best done in the operating room. Profuse bleeding is defined as bleeding in excess of 1500 mL upon insertion of the tube. Other indications are persistent bleeding over 3 to 4 h of 200 to 300 mL/h, and falling vital signs, despite rapid repletion of volume.

If an abdominal injury is present and vital signs continue to fall despite volume repletion and MAST application, then emergency thoracotomy may be indicated in order to cross-clamp the descending aorta where it enters the diaphragm. In at least one experimental study, this procedure was demonstrated to improve ventricular contractility and cardiac function. The procedure is not always successful, but is probably worth the attempt in the moribund patient.

Indications for emergency thoracotomy are shown in Table 118-2.

Airway and Ventilation

The single most important factor in the establishment of the airway in the trauma patient, either in the field or in the emergency department, is protecting the neck while not allowing the patient to succumb to airway obstruction. Patients with significant cervical spine injury can still move their necks and extremities. The presumption must be that significant injury is present, even in the absence of clinical signs, until confirmed by x-ray examination.

The simplest and quickest method of establishing the airway,

Table 118-2. Indications for Emergency Thoracotomy

Cardiac tamponade
Cardiac arrest as a result of trauma
Penetrating wound in proximity of the heart
Massive/persistent chest bleeding

even temporarily, is the bag mask over a simple plastic oral airway or nasopharyngeal tube. Use of this method is precluded if it cannot be done while protecting the neck, if hypopharyngeal injury or bleeding is present, gastric distention is already significant, or if foreign bodies are present in the upper airway and cannot be easily removed. Penetrating neck injuries may be associated with paratracheal hematoma, producing upper airway obstruction.

Oral endotracheal intubation is possible, if one person maintains stability of the neck while the other inserts the tube. This is difficult even in controlled circumstances and may be virtually impossible in the field. The esophageal obturator airway (EOA) has brought new possibilities to airway control in the arrested patient in the prehospital setting. It can be used in the emergency department, especially when the neck has not yet been completely evaluated. The tube can be inserted without movement of the neck. Meislin has demonstrated that, at least in the emergency department, blood gases can be successfully maintained, and are equal to oral endotracheal intubation.

One method that can be used in the patient with suspected neck injury is nasopharyngeal intubation. However, the patient must be breathing spontaneously. Complication rates reported range from 3 to 21 percent and consist of improper tube placement, bleeding, and laceration of the posterior pharynx so the procedure is not entirely benign. The only contraindications, other than operator inexperience, are a bleeding diathesis and nasal or midface fractures.

Cricothyroid puncture is still another alternative in the patient with suspected neck injury or in the patient in whom intubation fails. The complication rate of cricothyrotomy has been reported as high as 32 percent, with the most common complication being improper tube placement. Other complications include prolonged bleeding and fracture of the thyroid cartilage.

Indications for emergency tracheostomy are virtually nonexistent. This procedure is best done after resuscitation if necessary, and in the controlled environment of the operating room.

Oxygen in trauma patients should be administered at high flow rates, at least 10 to 12 L/min. The possibility of oxygen toxicity in these patients is minimal, and oxygen-carrying capacity is compromised by the blood loss.

Airway management, upper airway obstruction, ventilatory insufficiency, and thoracic trauma are discussed in greater detail elsewhere. The major causes of ventilatory insufficiency in the trauma patient are laryngotracheal trauma, facial injuries, hemothorax, pneumothorax, and flail chest. Rupture of the diaphragm, with herniation of the abdominal contents into the pleural space, impinges on the ability of lung expansion to occur. Subcutaneous emphysema is a pathologic sign, and indicates the presence of pneumothorax until proved otherwise. It can occur whenever a hollow abdominal viscus ruptures and the air dissects up the mediastinum into the neck.

Control of External Bleeding

All external bleeding must be controlled without doing any additional harm to the patient. This can most safely be done by applying direct digital compression or a compressing dressing. A blood pressure cuff can be used as a tourniquet, with inflation of the cuff pressure above the patient's systolic pressure. The duration of such inflation must be monitored to limit the possibility of

damage to the extremity. In general, deflation should occur every hour for 15 to 20 min.

Blind clamping of arterial bleeding should not be done. Prior to any clamping the bleeder should be clearly visible. In any case, noncrushing clamps should be used to minimize any possibility of permanently damaging any vessels.

Fluid Repletion and Correction of Shock

In general, two or more large-bore intravenous lines should be established, although as many as four may be necessary to administer fluids fast enough. Correction of shock and hypovolemia will not occur, however, unless bleeding has been stopped. Patients in shock may not bleed until the shock has been corrected, at which time bleeding will reoccur.

When abdominal injury is present, intravenous lines should always be started in the upper extremities or in the neck (internal or external jugular veins). Hematoma from internal jugular vein catheterization is a possibility and may be significant enough to cause upper airway obstruction.

A central line is necessary, not to measure current volume, but to estimate the rapidity of volume repletion. In addition, insertion of the line and measurement of the central venous pressure (CVP) enables one to diagnose the presence of cardiac tamponade. A sudden increase in CVP indicates that repletion is occurring rapidly and pulmonary edema may occur. Using the CVP response as an endpoint, 200 mL of fluid are administered in less than 20 min. If the patient's CVP remains the same or fails to rise at least 5 mm, the patient is hypovolemic, and fluids can be administered rapidly. Use of the subclavian route in an emergency situation has been associated with pneumothorax in 5 to 7 percent of cases. Therefore, subclavian insertion should be followed by chest x-ray. Other complications are listed in Table 118-3.

In patients with chest injuries there are two schools of thought on placement of subclavian lines. One says the line should be placed on the same side as the injury to avoid compounding existing injury; the other says that placement on the same side increases the likelihood of extravasation of fluids into the pleural space. A saphenous vein cutdown is a reasonable alternative in the patient with chest injury, but it should only be considered a temporary expedient; prolonged catheterization may lead to thrombophlebitis.

The flow rate of fluids is related to both the length and diameter of the catheters used, as well as the viscosity of the fluids used. To most rapidly correct the patient's fluid deficits, therefore, the shortest possible catheter should be inserted into the widest possible vein. A basilic or saphenous vein cutdown and insertion of sterile IV extension tubing offer a method of very rapid fluid insertion. Sterile pediatric feeding tubes can be used in the same fashion. Recently, large-bore catheter introducers have been recommended. Catheters in saphenous or femoral veins for prolonged

Table 118-3. Complications of subclavian vein catheterization

Catheter embolization
Pneumothorax
Venous air embolism
Laceration of the subclavian artery or vein
Infusion of fluids into the pleural cavity

periods of time are associated with a high incidence of thrombophlebitis.

Initial fluid resuscitation should be done with balanced electrolyte solutions, either normal saline or Ringer's lactate without dextrose. Two liters should be run in as rapidly as possible while monitoring the vital signs, including the CVP. Fluids should be administered to correct blood pressure, pulse, and CVP and to maintain urinary output.

If tachycardia persists, blood replacement is indicated. Although fully cross-matched blood is the best choice, in the emergency situation this is not always possible. Type-specific blood is the second choice and this can usually be ready in a matter of minutes. If neither is available, low Rh titer O negative blood can be used. The use of plasma expanders may be helpful but the typing of blood may be complicated and bleeding problems can occur.

The addition of albumin remains controversial at this time. Detractors claim that there is no benefit to the patient with the use of this costly material. Retention of fluids, prolonged respiratory support, and clotting problems may develop after resuscitation. Proponents of albumin point to a diminished need for fluids during resuscitation and less third-spacing.

Hetastarch has recently come to the forefront in resuscitation. In hypovolemic shock patients, there appears to be an increase in pulmonary wedge pressure, cardiac index, and mean arterial pressure with a reduction in arteriovenous shunting. If albumin is of benefit, hetastarch appears to be at least as good. More studies are necessary to assess its effects in the postinjury period.

Autotransfusion appears to be a valuable addition to the management of fluid replacement in the hypovolemic patient with pleural bleeding. Although some have used blood from the abdominal cavity, this is fraught with danger. Blood utilized for autotransfusions should not be contaminated. There are several commercially available devices for autotransfusion. The procedure is especially cost-effective in facilities with limited blood banking capabilities.

Nasogastric Tube Insertion

Insertion of a nasogastric tube is part of the initial resuscitation for a variety of reasons. Gastric distention as a result of the trauma itself, from attempts at intubation, or from using a bag breathing device on the patient, may be sufficient to impinge on the patient's ability to ventilate adequately. Patients who have sustained trauma may have either eaten or drunk recently; the nasogastric tube will empty the stomach and minimize the chances for aspiration. The presence of blood in the gastric aspirate in a patient who has sustained abdominal injury may indicate that stomach injury has occurred.

There are several conditions in which the location of the nasogastric tube is helpful in diagnosis. In diaphragmatic rupture, when the stomach has herniated into the left pleural space, the nasogastric tube may be seen coiled in the left chest on x-ray. When thoracic aortic rupture is present, the nasogastric tube will be deflected to the right on chest x-ray. Splenic rupture or hematoma may push the gastric bubble medially and the nasogastric tube will be seen pushed to the right on abdominal x-rays. Finally, much trauma is associated with ileus. The nasogastric tube will minimize ileus development and abdominal distention.

Catheterization

Since the presence of hematuria, either microscopic or gross, in patients with abdominal injury requires urologic evaluation, placement of the Foley catheter should be left until the volume is repleted and the patient has had an opportunity to adjust to the stimuli. The number of red cells in the urine does not correlate with the severity of the urologic injury. Although urologic injury is discussed in greater detail elsewhere, all hematuria requires evaluation when suspected as a result of trauma.

Multisystem Evaluation

Once the airway and circulation have been established and external bleeding controlled, rapid, complete evaluation of the patient may proceed. The objective is to evaluate head and neck injury, determine the presence of hidden blood loss, identify vascular injury, evaluate the possibility of significant abdominal and genitourinary injury, splint fractures, and obtain consultations.

A physical examination must be complete and the patient completely undressed. A rectal examination and pelvic examination must always be done. These examinations are frequently omitted in the press of other matters. The presence of blood on the gloved hand, the location of the prostate gland, and the evaluation of sphincter tone are mandatory. When a fractured pelvis is present, bone fragments may be palpated.

The patient should never be moved from the emergency department, except to the operating room, until he or she is stable. If possible, portable equipment should be brought to the bedside if necessary.

Injuries to specific systems are discussed separately in other sections of this book. Hidden blood loss must be sought diligently. Common injuries include fractures, especially pelvic fractures, and retroperitoneal injuries. The amount of blood lost from fracture sites can be estimated (see Table 118-4). In general, blood loss from fractures is 80 percent complete within 6 h of injury. Pelvic fractures produce extremely large volumes of blood loss and are frequently not considered as a source until the patient is in frank shock.

Patients with retroperitoneal blood loss frequently have unexplained shock, i.e., shock and no apparent bleeding. Abdominal expansion is late and peritoneal lavage may be negative or "weakly" positive. Routine x-rays of the abdomen may have a ground-glass appearance with loss of the psoas shadows. An intravenous pyelogram, CT scan, ultrasonogram, and arteriogram may be necessary to completely assess the retroperitoneum.

Splinting of fractures is the last step in stabilizing the patient. Neurovascular evaluation of the extremity should be done prior to splinting. If pulses are absent, then reduction of the fracture should occur as part of the splinting. If, after splinting, they do not return to completely normal, arteriography is mandatory to assess the

Table 118-4. Blood Loss From Fractures

Location	Amount (mL)
Pelvis	1500–2000
Femur	800–1200
Tibia	350–500
Humerus	200–500
Rib	100–150

vascular supply of the extremity. Vascular injury in an extremity or in the neck should be considered to have occurred when the patient is in shock, when active bleeding is present, when a hematoma of a major vessel is present and expanding, when a bruit is present, when pulses are absent distal to the injury, or when a neurologic deficit has developed.

Consultations

The patient is entitled to a single physician, in control of his or her care. During the initial phase of this care, it is the emergency physician who must determine the priority of consultations and of diagnostic studies, and who must monitor administration of fluids and drugs. Only when an appropriately trained trauma surgeon is on the scene should care be relinquished. The emergency physician then continues to act as part of the trauma team. It is only with a team approach and attention to detail that the morbidity and mortality of trauma can be changed.

BIBLIOGRAPHY

Bressler MJ, Rich GH: Occult cervical spine fracture in an ambulatory patient. *Ann Emerg Med* 11:440–442, 1982.

Calaham M: Acute traumatic tamponade: Diagnosis and treatment. *JACEP* 7:306–312, 1978.

Civetta JM, Nussenfeld RR, Rowe TR, et al: Prehospital use of military antishock trousers (MAST). *JACEP* 5:581–587.

Cogbill TH, Moore EE, Dunn EL, et al: Coagulation changes after albumin resusciation. *Crit Care Med* 9:22–26, 1981.

Dahn MS, Lucas CE, Ledgerwood AM, et al: Negative inotropic effect of albumin resuscitation for shock. *Surgery* 86:235–241, 1979.

Danzl DF, Thomas DM: Nasotracheal intubations in the emergency department. *Crit Care Med* 8:677–682, 1980.

Druy EM, Rubin BE: Computed tomography in the evaluation of abdomninal trauma. *J Comput Assist Tomography* 3:40–44, 1979.

Dunn EL, Moore EE, Moore JB: Hemodynamic effects of aortic occlusion during hemorrhagic shock. *Ann Emerg Med* 11:238–241, 1982.

Flynn TC, Ward RE, Iller PW: Emergency department thoracotomy. *Ann Emerg Med* 11:413–416, 1982.

Harrison EE, Nord NJ, Beeman RW: Esophageal perforation following the use of esophageal airway. *Ann Emerg Med* 9:21–25, 1980.

Herbst CA: Indications, management, and complications of percutaneous subclavian catheters. *Arch Surg* 113:1421–1425, 1978.

Johnson BE: Anterior tibial compartment syndrome following use of MAST suit. *Ann Emerg Med* 10:209–210, 1981.

Johnson KR: Genovesi MG, Lassar KH: Esophageal obturator airway: Use and complications. *JACEP* 5:36–39, 1976.

Johnson SD, Lucas CE, Gerrick SJ, et al: Impaired coagulation and increased need for transfusion in patients resuscitated from oligemic shock with supplemental albumin. *Arch Surg* 114:379–383, 1979.

Kay CJ, Rosenfield AT, Armm M: Gray-scale ultrasonography in the evaluation of renal trauma. *Radiology* 134:461–466, 1980.

Lucas CE, Ledgerwood AM, Higgins RF: Impaired salt and water excretion after albumin resuscitation for hypovolemic shock. *Surgery* 86:543–549, 1979.

Mattox KL, Allen MK, Feliciano DV: Laparotomy in the emergency department. *JACEP* 8:180–183, 1979.

Maull KI, Capehart JE, Cardea JA, et al: Limb loss following military anti-shock trousers (MAST) applications. *J Trauma*.

McGill J, Clinton JE, Ruiz E: Cricothyrotomy in the emergency department. *Ann Emerg Med* 11:361–364, 1982.

Meislin HW: The esophageal obturator airway: A study of respiratory effectiveness. *Ann Emerg Med* 9:54–59, 1980.

Puri VK, Paidipaty B, White L: Hydroxyethyl starch for resuscitation of patients with hypovolemic shock. *Crit Care Med* 9:833.

Ransom KJ, McSwain NE: Metabolic acidosis with pneumatic trousers in hypovolemic dogs. *JACEP* 8:184–187, 1979.

Siemens R, Polk HC, Gray LA, et al: Indications for thoracotomy following penetrating thoracic injury. *Trauma* 17:493–500, 1977.

Standards and Guidelines for Cardiopulmonary Resuscitation and Emergency Cardiac Care. *JAMA* 244:453–512, 1980.

Thurer RL, Hauer JM: Autotransfusion and blood conservation. *Curr Probl Surg* 19, 1982.

Tintinalli JE, Claffey J: Complications of nasotracheal intubation. *Ann Emerg Med* 19:142–144, 1981.

CHAPTER 119

HEAD INJURY

Neal Little

INTRODUCTION

The evaluation of head injury is one of the essential skills of any emergency physician. It becomes imperative to manage head injury correctly from the outset because, unlike compensating for blood loss from a liver laceration by transfusing blood and fluids, one cannot compensate for ongoing neurological damage. Head injury is a significant part of most multiple trauma, and the most important cause of long-term morbidity. In hospitals without neurosurgical coverage the emergency physician must be unusually expert in the evaluation of head injuries, for he or she will likely be the only physician to evaluate the patient, begin early treatment, and make critical decisions concerning the patient's potentially most significant injury. This chapter will first consider the pathophysiology of intracranial lesions in the head-injured patient, early complications of head injury, and then the clinical management of head-injured patients. Early diagnostic and therapeutic modalities will be discussed.

PATHOPHYSIOLOGY OF TRAUMATIC UNCONSCIOUSNESS

The usual first consideration of the physician in dealing with head injury is loss of consciousness. The underlying pathophysiology of traumatic loss of consciousness is intertwined with the mechanisms producing the alert, wakeful state. The ascending reticular activating system (ARAS) located in the core of the brainstem extends from the caudal medulla to the upper midbrain. This system is not a specific anatomic structure but rather a network of neurons that serves to keep the cerebral cortex "awake" and able to process information. Any pathologic entity causing unconsciousness must then affect either this ARAS or profoundly affect both cerebral hemispheres.

In traumatic unconsciousness, it is believed that shearing forces in the brainstem serve to temporarily cause cessation of activity in the ARAS and thus cause unconsciousness.

When acceleration forces are applied to the head, the brain actually moves a great deal within the skull. This movement twists and distorts the brainstem. Concussion is defined as temporary loss of neurological function as a result of trauma. The neurological function lost is usually consciousness, but other temporary losses such as visual loss ("seeing stars") can also qualify. Other than posttraumatic amnesia, headache, and possibly nonspecific slowly subsiding symptoms such as giddiness, there are no im-

mediate sequelae to concussion. The most clinically important fact concerning concussion is that it implies significant force applied to the head and thus the potential for the other lesions. The brief anterograde and retrograde amnesia that is a comcomitant of concussion usually contracts with time so that the lost time becomes less and less. It is not uncommon, however, to never develop recall of the instant surrounding impact.

Traumatic coma exists when this traumatic unconsciousness persists. Many other pathological processes occur in addition to the ones cited above. Axons in the brainstem and hemisphere are subjected to shearing forces and sustain damage documented anatomically and physiologically. Many factors combine in rapidly fatal traumatic coma. These include hemorrhage, vasomotor paralysis, elevated intracranial pressure, and edema formation. These will all be discussed separately.

LESIONS IN CLOSED HEAD INJURY

Closed injury to the head can potentially result in many pathological lesions. While it is convenient for the purposes of discussion to describe each as a separate entity, it must be understood that several lesions can occur in the same patient. It is because the head and brain are mobile that they are susceptible to acceleration forces. The brain can move within the skull, and when the skull suddenly starts or stops moving, the brain and skull impact on one another. The brain can be injured directly under the site of injury to the skull, termed a *coup injury*. The brain can impact on the skull opposite the site of injury, termed a *contre-coup injury*.

Cerebral Contusion

When the brain and skull impact upon each other, the cortical surface involved may sustain a contusion. There are small hemorrhages and local edema formation. There may be hemorrhagic necrosis of the brain. The area is usually wedge-shaped, with most destruction at the surface. Necrotic tissues become phagocytized later and a glial scar may develop. Areas where the brain is most susceptible to contusion are over the crests of gyri and where the inner table of the skull has an irregular contour, such as the orbital plate and sphenoid ridges. This is why subfrontal and temporal lobe tip contusions are common. The functional loss of activity may produce focal neurological symptoms, and the contused area may become a seizure focus. The hemorrhage in the brain substance may leak into the subarachnoid space.

Subdural Hematoma

Traumatic subdural hematoma usually occurs from veins which bridge between the cerebral cortex and dural venous sinuses. The motion of the brain inside the skull produces stretching and tearing of these veins with resultant venous bleeding. The blood accumulates and then begins to exert diffuse pressure on the adjacent brain. If the progression of bleeding is slow or ceases, the brain may accommodate the mass of clot by shifting and faster absorption of CSF. Faster rates of bleeding or concomitant cerebral swelling may exhaust the ability of the brain to accommodate the mass and herniation may occur. If the mass of clot is small and well tolerated, it may become an organized clot and form the membranes of a chronic subdural hematoma. A chronic subdural hematoma undergoes change based upon opposing factors. The fragile vessels in the capsule of the hematoma tend to rebleed and cause enlargement. This tendency is worse in the presence of any defect in coagulation, especially in the presence of Coumadin. The opposing factor is the tendency of the body to liquefy and absorb the hematoma. Rarely, a subdural hematoma can result from arterial bleeding on the surface of the brain from laceration.

Several factors place the patient at risk for development of subdural hematoma. Brain atrophy, commonly present in the elderly and alcoholics, results in a longer course for the bridging veins and thus easier rupture with minimal trauma. Minimal trauma, such as vigorous shaking, can result in subdural hematoma in infants and elderly patients with fragile vessels.

Several common clinical presentations occur with subdural hematoma. There may be sudden traumatic unconsciousness, focal deficit or seizures, and catastrophic herniation from acute subdural hematoma. Death commonly results. There may be head injury, with or without unconsciousness, followed by progressive headache and decreased level of consciousness. Focal hemiparesis, aphasia, or seizures may occur and symptoms may become gradually progressive with a subacute subdural hematoma. With this presentation there may be a lucid interval between the traumatic unconscious episode and the subsequent deterioration.

In patients with a chronic subdural hematoma, the initial trauma may not be very dramatic, and can be as trivial as vigorous head shaking in the elderly. This initial trauma may have been unrecognized or forgotten. The hematoma may be bilateral and its progressive enlargement may give gradual obtundation or loss of previously acquired intellectual functions (dementia) without focal signs. Decompensation may be sudden and simulate a cerebral thrombosis. Headache may or may not be a prominent symptom. Patients with significant cerebral atrophy may tolerate a very large hematoma with minimal signs and symptoms. Other patients may present with a course suggestive of tumor, i.e., progressive headache, dulling of mental functions, possibly hemiparesis or seizures, and papilledema. Patients may present with stupor or coma. This wide variability in clinical presentation of chronic subdural hematoma should be cause to consider it in a wide variety of clinical syndromes, especially in the elderly, alcoholics, and those with impaired coagulation. The symptoms and signs may fluctuate from day to day, or even hour to hour, making diagnosis difficult.

Epidural Hematoma

Bleeding into the epidural space is almost always arterial and usually from the middle meningeal artery. There is an associated fracture across the middle meningeal artery in 75 to 90 percent of cases. The rapidly expanding hematoma strips the dura off the inner aspect of the skull and locally compresses the brain. Epidural bleeding can occur from venous sinuses or from the bone of the skull. These hematomas are less common in the elderly. This is attributed to the tight bonding of the fibrous dura to the skull.

The classic clinical picture is traumatic unconsciousness, then a lucid interval with awakening and normal or near normal behavior followed by rapidly progressive lethargy, stupor, and coma, hemiparesis, and an ipsilateral dilated pupil. The lucid interval may be absent if the initial traumatic unconsciousness is prolonged and the onset of arterial bleeding swift. It may last from 15 min to days, very rarely a month. Seizures may occur. The hemiparesis is usually contralateral; however, herniation may cause the opposite cerebral peduncle to be compressed against the edge of the tentorium, resulting in ipsilateral hemiparesis. This is known as Kernohan's notch.

Intracerebral Hematoma

Trauma may cause shearing forces in the brain substance as it moves within the cranium. These forces may produce tears in the brain and blood vessels, resulting in intracerebral hematoma. The coagulation necrosis that accompanies cerebral contusion can also result in intracerebral hematoma. These effects are worse in the elderly with more fragile blood vessels. These hematomas are more common in the frontal and temporal lobes, and extremely uncommon in the cerebellum. There may be multiple lesions.

A typical history is similar to that of subdural hematoma. Pupillary inequality is uncommon. These hematomas are common contralateral to a skull fracture. If they are deep in the brain parenchyma they are termed *intermediate coup*.

Subarachnoid Hemorrhage

Traumatic subarachnoid hemorrhage usually occurs associated with a cerebral cortical contusion. Some blood from the contused area leaks into the subarachnoid space. The amount of blood can vary from minute to major. Significant hemorrhage may occur from laceration of a major vessel, especially the vertebral artery where it enters the dura.

Cerebral Laceration

Shearing forces in the moving brain can result in laceration of the cerebral substance. Frequently there is associated hemorrhage from vascular disruption, but there may not be. Fiber tracts in the corpus callosum, superior cerebellar peduncle, and pontomedullary junction are common sites of injury. Some of these injuries, particularly to the corpus callosum, arise because of laceration by a nearby rigid structure, the falx.

Cerebral Edema

Cerebral edema is a common occurrence with head injury. As elsewhere in the body, it is a nonspecific reaction to a wide variety of insults. It commonly occurs in the white matter and is associated with contusions and lacerations. Cerebral edema on a more widespread basis may accompany intracranial hematomas, possibly due to venous obstruction. Other mechanisms invoked for the development of diffuse edema include a loss of cerebral autoregulation (the ability of the cerebral vasculature to maintain constant flow in the face of hyper- or hypotension), dilatation of the resistance arterioles, and increased cerebral flow resulting in increased capillary pressure and the transudation of edema fluid. This results in a rise in intracranial pressure, due to the closed box effect of the skull. This is the substance of vasogenic theory.

Another theory emphasizes venous dilatation and stasis and a decrease in cerebral blood flow, and thus hypoxia of glial cells. These injured glial cells cannot maintain gradients of sodium and water and thus edema forms. This cytotoxic theory is more commonly accepted.

Regardless of the underlying pathophysiology, hypoxia and hypercarbia exacerbate the problem. Traumatic cerebral edema, without other lesions being present, can elevate intracranial pressure to high levels. The resultant decrease in cerebral flow can exacerbate cellular anoxia and produce more edema in a vicious cycle. Intracranial hypertension, commonly occurring in waves, can thus be a cause and effect of cerebral edema. Localized cerebral edema can also result in localized but not generalized increased intracranial pressure.

The relationship of intracranial pressure to the P_{CO_2} is critical to the understanding of traumatic intracranial hypertension. The P_{CO_2} is the chief regulator of cerebral blood flow. Increases in P_{CO_2} increase flow, and thus cerebral blood volume and pressure. At relatively low or normal levels of intracranial pressure, changes in P_{CO_2} have little effect on intracranial pressure. At elevated levels of intracranial pressure, however, P_{CO_2} changes exert a dramatic effect on intracranial pressure. This is summarized in Figure 119-1, and constitutes the rationale for hyperventilation as therapy for intracranial hypertension. Treatment of elevated intracranial pressure is covered in the section on therapy.

Children with head injury may have a rather unique syndrome of diffuse cerebral swelling. The clinical history is that of traumatic unconsciousness followed by a lucid interval and subsequent neurological deterioration. Analysis by CT scan at the time of deterioration reveals diffuse cerebral swelling, not on the basis of increased cerebral water content, but on the basis of cerebral hyperemia and increased blood volume. Treatment of this rather common syndrome differs from that of the usual cerebral edema in that mannitol, which further increases cerebral blood flow, is not used. The section on therapy covers other aspects of treatment.

LESIONS IN OPEN HEAD INJURY

When the cranial vault has been opened, either as a result of localized blunt trauma or by missile injury, many of the same pathological conditions can develop as with closed head injury. In addition to those, there are a few unique elements in open brain injury. These occur because not only can blood and CSF leak out, but bacteria can find an entrance to the cerebral contents.

Cerebral Contusion

Cerebral contusion with open brain injury is common. The brain area under an open depressed skull fracture is commonly contused.

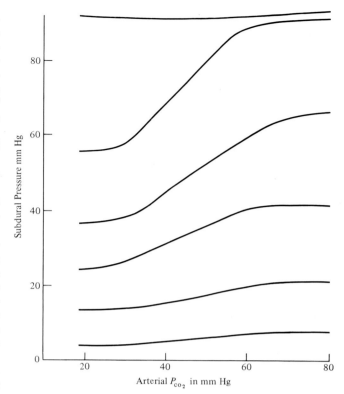

Figure 119-1. Intracranial (subdural) pressure vs. P_{CO_2}. (From Kent and Gosch, 1972, courtesy of Springer-Verlag.)

Likewise, any missile or object entering the brain can cause contusion on the entering surface.

Subdural Hematoma

The pathological considerations with open brain vs. closed head injury with subdural hematoma are identical except that subdural bleeding can also commonly occur from cerebral laceration and bleeding from the bone, in addition to the usual bridging vein tear. Injuries to the major venous sinuses may result in subdural or epidural bleeding.

Epidural Hematoma

Small amounts of blood in the epidural space can occur even from the scalp laceration or bone when the calvarium is open, and may decompress themselves due to the opening in the skull.

Cerebral Laceration

Laceration of the cerebral substance can occur directly from bone fragments or missile wounds with open brain injury, and one need not invoke shearing effects to explain their occurrence.

Subarachnoid Hemorrhage

As with closed head injury, this is a common concomitant of contusion. It may, however, occur from leakage of blood from the scalp or bone into the subarachnoid space.

Intracerebral Hematoma

Bone fragments or a missile can disrupt cerebral vessels and result in intracerebral hematoma. The blast effect of high-velocity bullets can disrupt vessels at some distance from the path of the bullet and result in extensive hemorrhage and hemorrhagic necrosis.

Intracranial Infections

While not an immediate occurrence, CNS infections after open head injury are of primary concern. Leakage of CSF can occur through a pathway that allows for entrance of bacteria and development of meningitis. Penetrating trauma can deposit bacterially contaminated bits of scalp, bone, and missile in the cerebral substance, and these then serve as a focus for abscess formation. Leakage of CSF after head injury with fracture of the basal skull or with penetrating trauma is felt to be a common occurrence and may accompany 2 percent of all cases of head trauma. Because of the closely adherent arachnoid, these rents usually seal quickly, usually in 24 to 48 h, and may not be detectable because of other injuries, particularly bleeding. Leakage of CSF may be intermittent or delayed. CSF may leak from the ear from temporal bone fracture, or the tympanic membrane may not be injured or seal and fluid develop in the middle ear. This may cause conductive hearing loss and a feeling of bubbles in the ear. Fluid from temporal bone fracture may also find its way to the nose and present as a clear or serosanguineous discharge. Basilar frontal fossa fractures may also cause CSF rhinorrhea. Intracranial air is present in 20 percent of cases.

If the fluid is thin, watery, and crystal-clear and tests positive for glucose on glucose test strips, it is likely to be CSF. Any contamination by blood will add glucose to it and invalidate the test.

PATHOPHYSIOLOGY OF HERNIATION SYNDROMES

Many of the pathological entities discussed can result in a "mass effect" on the brain. Addition of a new mass (e.g., blood clot, edema fluid, additional blood volume) can have several consequences. First, because of the closed nature of the skull, intracranial pressure rises. This can, to some extent, be accommodated by more rapid resorption of CSF or by decreased cerebral blood volume. Second, local mass effect may cause displacement of cerebral substance. Movement of the brain can result in dysfunction of critical brainstem centers controlling respiration and circulation and result in death. This secondary dysfunction of previously functioning brainstem centers can occur in several ways.

First, a unilateral mass such as a subdural or epidural hematoma over the cerebral surface may push on the hemisphere, forcing the medial aspect (uncus) of the temporal lobe across the opening of the tentorium. This is called uncal or tentorial herniation of tentorial pressure cone (see Fig. 119-2). The immediately adjacent structures at the opening of the tentorium are affected. These structures are the third nerve, ipsilateral cerebral peduncle, posterior cerebral artery, and midbrain. The clinical effects can then be ipsilateral third nerve paralysis, (dilated pupil, ptosis, externally deviated eye) contralateral hemiparesis and possibly contra-

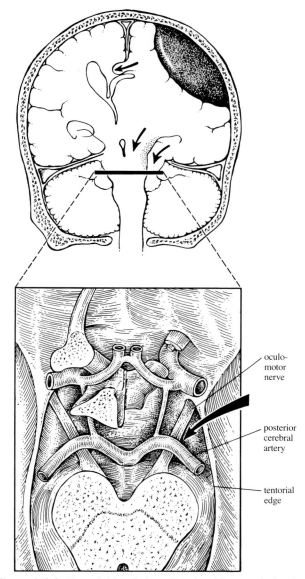

Figure 119-2. Tentorial herniation. (Reprinted by permission from Milhorat, 1978.)

oculo-motor nerve

posterior cerebral artery

tentorial edge

lateral visual field loss (from posterior cerebral artery compression affecting occipital lobe), and decreasing level of consciousness.

In rare circumstances the medial aspect of the temporal lobe may push the midbrain to the opposite edge of the tentorium which then can compress the contralateral cerebral peduncle (Kernohan's notch) and result in a hemiparesis ipsilateral to the mass.

More diffuse mass effect in the supratentorial space may cause the midline structure of the brain to herniate "centrally" through the opening of the tentorium. This central herniation syndrome has several stages which are summarized in the chapter on coma. For a more thorough discussion of these effects, refer to Chapter 10D.

Mass effect in the posterior fossa may cause herniation of posterior fossa contents (especially cerebellar tonsils) through the foramen magnum, as tonsillar herniation. When the cerebellar tonsils compress the medulla there is usually sudden fatal respiratory and circulatory arrest.

SKULL FRACTURES

Fractures of the skull are classified as linear, comminuted, or depressed, and further classified as open or closed. A fracture of the skull has significance under the following circumstances: An open skull fracture or basilar skull fracture can allow leakage of cerebral contents—brain and CSF—and allow for contamination of the intracranial space. A depressed skull fracture, in addition to the local trauma and potential for bleeding caused by it, may make the underlying brain more susceptible to seizures. Fractures into the paranasal sinuses may set up conditions for sinus infection.

The other primary significance of skull fractures is that the forces necessary to produce them may cause significant concomitant injuries, such as intracranial hematomas. Epidural hematoma, usually caused by laceration of the middle meningeal artery, is associated with a skull fracture between 75 and 90 percent of the time. The dural venous sinuses may be directly lacerated by overlying bone fragments from skull fracture. Fractures involving temporal bone may directly involve the middle and inner ear. Subdural hematoma occurs as often with or without skull fracture. Simple linear skull fracture by itself has little significance and no treatment. Significant intracranial lesions occur with or without it. A discussion of indications for skull x-rays will be covered under the evaluation of the head-injured patient.

IMMEDIATE COMPLICATIONS OF HEAD INJURY

In addition to the intracranial lesions previously discussed, several complications of significance can affect the patient with head injury. Seizures can occur at the time of trauma or very shortly thereafter, or their onset can be delayed by days, weeks, or years. Penetrating trauma to the brain has the highest incidence of seizures, approaching 50 percent. Minor closed head injury without cerebral laceration or coma has a 2 to 5 percent incidence of seizures. One of the great difficulties arises in evaluating the head-injured patient immediately after a seizure where the lethargy and possibly postictal paralysis could be either due to the seizure itself or a developing intracranial hematoma.

A potential early complication of head injury is diffuse intravascular coagulation. It is much more common in patients with severe head injury (49 percent) and virtually nonexistent in mild head injury. The brain is a rich source of thromboplastin and it is felt that the injured brain releases thromboplastin and initiates the coagulation cascade. Both open and closed head injury are associated with this abnormality.

Pulmonary edema can occur in the head-injured patient on a neurogenic basis. It is felt, based on clinical and animal studies, that the pulmonary vascular system responds to intracranial pressure like the systemic vasculature, and that the pulmonary edema is due to pulmonary venous hypertension.

The syndrome of inappropriate secretion of antidiuretic hormone may occur as a result of head injury. It occurs in 5 to 10 percent of patients with moderate to severe injury. One finds low serum sodium and osmolality, high urine sodium, and urine osmolality greater than serum, and urinary sodium loss not due to renal, cardiac, hepatic, or adrenal disease. The resulting hypotonic extracellular fluid volume expansion may exacerbate cerebral and other edema.

DELAYED COMPLICATIONS AFTER HEAD INJURY

Many complications can occur in a delayed fashion after head injury. Seizures have been discussed. CSF leak and infectious complications can occur days to weeks to years later. Hydrocephalus can develop. This can be on an obstructive basis from blockage of CSF pathways or from diffuse brain injury with subsequent atrophy.

Subdural hygroma, the presence of excess fluid in the subdural space, can develop, and while rarely causing focal deficit, can halt neurological recovery. Subdural hematomas have been discussed.

A posttraumatic syndrome or postconcussion syndrome may develop. Commonly this includes headache, dizziness, nervous instability, and difficulty with concentration. There may be no correlation with the severity of trauma or duration of coma. The syndrome is extremely common, and some components of it may be present in 80 percent of patients with minor head trauma 3 months after injury. The syndrome can occur over an extended period of time, and be very resistant to treatment. The exact basis of the syndrome is a subject of great debate. Early symptoms of headache can be due to intracranial damage from the lesions previously described, but late or persistent headache rarely so. Migraine, however, is not felt to be precipitated or aggravated by trauma. Many mechanisms, both organic and psychogenic, have been invoked to explain posttraumatic headache, which has many and varied clinical characteristics. The dizziness that usually accompanies the syndrome is rarely described as true vertigo, but is usually described as a feeling of giddiness, faintness, or unsteadiness, or a dazed feeling. The pathogenesis may involve disturbances of equilibrium on an organic basis, but the site of involvement is a subject of debate. The "realness" or organicity of the psychogenic symptoms centers more on a debate on mind-brain-psyche and on the many social–financial-compensation factors involved. Regardless, the syndrome is associated with significant morbidity and lost work time.

Injuries Associated with Head Injury

It is uncommon for head injury to occur as a totally isolated event. Associated injuries are common. Injury to the cervical spine is a concomitant to 15 to 20 percent of head and facial injuries, and should always be considered in the head-injured patient. Other injuries are well covered in other chapters and clearly may take precedence in their potential for life threat. However, injury to the nervous system is extremely important and different from that of other systems in that one can rarely compensate for its injuries as by blood transfusion or MAST trousers for intraabdominal bleeding, or supplemental oxygen or controlled ventilation for lung injury.

DIAGNOSTIC TESTS IN THE HEAD-INJURED PATIENT

For most of the pathological entities described, one will need a diagnostic test for definitive diagnosis prior to specific therapy. When to consider doing these tests will be covered in the section on patient management.

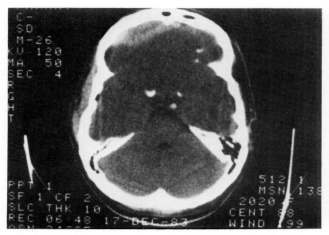

Figure 119-3. Frontal epidural hematoma. The localized lenticular-shaped blood density in the frontal region is the common configuration of an epidural hematoma.

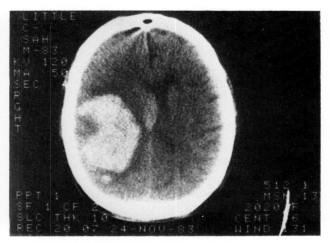

Figure 119-5. Intracerebral hematoma. The localized blood density mass in the parietal region has associated edema surrounding it, seen as a darker band.

Computerized Tomography

The CT scan has revolutionized the management of head trauma. All the surgically treatable conditions described can usually be diagnosed, especially acute conditions. This is because most of the surgically treatable conditions involve hematomas (epidural, subdural, intracerebral) and acute bleeding can be seen well on CT scans (see Figs. 119-3, 119-4, and 119-5). If one is going to perform a contrast procedure such as angiography or intravenous pyelography, it is best if the CT scan can be done first so that areas of cerebral contusion, which may contrast enhance, do not appear as blood. One should have completed a reasonable evaluation of the cervical spine (lateral, AP, and odontoid) prior to CT scan because of potential head positioning required.

CT scans may be less reliable for chronic subdural hematomas, especially bilateral. Contrast enhancement improves the yield. CT scan can reveal subarachnoid hemorrhage (Fig. 119-6), either spontaneous or traumatic, but may be false negative with small amounts of blood or with hemorrhage only near bone. Some lesions which can occur in a delayed fashion may not show on an initial CT scan. CT scan can be used for detection of bony abnormality. However, clinical suspicion of the bony abnormality must be communicated to the radiologist so that special attention can be directed to it. A lesion not well seen routinely might be a high parietal depressed fracture. However, CT may be as sensitive as skull x-ray. With this consideration, skull x-rays add nothing therapeutically significant to CT scan and need not be done if CT scan is to be performed and special clinical attention to suspected areas is achieved. Facial bone injury does not fall into this category.

Cerebral Angiography

Cerebral angiography can also detect most significant and surgically treatable posttraumatic hematomas but is not as sensitive as CT scan and subjects the patient to the risks of an invasive procedure. However, it will detect injuries to the carotid and vertebral arteries. If other arteriography is being performed, such as arch

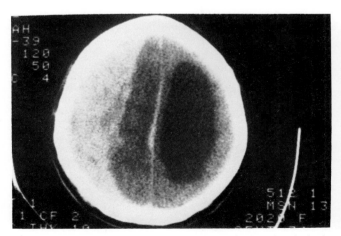

Figure 119-4. Subdural hematoma. This massive, panhemispheric collection of blood assumes a typical shape as it outlines the cortex. There is also ventricular enlargement.

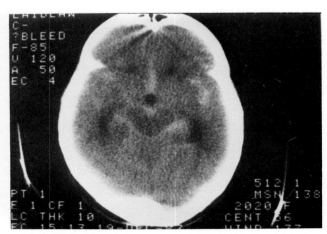

Figure 119-6. Subarachnoid hemorrhage. Blood in the subarachnoid spaces appears as faint white lines in the major fissures.

aortography, it may be quick and efficacious to perform cerebral angiography for head injury. It is second best to CT, but a reasonable alternative if CT is not available or is malfunctioning. When there is doubt about whether a subarachnoid hemorrhage seen on CT is traumatic or caused by an aneurysm, angiography will be needed.

Nuclear Brain Scan

This test is listed only to point out that it has no place in the evaluation of head trauma as it may not detect most of the lesions under consideration.

Skull X-Rays

Skull x-rays rarely make a definitive, therapeutically significant diagnosis in head trauma with the exception of depressed skull fracture. In other circumstances, e.g., linear skull fracture, they serve only to raise one's level of suspicion about concomitant intracranial lesions such as hematomas. They may cause further testing to be done but cannot exclude intracranial lesions. If one has made the clinical decision to pursue a suspected intracranial hematoma, CT scan would be preferred. As discussed under CT scan, skull x-rays add little to CT. The subject of skull x-rays with minor head trauma is discussed under patient management. Basilar skull fractures, a potentially therapeutically significant entity (e.g., CSF leak), rarely show on x-rays.

Cervical Spine X-Rays

Because of the movement of the neck that accompanies head injury, concomitant cervical spine injury detection is an important part of head trauma evaluation. The cross-table lateral film, including all seven vertebrae, is the most productive and revealing, but may miss 20 percent of cervical spine injuries. AP and odontoid films should always be done. Special techniques such as "swimmer's view," pulling down the shoulders, or tomography may be needed to visualize all seven vertebrae. Additionally, tomography may further clarify or identify abnormalities suspected or poorly defined on plain films. Normal plain x-rays do not exclude significant ligamentous injury, and at times carefully controlled flexion-extension views may be necessary.

CLINICAL MANAGEMENT OF HEAD INJURIES

For the purposes of discussion, patients with head injuries will be divided into three arbitrary categories. *Severe head injury* will be used to describe those patients with coma or a profoundly altered level of consciousness. *Moderate head injury* will be used for those with alteration of consciousness short of coma and/or focal neurological signs. *Mild head injury* categorizes patients with very brief or no loss of consciousness, who are alert and have a normal neurological examination.

Injury severity scales such as the Glasgow coma scale can be used for studying populations of head-injured patients or charting the course over time of an individual patient. The initial diagnosis and disposition of any given head-injured patient is more complex than any simple scale can encompass.

Severe Head Injury: Examination

The most important parts of the neurologic examination in patients with severe head injury are the examination of the pupils and the best motor response. A summary of the initial examination and stabilization priorities is given in Table 119-1. Although in more traditional textbooks on coma the respiratory pattern has been emphasized as an important sign in localizing the level of involvement of the nervous system, in the setting of severe acute head injury and potentially multiple associated injuries, the respiratory pattern loses its significance for several reasons. Associated injuries may produce a degree of shock or acidosis or severe pain which may alter the respiratory status. Indeed, 50 percent of patients with severe head injuries have additional major injuries. Second, immediate control of the airway is such an important intervention in the early care of these patients that they are not allowed to fully develop what might be an otherwise unhindered respiratory pattern. Control of the airway and ventilation has therapeutic value and therefore the localizing value of the respiratory pattern is less useful in this setting than it is in other causes of coma. One of the standard diagnostic tests used in the comatose patient, that of doll's eye maneuvers, is likewise not utilized in these patients because of the likelihood of concomitant cervical spine injury. One must always treat a patient with a severe head injury as having a concomitant cervical spine injury until proved otherwise. To obtain the information learned by doll's eye maneuvers, cold water calorics are far more reliable and safer.

In the initial evaluation of these patients it is obvious that the standard ABCs of acute care must be followed first; that is, management of the airway, assurance of breathing, and a guarantee of effective cardiac output. In addition, one must immediately pay attention to stabilization of the cervical spine and compression of obvious hemorrhage. Then in standard fashion a rapid screening general examination is done to detect obvious associated injuries such as chest, trunk, and extremity injuries, and then after assurance of intravenous access and initial obtaining of cross-table cervical spine x-rays, one proceeds with the rest of the simultaneous evaluation and care of the patient based upon the screening evaluation as to which injuries will take priority. It cannot be emphasized strongly enough that the neurologic examination at times must take second place to the evaluation and treatment of shock or potential shock and blood loss in multiple trauma patients.

Once the ABCs have been assured and a quick review of the patient's injuries has been obtained, one must then perform a rapid screening neurologic examination. This should take less than a minute. One looks for obvious external signs of head injury, palpates the head and the face, examines the pupillary response, observes spontaneous extraocular movements, establishes the level of consciousness, and obtains the best motor response from the extremities, usually in response to pain, or spontaneously.

Table 119-1. Initial Examination and Stabilization in Severe Head Injury

Airway, breathing, circulation, cervical-spine immobilization, compression of hemorrhage
Pupils, best motor response
Establish IV access, x-ray cervical-spine, intubate
Secondary screening exam for associated injuries, included peritoneal lavage or other study to exclude intraabdominal bleeding
Secondary, more detailed neurological examination
Pupils, best motor response repeatedly

Pitfalls in Severe Head Injury

It is worth mentioning several potential pitfalls in the management of the severe CNS injury at this point. These are listed in Table 119-2. While in the older literature Cushing's sign was used to correlate with a severe head injury or the presence of an intracranial mass, it is currently felt that its presence is a very late and/or unreliable finding with an expanding intracranial mass, and that the classical elevation of blood pressure and slowing of pulse may never be seen with a large intracranial mass, or it may be such a late finding as to be useless in directing therapy. Likewise, papilledema is a sign that one should never see in an acute head injury. Many hours and potentially several days are required for papilledema to develop, even in the presence of severe intracranial hypertension. Subhyaloid hemorrhages indicate severe intracranial hypertension. These hemorrhages occur because the sudden rapid increase in intracranial pressure is transmitted to the venous system inside the eye with resultant sudden hemorrhage in the pre-retinal, or subhyaloid region. Otherwise, examination of the fundus is a relatively unimportant part of the neurologic examination and one should not waste a great deal of time on it when there are other more important priorities in the initial examination.

There are several purposes to the initial screening neurologic examination. The first is to establish the severity of neurologic injury, the second is to obtain a reliable baseline examination, and the third is to establish whether the patient has signs of a focal intracranial mass lesion or signs of severe neurologic deficit which could potentially be due to either lateralized or nonlateralized mass intracranial lesions. While the traditional sign of an expanding mass intracranial lesion, that of the unilateral dilated and fixed pupil (Hutchinson's pupil) with contralateral hemiparesis, is the most common classic sign of an expanding mass lesion, the tentorial pressure cone, one must be aware of a less common phenomenon already described as Kernohan's notch.

A final word on penetrating trauma: Penetrating bodies protruding from the head should never be removed. While the foreign body is still lodged in the head it provides tamponade of bleeding vessels. Release of the tamponade can cause catastrophic bleeding and deterioration of the patient. Penetrating foreign objects should only be removed in the operating room under controlled conditions.

Intracranial Lesions in Severe Head Trauma

Approximately 50 percent of the patients in this category will have an intracranial hematoma. These have previously been described. In addition to these entities, intracranial hypertension is a critical problem, as it is for the remaining 50 percent without a hematoma. All the patients in this category will require a CT scan or cerebral angiogram to rule out mass lesion and many may benefit from monitoring intracranial pressure. This is described in the section on therapy. They will need, as a minimum, baseline CBC, elec-

Table 119-2. Pitfalls in Severe Head Injury

Cushing's sign
Shock
Papilledema
Dilated pupil from local trauma
Brachial plexus injury
Kernohan's notch

trolytes, BUN, glucose, coagulation, screen, and arterial blood gases.

Moderate Head Injury

Moderate head injury means a patient with some alteration of level of consciousness short of coma and/or focal neurological signs. Concussion, as discussed, means transient loss of a neurological function as a result of trauma, with rapid return to normal. One must be sure very early in the interaction with the patient that a mild change in mental status is not due to shock or hypoxia from other injuries. One can never ascribe shock or hypotension to head injury alone as one cannot lose enough blood into the head to cause hypovolemia. Rare exceptions can occur only in infants.

One may attribute altered mental status to intoxicants such as alcohol or other drugs; however, one must be wary in ascribing altered mental status purely to the effects of alcohol in a patient who has had a head injury. This is obviously one of the most difficult and challenging diagnostic problems of the clinician. These patients are the ones to watch extremely closely for progressions of signs that may indicate the development of a mass intracranial lesion. As discussed above, the ABCs and screening neurologic examination are done rapidly with assurance of immobilization of the cervical spine. Obviously, an examination of pupils, extraocular movements, tympanic membranes, physical examination of the head, motor status, and mental status are the most important. One may be seeing the patient in a lucid interval prior to the development of signs of a mass intracranial lesion.

In this group of patients skull x-rays may have some moderate usefulness. A fracture across the middle meningeal groove or venous sinuses would prompt one to be very aggressive in the management of the patient. Fractures across the sinuses, particularly the frontal sinus, may require management in and of themselves. As in all tests, a negative skull x-ray does not exclude the presence of significant intracranial injury. In this category of patients the most useful test is serial neurologic examinations, separated by short intervals of time. It will be the progression or regression of signs and symptoms that will allow for the more precise management and decision about CT scan for these patients. Those patients progressing rapidly need consideration of a definitive diagnostic test for an intracranial mass lesion and/or preparation for surgery. When one has been assured that there is no sign of blood loss or decreased circulating blood volume, these patients should have minimal to no IV fluids and the intravenous line should be placed only for access in case medications are needed. One of the ways to ensure that large amounts of fluid cannot be given to those patients accidentally or when they are being x-rayed or cannot be watched closely, is to use relatively small-caliber IV lines with mini-drippers and small bottles of fluid so that they cannot inadvertently receive more fluid than one would desire.

Patients bleeding profusely from scalp wounds should have traction placed on the galea to help obtain hemostasis. Sometimes several sutures put through the galea and then tight closure of the galea will slow the bleeding to the point where it can be otherwise controlled easily. In general, in a noncosmetic area the best closure of the scalp is in a single layer using a large 2 or 3-0 synthetic monofilament suture.

Some patients with moderate head injury may need to be observed in a hospital setting. While this is an individualized decision in each case, several classes of patient should be considered for admission. These include: any patient with a skull fracture (especially across the middle meningeal artery, venous sinuses, or basilar skull), infants, the elderly, those unlikely to be observed closely at home, and any patient with neurological deficit. This is most appropriately done on a neurosurgery service or on a service where definitive care can be rendered quickly should progression of signs and symptoms develop, indicating a mass intracranial lesion. For this reason it is not appropriate to observe such patients on a service or in a hospital where access to the necessary resources is not quickly available.

Mild Head Injury

Mild head injury means either no loss of consciousness or a very brief loss of consciousness and a normal neurologic examination. One must exclude those with signs of or suspicion of penetrating injury to the head or depressed skull fracture. A very common example of this would be a young child with a minor head injury at school brought in by parents for evaluation. Obviously the disposition of these patients will depend a great deal on the assessment of the severity of injury and the time lag between injury and examination. In these patients there is nothing more useful than a very thorough neurologic examination. A great deal of reassurance can be communicated to the family by a thorough professional neurologic examination testing such things as gait, tandem walking, and finger-to-nose testing. This sense of thoroughness does a great deal more for reassurance and establishment of true normality than such things as skull x-rays. It is important in these patients, as with others, to palpate the head. As a general rule in children older than several years old, if there is no clinical sign of a skull fracture, that is, there is no particular spot on the head that is very tender and none of the other signs that suggest skull fracture such as CSF rhinorrhea or otorrhea, Battle's sign, or depressed skull fracture, the usefulness of a skull x-ray in this setting is extremely limited. There is a large volume of literature concerning usefulness of skull x-rays in this setting. The findings are that, in general, x-rays have been found to be useless. One can always find an exception to this rule; however, thorough documentation of a normal examination and assurance of competent neurologic observation is much more useful disposition for the patient than detection of an occult skull fracture. It is a difficult question in these patients as to when to x-ray. Mentioned above are some of the criteria that are useful. Other factors that might be considered would be significant injury directly over the region of the frontal sinus, which could have resulted in at least outer table depressed fracture of the frontal sinus, which might require ENT evaluation, or the presence of a ventricular shunt.

Another question in these patients is how long to observe them, and who should observe them. As a general rule most of these patients can be discharged from the emergency department. If there is a question as to the reliability of someone to observe them, keeping them around the emergency department for somewhat extended periods of time may be in order, especially until a reliable observer can be found. In rare instances they may need hospitalization for observation. A more significant question is that of admission for all skull fractures. Frequently, patients with skull fractures are admitted to the hospital for neurological observation. However, it is unusual in the patient who has a relatively benign history, a normal examination, and a skull fracture not in a "dan-

gerous area," to find progression of neurologic symptoms suggesting a developing intracranial mass. Areas of high danger include fracture across the middle meningeal artery or venous sinus, and at times fractures posteriorly in the skull, as posterior fossa hematomas may present with catastrophic suddenness. There is no hard and fast rule concerning when and whether these patients should be admitted for observation, but an individual decision must be reached concerning each case. CT scanning may be less expensive and more reliable than admission.

Evaluation After Head Injury

Patients may present themselves for evaluation days to weeks or more after head injury. Commonly, they have components of the postconcussion syndrome described. This syndrome can be extremely disturbing to the patient and family. The extent of emergency evaluation for organic factors such as chronic subdural hematoma or hygroma, hydrocephalus, etc., must be a very individualized judgment. Factors weighing on the side of immediate CT scan include impaired coagulation, especially in the presence of Coumadin, preexisting shunt for hydrocephalus, unreliability of observation or followup, or frequency of presentation for evaluation.

Pediatric Head Injury

When dealing with very young children with head injury, that is, under the age of 2 years, one must include in the history and examination several factors that would not be considered in adults. It is rare to find in the history a reliable reporting of neurologic deficits such as weakness, numbness, or double vision. The examination of children is rarely as formal as that in adults. Observation of behavior and normal coordinated motor acts constitutes the bulk of the examination. As mentioned in the section on severe head injury, at times a subhyaloid hemorrhage in children is indicative of a rapidly expanding intracranial lesion or massive intracranial pressure. By far the most sensitive indicator of intracranial pressure in a child with an open fontanel is the pressure on the fontanel. A sunken fontanel with the child in the sitting position and not crying is the best and most reliable indicator that intracranial pressure is not high. If one needed to follow any particular sign in children with head injury, the fontanel is the most sensitive and early indicator. Also, because of the open fontanel and the expansion of the intracranial sutures, it is rare to find focal neurologic signs in children, even with an expanding hematoma.

The history of an expanding hematoma may reveal a head injury with a sudden loss of consciousness followed by a relatively more alert period, which is then followed by subsequent deterioration consisting of such nonspecific symptoms as lethargy, poor feeding, irritability, and then catastrophic respiratory arrest and death. One rarely progresses through the focal findings of unilaterally dilated pupil, focal hemiparesis, etc. This should also make one aware that these signs should not be looked for to assess the severity of head injury. The level of consciousness and arousability remain the most sensitive indicators. Children who have a ventricular shunt for hydrocephalus for whatever reason are more at risk for the development of sudden deterioration from subdural hematoma because they have an additional pressure release system whereby the brain can shift an enormous amount without development of signs of intracranial mass. Then, when the capacity of the brain to shift has been expended, a sudden catastrophic demise occurs. Those patients should be treated as a special category and more aggressive management would be in order.

Because of the nonspecificity of signs of neurological deterioration in young children, one must be assured that if the child is released from the emergency department that the observers are competent and concerned and can return the child promptly for reevaluation. Child abuse cannot only take the form of direct blows to the head, but also vigorous shaking, which can produce a subdural hematoma.

Pediatric patients can develop a syndrome of sudden, massively elevated intracranial pressure with increased cerebral blood flow and increased cerebral blood volume as described. One is more liberal in ordering skull x-rays in children under 1 year as fracture may be present without the clinical criteria already mentioned, particularly if a shunting tube is in place. Also, children who have suffered a very localized force to the head (such as from a baseball bat) should be x-rayed to detect depressed fracture.

Other Considerations

A hospital that does not have neurosurgery capability is in a particularly difficult position regarding all forms of head injury. Frequently, patients with severe head injury have other severe injuries and the timing of transfer to a center with a neurosurgeon becomes an extremely difficult judgment. One must try to stabilize the patient hemodynamically and prevent further harm. One must in some way discover some injuries so as to prevent further harm, but on the other hand, one cannot take a great deal of time assessing those patients where definitive care for head injury will be rendered elsewhere. The timing of various interventions in these patients must be determined by the minute details of the injury, the patient's presentation, distance to other hospitals, availability of specialists, etc. As a general rule, if the physician cannot exclude the development of an intracranial mass lesion and he or she will have to send a patient elsewhere for that, all speed should be used in the transfer, with only the establishment of an intravenous line, stabilization of the cervical spine and assurance of the airway, and splinting of suspected fractures. Intubation may be needed. Detection of occult intraabdominal bleeding is relatively useless in this setting unless it can be dealt with quickly enough so that the head injury would not deteriorate. This is obviously a difficult judgment. Patients with moderate head injury, as discussed above, who will need neurologic observation, should not be observed in a setting or on a service that cannot render definitive treatment should a mass intracranial lesion develop.

Pitfalls in Diagnosis

There are several findings on neurologic examination that could be potentially misleading. While one usually associates the presence of a dilated, fixed pupil with compression of the third nerve as from a mass intracranial lesion, a dilated, fixed pupil can occur from local trauma to the eye. The ciliary ganglion of the eye can be contused, thereby affecting the pupilloconstrictor fibers, resulting in a dilated pupil. Therefore, local trauma can produce a dilated, fixed pupil. However, the examiner ought to have a high

level of suspicion that it potentially could be caused by a mass intracranial lesion and that likely should be ruled out. In a comatose patient with an unreactive pupil one may be misled by the presence of a blind eye. A blind eye will have a consensual light reaction. Another potential focal neurologic finding which could be from a peripheral injury is that of brachial plexus lesions. The comatose patient who is not using one upper extremity may have an injury to his or her brachial plexus. The usual mechanism of injury is a stretching of the brachial plexus from force to the side of the head and on the shoulder. This is a difficult diagnosis to make in a comatose patient and is usually definitively diagnosed only later. At times, fractured extremities or restrained extremities may not move quite as well as unrestrained or uninjured extremities, and may therefore give the false impression of a localizing sign. Another finding on physical examination that tends to be misleading is that the margin of a subgaleal hematoma almost always feels as if the area is depressed. One should be aware of this and not pursue further what may seem to be an obvious clinically depressed skull fracture when the x-rays are negative.

CLINICAL MANAGEMENT—SUMMARY

To summarize, the most useful parts of the neurologic examination in patients with head injury are as follows: In the comatose patient attention should be paid to the pupils, extraocular movements, and best motor response. In those with moderate head injury the level of unconsciousness, repeated mental status examinations, any drift of the outstretched extremities on the motor examination, and the pupillary examinations are the most important. Less useful parts of the neurologic examination in the setting of acute injury are examination of the fundus, detailed sensory exams, reflexes, and Babinski signs.

Initial Therapy in Head Injury

In the emergency setting, initial evaluation and therapy proceed simultaneously. Some initial therapeutic interventions, such as cervical immobilization, take place routinely. Others, such as surgery, usually await definitive diagnosis. The following are early therapeutic maneuvers to consider.

Patient Positioning

If no contraindications such as spine fracture or hypotension exist, the head-injured patient should be placed 30 to 45° upright. This may lower intracranial venous pressure and thus intracranial pressure. It is not universally efficacious, however.

Hyperventilation

The manner in which hyperventilation reduces intracranial pressure has been discussed. It is one of the most efficacious, rapidly acting, and safe tools the emergency physician has in early management of severe head injury. The optimum P_{CO_2} is 25 mmHg. Intubation further protects the airway against aspiration.

Oxygenation

Oxygenation may be impaired in the head-injured patient from concomitant chest and lung injury, neurogenic pulmonary edema, retained secretions, and atelectasis or shock lung. Supplemental oxygen should be supplied to provide the brain with an optimum environment for metabolic needs.

Osmotic Diuretics

Osmotic diuretics reduce intracranial pressure through dehydration of the brain, improve intracranial compliance (ability to withstand a volume change without pressure change), and increase cerebral blood flow. Mannitol is the most commonly used osmotic diuretic. The dose is 0.5 to 1 g/kg. It should be avoided if anuric renal failure is suspected. Other agents used include hypertonic glucose (50 mL of 50% glucose), urea, and glycerol. The advantage to glucose is its ready availability and correction of hypoglycemia (as from insulin shock or drug overdose). Urea takes time to mix and is not readily available.

While osmotic diuretics are efficacious in reducing intracranial pressure, they should not be used blindly as they may obscure potentially significant neurological signs and thus delay diagnosis and therapy. The physician should have a plan for either CT scan or surgery once they are given.

To use osmotic diuretics on a long-term basis is to substitute one disease for another, i.e., dehydration and hypovolemia for intracranial hypertension. To justify this use, one should have a means of measuring intracranial pressure.

Mannitol, because it enhances cerebral blood flow, is felt to be contraindicated in the pediatric syndrome of cerebral edema, as discussed.

Furosemide

Furosemide has been used to lower intracranial pressure in patients with brain tumors. Some authors believe it is useful in trauma, particularly in the elderly or children, while others question its usefulness. Doses advocated are 0.5 to 1 mg/kg.

Antibiotics

Antibiotics have been advocated as prophylaxis for basilar skull fracture and CSF leak. Their use is controversial, as some studies report a benefit and some do not.

Glucocorticoids

Potent glucocorticoids have a long history of use in neurological conditions. Their use in traumatic cerebral conditions is not as popular as in the past, and their efficacy in improving outcome or decreasing intracranial pressure is doubtful.

Barbiturates

Intermediate-acting (pentobarbital) and short-acting (thiopental) barbiturates reliably lower intracranial pressure. Cerebral blood flow is reduced. Whether this is a primary effect or secondary to reduced metabolic needs is controversial. Barbiturates are not used as a first-line drug, but usually in the setting of intracranial hypertension refractory to hyperventilation (and possibly mannitol), and as an adjunct to hypothermia. One needs reliable intracranial pressure monitoring and assurance of no surgically treatable hematoma. Because of the coma induced by barbiturates, the value of the clinical examination is lost and one must rely on intensive monitoring.

Hypothermia

Hypothermia lowers intracranial pressure and metabolic needs. It has been used in a variety of insults to the brain such as trauma, anoxia from drowning, and Reye's syndrome. Because of cardiac arrhythmias and pulmonary insufficiency, temperatures are rarely below 32°C (90°F). Commonly, barbiturates and agents which initially abolish shivering, such as chlorpromazine, are used. Because of the induced coma, one must rely on intensive monitoring. Use of hypothermia is not a primary modality, but is adjunctive in the case of refractory intracranial hypertension. Hyperthermia should be avoided as it exacerbates cerebral edema.

Paralyzing Agents

Agents such as curare and pancuronium which paralyze skeletal muscle are used as adjuncts in management of severe head injury in several ways. They are used to facilitate compliance with the respirator to induce hyperventilation and prevent "bucking" the respirator, and elevating intrathoracic venous and thus intracranial pressure. One must be assured that no surgical lesion exists and that continuous access to artificial ventilation is assured. Their place is mostly in the intensive care of the patient and rarely to facilitate intubation and CT scanning.

Anticonvulsants

Seizures in the setting of head injury are common, particularly with penetrating trauma. Their occurrence may signal decompensation and obscure the significance of the neurological examination. Many centers treat all patients with severe head trauma, especially those with penetrating trauma, prophylactically with anticonvulsants. Despite this, seizures may still occur. The drug of choice is diphenylhydantoin, 15 to 18 mg/kg intravenously as a loading dose at 25 mg/min.

Fluid Restriction

Once one is assured that there is no source or suspicion of blood loss, one should restrict the usual large volumes of fluid given to trauma patients. The brain participates with the rest of the body in extracellular fluid volume, and generalized expansion affects it, especially in the face of cerebral edema. Fluid restriction may be the only treatment needed for the syndrome of inappropriate antidiuretic hormone secretion (SIADH) or its prophylaxis. It is not the particular IV fluid composition that is as important as the restriction of volume. Whether fluid restriction is used on a long-term basis or not, initial restriction and certainly avoidance of large volumes are indicated.

Surgery

Surgery is indicated for removal of subdural, epidural, and at times intracerebral hematomas, and for elevation and repair of depressed skull fracture. In a delayed fashion it may be needed for repair of a CSF leak. Whether intracranial pressure monitors are placed in the operating room or at the bedside is subject to individual preferences. When considering evacuation of acute subdural or epidural hematomas, the sooner surgery is accomplished, the better.

There are few indications for placement of a burr hole in the emergency department. In the setting of uncal herniation where there will be any delay in obtaining the services of a neurosurgeon and modalities to reduce intracranial pressure fail, one should consider a burr hole on the side of the dilated pupil, 1 in above the zygoma and 1 in anterior to the ear, avoiding the temporal artery. Relief of an acute epidural hematoma may be lifesaving. A decision to proceed with this must be highly individualized.

Intracranial Pressure Monitoring

Elevated intracranial pressure is a common occurrence in head trauma. As there are no specific clinical parameters resulting from elevated intracranial pressure, it must be monitored on a continuous basis if one is going to aggressively treat it. There are several ways to monitor pressure, with advantages and disadvantages to each. A catheter placed in the ventricle can both record pressure and remove CSF to lower it. However, the ventricles may be small and collapsed with high pressure, and the procedure itself is invasive. Subdural pressure monitoring can be done by placing a bolt or stopcock through a twist drill hole in the skull and piercing the dura. This simple, effective technique can be done at the bedside. CSF cannot be removed, however. Various types of strain gauges can be placed in the subdura or epidural space; however, drifting of baseline and calibration are at times unreliable.

Selection of patients for monitoring involves judging those at risk for elevated intracranial pressure. Some advocate monitoring all patients with severe head injury (unable to obey simple command). Some reserve intensive monitoring for those whose neurological examination is so bad (the patient is decerebrate or flaccid) that clinical worsening would be difficult to detect. Some advocate monitoring all severe head-injured patients with an abnormal CT scan, or with a normal CT scan and several "risk" factors—hypotension on admission, pathologic posturing, or age over 40.

Like intraarterial pressure monitoring, pulmonary capillary wedge pressure monitoring, and cardiac output measurements, intracranial pressure monitoring opens up the intensive management of severe head injury to scientific treatment on a rational basis.

BIBLIOGRAPHY

Anderson DW, McLaurin RL (eds): National head and spinal cord injury survey. *J Neurosurg* 53:S1–S43, 1980.

Annegers J, et al: Seizures after head trauma: A population study. *Neurology* 30:683–689, 1980.

Balasubramaniam S, et al: Efficacy of skull radiography. *Am J Surg* 142(3):366, 1981.

Becker DP, et al: The outcome from severe head injury with early diagnosis and intensive management. *J Neurosurg* 47:491–502, 1977.

Bligh AS, et al: A patient selection for skull radiography in uncomplicated head injury: A national study by the Royal College of Radiologists. *Lancet* 8316:115, 1983.

Braakman R, et al: Megadose steroids in severe head injury: Results of a prospective double-blind clinical trial. *J Neurosurg* 58(3):326, 1983.

Bruno PO, Longlob JT: Diagnosis and management of thoracolumbar spine fractures. *Curr Conc Trauma Care* Winter, 1979, pp. 13–18.

Bruce, DA et al: Diffuse cerebral swelling following head injuries in children: The syndrome of "malignant brain edema." *J Neurosurg* 54(2):170, 1981.

Bruce DA, et al: Resuscitation from coma due to head injury. *Crit Care Med* 6(4):254, 1978.

Bruce DA, et al: The value of CAT scanning following pediatric head injury. *Clin Pediatr* 19(11):719, 1980.

Byrnes D: Head injury and the dilated pupil. *Am Surg* 45(3):139, 1979.

Chandler J: Traumatic cerebrospinal fluid leakage. *Otolaryngol Clin North Am* 16(3):623–632, 1983.

Clark JA, et al: Disseminated intravascular coagulation following cranial trauma. *J Neurosurg* 52(2):266, 1980.

Cooper PR, et al: Dexamethasone and severe head injury: A prospective double-blind study. *J Neurosurg* 51(3):307, 1979.

Cordobes F, et al: Observations on 82 patients with extradural hematomas. *J Neurosurg* 54:179–186, 1981.

Cottrell JE, et al: Furosemide and head injury. *J Trauma* 21(9):805, 1981.

Cumins RO, et al: High yield referral criteria for post-traumatic skull roentgenography. *JAMA* 244(7):673, 1980.

De Campo T, et al: How useful is the skull x-ray examination in trauma? *Med J Aust* 2(10):553, 1980.

de Lacey G, et al: Mild head injuries: A source of excessive radiography? *Clin Radiol* 31(4):32, 1980.

Dempsey RJ, Kindt G: Experimental augmentation of cerebral blood flow by mannitol in epidural intracranial mass. *J Trauma* 22(6):449–454, 1982.

DeSmet AA, et al: A second look at the utility of radiographic skull examination for trauma. *Am J Radiol* 132:95, 1979.

Dick A: The role of steroids in head trauma. *Curr Conc Trauma Care* 1(1):5, 1977.

Einhorn A: Basilar skull fractures in children. *Am J Dis Child* 132(11):121, 1978.

Enevoldsen E, Jensen F: Autoregulation and CO_2 response of cerebral blood flow in patients with acute severe head injury. *J Neurosurg* 48:689–703, 1978.

Eyes B, et al: Post-traumatic skull radiographs. Time for reappraisal. *Lancet* 2(8080):85, 1978.

Fischer RP, et al: Post concussive hospital observation of alert patients in a primary trauma center. *J Trauma* 21(11):920, 1981.

Gentleman D, Jennett B: Hazards of inter-hospital transfer of comatose head-injured patients. *Lancet* 853–856, 1981.

Gudeman SK, et al: Failure of high-dose steroid therapy to influence intracranial pressure in patients with severe head injury. *J Neurosurg* 51(3):301, 1979.

Gudeman SK, et al: Computed tomography in the evaluation of incidence and significance of post-traumatic hydrocephalus. *Radiology* 141:397–402, 1981.

Healy JF, et al: Computed tomographic evaluation of depressed skull fractures and associated intracranial injury. *Comput Radiol* 6(6):323, 1982.

Jennett B: Skull x-rays after recent head injury. *Clin Radiol* 31(4):463, 1980.

Jones PW: Hyperventilation in the management of cerebral oedema. *Intens Care Med* 7(5):205, 1981.

Karpman RR, et al: Observation of the alert, conscious patient with closed head injury. *Ariz Med* 37(11):772, 1980.

Kenning JA, et al: Upright patient positioning in the management of intracranial hypertension. *Surg Neurol* 15(2):148, 1981.

Kent G, Gosch H: Aterial P_{CO_2} effect at various levels of intracranial pressure, in Brock M, Dietz H (eds): *Intracranial Pressure*. Berlin, Springer-Verlag, 1972.

Kirkpatrick J: Neuropathology of head injury in neurology clinics. Vol. IV, No. 3, Baylor College of Medicine, Geigy Pharmaceuticals, 1982.

Larsen KT, et al: High yield criteria and emergency department skull radiography: Two community hospitals' experience. *JACEP* 8(10):393, 1979.

Leonidas JC, et al: Mild head trauma in children: When is a roentgenogram necessary? *Pediatrics* 69(2):139, 1982.

Levan AB, et al: Treatment of increased intracranial pressure: A comparison of different osmotic agents and use of thiopental. *J Neurosurg* 5(5):570, 1979.

Mahoney BD, et al: Emergency twist drill trephination. *J Neurosurg* 8(5):551, 1981.

Marshall L, et al: The outcome with aggressivetreatment in severe head injuries. Part I: The significance of intracranial pressure monitoring. *J Neurosurg* 50:20–25, 1979.

Marshall L, et al: The outcome with aggressive treatment in severe head injuries. Part II: Acute and chronic barbiturate administration in the management of head injury. *J Neurosurg* 50:26–30, 1979.

Masters SJ: Evaluation of head trauma: Efficacy of skull films. *Am J Roentgenol* 135(3):539, 1980.

Mendelow AD, et al: Admission after mild head injury: Benefits and costs. *Br med J* 285(6354):1530, 1982.

Milhorat TH: *Pediatric Neurosurgery*. Contemporary Neurosurgery Ser. Philadelphia, Davis Co, 1978, vol 16.

Mill J, Douglas, et al: Early insults to the injured brain. *JAMA* 240(5):439–442, 1978.

Miller J Douglas, et al: Significance of intracranial hypertension in severe head injury. *J Neurosurg* 47:503–516, 1977.

Miner ME, et al: Disseminated intravascular coagulation fibrinolytic syndrome following head injury in children: Frequency and prognostic implications. *J Pediatr* 100(5):687, 1982.

Narayan RK, et al: Intracranial pressure: To monitor or not to monitor? A review of our experience with head injury. *J Neurosurg* 56(5):650, 1982.

Nelson S: Review of therapeutic agents used in head injuries. *Curr Conc Trauma Care* 1(1):3, 1977.

Obisesan AA, et al: The uses and abuses of skull x-rays in head injury. *Nigerian Med J* 9(1):65, 1979.

Parkinson D: Concussion. *Mayo Clin Proc* 52:492–496, 1977.

Phillips LA: Comparative evaluation of the effect of a high yield criteria list upon skull radiography. *JACEP* 8(3):106, 1979.

Poczi T, et al: Syndrome of inappropriate secretion of antidiuretic hormone (SIADH) after head injury. *J Neurosurg* 10(6):685–688, 1982.

Raphaely RC, et al: Management of severe pediatric head trauma. *Pediatr Clin North Am* 27(3):715, 1980.

Rimel RW, et al: Disability caused by minor head injury. *J Neurosurg* 9(3):221, 1981.

Ropper AH, et al: Head position, intracranial pressure and compliance. *Neurology* 32(11):1288, 1982.

Rowbotham, GF, Whalley N: Prolonged compreession of brain resulting from extradural hemorrhage. *J Neurol Neurosurg Psychiat* 15:64, 1952.

Royal College of Radiologists: A study of the utilization of skull radiography in 9 accident-and-emergency units in the U.K. *Lancet* 2(8206):1234, 1980.

Rutherford W: Sequelae of concussion caused by minor head injury. *Lancet* January 1, 1977, 8001.

Saul TG, et al: Effect of intracranial pressure monitoring and aggressivetreatment on mortality in severe head injury. *J Neurosurg* 56(4):498, 1982.

Seelig J, et al: Traumatic subdural hematoma. *N Engl J Med* 304(25):1511–1518, 1981.

Singer HS, et al: Head trauma for the pediatrician. *Pediatrics* 62(5):819, 1978.

Stone JL, et al: Traumatic subdural hygroma. *J Neurosurg* 8(5):542–550, 1981.

Tress BM: The need for skull radiography in patients presenting for CT. *Radiology* 146–87–89, 1983.

Van der Sande JJ, et al: Head injuries and coagulation disorders. *J Neurosurg* 49(3):357, 1978.

Weston PAM: Admission policy for patients following head injury. *Br J Surg* 68:663–664, 1981.

Wintzen AD, et al: Subdural hematoma and oral anticoagulant therapy. *Arch Neurol* 39(2):69, 1982.

Wrightson P, et al: Time off work and symptoms after minor head injury. *Injury* 12(6):445, 1981.

Young B, et al: Failure of prophylactically administered phenytoin to prevent early post-traumatic seizures. *J Neurosurg* 58(2):231, 1983.

CHAPTER 120
CERVICAL
SPINE INJURIES

Robert Swetnam

INTRODUCTION

Trauma is the leading cause of death from ages 2 to 40. Approximately 70 percent of all severe motor vehicle accident victims have significant central nervous system trauma, with approximately 10 percent of those having cervical spine injury. It is estimated that there are between 4000 and 5000 new quadriplegics in the United States every year. This number is in addition to the almost 75,000 who are presently alive in the United States.

A cervical spinal cord injury is devastating, both psychologically and economically. The average new quadriplegic is 22 years of age. Due to ever-improving medical technology and treatment, a significant percentage of these individuals are living many years after their injury. The initial cost of resuscitation and rehabilitation has been estimated at between $50,000 and $250,000. Total direct and indirect costs of all spinal cord victims throughout the United States is between $1 and 2 billion per year.

Until very recently, the general consensus in the medical community was that very little, if anything, could be done once the patient had developed quadriplegia from a cervical spine injury. Many physicians still believe this to be true. There is, however, growing evidence that early treatment, including prompt immobilization and reduction, along with various pharmacologic agents, may decrease dramatically the morbidity and mortality which this group of individuals now experience. It is possible that many of the patients who up until now we would have considered "hopeless" will, in the near future, be able to return to society with a complete, or nearly complete, recovery.

CLASSIFICATION OF CERVICAL SPINE INJURIES

Vertebral Fractures

Injuries to the vertebral column may be classified as fractures, dislocations, or a combination of both. Fractures may involve the pedicles, spinous process, body, or lamina. Some are considered to be stable while others, due to the potential for disruption of the spinal ligaments, are inherently unstable (see Table 120-1).

Fractures of the vertebral body are by far the most common type of bony injury. Most occur as a result of the force being applied along the long axis of the vertebral canal. This is most commonly seen as a result of falls or during dives into shallow water.

Fractures of the body are classified according to their appearance:

Type 1: Fracture of the anterior/superior portion of the vertebral body. The remainder of the vertebral body is intact and there is no bony displacement into the vertebral canal. Ligaments are usually intact.

Type 2: Teardrop fracture. Entire upper portion of the body is crushed. Generally considered unstable.

Type 3: The upper and lower portion of the anterior vertebral body is involved. The posterior vertebral body is intact, although it may be displaced somewhat posteriorly into the canal. Unstable.

Type 4: Crush injury to the entire vertebral body. There is usually marked impingement into the vertebral canal by posteriorly displaced fracture fragments. Unstable.

Table 120-1. The Spectrum of Acute Instability in Cervical Spine Injuries

Most Unstable

1. Rupture of transverse atlantal ligament
2. Fracture of dens
3. Burst fracture with posterior ligamentous disruption ("flexion teardrop")
4. Bilateral facet dislocation (or equivalent posterior disruption)
5. Burst fracture of vertebral body without posterior ligamentous disruption
6. Hyperextension fracture dislocation
7. Hangman's fracture
8. Extension teardrop fracture (stable in flexion)
9. Jefferson fracture (burst of C1)
10. Unilateral facet dislocation (or equivalent posterior disruption)
11. Anterior subluxation
12. Simple wedge compression fracture without posterior disruption
13. Pillar fracture
14. Fracture of posterior arch of C1
15. Spinous process fracture ("clay shovelers")

Least Unstable

Source: Reprinted with permission from Trafton G: Spinal cord injuries. *Surg Clin North Am* 62(1):61–72, 1982.

Incomplete (Partial) Cord Lesions

It is now estimated that approximately 55 percent of all patients entering the emergency department with a cervical neurologic injury have incomplete cord involvement. Recognition of these types of lesions is imperative for proper management. Even minimal neurologic sparing below the level of injury alters the outlook for potential recovery dramatically.

Central cord lesions occur primarily as a result of hyperextension injuries. Both anterior and posterior cord functions are involved. Neurologic deficits will be more pronounced in the arms than in the legs. It is therefore imperative that the neurologic examination include a thorough evaluation of function in both the upper and lower extremities.

Anterior cord syndrome occurs either as a result of impingement in the canal of bony fragments, or occasionally as a result of spasm of the anterior spinal artery. In this type of injury the anterior cord functions (motor, pain) are disrupted. Posterior cord function, such as vibratory and tactile sensation, are intact. The presence of this type of lesion is considered by many to be an indication for surgical intervention.

Brown-Séquard's syndrome is described as a hemisection of the spinal cord. Although it generally occurs as a result of penetrating trauma to the central canal, it may occasionally result from blunt trauma. Pain and temperature sensation are lost on the opposite side of the lesion, while tactile and vibratory deficits occur on the side of the lesion.

PATHOPHYSIOLOGY OF SPINAL CORD INJURY

When an individual develops neurologic dysfunction from spinal cord injury, it is rarely due to actual transection of the cord. The cord and its tough outer covering are generally left intact. Ultimate destruction seems to result from internal dysfunction of the cord and disruption of the blood supply.

Research by Lohse and associates has shown that in experimental transient traumatic paralysis, spinal cord blood flow (SCBF) rose above pretraumatic levels, and maintained that level throughout the experimental time. Several others have shown that when an animal is subjected to a force which causes permanent neurologic dysfunction, the flow first rises, and then falls to 70 to 80 percent of pretrauma levels. The resultant cord ischemia appears to be the final common pathway to neurologic cell death.

The apparent cause of loss of autoregulation of the cord following injury is still a mystery. Some investigators believe that this is due to a release of vasoconstricting substances within the cord matrix. An abnormally high level of norepinephrine in the spinal cord immediately following trauma has been demonstrated by some investigators. Other investigators, however, have been unable to reproduce these results. Antagonists to many naturally occurring vasoconstrictive substances (angiotensin II, adrenaline, histamine, serotonin) have been studied with little apparent success as yet.

Faden and associates have been using massive doses of naloxone in treating spinal cord trauma. By (apparently) blocking endogenous endorphins they have significantly improved mean arterial pressure and have had encouraging results. It is possible, by simply blocking or reversing the neurogenic shock which follows immediately after spinal cord injury, we may eventually improve dramatically the morbidity of cases which we now consider "hopeless."

PATIENT EVALUATION

Physical Examination

Many patients with spinal cord injuries are victims of multiple trauma. It is easy to overlook the neck in initial evaluation when there are other obvious critical areas of injury. It is extremely important to consider the possibility of cervical spine or spinal cord injury in any patient with trauma to the head or in any patient sustaining multiple injury. Failure to do so may lead to tragic results.

Any patient with one or more of the following should be considered to have a spinal cord injury until proved otherwise:

1. Impaired consciousness
2. Any obvious neurologic deficits
3. A consistent history
4. Head or facial injury
5. Localized deformity or swelling
6. Unexplained hypotension

A physical examination must include a complete neurologic evaluation. A cursory "look" may cause a physician to fail to recognize an important, but not necessarily obvious, finding.

Evaluation of level of consciousness, orientation, and of cranial nerve functions is mandatory. Evaluation of both anterior and posterior cord functions by testing position, motion, pain, temperature, and touch is necessary to diagnose partial cord lesions. Motor strength and deep tendon reflexes should be evaluated. Observance of the patient's respiratory status may reveal abdominal breathing only. Priapism should be looked for. Either of these is a strong indicator of spinal cord dysfunction.

A sensory examination will easily determine the upper level of cord involvement (see Table 120-2). A strong handshake indicates that motor function is normal through the T1 level. The value of determining the initial level of cord involvement cannot be underestimated. Determination of the level of involvement not only provides an indicator of ultimate prognosis, but it also serves as a baseline for subsequent neurologic assessments. Occasionally, due to cord edema, the patient will experience ascending cord dysfunction. When the initial involvement is in the C4, C5 level, any deterioration of neurologic status will result in respiratory embarrassment and potential cardiopulmonary arrest.

In a patient with obvious neurologic deficits, local spinal cord function must be determined. The absence of bubble cavernosis or "anal wink" indicates spinal shock. Until these return (these are cord-mediated reflexes), determining prognosis for neurologic recovery is impossible.

Table 120-2. Motor, Sensory Levels of Cervical Nerve Roots

Nerve Root Level	Motor	Sensory
C3		Lower neck
C4	Diaphragm	Clavicular area
C5	Deltoid, biceps	Lateral upper arm
C6	Extensor carpi radialis	Thumb and lateral forearm
C7	Triceps, wrist flexors, finger extensors	Middle finger
C8	Finger flexors	Little finger
T1	Hand intrinsics	Medial forearm

Radiology of Spinal Cord Injury

Radiologic evaluation of the cervical spine has become a relatively complex undertaking over the years. Although routine radiographs are still by far the most commonly used diagnostic tool, laminography along with CT scanning have dramatically increased the accuracy in evaluating spine and spinal cord injuries.

Routine Radiographs

Routine radiographs include (1) a cross-table lateral (which should be done first), (2) AP views, and (3) open-mouth views. In one study, over 90 percent of all abnormalities were diagnosed with these views only. Oblique x-rays may be taken if necessary to better evaluate vertebral foramina and bony alignment.

Indications for x-rays of patients with suspected spinal cord injury include any of the following:

1. Localized pain
2. Deformity
3. Neurologic dysfunction
4. Crepitance
5. Edema
6. Altered mental state

When viewing the lateral projection, several areas are of particular importance:

1. Alignment of the upper portion of the cervical spine.
2. Normal alignment of the anterior and posterior borders of the vertebral body, and normal joint space between the odontoid process in the posterior surface of the arch of the atlas.
3. Bony structures of the vertebral body.
4. Alignment of the posterior margin of the articular process.
5. Disc spaces.
6. Facet joints.
7. Prevertebral soft tissue.
8. AP diameter of the cervical neural canal.
9. The spinous process and inner spinous process distance.

In evaluating the open-mouth view, the emergency physician should pay particular attention to (1) The atlantooccipital joint, (2) the atlantoaxial joint, (3) the odontoid process, (4) alignment of the lateral edges of the articular masses of the atlas with C2, and (5) midline position of the odontoid process.

Flexion-Extension Views

Flexion-extension views may be necessary in cases where routine radiographs are normal, but there is still a question of cervical spine instability. CT scans and/or laminograms are not useful when there is a question of ligamentous disruption.

All flexion and extension x-rays should be controlled by a physician (emergency department physician, neurosurgeon, radiologist). The procedure should be performed under fluoroscopy. The onset of any neurologic symptoms or abnormal fluoroscopic findings should cause the physician to immediately terminate the procedure.

Pitfalls of Radiographs

Accurate evaluation of cervical spine radiographs is extremely difficult. Several normal variances which are commonly seen make correct assessment even more perplexing.

In the younger population, a 2½-to-3-mm C2/C3 subluxation is frequently seen. This is usually observed on the lateral film when the neck is in a neutral or flexed position (Fig. 120-1). If there are no localized bony tenderness, neurologic deficits, or other radiographic findings, this should be considered a normal variant. In juveniles there also may be a wedging of the body of C3. This usually will resolve by the age of 12 and should never be considered normal in the adult.

When the open-mouth view is performed, rotation of the patient's head may occasionally prevent accurate interpretation. An odontoid fracture may be diagnosed due to the dissymmetry between the odontoid process and the body of C1. Confusion may also result from overlapping of maxillary incisors or the anterior arch of the atlas (Fig. 120-2). If these occur and there are no physical findings to suggest an odontoid fracture, the x-rays should be repeated or a laminogram be performed.

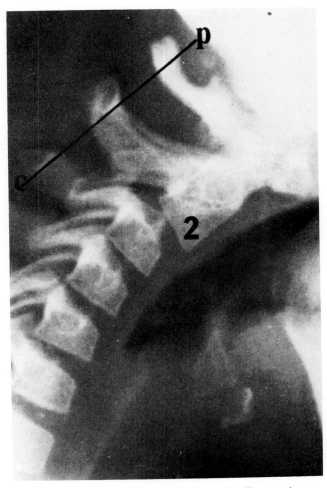

Figure 120-1. Pseudosubluxation of C2 on C3. The anterior cortical surface of the posterior arch of C2 touches the posterior cervical line (*pc*). (Reprinted by permission from Harris JH, Jr: The radiology of acute cervical spine trauma. Baltimore, The Williams & Wilkins Company, 1982.)

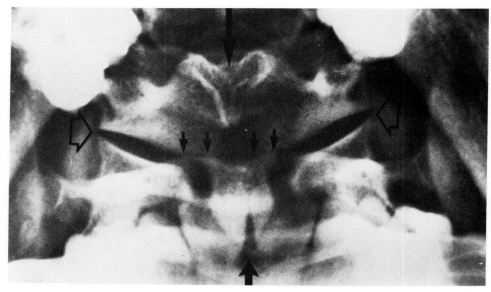

Figure 120-2. The atlantoaxial articulation seen in the open-mouth view. The dens is centrally located between the lateral masses of the axis. The lateral margins of the lateral atlantoaxial joints are precisely symmetrical (open arrows), and the spinous process of C2 (stemmed arrow) is in the midline. Two frequently perplexing natural artifacts are illustrated. The space between the central maxillary incisor teeth (large arrow) simulates a vertical defect in the dens. The thin, curvilinear, transverse lucent band at the base of the dens (small arrows) is caused by the Mach effect of the superimposed anterior arch of the atlas. This may be mistaken for a fracture line. (Reprinted by permission from Harris JH Jr: Acute injuries of the spine. Semin Roentgenol 13:53, 1978.)

CT Scan

The new generation of CT scanners may provide valuable information without movement of the spine. Bony alignment can be evaluated, along with spinal canal integrity. The presence of fracture fragments and herniated disc material may also be more easily demonstrated by this procedure. Occasionally, however, a subtle fracture may best be demonstrated by routine radiographs or laminograms. The integrity of ligaments and the stability of the spine is still best determined by "dynamic radiographs" (flexion-extension views under fluoroscopy).

MANAGEMENT OF CERVICAL SPINE INJURIES

Management of cervical spine and cervical cord injuries is an extremely complex and controversial subject. Few authors or investigators agree completely on the proper management of this type of trauma. One point of agreement among most, however, is that early intervention is necessary to provide the patient with the best chances for recovery. According to European studies, those patients who were treated within 4 h had a significantly better rate of neurologic recovery than individuals treated after 4 h.

Airway Management

During the excitement and confusion surrounding the evaluation and treatment of a critically injured patient, it is easy for the physician to overlook the possibility of a spinal cord injury. Airway management may be simply an oral tracheal or endotracheal tube without consideration of the patient's neurologic status. This is a potentially tragic mistake and should be avoided at all costs.

Nasotracheal intubation is the ideal method for securing the airway. In most instances, this can be done with relative ease and without compromising the patient's neurologic status. An oral tracheal intubation may be attempted, if necessary, with careful traction on the patient's head and avoidance of hyperextension of the neck.

If nasotracheal intubation is unsuccessful due to technical difficulties or significant facial trauma, a cricothyroidotomy should be performed. This is considered the ideal method for emergency airway management in those patients where nasotracheal intubation is unsuccessful. This surgical technique is discussed in Chapter 3, "Advanced Airway Support."

In patients who require immediate airway management, transtracheal ventilation may be an ideal temporizing method. This entails simply placing a 14-guage catheter through the cricothyroid membrane and attaching it to high-pressure jet insufflation (50 psi). This is not considered for long-term use and should be followed as soon as is feasible with either a tracheostomy or a cricothyroidotomy.

The mainstay of surgical airway management, the tracheostomy is fraught with complications and an attempt by inexperienced personnel only leads to serious complications both immediate and delayed. The procedure may also be time-consuming, and when the airway is completely obstructed, the patient may not survive the attempt.

Immobilization and Traction

Proper immobilization is necessary to enhance the potential for neurologic recovery and to prevent further damage to the cord.

Positioning a patient on a spine board with sandbags and proper restraints is a necessary measure to prevent further cord injury. A hard cervical cord collar (Philadelphia collar) may also be of benefit, both in the field and in the emergency department.

The soft cervical collar, ubiquitous in emergency departments and EMS vehicles across the United States, has two basic functions:

1. It provides a false sense of security to the medical team.
2. It acts as an excellent tourniquet for those patients with expanding neck hematomas. It does not, in fact, prevent movement of the cervical spine and should not be relied upon to do so.

Traction is an almost universally used form of therapy in spinal cord injuries. It is used, generally, to either stabilize the spinal cord or to affect a reduction of a subluxed cervical vertebra. A weight of 2.25 kg (5 lb) per vertebral space [i.e., a C4–C5 lesion would require 9 to 11.5 kg (20 to 25 lb) of traction] is generally considered adequate. Increased traction can be added in the form of 2.25 to 4.5 kg (5 to 10 lb) every 15 min until a reduction is achieved or the initial weight has been doubled. The procedure should be monitored closely to prevent undue distraction and increased injury to the spinal cord. A C5–C6 vertebral space of 5 mm or greater is an indication of excessive traction and the necessity to alter therapy. The reduction of a subluxed vertebra can be facilitated by the use of IV Valium and/or analgesics.

Traction is generally provided by the use of either a halter device or Gardner-Wells tongs. (Cruchfield tongs are no longer in general use.) For supplying traction while transporting a patient a spring type device is available which will maintain the desired amount of "pull."

Drug Therapy

Corticosteroids

The use of dexamethasone or other corticosteroids in spinal cord injuries is extremely controversial. Their use is based largely on theory and there is little actual clinical evidence to prove their efficacy. Most neurosurgeons and emergency physicians continue to treat spinal cord injuries with steroids, at least initially. Some, however, have discontinued their use entirely.

Controversy also surrounds the dosage of dexamethasone. Recommendations range from a 4-mg initial bolus up to a 1.5 to 2 mg/kg starting dose. Until further evidence becomes available, 50 to 100 mg of dexamethasone is recommended to start, followed by 50 to 100 mg every 6 h for 3 days. If no improvement is seen by that time, the steroids should be discontinued. No tapering is necessary. There is no evidence whatsoever to indicate that continued use beyond this point is of any benefit to the patient who has not shown improvement initially. The increased incidence of complications, however, is substantial.

Diuretics

Osmotic diuretics have been used sporadically in treating spinal cord injuries for many years. As with many other forms of therapy, their efficacy is in doubt. Many spinal cord centers, however, continue to use this class of drugs in the initial management of spinal cord injury.

Narcan[1]

Since 1981, naloxone has been used experimentally in the treatment of various conditions. There has been some (apparent) success when using this drug in the treatment of cerebral/vascular accidents, shock, and sepsis. Its use in experimental spinal cord trauma has also elicited encouraging initial results.

Faden et al. have used large doses of Narcan in the initial management of experimental spinal cord injury. Test animals who received Narcan showed dramatically better neurologic recovery than controls treated with saline. In their work, mean arterial pressure was measured and found to be significantly increased over controls. Unfortunately, however, direct measurement of the spinal cord blood flow was not obtained in these animals. It remains to be seen whether the improvement in spinal cord function is a direct result of maintaining spinal cord blood flow, or is due to another as yet unknown mechanism.

The dose of Narcan presently recommended is massive by present standards. An initial bolus of 1 to 2 mg/kg is given, followed by an infusion of 1 to 2 mg/kg per hour.

Surgical Indications for Spinal Cord Trauma

There appears to be little agreement as to the exact indications for surgery when a patient sustains a spinal cord injury. There are many gray areas where the decision of whether or not to operate is a most difficult one. If the result following surgery is permanent quadriplegia, the decision to operate will surely be viewed by the patient (and his or her attorney) as an incorrect one. Conversely, the decision not to operate and treat the patient conservatively will be interpreted as improper by the individual who does not improve or who develops complete quadriplegia.

Most authorities, however, do agree that there are some very strong indications for surgical intervention. Any patient who has a rapidly progressing neurologic deficit is considered a surgical candidate. Complete obstruction of the canal seen either on myelography or CT scanning is also considered by most to be an indication for decompression laminectomy. Those individuals with open spinal fractures or radiographic evidence of bony fragments within the canal will also usually require early operative intervention.

Those trauma victims who display rapid neurologic improvement are generally not considered candidates for surgical intervention. Other contradindications include evidence of central cord injury, fluctuating paraparesis and quadriparesis, or shock from other associated injuries.

Other Therapeutic Measures

Due to the poor success rate of most present forms of therapy, research with numerous other treatment modalities continues. Among them are included local cooling of the cord, thyrotropin releasing hormone (TRH), gamma hydroxide butyrate, and dimethyl sulfoxide (DMSO). Very recently, the use of clonidine in the animal laboratory has shown promising results. None of these therapeutic measures has been proved, as yet, to be effective

[1]This drug has not been approved for this purpose by the FDA at the time of publication.

clinically. Some have been abandoned, others are being used only in the laboratory. A search for the panacea continues.

SUMMARY

Spinal cord injuries from cervical spine trauma are tragic events. The cost both in monetary values and in human resources is enormous. As the medical community develops an ever-increasing awareness of the possibility of this type of injury, the patient's chances for neurologic recovery will continue to improve.

Early treatment, including prompt reduction of dislocations and stabilization of fractures, has been shown to be most effective in reducing morbidity and mortality. The standard forms of pharmacologic therapy (i.e., steroids, osmotic diuretics) are controversial at best. Present research with naloxone, thyrotropin-releasing factor, clonidine, and others, may eventually lead to a treatment regimen that will dramatically improve neurologic function.

BIBLIOGRAPHY

Albin MS: Resuscitation of the spinal cord. *Crit Care Med* 6(4):270–276, 1978.

Bucholz RW, Burkhead WZ, Graham W et al: Occult cervical spine injuries in fatal traffic accidents. *J Trauma* 19(10):768–771, October, 1979.

Cloward RB, Netter FH: Acute cervical spine injuries. *Clinical Symposia,* 32(1), 1980.

Colohan DP: Emergency management of cervical-spine injuries. *Emerg Physician Series,* 1977.

Dolan EJ, Tator CH, Endrenyi L: The value of decompression for acute experimental spinal cord compression injury *J Neurosurg* 53:749–755, 1980.

Ducker TB, Saleman M, Daniell H: Experimental spinal cord trauma, III: Therapeutic effect on immobilization and pharmacologic agents. *Surg Neurol* 10:71–76, 1978.

Dula DJ: Trauma to the cervical spine. *JACEP* 8(12):504–507, 1979.

Faden AI, Jacobs TP, Mougey E, et al: Endorphins in experimental spinal injury: Therapeutic effect of naloxone. *Ann Neurol* 10(4):326–332, 1981.

Faden AI, Jacobs TP, Holaday JW: Comparison of early and late naloxone treatment in experimental spinal injury. *Neurology* 32(6):677–681, 1982.

Feuer H: Management of acute spine and spinal cord injuries. *Arch Surg* 111:638–645, 1976.

Green BA, Callahan RA, Klose KJ, et al: Acute spinal cord injury: Current concepts. *Clin Orthop* 154:125–135, 1981.

Hansebout RR, Kuchner EF, Romero-Sierra C: Effects of local hypothermia and of steroids upon recovery from experimental spinal cord compression injury. *Surg Neurol* 4:531–534, 1975.

Holaday JW, Faden AI: Naloxone reversal of endotoxon hypotension suggests role of endorphins in shock. *Nature* 275:450–451, 1978.

Kuchner EF, Hansebout RR: Combined steroid and hypothermia treatment of experimental spinal cord injury. *Surg Neurol* 6:371–375, 1976.

Lohse DC, Senter HJ, Kauer JS, et al: Spinal cord blood flow in experimental transient traumatic paraplegia. *J Neurosurg* 52:335–345, 1980.

Markowski J, Berg E: Critical management and outcome of acute cervical spine injuries and quadriplegia. *Curr Concepts Trauma Care* 00:11–18, 1982.

Meyer PR Jr: New focus on spinal cord injury. *JAMA* 245(12):1201–1206, 1981.

Naftchi NE: Functional restoration of the traumatically injured spinal cord in cats by clonidine. *Science* 217:1042–1044, 1982.

Pope TL Jr, Riddervold HO: Pitfalls in interpreting cervical films. *Diagnosis* 23–32, 1980.

Roub LW, Drayer BP: Spinal computed tomography: Limitations and applications. *Spinal Computed Tomography* 267–273, 1979.

Scher AT: Unrecognized fractures and dislocations of the cervical spine. *Paraplegia,* 25–30, 1981.

Senter HJ, Venes JL, Kauer JS: Alteration of posttraumatic ischemia in experimental spinal cord trauma by a central nervous system depressant. *J Neurosurg* 50:207–216, 1979.

Senter HJ, Venes, JL: Loss of autoregulation and posttraumatic ischemia following experimental spinal cord trauma. *J Neurosurg* 50:198–206, 1979.

Shaffer MA, Doris PE: Limitation of the cross table lateral view in detecting cervical spine injuries: A retrospective analysis *Ann Emerg Med* 508–513, 1981.

Simon RR, Brenner BE: Emergency cricothyroidotomy in the patient with massive neck swelling: Part 1: Anatomical aspects. *Crit Care Med* 11(2):114–118, 1983.

Simon RR, Brenner BE: Emergency cricothyroidotomy in the patient with massive neck swelling. Part 2: Clinical aspects. *Crit Care Med* 11(2):119–123, 1983.

Sonntag VKH: The early management of cervical spinal cord injury. *Ariz Med* 664–647, 1982.

Stauffer ES: Diagnosis and prognosis of acute cervical spinal cord injury. Acute Cervical Spinal Cord Injury, pp. 9–15, No. 112, 1975.

Tadmor R, David KR, Roberson GH, et al: Computed tomographic evaluation of traumatic spinal injuries. *Technical Notes* 825–827, 1978.

Trafton PC: Spinal cord injuries. *Surg Clin North Am* 62(1):61–72, 1982.

Wagner FC Jr: Management of acute spinal cord injury. *Surg Neurol* 7:346–350, 1977.

Wales LR, Knopp RK, Morishima MS: Recommendations for evaluation of the acutely injured cervical spine: A clinical radiologic algorithm *Ann Emerg Med* 9(8):422–428, 1980.

Williams CF, Bernstein TW, Jelenko C: Essentiality of the lateral cervical spine radiograph. *Ann Emerg Med* 10(4):198–203, 1981.

CHAPTER 121
THORACIC INJURIES

Robert F. Wilson, Zwi Steiger

Chest injuries are directly responsible for over 25 percent of the 50,000 to 60,000 fatalities that result annually from automobile accidents, and they contribute significantly to another 25 percent. Not only are thoracic injuries increasing in number, but more rapid and better transportation by trained ambulance personnel are bringing critically injured patients to the emergency department who previously would have died before arriving at the hospital.

INITIAL RESUSCITATION

Ensuring the Adequacy of Ventilation

The initial step in resuscitation is to ensure the adequacy of ventilation. With trauma or sepsis, the minute ventilation should be about one-and-one-half to two times normal (i.e., 9 to 12 L/min). If it is not, one should rapidly and systematically examine the patient for the possible cause(s) and begin therapy immediately (see Table 121-1).

Patients with chest trauma who are in or who develop respiratory distress have a high mortality rate. In one series of patients admitted with chest trauma, 11 percent required endotracheal intubation on or soon after admission to the emergency department. Of these patients, 58 percent died. If shock was present with respiratory distress, the mortality rate rose to 73 percent. Acute respiratory distress was more frequent in patients with blunt trauma (17 percent) than in those with penetrating injuries (8 percent) (Table 121-2).

Etiology

In patients with blunt trauma who require tracheal intubation, the most frequent factors causing respiratory distress include shock, coma, multiple rib fractures, and hemothorax or pneumothorax. In patients with penetrating trauma, the most frequent injuries associated with inadequate ventilation are severe shock and lung damage with hemopneumothorax.

Cardiac Arrest with Ventilatory Assistance

Although early intubation and positive pressure ventilation of critically injured patients with severe respiratory distress is indicated, the most frequent time for cardiac arrest in such patients is just after intubation. Possible causes for cardiac arrest include:

1. Conversion of a simple pneumothorax to a tension pneumothorax.
2. Reduction of venous return below a critical value in severely injured patients.
3. Intubation of the esophagus.
4. Migration of the endotracheal tube into the right mainstem bronchus.

Table 121-1. Causes of Inadequate Ventilation

CNS dysfunction
  Due to trauma
    Concussion
    Direct trauma to the medulla
    Increasing intracranial pressure
  Due to drugs
    Narcotics
    Sedatives
    Poisons
Airway obstruction
  Pharynx
    Vomitus
    Foreign bodies
    Relaxed tongue
  Larynx
    Foreign bodies
    Direct trauma
  Trachea
    Foreign bodies
    Direct trauma
Chest wall injury
  Pain from fractures
  Flail chest
  Open (sucking) wounds
Pleural collections
  Hemothorax
  Pneumothorax
    Simple
    Tension
Diaphragmatic injuries
Parenchymal dysfunction
  Contusion
  Aspiration
  Intrabronchial hemorrhage
  Previous disease

Table 121-2. Injuries Associated with Respiratory Distress after Trauma

Trauma	Incidence, %
Blunt	
Rib fractures/flail chest	75
Hemothorax, pneumothorax	55
Lung contusion	39
Intracranial injuries	39
Diaphragmatic injury	9
Spinal cord injury	4
Penetrating	
Pulmonary damage with hemopneumothorax	55
Cardiac injury	29
Diaphragmatic injury	17
Chest wall defects	7

Source: Wilson RF, Gibson DB, Antonenko D: Shock and acute respiratory failure after chest trauma. *J Trauma* 17:697–705, 1977.

5. Systemic air emboli in patients with lung tears and hemoptysis.
6. Abrupt change in pH by excess hyperventilation.
7. Vagal response (rare).

In one recent series 28 percent of patients receiving cardiopulmonary resuscitation were found to have the tip of their endotracheal tube in the right mainstem bronchus.

Diagnosis

Clinical Features

If the patient is making little or no effort to breathe, central nervous system dysfunction due to head trauma or drugs should be suspected. If the patient is attempting to breathe but is moving little or no air, upper airway obstruction, particularly if there is inspiratory stridor, should be suspected. Other causes of upper airway obstruction are dentures or vomitus in the pharynx, larynx, or upper trachea. In comatose patients, particularly alcoholics and those with fractures of the mandible, the tongue may fall back and occlude the pharynx. Occasionally, rapid, direct trauma may cause fracture of the larynx or transection of the upper (cervical) trachea. If the patient is attempting to breathe and the upper airway appears to be intact, flail chest, hemothorax or pneumothorax, diaphragmatic injury, or parenchymal damage due to contusion should be sought.

Treatment

Airway Control

If there is any hint of obstruction of the upper airway, the pharynx, larynx, and trachea should be aspirated with a suction catheter and examined digitally or endoscopically. If the tongue is falling back into the pharynx, the jaw should be pulled forward and an oral airway inserted (if the patient will tolerate it without gagging and vomiting). If there is laryngeal damage, a cricothyroidotomy or tracheostomy may be required. A cricothyroidotomy is performed more rapidly than a tracheostomy but may not correct an airway problem due to upper tracheal avulsion. Cricothyroidotomy

is increasingly recognized as the airway of choice in emergency situations where endotracheal intubation is difficult or dangerous to accomplish. Recently, a technique has been developed to facilitate emergency cricothyroidotomy in patients with massive neck swelling. The hyoid bone is used to localize the midline and provide traction on the larynx.

Relief of Hemopneumothorax

If a hemothorax or pneumothorax is suspected in a patient with acute respiratory distress, a chest tube should be inserted, without waiting for a chest roentgenogram, through the fourth or fifth intercostal space in the midaxillary line on the affected side. Digital examination of the pleural cavity through the intended site of the chest tube before it is blindly inserted will reduce the chances of inserting the tube into the lung parenchyma if the lung is stuck to that area by adhesions.

Once a properly functioning chest tube is in place, it should be connected to 20 to 30 cmH$_2$O suction. If a tension pneumothorax is present, a large needle can be inserted into the pleural space through the second intercostal space in the midclavicular line to produce temporary decompression while a chest tube is being inserted.

If a sucking chest wound is present, it should be sealed with petrolatum gauze and a sterile dressing. A chest tube should then be inserted at another site.

Intercostal Nerve Blocks

The severe pain of multiple fractured ribs can greatly impair ventilation. In such circumstances, blocking the intercostal nerves of the ribs involved and two ribs above and two ribs below with a long-acting local anesthetic such as 0.5% bupivacaine hydrochloride (Marcaine) mixed with an equal quantity of 1% lidocaine with epinephrine may dramatically relieve pain and improve ventilation.

Endotracheal Intubation and Ventilatory Support

In patients with chest trauma, impairment of ventilation is an obvious indication for ventilatory support. Extensive flail chest, parenchymal damage involving more than one lobe, and diaphragmatic rupture are best treated by endotracheal intubation and ventilatory assistance, particularly if there are associated injuries, even if the patient's ventilation temporarily seems adequate. Ventilatory assistance should be considered with marginally adequate ventilation if the patient is in shock, has had other multiple injuries, is comatose, will probably require multiple transfusions, is elderly, or has an underlying pulmonary problem.

In marginal situations, a respiratory rate greater than 30 to 35/min, a vital capacity less than 10 to 15 mL/kg, a negative inspiratory pressure less than 20 to 25 mmHg, and an increased respiratory effort can be considered indications for ventilatory support. Serial blood gas values are more informative than isolated values. Consequently, an arterial sample should be drawn soon after admission and at frequent intervals. An arterial P_{CO_2} above 45 mmHg in a patient with trauma is evidence of a significant reduction in pulmonary function and indicates the need for ventilatory support. Excessive ventilation producing an arterial P_{CO_2} less than 25 mmHg may also be an indication for ventilatory assistance.

If the arterial P_{O_2} is less than 50 mmHg while the patient is breathing room air, or less than 80 mmHg while he or she is breathing supplemental nasal oxygen (equivalent to an Fi_{O_2} of 0.4 or more), he or she should probably be placed on a ventilator.

If the patient is awake and has only marginal ventilation, nasotracheal intubation should be attempted. With adequate nasal anesthesia, a nasotracheal tube can generally be inserted easily and is much better tolerated than an orotracheal tube. Insertion of an orotracheal tube in an awake patient can be a major struggle and often requires the patient to be sedated with 5 to 10 mg of diazepam IV or paralyzed with 40 mg (2.0 mL) of succinylcholine.

Shock

Once adequate ventilation has been attained, efforts should be directed toward rapidly restoring tissue perfusion, particularly if there is any respiratory distress. In a study at Detroit General Hospital, chest trauma patients who were in shock in the emergency department had a mortality rate of 7 percent. If respiratory distress was also present, the mortality rate increased tenfold to 73 percent.

Etiology

The most frequent sources of bleeding that can cause or contribute to shock in patients with *blunt* chest trauma are pelvic or extremity fractures (59 percent), intraabdominal injuries (41 percent), and intrathoracic bleeding (26 percent). In addition, 15 percent had myocardial contusion and 7 percent had spinal cord injuries. These can contribute to the hypotension because of decreased myocardial contractility and decreased sympathetic tone, causing increased vascular capacitance.

In patients with *penetrating* chest trauma and shock, the cause of shock was intrathoracic injury in 74 percent. In these patients, the intrathoracic injuries, which were often multiple, included massive bleeding from the lung, 36 percent; cardiac injuries (usually with tamponade), 25 percent; large-vessel damage, 14 percent; and chest wall vessels (intercostal or innominate arteries), 10 percent. This finding conflicts with statements that continued severe bleeding in the chest is more apt to come from damage to chest wall vessels than from injuries to the lung. In addition, 40 percent of patients with chest trauma had extrathoracic injuries contributing to shock. These included intraabdominal bleeding, 34 percent; bleeding from extremity vessels, 12 percent; and spinal cord injuries, 5 percent.

Diagnosis

In patients with blunt chest trauma and shock, the most likely site of continued severe bleeding is the abdomen, particularly if the patient does not have fractures involving the pelvis or large extremity bones. Peritoneal lavage is generally a very accurate technique for ruling out massive intraperitoneal bleeding.

Treatment

Correction of hypotension within 30 min is essential, particularly if the patient has severe bleeding requiring massive transfusion. In previously healthy patients requiring massive transfusion, those in whom the duration of hypotension was less than 30 min had a mortality rate of only 11 percent. If the hypotension was more prolonged, the mortality rate rose to 40 percent to 50 percent. If the patient had underlying disease or was over 65, the mortality with hypotension for more than 30 min was 91 percent.

Occasionally, a large hemothorax or pneumothorax can interfere with venous return and, consequently, it should be evacuated as rapidly as possible. However, if blood is pouring rapidly out of the chest tube, the chest tube should be clamped and the response of the vital signs noted after each increment of 200 mL of blood is removed. If vital signs are improving, the blood can continue to be evacuated rapidly. However, if the patient deteriorates as blood is being removed, a tamponade of bleeding from the lung may be removed and the patient may be exsanguinating into his or her chest. In these unusual circumstances, the chest tube should be clamped and the patient should have an immediate thoracotomy.

In patients with chest trauma, external cardiac massage is of little value. The trauma patient suffering a cardiac arrest is generally hypovolemic and, consequently, external massage is usually ineffective and may cause additional bleeding or tissue damage. External massage may be harmful in patients with injuries to the heart, thoracic aorta, or other great vessels. In one series, major cardiovascular disruption was found in all patients receiving external cardiac compression after truncal trauma. In 12 percent of the patients receiving forced ventilation and prehospital external cardiac compression, air embolism to the coronary arteries was the cause of death.

Open cardiac massage is usually performed through an anterior fifth intercostal space incision on the left (or right if the penetrating injury is present on that side). The pericardium is opened vertically anterior to the phrenic nerve. The thoracic incision allows direct inspection of the heart, direct control of bleeding sites in the chest, and complete evacuation of any pericardial tamponade, hemothorax, or pneumothorax on that side. In addition, it allows the physician to compress or clamp the descending thoracic aorta. Since about 60 percent of the cardiac output normally passes below the diaphragm, clamping the descending thoracic aorta can increase coronary and carotid blood flow almost threefold. This has been shown to significantly improve cardiac function.

Recently, there has been increased interest in "emergency department thoracotomies." It is becoming increasingly clear from our own experience and the experience of others that emergency department thoracotomy can be very helpful in patients with isolated penetrating wounds of the chest. However, patients requiring CPR for blunt trauma or abdominal injuries, and patients "dead" at the scene, do very poorly.

INJURY TO THE CHEST WALL

Soft Tissue Injuries

Probing of chest wounds to determine their depth is inadvisable because it may damage underlying structures and cause severe recurrent bleeding, pneumothorax, or a sucking chest wound.

Bleeding from some of the larger muscles can be rather brisk at times and is best controlled by individual ligatures and careful closure of all layers.

Open (Sucking) Chest Wounds

Small open chest wounds can act as one-way valves, allowing air to enter during inspiration, causing an expanding pneumothorax. This not only reduces effective tidal volume but also interferes with venous return. With large chest wall wounds, air tends to come into the pleural cavity through the wound rather than through the tracheobronchial tree. If the open chest wound is larger than the trachea, effective ventilation may cease.

Sucking wounds of the chest should be covered immediately by a sterile airtight dressing, such as petrolatum gauze, and a chest tube inserted at a separate site to relieve the pneumothorax. The chest tube is not inserted through the wound because it is then apt to enter any associated wound of the lung or diaphragm.

Massive Chest Wall Loss

Injuries caused by close-range shotgun blasts or high-powered rifles may destroy such large quantities of chest wall that it may be impossible to close in the usual manner. It is important, however, to cover the lungs and heart and close the diaphragm. For small defects, resection of adjacent ribs and a thoracoplasty may be adequate. With large defects rotated muscle flaps and/or Marlex mesh may be required.

Massive Subcutaneous Emphysema

Subcutaneous emphysema usually develops because air from lung parenchyma or the tracheobronchial tree has gained access to the chest wall through an opening in the parietal pleura. The air may reach the chest wall by dissecting back along the bronchi into the hilum and mediastinum and then into the extrapleural spaces. Rarely, subcutaneous emphysema may be caused by injury to the esophagus.

Swelling from subcutaneous emphysema may occasionally reach massive proportions, swelling the eyelids shut and, in males, swelling the scrotum to several times normal. Although the patient's appearance may be greatly distorted and he or she may have moderate or severe discomfort, the subcutaneous emphysema itself does not cause any significant ventilatory or hemodynamic problem unless there is an associated pneumothorax.

Patients with subcutaneous emphysema should be thought to have an underlying pneumothorax, even if it is not visible on the chest film. If the patient requires a general anesthetic for associated injuries or is to be placed on a ventilator, it is prudent to insert a chest tube on the involved side(s). If the subcutaneous emphysema is severe or develops rapidly, a major bronchial injury should be suspected and sought for by bronchoscopy.

If there is any respiratory difficulty, a tracheostomy around which the skin and fascia are closed very loosely serves to maintain adequate ventilation and also allows a route for air to escape from the mediastinum and subcutaneous tissue. Occasionally, linear incisions into the subcutaneous space of the chest wall may

be required to relieve massive subcutaneous emphysema. Once the initiating cause is controlled, the subcutaneous emphysema usually disappears gradually over a period of days.

Clavicular Fractures

Isolated clavicular fractures due to blunt trauma are usually quite harmless. Occasionally, however, direct trauma produces sharp fragments that may injure the subclavian vein and produce a moderately large hematoma or venous thrombosis. Rarely, excess callus forming at the site of a clavicular fracture may press against the subclavian artery or brachial plexus, producing a thoracic outlet syndrome.

Rib Fractures

Simple Fractures

Rib fractures should be assumed to be present in any patient who has pain and tenderness localized over one or more ribs after chest trauma. However, at least 10 percent of rib fractures (particularly the anterior and lateral portions of the first 4 ribs) will not visualize for 7 to 14 days after the injury. Furthermore, injuries to the cartilaginous portions of the ribs may never be seen on x-ray.

Rib injuries most frequently result from direct trauma but occasionally may be caused by rapid flexion or extension, particularly in the elderly. If there is concern about pneumothorax, the patient should have both inspiratory and expiratory posteroanterior (PA) roentgenograms. If the patient had severe trauma, if the rib fractures have sharp fragments, or if the patient had other injuries, serial chest roentgenograms should be obtained. Delayed pneumothorax or hemothorax (due to trauma to the lung parenchyma or intercostal vessels by rib fragments) may develop 6 to 24 h after the initial injury.

Even if the rib fragments do not damage the underlying lung or cause a hemopneumothorax, the fractures can greatly interfere with ventilation because of pain produced by motion of the bone fragments or spasm of adjacent muscles in an effort to splint that portion of the chest wall.

Strapping the chest with adhesive tape to relieve the pain may be effective in young, athletic individuals with few rib fractures, but in less vigorous patients strapping may significantly reduce ventilation and cause progressive atelectasis. Rib belts are more pleasant to use than adhesive tape, do not blister the skin, and can be adjusted by the patient. Mild to moderate chest wall pain is best treated by 30 to 60 mg of codeine every 3 to 4 h. Severe pain is best relieved by intercostal nerve block using a long-acting anesthetic such as 0.5% Marcaine.

First and Second Rib Fractures

First and, to a certain extent, second rib fractures should make one look closely for injuries to the myocardium, thoracic aorta, and major bronchi. In one series, 33 percent of patients with fracture of the first or second ribs had myocardial contusion and 6 percent had a major vascular injury. These fractures have special significance since they are usually caused by severe trauma and are associated with higher mortality rates than any other rib fractures, primarily because of the frequent, severe associated injuries.

Multiple Rib Fractures

Severe pain from multiple rib fractures is best controlled with repeated intercostal nerve blocks. To achieve adequate relief of pain, the intercostal block must usually include two intercostal nerves above and two below the injured ribs. Any residual tender spots should be injected individually. This will often produce dramatic pain relief for several hours. Since it is easy to puncture the lung during an intercostal block, it is wise to obtain a chest x-ray after the procedure.

If the patient with fractured ribs following blunt trauma becomes hypotensive and does not have a large hemothorax or tension pneumothorax to account for the fall in blood pressure, intraabdominal bleeding must be suspected. In one series of 783 patients with blunt chest trauma, 71 percent of the patients admitted in shock had a ruptured intraabdominal viscus.

In general, it is wise to hospitalize any patient with three or more fractured ribs for at least 24 to 48 h, especially if the ninth, tenth, or eleventh ribs are involved. Such fractures are apt to be associated with spleen or liver injuries, and admitting the patient provides ample time to observe the patient for additional injuries that might not be apparent initially.

Costochondral separation results in substantial morbidity since the relatively poor blood supply to costal cartilage frequently results in delayed healing and an inordinate amount of pain. If attempts at nonoperative therapy are ineffective, surgical excision of the involved costal cartilage is often curative. A rare posttraumatic intercostal neuroma may require local alcohol injection or excisional therapy.

Flail Chest

Pathophysiology

Segmental fractures (i.e., fracture in two or more locations on the same rib) of three or more adjacent ribs anteriorly or laterally often result in an unstable chest wall and a flail chest. This is characterized by a paradoxical inward movement of the involved portion of the chest wall during inspiration and outward movement during expiration. The underlying lung damage, together with the reduced ventilatory efficiency and increased ventilatory work, may cause progressive respiratory insufficiency.

In the past *pendelluft* (a ventilatory phenomenon referring to movement of air back and forth between the injured and uninjured lungs with each breath) was considered to be an important cause of the ventilatory impairment seen with flail chest. However, *pendelluft* is clinically significant only in rare circumstances when the upper airway is obstructed.

Immediately after the injury, little flail may be apparent. Later, as lung compliance falls and more pressure is needed to inflate the lungs, the differential between intrathoracic and atmospheric pressure may overcome the resistance of the muscles attached to the fractured ribs, thereby allowing the involved chest wall to move paradoxically. In addition, the patient may tire rapidly because of decreased efficiency of ventilation and increasing muscle

effort. Thus, a vicious cycle of decreasing efficiency of ventilation, increasing fatigue, and hypoxemia may develop.

Treatment

A flail chest can be most quickly managed initially by applying a sandbag or pressure over the unstable portion of the chest wall. This is of particular value at the roadside when hospital facilities are not available. Although this reduces vital capacity, it increases effective tidal volume and the efficiency of ventilation.

Probably the major advance in the therapy of severe flail chest has been the increasing use of early ventilatory assistance to internally splint the chest wall and maintain optimal expansion. Nevertheless, patients with a mild-to-moderate flail chest and little or no underlying pulmonary contusion or extrathoracic injury can often be managed well without ventilator assistance. Careful selection, observation, and treatment of such patients is extremely important.

Trinkle and co-workers started a storm of controversy by reporting a study which indicated that internal mechanical stabilization of the thorax was not necessary in all patients with flail chest and might even be deleterious. However, ventilatory support was provided if and when the arterial P_{O_2} was less than 60 mmHg on room air or less than 80 mmHg on supplemental oxygen. They also pointed out that the extensiveness of the underlying pulmonary contusion was the main indication for ventilatory assistance.

Some of the prominent features of therapy used by those who advocate nonventilator therapy include:

1. Adequate relief of pain by analgesics or intercostal nerve block.
2. Frequent coughing and chest physiotherapy.
3. Restriction of intravenous fluids to 50 mL/h to prevent fluid overload.
4. Methylprednisolone, 30 mg/kg, immediately, and then every 6 to 8 h for 48 to 72 h, to help return the increased capillary permeability toward normal. This may be particularly helpful if any element of fat embolism is present.
5. Salt-poor albumin (25 g) daily to maintain plasma oncotic pressure.
6. Blood loss replaced with whole blood or plasma, not with crystalloids.
7. Furosemide as needed to prevent fluid overload.
8. Supplemental nasal oxygen to maintain the arterial P_{O_2} above 80 mmHg.

Ventilatory Support

A patient with flail chest should be given ventilatory assistance immediately (even with relatively normal blood gases) if he or she has shock, three or more associated injuries, severe head injury, previous severe pulmonary disease, fracture of eight or more ribs, or is older than 65 years. Such patients usually require assisted ventilation for 10 to 14 days. Early ventilatory assistance in patients with a flail chest and significant associated injuries was associated with a mortality of 7 percent. This was in contrast to a mortality rate of 69 percent in similar patients in whom ventilatory assistance was delayed until there was clinical evidence of acute respiratory failure.

In the patient with flail chest who has marginal clinical indications for ventilatory assistance, any deterioration in pulmonary function (as reflected by increasing tachypnea, decreased tidal volume, falling arterial P_{O_2} or rising $P(A - a)_{O_2}$ or physiologic shunt) is an indication for tracheal intubation and mechanical support. Ventilated patients seem to do better if intermittent mandatory ventilation is used rather than controlled mandatory ventilation (CMV).

Recently, there has been increased interest in operative stabilization of the chest wall after trauma if a thoracotomy is performed or when mechanical ventilation is difficult or undesirable.

Sternal Fractures

Sternal fractures are frequently associated with cardiovascular injury, particularly myocardial contusions. Consequently, serial ECGs should be performed for the first 48 h. The fractures are usually transverse and so unstable that a significant flail is often present. Treatment usually includes ventilatory support for at least a few days. Operative fixation is often unsatisfactory and should be delayed for several days because of severe associated injuries. Painful pseudoarthrosis and permanent overlap deformities are not uncommon and may require later reconstruction.

INJURIES TO THE LUNGS

Pulmonary Contusions

Etiology

Most frequently, pulmonary contusion follows rapid deceleration injuries. Pulmonary contusions may also result from high-energy shock waves propagated through air or water or by high-velocity missiles hitting adjacent tissue. Three basic phenomena are important in the etiology of pulmonary contusion: (1) the *spalling* effect, in which the liquid-gas interface is disrupted by a shock wave; (2) overexpansion of alveoli following the implosion effect caused by the pressure wave; and (3) the inertial effect as low-density alveolar tissue is stripped from heavier hilar structures.

Pathophysiology

The pathologic changes in pulmonary contusion include alveolar capillary damage, with interstitial and intraalveolar extravasation of blood as well as interstitial edema. Later, increasing interstitial edema and peribronchial extravasation of red blood cells cause a progressive decrease in compliance and increase in physiologic shunting with resultant hypoxemia.

Diagnosis

The diagnosis of pulmonary contusion is usually made from the history and the finding of localized opacifications on the initial chest roentgenogram. Many of the worst contusions occur in patients without rib fractures. These parenchymal lesions tend to increase in severity during the first 24 to 72 h after trauma so that a negative chest roentgenogram on admission may be misleading.

Significant hypoxia may be delayed for 4 to 6 or more h after the episode of trauma. Arterial blood gases may then deteriorate progressively over the next 24 to 72 h as the parenchymal lung injury increases. Therefore, blood gases should be repeated in 6 to 12 h.

A distinction should be drawn both conceptually and clinically between pulmonary contusion and the adult respiratory distress syndrome (ARDS) with which it is often confused. Pulmonary contusion occurs at the time of injury, is usually fairly well localized to a segment or lobe, and tends to progress for 48 to 72 h. In contrast, ARDS occurs later, usually 48 to 72 h after the injury, and tends to be diffuse. Both problems can be complicated by pulmonary infections, and ARDS may itself be caused by severe pulmonary infections or fat emboli.

Treatment

Treatment of pulmonary contusions includes maintenance of adequate ventilation to all parts of the lung. Chest physiotherapy, intercostal nerve blocks, and coughing or nasotracheal suction are used as needed. The use of steroids is controversial and their use is not recommended except with smoke inhalation, aspiration of gastric contents, or fat embolism. One recent report suggests that large doses of steroids will reduce the size of experimental contusions, presumably by lysosome preservation, decreased capillary permeability, and anti-inflammatory properties.

Pulmonary Hematoma

Pulmonary hematomas consist of a rather large parenchymal tear filled with blood and localized to a lobe or one or more segments. The hematomas generally resolve spontaneously over a few weeks; however, if they become infected, they may cavitate and form lung abscesses that are difficult to manage.

Pulmonary Laceration with Hemopneumothorax

Major hemorrhage from lacerations of the lung following blunt trauma is usually caused by the sharp ends of fractured ribs, but occasionally it may be caused by tearing of the lung at previous pleural adhesions as the lung moves away from the chest wall during rapid deceleration. In some instances, the adhesions themselves are quite vascular, and bleeding from torn adhesions alone can cause shock.

Tube thoracostomy and suction drainage of the pleural cavity is the treatment of choice for hemopneumothorax. If blood is present, a large-bore (no. 32 or 36 French) chest tube is required. If the bleeding or air leak cannot be controlled or the lung cannot be expanded with chest tubes and suction, thoracotomy may be required.

Systemic Air Embolism

In patients with penetrating chest wounds, particularly those caused by high-velocity missiles, assisted ventilation must be used with care since high ventilatory pressures may force air from an injured bronchus into an adjacent open pulmonary vein, producing systemic air embolism. Such bronchovenous fistulas may account for the severe arrhythmias and sudden deaths that occur soon after the induction of general anesthesia or ventilatory assistance in patients with severe penetrating chest wounds. If cerebral air embolism occurs, hyperbaric therapy may be curative.

Intrabronchial Bleeding

Intrabronchial bleeding is poorly tolerated and can rapidly cause death by flooding the alveoli. These patients almost invariably die from ''drowning'' and not from hypovolemic shock; however, the combination is lethal. The noninvolved lung must be kept as free of blood as possible, and nasotracheal suction or bronchoscopy should be used as often as necessary.

If the bleeding is severe, a double-lumen endotracheal (Carlen's) tube can be used to confine the blood to one lung. If a Carlen's tube is not available or cannot be inserted, one may insert a long endotracheal tube over a flexible bronchoscope into the left mainstem bronchus. The balloon on the endotracheal tube can then be inflated. If the bleeding is from the left lung, the endotracheal tube will prevent blood from passing into the right lung, and ventilation of the right lung may then be maintained spontaneously or via another endotracheal tube. In some instances, the bleeding can be controlled only by occluding the involved bronchus with a Fogarty arterial balloon catheter or packing it with gauze. Obviously, these are temporary measures until the bleeding can be controlled surgically.

If severe intrabronchial bleeding continues, a thoracotomy may be required. This should be done with the patient supine or only slightly turned to reduce drainage of blood into the dependent lung. The bronchus should be occluded at the hilum with an atraumatic clamp as soon as possible. If the bleeding site within the lung cannot be controlled with direct ligation or suture of the bleeding vessels, the involved lobe should be resected.

Arteriovenous Fistulas

Arteriovenous fistulas following penetrating chest trauma are uncommon because of the small pressure differential between the pulmonary arteries and veins. A high degree of shunting in the lung with a residual pulmonary density, however, should make one suspect this problem.

Aspiration

Aspiration of gastric contents is common after severe trauma, especially if the patient is unconscious. If not recognized immediately and if thorough irrigation of the tracheobronchial tree is not performed with buffered saline or bicarbonate solution within 5 to 10 min, a severe chemical pneumonitis may develop. The physician should suspect this problem if there is vomitus in the mouth or on the clothes of an unconscious trauma victim.

If a foreign body is aspirated into the tracheobronchial tree, it is usually readily diagnosed if radiopaque. However, radiolucent foreign bodies have remained lodged in various bronchi, causing repeated pulmonary infections or hemoptysis for years before being discovered. Persistent or recurrent cough, atelectasis, or pneu-

monia after trauma should be an indication for bronchoscopy and/or bronchography.

Signs, symptoms, and radiologic changes characteristic of aspiration pneumonitis are often delayed for 6 to 24 h. Aspiration of food particles, bile-stained fluid, or coffee-ground-colored material from the trachea should be an indication for urgent bronchoscopy. The gastric acid will have already caused much of its damage but any remaining food particles can be removed.

The use of corticosteroids in doses equivalent to 100 to 200 mg of hydrocortisone every 4 to 6 h IV is controversial. Corticosteroids may help to reduce inflammatory changes in the lungs, but they will be of value only if started within 1 to 2 h of the aspiration.

PLEURAL COLLECTIONS

Hemothorax

Etiology

Hemothorax is most frequently caused by bleeding from lung parenchymal injuries. The compressing effect of the shed blood, the large concentration of thromboplastin in the lungs, and the low pulmonary arterial pressure combine to favor clotting and an early cessation of bleeding from lung parenchyma. Consequently, continued significant bleeding inside the chest may often come from severe lung injuries or damage to intercostal vessels. Because all the intercostal vessels (except the first two) arise directly from the aorta, bleeding from them may be brisk and persistent.

Diagnosis

Hemothorax should be suspected following trauma if the breath sounds are reduced and the chest is dull to percussion on the involved side. Fluid collections greater than 200 to 300 mL can usually be seen on good upright roentgenograms of the chest. Occasionally, however, blood may collect between the lung and diaphragm. This so-called subpulmonic hemothorax may not be appreciated on routine upright films. A decubitus x-ray, however, may show a large quantity of fluid layering out against the dependent lateral chest wall.

Each side of the chest can hold up to 3000 mL of blood. If the chest cavity is half filled with blood, it can be assumed that at least 1500 mL of blood is present and that a thoracotomy should be performed.

Treatment

Blood in the pleural cavity should be removed as completely and rapidly as possible. The hemothorax not only restricts ventilation and venous return, but the clots also release fibrinolytic and fibrinogenolytic substances. These substances may cause troublesome continuing bleeding from relatively small vessels. Such bleeding often stops rapidly if the hemothorax (clot) is removed.

Closed Thoracostomy (Chest Tube) Drainage

A very small hemothorax that is not seen to be increasing on serial x-ray films does not always have to be removed but should be carefully observed. If the hemothorax is large enough to drain, avoid needle aspiration and rely on chest tubes. On several occasions, repeated needle aspiration has resulted in a pneumothorax or an infected hemothorax.

A large (no. 32 to 36 French) catheter is the ideal chest tube for draining a hemothorax. It should be inserted in the midaxillary line at the fifth or sixth intercostal space. The patient should be sitting up if possible and the catheter directed posteriorly and toward the apex to reduce the chances of damaging a high-lying diaphragm. If hemothorax persists and there is minimal chest tube drainage, the chest tube is either occluded by clots or is not inserted into the proper area. A chest tube that is not functioning properly should be replaced rather than irrigated. Irrigation to remove clots is seldom successful for more than a few minutes and may introduce serious contamination. If minimal drainage persists, the hemothorax is probably partially clotted or loculated. Decubitus films of the chest showing a fluid shift indicate that some of the blood is unclotted and may be at least partially removed by another chest tube.

Thoracotomy

Most patients with intrathoracic bleeding can be treated adequately by administration of IV fluids and evacuation of the hemothorax with a chest tube; only 9 percent of our patients with penetrating chest wounds require thoracotomy for continuing hemorrhage.

Thoracotomy is generally indicated when (1) the patient's vital signs remain unstable, (2) more than 1500 mL of blood is lost from the chest, or (3) drainage of blood from the chest tubes exceeds 200 mL/h for 3 to 4 h or longer. A thoracotomy may also be needed if the patient's condition deteriorates rapidly after rapid infusion of 2 to 3 L of fluid. In these circumstances, continued severe bleeding from a large vessel or large lung laceration is assumed.

Occasionally, when the chest tube is initially inserted, blood will emerge at an alarmingly rapid rate. If the patient's condition improves as the blood is removed, continuing drainage and observation of the patient is in order. However, if the patient's condition deteriorates as the blood is removed, the chest tube should be clamped and the patient taken immediately to the operating room.

A median sternotomy incision is preferred for penetrating wounds of the thoracic outlet or injuries involving the proximal portions of the aortic arch vessels. For the right subclavian artery, an extension into the right neck is preferred. For injury to the distal left subclavian artery, a left anterolateral thoracotomy with a supraclavicular incision and possible clavicular resection provides the best exposure.

Antibiotics

Although controversial, recent studies suggest that prophylactic antibiotics decrease the incidence of pneumonia, fever, and positive pleural and wound cultures after penetrating chest trauma requiring a chest tube.

Autotransfusion

In patients with massive bleeding into a body cavity, autotransfusion may greatly reduce the need for bank blood and decrease the risks associated with its use. Intrathoracic bleeding is ideal for this technique because there is usually no contamination of the blood by bile or intestinal fluid. Although not practiced widely, advocates of this technique are extremely enthusiastic and have pointed out that its advantages far outweigh the risks of anticoagulation and any contamination that may occur. Air embolism can be a very serious complication. However, this is avoidable and the use of proper equipment should preclude its occurrence.

Decortication

Recently there has been some enthusiasm for early decortication of any hemothorax remaining after chest tube drainage to prevent later empyema. However, most thoracic surgeons still manage most small- to moderate-sized residual hemothoraces in an expectant manner because they usually disappear spontaneously within 4 weeks.

Occasionally a retained hemothorax should be decorticated because it (1) occupies more than a third of one side of the chest, (2) causes atelectasis of a lobe or segments, or (3) is associated with fever. Delay under such circumstances may result in an infected pleural space or a thick peel, both of which increase the difficulty of decortication.

Some errors that may lead to a need for decortication include (1) delay in chest tube insertion (often because the first roentgenogram appeared to be relatively normal), (2) improper positioning of the chest tube, (3) early occlusion of the chest tube with clots, (4) continued or late bleeding from the chest wall or from a pulmonary contusion, and (5) communication with the abdominal cavity through a diaphragmatic injury.

Pneumothorax

A pneumothorax is not apt to cause severe symptoms unless it (1) is a tension pneumothorax with pressure equal to or greater than atmospheric pressure, (2) occupies more than 40 percent of one hemithorax, or (3) occurs in a patient with preexisting cardiopulmonary disease.

Pathophysiology

Collections of air or blood within the pleural cavity reduce vital capacity and raise intrathoracic pressure, reducing ventilation and venous return to the heart. During inspiration, the negative intrapleural pressure increases the tendency for air or blood to leak into the pleural cavity through any wound in the lung or chest wall. If there is any obstruction to the upper airway or if the patient has chronic obstructive lung disease, additional air may be forced into the pleural cavity during expiration, causing a tension pneumothorax with intrapleural pressures equal to or exceeding atmospheric pressure. Any delay in relieving a tension pneumothorax, particularly in a hypovolemic patient, may result in severe hypoxemia, cardiovascular collapse, and death.

Diagnosis

If there is a suspicion of a pneumothorax, but it is not clearly seen on the first chest roentgenogram, repeat films during expiration may be helpful. Apical lordotic films will also allow better visualization of the apex of the chest where the pneumothorax is usually worst. Occasionally a hemopneumothorax after a stab wound is delayed, but seldom beyond 6 h.

If a tension pneumothorax is suspected because the patient is in severe respiratory distress with decreased breath sounds and hyperresonance on one side, insertion of a large needle into the involved side may help confirm the diagnosis and provide some temporary relief until a chest tube can be inserted. Delay in the insertion of a chest tube until chest films are obtained may be fatal.

Treatment

Although a very small pneumothorax that is unchanged on two chest roentgenograms taken 4 to 6 h apart in an otherwise healthy individual can often be treated by observation alone, a chest tube or small catheter should probably be inserted as a precautionary measure, especially if general anesthesia or ventilatory assistance is contemplated.

If at all possible, chest tubes should be inserted while the patient is sitting upright. When the patient is lying down, the diaphragm may occasionally rise as high as the second to third intercostal space, especially if the abdomen is distended. If only a pneumothorax is present, a small-to moderate-sized (no. 24 to 28 French) chest tube may be inserted anteriorly in the second intercostal space in the midclavicular line. However, a hemothorax usually requires a large (no. 32 to 40 French) chest tube inserted in the fifth intercostal space in the midaxillary line.

Although some physicians insert chest tubes over trocars, we prefer to insert them using a large blunt hemostat. The skin incision for the chest tube should be at least an inch below the interspace through which the tube will be placed. The resulting oblique tunnel through the chest wall usually closes promptly after the tube is removed, reducing the chances of recurrent pneumothorax when the tube is removed. Once the tube has been inserted, the physician should ascertain that it is functioning properly. It may then be secured in position with heavy sutures and tape.

The intrathoracic position of the chest tube and the amount of air or fluid remaining in the pleural cavity should be checked with upright posteroanterior and lateral chest films as soon as possible after the tube is inserted. While the patient is en route to the radiology department, the chest tube should *not* be clamped because a continuing air leak can collapse the lung or cause a tension pneumothorax. While the tube is unclamped, the water-seal bottle should be kept 1 to 2 ft lower than the patient's chest.

Serial chest films and careful recording of the volume of blood loss and the size of the air leak are important guides to the functioning of the chest tubes. If a chest tube becomes blocked and a significant pneumothorax or hemothorax is still present on the film, the tube should be replaced. This can be done easily through the same hole that the previous chest tube occupied.

In general, patients can tolerate a small or moderate-sized pneumothorax without complications if there is no continuing air leak. An air leak will usually stop within 24 to 48 h if the lung can be completely expanded. However, if a combination of pneumothorax and continued air leak is not corrected within 24 to 48 h, the incidence of empyema and bronchopleural fistula is greatly increased.

The most frequent reasons for failure to evacuate a pneumothorax rapidly and completely are (1) improper position of the chest tube(s), (2) an inadequate number of chest tubes, or (3) inadequate suction. An air leak and pneumothorax persisting in spite of two well-placed chest tubes attached to 20 to 30 cmH$_2$O suction are generally due to occlusion of the bronchi with secretions, a tear of one of the larger bronchi, or a large tear of the lung parenchyma. Under such circumstances, emergency bronchoscopy should be performed to clear the bronchi and identify any damage to the tracheobronchial tree, with particular attention to the origins of the mainstem bronchi.

Pneumomediastinum

Occasionally, air will accumulate in the mediastinum, with or without a pneumothorax. The diagnosis of pneumomediastinum should be suspected from the presence of a crunching sound (Hamman's sign) over the heart during systole. This is present in about 50 percent of patients with pneumomediastinum and is accentuated when the patient is in the left lateral decubitus position. Subcutaneous emphysema in the neck should make one look closely for this problem. Air along the pericardium or inner border of the pleura on the chest roentgenogram is diagnostic.

There is little or no disability from a pneumomediastinum, except perhaps in the newborn. In many instances no obvious source can be found. One should, however, look particularly carefully for injury to the central tracheobronchial tree, pharynx, or esophagus, as well as for an associated pneumothorax.

TRACHEOBRONCHIAL INJURIES

Distal (Thoracic) Trachea and Major Bronchi

Etiology

Most injuries to the lower trachea or larger bronchi are due to rapid deceleration and shearing of the more mobile distal bronchi from the relatively fixed proximal structures. However, forced expiration against a closed glottis or compression against the vertebral column may also play a role, particularly in tracheal lacerations.

Diagnosis

Injuries to the trachea or major bronchi should be suspected if there is massive subcutaneous or mediastinal emphysema or if there is a pneumothorax with a continuing large air leak that is not corrected by two large chest tubes attached to 20 to 30 cmH$_2$O suction. Most of these injuries occur within 2 cm of the carina in the distal trachea or at the origin of the upper lobe bronchi. On bronchoscopy the characteristic injury in the trachea is a vertical tear in the membranous portion near its attachment to the tracheal cartilages. The tears of the major bronchi are usually transverse at the origins of the upper lobes. If bronchoscopy is either not available or not conclusive, bronchography may be of value, particularly if the diagnosis has been delayed.

If the lung somehow expands and the air leak stops, partial lacerations of the bronchi will often result in repeated infections and eventual severe bronchial stenosis and atelectasis. Complete laceration of a bronchus causes a rapid, complete atelectasis of the distal parenchyma; however, the incidence and severity of distal infection is reduced. Persistent tracheal tears may result in severe mediastinitis.

Treatment

Any delay in repair of a bronchial tear may cause severe pulmonary infection with later stricture formation. Lower tracheal and bronchial lacerations, particularly if they involve more than a third of the circumference, require thoracotomy and direct repair as soon as feasible. Linear tears of the pulmonary artery may accompany some of these injuries, especially if the middle lobe bronchus is involved.

High (Cervical) Tracheal Injuries

Injuries to the cervical trachea usually occur at the junction of the trachea and cricoid cartilage. This is most frequently caused by striking the anterior neck against the dashboard in an auto accident. A karate chop to the neck may also cause this injury with or without fracture of laryngeal cartilages. In the past these were referred to as "clothesline injuries" because many of them occurred in individuals running into a clothesline at neck level.

Evidence of trauma to the neck with subcutaneous emphysema should arouse suspicion. Inspiratory stridor is apt to occur only with a 70 percent to 80 percent upper airway obstruction. Often, however, a high tracheal injury is only suspected if an endotracheal tube or bronchoscope cannot be inserted past the cricoid cartilage. Bronchoscopy or surgical exploration will usually confirm the diagnosis.

If the laceration of the trachea is small and high, it may be managed simply by performing a tracheostomy below the injury. If the laceration involves more than a third of the circumference, it should be repaired and protected with a lower tracheostomy.

DIAPHRAGMATIC INJURIES

Diaphragmatic injuries are caused most frequently by penetrating trauma, particularly gunshot wounds of the lower chest or upper abdomen. Rupture due to blunt trauma is much less frequent and occurs in only 4 to 5 percent of admitted patients. If there is a fracture of the pelvis, the incidence is doubled.

The mechanisms producing diaphragmatic injuries are probably multiple and include sudden increases in intraabdominal or intrathoracic pressure while the diaphragm is fixed by a crushing force. Because of the protective effect of the liver on the right and the possible increased weakness of the left posterolateral diaphragm, it was felt that almost 90 percent of the diaphragmatic injuries following blunt trauma occurred on the left. Recently, however, it has been noted that the incidence of right- and left-sided diaphragmatic rupture may be equal, but it is more difficult to diagnose right-sided tears.

Natural History

Diaphragmatic injuries may present in any of three phases: (1) an early or acute phase usually associated with cardiovascular or respiratory symptoms due to associated injuries; (2) a latent asymptomatic phase that may persist for days, months, or years;

and (3) a late phase associated with obstruction or strangulation of the bowel, or occasionally with respiratory distress. Even small diaphragmatic injuries may result in a rather large amount of viscera gradually working its way into the chest because of the negative pressure there.

Since 60 to 80 percent of normal ventilation depends upon proper function of the diaphragm, extensive damage to this structure can cause serious ventilatory problems. However, the initial signs and symptoms are often masked by other injuries. Unless the diaphragmatic lesion is quite large, symptoms due to obstruction or strangulation of abdominal viscera in the thoracic cavity usually occur late.

Diagnosis

With penetrating trauma, the diagnosis of diaphragmatic injury is usually only made intraoperatively. However, if the entrance wound is in the abdomen and there is evidence of an intrathoracic injury or foreign body, one should assume that the missile or knife has transgressed the diaphragm. If there are both chest and abdominal injuries, aspiration of abdominal lavage fluid through a previously placed chest tube is diagnostic.

With blunt trauma, any abnormality of the diaphragm or left lower lung field should arouse suspicions of a diaphragmatic tear. If a nasogastric tube enters the abdomen and its tip is present in the chest, it is apparent that a portion of the stomach has herniated through a diaphragmatic lesion. A dilute barium swallow or enema may also demonstrate proximal intestine or colon in the chest.

Not infrequently, a preexisting diaphragmatic eventration may be mistaken for diaphragmatic rupture. If suspected, a pneumoperitoneum (with carbon dioxide) may be helpful. It may be difficult at times to differentiate injuries to the phrenic nerve, causing eventration of the diaphragm, from traumatic diaphragmatic hernias. Modified peritoneal lavage, CT scan with contrast, and intraperitoneal technetium sulfur colloid have been suggested recently for diagnosing diaphragmatic rupture, especially on the right.

Treatment

Repair of acute diaphragmatic injuries using a transabdominal route is recommended because associated intraabdominal injuries are present in up to three-quarters of the cases. If the diaphragmatic injury is not recognized for several weeks or if the hernia is on the right side, a transthoracic approach is preferred.

A chest tube should be inserted after the diaphragmatic repair, even if there is no apparent pulmonary injury or residual hemopneumothorax. If bile drains from the chest tube, early transthoracic repair of the bronchobiliary fistula has been recommended. However, we have done better with an abdominal approach.

CARDIAC INJURIES

Penetrating Wounds

Etiology

Gunshot wounds of the heart are becoming more frequent than stab wounds and cause greater morbidity and mortality. Stab wounds of the heart usually involve only one chamber, seldom cause damage to intracardiac structures, usually have an obvious tract, and often seal so that relief of the tamponade in itself may be lifesaving. However, gunshot wounds are much more likely to cause through-and-through injuries that continue to bleed, and are more likely to cause intracardiac injuries. In addition, the tract of a bullet is unpredictable and other organ damage is much more likely to occur.

Pathophysiology

The main hemodynamic problems caused by penetrating cardiac wounds are hemorrhage and tamponade. Bleeding may rapidly progress to hypovolemic shock or death. The tamponade results in impaired diastolic filling of the heart; however, it also limits the amount of bleeding from the myocardial wound and may be lifesaving, at least temporarily. Damage to the proximal portion of a major coronary artery is uncommon, but it may result in arrhythmias or myocardial infarction with resultant cardiogenic shock.

If the pericardial and myocardial wounds are small, which is the usual situation in patients who arrive at the hospital alive, the main problem is tamponade. With pericardiocentesis, these patients will usually improve rapidly, at least temporarily.

Diagnosis

Clinical Features

All patients in shock with a penetrating wound of the middle or lower chest between the midclavicular line on the right and midaxillary line on the left should be considered to have a cardiac injury until proved otherwise. Virtually all patients with a penetrating wound of the heart will have some tamponade, with varying degrees of hypovolemia. If the only problem is tamponade, the neck veins will often be distended, the blood pressure (particularly the pulse pressure) will tend to be low, and the heart tones occasionally faint or muffled. This combination, often referred to as Beck's triad, can be very deceptive and many false-positives and -negatives occur. With hypovolemia, the neck veins will usually not be distended until or unless the blood volume is adequately restored. Furthermore, chest injuries can cause the patient to breathe abnormally or strain, raise the central venous pressure, and distend the neck veins in the absence of tamponade. Even with a large tamponade, the heart tones are usually fairly clear, thus muffled heart sounds is the least reliable sign in Beck's triad. Paradoxical pulse characterized by a drop in systolic blood pressure of more than 10 to 15 mmHg during normal inspiration, should suggest tamponade.

Pericardiocentesis

All patients with a possible cardiac injury and shock should have pericardiocentesis. This is primarily a diagnostic procedure, but removal of as little as 5 to 10 mL of blood from the pericardium may increase stroke volume correspondingly, with a dramatic improvement in cardiac output and blood pressure.

The main approaches for pericardiocentesis are precordial and paraxiphoid. With the precordial approach, a 16- or 18-gauge needle is inserted into the fifth intercostal space 2 to 3 cm lateral to the sternal border, so as to avoid the internal mammary vessels that lie 0.5 to 1.0 cm from the sternum. This precordial approach is more direct, but more apt to result in false-negative or false-positive results and can easily lacerate the midportion of the anterior descending coronary artery.

It is much safer to use the paraxiphoid approach. An 18-gauge (10-cm) spinal needle should be used. The skin is punctured with a knife blade 2 cm below the costal border adjacent to the xiphoid. If a metal needle is used, pericardiocentesis should be done with constant ECG monitoring provided such monitoring will not delay the pericardiocentesis. The ECG monitoring is best done by attaching the V lead of the ECG to the metal needle with an insulated wire with alligator clips.

The needle is passed upward and backward at an angle of 45° for 4 or 5 cm until the point seems to enter a cavity. Most physicians direct the needle toward the left shoulder; however, directing the needle toward the right shoulder is less likely to result in penetration into a cardiac chamber. One should aspirate frequently as the needle is advanced and, if no blood is obtained, periodically insert a stylet or inject 0.5 to 1.0 mL of saline to be certain that the needle is not plugged. The needle is then carefully passed further until blood is obtained, cardiac pulsations are felt, or the ECG shows an abrupt change.

Generally, most of the blood in the pericardial cavity is clotted and, consequently, one can usually remove only 3 to 4 mL at a time and in a rather erratic fashion. Easy removal of large quantities of blood usually indicates that the blood is being aspirated from a cardiac chamber. If a plastic catheter or needle is used for the pericardiocentesis, it should be left in place for continuous drainage of the intrapericardial blood until the wound is surgically repaired.

About 25 percent of patients with acute tamponade will have a negative pericardiocentesis; therefore, if no blood is aspirated, this does not rule out tamponade. If there is a strong suspicion of tamponade in a stable patient, but the pericardiocentesis is negative, a small subxiphoid incision can be made under local anesthesia to make a pericardial window. Dissection is continued down to the diaphragmatic portion of the pericardium and this area is opened under direct vision. If blood is found, the incision can be extended up as a midsternotomy to repair the cardiac wound. In patients with thoracic and abdominal injuries with possible cardiac damage, a transdiaphragmatic pericardiotomy can be done through the abdomen.

X-Ray Films

Roentgenograms may delay needed surgery and are of little assistance in diagnosing a cardiac lesion except in the unusual case with intrapericardial air. Since the average acute tamponade has only 200 mL of blood and clots, significant enlargement of the cardiac shadow by an acute tamponade is unusual.

ECG and Echocardiography

Electrocardiographic changes are usually nonspecific. ST-T wave changes may indicate pericardial irritation or may merely reflect associated ischemia or hypoxia. Echocardiography can be helpful in diagnosing the presence of pericardial fluid. However, it is usually not immediately available, and there are occasional false-positive and false-negative results.

Treatment

Fluid Replacement

Patients with penetrating wounds of the chest should have two or more large intravenous lines in place with at least one in a leg vein in the event that the superior vena cava or one of its major branches is injured. It is particularly important to have adequate or increased blood volume if tamponade is present.

Cardiorrhaphy

All patients with suspected injury to the heart should have an emergency thoracotomy to accurately assess the injuries, to completely relieve tamponade, and to repair any injuries found. An almost immediate thoracotomy is particularly important if the patient has persistent shock and is deteriorating.

After an endotracheal tube has been inserted, the chest is opened either through an anterior thoracotomy or midsternotomy. The transpleural approach through a long incision in the fourth left anterior intercostal space is usually preferred. If additional exposure is necessary, the adjacent cartilages may be divided at the sternum. It may be necessary to divide the sternum transversely so that the incision may be extended into the right thorax. Some surgeons prefer a sternal splitting approach, particularly if the injury is likely to be in the anterior mediastinum or if cardiopulmonary bypass may be needed.

If an anterior thoracotomy incision is used, and the internal mammary vessels are cut they should have suture ligatures proximally and distally. The pericardium is incised anterior and parallel to the phrenic nerve to provide ample exposure of the heart. All pericardial blood is removed and the wound in the heart is located. Bleeding is controlled by pressure over the wound with a finger. Repair of the myocardial injury is best done with interrupted, pledgetted horizontal mattress sutures using 2-0 nonabsorbable material swedged onto a long, slender, curved needle. If bleeding persists, one must look at the back of the heart for a through-and-through injury. After hemostasis is established, the pericardium is either approximated loosely with a few widely spaced sutures or it is left completely open to prevent recurrent tamponade.

Open Cardiac Massage

If cardiac arrest occurs before transport to the operating room, an endotracheal tube should be inserted and an emergency left anterolateral thoracotomy performed in the emergency department to provide open cardiac massage. Closed massage is ineffective and may cause additional damage in these patients. The bleeding site can usually be controlled with a fingertip while the massage is being performed. In addition, clamping or compressing the descending thoracic aorta increases almost threefold the blood flow to the heart and brain.

Coronary Artery Injuries

Ligation of the cut ends is the treatment of choice for lacerations of small or distal coronary vessels. Suture ligation may also be applied to injuries of the proximal coronary arteries if there is no evidence of cardiovascular dysfunction. However, such patients must be observed closely. If arrhythmias, myocardial infarction,

or impaired hemodynamic function develop, an aorto-coronary bypass with saphenous vein should be performed. Standby cardiopulmonary bypass equipment is essential for such surgery.

Occasionally, a fistula between a coronary artery and cardiac chamber may develop long after hospitalization and should be suspected if a murmur develops. Such murmurs can also be due to a ventricular septal defect, valve injury, or papillary muscle infarction.

Intracardiac Injuries

If heart failure is not present at the time of injury, valvular or septal injuries are best repaired electively after complete cardiac catheterization 6 to 8 weeks later.

Emboli

Rarely a bullet or other foreign body may embolize to the heart. Most of these should be surgically removed to reduce the chance of later thromboembolism and infection with endocarditis.

Blunt Trauma

An increasing incidence of cardiac damage from blunt trauma is being recognized. Cardiac injury is the most frequent unsuspected visceral injury responsible for death in fatally injured accident victims.

The mechanisms involved in cardiac damage from blunt trauma include acceleration-deceleration, compression, and a sudden increase in intrathoracic or intraabdominal pressure. The spectrum of cardiac injuries that may result from blunt trauma include myocardial contusion, pericardial effusions, septal defects, and rupture of valvular structures or cardiac chambers.

Myocardial Contusion

Incidence

Myocardial contusion occurs much more frequently than is generally recognized. In carefully monitored patients admitted to the hospital with severe blunt chest trauma, the incidence is probably at least 20 to 25 percent and has been reported to be as high as 76 percent.

Pathology

The pathologic changes usually consist of subendocardial hemorrhage and a much larger area of myocardial damage with focal myocardial edema, interstitial hemorrhage, myofibrillar degeneration, and focal myocytolysis. The boundaries of damage are usually sharply demarcated in contrast to the lesions usually seen with myocardial infarction. Shock, hypovolemia, and excessive catecholamine release may greatly aggravate these changes and increase the likelihood of dangerous arrhythmias.

In some instances, the myocardial lesion may closely resemble an infarction. This is most apt to occur if there is concomitant coronary vascular occlusion caused by arterial spasm, intimal tears producing a flap, or compression from adjacent hemorrhage and edema. Occasionally, transient hypotension may cause complete occlusion of a previously diseased vessel.

Usually there is complete clinical recovery with minimal residual scarring following a myocardial contusion. However, in some cases, softening and fibrotic replacement of the contused myocardium are followed by thinning of the scar, leading to ventricular dilatation and aneurysm formation.

It has been shown that contusion with hemorrhage around major coronary arteries following severe cardiac trauma in dogs can significantly narrow coronary arteries.

Diagnosis

Cardiac contusions are among the most frequently missed or delayed diagnoses in hospitalized injured patients. The reasons for delay in diagnosis are often related to (1) attention directed toward other severe injuries, (2) lack of evidence of thoracic injury, or (3) lack of evidence of cardiac injury on initial examination.

Clinical Features

In some patients, a tachycardia completely out of proportion to the degree of trauma or blood loss may be the first clue to the diagnosis. Aside from evidence of significant chest wall injury, the only other physical signs helpful in establishing the diagnosis are the presence of a friction rub or an abnormality in heart sounds.

ECG

The diagnosis of myocardial contusion is usually made by ECG; however, this will miss about two thirds of patients with ventricular dyskinesia following trauma. Myocardial contusion must be suspected in all patients with significant blunt injury to the chest (particularly by a steering wheel) and serial ECGs should be done for at least 48 h. The most frequent arrhythmias are sinus tachycardia, atrial fibrillation, and ventricular and atrial premature beats. Sinus node dysfunction due to blunt trauma may be much more common than formerly suspected.

ST-T wave abnormalities present on admission or developing after 24 to 48 h and persisting for several days can usually be accepted as evidence of myocardial contusion. The development of a bundle branch block or arrhythmia is also highly suggestive. Persistent ECG changes or development of significant Q waves indicate extensive myocardial scarring with possible formation of a ventricular aneurysm.

Enzymes

Serum glutamic-oxaloacetic transaminase (SGOT), lactic dehydrogenase (LDH), and creatine phosphokinase (CPK) levels are usually elevated in patients with severe blunt chest trauma because of injuries of liver, lung, bone, brain, and skeletal muscle. Consequently, they are of little value in diagnosing cardiac injuries. Myocardial (CPK-MB) isoenzymes should be much more accurate but have also tended to be elevated along with the other fractions in individuals with no other evidence of myocardial injury.

Other Studies

The technetium scan has been suggested as a possible diagnostic technique to detect cardiac contusion. In one recent series, tech-netium pyrophosphate scans were much more sensitive than ECG or CPK-MB studies. Low cardiac output as measured by impedance cardiography or impaired wall motion on radionuclide angiography may be the most sensitive index of cardiac contusion. However, these techniques may be difficult to apply in patients with acute, severe thoracic injury.

Insertion of a pulmonary artery catheter and determination of ventricular function before and after a fluid load have revealed a high incidence of biventricular failure. Patients with biventricular dysfunction had a 40 percent incidence of morbidity and mortality.

Cardiac catheterization and coronary angiography may be useful in patients who appear to have an acute myocardial infarction with cardiospecific enzyme and ECG changes. These studies should also be performed in patients in whom cardiac symptoms persist after injury and in those suspected of having preexisting coronary artery or other cardiac disease.

Treatment

If a myocardial contusion is suspected, the patient should be treated as if an acute myocardial infarction had occurred. Particular attention must be directed to prevention and treatment of complications, especially arrhythmias and congestive heart failure. Continuous cardioscopic monitoring and careful avoidance of fluid overloading are important. If cardiogenic shock develops and is refractory to pharmacological therapy, intraaortic balloon counterpulsation may be effective.

Anticoagulants should be avoided in patients with cardiac contusion. Most of these patients have other significant injuries that may be complicated by anticoagulants. Furthermore, anticoagulation may increase bleeding into the contused myocardium or pericardial cavity.

Pericardial Effusions or Tamponade

Pericardial injury should be suspected in patients with severe blunt trauma to the chest, particularly if there is ECG evidence or other evidence of myocardial damage. Hemopericardium can lead to tamponade within minutes or as late as a week or more after the injury. Retained pericardial blood can also cause later constrictive pericarditis.

Pericardial lacerations usually occur across the base of the heart near the junction of the visceral and parietal pericardium. Recently, it has been shown that traumatic rupture of the pericardium is more frequent than previously thought and should usually be repaired.

If cardiac tamponade is suspected, pericardiocentesis should be performed. If the diagnosis of tamponade is established and the patient is hemodynamically unstable a thoracotomy should be performed to relieve the tamponade and correct any underlying injury.

Septal Defects

Septal defects after blunt chest trauma are rare. The muscular interventricular septum near the apex is particularly susceptible to perforation. Diagnosis may be difficult because rupture of chordae tendineae and/or papillary muscles causing mitral or tricuspid insufficiency may closely mimic a septal perforation.

The murmurs of traumatic ventricular septal defect are usually only detected several days or weeks after the injury. In most cases abnormal ECG findings (especially supraventricular arrhythmias, conduction disturbances, or QRS abnormalities) may be the first signs of significant cardiac injury. The triad of chest trauma, systolic murmur, and an infarct pattern on the ECG should suggest intraventricular septal defect.

Although small traumatic ventricular septal defects may close spontaneously, surgical repair—preferably 6 to 8 weeks after the trauma—is the treatment of choice. The presence of congestive heart failure may require earlier operation. Occasionally the patient may develop an acute bacterial endocarditis.

Isolated atrial septal defects due to blunt trauma are extremely rare and most of these patients die rapidly.

Valve Injuries

Rupture of the aortic valve is the most common valvular lesion in patients who survive nonpenetrating cardiac injury. Blunt trauma rarely may also lacerate the papillary muscles or chordae tendineae of the mitral valve. The prognosis for rupture of the mitral papillary muscle or mitral valve leaflet is grave, and death usually occurs within a few days after the injury. The tricuspid valve is rarely involved in blunt trauma and tricuspid insufficiency does not usually cause a significant hemodynamic problem unless the patient has pulmonary hypertension.

Any patient without a history of heart disease who presents with heart murmurs after severe blunt trauma to the chest should be suspected as having aortic valve damage. The diagnosis of traumatic aortic valvular insufficiency is usually made when a diastolic murmur is heard in a dyspneic trauma patient who has chest pain and previously had no murmur. As the lesion worsens, the diastolic pressure decreases. Peripheral signs of aortic insufficiency, such as visible capillary pulse, Corrigan's pulse, pistol-shot sounds over the brachial and femoral vessels, and Duroziez's murmur (biphasic arterial bruit) may also become evident. Echocardiography may occasionally be diagnostic, but cardiac catheterization is essential prior to surgical therapy. The avulsion-type valve injury most frequently seen after blunt chest trauma makes leaflet repair difficult and tenuous. Consequently, valve replacement is the recommended procedure.

Chamber Rupture

Rupture of a cardiac chamber is the most common injury noted in autopsy examinations of patients after blunt cardiac trauma. Most of these patients die rapidly from exsanguination or tamponade. Shock not responding properly to fluid replacement and/or transfusions after blunt chest trauma may represent cardiac tamponade from a ruptured cardiac chamber. A positive pericardiocentesis under such circumstances is an indication for immediate surgery, preferably with cardiopulmonary bypass support.

Followup

It is important that patients with proven or suspected cardiac injury be closely observed, not only throughout their hospital stay but also later for initially undiagnosed injuries or complications. One must look particularly for posttraumatic pericarditis, ventricular septal defect, valvular defects, and ventricular aneurysms; and aortic, pulmonary, or coronary artery fistulas or chamber communication. When such problems are found and it appears that the defect endangers the patient's life, cardiac catheterization should be performed as soon as possible followed by surgical repair. However, if the patient tolerates the lesion well, cardiac catheterization should be performed electively 6 to 8 weeks later.

INJURY TO THE GREAT VESSELS

Traumatic Rupture of the Aorta

Mechanisms of Injury

The mechanisms for traumatic rupture of the aorta include (1) horizontal deceleration shearing of the aorta where its mobile portion meets the more fixed portion; (2) marked compression, causing bursting of the aorta; or (3) a combination of the above. Acute flexion with stretching of the aorta or its branches may contribute to the ease of rupture.

Location

The majority (95 to 99 percent) of aortic injuries after automobile accidents occur in the aortic isthmus, just distal to the left subclavian artery. The next most common intrathoracic great vessel injury with automobile accidents is laceration of the subclavian artery at the thoracic inlet. With falls from heights or in plane crashes, there is a significant incidence of injury to the ascending aorta. Another injury that may occur is laceration or avulsion of the innominate artery.

Natural History

In decreasing order of frequency, the aortic tear may result in (1) complete disruption of the circumference of the aorta with exsanguinating hemorrhage; (2) incomplete disruption, with an expanding hematoma contained by the adventitia of the aortic wall with gradual development of a saccular aneurysm; or (3) dissection with partial aortic obstruction producing late findings similar to those found with coarctation of the aorta.

Of the estimated 8000 patients who have a traumatic rupture of the thoracic aorta annually, 80 to 90 percent die within a few minutes of their injury. Of those who survive for 1 h, 30 percent die within 6 h, 40 percent within 24 h, 72 percent within 8 days, 83 percent within 3 weeks, and 90 percent within 10 weeks.

Diagnosis

Clinical Features

Early diagnosis of traumatic rupture of the thoracic aorta depends primarily upon a high index of suspicion. Although great force is usually needed to tear the aorta, about one-third of these patients have little or no external evidence of chest trauma. Furthermore, the majority have multiple severe extrathoracic injuries that tend to distract the physician. Consequently, if aortic transection is to be diagnosed early, it must be suspected in any patient who has been in an automobile accident at speeds exceeding 30 mph.

Findings that suggest the diagnosis of traumatic rupture of the aorta include (1) a systolic murmur over the precordium or on the back, medial to the left scapula; (2) hoarseness or voice change because of pressure of the hematoma on the left recurrent laryngeal nerve; (3) hypertension in the upper extremities; or (4) hypotension or weak pulses in the lower extremities. In rare instances in which the injury involves the ascending aorta, the resulting aneurysm or hematoma may produce a clinical picture of superior vena caval obstruction.

Chest Roentgenogram

Although the circumstances of the accident and the physical findings are helpful, the diagnosis is usually made or suspected from findings on the routine chest roentgenogram. Since over 95 percent involve the aorta near the attachment of the ligamentum arteriosum, the characteristic and most accurate radiologic finding is blurring or obliteration of the aortic knob. The most frequently described radiologic finding is widening of the superior mediastinum adjacent to the aortic knob. However, a ratio of mediastinal width to chest width greater than 0.28 on erect PA films is considered to be a more specific and sensitive roentgenographic sign. Other x-ray signs include apical cap, downward displacement of the left mainstem bronchus, obliteration of the usual clear space between the aortic knob and left pulmonary artery, and displacement of the trachea or esophagus to the right. Although fractures of the first or second ribs have been thought to be associated with an increased incidence of traumatic aortic rupture, this assumption is being increasingly questioned. Unfortunately, the widened mediastinum and other radiologic changes may not be apparent on the chest roentgenogram for several hours on up to a third of patients. Consequently, serial chest films should be taken in any patient with severe chest or upper abdominal trauma at 4-to-8-h intervals during the first day and then daily for at least the next 3 days. Some patients with traumatic rupture of the aorta may never have a widened mediastinum; up to two-thirds of patients over 65 may not show mediastinal widening.

A false appearance of mediastinal widening can easily be obtained if the chest roentgenograms are taken anteroposterior (AP) instead of PA less than 100 cm from the x-ray machine, with the patient lying flat, and with poor inspiration. The optimal chest x-ray is an upright PA film taken at 6 ft with good inspiration.

Aortography

If an aortic rupture is suspected on clinical or radiologic grounds, an aortogram should be performed. Widening of the superior mediastinum does not always indicate disruption of the aorta or its branches. In 50 to 85 percent of patients with a widened mediastinum after blunt trauma, the aorta and its branches are normal on aortography. The widening of the mediastinum has been found at surgery and autopsy to consist primarily of bleeding from disruption of mediastinal veins. These venous injuries usually resolve spontaneously.

Aortography is usually performed using a percutaneous femoral artery catheter. If the femoral artery pulse is weak, right axillary arterial catheterization may provide good visualization of the thoracic aorta. In addition to getting a good view of the aortic isthmus with LAO views, the entire aorta and its branches should be visualized to rule out unusual traumatic ruptures that might otherwise be missed. Recently, increasing attention has been given to subclavian artery injuries after blunt trauma.

If the patient appears to be in shock from an aortic rupture, or has a rapidly expanding mediastinal hematoma, he or she should be taken directly to the operating room without aortography.

Computed Tomography

Although aortography has been considered the ideal method for diagnosing traumatic aortic rupture, contrast-enhanced computed tomography (CT scan) may demonstrate an aortic dissection which was not revealed by biplane thoracic aortography.

Treatment

The chances of successful management of a rupture of the thoracic aorta depend largely on the number and severity of associated injuries. The decision to repair the thoracic aorta immediately in the poor-risk patient with other multiple severe injuries is difficult and must be individualized. It may be preferable to carefully observe some poor-risk patients with multiple severe injuries. This should be done in or adjacent to the operating room, until the risk of surgery is reasonable.

Surgery without Bypass

Repair of traumatic tears of the thoracic aorta are usually performed with maintenance of blood flow to the lower part of the body with an external shunt or cardiopulmonary bypass. In a few centers, however, aortic repair is preferentially performed without an external shunt or cardiopulmonary bypass because it is believed to be quicker and safer. Under such circumstances an intravenous infusion of trimethaphan camsylate (Arfonad) is often used to reduce the blood pressure in the upper portion of the body to diminish the chances of intracerebral hemorrhage or left heart failure while the aorta is clamped. The operation must be rapid and precise because clamping of the descending aorta for more than 20 min without perfusion of the distal aorta invites serious risk of damage to the spinal cord and abdominal viscera.

External Shunt

An increasingly used alternative to cardiopulmonary bypass is a tube or graft to divert blood around the involved aorta. This greatly reduces the danger of distal ischemia (particularly to the spinal cord), and proximal hypertension. The proximal end of the tubing (filled with heparinized saline) can be inserted into the ascending aorta, the aortic arch, or the apex of the heart. The distal end can be inserted into the middle or lower descending thoracic aorta or femoral artery. Studies have shown that flow through a 7.5-mm cannula is about 2000 mL/min, while flow through a 9-mm cannula is about 4000 mL/min. If special heparin-coated polyvinyl tubing is used, the patient does not have to be exposed to the risk of systemic heparinization; this consideration is especially important in patients with intracranial injuries.

Interestingly, the aortic tear can be missed on direct visual examination or palpation because the aorta may look and feel surprisingly normal at surgery except for some subadventitial hemorrhage. A transverse incision into the suspected area, after proximal and distal aortic clamping, may be required to confirm the diagnosis and the location and extent of injury.

Although a recent incomplete tear of the aorta can often be repaired directly, complete, tears, particularly if more than 2 to 3 days old, usually require insertion of a short prosthetic graft.

Surgery with Cardiopulmonary Bypass

Repair of traumatic rupture of the thoracic aorta is often performed under partial bypass because it allows increased time for a meticulous, unhurried repair and reduces the risk of ischemic damage to the spinal cord and abdominal viscera. The usual circuit, from the femoral vein to the femoral artery, requires an oxygenator. Left atrial–femoral artery bypass does not require an oxygenator. If the patient's condition is stable, transfer to a hospital where cardiopulmonary bypass is available is wise.

ESOPHAGEAL INJURIES

Isolated Injuries

Lacerations of the esophagus are caused most frequently iatrogenically by endoscopy or biopsy of a narrowed or obstructed esophagus. The esophagus can also be injured by swallowed foreign bodies that perforate the wall at the time of swallowing or that may, if left in situ, cause deep ulceration with later perforation. Injury to the esophagus by external trauma is extremely rare and was noted in only 3 (0.4 percent) of 796 patients with penetrating chest injuries.

If esophageal injury is suspected, an esophagogram should be performed. Many physicians prefer a water-soluble radiopaque material, such as Gastrografin, because it causes less reaction than barium in the surrounding tissues. However, with such contrast material there is at least a 25 percent incidence of false negative results, which are rare with dilute barium. Even when extravasation is noted, the exact site of perforation may be missed unless the fluoroscopy is done very carefully. The esophagogram is usually performed prior to esophagoscopy to warn the endoscopist of any unusual injury, constriction, or anomaly that may be present. Bronchoscopy should be performed to rule out concomitant tracheobronchial injuries.

Although esophageal perforations should be repaired within 6 to 12 h of injury, the ability to do this depends on early diagnosis. If treatment is delayed beyond 24 h, a primary closure is not advisable because local edema, tissue necrosis, and infection make secure suturing and primary healing unlikely. The mediastinitis is usually severe and may be rapidly fatal in such patients unless the site is drained adequately.

Whether or not a repair is attempted, continuous complete drainage of the stomach (preferably with a gastrostomy tube) and the adjacent mediastinum (with a chest tube) is extremely important and may be necessary for several weeks or longer. Some believe that complete defunctionalization of the esophagus with a gastrostomy and cervical esophagostomy provides the greatest safety.

Tracheoesophageal Fistula

Although traumatic tracheoesophageal fistulas are occasionally caused by gunshot wounds of the neck or upper mediastinum, the most frequent cause of this lesion in patients without malignancies is erosion of a rigid tracheostomy tube through the posterior tracheal wall into the esophagus. If there is only partial disruption of the esophageal wall, the immediate consequences of the fistula may not be severe. However, chronic strictures have been reported. Because such fistulas are frequently found in patients with long-term nasogastric drainage, the pathogenesis may involve acid-peptic reflux as well as localized pressure or trauma. Early repair with insertion of a flap of pleura, pericardium, or intercostal muscle should be performed if possible. However, many of these repairs will break down and result in severe mediastinitis.

THORACIC DUCT INJURIES

Chylothorax is usually the result of thoracic surgery or penetrating trauma. Because the major portion of the thoracic duct is on the right, injuries to the thoracic duct usually cause a right chylothorax. Adequate drainage of the pleural cavity with a chest tube for several days usually results in spontaneous closure of the fistula. Intravenous hyperalimentation may help, not only by reducing the flow of chyle but also by preventing the protein malnutrition that can rapidly develop in some of these patients because of the loss of protein with the chyle. If the patient is allowed to eat, nonoperative therapy may be more successful if a strict no-fat diet or one with medium-chain triglycerides is followed.

Surgery may be required if the leak is large and persistent. Lymphangiograms preoperatively may occasionally help to locate the site of injury since it is often extremely difficult to identify the torn ends at the time of surgery. At surgery, the duct injury can occasionally be visualized after running saline into the subcutaneous tissue of both thighs. After a few minutes, a trickle of fluid may be seen at the site of the injured duct. Injection of dye, such as methylene blue, usually discolors the entire operative area very quickly and makes it difficult to identify the duct. Once the ends of the duct are identified, they should be ligated.

SUMMARY

Diagnosis and treatment of penetrating thoracic injuries depend primarily upon repeated physical examination and serial chest roentgenograms. Most patients with penetrating chest trauma can be treated conservatively by the judicious use of chest tubes (to remove air or blood that may have accumulated in the pleural cavity), and by maintaining adequate ventilation. Keeping the airway open by encouraging frequent deep coughing or using nasotracheal suction or bronchoscopy is essential. If there is any indication that a ventilator will be needed, it should be used early.

Emergency thoracotomy is only needed for about 10 to 15 percent of patients with penetrating trauma. When a thoracotomy is required for certain specific problems such as severe, continuing intrathoracic bleeding or suspected injury to the heart or great vessels, the surgery must be performed promptly and expeditiously.

In patients with nonpenetrating thoracic trauma, rib fractures and other chest wall lesions may distract the physician from suspecting dangerous extrathoracic injuries, which occur quite frequently. In addition, important intrathoracic injuries may not be diagnosed unless looked for very carefully. Shock is frequently due to extrathoracic injuries, particularly intraabdominal bleeding.

The flail associated with multiple segmental rib fractures may seem mild initially, but severe underlying pulmonary contusion or associated extrathoracic injuries, or both, make early ventilatory assistance critical.

Myocardial contusion occurs quite frequently, but is often missed unless serial ECGs are taken. Rupture of the thoracic aorta is usually suspected because of widening of the superior mediastinum on the chest roentgenogram. Aortography to confirm the aortic tear should be done if time permits, and early repair of the injury provides the best results.

BIBLIOGRAPHY

Abbott JA, Cousineau M, Cheitlin M, et al: Late sequelae of penetrating cardiac wounds. *J Thorac Cardiovasc Surg* 75:510–518, 1978.

Allmendinger PD, Low HB, Takata H, et al: Deceleration injury: Laceration of the thoracic aorta. *Am J Surg* 133:490–491, 1977.

Alter BR, Wheeling Jr, Martin HA, et al: Traumatic right coronary artery–right ventricular fistula with retained intramyocardial bullet. *Am J Cardiol* 40:815–819, 1977.

Anayanwu CH: Mitral incompetence and ventricular septal defects following nonpenetrating injury. *Thorax* 31:133–117, 1976.

Arom KV, Richardson JD, Webb G, et al: Subxiphoid pericardial window in patients with suspected traumatic pericardial tamponade. *Ann Thorac Surg* 23:545, 1977.

Asfaw I, Arbulu A: Penetrating wounds of the pericardium and heart. *Surg Clin North Am* 57:37–48, 1977.

Ayella RJ, Hankins JR, Turney SZ, et al: Ruptured thoracic aorta due to blunt trauma. *J Trauma* 17:119–205, 1977.

Bassett JS, Gibson RD, Wilson RF: Blunt injuries to the chest. *J Trauma* 8:418–429, 1968.

Bayer MJ, Burdick D: Diagnosis of myocardial contusion in blunt chest trauma. *JACEP* 6:238–242, 1977.

Berkoff HA, Rowe GG, Crummy AB, et al: Asymptomatic left ventricular aneurysm: A sequela of blunt chest trauma. *Circulation* 55:545–548, 1977.

Blair E, Topuzlu C, Deane RS: Major blunt chest trauma. *Curr Probl Surg* 6:1–64, 1969.

Bodai BI, Smith JP, Blaisdell FW: The role of emergency thoracotomy in blunt trauma. *J Trauma* 22:487, 1982.

Bognolo DA, Rabow FI, Vijayander RR, et al: Traumatic sinus node dysfunction. *Ann Emerg Med* 11:319, 1982.

Cheney FW Jr, Huang TH, Gronka R: Effects of methylprednisolone on experimental pulmonary injury. *Ann Surg* 190:236–242, 1979.

Chi S, Blair TC, Gonzalez-Lavin L: Rupture of the normal aortic valve after blunt chest trauma. *Thorax* 32:619–622, 1977.

Chilimindris CP: Rupture of the thoracic esophagus from blunt trauma. *J Trauma* 17:968–971, 1977.

Clark DE, Wiles CS III, Lim MK et al: Traumatic rupture of the pericardium. *Surgery* 93:495, 1983.

Collins MP, Shuck JM, Wachtel TL, et al: Early decortication after thoracic trauma. *Arch Surg* 113:440–445, 1978.

Coselli, JS, Mattox KL: Traumatic bronchobiliary fistula. *J Trauma* 23:161, 1983.

Das PB: Penetrating injury of the diaphragm with herniated colon leaking into the left pleural space. *Int Surg* 62:463–464, 1977.

De la Rocha AG, Creel RJ, Mulligan GW: Diaphragmatic rupture due to blunt abdominal trauma. *Surg Gynecol Obstet* 154:175, 1982.

DeMuth WE, Baue AE, Odom JA: Contusions of the heart. *J Trauma* 7:443–445, 1967.

Dronen S, Chadwick O, Novak R: Endotracheal tip position in the arrested patient. *Ann Emerg Med* 11:116, 1982.

Ekstrom D, Weiner M, Baier B: Pulmonary arteriovenous fistula as a complication of trauma. *Am J Roentgenol* 130:1178–1180, 1978.

Enders GC, Graeber GM, Poirier RA: Wounds traversing two or more cardiac chambers: Case presentation of two survivors and review of the literature. *J Thorac Cardiovasc Surg* 76:83–89, 1978.

Espada R, Whisennad HH, Beall AC Jr, et al: Surgical management of penetrating cardiac injuries. *Thoracic Cardiovasc Surg* 17:97, 1976.

Fallah-Nejad M, Wallace HW, Su CC, et al: Unusual manifestations of penetrating cardiac injuries. *Arch Surg* 110:1357–1362, 1975.

Flynn TC, Ward RE, Miller PW: Emergency department thoracotomy. *Ann Emerg Med* 11:413, 1982.

Fordham SD: Bullet embolism. *Int Surg* 61:481–483, 1976.

Garrison, RN, Richardson JD, Fry DE: Diagnostic transdiaphragmatic pericardiotomy in thoracoabdominal trauma. *J Trauma* 22:147, 1982.

Grover FL, Richardson D, Jewel JG, et al: Prophylactic antibiotics in the treatment of penetrating chest wounds: A prospective double-blind study. *J Thorac Cardiovasc Surg* 74:528–536, 1977.

Gundry SR, Williams S, Burney RE: Indications for aortography in blunt thoracic trauma: A reassessment. *J Trauma* 22:664, 1982.

Harada M, Osawa M, Kosukegawa K, et al: Isolated mitral valve injury from nonpenetrating cardiac trauma: Report of a case with successful repair. *J Cardiovasc Surg* 18:459–464, 1977.

Harrison WH, Gray AR, Couves CM, et al: Severe nonpenetrating injuries to the chest: Clinical results in the management of 216 patients. 100:715–722, 1960.

Hellman RM, Rufty AJ Jr: Left ventricular aneurysm caused by blunt chest trauma. *South Med J* 71:652–655, 1978.

Iverson LI, Mittal A, Dugan DJ, et al: Injuries to the phrenic nerve resulting in diaphragmatic paralysis with special reference to stretch trauma. *Am J Surg* 132:263–269, 1976.

Jancu J, Marvan H: Traumatic rupture of right diaphragm presenting as pleuropneumonia. *South Med J* 69:1226–1227, 1976.

Jones, JW, Hewitt RL, Drapanas T: Cardiac contusion: A capricious syndrome. *Ann Surg* 181:567–574, 1975.

Karrel R, Shaffer MA, Franaszek JB: Emergency diagnosis resuscitation and treatment of acute penetrating cardiac trauma. *Ann Emerg Med* 11:504, 1982.

Katz S, Gimmon Z, Lewis BS: Coronary angiography after traumatic myocardial contusion. *J Trauma* 19:126–128, 1979.

Kessler KM, Foianin JE, Davia JE, et al: Tricuspid insufficiency due to nonpenetrating trauma. *Am J Cardiol* 37:442–444, 1976.

Kimbler, RW, Stokes JP, Barnhorst DA: The surgical treatment of traumatic rupture of the aortic valve: Report of a case after blunt chest trauma. *J Trauma* 17:168–170, 1977.

Kirsh MM, Orringer MB, Behrendt DM, et al: Management of unusual traumatic ruptures of the aorta. *Surg Gynecol Obstet* 146:365–370, 1978.

Kleinerman J, Gerblich AA: Blunt chest trauma and the lung, editorial. *Am Rev Respir Dis* 115:369–370, 1977.

Krajcer Z, Cooley DA, Leachamn RD: Ventricular septal defect following blunt trauma: Spontaneous closure of residual defect after surgical repair. *Cathet Cardiovasc Diagn* 3:409–415, 1977.

Kress, TD, Balasubramanian S: Cricothyroidotomy. *Emerg Med* 11:197, 1982.

Kumar SA, Puri VK, Mittal VK, et al: Myocardial contusion following nonfatal blunt chest trauma. *J Trauma* 23:327, 1983.

Layton TR, Dimarco RF, Pellegrini RV: Rupture of the left atrium from blunt trauma. *J Trauma* 19:117–118, 1979.

Lasky II, Nahum AM, Siegel AW: Cardiac injuries incurred by drivers in automobile accidents. *J Forensic Sci* 14:13–33, 1969.

Leamon PL: Rupture of the right hemidiaphragm due to blunt trauma. *Ann Emerg Med* 12:351, 1983.

Liedtke AJ, DeMugh WE: Nonpenetrating cardiac injuries: A collective review. *Am Heart J* 86:687–697, 1973.

Lukacs L, Lonyai T: Successful repair of left ventricular aneurysm due to blunt trauma. *J Cardiovasc Surg* 19:407–410, 1978.

Manzano, JL, Bolanos J, Lubillo S, et al: Internal costal fixation of fractured ribs in a 6 year old patient. *Crit Care Med* 10:67, 1982.

Markovchik VJ, Evans GT, Rosen P, et al: Traumatic acute pericardial tamponade. *JACEP* 6:562–567, 1977.

Marsh DG, Sturm JT: Traumatic aortic rupture: Roentgenographic indications for angiography. *Ann Thorac Surg* 21:337–340, 1976.

Mattox KL, Feliciano DV: Role of external cardiac compression in truncal trauma. *JACEP* 7:12–15, 1978.

McIlduff JB, Foster ED, Alley RD: Traumatic aortic rupture: An additional roentgenographic sign. *Ann Thorac Surg* 24:77–29, 1977.

Miller MS, Scott FC: Cardiac contusion and right bundle branch block. *JACEP* 6:504–505, 1977.

Munim A, Chodoff P: Traumatic acute mitral regurgitation secondary to blunt chest trauma. *Crit Care Med* 11:311, 1983.

Naclerio EA: Chest trauma. *Clin Symp* 22:75–109, 1970.

Parmley LF, Manion WC, Mattingly TW: Nonpenetrating traumatic injury of the heart. *Circulation* 18:371–396, 1958.

Pearce W, Blair E: Significance of the electrocardiogram in heart contusion due to blunt trauma. *J Trauma* 16:136–140, 1976.

Pezzella AT, Todd EP, Dillon ML, et al: Early diagnosis and individualized treatment of blunt thoracic aortic trauma. *Am Surg* 44:699–703, 1978.

Pinilla JC: Acute respiratory failure in severe blunt chest trauma. *J Trauma* 22:221, 1982.

Popovsky J, Lee YC, Berk JL: Gunshot wounds of the esophagus. *J Thorac Cardiovasc Surg* 72:609–612, 1976.

Rajs J, Jakobsson S: Severe trauma and subsequent cardiac lesions causing heart failure and death. *Forensic Sci* 8:13–21, 1976.

Ramzy AI, Rodriguez A, Cowley RA: Pitfalls in the management of traumatic chylothorax. *J Trauma* 22:513, 1982.

Rao G, Garvey J, Gupta M: Atrial septal defect due to blunt thoracic trauma. *J Trauma* 17:405–406, 1977.

Rowland TW: Traumatic aortic insufficiency in children: Case report and review of the literature. *Pediatrics* 60:893–895, 1977.

Rubio PA, Bahadorzadeh K, Waisser E, et al: Acute bacterial endocarditis following traumatic ventricular septal defect. *J Cardiovasc Surg* 19:433–436, 1978.

Sabbah HN, Stein PD, Hawkins ET, et al: Extrinsic compression of the coronary arteries following cardiac trauma in dogs. *J Trauma* 22:937, 1982.

Sacchetti AD, Beswick DR, Morse SD: Rebound rib: Stress induced first rib fracture. *Ann Emerg Med* 12:177, 1983.

Sankaran S, Wilson RF: Factors affecting prognosis in patients with flail chest. *J Thorac Cardiovasc Surg* 60:402–410, 1970.

Schaff HV, Brawley RK: Operative management of penetrating vascular injuries of the thoracic outlet. *Surgery* 82:182–191, 1977.

Schick, TD, van der Zee H, Powers SR Jr: Detection of cardiac disturbances following thoracic trauma with high frequency analysis of electrocardiogram. *J Trauma* 17:419–424, 1977.

Shier MR, Wilson RF, James RE, et al: Fat embolism prophylaxis: A study of four treatment modalities. *J Trauma* 17:621–629, 1977.

Siemens R, Polk HC Jr, Gray LA Jr, et al: Indications for thoracotomy following penetrating thoracic injury. *J Trauma* 17:498–500, 1977.

Silverman EM, Littler ER: Bullet in the left ventricle from a remote gunshot wound to the heart. *Chest* 71:234–236, 1977.

Simon RR, Brenner BE, Rosen MA: Emergency cricothyroidotomy in patients with massive neck swelling. Part 2: Clinical aspects. *Crit Care Med* 11:119, 1983.

Smith JM III, Grover FL, Marcos JJ, et al: Blunt traumatic rupture of the atria. *J Thoracic Cardiovasc Surg* 71:617–620, 1976.

Snow N, Lucas AE, Richardson JD: Intra-aortic counterpulsation for cardiogenic shock from cardiac contusion. *J Trauma* 22:426, 1982.

Splener CW, Benfield JR: Esophageal disruption from blunt and penetrating external trauma. *Arch Surg* 111:663–667, 1976.

Sturm JT, Cicero JJ: The clinical diagnosis of ruptured subclavian artery following blunt thoracic trauma. *Ann Emerg Med* 12:45, 1983.

Sturm JT, Points BJ, Perry JF Jr: Hemopneumothorax following blunt trauma of the thorax. *Surg Gynecol Obstet* 141:539–540, 1975.

Subramanian VA, Berger RL: Transection of the innominate artery due to blunt chest trauma: Successful immediate repair in two consecutive patients. *Ann Thorac Surg* 21:357–360, 1976.

Symbas PN, Harlaftis N, Waldo WJ: Penetrating cardiac wounds: A comparison of different therapeutic methods. *Ann Surg* 183:377–381, 1976.

Szentpetery S, Lower RR: Changing concepts in the treatment of penetrating cardiac injuries. *J Trauma* 17:457–461, 1977.

Tector AJ, Reuben CF, Hoffman JF, et al: Coronary artery wounds treated with saphenous vein bypass grafts. *JAMA* 225:282–284, 1973.

Torres-Mirabal P, Gruenberg JC, Talbert JG, et al: Ventricular function in myocardial contusion: A preliminary study. *Crit Care Med* 10:19, 1982.

Trinkle JK, Richardson JD, Franz JL, et al: Management of flail chest without mechanical ventilation. *Ann Thorac Surg* 19:355, 1975.

Weigelt JA, Aurbakken CM, Meier DE, Thal ER: Management of asymptomatic patients following stab wounds to the chest. *J Trauma* 22:291, 1982.

Wilson JM, Borden CH Jr, Peterson SR, et al: Traumatic hemothorax: Is decortication necessary? *J Thorac Cardiovasc Surg* 77:489–495, 1979.

Wilson JM, Thomas AN, Goodman PC, et al: Severe chest trauma: Morbidity implication of first and second rib fracture in 120 patients. *Arch Surg* 113:846–849, 1978.

Wilson RF, Arbulu A, Bassett J, et al: Acute mediastinal widening following blunt chest traum: Critical decisions. *Arch Surg* 104:551–558, 1972.

Wilson RF, Bassett JS: Penetrating wounds of the pericardium or its contents. *JAMA* 195:513–518, 1966.

Wilson RF, Gibson DB, Antonenko D: Shock and acute respiratory failure after cest trauma. *J Trauma* 17:697–705, 1977.

Wilson RF, Mammen E, Walt AJ: Eight years of experience with massive blood transfusions. *J Trauma* 11:275–285, 1971.

Wilson RF, Murray C, Antonenko D: Nonpenetrating thoracic injuries. *Surg Clin North Am* 57:17–36, 1977.

Wilson RF, Sarver EJ, Arbulu A, et al: Spontaneous perforation of the esophagus. *Ann Thorac Surg* 12:291–296, 1971.

Zaplonski A, Ilves R, Todd TRJ: Injury to the middle lobe bronchus and pulmonary artery: An unusual pattern. *Ann Thorac Surg* 35:156, 1983.

CHAPTER 122
ABDOMINAL TRAUMA

Ronald L. Krome

The critical issue in the management of patients with abdominal trauma is the presence of significant injury to an intraabdominal or retroperitoneal structure. All diagnostic and therapeutic decisions must be made with this in mind. Surgical intervention may be part of resuscitation and stabilization. Indications for immediate surgical intervention are listed in Table 122-1. The development and refinement of peritoneal lavage, and the development of CT scanning have had significant impact on the treatment of these injuries.

PENETRATING WOUNDS

Until recently, it was standard practice to take any patient with a penetrating wound to the operating room. Currently, it is becoming standard to attempt a more specific definition of the injury prior to making a decision. Still, patients who have sustained a penetrating gunshot wound should be taken to the operating room as soon as possible for the completion of stabilization and exploration, while those with stab wounds can be assessed more slowly and deliberately, provided their vital signs remain stable. Patients with penetrating abdominal wounds and shock, or unstable vital signs, are candidates for rapid surgical intervention.

Although penetrating wounds can occur as isolated injuries, they may be associated with extraabdominal injuries. Penetrating abdominal injuries may cross the diaphragm and enter the chest. The opposite can also occur, so that thoracic injuries can present with predominantly abdominal findings. This is especially true if the injury is in the lower chest or upper abdomen.

After the airway is established and multiple IV lines are in place, more careful attention can be paid to the wounds to assess the possibility of penetration. If a gunshot wound is present, the assumption should be that the peritoneum has been violated and significant organ injury has occurred. Missiles such as bullets do not have a predictable trajectory. Injury from a high-velocity missile may occur at a distance from its path because of the transmission of shock waves through organs. For these reasons, gunshot wounds usually require surgical exploration.

If a stab wound has been sustained, peritoneal lavage may be indicated. The wound should be anesthetized and probed gently with a gloved finger after the patient is prepped and draped. If penetration is confirmed or if evisceration is present, this may be all that is required prior to continued exploration of the patient in the operating room. In any case, peritoneal penetration is an indication for surgical consultation.

Patients with wounds of the back or flank are difficult to assess. Penetration cannot be determined by probing with any accuracy. If the base of the wound can be seen or felt, then operative exploration may not be necessary. If not, then other diagnostic adjuncts are necessary, including peritoneal lavage, intravenous pyelogram (IVP), CT scan, or all these. Arteriography also may be helpful.

BLUNT TRAUMA

Anatomic Contents

On the right, the seventh through tenth ribs overlie the liver, so that blunt injuries in this area can result in liver damage. This may occur either primarily, or secondarily as a result of rib fracture with subsequent penetration and/or laceration of the liver.

On the left, the ninth and tenth ribs overlie the spleen, so that fracture of these ribs may produce splenic injury. The eleventh and twelfth ribs on the left and the twelfth rib on the right cover the kidneys; fracture of these ribs can result in injury to the kidneys.

When three or more ribs are fractured, either on the same side or in total, associated extrathoracic injury is common. Often this involves intraabdominal injury. Abdominal injury, as well as thoracic injury, may accompany fractures of the first and/or second rib because of the force necessary to fracture them.

Significant peritoneal signs may not be present when retroperitoneal organs are injured—the duodenum, kidneys, adrenals, ureters, and portions of the ascending and descending colon. Rupture of a hollow retroperitoneal viscus does not produce free intraperitoneal air. Air that is released is located in the retroperitoneum and should be sought on abdominal films. Because the aorta and vena cava are located in the retroperitoneum, major bleeding from

Table 122-1. Indications for Surgical Intervention in Abdominal Trauma

Failure of vital signs to respond to fluid administration
Deterioration of vital signs during observation and stabilization
Expansion of the abdomen
Free air under the diaphragm
Retroperitoneal air
Positive peritoneal lavage
Falling hemoglobin despite adequate blood replacement

trauma to these vessels may not produce early abdominal distention.

The mesentery, the jejunum at the ligament of Treitz, and the renal pedicles are all points of fixation of abdominal organs. Acceleration-deceleration injuries may result in a shearing effect at these fixed points, producing significant visceral injuries without obvious external signs of trauma. The rectum and bladder are also retroperitoneal organs that when injured produce few, if any, peritoneal signs.

INITIAL TREATMENT

The initial approach is outlined in Table 122-2. Every patient who is even suspected of having significant intraabdominal injury should have at least two large-bore intravenous lines inserted, at least one of which should be placed in a central venous location. Fluids should be rapidly infused in an attempt to return vital signs toward normal. Because ileus and gastric distention frequently accompany abdominal trauma, a nasogastric tube should be inserted. This will serve to empty the stomach, relieve gastric distention, minimize the possibility of vomiting and aspiration, improve tidal volume, and facilitate abdominal evaluation. In addition, the presence of a bloody gastric return may indicate injury to the stomach or esophagus.

When the intravenous lines are inserted, baseline laboratory studies should be obtained. Although some will not be helpful initially, they do provide an opportunity for monitoring which may be necessary during the preoperative and/or the postoperative periods. Even though we recommend that a serum amylase level should be obtained initially, recent studies indicate that it is of limited usefulness. It is said to be elevated in pancreatic and small bowel injuries. Blood for transfusion should be available.

Foley catheter placement should be left until the last part of the patient's evaluation and following placement of IV lines. This is especially true when the patient has sustained blunt abdominal trauma. The presence of hematuria following trauma may be an indication for urologic evaluation. Since the passage of the catheter, especially in men, is almost always accompanied by hema-

Table 122-2. Initial Approach to Abdominal Trauma

1. ABCs (patent *a*irway, control *b*leeding, ensure *c*irculation)
2. IVs—at least two
3. Nasogastric tube
4. Foley catheter (late)
5. Complete physical examination
6. Laboratory studies
   CBC
   BUN
   Electrolytes
   Amylase
   Type and crossmatch
7. Roentgenograms
   Chest
   Flat and upright of abdomen
   Lateral decubitus of abdomen
   Cross-table lateral of abdomen
8. If indicated,
   Peritoneal lavage
   IVP
   Arteriography
   Scanning

turia, urologic evaluation may be obviated if a spontaneously voided specimen can be obtained. The patient may be more cooperative if time has passed and if fluid volume is replaced. If fracture of the pelvis is suspected, a catheter should not be passed until the integrity of the urethra is assured.

PHYSICAL EXAMINATION

Following stabilization of the neck and airway, should that be indicated, the patient should be completely undressed. The local area of abdominal trauma should be assessed and, if a penetrating wound is present, it should be evaluated. Flank discolorations should be sought. Grey Turner's sign develops late and is associated with a retroperitoneal hematoma. A rectal examination should be done in all patients, and a pelvic examination in all women. Blood on the gloved finger is indicative of trauma until proved otherwise. The absence of a prostate gland, or its abnormal location, indicate urethral trauma, usually associated with pelvic fracture. On rectal and/or pelvic examination bone fragments from a fractured pelvis may be palpated.

Groin tenderness on direct pressure or on compression may be present with a fractured pelvis. Lower rib tenderness and tenderness of the lumbosacral region may indicate a fracture, which can be associated with intraabdominal injury.

CLINICAL FEATURES

Tenderness and Rigidity

Because almost all patients have tenderness over the injured area, this is a difficult sign to use initially. If, however, during the repeated examinations that follow, the tenderness progresses, it may indicate a continuing intraabdominal process. Rebound tenderness does not usually develop until 6 to 12 h after the initial injury, because it takes that long for peritoneal irritation and inflammation to occur.

Guarding, the patient's response to tenderness, is a voluntary muscular effort in which the abdominal muscles are splinted to protect the patient from being hurt by the examiner. Guarding, therefore, is a difficult sign to evaluate in trauma.

Rigidity, which indicates generalized inflammation of the visceral and parietal peritoneum, has much more significance. This is a reflex indicating that generalized peritonitis is present, and therefore surgical intervention is necessary. This will not usually occur until 6 to 12 h have elapsed from the time of the initial injury. Shortly after abdominal trauma, gastric distension and/or ileus may occur even though there is no viscus injury. Ileus can result from thoracic or lumbosacral injuries. Abdominal distention can result from either the accumulation of swallowed air, ileus, or intraperitoneal bleeding.

Bowel Sounds

Bowel sounds are, at best, of limited value in assessing the severity of intraabdominal injury. There is no way to predict what the sounds may be like. When ileus is present, bowel sounds are diminished or absent.

Deterioration of Vital Signs

Any patient who has sustained abdominal injury and has deteriorating vital signs during resuscitation belongs in the operating room, and surgical intervention becomes a part of stabilization. A patient with poor vital signs that do not respond to rapid fluid and blood replacement, a patient with falling hemoglobin or an abdomen increasing in girth, all require surgical intervention.

Virtually all patients who have sustained abdominal trauma will complain of pain; therefore, it is difficult to use this symptom to assess the need for surgical intervention. The presence of rebound tenderness and boardlike rigidity, with or without a rapidly expanding abdomen, and despite the presence of a nasogastric tube, are all indications that significant intraabdominal injury may have occurred.

RADIOLOGIC EVALUATION

The following should be obtained: flat and upright films of the abdomen, a lateral decubitus film of the abdomen, and an upright film of the chest to include the diaphragm. The latter is obtained because free air under the diaphragm is most easily detected on this view. Other films may be indicated. Retroperitoneal air may be seen if a tear of the duodenum allows air to track along the biliary tree, so that the air will appear to be in the biliary tree itself.

Fluid or blood in the peritoneal cavity may give the abdominal films a ground-glass appearance, with a paucity of gas-filled loops of bowel. Retroperitoneal bleeding or intraabdominal bleeding may obscure the psoas shadows so that they are not seen on views of the abdomen. If a splenic injury has occurred and blood is present in the left upper quadrant, the gastric bubble may be displaced medially. This same thing can occur if there is a subcapsular hematoma of the spleen.

A cross-table lateral film of the abdomen may be helpful by demonstrating anterior displacement of the stomach and/or small bowel as a result of pancreatic hematoma, retroperitoneal hematoma, or subcapsular hematoma of the spleen. Intramural hematomas of the small bowel, especially the duodenum, may produce partial or complete obstruction. Routine films, then, may show local areas of dilatation of the bowel, a "sentinel loop." If the intramural hematoma of the duodenum involves the area of entry of the common duct, then elevation of the serum amylase level may be present, and the nasogastric aspirate will not contain bile.

PERITONEAL LAVAGE

No other single diagnostic procedure has made as significant an impact on the management and treatment of abdominal injury as peritoneal lavage. Even the changes we are seeing with the advent of CT scans in this area have not been as significant.

Indications for peritoneal lavage include (1) the presence of signs and symptoms associated with blunt abdominal trauma, (2) penetrating abdominal trauma with inconclusive signs, (3) the presence of an altered sensorium making abdominal evaluation difficult, (4) unexplained shock. Contraindications are relative, and the procedure can generally be modified to account for their presence. They include (1) a full bladder, (2) previous abdominal surgery, and (3) a gravid uterus.

A full bladder should be emptied by either having the patient void, or by inserting a Foley catheter. If the patient has had previous abdominal surgery, the peritoneal lavage can be done in an area free of scar. It need not be done in the midline. There are reports of pregnant patients having peritoneal lavage without any complications. The risks of the procedure must be weighed against the risks of an undetected abdominal injury, or doing an unnecessary exploratory laparotomy. In women who have had previous surgery, in whom a peritoneal lavage may be difficult to perform, culdocentesis should be considered.

If the patient has clear-cut signs of intraabdominal injury, peritoneal lavage is not indicated because it is unnecessary and will delay definitive therapy. Complications include perforation of a hollow viscus, laceration of major vessels, and the production of a false-positive study because of bleeding caused by the procedure itself.

Technique

The bladder must be emptied. The skin is prepped and draped and local anesthetic used. A small transverse skin incision is made 2 cm below the umbilicus in the midline and carried down to, but not through, the peritoneum (see Fig. 122-1). All bleeding should be controlled prior to entering the peritoneum. Two small hemostats are used to pick up the peritoneum, and the lavage catheter is poked through, aiming at the pelvis. Some physicians make a small nick in the peritoneum through which the catheter is inserted,

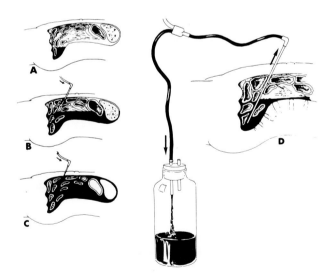

Figure 122-1. Diagnostic peritoneal lavage. *A:* Small amount of free intraperitoneal fluid gravitates toward cul-de-sac because it is the most dependent portion of the peritoneal cavity. *B, C:* Intraperitoneal administration of Ringer's lactate solution. The fluid has a tendency to collect posteriorly as the air-containing viscera move anteriorly. The intraperitoneal fluid gives the intestines more mobility. *D:* Catheter directed toward cul-de-sac. In theory the amount of blood in the last 50 mL of dialysate removed is most apt to represent the amount of blood in the peritoneal cavity. (From Sachatello CR, Bivins B: Technic for peritoneal dialysis and diagnostic peritoneal lavage. *Am J Surg* 131:638, 1976. Used by permission.)

to ensure that no viscus is inadvertently entered. The central stylet is then removed.

Immediate aspiration of 20 mL or more of blood is considered a positive test and the procedure terminated. If less than 20 mL is obtained or if no blood is obtained, the procedure is continued. The lavage fluid, Ringer's lactate, is administered at a volume of 20 mL/kg, to a maximum of 1000 mL, as rapidly as possible. The fluid is allowed to stay in the peritoneal cavity for 5 to 15 min and then is allowed to return, using gravity drainage (Fig. 122-1). If less than 500 mL is returned, an additional 10 mL/kg, up to 500 mL, is inserted.

If the fluid return in the tubing and in the drainage bottle is clear, then the chance of a significant injury is less than 1 percent. If the fluid is clear in the tubing, but red in the bottle, then the chance of significant injury is considered to be 24 percent. If the return in both is red and tubid, the chance of significant injury is said to be in the range of 96 percent.

If the peritoneal lavage effluent is not obviously positive, it should be submitted for white and red cell determination; amylase determination; and examination for intestinal contents, bile, and bacteria. When these results are added to the inspection of the fluid and are positive, the chance of significant injury is about 98 percent. The study is positive if the white blood cell count exceeds 500/mL, if the red blood cell count is greater than 100,000/mL; if the amylase level is greater than 100 Somogyi units/100 mL; or is positive for bile, intestinal contents, or bacteria.

If a stab wound has occurred, then the lavage is considered positive if the red blood cell count is greater than 50,000/mL or the white blood cell count is greater than 250/mL. In addition there are recent studies which show that more injuries can be detected if an initial negative peritoneal lavage is repeated at 6 h ("sequential peritoneal lavage").

False-positive results can occur, especially if retroperitoneal bleeding is present as, for example, from pelvic fracture. These are minimized if the lavage technique utilized is open, as described above. Some recommend doing a supraumbilical incision, if pelvic fracture is suspected, to avoid putting the lavage catheter through extraperitoneal hematoma.

The classic use of peritoneal lavage is outlined in Table 122-3. If at the time of initial evaluation the patient's vital signs are unstable, and if the patient cannot be resuscitated with rapid infusion of volume, he or she should be taken to the operating room. Peritoneal lavage is not indicated if the abdomen is expanding; if

Table 122-3. Use of Peritoneal Lavage in Blunt Abdominal Trauma

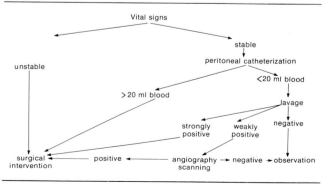

for any reason the patient is deteriorating, surgical intervention is necessary, not peritoneal lavage.

If, on the other hand, the patient's vital signs are stable but abdominal injury is suspected, then lavage is carried out. If the initial lavage is negative or not clearly positive, it should be repeated 6 h later. If the initial aspirate consists of 20 mL or greater of nonclotting blood, the patient belongs in the operating room.

If lavage is negative, and again negative at the sixth hour and the patient continues to remain stable, then further diagnostic studies can be carried out. In any case, the patient should be kept for prolonged observation to ensure that no injury has occurred as a result of the study.

OTHER DIAGNOSTIC STUDIES

CT scanning is being increasingly utilized in assessing blunt abdominal injuries. Studies to date would seem to indicate that its best utilization is in detection of retroperitoneal hematomas and organ injuries. It has also been useful in assessing the presence of splenic, pancreatic, liver, and renal injuries. It may well be that, in patients with a negative peritoneal lavage, the next study will be an abdominal CT scan. Scanning of the liver and/or spleen using isotope injection has been found helpful in some institutes.

Arteriography, when occult injury is present, is also useful. After a catheter is threaded into the aorta, specific arterial studies can be done to detect vascular (arterial) injury, or to assess the presence of subcapsular bleeding in the liver, kidney, or spleen.

If retroperitoneal or renal injury is suspected, drip infusion IVP may be indicated. If renal artery compromise is present, then nonfunctioning kidney(s) may be found. Depending on the injury, extravasation of dye may be seen. Retroperitoneal bleeding may distort the path of the ureters, the shape of the kidneys, or the shape of the bladder.

SPECIFIC ORGAN INJURY

Liver

The liver is frequently injured when there are penetrating injuries of the right upper quadrant or the right lower chest. In blunt injuries to the right lower chest, when fractures of the ribs occur, subsequent injury to the liver is not uncommon. In one study, injuries to the liver were associated with other injuries in 37 percent of cases. If the liver laceration is small, bleeding may stop spontaneously. There is, obviously, no way of knowing this in advance. Subcapsular hematomas of the liver may rupture later; the same can happen with the spleen. Therefore, a remote history of trauma should be sought in any patient with abdominal distention and a low hemoglobin, or in unexplained shock.

Traumatic hematobilia is rare; generally it is a result of a penetrating injury to the liver in which intraperitoneal bleeding has not been significant, or even detected. Patients may present with complications of this problem at some time distant from the initial traumatic insult. The classic triad for this syndrome is gastrointestinal bleeding (hematemesis or melena), biliary colic, and jaundice. The diagnosis is established by selective angiography. Treatment is surgical. CT scanning or radioactive scanning may be helpful in establishing the diagnosis.

Pancreas

Pancreatic trauma is most often associated with severe vascular injury, duodenal injury, or gallbladder injury. It can result from either blunt or penetrating causes. Isolated injuries are rare but do occur. They are difficult to diagnose, although the increasing use of CT scans in this area may be extremely helpful. A sentinel loop may be present on routine x-rays. Retroperitoneal air may also be present and the serum amylase level may be elevated, but the latter is not reliable. Pancreatic pseudocysts may develop as a result of injury to a distal duct.

Duodenum

Injuries to the retroperitoneal duodenum may produce air on routine radiographs. If the injury results in an intramural hematoma, then a sentinel loop may be seen, and duodenal obstruction, either partial or complete, may result. Generally, these hematomas produce gastric outlet obstruction. They usually resolve without surgical intervention, but with prolonged nasogastric suction. In this case, the gastric return will be voluminous, positive for blood, and free of bile.

Stomach

Injuries to the stomach should be suspected whenever the nasogastric return contains blood, usually gross blood. The stomach is much more commonly injured as a result of penetrating trauma than as a result of blunt injuries. A gastric return that contains gross blood in a patient who has sustained a penetrating wound to the upper abdomen is a clear indication that surgery will be necessary.

Intestines, Including the Rectum

The small intestines are the most commonly injured organ as a result of penetrating injury. Predisposing factors include recent ingestion of food, small bowel incarceration, hernias, anatomic points of fixation, adhesions, and improperly worn lap seat belts. Small bowel perforation results in the spillage of intestinal contents with subsequent development of sepsis and shock. If bleeding is minimal, the first peritoneal lavage will be negative. The subsequent 6-h lavage may be positive.

Free air under the diaphragm may be detected. Avulsion of the mesentery may occur with intraperitoneal bleeding. When intestinal perforation is even considered possible, antibiotics should be started in the emergency department.

Perforating injuries of the colon and rectum may occur secondary to pelvic fracture. They may be detected by finding stools positive for blood on rectal examination. Since the rectum is retroperitoneal, peritoneal signs do not accompany injuries to this organ.

Blunt injuries to the colon are rare, but when they do occur they occur in the transverse colon. They are usually diagnosed at the time of surgery. X-ray studies and sequential peritoneal lavage may be helpful.

Colon injuries consist of one of four types: lacerations or perforations, avulsions of the mesentery, intramural hematomas, and stenosis, as a late complication.

Kidneys, Ureters, Bladder

Although injuries to these organs are dealt with in much greater detail in Chapter 123, "Genitourinary Trauma," it should be emphasized that associated genitourinary injuries should be considered in every abdominal trauma event when hematuria is present, either microscopic or gross. Such injuries also should be considered when there is a flank mass, obliteration of the psoas shadows or renal outlines, or fracture of a lumbar transverse process on routine abdominal studies. The drip infusion intravenous pyelogram is the classic study for determining renal injury; CT scanning is rapidly entering this field of diagnosis.

Spleen

The spleen is the most commonly injured organ as a result of blunt trauma. There may be early left upper quadrant tenderness with some guarding, and occasionally some rigidity. There may be associated left shoulder and/or scapular pain. Shock may occur early if bleeding is voluminous. Lower rib fractures may produce injuries to the spleen and a penetrating left lower chest wound may violate the abdomen and enter the spleen.

Splenic injuries may not manifest themselves at the time of injury, but sometime later. So-called delayed rupture of the spleen or ruptured subcapsular hematoma should be suspected in any patient with left upper quadrant pain and/or tenderness, tachycardia, a low hemoglobin, and a remote history of trauma. Occult splenic rupture occurs in only 1 percent of cases. Most commonly it is manifested only by vague symptoms. Abdominal films may show displacement of the gastric bubble to the right (medial). Chest x-ray may show an elevated left diaphragm. CT scans may be helpful.

Vascular Injuries

Injuries to the major vessels in the abdomen usually are the result of retroperitoneal trauma. They should be suspected in any patient who sustains a penetrating injury of the flank or back. Penetrating injuries of the abdomen can lacerate the aorta and/or the vena cava. If the latter is injured, then a rapidly expanding abdomen will present. If the former, bleeding is mostly retroperitoneal and expansion of the abdomen occurs later. In a patient with a penetrating abdominal wound and a rapidly expanding abdomen, especially with a falling blood pressure, the military antishock trousers (MAST) should be applied. Emergency thoracotomy may be necessary in order to clamp the descending aorta just above the diaphragm, to limit bleeding.

Diaphragmatic Injuries

Diaphragmatic injuries are often difficult to diagnose, but should be suspected anytime there is a lower chest or upper abdominal penetrating injury. Suspicion should also be aroused when there is an apparent effusion in the left chest, or if the diaphragm is elevated. Blunt abdominal trauma can also produce rupture of the diaphragm.

Delays in diagnosis are not unusual. Although classically described as occurring on the left side, the right diaphragm can be involved. Air-fluid levels may be seen if abdominal contents have herniated up into the chest cavity and bowel sounds may also be heard. Insertion of a nasogastric tube may be both diagnostic and therapeutic: diagnostic if seen coiled in the left chest, and therapeutic because the tube will reduce gastric distention and minimize ileus, permitting expansion of the lung.

The liver appears to protect the right diaphragm and prevent herniation. If the rupture involves the left side, abdominal contents may enter the pleural space, limiting the patient's ability to ventilate.

Evisceration

Evisceration can occur whenever the abdominal wall has been lacerated and the peritoneum violated. Any abdominal organ, except for those in the retroperitoneum, can then herniate through the opening. In general, any eviscerated organ should be covered with moist sterile drapes and towels, and left to be replaced in the operating room. This same treatment should be instituted in the prehospital care area as well.

However, if the evisceration is through a small opening and the color of the organ is such that vascular compromise appears to have been present, then it should be replaced in the peritoneum, as long as gangrene is not present. If in doubt, it should be left out.

All patients with an evisceration have peritonitis and the appropriate antibiotics should be started.

BIBLIOGRAPHY

Breen PC, Rudolph LE: Potential sources of error in the use of peritoneal lavage as a diagnostic tool. *JACEP* 3:401–403, 1974.

Budd DC, Fouty WJ Jr, Johnson RB, et al: Occult rupture of the spleen: A dilemma in diagnosis. *JAMA* 236:2884–2886, 1976.

Burney RE, Mueller GL, MacKenzie JR: Evaluation of experimental blunt and penetrating hepatobiliary trauma by sequential peritoneal lavage. *Ann Emerg Med* 12:279–289, 1983.

Defore WW, Mattox KL, Jordan GL Jr, et al: Management of 1,590 consecutive cases of liver trauma. *Arch Surg* 111:493–497, 1976.

Druy EM, Rubin BE: Computed Temography in the Evaluation of Abdomninal Trauma *J Comput Assist Tomography* 3:40–44, 1979.

Harlaftis NN, Akin J: Hemobilia from ruptured hepatic artery aneurysm: Report of a case and review of literature. *Am J Surg* 133:229–232, 1977.

Haycock CE, Machiedo G: The use of peritoneal lavage as a diagnostic tool in emergencies. *JACEP* 3:397–400, 1974.

Hegarty MM, Bryer JV, Angorn IB, et al: Delayed presentation of traumatic diaphragmatic hernia. *Ann Surg* 188:229–233, 1978.

Howell SH, Bartizal JF, Freeark RJ: Blunt trauma involving the colon and rectum. *J Trauma* 16:624, 1976.

Jackson FL, Thal ER: Management of stab wounds of the back and flank. *J Trauma* 19:660–664, 1979.

Leaman PL: Rupture of the right hemidiaphragm due to blunt trauma. *Ann Emerg Med* 12:531–357, 1983.

Lucas CE, Ledgerwood AM: Factors influencing outcome after blunt duodenal injury. *J Trauma* 15:839–846, 1975.

Mueller GL, Burney RE, MacKenzie JR: Leukocytosis in peritoneal lavage effluent after selected abdominal organ injury in an experimental model. *Ann Emerg Med* 11:343–347, 1982.

Olsen WR: Peritoneal lavage in blunt abdominal trauma. *JACEP* 2:271–275, 1973.

Walt AJ (ed): Symposium on trauma. *Surg Clin North Am* 57:1–226, 1977.

CHAPTER 123
GENITOURINARY
TRAUMA

Brooks F. Bock

The evaluation and treatment of an acutely injured patient present a serious challenge to the emergency physician. Although hematuria is the finding that frequently leads to a urologic evaluation, 2 to 20 percent of patients with renal injuries may not show any microhematuria on initial evaluation. Evaluation for urologic injury necessitates a thorough understanding of blunt and penetrating injuries to the kidney, ureter, bladder, urethra, and genitalia. Most patients with genitourinary trauma are seen initially by the emergency physician, who must be skilled in evaluating the initial intravenous pyelogram (IVP) and cystogram. This chapter discusses these areas of concern.

If the patient suspected of having a urologic injury is stable initially, evaluation begins with a urinalysis. The urine specimen should be obtained without catheterization if possible, since catheterization can result in iatrogenic microhematuria. If the patient is unable to void, a fluid challenge is given to initiate a diuresis. If a voided specimen still cannot be obtained, a small-caliber no. 16 French Foley catheter is gently inserted using aseptic technique to obtain urine. (See the exception to this under the section on urethral trauma.)

BLUNT RENAL TRAUMA

In a study of 115 patients with blunt renal trauma seen over a 10-year period at Parkland Memorial Hospital, motor vehicular accident was the cause of injury in 86 of the patients. Other causes and the number of patients affected were as follows: falls, 15; fights, 7; football injury, 4; crush injury, 2; swing injury, 1. It is significant that 44 percent of these patients had associated injuries most often involving the liver, spleen, or pancreas. Thus, the mortality rate for patients with blunt injury to the kidney is generally attributed to associated injuries. There were 11 deaths: two due to isolated injury to the renal pedicle, and nine associated with head injury, shock, renal failure, and laceration of the liver.

The common mechanism of injury in these cases is either direct trauma or deceleration. Direct renal trauma has many causes while deceleration injury is most commonly caused by automobile accidents or falls from heights. Direct renal trauma is often associated with fractures of the posterolateral aspect of the eleventh or twelfth ribs, or the transverse processes of the first, second, or third lumbar vertebra. Deceleration injury occurs when the patient's body is brought to a sudden stop, while the kidney, which

can rotate on the renal hilum, continues moving within the retroperitoneal space. This results in a stretch injury to the renal artery or to the renal pelvis. Stretching of the renal artery results in an intimal tear with platelet aggregation, thrombus formation, and potential occlusion of the renal artery. Injury to the renal pelvis is especially common in children and most often involves disruption at the ureteropelvic junction.

Clinical Features

Pain is a frequent symptom and generally is localized in the flank, upper abdomen, or both. It ranges from dull to intense and is relatively constant.

Microscopic or macroscopic hematuria is found in 80 to 98 percent of patients with blunt renal trauma. The absence of hematuria, then, does not exclude blunt renal trauma. In an analysis of 41 patients suffering blunt renal trauma and revealing no hematuria, the following injuries were reported: pedicle injury, 32 percent; major parenchymal injury, 24 percent; and minor parenchymal injury, 44 percent. In addition, the degree of hematuria does not correlate with the degree of injury.

Fractures are often associated with blunt renal trauma and in the study done at Parkland Memorial Hospital, it was found that of the 115 patients evaluated, 59 had associated rib fracture, 11 had associated pelvic fracture, 8 had associated vertebral fracture, and 8 had associated skull fracture.

After careful history, physical examination, and urinalysis, radiologic examination is the next appropriate diagnostic modality. First, the examiner should obtain a scout or plain film to evaluate the abdomen prior to contrast material injection.

The following findings may indicate underlying renal injury:

- One renal shadow
- Abnormal bowel gas pattern
- Obliteration of the psoas shadow by retroperitoneal blood or urine
- Scoliosis away from the injured side
- Calcifications indicating tumor, cyst, calculus, or aneurysm

Intravenous pyelography is indicated whenever a patient has hematuria with even a minimal amount of abdominal trauma because of the high incidence of urinary tract abnormalities such as horseshoe kidney, hydronephrotic kidney, or carcinoma of the kidney seen in these situations. In the absence of hematuria, intravenous pyelography should be performed when there are associated rib or vertebral fractures, or both, or when genitourinary injuries are suspected because of retroperitoneal fullness, absent psoas shadows on radiography, or severe abdominal or costovertebral tenderness. An unexplained ileus with associated abdominal pain is yet another indication for a pyelogram in blunt abdominal trauma.

An IVP should be performed using a 60 percent iodine-containing contrast material as a bolus at a dose of 1 mL/kg body weight. The dose should be infused through an indwelling intravenous catheter, in 1 to 2 min. If bladder injury is suspected, the IVP should be performed prior to a cystogram. This avoids the problem of residual contrast material in the pelvis obscuring the lower ureters or suggesting ureteral disruption while the IVP is being performed.

Following contrast injection, 1-min, 5-min, 10-min, and 20-min films should be obtained if time permits. The 1-min film is particularly useful for demonstrating the nephrographic phase in which the kidney appears as a brightly highlighted structure containing contrast material. The 5-min films are to evaluate the upper collecting system, and the 10- and 20-min films are useful in evaluating the ureter. If the entire length of the ureter is not seen, films in the oblique position will sometimes enable visualization of the full length. If immediate surgery is contemplated a single film taken 5 min after contrast injection will provide valuable information to the operating surgeon regarding presence and function of both kidneys.

Of all patients who have significant blunt renal trauma, 70 percent have an abnormal IVP. The most common abnormal findings are delayed visualization (nephrographic phase) of one or both kidneys, extravasation from the upper collecting system or the ureter, and nonvisualization of a kidney. Delayed visualization or nonvisualization of a kidney generally means there has been compromise or interruption of the renal vasculature. Extravasation generally indicates a direct injury to the renal parenchyma or to the collecting system itself (Fig. 123-1).

Blunt renal injuries are classified as minor parenchymal, major parenchymal, or pedicle injuries. Studies suggest that of all blunt renal injuries, approximately 47 percent are minor parenchymal injuries, 31 percent are major parenchymal injuries, and 22 percent are pedicle injuries. A renal contusion is an example of the minor parenchymal type while a renal artery occlusion is an example of the pedicle injury.

Treatment

A flow chart for the therapeutic management of patients with blunt renal trauma is shown in Table 123-1.

The most common serious complication resulting from blunt renal injury is hypovolemic shock secondary to blood loss. Other complications include acute tubular necrosis, renal infarction, and hypertension. Hypertension is a relatively infrequent finding and

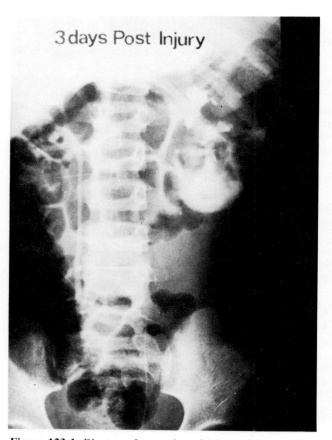

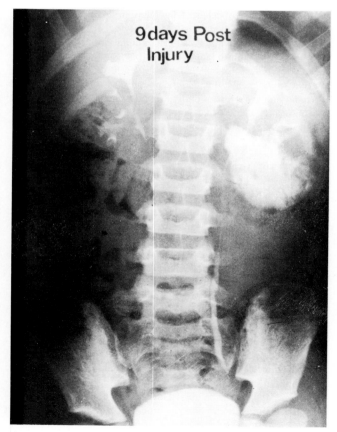

Figure 123-1. Blunt renal parenchymal injury with contrast extravasation at left lower pole as seen by IVP. Treated nonoperatively with complete healing. (Courtesy of Detroit General Hospital.)

Table 123-1. Flow Chart for Management of Renal Injuries

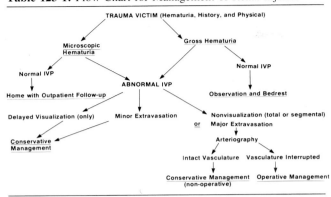

Source: From Peters PC, Bright TC III: Blunt renal injuries. *Urol Clin North Am* 4:22, 1977. Used by permission.

is generally a late sequela, occurring because of unilateral vascular occlusion.

Diagnostic Imaging in Urologic Trauma

Diagnostic imaging is a useful adjunct in evaluating the stable patient with blunt trauma to the abdomen who is not in need of emergency exploratory laparotomy. This assumes that the appropriate plain radiographs have been obtained and that additional information is necessary for the management of the patient.

Ultrasound is particularly useful in diagnosing and following posttraumatic complications by identifying and localizing hematomas and other fluid collections. Radionuclide scintigraphy is a reliable screening method for injuries to the kidneys but, most importantly, scans are useful in serial observation of the vascular supply in patients treated without an operation. Computed tomography (CT) is the roentgenologic screening method of choice in the stable multitrauma patient with blunt abdominal injury. It is both sensitive and specific in the evaluation of renal injuries. Most studies reporting on the use of these techniques in trauma evaluation are small. Their use in the future will increase as clinicians become more familiar with their appropriate utilization and interpretation. It is anticipated that the use of CT in patients with penetrating trauma to the abdomen will increase with shortening of exposure times and with increasing availability.

PENETRATING RENAL TRAUMA

Penetrating trauma to the kidney presents a complicated management protocol for the emergency physician because it is not often found in an isolated state. In a series of patients seen over a 5-year period at Detroit General Hospital, 80 percent of all penetrating renal injuries were associated with other intraabdominal injuries that required surgery. Approximately 7 percent of gunshot wounds to the abdomen involved direct penetration to the kidney or its attendant structures, and about 6 percent of all abdominal stab wounds involved a similar type of injury. Consequently, back and flank wounds should be carefully evaluated through urinalysis and IVP to rule out renal injury.

Penetrating injury to the kidney parenchyma alone is not at-tended by a terribly high mortality rate. However, because of the large number of associated injuries, often involving major vessel trauma, penetrating renal injury can pose a grave problem. If penetration to the kidney is associated with disruption of the inferior vena cava or aorta, the mortality rate is 55 to 60 percent. Injury from direct penetration to the renal pedicle is relatively uncommon but, when present, is frequently associated with the loss of a kidney. Twelve of 33 patients seen at Ben Taub Hospital with renal vascular injury secondary to penetrating trauma died. Eleven patients who survived required nephrectomy.

Clinical Features

The single most useful laboratory test is the urinalysis. The above study revealed microscopic or macroscopic hematuria in 70 to 88 percent of the patients. Again, we must repeat the caution to thoroughly evaluate the patient with suspected penetrating renal injury and no hematuria.

Radiologic evaluation by IVP is most often diagnostic in revealing either extravasation or delayed visualization. Should there be nonvisualization of a kidney, renal arteriography is helpful in evaluating the pedicle injury and provides information for the surgeon in the event of a nephrectomy.

Treatment

Penetrating wounds of the kidney are classified as either major or minor. Major wounds include those that involve multiple lacerations, major pole damage, or complete shattering of the renal parenchyma. Minor injuries generally include a single simple puncture or stab wound of the kidney. A major injury, such as a gunshot wound to the pedicle, is generally treated by primary surgical repair of the kidney, or nephrectomy. Injuries classified as minor, such as a single stab wound to the upper pole, are usually observed and followed with repeat IVP. Many urologic and trauma surgeons believe that any retroperitoneal hematoma, which is not expanding even though extravasation is demonstrated, should not be explored surgically.

URETERAL INJURY

The ureter courses through the retroperitoneum, and its attachment to the kidney is delicate and unsupported by fascia. It may be injured by extreme blunt abdominal trauma, and vertebral or pelvic fractures. In children, a sparsity of retroperitoneal fat allows more frequent injury.

Injury to the ureter is generally a result of external violence or a complication of a surgical procedure. In the case of external violence, 95 percent of ureteral injuries are the result of gunshot wounds. Those that result from a high-velocity missile are the most difficult to treat and have the worst prognosis. Stab wounds to the ureter are rare. One report lists only two ureteral injuries seen in 947 patients suffering stab wounds to the abdomen. Blunt injury occasionally causes ureteral disruption, usually by avulsion, and is most often associated with falls or accidents involving rapid deceleration.

Gynecologic, obstetric, and urologic procedures are associated with a 0.5 to 10 percent incidence of ureteral damage. This incidence is present in patients who have had surgery involving the pelvis, abdomen, or both.

Clinical Features

On examination of the trauma patient, again hematuria is the most consistent finding. In a review of 29 ureteral injuries, 10 caused by external violence and 19 by surgical trauma, hematuria was present 90 percent of the time in those suffering external violence, while it was present only 11 percent of the time in those suffering surgical trauma.

Intravenous pyelography in all categories of patients with ureteral injury demonstrates extravasation of contrast material in about 42 percent and obstruction in about 58 percent (Fig. 123-2). The high incidence of obstruction is certainly due to the many injuries caused by intraoperative ligation of the ureter. Retrograde pyelography evaluated by a urologist is often helpful in localizing the exact site of injury.

Injuries to the ureter are never life-threatening on their own but are almost always associated with a life-threatening injury. Because of this, injury to the ureter must be suspected and looked for if it is to be diagnosed.

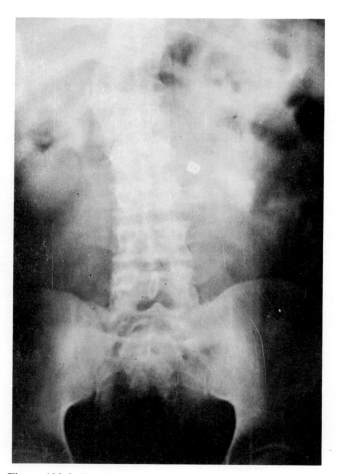

Figure 123-2. Gunshot wound of left ureter with extravasation of contrast material into retroperitoneal space as seen by IVP. (Courtesy of Detroit General Hospital.)

Treatment

Therapy for ureteral injury remains somewhat controversial but often involves construction of a water-tight anastomosis and the placing of a ureteral stent. This stent is generally a small Silastic tube placed within the lumen of the ureter. This allows the ureter to heal over the stent, which is then generally removed through the bladder. More extensive injury may require reimplantation or a transureteroureterostomy. If all or nearly all the ureter is damaged, renal autotransplantation into the pelvis must be performed. The prognosis for a patient suffering ureteral injury is generally good if the injury is recognized early and treated appropriately.

BLADDER TRAUMA

Patients who have lower abdominal or pelvic injury must be carefully evaluated for injury to the bladder. Blunt trauma is the cause of 75 to 90 percent of all bladder injuries. In patients with blunt trauma that results in a ruptured bladder, about 70 percent have a pelvic fracture. The converse is that about 10 percent of patients with a pelvic fracture have a ruptured bladder. Therefore, the association between these two injuries is extremely important. Although less frequent than blunt trauma, penetrating trauma causes between 10 and 25 percent of all bladder injuries.

Clinical Features

The infant bladder is entirely an abdominal organ and, therefore, when it is injured, peritoneal signs and findings will be present. The adult bladder is a pelvic organ that is protected by the bony pelvis and rises out of the pelvis only when distended. This means that peritoneal signs are infrequent and diagnosis must depend on other historical and physical findings.

The types of bladder injuries and attendant frequencies are as follows:

- Contusion, 20 to 44 percent
- Extraperitoneal rupture, 28 to 44 percent
- Intraperitoneal rupture, 13 to 48 percent
- Combined, 10 to 14 percent

Microscopic or macroscopic hematuria, dysuria, lower abdominal pain, and occasionally shock are associated with injury to the bladder.

The cystogram is the most helpful diagnostic study available to the emergency physician when trauma to the bladder is suspected (Fig. 123-3). The cystogram is obtained by filling the bladder by gravity flow through a Foley catheter with a 30 to 60 percent iodine-containing contrast material (generally 200 to 300 mL). After gravity flow is completed, another 50 mL of contrast material may be added to the bladder and the catheter clamped. Roentgenograms are obtained in the oblique and anteroposterior positions (Fig. 123-4). It is important to obtain a postevacuation film of the bladder to assess the posterior aspect of the pelvis, where extravasation may occur. Note that, as previously mentioned, the cystogram should be performed after the IVP has been done.

The use of an IVP to diagnose a ruptured bladder is unreliable. Only 11 percent of patients with a proven bladder rupture demonstrate extravasation on intravenous pyelography.

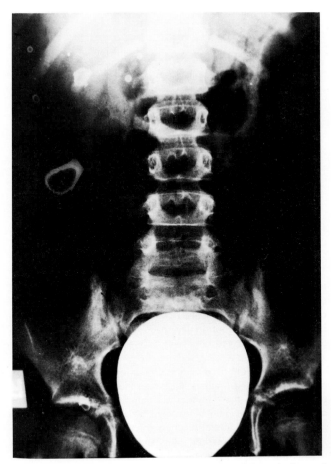

Figure 123-3. Normal cystogram. (Courtesy of Detroit General Hospital.)

Abnormal findings on cystogram include a teardrop-shaped bladder, elevation of the bladder, and extravasation of contrast material into the pelvis or into the peritoneal cavity.

Bladder injuries causing rupture are classified as extraperitoneal and intraperitoneal. Of all blunt injuries to the bladder, 75 percent are extraperitoneal and are generally associated with fractures of the pubis or the pubic rami. Twenty-five percent are intraperitoneal and generally secondary to direct trauma to the distended bladder such as that suffered from a kick or blow. This type of injury is frequently seen with lap seat belts worn in automobiles. Injury from penetrating wounds depends on the site of entry and the trajectory of the penetrating missile or instrument.

Other bladder injuries the emergency physician may see include (1) injury following a procedure done in the urologist's office, such as instrumentation to remove a bladder calculus; and (2) rupture of the bladder from long-term use of an indwelling Foley catheter. One should also be aware of a condition called "spontaneous" bladder rupture. This is not entirely spontaneous in that all such patients demonstrate preexisting bladder wall disease or abnormality. Minor trauma can precede rupture and the physician must maintain a high level of suspicion to make the diagnosis. The patient has lower abdominal pain and hematuria and the diagnosis is confirmed by cystogram. Because of the difficulty in making the diagnosis and the general debilitated state of the patient, spontaneous bladder rupture has a 50 percent mortality rate.

URETHRAL TRAUMA

Urethral trauma in the male is classified into anterior urethral injury, occurring distal to the urogenital diaphragm; and posterior urethral injury, occurring proximal to the urogenital diaphragm. The anterior urethra is comprised of the penile and bulbous urethra, whereas the posterior urethra is comprised of the membranous and prostatic urethra (Fig. 123-5).

The urogenital diaphragm is a 1.5-cm fascial layer that lies between the ischial rami. It is traversed by the membranous urethra. Injury to the urogenital diaphragm may damage the urinary continence mechanism or may disrupt the autonomic nerves involved in sexual potency in the male.

Posterior Urethral Injury

Ten to 20 percent of all pelvic fractures in the male are associated with posterior urethral injury. Fracture of the pelvis is by far the most common cause of this type of injury; however, it can be caused by gunshot wounds, shotgun blasts, or stab wounds. Fracture of the pubic rami or the ischium most particularly involves severance of the urethra just above the urogenital diaphragm. When this occurs, there is an upward and posterior displacement of both the prostate and the bladder. This displacement can be felt on

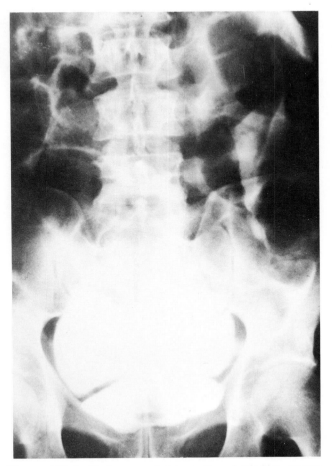

Figure 123-4. Cystogram of intraperitoneal bladder rupture. (Courtesy of Detroit General Hospital.)

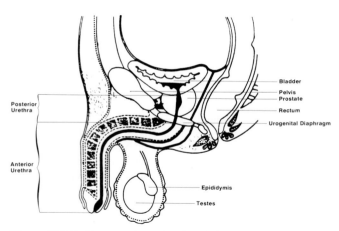

Figure 123-5. Cross section of male pelvis revealing penile urethra, bulbous urethra, membranous urethra within the urogenital diaphragm, and the prostatic urethra.

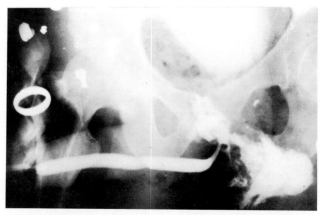

Figure 123-7. Shotgun blast injury of the prostatic urethra with contrast extravasation as seen in retrograde urethrogram.

rectal examination in that the prostatic fossa becomes boggy and quite edematous.

The patient suffering posterior urethral trauma is generally unable to void, and may have blood present at the urethral meatus. Under no circumstances should the patient be catheterized because this type of instrumentation can cause further injury. Intravenous pyelogram may be helpful in pointing the emergency physician to the diagnosis of posterior urethral trauma when a teardrop-shaped bladder is present or when the bladder is significantly elevated off the symphysis pubis.

The most helpful diagnostic study is the retrograde urethrogram which involves the retrograde injection of 8 to 10 mL of a 20% aqueous iodine-containing contrast material (Fig. 123-6). The contrast mixture is injected into the urethral meatus with a sterile 50-mL, catheter-tip syringe. X-ray films are obtained in the oblique position and readily reveal the disruption of the posterior urethra (Fig. 123-7).

In the past, primary repair was attempted on patients with posterior urethral injury but it was found to have a very high incidence of impotence and incontinence. At the present time, suprapubic cystostomy is the treatment of choice and no attempt is made to explore or drain the retropubic space. If healing results in a urethral stricture, delayed urethroplasty is performed 3 to 4 months after injury.

Several areas of special consideration exist when dealing with pelvic fracture and urethral injuries in the male child and in the female, although these injuries are unusual. In the male child, a urethral catheter should be avoided because it results in a high incidence of penal-scrotal junction stricture.

In the female with urethral injury and pelvic fracture, the urethra tears at the bladder neck and is therefore associated with vaginal rupture. This requires operative intervention because of the high incidence of urethral-vaginal fistulae.

Anterior Urethral Trauma

Trauma to the anterior urethra is generally the result of a blunt or straddle injury. However, it may be the result of a gunshot wound, a shotgun blast, or a stab wound, and can even be self-inflicted. Penetrating injury is fairly easy to evaluate by retrograde urethrography. Presenting features of blunt injury will often include pain, swelling, and ecchymoses in the perineum, and blood at the urethral meatus. This again should be evaluated by retrograde urethrography. The therapeutic modalities for handling anterior urethral injury are somewhat controversial. Generally a minimal urethral tear with no extravasation is treated with an indwelling urethral catheter for 7 to 10 days. A complete tear of the anterior urethra is generally treated by initial exploration and primary anastomosis. Stricture formation following either treatment is seen in approximately 15 to 25 percent of all cases.

GENITAL TRAUMA

Penile Trauma

Injury to the penis is caused by penetrating objects such as a gunshot or knife wound, by avulsion as in industrial injury, or by strangulation as may occur when a ring is placed on the penile

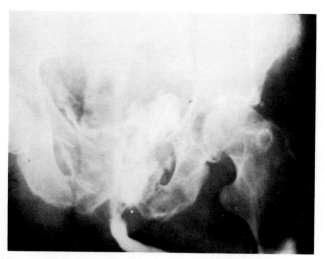

Figure 123-6. Retrograde urethrogram revealing pelvic fracture and rupture of the membranous urethra. (Courtesy of Detroit General Hospital.)

shaft. The types of injury seen include complete transection or amputation of the penile shaft, incomplete amputation, and avulsion of the penile skin. Injury is usually easily seen on physical examination, but strangulation injury may result in delayed necrosis from ischemia. The integrity of the penile urethra should be evaluated by retrograde urethrography.

The aim of initial therapy is to do everything possible to maintain penile length. Urologic consultation is mandatory if debridement or penile shortening is anticipated. The therapeutic goal is to preserve cosmetic appearance while maintaining fertility and sexual potency.

Scrotal and Testicular Trauma

Injury to the scrotum and its contents may be caused by penetrating or blunt trauma. A superficial laceration requires cleansing and primary closure by the emergency physician. When evaluating deep penetrating wounds in which testicular injury is suspected, immediate operative exploration and repair is indicated.

A scrotal hematoma should be treated with ice packs, scrotal elevation, analgesia, and observation for increase in size. If there is avulsion of the scrotum or the testes one should obtain hemostasis, cover the avulsed area with pads moistened with saline solution, and refer the patient to the urologist.

Vulvar Trauma

Vulvar injury occurs secondary to a fall on a sharp object, direct blunt trauma, or missile penetration. Injuries involving the vulva often extend into contiguous structures such as the vagina, rectum, bladder, or urethra.

Careful examination of the perineum, pelvis, and rectum are necessary for correct diagnosis. It may be necessary to examine children under anesthesia, while radiologic evaluation is generally needed to detect a foreign body. Again, retrograde urethrography is indicated to assure urethral continuity. The management goal is to restore normal anatomic relationships and function.

BIBLIOGRAPHY

Bright TC III, Peters PC: Ureteral injuries due to external violence: Ten years' experience with 59 cases. *J Trauma* 17:616–620, 1977.

Brosman SA, Fay R: Diagnosis and management of bladder trauma. *J Trauma* 13:687–694, 1973.

Brower P, Paul J, Browman SA: Urinary tract abnormalities presenting as a result of blunt abdominal trauma. *J Trauma* 18:719–722, 1978.

Cass AS: Bladder trauma in the multiple injured patient. *J Urol* 115:667–669, 1976.

Del Villar RG, Ireland GW, Cass AS: Management of bladder and urethral injury in conjunction with the immediate surgical treatment of the acute severe trauma patient. *J Urol* 108:581–585, 1972.

Eickenberg H, Amin M: Gunshot wounds to the ureter. *J Trauma* 16:562–565, 1976.

Jones TK, Walsh JW, Maull KD: Diagnostic imagining in blunt trauma of the abdomen. *Surg Gynecol Obstet* 157:389–398, 1983.

MacMahon R, et al: Management of blunt injury to the lower urinary tract. *Can J Surg* 26:415–418, 1983.

McDonald EJ, Korobkin M. Jacobs RP, et al: The role of emergency excretory urography in evaluation of blunt, abdominal trauma. *Am J Roentgenol* 126:739–742, 1976.

McElfresh EC, Bryan RS: Power take-off injuries. *J Trauma* 13:775–782, 1973.

Peters PC (ed): Symposium on urologic emergencies. *Urol Clin North Am* 9:251–254; 285–296, 1982.

Pontes JE: Urologic injuries. *Surg Clin North Am* 57:77–96, 1977.

Thompson IM, Carlton EC Jr (eds): Symposium on genitourinary trauma. *Urol Clin North Am* 4:1–163, 1977.

Wein AJ, Arger PH, Murphy JT: Controversial aspects of blunt renal trauma. *J Tauma* 17:662–666, 1977.

CHAPTER 124
BASIC MANAGEMENT
OF FRACTURES
AND DISLOCATIONS

Joseph F. Waeckerle

INTRODUCTION

The following is a brief synopsis of the pathophysiology and treatment of fractures and dislocations. Its purpose is to supplement the knowledge of the emergency physician with regard to some orthopedic problems often seen in the emergency department. It is not intended to be a complete discussion of fractures or their treatment. Recommended readings are offered at the end of the synopsis.

Definitions

Fracture—A fracture is a complete or incomplete break in the continuity of a bone.

Complete fracture—A fracture which extends all the way through the bone and involves both cortexes as well as the medullary system.

Incomplete fracture—An incomplete fracture or torus, buckle, or greenstick fracture is a fracture in which only one cortex and possibly the medullary system is involved but the opposite cortex remains intact.

Closed fracture—A closed fracture does not communicate with the external environment through overlying soft tissue injuries.

Open fracture—An open fracture communicates with the external environment through a soft tissue injury. It may be produced by a force from outside such as a projectile or by the bone itself damaging the soft tissue and puncturing the skin.

Comminuted fracture—A comminuted fracture has three or more fragments.

Impacted fracture—An impacted fracture has one of the fragments driven into the cancellous opposite fragment.

Avulsion fracture—An avulsion fracture, or pull-off fracture, most commonly is due to a ligament or tendon being stronger than the bone and pulling off a fragment of the bone at its attachment.

Description

Fractures may be described in several ways: (1) by anatomic location—that is, whether they occur at the proximal, middle, or distal area of the bone or whether they are supracondylar or subtrochanteric, etc.; (2) by the direction of the fracture line—a transverse line, an oblique line, which is usually less than 45°, and a spiral line, which is an oblique fracture combined with a rotatory component; (3) by the number of fragments present—a linear fracture, two components, or a comminuted fracture, three or more fragments; (4) by complete or incomplete defects in the bone; (5) by the presence of impaction or angulation, i.e., alignment; and (6) by the fact that the fracture is open or closed.

CLASSIFICATION OF FRACTURES BY MECHANISM OF INJURY

Direct Trauma

Fractures which are the result of the direct application of a force over the fracture site are divided into three classifications. The first is the *"tapping"* fracture, which is more commonly understood as a nightstick fracture. This is a linear fracture through the bone with little or no soft tissue involvement. The second fracture seen with direct trauma is a *crush fracture*. The bone is usually comminuted or transversely fractured due to such forces. There is also extensive soft tissue injury associated with this fracture. The third fracture encountered with direct forces is *penetrating*. Emergency physicians often see such injuries associated with missile wounds. It must be kept in mind that such projectile injuries are usually classified into high- and low-velocity injuries as determined by the kinetic energy of the bullet which varies directly with the square of its velocity and with its mass ($\frac{1}{2} mV^2$). High-velocity projectiles, greater than 650 to 800 meters/s, cause extensive soft tissue injuries due to fragmentation of bone which produces secondary missiles and a cavitation phenomenon. In contrast, low-velocity missiles produce little in the way of soft tissue injury and fragmentation of the bone. The treatment and prognosis vary considerably for the two types of missile wounds so an attempt must be made to document the source as best as possible.

Indirect Trauma

Fractures produced by loads acting at a distance from the fracture site are the result of indirect trauma. They are classified into traction or tension, angulation, rotational, compression, and combinations of the above. *Traction* or *tension* fractures are usually transverse fractures which are the result of the bone being pulled apart. *Angulation* fractures are the result of the long axis of the bone being angulated so that the convex portion is under tension stress and the concave portion is under compression stress. As a result, a transverse fracture occurs with frequent splintering of the cortex under compression. *Rotational* stress or torque produces spiral fractures. Pure rotational stress or torque is rare and it is more commonly associated with an axial load or force. The result is an oblique fracture which is usually equal to or less than 45°. *Compression* forces act on the longitudinal axis of the bone and produce axial loading. The result of such forces is "T" or "Y" fractures.

Any combination of the above forces can be seen as one would expect. Angulation and axial loading produce oblique fractures with splintering. A common example of this is a butterfly fragment associated with an oblique fracture. Fractures may also be produced by angulation with a rotational load. Such fractures are long and sharp spiral fractures. As mentioned above, rotational fractures are commonly associated with compression injuries and usually cause oblique fractures of less than 45°.

Pathologic Fractures

Pathologic fractures are due to a weakness in the bone secondary to a disease process but are not necessarily associated with any recognized force or injury. It is essential that, when an emergency physician sees a fracture without any discernible cause, a pathologic fracture be considered and the underlying etiology pursued. The etiologies may be divided into general and local causes. Some common examples of general diseases of the bone that cause pathologic fractures are osteoporosis, developmental abnormalities, nutritional and hormonal disorders, hematopoietic diseases, and Paget's disease of the bone. There are many causes for a localized disease of the bone such as cysts, benign and malignant tumors, infections, irradiation, and neurotrophic problems such as syphilis, diabetes, osteomyelitis, and syringomyelia.

Another commonly seen fracture in today's athletic society is the *stress* fracture. As mentioned previously, repeated or cyclic stresses will cause fatigue on all tissues which bear those forces. As the tissues absorb the forces acting upon them, they must store some of these forces. When the muscle and soft tissue, which are absorbing the loads along with the bone, begin to fatigue, there is a greater concentration of load upon the bone itself. After the bone becomes sufficiently fatigued, it will fail, resulting in a stress fracture. Stress fractures may be difficult to see on x-ray yet are very painful. They should be suspected in any athletic person who presents with appropriate history and clinical findings. These fractures frequently are not seen on the first x-ray examination and may require a second examination 10 to 14 days later, or a bone scan.

COMPLICATIONS OF FRACTURES

There are many complications of fractures of which the emergency physician should be aware. The immediate complications of fractures are damage to the neurovascular system and associated soft tissue or visceral injuries. All patients who present to the emergency department with possible fractures should have an assessment of the neurovascular status above and below the fracture site recorded on the medical record. An intermediate complication is fat embolism. Long-term sequelae of fractures include nonunion, avascular necrosis, angulation deformities, shortening, overgrowth, infection, joint stiffness, posttraumatic ossification, and posttraumatic arthritis.

HEALING

Primary healing is defined as *union*. Once primary union takes place, consolidation and remodeling, which are determined by the stress loads acting upon the bone, will take place. Healing is affected by a number of conditions. Favorable conditions for healing include: fractures through cancellous bone; adequate blood supply, which is especially prevalent at the ends of bones; minimal soft tissue injuries adjacent to the bone; minimal hematoma surrounding the fracture site; impaction, spiral, or oblique fractures with good apposition; and absence of infection.

In contrast, there are unfavorable conditions which retard bone healing. These include poor apposition with separation or distraction of the fragment ends; severe comminution; severe soft tissue damage with large fracture hematomas; shearing or rotatory forces producing the fracture; loss of blood supply to the area; infection of the fracture site; and metabolic or systemic disorders which affect the patient's ability to heal.

CLINICAL FEATURES OF FRACTURES

The history is of the utmost importance in evaluating any fracture. If the patient is able to recall the mechanism of injury, it is of great help to the physician as it may have diagnostic and therapeutic implications. Keep in mind that there may not be a good history of mechanism of injury obtainable with a pathologic or fatigue fracture. The past medical history is helpful in determining whether the patient has had prior injury to the area and has been in good health prior to the injury, and to elicit any known allergies, medical problems, and medications, if any, including the use of aspirin.

PHYSICAL EXAMINATION

The physical examination usually demonstrates some or all of the classic findings associated with fractures. These include local swelling, deformities seen or felt due to muscle spasm or angulation of the bone, ecchymoses, tenderness and pain (provided the patient's neurological status is intact), loss of function of the extremity secondary to the pain and loss of the lever arm (this is not necessarily seen with greenstick, impaction, or fatigue fractures), crepitus, abnormal mobility, and lastly, the patient's attitude. Crepitus with abnormal mobility is pathognomonic for fractures. The patient's attitude may be very helpful, as the physician can ascertain how the patient guards the injured area and carries himself or herself to protect the injured area. An appropriate clinical evaluation must always include a primary survey with attention to the ABCs of resuscitation to rule out any life-threatening emergencies. A fractured spine, some pelvic fractures, and, rarely, a fractured femur may produce life-threatening emergencies but, again, this is an exception.

Once the primary survey is completed and the patient is stabilized, the secondary survey can be carried out, at which time a careful physicial examination of the affected area should be performed to ascertain the presence of a fracture. During the secondary survey, a detailed neurovascular assessment above and below the injured area must be done and documented. Associated soft tissue injuries, especially the presence of an open wound, also should be documented. Any visceral damage, especially when the fractures involve areas such as the scapula, ribs, clavicle, and pelvis, should be ruled out. Lastly, examination of adjacent bone and joints should always be done. If there was enough force produced to fracture one bone, there might be enough force to fracture other bones or damage the joints. Neighboring fractures or joint injuries are often overlooked, i.e., a fractured femur with a dislocated hip joint or a fractured tibia with a posterior cruciate ligament injury.

RADIOGRAPHIC EXAMINATION

X-rays are always essential in the appropriate evaluation of an orthopedic complaint. They aid the physician in detecting fractures and evaluating their seriousness, indirectly assessing ligamentous integrity, looking for complicating factors, and following results of treatment. There are times when the clinical findings and the x-rays are both positive; conversely, there are times when the clinical findings are negative but the x-rays are positive; and there are times when the x-rays are negative but the clinical findings are suspicious enough to warrant therapy. It should always be remembered that at least two views showing trabecular detail taken at right angles to each other are required to properly assess any bony injury. Special views may be needed to determine the angulation and severity of injury of some fracture sites. Comparison views of the opposite side may be helpful, especially in children with open epiphyses. Another point to remember in x-raying long bones is that the joints above and below must be included to have a complete radiographic examination. Often there are associated injuries to the joints when a long bone is fractured. If no fracture is visible but the patient has positive clinical findings, the patient should be treated conservatively and subsequent x-rays ordered after a 7-to-10-day wait to see if a fracture line appears.

In determining primary healing of a bone, that is, bony union, one must evaluate the patient clinically and radiographically. Clinically, there should be no motion, crepitus, or tenderness at the fracture site. On x-ray, the physician should see bony trabeculae across the fracture. Such trabeculation demonstrates that the fracture union is mature. Earlier in the course of healing, a visible callus bridging the fragments is seen. This callus should start to form within 5 to 7 days after the injury but may not be seen on x-ray for several weeks depending on the bone involved.

GENERAL PRINCIPLES OF TREATMENT

The proper handling of a patient with a possible fracture is important. The patient's area of injury should be immobilized in a comfortable position which causes no impingement upon the neurovascular status. Moreover, such immobilization should prevent further movement, soft tissue or neurovascular injuries, and pain; help decrease the incidence of shock and fat embolism; and lastly, ease the transportation of the patient.

Definitive Treatment

Once the patient is stabilized, the physician is ready to treat the fracture. The physician should attempt to achieve as close-to-perfect an anatomical alignment of the fracture site as possible with the hope of returning normal function and appearance to the patient within the shortest period of time. As the human body will remodel and reshape with time, accurate apposition of fragments is not always necessary, especially if no angular or rotational deformities exist and shortening is not too great. However, it is essential that the physician attempt to restore the normal planes of functions of the joints above and below the fracture site. It is also important that articular fractures be near-perfectly repositioned. Two other principles should be kept in mind: the reduction should be done as soon as possible without jeopardizing the patient; and the physician should never forcefully manipulate a fracture to attain anatomic alignment.

Closed Reduction

There are certain times when closed reduction is not indicated: when there is no displacement of significance, when no reduction is possible for whatever reason, when the physician is unable to hold the reduction, when the fracture is the result of a traction stress, and when there is no soft tissue bridge to act as a hinge to reduce the fracture. Fractures are reduced by traction or traction and manipulative measures. Traction requires a soft tissue bridge to act as a hinge and hold the fracture site in apposition. Reduction by traction may be obstructed or inhibited if there is a large hematoma present at the fracture site, if some soft tissue is obstructing apposition of the bone, or if the bone has "buttonholed" through the soft tissue. Traction is always in the longitudinal axis of the bone. When one attempts to manipulate a fracture while traction is being applied, the physician should manipulate the distal fragment, which is the fragment that can be moved and controlled, rather than the proximal fragment, which usually cannot be moved or controlled.

Anesthesia is essential for the comfort of the patient and the attainment of an anatomic reduction. There are a number of ways of anesthetizing an area to achieve reduction. These include local infiltration into the fracture hematoma with an anesthetic agent, regional intravenous anesthesia into the extremity, a regional nerve block, and intravenous sedation, which causes some amnesia. General anesthesia may be required, especially in children.

Immobilization

Immobilization of a fracture site, once reduction has taken place, is utilized to relieve the pain, help prevent further stresses on the fracture site, and maintain the reduction. It must be kept in mind that immobilization should be done so that the joints which are not involved are free to move, especially in adults, and that the patient is able to ambulate and move about as much as possible and as soon as possible. Immobilization of a fracture site may be done by plaster or synthetic casting, traction, or internal fixation. Only immobilization using plaster or synthetic casting will be discussed in this synopsis.

Plaster is a muslin cloth impregnated with dextrose or starch and a calcium sulfate hemihydrated salt. The plaster, when combined with water, adds another water molecule to the calcium sulfate, which causes crystallization and an exothermic reaction. If the physician wishes to retard the crystallization of the plaster, he or she may either use colder water or add salt to the water. The setting time of the plaster is directly proportional to the temperature of the water and to the amount of heat produced by the reaction of the calcium taking on another water molecule. The hotter the water, the shorter the setting time and the more heat produced. Enough heat can be produced to cause discomfort to the patient and burns can occur without proper protection.

There are some basic rules when applying either a circular or splint cast. Usually one immobilizes the joint above and below a fracture site. Also, one should hold the reduction with the plaster, which requires an appropriately snug fit utilizing stockinet, wadding, and the plaster as the three layers of the cast. More wadding should be utilized if the physician anticipates swelling, and all bony prominences should be well padded before applying the plaster.

Application of a Circular Plaster Cast

There are some helpful hints in applying a circular cast to a patient. Before the physician dips the plaster, the first 2 to 3 in should be unwrapped so that the end is easily found. Lukewarm water is used in most instances. The plaster roll should be the largest size possible to apply to the affected area. It should be dipped in the water until no bubbles come from the plaster. While it is in the water or once removed, the physician should pinch both ends of the plaster and allow the excess water to drain, but should not twist the plaster. By pinching the ends, the unwanted "roll off" of the plaster will be inhibited.

The plaster should always be applied in the same direction as the wadding, and should be rolled by the dominant hand without taking the roll off the patient at any time. There should be a 50 percent overlap as one applies the plaster, and the roll should always be moving. The physician should use the palms and thenar eminences and not the fingers in applying the plaster. As the extremity changes circumference, "tucks" may be employed by the physician to ensure there are no irregularities in the plaster. This should be done at the lower border where the circumference change is the greatest and should be done by the nondominant hand. The plaster should be applied with minimal tension and at no time should the direction of the plaster be reversed. Once a roll is applied it should be smoothed and molded in the opposite direction of the application with the palm and thenar eminences of the hands so that a homogeneous plaster cast is produced.

Once the appropriate number of layers are utilized to immobilize the joint, further manipulation of the fracture site to ensure appropriate reduction may be done while the plaster is still wet. As mentioned above, it should be done with the palms and thenar eminences and must be done before crystallization occurs because

if the plaster sets up and then is fractured, it will not recrystallize and the benefits of the plaster cast are lost. The plaster cast should be applied so that it is slightly too long on the patient. It then can be trimmed and cut back to the appropriate length, after which the stockinet may be rolled or turned back and smoothed with one small layer of plaster roll. Once the plaster is applied, manipulated, and smoothed, it must be allowed to set up. Plaster will harden within 15 to 30 min but will not totally set up for approximately 24 h. No weight-bearing should be allowed during that time nor should the cast be made wet after it has set.

Splints

Splints are utilized in certain situations, especially by the emergency physician, to treat fractures. They allow for swelling and the area surrounding the fracture site to be visualized and treated as needed; and they allow for appropriate immobilization without the feared sequelae of neurovascular compromise. There are also a number of ways of making a splint, but basically a splint is a layer of stockinet, with or without wadding, and approximately 10 layers of plaster cut to the proper length. The ends of the splint should be molded and smoothed so as to prevent harm to the patient. The splint should be applied dripping wet, affixed by a cotton or elastic bandage. It must be emphasized that the cotton or elastic bandage should not be wrapped too tightly. One does not wish to compromise neurovascular status by the cotton or elastic wrap, which is why the physician put the splint on in the first place. Numerous premade splints are available and useful, if they serve to comfortably immobilize the desired area.

Synthetic Materials

Synthetic casts have been on the market for a period of time. In the past, they have required a special light source or other mechanism to initiate their conforming to the fracture site. Recently, new materials have been introduced which can be dipped into cold water, rolled similar to plaster, and easily molded. The advantages of a synthetic cast are many: It is light and comfortable, long-wearing; water-resistant; and the patient may bear weight within 20 min of application. It is especially useful as the second cast. As mentioned above, the new products are much more easily utilized and convenient than older ones, but application and use still takes some practice.

Complications of Immobilization by Plaster

There are obviously complications with any form of treatment, and the use of plaster is no exception. Any loose-fitting cast which allows movement will produce plaster sores, abrasions, and possibly infection, as well as possible loss of reduction. On the other hand, any tight-fitting cast which does not allow the limb to swell, especially if applied acutely, may compromise neurovascular status. The patient should always be instructed to return to the emergency department or call the physician should the area distal to the fracture site or encompassed by the cast hurt an increasing or inordinate amount, or tingle. Moreover, the physician should perform a cast check within the first 24 to 36 h to assess the neurovascular status of the patient, keeping in mind the five P's: pain, pallor, paresthesia, pulselessness, and paralysis. A good rule to follow to avoid such complications is that no circular cast should be applied to a fracture site with excessive swelling or circulatory insufficiency, or to patients with impaired sensation from any cause. It should be reiterated that the amount of wadding or padding utilized prior to the application of the plaster is somewhat determined by the anticipated swelling, as well as by the need to protect the bony prominences. As the swelling subsides and the second cast is applied, less padding will be utilized, so that the immobilization is continued over the fracture area. All fractures, whether splinted or cast, should be elevated, iced, and rested during the first 2 to 3 days.

If a patient presents in the emergency department with evidence of severe swelling causing any neurovascular impingement or hint of neurovascular impingement, the circular cast should be split throughout its entire length. The padding and stockinet are then divided with scissors and the entire cast is spread to decrease the edema and hopefully restore circulation. If the physician must divide the cast the cast, wadding, and stockinet are split on opposite sides of the cast and the cast is fixed with cotton elastic bandages.

It is appropriate to inform the patient of not only what to look for in the way of neurovascular compromise should swelling occur, but also that some movement at the fracture site may be experienced until a callus begins to form. Also, it is wise to inform the patient that some itching will occur under the cast during the course of healing; it is dangerous to utilize hangers or wires or other instruments to scratch, as it could induce injury and infection.

Open Fractures

Possibly the single most important factor in management of the fracture is the treatment of the overlying soft tissues. If the soft tissue over a fracture is violated, then attention should be paid to this injury first. It should be appropriately cleaned and debrided and a decision made as to whether a primary or secondary closure is required. If the wound communicates with the fracture, surgical irrigation and debridement is required. The decision on prophylactic antibiotics as well as the use of tetanus and tetanus immune globulin should be made within 3 h of the time of injury so that maximum benefits may be achieved. If a cast is needed to immobilize the fracture, a window may be incorporated into it so that the healing of the soft tissue injury can be monitored. A helpful hint to determine the location of the soft tissue injury is to apply an increased amount of dressing over the soft tissue injury prior to the casting so that a bulge is visible once the cast is completed. This bulge can then be cut out with the cast saw, creating a properly placed window.

Dislocations

Dislocation is a complete disruption of a joint so that no articular surfaces are in contact. A subluxation, in contrast, is a partial disruption of the articular surface; it is more commonly associated with a fracture.

Clinical features of dislocation are similar to those of a fracture. The patient experiences pain, loss of normal anatomy and motion, as well as guarding the joint. To appropriately evaluate an injured joint requires radiographic examination. Two views at right angles are especially essential in the correct evaluation of a joint. Neurovascular examination is also very important, as there is an in-creased incidence of neurovascular injuries with dislocations, especially in the knee and shoulder. Postreduction films, as well as postreduction examination, should be completed and charted.

Children's Fractures

Children's fractures differ from adult fractures. While adults are exposed to a great variety of injuries which can fracture bones, the causes of fractures in children are usually very simple, i.e., direct forces. Bone changes and outcome of these fractures are usually predictable as long as the basic principles of treatment are followed.

The history, especially the mechanism of injury, is obviously more difficult to obtain in infants and children. Clinical findings do not differ greatly but the physician should be especially aware of the child's attitude. Infants and children will not assume any position or will not move in any way which causes pain. This should always be kept in mind by the physician when examining the infant or child.

X-rays are essential but more difficult to interpret in infants and children as ossification may not have occurred. Fractures through the epiphyseal plate (which are 15 percent of all children's fractures) require expertise in evaluation. It is, therefore, always prudent to x-ray the opposite (hopefully normal), corresponding area for comparison. Any defect is suspicious. A wrinkle or change in contour of the cortex (torus or buckle fracture) may be easily missed if one does not pay careful attention to the x-rays. Moreover, missing an epiphyseal fracture, which may subsequently cause growth disturbances, can produce permanent disability to the patient.

As mentioned, the principles of treatment are simple, with alignment being the most important factor. Although some angulation is acceptable in children, rotational deformities are not! Childrens' bones remodel in response to the lines of stress, thus making accurate anatomical reduction less important. The younger the child, the more proximal the fracture to the epiphyseal plate, the more remodeling will occur so more angulation is acceptable. This is especially true when the fracture is proximal to one of the body's hinge joints. As bone growth is often stimulated, some degree of overriding or side-to-side apposition is desirable in certain age groups, particularly in lower-extremity fractures.

Principles of treatment are similar to the adult but techniques do differ. Reduction is always gentle and may require general anesthesia. Immobilization of a child's fracture should be sufficient to prevent any deformity without causing discomfort. Sometimes in children, joints above and below fracture sites need to be immobilized due to the patient's activity. Permanent joint stiffness is virtually unknown in children in contrast to adults. Therefore, such joint immobilization is acceptable. The period of immobilization is less, as bone healing is rapid in children. Bone healing is inversely proportional to the age. The younger the patient, the faster the bone healing. Nonunions in children are uncommon and open reductions are rarely employed.

If there are clinical findings suggestive of a fracture, but none is seen on the x-ray, it is always wiser to treat the child conservatively with immobilization such as a volar splint. The job of the orthopedic surgeon or pediatrician who follows the patient is made easier due to the appropriate immobilization, ice, elevation, and rest.

CONCLUSION

In conclusion, the principles of caring for fractures require knowledge and experience. Understanding the basics of how fractures occur, how to diagnose and treat such injuries, how bones heal, and reduction and immobilization techniques, make the emergency physician competent and comfortable in evaluating the patient who presents to the emergency department. Moreover, proper evaluation and disposition is what every patient deserves, and our orthopedic colleagues greatly appreciate such competency as well.

BIBLIOGRAPHY

Blount WP: *Fractures in Children.* Baltimore, Williams & Wilkins Co, 1965, pp 1–8.

DePalma AF: Principles, in *The Management of Fractures and Dislocations,* ed 2. Philadelphia, WB Saunders Co, pp 1–116.

Eriksson E: *Illustrated Handbook in Local Anesthesia.* Chicago, Year Book Medical Publishers, 1969.

Lamid S, Wang R: The range of local anesthesia. *Drug Ther* 5:103–106; 115–118, August 1975.

Moore DC: *Regional Block: A Handbook for Use in the Clinical Practice of Medicine and Surgery,* ed. 4. Springfield, CC Thomas, 1978.

Patzakis MJ, Harvey JP Jr, Ivler B: The role of antibiotics in the management of open fractures. *J Bone Joint Surg* 56–A:532–541, 1974.

Rockwood CA Jr, Green DP (eds.): Principles of fractures and dislocations, in *Fractures,* ed 2. Philadelphia, JB Lippincott, 1984.

Salter RB, Harris WR: Injuries involving the epiphyseal plate. *J Bone Joint Surg* 45–A:587–622, 1963.

Schiller MG: Intravenous regional anesthesia for closed treatment of fractures and dislocations of the upper extremities. *Clin Orthop* 118:25–29, 1976.

Simon RR: *Orthopedics in Emergency Medicine: The Extremities.* New York, Appleton-Century-Crofts, 1982.

Tachdijian MO: Fractures and dislocations, in *Pediatric Orhopaedics.* Philadelphia, WB Saunders Co, 1972, pp 1532–1769.

CHAPTER 125
UPPER EXTREMITY
TRAUMA

John W. Packer

SHOULDER

The shoulder is made up of the clavicle, scapula, and humerus, and attached to the thorax by sternoclavicular joint and multiple muscle attachments. The ratio of motion between the glenohumeral joint and the thoracoscapular junction is 2:1 so that abduction and elevation of the shoulder is carried out as a combination of motions between the shoulder joint and the scapula.

Clavicle Fracture

The clavicle, the most commonly fractured bone at birth, is a bone frequently fractured in children by a fall on the point of the shoulder or on the outstretched arm. In children, the fracture is usually in the middle third of the clavicle with angulation in a greenstick fashion pointing superiorly. There is sometimes over-riding of the fracture fragments with shortening of the clavicle, necessitating a mechanism for pulling the clavicle back to its normal length. Length is restored by application of a figure-of-eight bandage or clavicle strap for protraction of the scapulae. In the adult, the fracture often occurs beyond the coracoclavicular ligaments toward the lateral end of the clavicle. These fractures must be treated quite similarly to an acromioclavicular (AC) dislocation.

Scapula Fracture

When seen early, fractures of the body of the scapula can often be diagnosed by localizing swelling outlining the triangular configuration of the scapula. Rib fractures and pulmonary contusions frequently accompany fractures of the scapula.

Sternoclavicular Joint Dislocation

Sternoclavicular joint dislocations occur in anterior and posterior directions. The anterior dislocation is treated with a clavicle strap and sling. The posterior dislocation can be an emergency because of encroachment upon vital structures in the mediastinum (trachea, esophagus, great vessels). The posterior dislocation can be reduced with retraction of the shoulders using a sandbag between

the shoulders, by applying a clavicle strap, or by grasping the clavicle with a towel clip and pulling it forward.

Acromioclavicular Joint Sprain (Dislocation)

Acromioclavicular joint injuries are classified by the degree of injury to the AC and coracoclavicular ligaments. In a first-degree sprain, the AC ligament is partially torn without subluxation of the joint. In a second-degree sprain, the AC joint is torn, allowing subluxation, but the coracoclavicular ligaments are not torn. In a third-degree sprain, both sets of ligaments are torn and there is a complete dislocation of the AC joint (Fig. 125-1).

Acromioclavicular injury can best be diagnosed clinically by localizing tenderness over the AC joint and over the coracoid process. With slight downward traction of the upper arm there is upriding of the clavicle in relation to the acromion. The upriding of the clavicle can be confirmed by anteroposterior roentgenograms of both clavicles, preferably in the same film, taken while the patient is standing and holding equal amounts of weight in both hands. Measurement between the coracoid process and the clavicle should be the same unless there is upriding of the clavicle. A patient with an AC dislocation can usually be treated with a sling and swathe. With marked upriding, special AC splints and straps may be necessary to hold the dislocation reduced, or surgical fixation should be used. Late excision of the distal clavicle will relieve symptoms of AC joint arthritis or excessive upriding of the clavicle.

Shoulder Dislocation

Dislocation of the shoulder is a common injury, particularly in young athletes. The most common direction for dislocation (95 percent) is the anterior or subcoracoid dislocation. The mechanism of injury is usually one that forces the shoulder into marked abduction and external rotation, simultaneously levering the head of the humerus out of the glenoid, tearing the anterior capsule and glenoid labrum with dislocation of the humeral head anteriorly. When the arm is brought to the side, the humeral head rests in a subcoracoid, anteriorly dislocated position. Marked muscle spasm causes pain and prevents easy reduction.

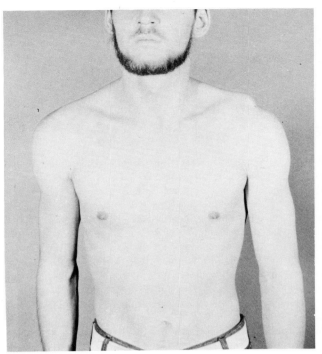

Figure 125-1. Third-degree sprain of acromioclavicular joint with upriding of the distal clavicle due to complete tear of acromioclavicular and coracoclavicular ligaments.

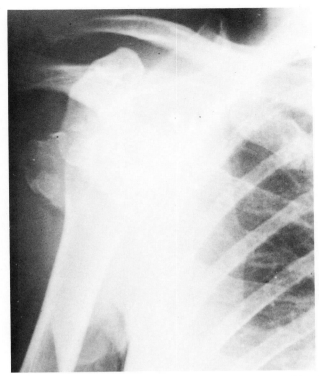

Figure 125-2. Anterior dislocation of the shoulder. Humeral head is in subcoracoid position. Note the fracture of the greater tuberosity.

The patient will have a history of a mechanism of injury usually into abduction and external rotation. There will be flattening of the normal contour over the deltoid muscle, prominence of the acromion, and sometimes the humeral head can be palpable anteriorly.

Roentgenograms will show the humeral head in a subcoracoid position (Fig. 125-2). An axillary view and a tangential scapular view will confirm that the head is anterior to the glenoid. It should be ascertained whether the greater tuberosity has been avulsed at the time of the dislocation. Any associated fracture, particularly of the surgical neck or humeral head, can complicate attempted reduction. If recognized, manipulation should be carried out under appropriate general or regional anesthesia to prevent disimpaction of such a fracture.

There is a much higher incidence of recurrent dislocation in young adults who have severe initial trauma or who have not had adequate initial immobilization. In a patient under the age of 30, the initial treatment should consist of closed reduction and immobilization of the shoulder in adduction and internal rotation by use of a Velpeau's bandage or shoulder immobilizer for at least 4 and usually 6 weeks.

In spite of this treatment, the chance of recurrent dislocation is great if there has been a tear of the glenoid labrum resulting in the Bankart lesion so that the glenoid labrum does not reattach to the glenoid rim during the healing process. In recurrent dislocation, the treatment is symptomatic and the long immobilization advised for the initial treatment is not necessary. Once the shoulder has had a recurrent dislocation, the chances of repeated dislocations are so great that surgical repair is advised.

Posterior dislocation of the shoulder is rare. The most common cause is a tonic-clonic seizure with violent internal rotation of the humerus. Posterior dislocation of the shoulder should be suspected in any patient who complains of shoulder pain following a seizure or electrical shock phenomenon. Dislocation is often unrecognized because of inadequate radiologic investigation. A true AP film of the scapula should not show overlapping of the humeral head at the glenoid (Fig. 125-3). A tangential scapular view will show posterior displacement of the humeral head in relation to the glenoid. A transthoracic lateral view is often confusing and not helpful in this diagnosis. The best view for demonstrating anterior or posterior dislocation of the shoulder is a good axillary view. Clinically, the patient with a posterior dislocation of the shoulder has pain, inability to passively externally rotate the arm, prominence of the humeral head posteriorly, and a relatively flat shoulder anteriorly.

The secret to successful reduction of anterior or posterior dislocation of the shoulder is patient relaxation. A dislocated shoulder can usually be reduced by any of the methods described if the patient is given adequate analgesics, is cooperative, and gives as much voluntary relaxation as possible.

The technique of having the patient lie in a prone position with a weight suspended from the wrist (not held in the hand) is an atraumatic way of reducing the shoulder. Another method is to have an assistant apply countertraction with a sheet and pull from the axilla toward the patient's opposite shoulder. Then the person reducing the shoulder can give gentle constant traction in a longitudinal manner with the shoulder abducted approximately 45°. With prolonged constant traction, this method is usually successful. Occasionally, increasing the abduction to more than 90° while the traction is maintained is necessary to help lever the shoulder back into the proper position. More vigorous methods such as the Kocher maneuver can force the humerus into positions that might

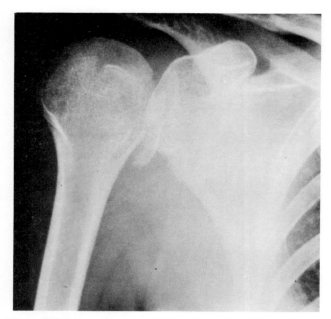

Figure 125-3. Posterior dislocation of the shoulder. Note the marked internal rotation of the humeral head with the fracture locked on the posterior glenoid rim.

result in fracture of the head, neck, or shaft of the humerus. If an associated fracture is noted, a decision should be made prior to manipulation whether the patient will need a general anesthetic for maximum muscle relaxation.

Open reduction and internal fixation are often necessary if the patient has a displaced fracture of the neck of the humerus and a dislocation of the humeral head (Fig. 125-4).

In treating dislocations of the shoulder, brachial plexus injuries are sometimes evident; however, paralysis of the deltoid and hypesthesia over the deltoid region, as a result of stretching of the axillary nerve, are more common injuries. Prior to any manipulation attempts, the neurological status of the extremity should be documented, as well as the vascular status, condition of the rotator cuff, or presence of any associated fracture.

Rotator Cuff Tears

Rotator cuff tears result from an indirect force applied to the shoulder. The rotator cuff is made up of tendinous insertions of the subscapularis, supraspinatus, infraspinatus, and teres minor muscles. These tendons blend together and attach to the lesser and greater tuberosities to help initiate abduction and to control internal and external rotation of the shoulder. Many adults over age 50 will have degeneration of the rotator cuff. A fall with indirect force applied to the rotator cuff will produce a tear that can prevent active abduction of the shoulder. The lesion can occur in younger persons but greater force is required.

Rotator cuff tendinitis and degeneration are often confused with bursitis or calcific tendinitis but are rarely associated with calcification in the rotator cuff. The radiologic appearance of calcification is a diagnostic sign of calcific tendinitis. The patient with restricted painful motion but without calcification should be considered to have a degenerative tear and tendinitis due to rotator cuff degeneration.

The patient with acute rotator cuff tear has pain, cannot abduct the shoulder at the glenohumeral articulation, is able to shrug the shoulder, and abducts only at the thoracoscapular area. Arthrography of the shoulder is diagnostic of a rotator cuff tear when it demonstrates extravasation of dye from the shoulder joint (Fig. 125-5). Differentiation in the emergency department can often be

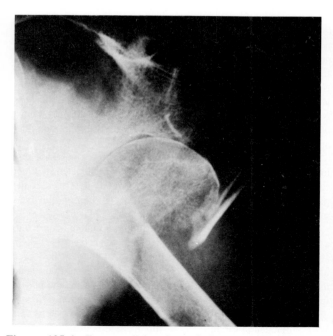

Figure 125-4. Fracture-dislocation of the proximal humerus. Humeral head is dislocated anteriorly with the shaft displaced. Always obtain a roentgenogram of the shoulder before attempting reduction of a dislocation.

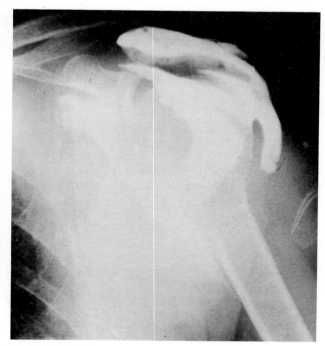

Figure 125-5. Shoulder arthrogram of rotator cuff tear demonstrating extravasation of contrast material into the subdeltoid bursa.

made by infiltrating a local anesthetic into the area of tenderness in the shoulder. If active abduction can be demonstrated in the absence of pain by local infiltration, the patient does not have a significant rotator cuff tear. If the pain is eliminated and the patient does not have active abduction but has passive abduction, the diagnosis of a rotator cuff tear should be strongly considered. Small rotator cuff tears can often be treated by sling immobilization. Larger rotator cuff tears require surgical repair.

Tendinitis and Tenosynovitis

Tendinitis and tenosynovitis occur about the shoulder area because of degenerative changes that take place in this relatively avascular tissue, as well as repetitive trauma to which the tendons are subjected. Calcific deposits often form in the reparative process along with inflammatory cells.

Calcific tendinitis occurs most frequently in the supraspinatus tendon. The patient complains of a deep ache in the shoulder, a painful arc of motion, and has point tenderness over the site of inflammation. Tenosynovitis of the long head of the biceps has similar symptoms with tenderness localized to the bicipital groove anteriorly.

Internal and external rotation films of the shoulder best demonstrate calcification. Lack of calcification should suggest the possibility of a rotator cuff tear.

Nonsteroid anti-inflammatory agents are effective in most cases. For resistant cases, attempts at aspiration of the calcification, and injection of a local anesthetic and a steroid into the most tender area will often relieve symptoms.

The patient who does not move his or her shoulders because of conditions that cause pain or because of therapeutic immobility will often develop adhesive capsulitis. This painful condition can be overcome only by exercises to stretch the capsule, restoring its length and allowing the shoulder joint to resume its extensive range of motion.

Humeral Fractures

Proximal humeral fractures. Fractures of the proximal humerus have been classified by Neer according to displacement (Fig. 125-6). The muscle attachments determine the amount and type of displacement occurring in fractures of the proximal humerus. The lesser and greater tuberosities are separated by the bicipital groove through which the long head of the biceps travels. The subscapularis muscle attaches to the lesser tuberosity and internally rotates the humerus. The supraspinatus attaches to the greater tuberosity superiorly, resulting in abduction of the humerus. The infraspinatus and teres minor attach posteriorly to the greater tuberosity, initiating external rotation. The deforming force on the shaft of the humerus in a fracture about the surgical neck is the pectoralis major which pulls the humeral shaft into adduction. Fractures through the anatomical neck cause separation of the humeral head from the shaft. It is left without blood supply or tendinous insertion. Neer's classification shows that fragments can be displaced in predictable directions by the attachment of soft tissue: two-part, three-part, or four-part fractures, or anterior or posterior dislocation of the humeral head.

Recognition of fractures of the proximal humerus is important in the emergency department. In those fractures that are not sig-

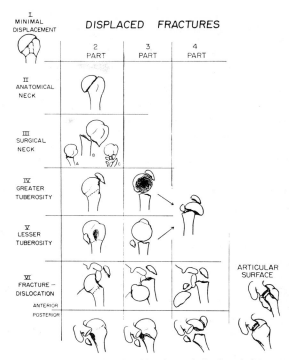

Figure 125-6. Anatomic classification of displaced fractures of the proximal humerus. (Neer CS II: Displaced proximal humeral fractures. Part I. Classification and evaluation. *J Bone Joint Surg* 52A:1079, 1970. Used by permission.)

nificantly displaced, immobilization by a shoulder immobilizer, a Velpeau's bandage, or sling and swathe is usually adequate until rehabilitation is initiated after 1 to 2 weeks. Open reduction and internal fixation are often required if the fracture is significantly displaced or irreducible. The patient should be referred to an appropriate surgeon. Neurovascular status can be impaired in fractures and dislocations about the proximal humerus. The neurovascular status should be documented before and after manipulation of the fracture.

Children with open epiphyses will have significant displacement and angulation of epiphyseal separations in the proximal humeral epiphysis. The anterior angulation accompanying these injuries will usually remodel over a period of 2 to 3 years. If the patient is near skeletal maturity, however, more exact reduction must be carried out.

The possibility of pathological fractures of the humerus should be considered in the patient who has metastatic carcinoma, multiple myeloma, the child with unicameral bone cysts, or other bone lesions, because fracture can occur with less than usual violence in these conditions (Fig. 125-7).

Humeral shaft fracture. Closed fractures of the shaft of the humerus are frequently associated with radial nerve paralysis. The nerve is usually stretched, resulting in neuropraxia. Rarely is the nerve lacerated. If the radial nerve paralysis has an onset immediately following the injury, the prognosis for return of function of the nerve is good. Prior to manipulation of a fracture of the shaft of the humerus, documentation of extension of the wrist, thumb, and fingers is mandatory (Fig. 125-8). If, after manipulation, the patient can no longer extend the wrist and fingers, exploration of the fracture with removal of the nerve from entrapment is indicated.

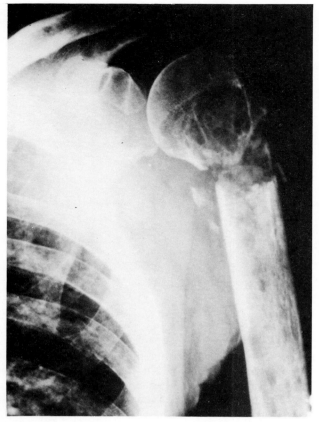

Figure 125-7. Pathologic fracture of the proximal humerus in multiple myeloma.

Fractures of the humeral shaft are usually treated in the emergency department by applying a coaptation splint, a hanging arm cast, or other device for external immobilization. Swelling of the elbow and hand are to be expected after this fracture. The patient is more comfortable in a semisitting position so that the fractured humerus is aligned by traction from the weight of the arm. If no distraction occurs, healing is usually complete in 6 to 8 weeks. Fractures of the humerus are frequently associated with delayed

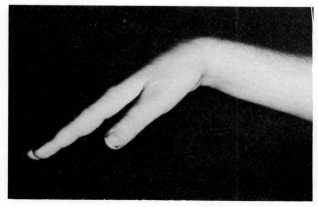

Figure 125-8. Inability to extend wrist, fingers, and thumb in radial nerve paralysis associated with fracture of the humeral shaft. Do not be fooled by interphalangeal extension by ulnar innervated interosseous muscles.

union and they must be immobilized until adequate clinical and roentgenographic union have occurred.

ELBOW

Supracondylar Fracture

The displaced supracondylar fracture in a child is a true emergency. This injury often results in vascular compromise of the musculature in the forearm and hand (Fig. 125-9).

The most common mechanism of injury is a fall on an outstretched arm resulting in a posterior displacement of the supracondylar fragment of the distal humerus and anterior displacement of the knife-like edge of the distal portion of the proximal humeral fragment. Tearing of muscles and occasionally entrapment of the brachial artery or median nerve accompanies this injury. Careful assessment of neurovascular status is mandatory.

Treatment consists of closed reduction under appropriate anesthesia, overhead traction with an olecranon pin, or skin traction in a side-arm position. Hospitalization with close nursing and physician observation is indicated for supracondylar fractures.

Careful monitoring of radial pulse and finger motion prior to definitive treatment is necessary. Prevention of Volkmann's ischemic contracture by timely fasciotomy is occasionally necessary. Maintenance of fracture reduction is sometimes difficult because of the inability to adequately flex the elbow without further compromising circulation. Management of this dangerous and difficult fracture should be in the hands of a well qualified surgeon.

Undisplaced supracondylar fractures will often swell a great deal but can be treated on an outpatient basis with adequate flexion of the elbow to prevent further displacement. Close neurovascular

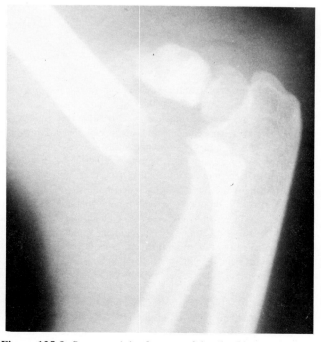

Figure 125-9. Supracondylar fracture of the distal humerus causes extensive soft tissue damage. Careful monitoring of the neurovascular status is mandatory.

observation by responsible parents or medical personnel is essential.

Elbow Dislocation

Dislocation of the elbow joint results from a hyperextension injury. The resulting posterior dislocation can be associated with either medial or lateral displacement. Roentgenograms should include a lateral view of the elbow and an AP view of both the forearm and humerus to prevent distortion of the articular surface due to flexion deformity (Fig. 125-10).

Reduction is accomplished by traction and gentle manipulation. Examination for ligamentous stability will help determine the length of immobilization. Postreduction films are necessary to document complete reduction. If reduction is incomplete, there is usually soft tissue interposition, frequently a nerve. Immobilization in a posterior splint for 2 to 3 weeks is followed by a gradual increase in active motion. Excessive passive motion in the elbow increases the risk of developing myositis ossificans.

Epiphyseal Injuries

Epiphyseal injuries in children are common. Anatomical reduction is mandatory for displaced fractures of the articular surface of the distal humerus. When the lateral epicondyle and capitellum are fractured, they are pulled into a rotated, displaced position by the extensor muscle origin. Medial epicondyle fractures that do not involve the articular surface of the distal humerus can often be left in their displaced position if the displacement is less than 1 cm. Medial epicondyle fractures are occasionally associated with

ulnar nerve irritation, requiring exploration, internal fixation, and sometimes anterior transposition of the nerve.

Olecranon and Coronoid Process Fractures

Undisplaced fractures of the olecranon and coronoid processes can be treated by appropriate immobilization in extension or flexion, respectively. Displaced fractures of the olecranon require internal fixation to restore active extension of the elbow.

RADIUS AND ULNA

Radial Head

Fractures of the radial head commonly occur from a fall on the outstretched hand. Most of these fractures are undisplaced or impacted. Aspiration of the hemarthrosis will often give good pain relief and allow early motion. Radial head excision should be considered if there is marked comminution of the fracture, angulation of the articular surface of more than 30° or more than 2 mm offset in a two-part fracture. The fat pad sign with fat density radiolucency just anterior to the distal humerus is indicative of effusion or hemarthrosis within the elbow joint, and is often a tipoff to an occult radial head fracture.

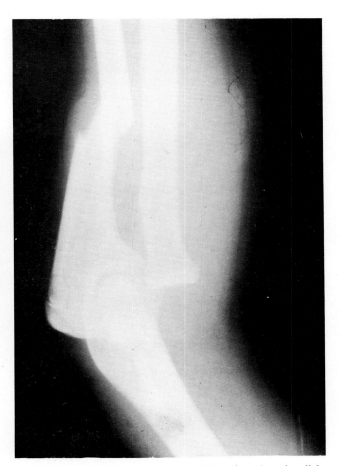

Figure 125-11. Monteggia's fracture-dislocation: Anterior dislocation of the radial head and fracture of the proximal ulna.

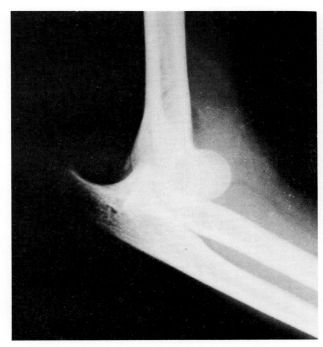

Figure 125-10. Posterior dislocation of the elbow is best demonstrated on lateral roentgenogram.

Monteggia's Fracture-Dislocation

The Monteggia fracture-dislocation occurs with fracture of the proximal third of the ulna and dislocation of the radial head. In the more common type, there is anterior dislocation of the radial head with anterolateral angulation of the ulna fracture (Fig. 125-11). Posterior dislocation of the radial head is less common. Closed reduction is successful in most children but open reduction with internal fixation is advised in adults. In any fracture of the proximal half of the ulna, special attention should be paid to the radial head to rule out Monteggia's fracture-dislocation.

Galeazzi's Fracture

An isolated fracture of the shaft of the radius is commonly associated with dislocation of the distal radioulnar joint, the Galeazzi fracture. Both the Monteggia and Galeazzi fractures often require open reduction and internal fixation for stability of the shaft fracture and to maintain appropriate reduction of the accompanying dislocation. Roentgenograms of both the elbow and wrist in fractures of the forearm will ensure that associated dislocation is not overlooked.

Shaft of Radius and Ulna

Fractures of both bones of the forearm in children are often greenstick fractures with marked deformity and angulation, but they are easily reduced by straightening the angulation and cracking through the intact cortex. Failure to crack through the intact cortex will often result in some recurrence of the deformity. Overriding and displaced fractures frequently require regional or general anesthesia for satisfactory reduction.

Fractures of the shaft of the radius and ulna in adults, when displaced, usually require open reduction and internal fixation with compression plates.

A nightstick fracture, or fracture of the shaft of the ulna from a direct blow, requires immobilization in a long arm cast to prevent rotation of the forearm. This fracture heals quite slowly and must be immobilized until solid clinical union has been accomplished.

BIBLIOGRAPHY

Bateman JE: The diagnosis and treatment of ruptures of the rotator cuff. *Surg Clin North Am* 43:1523–1530, 1963.

Bruce HE, Harvey JP, Wilson JC: Monteggia fractures. *J Bone Joint Surg* 56A:1563–1576, 1974.

Dameron TB Jr, Reibel DB: Fractures involving the proximal humeral epiphyseal plate. *J Bone Joint Surg* 51A:289–297, 1969.

Heinig CF: Retrosternal dislocation of the clavicle: Early recognition, x-ray, diagnosis, and management. *J Bone Joint Surg* 50A:830, 1968.

Hughston JC: Fractures of the distal radial shaft. Mistakes in management. *J Bone Joint Surg* 39A:249–264, 1957.

McLaughlin HL: Posterior dislocation of the shoulder. *J Bone Joint Surg* 44A:1477, 1962.

Neer CS II: Displaced proximal humeral fractures. Part I. Classification and evaluation. *J Bone Joint Surg* 52A:1077–1089, 1970 (23 refs).

Neer CS II: Displaced proximal humeral fractures. Part II. Treatment of three-part and four-part displacement. *J Bone Joint Surg* 52A:1090–1103, 1970.

Packer JW, Foster RR, Garcia A, et al: The humeral fracture with radial nerve palsy: Is exploration warrented? *Clin Orthop* 88:34–38, 1972.

Rockwood CA, Green DP (eds): *Fractures,* ed 2. Philadelphia, JB Lippincott, 1984.

Rowe CR, Sakellarides HT: Factors related to recurrences of anterior dislocations of the shoulder. *Clin Orthop* 20:40–48, 1961.

Smith L: Deformity following supracondylar fractures of the humerus. *J Bone Joint Surg* 42A:235–252, 1960.

Smith L: Deformity following supracondylar fractures of the humerus. *J Bone Joint Surg* 47A:1668, 1965.

CHAPTER 126
INJURIES OF WRIST
AND HAND

Peter Carter

A. Fractures and Dislocations of the Wrist

As a prologue to a discussion of wrist injuries, it is helpful to review the technique and significance of proper x-ray views of the wrist. A roentgenographic study of the wrist that does not include a true lateral and AP view is not acceptable. When in doubt, comparison views of the normal side may be useful.

In a true lateral view the radius and ulna are superimposed and only one forearm bone is readily seen. In the normal person, the lateral x-ray film shows the lunate in the radius and the capitate in the lunate (Fig. 126A-1). Look at this relationship in every injured wrist. Note also that when the wrist is not flexed or extended, but aligned with the forearm, the moon-shaped lunate is like a cup filled with the capitate and resting in the radius. The face or mouth of this cup points directly away from the face of the radius.

On an AP view of the wrist, the bones more or less make up two rows with the scaphoid (navicular) forming the link between the two rows of bones. In the normal film, all bones show about the same 2-to-3-mm joint space. When the space between the lunate and scaphoid is greater than this, scapholunate dissociation is present and represents severe ligamentous disruption in the wrist.

The normal lunate is square or rectangular in shape. If it is triangular or pie-shaped, lunate dislocation is present.

CARPAL INJURIES

Fractures

By far the most common fracture in the carpals is fracture of the scaphoid. Frequently, the patient does not seek medical attention and assumes the wrist is sprained. If the patient has pain or tenderness in the anatomist's snuffbox (on the radial side of the wrist), or if swelling in this area is present, the emergency physician should splint the wrist and warn the patient of a possible fracture, even though the initial x-ray film may be normal. Reex-

amine the patient and repeat roentgenograms in 1 or 2 weeks, because occasionally a fracture will not be seen initially but will be visible at this time.

Fractures of all other carpal bones have been reported, but because they are infrequent, they will not be covered in this discussion. The patient with this type of injury should be referred to an orthopedic surgeon.

Dislocations

Basically, there are only two carpal dislocations. They are frequently missed at the initial examination, even though x-ray films are taken. If a good lateral film is made and the relationship of the radius, lunate, and capitate carefully studied, the dislocation should rarely be missed.

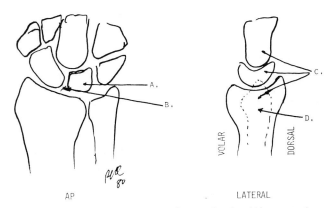

Figure 126A-1. Roentgenogram of normal wrist: (A) square shape of lunate; (B) space between lunate and scaphoid (navicular) equal to other bones; (C) the capitate sits in the lunate, the lunate in the radius; (D) a good lateral film with radius and ulna superimposed.

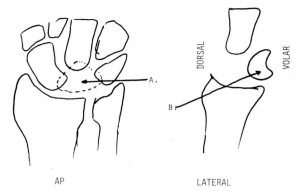

Figure 126A-2. Lunate dislocation: (A) pie-shaped lunate; (B) volar tilt of lunate (cup spilling water).

Lunate Dislocation (Volar)

Almost all dislocations of the lunate are volar (Fig. 126A-2). Clinically, there is a vague and painful swelling of the wrist. Occasionally, the patient complains of tingling in the radial three digits (acute carpal tunnel syndrome). On examination, the patient has a marked loss of flexion of the wrist, but the diagnosis is confirmed by a good lateral x-ray view. The lunate no longer cradles the capitate but is tilted volarly. If you imagine the lunate as a moon-shaped cup, the dislocated cup is spilling water out the volar side of the wrist. Once the diagnosis is made, an orthopedic surgeon should treat this injury.

Perilunate Dislocation

Perilunate dislocation may be seen either with or without a fracture of the scaphoid (Fig. 126A-3). Although frequently overlooked on initial x-ray examination, the diagnosis is again made by the true lateral x-ray film. The lunate and the radius are in normal position, but the capitate (and the remainder of the distal carpal row) has dislocated dorsally around the lunate (hence the name, perilunate dislocation). Perilunate dislocation requires treatment by an orthopedic surgeon.

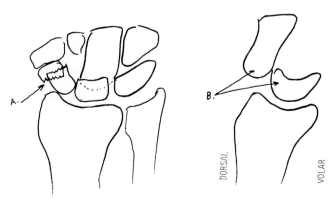

Figure 126A-3. Perilunate dislocation and fracture of scaphoid: (A) fracture of scaphoid (may dislocate instead of fracture); (B) lunate in radius but capitate dorsally displaced.

Scaphoid Dislocation

Rotatory subluxation of the scaphoid goes by several names. Scapholunate dissociation, dorsiflexion intercarpal instability, or DISI deformity, although slightly different, are in this discussion essentially the same. The patient may have a snapping wrist in which a click is felt in the wrist by the patient and occasionally by the examining physician. In other cases, no snapping in or out of reduction is present.

Radiologic signs of scaphoid dislocation are as follows:

1. The scaphoid is foreshortened on the AP view.
2. The scaphoid is vertically oriented on the lateral view.
3. The AP film shows a widening of over 3 mm in the space between the lunate and the scaphoid.

INJURIES OF THE DISTAL FOREARM BONES

Colles' Fracture—Smith's Fracture

Fracture of the distal end of the radius (often with ulnar styloid fracture) is termed Colles' fracture when the face of the distal fragment tilts dorsalward (the most common) (Fig. 126A-4). The diagnosis is confirmed by x-ray film. This fracture often occurs in an elderly patient who has fallen on the outstretched arm. Smith's fracture is volar displacement of the distal radius and results from a fall on the volar flexed wrist.

The fracture should be splinted and the patient referred to an orthopedic surgeon for treatment. Swelling is frequently a problem and strict elevation of the extremity is necessary.

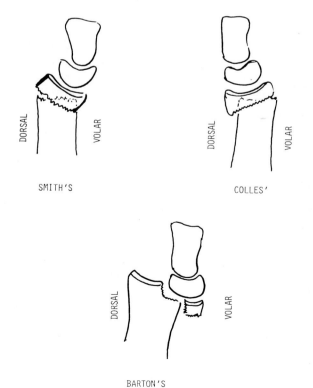

Figure 126A-4. Fractures of distal forearm bones.

Barton's Fracture

Barton's fracture, although similar in clinical deformity to Smith's fracture, is a much more serious injury and frequently requires open reduction and internal fixation (Fig. 126A-4). An intraarticular fracture is present on the volar lip of the radius and the remainder of the carpal bones are dislocated volarly. Orthopedic consultation is mandatory in this injury.

BIBLIOGRAPHY

Bell MS: Linear tomography and the injured wrist. *Injury* 8:303–306, 1977.

Boyes JG Jr: Wrist sprain with subluxation of the scaphoid. *Am Fam Physician* 15:149–151, 1977.

Carter PR: *Common Hand Injuries and Infections: A Practical Guide to Early Treatment.* Philadelphia, Saunders, 1983.

Collert S, Isacson J: Management of redislocated Colles' fracture. *Clin Orthop* 135:183–186, 1978.

Dobyns JH, Sim FH, Linsheid RL: Sports stress syndromes of the hand and wrist. *Am J Sports Med* 6:236–254, 1978.

Ganel A, Engel J, Ditzian R: Arthrography as a method of diagnosing soft-tissue injuries of the wrist. *J Trauma* 19:376–380, 1979.

Gilula LA, Weeks PM: Post-traumatic ligamentous instabilities of the wrist. *Radiology* 129:641–651, 1978.

Green DP: The "sprained wrist." *Am Fam Physician* 19:114–122, 1979.

Hamlin C: Traumatic disruption of the distal radioulnar joint. *Am J Sports Med* 5:93–97, 1977.

Hartwig RH, Louis DS: Multiple carpometacarpal dislocations. A review of four cases. *J Bone Joint Surg* 61:906–908, 1979.

Hollingsworth R, Morris J: The importance of the ulnar side of the wrist in fractures of the distal end of the radius. *Injury* 7:263–266, 1976.

Kaye JJ: Fractures and dislocations of the hand and wrist. *Semin Roentgenol* 13:109–116, 1978.

King RE: Barton's fracture-dislocation of the wrist. *Curr Pract Orthop Surg* 6:133–144, 1975.

McCue FC III, Baugher WH, Kulund DN, et al: Hand and wrist injuries in the athlete. *Am J Sports Med* 7:275–286, 1979.

Morawa LG, Ross PM, Schock CC: Fractures and dislocations involving the navicular-lunate axis. *Clin Orthop* 118:48–53, 1976.

Palmer AK, Dobyns JH, Linscheid RL: Management of post-traumatic instability of the wrist secondary to ligament rupture. *J Hand Surg* 3:507–532, 1978.

Posner MA: Injuries to the hand and wrist in athletes. *Orthop Clin North Am* 8:593–618, 1977.

Vance RM, Gelberman RH, Braun RM: Chronic bilateral scapholunate dissociation without symptoms. *J Hand Surg* 4:178–180, 1979.

Van Herpe LB: Fractures of the forearm and wrist. *Orthop Clin North Am* 7:543–556, 1976.

Weeks PM, Young VL, Gilula LA: A cause of painful clicking wrist: A case report. *J Hand Surg* 4:522–525, 1979.

Woodward AH, Neviaser RJ, Nisenfeld F: Radial and volar perilunate transscaphoid fraction dislocation. *South Med J* 68:926–928, 1975.

B. Hand Injuries and Infections

Hand emergencies are everyone's problem. Those of us who take care of patients in the emergency department are faced with the problem daily. In fact, the hand is the most commonly injured part of the body. In a 1975 study of emergency patients at The Roosevelt Hospital in New York, 9 percent had a complaint referable to the hand. The majority of these complaints can be superbly treated by the emergency physician who has a basic knowledge of the anatomy and physiology of the hand.

Although the combined anatomy of the hand is complex, it is built on a series of simple functional units. Armed with a basic understanding of the anatomy and frequent reference to an atlas, the physician should be able to recognize the potential problems of almost every hand injury. By and large, the diagnosis is made by clinical examination and correlation between the evidence of injury, known anatomical structures, and loss of function. Topographical anticipation and the logical interpretation of clues can bring out the Sherlock Holmes in most of us.

What follows are didactic suggestions made rigid by the scope of the problem. These suggestions are certainly not the only possible mode of treatment, but they do represent an acceptable method that for the most part has been developed by others but tested by me in clinical practice.

REGIONAL ANESTHESIA OF THE INJURED HAND

Two types of regional blocks are useful in both examining and treating emergency patients. Almost any emergency hand problem can be handled with either a digital (intermetacarpal) regional block, or a wrist block of one of the three major nerves: median, ulnar, or radial. Remember that regional anesthesia is not as immediate as infiltrating the wound directly and must be given time to take effect, which usually takes 5 to 10 min. On occasion, another 10- to 15-min wait may be necessary.

Do not administer anesthesia until an adequate sensory examination has been carried out. Once the hand is anesthetized, it is impossible to check the patient for sensation for several hours. Anesthetic agents used for either the digital or wrist block are a 2% solution of lidocaine or mepivacaine. Epinephrine is contraindicated for anesthesia of the hand or digits. Use a 10-mL syringe and a needle no larger than 27 gauge.

Digital or Intermetacarpal Block

If the injection is made in the web space between the fingers, there is less pain associated with it. Because aspiration with a 27-gauge needle is ineffective, slowly inject the solution moving the needle back and forth to prevent intraarterial injection. Even if intraarterial injection is inadvertently done, the only complication is a hematoma, as mepivacaine is not toxic to the vascular tree and it is unusual to inject a bolus large enough to result in a toxic blood level. The digital or intermetacarpal technique is best suited for injuries of the long and ring fingers. The thumb or border digits are more painlessly anesthetized by wrist block anesthesia.

Wrist Block Anesthesia

The key to wrist block anesthesia is an accurate understanding of the topographical anatomy of the three nerves at the wrist level (Fig. 126B-1).

Median nerve block. The median nerve lies just deep to the palmaris longus tendon (present in 85 percent of patients). Slowly inject about 3 to 5 mL of 2% mepivacaine and do not puncture the patient more than once, as multiple punctures of the nerve can lead to permanent paresthesias and nerve damage. The patient should feel a deep fullness develop in the region of the wrist. If the fullness is superficial, the main portion of the median nerve will not be adequately anesthetized and only the superficial branch will be blocked.

Ulnar nerve block. The ulnar wrist block can be given in one of two ways. The ulnar nerve is just radial and deep to the flexor carpi ulnaris tendon, and can be approached from the volar or ulnar side. If approached from the ulnar side, inject extremely distally, or at the level of the wrist flexion crease. The flexor carpi ulnaris muscle extends very distally at this point and if mepivacaine is injected intramuscularly, satisfactory block will not develop. A second injection is necessary to block the superficial branch of the ulnar nerve. This branch takes off from the nerve approximately 8 cm proximal to the wrist and heads dorsally. It may be easily blocked by subcutaneously injecting 1 to 2 mL dorsal to the ulnar styloid.

Superficial radial nerve block. The superficial branch of the radial nerve is the only portion of the radial nerve that extends into the hand. Subcutaneously inject 3 to 4 mL of 2% mepivacaine 2 fingerbreadths proximal to the radial styloid on the palmar or volar side.

BASIC TENETS OF HAND CARE

Position of Function

The exquisite anatomical design of the hand has impressed humanity for centuries. It is based on the balanced gliding of joints and tendons powered by muscles under the control of the cerebral cortex. Anything that interferes with this gliding compromises hand function.

Following any hand injury of significance, the structures must be placed at rest so they can heal rapidly with minimal scar tissue formation. When the inevitable stiffness does occur, the arc of motion must be in the most favorable position for use. Forcing the patient to move the injured hand in the first week does not protect against scar formation. On the contrary, the pain and swelling frequently are associated with excess fibrosis and stiffness. When in doubt, splint the hand and allow it to rest.

The optimum position for hand immobilization is to extend the wrist approximately 30° (with the long axis of the forearm roughly lined up with the long axis of the relaxed thumb). The metacarpophalangeal (MP) joints should be immobilized in 60 to 70° of flexion and the interphalangeal (IP) joints in 15 to 20° of flexion. The thumb should be abducted away from the palm (Fig. 126B-2).

The tendency for the injured hand is to fall into wrist flexion and MP joint hyperextension. This must be counteracted because severe permanent joint contractures can develop within 3 to 4 weeks in adults (Fig. 126B-3). In general, this tendency can be avoided by applying a volar plaster slab held in place by a conforming gauze dressing. Do not apply the volar plaster slab with an elastic bandage because it can constrict venous return if swelling develops, and it also encourages the patient to depend on the elastic wrap later in rehabilitation, a habit that is hard to break.

Hand Dressing

Although there are many different hand dressings, they all have similar objectives: to immobilize the hand in the position of function; to allow elevation; to be serviceable and durable; and, insofar as possible, to allow as close to normal use of the uninjured parts of the hand.

For those not familiar with the use of plaster, the circumferential plaster dressing can be modified to one of plaster splints and gauze bandages (Fig. 126B-4).

Child's hand dressing. Children represent a special problem because their small size prevents the application of a plaster that

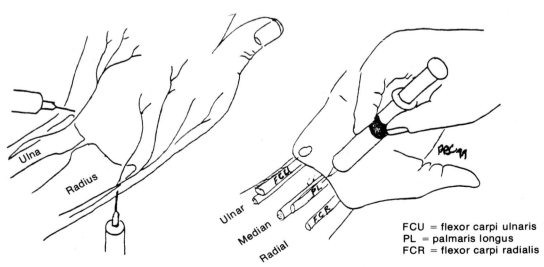

Figure 126B-1. Simple hand anatomy.

FCU = flexor carpi ulnaris
PL = palmaris longus
FCR = flexor carpi radialis

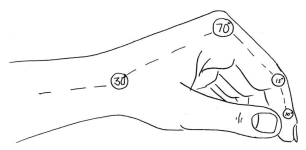

Figure 126B-2. Position of function.

fits the chubby contour of the extremity. The so-called turtle sign (Fig. 126B-5A) or disappearing finger act (Fig. 126B-5B) is a frequent complication and follows the child's attempts to wiggle out of what was previously a well-fitted dressing. Because of this, we adhere to the dictum: ''The smaller the child, the bigger the dressing'' (Fig. 126B-5C).

Elevation and Prevention of Edema

After the injured hand has been adequately immobilized, instruct the patient to elevate it. Because this is so important, it cannot be overstressed. Faithfully elevate for two reasons: (1) to prevent swelling, because the protein-rich fluid of edema acts as glue around the tendons and joints of the hand and increases stiffness; and (2) to provide more comfort and lessen the need for pain medication. When standing, the patient can elevate his or her hand by resting it on the head. When sitting, the patient can sit next to a table and rest the hand and arm on a stack of magazines so that the hand is higher than the elbow and the elbow is higher than the shoulder. Perhaps the best way to check whether the hand is appropriately elevated is to imagine a drop of water beginning at the fingers and running downhill onto the chest. If the position of elevation is proper, this drop of water will not have to run uphill at any point on the upper limb.

BONE AND JOINT INJURY

When evaluating injured bones and joints in the hand, carefully localize the site of maximum pain and tenderness. Swelling and ecchymoses are often more generalized. Try to localize tenderness to the specific joint, and then identify a specific area about the

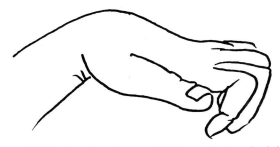

Figure 126B-3. A volar plaster splint is applied to the injured hand to prevent contracture due to wrist flexion and extension of the MP joint.

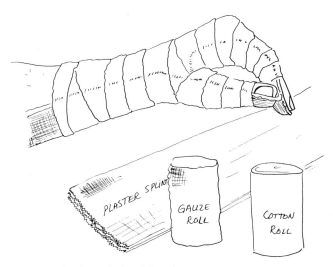

Figure 126B-4. Basic hand dressing.

joint that is most tender. Testing for joint stability may require some form of regional anesthesia, as described earlier. Grossly unstable joints, particularly in the thumb, may require early surgery for optimal results. While the hand is anesthetized, the active motion test allows one to be sure that a full arc of smooth gliding motion is present in the fingers rather than the teeter effect of a dislocated joint.

Roentgenographic examination is mandatory to rule out fracture. Occasionally, if an inadequate view is accepted, a subtle fracture or dislocation may be missed (Fig. 126B-6). Particularly in the digits, a true anteroposterior (AP) and lateral films are important for assessment. When AP and lateral films of the hand are ordered for a finger injury, the views of the finger are usually oblique. True lateral and AP films of the finger will be made if the fingernail is used as a landmark (Fig. 126B-7). When an AP film of the proximal interphalangeal (PIP) joint to examine the joint space is desired, the bone distal to the joint must be used as a reference. Other trouble areas are the carpometacarpal (CMC) joint areas of the ring and small fingers. The CMC joints form a seimcircular arch. Obtaining a lateral film of the small finger CMC joint requires that the wrist be oblique.

FRACTURES

If a fracture is present, it should be categorized using the following criteria: Is the fracture open or closed; complete or incomplete; displaced or nondisplaced; comminuted or noncomminuted; transverse, oblique, or spiral? Reduction can be evaluated by determining if length has been restored, if the bones are in contact, and if both linear and rotational alignment are satisfactory.

The open fracture in the hand must be thoroughly cleansed and debrided. This is best done in an operating room if there are multiple compound fractures, severely contaminated wounds, or wounds with poor skin coverage. In any case, complete regional anesthesia, tourniquet, hemostasis, and fastidious sterile technique are paramount. Copious saline lavage is warranted after a thorough scrub with surgical soap. Loose closure to prevent desiccation of tendons and joints is acceptable. Although somewhat controversial, a short 2- to 4-day course of a broad-spectrum antibiotic in

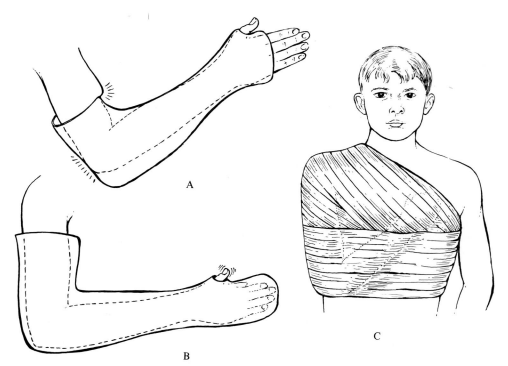

Figure 126B-5. (A) The turtle sign; (B) disappearing finger act; (C) appropriate child's hand dressing.

conjunction with, but not in lieu of, good surgical technique and debridement is valuable.

Although uncommon, tetanus may follow an open-hand wound, particularly those caused by lawn mowers. Tetanus-prone wounds should be closed secondarily and all patients with open wounds should receive tetanus prophylaxis.

Phalanx Fractures

Foam splints applied to the fingers are best fitted to the dorsal surface because the bone is closer to the skin and therefore better immobilized.

Distal phalanx. Unless grossly displaced, an external splint for 10 to 14 days, combined with elevation, is adequate treatment of a fractured distal phalanx. Gross displacement may require open reduction and internal fixation. Since crush injury to the soft tissue is usually present, the importance of elevating the limb to prevent swelling should always be stressed to the patient. Usually, oral

analgesics as an adjunct to, and not as a replacement for, elevation are frequently required for 24 to 48 h.

Middle phalanx. This densely cortical bone requires 3 to 4 weeks of immobilization for clinical union. Linear malalignment is usually obvious clinically, since this bone is close to the skin. However, rotational deformities may be subtle but disabling, and must be suspected if they are to be detected (Fig. 126B-8).

Proximal phalanx. Fractures of the proximal phalanx are among the most disabling injuries of the hand, and are best referred to a hand surgeon. Some displaced fractures require open reduction, and many are complicated by PIP joint contractures and significant loss of function.

In general, these fractures tend to angulate apex volarly. After an adequate wrist block is done, longitudinal traction and more flexion are required to reduce the fracture. Since the bone is subcutaneous dorsally, palpation can be helpful in the immediate assessment of the reduction, but a good lateral roentgenogram is

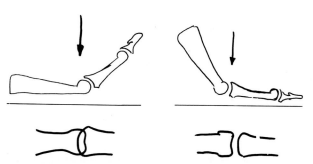

Figure 126B-6. Joint space varies with changes in finger position.

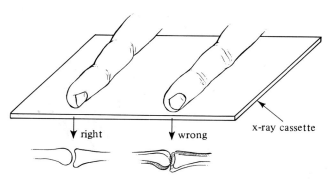

Figure 126B-7. Align the fingernail perpendicular or parallel to the horizontal for a good lateral or AP film of the finger.

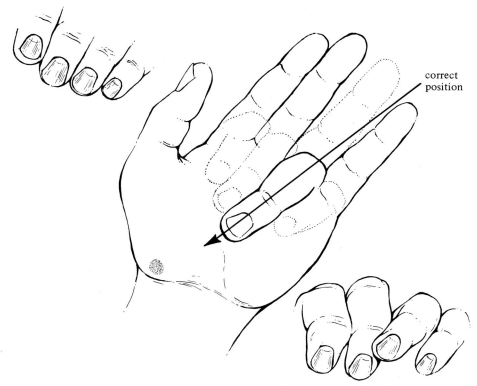

correct
position

Figure 126B-8. To examine for rotational deformities of the phalanges, flex the fingers upon the palm. The fingernails should point to the radial styloid.

important for verification. Apply a dorsal foam splint with the wrist at 30° of extension, the MP joint flexed from 30 to 50° and the IP joints flexed from 10 to 15°.

Metacarpal Fractures

Boxer's fracture is the fracture and volarward angulation of the fifth metacarpal neck. The bone is frequently so strongly impacted that it cannot be disimpacted by closed technique even under general anesthesia. Up to 40 to 50° of angulation is acceptable in a *stable* fracture, providing rotational alignment is satisfactory. The ring finger metacarpal is also like the fifth in this regard. Splinting the hand in the functional position for 3 weeks, followed by a period of rehabilitation to regain motion, usually results in normal hand function with the "knocked down knuckle" cosmetic defect.

Metacarpal neck fractures of the index and long fingers demand more accurate restoration of alignment because of limited motion at the base of the metacarpal. Over 20° angulation is not acceptable here.

Spiral fracture of the metacarpal shaft is most likely to cause rotational malalignment. In transverse fractures, apex dorsal angulation may be so difficult to control that temporary pin fixation may be required.

JOINT INJURY

Fracture

Fractures of the small joints of the hand involving a large portion of the articular surface often require temporary pin fixation, par-

ticularly if the fracture pattern is an unstable one. If splinted, such fractures tend to angulate insidiously.

Dislocations

Distal interphalangeal joint. Because of the tight skin envelope, many dislocations of the DIP joint are open and the treatment described for open fractures is appropriate. Occasionally a temporary transfixion pin is helpful to treat a ruptured extensor tendon.

Proximal interphalangeal joint. Dislocations of the PIP joint are common. Once reduced, the active motion test will rule out a trapped collateral ligament. If not trapped in the joint, the torn collateral ligament need not be repaired. Postreduction, true AP and lateral films should be made to rule out fracture of the joint and to confirm that a truly concentric reduction has been accomplished.

Metacarpophalangeal joint. Dislocations of the MP joint are usually irreducible by closed means, and open reduction is necessary. In the thumb, dislocations of the MP joint can often be reduced by hyperflexion of the IP joint, followed by pushing the dorsally displaced proximal phalanx back over the metacarpal head. After reduction, stability of the collateral ligaments of this joint should be checked and if unstable, the dislocation should be repaired surgically.

TENDON INJURY

Tendon injuries occur frequently and many occur with a deceptively small penetrating wound, or as a result of a blunt injury.

Examples are the cook separating frozen meat patties with a knife that slips; the child who grabs a knife or falls through a window; the football player whose ring finger flexor profundus tendon avulses when he grabs an opposing player's jersey, or whose extensor tendon is crushed when his finger is stepped on.

It is critical to consider the stance of the finger when the tendon was lacerated. If the finger was being actively flexed (such as the child grabbing a knife), the tendon laceration will be distal to the skin laceration (Fig. 126B-9A and 9a). If the finger was lacerated in extension (as a fall on a sharp object with the outstretched hand), the tendon laceration will be at the same level as the skin laceration (Fig. 126B-9B and 9b). This, of course, is because the finger is usually examined in full extension.

Diagnosis of Complete Tendon Injury

The complete laceration of a flexor or extensor tendon can be identified by the active motion check and by observation of an altered stance of the digit.

Active motion tests. To test motion in flexor profundus lacerations and ruptures, stabilize the PIP and MP joints while asking the patient to flex only the tip. Take care not to be fooled by the patient who can willingly extend the joint maximally and then relaxes it just as the examiner asks him or her to flex it. This test may be modified for the flexor pollicis longus, as well.

The flexor sublimis test is done by having the patient flex the finger while you hold the other fingers extended. This blocks the action of the profundus tendon and allows an isolated test of sublimis function. This is best for evaluating injuries of the long and ring fingers.

Extensor tendons are frequently lacerated because of their vulnerability over the dorsum of the hand and digits. Even though the tendon can be seen to be completely lacerated in the wound, the patient often can extend the digit fully. This is because the uncturae tendinae over the back of the hand, and the extensor hood over the dorsum of the digit can maintain function. Occasionally, if the laceration is in exactly the right place, these evolutionary fail-safe mechanisms are inadequate and the patient cannot actively extend the joint.

Altered stance of the digit. This clinical test is important because it requires no active participation on the part of the patient and is especially useful in patients who are not able to cooperate with active motion testing (children, or comatose, aged, or retarded patients). Normally the hand at rest shows a cascade of progressively increasing flexed position of the digital segment (Fig.

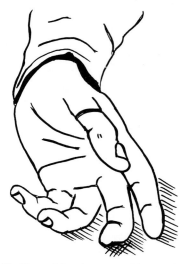

Figure 126B-10. Normal hand stance—Pieta, Michelangelo.

126B-10). The lacerated tendon may alter this in an obvious or subtle way. Recognition of a tendon laceration by this test alone requires careful observation and topographical anticipation.

Treatment

Treatment of tendon injuries is one of the most difficult and unpredictable problems in hand surgery. The inappropriate early treatment of these injuries often leads to permanent disability for the patient.

Extensor tendon. Extensor tendon injuries in which the extensor tendon ends can both be seen without lcoal exploration can be repaired with a near-far near-far suture technique (Fig. 126B-11). The suture material should be strong (3-0 wire or polypropylene) and not reactive. If the tendon ends are not easily located in the wound, exploration of the wound and location of the tendons should be done in the operating room.

Flexor tendon. Flexor tendons should *never* be repaired in the emergency department under any circumstance. If a hand surgeon is not immediately available, flexor tendon injuries should be repaired secondarily, and the emergency physician should cleanse the wound and suture the skin laceration only. Errors of commission are much more disabling here than simple wound closure and later repair. When in doubt, close the skin and splint appropriately.

Mallet finger. This is a partial tendon injury at the DIP joint. The clinical deformity usually develops 5 to 7 days after injury.

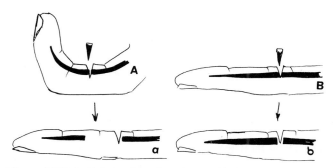

Figure 126B-9. Relationship of tendon to skin laceration depending on finger position at time of injury.

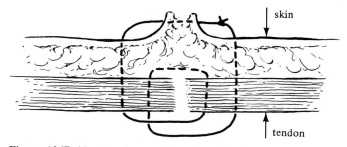

Figure 126B-11. Near-far near-far suture technique.

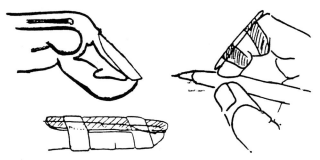

Figure 126B-12. Splinting technique for mallet finger. A dorsal splint that avoids forced hyperextension, especially until initial swelling subsides, is closer to the bone, and provides immobilization. Also, the patient is more likely to wear it faithfully for the full 6 weeks of treatment.

Even if accompanied by a small avulsion fracture, it can be managed by the primary physician using the splinting technique described in Figure 126B-12. Splint the finger for 6 full weeks and then wean the patient out of the splint slowly over 7 to 10 days. If there is a large fracture fragment, internal fixation is generally necessary.

Partial Tendon Injury

Partial tendon injuries can become complete tendon injuries if the injury is not recognized and splinted properly. The three cardinal diagnostic points of a partial tendon laceration are as follows:

1. Pain when the patient attempts to use the partially lacerated tendon
2. A slightly decreased tone resulting in an altered stance of the hand at rest
3. Weakness of the tendon when it is actively flexed

If any of these signs or symptoms are present or if you suspect a tendon injury, especially in a child who is hard to examine, no harm can be done by splinting the hand in a relaxed position for 3 weeks until the partial tendon laceration has had an opportunity to heal.

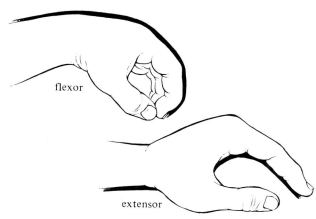

Figure 126B-13. Splinting position for flexor and extensor injuries.

Splint the flexor tendons with the wrist flexed 30 to 45° and the fingers gently flexed. Extensor tendons can be splinted in the functional position (wrist extended 40°, MP joints flexed 40 to 60°, and IP joints flexed 5 to 10°) as shown in Figure 126B-13. Flexor tendons should be splinted for 3 weeks and extensor tendons 4 to 5 weeks. Time for healing is increased in extensor tendon injuries, since late stretching of the extensor tendon can occur because the opposing flexor tendons are more powerful than the extensors. The newly formed collagen has a tendency to stretch until the collagen molecules are aligned.

Boutonniere deformity. A common partial tendon injury is the dorsal crush to the top of the PIP joint received in football when the finger is stepped on. Five to seven days later the patient develops a boutonniere deformity.

NERVE LACERATION

Neurological Examination of the Hand

The hand has three major nerves: the median, ulnar, and radial. Clinically, tests for sensation and motor function can be done that will establish the integrity of the nerve. Nonfunctional nerves do not always require treatment, but they should be identified and recorded as early in the patient's treatment as possible.

Sensory examination. One of the best clues to loss of sensation in the hand is loss of sweating. In the unconscious or uncooperative patient or child, this is a most helpful sign. If the patient can cooperate, the two-point discrimination test is quick and reliable. This is best performed using a paper clip. Pinprick is frequently misleading. The normal individual should recognize two stimuli at 5-mm distance apart or greater.

Motor examination. In testing for motor function, always feel the muscle belly contract. There are many trick motions in the hand, and the examiner can be easily fooled.

Ulnar nerve. Test the first dorsal interosseus muscle. Ask the patient to abduct the extended index finger *against resistance* and palpate the muscle in the web space on the radial side of the index metacarpal (Fig. 126B-14).

Median nerve. Check the ability to contract the abductor pollicis brevis by asking the patient to bring the thumb perpendicularly out of the palm while you palpate the thenar eminence (Fig. 126B-4).

Radial nerve. See if the patient can completely extend the fingers with the wrist extended. Don't just ask the patient to extend the fingers because, with marked wrist flexion, the normal tenodesis effect of the extensor tendons is enough to cause finger extension (Fig 126B-14).

Treatment

The repair of a lacerated nerve is beyond the scope of most emergency physicians and the patient should be referred. A few pertinent comments may be helpful to the physician referring the case.

Isolated lacerations of digital sensory nerves are best treated in a delayed fashion because sensation will often return within 3 to 4 days, even though the finger lacked sensation right after injury. A more accurate examination can also be done when the patient is seen 2 to 3 days later in a quiet examining room.

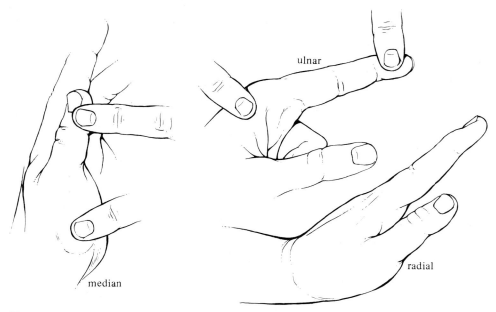

ulnar

median

radial

Figure 126B-14. Maneuvers for testing motor function in the hand.

However, for optimal results, any laceration of a mixed sensory and motor nerve, such as a median or ulnar nerve laceration at the wrist, should be repaired primarily if the wound conditions and status of the patient's general health allow it. Never tag nerve ends for the reconstructive surgeon since this merely leads to more scarring.

ARTERIAL INJURY

Control of Hemorrhage

Repair of injured vessels is a specialized operating technique. The responsibility of the emergency physician is to control the hemorrhage in such a way that vascular repair may be possible. Initially, use pressure to control bleeding and elevate the extremity.

Bleeding can be easily controlled by applying a blood pressure cuff or tourniquet on the upper portion of the arm, and inflating the cuff to 250 to 300 mmHg. Then, inspect the wound. *Never* control bleeding by blindly grabbing with a hemostat in any portion of the upper extremity because such crush injuries to nerves and vessels will severely compromise the repair in the operating room.

COMPARTMENT SYNDROME: VOLKMANN'S ISCHEMIC CONTRACTURE

This devastating complication requires early recognition, since prompt operative intervention frequently may save the function of the limb. Although this syndrome classically follows a supracondylar fracture of the humerus in a child, it may follow other injuries in a child or adult. Always maintain a high index of suspicion for compartment syndrome when evaluating injuries of the forearm or leg. In the extremities, the fascial sleeves are unyielding and tissue death will occur if the pressure is not relieved.

There is no single clinical test to rule out impending Volkmann's ischemic contracture.

The following are some common conditions with the potential for development of a compartment syndrome:

• Any fracture of the elbow
• Both bone forearm fractures
• Crush injury to the forearm muscles
• Extravasation of blood (e.g., transfusion) in the forearm
• Inadvertent arterial injection of drugs (barbiturates)

Classically, the patient complains of excruciating pain (often unrelieved with morphine) in the forearm muscles. This may diminish late in the course of the syndrome. Severe forearm pain should make the physician as anxious as it makes the patient. Passive stretching of the fingers causes severe pain in the forearm muscle region. Although the pulse is frequently absent, it may be present and frequently the skin circulation is unimpaired. The patient may complain of stocking-glove anesthesia. This is not a hysterical complaint, but is related to ischemia.

When the physician suspects an impending Volkmann's contracture, a surgeon capable of complete forearm decompression should be called promptly. Only a few hours are required to seal the fate of the ischemic muscle.

SKIN INJURY

Fingertip Amputation

The object of treatment is early rehabilitation of the hand with a painless, durable skin cover. Description of the plethora of complicated, tricky, and novel pedicle flaps for these injuries as a rule has no indication here, but when done, repair is best done in the operating room. With few exceptions, the most rapid rehabilitation of the fingertip injury is by a free skin graft. Unless the wound is extremely clean and tidy, it is best to delay the skin graft for 3 to

5 days to allow the wound to clean itself via dressing changes, and to obtain satisfactory hemostasis so that the graft will not be lifted off by hematoma. Placing the skin graft in the operating room usually results in a technically superior skin graft and a better percentage of graft take. For the rare patient for whom a simple skin graft proves inadequate, a pedicle flap skin graft can be provided later.

In small children (less than 5 years old) small tip amputations (0.5 cm to 0.75 cm) do not need skin grafts. They usually heal nicely with serial dressing changes every 3 to 5 days.

It is generally better to refrain from reattaching a completely amputated tip. In adults, the injured tip usually does not survive due to infection, and achievement of the primary goal, a mobile digit with a healed wound and rapid return to function, is delayed. In children if a small amount of tissue is involved, the finger will heal with serial dressing changes alone. If more tissue is involved, delayed skin grafting produces the best results.

Partial Amputation—Screen Door Finger

A partial amputation leaving a volar skin bridge often follows the slamming of a door on a finger. The fingernail plate is avulsed from the sulcus and prevents reduction of the bone or soft tissue or both. This may be handled by trimming off the torn proximal edge of the nail (a new one grows back in 3 months) and repairing the nail bed with 6-0 gut sutures (Fig. 126B-15).

HAND INFECTION

Infections in the hand pose a serious threat to function. A hand infection in a diabetic, even if trivial, is potentially life-threatening. Treatment is early initiation of appropriate antibiotics, and operative drainage if an abscess is present. Always place the patient on a penicillinase-resistant antibiotic until culture reports are obtained. Ampicillin is an unacceptable antibiotic for the treatment of hand infections. Elevation and immobilization in the position of function combined with intravenous antibiotic therapy frequently will lead to resolution within 24 to 48 h. At the end of this time, if an abscess is evident, incision and drainage are necessary.

Incision and drainage of the hand should always be along the accepted lines of skin incisions. In addition, excise a wedge of

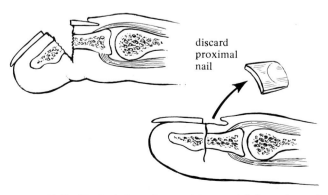

Figure 126B-15. Technique for repairing partial fingertip avulsions involving the nail.

discard proximal nail

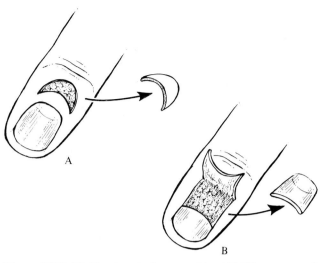

Figure 126B-16. Treatment of paronychia. (A) When *no* pus is present under the nail; (B) when pus is present under the nail.

palmar skin tissue so that as the swelling recedes, the wound will remain open and drain freely. Incisions made along the appropriate lines will close rapidly without evidence of increased scar formation especially if made on the palmar side.

Paronychia

Do not drain a paronychial abscess unless gross pus is evident. It will resolve with elevation, antibiotics, and repeated soaks in warm water for 5 to 10 min at a time, 5 to 6 times a day when the patient is not elevating the hand. If pus is present but not under the nail, excision of a crescent-shaped ellipse of tissue provides drainage and rapid healing. The more extensive subungual abscess is best drained by removal of part or all of the nail (Fig. 126B-16).

Felon

A felon is an extremely painful infection that frequently follows a wound in the digit. The patient not infrequently gives a history of having got a splinter in the finger and then picked at it with a needle. Proper drainage requires an understanding of the anatomy of the pad of the fingertip. The fibrofatty structure is oriented much like a grapefruit in the way the fibrous septa radiate out to the skin from the distal phalanx. Although there are many different ways to drain a felon, the majority of complications come from inadequate drainage. I prefer the fishmouth incision described in Figure 126B-17. Great care must be taken to place the incision just under the fingernail because an incision more palmar by only 2 to 3 mm will cause sloughing and a painful scar.

This procedure should be done under digital or wrist block anesthesia, and tourniquet technique is necessary for adequate visualization and to prevent exsanguination. After the incision has been made, the volar pad of the finger should fall volarly somewhat and a strip of nonadherent gauze, such as Xeroform gauze, can be placed over the incision. The gauze should be removed in 5 days; following this, the patient can begin soaking the finger.

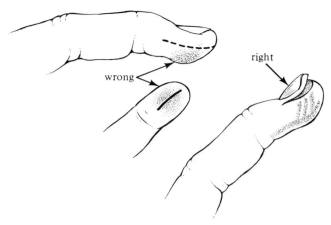

Figure 126B-17. Method of incision and drainage of a felon.

Antibiotic therapy and strict elevation of the hand are also necessary.

Human Bite Infection

The cause of this lesion is usually a fist to the mouth in some pugilistic encounter. Suspect a human bite if there is any laceration over a knuckle, because the patient often gives an incorrect history.

Open the wound, profusely irrigate it, and do not suture it. Apply a splint with the MP joint flexed to allow drainage from the MP joint. The proximity of the MP joint to the skin makes it vulnerable to bacterial inoculation and its moist avascular environment provides a fortuitous culture media for the organisms of the mouth. Most infections respond to penicillin therapy.

Flexor Tendon Tenosynovitis and Subcutaneous Finger Infection

Flexor tendon tenosynovitis is uncommon, but it is catastrophic because it erodes and ruins the delicate flexor tendon mechanism (Fig. 126B-18).

The three cardinal signs of tenosynovitis according to Kanavel are:

1. There is tenderness along and limited to the course of the flexor sheath

2. Flexion stance of the finger—as the closed space is distended with pus, the finger is drawn into flexion
3. There is pain on passive extension of the finger, most marked at the base of the digit

These signs help in distinguishing between a true flexor tendon tenosynovitis and the more common subcutaneous infection. If these signs are equivocal, hospitalize the patient for hand elevation and immobilization, and intravenous antibiotics. The infection should be incised and drained as an urgent procedure in the operating room if all three signs are present and if there is a fullness palpable at the base of the finger, at the cul-de-sac of the flexor tendon synovial sheath.

Deep Palmar Space Infection

Palmar space infections are fortunately rare. They are characterized by exquisite swelling and tenderness localized to the area of the palmar space (Fig. 126B-19). Lymphatic drainage from the palmar side is toward the dorsal surface, so swelling of the dorsal hand is prominent. Always turn the hand over and check the palm for abscess. Treatment is surgical drainage and intravenous antibiotic therapy.

INJECTION INJURY

Injury by a high-pressure grease or paint gun is one of the most deceptive of all hand injuries, and devastating in its effect. Usually a small 1-to-3-mm wound over the finger is all that is apparent immediately after injury. However, the injected fluid travels along the path of least resistance, down the tendon shaft. Paint solvents are highly noxious to the delicate and vulnerable environment of the flexor tendon. This injury demands the attention of a surgeon competent to decompress the entire hand and fingers, but it must first be recognized by the emergency physician as a true emergency.

REIMPLANTATION

Several years ago, reports from a group of American surgeons visiting Communist China revived interest in reimplantation of extremities and digits. In a few centers of the United States mi-

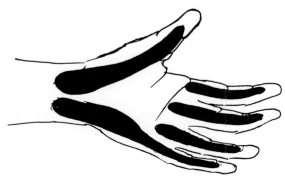

Figure 126B-18. Synovial sheaths of flexor tendons.

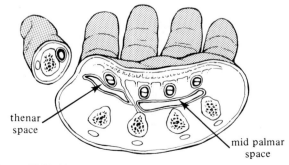

thenar
space

mid palmar
space

Figure 126B-19. Midpalmar and thenar spaces. (Adapted from Netter FH, in Lampe EW: Surgical anatomy of the hand. *Clin Symp* 21:25, 1969.)

crosurgeons have replaced severed digits and have obtained survival. Many, if not most, of these surviving fingers are stiff, anesthetic, painful, and nonfunctional. In addition, the costs involved for surgery and rehabilitation can be enormous. Unfortunately, the health consumer may often expect referral by the emergency physician for reimplantation.

The following are suggested criteria for reimplantation of digits and the upper extremity, and suggestions for transportation of the severed part. This field is rapidly changing and the physician is advised to contact his or her regional reimplantation center for more specific instructions. Criteria for reimplantation that may yield satisfactory results include:

- A sharply incised wound
- A young, stable patient
- An amputated thumb
- Multiple-digit amputations
- Proximal rather than distal level of amputation

Contraindications to reimplantation include treatment of major life-threatening injuries that take priority over reimplantation; technically unfeasible or impractical reimplantation, such as an amputation distal to the PIP joint or distal to the IP joint of the thumb; single digit amputations except possibly the thumb; an aged or emotionally unstable patient.

When a patient is referred for reimplantation, be sure to notify the center before transfer, and always warn the patient that reimplantation may not be possible after the surgeon has evaluated the injury. The digit should be placed in a dry, clean or sterile plastic bag, which is then tightly sealed. Place the plastic bag in ice water. Do not use dry ice. Do not place the part in formalin, water, or saline, and do not tag the vessels or nerves. Make no attempts to perfuse the part.

BIBLIOGRAPHY

Carter PR: *Common Hand Injuries and Infections: A Practical Guide to Early Treatment.* Philadelphia, W.B. Saunders, 1983.

Dommisse IG, Lloyd GJ: Injuries to the fifth carpometacarpal region. *Can J Surg* 22:240–244, 1979.

Eaton RG, Little JW: Joint injuries and their sequelae. *Clin Plast Surg* 3:85–98, 1976.

Frazier WH, Brand DA: Quality assessment and the art of medicine: The anatomy of laceration care. *Med Care* 17:480–490, 1979.

Miller M, Fox RS, et al: Hand injuries: Incidence and epidemiology in an emergency service. *JACEP* 7:265–268, 1978.

The Hand. American Society for Surgery of the Hand, 2d ed. Churchill-Livingstone, New York, 1983.

Haury B, Rodeheaver G, Vensko J, et al: Debridement: An essential component of traumatic wound care. *Am J Surg* 135:238–242, 1978.

Hentz VR: Common hand problems. *Surg Clin North Am* 57:1103–1132, 1977.

Holden CE: Compartment syndromes following trauma. *Clin Orthop* 113:95–102, 1975.

Kaye JJ: Fractures and dislocations of the hand and wrist. *Semin Roentgenol* 13:109–116, 1978.

Lister GD, Kleinert HE, Kutz JE, et al: Primary flexor tendon repair followed by immediate controlled mobilization. *J Hand Surg* 2:441–451, 1977.

Posner MA: Injuries to the hand and wrist in athletes. *Orthop Clin North Am* 8:593–618, 1977.

Roberts AH, Teddy PJ: Retrospective trial of prophylactic antibiotics in hand infections. *Br J Surg* 64:394–396, 1977.

Tsuge K, Ikuta Y, Matsuishi Y: Repair of flexor tendons by intratendinous tendon suture. *J Hand Surg* 2:436–440, 1977.

CHAPTER 127
TRAUMA TO THE
PELVIS AND HIP

A. Trauma to the Pelvis

Joseph F. Waeckerle

Pelvic fractures comprise 3 percent of all skeletal fractures. These fractures and their associated injuries are the third most frequent cause of death from blunt trauma sustained in automobile accidents. Most pelvic fractures are secondary to automobile passenger or pedestrian accidents, but about one-third are the result of minor falls in older persons and from major falls or industrial accidents. This chapter discusses the most common fractures of the pelvis and hips, the mechanism of injury, radiologic evaluation, and treatment.

Anatomy

The major functions of the pelvis are protection, support, and hematopoiesis. The pelvis consists of the innominate bone, which is made up of the ilium, ischium, and pubis; the sacrum; and the coccyx. The iliopectineal or arcuate line divides the pelvis into the upper or false pelvis, which is part of the abdomen, and the lower true pelvis. In addition, this line constitutes the major portion of the femorosacral arch, which, along with the subsidiary tie arch (bodies of pubic bones and superior rami), supports the body in the erect position. In the sitting position the weightbearing forces are transmitted by the ischiosacral arch augmented by its tie arch, the pubic bones, inferior pubic rami, and ischial rami. When traumatized, the tie arches fracture first, especially at the symphysis pubis, pubic rami, and lateral to the sacroiliac (SI) joints. Incorporated in the pelvic structure are five joints that allow some movement in the bony ring. The lumbosacral, sacroiliac, and sacrococcygeal joints and the symphysis pubis allow for little movement. The acetabulum is a ball and socket joint that is divided into three portions: the iliac portion, or superior dome, is the chief weight-bearing surface; the inner wall consists of the pubis and is thin and easily fractured; and the posterior acetabulum is derived from the thick ischium.

The pelvis is extremely vascular, a fact that is significant in pelvic fractures (Fig. 127A-1). The nerve supply through the pelvis is derived from the lumbar and sacral plexi. Injury to the pelvis may produce deficits at any level from the nerve root to small peripheral branches (Fig, 127A-2).

The lower urinary tract is contained in the pelvis (Fig. 127A-3). In the adult, the bladder lies behind the symphysis and pubic bones, and the peritoneum covers the dome and base posteriorly. The location of the bladder and the degree of peritoneal reflection are determined by urine content. The lower gastrointestinal tract housed in the pelvis includes a small portion of the descending colon, the pelvic or sigmoid colon, the rectum, and the anus.

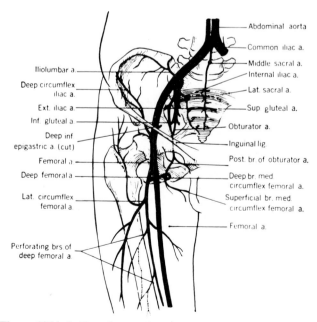

Figure 127A-1. Vascular supply to pelvis. (From *Stedman's Medical Dictionary*, ed. 23. Baltimore, The Williams & Wilkins Co, p 792. Used by permission.)

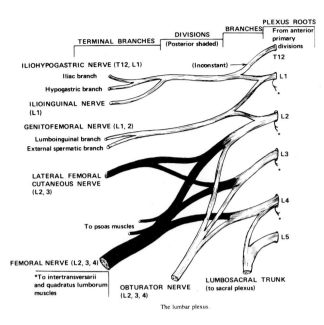

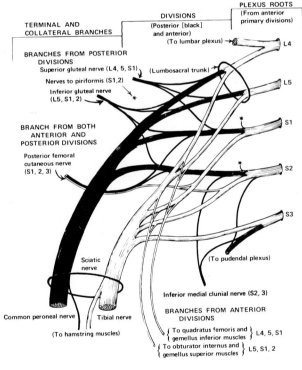

Figure 127A-2. The nerve supply to the pelvis is provided by the lumbar and sacral plexuses. (From Chusid JG: *Correlative Neuroanatomy & Functional Neurology*, ed 17. Los Altos, Lange Medical Publications, 1979, p 123, 126. Used by permission.)

CLINICAL EVALUATION

History

The emergency physician should assume that all victims of serious or multiple trauma, or both, have fractures of the pelvis. A patient with a suspected pelvic fracture should be questioned about details

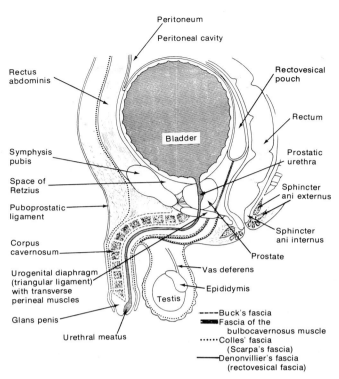

Figure 127A-3. Sagittal section of the male pelvis showing the relationship of the full bladder. [From Kane WJ: Fractures of the pelvis, in Rockwood CA, Jr, Green DP (eds): *Fractures*, vol 2. Philadelphia, JB Lippincott, Co, 1975, p 916 and 917. Used by permission.]

of the accident to determine the mechanism of injury. The patient should be asked about prehospital evaluation and treatment, and specifically questioned to determine areas of pain, last urination or defecation, present bladder sensation, and the last solid or fluid intake. In addition, time of the last menses or the presence of pregnancy, current medications, and allergies should be determined.

Physical Examination

Symptoms and signs of pelvic injuries include local pain and tenderness, especially pain upon walking; abdominal pain; and pelvic crepitus. On inspection look for perineal and pelvic edema, ecchymoses, lacerations, and deformities. Roll the patient over if appropriate and examine the areas overlying the sacrum and coccyx. Look for hematomas above the inguinal ligament or over the scrotum (Destot's sign). On palpation feel for irregularities, crepitus, or movement at the iliac crests, pubic rami, and ischial rami. Palpation of a bony prominence or large hematoma or tenderness along the fracture line is possible (Earle's sign). Compress the pelvis lateral to medial through the iliac crests, anterior to posterior through the symphysis pubis, and anterior to posterior through the iliac crests. Compress the greater trochanters and determine the range of motion of the hips. Always perform a rectal examination. Superior or posterior displacement of the prostate, or rectal injuries are indicative of intraperitoneal and urologic injury. Decrease in anal sphincter tone may suggest spinal cord injury. Check all pulses and determine neurologic function. If a pelvic fracture is found, assume intraabdominal, retroperitoneal, and urologic injuries until proved otherwise.

Radiologic Evaluation

Stabilization of the patient takes priority over obtaining x-ray films. Unnecessary movement may produce further injury or cause more blood loss. After stabilization, roentgenographic evaluation of the pelvis is a must in all unconscious patients who have sustained multiple injuries. Lower extremity long-bone fractures as well as pelvic symptoms or signs are also indications for roentgenograms. A standard anteroposterior (AP) view of the pelvis is necessary as a baseline. If additional studies are needed, lateral views, AP views of either hemipelvis, internal and external oblique views of the hemipelvis, or inlet and tilt views of the pelvis may be done. Angiography may be necessary to determine a source of bleeding. The patient's condition must dictate what is done and when.

CLASSIFICATION OF PELVIC FRACTURES

Fractures of the ilium and ischium comprise about two-thirds of pelvic fractures, while acetabular, coccygeal, and sacral fractures comprise the remainder.

Pelvic fractures are classified into types I, II, III, and IV, depending on the degree of disruption of the pelvic ring (Table 127A-1 and Fig. 127A-4).

Table 127A-1. Classification of Pelvic Fractures*

I. Fractures of individual bones without a break in the continuity of the pelvic ring.
    Avulsion fractures
        Anterior superior iliac spine
        Anterior inferior iliac spine
        Ischial tuberosity
    Fracture of the pubis or ischium
    Fracture of the wing of the ilium (Duverney)
    Fracture of the sacrum
    Fracture or dislocation of the coccyx
II. Single break in the pelvic ring
    Fracture of two ipsilateral rami
    Fracture near or subluxation of the symphysis pubis
    Fracture near or subluxation of the SI joint
III. Double breaks in the pelvic ring
    Double vertical fractures or dislocation of the pubis or both
        (straddle fractures)
    Double vertical fractures or dislocation or both (Malgaigne)
    Severe multiple fractures
IV. Fractures of the acetabulum
    Undisplaced
    Displaced

*Classification of pelvic fractures as adapted by Kane WJ: Fractures of the pelvis. In Rockwood CA, Jr. Green DP (eds): *Fractures*, vol 2. Philadelphia. JB Lippincott Co. 1975, p 925 from the classification by Key JA, Conwell HE: *The Management of Fractures, Dislocations, and Sprains.* ed 4. St. Louis, CV Mosby CO. 1946, p. 857. Used by permission.

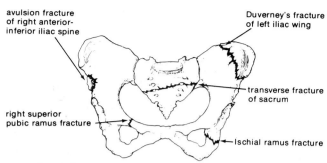

Type I: Fracture of individual bones without break in pelvic ring. Examples shown above.

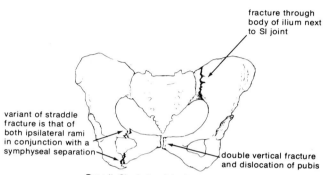

Type II: Single break in the pelvic ring. See examples above.

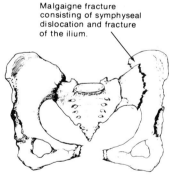

Type III: Double break in pelvic ring.

Figure 127A-4. Pelvic fractures (type I, II, and III) according to classification by Key JA, Conwell HE: *The Management of Fractures, Dislocations, and Sprains*, ed 4. St. Louis, CV Mosby, Co, 1946, p 857, as adapted by Kane WJ: Fractures of the pelvis, in Rockwood CA, Jr, Green DP (eds): *Fractures*, vol 2. Philadelphia, JB Lippincott Co, 1975, p 925. Illustrations adapted from *Fractures*, pp 926, 931–2, 934–5, 943, 947, 949).

Type I Fractures

Type I consists of fractures of individual bones without a break in the pelvic ring (Fig.127A-4). These fractures are usually stable and heal well with bed rest.

Avulsion fracture of anterior superior iliac spine. Avulsion occurs due to contraction of the sartorius muscle. Symptoms and signs are local pain, tenderness, and swelling and pain with flexion or abduction of the thigh. There is minimal displacement of the anterior superior iliac spine visible on the AP film of the pelvis.

Avulsion fracture of anterior inferior iliac spine. Avulsion occurs due to forceful contraction of the rectus femoris muscle. Symptoms and signs are sharp pain in the groin, difficulty with ambulation, and inability to flex the hip. The AP film shows downward displacement of the fragment, but this must be differentiated from the epiphyseal line of the os acetabuli.

Avulsion fracture of ischial tuberosity. The mechanism of injury is due to contraction of the hamstrings and the fracture is seen in youths whose apophyses are not united. Symptoms and signs include acute or chronic pain with sitting, or upon flexing the thigh with the knee extended. Rectal examination reveals tuberosity tenderness. The roentgenogram shows detachment of the apophysis from the ischium with minimal displacement. The apophysis closes between ages 20 to 25.

Fracture of single ramus of pubis or ischium. These injuries are commonly seen in the elderly and the mechanism of injury is usually a fall with direct trauma. Symptoms and signs include local pain and tenderness and inability to ambulate.

Examination of the pubic bones will usually distinguish a fracture of the pubis from a femoral neck fracture but a lateral film of the injured hip is recommended to rule out femoral neck injury. The AP roentgenogram of the pelvis shows nondisplaced fracture of the ramus.

Ischium body fractures. The incidence of ischial body injury is very low. The mechanism of injury is violent, external trauma, such as a fall in a sitting position. Symptoms and signs include local pain and tenderness, and pain with hamstring movement.

The x-ray film shows fracture of the body or tuberosity of the ischium. There may be a large fragment with comminution or a butterfly pattern seen on the AP film of the pelvis.

Iliac wing (Duverney) fractures. The mechanism of injury in an iliac wing fracture is direct trauma, usually lateral to medial. Symptoms and signs include pain, swelling, and tenderness over the iliac wing. There is severe pain on ambulation and Trendelenburg's sign is present. Although accompanying abdominal injuries are infrequent, abdominal rigidity, lower quadrant tenderness, and ileus are common findings. The AP film of the pelvis shows minimal displacement of fragments.

Sacral fractures. Transverse fractures of the sacrum are more common with massive pelvic injuries. The mechanism of injury is direct trauma by a posterior to anterior force, producing a transverse fracture. A rectal examination with the other hand on the sacrum causes pain and movement at the fracture site.

Roentgenogram interpretation may be difficult, and exactly aligned AP views are necessary to show the fracture. Look for a transverse fracture line at the level of the lower SI joint, and irregularity, buckling, or sharp angulation of the foramina. Examine the body and wings closely. A lateral view may show displacement anteriorly. Sacral root injury, especially S1 and S2, may be present.

Coccyx fractures. Coccygeal fractures are more frequent in women and are generally caused by direct violence or a fall in the sitting position. Symptoms and signs include pain, tenderness, and swelling and ecchymoses over the lower sacral region. There may be pain upon getting up from a sitting position or straining at stool. The rectal examination reveals pain and movement of the coccyx.

The roentgenogram is of questionable value, but AP and lateral views with sharp flexion of the thighs may demonstrate the fracture.

Type II Fractures

Type II fractures consist of a single break in the pelvic ring (Fig. 127A-4). These are by definition stable fractures with little or no displacement and are treated with bedrest. However, about one-fourth of patients with type II fractures have major associated soft tissue visceral injuries, especially genitourinary injuries.

Fracture of two rami ipsilaterally. The mechanism of injury is direct trauma, but forces through the femur can also cause fractures. Deformity, ecchymoses, and hematoma formation may be detected by palpation, and pain and motion at the fracture site are elicited by compression maneuvers. Flexion, abduction, external rotation, and extension of the hip (Patrick's test or Fabere sign) elicit pain. An AP x-ray film of the pelvis reveals fractures with no or minimal displacement.

Fracture near or subluxation of the symphysis pubis. The mechanism of injury to the symphysis pubis is usually direct anteroposterior trauma. These injuries may occur during or after childbirth. Symptoms and signs include severe pain with some external rotation of the lower extremities. Compression and palpation produce displacement pain. Bruising is generally absent.

The x-ray film shows fracture, subluxation, or dislocation. Subluxation may occur in either the sagittal or coronal plane. Dislocation occurs by overlapping in the midline, by superoposterior or inferoanterior displacement of one articulating surface in relation to the other. Complications include genitourinary injuries and SI joint disruption.

Fracture near or subluxation of the SI joint. The mechanism of injury to the SI joint is direct trauma from behind, or from behind and laterally. Symptoms and signs include local pain, pain with ambulation, and pain by compression maneuvers and Patrick's test. The posterior superior iliac spine appears more prominent on the injured side.

Radiologic views of the pelvis, sacrum, and SI joints are required. The films most often show fracture through the weak areas of the sacrum (first and second foramina), fracture through the ilium, overlapping of the ilium on the sacrum, or loss of regular joint space. In addition, carefully check for accompanying anterior pelvic ring injuries.

Type III Fractures

Type III fractures are characterized by a double break in the pelvic ring (Fig. 127A-4). They are unstable fractures and are frequently associated with visceral or soft tissue injuries.

Double vertical fracture or dislocation of the pubis (straddle fractures). The mechanism of injury in the straddle fracture is direct trauma to the arch, or lateral compression of the pelvis. Symptoms and signs include pain, deformity, bruising, and swelling. The fracture can be seen in the AP view.

Treatment is conservative, but the incidence of complications is high. In the series by Peltier, 20 percent of patients had lower genitourinary injuries and 38 percent had visceral abdominal injuries.

Double vertical fracture or dislocation (Malgaigne's fracture). Malgaigne's fracture consists of fractures of the superior and inferior rami or dislocation of the symphysis in association with sacral or iliac fracture, or SI joint dislocation. The mechanism of injury is debatable, but direct AP trauma is probably the most common cause.

Symptoms and signs include pain, crepitus, contusion, swelling, and decreased range of motion of the lower extremity. Middle fragment movement or displacement is seen, and there is pain and movement with compression maneuvers. The ipsilateral leg appears shortened.

Anteroposterior radiologic views may be sufficient but other views may also be required. All complications associated with pelvic trauma are frequently seen with this injury. Sacroiliac joint reduction is difficult and may result in chronic problems.

Severe multiple pelvic fractures. The mechanism of injury is exceptional trauma to the pelvis with strain on the weakest portion, or anterior tie arches that causes them to fracture along with the posterior ring. The incidence of sacral fractures ranges from 4 to 74 percent (Furey, 1942) and the injury is due to forces generated by rotation, leverage, and shearing.

Multiple fractures are easily seen on x-ray, but acetabular and sacral fractures are difficult to see, so special views may be necessary. To recognize sacral fractures, compare the distance between the upper and lower borders of the SI joint (the lateral sacral

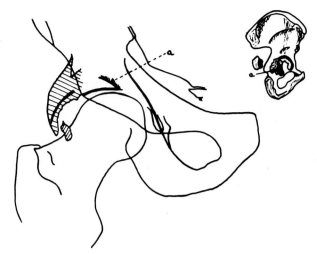

Figure 127A-6. Fracture of posterior lip with some impaction and comminution. (From Judet R, Judet J, Letournel E: Fractures of the acetabulum: Classification and surgical approaches for open reduction. *J Bone Joint Surg* 46A:1623, 1964. Used by permission.)

promontory) and the midline on both sides. These should be equal. Also, inspect and compare the sacral foramina.

Complications include genitourinary, gastrointestinal, vascular, and neurologic injuries. Treatment is conservative but requires adequate reduction of the ilium.

Type IV Fractures of the Acetabulum

Type IV acetabular fractures are increasing in frequency with an increase in automobile accidents. They are seen commonly with other pelvic injuries. The roentgenographic anatomy of type IV fractures is shown in Fig. 127A-5. There are four anatomical types of fractures, and all are associated with hip dislocations: posterior (Fig. 127A-6 and Fig. 127A-7), ilioischial column (Fig. 127A-8), transverse (Fig. 127A-9), and iliopubic column (Fig. 127A-10). In addition, combinations of any of these fractures can occur.

Posterior fracture. The mechanism of injury in a posterior fracture is direct trauma to a flexed knee and hip. Anteroposterior and lateral radiologic views easily demonstrate the posterior acetabular fracture with the posterior hip dislocation. Complications are sciatic nerve injury and femoral fractures.

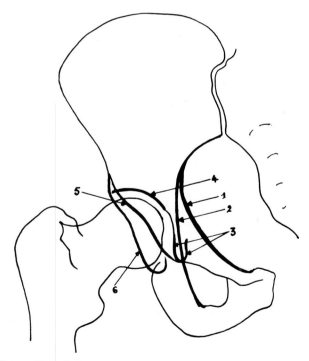

Figure 127A-5. Roentgenographic anatomy of type IV acetabular fractures. The AP view shows (1) arcuate (iliopectineal) line, (2) ilioischial roentgenographic line, (3) roentgenographic U, (4) roof, (5) anterior lip, and (6) posterior lip. (From Judet R, Judet J, Letournel E: Fractures of the acetabulum: Classification and surgical approaches for open reduction. *J Bone Joint Surg* 46A:1616, 1964. Used by permission.)

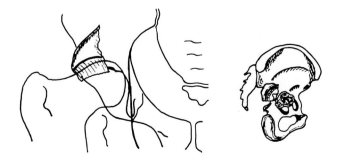

Figure 127A-7. Posteriosuperior rim fracture. (From Judet R, Judet J, Letournel E: Fractures of the acetabulum: Classification and surgical approaches for open reduction. *J Bone Joint Surg* 46A:1624, 1964. Used by permission.)

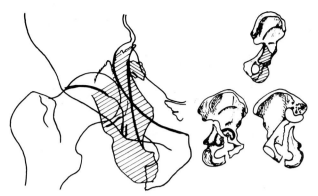

Figure 127A-8. Ilioischial fracture. (From Judet R, Judet J, Letournel E: Fractures of the acetabulum: Classification and surgical approaches for open reduction. *J Bone Joint Surg* 46A:1625, 1964. Used by permission.)

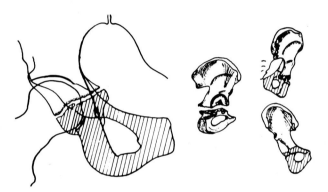

Figure 127A-9. Transverse fracture without displacement. (From Judet R, Judet J, Letournel E: Fractures of the acetabulum: Classification and surgical approaches for open reduction. *J Bone Joint Surg* 46A:1627, 1964. Used by permission.)

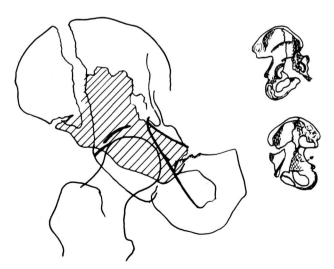

Figure 127A-10. Iliopubic fracture. (From Judet R, Judet J, Letournel E: Fractures of the acetabulum: Classification and surgical approaches for open reduction. *J Bone Joint Surg* 46A:1632, 1964. Used by permission.)

Ilioischial column fracture. The mechanism of injury is posteriorly directed force to a knee with the thigh abducted and flexed. The AP x-ray film demonstrates a large, medially displaced fragment with central dislocation of the femoral head. The most common complication is sciatic nerve injury.

Transverse fracture of acetabulum. The mechanism is force lateral to medial over the greater trochanter, or force posterior to anterior on the posterior pelvis with the hip flexed. An AP x-ray film clearly demonstrates the fracture with a central hip dislocation.

Iliopubic column fracture. The mechanism of injury is a lateral force to the greater trochanter with the hip externally rotated. On roentgenography, there is marked external rotation of the hip. The ilioischial line is disrupted and the anterior lip is fractured.

Further discussion on acetabular fractures appears in Section 127B, ''Trauma to the Hip.''

Treatment

Anatomical restoration is required for hip fractures. If the difficult task of reduction of the femoral head and exact restoration of the displaced fractured acetabulum cannot be done quickly and safely, surgery is indicated. If there is no displacement, bed rest is the treatment of choice. If redislocation occurs, the hip is unstable and surgery is necessary.

Failure to recognize pelvic trauma leads to nonstabilization of the fracture which, in turn, enhances blood loss and causes further injuries. It may also lead to an incomplete evaluation of pelvic injury.

It is imperative that the physician recognize associated injuries, especially those requiring immediate workup.

Complications

Complications include hemorrhage, myositis ossificans, infection, thrombophlebitis, and sciatic nerve injuries.

Hemorrhage. Hemorrhage is a major cause of death in pelvic injuries. Hauser and Perry (1966) reported that patients with type III fractures required blood replacement two-and-one-half times more often than type I, II, or IV and needed two-and-one-half times more blood than patients with types I, II, or IV fractures who received transfusions. Retroperitoneal bleeding is an inevitable complication and up to 4 L of blood can be accommodated in this space. Both small and large vessels, especially the superior gluteal and internal pudendal branches of the internal iliac artery, can be disrupted.

General resuscitative measures include massive crystalloid, colloid, and blood replacement.

An antishock garment provides stabilization, shifts intravascular volume, and may be helpful in controlling bleeding sites.

If the patient is exsanguinating, angiography can be done and small bleeding sites controlled by selective embolization. Most authorities agree that aggressive fluid and blood replacement is best. Laparotomy is a last measure.

Urinary tract injuries. Urinary tract injuries are discussed in Chapter 123, ''Genitourinary Trauma.''

Gynecological injury. Gynecological injuries are usually associated with anterior trauma, and vaginal laceration is the most common injury. Treatment is repair of wounds and antibiotic therapy.

There is a high fetal death rate associated with pelvic trauma in the last trimester of pregnancy if the mother is in shock; if there is placental, uterine, or direct fetal injury; or if the mother dies. Immediate cesarean section must be considered.

Rectal injuries are rare, and are usually associated with urinary injuries and ischial fractures. Diagnosis is by rectal examination; treatment is by surgical repair.

Ruptured diaphragm. Ruptured diaphragm associated with fracture of the pelvis may be more common than previously thought. It may be associated with rib injuries. Diagnosis is by physical findings, such as displacement of the heart toward the right, absent breath sounds, presence of bowel sounds in the chest, and a positive chest x-ray film if the defect is large. Diagnosis may be difficult if the defect is small.

Nerve root injury. Nerve root or peripheral nerve injuries can occur due to traction, pressure from hemorrhage, callus or fibrous tissue, and impingement-laceration by bone fragments. The onset of symptoms and signs may be delayed, but deficits usually follow a nerve root pattern. Lumbar nerve root injuries are associated with SI joint dislocation or fracture. Sacral root injuries are associated with sacral fractures, especially fractures of S1 and S2.

Pelvic Fractures in Children

Commonly caused by auto-pedestrian accidents, pelvic fractures in children have a high incidence of associated injuries due to less protection afforded by the developing pelvis. Genitourinary injury is frequent but hemorrhage determines mortality. Children in shock who respond poorly to fluid replacement have the highest mortality.

Postponement of surgery until stabilization of circulation is recommended unless the patient is exsanguinating despite treatment. If the child does not respond to transfusions equal to the estimated total blood volume (TBV) (88 mL/kg × wt [kg] = TBV) within 1 h, suspect major vascular injury and operate. Both arterial and venous injuries are associated with significant SI joint injury.

BIBLIOGRAPHY

Baylis SM, Lansing EH, Glas WW: Traumatic retroperitoneal hematoma. *Am J Surg* 103:477–480, 1962.

Bonnin JG: Sacral fractures and injuries to cauda equina. *J Bone Joint Surg* 27:113–127, 1945.

Brooks DH, Grenvik A: G-suit control of massive retroperitoneal hemorrhage due to pelvic fracture. *Crit Care Med* 1:257–260, 1973.

Coffield KS, Weems WL: Experience with management of posterior urethral injury associated with pelvic fracture. *J Urol* 117:722–724, 1977.

Dunn W, Morris HD: Fractures and dislocations of the pelvis. *J Bone Joint Surg* 50A:1639–1648, 1968.

Epstein HC: Traumatic dislocations of the hip. *Clin Orthop* 92:116–142, 1973.

Froman C, Stein A: Complicated crushing injuries of the pelvis. *J Bone Joint Surg* 49B:24–32, 1976.

Furey WW: Fractures of the pelvis with special reference to associated fractures of the sacrum. *Am J Roentgenol* 47:89–96, 1942.

Goodell CL: Neurologic deficits associated with pelvic fractures. *J Neurosurg* 24:837–842, 1966.

Gourin A, Garzon AG: Diagnostic problems in traumatic diaphragmatic hernia. *J Trauma* 14:20–31, 1974.

Harris WR: Avulsion of lumbar roots complicating fractures of the pelvis. *J Bone Joint Surg* 55A:1436–1449, 1973.

Hauser CW, Perry JF Jr: Massive hemorrhage from pelvic fractures. *Minn Med* 49:285–290, 1966.

Hawkins L, Pomerantz M, Eiseman B: Laparotomy at time of pelvic fracture. *J Trauma* 10:619–623, 1970.

Judet R, Judet L, Letournel E: Fractures of the acetabulum: Classification and surgical approaches for open reduction. *J Bone Joint Surg* 46A:1615–1646; 1675, 1964.

Kane WJ: Fractures of the pelvis, in Rockwood CA Jr, Green DP (eds): *Fractures*. Philadelphia, JB Lippincott Co, 1975, vol 2, pp 905–1011.

Levine JI, Crampton RS: Major abdominal injuries associated with pelvic fractures. *Surg Gynecol Obstet* 116:223–226, 1963.

Lucas GL: Missile wounds of the bony pelvis. *J Trauma* 10:624–633, 1970.

McAvoy JM, Cook JH: A treatment plan for rapid assessment of the patient with massive blood loss and pelvic fractures. *Arch Surg* 113:986–990, 1978.

Patterson FP, Morton KS: The cause of death in fractures of the pelvis. *J Trauma* 13:849–856, 1973.

Patzakis MJ, Harvey JP JR, Ivler D: The role of antibiotics in the management of open fractures. *J Bone Joint Surg* 56A:532–541, 1974.

Peltier LF: Complications associated with fractures of the pelvis. *J Bone Joint Surg* 47A:1060–1069, 1965.

Pokorny M, Pontes JE, Pierce JM Jr: Urological injuries associated with pelvic trauma. *J Urol* 121:455–457, 1979.

Quinby WC Jr: Fractures of the pelvis and associated injuries in children. *J Pediatr Surg* 1:353–364, 1966.

Quinby WC Jr: Pelvic fractures with hemorrhage, editorial. *New Engl J Med* 284:668–669, 1971.

Ravitch MM: Hypogastric artery ligation in acute pelvic trauma, editorial. *Surgery* 56:601–602, 1964.

Reynolds BM, Balsano NA, Reynolds FX: Pelvic fractures. *J Trauma* 13:1011–1014, 1973.

Rothenberger DA, Velasco R, Strate R, et al: Open pelvic fracture: A lethal injury. *J Trauma* 18:184–187, 1978.

Rothenberger D, Quattlebaum FW, Perry JF Jr, et al: Blunt maternal trauma: A review of 103 cases. *J Trauma* 18:173–179, 1978

Wakeley CPG: Fractures of the pelvis: An analysis of 100 cases. *Br J Surg* 17:22–29, 1930.

B. Trauma to the Hip

Joseph F. Waeckerle, Martin Weissman
Harry Herkowitz, Kenneth Gitlin

ANATOMY

The hip is a ball and socket joint made up of the acetabulum and femur (Fig. 127B-1). The hip includes the acetabulum and the proximal femur 2 to 3 in below the lesser trochanter. The functions of the hip are weight bearing and movement. The fibrous capsule that surrounds the joint on all sides is exceedingly strong. It attaches around the acetabulum proximally and runs to the intertrochanteric line distally on the anterior surface. Posteriorly, it falls short of the intertrochanteric crest and inserts on the neck of the femur. It is weakest posteriorly.

The blood supply of the femoral head is derived from nutrient branches of the obturator, medial femoral circumflex, and superior and inferior gluteal arteries. These course beneath the reflection of the capsule on the neck of the femur, and also along the ligamentum teres. The capsular vessels are much more important than those of the ligamentum teres.

PHYSICAL EXAMINATION

General examination includes a detailed history and complete examination with careful evaluation of the hip. Inspection of the unclothed, erect patient is done looking for a list, asymmetry of the muscles, and injuries or scars. If possible, test the gait for abnormalities such as Trendelenburg's sign, a waddling gait due to paralysis of the gluteal muscles in which the trunk lists to the affected side with each step. With the patient supine, inspect the position of the extremities for rotation and shortening. Test for range of motion (ROM) beginning with rotation of the hip with the leg in extension. If this maneuver is painful, all other maneuvers should be done cautiously, if at all. Palpation of the hip is helpful but requires practice to interpret findings. A small portion of the femoral head may be palpated below the inguinal ligament and lateral to the femoral artery. Direct pressure may elicit pain, rocking the femur may cause crepitus, and if the head does not move, a fracture of the femoral neck is possible. If the femoral head is not felt, dislocation is suggested. Always rule out associated femoral shaft injuries.

CLASSIFICATION OF HIP FRACTURES

Hip fractures are classified as femoral neck, trochanteric, intertrochanteric, and subtrochanteric. For purposes of this discussion, fractures in the region of the hip are divided into two major groups: (1) those that occur within the capsule of the joint, and (2) those that occur at the base of the femoral neck with involvement of one or both trochanters. The prognosis for successful union and restoration of normal function varies considerably with the two groups.

In intracapsular fractures with displacement, the femoral neck vessels will be torn, and the blood supply through the ligamentum teres may not be sufficient to nourish the entire femoral head. Therefore, aseptic necrosis will inevitably result unless some of the capsular vessels remain intact. Basilar neck and intertrochanteric fractures below the capsule rarely sever important arteries.

Slipped Femoral Capital Epiphysis

The acute slipped femoral capital epiphysis, which occurs in adolescence, takes place within the capsule and may leave the ligamentum teres as the only available blood supply. The vessels in this ligament are larger in children and hence supply more blood to the femoral head than in adults. Therefore, comparable fractures in young persons seem to carry a more favorable prognosis. Gradual slipping of the femoral capital epiphysis might possibly permit readjustment of the blood supply by the capsular vessels, and along with the supply to the ligamentum teres, accounts for the low incidence of delayed aseptic necrosis resulting from this lesion.

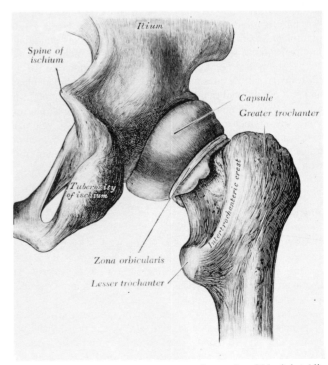

Figure 127B-1. Synovial membrane of capsule of hip joint (distended). Posterior aspect. (From Goss CM (ed): *Anatomy of the Human Body* by Henry Gray, ed 29. Philadelphia, Lea & Febiger, p 344. Used by permission.)

Slipping of the femoral capital epiphysis in adolescence should be recognized early before any marked displacement has occurred. Clinically, the patient complains of either groin pain with weight-bearing, pain on external rotation of the hip, or knee pain that is referred from the hip.

This condition should be treated with multiple threaded pins that allow early hip motion and ambulation with crutches without weight-bearing on the affected hip. Weight-bearing may be resumed when roentgenograms reveal bony fusion between the head and neck. Subsequent development of pain with radiologic evidence of altered contour of the head suggests the possibility of aseptic necrosis or cartilage necrosis. The patient should be treated accordingly by prolonged protection against weight-bearing.

Femoral Neck Fractures

Femoral neck fractures are classified as stress, impacted, displaced, and comminuted. The mechanism of injury is most often minor torsion, generally with osteoporosis or osteomalacia, and is believed to be pathological in origin.

Fractures of the femoral neck are quite common among elderly persons, who are susceptible to falls. In fact, it may be that a stress fracture occurs first, resulting in the fall. Stress fractures may not be evident immediately on x-ray so repeat films are done 10 to 14 days after the injury.

Clinical Features

The patient with an impacted fracture may be able to walk without severe difficulty, but may have a limp. However, unless the fracture is recognized and adequately treated within a few days, displacement occurs and the prognosis is generally poor. Minor pain, minimal muscle spasm, and slightly decreased range of motion are usual physical findings in stress or impacted fractures. In contrast, displaced fractures cause severe pain, inability to ambulate, and severely limited range of motion. The classic position of the affected limb is one of shortening, abduction, and external rotation. Any attempt to internally rotate the hip causes severe pain. The displaced fracture is detected on AP and lateral x-ray films. Impacted fractures should be easily seen on AP and lateral films, with disruption of Shenton's line.

Treatment

During the first 24 h after admission, Buck's traction may be applied to the leg. Treatment for stress fractures is no weight-bearing in the young, and possible surgery in the elderly. The treatment of choice for impacted and displaced fractures is prompt, early internal fixation or prosthetic arthroplasty.

For the elderly and debilitated patient, primary prosthetic replacement of the femoral head with a metal stem prosthesis is now a successful and commonly used procedure. Bed rest or cast application has long been abandoned because of the associated incidence of pneumonia and phlebitis. Early weight-bearing is permitted and encouraged with reduction of postoperative morbidity.

The prognosis for a good, functional result with bony union is markedly improved when internal fixation is skillfully applied following an accurate reduction. An undisplaced impacted fracture has a higher incidence of union and markedly decreased likelihood of aseptic necrosis. Weight-bearing after surgical fixation is not permitted until solid union is demonstrated radiologically. This usually requires at least 3 to 6 months.

Complications

The most significant complications are nonunion and avascular necrosis. Nonunion is usually the result of poor reduction or inadequate immobilization of the fracture and frequently accompanies aseptic necrosis of the femoral head. Not infrequently it occurs in spite of good reduction or adequate immobilization and is secondary to a diminished blood supply to this area. Many methods have been described for treating nonunion of femoral fractures by techniques such as bone grafts driven through the femoral neck, trochanteric osteotomies, or subtrochanteric osteotomies.

Every attempt should be made to save the femoral head in a young, healthy patient with no evidence of aseptic necrosis or collapse of the femoral head and no loss of articular congruency. If these complications occur, an endoprosthesis or, if necessary, total hip replacement is indicated. Nonunion with or without a viable head occurring in an elderly patient is an indication for prosthetic replacement.

Although avascular necrosis usually presents within 3 years of injury, changes may occur up to 20 years later. The incidence of avascular necrosis is higher with severe fractures or fractures that are not surgically reduced to the anatomic position within 48 h.

Femoral Head Fractures

Shear fractures of the superior aspect of the femoral head are associated with anterior dislocation, and inferior head fractures are associated with posterior dislocation. Symptoms and signs are those of the associated dislocation. X-ray films, especially the postreduction films, demonstrate the fragment.

Treatment is reduction of the fracture and possible surgery to fix fragments, especially if they are large. If a significant portion of the superior weight-bearing surface is involved, a total joint replacement gives excellent results.

Comminuted fractures are usually due to severe trauma and may be associated with other injuries. Hip replacement is the treatment of choice unless the acetabulum is involved. In that case, the fracture is treated by traction and delayed surgery.

Trochanteric Fractures

Greater trochanter. Greater trochanter avulsions are occasionally seen and the displaced or comminuted fragment is shown by an AP film. If displacement is greater than 1 cm, fixation is advisable in the young but not in the old patient.

Lesser trochanter. Lesser trochanter fractures are seen in children and young, athletic adults. If there is a greater than 2 cm displacement as seen on the AP film, screw fixation is indicated.

Intertrochanteric and subtrochanteric. An intertrochanteric or basilar neck fracture is an extracapsular fracture occurring in a line between the greater and lesser trochanters.

Subtrochanteric fractures, or fractures below the intertrochanteric line without an associated fracture of either the lesser or greater trochanter, will also be considered in this group of fractures.

Fractures that involve the intertrochanteric region may be oblique along the intertrochanteric line, or extremely comminuted with fragments of both trochanters and the proximal end of the shaft of the femur. These fractures are usually produced by direct trauma, commonly falls or automobile accidents. The mechanism of injury in a subtrochanteric fracture is direct trauma, or occasionally an extension of an intertrochanteric fracture.

Clinical Features

Symptoms and signs include hip pain, swelling, and ecchymoses. There is marked external rotation and shortening of the extremity in contrast to the minimal deformity associated with femoral neck fractures. Symptoms and signs of subtrochanteric fractures are similar to those of trochanteric or femoral fractures. Hypovolemic shock can result if large amounts of blood are lost into the thigh.

Treatment

The use of closed treatment has long been abandoned and it is generally accepted that open reduction and internal fixation with a Jewett nail and side plate, or a compression screw and side plate, is indicated in a comminuted intertrochanteric or basilar neck fracture.

Complications include malunion of the fracture, infection, and thromboembolism. Avascular necrosis is rare because the bone in the region of the greater trochanters is predominantly cancellous and possesses a rich supply of blood derived from many nutrient arteries. Nonunion of fractures in this region is exceedingly rare. Malunion with coxa vara deformity, however, is not infrequent.

Anteroposterior and lateral roentgenograms of the hip and knee are necessary to assess the patient. Traction is required to reduce the fracture.

Complications of subtrochanteric fractures are similar to those seen with intertrochanteric fractures, except there is a high incidence of nonunion.

HIP DISLOCATIONS

Hip dislocations can be classified as anterior, posterior, and central. Acetabular fracture with central hip dislocation has been discussed under type IV pelvic fractures.

Anterior Dislocations

About 10 percent of hip dislocations are anterior, and the majority are secondary to auto accidents, but they may also result from a fall, or a blow to the back while squatting. The mechanism of injury is forced abduction that causes the head to be levered out through an anterior capsular tear. The affected extremity is in abduction and external rotation. Neurovascular compromise is an unusual, but possible, complication.

An AP film of the pelvis easily demonstrates the head to be inferior and medial to the acetabulum. A lateral view illustrates the anterior dislocation more clearly, although it may be difficult to obtain because of the patient's pain.

Treatment for the dislocation is early closed reduction, usually under general anesthesia. Strong, in-line traction is done while flexion and internal rotation are carried out. Finally, the hip is abducted once the head clears the rim of the acetabulum. The dislocation should be reduced quickly, within a few hours, because the longer the delay in reduction, the higher the incidence of aseptic necrosis.

Posterior Dislocations

Posterior dislocations comprise 80 to 90 percent of hip dislocations. They are caused by force applied to a flexed knee, directed posteriorly. Acetabular fractures may result as well. On examination, the extremity is shortened, internally rotated, and adducted.

Anteroposterior and lateral x-ray films of the pelvis and hip will reveal the dislocation but further assessment of the acetabulum and femur must be done to rule out fractures. The oblique views of Judet will reveal an acetabular fracture. Also, inferior femoral head fracture will be seen on the AP or oblique view. Hip dislocations are difficult to recognize with femoral shaft fractures so roentgenograms of the pelvis and hips should be routinely obtained in such cases.

The treatment of posterior dislocation without fracture is closed reduction, preferably under general anesthesia, as quickly as possible and always within 48 h. In-line traction, gentle flexion to 90°, and then gentle internal-to-external rotation is done (Allis maneuver). The Stimson maneuver may prove useful in certain situations.

Complications include sciatic nerve injury in about 10 percent of the patients, and avascular necrosis that increases in direct proportion to the delay in adequate reduction.

HIP INJURIES IN CHILDREN

Fractures of the proximal end of the femur are rare in children. Trauma may produce a displaced epiphysis or a fracture of the neck, trochanteric, or subtrochanteric region. Traumatic epiphyseal separation is probably less common than the previously mentioned fractures, but is more common than dislocation. The treatment is anatomical reduction usually best obtained by surgery.

Traumatic dislocations in children are rare. They are more common in boys (4:1) and more common between ages 4 to 7 and 11 to 15. The frequency of left versus right is equal, and bilateral dislocations are reportable. Posterior dislocations occur with an 80 to 85 percent frequency. The mechanism of injury and the clinical picture are similar to that seen in traumatic dislocation in the adult. The presence of an associated fracture is rare.

The treatment is closed reduction. Dislocation is an orthopedic emergency and reduction should be done within 12 h. Delay in reduction past 24 h is associated with a much higher incidence of complications.

FEMORAL SHAFT FRACTURES

Fractures of the shaft of the femur most often occur in men during their most active period in life. Falls, and industrial and automobile accidents account for the majority of these fractures.

Severe, direct trauma may result in transverse fractures with displacement, oblique or spiral oblique fractures, or badly comminuted segments.

The femur is surrounded by large muscle groups with a rich vascular supply (Fig. 127B-2). Therefore, femoral fractures may result in the loss of at least 1 L or more of blood into the soft tissues of the thigh, producing clinical shock. The initial evaluation should always include careful neurovascular examination of the extremity.

It is best to splint the leg at the time of injury as it lies. Frequently, Hare traction or Thomas' splint can be placed over the trousers, applying traction by means of a twisted rope extending from a sling around the ankle.

Treatment

In infants and children up to 3 or 4 years of age, fractures of the shaft of the femur are treated by direct overhead traction applied to both legs. The infant should be lifted up until no weight is borne by the sacrum. This technique is not used in older children since hydrostatic pressure makes it difficult for blood to reach the

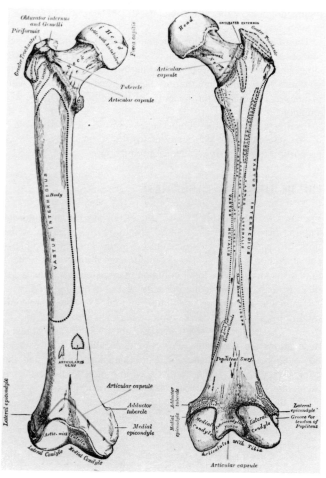

Figure 127B-2. Anterior and posterior surfaces of right femur. [From Goss CM (ed): *Anatomy of the Human Body* by Henry Gray, ed 29. Philadelphia, Lea & Febiger, p 241. Used by permission.]

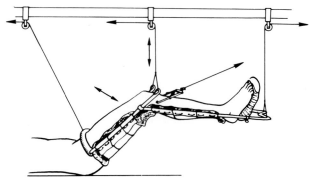

Figure 127B-3. Fisk traction achieves suspension by a half Thomas ring and Pearson attachment. Mobilization of the knee is assisted by traction to the cut ends of the Thomas ring, which can be moved up and down by the patient. [From Mooney V: Fractures of the shaft of the femur, in Rockwood CA Jr, Green DP (eds): *Fractures,* Philadelphia, JB Lippincott Co, 1975, vol 2, p 1087. Used by permission.]

foot in the overhead position and perfusion of the extremity may be impaired.

In an older child or adult, the Fisk type of traction by means of a half Thomas ring and Pearson attachment, to allow for flexion of the knee, is satisfactory if sufficient traction is applied to reduce overriding and thus prevent shortening (Fig. 127B-3). The traction must be skillfully adjusted so that the lower fragments line up with the upper fragments. A Steinmann pin or Kirschner wire inserted through the femur, high enough not to endanger this growth plate in children, or the knee joint in either children or adults, provides the best means for obtaining skeletal traction. This is much more efficient than Buck's or Russell's traction.

The intramedullary rod is frequently the method of choice for the treatment of uncomplicated fractures of the midshaft and junction of the upper and middle thirds of the femur, except where comminution is so extensive that stability with the rod cannot be maintained. The rod gives excellent immobilization, maintains the reduction, and permits ambulation with active exercise of both the hip and the knee joint. It is the preferred method from the standpoint of functional recovery and obtaining excellent reduction with decreased hospital cost. It should be reserved for use by orthopedic surgeons who have had special training in its insertion and who are sufficiently skilled to apply it without undue risk to the patient. Complications include thrombophlebitis, infection, bending or breaking of the rod, splitting of the bone from too large a rod, and nonunion.

In cases where comminution is severe, either dual plating or the use of a compression plate device can result in excellent fixation.

Lower Femoral Epiphyseal Fractures

Displacement of the lower femoral epiphysis, or slippage at the line of the epiphyseal growth cartilage plate, can occur during childhood. Most often the epiphysis is pushed anteriorly onto the anterior surface of the distal end of the shaft of the femur. Compression of the femoral artery and vein over the sharp edge of the distal end of the femoral diaphysis may result in a serious circulatory disturbance of the foot.

Treatment

If the slip is not complete, reduction may be obtained by applying adhesive skin traction and extending the leg. Dislocations of this type can also be reduced by manipulation under anesthesia. The procedure requires traction with the knee held in flexion, and reduction is maintained by immobilization of the leg with the knee flexed at approximately 90°. When the swelling has subsided after 2 or 3 weeks, the flexion can be gradually decreased. Since this injury occurs in children, there is usually little danger of permanent stiffness in the knee joint.

BIBLIOGRAPHY

Aadalen RJ, Weiner DS, Hoyt W, et al: Acute slipped capital femoral epiphysis. *J Bone Joint Surg* 56A:1473–1487, 1974.

Bentley G: Impacted fractures of the neck of the femur. *J Bone Joint Surg* 50B:551–561, 1968.

Boyd KS, Burke JF, Colton T: A double-blind clinical trial of prophylactic antibiotics in hip fractures. *J Bone Joint Surg* 55A:1251–1258, 1973.

Brav EA: Traumatic dislocation of the hip. *J Bone Joint Surg* 44A:1115–1133, 1962.

Casey MJ, Chapman MW: Ipsilateral concomitant fracturees of the hip and femoral shaft. *J Bone Joint Surg* 61A:503–509, 1979.

Clawson DK, Melcher PJ: Fractures and dislocations of the hip, in Rockwood CA Jr, Green DP (eds): *Fractures.* Philadelphia, JB Lippincott Co, 1975, vol 2, pp 1012–1074.

Clawson DK, Smith RF, Hanson FT: Closed intramedullary nailing of the femur. *J Bone Joint Surg* 53A:681–692, 1971.

De Palma AF, Danryo JJ, Stose WG: Slipping of the upper femoral epiphysis. *Clin Orthop* 37:167–183, 1964.

Deyerle WM: Multiple-pin peripheral fixation in fractures of the neck of the femur: Immediate weight-bearing. *Clin Orthop* 39:135–156, 1965.

Duncan CP, Shim S-S: Blood supply of the head of the femur in traumatic hip dislocation. *Surg Gynecol Obstet* 144:185–191, 1977.

Elliott RB: Fractures of the femoral condyles: Experiences with a new design femoral condyle blade plate. *South Med J* 5:80–95, 1959.

Epstein HC: Traumatic dislocations of the hip. *Clin Orthop* 92:116–142, 1973.

Evarts CM: Endoprosthesis as the primary treatment of femoral neck fractures. *Clin Orthop* 92:69–76, 1973.

Gartland JJ, Benner JH: Traumatic dislocations in the lower extremity in children. *Orthop Clin North Am* 7:687–700, 1976.

Jacobs R, Niemann K: Fractures of the hip in childhood. *South Med J* 69:629–631, 1976.

Key JA, Conwell HE: *Management of Fractures, Dislocations, and Sprains.* St Louis, CV Mosby Co, 1951.

Korn NW, States JD: Slipping capital femoral epiphysis: A long-term follow up and review of cases in Rochester, New York. *Clin Orthop* 48:119–128, 1966.

Seinsheimer F: Subtrochanteric fractures of the femur. *J Bone Joint Surg* 60:300–306, 1978.

Thaggard A III, Harle TS, Carlson V: Fractures and dislocations of bony pelvis and hip. *Semin Roentgenol* 13:117–134, 1978.

Tronzo RG: Hip nails for all occasions. *Orthop Clin North Am* 5:479–492, 1974.

CHAPTER 128
KNEE INJURIES

Joseph F. Waeckerle, Robert J. Rothstein

Injuries to the knee are becoming increasingly more common in our sports-oriented society. It is essential that the emergency physician become familiar with the examination of the normal and abnormal knee, to be able to recognize specific injuries, and to treat and appropriately refer these injuries. This chapter will deal with examination of the knee and recognition of fractures and dislocations of the patella; fractures of femoral condyles; fractures of the tibial spines, tuberosity, and plateaus; ligamentous and meniscal injuries of the knee joint; knee dislocation; and osteochondritis dissecans.

As with all orthopedic injuries, the accurate diagnosis of the injured knee is required before proper treatment can be instituted. However, with the knee it is particularly important to do a complete and careful examination in a logical stepwise manner since the knee is so essential for ambulation. As with many other problems, the emergency physician has the unique opportunity, in most instances, to be the first to see the patient with a knee injury. This allows the emergency physician the first examination, which is usually the easiest to perform, since the patient does not anticipate the pain and, therefore, does not guard and muscular spasm causing further guarding may not yet have occurred. It is imperative that the emergency physician understand the reasons for the various tests performed in the examination of the knee and develop a technique so that he or she is comfortable with the examination and thereby renders proper treatment.

The appropriate x-rays of the knee should be done as early as possible in the examination of the knee. Once the neurovascular status of the knee has been evaluated, x-rays should be taken. This is usually done prior to the palpation and inspection of the knee. There are a few exceptions to this rule, one of which is examination of the knee on the field or on the sidelines after the injury. Another might be some palpation of the knee to localize specific problems so that special views might be ordered such as the sunrise or sunset view of the patella for possible subluxation or fractures, or for stress testing under fluoroscopy, which is especially applicable in the child with a possible epiphyseal injury.

EXAMINATION

The examination of the knee is divided into five phases: history, observation, inspection, palpation, and stress testing.

History. The mechanism of injury as well as any serious problems frequently clarifies subtleties in the examination, allowing a more accurate diagnosis and appropriate treatment.

Observation. The patient should be examined while walking, if possible, and in both the sitting and lying positions. The physician should take note of the gait, muscular development, and functional range of motion at this time.

Inspection. The knee should be inspected for swelling, ecchymoses, effusion, masses, patella location and size, muscle mass, erythema, and evidence of local trauma. Also, the physician should note at this time, with the patient in a supine position, leg lengths (equal or unequal). Lastly, the physician should ask the patient to perform the best possible active range of motion.

Palpation. Initially the neurovascular status of the leg should be noted. As with all orthopedic examinations, the noninjured or normal knee should be compared to the injured knee during all aspects of the examination but especially during palpation and stress testing. When the physician palpates the knee, he or she should begin in the nontender areas and work lastly toward the tender area so that the patient does not guard or become apprehensive. The examiner should always palpate the knee joint in a systematic manner. Effusion, tenderness, increased temperature, strength, sensation, and location of pulses should be noted.

The physician should examine the patella for size, shape, and location with the knee in flexion, while mobility should be checked in extension. It should also be compressed to check for pain as well as moved laterally and medially to ascertain possible subluxation. The popliteal space should also be palpated for masses, swelling, and circulation status.

Stress testing. The final phase of the examination of the knee is stress testing. This is the most controversial and difficult aspect of the examination of the knee, although potentially it is the most informative. A brief summary of the instabilities and tests performed to demonstrate them are presented in the section on ligamentous and meniscal injuries.

FRACTURES

Fractures of the Patella

Fractures of the patella occur from a direct blow, a fall on the flexed knee, or from forceful contraction of the quadriceps muscles. Fractures may be transverse, comminuted, or of the avulsion type (when the quadriceps muscle pulls off a small portion of the patella) (Fig. 128-1). Any fracture may be open or closed. A nondisplaced transverse fracture of the patella should be treated with a cylinder cast from ankle to groin, molded firmly over the

UNDISPLACED   TRANSVERSE   COMMINUTED

Figure 128-1. Types of patellar fractures. [From Hohl M, Larson RL: Fractures and dislocations of the knee, in Rockwood CA Jr, Green DP (Eds): *Fractures*. Philadelphia, JB Lippincott Co, 1975, vol 2, p 1149. Used by permission.]

condyles of the femur, for 6 weeks. During this time the patient should be encouraged to walk on crutches, with partial weight-bearing, progressing to full weight-bearing as tolerated.

If the transverse fracture is separated slightly, a cylinder cast may be sufficient, assuming adequate reduction occurs. However, this usually requires open reduction and wire fixation. If the fragments are widely separated, most often there is associated knee joint injury. The patellar injury can be treated with delayed open reduction once the swelling from the associated injuries resolves.

Comminuted fractures must be treated surgically by removal of smaller fragments (or all fragments if they are small) and suturing of the quadriceps tendon and patellar ligaments.

All open fractures must be debrided and irrigated.

Dislocation of the patella usually occurs from a twisting injury on the extended knee. The patella is displaced laterally over the lateral condyle resulting in pain and deformity of the knee. Reduction is accomplished by hyperextending the knee, flexing the hip and sliding the patella back into place. This is accompanied by immediate relief of pain but further soreness from capsular injury will persist for a period of time. The knee should be immobilized in a long leg cast for 6 weeks after reduction and the patella and knee should be x-rayed to rule out bony injury. Recurrent lateral dislocations of the patella and superior, horizontal, and intercondylar dislocations require referral to an orthopedic surgeon for possible surgical intervention.

Fractures of Femoral Condyles

Fractures of the femoral condyles include supracondylar, intercondylar, condylar, and distal femoral epiphyseal fractures (Fig. 128-2). Most often, these injuries are secondary to direct trauma from a fall or blow to the distal femur. Examination reveals pain, swelling, deformity, rotation, and shortening. Although neurovascular injuries are uncommon, status of distal sensation and pulses must be checked. The space between the first and second toe, innervated by the deep peroneal nerve, should be tested for sensation. In addition, search for ipsilateral hip dislocation or fractures and damage to the quadriceps apparatus must be made. Depending on the type of fracture, closed or open reduction, skeletal traction and cast immobilization may be necessary. Therefore, orthopedic consultation is essential.

Fractures of the Tibial Spines and Tuberosity

Although isolated injuries of the tibial spine are uncommon, they usually result in damage to the cruciate ligaments. The injury is

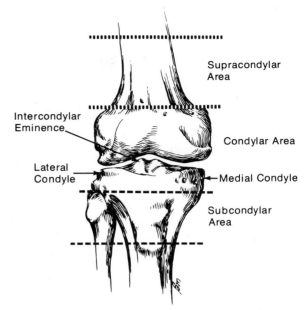

Figure 128-2. The supracondylar and condylar areas of the femur, and the medial and subcondylar areas of the tibia. [Modified from Hohl M, Larson RL: Fractures and dislocations of the knee, in Rockwood CA Jr, Green DP (eds): *Fractures*. Philadelphia, JB Lippincott Co, 1975, vol 2, pp 1132, 1147. Used by permission.]

most often caused by a force directed against the flexed proximal tibia in an anterior or posterior direction resulting in incomplete avulsion of the tibial spine, with or without displacement, or complete fracture of the spine. Examination will show a painful, swollen knee, 2° hemarthrosis, inability to extend fully, and a positive drawer sign. If the fracture is incomplete or nondisplaced, closed reduction by an orthopedic surgeon may be attempted. Complete, displaced fractures often need open reduction.

The quadriceps mechanism inserts on the tibial tubercle. A sudden force to the flexed knee with the quadriceps muscle contracted may result in a complete or incomplete avulsion of the tibial tubercle. The fracture line may extend into the joint. Examination will reveal pain and tenderness over the proximal anterior tibia with pain on passive or active extension. If the avulsion is small or nondisplaced, the fragment may be maintained in position by plaster cast immobilization; otherwise, open reduction and internal fixation is necessary.

Fractures of the Tibial Plateaus

Fractures of the tibial plateaus are produced by direct force which drives the femoral condyles into the articulating surface of the tibia. Both medial and lateral plateaus may be fractured simultaneously although the lateral plateau is more often fractured. Direct trauma to the lateral aspect of the knee may account for the preponderance of lateral tibial plateau fractures. The patient presents with painful swelling of the knee and limitation of motion. Ligamentous instability may also be demonstrated. If one or both plateaus are fractured but not displaced, treatment in a long leg plaster cast, without weight-bearing, for 6 weeks should be adequate. Depression of the articular surface necessitates open reduction and elevation of the bony fragment.

RECOGNITION AND MANAGEMENT OF LIGAMENTOUS AND MENISCAL INJURIES

The knee joint depends upon surrounding ligaments and muscle for stability (Fig. 128-3). Although most stable in full extension, it is frequently subjected to injuries from various forces while extended or in stages of flexion. Such forces may result in strain or rupture of the medial and lateral collateral ligaments, the anterior and posterior cruciate ligaments, and the medial and lateral menisci, singly or in combination. It is with injuries to the ligaments and menisci that examination with stress testing is so crucial to determine stability of the joint.

Instability of the knee can be divided into two categories: straight and rotatory. Straight instabilities of the knees are further subdivided into medial, lateral, posterior, and anterior. The physician should remember that often the first examination will be the only valid one because pain causing voluntary and involuntary guarding will not allow the next physician to examine the knee with great precision and care. In examining the knee for instabilities, the patient should have the test performed with the knee in 20 to 30° of flexion because full extension is often impossible to achieve and is uncomfortable. The patient must be reassured and relaxed and made as comfortable as possible, which may require allowing the leg to hang over the side of the bed with the bed supporting the posterior thigh rather than the physician holding the leg up in the air.

The initial stress testing, once the patient is ready, is an abduction or valgus deformity applied to the knee, with 20 to 30° flexion, to give the physician some idea of the integrity of the medial joint line, and a varus or adduction force applied to the lateral aspect of the knee, again with 20 to 30° of flexion, to ascertain the integrity of the lateral structures of the knee. If the patient is unstable with 20 to 30° of flexion, then he or she should be brought into full extension, if possible, and the specific maneuver carried out again. If there is straight medial instability in

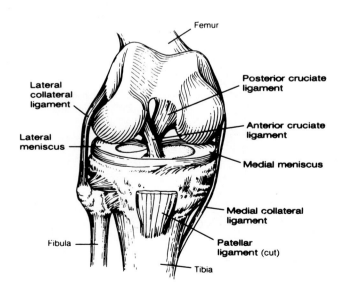

Figure 128-3. Ligaments of the right knee joint. The articular capsule and the patella have been removed. (From Spence AP, Mason EB: *Human Anatomy and Physiology*. Menlo Park, The Benjamin/Cummings Publishing Co, Inc, 1979, p 174. Used by permission.)

full extension, this indicates a severe lesion; that is, the posterior cruciate ligament is torn along with the medial ligaments and frequently the anterior cruciate. If there is straight lateral instability with the knee in full extension, then this likewise indicates a severe injury in the lateral collateral ligament, posterior lateral corner of the knee, as well as the anterior and posterior cruciate ligaments. Peroneal nerve injury may also be seen here.

It must be emphasized that straight instability is established only if the valgus or varus tests are positive in full extension. If the tests are negative in full extension but positive with 20 to 30° of flexion, then a rotatory instability exists. It must also be remembered that if the tests are positive in full extension, then they will also be positive with 20 to 30° of flexion.

Straight posterior instability indicates a deficit in the posterior cruciate ligaments. This is done by the standard posterior drawer test with the knee in neutral position. If the knee is examined with flexion at the hip and knee, that is, the appropriate position for performing the posterior and anterior drawer signs, then the physician might sometimes see posterior sag or dropback of the tibial tubercle due to loss of the integrity of the posterior cruciate. If there is straight anterior instability, the knee might sublux forward, which would then give the physician the false impression of too much posterior play. The straight anterior instability is the only straight instability that does not require loss of posterior cruciate ligament function. It is ascertained by the anterior drawer sign and is due to a tear in the anterior cruciate ligament, often in conjunction with a tear in the posterior medial and/or posterior lateral structures of the knee.

Anteromedial rotatory instability, which was the first rotatory instability to be described in 1968 by Slocum and Larson, is the best understood and least controversial. The injury that causes such instability is usually a tear in the deep portion of the medial collateral ligament which may be associated with a tear in the superficial portion of the ligament as well as the anterior cruciate. The test is conducted with the patient in a supine position, the hip flexed to 45° and the knee flexed approximately 80° with the foot resting on the examination table, similar to the drawer test. The examiner then assesses the movement of the medial tibial condyle and lateral tibial condyle when pulling on the upper third of the calf as he or she sits on the foot. The test is performed with the foot in neutral position, then with the foot in progressive degrees of external rotation, and with the foot in progressive degrees of internal rotation. The internal rotation tests the anterior lateral structures and the external rotation stresses the anterior medial structures. The initial instability should decrease as one rotates in either direction as the opposite side's intact structures begin to support the knee.

It must be emphasized that the posterior cruciate must be intact for any rotatory instability tests to be valid. The anteromedial rotatory instability test is associated with a positive abduction or valgus stress test with the knee in 20 to 30° of flexion. The anterolateral rotatory instability is characterized by anterior-internal rotational subluxation of the lateral tibial condyle on the femur, which is the result of anterior cruciate insufficiency along with lateral compartment laxity. There are three tests described to aid in the diagnosis of such instability: the lateral pivot shift, the anterolateral rotatory instability test, and the jerk test. The lateral pivot shift is easily performed once the examiner is comfortable with it but may be somewhat painful to the patient. While the patient is supine and relaxed, the examiner lifts the heel of the foot to 45° of hip flexion with the knee fully extended. The other hand grasps the knee with the thumb behind the fibular head. The examiner internally rotates the ankle and knee, applies a valgus force to the knee and then flexes the knee. If an anterior subluxation of the tibia is present, a sudden visible, audible, and palpable reduction of the subluxation occurs about 20 to 40° of flexion. The remaining two tests can be reviewed in an orthopedic text or any symposium on knee injuries.

Posterior lateral rotatory instability which usually involves a tear of the arcuate ligament complex (posterior lateral capsule) is evaluated by using the adduction or varus stress test as well as hyperextension and external rotation recurvation when lifting the leg off the bed holding only the toes. It is important to differentiate this instability from straight lateral instability, which is easily done by putting the knee in full extension and redoing the adduction or varus stress test. If the test is positive in flexion and extension, then the posterior cruciate is torn. If, however, it is positive only in 20° of flexion, then the posterior lateral structures are torn.

Lastly are combined instabilities. Because of the nature of the injuries which occur to the knee, anteromedial-anterolateral instability occurs most frequently and is usually classified separately. It is usually the result of an external rotation-abduction force. The physician should remember, however, that virtually any combination of medial and lateral instabilities of the knee can occur.

The authors would like to mention briefly a few specific points in examination of the knee. Traumatic effusions (hemarthroses) of the knee are secondary to three events: ligamentous tears, osteochondral fractures or fractures into the joint line, and peripheral meniscal tears. Traumatic effusions of the knee always occur within 24 h and most of the time occur within 1 to 6 h. This is in contrast to chronic effusions of the knee due to synovial fluid proliferation, which occur 24 to 48 h after strenuous use of the joint. The significance of that is that the physician does not need to tap a sudden effusion which occurs after an injury to ascertain whether it is bloody or not in almost any instance. To do so *needlessly* exposes the patient to the possibility of contamination and/or infection. The possible indication for tapping a knee would be to relieve the pressure and pain caused by the fluid distention. If one chooses to tap the knee and fat globules are present in the bloody effusion, then an osteochondral fracture is almost a certainty. It is also important to remember that children who present with knee injuries may have epiphyseal separation rather than a ligamentous tear, which is not demonstrated by standard x-rays. Upon examination, the physician will note that there is some instability or that the patient guards and hurts when the maneuvers are performed. Such children should be stressed under x-ray to ascertain possible separation of the epiphyseal plate.

Stable injuries involving a single ligament with minor strain can be managed with a compression dressing, ice packs, elevation, and ambulation as soon as comfortable for the patient. More severe, but stable, ligamentous injuries necessitate ice, elevation, and immobilization. These injuries should be referred to an orthopedic surgeon for followup. Unstable injuries necessitate immediate orthopedic consultation for definitive management.

Meniscal Injuries

Meniscal tears often present with joint or groin pain, locking of the knee, and effusion, although the effusion may be delayed by 6 to 12 h. Acute effusions are often accompanied by ligamentous injury. Possible meniscal damage is assessed by eliciting joint line tenderness to palpation and with the McMurray's maneuver. This maneuver is done by bringing the knee from full flexion to mild flexion while rotating the foot externally and palpating the medial joint line, then rotating the foot internally and palpating the lateral joint line. Locking of the knee can be treated by having the patient positioned with the leg hanging over the edge of the table and the knee in 90° of flexion. After a period of relaxation, the knee can be rotated with careful traction on the leg. If reduction is unsuccessful, immediate referral to an orthopedic surgeon is warranted. In any case, such injuries should be treated with a compression dressing, ice, and splinting, followed by orthopedic referral. Arthrography and arthroscopy with arthroscopic surgery may be necessary.

Knee Dislocation

Knee dislocation is a result of hyperextension, direct posterior force applied to the anterior tibia, force to the fibula or medial femur, force to the tibia or lateral femur, or a rotatory force resulting respectively, in anterior, posterior lateral, medial, or rotatory dislocation. Very often reduction occurs spontaneously because of the tremendous ligamentous disruption. However, suspicion of the injury is important because of the high incidence of associated complications, including popliteal artery injury and peroneal nerve injury, in addition to ligamentous and meniscal injury. Early reduction of the dislocation is essential; orthopedic and perhaps vascular surgery consultation should be obtained acutely.

Osteochondritis Dissecans

Osteochondritis dissecans is a loose body in a knee joint which may cause locking, effusion, and buckling of the knee. X-ray may be negative or reveal a calcified body in the joint. Immobilization of the child under 12 is appropriate while older children and adults require surgery to prevent degenerative arthritis.

Summary

In summary, the knee is a complex joint. Understanding the anatomy and physiology of its motion, mechanism of the forces producing injuries, and facility in examination of the knee are essential for the emergency physician who will be confronted relatively often by injuries to this joint. Thorough and careful examination on initial presentation, recognition of significant abnormalities, thoughtful initial care, and appropriate referral are the goals in management of knee injuries for the emergency physician.

BIBLIOGRAPHY

Ahstrom JP Jr: Osteochondral fracture in the knee joint associated with hypermobility and dislocation of the patella: Report of 18 cases. *J Bone Joint Surg* 47A:1491–1502, 1965.

Cave EF: Calcification in the menisci. *J Bone Joint Surg* 25:53–57, 1943.

Duthie HL, Hutchinson JR: The results of partial and total excision of the patella. *J Bone Joint Surg* 40B:75–81, 1958.

Hand WL, Hand CR, Dunn AW: Avulsion fractures of the tibial tubercle. *J Bone Joint Surg* 53A:1579–1583, 1971.

Hohl M, Luck JV: Fractures of the tibial condyle: A clinical and experimental study. *J Bone Joint Surg* 38A:1001–1018, 1956.

Hohl M: Tibial condylar fractures. *J Bone Joint Surg* 49A:1455–1467, 1967.

Hughston JC: Subluxation of the patella. *J Bone Joint Surg* 50A:1003–1026, 1968.

Jones KG: Reconstruction of the anterior cruciate ligament: A technique using the central one-third of the patellar ligament. *J Bone Joint Surg* 45:925–931, 1963.

Kaufer H: Mechanical function of the patella. *J Bone Joint Surg* 5:1551–1560, 1971.

Kennedy JC, Granger RW, McGraw RW: Osteochondral fractures of the femoral condyles. *J Bone Joint Surg* 48B:436–440, 1966.

Myers MH, Harvey JP Jr: Traumatic dislocation of the knee joint: A study of 18 cases. *J Bone Joint Surg* 53A:16–29, 1971.

Rockwood CA, Green DP (eds): *Fractures*, ed 2. Philadelphia, Lippincott, 1984.

Simon RR: *Orthopedics in Emergency Medicine: The Extremities*. New York, Appleton-Century-Crofts, 1982.

Smith FB, Blair HC: Tibial collateral ligament strain due to occult derangements of the medial meniscus: Confirmed by operation in 30 cases. *J Bone Joint Surg* 36A:88–93, 1954.

Willner P: Recurrent dislocation of the patella. *Clin Orthop* 69:213–215, 1970.

CHAPTER 129
LEG INJURIES

Joseph F. Waeckerle

INTRODUCTION

Although the fractured tibia is the most common of all long bone fractures, its treatment is varied and sometimes controversial. Because of the many fractures seen and the frequency of open fractures, tibial fractures are associated with a high complication rate. The frequency of fractures as well as the complication rate are due to the fact that the tibia, and fibula as well, have minimal protection from surrounding soft tissues, which makes them vulnerable to injurious forces.

As with most fractures, the leg is susceptible to direct and indirect mechanisms of injury. Direct blows usually cause tibial shaft fractures which are associated with fibular shaft fractures. Because the violence is directly to the bone, soft tissue injury with initial displacement of fracture site and comminution of the fracture often result. In contrast, indirect forces such as rotation and compression usually cause spiral or oblique fractures of the tibia, sometimes associated with fibular shaft fractures. Isolated fibular shaft fractures are, in fact, uncommon injuries.

ANATOMY

The tibia and fibula run parallel and are tightly connected by the interosseous ligament. The surrounding soft tissue is divided into three compartments. The first, the anterior compartment, consists of the muscles (tibialis anterior, extensor digitorum longus, extensor hallucis longus, and peroneus tertius), the anterior tibial artery, and the deep peroneal nerve. Because this compartment is bound by the tibia, fibula, and fascia, there is little room for swelling. The second compartment is the lateral compartment which consists of the peroneus brevis and peroneus longus muscles, along with the superficial peroneal nerve. The superficial peroneal nerve is at risk when an injury occurs high up the fibular shaft or at the neck of the fibula. The third compartment is the posterior compartment which consists of the soleus, gastrocnemius, tibialis posterior, flexor hallucis longus, and flexor digitorum longus muscles, the posterior tibial nerve, and the posterior tibial artery.

Injuries to the anterior compartment from swelling are more often seen than to the lateral or posterior compartments. The latter two are also bound compartments and if a significant amount of swelling occurs a compartment syndrome may also be seen there.

There are multiple classifications for describing leg fractures. Probably the easiest is to classify tibial fractures as stable or unstable, which would help with regard to treatment. Some classifications, by describing the fractures with regard to displacement, comminution, and soft tissue injuries, can predict the healing potential somewhat.

CLINICAL EVALUATION

As with all orthopedic injuries the symptoms and signs the patient presents with are directly proportional to the severity of the injury. Pain is usually severe and localized with leg fractures. Crepitus in motion as well as obvious deformity are often present. Usually the deformity is external rotation and valgus in nature. Local swelling and discoloration as well as the presence of wounds may aid the physician in diagnosing a fracture. Any wound which violates the integrity of the skin associated with a leg fracture must be considered an open fracture. Although direct neurovascular injury is not a common complication of leg fractures, neurovascular assessment should always be done and recorded on the chart. This consists of documentation that both the vascular supply to the foot as well as the motor and sensory supply to the leg, especially the functions of the peroneal nerve, are intact.

In evaluating leg fractures, AP and lateral x-ray views are generally adequate to demonstrate the fracture, as well as the position of the fragments. As always, the x-rays require good trabecular detail to demonstrate the smaller, nondisplaced fractures, especially those seen in the fibula. Also, the x-rays should demonstrate both the knee and ankle articular surfaces.

Treatment

Leg fractures are usually not difficult to treat with regard to emergency department management. Once the initial examination is completed and the fracture is identified and defined, closed reduction, an immobilization long leg splint, and referral are appropriate. Difficulty in managing such fractures in the emergency department occurs when the physician is not able to obtain an adequate reduction or there are severe associated soft tissue injuries with an open fracture. Although mentioned in previous chapters, it is emphasized to the reader again that it is, in fact, more important to treat the soft tissue injuries properly than the fracture itself. This requires that the physician gently but thoroughly cleanse the soft tissue by debridement and irrigation and provide appropriate tetanus prophylaxis and antibiotic coverage.

The immobilization must allow the physicians treating the patient to view the soft tissue wounds. Another important point regarding fractures of the leg is that occasionally emergency reduction of a fracture may be required due to the fact that the fracture has compromised vascularity distal to the fracture site. Although this is not common, such reduction might be needed prior to x-ray evaluation when the compromise threatens the limb blood supply.

Complications

The most common complication associated with leg fractures is the soft tissue injury with secondary infection. As with any orthopedic injury, an infection can be disastrous. Also as mentioned earlier, the anterior compartment syndrome, seen some 24 to 48 h after injury, can occur. The patient should be specifically warned to avoid any actions which might precipitate a compartment syndrome and to seek help if there are any of the symptoms or signs of such (i.e., delayed signs and symptoms of neurovascular compromise). Nerve damage is usually uncommon with leg fractures but may occur if there is an injury to the fibular head. This involves the superficial peroneal nerve. Damage to the vascularity is also not usual but can occur in upper tibial fractures with injury to the anterior tibial artery as it passes through the interosseous membrane. As with all orthopedic injuries, nonunion or delayed union is common if the fracture site is complicated by a severe displacement or comminution. Also, arthritis may occur in some individuals.

Fibular Fractures

As mentioned in the introduction, isolated fibular fractures, especially of the shaft, are uncommon. The more common injury to the fibula is fracture at the ankle joint and is addressed in Chapter 131, ''Ankle Injuries.'' Occasionally, however, fractures do occur to the fibular shaft due to direct and indirect trauma. The patient may present with local swelling and tenderness over the fracture site itself and pain on ambulation. Because of the difficulty in sometimes seeing fractures of the fibula (especially if it is a stress fracture, which is commonly seen in the distal third), x-rays which show good trabecular detail are required. AP and lateral views are generally adequate.

Treatment of fibular fractures is usually designed to give the patient comfort. Very often the patient does not require immobilization. However, in some instances the patient may be more comfortable in a short leg walking cast and crutches for approximately 2 weeks.

CHAPTER 130
FOOT INJURIES

Joseph F. Waeckerle

INTRODUCTION

The foot bears the weight of the body, and any injuries to it are magnified because of tremendous stress. The patient with an injured foot becomes debilitated to the point of not being able to bear any weight, or function properly. Loss of mobility of the joints of the foot as well as pain at the fracture site and subsequent arthritis may cause the patient discomfort and disability seemingly out of proportion to the injury sustained. It behooves the physician treating the patient with a foot injury to keep this in mind in order to minimize disability by appropriately treating the bone and soft tissue injuries from the beginning.

The mechanisms of injury resulting in fractures and soft tissue damage to the foot include direct and indirect trauma as well as overuse or stress injuries. An adequate history will often help the physician determine the location of the injury and predict what injuries might be seen. This is important because radiographic evaluation of the foot is sometimes very difficult due to the many overlying bony shadows, secondary ossification centers, and sesamoid bones. Comparison views with the opposite foot are often essential to properly evaluate an injured foot.

Classification

Classification of the fractured foot is complex, and it is beyond the scope of this chapter to present a detailed classification or complete discussion of all fractures of the foot. The following discussion will touch upon the more common injuries seen. For more detail the reader is referred to the texts which discuss fractures and dislocations.

Anatomy

The foot consists of the hindpart, which is made up of the calcaneus and talus; the midpart, which is separated from the hindpart by Chopart's joint and consists of the navicular, cuboid, and cuneiforms; and the forepart, which is separated from the midpart by Lisfranc's joint and consists of the metatarsals and phalanges. There are 28 bones, 57 major articular surfaces, and many ligaments as well as tendons and other soft tissues that contribute to the stability and integrity of the foot.

Some major points to keep in mind are: (1) The long arch of the foot depends upon the position and alignment of the bones and not the soft tissue as commonly believed. (2) Weight-bearing on the foot causes an equal distribution of forces between the heel and forepart. (3) The first metatarsal head bears two times as much weight as the other metatarsal heads. This is important because treatment of great toe injuries, especially of the metatarsal head, requires a more conservative approach. (4) Lastly, an anatomical note of importance is that when a push-off force on the foot occurs, the maximum load is borne by the second metatarsal. With repeated pushing off, stress fractures of the second metatarsal may be seen. Some stress fractures of the third metatarsal may also be seen because after the second it bears more weight than the other metatarsals during the push-off or acceleration phase to which runners commonly subject their feet.

CALCANEAL FRACTURES

The calcaneus is the largest of the tarsal bones in the foot and functions as the base for locomotion and support of the weight of the body. It is the most often fractured of the tarsal bones, being involved in some 60 percent of such injuries. The difficulty with calcaneal fracture is that there is no optimal treatment and, therefore, a good result is not often obtained. Calcaneal fractures are usually classified as fractures involving the process or tuberosity, and fractures involving the body. The mechanism of injury is usually one of compression.

Because of the fact that the patient must sustain a significant compression force to fracture the calcaneus, associated injuries are not uncommon; 10 percent of all calcaneal fractures are associated with lumbar compression injuries and 26 percent are associated with other injuries to the extremity. This points out that it is important to get a good history of the mechanism of injury. Also, the physician must examine the patient for injuries associated with the calcaneal fracture, including back, pelvic, hip, and knee injuries. The symptoms and signs associated with calcaneal fractures are directly proportional to location and severity of the injury to the calcaneus as well as other associated injuries. Generally, the patient will experience swelling, pain, and ecchymoses at the fracture site. Often the fracture site will be exquisitely tender locally, with decreased range of motion and the inability to bear any weight on the fracture.

Standard radiographic views of the foot which consist of three different views may not be sufficient in evaluating calcaneal fractures, but should be ordered initially. Besides the PA, lateral, and axial views, certain "scout films" may be required to specifically delineate various fracture sites of the calcaneus. It is essential that, in evaluating calcaneal fractures, the x-rays demonstrate good trabecular detail.

Treatment

As with all fractures, the objective in treating the patient is to restore normal anatomy and function as quickly as possible. This requires a great deal of skill and expertise with most calcaneal fractures; therefore, a consultant should be called in early in the management of the case. If the patient has gross swelling or is unstable, conservative treatment with a posterior splint providing immobilization, as well as attention to the soft tissue swelling and injuries, is imperative. In all instances, reduction of the calcaneal fracture to the closest anatomical position should be done as soon as possible by the consultant.

TALUS FRACTURES

Although talus fractures are the second most common foot fracture, they are still relatively uncommon. The talus is held in place by ligaments surrounding it and has no muscular attachments. Because of the fact that most of the talus is covered by articular cartilage, the blood supply is tenuous and enters by way of the ligamentous and capsular support to the bones. Therefore, fractures of the talus, especially of the neck, associated with body dislocations, may cause avascular necrosis of the bone. The mechanism of injury which produces a talus fracture dislocation is usually one of hyperextension. The patient complains of intense pain and is unable to bear weight. There is localized swelling, discoloration, and tenderness to palpation. Moreover, there is an obvious loss of the normal contour of the foot. Any range of motion is intensely painful to the patient. X-ray evaluation for suspected talus fractures usually requires routine views of the foot. In certain instances, more detailed and specific x-rays may be ordered.

Treatment

Treatment for talus injuries depends somewhat upon the extent of the fracture. Simple, nondisplaced minor chips or avulsion fractures require immobilization as well as ice, elevation, and followup. These patients do not usually have long-term complications. In contrast, fractures of the neck and body, or fracture-dislocation of the talus, may be very difficult to treat, causing extensive problems to both the patient and the physician in the long run. In such instances, besides assessing neurovascular status of the foot and adequately evaluating and immobilizing the injury, the emergency physician should seek consultation for further care.

MIDPART FRACTURES

The midpart of the foot is infrequently fractured but if it is injured, multiple fractures may occur. Fracture is usually the result of direct trauma to the midpart of the foot. This area of the foot is most susceptible to direct trauma because it is the least mobile portion of the foot and includes five tarsal bones and all their articular surfaces and ligamentous support. Because of the many articulating surfaces, injuries to the midpart of the foot are associated with subluxation and/or dislocation. If the physician encounters an isolated midfoot fracture, it is most often of the navicular bone. Injuries to the cuboid and cuneiforms occur in combination with injuries to the navicular or one another and are usually the result of a crushing type injury. Various classifications are used to describe injuries to the midfoot. Such injuries are divided into those to the navicular and those to the other bones.

Symptoms and signs are similar to other orthopedic type injuries. That is, the patient presents with pain, swelling, and tenderness over the involved area. The standard x-ray views (AP, lateral, and oblique) are generally adequate to demonstrate most injuries in this area.

Treatment

The treatment is ice, elevation, and immobilization if there is no displacement and the anatomical position is acceptable. If not, then consultation for further closed reduction or open reduction–internal fixation are required so that the patient can achieve and maintain as close to anatomical reduction as possible.

TARSAL-METATARSAL FRACTURE DISLOCATIONS

As defined earlier, the tarsal-metatarsal joint is referred to as Lisfranc's joint. Injuries to this area are uncommon, and are usually caused by automobile accidents. The mechanism of injury is complicated and varied but is usually a severe hyperextension of the forefoot on the midfoot, causing dorsal dislocation. There may be associated fractures. Such injuries occur because ligamentous support is the stabilizing support to this joint. The keystone of this joint is the second metatarsal; it is the locking mechanism of the midpart of the foot. Therefore, a fracture at the base of the second metatarsal is almost pathognomonic of a disrupted joint. Symptoms and signs are routine pain, swelling, discoloration, loss of range of motion, loss of weight-bearing, and possibly some paresthesia in the midpart of the foot. X-rays needed are the standard three views, but a comparison view with the opposite side is almost mandatory to properly evaluate the patient.

Treatment

The treatment of this fracture-dislocation is very difficult because complete restoration of position by closed reduction requires strong traction. In fact, correction of this deformity may require open reduction and internal fixation. Therefore, it is important to get the consulting surgeon involved in the case as early as possible.

METATARSAL FRACTURES

As mentioned earlier, the second and third metatarsals are relatively fixed due to their anatomical configuration position and are subjected to a great deal of stress, especially during the push-off phase of running or walking. In contrast, the first, fourth, and fifth metatarsals are relatively mobile. The significance of this is that excessive stress over a period of time can result in the development of stress fractures usually occurring in the second and third metatarsals. Other mechanisms of injury to the metatarsals are direct trauma or crush injuries and occasionally indirect force such as twisting type injury. Because the direct trauma or crush injury is usually fairly significant there is frequently more than one metatarsal fractured. Moreover, associated soft tissue injuries with severe swelling and possible vascular compromise may occur.

Metatarsal fractures are divided into neck fractures and shaft fractures. Specific mention should be made of the pulloff fracture of the base of the fifth metatarsal, which is commonly called the Jones ballet dancer's fracture. This injury is usually due to plantar flexion and inversion resulting in the peroneus brevis tendon pulling off a portion of the bone where it inserts. This specific fracture may often be confused with a ligamentous injury to the ankle. It behooves the physician, when evaluating lateral ankle injuries, to include in the x-rays the base of the fifth metatarsal to ensure that this fracture has not occurred.

Patients who experience metatarsal fractures present with typical findings but especially local tenderness. The x-ray evaluation consists of the three standard views of the foot and usually does not require any further x-ray evaluation.

Treatment

Treatment for metatarsal fractures is ice, elevation, analgesics, and noncircumferential immobilization. A cast should not be applied to these patient before 24 to 48 h because there may be severe swelling associated with the crushing type injury which caused the fracture. Once the swelling goes down, a short leg cast should be applied for 4 to 6 weeks.

Jones Fracture

Regarding the Jones fracture at the base of the fifth metatarsal, this is by far the most common of the metatarsal fractures. These patients will specifically present with local tenderness over the fracture site. As mentioned earlier, this injury is often confused with lateral ligamentous sprain to the ankle and it is important that the base of the fifth metatarsal be visualized in x-rays of the ankle to rule out such fracture. Moreover, the physician must keep in mind that this is a secondary growth center or apophysis and that oblique and transverse fractures may be confused with the growth center. The treatment for the Jones fracture is usually conservative and consists of taping, a postoperative or fracture shoe, and crutches for a short period of time.

Stress Fractures

Brief mention should be made of stress fractures to the second and third metatarsal which usually occur proximal to the head. These fractures are usually insidious in onset and may not appear on x-ray for 2 to 3 weeks after their occurrence. The physician may treat the patient as if he or she has a stress fracture, even though it is not present on x-ray, and then re-x-ray the patient or perform a bone scan 2 or 3 weeks later, which will usually delineate the fracture site. Treatment for stress fractures is rest or, occasionally, immobilization.

PHALANGEAL INJURIES

Injuries to the phalanx are common and usually result from direct trauma. Such injuries consist of both fractures and fracture-dislocations. The majority of phalanx fractures are the result of a direct trauma, such as dropping a heavy object on the toes. An indirect mechanism causing fractures is hyperextension; an indirect mechanism causing dislocations is compression with dorsiflexion of the proximal phalanx.

The patient presents with pain, swelling, and discomfort, especially when wearing shoes and walking, within a few hours after an injury to the phalanx and/or its joints. In some instances when a dislocation or subluxation has occurred there is obvious deformity but this may not always be the case because swelling may be significant enough to mask the deformity. X-ray evaluation is usually best in the AP and oblique views.

Treatment

Treatment is similar to all other fractures, that is, reduction of the subluxation-dislocation and reduction of the fracture to its most anatomically correct position then ice, elevation, and immobilization. Immobilization can occur through dynamic splinting (so-called ''buddy taping''), a postoperative shoe, or in certain instances a walking boot cast. Due to the fact that the great toe bears one-third of the body weight of that side, it sometimes may need more extensive immobilization such as is provided by the walking boot cast. Displaced phalangeal fractures which are irreducible because of their instability may require internal fixation and, therefore, early referral. Open phalangeal fractures demand adequate soft tissue treatment and early referral is strongly recommended for them as well. If the injury, whether it be a fracture or dislocation, is resistant to attempts at closed reduction to achieve anatomic position, referral to the orthopedic specialist is recommended because of the possible long-term sequelae.

CHAPTER 131
ANKLE INJURIES

Joseph F. Waeckerle

The ankle bears as much or more weight than any other joint in the body per unit area. Its anatomical design and weight-bearing function predispose it to a wide variety of injuries. To recognize and appropriately treat ankle injuries, the physician must understand the anatomy and mechanisms of injury. Treatment should be designed so that no prolonged disability or irreparable damage results.

Anatomy

The ankle consists of three bones, the tibia, fibula, and talus, which are bonded together by ligaments to form a hingelike joint. Groups of muscles cross the joint and produce movement, mostly through dorsiflexion and plantar flexion.

Bones. Bony stability is provided by the shape of the talar bone in the lower end of the tibia and intermalleolar distance. The talus is interposed between the tibia and fibula. It is wider anteriorly than posteriorly to provide for articulation with the distal tibia and the medial and lateral malleoli. In dorsiflexion, more of the anterior, wider portion of the talus fits into the slightly concave undersurface of the tibia. This tighter fit allows the malleoli of the tibia and fibula to bear more stress if any twisting motion occurs. In plantar flexion, the narrower, posterior portion of the talus occupies the mortise so that there is more play in the ankle joint. It is therefore easier for twisting motions to result in injury with the ankle in plantar flexion. Due to the inherent joint design, dorsiflexion is accompanied by eversion and plantar flexion with inversion.

Ligaments. Three groups of ligaments unify the bony structures of the ankle. The medial collateral or deltoid ligament is a thick triangular band that provides medial support to the ankle joint. It consists of a superficial and deep set of fibers. Both sets of fibers originate from the broad, short, and strong medial malleolus. The superficial fibers run in a sagittal plane and insert on the navicular and talus. Deep fibers run more horizontally and insert on the medial surface of the talus.

The lateral support of the ankle is provided by the anterior talofibular, calcaneofibular, and posterior talofibular ligaments (Fig. 131-1). They originate and insert as their names suggest. Along with the lateral malleolus, these ligaments prevent lateral movement of the talus.

The lower portions of the tibia and fibula are bound together by the ligaments of the syndesmosis. These ligaments consist of the anterior and posterior tibiofibular ligaments, the interosseous

ligament, and the inferior transverse ligament. The anterior and posterior tibiofibular ligaments are bands of fibers running between the margins of the tibia and fibula anteriorly and posteriorly. The inferior transverse ligament is a strong group of fibers that support the posterior inferior portion of the ankle joint. Finally, the interosseous ligament is simply the lower portion of the interosseous membrane. It provides the strongest bond between the tibia and fibula at the joint.

Muscles. There are basically four compartments of muscles that traverse the ankle joint (Fig. 131-2). Anteriorly, the tibialis anterior, extensor digitorum longus, and extensor hallucis longus run over the ankle joint and contribute to dorsiflexion of the ankle. Medially, the tibialis posterior, flexor digitorum longus, and flexor hallucis longus run behind the medial malleolus and contribute to inversion of the foot. Posteriorly, the soleus and gastrocnemius muscles provide plantar flexion. Laterally, the peroneus longus and brevis muscles run in a sheath directly behind the lateral malleolus. These muscles contribute to eversion and plantar flexion.

Nerves and blood supply. The vascular supply to the area of the ankle is a continuation of the external iliac, femoral, and popliteal arterial system. The anterior and posterior tibial arteries as well as the peroneal artery are continuations of the popliteal artery and supply the ankle and foot. Nervous supply is from the sciatic nerve.

In summary, the ankle joint is a ring consisting of the tibia, fibula, and talus bound together by three major groups of ligaments. Almost all injuries to the ankle are due to the abnormal motion of the talus as it sets in the mortise. The talar motion causes direct or indirect stress on the malleoli or lower portion of the tibia, resulting in injury. If there is a single break in the ring, talar shift may not occur due to the ligamentous support. However, if there are two breaks in the ring, either a fracture of the malleoli or a fracture of one malleolus and a ruptured ligament, or two ruptured ligaments, then integrity of the ring is violated and talar shift will occur. This anatomical fact is important in assessing the stability of any injured ankle.

History of Injury

As with all orthopedic injuries a careful history of the mechanism of injury is essential and should always precede clinical and roentgenographic examination. The physician should attempt to ascertain the position of the foot, the direction of the stresses, and all

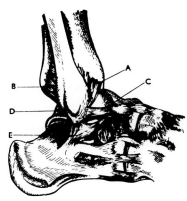

Figure 131-1. Lateral ligaments of the ankle. (From Bonnin JG: Injuries to the Ankle. Darien, Conn, Hafner Publishing Co, 1970, p. 36. Used by permission.)

other pertinent data to reconstruct the injury. This will aid in the determination of what bones or ligaments are most likely to be injured. It is also helpful to ask if any noise occurred during the time of injury that might indicate that a ligament popped, a bone subluxed or dislocated, or a tendon snapped. The physician should ask if the onset of pain was immediate, if swelling occurred right after the injury, and if disability was immediate or delayed. A history of previous ankle injury and its treatment may affect physical findings and treatment.

Clinical Examination

A partial clinical examination should always precede roentgenographic examination. If the ankle is grossly deformed, the diagnosis of an unstable joint is obvious and radiologic evaluation should occur after the physician ensures that neurovascular status is not compromised. In the absence of a gross deformity, inspect

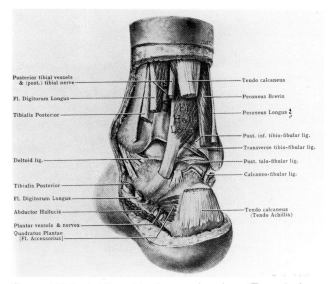

Figure 131-2. Ankle and heel, posterior view. (From Anderson JE: Grant's Atlas of Anatomy, ed 7. Baltimore, The Williams & Wilkins Co, 1978, p 4-89. Used by permission.)

for local swelling and the loss or prominence of anatomical landmarks. Look for ecchymoses, although subcutaneous bleeding may occur either with fractures or sprains. Palpation can localize the area of maximal tenderness, crepitus, and loss or distortion of anatomical landmarks. Gently put the ankle through a range of motion to evaluate stability and to determine positions that produce or relieve pain. Manipulation must be gentle to avoid further injury. After examining the injured ankle, examine the opposite and supposedly normal joint. This will give an idea of the range of motion and laxity of the normal ankle joints. Again, the physician must keep in mind past history because a prior injury to the uninjured joint will prevent proper comparison.

Roentgenographic Examination

Roentgenograms are ordered to detect fractures and evaluate their severity. Although ligamentous injuries are not seen on x-ray films, improper anatomical relationships give a hint that ligamentous injury has occurred. The roentgenogram also allows the physician to look for further complicating factors such as foreign bodies or diseases of the bone. Lastly, the physician can utilize radiologic evaluation to follow the results of treatment of the patient with the ankle injury.

Proper radiologic evaluation of any ankle injury is essential. The examination should consist of an AP film in which the ankle is in 5 to 15° of adduction; a true lateral view that includes the base of the fifth metatarsal; and a 45° internal oblique film with the ankle in dorsiflexion. The roentgenogram should be of sufficient quality that trabecular detail is seen in all views. A comparison view of the opposite side can be helpful, especially in children. Also, a cone-down view or stress view of an area with questionable findings may be helpful. The physician should use the bright light to properly examine the outline of the bony detail and to detect soft tissue swelling.

LIGAMENTOUS INJURIES OF THE ANKLE

Approximately 75 percent of all ankle injuries are sprains. More than 90 percent involve the lateral ligaments, less than 5 percent involve the deltoid ligament, and less than 5 percent involve the anterior or posterior tibiofibular ligament and anterior and posterior capsule. Of lateral ligament injuries, 90 percent involve the anterior talofibular ligament, with 65 percent of these sprains being isolated, and 25 percent with concomitant injuries to the calcaneofibular ligament. The posterior talofibular ligament or third component of the lateral collateral ligament is stabilized against posterior displacement of the talus and is therefore rarely injured except in cases of complete dislocation. Because the anterior talofibular ligament and calcaneofibular ligament are two separate structures, the standard classification of first-degree, second-degree, and third-degree sprains is difficult to apply. Hence, injury to these ligaments is classified as either a single or double ligament injury. Only one ligament may be torn so that the integrity of the joint is weakened in one plane of direction, but it is not necessarily unstable. These ligaments usually tear in sequence from anterior to posterior, so that the anterior talofibular ligament tears first, followed by the calcaneofibular ligament.

Anterior Talofibular Ligament Injuries

Laxity of the anterior talofibular ligament may be adequately assessed by physical examination. The most helpful test is the anterior drawer maneuver. If the ligament is torn, the talus will sublux anteriorly and laterally out of the mortise with observable movement and crepitation at the limit of excursion. This maneuver should be performed on all patients with suspected lateral ligamentous injuries.

With one hand, grasp the calcaneus with the finger and thumb behind the malleoli, and with the opposite hand stabilize the extreme distal tibia and fibula. The foot should be slightly plantar flexed and inverted, which is its normal relaxed position. Next, apply a forward anterior force to the calcaneus, keeping the distal tibia and fibula fixed. Movement of the talus anteriorly more than 3 mm *may* be significant, but movement greater than 1 cm *certainly* is significant. There are both false-positive and false-negative results with this test but the most common difficulty is the physician's unfamiliarity with the examination.

If the tear extends further posteriorly into the calcaneofibular portion of the lateral ligament, talar tilt occurs, since the lateral ankle is now unstable, not only in the anterior posterior plane but in the medial lateral plane as well. Place the foot at 20 to 30° of plantar flexion with slight adduction, and apply inversion stress upon the calcaneal forefoot. Talar tilt or movement of the talus in the mortise is clinically felt due to tilting of the talus in relation to the distal articular surface of the tibia. This is then compared to the normal side.

Good muscle relaxation is important for proper evaluation. If diagnostic maneuvers are painful, voluntary and involuntary muscle contractions, to guard against further movement, will prevent assessment. The use of ice packs or local anesthetic infiltration can be helpful.

If the posterior talofibular ligament is involved, the ankle is obviously unstable, with both a positive anterior drawer sign and marked talar tilt. In most posterior talofibular ligament injuries, the ankle is dislocated and neither test need be performed.

Medial Collateral Ligament Injuries

The medial collateral ligament is rarely injured alone. Its injury is usually accompanied by a fracture of the fibula or tear of the tibiofibular ligaments anteriorly or posteriorly. This injury is usually the result of a significant eversion stress. It is almost impossible to tear the deltoid ligament without an accompanying fracture of the fibula or separation of the tibiofibular syndesmosis. Evaluation of the medial collateral ligament is done by stressing the ankle with a medial to lateral force. This is simply a talar tilt sign for evaluating the medial aspect of the ankle.

Tibiofibular Syndesmotic Ligament Injuries

Tibiofibular syndesmotic ligaments are a continuation of the interosseous ligaments at the distal tibia and fibula. Injuries to this ligament system occur secondary to hyperdorsiflexion and eversion. The talus usually pushes superiorly, separates the tibia and fibula, and displaces the fibula laterally, resulting in a partial or complete rupture. Diastasis will not necessarily be evident on radiologic or physical examination because the interosseous membrane above the ligament system will usually keep the tibia and fibula together.

The history is often nonspecific, but frequently the patient will complain that he or she felt something pop or give during a movement which caused dorsiflexion and eversion. There is little swelling, and the patient will complain of pain over the anterior and posterior superior aspects of the ankle. The patient will prefer to walk on the toes. On examination there is point tenderness over the anterior or posterior ligaments. There may be some tenderness over the medial malleolus secondary to a concomitant medial collateral ligament injury. In severe injury, there is also point tenderness over the distal tibia and fibula. Bilateral compression of the malleoli also causes pain as it causes movement in the injured area. Radiologic changes may only include soft tissue swelling at or below the medial malleolus and above the lateral malleous up to the midshaft fibula. This is a serious injury with significant long-term sequelae. A stress test of sorts may be helpful: Dorsiflex the foot with the patient supine or standing. This will cause pain and separation of the tibia and fibula.

Roentgenographic Findings in Ankle Sprains

The physician should always order standard x-ray views to evaluate an ankle injury, for radiologic findings can be surprising. If the standard views show avulsion or pull-off fracture, oblique or spiral fracture, transverse fracture, diastasis of the tibia, fibula, or a fractured fibular shaft, there is also rupture of the concomitant ligament. In such instances, no stress films are needed. However, stress films are indicated if instability is suspected or demonstrated by abnormal talar positioning, or if the joint line between the talus and mortise of the ankle is not symmetrical.

The anterior drawer sign as explained earlier may be done under x-ray or fluoroscopy. There is some difficulty in establishing reference points for measuring the movement of the talus anteriorly in relation to the mortise of the ankle. Although different authors have utilized different reference points, the current literature suggests that greater than 3-mm movement of the talus anteriorly to the posterior border of the calcaneus may be significant. Greater than 1 cm is certainly indicative of disruption. If there is some question as to the findings, the opposite ankle should be stressed in a similar manner and measured for comparison, providing the opposite ankle has not been injured in the past.

The talar tilt test, whether done in the medial or lateral ligamentous system, is also not extremely sensitive because there is variability of tilt among normal individuals and even between a pair of normal ankles. Moreover, pain, spasm, and edema may prevent adequate evaluation. As with the anterior drawer maneuver, there is no way to standardize the amount of force used by the physician during the test. However, the test may be positive if there is greater than 5° of talar tilt. If there is greater than 25° talar tilt, the examination is definitely abnormal. A difference of 5 to 10° talar tilt between the injured and uninjured side is probably significant in most instances.

In experienced hands, ankle arthrography is quick and simple to perform. It should be done within 24 to 48 h since clot formation after that time may prevent leakage of dye. Extraarticular leak of contrast material is generally indicative of a tear. However, the flexor hallucis longus and flexor digitorum longus tendon sheath fills in 20 percent of normal individuals, the peroneal tendon sheath fills in 14 percent, and the talocalcaneal joint space fills in 10 percent. Evaluation of the calcaneofibular ligament by standard arthrography techniques is associated with a high incidence of false-negative results.

Classification of Sprains

Ligamentous injuries are classified into first-, second-, and third-degree sprains. A first-degree sprain is stretching or microscopic tearing of a ligament, causing local tenderness and minimal swelling. Weight-bearing is possible and x-ray films are normal.

In a second-degree sprain, there is severe stretching and partial tearing of a ligament, causing marked tenderness, moderate edema, and moderate pain with weight-bearing. Radiologic evaluation with standard views will not demonstrate bony abnormality. However, if the ankle is stressed, loss of ligamentous function will be demonstrated by the abnormal relationship of the talus and mortise.

Third-degree sprain is due to complete rupture of ligaments. The patient is unable to bear weight, and there is marked tenderness and swelling, and often an obviously deformed joint. Standard radiologic evaluation will reveal an abnormal relationship of the talus and mortise. Usually, stress films are not needed but with a complete rupture they are almost always positive if the test is performed properly.

Treatment

There is much debate with regard to the treatment of ankle injuries. First-degree sprains may be treated by compression dressings, elevation, and ice. Fifteen minutes of ice application to produce local anesthesia, followed by range of motion exercises to the development of pain, followed again by 15 min of ice application, is beneficial. This should be done approximately four times a day until the patient can resume normal function without pain. The decision to institute nonweight-bearing or partial weight-bearing is an individual one. In the case of an athlete with a first-degree sprain, full athletic activity should not be resumed until that person can sprint without limping, run circles and figures of eight at full speed without pain, and, finally, cut at right angles off the affected joint without pain.

Second-degree sprains of the ankle are best treated with the ice method as described above, and immobilization. If there is extensive edema, a posterior splint, ice, and elevation are utilized until swelling diminishes; then, immobilization for 4 to 6 weeks in a walking cast and a walking hinge cast is usually recommended.

The treatment of third-degree sprains of the ankle is debatable. The decision whether to immobilize or to operate is not made easily and a number of considerations are important. The emergency physician is not usually asked to advise treatment for third-degree sprains because orthopedic consultation should be obtained for such injuries.

It is always prudent to maintain good liaison and communication with the patient's orthopedic surgeon. Patients with ankle injuries need appropriate diagnosis and treatment. Long-term sequelae of misdiagnosis and mistreatment are significant. Appropriate followup of ankle injuries is an absolute necessity.

ANKLE FRACTURE

Fractures are caused by forces acting upon the ankle joint that produce disruption of the joint ring. After ascertaining the mechanism of injury, standard roentgenograms are necessary for fracture diagnosis. Ligamentous avulsions will usually cause transverse malleolar fractures or small chip or pull-off fractures of the

malleolus below the joint line. Shifting of the talus causes it to strike the opposite malleolus and may cause an oblique fracture, often with comminution on the side of the bone subjected to the compression force. This evidence allows for prediction of the mechanism of injury, which is important because injuring forces must be reversed for fracture reduction.

Ligamentous injuries often occur with fractures, and have a more serious prognosis than the fracture itself.

Classification of Fractures

Wilson classifies ankle fractures by mechanism of injury, according to four primary forces: external rotation, abduction, adduction, and vertical compression (Fig. 131-3). Although convenient, this classification is limited in usefulness in that almost all ankle fractures occur as a result of a combination of the four forces.

External rotation. External rotation is usually associated with abduction, but it may be associated with other forces as well. Rotation at the ankle joint causes sequential injuries that are initiated on the medial side and extend laterally. Therefore, the first injury to occur is either a pull-off or a transverse fracture of the medial malleolus or rupture of the deltoid ligament. As the forces continue, the anterior tibiofibular ligament is ruptured. The talus then impacts upon the fibula and fractures it. Finally, the posterior tibial tubercle fractures, and the interosseous, posterior inferior tibiofibular, and the inferior transverse ligaments tear.

Abduction. Injuries to the ankle from abduction alone are less

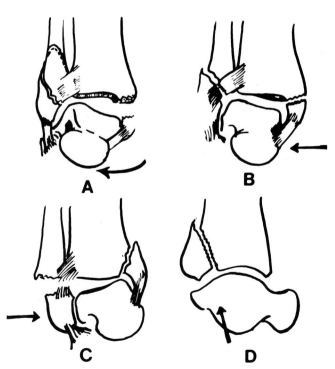

Figure 131-3. Basic mechanisms of ankle injury with the characteristic fractures produced by each: (A) external rotation, (B) abduction, (C) adduction, and (D) vertical compression. [Wilson FC: Fractures and dislocations of the ankle, in Rockwood, CA Jr, Green DP (eds): Fractures. Philadelphia, JB Lippincott Co, 1975, vol 2, p 1369. Used by permission.]

common but do occur. Again, the sequence of injury is medial to lateral but without a rotatory component. The initial injury is either a transverse or pull-off fracture of the medial malleolus or rupture of the deltoid ligament, which is the rarer of the two, followed by a fracture of the fibula below the syndesmotic ligaments or a rupture of the syndesmotic ligaments. If the ligaments rupture before the fibula fractures, the fibula will fracture near the junction of the middle and distal third of the fibula. Therefore, the shaft of the fibula must be visualized upon radiologic evaluation of such an injury.

Adduction. The third primary force is that of adduction, lateral to medial. This force is frequently an isolated event in contrast to the preceding two. The lateral collateral ligaments will rupture, or cause a pull-off or a transverse fracture of the lateral malleolus. With the continuation of the force the talus impacts upon the medial malleolus and causes a spiral fracture.

Vertical compression. Vertical compression is most often associated with the other forces in the production of ankle fractures, however, it may occasionally cause an isolated fracture. Depending upon the position of the talus in the mortise, vertical compression can cause an anterior or, rarely, a posterior marginal fracture of the tibia. Radiologic evaluation may demonstrate small fractures of the anterior or posterior lip of the tibia due to ligamentous pull-off, or larger vertical fractures through the articular surface of the tibia. Comminution is common with both anterior and posterior fractures, making anatomical reduction very difficult.

Other ankle fractures are intraarticular or osteochondral fractures of the talus, and avulsion fractures of the base of the fifth metatarsal that usually occur on the lateral aspect of the talus. If undetected, intraarticular fractures of the talus or osteochondritis dissecans can lead to loose bodies floating in the joint, and early degenerative arthritis.

Avulsion fractures of the base of the fifth metatarsal are probably one of the most commonly missed fractures. The history is an ankle injury due to plantar flexion and inversion. The peroneus brevis insertion at the base of the fifth metatarsal is stressed, resulting in a pull-off fracture. The base of the fifth metatarsal should be evident in proper radiologic examination of the ankle, but this is not necessarily always the case. The physician may not see the fracture if he or she does not suspect it. The epiphyseal plate of the base of fifth metatarsal can be differentiated from a pull-off fracture since the epiphyseal plate is usually oblique or longitudinal, while the fracture line is transverse.

Treatment

The goals of treatment of all ankle injuries, including fractures, are to restore the anatomic position of the talus in the mortise, return the joint line parallel to the ground, and ensure a smooth articular surface. These goals are achieved by immobilization or surgery. Most ankle injuries can be appropriately and adequately treated by immobilization. The primary indication for operative treatment is the inability to maintain anatomical positioning of the talus in relation to the ankle mortise.

Anatomical reduction is usually done by reversal of the injuring forces. Plantar flexion of the ankle in reduction of medial malleolar injuries should be avoided since the anterior fibers of the deltoid ligament are taut in this position, preventing positioning of the medial malleolus.

OTHER INJURIES OF THE ANKLE

Contusion

Direct trauma can produce contusion of the soft tissues or periosteum with swelling, discoloration, and point tenderness. Radiologic evaluation may demonstrate a cortical fracture in addition to soft tissue swelling. Treatment is symptomatic and consists of ice, a compression dressing, rest and elevation, and analgesics.

Tenosynovitis

Tenosynovitis is usually secondary to direct trauma or overuse of the tendons. The patient will have tenderness and swelling in the localized area but may have crepitus of the tendon as it moves through the sheath. X-ray films are negative. Treatment is ice and rest, but partial immobilization and anti-inflammatory medication may be necessary.

Subluxation. Peroneal tendon subluxation or tear may result from a direct blow, with or without dorsiflexion and eversion. The peroneal retinaculum tears and the tendons slip from their anatomical position. There may be an associated tenosynovitis. The patient usually complains of a clicking, slipping sensation, with pain and tenderness at the posterior lateral malleolus. The examining physician may feel or see displacement of the peroneus musculature upon contraction of the muscle group.

Achilles tendon injuries are common in runners and joggers. They are usually seen in the older individual but may be seen in the young. The patient will give a history of direct trauma or repetitive irritation to the area with symptoms of swelling and tenderness over the Achilles tendon or at its insertion. Treatment is rest, shortening of the Achilles tendon by heel elevation, and anti-inflammatory medication. In the younger individual, the Achilles tendon may rupture due to intense athletic activity. Such an injury is disabling and requires immediate orthopedic consultation and surgery in most instances.

Complications

There are a number of complications associated with ankle injuries, especially if they are improperly treated.

Nonunion occurs in 10 to 15 percent of fractures of the medial malleolus treated by a closed method. If it occurs, surgical correction is required.

Malunion can occur at any fracture site. If the patient is symptomatic and arthritic changes are not significant, surgery to correct the malunion may be done. Such surgery is often unsuccessful. Fusion may be the treatment of choice if there is degenerative or traumatic arthritis, or if the surgery has not been successful.

Infections are a complication of open fractures or the surgical treatment of closed fractures.

Traumatic arthritis occurs in 20 to 40 percent of ankle fractures regardless of the methods of treatment, but it is more common in inappropriately treated injuries. Loss of either the anterior or posterior tibial vessels may result in tissue destruction. The best treatment of possible neurovascular injuries is prophylaxis. Sudeck's atrophy secondary to sympathetic dystrophy is a complication of ankle injuries. Synostosis or ossification of the interosseous membrane may follow injuries to the syndesmotic ligaments, resulting in stiffness of the ankle joint. Finally, instability of the talus in the mortise is the most feared sequela. The loss of the support function of the ligaments predisposes the patient to recurrent sprains, resulting from progressively less trauma. This is especially disabling in athletes.

BIBLIOGRAPHY

Anderson JE: *Grant's Atlas of Anatomy,* 7 ed. Baltimore, Williams & Wilkins, 1978.

Black HM, Brand RL, Eichelberger MR: An improved technique for the evaluation of ligamentous injury in severe ankle sprains. *Am J Sports Med* 6:276–282, 1978.

Bonnin JG: *Injuries to the Ankle.* Darien, Conn, Hafner Publishing Co, 1970.

Johannsen A: Radiological diagnosis of lateral ligament lesion of the ankle: A comparison between talar tilt and anterior drawer sign. *Acta Orthop Scand* 49:295–301, 1978.

Starkey JA: Treatment of ankle sprains by simultaneous use of intermittent compression and ice packs. *Am J Sports Med* 4:142–144, 1976.

Turco VJ: Injuries to the ankle and foot in athletics. *Orthop Clin North Am* 8:669–682, 1977.

Wilson FC: Fractures and dislocations of the ankle, in Rockwood CA Jr, Green DP (eds): *Fractures,* Philadelphia, JB Lippincott Co, 1975, vol 2.

SECTION 17
NEUROLOGY

CHAPTER 132
THE NEUROLOGICAL
EXAMINATION

Gregory L. Henry

The individual components of the nervous system can be easily tested and analyzed in a simple but structured fashion. It is easy for the less organized examiner to spend a vast amount of time and yet obtain little information. The object of this discussion is to lay the groundwork for the diagnosis and treatment of neurological problems in the emergency department.

A systematic approach for doing the neurological examination must be accompanied by an equally thorough method for recording the examination findings. It is not adequate to write, "Neuro within normal limits." The pertinent positive and negative findings should be recorded on the chart, depending on the patient's chief complaint.

The press of patient care duties in the emergency department mandates that the basic areas of examination are approached quickly and directly. Further tests in any specific area should only be prompted by positive findings.

The object of the neurological examination is to answer two questions: (1) Where is it? and (2) What is it? The first question usually refers to the level of the nervous system involvement: peripheral nerve, spinal cord, cerebellum, brainstem, or cerebral hemisphere. A disease can involve a number of these areas, and a patient can have more than one disease, so that all data must be synthesized before any conclusions are reached. For example, the chronically demented patient is the one most likely to fall and develop an acute subdural hematoma. The answer to the question, Where is it?, is obtained chiefly by objective data from the neurological examination.

The question, What is it?, is asked to determine the mechanism by which the nervous system is being compromised. As a general rule, this question is best answered by history.

HISTORY

Entities that come on suddenly, within seconds to minutes, with distinct neurological signs and symptoms are almost invariably vascular in nature. Such vascular events may be large with huge deficits at the onset or may represent multiple small infarcts with accumulation of deficits which lead to more and more progressive neurological decline.

The nervous system, however, frequently has warning that a vascular catastrophe is imminent. The transient ischemic attack is such a warning signal. Transient ischemic attacks should be viewed as prestroke lesions and treated aggressively as an emergency medical problem.

A history obtained from family and friends is essential to determine the patient's premorbid level of function. It is not adequate to ask the family if the patient was "all right" prior to presentation to the emergency department. Many families have an unusual perception of what normal mental status and function is and these perceptions must be carefully determined. It is helpful to have a family member in the room with the patient to assist in monitoring the veracity of the patient's statements. Most patients with a history of progressive downhill function over weeks to years are affected with degenerative disease or some chronic dementing process. If the patient has had a slow downhill course with little change in mental status, it is unlikely that a definitive diagnosis will be made in the emergency department. The emergency physician should always beware of the patient with mild to moderate CNS impairment who presents with sudden deterioration over 2 or 3 days. Such a patient is a prime candidate for a subdural hematoma, CNS infection, dehydration, or some other toxic metabolic condition, including overmedication. Patients with rapidly fluctuating, nonfocal neurological signs should be considered to have a primarily metabolic insult until proved otherwise.

Multiple sclerosis is, as always, nebulous and difficult to diagnose. There is no definitive test for this disease, but it may be suspected in patients who have rapidly changing multiple focal neurological findings which are unrelated to a specific anatomic site.

SCREENING EXAMINATION

A basic neurological screening examination should be employed for all patients with general neurological complaints. It consists of evaluating six areas: (1) mental status, (2) cranial nerves, (3) motor response, (4) sensory response, (5) coordination (cerebellar function and gait), and (6) reflexes. Each area is described below, and the areas evaluated and tests employed are summarized in Table 132-1.

Mental Status

Examination of mental status is performed simply by speaking with the patient. In the emergency department detailed tests for

Table 132-1. Neurological Screening Examination

Area	Test
Mental status	Normal orientation, speech
Cranial nerves	Funduscopic, extraocular movements and pupillary response, visual fields, corneal reflexes, and facial muscular strength
Motor	Four basic muscle groups, tone, drift, heel-and-toe walking
Sensory	Cold and vibration on areas indicated by patient or on distal extremities
Coordination (gait)	Observation of gait, and finger-to-nose testing
Reflexes	Deep tendons—knees, ankles, elbows, and wrists; degenerative reflexes—Babinski's, snout, grasp, and root

hemispheric function are not necessary in a patient who is conversing normally, is making reasonable responses to questions, and is well oriented. Anything more than observation of simple speech, reasoning power, and normal communications skills is out of the realm of a screening examination. If subtle mental status changes are suspected, more involved testing is required. The brain is divided into a right and left half. In the vast majority of human beings, the left-sided brain is dominant. Dominant functions include speech, mathematical ability, and certain other communications skills. Physicians are usually less adept at testing nondominant hemisphere functions. The nondominant hemisphere is involved with spatial orientation, sound localization, and body self-image. Specific tests for these areas need only be performed if initial screening evaluation reveals difficulties.

Cranial Nerves

Tests for intact brainstem function are concerned chiefly with the second through seventh cranial nerves.

Mass lesions that are causing pressure either directly or indirectly on the diencephalon can alter the visual fields and pupillary response to light. Insidious tumors of the cerebral hemispheres which may have very few gross neurological findings, can cause early changes in the visual fields. An intact pupillary response to light requires both reception by the second cranial nerve and motor outflow from the third cranial nerve. Visual fields can be tested simply by having the patient look at the examiner's nose from an arm's length distance. With both arms extended and the elbows at right angles, the examiner quickly flicks both index fingers at the same time. The patient is then asked which finger moved. If the patient responds that both fingers moved, gross bitemporal lesions can be eliminated. This test should be performed to evaluate all four quadrants of vision.

Midbrain and pontine dysfunction can be detected by following extraocular movements. The patient is asked to follow the examiner's light into the six cardinal positions of gaze, making sure that the eyes are put through the full range of motion. The patient can also be observed simultaneously for nystagmus. Any abnormal findings should prompt a more detailed examination.

The fifth cranial nerve has extensive motor and sensory functions. The corneal reflex is often affected in hemispheric disease long before general facial sensation or the muscles of mastication are involved. Corneal sensation is tested by lightly touching the cornea with a small wisp of cotton. To do this, the patient must look opposite to the direction from which the examiner approaches. Scleral or lid response does not count, and only by touching the cornea can this sensation be tested. Unilateral depression of the corneal reflex is objective evidence of intracranial disease.

Seventh nerve function is commonly tested by having a patient smile or show the teeth. While considerable emphasis has been placed on the significance of asymmetry of the nasolabial folds, many people have slight asymmetry. A better test for facial strength is to ask the patient to squeeze the eyes tightly, and observe the degree to which the eyelashes are buried. Then, try to open the patient's eyes against such resistance. Another test is to have the patient purse the lips as in a whistle. Upper motor neuron lesions are characterized by unilateral weakness of the lower half of the face, while peripheral lesions involve the entire half of the face.

The eighth cranial nerve rarely requires testing in the emergency department unless there are specific complaints related to vertigo or hearing difficulties. Whenever questions with regard to the eighth cranial nerve function are raised, tests of both the vestibular and cochlear portions of the nerve are necessary. Speech reception testing by whispering numbers and words, as well as tuning fork evaluation for both the standard Weber and Rinne responses is usually sufficient to separate out gross hearing abnormalities.

Tests for the ninth, tenth, eleventh, and twelfth cranial nerves are essentially useless in the emergency department. There are no acute diseases which will manifest themselves with findings only in these areas, and in a rapid neurological screening examination they are of little value. Lower cranial nerve testing is important, however, if screening examination findings are referable to other cranial nerves.

Motor Response

Evaluation of general muscle strength, tone, and symmetry is the objective of the screening examination. Have the patient lie on the back so that the legs and arms can be observed. To check tone, quickly lift the knee off the cot and observe the actions of the foot. The normal response is to drag the heel along the bed as the knee is quickly jerked upward. If the leg comes up as a single unit, tone is probably increased. Gross bulk is estimated by observing the muscles of the calf and upper arm for mass, asymmetry, or fasciculations.

As a general rule, muscles essential in maintaining the body's normal posture have bilateral innervation and are less useful for determining lateralized weakness. In the upper extremities, the dorsiflexors of the wrist and the extensors of the forearm at the elbow have sufficiently uncrossed fibers to be useful in examination. In the lower extremities, evaluation of the dorsiflexors of the great toe and the flexors of the lower leg at the knee is all that is required to get a general idea of focal weakness.

An extremely sensitive indicator of focal weakness is testing for drift. In this examination, the patient is asked to extend both arms in front of the body, with the palms up and eyes closed. The patient is then carefully observed to see if there is any movement of one arm downward while the eyes remain closed. This test can be especially helpful in the minimally cooperative patient who is exhibiting give-way weakness on specific muscle testing. Another exceptionally good test for gross strength is to have the patient walk on the heels and then on the toes. This requires intact muscular strength.

Sensory Response

Testing sensation is the least exacting and least informative part of the neurological screening examination. If the patient has an area of decreased sensation, it is probably best to have the patient outline that area before attempting to isolate the lesion. If a definitive nerve root or peripheral nerve is outlined, direct testing for sensation should confirm the diagnosis.

A much more useful system in the emergency department is to think of sensory and motor loss in terms of patterns. Whenever sensation is found to be lacking in the "stocking glove" distribution, peripheral nerve lesions should be considered. Loss of either motor or sensory response in the upper extremities and across the chest in a cloak or capelike distribution is often asso-

ciated with lesions in the spinal column. Syringomyelia, a degenerative disease process, may present in such a fashion. More important to the emergency physician is that traumatic central cord syndrome with spreading inoxia of the cervical cord may likewise present with a capelike distribution. Loss of all sensation below a specific vertebral level defines a spinal cord injury. A mixed picture may be seen with only partial cord involvement, as in the Brown-Séquard syndrome. Loss of sensation on one side of the body or the other denotes a lesion high in the central nervous system before entering into brainstem structures. Areas of alternating hemianesthesia or hemiplegia, that is, facial findings on one side and lower body findings on the opposite side, always indicate a lesion in the brainstem itself.

In the patient who does not have a specific sensory complaint,

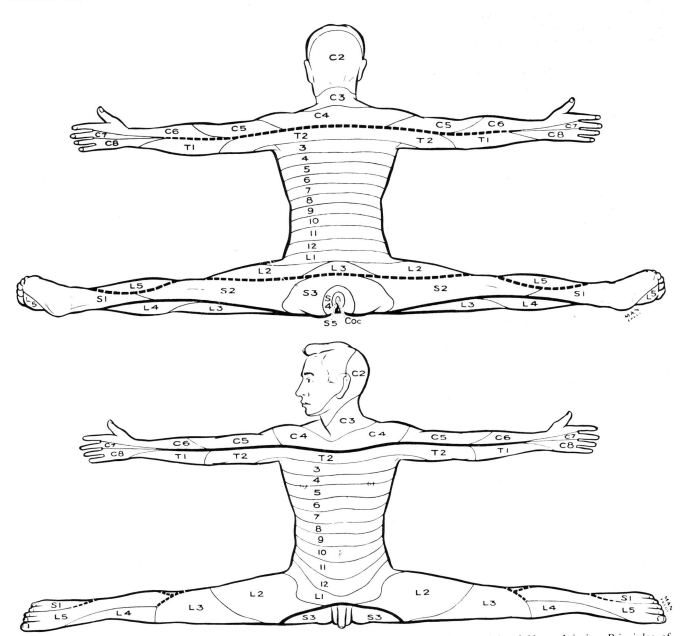

Figure 132-1. Nerve root origin of various reflexes. (From Haymaker W, Woodhall B: Peripheral Nerve Injuries: Principles of Diagnosis, ed 1. Philadelphia, Saunders, 1945, p 16. Used by permission.)

testing with a cold stethoscope, reflex hammer, or tuning fork is probably as accurate as any other method. Remember that sensory loss confined to one-half of the body usually involves a CNS lesion and most often is a hemispheric problem. If there is some decrease in response to vibratory sensation or hot and cold in either the hands or the feet, compare the lower extremities with each other, and against the upper extremities. Peripheral neuropathies tend to be symmetrical and show increasing sensation as one moves proximally along the limb. In symmetrical metabolic peripheral neuropathies there should be approximately the same level of nerve loss in both lower and upper extremities, and the legs tend to be involved earlier than the hands and arms.

The Romberg test requires explanation. A properly performed Romberg examination should be done with the patient standing and unsupported by any aids. With the feet together and arms at the side, the patient is asked to stand with the eyes open. If a patient cannot stand with the eyes open, the problem is usually related to one of cerebellar coordination. If the patient is able to stand with the eyes open but has difficulty in holding this position with the eyes closed, the problem is not one of coordination but one of sensation, with abnormality in position sense. This usually indicates involvement of posterior column function or may be seen as an isolated finding or as part of a general peripheral neuropathy.

Coordination (Gait)

This part of the neurological examination is frequently referred to as cerebellar testing. In truth, it is difficult to isolate the cerebellum because many areas are responsible for coordinating motor activity. Observing the patient's stance and gait is useful for testing both motor function and coordination. A broad-based, unsteady gait suggests cerebellar dysfunction. Patients with midline cerebellar lesions may have difficulty sitting up in bed without help. One good test for peripheral cerebellar lesions is finger-to-nose testing. Ask the patient to be precise, and to touch the tip of your finger and the tip of his or her nose in rapid sequence. Development of oscillation the last few inches before touching the target is abnormal. Hysterical patients commonly produce wide

Table 132-2. Diagnostic Neurological Tests Correlated with Specific Abnormal Neurological Complaints

Presenting Signs, Symptoms	Accessory Tests	Presenting Signs, Symptoms	Accessory Tests
Confusion, delirium, paucity of affect	Basic neurological examination plus: Formal mental status testing Aphasia testing Psychological testing Thought process and content evaluation (remember the patient with decreased affect may be psychologically depressed, so try to obtain a measure of thought content) Snout, grasp, root, Babinski's reflexes Physical examination of head, supple neck	Coma	Enough history should be taken to divide the patients into those with: Vertigo—All vertiginous patients should have positional testing and cold water caloric testing Syncope—patients require cardiac examination with ECG and perhaps in-house monitoring Completely separate examination: Level of consciousness Respirations Doll's eye movements or caloric testing Pupillary responses Motor responses and general physical examination
Blurred, dim, absent, or double vision	Basic neurological examination plus: Visual acuity and light perception Optokinetic nystagmus—in blindness Red glass testing—diplopia Careful funduscopic examination Careful auscultation of head and eyes	Trauma	Coma: Go directly to coma protocol Awake: Do limited examination Fine motor movements Drift Do not put patients through major testing until cervical spine x-ray films are reviewed. Remember, the order of the examination never changes, and the ABCs (airway, breathing, and circulation) precede all else in traumatized patients
Headache	Basic neurological examination plus: Auscultation of head and neck Careful palpation of the head and neck, particularly the temporal arteries		
Focal weakness	Basic neurological examination plus: Systematic testing of each nerve root or peripheral nerve involved in both motor and sensory function Hemispheric testing	Back pain without history of direct trauma	Basic neurological examination. If negative, do a cranial nerve examination, plus: Straight leg raising Anal wink Expanded motor sensory Reflex examinations Gait
Nonfocal weakness	Basic neurological examination plus: Test for muscle fatigue, including lid lag and drift (suspect myasthenia gravis, Lambert-Eaton syndrome, alcoholic myopathy)		
Dizziness	Basic neurological examination plus: Orthostatic vital signs taken on both arms		

oscillations from the moment they begin the motor task, or always touch precisely off the target.

Reflexes

Both deep tendon and regressive reflexes can be rapidly tested. Asymmetry of response is the significant finding. The patient with brisk reflexes in all extremities, and no other signs of neurological disease, probably has a normal variant. Likewise, the patient who essentially has no deep tendon reflexes without other neurological findings is probably exhibiting a baseline state. A change, however, in the threshold required to elicit a reflex or clonus on one side of the body suggests a lateralizing lesion high in the CNS. A difference in reflexes between the arms and the legs suggests a lesion involving the spinal cord. Depression of reflexes in only one limb, while the other is symmetrical, is consistent with a root or peripheral nerve lesion. The various reflexes and their nerve roots of innervation are listed in Figure 132-1.

Pathological reflexes, such as Babinski's reflex and snout, root, and grasp reflexes, indicate a lack of inhibition from higher cortical centers to primitive stereotype responses. Babinski's reflex, which is elicited by stroking the lateral aspect of the foot, is the most commonly used, and is a good lateralizing sign. The presence of snout, root, and grasp reflexes indicates diffuse, bilateral hemispheric disease.

Depending on the chief complaint of the patient and positive findings in the neurological examination, a more thorough examination may be necessary. Some aspects of such an examination require special training, but frequently you can further delineate the patient's problems by just a few simple testing procedures. Listed in Table 132-2 are various presenting complaints and the accessory tests that can aid the emergency physician in making a diagnosis.

BIBLIOGRAPHY

Brust JM: Transient ischemic attacks: Natural history and anticoagulation. *Neurology* 27:701–707, 1977.

Dalessio DJ, Otis SM, Smith RA: Cerebrovascular disease: Concepts and management. *Compr Ther* 3:33–41, April 1977.

Daly DD: Cerebral localization, in Baker AB, Baker LH: *Clinical Neurology*. Hagerstown, Harper & Row, 1976, vol 1, pp 1–42.

De Jong RN: Case taking and the neurological examination, in Baker AB, Baker LJ: *Clinical Neurology*. Hagerstown, Harper & Row, 1977, vol 1, chap 1, pp 1–83.

Haymaker W, Woodhall B: *Peripheral Nerve Injuries: Principles of Diagnosis*, ed 1. Philadelphia, Saunders, 1945.

Katzman R, Clasen R, Klatzo I, et al: Brain edema in stroke. Report of Joint Committee for Stroke Resources. *Stroke* 8:512–540, 1977.

Little JR, Tubman DE, Ethier R: Cerebellar hemorrhage in adults: Diagnosis by computerized tomography. *J Neurosurg* 48:575–579, 1978.

Merritt H: *A Textbook of Neurology*, ed 6. Philadelphia, Lea & Febiger, 1979.

Plum F, Posner JB: *The Diagnosis of Stupor and Coma*, ed 2. Philadelphia, Davis, 1972.

Schaffner MH, Jelenko C III: Rapid orthopedic and neurologic evaluation. *Ann Emerg Med* 9:103–104, 1980.

Toole JF, Cole M: Ischemic cerebrovascular disease, in Baker AB, Baker LH: *Clinical Neurology*. Hagerstown, Harper & Row, 1976, vol 1, pp 1–45.

Weiner HL, Levitt LD: *Neurology for the House Officer*, ed 2. Baltimore, Williams & Wilkins, 1978.

This bibliography contains references for both this and the following chapter.

CHAPTER 133
STROKE SYNDROMES
AND LATERALIZED
DEFICITS

Gregory L. Henry

Patients frequently present to the emergency department with an acute specific loss of neurologic function. When such lesions are specific to a region or side of the body, the patient is considered to have a lateralized neurologic deficit. Lateralized deficits of the central nervous system may be caused by multiple diseases but are usually mediated through compromise of vascular supply or acute bleeding. The systematic approach to these patients quickly rules out peripheral nerve involvement or spinal cord disease. Since compromise of vascular supply and neurovascular accidents compose the majority of the lateralized deficits, the stroke syndromes will be used as the prototype for the discussion. Later in the chapter differential diagnosis of lateralizing lesions will be discussed.

STROKE

Stroke is one of the most common neurologic problems seen in an emergency department. The full-blown anterior circulation stroke syndromes are usually recognized without difficulty, but the more subtle forms of stroke, often characterized by a confusing and unpredictable picture, may baffle even the most experienced examiner. A careful delineation of the underlying mechanism involved and the regions of the brain affected are of absolute necessity for both initiating treatment and making reasonable judgments with regard to prognosis.

In truth, cerebrovascular disease of any type is not a neurologic disease, in the strictest sense of the term. Stroke syndromes include not only infarcts and hemorrhages, but also the entire gamut of local or systemic vascular and perivascular disease. Any disease process that impedes regional cerebral blood flow may present as a typical stroke. Examples of diverse entities resulting in stroke are malaria, trichinosis, intracerebral hematoma, and neoplasms.

As with most neurologic problems, with stroke a thorough history is important to define the etiology, and the physical examination will be the best guide to the anatomic location. Because of the waxing and waning character of cerebrovascular disease, it is essential to question both the patient and the patient's family members for an accurate description of the signs and symptoms. Frequently, signs and symptoms will change or disappear by the time the patient is seen in an emergency department, and many decisions will have to be made on the basis of history alone. A good example is the patient with a transient ischemic attack (TIA). This disorder is characterized by the absence of permanent neurologic deficits, but can be amenable to a number of modes of therapy. Failure to make the diagnosis because of a lack of hard physical findings may result in a return visit because of a completed stroke.

The first part of this discussion will relate the various disease entities that affect the vasculature of the brain. The second part will describe the most common presenting complaints and specific syndromes with which the emergency physician is most often confronted. It will also include a differential diagnosis, and historical and physical examination tips that may lead to the correct diagnosis for each presenting complaint.

CEREBROVASCULAR LESIONS

Pathophysiology

The neurons of the brain require an uninterrupted supply of glucose and oxygen for metabolism because the brain cannot store these substances to any great degree. A decrease in the cerebral circulation will cause neuron dysfunction due to a decrease in supply of these two basic nutrients.

Blood reaches the brain through the four major vessels in the neck: two carotid and two vertebral arteries. Approximately 80 percent of the cerebral blood volume, referred to as the anterior supply, is handled by the carotid arteries. The remaining 20 percent, referred to as the posterior circulation, comes through the vertebral-basilar system. The anterior circulation is generally considered to supply most cortical and deep gray matter structures, as well as the optic nerves and retinas. The vertebral arteries, which are branches off the subclavian arteries, enter the skull through the foramen magnum and then combine near the pontomedullary junction to form the basilar artery, which has multiple fine branches. The vertebral-basilar system supplies nourishment to the upper spinal cord, brainstem, cerebellum, and certain deep gray matter structures. These two systems are interconnected at various levels, the principal one being the arterial circle of Willis.

There is considerable individual variation in collateral blood supply, a fact that accounts for individual variation in symptoms with similar anatomic lesions.

Ischemia and Infarct

In the emergency department, the physician is usually confronted with two types of ischemic problems: thrombotic occlusion of a vessel as a primary process, and occlusion of a vessel due to an embolus from a distant source. A third mechanism is external compression of a vessel due to hemorrhage or due to the progressive enlargement of a mass lesion. Compressive occlusion, however, usually is associated with a long history and does not result in sudden onset of symptoms.

Thrombotic Ischemia

Primary thrombotic ischemia may be due to atherosclerosis or vasculitis, such as giant cell arteritis or systemic lupus erythematosus. Thrombosis may also develop when constituents of blood are too viscous to traverse the arteriolar and capillary systems. Acute infectious process characterized by arteritis, such as syphilis or trichinosis, may mimic the atherosclerotic-type ischemic syndrome. Arterial occlusive disease outside the central nervous system or low-cardiac-output states may cause decreased cerebral blood flow. Disease of the aorta or cranial arteries, such as Takayasu's aortitis and aortic arch aneurysms, as well as mechanical problems, such as arthritis of the cervical spine, may contribute to cerebral ischemia.

On a statistical basis, however, the most common causes of infarction are atherosclerosis and embolism. There is still considerable debate over what the most common source of cerebral ischemic lesions is, but the emboli from atherosclerotic plaques in the internal carotid arteries may be the most common source of vascular occlusive disease. It is clear from autopsy studies that small cystic or lacunar infarcts are the most common form of cerebral infarction. The brain receives approximately 20 percent of the entire cardiac output and therefore is continually showered with any and all foreign material that may be present in the bloodstream. Many of these very minute infarcts are in relatively silent areas of brain function and may therefore go unnoticed.

Cerebral Embolism

Cerebral embolism is the term used to describe the occlusion of any intracranial vessel by a fragment of foreign substance arising outside of the CNS. The reason for occlusion may vary tremendously, but once it has taken place, the pathologic process is the same. Vascular stasis is followed by edema, which, in a short time, leads to cell death and necrosis. The majority of emboli that reach the brain are sterile, and are believed to arise from the large vessels of the neck and the heart. Air embolism following thoracic injury, and fat embolism following long bone injuries, are well documented. Bacterial and fungal emboli may result from endocarditis, sepsis, or from a focus of infection anywhere in the body. In adults, a mural thrombus from atrial fibrillation or myocardial infarction can result in an embolus. Transient ischemic attacks are most likely due to showers of microemboli from plaques in the great vessels of the neck.

Intracranial Hemorrhage

Intracranial hemorrhage may be the result of bleeding in multiple locations anywhere in the cranial vault. Bleeding can develop in the epidural, subdural, subarachnoid, intraparenchymal, and intraventricular spaces. Traumatic lesions of the middle meningeal artery are the usual source of epidural or extradural hematomas. Subdural hematomas may be the result of either traumatic or spontaneous bleeding from the veins that lie in the subdural space. Subarachnoid bleeding is usually due to rupture of a saccular aneurysm in the cerebral network, or less often, an arteriovenous (AV) malformation.

The majority of hemorrhages into the brain substance are produced by rupture of the arteriolar aneurysms that may be the result of hypertension or congenital malformations. Cerebral hemorrhages have been, to a much lesser extent, associated with certain blood dyscrasias, neoplasms, infections, and anticoagulants. Unlike embolic or thrombotic strokes, intracerebral hemorrhages, particularly the hypertensive variety, may be fatal in up to 80 percent of cases.

Incidence of CVA

Cerebrovascular accidents (CVAs) of all types occur in definable patient populations. Embolic and thrombotic lesions are more likely to occur in patients with the following problems:

- TIAs
- Hypertension
- Clinical evidence of atherosclerosis
- Cardiac abnormalities
- Diabetes mellitus
- Elevated blood lipids, cigarette smoking, erythrocytosis, and gout

There is good evidence that up to 70 percent of patients who have anterior circulation TIAs will develop cerebral infarction within 2 years. The TIA should be considered presumptive evidence of an impending cerebrovascular accident and should be treated aggressively. Hemorrhagic lesions such as aneurysmal bleeding and spontaneous interparenchymal rupture have a strong correlation with hypertension. Since atherosclerosis is a systemic illness, it can be assumed that the process is occurring in cerebral vessels as well.

Those patients with angina pectoris and intermittent claudication of the legs are at increased risk for stroke. Arterial bruits over the carotid arteries can be associated with a hemodynamically significant stenosis (i.e., greater than 70 percent) in 90 percent of cases, making this a significant finding. Patients with congenital heart disease, such as septal defects and valvular disease, and those with atrial fibrillation have a higher incidence of embolic stroke, particularly in conjunction with thyroid disease. Diabetics are prone to stroke because of accelerated atherosclerosis, hypertension, and peripheral vascular disease. Patients with elevated lipid levels, a history of cigarette smoking, erythrocytosis, and gout are also predisposed to stroke.

Clinical Features

When evaluating a patient with an acute lateralizing lesion, the emergency physician should be able to define the time course of the illness and current status of the disease, and be able to establish a time frame under which the rest of the workup should be accomplished.

Emergency department evaluation of the potential stroke victim should include a general physical examination, with particular attention to the patient's neurologic status. A patient's vital signs are paramount and may suggest that a hypertensive hemorrhage has occurred. A thorough examination of the patient's head and neck is important to rule out trauma. By careful auscultation of the head, eyes, and carotid arteries, bruits suggestive of AV malformations or vascular stenosis may be detected. A good cardiac examination is necessary to evaluate valvular disease or atrial fibrillation.

The neurological examination should be directed toward determination of the anatomic regions involved. Even in the comatose patient, signs of lateralization should be sought by checking the patient's withdrawal response to noxious stimuli. Hemiparesis, paraparesis, or even quadriparesis can be detected by noting whether the motor response is unilateral, whether the upper extremity responses are greater than those of the lower extremities, or whether facial grimacing and head and neck movement are present but movement of the extremities is absent. Conjugate deviation of the eyes and pupillary changes will help to determine if lateralization is present. Conjugate deviation of the eyes is often present in patients with large cerebral lesions. Remember that the eyes look toward the lesion in major hemispheric abnormalities, and away from the lesion in brainstem abnormalities. Check for nuchal rigidity and abnormal plantar responses.

A reasonable clinical impression can usually be formulated after initial history taking and physical examination. It is of utmost importance to try to distinguish hemorrhage from infarct, as the therapy for these two lesions is markedly different.

Obtain baseline laboratory studies, including ECG, CBC, PT, and PTT. Skull roentgenograms are usually obtained, but are generally of little value in diagnosis of the lesion.

Computerized tomography (CT) scanning has become the procedure of choice in differentiating the acute bleed from the cerebral infarct. It demonstrates virtually all instances of supratentorial hemorrhage and most cerebellar hemorrhage as well. The CT scan is not without error in detecting smaller hemorrhages, but in those circumstances where spinal tap may be hazardous, such as in the patient with a large supratentorial mass lesion, it may be of great value to the patient.

Angiography is an alternative for those patients in whom there is a question about the etiology of the lesion. If hemorrhage is not suspected, and if no specific therapy such as anticoagulation or surgery is anticipated, angiography is probably not indicated.

Traditionally, the examination of CSF obtained by lumbar puncture has been carried out early in suspected cases of intracerebral and subarachnoid hemorrhage due to the high incidence of blood in the CSF. A negative finding was thought to reassure the treating physician about to begin anticoagulant therapy on a stroke in progress. This is not necessarily true, as some intracerebral bleeding does not communicate with the subarachnoid space.

A suspected acute vascular event requires an acute vascular diagnosis either by CT scan or angiography. Even in the case of the patient with rapid onset of headache, nuchal rigidity, and obtundation, and with no lateralizing findings and no history of trauma, a lumbar puncture is probably not needed to confirm the diagnosis of subarachnoid hemorrhage. If a patient has focal findings that strongly suggest a mass CNS lesion, such as subdural hematoma or brain abscess, the lumbar puncture should be deferred if other studies are available. A lumbar puncture is also contraindicated if cerebellar hemorrhage is suspected. In that case, a CT scan or angiogram should be obtained.

Treatment

Thrombotic and Embolic Stroke

Definitive diagnosis and therapy of thrombotic and embolic vascular problems are usually not initiated in the emergency department. There are some general measures, however, that all emergency physicians can take to expedite patient recovery.

Avoid rapid lowering of the blood pressure in the first 10 days, unless the pressure is in a critically high range, usually a diastolic pressure above 120 mmHg. Then it is advisable to lower the patient's diastolic pressure to only the 100-mmHg range. If hypotension is present on initial examination, it should be corrected by the appropriate means.

Carefully monitor the routine use of intravenous fluids in stroke patients. Excessive amounts of free water may increase cerebral edema and actually add to the area of infarction. Standard nursing care, such as protecting the patients from aspiration and frequent turning to prevent decubiti, is as important in the emergency department as in nursing units.

The specific therapy for thrombotic and embolic stroke includes anticoagulation and various surgical procedures. There is much controversy about the role of anticoagulant therapy in stroke patients, but the following guidelines may be helpful:

1. Patients experiencing TIAs are highly prone to developing completed strokes. This group of patients should be aggressively investigated, and if no surgically correctible lesions are found, an indefinitely long course of oral anticoagulants should be instituted.
2. For the stroke in evolution, defined as documented progressive neurological involvement, most authorities advocate the immediate institution of intravenous heparin therapy to prevent further damage. Of course, it must be certain that a mass intracerebral lesion or hemorrhage is not present. Computerized tomography scanning or angiography may be done, and if no surgically correctible lesions are found, the patient may be switched to oral anticoagulants.

Vasodilators have long been used in the treatment of cerebrovascular disease without convincing evidence of their benefit. Amyl nitrate, papaverine hydrochloride, isoxsuprine hydrochloride, acetazolamide, carbon monoxide, and several other agents increase cerebral blood flow in normal tissue, but there is no evidence that these agents alter the course of ischemic strokes or prevent TIAs. Many investigators believe that the dilation of blood vessels in the remaining normal tissue may actually cause an intracerebral "steal" syndrome, thus reducing the perfusion pressure to already ischemic areas.

A certain percentage of patients with cerebral infarction will develop seizures, but there is no reason in the emergency department to give prophylactic anticonvulsants to these patients.

Corticosteroids have been found to be of little benefit in cerebral infarction states. It is usually wise to withhold corticosteroids unless the patient has definite signs of increased intracranial pressure or evidence of uncal herniation.

Surgery for embolic and thrombotic lesions is certainly not the province of the emergency physician, but remember that carotid endarterectomy is still the most commonly performed surgical procedure for ischemic cerebrovascular disease. In many series, if surgically approachable lesions of the carotid arteries are corrected, the incidence of completed stroke can be markedly reduced. Newer procedures for cerebral artery revascularization, such as anastomosis of the temporal artery to the middle cerebral artery, or saphenous vein bypass of various cerebral arteries, have not yet been shown to be effective.

Hemorrhagic Stroke

Emergency treatment of hemorrhagic strokes follows the same basic rules for therapy of thrombotic and embolic lesions. It is perhaps of even greater importance in hemorrhagic stroke, however, to ensure that the blood pressure is lowered to 90 to 100 mmHg diastolic within a reasonable period of time, without subjecting the patient to hypotension. Unlike thrombotic strokes, where blood pressures above the normal range can be allowed to persist, it is generally considered that blood pressure in hemorrhagic stroke should be brought within the acceptable levels of normal, depending upon the patient's age.

Generally there is considerable cerebral edema with hemorrhagic lesions and antiedema agents should not be withheld if there is evidence of herniation or progressive obtundation. Because of their transient effects, mannitol and urea are not useful in the longterm management of cerebral edema secondary to intercerebral hemorrhage. These agents are beneficial when given just before neurosurgery in an effort to reverse herniation.

Clotting abnormalities, either intrinsic or secondary to anticoagulant therapy, should be vigorously sought and corrected by administering the appropriate clotting factors or by reversing the chemical anticoagulants present.

Surgical therapy for intracerebral hematomas is an investigative procedure at this point. There is clear evidence, however, that evacuation of a hematoma in the cerebellum can be lifesaving to the patient. If an intracerebellar hematoma is suspected, a CT scan should be obtained immediately and a neurosurgeon consulted. Under no circumstances should a lumbar puncture be performed on a suspected cerebellar hematoma.

In many centers it is standard therapy to administer antifibrinolytic agents to patients with subarachnoid hemorrhage. ε-Aminocaproic acid (Amicar) is the agent of choice and is usually given intravenously in amounts of 30 to 36 g/day.

SPECIFIC CEREBROVASCULAR SYNDROMES

Now that we have considered the pathophysiology of the various types of lesions that can compromise the cerebrocirculation and have described a general approach to assessment and management of these problems, we will review the most common presenting syndromes with which the emergency physician will be confronted. The vascular anatomy of the brain varies minimally from patient to patient, but the collateral circulation is variable. Therefore, a specific patient may have only a portion of the syndromes herein discussed.

Ischemic Stroke Syndromes

Middle Cerebral Artery Syndromes

Occlusion of the middle cerebral artery is usually by embolic phenomena. The clinical picture includes contralateral hemiplegia and hemianesthesia, contralateral homonymous hemianopsia with impairment of conjugate gaze in the direction opposite the lesion, aphasia with dominant involvement, and constructional apraxia and anosognosia with nondominant hemisphere involvement. The usual occlusion, however, involves only the branches of the middle cerebral artery, resulting in incomplete syndromes. Arm involvement is usually greater than leg involvement, and varying forms of aphasia occur with the involvement of the dominant hemisphere.

Anterior Cerebral Artery Syndromes

With the involvement of the anterior cerebral artery, there are frequently paralysis of the contralateral foot and leg and contralateral center loss, with contralateral gegenhalten, abulia, gait apraxia, and urinary incontinence.

Posterior Cerebral Artery Syndromes

The posterior cerebral artery supplies blood to the occipital cortex and branches that supply upper midbrain structures. These patients may have contralateral homonymous hemianopsia or quadrantanopsia, memory loss, dyslexia without agraphia, contralateral hemiparesis, contralateral hemisensory loss, and ipsilateral third nerve palsy with contralateral hemiplegia.

Vertebral-Basilar Artery Syndromes

Vertebral-Basilar Lesions

The vertebral basilar arteries are subject to both atherosclerotic narrowing and embolic phenomena. Since the vertebral system supplies the posterior portions of the brain, including the cerebellum and brainstem, deficits resulting from occlusion of these arteries are predictable. These include ipsilateral ataxia, contralateral hemiplegia with sensory loss, ipsilateral horizontal gaze palsy with contralateral hemiplegia, ipsilateral peripheral seventh nerve lesions, intranuclear ophthalmoplegia, nystagmus, vertigo, nausea and vomiting, and deafness and tinnitus.

Basilar Artery Occlusion

Occlusion of the basilar artery in itself usually gives rise to such severe bilateral signs as quadriplegia and coma, and the locked-in syndrome. In the locked-in syndrome, the patient has a lesion of the tectual pons that knocks out all motor function except upward gaze.

Cerebellar Infarcts

Cerebellar infarcts usually produce dizziness, nausea, vomiting, and nystagmus, and the inability to stand or walk if midline cerebellar functions are involved. The patient should be observed carefully, and if cerebellar swelling is causing a rapid downhill course, the patient should undergo emergency decompression of the posterior fossae.

Lacunar Infarction

In 1967, Fisher outlined a series of specific brainstem infarctions that were due to small microinfarcts referred to as *lacunar infarctions*. These small cystic infarcts occur principally in the deep gray matter and brainstem and result in some discernible patterns. There are four specific lacunar infarct states that have been delineated. They are:

1. The clumsy hand dysarthria syndrome due to a small lesion in the midpons.
2. Leg paresis and ataxia due to a lesion in the pons or internal capsule resulting in ataxia and weakness in one leg.
3. A pure sensory stroke, resulting from a lesion in the thalamus. This usually results in a sensory loss in the face, arm, or leg with no hemiplegia or other signs.
4. Pure motor hemiplegia due to a lesion in the pons or internal capsule with paralysis of the arm, face, and leg without sensory loss. In a right hemiplegia, no aphasia is found. In a left hemiplegia, no parietal lobe findings are evident.

Lacunar infarct states are found in hypertensive patients, and control of hypertension is the principal mode of therapy. Many of these patients have relatively transient deficits, and with proper care return to good function.

The scope of this text does not permit a thorough review of all the various brainstem stroke syndromes. Suffice it to say, the majority of brainstem stroke lesions are due to lesions in the vertebral-basilar system, and accurate anatomic localization is possible because of the relatively precise and localized neuroanatomy of the region. There are multiple eponymic syndromes, such as Wallenberg's, Weber's, and Parinaud's syndromes, that are associated with the brainstem, but the important feature to remember is that whenever you have alternating symptoms, i.e., lesions on one side involving the cranial nerves on one side of the brainstem, and sensory or motor problems on the opposite side of the body, the lesion must be involving descending tracts after they have left the cortex and internal capsule and before they have decussated in the lower medulla. In this way, a patient may exhibit findings of the cranial nerves on one side of the body and motor and sensory findings below the level of the foramen magnum on the opposite side of the body. Finer articulations than these are not usually necessary in the emergency department setting and they are amply discussed in currently available texts.

Transient Global Amnesia

Ischemia to hippocampal and amygdaloid structures may result in a much underdiagnosed syndrome known as transient global amnesia. This syndrome usually occurs in patients who are over 60 and is characterized by an abrupt loss of the ability to recall recent events or record new memories; however, there is usually very good memory of past events. During the episode, the patient is usually able to perform highly complex tasks, even arithmetic, and speech is usually unimpaired. The majority of these patients recover completely, and it is questionable whether their symptoms represent the same prognostic values as do other TIAs.

Hemorrhagic Syndromes

Subarachnoid Hemorrhage

Subarachnoid hemorrhage usually results from rupture of a saccular aneurysm. It occurs at sites of arteriolar bifurcation or branching. The majority of patients who experience ruptured aneurysms are between the ages of 36 and 65 years of age. Patients with polycystic kidneys and coarctation of the aorta are known have a higher incidence of subarachnoid aneurysmal bleeds. Unlike thrombotic and embolic lesions that frequently present with TIAs, aneurysms are usually asymptomatic until they rupture.

Typically, the onset is marked by an extremely severe headache that the patient describes as the worst headache he or she has ever experienced. The patient usually does not lose consciousness at this point, but may have a rapid onset of stupor progressing to coma, without focal lateralizing signs. The patient's general physical examination and neurological examination may be normal, except for signs of increased meningeal irritation.

Hypertensive Intracerebral Hemorrhage

The hypertensive intracerebral hemorrhage syndromes likewise have a fairly characteristic presentation. Hypertensive hemorrhage almost always proceeds from the small penetrating vessels of the brain that have been damaged by hypertension and usually arises in the following locations, in decreasing order of frequency: putamen, thalamus, pons, and cerebellum. Hemorrhages that are due to anticoagulants or a bleeding diathesis usually involve areas such as the frontal, temporal, parietal, or occipital lobes, which are sites rarely involved with hypertensive hemorrhage.

Hemorrhage of the putamen often presents a picture indistinguishable from middle cerebral artery occlusion, with contralateral hemiplegia, hemianesthesia, homonymous hemianopsia, aphasia, or hemineglect, depending upon the hemisphere involved. There is usually greater depression of consciousness in the patient with putamenal hemorrhage than in the patient with standard middle cerebral artery occlusions.

Thalamic hemorrhage produces contralateral hemiparesis with contralateral hemianesthesia. The sensory loss is usually considerably greater than the motor deficit. Occasionally there is restriction of the upward gaze or skewed deviation of the eyes without visual field defect.

Pontine hemorrhage usually results in pinpoint pupils that are minimally reactive to light, and decerebrate posturing. These patients rapidly progress to coma and lack normal oculovestibular reflexes when caloric testing is performed.

Of all the hemorrhagic or occlusive diagnoses, cerebellar hemorrhage is the most important to make. The patient typically develops sudden dizziness and vomiting, with marked truncal ataxia. The patient is unable to stand and walk, but is otherwise alert and oriented. No hemispheric abnormalities are noted. There may be findings associated with compression of the ipsilateral pons, such as ipsilateral sixth nerve palsy and parapontine gaze center abnormalities, and facial weakness. The patient rapidly progresses to coma, and frequently death results from brainstem compression. This is a treatable form of hemorrhage, and if diagnosed early, it may be relieved by surgical decompression and evacuation of the hematoma, which may restore the patient to near normal function.

DIFFERENTIAL DIAGNOSIS OF PRESENTING COMPLAINTS

Few patients present to an emergency department complaining of a specific disease. Therefore, a standard system of evaluation is necessary to take a general symptom complaint unrelated to a specific etiology. This section will be presented in a schematic form to make it more useful in the emergency department.

Right-Sided Weakness

Cortical Localization

If aphasia is present, the lesion must have a cortical component. Check the patient's ability to name objects, repeat sentences, read, and comprehend and carry out commands. Remember that all right-handed patients, and perhaps 70 to 80 percent of all left-handed patients, are left hemisphere–dominant.

Cortical sensory loss. Cortical sensory loss manifests as loss of two-point discrimination, graphesthesia, stereognosis.

Loss of sensation in the face and arm more than in the leg strongly suggests middle cerebral artery distribution in the cortex.

Eye deviation. Eyes deviate toward the hemisphere involved and away from the hemiparesis.

Field defect is usually present.

Subcortical Localization

Examples of subcortical lesions include lesions of the internal capsule, basal ganglion, or thalamus. The face, arm, and leg are equally involved.

Signs of subcortical localization include the following:

No aphasias
Abnormal posturing
Extremely dense sensory loss
Eye deviation may be the same as in cortical lesions

Left Brainstem

Right hemiplegia with left-sided brainstem signs, such as cranial nerve palsies on the left side of the face
Cerebellar signs with abnormal finger-to-nose and rapid alternating movement testing on the left, with weakness on the right
Nystagmus that is most marked when the patient looks toward the side of the lesion
Possible hearing loss
Alternating sensory findings, with sensory loss and weakness on the right side of the body, and sensory loss on the left side of the face, due to involvement of the different tracts for each area.
Dysarthria
Tongue deviation, and abnormal gaze palsies resulting in difficulty looking to the left; due to left brainstem involvement.

Spinal Cord Lesions

With spinal cord lesions, there is no involvement of the face, and no aphasias, dysphasias, or dysarthrias. Paralysis is on the same side as the lesion, but pain and temperature sensation may be on the opposite side of the weakness, i.e., Brown-Séquard syndrome.

A sensory level to pinprick is evident.

Bladder and bowel disturbances may be noted.

Differential Right-Sided Weakness—Numbness

1. Vascular—Thrombotic, hemorrhagic, AVM, subarachnoid hemorrhage, transient ischemic attack, venous infarct, carotid or intracerebral lesion
2. Subdural hematoma, epidural hematoma
3. Tumor, primary or metastatic
4. Brain abscess
5. Cardiac disease—Low flow states and arrhythmias
6. Seizure disorder—Postictal paralysis (Todd's paralysis)
7. Bell's palsy—Peripheral seventh nerve, face
8. Vascular migraine headache
9. Metabolic—Rare cause of focal findings
10. Functional—Psychiatric

Left Hemiplegia

In the majority of patients, the nondominant hemisphere is the right hemisphere, which controls the left half of the body. Therefore, assessment of the left hemiplegia basically involves testing of nondominant, or right hemispheric, function. If the lesion is cortical, check for denial of the lesion by answering the following questions:

Does the patient ignore the left side? Or does the patient fail to recognize body parts as being his or her own?
Does the patient extinguish double simultaneous stimulation by suppressing one part of the body?

Additional questions that are helpful in evaluating nondominant hemisphere function are as follows:

Does the patient exhibit constructional apraxia? Can the patient draw a simple map, and name and locate areas on it? Can the patient also draw a clock and fill in the numbers?
Does the patient have spatial disorganization with respect to the room?
Is there a decrease in persistence of tasks that are assigned?

All of the above indicate involvement of the nondominant hemisphere. In addition, note findings that are common to both hemispheres, such as quadrantanopsias and weakness in the arm greater than the leg. Subcortical, brainstem, and spinal cord findings are the same as noted in the section on right-sided weakness, except they would be on the left side.

Left-Sided Weakness and Numbness

The entire list of differential diagnoses listed under right-sided weakness are applicable to left-sided weakness.

The bibliography for this chapter may be found at the end of Chapter 132, page 899.

CHAPTER 134
SEIZURES AND
STATUS EPILEPTICUS

Carl Sacks

A seizure is a symptom of disturbed neuronal function. It is a condition of cerebral origin in which there is a dusturbance of movement, behavior, sensation, or consciousness. Epilepsy is seizures with spontaneous recurrence. Status epilepticus is seizure activity that is prolonged and repetitive. It has been widely accepted that two or more seizures without regaining consciousness, or a single seizure lasting for 20 min or longer, constitutes status epilepticus.

PATHOPHYSIOLOGY

A seizure seems to occur when constitutional or extraneous factors or both result in hyperirritability and an abnormally excessive discharge of neurons. These factors may defeat the normal defense mechanisms that guard against excessive discharge by altering the sodium-potassium pump that holds the neurons in a state of polarization. Hydration, dehydration, adrenal insufficiency, and other factors may lower interneural potassium and raise interneural sodium, potentiating instability.

Some neurons release chemical substances that induce a state of hyperpolarization and reduced irritability. Others release substances that induce depolarization and hyperirritability. Finally, it is thought that collections of neurons exist that are capable of exerting direct inhibitory effects on other parts of the nervous system, preventing repeated discharge. If the inhibitory pool is damaged, a seizure may originate in the area it governs. The seizure focus may remain localized, or spread locally or centrally. Once established, the seizure focus can evolve in three different manners. It may remain static and cause aberration of motion or sensation of one part of the body, such as the hand. It may spread locally along a gyrus as in the early stages of a Jacksonian seizure and become generalized only when the corpus callosum has been crossed. The focus may also spread immediately down the corticothalamic pathway in an immediate generalized seizure.

Given the appropriate stimulus, anyone can have a seizure. In normal individuals the seizure threshold is so high that a seizure occurs only if the subject undergoes electroshock, or is given a convulsant drug. There is a continuum ranging from the normal individual who has never had a seizure; to the individual who will have a seizure precipitated by fever, by metabolic or physical stress, or by sensory stimuli such as emotional stress or a flickering light; and terminating with the person who has recurrent attacks without demonstrable cause.

Primary and Secondary Epilepsy

Primary, or idiopathic, epilepsy is epilepsy of unknown etiology. Primary epilepsy may be a major seizure (grand mal), a minor seizure (petit mal), a myoclonic seizure (myoclonic jerks), or an aberrant seizure (dog attack). The age of onset is almost always during the first or second decade. There is frequently a familial incidence. There are no abnormal interictal neurological signs, and a characteristic electroencephalogram (EEG) is commonly, but not always, present.

Secondary, or symptomatic, epilepsy is due to an irritating neural disturbance, either of intracranial or extracranial origin (Table 134-1).

Table 134-1. Causes of Secondary Epilepsy

Intracranial etiologies:
  Trauma
  Infection
  Degeneration
  Vascular lesions
  Intracranial space-occupying lesions (subdural hematoma)
Extracranial etiologies:
  Anoxia:
    Cardiac
    Respiratory
  Endocrine-electrolyte disorders:
    Hypoglycemia
    Hypocalcemia
    Hyponatremia
    Hypomagnesemia
  Toxins and poisons (withdrawal or intoxication or both):
    Alcohols
    Phenobarbital
    Phenytoin
    Lead
    Chlorinated hydrocarbons
  Febrile seizures
  Eclampsia of pregnancy

Intracranial causes may be focal or general. The cerebral cortex differs in its susceptibility to the development of seizures. The frontal, temporal, and parietal lobes are the most vulnerable, while the occipital lobe is the least vulnerable. Focal seizures may be triggered by congenital malformations such as aneurysms or arteriovenous malformations. They may also result from cerebral abscess, cerebral tumor, ischemic lesions, parasitic cysts, trauma, and cerebral edema. Trauma may induce a focus either at the site of the blow or in the frontal cortex. A blow to the head causes the soft brain to be oscillated rapidly in the bony vault, where the frontal cortex is vulnerable because of its intimate contact with the sharp surfaces of the sphenoid bone. As they are so prone to damage by herniation, the temporal lobes are the immediate victims of cerebral edema. They are also extremely vulnerable to anoxia or hypoglycemia.

Some diffuse intracranial causes of seizures are maturational defects, neurosyphilis, cerebral atrophy, cerebral atherosclerosis, and lipoid storage disease.

Pathology of extracranial origin, through its ability to alter neural function at the cortical or interlaminar thalamic regions, may induce secondary seizures.

Secondary (nonidiopathic) cortical focal seizures indicate underlying abnormalities. The treating physician is lax toward the patient by merely trying to beat the seizure into pharmacological submission with pills, capsules, and syringes, while abandoning or ignoring the search for the possibly life-threatening or curable cause.

Major Motor Seizure

A major seizure may be characterized by a prodromal period of irritability or tension lasting for hours or days. An aura is rare in a seizure of thalamic interlaminar origin, but it is not uncommon in a seizure of cortical origin. The victim loses consciousness, usually without warning, becomes rigid in extension, falls to the ground, becomes apneic, and may urinate and defecate. In a short time there are facial spasms, and the tonus slackens only to be succeeded by generalized tonic contractions. After a variable and seemingly interminable period, the clonus slackens, rendering the patient comatose and flaccid. Consciousness slowly returns, often with the postictal symptoms of confusion, headache, and fatigue.

Petit Mal Seizure

Minor, or petit mal, seizures are transient in nature, rarely lasting more than a few seconds, and the comportment and consciousness are characteristically altered during this time. Subjects abruptly cease their current activity. They may stare, roll the eyes up, and quite frequently rapidly flutter the eyelids. For this short time, although they do not fall or exhibit tonic or clonic phenomena, they are unconscious and unresponsive, and are unable to speak or respond to the spoken word. They then resume their current activity and are frequently unaware of the transpired attack. These episodes may be very frequent, occurring up to 100 or more times a day. The attacks are characterized by bursts of symmetric and simultaneous 3-s^{-1} spike and slow wave activity on the EEG. The attacks may occur as isolated phenomena or be associated with major seizures. To complicate the matter the 3-s^{-1} spike slow wave EEG pattern may be associated with kinetic and myoclonic attacks. The term *petit mal triad* describes the associated characteristic seizures and myoclonic attacks with the above-mentioned EEG pattern.

Partial seizures of a temporal focal origin may mimic a petit mal attack, but observation and electroencephalographic investigation will often reveal the true nature of the seizure. Differentiating features of petit mal and minor temporal seizures are listed in Table 134-2.

Focal Seizure

A focal cortical discharge may produce only focal manifestations, or it may be responsible for the aura preceding a generalized seizure. As the functional architecture of the cortex is well established, one can often correlate focal symptoms of a seizure with the probable cortical focus. Foci originating in the prerolandic or motor cortex result in unilateral clonic or tonic contractions. In emergency patients, the occurrence of a focal motor seizure should arouse suspicion of a mass CNS lesion, especially a subdural hematoma, until proved otherwise. Foci originating in the postrolandic or sensory parietal cortex result in paresthesia or dysesthesia. Frontal lobe seizures are frequently devoid of focal manifestations, thus tempting a diagnosis of idiopathic epilepsy. However, if the focus encompasses the frontal lobe field area (Broca's area 8) or is in the supplementary motor area, there may be adverse turning of the eyes and head. Foci of the occipital lobe may produce negative seizures, sudden brief impairment of vision or positive seizures, flashing lights, or sometimes a complex visual scene.

Temporal Lobe Seizures

The psychic content of temporal lobe seizures renders them especially susceptible to misdiagnosis. The extremely varied symptoms include visceral sensations, hallucinations, memory

Table 134-2. Differentiating Features of Petit Mal and Minor Temporal Lobe Seizures

	Petit Mal	Temporal Lobe Seizures
Age	Occurs mainly in children and usually disappears by adulthood	Any age
Etiology	Idiopathic, primary	Secondary: trauma, anoxia, fever, tumor, infection, etc.
Frequency	Frequent to very frequent	Less frequent
Postictal phenomena	None	Confusion not unusual
EEG	Bilaterally synchronous and symmetrical 3-s^{-1} spike and slow waves	Often temporal focal activity. May need sphenoid or nasopharyngeal electrodes
Duration	Few seconds	Often longer
Physical manifestations	Often fluttering of eyelids	Often lip smacking or stereotyped movements
Other investigations	Usually not indicated	Desirable

disturbances, dream state, automatism, and affective disorders. One common visceral sensation, usually unpleasant, is often described as fear commencing in the epigastrium and rising up to the chest, throat, mouth, and lips.

Hallucinations may affect smell, taste, hearing, vision, and movement (vertigo). Sometimes objects appear distorted, larger smaller, closer, or more distant than they are.

Disturbances of memory are characterized as *déjà vu*—a sense of familiarity with an unfamiliar environment—or *jamais vu*—a sense of unfamiliarity with a familiar environment, a sense of time standing still or rushing past. Feelings of derealization and depersonalization can also occur.

Primary automatism may be the only manifestation of a focal temporal seizure or it may be the prelude of a major seizure secondary to spread from the temporal focus. Secondary automatism, however, commonly follows major seizures.

The inner surface of the temporal lobe includes the limbic system, so it is not surprising that disturbances of emotion such as anxiety, fear, ecstasy, depression, or paranoid feelings may occur.

CONDITIONS THAT MAY SIMULATE EPILEPSY

All disturbances of movement, sensation, behavior, or consciousness are not due to seizures. Myoclonia may be associated with Creutzfeldt-Jakob disease, benign essential myoclonus, and nocturnal myoclonus. Disturbances of sensation may originate from the cranial nerves, spinal nerves, peripheral nerves, or spinal cord. Disturbances of behavior and consciousness may be of toxic, psychiatric, metabolic, or hysterical etiology. Drug-induced dystonia, tetany, tetanus, and strychnine poisoning can also cause movement disorders.

Some conditions that alter consciousness and mimic epilepsy are narcolepsy, cataplexy, sleep paralysis, and syncope. Narcolepsy is characterized by episodes of uncontrollable sleep lasting for minutes or hours. Males are affected more than females. Subjects are generally extremely obese, and they may also experience nocturnal apnea.

Cataplexy consists of a sudden loss of postural tone and feeling of weakness. The subject falls to the ground, consciousness intact. The episode is triggered by violent emotion such as laughter, anger, and excitement.

Sleep paralysis is characterized by complete loss of muscle power, usually upon awakening from sleep and occasionally just before dropping off to sleep. Consciousness remains intact. These episodes occur primarily in males.

Reduced blood flow to the brain may impair consciousness. Common causes of syncope are vasovagal attack, heart disease, basilar migraine, vertebrobasilar insufficiency, blood loss, hypotensive drugs, and Valsalva-related maneuvers.

While the EEG is normal during the phenomena that mimic seizures, it is generally pathological in the ictal and interictal phase of seizures. Careful physical and neurological examination should usually enable one to arrive at the proper diagnosis. The characteristic hysterical major seizure (pseudoseizure) usually does not conform to the classic pattern hitherto described (Table 134-3). Unfortunately, true epileptics can also exhibit pseudoseizures that are almost impossible to differentiate from the true ones. Hysterics who have had the occasion to witness true seizures often give remarkable imitations. When in doubt, assume the seizure is real and act appropriately.

Table 134-3. Differential between True and Hysterical Seizures

	True Seizure	Hysterical Seizure
Occurrence	Night or day, alone or in company	Usually related to emotional upset, usually in company
Pattern	Usually conforms to a classic type. Patient may bite tongue, or otherwise injure self	Often bizarre pattern, tongue biting and injury rare
Incontinence during seizure	Common	Rare
Corneal reflexes during seizure	Absent	Present
Plantar responses during seizure	Often extensor	Flexor
EEG	Abnormal epileptic pattern; almost always occurs during attack and usually occurs interictally	Tracing is abnormal but not epileptic

CLINICAL FEATURES

Correct unstable vital signs immediately. Determine by history or observation whether the alleged seizure was indeed a true seizure. If the patient appears postictal, has a bitten tongue, or was incontinent, it is likely he or she had a seizure.

Look for evidence of extracranial pathology that could provoke a seizure: hypothermia or hyperthermia, alcohol withdrawal, hypoglycemia, acid-base or electrolyte disorders, anoxia, hyperosmolar states, toxins, or drugs.

Determine if there is any evidence of intracranial pathology that could provoke a seizure, such as recent trauma, meningitis, tuberous sclerosis, Sturge-Weber syndrome or von Recklinghausen's disease, or facial hemiatrophy.

Look for evidence that the patient has a long history of seizures such as old scars on the face and tongue, old fractures, gingival hypertrophy secondary to chronic phenytoin therapy, or the presence of anticonvulsants in the patient's possession.

Neurological Examination

The neurological examination should be directed to determine the level of CNS functioning and the presence of focal signs. Check the state of consciousness, pupillary reflexes, corneal reflex, caloric response, and gag reflex.

Signs of secondary seizures due to intracranial etiology include unequal pupils; retinal exudates, hemorrhage, or papilledema; bruits over the head or neck to suggest an arteriovenous malformation; plantar extensor responses; asymmetry of deep tendon reflexes or muscle tone; and asymmetry of rapid alternating movements and pain response.

Obtain a history from the patient, family, or friends. Determine the general medical history and allergy to medications; age at first seizure; and time of the last seizure before the one in question. Determine if the patient is compliant or noncompliant, or had a recent change of dosage in medication.

Once the patient is responsive, inquire about a prodrome, aura, and focal onset. Ask witnesses how the seizure began, for example, by staring into space, vacant expression, cry, paling or flushing, breath holding, irritability, clenching or grinding of teeth, smacking of lips, or swallowing.

Ask about motor movements as the seizure progressed. In particular, determine if both sides of the body were involved, or if movements were more marked on one side than on the other, or if the seizure involved both the upper and lower extremities, and, if so, if both were equally involved.

Ask how long the seizure lasted, if there was any difference in behavior before, after, or during the seizure, and if the patient remembered anything about the seizure.

Laboratory Examination

Laboratory and radiologic evaluation of special procedures will not be necessary if the patient is a known seizure patient; has a simple seizure that follows the normal pattern; quickly regains consciousness; does not have any evidence or history of trauma, drugs, alcohol, or diabetes; and if the neurological examination is normal. However, even in such patients, it may be useful to obtain anticonvulsant drug levels.

If this is a first seizure, or if the above criteria are not present, obtain a CBC, as well as blood glucose, sodium, potassium, chloride, carbon dioxide, BUN, calcium, magnesium, creatinine, and alcohol levels. Osmolarity, blood gases, toxicology, and anticonvulsant drug levels may be indicated depending on the results of examination and history.

Radiologic Examination

A skull roentgenogram may reveal a fracture; intracranial hypertension as manifested by a shift in a calcified pineal, erosion of the clinoid processes of the dorsum sellae, beaten silver appearance of the skull, or widening of the sutures in an infant; or an intracranial space-occupying lesion by shift of the calcified pineal, local erosion of the inner table, or calcification of a neoplasm, cyst, or arteriovenous malformation.

The chest roentgenogram may reveal a primary pulmonary neoplasm that may have metastasized to the brain or a pneumonia that may have seeded meningitis.

Ultrasonic echoencephalography may show a shift of the midline of the brain, suggesting the presence of an asymmetric intracranial space-occupying lesion.

More sophisticated techniques that can be utilized for evaluation are radioisotope techniques, arteriography, computerized tomography (CT), air encephalography, or electroencephalography.

The radioisotope (commonly, technetium 99) is injected by vein, passes up into the cerebral circulation, and tends to accumulate where there are many small blood vessels and breakdown of the integrity of the cerebral vasculature. Up to 85 percent of all tumors, arteriovenous malformations, and leaking aneurysms may be detected by radioisotope technique.

Arteriography gives a precise picture of the arterial and venous blood supply. It may detect atheromas, aneurysms, arteriovenous malformations, the displacement of vessels by a space-occupying lesion, and a blush as it passes through the abnormal vasculature of a neoplasm.

Briefly, CT scanning involves a narrow beam of x-rays that traverses the skull in a series of steps. A pair of accurately aligned detection units follows the beam across the head and sends the transmitted rays to a computer that provides a printout. In this way, and by adjusting the sensitivity of the computer, small percentage variations of the x-ray penetration can be perceived. The size and shape of the ventricles, atrophy of the gyri, and the size and position of a brain tumor, hematoma, or bleed may be discovered without invasive technique.

Changes in the frequency amplitude and pattern of change in electrical potential of the cerebral cortex are explored by the recording electrodes of the EEG. The patterns may indicate the presence and type of epileptic activity, if the activity is focal or diffuse, if it radiates from one site to another, and if it is associated with destructive or toxic metabolic changes. One can have epileptic discharges without clinically apparent seizure activity. One can rarely have clinically certain seizures without typical EEG changes, presumably because the discharge is originating from a site that cannot be explored by the electrodes.

The only solid indication for an immediate spinal tap is to rule out meningitis. When there is strong evidence of an intracranial bleed or space-occupying lesion, a tap is dangerous and generally will not yield information that cannot be found more effectively by a lower risk process. If a tap is necessary, it should be preceded by fundoscopy, a skull roentgenogram, and careful neurological examination to rule out focal signs.

TREATMENT

First secure vital functions. If there are signs of anoxia, open the airway with a jaw lift, suction secretions, and explore the mouth for a foreign body if spontaneous respiration is not reestablished. Secure the airway with a nasotracheal tube or by endotracheal intubation, whichever is most appropriate. Administer supplementary oxygen if indicated, and correct hypotension.

Pass a nasogastric or Ewald tube and empty the stomach both to avoid regurgitation and possible aspiration, and to empty the stomach of possible toxins.

Every comatose or stuporous patient should receive 100 mL of 50% dextrose intravenously after blood has been drawn for electrolytes and other studies. If ethanolism is suspected, follow this with 200 mg of thiamine intravenously.

Protect the patient from physical harm by gentle but firm restraint to prevent a fall from the stretcher.

Have a bite block ready at the bedside in anticipation of recurrence of seizures.

Search for and treat all signs of secondary seizures.

Administer appropriate anticonvulsant therapy if indicated. Anticonvulsants should not be administered and certainly not prescribed for a first single seizure. These medications are indicated only after investigations have proved there is a tendency for spontaneous recurrence. Anticonvulsants can interfere with the electroencephalographic studies. By giving patients a prescription for an anticonvulsant, you have, appropriately or not, labeled them epileptics and condemned them to all the related legal, insurance, employment, and medical complications. Any person, epileptic or not, may have a seizure or even status epilepticus after acute withdrawal from maintenance phenobarbital or phenytoin.

On the other hand, the administration of phenytoin and phenobarbital to a patient with a history of treated recurrent seizures, old facial scars, gingival hypertrophy, and an empty prescription bottle in the pocket makes sense.

Phenobarbital is the only effective medication for febrile seizures

Table 134-4. Primary Antiepileptic Drugs

Class	Indications	Generic Name	Trade Name
Hydantoins	Generalized convulsive seizures; all forms of partial seizures	Phenytoin	Dilantin
		Mephenytoin	Mesantoin
		Ethotoin	Peganone
Barbiturates, desoxybarbiturate	Generalized convulsive seizures; all forms of partial seizures	Phenobarbital	Luminal
		Mephobarbital	Mebaral
		Metharbital	Gemonil
		Primidone	Mysoline
Oxazolidinediones	Generalized nonconvulsive seizures (absences)	Trimethadione	Tridione
		Paramethadione	Paradione
Succinimides	Generalized nonconvulsive seizures (absences)	Phensuximide	Milotin
		Methsuximide	Celontin
		Ethosuximide	Zarontin
Acetylurea	Partial seizures with complex symptoms	Phenacemide	Phenurone
Dibenzazepine	Partial seizures with complex symptoms; generalized convulsive seizures	Carbamazepine	Tegretol
Benzodiazepine	Generalized nonconvulsive seizures (absences)	Clonazepam	Clonopin
Branched-chain carboxylic acid	Clonic seizures; absences; generalized tonic-clonic seizures; all forms of partial seizures	Valproic acid	Depakene

Source: Penry JK, Newmark ME: The use of antiepileptic drugs. *Ann Intern Med* 90:208, 1979. Used by permission.

and ethanol-related seizures. Phenytoin is not indicated. The primary antiepileptic drugs, their uses, and their elementary pharmacological properties are listed in Tables 134-4 and 134-5.

STATUS EPILEPTICUS

To treat grand mal status epilepticus, one must know what it is and how it kills. Status epilepticus is characterized by generalized tonic-clonic seizures that are so prolonged or so frequent that they create a fixed and lasting epileptic condition. The reported frequency of tonic-clonic status varies from 1 to 5 percent. The reported mortality is currently 6 to 18 percent. Death during tonic-clonic status may be due to anoxia associated with postictal or interictal apnea, aspiration, and iatrogenic respiratory depression. It may be due to circulatory collapse because of exacerbation of preexisting cardiovascular disease or, again, an iatrogenic cause. Death may ensue because of trauma from falling off the stretcher, renal failure, or the factor that precipitated the seizure. There is considerable evidence that aberrant critical discharges, with their increased metabolic demands, may lead to permanent neuronal damage if not terminated in 1 h. Also, the longer seizures persist, the more aberrant circus-rhythm pathways are potentiated.

To protect against anoxia, the patient should undergo endotracheal intubation, ideally by the more stable nasotracheal technique or by the orotracheal route if necessary. A patent airway is guaranteed, and aspiration is minimized (and further reduced by gastric suction). If respiratory depression results from medication, mechanical ventilation guarantees adequate oxygenation.

Proper restraint guards against trauma. Cardiac and blood pressure monitoring and cautious administration of the appropriate anticonvulsant will help thwart cardiovascular collapse. Appropriate fluid and electrolyte therapy should protect the kidneys. By giving 50 g of dextrose intravenously, and by conducting appropriate physical, neurological, radiological, and chemical investigations, hopefully the tractable secondary precipitating factors will be discovered and nullified.

The best and most stable intravenous line is a large-bore, through-the-needle catheter.

There is considerable variation in sequence, but the drug of choice for initial control of tonic-clonic status epilepticus is intravenous diazepam at a dose of no more than 5 mL/min with careful monitoring of respiration and blood pressure. Diazepam acts rapidly, reaching maximum brain concentration 1 min after intravenous injection. It has a limited duration of action with a half-life of 15 to 90 min. Serum concentrations of at least 0.5 μg/mL are needed for seizure control. These concentrations are not attainable with diazepam given intramuscularly. From 68 to 74 percent of

Table 134-5. Pharmacologic Properties of Six Antiepileptic Drugs

Drug	Oral Dosage, mg/day	Expected Blood Level		Time to Reach Steady-State Blood Levels, days	Serum Half-Life, h	Effective Blood Level, μg/mL	Toxic Blood Level, μg/mL
		Average, μg/mL	Range, μg/mL				
Phenytoin	300	10	5-20	5–10	24 ± 12	> 10	> 20
Phenobarbital	120	20	10-30	14–21	96 ± 12	> 15	> 40
Primidone	750	8	5-15	4–7	12 ± 6	> 5	> 12
Phenobarbital	Derived	24	5-32	14–21			
Carbamazepine	1200	6	3-12	2–4	12 ± 3	> 4	> 8
Valproic acid	1500	50	40-70	2–4	12 ± 6	> 50	> 100
Ethosuximide	1000	60	40-100	5–8	30 ± 6	> 40	> 100

Source: Penry JK, Newark ME: The use of antiepileptic drugs. *Ann Intern Med* 90:215, 1979. Used by permission.

grand mal status cases have been lastingly controlled by intravenous diazepam.

Generally, the second drug of choice is phenytoin administered intravenously at a rate of 40 mg/min or less in a concentration of 6.7 mg/min or less. The loading dose, calculated from its volume of distribution of 0.64 L/kg necessary to obtain serum levels of 10 to 20 μg/mL (approximately 750 to 1000 mg), is dissolved in normal saline and piggy-backed via IVAC into the main IV line of normal saline, in which it is used to prevent precipitation. Brain tissue levels will be approximately 90 percent of maximum at the end of infusion and at maximum 1 h after the infusion. As phenytoin increases the refractory period of the AV mode and slows conduction through the bundle of His, it may cause AV block or aggravate a preexisting AV block. It may also diminish myocardial contractility; thus phenytoin should only be administered when a patient is on a cardiac monitor, and should be slowed or stopped at any sign of hypotension, bradycardia, or PR interval prolongation.

Phenytoin is contraindicated in the presence of second- or third-degree heart block. Intramuscular phenytoin has no place in the treatment of epilepsy. Absorption is prolonged, incomplete, and erratic, and involves considerable pain and rhabdomyolysis.

The third drug of choice is phenobarbital. It may cause profound circulatory and respiratory depression, but has very little effect on cardiac automaticity. Unlike phenytoin, which primarily inhibits spread from an epileptogenic focus, phenobarbital inhibits the focus itself. It may be used in the patient who is allergic to or refractory to a full loading dose of phenytoin, as well as in the presence of significant heart block. Therapeutic serum levels are from 10 to 30 μg/mL, and the volume of distribution is 0.64, as with phenytoin. Thus, the average loading dose is 15 to 20 mg/kg, and not the total of 2 to 4 grains often and wrongly encountered in the literature. The total dose can be diluted in 100 mL of normal saline and administered IV piggyback via infusion pump at a rate of from 25 to 50 mg/min, while the patient is frequently monitored for signs of cardiovascular or respiratory depression, which may be much more readily provoked by a combination of valium and phenobarbital. Maximum brain tissue levels are attained approximately 1 h after infusion.

If the foregoing drugs are unsuccessful, it may be because suboptimal doses of medication have been used, the etiological cause of the seizure has not been isolated and eliminated, acid-base and electrolyte problems remain uncorrected, the patient is hypoxic, the patient has become hyperosmolar, or finally, because the seizures are refractory to the agents used.

Lidocaine administered by the intravenous route has been found effective in controlling grand mal and focal motor status. One must be aware that it has not been approved by the Food and Drug Administration for this purpose and that in toxic doses lidocaine itself may induce seizures. The problem is compounded by the fact that some of the dosage regimens used exceed that recommended by the American Heart Association for the treatment of the cardiac arrhythmias. Bernard and Bohn recommend starting treatment with a bolus of 2 to 3 mg/kg. If the seizures do not stop, they are probably refractory to lidocaine. If they stop and then recommence, Bernard and Bohn recommend a lidocaine infusion of 3 to 10 mg/(kg·h). This latter approach seems quite illogical in view of our knowledge of the pharmacokinetics of lidocaine. The half-life of an IV bolus of lidocaine is approximately 10 min. The therapeutic level for cardiac arrhythmias (1.2 μg/mL) is only maintenance for about 20 min after the

single bolus. It is thus recommended that the normal cardiac therapeutic blood level of lidocaine (1.2 to 5.0 μg/mL) be maintained by a loading dose of 1 μg/kg followed by an infusion of 20 to 50 mg/(kg·min) or its equivalent 1.2 to 3.0 μg/(kg·h).

A conservative protocol for the initiation of therapy would be the following. An IV lidocaine bolus of 1 mg/kg is given. There are two possible responses: (1) The status is broken and there is no exacerbation. Lidocaine therapy is terminated. (2) The seizures do not stop, or there is only a transient cessation. Give another bolus, this time 0.5 mg/kg, and start a lidocaine drip of 2 mg/min. If the seizures are not permanently terminated, give another bolus of lidocaine of 0.5 mg/kg and increase the drip rate to 3 mg/min. If seizure activity still persists, one last lidocaine bolus of 0.5 mg/kg is given, and the IV drip rate of lidocaine is increased to 4 mg/min. If the status persists, an alternate therapy is pursued. If the seizure activity is terminated, try to gradually taper the drip rate to zero as other long-term anticonvulsants are added to control the seizures.

A continuous IV drip of valium can also be used to treat refractory status epilepticus until other definitive measures are instituted; 100 mg is diluted in 500 mL of D_5W and administered IV at a rate of 40 mL/h on an infusion pump. The serum levels will be from 0.2 to 0.8 μg/mL. The patient must be intubated, as laryngospasm may occur. The combination of valium and phenobarbital may result in severe respiratory and/or cardiovascular depression.

Paraldehyde, although once quite commonly used for status epilepticus, has become much less popular, because, in large doses, it has been associated with hepatitis, respiratory depression, hypotension, and metabolic acidosis. As a powerful sedative, it can cause a state that may be easily confused with a prolonged postictal depression. Intravenous paraldehyde can, in addition, cause severe phlebitis, pulmonary edema, and hemorrhage. Intramuscular paraldehyde is extremely painful and can cause a sterile abscess, local nerve damage, and severe rhabdomyolysis. The most benign method of administration is a rectal enema at a dose of 0.2 mL/kg diluted in twice the volume of milk or mineral oil. If all else fails, seizures may respond to general anesthesia, using secobarbital (Seconal), amobarbital, or halothane with a neuromuscular junction blockade. If status recurs upon cessation of anesthesia, selective neurosurgery, with removal of an isolated epileptogenic focus, or implantation of a cerebellar stimulator, may be the only hope.

Sodium valproate is not available for parenteral administration. However, status epilepticus has been reportedly controlled by the administration of 600 mg of the crushed tablets in water, administered qid by nasogastric tube. It has been reported that the substance can be made into lipid-based suppositories and administered in doses of 400 to 800 mg every 6 h. Blood levels above 40 μg/mL generally give good results. Sedation and ataxia are secondary effects, and there have been reports of hepatic failure as well.

TODD'S PARALYSIS

Todd's paralysis is a transient nonprogressive focal paralysis that occurs in the postictal period of a seizure and is generally of focal onset. The etiology has generally been attributed to a transient exhaustion of the most used neurons. While the usual duration of the focal paralysis is 1 or 2 h, it can, exceptionally, last for 1 or

2 days, and has been alleged in the neurological folklore to last up to a week.

As it is not at all uncommon for irritative and destructive intracranial foci to coexist in close proximity to one another, one cannot automatically assume that all postictal focal paralysis is benign.

A destructive focus should be suspected if the postictal paralysis is progressive, or if it is accompanied by cranial nerve signs that are known not to have predated the ictus.

Head trauma, meningismus, signs of intracranial hypertension, or a change in the duration and/or pattern of a previously documented Todd's paralysis are indications for further investigation.

The scope and intensity of the follow-up investigations are determined by the clinical presentation and progression of the individual patient.

BIBLIOGRAPHY

Bernhard CG, Bohm E: *Local Anaesthetics as Anticonvulsants: A Study on Experimental and Clinical Epilepsy*. Stockholm, Almqvist and Wiksell, 1965.

Delgado-Escueta AV, Westerlain C, et al: Management of status epileptics. *N Engl J Med* 306:1337–1340, 1982.

Ernest MP, Marx JA, et al: Complications of intravenous phenytoin for acute treatment of seizures. *JAMA* 249:762–765, 1983.

Epstein MH, O'Connor JS: Destructive effects of prolonged status epilepticus. *J Neurol Neurosurg Psychiatry* 29:251–254, 1966.

Glaser GH, Perry JK, Woodbury DM: Antiepileptic drugs: Mechanisms of action, in *Advances in Neurology*. New York, Raven Press, 1980, vol. 27.

Greenblatt DJ, Bolognini V, Koch-Weser J, et al: Pharmacokinetic approach to the clinical use of lidocaine intravenously. *JAMA* 236:273–277, 1976.

Hillestad L, Hansen T, Melsom H, et al: Diazepam metabolism in normal man: Serum concentrations and clinical effects after intravenous, intramuscular, and oral administration. *Clin Pharmacol Ther* 16:479–484, 1974.

Hunter RA: Status epilepticus: History, incidence, and problems. *Epilepsia* 1:162–188, 1959.

Janz D: Conditions and causes of status epilepticus. *Epilepsia* 2:170–177, 1961.

Katt H, Penry J: Usefulness of blood levels of antiepileptic drugs. *Arch Neurol* 31:283–288, 1974.

Manhire AR, Espir M: Treatment of status epilepticus with sodium valproate, letter to editor. *Br J Med* 3:808, 1974.

Mayeux R, Leuders H: Complex partial status epilepticus: Case report and proposal for diagnostic criteria. *Neurology* 28:957–961, 1978.

Meldrum BS, Vigouroux RA, Brierly JB: Systematic factors and epileptic brain damage: Prolonged seizures in paralyzed, artificially ventilated baboons. *Arch Neurol* 29:82–87, 1973.

Neophytides AN, Nutt JG, Lodish JR: Thrombocytopenia associated with sodium valproate treatment. *Ann Neurol* 5:389–390, 1979.

Oxbury JM, Whitty CWN: Causes and consequences of status epilepticus in adults: A study of 86 cases. *Brain* 94:733–744, 1971.

Penry JK, Newark ME: The use of antiepileptic drugs. *Ann Intern Med* 90:207–218, 1979.

Perrier D, Rapp A, Young B, et al: Maintenance of therapeutic phenytoin plasma levels via intramuscular administration. *Ann Intern Med* 85:318–321, 1976.

Roger J, Lob H, Tassinari CA: Status epilepticus, in Vinken PJ, Bruyn GW (eds): *Handbook of Clinical Neurology*. New York, American Elsevier, 1974, vol 15, pp 145–188.

Sturdee DW: Diazepam: Routes of administration and rates of absorption: A study of women with preeclampsia. *Br J Anaesth* 48:1091–1096, 1976.

Sussman NM, McLain LW Jr.: A direct hepatotoxic effect of valproic acid. *JAMA* 247:1173–1174, 1979.

Svensmark O, Buchthal F: Accumulation of phenobarbital in man. *Epilepsia* 4:199–206, 1963.

Taverner D, Bain WA: Intravenous lidocaine as an anticonvulsant in status epilepticus and serial epilepsy. *Lancet* 2:1145–1147, 1958.

Vajda FJ, Mihaley GW, Miles JL, et al: Rectal administration of sodium valproate in status epilepticus. *Neurology* 28:897–899, 1978.

Wilder BJ, Ramsay RE, Willmore LJ, et al: Efficacy of intravenous phenytoin in the treatment of status epilepticus: Kinetics of central nervous system penetration. *Ann Neurol* 1:511–518, 1977.

CHAPTER 135
ACUTE PERIPHERAL
NEUROLOGICAL
LESIONS

Gregory L. Henry

There is no problem more frustrating or confusing for the busy emergency physician than a patient who is complaining of generalized weakness or nonspecific ailments in an extremity. These types of problems can be extremely time-consuming and produce very few results unless the physician has a logical and systematic approach to examination and treatment. Four basic guidelines for evaluation are given below.

First, most peripheral neuropathies and myopathies are slowly developing processes with a good history of downhill progression. Family members and the patient should be consulted to determine if the process is acute or chronic. Diffuse, bilateral nerve-muscle lesions are those that evolve over a few hours to days (or at least worsen acutely) and that do not involve severe changes in mental status, at least as their predominant symptomatology.

Second, peripheral nerve lesions must be separated from central nervous system disease. For example, patients with numbness and aching in the right hand may be so occupied with this symptom that they fail to realize they are also having trouble with word finding and facial numbness. It is absolutely essential that by history and physical examination a search is made which will exclude lesions of the central nervous system.

Third, of all examinations done in medicine, motor and sensory examinations are often the most imprecise. When unsure as to the cause of a specific symptom, it is prudent to advise the patient to return should the symptoms worsen. A brief emergency department evaluation is not the basis for a diagnosis of hysteria or functional disorder.

Fourth, reflexes are notoriously difficult to evaluate in the amount of time generally available in the emergency department. A few general statements, however, can be made.

Hyperreflexia in the face of down-going toes and no other pathologic reflexes is probably a normal variant. Lesions such as a previous stroke, multiple sclerosis, cerebral palsy, and amyotrophic lateral sclerosis may all give hyperreflexia, but these lesions are usually quickly separated out by history and physical examination.

In the hyporeflexic patient the situation is more difficult. *The patient who is truly areflexic—that is, no reflexes—usually has a neuropathic as opposed to a myopathic disorder.* However, hyporeflexia may be a normal variant, a sign of spinal shock, a sign

of acute cerebral vascular accident, or may accompany a variety of myopathies and neuropathies, and is therefore a nonspecific finding.

Keeping in mind the order and extent of the physical examination described in Chapter 132, "The Neurological Examination," and with the above basic guidelines, we are ready to construct the differential diagnosis of acute peripheral problems.

It is beyond the scope of this chapter to discuss the myriad diseases that produce myopathies and neuropathies. We will concentrate on those entities that are both common and acute. No attempt will be made to describe the chronic disease processes that can usually be segregated out by history.

ACUTE TOXIC NEUROPATHIES

Bacterial Illnesses

Overwhelming bacterial sepsis may cause generalized weakness and lack of motor coordination, but only a limited number of bacterial illnesses will present early with severe peripheral neurologic findings. These are diphtheria, botulism, and tetanus.

Diphtheria

Infections with *Corynebacterium diphtheriae* are usually characterized by an acute onset, exudative pharyngitis, high fever, and malaise. The organism gives off a powerful exotoxin that acts directly on the heart, kidneys, and the nervous system. The most common presenting neurologic problem with diphtheria is mononeuritis or a mononeuritis multiplex. For example, neurologic involvement of the palate with difficulty in speaking and changing quality of voice can occur. The most commonly observed paralyses, however, involve the intrinsic and extrinsic muscles of the eye, producing ptosis, strabismus, and problems in accommodation. When the limbs are involved, the patient is critically ill and has bilateral flaccid weakness or paralysis accompanied by absent deep tendon reflexes and, in long-standing cases, atrophy. Sensory involvement is rare. However, bladder and rectal sphincter muscles may be involved, producing urinary retention, overflowing incontinence, and incompetent anal sphincter tone. The ascending transverse myelitis of the Guillain-Barré type has been recorded with cases of diphtheria.

Botulism

Botulism toxin is a preformed toxin, elaborated by *Clostridium botulinum,* an anaerobic gram-positive bacillus that affects both striated and smooth muscle. The toxin exerts its effect principally at the myoneural junction, without direct toxicity to the muscle fibers or the peripheral nerve itself. The principal mode of action is in prevention of the release of acetylcholine. There are at least seven major toxins, but toxins A, B, and E are the ones primarily causing disease in humans.

The principal source of botulism in the United States is food which has been inadequately prepared. There are no definitive telltale signs or smells of the organism so that it may exist in foods which are normal on inspection. The neurologic symptoms usually appear in 24 to 48 h after ingestion of contaminated foods and may or may not be preceded by nausea, vomiting, and diarrhea. The most common early presenting neurologic complaints are related to eye and bulbar musculature. Symptoms spread very rapidly, however, to involve all the muscles of the trunk and extremities. The smooth muscle of the intestine and the bladder may occasionally be involved, resulting in ileus and acute urinary retention. Good mental status is maintained until the patient is terminal.

It is important to differentiate botulism from diphtheria or Guillain-Barré syndrome. Guillain-Barré syndrome is an ascending transverse myelitis and does not usually begin with involvement of bulbar musculature. Diphtheria is an acute febrile illness, with pseudomembranous oropharyngitis and cardiac involvement. With rapid deterioration botulism may occasionally be confused with undiagnosed myasthenia gravis. The two are easily differentiated with the edrophonium chloride (Tensilon) test. Botulism should not improve with the administration of cholinesterase inhibitors.

A variant form of botulism, infant botulism, has recently had a resurgence. In almost 40 percent of affected infants, the source of the botulism can be traced to raw honey containing botulinum spores. Children affected with this disease may exhibit lethargy and failure to thrive, eventually leading to paralysis and death. It is almost always insidious in infants, due to the extremely small amounts of botulinum toxin ingested along with the honey.

After diagnosis and respiratory support, further treatment of botulism patients is usually carried out in the intensive care unit. As with all ingested toxins, removal of the remaining offending agent by gastric lavage, activated charcoal, and instillation of cathartics is advised. The decision to use botulinum antitoxin is usually made following consultation with infectious disease specialists.

Tetanus

Clostridium tetani is an ubiquitous organism that is present in animal excrement and fertilized soil. Common medical practice is based upon the belief that tetanus infections are the result of entry of the organism through puncture wounds in the human body. Indeed, tetanus prophylaxis following childhood immunization generally consists of toxoid boosters in association with fresh wounds. However, half the reported cases of tetanus in the last 10 years were not associated with a history of injury or accident. The emergency physician should never exclude the diagnosis of tetanus because of the lack of antecedent trauma.

The symptoms of tetanus are due to the toxin elaborated by the organism. Tetanus is unusual in that it has both a local and systemic effect. It may cause local tetany where it diffuses through the perineural tissues at the site of inoculation. More commonly, however, the patient will have generalized tetanus 5 to 10 days after inoculation. The most common presenting symptom is trismus, but it is usually rapidly followed by neck stiffness, rigidity of the back muscles to the point of opisthotonos, and a characteristic tight rigid facial expression that is referred to as risus sardonicus.

Temperature elevations between 38.3°C (101°F) and 39.4°C (103°F) are the rule, but an occasional case of afebrile tetanus has been reported. There are no specific blood, urine, or cerebral fluid abnormalities that will confirm the diagnosis. The combination of rapidly progressive trismus, persistent truncal and extremity tetany, risus sardonicus, and intermittent convulsions give little problem in formulating a differential diagnosis. Strychnine can produce tetany and convulsions, but pronounced muscle relaxation between convulsions is characteristic of strychnine poisoning.

Metallic Poisons

Poisoning by metallic compounds usually results in prominent central nervous system as well as peripheral nervous system findings. It is impossible to mention all the various types of metallic poisoning syndromes but arsenic and lead poisoning are worth reviewing. Arsenic is still found in insecticides, rat poisons, and herbicides, and in certain medicinal compounds. Acute gastrointestinal irritation with vomiting and diarrhea are usually presenting signs following ingestions of large amounts of arsenic. In patients receiving lower doses, however, polyneuritis may be one of the presenting complaints. In such cases, a history of occupational exposure is absolutely necessary.

Lead poisoning usually results from accidental and industrial, toxic exposure. Lead may be absorbed through the skin or the lungs, or ingested through the gastrointestinal tract. In severe acute lead poisoning the principal symptoms are acute weakness, prostration, and abdominal pain. In those patients who have received chronic smaller doses of lead, a peripheral motor neuropathy is common. These patients will have sensory findings but may have pronounced distal weakness.

Organic Compounds

Neuromuscular toxic effects can result from a wide variety of organic compounds. The alcohols, phenothiazines, and aminoglycoside antibiotics are discussed here.

Ethanol, methanol, and other alcohols may produce long-standing, slowly progressive peripheral neuropathies, predominantly sensory. Myopathies can be present as well. Acute intoxication with these agents usually causes pronounced central nervous system effects.

The phenothiazines may produce local dystonias even though the mechanism is central. Buccolingual dyskinesias caused by phenothiazine derivatives should be well known to emergency physicians. Often these are not seen in persons taking chronic psychiatric medication, but in those receiving small amounts of phenothiazines for symptoms such as nausea and vomiting, or in those who abuse street drugs.

Neuromuscular blockade can be enhanced by aminoglycoside antibiotics. This is usually encountered in hospitalized patients, especially postoperatively.

Tick Paralysis

Tick paralysis is a reversible, rapidly progressive motor weakness in which the site of action of the toxin is not completely known. Neuromuscular end-plate conduction is affected without morphologic changes. Two varieties of ticks, the wood tick, *Dermacentor andersoni,* and the dog tick, *D. variabilis,* have been responsible for the reported cases in the United States and Canada.

The tick must be present on a person for at least 5 days before symptoms develop. The symptoms of tick paralysis are almost identical to those of Guillain-Barré syndrome. Flaccid paralysis begins at the extremities and trunk, and moves up to involve the bulbar musculature. The patient is generally afebrile and there is usually no loss of consciousness. There are no specific blood, urine, or cerebrospinal fluid changes to aid in the diagnosis. The diagnosis of tick paralysis is made by finding the tick after a thorough examination of the body, including the hairy areas. Formerly, acute poliomyelitis would also be considered in the differential diagnosis of tick paralysis and Guillain-Barré syndrome. However, polio can usually be differentiated from the other two types of paralysis by their lack of fever or neck stiffness, or of cellular and protein changes in the cerebrospinal fluid.

Metabolic Neuropathy

The majority of nutritional and metabolic neuropathies have a slow onset, are progressive, and are clearly beyond the scope of the emergency physician. There are, however, several variants that may occur in a rapid fashion and are thus worth considering in a differential diagnosis: hyperinsulinism, gout, and acute intermittent porphyria. In contrast to diabetic neuropathy, which is symmetric and slow in onset, hyperinsulinism associated with pancreatic tumors may produce acute paresthesias, impaired sensation, muscle weakness, and hyporeflexia. It is usually seen in conjunction with symptomatic hypoglycemia.

During gouty attacks there may be a sudden onset of generalized extremity neuropathy or neuropathies, particularly of the lumbar plexus. The neuropathies seem to disappear when symptoms of gout are controlled.

Acute intermittent porphyria is characterized by psychosis, abdominal pains, and polyneuropathy of the Guillain-Barré type.

Neuropathy of Guillain-Barré

Today, the neuropathy of the Landry-Guillain-Barré disease is thought to be not a disease but a symptom complex that may follow many infectious diseases, exposure to toxins, and collagen vascular diseases. This syndrome usually follows an acute febrile episode or an acute metabolic problem by days or weeks and may be rapidly progressive. Persons in the third to fourth decades are most frequently affected, but it may occur in young children and in older adults.

The usual pattern of presentation is that of an ascending transverse myelitis. The lower extremities are usually involved first, and are more severely affected than the upper extremities. The bulbar musculature, however, may be involved partially or totally. Although paralysis usually reaches the maximum within a week, in some patients maximum paralysis is reached within hours. This is considered to be a motor neuron disease, but sensory symptoms are not uncommon and radicular pain is often noted. Although paralysis is rapid in onset, recovery may take a month to years but it is usually complete.

In the emergency department differential diagnosis is difficult. Frequently the patient gives a vague history of weakness in the lower extremities without any other antecedent history. Since this is a motor neuron disease, reflex arcs are often affected early. A patient who has weakness and loss of lower extremity reflexes should be considered to have Guillain-Barré disease until proved otherwise. Acute exacerbations of lead poisoning, porphyria, botulism, and diphtheria may all enter into the differential diagnosis and must be separated out by history and other pertinent clinical findings.

ACUTE MYOPATHIES

Like neuropathies, most myopathies, particularly in young people, progress slowly. The rapidly progressive acquired myopathies are relatively few in number and a reasonable differential diagnosis can be made in the emergency department.

The first task is to differentiate neuropathies from myopathies. Neuropathies tend to give distal symptoms, first with pronounced distal weakness progressing proximally. With myopathies, large muscle and central muscle groups are frequently affected at the same time as distal muscle groups, so diffuse or predominantly proximal weakness is a striking finding. A second important clue in differentiating neuropathies and myopathies is that myopathies rarely include sensory symptoms. There may be aching in the involved musculature, but the paresthesias and decreased sensation are not noted. A third differentiating feature is the fact that in myopathies, despite rather pronounced weakness, the patient will maintain deep tendon reflexes until the disease process is extremely advanced.

Laboratory testing is usually more fruitful for the emergency physician in myopathies as opposed to neuropathies. An elevated leukocyte count, sedimentation rate, and elevated muscle enzymes along with normal spinal fluid parameters characterize myopathies.

Polymyositis Syndrome

It is of little value for the emergency physician to subclassify acute polymyositis into its multiple causes. Polymyositis is more a syndrome than a specific disease. This form of myopathy, however, usually evolves rapidly, and, within weeks of onset, the patient has pronounced symptoms. In severe cases, however, severe weakness may develop over several days. Most patients have muscular pain and tenderness. A significant number also have dysphasia. Accompanying signs and symptoms, such as arthralgia, fever, and Raynaud's phenomenon all lend credence to the diagnosis of polymyositis. After the polymyositis syndrome is suspected, investigation is necessary to isolate the various treatable causes. Such a complex workup is beyond the scope of emergency diagnosis.

Many infections, including trichinosis and toxoplasmosis, and many viral entities have been associated with polymoysitis. All the collagen vascular diseases except periarteritis nodosa have also been implicated. Endocrinopathies, including both hyperthyroidism and hypothyroidism as well as adrenal cortical and parathyroid lesions, are part of the differential diagnosis. Steroids, which are used in treating many forms of polymyositis, can actually exacerbate the problem. Several of the drugs used to treat malaria and other protozoan infection have been associated with polymyositis. This can be confusing, as malaria itself can cause polymyositis. In approximately 10 percent of adults, polymyositis is a remote manifestation of carcinoma. There is no specific emergency department therapy for polymyositis, and use of steroids should await correct diagnosis.

Alcoholic Myopathy

Along with the well-known alcoholic peripheral neuropathy and the propensity to develop other skeletal disorders, alcoholics are prone to at least one type of unique myopathic syndrome. During prolonged periods of heavy alcohol intake, an alcoholic may have severe muscle tenderness and swelling, muscle cramps, and severe weakness. Signs and symptoms may be generalized or focal. This syndrome represents the acute diffuse necrosis of skeletal muscle fibers all in one stage of degeneration, or acute rhabdomyolysis. Muscle degeneration can lead to life-threatening hyperkalemia or hypocalcemia and secondary binding without released intracellular PO_4, and myoglobinuria can cause renal failure. In the alcoholic with acute muscle pain and weakness, serum electrolyte levels, muscle enzymes, and urinalysis for myoglobin are necessary. Although most patients recover within weeks, return to normal motor functions may take many months.

Myasthenia Gravis

Myasthenia gravis is not a true myopathy, but the presenting symptoms and examination features closely resemble those of the other myopathic diseases. It is discussed in detail in the following chapter.

Acute Periodic Paralysis

The most bizarre of the acute weakness syndromes are those that comprise the acute periodic paralyses. There are three basic types of primary forms: hyperkalemic, hypokalemic, and normokalemic. The exact mechanisms of these types have not been fully delineated, but by electron microscopy an abnormal number of mitochondria and abnormalities in the sacroplasmic reticulum have been noted.

There is no group of patients more likely to be turned out of the emergency department with a diagnosis of hysteria than patients with periodic paralysis. This disease is rarely suspected before the ninth or tenth attack. Periodic paralysis occurs predominantly in males (by 4 or 5 to 1 ratio), and generally the onset is between the seventh and twenty-first years of life.

Interestingly enough, the patient may often be awakened from sleep by the weakness. A history of extreme physical exertion on that day is important in establishing the diagnosis. Cold weather, large meals, trauma, and surgery may provoke an attack. Some patients will have the attacks on a regular basis, almost daily; others will have only a limited number throughout their lifetime. But the usual story is one of sudden extreme weakness without associated pain. These patients will give a history of being normal prior to and after the episodes, which usually last 1 or 2 h, and may be so severe that these patients will fall while walking or gag while eating.

An in-depth discussion of the various forms of periodic paralysis and paramyotonia congenita is beyond the scope of this basic review, but an understanding of these attacks should alert the emergency physician to consider the diagnosis, obtain a serum potassium level, and provide neurologic referral.

NONMYASTHENIC SYNDROMES OF MALIGNANCY

As the average age of the population increases, there will by sheer weight of numbers be more interaction between emergency physicians and patients suffering from or being treated for various forms of cancer. Many acute side effects of cancer or its treatment are due to local disease extension or metastasis. The following entities, however, are unrelated to the tumor mass itself but represent the remote effects of the tumor or its treatment: Eaton-Lambert syndrome, effects of drugs and radiation, cerebellar degeneration, polymyositis, and acute dementia.

Eaton-Lambert syndrome. For a number of years it has been recognized that there is abnormal neuromuscular transmission associated with certain malignancies, particularly oat-cell carcinoma of the lung. This syndrome, when first described by Eaton and Lambert, was thought to be a mild variant form of myasthenia gravis. However, as the syndrome became more fully delineated, it was clear that the differences between the two were multiple. In the Eaton-Lambert syndrome the patient will occasionally have aching muscle pain and will rarely be as weak as the patient with myasthenia gravis. There is less fluctuation of weakness and strength than found in myasthenia gravis. The cranial nerves are almost always spared in the Eaton-Lambert syndrome.

A rather remarkable finding is the fact that unlike myasthenia gravis, which gets worse with repetitive activity, with the Eaton-Lambert syndrome grip strength actually improves with repeated activity. There is no response to edrophonium.

Drugs and radiation therapy. For cancer patients currently under treatment, medications and dosage schedules must be carefully reviewed to determine the cause of weakness. Many chemotherapeutic agents are metabolic poisons and it can be on this basis that the patient is weak. *Steroids may produce a polymyositis syndrome.* Many tumors are treated with radiation. If the spinal column is involved, transverse myelitis may develop very suddenly from months to even years later. This is a true medical emergency. The differential diagnosis is radiation myelitis, or a compressive lesion due to metastasis. Emergency neurosurgical consultation and myelography are often necessary.

Another and yet unexplained remote effect of cancer is acute weakness and cerebral degeneration. Patients have a rapid history of deterioration with inability to walk and control the upper extremities, and there is evidence of pancerebellar involvement.

Polymyositis. Polymyositis may be a remote effect of carcinoma. Occult malignancy will be discovered in about 10 percent of adults with polymyositis.

RANDOM, ASYMMETRIC MULTIPLE LESIONS

Mononeuritis Multiplex

Acute temporal arteritis is probably the prototype for this disorder. The principal lesion is infarction of peripheral nerves due to arteritis in the vasa vasorum of the peripheral nerves. It occurs in diabetic patients and those with collagen vascular disease. The patient may complain of a specific peripheral nerve lesion in the right arm, another one in the left leg, and still another in the region of the cervical plexus. On specific testing, perfectly anatomic localizations can be delineated and usually the underlying disease has already been diagnosed. Treatment with steroids may be indicated.

Multiple Sclerosis

Multiple sclerosis is, of course, not a peripheral neurologic problem. However, its presentations are often related to peripheral symptomatology.

Multiple sclerosis is a patchy degenerative disease involving the myelin material of the central nervous system. This disease usually presents between 20 and 40 years of age and it may have a markedly waxing and waning course throughout the patient's life. Frequently patients with multiple sclerosis will relate that during hard work or strenuous physical activity they noted mild diplopia or weakness in an extremity. On examination, there is often no specific abnormality and the patient may be dismissed as having hysterical symptoms. It is well recognized that as a patient engages himself in physical exertion and raises the body temperature, temporal differences in nerve conduction develop and result in symptomatology. Many patients will have episodes only during periods of exertion for several years. The diagnosis is more obvious when signs and symptoms of decreased vision along with numbness, weakness, or incoordination develop. Between 50 and 75 percent of patients with acute retrobulbar neuritis will develop multiple sclerosis. The diagnosis of multiple sclerosis depends on the appearance of multiple lesions through space and time. It is therefore important that the patient with widely diffuse symptoms be referred for follow-up whether or not positive findings are present on initial examination. For those patients whose symptoms are not transitory, or those with functional difficulties, admission and inpatient therapy may be required.

SPECIFIC ISOLATED PERIPHERAL NERVE LESIONS

Infections

Herpes zoster represents the most important infection that clinically presents as an isolated peripheral nerve lesion. Herpes as a whole tends to present as an independent condition, but it may be associated with surgical procedures, diabetes, and occasionally trauma. Extreme pain, which is generally in a dermatomal distribution, usually precedes the skin lesions by several days. The dermatomes most often affected are the thoracic, followed by the trigeminal nerve, lumbar plexus, and finally the cervical plexus. Although herpes produces principally sensory involvement, motor dysfunction may be seen in up to 25 percent of patients. Although the sensory disturbances and skin lesions usually abate with time, the motor disturbances seen with herpes do not usually completely resolve.

Allergic Neuropathy

An unusual phenomenon that is seen approximately nine times more in males than in females is an allergic neuropathy following the injection of immunologic materials, usually tetanus toxoid. The neurologic complications usually develop about 2 days after signs of generalized serum sickness. Although central nervous system signs are reported, the most common neurologic complication is a motor peripheral neuropathy involving the brachial plexus. It may or may not be bilateral. A single nerve such as the radial or optic nerve may be involved.

Vascular Peripheral Nerve Lesions

Volkmann's Paralysis

Volkmann's ischemic paralysis is the prototype for vascular peripheral nerve lesions. The paralysis is primarily due to injury to the nutrient vessels of a peripheral nerve, but it can be iatrogenically induced by a tight-fitting cast. During the first few hours, severe pain is the principal symptom. As the disease process progresses, nerves and muscles undergo extensive fibrosis with resultant contractures and impairment of both motor and sensory functions.

Tic Douloureux

Tic douloureux, or trigeminal neuralgia, should be mentioned here. There is probably no one explanation for the source of pain in trigeminal neuralgia. It is believed by many that pulsations from a branch of the basilar artery serve as irritants and decrease the trigeminal nerve's threshold for pain. The symptom is severe lancinating pain usually confined to the area of distribution of the third portion of the trigeminal nerve. Often multiple portions of the trigeminal nerve will be involved, but bilaterality is unusual. Such pain usually presents little problem in differential diagnosis, but treatment may be difficult. During acute attacks opiates are helpful. It is inappropriate for the emergency physician to initiate chronic therapy without consulting the physician who will follow the patient.

Ninth nerve neuralgia, or glossopharyngeal tic, is less common. Although rare, this disorder is characterized by intense pain localized to the area of the ear and throat on the affected side. Pain may radiate to the posterior third of the tongue, tonsillar pillars, and the oropharynx and larynx. The most common irritants that initiate this unusual pain are swallowing, talking, or chewing. Unlike tic douloureux, the pain of glossopharyngeal neuralgia may last for longer periods of time and usually tends to come in waves or clusters at a particular time of the year. There is no single theory as to the cause of glossopharyngeal neuralgia, but a vascular etiology is hypothesized.

Cranial Nerve Neuropathy

The cranial nerve neuropathies represent a separate subcategory of specific isolated nerve lesions. The general maxim from neurology and ear, nose, and throat surgery is that any cranial nerve neuropathy may represent a tumor until proved otherwise. In all practicality, however, most cranial nerve neuropathies seen by the emergency physician are more likely to be vascular or idiopathic lesions of sudden onset. It is beyond the scope of this discussion to detail each cranial neuropathy, but because the seventh nerve is frequently involved in both traumatic and infectious conditions and is the most commonly involved with idiopathic dysfunction, it will be discussed here.

The seventh cranial nerve, or facial nerve, has two principal divisions as it leaves the brain stem. These are a motor root and the nervus intermedius, which functions to supply taste to the anterior two-thirds of the tongue and automatic fibers to the salivary and lacrimal glands. Above the brainstem, the seventh nerve has both crossed and uncrossed fibers, while below the seventh nerve nucleus fibers are uncrossed. If a patient retains muscular strength in the forehead and upper face but not the lower face, the lesion is probably central, i.e., in the brainstem or above. If the patient has weakness of the forehead, around the eyes, and lower face, this probably represents a lower neuron involvement of type usually seen with Bell's palsy.

Bell's Palsy

Bell's palsy is not a specific disease but represents a constellation of symptoms of multiple etiologies. The exact location of the disorder along the seventh nerve or in the brainstem can often be ascertained by careful physical examination. It is important to localize the level of involvement to determine if a structural lesion or idiopathic Bell's palsy is present. Lesions in the tegmentum of the brainstem involve the nucleus of the seventh nerve and almost invariably have an accompanying sixth nerve palsy. Lesions of the seventh nerve at the point of emergence from the brainstem frequently have associated auditory components due to involvement of the eighth nerve as well. If the lesion is peripheral to the lateral geniculate ganglion, lacrimal fibers are spared and there is usually an excess collection of tears in the conjunctival sac on that side. Beyond the point where the chorda tympani nerve arises, autonomic functions are no longer involved, and a lesion beyond the stylomastoid foramen results only in motor weakness and is characteristic of Bell's palsy.

Once the diagnosis of idiopathic Bell's palsy has been established, the next problem is treatment. There is a considerable growing body of evidence that high-dose steroid therapy in short bursts may be of benefit in treatment of Bell's palsy. If steroids are given, they should be prescribed in consultation with an otolaryngologist or neurologist who can also initiate electrostimulatory therapy for the patient's muscles while waiting for recovery of the seventh nerve. There is a small but firm group who advocate unroofing the canal of the seventh nerve if recovery has not oc-

curred after approximately 6 weeks. However, 98 percent of patients with Bell's palsy recover at least partial function, and operative intervention should be saved for those patients with prolonged or severe difficulty.

TRAUMA AND NERVE COMPRESSION SYNDROMES

Spinal Cord Compression

Lesions along the cord may produce distinct isolated neurologic syndromes. One of the emergent problems is compression of the spinal cord. This may occur as a result of trauma, herniation of intervertebral disks, primary or metastic tumors, AV malformations, radiation myelitis, or cysts. It is important to remember that acute spinal cord compression is often associated with areflexia. Cremasteric reflexes, anal sphincter tone, and motor activity in the extremities all help to localize the lesion. Emergency neurosurgical consultation and myelography are indicated.

Root and Trunk Syndromes

The peripheral nerve is the endpoint in a long process of combinations and divisions of nervous tissues. After exiting the cord in the cervical upper thoracic and lumbar regions, nerve roots at each particular level combine with other nerves to form plexuses. Plexuses then form major and minor trunks which divide to form specific peripheral nerves. Therefore, depending on the lesion along the nerve, different symptoms can result. The patient with a C-6 root lesion will have a different distribution in the hand than a patient with a medial nerve injury. When evaluating isolated complaints, do not overlook the possible multiple levels at which a nerve might be involved.

Specific Peripheral Nerve Neuropathies

There is not adequate room to list all the various nerve root compression syndromes that the emergency physician might encounter. Two texts are absolutely essential: *Aids to the Investigation of Peripheral Nerve Injuries,* which was first published in 1942 as an aid to British trauma surgeons and has stood the test of time as an excellent reference for acute neuromuscular problems; the other, *Peripheral Entrapment Neuropathies,* by H. P. Kopel and W. A. Thompson, carefully reviews not only the physical findings in entrapment disorders but lists possible locations on the nerve where they are involved.

Common Nerve Entrapments

The most common causes of acute mononeuropathies are usually traumatic, following fractures, dislocations, or acute soft tissue swelling. A mononeuropathy can be a result of repetitive motor activity that causes increased connective tissue in small spaces. It should be remembered that with high-velocity missile injuries, direct contact with a nerve is not necessary to produce palsy. Besides trauma, causes of entrapment neuropathies include any inflammation or degeneration in and around tight canals where nerves must pass. This is frequently seen in patients with rheumatoid arthritis, myxedema, thyroid disease, amyloidosis, and pregnancy.

BIBLIOGRAPHY

Aids to the Investigation of Peripheral Nerve Injuries. London, HM Stationery Office, 1942.

Drachman DB: Myasthenia gravis. *N Engl J Med* 298:136–142, 186–193, 1978.

Engel WK, Festoff BW, Patten DM, et al: Myasthenia gravis. *Ann Intern Med* 81:225–246, 1974.

Hoffman E: Carpal tunnel syndrome: Importance of sensory nerve conduction studies in diagnosis. *JAMA* 233:983–984, 1975.

Kopel HP, Thompson WA: *Peripheral Entrapment Neuropathies*. Baltimore, William & Wilkins, 1963.

Mazui MH, Dolin R: Herpes zoster at the NH: A 20 year experience. *Am J Med* 65:738–744, 1978.

Soffer D, Feldman S, Alter M: Epidemiology of Guillian-Barré syndrome. *Neurology* 28:686–690, 1978.

CHAPTER 136
MYASTHENIA GRAVIS

Carl Sacks

Myasthenia gravis is a condition, probably of multiple etiologies, that is characterized by episodic weakness or paralysis of voluntary musculature with preservation of deep tendon reflexes and pupillary responses, and by partial or complete recovery after rest or anticholinesterase drugs. The condition is usually associated with circulating antiacetylcholine receptor antibodies that affect postsynaptic acetylcholine receptor sites.

The incidence of myasthenia gravis is from 2 to 10 per 10,000 population. There does not seem to be a geographic or climatic distribution. Females are affected two to three times more frequently than males, but the peak incidence for females is in the third decade. After the age of 40, males are afflicted as frequently as females. The peak incidence for males is in the sixth and seventh decades.

The mortality rate is approximately 20 percent, with the majority of deaths due to failure of the respiratory muscles or to aspiration.

Spontaneous remissions and exacerbations occur in 25 to 50 percent of all patients, and are far more frequent in the first 2 years of the disease. Exacerbation is frequently secondary to fatigue, illness, and alcohol or high carbohydrate ingestion.

PATHOPHYSIOLOGY

Although there are few if any pathological findings that are absolutely pathognomonic of myasthenia gravis, there is a highly suggestive constellation. There is a reduction in the postsynaptic folds and an increase in the width of the synaptic clefts of the motor end plates of the chronically afflicted muscles. The number of postsynaptic acetylcholine receptors is greatly reduced. Antinuclear antibodies, antistriated muscle antibodies, and acetylcholine receptor antibodies have been demonstrated. A condition analogous to myasthenia has been experimentally created by immunizing an animal against its own motor end-plate acetylcholine receptors. The temptation to conclude that the condition is a postsynaptic autoimmune phenomenon must be temporized by evidence showing that acetylcholine antibodies have not been demonstrated in all cases, and that they have been demonstrated in humans without clinical symptoms of myasthenia.

Light microscopy of afflicted muscle often shows sizable fiber atrophy, degeneration, and necrosis. There are characteristically round cell infiltrations surrounding the affected fibers and the venules. The changes are not pathognomonic for myasthenia and can also be seen in polymyositis.

About 10 percent of patients have a tumor of the thymus, and 50 percent of all thymomas are associated with myasthenia gravis. Another 70 to 75 percent of patients may have lymphoid hyperplasia of the germinal centers. Again, both conditions exist without myasthenia.

Approximately 5 percent of patients with myasthenia develop hyperthyroidism at some time, and symptoms may not occur simultaneously or they may complicate each other. The exact causal relationship, if any, is not known, and each entity should be treated individually.

Also, a more random association has been suggested between myasthenia and diseases of established autoimmune origin such as systemic lupus erythematosus and rheumatoid arthritis.

Any substance that affects the myoneural junction can exacerbate myasthenia gravis (Table 136-1). The patient with myasthenia is exquisitely sensitive to succinylcholine chloride and decamethonium bromide, which also bind to the end-plate receptor and cause prolonged depolarization. This extreme sensitivity to subminimal doses is also exhibited by curare (d-tubocurarine), which binds preferentially to the end-plate receptors, denying access to acetylcholine molecules and causing a nondepolarizing block. Aminoglycoside and polymyxin antibiotics have curare-like properties and may cause paralysis in patients with myasthenia.

CLINICAL FEATURES

Neonatal Myasthenia

There is some evidence for a true congenital form of myasthenia. A transient neonatal myasthenia of 2 or 3 weeks duration, caused by transplacental transfer antiacetylcholine receptor antibodies, may affect up to 30 percent of infants born to mothers with myas-

Table 136.1 Some Agents that Exacerbate Myasthenia

Muscle paralyzers:	Antibiotics:
Succinylcholine	Aminoglycosides
Decamethonium	Polymyxins
d-Tubocurarine	Oxytetracycline
Antipsychotics:	Alkalizing agents:
Lithium	Thiotepa
Antiarrhythmics:	Anticonvulsants:
Quinidine (quinines)	Trimethadione
Procainamide	Phenytoin

thenia gravis. Neonatal myasthenia is characterized by a general paucity of movements and facial expression. The eyes do not move, the lids sag, the mouth remains open, and sucking is weak or absent.

Adult Myasthenia

Myasthenia gravis may affect the extraocular muscles, the bulbar muscles, and the entire cranial trunk and limb muscles either singly, in a group, or in any possible combination. The onset may be symmetric or asymmetric.

Weakness or paralysis of the extraocular muscles, manifested by ptosis, diplopia, and asymmetric following movements of the eyes, is the initiating symptom in the 40 to 70 percent of cases of myasthenia, and will eventually develop in 90 percent of all cases. A provocative test is to see if diplopia or ptosis develops after prolonged upward gaze.

The bulbar musculature is affected to some degree in 40 to 70 percent of all patients. Weakness of the facial muscles creates a toneless, ironed-out, expressionless look. The eyes cannot completely close, the lips retract, and masseter weakness causes the jaw to hang open. Weakness of the tongue and laryngeal muscles causes dysarthria, dysphagia, and not infrequently aspiration. Weakness of the pharynx causes a nasal voice and regurgitation of food. Masseter strength may be tested by seeing how long it takes or how easy it is to pull a tongue blade from between clenched jaws. The amount of time that a person can count aloud before dysarthria or dysphonia appear is another widely used provocative test.

Although up to 50 percent of all myasthenia victims may have weakness of the limb and trunk musculature, only 15 percent or less have had previous weakness of cranial nerve enervated muscles. There is a tendency for proximal musculature to be affected before distal musculature. The onset may be symmetrical or asymmetrical. Occasionally, only isolated muscle groups are involved. In advanced cases all muscle groups may be involved and there may be signs of muscle atrophy. The deep tendon reflexes are preserved.

The weakness-fatigue pattern is a variable expression of the development and evolution of the process. The patient may be unable to climb up a flight of stairs, or may stumble while descending them. He or she may no longer be able to eat a full meal or comb the hair without becoming weak in the shoulder girdle. A few other provocative tests are to observe the number of situps or pushups the patient can do or, on a more moderate scale, how many times the patient can raise the hands above the head, cross and uncross the legs, or rise up and down on the toes before weakness sets in.

A widely accepted clinical classification of myasthenia gravis, based on severity, prognosis, and response to medication is as follows:

Group 1: Localized nonprogressive form of myasthenia with perhaps only ptosis or diplopia. An anticholinesterase drug corrects the defect in the majority of patients. Drug resistance is rare. The prognosis is excellent.

Group 2: Generalized myasthenia involving more than one group of striated muscles, of both cranial and skeletal origin. The onset is gradual. This moderate form may remain static for long periods of time. Early or late spontaneous remission may occur.

This group is usually amenable to drug therapy. The prognosis is fairly good.

Group 3: Acute fulminating onset of generalized myasthenia with severe bulbar manifestations. Usually there is early involvement of the respiratory system. In a short time from onset the patient may develop myasthenic crisis. The response to drug therapy is poor, as is the prognosis.

Group 4: Late severe myasthenia that usually develops at least 2 years after the onset of group 1 or group 2 symptoms. The prognosis is poor.

Group 5: Muscle atrophy. Most of these patients start as group 2, but 6 or more months later begin to show muscular atrophy unrelated to the disease. This group is descriptive and the prognosis is dependent on other features, as stated above.

Diagnosis Confirmation

While a history of episodic weakness exacerbated by exercise, fatigue, sleeplessness, and alcohol, and temporarily ameliorated by rest, is highly suggestive of myasthenia gravis, electrophysiological and chemical tests can confirm the diagnosis.

In normal muscle, when an electromyogram is used to record the action of a muscle receiving a supramaximal electrical stimulation at a frequency of 3 cycles per second, the amplitude of the evoked action potential remains maximal over multiple stimuli and then slowly declines. When a myasthenic muscle is so treated, there is an immediate stepladder decline in the action potential in almost all cases.

Any substance that increases the concentration of acetylcholine at the synaptic cleft, such as an acetylcholinesterase inhibitor, may partially reverse the symptoms of myasthenia. The subject undergoes intravenous catheterization and then is asked to exercise the suspect muscle groups, i.e., look up until ptosis develops or count until there is dysarthria. Then 2 mg of edrophonium (Tensilon), a fast-acting acetylcholinesterase inhibitor, is administered intravenously. Objective improvement of symptoms should start 20 to 30 s after injection and last 4 or 5 min. If there is no improvement within 30 s, an additional 8 mg, in two 4-mg increments, should be administered. If there is again no response, the test is considered negative. The test should be done with caution in patients with asthma or cardiac disease, and 0.5 mg of atropine should be available for immediate intravenous administration if profound bradycardia, hypotension, salivation, or fasciculation appear.

An intramuscular injection of 1.5 mg of neostigmine combined with 0.5 mg of atropine to reverse muscarinic symptoms has equivalent but longer-lasting results. The first effects are noticeable in about 10 min; the maximal response is in 30 min, and the duration is about 4 h.

Provocative tests, such as the exacerbation or worsening of symptoms by supraminimal doses of curare or guanidine hydrochloride, are exceedingly dangerous, and should not be used under any circumstances.

In addition to the tests specifically diagnostic for myasthenia gravis, roentgenograms, laminograms, tomograms, and CT scans of the thymus may reveal the associated thymoma.

There should also be a search for associated thyroid and autoimmune diseases. If clinically indicated, blood gases and spirometry can be used to evaluate respiratory function. Any febrile episode that may exacerbate myasthenia should be fully investigated.

TREATMENT

Myasthenia is treated by drugs, surgery, or both. The drugs used are cholinergics, and steroids or immunosuppressants. The surgery is thymectomy.

The effects of cholinergics are purely symptomatic. The established cholinergics are all reversible acetylcholinesterase inhibitors and rarely is one more clinically efficacious than the other. They are not used in combination, and the one that is selected is usually that which has the fewer gastrointestinal and muscarinic side effects.

The dosage of the cholinergics is determined by a combination of both clinical observation and the briskness of response to the Tensilon test. Persistent weakness may be due to inadequate medication, depolarizing block secondary to overmedication, or a refractory state to medication.

Once the diagnosis is suspected or determined, neurological consultation is necessary to institute appropriate medication. Medication is usually started at a moderate dose tid, and rapidly increased by decreasing the time between doses and then by incrementing each individual dose. Unwanted muscarinic effects may be controlled by the judicious use of 0.4 mg of atropine orally.

Oral cholinergics used are neostigmine bromide and pyridostigmine bromide. The maximum effect is seen in approximately 2 h, and the duration of action can vary from 2 to 6 h.

Neostigmine comes in 15 mg tablets. The low to average adult starting dose is 2 tablets PO tid with meals and may range up to 16 or more tablets a day with an interval of 3 h between doses.

Pyridostigmine comes in 60-mg regular tablets. It is usually less muscarinic than neostigmine. The dosage may range from one tablet tid to three tablets every 3 h. A 180-mg sustained-release tablet also exists, but it may have variable absorption and is best reserved for nocturnal dosage.

Adjuncts such as ephedrine, guanidine, and potassium chloride have been used empirically to supplement the cholinergics with variable results. Steroids are quite effective, but their marked side effects dictate their use only after failure of cholinergics and thymectomy.

Other immunosuppressives such as 6-mercaptopurine, azathioprine, glycophosphamide, and antilymphocyte antibody have been used in experimental centers and have occasionally been associated with remission when all else failed. Plasma exchange therapy has also been attempted.

While there are no universally accepted criteria, most authorities believe that an established diagnosis of thymoma is an almost absolute indication for thymectomy and radiation. Many believe thymectomy is indicated in significantly debilitating myasthenia that is unresponsive to medical therapy for a period of 6 months, especially if the patient is not a candidate for steroids.

Myasthenic and Cholinergic Crisis

Myasthenic crisis and cholinergic crisis, although of different causality, have many clinical similarities. The paralysis of myasthenic crisis is due to sudden exacerbation of the basic process that has become refractory to medication. The paralysis of cholinergic crisis is due to depolarizing block secondary to cholinergic overdosage. Not uncommonly, a patient in myasthenia crisis is believed to be weak because he or she is under-medicated, and is

given an inordinate dose of a cholinergic, thus combining the two unfortunate states. In either case life-threatening paralysis is the cardinal problem and further administration of cholinergics is useless.

Weakness of the respiratory musculature leads to hypoventilation and anoxia. If there is a cholinergic excess, bronchospasm will further compromise ventilation. If the clinical picture, spirometry, or blood gases indicate a dubious state of oxygenation, immediate endotracheal intubation and respiration assistance are necessary.

Serious weakness of the bulbar musculature will compromise swallowing. The patient can no longer meet minimal fluid and nutritional needs orally, and any attempt to do so will lead to aspiration. If there is a cholinergic override, the oral as well as the pulmonary secretions are greatly increased.

Fluid and mineral balance are maintained by an intravenous line that can also be used for drug administration. Feedings can be provided by a nasal feeding tube to supply nutrition needs. A cuffed endotracheal tube plus frequent oral and endotracheal suction will minimize aspiration.

Although myasthenia does not affect the detrusor muscle, profound weakness may make it impossible to use a bedpan or urinal. A condom or foley catheter may be required. Care must be taken to avoid decubitus ulcers.

If the diagnosis is cholinergic crisis, cholinergics are withheld for several days, and are not to be started again until the intravenous Tensilon test is positive. Initial treatment is 1 mg of neostigmine, which is repeated every 3 h and may be increased to 2 mg as dictated by the Tensilon test. As strength improves, the patient can be weaned off the respirator, extubated, and started on oral medication.

If the weakness is attended by marked ventilatory resistance and bronchospasm, and profound bradycardia and hypotension, one should suspect at least an element of cholinergic excess, especially if fasciculation, myosis, and hypersalivation are also seen. If there is a rapid and favorable response of the life-threatening manifestations to 1 mg of intravenous atropine, the suspicion is practically confirmed, and atropine should be continued as long as such symptoms recur. Under no circumstances should one use a strong acetylcholinesterase reactivator such as pralidoxime (2-PAM) chloride, for this may aggravate the myasthenia process.

DIFFERENTIAL DIAGNOSIS

There are some conditions that because they are characterized by transient recurrent weakness or by weakness associated with diplopia may be confused with myasthenia gravis.

Eaton-Lambert syndrome. Eaton-Lambert syndrome is characterized by fluctuating weakness, recovery with rest, and extreme sensitivity to *d*-tubocurarine. Cranial muscles are almost always spared or have minor transient involvement. Deep tendon reflexes are depressed and the muscles tend to ache. The rapid decline in action potential of the muscle when stimulated at 3 cycles per second is similar to that of myasthenia gravis. However, at higher-frequency stimulation, about 20 cycles per second, the pattern change in action potential in Eaton-Lambert syndrome is incremental rather than decremental, while that of myasthenia gravis is unchanged.

Myasthenia gravis may be a paraneoplastic syndrome, and most often is associated with oat-cell tumors of the lung. The basic defect is in the calcium-mediated release of acetylcholine. The response is excellent to guanidine and poor to neostigmine.

Botulism. Botulism is characterized by a progressive nonremitting weakness starting with the extraocular and bulbar musculature. It may be superficially similar to group 3 myasthenia and is usually even more fulminating. Unlike myasthenic or cholinergic crisis, there is loss of deep tendon reflexes in botulism. There may be autonomic cholinergic inhibition with fixed dilated pupils, dry mouth, dry eyes, and inability to urinate. The culprit is, of course, the toxin released by *Clostridium botulinum*, which blocks the release of acetylcholine. There is therapeutic response to guanidine. When confronted with a patient with diplopia, weakness, and respiratory compromise, intubation and respirator assistance should be initiated before contemplating a differential diagnosis and searching for improperly canned foods.

Tick paralysis. Tick paralysis is characterized by a progressive ascending flaccid paralysis with early diplopia, bulbar muscle weakness, and eventually respiratory paralysis. The pathogen is a potent neurotoxin elaborated by the engorged tick. Because of the transient half-life of the toxin, symptoms start to reverse soon after the tick is removed from the victim.

Familial periodic paralysis. Familial periodic paralysis is a dominant mendelian disorder characterized by recurrent episodes of flaccid, generally nonprogressing, paralysis with loss or reduction of deep tendon reflexes. Usually only the limb musculature is involved. Paralysis may last for minutes to days, and individual recurrences are usually a month or more apart. Acute hypokalemia coincides with the onset of symptoms, and a heavy ingestion of carbohydrates may be provocative. Treatment is with intravenous potassium.

Adynamia episodica hereditaria. Adynamia episodica hereditaria has clinical features and hereditary characteristics similar to familial periodic paralysis, but, contrary to the latter, the acute episode is characterized and may be provoked by an acute elevation in potassium. Ingestion of carbohydrates is curative, not provocative. These two entities may represent forms of extreme sensitivity to changes in membrane resting potential, secondary to shifting of potassium from the surroundings into the cell, and vice versa, causing a polarizing and depolarizing block.

Sleep Paralysis. Sleep paralysis, which occurs predominantly in males, is characterized by complete loss of strength of the limbs usually upon awakening but occasionally just before falling asleep. Breathing is not compromised. The paralysis usually lasts only for minutes, exceptionally up to an hour. The state can be reversed by touching the person. Speaking or shouting is ineffective. Sleep paralysis may exist as an isolated entity or be associated with narcolepsy, catalepsy, or hypnagogic hallucination.

BIBLIOGRAPHY

Aharnov A, Abramsky O, Tarrab-Hazdia R, et al: Humoral antibodies to acetylcholine receptor in patients with myasthenia gravis. *Lancet* 1:340–342, 1975.

Aita JF, Wanamaker WM: Body computerized tomography and the thymus. *Arch Neurol* 36:20–21, 1979.

Appel SH, Almon RR, Levy N: Acetylcholine receptor antibodies in myasthenia gravis. *N Engl J Med* 293:760–761, 1975.

Booker HE, Chum RWM, Sanguino M: Myasthenia gravis syndrome associated with trimethadione. *JAMA* 212:2262–2263, 1970.

Castleman B: The pathology of the thymus gland in the myasthenia gravis. *Ann NY Acad Sci* 135:496–503, 1966.

Clement JG: Neuromuscular blockade by nitrogen mustard, letter to the editor. *Anesthesiology* 47:317, 1977.

Conti-Tronconi BM, Morgutti M, Sghirlanzon A, et al: Cellular immune response to acetylcholine receptor in myasthenia gravis, I: Relevance to clinical course and pathogenesis. *Neurology* 29:496–501, 1979.

Cuenoud S, Feltkamp TEW, Fulpius BW, et al: Antibodies to acetylcholine receptor in patients with thymoma but without myasthenia gravis. *Neurology* 30:201–203, 1980.

Czlatowski A: Myasthenia syndrome during penicillamine treatment. *Br Med J* 2:726–727, 1975.

Drachman DB: Myasthenia gravis. *N Engl J Med* 298:136–142, 186–193, 1978.

Eaton LM, Lambert EH: Electromyography and electric stimulation of nerves in diseases of motor unit: Observations on myasthenic syndrome associated with malignant tumors. *JAMA* 163:1117–1124, 1957.

Engel AG, Santa T: Histometric analysis of the ultrastructure of the neuromuscular junction in myasthenia gravis and in the myasthenic syndrome. *Ann NY Acad Sci* 183:35–58, 1971.

Fambrough DM, Drachman DB, Satyamurti S: Neuromuscular junction in myasthenia gravis: Decreased acetylcholine receptors. *Science* 182:293–295, 1973.

Fenichel GM: Clinical syndromes of myasthenia in infancy and childhood. *Arch Neurol* 35:97–103, 1978.

Granacher RP: Neuromuscular problems associated with lithium, letter to the editor. *Am J Psychiatry* 134:702, 1977.

Howard FM Jr, Drake DD, Lambert EH, et al: Alternate-day prednisone: Preliminary report of a double-blind controlled study. *Ann NY Acad Sci* 274:596–607, 1976.

Jaretzki A III, Bethea M, Wolff M, et al: A rational approach to total thymectomy in the treatment of myasthenia gravis. *Ann Thorac Surg* 24:120–130, 1977.

Jenkins RB: Treatment of myasthenia gravis with prednisone. *Lancet* 1:765–767, 1972.

Lake KB, VanDyke JJ: Prolonged nasotracheal intubation. *Heart Lung* 9:93–97, 1980.

Lindstrom JM, Seybold ME, Lennon VA, et al: Antibody to acetylcholine receptor in myasthenia gravis: Prevalence, clinical correlates, and diagnostic value. *Neurology* 26:1054–1059, 1976.

McQuillen MP, Cantor HE, O'Rourke JR: Myasthenic syndrome associated with antibiotics. *Arch Neurol* 18:402–415, 1968.

Miller RD, Way WL, Katzung BG: The potentiation of neuromuscular blocking agents by quinidine. *Anesthesiology* 28:1036–1041, 1967.

Neil JF, Himmelhoch JM, Licata SM: Emergence of myasthenia gravis during treatment with lithium carbonate. *Arch Gen Psychiatry* 33:1090–1092, 1976.

Osserman KE: Myasthenia gravis. *Ann NY Acad Sci* 135:1–679, 1966.

Osserman KE, Tsairis P, Weiner LB: Myasthenia gravis and thyroid disease: Clinical and immunological correlation. *J Mount Sinai Hosp NY* 34:469–483, 1967.

Perlo VP, Arnason B, Poskanzer D, et al: The role of thymectomy in the treatment of myasthenia gravis. *Ann NY Acad Sci* 183:308–315, 1971.

Pinching AJ, Peters DK, Davis JN: Remission of myasthenia gravis following plasma-exchange. *Lancet* 2:1373–1376, 1976.

Pirofsky B, Reid RH, Bardana EJ Jr, et al: Myasthenia gravis treated with purified antithymocyte antiserum. *Neurology* 29:112–116, 1979.

Pittinger CB, Eryasa Y, Adamson R: Antibiotic-induced paralysis. *Anesth Analg* 49:487–501, 1970.

Robertson WC, Chun RW, Kornguth SE: Familial infantile myasthenia. *Arch Neurol* 37:117–119, 1980.

Vincent A, Newson-Davis, J, Martin V: Antiacetylcholine receptor antibodies in *d*-penicillamine-associated myasthenia gravis, letter to the editor. *Lancet* 1:1254, 1978.

Warmolts JR, Engel WK: Benefit from alternate day prednisone in myasthenia gravis. *N Engl J Med* 286:17–20, 1972.

Wolf SM, Barrows HS: Myasthenia gravis and systemic lupus erythematosus. *Arch Neurol* 14:254–258, 1966.

SECTION 18
PSYCHIATRIC
EMERGENCIES

CHAPTER 137

EMERGENCY

PSYCHIATRIC

EVALUATION

A. The Psychiatric Patient

Beverly Fauman

The emergency department should be designed and staffed with the behavioral emergency in mind. The emergency department staff must be able to stabilize and provide initial assessment for the patient who is unable to control his or her behavior, or who may be suicidal. This section will cover the initial approach to the patient who is thought to have an acute psychiatric problem, the technical aspects of restraining, evaluating, and stabilizing the psychiatric emergency, and some common psychiatric problems that present to the emergency physician.

A patient may be self-identified as a psychiatric patient, or may be so identified by family or friends, or by physicians, police officers, fire fighters, emergency medical technicians, or employers. A behavioral emergency may be the sole reason for the patient's appearance in the emergency department, or may compound and complicate the primary reason for the patient's visit. Because there is a relative separation in our health care delivery system between psychiatric care and general medical care, the emergency physician must differentiate the patient with a pure psychiatric problem from one with a mixed psychiatric-medical problem, or from one with a medical problem masked by a psychiatric illness. The emergency physician must be sensitive to the meaning of psychiatric symptoms because of the relative unavailability of psychiatric consultation and the dangers of transferring an unrecognized medical emergency to a psychiatric hospital, and because much of the practice of emergency medicine is affected by the emotional impact of life-threatening illness or serious trauma.

Obvious psychiatric emergencies include acute grief reactions, anxiety or panic, acute psychosis, or overt suicidal threats. Less easily recognized emergencies may include depression, ''accidental'' injury, and drug reactions. Other psychiatric problems that may come to the attention of the emergency physician are conversion reactions; psychophysiologic reactions; responses to crises such as job or school changes, pregnancy, medical illness, and/or major disaster; or reactions to personal abuse or violence. In addition, people may come to the emergency department for solutions to problems of housing, finances, violent or criminal behavior, abuse of drugs or alcohol, or inability to get along with others. In many of these instances, the patient may be considered to be a psychiatric patient.

Less frequently, a patient may be recognized as a psychiatric emergency by an astute emergency physician who notices more subtle clues of disturbance: any accident, such as an accidental drug overdose, auto accident, or an unexplained unusual injury, should be considered potentially as self-destructive behavior and pursued to be certain a suicidal patient isn't discharged. Finally, recurrent visits to an emergency department, or to multiple physicians or hospitals, even when it appears to be for a valid medical reason, should prompt the emergency physician to conduct a brief psychiatric interview. Asthma, sickle cell anemia, angina, and ulcer disease, for example, are exacerbated with psychological stress. At the very least, patients with recurrent, chronic, or slowly healing illnesses become discouraged, and an opportunity to talk to an empathic physician may renew their hopes and cooperativeness. However, patients should be discouraged from using the emergency department as a drop-in psychiatric clinic.

As in the general practice of emergency medicine, the primary determination to be made is the presence of a life threat. In psychiatric patients, this assessment is complicated by the fact that there are fewer clear data to evaluate than in a medical emergency. That is, ''vital signs'' are not obtained solely with a sphygmomanometer and a watch, but with a clinical appreciation for acuteness of the illness.

There are two truly urgent psychiatric problems that require a rapid response: the patient who is violent or potentially so, and the patient with a life-threatening medical illness which presents

The bibliography for all chapters in Section 18, ''Psychiatric Emergencies,'' may be found at the end of Chapter 139, page 949.

as a psychiatric disorder. In these cases one or more of the following behaviors are usually present:

1. The patient exhibits or threatens violence.
2. The patient, for less well defined reasons, makes the emergency department staff distinctly anxious.
3. The patient's behavior alternates rapidly or changes abruptly during evaluation, e.g., shouting alternating with dozing off, or cooperativeness alternating with belligerence.
4. The patient expresses a fear of losing control.
5. The patient is unable to cooperate with the evaluation, or appears confused and forgetful.
6. The patient has signs of injury, acute illness, or abnormal vital signs, and exhibits odd behavior as well.

Some of these behaviors are also seen in less acute patients, notably those patients who are intoxicated, have chronic psychiatric illness, or who suffer from a chronic organic brain disorder. Failure to appropriately evaluate the above behaviors may mean that some intoxicated patients or those with chronic organic disease who also have acute life-threatening illness will be misdiagnosed, or that medical patients who present with psychiatric symptoms will be mismanaged.

In order to assess the patient with disordered behavior, staff should be familiar with the indications and methods for applying restraints. The physical facilities should include an area for isolating psychiatric patients. Ideally, a combined medical-psychiatric area would allow behavioral control of a patient with medical evaluation in progress. Triage personnel should be able to differentiate simple and severe psychiatric problems, and be able to direct the patient to the appropriate area for treatment.

Restraints

It is necessary to physically restrain the dangerous, agitated patient who cannot cooperate for adequate evaluation in order to protect the physician, emergency department personnel, and other patients in the emergency department. The premature use of drugs to control behavior may obliterate the signs of mental illness, so that psychiatric evaluation is later difficult. Thus, the physician and paramedical personnel should not hesitate to restrain a patient if the safety of the patient or others is in jeopardy.

Use of Physical Restraints

Establish need for restraints
Attempt verbal control
Call for adequate support personnel
Apply necessary restraints
Explain why restraints are applied
Search patient for weapons or drugs
Determine cause of patient's behavior
Determine continuing need for restraints

The effective use of restraints in the emergency department consists of establishing the need for restraints, applying them appropriately, evaluating the patient, and assessing the continuing need for restraints.

The need for restraints exists if no one, including the patient, seems to be in control of the patient's behavior, and that behavior threatens the patient or others. The need continues until adequate assessment is completed and control can be maintained by other means.

The patient who is treated as helpless or crazy will frequently behave according to those expectations. Conversely, if personnel act as if they expect the patient to behave and exercise self-control the patient may try to comply. Talk to the patient about his or her behavior and its effect on others: "Your actions are frightening others, and we cannot allow such behavior here. Can we talk about whatever is bothering you?"

If the patient does not respond to verbal requests, do not try to restrain the patient unless you have enough help. Struggling with an out-of-control patient may escalate the patient's anxiety (as well as your own) and may result in injury to the patient, yourself, or someone else. If you have to make a choice between struggling with a potentially dangerous, though ill, patient without adequate help, or letting the patient go, you must choose to protect yourself. Do not try to be a hero. On occasion, the mere demonstration of sufficient staff adequately controls the patient. In restraining a patient, it is useful to use a team approach: a leader should assign five staff members to immobilize the limbs and the head, while a sixth applies the restraints.

Strong leather limb restraints should be available in every emergency department for the control of violent psychiatric patients. Bandages and sheets are not suitable for use as restraints because they chafe and bind, and are easily ripped or cut. It is also desirable to have a trunk restraint such as a Posey belt, and a large, thin, flexible mattress that can be used to pin the excited or violent patient against the wall.

Restrain the patient so he or she cannot remove the restraints, but make sure the airway is patent and rapid access to an intravenous route is preserved. A patient restrained in a supine position, with each limb in a different corner, may feel threatened or vulnerable to attack. This position also favors aspiration. It is better to restrain the patient so that sideways movement is permitted. Whatever position is used, restraints should be checked frequently so they are not uncomfortable or injurious to the patient. Never apply only one restraint. If two are used, they should be applied to one arm and the contralateral leg. Restraints should be periodically switched to the opposite extremities for patient comfort. Violent patients generally need four limb restraints. After being restrained, the patient should be placed in an area that allows direct observation, such as the hall near the nursing station, a room directly visible to the nursing station, or in an area monitored by camera or in person. Violent patients can rock the stretcher and overturn it, even when all limbs are restrained.

Even if you believe the patients cannot understand you, explain that restraints are being applied for their protection and to help them control their behavior. Repeat this explanation after they are restrained. Patients are generally frightened when they cannot control their behavior and are relieved when someone else controls it for them. Furthermore, other patients and ancillary staff within earshot need to hear that the restraints are therapeutic and not punitive.

After the restraints are applied, carefully search the patient and all clothing, including underwear, for hidden weapons such as knives or razor blades, or for drugs.

Periodically assess whether the patient's condition has improved so that physical restraint is no longer necessary. Checking the restraints for comfort and integrity, as well as checking the status of the restrained patient at least every 20 to 30 min, is reasonable. The decision to release the patient from physical restraints should be made by the physician or paramedical personnel on the basis of judgment of the patient's condition and behavior, and not on the patient's pleas, promises, bargains, or threats. Restraints should be removed stepwise over a period of time; that is, if all four limbs are restrained, restraints should first be reduced to two limbs, and finally to none.

Restraints are indicated if patients exhibit behavior that is dangerous to themselves or others, and they cannot be safely contained in any other fashion.

Isolation Room

The emergency department should have a designated area for evaluating patients with major behavioral symptoms. The following requirements should be met.

- Resuscitation equipment should be immediately available.
- Leather restraints that can be used on the stretchers in the area should be available.
- The area should be designed so that all patients are under direct observation at all times.
- The area should be readily accessible to staff members, both for behavioral control and emergency medical management.
- The room should have minimal or no portable items which might be converted into weapons, such as ashtrays, lamps, small tables, small chairs, or footstools.
- A telephone, preferably a wall unit, with direct access to an outside line should be available.
- The room should not have windows; or if they are present, plexiglass or wire glass barriers should be installed.

In addition, a number of amenities can make the task of dealing with psychiatric emergencies easier and less anxiety-provoking. Additional suggestions for the isolation room are:

- It should be large enough to provide for chair and stretcher space for each patient, so that patients can lie down or sit up if they are able.
- It should be partially soundproof to diminish stimuli coming to the patient as well as sound emanating from the patient.
- It should have a light source that can be controlled by rheostat, also to allow decrease of stimuli.
- It should have a "panic button" which alerts staff outside of the area to the need for assistance.

An emergency department with 60,000 to 80,000 patient visits annually probably sees an average of 5 to 10 percent psychiatric patients. Although this is a relatively small number, psychiatric patients take a disproportionate amount of time, up to three times the average length of stay for other patients in the emergency department. The minimal physical needs to handle such a caseload are two isolation rooms and one interview room, and more space is necessary if a sizable number of patients have severe alcohol or drug-related behavioral disturbances. Patients who are marginally under control may be better managed if they can be held in a separate psychiatric waiting area which is monitored by psychiatric staff.

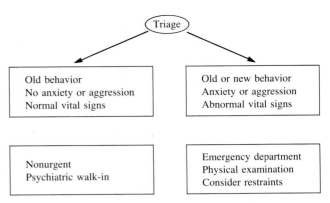

Figure 137A-1: Triage of the psychiatric patient

Triage

Rules should be applied to psychiatric patients that are comparable to those for the triage of all other patients. Treatment priorities must be considered (Fig. 137A-1). Thus, not all psychiatric patients can wait, nor must they all be immediately directed to the psychiatric area proper.

All patients should have vital signs taken. If the patient's complaint does not make the triage officer or the patient anxious, if the patient has felt this way before and is not suicidal or homicidal, and if vital signs can be obtained and are normal, the patient can be considered "ambulatory" or nonurgent.

The patient should be escorted to the emergency department and evaluated by a physician as soon as possible if vital signs are abnormal, if the triage officer feels anxious, or if the patient or family is unable to deal with the patient's behavior. In these cases not only may delay be life-threatening but also everyone's anxiety may impair the functioning of the emergency department.

If the patient's behavior or complaint is new and everyone is uncomfortable about it—in particular, if anyone is concerned about a suicidal or homicidal threat—the patient should be taken to an area where a good medical evaluation can proceed without concern about the patient "escaping" or hurting someone. Restraints should be considered at the first indication of their need, before the situation gets out of hand. These "vertical" emergencies, i.e., where the patient is able to ambulate but in fact has potential life-threatening illness, are often difficult to recognize. Often they are missed because vital signs have not been obtained, or if obtained, have been ignored.

After placement of a psychiatric patient has been decided upon, evaluation should proceed as follows:

Nonurgent

- Take a medical history and, in particular, ask about depression and suicidal thoughts.
- Do the indicated medical evaluation.
- If there are no medical problems, and no suicidal ideation or destructive behavior, advise appropriate referral.
- If there are medical problems, suicidal thoughts, or destructive, aggressive behavior, explore these further.
- If there is a potential life threat, detain the patient, obtain a consultation, or hospitalize.

Urgent

- Consider whether restraints are indicated.
- Talkdown: Orient the patient, reassure that you will try to help, offer an explanation of what's going on as far as you can tell, and describe what you expect to be the course of the emergency visit.

- If talkdown is unsuccessful, try placing the patient in a quiet area where there is minimal stimulation and disturbance, monitoring the patient's behavior and vital signs frequently.
- Obtain history from any other sources.
- Proceed with medical assessment as well as you can.

B. Medical History and Physical Examination
Judith E. Tintinalli

INTRODUCTION

It is preferable to have a separate area in the emergency department for the observation and treatment of psychiatric patients. However, certain patients, such as those with possible medical problems, the elderly, and those with drug or alcohol intoxication, are better examined where medical observation and treatment can be done. Patients who may need intravenous infusions should not be sent to the psychiatric area.

Psychiatric patients in a medical area need close observation and reliable restraining procedures (see section on restraints in Chapter 137A). Violent, loud behavior is not only upsetting to patients and staff, it also makes it impossible to evaluate the patient medically. Therefore, after the initial evaluation has ruled out immediate life-threatening causes of violent behavior such as hypotension, hypoxia, hypoglycemia, psychomotor seizures, or head injury, sedation should be considered if the patient has not calmed down sufficiently (see Chapter 137D on antipsychotic drugs). Antipsychotic drugs or sedatives with ganglionic blocker or cardiac effects should be avoided. One of the diazepines is safest, although it will not sedate the truly psychotic patient.

DIFFERENTIAL DIAGNOSIS

Functional Disorders

Functional disorders are those in which impairment of brain tissue function by either neurologic or physiologic parameters cannot be identified. Schizophrenia is the most common example; it usually becomes evident before the age of 40, commonly around 20. In the emergency department, the diagnosis of a functional disorder is generally made after an organic brain syndrome has been excluded.

Organic Brain Syndrome

Organic brain syndrome is characterized by behavioral disturbances due to an underlying pathophysiologic central nervous system or systemic process. The psychiatric classification of organic brain syndromes is not particularly helpful to clinicians because the differential diagnoses are organized according to psychopathology (delirium, dementia, amnestic syndrome, organic delusional syndrome, organic hallucinosis, organic affective syndromes, organic personality syndromes). The clinician's perspective is from an anatomic or physiologic standpoint.

The major abnormalities on mental status exam which suggest the presence of an organic brain syndrome are (1) impairment of orientation to time, person, or place; (2) impairment of consciousness, with a loss of awareness of the environment and inability to sustain attention; (3) memory impairment; (4) cognitive impairment; (5) visual hallucinations. Dubin et al. include abnormal vital signs and patient's age over 40 as additional strong criteria for organic brain syndrome.

HISTORY

Individuals over age 40 with no previous psychiatric history are more likely to have an organic brain syndrome as opposed to a functional illness. Medical records of local psychiatric hospitals should be checked for prior psychiatric admissions. In many cases, the history as related by the patient may not be helpful or may be misleading. Family and friends should be carefully interviewed to obtain a clear idea of the level and rate of onset of symptoms. Reports of acute changes in behavior or functioning should be regarded as organic. Urine or stool incontinence point to the presence of an organic brain syndrome. History of drug or alcohol abuse by the patient should be obtained, since both are common in psychiatric patients. The signs and symptoms of intoxication may mask the underlying psychiatric disorder. Past medical history, including medications, allergies, and last menstrual period, should be determined and recorded (Table 137B-1). A large number of medications, including over-the-counter medications, can produce behavioral changes, especially in the elderly, and should be considered as etiologic agents for acute organic brain syndromes (Table 137B-2).

Table 137B-1. Major Organic Causes of Disturbed Behavior

Metabolic and endocrine disorders	Shock
	Hyper- or hypoglycemia
	Hyper- or hypothyroidism
	Hypercalcemia
	Hyper- or hyponatremia
	Hypoxia
	Sepsis
	Uremia
	Hepatic encephalopathy
	Steroid "psychosis"
	Hyperpyrexia
CNS disorders	Encephalitis
	Meningitis
	Head injury
	Stroke
Drug or alcohol abuse	Hallucinosis
	Intoxication
	Withdrawal
	Overdose
Seizure disorders	Psychomotor seizures
	Postictal states
	Postictal psychosis

PHYSICAL EXAMINATION

The examining physician should make sure the patient has been completely disrobed and gowned, and searched before examination. This is necessary for a complete examination as well as to ensure that objects which can be used as weapons are removed. Seemingly innocuous objects such as belt buckles can injure staff or other patients.

Vital signs are important screening tools for the physician. Fever or hypothermia indicate a medical problem. Hypertension could be incidental or secondary to agitation, or if malignant hypertension is present, cerebral edema could account for behavior changes. If hypertension is suspected secondary to agitation, the patient should be sedated and then completely reevaluated when calm. Likewise, tachycardia could be secondary to panic or agitation, or could be a sign of underlying medical illness, hypovolemia, or endocrine disorder. Tachypnea could be secondary to fright and agitation, or could be present because of hypoxia, salicylate intoxication, or metabolic acidosis.

On general physical inspection, the patient should be carefully checked for signs of trauma. Contusions or abrasions about the head, face, and neck are especially common if the patient is argumentative or bellicose. Check for frostbite on the extremities. Since most psychiatric patients will be restrained, it is more difficult, but still necessary, to check extremities carefully. Check for "hesitation" marks on the wrists of suicidal patients. Look for evidence of physical abuse in the elderly, who may have been subject to forceful restraint by exasperated family or caretakers. If trauma is demonstrated or suggested by the history, the mechanism of injury should be carefully reconstructed. Psychiatric patients are notoriously insensitive to or unconcerned with pain.

Chest, cardiac, and abdominal examination should be carefully done. Breast examination is necessary in females. Examination of the abdomen is quite difficult in psychiatric patients for several reasons. Patients are generally uncooperative, and mild or moderate tenderness may not be reproducible from examiner to examiner.

Table 137B-2. Medications Resulting in Behavior Changes

	Mental Status/Mood Alteration	Hallucinations	Depression	Psychosis	Seizures
Cardiac:					
Digitalis	x	x	x		
Reserpine			x		
Pronestyl	x	x	x	x	
Propranolol (β-blockers)		x	x	x	
Hydralazine	x		x		
α-Methyldopa			x		
Anti-infective:					
Isoniazid	x	x		x	x
Sulfonamides	x				
Penicillins				x	x
Neuropharmacologics:					
Lithium	x				x
Phenytoin	x	x		x	x
Antihistamines	x	x	x	x	x
Anticholinergics (antidepressants)	x	x		x	x
L-Dopa	x	x	x	x	
Phenothiazine	x				x
Miscellaneous:					
Clonidine				x	
Acetylsalicylic acid	x				x
Steroids	x		x	x	
Nonsteroidal allyso-propylacetamide	x	x	x	x	x
Aminophylline		x		x	x
Cimetidine	x	x		x	

Source: Adapted from Fauman MA, Fauman BJ: The differential diagnosis of organic based psychiatric disturbance in the emergency department. *JACEP* 6:317–318, 1977.

Even mild pain may indicate the presence of a severe intraabdominal abnormality. Prior medication with antipsychotics, especially haloperidol, may be associated with relative insensitivity to pain.

Finally, the neurologic exam should focus on the detection of focal neurologic signs, evaluation of motor function, and reflex changes. Seizure activity always indicates an organic abnormality. Dystonias are sometimes mistaken for seizures. Dystonias with involvement of every major muscle group, often mimicking musculoskeletal or focal neurologic disease, have been reported. The presence of dystonias or cogwheel rigidity point to previous administration or misuse of drugs with extrapyramidal effects.

LABORATORY EVALUATION

Laboratory evaluation should include simple screening tests such as CBC, glucose, BUN, and electrolytes. In a review by Purdie et al. fluid and electrolyte disorders were found in 12 percent of emergency patients with an acute organic brain syndrome. Gleadhill et al. noted a 15-fold greater incidence of hyponatremia in schizophrenic patients with an acute organic brain syndrome than in nonschizophrenic patients. In a review in our own institution of 500 consecutive psychiatric patients who did not have clinical evidence of an acute organic brain syndrome, the only laboratory studies which were found to be of value were the blood glucose and white blood cell count. Elevation of the blood urea nitrogen was detectable as clinical dehydration. Electrolyte abnormalities were not detected unless there was a prior history of diuretic administration, or evidence of edema on physical examination. Regardless of which tests are done, abnormalities should be treated seriously. If the white count is elevated, careful reevaluation for signs of occult infection, such as otitis or periodontitis, should be done. In our institution, elevations of the white count are treated by reevaluation, chest x-ray, and urinalysis, and a repeat white count. Often agitation results in demargination of white cells, and a repeat count 4 to 6 h after the patient has been calmed, will be within normal limits. Further laboratory or x-ray evaluations may be necessary, depending on the results of history and physical examination.

Table 137B-3. Factors Used to Differentiate Acute Organic Brain Syndrome from Functional Disorder

History, especially of alcohol or drug abuse
Medication and allergy history
Mental status examination
Physical examination
Screening laboratory studies

SUMMARY

In summary, the emergency department evaluation of patients with disturbed behavior should consist of (1) careful history from the patient, family, friends, and local psychiatric institutions; (2) determination of associated alcohol or drug abuse; (3) medication and allergy history; (4) mental status evaluation focusing on orientation, consciousness, memory, cognitive function, and detection of hallucinations; (5) physical examination with careful detection of trauma and thorough evaluation of any areas which elicit pain; (6) screening laboratory evaluation, consisting of at least a complete blood count and blood sugar (Table 137B-3). If the diagnosis of a functional disorder is made only *after* the exclusion of an organic brain syndrome, and if the patient is declared medically clear only after associated or complicating medical illnesses are ruled out, diagnostic errors will be kept to a minimum.

BIBLIOGRAPHY

Dubin WR, Weiss KJ, Zeccardi JA: Organic brain syndrome: The psychiatric imposter. *JAMA* 249:60–62, 1983.
Fauman MA, Fauman BJ: The differential diagnosis of organic based psychiatric disturbance in the emergency department. *JACEP* 6:315–323, 1977.
Fishbain, DA: Pain insensitivity in psychosis. *Ann Emerg Med* 11:630–632, 1982.
Gleadhill IC, Smith TA, Yium JJ: Hyponatremia in patients with schizophrenia. *South Med J* 75:426–428, 1982.
Lee AS: Drug-induced dystonic reactions. *JACEP* 6:351–354, 1977.
McEvoy JP: Organic brain syndromes. *Ann Intern Med* 95:212–220, 1981.
Petrie WM, Lawson EC, Hollender MH: Violence in geriatric patients. *JAMA* 248:443–444, 1982.
Purdie FR, Honigman B, Rosen P: Acute organic brain syndrome: A review of 100 cases. *Ann Emerg Med* 10:455–461, 1981.

C. The Psychiatric Interview

Beverly Fauman

The technique for the psychiatric interview differs from that for the usual history in that the physician must note the patient's mood, style, and feeling in addition to obtaining factual information. Psychiatric interviews can be time-consuming and must often be supplemented by history from the patient's family or other agencies.

Interview Technique

The emergency physician should initially approach the patient with open-ended questions that allow the patient to describe the problem. This provides an opportunity to observe the patient's behavior, appearance, speech, affect, thought processes, and content of thought.

During the interview, the physician should pay attention to his or her own emotional responses to the patient. The emotional reaction of a physician to a patient is known as *countertransference*, which is somewhat analogous to a "gut" reaction. The patient may engender in the physician feelings such as anger, anxiety, sexual arousal, warmth, or sympathy. If alert to such reactions, the physician is better able to deal with them and to take a logical approach in diagnosis and disposition.

Beginning the Interview

The psychiatric interview should begin in an atmosphere comfortable for both the patient and physician. If the emergency physician will be exploring the possibility of a psychiatric basis for the patient's symptoms after the physical examination, it is useful to make a clear distinction between the "medical" examination and the psychiatric interview. Generally, maneuvers that make the patient feel mature improve the interview. Having the patient get dressed rather than remain in an examining gown, having the patient sit in a chair rather than lie down, having the physician sit rather than stand over the patient, and asking other family members or friends to leave the interview room, at least initially, all give the patient an opportunity to be more in charge of the situation.

The patient who is in distress can sense if the physician feels rushed or is unenthusiastic about the interview. The patient may react by refusing to talk or by answering so vaguely that the interview is prolonged.

A useful technique is to ask an opening question such as "what can you tell me about what is going on?" and then to say nothing more for 2 min or so. The silence may be difficult for an active, busy physician to endure, but the patient is even more uncomfortable with it and will usually begin to volunteer more information than might be obtained by direct questioning. This technique indicates to the patient that you are interested and willing to take the time to listen. Paradoxically, this technique allows the physician to complete an evaluation in far shorter time than that afforded by direct questioning. This period of time is generally enough to assess how acute the problem is, how severe it is, and, in particular, how responsive the patient is to someone who takes the time to listen.

Some patients who are extremely agitated or psychotic may have to be physically restrained before they can be interviewed. If the patient is unable to exercise self-control, it may be comforting for the patient to be controlled by leather restraints and adequate security personnel. When the initial agitated or combative behavior is under control, the physician can then proceed with the interview. Remember that you are not required to be heroic or take risks; take whatever measures you need to feel comfortable with the patient. Do not bargain with the patient when external controls are necessary. For example, if the patient says "I'll talk to you only if you untie my wrists," you should answer: "I will decide in a while whether it is a good idea to release the restraints.

In the meantime, perhaps we can talk about what brought you here."

Content and Aims of the Interview

The emergency physician needs to determine four things when conducting an emergency department psychiatric interview: the nature of the problem, its duration, the patient's expectations, and the patient's disposition.

The patient should be asked about major concerns and difficulties. If there have been psychiatric problems in the past, their frequency, duration, and treatment should be determined.

For emergency purposes it is important not to get caught in a long recitation of the patient's difficulties. It is important to know if the patient has had any prior psychiatric intervention, and extremely important and useful to know why the prior treatment ended. This will give clues to the type of illness, to its chronicity, and to the appropriate disposition, since multiple failures at treatment in the past suggest a chronic illness such as schizophrenia or a personality disorder. Failure at outpatient treatment may indicate the need for inpatient care. A story of multiple misdiagnoses or prior inadequate or inconsiderate care may indicate a patient who is sociopathic or hysterical. In general, all hospitals and all physicians are as ethical and concerned as you are, and a patient's conviction that this is not so is more often a clue to the correct diagnosis than to anything else.

Confirmation of the patient's history with a family member, friend, prior records, or another hospital is usually very helpful, although again multiple details are not necessary. However, friends and family members should be consulted for details of the present illness, especially if the patient denies any problems or will not communicate.

A most important feature of the illness is the reason why and circumstances under which the patient or family decided to seek help. The interviewer needs to determine if the patient expects hospitalization, drug treatment, or follow-up care, or if the patient wants the physician to intercede in some situation that the patient is not handling well, such as difficulties at home or at work. Pursuing this question will not only allow you to approach the conclusion of the interview, it will often yield important diagnostic information you have not obtained previously. In the psychiatric encounter, the patient should know what you think the problem is, what you are recommending, and how he or she is to proceed to get help. This is analogous to a medical situation in which the patient understands the prescription and its purpose, knows where to fill it, and knows the instructions for follow-up.

It is not necessary for emergency department evaluations to be more elaborate than outlined, although an impression of the psychiatric diagnosis is useful for your own preciseness and for a psychiatric referral. If no psychiatric consultation is available, the question of hospitalization may have to be determined by the emergency physician. In most states there is an obligation to hospitalize a patient if there is an immediate danger to the patient or others, if the patient has committed an overtly dangerous act, and if the danger or dangerous act is related to a psychiatric illness.

Beyond the legal obligation to detain and hospitalize an acutely dangerous, psychiatrically ill patient, a patient may profit from hospitalization if the patient is young or has at most two prior psychiatric hospitalizations. If there have been more than two hospitalizations but the patient returns to a reasonable level of function between illnesses, the prognosis may also be quite good. It is useful to have some grasp of the indicators for a good prognosis, because a psychiatric consultant will be more responsive to your requests for help in these instances. Conversely, the patient's family should not be encouraged falsely when the patient has had a progressive, downhill course over several years.

If you cannot justify involuntary hospitalization and you have no convincing evidence that hospitalization will help the patient, the only criterion for hospitalization is lack of other available options: no place to stay, no social supports, a likelihood that the patient will deteriorate and that no psychiatric care will be obtained or is available on an outpatient basis.

Patients should not be allowed to sign out against medical advice just because they are hostile, demanding, or obnoxious. This type of behavior may be a symptom of the underlying mental or medical disorder that needs urgent attention.

Mental Status Examination

A brief evaluation of mental status should be part of the assessment of every emergency department patient. This information should be noted in the chart as rigorously as are vital signs, most importantly because it serves as a baseline. A more thorough formal examination is required for any patient who exhibits unusual behavior, appearance, speech, or affect; a thought disorder; or impairment of awareness, judgment, or cognitive function. In addition, the mental status examination is necessary to differentiate organic from functional illness. Areas that should be evaluated are affect, thought process and content, and cognitive function.

Observation

Important clues to the duration, severity of illness, and the relationship of the patient to others can be gained through observation. If the patient came to the emergency department alone, this may indicate a lack of concerned relatives or friends, or isolation from others. Chronic psychiatric patients may return to the psychiatric walk-in clinic rather than the emergency department. A disheveled appearance may indicate the patient's inability for self-care or lack of concern with appearance. The patient who is disruptive and demanding, or who will not wait for an evaluation is commonly regarded as uncooperative when, in fact, he or she may be unable to cooperate. Observation about general behavior should include an estimate of appropriateness to age and socioeconomic status. Other aspects to be noted include the patient's alertness and the presence of slurred or incoherent speech that may indicate alcohol or drug intoxication.

Feelings

Subtle clues to illness can be detected by experienced emergency department staff. Patients are able to evoke any number of negative or positive feelings among the hospital personnel. It is important that the staff ventilate appropriately the negative or uncomfortable emotions evoked by some patients, both to relieve some of the strain of the practice of emergency medicine and to recognize important clues to a patient's diagnosis. This is often done informally in the doctor's room or boardroom, via "gallows humor." The emergency physician can sometimes help the staff gain insight into a patient's behavior. For example, upon observing staff getting angry with a patient, the physician can initiate a brief discussion somewhere away from the patient.

Open-ended questions such as "How have things been going for you?" may elicit statements that reflect the patient's underlying feelings. In order to arrive at a diagnosis, feelings such as anger, sadness, apathy, anxiety, frustration, and helplessness should be correlated with other aspects of the mental status examination.

Affect

There are several elements to identify in describing a patient's affect. *Flat affect* is an overused description. The patient, in fact, may be withdrawn, depressed, or overwhelmed. Describe affect in terms of the prevailing mood during your interview. Note whether the patient is depressed, suicidal, or anxious, and how frequent, how intense, and how persistent the moods are. Affect can vary throughout the course of a week, day, or even during the interview. The patient's description of moods and feelings may or may not fit with your observation of the patient's affect. As above, a good clue to affect is how the patient makes you feel.

Thought Process and Content

Thought process describes how the patient tells his or her story. An appropriate coherent thought process is logical, chronological, and consistent. The interviewer should easily be able to follow the patient's train of thought and be comfortable with the patient's answers.

Thought content is the actual material the patient is relating. The presence of perceptual distortions, such as sensory or auditory hallucinations, or feelings of unreality or separation from the world, should be determined. The patient may have persistent concerns about something he or she has done or wants to do, or about self-worth. The patient may feel controlled, or may believe that he or she can control events or other people. The patient may be exceptionally concerned about physical symptoms or illnesses, or may even recognize that something is wrong with his or her thought processes.

Cognitive Function

When there is a medical cause of behavioral disturbance, the most striking area of change is in cognitive function. The patient's awareness of surroundings and orientation should be noted, as should ability to follow instructions, such as "Hold this thermometer under your tongue" or "Get undressed and put on this gown." Specific signs and symptoms that are highly suggestive of organic brain disorders are memory impairment, disorientation, and focal or generalized neurologic abnormalities. Some organic brain disorder often follows head trauma, stroke, or hypoxia, and may be an accompaniment to metabolic disturbances such as acidosis, hyponatremia, or hypoglycemia, or toxicities such as alcohol intoxication, carbon monoxide poisoning, or sedative overdose. Inability to use words or numbers also suggests organic impairment, not functional psychosis, although anxiety and depression can impair one's ability to concentrate and do simple calculations and memory tests.

Priority Assessment

The specific goal of the emergency psychiatric assessment is to determine the need for immediate management. The emergency physician is often faced with making a decision regarding hospitalization where there is no psychiatric consultation available, or may wish to transfer a patient to a psychiatric facility where associated medical problems may not receive appropriate care.

If there is an abnormality on mental status examination, and one suspects or knows this is a recent change, there is a need to rule out potential life-threatening organic disorders by appropriate laboratory tests, and medical history and physical examination. A change in mental status during the course of observation in the emergency department is highly significant, and virtually always indicates organic disease. In such a case, the patient should be kept in a medical facility, that is, a holding unit, or acute medical or neurology service, rather than be sent to a physically separate psychiatric hospital.

The physician's appreciation of a patient's mental status occurs throughout the emergency department evaluation, and it need not be formal, except to document deficits where there is concern about an organic disturbance. State of alertness, ability to respond to questions, the ability to relate to medical personnel and to familiar faces, ability to understand questions and instructions, and general appearance, mood, and manner are part of a mental status examination, and should be noted in the medical record, especially if there is anything out of the ordinary.

Concluding the Interview

The physician should define the problem. If the physician believes there is no acute psychiatric problem, this should be stated. The patient should be informed of any actions that will be taken and what is expected of the patient. There should be an allowance during this time for the patient to regain self-control. The physician should avoid the temptation to write a prescription merely because it is an easy disposition.

For medical record thoroughness, this conclusion should be documented, along with a specific statement about the physician's judgment of the patient's danger to self. If appropriate, the name and telephone number of a responsible adult who knows the patient could be included in the chart.

Access to a psychiatric consultation varies considerably from one emergency facility to the next. A good arrangement is to have available a resourceful social worker to handle dispositions to mental health clinics or other outpatient facilities, and to call the psychiatrist only if the physician feels uncomfortable about a particular patient or is unsure of the diagnosis or disposition. The emergency physician should become familiar enough with the basic techniques for handling the psychiatric emergency so that the psychiatrist is regarded as a consultant much in the same way as the otolaryngologist or cardiologist. Referrals and transfers should be handled in a similar manner.

D. Emergency Drug Therapy

Beverly Fauman

Most psychiatric emergencies do not require medication. The decision not to use drugs is as much a part of the role of the emergency physician as is the judicious use of psychopharmacologic agents.

Many psychiatric medications have side effects that bring patients to the emergency department; many are also used in suicide attempts. This chapter will discuss psychiatric medications, their side effects, and the psychiatric side effects of nonpsychiatric drugs.

The major classifications of psychopharmacologic agents are minor tranquilizers or antianxiety agents, major tranquilizers or antipsychotic agents, antidepressants, and lithium compounds.

MINOR TRANQUILIZERS

The benzodiazepines and meprobamate have been prescribed instead of barbiturates for a number of years for a myriad of conditions. Initially, it was believed that these agents were less addicting than barbiturates.

In low doses, the minor tranquilizers (Table 137D-1) are sedating, and will calm anxiety. In depressed patients, the minor tranquilizers may increase depression. Minor tranquilizers are the most common agents used in suicide gestures or attempts.

With chronic use some tolerance develops, and patients may complain of withdrawal symptoms—increased anxiety, irritability, hyperreflexia, decreased appetite, or nausea and vomiting. Seizures have been reported on sudden withdrawal from chronic high doses of benzodiazepines.

Table 137D-1. Common Minor Tranquilizers

Tranquilizer	Common Oral Dose, mg
Alprazolam* (Xanax)	0.25–1 tid
Chlordiazepoxide (Librium)	5–15 tid
Diazepam (Valium)	2–5 tid
Lorazepam (Ativan)	1–3 bid
Oxazepam (Serax)	10–15 tid

*Relatively short half-life of 10 to 12 h.

Minor tranquilizers have a high abuse potential and can be addictive. There is virtually no indication for an emergency physician to prescribe minor tranquilizers for the management of anxiety. If one is concerned about the possibility of abuse, it may be better to prescribe muscle relaxants other than diazepam for sprains and low back pain. As a general rule, emotional responses to ordinary life situations should not be treated by medication. It is generally not appropriate to prescribe minor tranquilizers for an acute grief reaction since there is evidence these drugs delay or interfere with the treatment of the grief reaction.

Chlordiazepoxide or diazepam may be helpful in the emergency department management of the acute alcohol withdrawal syndromes.

Subjective complaints of withdrawal from minor tranquilizers should be handled by referral to a drug treatment program. Symptoms such as vomiting or seizures should be managed by admission to the hospital or by treatment in the emergency department.

MAJOR TRANQUILIZERS

The phenothiazines were discovered to have potent antipsychotic effects in the early 1950s. Since then, a number of drugs with similar properties, classified as major tranquilizers, have been developed. The use of these drugs is in no small way related to the decline of chronically hospitalized psychiatric patients and to the growth of the community mental health movement.

Major tranquilizers (Table 137D-2) are potent drugs and have significant risks, including sudden death. They should not be used to silence an unruly patient, or when the diagnosis is uncertain. Agitated, disruptive patients can often be managed by the judicious use of restraints and a secluded room. For extremes of agitation, small amounts of amobarbital or alprazolam, intravenously, can be used for a temporary calming effect. In addition, this will not alter the manifestation of the psychosis, so that subsequent psychiatric evaluation is still meaningful.

Major tranquilizers used inappropriately in the nonpsychotic individual can cause severe central nervous system depression, hypotension, and tachycardia. Even when used appropriately, orthostatic hypotension and tachycardia are commonly seen with the intramuscular administration of the phenothiazines or thiothixene. Major tranquilizers used in the psychotic patient can treat symptoms so successfully that a unit receiving the patient in transfer may see no reason to admit the patient. This may result in the patient's return to the emergency department 4 to 8 h later, when the effect of the drug has worn off.

Major tranquilizers can be given in the emergency department when the patient is known to have a psychiatric disorder or an organic brain disorder, if the disorder is known to be responsive to major tranquilizers, and if the patient is psychotic and cannot be successfully managed by using verbal or physical restraints. The emergency department physician and the psychiatric unit should agree upon a drug treatment protocol for psychiatric emergencies.

A major tranquilizer the emergency department should be familiar with is haloperidol. It does not cause hypotension, but it often causes tachycardia. It is not unduly sedating and can be administered intramuscularly or by mouth in relatively low doses. For the appropriate patient, 2 to 5 mg IM initially will sufficiently control symptoms within 20 min. Haloperidol can lower the seizure threshold, as can all major tranquilizers. Parkinsonian tremor and rigidity are more common side effects with haloperidol than with lower-potency major tranquilizers.

Thorazine is not as good a drug for emergency use because it is very sedating; if given inappropriately, it can render the patient unresponsive for 4 to 12 h, making further evaluation impossible. Its hypotensive effect can be severe and has been known to cause cardiac arrest. Relatively large doses need to be given, compared with those of haloperidol and thiothixene, and the intramuscular injection is painful.

The thioxanthenes are structurally similar to the phenothiazines. Thiothixene (Navane) is a sedating agent which can be administered intramuscularly and in lower doses than chlorpromazine. The precautions that should be taken with chlorpromazine apply also to thiothixene.

Major tranquilizer is something of a misnomer, as many drugs in this class do not ''tranquilize.'' These drugs work by as yet not well understood mechanisms to decrease extreme anxiety and diminish psychotic thinking. They allow healthy aspects of a patient's behavior to maintain control. They are useful in the treatment of psychosis, whether the cause is organic illness or psychiatric illness. The phenothiazines and thiothixenes are chemically similar; the butyrophenones are distinctly different.

The patient who is not psychotic will generally be far more sensitive to the sedative effects of the major tranquilizers, and may fall into deep and prolonged sleep from doses that merely calm the acutely psychotic schizophrenic. Further, nonpsychotic individuals often experience profound dysphoria when given major tranquilizers—bad dreams, confusion, and muscle pains. The nonpsychotic patient who takes small doses of major tranquilizers, inadvertently or ill-advisedly, has disproportionately more Parkinson-like reactions than the schizophrenic patient on appropriate higher doses.

ADVERSE EFFECTS OF MAJOR TRANQUILIZERS

Dystonic Reactions and Extrapyramidal Effects

A drug-induced dystonic reaction is an extrapyramidal motor disturbance consisting of uncoordinated and involuntary spasmodic movement of certain muscle groups. Dystonic reactions can involve the following anatomical regions: eye muscles, resulting in an oculogyric crisis; neck muscles, resulting in torticolis; muscles of tongue and jaw; back muscles, resulting in opisthotonic posturing; and muscles of the abdominal wall, hips, and pelvis. Hallucinations or an increase in other psychotic symptoms may also occur.

Table 137D-2. Common Major Tranquilizers

Tranquilizer	Common Oral Doses, mg
Chlorpromazine (Thorazine)	100–200 bid/qid
Fluphenazine* (Prolixin, Permitil)	0.5–10 bid
Trifluoperazine (Stelazine)	1–10 bid
Haloperidol (Haldol)	0.5–2 bid
Thiothixene (Navane)	2–10 bid
Loxapine (Loxitane)	10–30 bid
Molindone (Moban)	25–50 bid

*Often used as depot, with effects lasting up to 2 weeks.

A drug-induced dystonic reaction is characterized by (1) abrupt onset, (2) intermittent and bizarre neuromuscular manifestations, (3) normal physical examination except for muscular findings, (4) recent medication history, and (5) rapid response to anticholinergic agents. Careful clinical evaluation and laboratory testing are necessary for those patients with abnormal vital signs or neurological findings, or with a poor response to anticholinergic agents within 30 min. In the differential diagnosis of extrapyramidal reactions, depending on the group of muscles involved, one should consider hysterical conversion reactions, acute psychosis, meningitis or encephalitis, Parkinson's disease, tetany, or hypocalcemia.

The incidence of drug-induced dyskinesias is increasing because major tranquilizers are still widely used in medical practice, occasionally without real indication. In addition, they are frequently abused by the general population. Individuals buying street drugs may often get haloperidol or thiothixene when they have asked for diazepam, THC, or various downers or uppers.

Extrapyramidal side effects such as dystonic reactions, tremors, and rigidity can be influenced by suggestion or emotion. This does not mean that the patient is faking or hysterical. Side effects occur more frequenlty on first exposures, often at low doses. Patients may not know that they have taken a major tranquilizer; ask patients if they have taken nerve pills, street drugs, or antiemetics. One of the phenothiazines, fluphenazine (Prolixin), is often given as a depot injection with effects lasting 2 to 3 weeks.

Dystonic reactions following ingestion of phenothiazines are more common in the naive user. Thus someone who takes a relative's "nerve pill," a single street drug, or an antiemetic phenothiazine such as prochlorperazine (Compazine) for nausea is more prone to experience an acute dystonic reaction. Because there is no psychiatric history in such patients, the diagnosis may be delayed.

Treatment is with diphenhydramine (Benadryl) 25 to 50 mg intravenously, or benztropine (Cogentin) 1 to 2 mg intravenously, administered slowly. Relief generally occurs in minutes, confirming the diagnosis. If medication is given intramuscularly, relief occurs in under 30 min. Because the duration of action of the aggravating drug can be several hours to 2 weeks, the patient must be given a prescription for an antiparkinsonian agent such as benztropine (1 to 2 mg PO bid) or diphenhydramine (25 to 50 mg PO bid) for the next 24 to 72 h.

If the patient has been placed on the major tranquilizers by an appropriate treatment facility, there is no need to stop the drugs because of these side effects, although it may be necessary to reduce the dose. In most cases, this sensitivity disappears with continued use of the drug, so it is not necessary to warn the patient of sensitivity or to stop its use if it has been prescribed for a psychiatric condition. Tolerance usually develops rapidly. In addition, the characteristics and natural course of these disturbing, and often terrifying, side effects, should be explained to the patient, and the patient should be urged to continue taking the antipsychotic medication which has been prescribed.

Hypotension

Orthostatic hypotension and tachycardia are frequent early side effects of chlorpromazine and haloperidol. Tolerance develops to many of the effects of major tranquilizers; for this reason, it is difficult for a patient to take a lethal overdose. High doses may

Table 137D-3. Common Antidepressants

Antidepressant	Type
Amitriptyline (Elavil)	Tricyclic
Doxepin (Adapin, Sinequan)	Tricyclic
Imipramine (Tofranil)	Tricyclic
Maprotiline (Ludiomil)	Tetracyclic
Phenylzine (Nardil)	MAO inhibitor
Tranylcypromine (Parnate)	MAO inhibitor

causes hypotension, central nervous system depression, and seizures. In addition, these drugs potentiate barbiturates, alcohol, and morphine. Blood dyscrasias such as pancytopenia, thrombocytopenic purpura, or eosinophilia, and ophthalmic problems such as pigmentary retinopathy are also occasional adverse effects of major tranquilizers.

Effects of Antidepressants

The two most common groups of antidepressant drugs (see Table 137D-3) are tricyclics and monoamine oxidase inhibitors. Side effects of the tricyclic group are predominantly anticholinergic: dry mouth, dry eyes, double vision, urinary retention. Some psychiatrists believe that these side effects must be evidenced to demonstrate a satisfactory blood level. Tolerance develops over time. These side effects are minimized by lowering the dose, and eliminated by stopping the drug.

Patients on monoamine oxidase inhibitors may experience an adrenergic crisis, including apprehension, chest pain, and pounding headache; a hypertensive crisis with cerebral hemorrhage may be precipitated by ingestion of tyramine-containing foods such as wine and some cheeses. This often represents a medical emergency, and must be treated symptomatically.

One frequently seen side effect of antidepressants is the development of a flagrant psychosis. This usually occurs in a patient for whom the antidepressants were inappropriately prescribed, particularly in a schizophrenic or in a patient with an organic brain disorder. Frequently, one clue is that the prescription was not written by a psychiatrist. This is a drug-induced psychosis, and the appropriate management is to discontinue the medication.

There is no emergency indication for the use of antidepressant medication. The management of antidepressant overdoses is discussed in Chapter 26, "Tricyclic Antidepressants."

PSYCHIATRIC SIDE EFFECTS OF NONPSYCHOTROPIC AGENTS

Frequently patients develop a symptom which they do not relate to ingestion of a medication. When these symptoms are behavioral, the patient or the family may become frightened and come to an emergency department. It is especially important for the emergency physician to identify these drug reactions, since administering an additional drug can complicate the diagnostic problem considerably, and a patient exhibiting psychiatric symptoms is quickly stigmatized.

As has been described above, most psychiatric medications may produce behavioral side effects. Over-the-counter (OTC) drugs for colds, sinus symptoms, allergies, or headache often contain antihistamines, which produce anticholinergic symptoms; many sedatives and pain relievers contain atropinic compounds, which are also anticholinergic. Diet aids, OTC mood elevators, and stimulants produce an amphetamine-like response, including irritability and paranoia. Major tranquilizers, antidepressants, and the antiparkinsonian agents which are frequently prescribed concomitantly with major tranquilizers in order to prevent extrapyramidal side effects all have anticholinergic properties which may be additive. Thus, a patient may be unable to recall the one cold tablet or the eye drops that finally provoked the atropine psychosis, and the family may discount it. The physician must remember to ask directly, and if suspicion remains, to ask repeatedly about any medications. Elderly patients are particularly susceptible, both because of a decreased tolerance and because of an increased likelihood that they will be on multiple medications.

Even if the physician has not observed the particular reaction that the patient is experiencing, discontinuance of a medication may nearly always be advised to see if the behavioral problem improves. Conversely, it is easy to see how administration of an anticholinergic major tranquilizer to a patient exhibiting unusual behavior could cloud the diagnostic picture.

Although all medications have side effects, there are some behavioral reactions commonly associated with prescription drugs. Oral contraceptives may produce depression, and estrogenic compounds may produce mild elevation of mood. Other hormones, such as thyroid hormone, may produce mood elevation, irritability, or psychosis.

Cardiac drugs are associated with a variety of psychiatric effects. Digitalis can produce depression, hallucinations, or a frank psychosis. Quinidine may produce delirium or dementia. Propranolol may produce a toxic psychosis which does not appear to be dose-related.

Antihypertensives may produce depression, which can be exaggerated by hypokalemia, commonly seen in hypertensive patients who are also on diuretics. Methyldopa, as well as guanethidine and clonidine, are known to produce depression. Incidentally, the mechanism of action for guanethidine and clonidine is blocked by the tricyclic antidepressants, which may lead to a frustrating cycle of increasing doses with repeated loss of control of either the blood pressure or depressive symptoms. Cimetidine has been reported to produce delirium, especially in elderly patients or in patients with kidney or liver disease.

Analgesics are frequently implicated in the production of psychiatric symptoms, and are commonly abused because of their effect on the central nervous system. Pentazocine may produce hallucinations; these may also occur during withdrawal. Propoxyphene may produce a psychotic reaction and hallucinations. Both these drugs produce a physiologic dependence. Indomethacin may produce depression; less commonly it also produces an acute psychosis with visual or auditory hallucinations.

Any hypoglycemic agent can produce hypoglycemic reactions with behavioral manifestations, which range from anxiety, irritability, and dysphoria to an acute psychosis.

CHAPTER 138
CRISIS INTERVENTION

Beverly Fauman

Immediate and adequate response to a psychologic crisis can minimize the subsequent morbidity. Precipitating causes can be varied, such as rape, violence or abuse, severe burns, the serious illness or death of a loved one.

Following major national losses, such as Kennedy's assassination, some people experience a threat to their own integrity and some may experience panic. This is not because of the loss itself, but because of the symbolic meaning of it.

Similarly, a seemingly minor loss, such as death of a distant cousin or rejection by a lover, loss of a pet, or a tooth extraction, may produce a feeling of crisis. It is imperative that the emergency physician recognize that the patient's inappropriate response to a crisis will require treatment.

A patient who comes to the emergency department in a panic state may not be able to give relevant information about precipitating factors because of anxiety, confusion, or disorganization.

The interviewer must gather information from family, friends, or observers to determine where and in what condition the patient was found. The first priority is to rule out serious medical illness or injury. Then, if unable to talk immediately, the patient should be taken to a quiet relaxed atmosphere. State that you realize something upsetting has happened to the patient and that you expect to be able to discuss it in a while. The most valuable thing you can do at this point is to tell the patient that you realize he or she has had a terrifying or terrible experience.

Management

Crisis theory maintains that people respond to crises according to their prior ability to cope and according to the meaning of the current crisis to them. While we can all appreciate that it is traumatic to lose a loved one in an accident, it is important to recognize that this trauma would be different for an invalid spouse with several children, for a career woman who was filing for divorce, or for an elderly man with grown, self-sufficient children. A crisis also would be handled differently by someone who had a history of several psychotic depressions following major losses and someone who had experienced a prior serious loss and recovered well.

Use common sense to decide what a normal response should be. If the patient is able to discuss the loss or trauma, responds to your concern and interest, has a reasonable history of dealing with usual life experiences, and is appropriate in manner and speech, you may need only provide an opportunity for the patient to talk. If the patient's concerns seem extreme or bizarre, or if the patient has had serious psychiatric problems in the past and does not respond to your involvement, consider psychiatric consultation.

Encourage the patient to talk about all aspects of the loss or injury: "How did you meet your spouse?" "Do you have any concern that you are responsible for what happened?"

Avoid reassurance. Your role is not to talk the patient out of guilt and grief, but to let the patient share those feelings with someone.

Avoid medication. Any medication in these circumstances delays and impairs the mourning that must be done. It also masks the healing that is occurring, so that you and the patient might come to believe it's the pills that have made the patient feel better, rather than the therapy, setting up a potential for abuse of drugs.

A. Acute Grief Reaction

Emergency physicians are likely to see a great number of acute grief reactions. The responsibilities of the emergency physician are to recognize and facilitate the process of grieving, and to refer patients with pathological grief reactions for appropriate consultation. Proper management and early intervention in severe reactions can result in more rapid adjustment by the patient.

Etiology

An acute grief reaction is the development of an awareness of a sudden loss. Specific events seen in an emergency department frequently resulting in acute grief reaction are sudden infant death syndrome (SIDS), death on arrival (DOA) or in the emergency department (DIE), and death in terminal patients. A patient may deny the actual loss for a time or, conversely, may anticipate the loss of a loved one because of factors such as aging or chronic illness. The loss of anyone or anything in which the patient has placed emotional energy may produce an acute grief reaction. The way that grief is expressed varies according to culture and to personal experience of grief and loss. The physician can gain an appreciation for the patient's way of expressing grief by asking the patient or family members how they mourn, what the rituals of funerals are for them, and what and when other important losses have occurred.

Clinical Features

The first stage of an acute grief reaction can be manifested by disbelief, denial, or a sense of being overwhelmed. Sometimes the loss is so sudden that a panic response occurs, with screaming, moaning, or collapse and inability to move. In some situations, this response may be heightened by the patient's guilt feelings.

The second stage is the sensation of powerlessness over what has happened. There is generally a lot of muscular hyperactivity in this stage, including pacing, handwringing, hair pulling, and crying. When the realization occurs that nothing can be done to restore the loss, the behavior may change to motionlessness, accompanied by despair and sorrow. Fatigue, loss of appetite, and frequent sighing may persist over several days to weeks.

The last stage is the separation reaction. During this stage the mourner acknowledges the loss and its meaning. The more important and complex a relationship, the more difficult it is to let go, or decathect. The major feelings experienced are anxiety and anger at being left behind, and these feelings may be transferred to the living, such as the physician or family members. Anger about the loss implies that the patient recognizes the fact of the loss, and in this sense is healthy. In a normal grief reaction this stage merges with mourning, and the patient gradually "lets go" and develops ways of dealing with the loss so that life can go on.

Assessment of Severity

The severity of a grief reaction is related to the suddenness and importance of the loss, and to the patient's ambivalence about it. Psychiatric consultation or referral should be considered in the following instances:

- Anorexia or fatigue resulting in significant weight loss, or impairment of social relations or ability to work, persisting over 1 month.
- Somatization that results in multiple visits to hospitals, doctors' offices, and emergency departments.
- Use of drugs or alcohol beyond prior habits.
- Poor reality testing such as denial of the loss over several days.
- Inappropriate emotional response to the loss.
- Frank psychosis.

Management

The normal response to an acute loss can be managed by any physician. Treatment consists of helping the patient identify the loss and vent feelings about it. The emergency physician's task is to be receptive to the patient's value system and expression of emotion, to be honest with the patient, and to avoid laying blame or suspicion. The physician should recognize the abnormal or excessive response that requires referral. If the circumstances surrounding a death are unclear, it is not the emergency physician's job to ask questions. Leave that for the police. On the other hand, the physician should not avoid the task of informing the family that their relative is dead, nor should the physician try to avoid the family's grief by sedating them first.

In most instances, use of sedatives or tranquilizers merely delays the necessary psychological tasks, and should be avoided. When the loss has been completely unanticipated or overwhelming, the physician should ensure that provision is made for follow-up care to be certain the patient has had an opportunity to ask questions and enter the states of mourning.

In the special case of SIDS, several issues should be kept in mind. If possible, talk to both parents together initially, assuring them that nothing they have done has caused their child's death. Educate your staff, paramedics, and public safety officials about SIDS, so they do not inadvertently make remarks that are judgmental. Refer the parents for follow-up counseling.

B. Depression

The emergency physician probably encounters depression more frequently than any other psychiatric condition in a usual emergency department population. It is necessary to know some of the differences and similarities between major depression, manic-depressive disorder, and dysthymic disorders.

Mood is the major feature of most depressive disorders. This is expressed in gloominess, hopelessness, loss of sense of humor, boredom, and loss of interest in events, other people, sex, and food. The patient may complain of lack of energy, fatigue, feeling "unwell," and having trouble thinking. Sleep is often disturbed, and waking behavior can often be characterized as restless. Depressive disorders may be recurrent or may consist of a single episode. Prior history of depressive episodes, family history of depression or alcoholism, and a good previous response to antidepressant medication all help to confirm this diagnosis.

Major depression is generally quite demarcated, results in great impairment, and is often characterized more by psychotic or delusional thinking than by the depression itself. A psychotic patient who dwells on physical symptoms, fears of "rotting" or widespread cancer, or thoughts of guilt or worthlessness is most likely suffering a major depression.

Manic-depressive disorder implies that there has been at least one full manic syndrome in the patient's history. This history is useful to obtain because the treatment and prognosis for manic-depressive disorder differs from that of the other depressive disorders.

Manic-depressive disorder is difficult to diagnose as such in the depressive phase on the first admission. There is often a family history of this disorder, and frequently a family history of alcoholism. This diagnosis does not suggest the degree of depression. That is, a patient with manic-depressive disorder may become psychotic and/or suicidal when depressed, or may suffer only moderate lows.

Depression is seen frequently in children as well as adults, and may be expressed as alternative behaviors that are an attempt to handle depressive feelings. Hyperactivity, drug taking, sexual promiscuity, and illegal activities are some behaviors that may be masking depression. Whenever these behaviors are new for the patient, the physician should explore the possibility of depression.

Dysthymic disorder is a depression which has been fairly constant for 2 years or more. It may become worse, but in general it persists as a mild to moderate depressive state which is often unresponsive to medication. Patients may report that they have tried "everything."

The psychiatric conditions that one may entertain in a differential diagnosis of depression include hysterical personality, manipulative personality, and psychosis with depression as one symptom. Remember that depressed patients frequently make the physician feel angry, and that both hysterics and manipulative patients often have an element of depression. The differentiating points include how recent, recurrent, and persistent the patient's symptoms are.

The emergency physician should be capable of assessing the severity of the depression and of making an appropriate disposition.

Failure to recognize the type and degree of depression may lead to unnecessary medical evaluation, or an inappropriate disposition for a potentially self-destructive patient.

Symptoms

Physical symptoms are usually the patient's major concern, and are often not recognized as psychiatric in origin, leading to unnecessary laboratory tests. These commonly include:

- Change in sleep pattern; usually early morning awakening but may be increased sleep.
- Change in appetite; usually a decrease but may be increased eating with weight gain.
- Change in bowel pattern; usually constipation.
- Change in activity, libido; usually fatigue and loss of interest but may be hyperactivity.

Less common symptoms include:

- Depressed mood.
- Inability to get pleasure out of work, hobbies, sex.
- Retardation of thought, speech, activity.
- Sense of worthlessness.
- Agitation, handwringing, pacing.
- False joviality, casualness.
- Psychotic symptoms, including paranoid delusions or delusions of severe bodily illness, damage, or decay.
- Improvement in the afternoons and evenings.
- Lack of concern about appearance, accident-proneness.
- Suicidal thoughts.

Medical History

Ask about any recent illness, especially life-threatening ones. After the initial flurry of activity around such disorders as myocardial infarct or cholecystectomy, the patient experiences a depression at the time when the relatives and physician may be expecting full recovery. The patient often misinterprets this depression as recurrence of the initial illness, and seeks medical attention for symptoms similar to the original ones.

Chronic illness, in particular that associated with alcoholism, often leads to depression. In addition, the patient who is under frequent or constant medical attention may look to physicians to solve life's problems. When a patient with a chronic illness comes to an emergency department with complaints of anything other than an obvious emergency, the emergency physician should determine whether the issue is a psychological problem rather than a medical one.

A careful drug history is important in connection with the medical history. Many drugs are recognized as potentially depressive: methyldopa (Aldomet), propranolol, reserpine, guanethidine, birth control pills. In addition, these give clues to medical conditions the patient may not have mentioned. Minor tranquilizers can exacerbate depression. Antidepressant prescriptions suggest a prior depression or another physician's recognition of depression.

Psychiatric History

The pertinent areas to explore in the emergency assessment of depression include prior psychiatric illness and treatment, prior history of depression, and history of suicide attempts. The physician should inquire about any recent or potential life change which may have precipitated the depression, such as illness or death of a relative, serious medical illness, divorce, job loss, graduation, or move.

In order to make a proper disposition, the physician must know what sort of support is available in the patient's environment. Family history of depression and suicide is important also.

Management

Both in determining the degree of depression and the appropriate disposition, the emergency physician should pay careful attention to the feelings engendered by the patient. If the patient is responsive to an empathic physician, and feels better after a brief interview, the patient is likely going to respond well to psychotherapy. Conversely, a sense of hopelessness and frustration hanging over the interview suggests the patient would be better off in a hospital. If for any reason you are uncomfortable letting the patient leave the emergency department when you have diagnosed a depression, obtain a specialty consultation, or if none is available, hospitalize the patient.

Giving a patient the diagnosis ''depression'' and explaining it as a genuine illness, usually self-limited, is a major aspect of emergency management. On the other hand, one should avoid rationalizing the patient's illness, trying to talk the patient out of it, making light of it, or prescribing drugs. Antidepressants take 2 to 3 weeks to work in those patients for whom they are appropriate, so should only be prescribed by the physician who will be following the patient. A patient often interprets the prescription as the physician's way to terminate the contact, especially when it is not given in the context of an ongoing therapeutic relationship.

Disposition

The two issues of concern to the emergency physician in the matter of depression are: (1) to diagnose it and identify it to the patient and family, and (2) to respond adequately to the life threat. Referral to a psychiatrist is indicated when the depression is repeated or prolonged, especially if it is affecting the patient's ability to work, interact socially, or function physically. Hospitalization is indicated when the physician feels that the patient is unable to follow through with referral recommendations, when the social supports are absent or destructive, when the patient's current or past history indicates that the illness will worsen without hospitalization, if there is evidence of inability to function in essential daily activities, or if there is evidence that the patient cannot control suicidal thoughts. Mild, reactive depression in a functioning adult will respond to an empathic initial interview and two to three follow-up visits with no medication.

C. Suicide

In the practice of emergency medicine, one of the most frequent and uncomfortable psychiatric problems encountered is the assessment of the patient who is self-identified as suicidal, makes an apparent suicide attempt, or is brought to the emergency department by others who believe the patient to be suicidal. Although there are some predictors of high or low suicide risk, these data may serve only to confirm one's concern, and not to decrease concern, for a particular patient.

Factors Associated with Suicide Risk

The following factors are associated with increased suicide risk.

Gender (male)
Age (older)
Marital status (divorced, widowed, estranged)
Home life (single, childless, socially isolated)
Substance abuse
Chronic illness, especially psychiatric illness
History of unemployment
Family history of suicide, depression, or alcoholism
Prior suicide attempt

Men *commit* suicide two to three times more frequently than women, generally by more violent techniques. Women *attempt* it three to four times more frequently. Although the risk for suicide increases with age, recently there have been an increasing number of suicides in males aged 15 to 30. The unemployed, unskilled worker is high risk, but persons who feel that they are not fulfilling their occupational role, even if their position may be that of a skilled, white-collar worker, are also at an increased risk. Although difficult economic conditions may contribute to depression

and difficulty in interpersonal relationships, a change in economic status rather than poverty itself is associated with a greater suicide risk. Single people, followed by the widowed, divorced, or separated, are at a higher risk than married persons, especially those with children.

Manic-depressive illness may lead to suicide more frequently than other psychiatric conditions, but this is an uncommon illness. Depression, on the other hand, is very common, and is frequently seen in association with suicidal thoughts and behavior. Schizophrenic patients may give bizarre warnings of their impending suicide, and are therefore harder to assess. When they do make suicide attempts, they frequently use unusual or bizarre means, sometimes with magical or symbolic ideas. The peculiar choices schizophrenics may use for suicide efforts, or the unusual explanations they give for the conditions in which they are found when attempting suicide, should not deter the physician from recognizing the seriousness of the attempt. Schizophrenics also often do not express depression in an easily recognizable way, further masking the intentions of their suicidal behavior.

There is a category of patients known commonly as ''borderlines''; that is, their symptoms lie somewhere between psychosis and neurosis. Certain characteristics of emergency medicine tend to appeal to this group, so that they may be disproportionately overrepresented in the emergency department. The transience of the doctor-patient relationship, the immediacy of response, and the implied power of an institution all satisfy needs of the borderline patient. Furthermore, these patients may be impulsive and dramatic, as well as exquisitely sensitive to changes in their environment, all of which may provoke suicide attempts. To complicate the picture still further, a number of these patients are ''cutters,'' and this cutting behavior must be understood in quite a different manner. Some borderline patients have difficulty maintaining their certainty about their own existence. Stresses such as termination of a relationship, failure on the job or in school, or physical injury may lead them to "need" an experience which proves to them that they exist. Cutting across a forearm or thigh to draw blood is such an experience for them, and does not constitute a suicide attempt. These patients may have scars from prior cutting or cigarette burns; they may be quite insistent that they are not suicidal, or that you just don't understand. They may also have a history of multiple unsuccessful attempts at psychiatric treatment, since these patients are very difficult to treat. The emergency physician must still make an effort to determine suicidal intent and the potential lethality of the attempt, and obtain a consultation when this effort is inconclusive.

Alcoholism and drug abuse are frequently associated with suicide. Unfortunately, because alcohol and many drugs used in suicide attempts are central nervous system depressants, the patient's behavior shortly after an ingestion is colored by the physiologic effect of the agent selected. Alcohol is quite commonly one of the drugs used when the patient takes an overdose of more than one drug. This may be related to one or more of the following. While alcohol is a depressant, it is also a disinhibitor, allowing a patient to overcome a normal reluctance toward self-inflicted harm. Alcohol impairs judgment, so that a patient might take more sedatives or analgesics than are appropriate (or than were intended). Finally, alcohol is synergistic with other CNS depressants, producing a lethal level faster than would alcohol or other depressants alone.

The act or threat of self-injury increases the risk of suicide. Patients who have made a previous suicide attempt are five to six times more likely to commit suicide. This is particularly true when the prior attempt was life-threatening. Similarly, patients who have had serious or frequent accidental injuries should be questioned about suicide intent. In one review of suicides, 47 percent had a history of a prior attempt, and 16 percent had been to an emergency department immediately before the suicide.

A family history of suicide, depression, or alcoholism is associated with an increased risk of depression and suicide.

Precipitating Causes

A patient who is depressed is more likely to commit suicide. Masked depression may be compounded if hypnotics, minor tranquilizers, or analgesics have inadvertently been prescribed to treat symptoms of depression.

Medical conditions that heighten the frequency of suicide attempts are recent surgery, intractable pain, and debilitating chronic illness.

A patient is at very high risk for suicide when he or she can see no other way out of a dilemma, or has no other way to vent feelings. A sense of hopelessness or helplessness, or an inability to communicate one's distress, may lead to a suicide attempt. Any recent life change, especially a loss, increases the possibility of suicide. A patient who is terminating relationships, who is putting affairs in order, or who seems to be withdrawing from responsibilities should be questioned about suicide. Further, a patient who has been depressed, or possibly psychotic, who suddenly appears to improve, should be watched closely for suicidal behavior. The apparent improvement may have occurred when the patient recognizes a solution for painful feelings, namely, suicide.

Patients Who Threaten or Attempt Suicide

Patients who talk about suicide, even casually, should be taken seriously, and evaluated for acute suicide risk and current psychiatric illness. Apparent lightheartedness may indicate anxiety, depression, uneasiness with the subject, or provocativeness. Manipulation, the so-called gesture, and attention seeking are cries for help just as much as suicide threats. Such a patient is trying to communicate something, even if it is not suicidal ideas.

The extent to which this communication is heard is frequently a measure of the remaining risk. A patient who has made a serious suicide attempt because of feelings that the spouse doesn't care, and whose spouse is present, very concerned and upset, and willing to engage in marital therapy, is now at a much lower risk. Conversely, a young woman who takes a few minor tranquilizers to show a boyfriend that she wants more affection, and whose boyfriend is uninvolved, cynical, or absent, may well make a more serious effort to harm herself. Unfortunately for the emergency department, the boyfriend who does respond to the overdose often reinforces that kind of attention-getting behavior.

Ask the patient about the reason for the visit to the emergency department, and determine what the patient is looking for as a response to the expression of suicidal thoughts, the overdose, the wrist-cutting, etc. Further evaluation should include the following:

1. Has the patient contemplated suicide before?
2. Are there current reasons for the patient to consider suicide? Ask specifically about changes in work, health, and intimate relationships. Is he or she a victim of abuse?
3. Is there a prior history of psychiatric illness? Ask about depressive symptoms, including weight loss, sleep disturbance, hopelessness, apathy, and helplessness.

In evaluating the seriousness of a suicide attempt, assess the intent and lethality of the method selected, note who rescued the patient, and observe the level of hope maintained by the patient. To determine intent, note whether the method selected was likely to work, and if it was a logical method for the patient's level of education and cultural background. Consider whether the patient's survival was sheer luck or reasonably predictable. Even if the patient claims not to realize the dangerousness of such actions, the lethality of the method chosen is an important measure of future suicide risk.

One way to get a feeling for the patient's intent is to ask about premonitions before an accident. A patient may be more willing to acknowledge these than to accept direct responsibility for driving too fast, being too casual around dangerous machinery, or mixing alcohol and a prescription drug.

Questions to Assess Suicide Intent

- Have you thought about suicide?
- How long have you been depressed and how hard is it to shake the feeling?
- How do you handle yourself socially, emotionally, and at work?
- How is your appetite?
- Are you sexually active?
- Do you have frequent backache or other physical complaints?
- Have you attempted suicide before, or do you know anyone who has committed suicide?
- What's stopping you?

Was the attempt made at a time when it was unlikely the patient would be found in time? Who discovered the patient? Note the patient's reaction to being found (i.e., angry or relieved).

Management of the Patient Who Threatens or Attempts Suicide

Any patient who talks about suicide should be taken seriously. It should be assumed that the patient who is talking about suicide wants to be stopped. The patient who wants to commit suicide won't be sitting in the emergency department. The emergency physician's responsibility is to listen to and acknowledge the patient's distress, not to try to talk the patient out of it. The patient should not be judged, chastised, or chided. The physician should avoid bargaining and not be intimidated by the patient's anger or threats. Suicidal patients may make a physician feel helpless, anxious, or angry. The physician must recognize these feelings so that they do not interfere with an objective assessment of suicide potential.

On the basis of the patient's response to your evaluation, you have the following choices. Hospitalization is indicated for the patient you believe is acutely suicidal, or who is unable to assume responsibility for controlling suicidal impulses. If the patient is unwilling to discuss suicidal thoughts, mood, or the events leading up to the suicide act, you might also consider hospitalization. Request a psychiatric consultation when you are not sure how acute the life threat is or you are unable to determine why the patient is talking about suicide, and you are unable to devote the time to such an exploration. If you are comfortable that the patient is not actually suicidal, you may discharge and refer to or recommend psychiatric help. If the patient seems responsive to your concern and experiences some relief during the interview, psychotherapy will probably be of benefit. Consider asking the patient to return for further evaluation in a day or two if the patient is unwilling to accept a referral. The patient's sense that you remain concerned, coupled with any sense of discomfort in the interim, may make a patient more willing to consider psychiatric evaluation. The opportunity for an emergency physician to see a depressed patient on no medication in follow-up 2 to 3 days later may also demonstrate the impact that this interpersonal encounter can have. In each instance, document your decision and the rationale for it.

Responsible family members should be told about the patient's potential for suicide, but only after the patient has been told that the family will be so informed. The patient should always know there is someone to talk to, but the emergency physician is generally not the individual who will provide long-term follow-up care.

A relative contraindication to hospitalization is the passive-dependent or borderline personality disorder. These patients often wish to be taken care of completely and do not understand that their behavior produces their problems. They find the staff on inpatient psychiatric units so giving, protective, and tolerant that they resist discharge and may say or do anything to achieve subsequent hospitalizations. One clue to these disorders is a history of an unusually brief (less than 3 days) or inordinately long (greater than 6 months) prior hospitalization. Another clue is that the hospital where the patient was previously hospitalized is unwilling to accept the patient for rehospitalization. However, even the borderline patient may become suicidal. If you believe the patient is acutely suicidal, you must hospitalize or obtain a psychiatric consultation.

If you are uneasy about discharging a patient who might be suicidal, consult with someone more experienced in the management of a suicidal patient, or hospitalize the patient.

Legal Issues

It is difficult to find the emergency physician at fault if he or she inadvertently discharges a patient who subsequently commits suicide. The lack of specialty psychiatric training, and the inability to gain in-depth knowledge about a patient through long-term care allows some leeway for judgment errors. Remember that the emergency physician does not commit a patient to a psychiatric hospital, but merely detains a patient until a psychiatrist can conduct an examination and start the proceedings for a legal, court-ordered commitment.

The emergency physician must document findings and recommendations in relation to suicidal patients. In the case of a patient who returns more than once, the physician should reassess suicide potential at each visit. A physician should never refuse to see or treat a self-destructive patient. The patient should not be allowed to sign out against medical advice. If a patient who may be suicidal wants to sign out before an adequate assessment has been made, the patient must be detained by whatever means are necessary until the physician can state that the patient is not likely to be acutely suicidal.

D. Psychophysiologic Reactions

A psychophysiologic reaction is a medical condition precipitated by an event with heavy emotional overlay. The medical symptoms may be short-lived, or require medical intervention that also addresses the psychologic aspects. Psychosomatic illness, an outdated term now included under psychophysiologic reaction, refers to symptoms or illnesses, such as peptic ulcer disease, that result in actual pathologic tissue changes.

Everyone experiences psychophysiologic reactions, such as diarrhea before an important examination, headache after an annoying encounter, or a dry mouth before giving a speech. The experience of a bodily change is real, and the emotional precipitant, which is usually helplessness or anger, can often be recognized. There are many symptoms and illnesses that are frequently considered psychophysiologic, such as irritable bowel, headache, asthma, ulcers, or neurodermatitis. The emergency physician should pursue a suspicion of such disease with appropriate questions. A patient who suggests or wonders if some event brought on the symptoms should be encouraged to talk about that possibility to see if there is a connection.

Medical evaluation should be pursued if there are indications that a disease may be present. Unlike conversion reactions (see Chapter 138E), where extensive medical evaluation may make the patient worse, psychophysiologic reactions do have physical components that may need treatment. As in a conversion reaction, the patient may escape an emotional stress by means of the symptom.

Clinical Features

The only absolute confirmation of a psychophysiologic reaction is repeated episodes of physiologic change after similar emotional stimuli. The probability is heightened when any of the following are true: (1) the patient has reacted similarly to the stimulus in the past, (2) the patient believes the symptom was stimulated by an emotional stress ("I got this headache after an argument with my boss"), (3) the patient has a history of one of the more typical psychophysiologic reactions such as asthma, neurodermatitis, or irritable bowel, and (4) there is a family history of one of the more typical psychophysiologic reactions.

Patients who somaticize, with real impairment of their ability to function, are not doing it consciously and do not have control over it. Because they are victims of their own bodies, they often present at the height of their illness as helpless and regressed. The reactions of the physician toward the patient can be varied. The physician who recognizes the probable psychologic etiology but does not appreciate the subconscious aspect may feel anger toward the patient, or may not take the medical component seriously. On the other hand, the physician may recognize the subconscious aspect but may become angry when the patient does not accept the diagnosis and refuses a psychiatric referral. Finally, the emergency physician may feel angry and manipulated when the patient shows up repeatedly in the emergency department with the same complaints.

Treatment

The patient who somaticizes, that is, who uses physical illness to express or resolve emotional conflicts, is frequently unable to see the connection. If it were possible to make such a connection, the patient would not need to get sick. Confrontation will only make such a patient angry, defensive, or sicker. The physician should first treat the medical condition. As that is being brought under control, the patient can be approached with questions about the possible emotional precipitant. For example, the time to take a few minutes to explore such questions with an asthmatic is after the wheezing has been relieved and the patient can breathe easily again. If such a patient begins to wheeze again during such a discussion, a dramatic demonstration will have occurred, for the physician at least.

The role of the emergency physician is to raise the question with the patient or to make the initial connection. However, the psychological issues behind psychophysiologic illness are so deep-rooted that they may require special intervention. The ideal long-term management of psychophysiologic illness is combined medical and psychiatric treatment. The patient needs the assurance that the medical problems will receive adequate attention before being able to explore the psychologic events that trigger them. There is no need for an emergency psychiatric consultation on these patients, but the consistent message from the emergency physician should be that the patient ought to seek psychiatric consultation.

E. Conversion Reaction

A conversion reaction is produced when a patient unconsciously converts a psychological conflict into a physical symptom that both expresses the conflict and helps resolve or avoid it. It is one of the most intriguing psychiatric syndromes that may be seen in the emergency department. The fact that such patients have to resort to a conversion reaction to deal with a difficult situation is a strong indication that they are not intuitive or insightful, and they will probably not be amenable to psychotherapy. The first physician to see such patients usually has the best chance of relieving them.

Two common misconceptions are that (1) conversion reactions occur only in young, hysterical females, and (2) that patients know they are faking.

A conversion reaction can occur in any person who feels trapped by a circumstance or by a strong feeling and has no other outlet.

The conversion symptom in some way gets the patient out of a difficult situation. For example, a man who is belittled by his employer but fears telling off the employer or quitting because he needs the job, may abruptly develop laryngitis. This enables him to keep working but prevents him from speaking up. Or a wife may suddenly develop paralysis of her legs because she is overwhelmed by her husband's demands in terms of housework, but feels she cannot ask him for help because he is studying for graduate exams. She is able to get around in a wheelchair and cook and care for the children, but she can no longer scrub floors and do other heavy housework.

The onset of a conversion reaction is sudden, usually in relation to a particular event and in an emotionally charged setting. The patient appears healthy and less concerned about the symptom that one would expect. The family does not appear insightful, and is often oversolicitous, in contrast to the patient's lack of concern. There is often a history of a curious undiagnosed prior illness that subsided spontaneously or even ''miraculously.'' Recurrence is not unusual and it may or may not be manifested by the same symptom.

Clinical Features

Conversion symptoms typically involve voluntary muscles, although they may, of course, take virtually any form. Pain is not a common conversion symptom. The most frequent complaints are motor disturbances, followed by sensory disturbances. The symptoms may either mimic physical illness or complicate existing physical illness. The symptom must have some explanation in terms of the dilemma it resolves. This can be determined by asking patients what they would do if they didn't have the symptom, what it keeps them from doing, or what they were doing or about to do when the symptom began. Such patients are not faking; that is, they do not have conscious control over the symptom, did not choose it, and are not aware or willing to accept that it is psychological. Therefore, questioning must proceed gently, that is, to gather information, not to confront patients or get them to admit or ''see'' what is really occurring.

A conversion reaction can mimic any condition. Therefore, the diagnosis should be made by suspecting or recognizing the symptoms rather than by excluding other possibilities. The most difficult differential diagnoses are organic neurologic or muscular disease, schizophrenia, and malingering or other factitious illnesses.

Malingering is the conscious complaining of a symptom that doesn't exist to avoid or get out of doing an unpleasant duty, excite sympathy, or gain compensation. The malingerer may have a great emotional investment in convincing the physician of an illness, in contrast with the conversion patient, who may appear relatively unconcerned over whether you find anything wrong. A more sophisticated type of factitious illness may be seen in the patient with Munchausen syndrome. This patient seems to have an investment in convincing the physician of the authenticity of the symptoms, can be quite sophisticated in medical terminology, diagnostic procedures, and physical findings, and usually has an extensive medical history. Hypochondriasis is not likely to be confused with conversion reaction because of the overconcern seen in the hypochondriacal patient.

A good history and physical examination, a thorough neurological examination, and the physician's ability to recognize an ill patient are the best diagnostic tools. The sooner a conversion reaction is identified, the more amenable it is to treatment. Conversely, multiple laboratory tests, specialty consultations, and other delays in defining the illness make it more entrenched and harder to treat.

Treatment

Once the physician has a reasonable idea why the patient has a particular conversion symptom, a solution can be prescribed. The solution must (1) respond to the dilemma, and (2) be face-saving for the patient. In the first example above, the physician helped the patient search for alternatives to deal with his boss when his voice got better. In addition, the physician prescribed a benign throat spray, emphasizing that it would provide relief over the next 3 days. In the second case, the wife was advised to take a rest period twice daily for the next week. She was informed she could expect gradual return of leg function and encouraged to plan realistic activities to avoid becoming overtired. The husband was cautioned that his wife's symptoms could recur if she became overtired.

F. Acute Anxiety Reactions and Panic Attacks

Anxiety reactions and panic attacks are somewhat similar to conversion reactions in that strong emotions are being expressed in physical terms. Variations of anxiety reactions include hyperventilation, panic attacks, and homosexual panic. Amnesia may also be an expression of severe acute anxiety. Patients who experience these syndromes commonly have serious psychological impairment which has been present for a long time. The immediate task is to stabilize such patients by helping them to relax and to master the current anxiety. You may also be able to help them recognize that there is a relationship between the symptoms they are now experiencing and a recent event.

Clinical Features

Patients experiencing an acute anxiety reaction or panic attack may believe they have an acute medical problem. In fact, they have converted a psychological conflict into physical symptoms and may complain of feeling fearful, being nauseous, feeling pressure in the chest, or suffocating. They may believe they are having a heart attack, stroke, or asthmatic attack. Tachycardia, tremors, diaphoresis, and hyperventilation may be present. As in a conversion reaction, if such patients recognized their emotional conflict, they wouldn't need to experience medical symptoms. It is important for the physician to realize that these patients are not in control of their symptoms, are not faking, and are not able to immediately identify the correct precipitant. Since such patients may be uncomfortable, uncooperative, impatient, and unreasonable, it is important for triage personnel to recognize that these patients believe they are truly ill and that they are not being consciously manipulative. If in fact the anxiety attack has been triggered by the phenomenon known as homosexual panic, it is additionally important that the emergency department staff not contribute to the problem by being too solicitous, too reassuring, or too friendly.

Assessment

The factors the emergency physician should ascertain from the patient, family, or old records include prior history of such attacks, prior psychiatric history, prior prescriptions for similar symptoms, and an obvious precipitant.

A patient who has repeated anxiety attacks may have an underlying depression or even a psychosis. A prior psychiatric history, particularly a hospitalization, lends more weight to this possibility. Incidentally, the most likely cause of acute anxiety in a patient who is currently under psychiatric care is the vacation or absence of the therapist for other reasons. A patient asking for diazepam may not be merely manipulative, since a fair number of patients with acute anxiety do well with minor tranquilizers. Homosexual panic occurs when someone is exposed to a number of individuals of the same sex and experiences sexual thoughts or feelings. Although these feelings are normal and may occur in anyone, they are usually repressed and may be intolerable for some people. Clues to the occurrence of a homosexual panic are that the patient was recently placed in a jail, dormitory, or barracks, and is now paranoid or loudly protesting that he or she is not homosexual.

The patient with no psychiatric history, no organic etiology, and for whom a likely precipitant can be elicited can be managed as an acute grief reaction, using as a focus a loss of self-esteem or a feeling of incompetence.

Management

A brief physical assessment, including vital signs, should precede the psychiatric evaluation. If the patient clearly perceives these anxiety reactions as foreign or abnormal, the physician should consider an organic etiology such as caffeinism, hyperthyroidism, hypoglycemia, or pheochromocytoma, which have similar signs and symptoms. An appropriate history and laboratory studies should be obtained to rule out these conditions. A number of drugs may produce anxiety, including, of course, many street drugs, stimulants, and antidepressants, as can withdrawal from any central nervous system depressant, including alcohol. If the patient is experiencing homosexual panic, it may be necessary to have a physician of the opposite sex perform the physical examination, or to defer all but the vital signs until later. Crowding, touching, or helpful overtures may provoke such a patient to violence.

After the physical examination, the physician should state that something has occurred in the patient's life that preceded the anxiety attack, and ask the patient what happened. A calm manner and willingness to listen will generally relieve the patient rapidly. An anxiety or panic reaction may be precipitated by loss of a significant other, a job or living situation, or self-esteem. If the patient mentions such a loss, the physician should restate it, adding empathic statements such as "You lost your (blank)? That really would have infuriated me!" This gives the patient authoritative approval for feelings that may be embarrassing and a model for future reference. Avoid trivializing responses, such as "So what are you so upset about? That's nothing to get so worked up over." A patient who has frequent anxiety reactions is usually quite suggestible and will respond to reassurance by and confidence in the caretaker. Conversely, an anxious or unorganized physician or other caretaker may only compound the patient's trouble.

Minor tranquilizers often relieve symptoms of an acute anxiety reaction but should not be given by the emergency physician for the following reasons:

- These drugs will often make the patient worse if the anxiety is only a surface symptom of an underlying severe depression or psychosis.
- A potential for abuse is set up if the anxiety is relieved by minor tranquilizers and the patient has not identified or mastered the precipitant. Furthermore, the patient will likely not accept follow-up and will repeatedly return to the emergency department for future attacks.
- Minor tranquilizers interfere with the working-through process. If the precipitant is identified, the patient needs to go through this process to master the anxiety.

If the patient has been treated often in the past with medication, he or she may be unwilling to talk at all. In this instance, after a genuine attempt to get the patient to talk, as the emergency physician you may call for a consultation or explain to the patient that although medication has been prescribed in the past, you do not think that is appropriate treatment for this condition at this time. A psychiatrist would often use a low dose of a major tranquilizer rather than a minor tranquilizer in this setting.

Patients should be encouraged to seek follow-up at a community mental health clinic or with a private psychiatrist, since the problem will most likely recur. A full homosexual panic may require emergency psychiatric hospitalization.

CHAPTER 139
ACUTE PSYCHOSIS
AND ORGANIC
BRAIN DISORDERS

Beverly Fauman

The concept of emergency psychiatry generally suggests that one will see primarily acutely psychotic and, therefore, dangerous patients. In fact, however, the acute psychotic patient is analogous to the severe multiple-trauma patient—exciting, somewhat frightening, but luckily not representative of the majority of emergency department patients. Patients who are acutely psychotic may be confused, hallucinating, or frankly disruptive. They must be managed and evaluated in a thoughtful manner, so that life-threatening conditions are not missed and no one is harmed.

Initial Management

The emergency physician should perform an adequate physical and mental evaluation before obtaining psychiatric consultation and before administering psychiatric medication.

Instruct triage personnel to handle patients with acute psychosis as a medical emergency. Although patients may be ambulatory, they are potentially injurious to themselves or others. The emergency department should have a designated area close to the regular treatment areas where such patients can be separated from other patients and where lights can be dimmed. Request that staff, family, or police who are too frightened to be useful move away from this area. Some staff members who are experienced with psychiatric patients and unafraid may achieve cooperation by "talking down," that is, calmly and repetitively orienting and reassuring the agitated patient. However, an anxious, frightened staff member may cause the patient to behave worse. If the talk-down is not sufficient, apply adequate physical restraints. Do not administer drugs before further assessment unless the patient's psychiatric history is known and it indicates that antipsychotic medication is warranted. In any case, give only enough medication to calm the patient, not induce sleep.

Perhaps the most important task of the emergency physician is to identify those psychotic patients whose behavior is caused or compounded by organic brain disease, for treatable causes of organic psychosis are multiple and delay in treatment can be dangerous. Numerous studies demonstrate that many patients who appear to have a psychiatric illness actually have an underlying medical disorder which is producing the behavioral symptoms.

There is no single pathognomonic sign or symptom that consistently distinguishes organic brain disorders from "functional" disease. In addition, it may be difficult to distinguish which aspects of a patient's abnormal behavior are the direct result of organic brain disorders, and which are psychological reactions to the organic impairment. Many patients become paranoid or angry when they are experiencing organic brain deficits. Depression is also a common reaction to impaired mental function. Usually, several clinical features in the history, behavior, and mental status examination alert the physician to the likelihood of organic illness. Sometimes only repeated observations may clarify the diagnosis.

In the history, note if this is the first episode, whether it began abruptly, and when it occurred, and describe the premorbid personality. Even if there were prior episodes, a thorough medical evaluation is indicated if this episode is different. Determine if there is any medical illness present such as diabetes, hyperthyroidism, hypertension, renal or hepatic disease, infection, epilepsy, or collagen disease. Look for evidence of precedent trauma; drug or alcohol intoxication; infection; pulmonary embolism; fat embolism; or anoxia on the basis of pulmonary or cardiovascular disease, hypovolemia, or carbon monoxide poisoning.

In eliciting information about the drug history, note if the patient is receiving any medications, and consider the possibility of illicit drug ingestion by noting whether there are needle track marks or odor of alcohol. A competent neurological examination including vital signs is necessary. Be sure to record this in as much detail as possible, since "soft" neurological signs may be the only clue to a diagnosis for several hours or days. A good mental status examination is also indicated.

Working Diagnosis

Clues that may be helpful in differentiating organic versus functional disorders are listed in Table 139-1. However, it is important to appreciate that organic mental disorders can mimic almost any psychiatric illness. It is particularly difficult to establish a diagnosis of either "functional" psychosis or organic brain disorder in a young, previously healthy individual on the basis of a single emergency department examination.

Table 139-1. Differentiation of Organic versus Functional Psychosis

Organic	Functional
Presence of medical illness or abnormal physical finding. Patient has seen a physician recently and may be taking medication, has had a recent change in dosage, or may have taken a street drug	No apparent medical cause
No prior psychiatric history	Prior psychiatric history
Confused, disoriented	
Disturbance of judgment, memory, or cognitive functioning	
Recognizes behavioral changes as abnormal	Acceptance of behavior as normal
	Aural hallucinations more common
Hallucinations	Visual hallucinations are uncommon

The young patient with an acute, functional psychosis, with a history of successful employment, ability to relate to other people, and ability for self-care, has a good prognosis if managed well. Outpatient management by a well-staffed psychiatric clinic or private psychiatrist who is comfortable with these patients may prevent not only this initial hospitalization, but also future hospitalizations. Aggressive psychiatric management at this point is invaluable, and it is worth every effort on the part of the emergency department to secure it. The patient who has had multiple psychiatric hospitalizations, is unable to hold jobs, has no interested family and a poor record of follow-up care is not going to get much better when the psychosis remits, and may do as well (if not better) in a state psychiatric facility.

The patient with an organic etiology or component to the psychiatric disorder must be managed in a medical setting, since psychiatric hospitals are neither equipped nor sufficiently well staffed to manage the medical aspects of patient care.

The emergency physician should not administer medication to the acute psychotic unless it is absolutely essential to the emergency department management of the patient. The physician who will ultimately care for the patient should be able to observe the patient unmedicated, and to decide what medication to use.

BIBLIOGRAPHY

Beck S, Blum HT, Gale MS, et al: Psychiatric training for emergency medicine residents on a multidisciplinary team. *JACEP* 5:694, 1976.

Denner LJ: Benzodiazepine withdrawal psychosis. *JAMA* 237:36, 1977.

Donlon PT, Hopkin J, Tupin JP: Overview: Efficacy and safety of the rapid neuroleptization method with injectable haloperidol. *Am J Psychiatry* 136:273, 1979.

Fauman BJ, Fauman MA: Recognition and management of drug abuse emergencies. *Comp Therapy* 4:38, 1978.

Fauman MA: The emergency psychiatric evaluation of organic mental disorders. *Psychiatr Clin of North Am,* 1983.

Fauman MA: Treatment of the agitated patient with an organic brain disorder. *JAMA* 240:380, 1978.

Fauman MA, Fauman BJ: The differential diagnosis of organic based psychiatric disturbance in the emergency department. *JACEP* 6:315, 1977.

Gardner ER, Hall RCW: Psychiatric symptoms produced by over-the-counter drugs. *Psychosomatics* 23:186, 1982.

Gerson S, Bassuk E: Psychiatric emergencies: An overview. *Am J Psychiatry* 137(1):1, 1980.

Glasscote R, Cummings E, Hammersley D, et al: *The Psychiatric Emergency: A Study of Patterns of Service.* Washington, DC, Joint Information Service (APA-NAMH), 1966.

Goodwin JM, Goodwin JS, Kellner R: Psychiatric symptoms in disliked medical patients. *JAMA* 241:1117, 1979.

Groves JE: Borderline personality disorder. *N Engl J Med* 305:259, 1981.

Guirguis EF: Management of disturbed patients: An alternative to the use of mechanical restraints. *J Clin Psychol* 39:295, 1978.

Hankoff LD, Mischorr MT, Tomlinson K, Joyce SA: A program of crisis intervention in the emergency medical setting. *Am J Psychiatry* 131(1):47, 1974.

Johnson R, Trimble C: The (expletive deleted) shouter. *JACEP* 4:333, 1975.

Kahn RL, Zarit S, Hilbert NM, Niederehe G: Memory complaint and impairment in the aged. *Arch Gen Psychiatry* 32:1569, 1975.

Kass F, Karasu TB, Walsh T: Emergency room patients in concurrent therapy: A neglected clinical phenomenon. *Am J Psychiatry* 136:91, 1979.

Kovacs M, Beck A, Weissman M: The communication of suicidal intent. *Arch Gen Psychiatry* 33:198, 1976.

Kresojevich R, Krome RL, Sellman G: The emergency department groupy. *JACEP* 3(2):81, 1974.

Lee A: Drug-induced dystonic reactions. *JACEP* 8:453, 1979.

Leeman CP: Diagnostic errors in emergency room medicine: Physical illness in patients labeled "psychiatric" and vice versa. *Intl J Psychiatry Med* 6(4):533, 1975.

Levy R, Gale MS: Interactional approach to the difficult emergency department patient. *JACEP* 7(1):7, 1977.

Lindemann E: Symptomatology and management of acute grief. *Am J Psychiatry* 101:141, 1944.

Mannon JM: Defining and treating "problem patients" in a hospital emergency room. *Med Care* 14:1004, 1976.

Mattsson EI: Psychological aspects of severe physical injury and its treatment. *J Traum* 15:217, 1975.

Nelson JC, Charney DS: The symptoms of major depressive illness. *Am J Psychiatry* 138:1, 1981.

Ott DA, Goeden SR: Treatment of acute phenothiazine reaction. *JACEP* 8:471, 1979.

Rada RT: The violent patient: Rapid assessment and management. *Psychosomatics* 22:101, 1981.

Robbins E, Stern M, Robbins L, et al: Unwelcome patients: Where can they find asylum? *Hosp Comm Psychiatry* 29:44, 1978.

Robbins ES, Hanin E, Moore A, et al: Transfers to a psychiatric emergency room: A fresh look at the dumping syndrome. *Psychiatr Q* 49:197, 1977.

Schnaper N, Cowley RA: Overview: Psychiatric sequelae to multiple trauma. *Am J Psychiatry* 133:883, 1976.

Slaby AE: Emergency psychiatry: An update. *Hosp Comm Psychiatry* 32:687, 1981.

Soreff S: Psychiatric consultation in the emergency department. *Psychiatr Ann* 8:189, 1978.

Surawicz FG: Alcoholic hallucinosis: A missed diagnosis. *Can J Psychiatry* 25:57, 1980.

Tupin JP: The violent patient: A strategy for management and diagnosis. *Hosp Comm Psychiatry* 34:37, 1983.

Weisman A, Worden W: Risk-rescue rating. *Arch Gen Psychiatry* 26:553, 1972.

Weissberg MP: Emergency room medical clearance: An educational problem. *Am J Psychiatry* 136(6):787, 1979.

Wilson LG: Viral encephalopathy mimicking functional psychosis. *Am J Psychiatry* 133:165, 1976.

SECTION 19
PHYSICIAN-PATIENT
INTERACTIONS

CHAPTER 140
PHYSICIAN-PATIENT
INTERACTIONS

B. Ken Gray, Peter Ostrow
Richard Ceyzyk, Ruth Beverly

Physician-patient interactions comprise a complicated set of verbal, written, and attitudinal communications that affect the patient's medical care and response to that care. This chapter defines the components of physician-patient interactions in both the concrete and abstract forms, and gives guidelines for these interactions. Areas to be discussed are patient expectations, physician attitude, privileged communications, the angry patient, and patient disposition.

PATIENT EXPECTATIONS

Patient expectations on entry to the emergency department generally encompass the following areas: quality of care, efficiency of treatment, and cost of care.

Quality of Care

The patient's criteria for quality of care involve a number of issues besides purely medical ones. Every patient, as well as those relatives or friends who bring the patient to the hospital, will have anxiety surrounding the acute illness or injury, and the emergency department visit. Their basic fears arise from a lack of knowledge about what will happen to them in the emergency department; the undetermined seriousness of their medical problems; and their fear of dependence upon individuals with whom they have not established a prior trust relationship.

It is important for members of the emergency department staff to listen to the patient's concerns, provide information and reassurance about the illness, and explain department procedures. In addition, family and friends waiting in the lobby should periodically receive information about the patient's condition.

Victims of violence experience a serious threat to their sense of security. Depending on their previous personality makeup, trauma victims may develop feelings of distrust, guilt, or irrational fears. Through sympathetic listening, the staff can help restore trust in others and allay fears and guilt. Calls to the family or other interested parties can play a part in this process. Sometimes repeated short visits by the staff to the patient throughout the emergency department stay will be useful. Providing the patient something to drink or communicating messages can help meet the traumatized patient's increased dependence needs.

Meeting with the families of dead or critically ill patients is an obligation for both the nurse and the physician. The necessity to devote attention to other critically ill patients can limit a physician's time with family members. The staff can be helpful in this process by giving time and support to the grief-stricken family.

Trained professionals can help survivors begin to cope with the emotional impact of their loss as well as guide them through the bureaucratic hurdles that these situations present, such as signing papers or contacting funeral homes. In an emergency department with limited staffing, in-service seminars for emergency department personnel can be scheduled, emphasizing the needs of the grieving family and designing a plan of intervention that can ease the burdens of surviving family members.

The patient expects to be educated about the illness or injury. The education includes explaining the diagnosis, interpreting symptoms and anxiety, instructing the patient about local wound or injury care and the course of the disease, and providing directions for when and how to obtain follow-up care.

Finally, the patient should receive treatment for symptoms, both in the emergency department and after discharge. Where indicated, pain medication can be given to make the patient more comfortable while awaiting the results of evaluation. If pain medication must be withheld, as in the evaluation of the acute abdomen, the patient should be told why this is necessary.

Efficiency of Treatment

By self-definition, the patient has come to the emergency department because he or she perceives the situation as an emergency. The patient expects to receive rapid treatment regardless of the patient load currently existing in the department. It should be made clear to the patient, by either signs posted in the department or verbal communication by admitting personnel, or both, that treatment priority is based on the degree of life threat present.

Cost of Care

Few patients are concerned with the cost of care at the time they need it. The degree of anxiety, the intensity of symptoms, and the convenience of receiving care whenever it is desired are uppermost in a patient's mind. However, patients should be informed in a general fashion about emergency department and hospital costs at discharge. If unduly concerned with costs, the patient may be referred to the social worker for reassurance and concrete information about how community agencies can ease the financial burden.

SPECIAL PHYSICIAN RESPONSIBILITIES

Physician Attitude

There must be a willingness and a commitment on the part of the emergency physician to meet the needs of all patients who come to the department for medical care, regardless of medical triviality or urgency.

Physician and staff attitudes can be shaped by the feelings elicited by patients or their complaints. For example, certain medical problems, such as rape or child or spouse abuse, evoke such a depth of emotional feeling in the staff that patient avoidance may result.

The victim of sexual assault needs especially sensitive handling. Fears about possible negative reactions of a loved one, impaired sexual functioning, possible pregnancy or venereal disease, demeaning contacts with police or courts, and possible future assaults are only some of the emotional and physical issues that need attention. Helping the patient through each step of the examination and with the police interview can do much to restore a badly shaken sense of self-confidence and self-worth. Special rape counseling units are ideally suited for this purpose.

No matter how difficult it may seem, the physician's attitude in the approach to these patients must be competent and caring. Unquestionably, the emergency department staff will follow the leadership set by the emergency physician. An empathetic attitude in dealing with these more unusual problems is bound to have a positive spin-off affecting the relationships of staff with each other, as well as with all patients in the emergency department.

Interaction between the emergency physician, nursing personnel, and the social worker, if one is available, is necessary to evaluate the psychosocial problems that may affect a patient's ability to respond to medical care. The ability of a patient to communicate rapidly and coherently with the examining physician may be impaired because of acute or chronic disease. In such a case, efforts are necessary to acquire prior history from untraditional sources such as neighbors, public health workers, police, relatives, drinking buddies, or caretakers.

Privileged Communications

Communications between patients and the emergency physician as well as other professional staff are privileged. There is, in effect, no difference in this responsibility from other patient-physician relationships. Two circumstances that should be of concern to the emergency department staff relate to this important responsibility.

First, the setting in which emergency care is provided is frequently not conducive to private communications. The use of curtained examining cubicles does not provide an adequate sound barrier. Discussions between professionals on the telephone, in hallways, or patient treatment areas may be overheard by other patients.

Second, the nature of emergency medicine is to deal with medical events that are surrounded by a considerable amount of anxiety. There may be conflicts between short-term and long-term consequences. Take, for example, a patient with a suicidal gesture such as a drug overdose which the patient wishes to keep from the family; or a minor who refuses to tell her parents she is pregnant. Such circumstances place the physician in conflict with the need to respect the patient's privacy and the need to provide appropriate care.

There are no easy resolutions of this dilemma; and each physician must determine which approach to take. It may be possible to justify involving family or friends simply by notifying them that the patient is in the emergency department.

Hostile or Angry Patient

Avoiding unnecessary provocation of a potentially hostile, angry patient in borderline control can reduce the likelihood and frequency of ugly physical confrontations in the emergency department.

A retrospective analysis of patients who have become physically threatening in the emergency department reflects three general classes of patients: (1) fear leading to anger; (2) grieving leading to anger; (3) delirious or intoxicated patients. About 90 percent of these patients fall into the latter category.

Fearful patients who respond to an initial feeling of anger do so as a gross emotional response. It is not meant personally and should not be interpreted as such by the emergency department staff. Anger can result because of a true or anticipated loss. An example of an anticipated loss would be the patient's fear of loss of control because of dependence on the staff. Delirious or intoxicated patients may have true organic brain syndromes and in such cases do not have voluntary control of their behavior.

The term *DICE* can be used as a mnemonic to address the following aspects of anger (adapted from Rockwell):

D—Direction of action. Determine if the anger is direct or diffuse. Encourage direct expressions of anger, and allow the patient to ventilate verbally. The important question here is whether the anger is self-directed or directed toward someone else.

I—Intent of anger. Is the patient serious with regard to action precipitated by the anger? For the emergency physician or staff, the specific question here is, Do you feel uneasy or threatened by the patient? This gut reaction is one of the most important keys to the evaluation of the patient.

C—Control. The patient should be asked if he or she is concerned about getting out of control. Most patients are eager to discuss this and are relieved by the question. Those patients who can indicate a concern over the loss of control usually are willing to accept intervention. A patient who considers him or herself to be in control is probably safe.

E—Expression. Determine how the patient expresses anger. Past behavior is usually the best predictor of future behavior. If the patient seems overly controlled as an individual but also expresses a worry over the possible loss of control, the patient should be considered a high risk.

The emergency department staff should provide a reduction in sensory provocation to the patient. For instance, if the patient is brought by the police, it is helpful when feasible to ask that the police remain out of the patient's view. Visual and aural sensations should be reduced as much as possible to reduce unnecessary provocation of the patient's fears.

Reassure patients that they will not be harmed, and that they are in a safe place where the staff and physician wish to help them. Do not be judgmental about a patient's feelings or opinions.

A single staff member should not try to subdue a patient alone. Such an approach will usually provoke the very attack you would like to avoid. When the decision is made to subdue a patient, the decision must not be ambiguous. On a single command word, the emergency department team must act in a coordinated fashion to restrain and quiet the patient.

Finally, there should be a formal department protocol for the methods of handling disruptive, disorderly patients, whether they be angry patients, those with alcohol or drug intoxication, or those who wish to leave against medical advice. The procedure should involve the emergency department physician, nursing and attendant staff, and hospital security personnel. Patients being discharged who refuse to leave, or who act in a voluntary, disorderly fashion on the premises, are liable for arrest and prosecution.

Patient Disposition

Most emergency physicians seek consultation for three basic reasons:

1. Hospital admission. To hospitalize a patient requires, at the least, a telephone conversation with a private physician who will accept the inpatient care of the patient.
2. Definitive treatment. Certain specialists such as orthopedic or plastic surgeons may be requested to provide care in the emergency department for patients who do not require admission.
3. Evaluation. Assistance in defining patient problems and disposition may be needed.

In most large private or community hospital emergency departments, approximately 10 to 15 percent of all patients seen are admitted to the hospital. This represents a group of patients that invariably receives a consultation. Most frequently, admitting consultations occur on the telephone with private attending staff physicians. In teaching institutions, consultations involve residents who evaluate patients in the emergency department as a part of their learning experience.

If the patient has no physician, the appropriate specialty staff physician must be selected by the emergency physician, using the referral system posted in the department. If the patient has a private physician on the staff of the hospital, that physician should be called. This practice maintains the professional relations between the emergency and private physician, and provides the opportunity for the private physician to assume responsibility for the direct care or the referral of the patient. If the private physician cannot be located, a discussion with the patient regarding medical needs is in order. The patient may have received similar primary or specialty care in the past, and may have the name of a physician who might be called. If not, a list of referral physicians can be provided by the emergency physician, and the selection made by the patient.

The skills of specialists, such as orthopedic and plastic surgeons, may be necessary to complete the patient's treatment in the emergency department before discharge. Finally, a consultation may be requested to determine appropriate patient disposition, such as admission versus discharge, or to define treatment for the discharged patient. Examples include surgical or gynecological consultation for patients with abdominal pain.

An emergency department usually has a list of specialists who have agreed to be available to the emergency department, customarily within a time frame of 30 min. Frequently a second list of backup specialists is also available. A protocol should be devised in conjunction with the hospital executive or emergency department committee in the event that the primary or secondary consultants are unavailable. In the unusual circumstance that the consultant cannot be located, transfer of the patient to another institution must be considered.

The determination for hospitalization is most commonly made on medical grounds. Occasionally, however, social factors affect the decision. Instances where this most commonly occurs relate to the elderly or resourceless patient, when admission for medical causes is necessary because the patient cannot cope with the environment. In these instances, the social environment is viewed as a complication affecting medical needs.

SPECIAL PROBLEMS AFFECTING PATIENT DISCHARGE

The rapid disposition of emergency patients is a major mode of operation in every emergency department. The recognition of factors that preclude simple treatment and discharge is not difficult. Most often, these are mental or physical impairments that either moderately or severely limit a patient's capacity to perform normal activities.

Hospital-based social workers, when available to the emergency department, can coordinate discharge planning in these cases. In most situations, social workers rather than physicians or nurses are familiar with community resources and have the time to develop working relationships with them. Unburdened with the incessant press of attending to acute trauma and illness, they can focus upon the psychosocial needs of patients and their families during the emergency department visit and upon discharge. In smaller or rural hospitals without social workers, emergency departments may contract for service or develop reciprocal relationships with local agencies. Ideally, the social worker will be a bridge linking the emergency department patient with the appropriate resources discussed below.

Postdischarge Care

There are many facilities and services available in all areas of the country that are licensed, supervised, and sometimes administered by federal, state, county, or metropolitan authorities. They provide a continuum of care and services for the patient discharged from the emergency department who is incapable of the normal activities of daily living. Categories of service and design will vary from location to location, but generally are as follows, ranked from most to least in services and functions provided.

Extended care facility. This category is meant to provide the same level of nursing care as the hospital but at a lesser cost. Most often, it is an adjunct to publicly supported and maintained facilities. Extended care facilities are few in number, and it is difficult to gain acceptance except for those few patients who have been treated in the affiliated emergency department or inpatient service. Transfer is generally made on a physician-to-physician level.

Skilled-care nursing homes. Skilled, in this instance, refers to nursing care, including the administration of intravenous or intramuscular injections, or controlled oral preparations; and very close nursing supervision.

Basic or intermediate nursing homes. These facilities provide a residential environment for those patients with chronic or acute disease who require simple supportive and nursing care. Most frequently, this involves the patient who is nonambulatory or incontinent, or whose mental functioning is grossly impaired.

Homes for the aged. As the name implies, these facilities are designed to provide residential supportive care for aged patients, usually restricted to those above the age of 60 to 65. Patients must be ambulatory and continent, and not in need of extensive nursing care. Physicians will visit at the patient's request. Patients generally have minimal to moderate mental impairment that limits full normal daily activities.

Adult foster care homes. These facilities are generally small capacity, converted private homes, licensed by the state to care for the mentally marginal patient. They are an outgrowth of the halfway house concept and are also known as community living facilities. Temporary or short-term placements may be arranged, but most often placements are viewed as permanent. Medications are not dispensed and are the responsibility of the individual patient, but they are monitored by residential supervisors. There is no capacity for physical nursing care beyond the most minimal level.

Room and board homes. These facilities are similar to aftercare homes, but are not required to provide close supervision. Basically, they provide a bed, sanitary facilities, and three meals a day. They supply a residential facility for the transient or down-and-out patient. No nursing care is provided, but the administration of medication may be supervised.

Emergency shelters. These facilities are usually established only in the larger metropolitan centers. They provide temporary shelter and sustenance for individuals and families who are catastrophically displaced from their homes by sudden, unforeseen events, or circumstances such as child or spouse abuse, or eviction. Provisions are for temporary assistance and sustenance without supervision or medical provision. The emphasis here is to plug the patient into the service delivery system provided by state or local welfare agencies, and to restore and maintain pretraumatic functioning.

The following categories of intervention are those that attempt to provide assistance and therapeutic regimens while minimizing or obviating physical displacement.

VNA or PH agencies. Visiting Nurse Association or public health agencies provide in-home assistance on a one-to-one basis of RN or LPN to patient and family. Routine services offered include administration of and instruction in the use of medication,

prostheses, and home health appliances; evaluation of medical progress; and institution of appropriate intervention. These agencies do not provide routine home maintenance services such as bathing, toilet assistance, or cooking. They are generally concerned with the medical aspects of a patient's care, but will evaluate the home situation and refer for appropriate assistance for the required service.

Homemaker service. These agencies provide certain nonmedical, in-home supportive services with trained and supervised homemakers to do those tasks of daily living that are beyond the patient's abilities. These include such functions as shopping, cooking, cleaning, and child care. Such services are generally viewed as part-time.

Meals on wheels. The name is self-explanatory. Such services are generally geographically limited and available only once a day, 5 days a week. They should not be considered as a substitute for normal adequate nutrition, but as an adjunct.

There are various additional outpatient services not universally available, such as geriatric psychiatric screening and counseling, geriatric police escort services, dial-a-ride, and home health aide service. An informed social worker can assist with up-to-date information in these areas and arrange appropriate referrals.

Major home care equipment problems are not usually encountered in the emergency department. These arrangements are usually made when the patient is hospitalized. However, the emergency department staff should listen for problems related to home equipment, or additions that could make the patient more functional. Equipment needs usually involve walkers, crutches, or wheelchairs. Sometimes, it is found that a hospital bed or air mattress makes it easier to maintain a confined patient in the home. Patients with special needs such as colostomy bags, wound dressings, or insulin syringes can be put in touch with a source of supply.

To ensure continuity of treatment, transportation needs are a major consideration. Lack of transportation is one of the prime reasons given for failure to follow through on clinic appointments. Staff members should determine the patient's own resources, and when they are sufficiently lacking, arrange transportation through church groups or welfare agencies.

Alcoholism

Alcoholics are perceived by the emergency staff as being disruptive to the hospital routine. Their intoxicated state makes it difficult to obtain a reliable medical history and can complicate physical examination. In addition, the alcoholic may overreact to real or imagined negative attitudes on the part of the hospital staff.

The social worker's first involvement with the alcoholic is usually an evaluation for placement. However, even if housing is not a concern to the patient, the patient should be involved in at least a brief discussion of alcohol dependence. After all, the patient who is intoxicated enough to be brought to the emergency department, or who suffers illness or injury as a result of alcohol intoxication, may have a serious drinking problem.

The alternative modes of treatment for alcoholic patients include hospital or custodial detoxification units; halfway houses; and self-help groups such as Alcoholics Anonymous. When discharged, the patient should know the medical follow-up plan, and be aware of the effects of alcohol on any medication that is prescribed.

Drug Abuse

The emergency department is an excellent site for identifying and confronting the problem of drug abuse. Great numbers of drug abuse patients, who might pass through other service agencies undetected, can be more readily identified in the medical setting. The geographic locale and the population served by each particular emergency department will determine the pattern of drug abuse encountered by hospital staff. With intravenous drug users, visible signs will be apparent to the experienced nurse or physician. Frequently, a history of drug abuse can be determined during the patient interview if the diagnosis itself, such as drug overdose or withdrawal, does not reveal the problem.

If supported by the emergency department staff, a social worker can develop an effective program of identification and initial treatment of the drug abuse patient. This service may be designed primarily to refer to community agencies or as a conduit to a hospital-based treatment unit, where one exists. It is necessary to take into account government regulations regarding disclosure of information of drug abuse patients. Timing is important: referrals should be made so that the patient can be interviewed within the treatment process. This may mean seeing the patient after the initial examination or while the patient is waiting for x-ray or laboratory results. If referral is made after the patient has been medically cleared, the patient may leave before the interview.

One must accept the fact that drug abusers make heavy use of denial, projection, and rationalization. It is very common for an experienced heroin user to deny any use since the most recent hospitalization, and later admit to interim use. One should not trap these patients in their lies but rather interpret that it may be hard for them to share their lifestyle with others. Reassurance about confidentiality is also important with many clients. Rewarding these patients for agreeing to seek help, or, if less motivated, at least for discussing their problems, is very helpful in building confidence.

When patients are highly resistant to reflecting on problem areas, the best means of breaking through their denial is by discussing the illness that brought them to the emergency room as a manifestation of their self-destructive behavior. This is more often the case with intravenous drug abusers, since they are reluctant to seek medical attention except when absolutely necessary. Rational thinking about their situation may be alien to addicts. As one heroin addict said to this author, "If you want to be a good junkie, you can't think about what you're doing to yourself."

In large urban areas, a wide range of referral facilities is generally available to the drug abuse patient: hospital inpatient detoxification units; residential drug-free programs, generally in the form of therapeutic communities; outpatient methadone detoxification maintenance clinics; and outpatient drug-free programs that may offer individual and group counseling.

Most of the above programs also have ancillary services relating to health care, continuing education, vocational training, and in some cases, child care. In a few cities there are even more specialized clinics targeted to subgroups such as women or ethnic minorities.

In most communities the options for treatment will be far fewer. In fact, it may be necessary to refer clients to community mental health centers or hospital psychiatric units.

BIBLIOGRAPHY

Ball M: Issues of violence in family casework. *Social Casework* 58:3–12, 1977.
Bennett MJ: Emergency medical services: The social worker's role. *Hospitals* 47:111, 114, 118, May 1973.
Bergman AS: Emergency room: A role for social workers. *Health and Social Work* 1:32–44, February 1976.
Berkman BG, Rehr H: Social needs of the hospitalized elderly: A classification. *Social Work* 17:80–88, 1972.
Chafetz ME, Blaine HT, Abram HS, et al: Establishing treatment relations with alcoholics. *J Nerv Ment Dis* 134:395–409, 1962.
Getz W, Altman DC, Berleman WC, et al: Paraprofessional crisis counseling in the emergency room. *Health and Social Work* 2:57–73, 1977.
Hankoff LD, Mischorr MT, Tomlinson KE, et al: A program of crisis intervention in the emergency medical setting. *Am J Psychiatry* 131:47–50, 1974.
Jacobsen PH, Howell RJ: Psychiatric problems in emergency rooms. *Health and Social Work* 3:88–107, 1978.
Johnson R, Trimble C: The (expletive deleted) shouter. *JACEP* 4:333–335, 1975.
Levinson VR, Struassner SLA: Social workers as "enablers" in the treatment of alcoholics. *Social Casework* 59:14–20, 1978.
Moffett AD, Bruce JD, Harvitz D: New ways of treating addicts. *Social Work* 19:389–397, 1974.
Moffett AD, Chambers CD: The hidden addiction. *Social Work* 15:54–59, July 1970.
Morehouse ER: Treating the alcoholic on public assistance. *Social Casework* 59:36–41, 1978.
Rockwell DA: An approach to fear and hostility. *Emerg Dig* 1:Ins 21, 1976.
Smith LL: A general model of crisis intervention. *Clin Soc Work J* 4:162–171, 1976.
St Pierre CA: Motivating the drug addict in treatment. *Social Work* 16:80–88, 1971.

CHAPTER 141
LEGAL ASPECTS OF
EMERGENCY MEDICINE

Warren Appleton

Medicine is the art and science that deals with the prevention, cure, and palliation of disease. Law is the enforced and binding customs of a community aimed at establishing social order and peace.

Medical professionals are acutely aware of the ever-increasing involvement of legal principles in the practice of medicine. The expanding role of government in regulation of health care, the recent surge of malpractice litigation, and physicians' growing role as administrators demonstrate the breadth of the legal-medical interface. This chapter focuses on specific areas within this interface: general principles, medical malpractice, medical records as evidence, confidentiality, reportable events, request for evidence, and staff interaction.

The goal of this chapter is to introduce basic concepts and terminology required to understand the legal ramifications of medical practice in the emergency department.

Disclaimer. A *disclaimer* is a legal concept that allows a person to repudiate certain legal responsibilities. The disclaimer for this chapter follows: The reader is instructed that an outcome of a case depends on its peculiar fact pattern. Changing one fact in a case may result in a different legal outcome. Also the reader must understand that state statutes and case rulings may vary considerably. The goal of this chapter is educational. It is not intended to function as legal advice. The reader should seek legal counsel from a competent professional if a potential need arises.

The concept of disclaimer is a contract principle and not applicable to negligence law. One cannot write a contract to disclaim responsibility for negligence.

GENERAL PRINCIPLES

The law is divided into two general categories, civil law and criminal law, both of which are subject to constitutional principles. The last two decades have seen the growth of a type of civil law called administrative law.

In criminal law, the plaintiff is the sovereign; the sovereign has a burden of proof of guilt beyond a reasonable doubt. The defendant's potential damage is measured as a misdemeanor or a felony, usually resulting in incarceration or loss of money. The measuring standard must be ascertainable through codified statute or regulation.

The emergency physician encounters criminal law in a variety of areas: prisoners, victims, reporting regulations, dangerous drug statutes, and government-based medical reimbursement.

In civil law, one party, who may be but is not necessarily a sovereign, seeks redress of disagreements arising from the parties' particular relationship. The burden of proof for the plaintiff is "more likely than not" rather than "beyond a reasonable doubt." Potential damage remedies are money or injunctions. The measuring standards may be contract, statute, regulation, or custom.

Administrative law is best characterized as procedural law. All governmental bodies by law and many private parties by contract are bound to certain procedural principles derived from constitutions, statutes, or bylaws. These principles apply to enforcement and judgment of existent rules and to promulgation of new rules.

In administrative law the legislature, by enabling statutes, delegates that the executive branch is to regulate. The judicial branch has the responsibility to review this executive process to ensure that the regulation is within the scope of the enabling statute and the application procedure is fair. Courts demonstrate a bias in favor of regulatory problem solving; the burden of proof is on the individual, who must usually prove the rule to be beyond the scope of legislation or that it is arbitrarily or capriciously applied.

Hospital privileges, medicaid rule making, and licensing law are examples of administrative law.

Underlying and watching over these areas of the law are certain constitutional guarantees. The major guarantee is that before a person loses life, liberty, or certain property rights, that person is entitled to due process. Due process is the right to notice of disagreement and the right to be heard by an unbiased tribunal prior to being subject to such a permanent loss.

The amount of process due is a function of the loss and the impact of the loss on individual and community. The greater the potential loss, the greater the due process protection. Due process is a major consideration in the areas of civil commitment, loss of governmental medical benefits, and administrative procedures.

Legal disputes are frequently settled through court action. This process can be envisioned as the determination of the true facts and application of these facts to the law. The court determines the law; either the court or a jury is the trier of fact. The application of facts to law is usually a function of the trier of fact, e.g., a jury.

MEDICAL MALPRACTICE

Although early medical malpractice was based on contract theory, it soon became apparent that most physicians' professional actions were best tested by tort theory. From the Latin *tortus* for "twisted," *tort* is defined as a breach of duties imposed upon parties by societal norms that results in damage. Torts are classically divided into intentional torts, negligence, and strict liability.

Intentional Torts

Four intentional torts are of special interest to the emergency physician.

Battery is the unconsented and intentional touching of another. *Assault* is the intentional placing of another in apprehension of an offensive touching. *False imprisonment* is the third intentional tort. It is defined as the total restraint of a person against that person's will and not conforming with specific societal exceptions. This is a potential liability when dealing with patients perceived as suffering psychiatric, sensory, or chemical impairment. The specific exceptions are in the main defined in each state's mental health code. These three actions are not only civil torts but also are potential criminal actions.

The fourth intentional tort is *infliction of emotional distress or outrage*. This tort is based on a principle that people should be free from mental as well as physical assault. Misidentifying a victim and notifying the wrong family with resultant emotional damage is an example of this tort.

Defenses

The intentional torts are subject to a variety of defenses or exceptions. Examples are necessity, such as in advanced cardiac life support, and self-defense or defense of others in cases of violent patients. In these cases, society defines a greater good to be achieved, saving a life and self-protection.

Consent is the expressed willingness that an act occur and is a defense to intentional torts if obtained correctly. Consent can be further divided into actual consent or implied consent. Actual consent is the verbal or written expression of willingness, such as a "yes" to the query, "Should we draw blood?"

Consent can be implied when based on an action that reasonably expresses a willingness that an act occur, for example, rolling up a sleeve for a tetanus shot. Society, in certain situations, deems an implied consent. For example, society deems consent on the part of unconscious and disoriented patients in order to save life and limb.

Minors present especially difficult consent issues. As a general rule minors are legally not capable of consenting; thus, when treatment is not necessary to save life or limb, the emergency physician should make reasonable attempts to obtain consent from the guardian. If the minor has effectively been abandoned by the guardian and no responsible adult is evident, the physician must weigh the particular facts. In questionable situations, it is better to err toward diagnosis and treatment. Those emancipated minors who by marriage or lifestyle have broken the bonds of parental control may consent for themselves.

In situations involving minors, disorientation, or unconsciousness, prudent medical care behooves the physician to inform next of kin and obtain consent when feasible and practicable.

On the basis of the individual's right of self-determination the doctrine of *informed consent* has evolved. Each individual in a free society has the right to know the extent of and need for an invasion of his or her body. Generally speaking, informed consent requires that the patient be competent to consent to and understand all the risks and benefits inherent in the proposed procedure, as well as the consequences of alternative methods of treatment or no treatment at all.

State courts have defined two standards upon which to test the scope of informed consent, standards of the reasonable patient and standards of the reasonable physician. Some states require the physician to tell the patient that which a reasonable patient would expect to be told under the same or similar circumstances. Other states require the physician to tell the patient what a reasonable physician would be expected to tell the patient under the same or similar circumstances.

Given that the informed consent doctrine is based on the precept of self-determination, the more logical application is the reasonable patient standard. Patients should be informed prior to consenting to manipulative procedures such as an IVP, suturing, casting, or culdocentesis. Documentation of such information sharing is standard practice; however, this does not replace the need for an informed oral conversation concerning the procedure, possible outcome, and alternatives.

Failure to obtain proper and informed consent exposes the physician to a charge of technical battery, and the physician may be responsible for all resulting damages if a patient is injured as a result of treatment and no informed consent was obtained. The patient may recover damages under these circumstances without having to prove the four elements of negligence. Defensive consent concepts only apply to intentional torts, not to negligent torts or strict liability.

Patients are capable of *refusing consent* to diagnosis and/or treatment. However, whether or not they are competent to refuse consent is a clinical question. Competence to refuse treatment must be assessed in the light of vital signs, mental status (both acute and chronic), age, toxins, and intoxicants. When a competent person refuses treatment, the physician should maintain a "welcome to return" attitude, try to obtain an against-medical-advice (AMA) receipt, and document the episode in the chart.

Negligence

Negligence is an act or omission that fails to meet a standard of care recognized by societal norms intended to protect people from *unreasonable* risk of harm. The societal-norm standard of care is variable and is a function of the role of the parties (citizen, EMT, physician), the milieu (crash site, ambulance, trauma center), and the potential for harm (runny nose, shortness of breath, dull chest pain). Greater expertise, a more advanced setting, and greater potential for harm dictate a higher standard of care.

Negligence is composed of three major elements: liability, causation, and damages. All must exist for a negligence action.

Liability

Potential liability attaches when a relationship between a doctor and a patient exists (duty) and there has been a breach of this duty of care. As a practical and judicial matter, a duty is incurred when a patient presents to the emergency room or dials 911. A classical and leading case in this area is *Wilmington General Hospital v. Manlove,* 174 A 2d 135.

The *Manlove* case involved an infant with fever and diarrhea brought to an emergency room by his parents. The child was under the care of an unavailable family physician; the child was sent home by the hospital nurse on the basis of the hospital's policy not to treat persons already under the care of a private physician because of a potential conflict of interest. Shortly thereafter the child succumbed to pneumonia. A main issue in the *Manlove* case was whether the hospital had a duty to provide emergency care. The Delaware Supreme Court quickly rejected the notion that patients belong to certain physicians and stated that the hospital could be held liable for refusal of service to a patient in the case of an unmistakable emergency if the patient had relied on well-established custom of the hospital to render aid in such a case. This evolved into the current definition of an *emergency:* any condition that the patient believes needs immediate medical attention, at any time of day or night.

Once the duty to diagnose and/or treat is established, the patient has the right to expect the physician to practice within the standard and not to abandon the patient in a precarious position.

Standard of care is usually defined in relative terms. The physician's duty is to act in the care of patients as a reasonable physician would act under similar circumstances. Given the potential for great harm in the case of emergency physicians, the standard at times is more definitive. The physician's duty is to ably exercise self-regulation and self-discipline through an accepted use of reason (differential diagnosis) and reasonably apply dictated interventions. This is the *standard of prudence.* Both standards are used by courts.

At times the standard of care is defined by statute. All states have child abuse statutes; many have disabled adult abuse statutes. These statutes internally define certain required interventions that must be taken by physicians. Breach of a statutory duty is termed *liability per se.* Reference to local statutes is mandatory.

The standard can be breached by performing an action poorly, or *malfeasance,* or by not performing an action required by the circumstances, or *nonfeasance.*

When the patient-physician relationship is unilaterally and prematurely terminated or disregarded by the emergency physician, the potential of *abandonment* arises. Abandonment can be both a negligence issue, and thus require expert testimony, or a legal action in itself which does not require expert opinion. The emergency physician must be aware of potential abandonment issues and take reasonable and prudent steps to avoid it. Especially critical areas are hospital admissions where the on-call physician does not respond promptly, patient transfers, and telephone dispositions.

Until the time when the consulted physician actually interviews and examines the patient, the emergency physician requesting consultation is responsible for the patient. Telephone orders without examination by the consultant do not alleviate this responsibility.

An effective protocol should be established between the emergency department and the medical staff to avoid this potential trouble area.

The risk of abandonment can also occur in transferring a patient from one emergency department to another. As a general rule, the transferring emergency department has primary responsibility for initial treatment and stabilization of the patient. Transfers should generally not be attempted unless the patient is capable of withstanding the transfer. The first receiving hospital is usually responsible for the safe transfer of the patient to the second receiving hospital. Transfer should not occur until the second receiving hospital has agreed to accept the patient. All appropriate records, x-rays, medications, and equipment should be sent with the patient. If the patient suffers serious damage because of the transfer, the transferring emergency physician and hospital might be liable for abandonment. Furthermore, if proper transferring procedures were not followed, the physician and hospital are also open to a charge of negligence in the manner of the transfer.

Patients can also suffer abandonment over the telephone. An example is the patient who is discharged from the emergency department, experiences a recurrence of symptoms, calls the emergency department, and is told not to worry about it until the morning. If the patient's condition worsens, the emergency department staff may well be liable for negligence and abandonment. A general telephone rule for the emergency department staff is never to diagnose or treat patients over the telephone. It may be a tempting convenience, but the medicolegal risks and hazards are many.

Causation

Liability not only must exist, it must also have been the cause of damage. Cause is divided into two categories, *causation in fact* and *proximate cause.* Lawyers and judges frequently misapply these concepts, often calling everything proximate cause.

As a matter of evidentiary proof, direct cause, or causation in fact, requires that the breach of duty was more likely than not the cause of the damage. When direct causes of damage are multiple, such as a forgotten sponge by Dr. A. and then application of an inappropriate antibiotic by Dr. B, courts test direct causation on a substantial factor scale. In this example, each factor could be found a substantial factor causing damage; thus, both tort-feasors caused the damage.

True proximate cause is based on public policy and is specifically the limitation which courts have placed upon the actor's responsibility for a breach of duty. A classic proximate cause example is whether or not a boat owner who negligently damages a drawbridge is responsible for damages incurred by people wanting but now not able to cross the bridge. True proximate cause deals with the foreseeability of the consequences of one's acts or omissions. Courts at times speculate on the *foreseeability* of danger, sometimes using the term *danger zones.*

Tarasoff v. Regents of the State of California, 551 P2d 334, is in part a proximate cause case. The California Supreme Court decided as an issue of public policy that it was foreseeable that a homicidal psychiatric patient was likely to attack a person after the patient named the victim. Following this realization the court stated the physician had a duty to inform that person of such an attack. When proximate cause is foreseeable, a duty is established.

The circular logic that one perceives in the proximate cause–duty area is one much discussed in legal literature. It confuses many.

Damage

Damage is classically divided into general damages and special damages. Characteristically general damages so naturally flow from a tortuous act that the defendant is automatically aware of their existence. Special damages must be pleaded in the complaint to give the defendant notice of the special demand. Pain and suffering are general damages; lost wages and hospital expenses are special damages. Courts allow the trier of fact to apportion damages among multiple tort-feasors. Damages can be apportionately reduced by actions attributable to the plaintiff.

Defenses

Legal defense to charges of medical negligence is based on: (1) a frontal attack on the basis and the credibility of the plaintiff's case; (2) collateral issues, e.g., statute of limitations, lack of jurisdiction, and Good Samaritan law; or (3) limitation of damages by patients' unreasonable actions.

A frontal defense attempts to break the negligence charge by showing no liability, no causation, or no damage. A frequent stumbling block in this defense is the physician's lack of adherence to the rationale of differential diagnosis. Diagnoses such as viral gastroenteritis and tension headache are examples of diagnoses of exclusion which short-circuit the concept of differential diagnosis and thus also destroy potential frontal defenses.

Good Samaritan laws based on the logic of Luke 10:30–37 exist in each state. Because Good Samaritan laws are not able to prevent the filing of a lawsuit, they are properly a collateral defense once a lawsuit is established. These laws, like statute of limitations laws, may form the basis for an accelerated judgment motion.

The goal of Good Samaritan laws (mostly passed on the wave of malpractice lawsuits) was to protect citizen responders from civil or criminal liability for acts directed at specified emergency settings, e.g., those attended by EMTs and paramedics. Each state statute is different and should be consulted. These statutes are a political matter and never a substitute for reasonable and prudent care. Currently many of these statutes are being eroded through legislative action.

Two types of the third defense pattern, limitation of damages defense, are contributory negligence and assumption of the risk; these are certainly tending to extinction, if indeed they ever existed. A third type, comparative negligence, or comparative damage, is the current concept. Frequently the trier of fact sets a percentage with regard to the plaintiff's and the defendant's liability for the result, in this case, the damage.

Discharge instructions, when prudent and reasonably within the capabilities of the discharged, can be evidence of the comparative negligence defense. By identifying certain signs and symptoms that indicate a reasonable need for reexamination or further communication, the physician effectively puts patients on notice that they have certain duties they must perform in care of their own bodies.

Many emergency departments have attempted to discharge their follow-up instruction responsibilities by the use of emergency department instruction sheets. These instruction sheets contain all appropriate instructions and are signed by the receiving patient. The instruction sheets have met with success but are by no means a panacea. The patient can always allege in court that nobody ever explained what was written on the instruction sheet. Furthermore, instruction sheets are simply another clinical tool for the emergency physician. If they are used improperly, they will not shield the physician from a negligence suit.

Each patient discharged from the emergency department should be invited to come back if the condition worsens and should also be given information to allow for proper follow-up.

Strict Liability

Certain activities are so dangerous that public policy dictates that the mere activity must compensate its damages. A lack of due care is not required as a matter of legal proof. A typical example is dynamite blasting. There is a trend favoring the expansion of this legal theory.

MEDICAL RECORDS: EVIDENCE

Evidence is defined as that which is legally submitted to a competent tribunal as a means of ascertaining the truth of any alleged matter. The measure of admissibility of evidence is a function of relevance and specific exceptions. The trier of law determines the admissibility of evidence.

The scope of medical records is defined by the Joint Commission on Accreditation of Hospitals (JCAH) and is viewed by many different groups for evidence of prior facts. These groups include physicians, peer reviewers, attorneys, juries, and patients. The medical record includes all pertinent documents, including discharge instructions.

The Joint Commission states that the "medical record shall be authenticated by the practitioner who is responsible for its clinical accuracy." Further emergency department records are a customary business practice and as such are recognized as exceptions to the hearsay rule and thus proper evidence in courts.

JCAH standard VII regulations also define basic standards of contents for records. Records should include patient identification, means and time of arrival, vital signs and cogent history of presenting complaint, prehospital care, therapeutic and diagnostic orders, test and procedure results, clinical observations, treatment results, diagnosis, disposition condition, instructions, and documentation of the facts concerning refusal of treatment.

Arguably, failure to maintain records as outlined above would violate the standard of care imposed by JCAH accreditation.

Medical records are legal evidence and should be viewed as such. Remarks or emphasis markings that seem appropriate at the time of writing the record may appear inflammatory at a judicial second look. When viewed by a trier of fact, a clear, concise record lends itself to more favorable interpretation than do scribbles.

The emergency record should also record significant negatives. For example, a chief complaint of chest pain with recorded patient denials concerning family history of heart disease, smoking, high blood pressure, and radiation is qualitatively different than a complaint of chest pain without mention of these factors. It is always wise to ask whether there is any other complaint and document that there is no further complaint.

Mistakes

On occasion errors occur on medical records. The proper technique to correct them is to put a single or double line through the mistake and to initial, date, and time the mistake. It is also good practice to insert a reason, e.g., wrong chart or false report from lab.

Transfers

A record should accompany a patient being transferred. Documentation of the condition of the patient at the time of transfer is of potential importance. Documentation of communication establishing the transfer and acceptance (including names and times) is appropriately put on the emergency department record since it is a form of disposition. It must be remembered that the transferring emergency department is responsible for the care and safety of the patient until the patient arrives at the receiving facility.

Prior Records

If prior emergency department records, inpatient records, or prior treating physicians are readily available and may shed light on the current complaint, every effort should be made to obtain this information. Comparison of prior and current ECGs, x-rays, and, at times, other evidence is very important in the care of patients. Patients frequently rely on specific emergency rooms because of this continuum of information resource. The physician that fails to make use of these prior sources creates potential negligent exposure.

Typical is the often-repeated pattern of the patient seen at several facilities with "migraines." In one case, the patient died with a subarachnoid hemorrhage 10 h after leaving the third physician consulted. Two phone calls—one to the private doctor and one to the prior treating emergency department for previous records—would have demonstrated that these migraines had never lasted for 3 days in this hard-driving computer wizard.

Changing Records

Once the medical record is finalized by signature or type proofreading, further records may add to but should not change the original medical record. An area of concern is the practice of signing charts prior to typing and not after proofreading. A phonetic or typing error can at times be very embarrassing. All medical records should be proofread before they are signed.

Changing records, which includes destroying records, is mentioned only to be condemned on the basis of both ethical and realistic reasoning. As a practical matter, changing records exposes one to much more severe consequences, including punitive damages. There are no defenses to such an action.

Res Ipsa Loquitur

The Latin phase *res ipsa loquitur* means "the thing speaks for itself" and is included here because it is a form of circumstantial evidence. There are three specific elements the plaintiff must prove to satisfy the requirements of the doctrine of *res ipsa loquitur*. First, the plaintiff must prove that the damages would not have occurred in the absence of somebody's negligence; second, that the instruments which caused the damage must have been under the exclusive control of the defendant at all times; and third, that the patient did not do anything which could in any way have contributed to his or her own injury.

An example is the totally functional patient who is admitted to the hospital from the emergency department for a routine appendectomy and awakens with an extremity palsy.

The legal effect and benefit of successfully invoking the doctrine of *res ipsa loquitur* is to shift the burden of proof from the plaintiff to the defendant. Now the plaintiff must no longer prove that the defendant was negligent. Rather, the defendant must now prove that he or she was not negligent. Thus in cases with multiple defendants, one defendant is now in the position of proving another defendant negligent. Proper medical record documentation of physical condition at transfer is a safeguard against this form of indirect proof.

CONFIDENTIALITY

Medical conversation and records are privileged and confidential. A right to privacy exists and is based on medical ethics and law. Discussing or relating private facts by oral or written communication to the press, unknown telephone callers, the police, and curious onlookers without consent is a transgression of a patient's right of privacy. An invasion of the right of privacy is compensable by law.

Certain exceptions to the privacy right exist. Minors and the mentally disabled are special cases in which the physician must frequently discuss facts with others. Laws requiring the reporting of epileptic drivers of cars, child abuse, venereal disease, animal bites, and communicable diseases functionally deem consent and allow the physician to report on these private matters.

A frequent trouble area is the neighbor or highly concerned parent of an adult patient. Although technically it is a breach of trust to discuss the patient's confidences with these people, as a practical matter it is at times required for good medical care. The closeness of the relationship between the patient and the third party and the need of the third party to know are the major factors in determining the extent of the discussion.

Patients have a right to the information on medical records, but not to the original record itself. In order to obtain a copy patients should effect a release of records in favor of themselves or a third party.

REPORTABLE EVENTS

Individual states have statute and agency regulations requiring the reporting of child abuse, disabled abuse, communicable disease including venereal disease, violent wounds, epileptic drivers, and those dead on arrival. Many of these statutes provide immunity to physicians concerning consent to treat and confidentiality issues; they do not provide immunity for negligence. Failure to report is often defined as a misdemeanor.

Abuse

There are over 2 million cases of child abuse per year in the United States. As a matter of public policy, society is willing to accept a degree of physical or emotional confrontation characterized as "corrective" but unwilling to accept "serious physical abuse or negligent care." Because studies indicate that many cases of abuse or neglect go unreported and undetected, child abuse laws typically encompass two points. First, health care professionals are given a collateral defense to a civil suit brought by a disgruntled reportee, thus hopefully fostering case reporting. Second, states may require reporting with sanctions against not reporting, essentially creating a per se civil standard of care. Breach of this standard of care may not only be negligent but also criminal. Individual state statutes should be read.

As a practical matter, the emergency physician must recognize that certain children are at immediate risk of harm and must be removed from the environment at once. Given a suspicion of potential future battering, the physician has the duty to involve the proper state agencies to effect a solution. The emergency physician is ethically bound to do the patient no harm. The parents' rights in this instance do not overshadow the patient's right not to be beaten. The emergency physician should try to avoid confrontation, but in the final event it is reasonable for the physician to hold a child who is at risk until proper authorities respond.

Whether or not a failure to report child abuse is a cause of subsequent damage to the child is a question of fact and as such is a jury question. Juries have found liability in these cases; see *Landeros v. Flood*, 551 P2d 389.

Several states have expanded their abuse reporting to include certain disabled groups. Although parental and spousal abuse is frequently seen in the emergency department, few reporting statutes currently exist. However, the potential for civil liability for missing a homicidal dance in a battering sequence is real. As a minimum, potential victims of homicide should be informed of their potential victimization, or police notified of the possible violence.

Violent Wounds

Gunshot and stab wounds require reporting to local authorities. Reference to local procedure is mandatory.

Communicable Diseases

Patients with communicable diseases often come to the emergency department for treatment, partially because of the constant availability of treatment, and also in part because of the relative anonymity available in the emergency department. All states have venereal disease reporting laws that require the emergency physician and other members of the staff to report these cases to the appropriate health agency.

Other areas of the hospital, such as the laboratory, might be a more appropriate reporting entity for cases of venereal disease. This is because the hospital laboratory ultimately determines whether the clinical specimens submitted are positive for venereal disease. If the laboratory interprets the test as positive, it seems reasonable for the laboratory to report its positive cases of venereal disease to the appropriate reporting agency. A formal protocol should be developed in each hospital.

Communicable diseases other than venereal diseases are also reportable in many states. Among these are acute infectious hepatitis, food poisoning, meningitis, and Rocky Mountain spotted fever. Reportable cases vary from state to state and should be reviewed by the emergency physician.

Animal Bites

Animal bite reporting laws also exist in all jurisdictions. These statutes usually require the emergency physician or the emergency department staff to report an animal bite to the appropriate local health official within a specified number of hours after the bite occurred or after it was seen. Such reporting is an obvious safeguard to protect the public from vicious animals and from the spread of animal-borne infections.

DOA

A person who arrives in the emergency department dead on arrival (DOA) is automatically reportable as a coroner's or medical examiner's case. Almost all states require that DOA cases be reported to the coroner or medical examiner for possible investigation of foul play and to determine the need for postmortem examination.

The emergency physician and the staff should tamper with the corpse as little as possible. Handling in the emergency department should be minimized so as not to interfere with the evidence-gathering function of the coroner or medical examiner. Nothing should be done by the emergency department staff to alter the appearance of the corpse since this only complicates the subsequent medical legal investigation. All blood and tissue specimens in such cases should be obtained by the coroner or medical examiner without the intervention of the emergency physician or other members of the emergency department staff.

REQUEST FOR EVIDENCE

Patients will come to the emergency department requesting that the physician collect evidence in two instances, rape and blood alcohol determinations.

There are no statutes which require the reporting of rape. In reality the "rape examination" is a response to a request by the patient for medical care and a request by society and the patient for the physician to make certain evidentiary observations and collect certain direct evidence. Once the clinical examination and evidence gathering is completed, the patient effects a medical record release in favor of the police department. The physician has a duty to respect the confidence and privacy of the patient.

A statutory definition of rape varies from jurisdiction to jurisdiction. Generally speaking, rape is defined as an unlawful carnal knowledge of a woman by a man forcibly, against her will, and with penetration, however slight, of the male genitalia into or upon the female. Statutory rape is sexual intercourse by a male with a female who is under statutory age, either with or without the female's consent.

It is important that the emergency physician and the emergency department staff recognize that rape is a legal conclusion and not a medical diagnosis. The legal conclusion of rape is customarily arrived at after a trial by jury with presentation of appropriate evidence and argument by the prosecution and the defense. The reader is asked to review Chapter 73.

Frequently the emergency department is involved in a controversy concerning blood alcohol. In the absence of a court order or an absolving statute a physician does not have a consent defense over an intoxicated person's denial of a blood alcohol drawing. Many states now allow for the forced drawing of a blood alcohol from the alleged defendant in a negligent homicide or potential negligent homicide case when drunk driving is the cause.

There would seem to be no ethical or medical consideration that requires a physician to draw blood alcohol as legal evidence at the potential defendant's request.

Whether or not a blood alcohol or drug screen is drawn on a medical diagnostic level should not be influenced by the above evidentiary considerations. If in fact, in good medical conscience, if it appears that a blood alcohol is required, it should be drawn.

In both the rape examination and legal blood alcohol determinations it is important to maintain the creditability of evidence by documenting a *chain of evidence.*

Specimens should be properly labeled and handed directly to the appropriate law enforcement official or examining pathologist. A receipt should be obtained from the receiving party. If no receiving party is available, the specimens should be placed in a locked receptacle and handed over at a subsequent date in order to prevent a break in the chain of evidence. Preserving the chain of evidence is extremely important when the matter goes to trial. If the chain is not preserved, the defense will invariably allege that someone tampered with the specimens along the way.

EMERGENCY DEPARTMENT AND MEDICAL STAFF INTERACTION

The unique position that emergency physicians fill in community medical care puts them in a position of potential conflict with the medical staff and/or hospital administration. Political situations vary and must be dealt with individually. However, certain frequent problems need special attention.

The emergency physician interacts in medical, ethical, practical, and personal levels with a variety of coprofessionals, health care providers, and administrators. The constant scrutiny and pressures of medical life are often cited as sources of professional impairment, both chemical and functional. Physicians must be aware of the potential of these disabilities to result in negligent practice in themselves and peers. Physicians have a duty to protect the patient from such malpractice and to help their peers through these crises.

At times physicians will be confronted with substandard practices by peers. The physician has a duty to the patient and should neither condone nor adopt another's substandard practices.

Four commonly recurring areas are a potential problem for the emergency department physician in relation to the medical and paraprofessional staff.

The first problem is the medical staff physician who instructs a patient to go to the emergency department for treatment and then fails to appear to treat the patient or fails to notify the emergency department of the patient's imminent arrival. The primary problem this creates for the emergency department is whether it should exercise clinical control over the patient and institute diagnosis and treatment. If the patient is a nonemergency patient and wishes to be seen only by the private physician, there is no difficulty. However, when the patient's clinical problems require immediate attention, emergency physicians are more likely to be sued for negligence if they do not render necessary emergency care despite the wishes of the private physician. As a general rule, it is better to err on the side of treatment when in doubt. An effort should be made to contact the patient's private physician, but administrative consideration should never interfere with appropriate patient care.

Another difficulty for the emergency physician is dealing with requests from the medical staff physician to write admission orders for patients admitted through the emergency department. If the emergency physician does not have admitting privileges at the hospital, the emergency physician should not write admission orders. The responsibility for writing admission orders rests with the medical staff physician to whose service the patient has been admitted. When emergency physicians write admission orders as a convenience for medical staff, the admitted emergency department patient is in danger of not being examined by the admitting physician as early as possible.

Another important medical staff question deals with the time period within which the emergency department patient must be examined by the medical staff physician to whose service the patient has been admitted. The answer depends on the clinical facts. If the patient's condition is serious, the patient should be seen as soon as possible after admission. When the patient's clinical condition is less serious, the admitting medical staff physician can be afforded a slightly longer time before seeing the patient. These time limits are arbitrary and depend on the particular clinical conditions of a case.

A fourth area of concern is the attending physician who attempts to observe the patient in the emergency department when good medical practice dictates that the patient be admitted forthwith. Some of the most controversial interstaff discussions concern this issue. The emergency physician must have the stamina to persevere in pointing out that it is poor medical practice to allow patients with serious illnesses to remain in the emergency department.

These problems between the emergency department and medical staff are politically delicate and difficult to resolve. They are a source of much anxiety for all involved. The emergency department and medical and paraprofessional staff must keep lines of communication open so that difficult areas can be discussed intelligently and calmly. Without open communication, personal and professional relationships are strained, and patient care is adversely affected; the result is a climate of confusion in which lawsuits arise.

CONCLUSION

Emergency care is based on three axioms and two principles:

Axioms. Each competent patient has a right of self-determination which dictates a requirement of informed consent. Every person has a right to expect professionals to use reasonable and standard practices. Each person presenting to an emergency department is legally deemed an emergency and should be seen by a physician.

Principles. When in doubt, err toward treatment, and above all else, take the most reasonable approach to the patient.

The legal aspects of emergency medicine constitute a broad subject with many variables. Each issue must be judged on its particular facts and merits. The emergency physician who can develop the ability to see medical-legal issues from the consumer's perspective will be best suited in a litigious environment. The reader is referred to the bibliography as a start in exploring the legal aspects of emergency medicine.

BIBLIOGRAPHY

Annas G: *The Rights of Hospital Patients*. New York, Discus Avon, 1975.
Annas G, Glaniz L, Katz B: *The Rights of Doctors, Nurses and Allied Health Professionals*. New York, Discus Avon, 1981.
George J: *Law and Emergency Care*. St Louis, Mosby, 1980.
King JH: *The Law of Medical Malpractice*. St Paul, Minn, West, Nutshell Series, 1977.
Lipp M: *Respectful Treatment; The Human Side of Medical Care*. New York, Harper & Row, 1977.
Prosser W: *Law of Torts*. St Paul, Minn, West, Hornbook Series, 1981.

CHAPTER 142
PHYSICAL VIOLENCE

Vera Morkovin

Increasing numbers of patients who present to emergency departments for treatment of injuries are victims of social or domestic violence. Because of the recurrent nature of many of these traumatic conditions, these victims are often in real danger of more serious or even fatal future injuries. Thus it is important that the situations which caused the injuries in these patients be identified in the emergency department, and preventive measures instituted when possible. The victims of human violence fall into several groups: children, battered women, the elderly, and victims of violent crime.

Child Abuse

The earliest type of physical violence to receive wide attention was child abuse, after the classic work of Kempe in 1962. The legal definition is "the physical or mental injury, sexual abuse, negligent treatment, or maltreatment of a child under the age of 18 by a person who is responsible for the child's welfare under circumstances which indicate the child's health or welfare is harmed or threatened thereby."

A high index of suspicion and thorough knowledge of the symptoms and signs of this condition are essential for emergency physicians, since these children are usually presented with a misleading history. It is essential that a detailed history be taken and meticulously documented, noting any discrepancies between accounts obtained separately from as many involved adults as are present, as well as from children. A complete examination should be carefully conducted, with the patient disrobed, whenever the injury or the circumstances suggest the possibility of abuse. Emergency personnel should never display doubt as to the veracity of the information offered, nor express judgmental attitudes toward the parents or caretakers. Subtle injuries may require radiographic and laboratory studies. Hospitalization should be arranged when any doubt exists, even for minor illness or injuries, to allow time for further investigation of the home, and the condition of siblings, if any.

Sexual abuse of children by adult relatives or household members has usually existed for some time before the problem is identified. These patients may be brought in when someone accidentally discovers the situation, or when the child has symptoms of vaginitis, proctitis, or behavioral disturbances. These children rarely present as victims of acute sexual assault.

It is essential for the emergency physician to be familiar with the local legal process for taking custody of children at risk, especially when parents or guardians are uncooperative, as this may need to be done very rapidly. Immediate reporting to appropriate agencies is the duty of all individuals who suspect child abuse or neglect. Many states have statutes granting immunity from civil liability to the reporting person. Where available, child abuse teams should be involved as early as possible.

The Battered Woman

Like child abuse, the problem of physically abused women has existed for centuries, and both were socially approved in earlier times when wives and children were considered chattels. With modern changing attitudes toward the rights of women, the problem is now receiving wide attention. The battered woman is defined as one who is repeatedly or seriously beaten by the man with whom she lives.

These patients, because of shame, guilt, or fear, often conceal the source of their injuries. Battered women can be found in every socioeconomic and ethnic group; however, the concealment may be more effective in the higher strata of society. Unless emergency department personnel are sensitive to the possibilities of this condition, they may overlook some real life threats. Some authors have claimed that husbands are also physically abused by their wives, but substantiation of this claim, except as a rare phenomenon, has not been forthcoming.

Most battered women fit into a typical pattern which can be elicited by interview and examination. Sometimes the mere sympathetic mention, by the examiner, of the possibility of abuse will open the floodgates, and a patient who has been bottling up her hidden problem will pour out her story. The beatings usually start very early in the marriage or relationship, and become more frequent and severe with time. Typically the husband has been abused as a child, and the wife's background may have conditioned her to expect physical abuse as normative. She usually has very low self-esteem, is completely dependent on her mate, and believes she lacks resources or skills to provide for herself or her children. Such families are often isolated and have few, if any, support systems. Contrary to the opinion previously held widely by psychiatrists, studies have shown that spouse abuse is not a type of erotic sadomasochism.

The most frequent injuries with which the victim presents result from blows to the head. Periorbital ecchymoses and fractured mandibles, nasal bones, and skulls are common, as well as partial strangulations, pulled hair, and injuries resulting from being thrown against walls or down stairs. Fractures of the forearms are sustained when the victim tries to shield her face. However, if she is pregnant, the punches or kicks frequently are directed toward the abdomen, and may result in a ruptured viscus or fractured pelvis. Women who come in for relatively minor trauma, or sometimes for unrelated problems, should be carefully examined for signs of old injuries in various stages of healing.

A victim of wife abuse knows that the beatings may occur when she is asleep, or after the flimsiest of provocations, being induced as often by passivity as by an action on her part. Thus she lives in a constant state of fear and tension. If she has in the past sought help from church, community, or law enforcement agencies, it is probable that she has met with rebuffs or misunderstanding. Any such attempts, even visits to a hospital, may have precipitated more severe beatings.

Thus the late complications of the syndrome are often self-destructive attempts to escape, such as alcohol, tranquilizers, or fantasies. She may then present to the emergency department with a behavioral abnormality, an overdose, or with alcohol or drug abuse. She may be seeking care for a battered child, since battering men often victimize their children as well as their wives. Eventually either partner in this desperate situation may kill the other. One study found that 8 percent of women who murdered their husbands had previously called the police for help several times. In another, over half of a series of women jailed for killing their mates had been battered wives.

Emergency physicians should use the resources of crisis intervention programs, social workers, and community agencies to mobilize support and to provide counseling for these families and shelter for victims when needed. Although many patients refuse to use these services, they are helped to take the first steps toward protecting themselves by the knowledge that such resources exist, and that their situations are not isolated ones.

Abuse of the Elderly

Physical abuse of the elderly, especially those handicapped or relatively immobile, is a phenomenon being reported with increasing frequency. The main abusers are family members who may be overburdened and stressed after caring for a ''difficult'' parent or grandparent, and caretakers in understaffed or poorly supervised extended care facilities.

The injuries of such patients are particularly difficult to attribute to violence. The very idea is repugnant. The victims are often confused by organic brain disease or drugs. The elderly fall frequently and bruise easily. Failing hearing or eyesight make them vulnerable to violence when they cannot identify their assailants. Osteoporotic bones fracture easily. Caretakers usually show appropriate concern when bringing aged patients to hospitals.

All these factors impinge on the physician's objectivity, and diminish the probability that injuries will be considered as possibly inflicted by violent persons. The elderly who live alone are understood to be at risk for criminal attacks. Those residing in homes or nursing centers are assumed to be relatively well protected.

It is important for the emergency physician to know that in recent times the incidence of documented violence against the elderly by caretakers has increased rapidly. Relatives and institution attendants who are poor, uneducated, and overworked can easily react with uncontrollable rage to the provocative or irritably passive behavior of their aged charges. Prevention of future abuse

in such cases can be initiated by having visiting nurses, competent social workers, or other advocates investigate the home or facility and work with the caretakers to improve conditions. The lack of adequate resources in many instances may be depressing to professionals, but even minimal intervention can produce positive changes.

Victims of Criminal Violence

The psychological aftereffects of rape have been well described by Burgess and Holstrum, and identified as the rape-trauma syndrome. It has been observed that very similar posttraumatic stress syndromes occur in victims of other types of criminal violence. The individual who has been mugged, robbed, shot, or stabbed may experience denial, delayed flashbacks, nightmares, psychosomatic symptoms, prolonged anxiety, and depression, often out of proportion to the actual injury sustained, and often completely disrupting the victim's life.

Victims have two basic emotions in common during the immediate period of the assault: fear of death, and helplessness due to loss of control. Later, to varying degrees, they experience feelings of guilt. According to Symonds, it is a primitive human instinct to blame the sufferer for any misfortune and thus protect one's own sense of invulnerability. Victims share this response, and turn it against themselves.

It is important to realize that for many injured patients who have just become victims, the emergency department or trauma room experience again evokes the fear of dying and the feelings of helplessness. It reenforces the self-blame when painful treatment may be perceived by the confused patient as punishment. Immediate supportive intervention by trained emergency personnel can minimize the delayed consequences of such psychological trauma. While treating the seriously injured, keep them in touch with reality and keep them informed. Counteract their ideas of self-blame, mobilize their support systems, validate their experiences, provide them opportunity to regain control by participating in their care whenever possible. The patient in crisis is in an extremely suggestible state. There is evidence that these techniques, applied early, can minimize the patient's panic and confusion, diminish the need for restraints or drugs, and do much to prevent the late posttraumatic stress syndromes.

BIBLIOGRAPHY

Burgess AW, Holmstrum LT: Rape trauma syndrome. *Am J Nurs* 131:981–986, 1974.

Gelles, R: *The Violent Home: A Study of Physical Aggression between Husbands and Wives.* Beverly Hills, Calif, Sage, 1979.

George JE (ed.): Child abuse reporting. *Emerg Phys Legal Bull* 3(2):4–10, 1977.

Kempe C: The battered child syndrome. *JAMA* 181:17–24, 1962.

Morkovin V: Care of the injured patient's emotional trauma, in Wilson and Marsden (eds): *Care of the Acutely Ill and Injured.* New York, Wiley, 1982, pp 179–182.

Morkovin V: The professional confronted with human violence. *Top Emerg Med* 3:9–14, 1982.

Reese RN: Child abuse and neglect. *Emerg Clin North Am* 1:207–216, 1983.

Symonds M: Victims of violence: Psychological effects and after-effects. *Am J Psychoanal* 35:19–26, 1975.

SECTION 20
EMERGENCY
MEDICAL SYSTEMS

CHAPTER 143
EMERGENCY
MEDICAL SERVICES

John H. van de Leuv

Emergency medical services (EMS) consist of several distinct components that together form a system of emergency services encompassing the entire spectrum of emergency medical care.

These components deal with emergency care rendered in the prehospital phase, in the emergency department, and in the inhospital phase. Prehospital emergency care is concerned with prevention, detection, communication, notification, rescue, initial stabilization, resuscitation, intervention, and transport. Emergency service in the emergency department is directed toward provision of general or special care, consultation, and transfer. The inhospital phase includes general care or special care in ICU or CCU, or for burns or spinal cord injuries, or neonatal or pediatric intervention. This chapter is chiefly concerned with the prehospital phase.

ORIGIN OF EMS

The Emergency Medical Services System (EMSS) Act of 1973 (Public Law 93-154) gave impetus to the development of local, state, and regional EMS systems. In addition, it presented guidelines for design and implementation of the systems.

State EMS System

Usually, a state EMS system is established under the wing of a supporting organization, such as the state department of public health, the state hospital or medical association or both, a regional planning council, or a combination of the above agencies.

Direct responsibility for planning, implementation, and operation of the EMS system generally rests with the regional EMS council, but some tasks may be delegated to county or local councils. The composition of the regional council, by law, consists of 49 percent providers (physicians, nurses, hospital administrators, paramedics, fire fighters) and 51 percent consumers.

The first order of business for the EMS council is planning. Generally, full-time staff assistance is necessary, preferably by individuals with expertise in planning, communications, transportation, public education, work force training, and medical care.

A specialist in the provision of emergency medical care is appointed director of the organization. Ideally, the director should be a full-time emergency physician.

A survey is done by the council to determine available resources: the number of vehicles in use as rescue units and ambulances; the number of radio units and telemetry units; hospitals with emergency departments and their categories; EMT and paramedic training programs; available physicians; advanced cardiac life support (ACLS), basic life support (BLS), and advanced trauma life support (ATLS) instructors, and paramedic and EMT personnel on active duty. With data from the survey, the council sets goals and objectives.

Short-term objectives are to organize an effective EMS council, survey available and needed components of the system, establish standing committees, and secure the greatest possible autonomy with the area council. Standing committees generally include emergency facilities, communications, transportation, public education, work force and training, data collection, and technical advisory committees.

Examples of long-term goals include continued improvement of the EMS system, public education in the use of the system, planning for a system of continued financial support, and devising a workable and lasting system. These objectives are plotted on a time schedule so that progress can be reviewed from time to time.

One of the first tasks of the council usually is to apply for a grant from the State Department of Health or other granting agents. Such grants may provide monies for planning and organization, purchase of communication equipment and transport vehicles, EMT training, and operation of the system. The monies available from the state department of health or other agents designated by that department allocate monies received from the federal government as block grants which include funds for the EMS system.

Early in the planning stage, the EMS council must also plan for sources of funding to augment the grant monies. An EMS program is not inexpensive. It is estimated that the cost per call is between $100 and $200. Reimbursement possibilities include (1) total tax support by geopolitical area residents, (2) support through continued grants, and (3) patient or third-party payment. The last alternative is probably too expensive. A compromise might be to have the public pay for the "availability" and the patient or insurer pay for the "use."

EMS AND ITS PREHOSPITAL CARE COMPONENTS

Prevention

Prevention of emergencies involves a widespread and concerted effort at education, such as the safety and accident prevention programs in industry. There must also be a determined effort by manufacturers to provide safe packaging and sufficient information concerning their products to facilitate initiation of measures to deal with unexpected overexposure.

Measures to improve the safety of vehicles and protective equipment are but one example of an industrywide attack on hazards facing the public. Another partially successful effort is found in the provision of "childproof" medication containers.

Training

Minimum training requirements for first responders, nurses, EMTs, physicians, and others involved in emergency care are described below.

First responders. Since first responders often are not EMTs, paramedics, or physicians, the EMS system must assume the responsibility for training the lay public and law enforcement personnel in basic life support. A considerable segment of the population can be trained by cardiopulmonary resuscitation (CPR) courses in public areas such as schools, fire stations, and hospitals.

Nurses. Nurses (RNs and LPNs or LVNs) who staff the emergency department must be trained to the highest degree possible. Just as nurses in the cardiac care units receive special training, so, too, must emergency department nurses be prepared for the role they assume. It is not unreasonable to expect all RNs to undergo a provider course in ACLS, and some should attain instructor status. Licensed practical nurses and emergency technicians should, as a minimum, have basic life support and preferably EMT basic training. The certificate of emergency nursing (CEN) sponsored by the Emergency Department Nurses Association (EDNA) has helped provide a higher level of competence and a sense of pride in the nurses of the emergency department.

Other good programs are the cardiac care and critical care courses. The EDNA core curriculum can serve as a guide to inservice materials.

Physicians. All hospital staff physicians should have CPR certification. Emergency physicians should have ACLS provider status as a minimum, and at least some should be ACLS instructors. In addition, the emergency department physician should be trained in and, if possible, be an instructor of advanced trauma life support.

Rescue squads. Standards for training levels of rescue squad members and time constraints for attaining these have been set forth by many EMS systems. The basic requirement is that of EMT (basic) status. EMT-A is in many states a step up from the EMT (basic). The nomenclature unfortunately is not uniform nationwide, but neither is reciprocity of certification. Each two- or three-person squad should have at least one paramedic on board.

Other personnel. All other personnel in the emergency department should have BLS certificates as a minimum.

Communications

The communication center is where most components of the EMS system are triggered into action. No matter how good the doctors, nurses, hospitals, and paramedics, no matter how modern the equipment, no matter how updated the training, the system has failed if it is unable to deliver the appropriate service to the correct location at the right time.

The first step in designing a communications system is the determination of the type of service to be provided. The prologue to a well-planned system is competent research to analyze factors such as demand for service, service area, existing facilities, and budget constraints.

Although individual communities have differing needs, certain aspects of a communications system are common to all areas, whether they are urban, suburban, or rural.

The basic elements comprising a communications system are as follows:

- Discovery and response
- Access: Notifying of and gaining entry into the system by the public
- Receiving and screening: Acquiring relevant data regarding emergencies and determining priorities
- Dispatch: Sending the closest appropriate aid to a location
- Hospital notification and participation: Provision of basic life support, medical control, and advanced life support

Discovery and Response

The discoverer is, by definition, any individual who first notices an emergency. He or she may or may not be able to do CPR. The first responder is an individual trained to perform CPR, while a second responder is trained to provide advanced cardiac life support. In some areas, the first and second response can be provided by the same unit, while in others, ACLS is provided by a second team at the scene or in the emergency department. Successful patient resuscitation depends on the rapidity and ease of notification and response of trained personnel. Eisenberg et al. have reported that the best results at resuscitation are obtained if basic life support is initiated within 4 min, and advanced life support within 8 min.

Access

The EMS system is triggered into action when a call is made for aid. The population covered by the service must be familiar with the means and the method to make contact. The contact can be by telephone, radio, telegraph, or fire alarm siren, although the telephone is the most convenient.

A single telephone number that is easy to remember is not only preferred but essential. A situation can only deteriorate when a citizen needs help fast, yet is faced with the difficulty of sorting out which of several numbers is the correct number for police, fire, and EMS. Often, the caller will in desperation dial 0 on the telephone and contact the operator for assistance. Unfortunately, the operator is not in the EMS system and has not been trained in medical screening. The operator may, of course, provide the correct number to EMS, but this wastes time.

The 911 concept is the most popular; 911 is an easily remembered, easily dialed telephone number that can be used for all emergencies. It is hoped by many EMS specialists that 911 will be adopted in all areas of the United States so that no matter where a person is, easy access to emergency care will be available. In 911 systems, all emergency calls are handled by one center, so that EMS and the police and fire departments need the same consideration.

Receiving and Screening

Once contact has been made, the receiving and screening responsibility begins. The individuals assigned to receive calls from the public must be capable of handling emergency demands. This capability includes the technical knowledge of the job, the ability to handle stress, and the ability to deal with hysteria and verbal abuse of the caller. The traditional technique of selecting candidates for this position by testing and interviewing should be augmented by the use of psychological profiles.

The difference in the size and scope of EMS systems begins to come into play at the receiving and dispatching stage of communications development. Some systems have the access-receiving and screening-dispatching functions at the same site, and use the same people to handle both. In larger systems, the access and receiving function is handled at one site, but the screening and dispatching function is handled at a different location. First and foremost, the site where calls are screened should be the same place from which EMS units are dispatched (see below).

Receiving and screening calls are two separate functions, although the receiver may also act as screener. Those assigned to EMS screening should be trained communicators with backgrounds in emergency medical care. In addition, they should be provided screening guidelines that have been developed with strong emergency physician involvement. Screeners must determine location information and gather important data about the urgency of the call. For example, if a call involves a victim of a shooting or heart attack, or an unconscious person, the screener can logically conclude that a high-priority emergency exists, and can have a unit dispatched without asking further questions other than to obtain location information. If, on the other hand, the caller's information suggests that a life-threatening situation does not exist, the guidelines should be flexible enough to allow the screener to continue with predetermined questions. For example, if a caller states that a boy fell off his bike and has pain in his right arm, the screener, according to guidelines, would ask if swelling, dislocation, or deformity is present. The screener who receives this information will then better be able to make an informed, intelligent decision regarding the dispatching of an EMS unit.

The need to have the screening site located with the dispatching site carries profound significance in the operation of an EMS system. In the provision of emergency care, the first-come–first-served adage carries much less importance than the policy of servicing first those with the most severe medical need. The screening done at the communications facility is nothing more than telephone triage. Triage results in the prioritization of calls, which in turn results in dispatch of units to the most serious conditions. If the screening and dispatching functions are separated, the likelihood of placing more serious cases behind less serious cases increases.

Dispatch

When the location of an emergency and the type and degree of distress have been determined, the decision to dispatch a unit is made. In many instances, this is comparatively simple. For the boy who fell off his bike and has a suspected simple arm fracture, the dispatcher will send the closest appropriate EMS unit, provided a more serious case does not occur in the same area. In other instances, the dispatching will be more complex. If there is a multiple-injury automobile accident, for example, it may be necessary to also dispatch police aid for traffic control and fire units for extrication or gasoline washdown.

When an EMS unit is dispatched, it is important to provide the crew with data related to the location, the type, and the degree of distress, as well as any other pertinent data. Such data may include diverse facts, such as a crowd is on the scene, a suspect in a shooting is still at the location, or a large fire is in progress in the area. Data like this are extremely helpful to the EMS crew in terms of preparation, securing the scene, and providing treatment.

A unit arriving on the scene will often find the situation to be quite different from that described to the communications facility. The screener cannot, and should not, be expected to receive complete information on each call. Screening can and should be expected to allow dispatchers to deploy resources intelligently, and to minimize inappropriate demands on the system.

Hospital Notification and Participation

Hospital emergency department involvement can begin once the unit arrives on the scene. Ideally, the hospital notification system may include the following components: (1) field unit to hospital, (2) communications center to hospital, and (3) hospital to hospital.

The nature of communications between hospitals and field unit varies depending on whether basic life support or advanced life support is being used in the field.

Communication between BLS personnel and the hospital is established via two-way radio, telephone, or both. Conversations between the emergency department and the BLS unit are generally limited to exchanges of information. This is acceptable because BLS personnel are not expected to provide advanced care. The radio hospital notification system should be separate from regular dispatching frequencies and all messages should be recorded on tape. The hospital must make certain that the frequency used for interface with BLS units is free from any other traffic such as hospital paging. This is necessary to ensure that lines of communication remain open for BLS functions.

In almost all life-threatening situations when an ACLS crew is on the scene, radio contact with a designated or receiving hospital must be established as soon as possible. Standing orders should be used when communication cannot be established for valid reasons, or if the system specifically allows standing orders to be used without medical control. It is not necessary for the medical control facility also to be the receiving facility. Neither is it mandatory for the system to use one facility for its medical control. Often geographic or geopolitical considerations play a role in determining the site or sites of medical control.

There are various valid reasons why a hospital cannot accept a particular patient. With a hospital notification system, field units can be advised to transport to a different facility if that is necessary. An additional benefit of hospital notification is the increased ability to coordinate resources in disaster planning. Effective communication can assure that multiple-casualty situations do not result in the overutilization of some hospitals and the underutilization of others. Obviously, apportionment of patients according to number and to type and degree of illness or injury adds to the quality of a health care delivery system.

Hospital Emergency Facility Categories

Hospitals and their emergency facilities can be categorized in three ways: horizontal, vertical, and circular. Horizontal categorization deals with the general capability of the hospital and its emergency department and the backup services for each facility (Table 143-1). Vertical categorization addresses the capabilities in seven special categories: poisoning, neonatal, burn, trauma, CNS, psychiatry, and cardiac. Circular categorization refers to agreements between hospitals with different levels of the horizontal and vertical categories to transfer and accept patients to an appropriate facility.

The Joint Commission on Accreditation of Hospitals (JCAH) is the first organization to attempt a nationwide categorization. This categorization has not met with nationwide acceptance but is a step in the right direction. Many EMS jurisdictions still use their own version or adopt parts of the process from other organizations (e.g., the trauma level designation as delineated by the American College of Surgeons).

Despite the well-intended attempts, categorization is still in a state of confusion. Also, too often categorization means self-categorization without attempts to verify the proclaimed status, or without clout to alter it, if needed.

Categorization should never be intended to guide the public to one facility or another but should serve as a guide for use by personnel in the prehospital phase and emergency department.

Medical Control

Simply stated, medical control is the entity accountable for the medical competence of an EMS system. Admittedly, medical control encompasses a universe of responsibility, including the training of physicians, nurses, paramedics, and EMTs; the performance of the system; and evaluation among others. Controversy occurs because medical control is usually centered upon an individual physician, a group of physicians, or a single hospital. Ideally medical control is vested in one institution but, as alluded to previously, this is not always possible.

If medical control is in one institution, this facility is called the resource hospital and other hospitals in the system are referred to as associate hospitals.

The resource hospital exists to coordinate the many and complex elements in the system. This does not mean that input from associate hospitals is not accepted. On the contrary, associate hospital input should be enthusiastically encouraged. Regular meetings with EMS administrators, medical control professionals, and associate hospital professionals make an outstanding forum for such areas as decision making, developing policies, and airing grievances.

Medical control also means quality review. It is mandatory to retain the credibility of an EMS that all ''runs'' of squads be reviewed by a knowledgeable body of representatives of components of the system. Problems thus unearthed should be discussed and proper measures taken to remedy the situation. It would be ideal if this reviewing body had disciplining authority.

Transport

Vehicle design. Essential equipment and medical requirements for ambulances and design of the ambulance and other rescue vehicles are set forth in publications of the government and of the American College of Surgeons. Ambulance design is guided by criteria developed by the National Academy of Engineering. The vehicles that have gained popularity are the van and modular units, with the latter being favored in recent years.

Equipment. Each rescue vehicle must have certain minimum equipment based on the purpose of the vehicle (BLS or ALS).

Life support measures have become more sophisticated, and the armamentarium of the providers in the field has become more complex and varied. It is impossible, given the scope of this chapter, to place dollar amounts on the cost of equipment.

Table 143-1. JCAH Categorization of Emergency Services (Horizontal Mode)

Level	Description	Physician Coverage	Hospital Facilities	Services Provided
I	Comprehensive emergency service	ED open 24 h/day; at least one experienced emergency physician on duty	Med, surg, ortho, peds, anesth available. Other specialties available in 30 min	Can manage physical and emotional problems on definitive basis
II	Major emergency service	ED open 24 h/day; one experienced emergency physician on duty	Specialty consultation available in 30 min	Can manage physical and emotional problems with provision for patient transfer to another facility when needed
III	General emergency service	ED open 24 h/day; physician available within 30 min by medical staff call roster		Specialty consultation available on request or by transfer to designated hospital for definitive care
IV	Limited emergency service	Mechanism for physician coverage defined by medical staff		Offers reasonable care in determining whether emergency exists. Renders first aid. Referral to nearest facility capable of providing necessary service

Source: Accreditation Manual for Hospitals. Chicago, Joint Commission on Accreditation of Hospitals, 1984, p 21.

Types of transport needed. Transport by land vehicles is most effective for ranges up to 30 mi or when the transport vehicle is expected to reach its destination in about 30 min. Much of this depends on notification, dispatch, availability, and terrain.

Helicopter transport is effective in favorable weather conditions, when the distance or time of transport is greater than mentioned in the above paragraph, or when terrain makes land transport ineffective or time-consuming. Many helicopter services provide a crew that includes a physician or specially trained nursing personnel to stabilize patients before transport and to monitor patients during the flight. The effective range of the helicopter is said to be between 50 and 150 mi. This mode of transport is also valuable in interhospital transfers. Helipads or otherwise secure landing areas must be available at or near the scene and at the destination.

Fixed-wing aircraft can be used for transport over distances greater than 100 mi. However, at each end of the flight, land or helicopter transport must supplement the use of this type of air transport.

BIBLIOGRAPHY

Accreditation Manual for Hospitals. Chicago, Joint Commission on Accreditation of Hospitals, 1984.

Ambulance Design Criteria. Washington, National Academy of Engineering, US Government Printing Office, 1971.

Committee on Emergency Medical Service, Division of Medical Sciences: National Academy of Science, National Research Council: *Medical Requirements for Ambulance Design and Equipment.* Publication No (HSM) 73-2035, US Dept of Health, Education, and Welfare, 1973.

Eisenberg MS, Bergner L, Hallstrom A: Cardiac resuscitation in the community: Importance of rapid provision and implication for program planning. *JAMA* 241:1905–1907, 1979.

Emergency Medical Services Act of 1973, 42 USC, 300d.

Essential equipment for ambulances. Bull Am Col Surg 62::7–12, September 1977.

Jelenko C III, Frey CF (eds): *Emergency Medical Services: An overview.* Bowie, Md, Brady, 1976.

Jenkins AL, van de Leuv JH (eds): *Emergency Department Organization and Management.* St Louis, Mosby, 1978.

Podgorny G: ACEP and UA/EM urge EMSS act extension, editorial. *JACEP* 8:170, 1979.

The prehospital care system. *Top Emerg Med* 1(4), January 1980.

CHAPTER 144
DISASTER PLANNING

Michael L. DeMars

Disaster planning is one of the most important issues the EMS community must address. Despite the development of sophisticated technological advances, humans still do not maintain control over their environment. Indeed, technology often leads to the occurrence of a disaster. With the establishment of an EMS network, plans must integrate the various agencies and services into a coordinated, working whole to provide efficient relief and care to those involved in a disaster.

A disaster is defined as the occurrence of any incident that produces casualties in numbers too great and at too fast a rate for a community's services to handle in its routine fashion. Disasters are of two major categories. *Natural* disasters include hurricanes, tornados, earthquakes, floods, and volcanic eruptions. *Human-made* or *human-related* disasters include road, rail, air, or water crashes; explosions and fires; chemical, nuclear, or microbiologic or toxic contamination of the environment; and riots, terrorism, and war.

Disaster planning must be done by all governmental entities. Cities, counties, and regions of substantial size should have workable written disaster plans. Airports are required to have such plans by Federal Aviation Agency regulations. Industries should conduct disaster planning both because of the large numbers of people they gather together and because of the increased risk of accidents at industrial sites. Facilities that house large numbers of persons, such as stadiums or arenas, should also plan for disaster management. Hospitals, of course, are required by the Joint Commission on Accreditation of Hospitals to have written disaster plans.

WRITING THE DISASTER PLAN

In writing a disaster plan, a number of factors must be considered. The plan must be comprehensive enough to include all necessary services. It must also be flexible enough to cover disasters of varying type and size. A plan should allow for minidisasters in which normal services are inadequate but full-scale mobilization of all services is not required. At the same time, simplicity must be sought because an overly complicated, voluminous plan will be too confusing for the participants to follow. To keep it simple, the plan should vary as little as possible from daily routine, since people function best if what they are doing is familiar. It has been suggested that separate disaster plans should be devised for special situations such as pediatric disasters. While this may sound de-

sirable, in reality it would defeat attempts at simplicity and result in a cumbersome, complicated package.

The plan must also be written with an eye to coordination with those of adjacent geopolitical areas. Since disasters do not honor local government boundaries, a community cannot afford to be insular in its planning, as agencies and services from other areas may have to be called for assistance.

Who should write the plan? Necessarily, a large number of organizations and services will be involved in the relief effort. Bouzarth and Mariano provide detailed lists of agencies and organizations that might be active. These lists need not be repeated here. It suffices to say that any organization or agency likely to contribute to providing disaster relief and rescue should be considered in writing the plan and their counsel and input sought. The actual writing of the plan will most likely be done by representatives of the major services in the planning process. This must include, at the minimum, representation from the police and fire departments, city or county health departments or both, public and private ambulance services, participating hospitals, local and regional EMS councils, and representatives of the medical community, in particular those involved in emergency medicine. The American College of Emergency Physicians promulgates the prominent involvement of emergency physicians in disaster planning and management and has published a position paper on the subject.

Essential Elements

Holloway, in his discussion of New York City's disaster preparations, outlines four essential components of areawide disaster care that must be considered. They are scene response, transportation, hospitals, and command and coordination.

Scene response. Scene response is that part of the plan dealing with activity primarily at the site of the disaster. This sets forth the procedure for the initial alert and activation of the plan, response by police, fire, and other rescue personnel, field medical care and triage, and on-site coordination of the rescue effort.

Transportation. Transportation deals, logically, with the movement of the victims from the scene to hospitals, shelters, and morgues.

Hospitals. The hospital component of the plan considers the part of the disaster operation occurring at or involving hospitals.

Since all hospitals have internal disaster plans which, hopefully, are coordinated with the area plans, this component of a community plan will deal with procedures for alerting the involved hospitals, classifying their capabilities for various levels of care, and obtaining up-to-date information on their status and capacity.

Command and coordination. The command and coordination component deals with the overall coordination of the disaster effort in the community and the provision of effective communication with and between the various agencies and services involved.

These, then, are the basic components of a disaster plan that must be considered and encompassed. They will be discussed in greater detail later.

Some states have provided guidelines for writing disaster plans which cities and counties follow. While some adjustment for local variations must be made, such guidelines can help provide uniformity among different geopolitical subdivisions.

THE DISASTER OPERATION

Although not an entirely complete division of activity, the disaster effort can be regarded in two parts: the prehospital phase, dealing with all aspects outside of the hospital, and the hospital phase, dealing with the intrahospital activity.

Prehospital Phase

Police

In the actual disaster situation, the police—along with the fire department—are usually the first responders. They will have multiple demands placed upon them, varying according to the type of disaster that has occurred. Prime consideration, of course, is given to assuring the safety of victims and bystanders. Persons in immediate danger of further injury should be removed to safety. The presence of danger factors such as fire near explosive or highly combustible materials must be identified so they can be corrected before further incident. Crowd control must be established and maintained. Panic may occur among those involved in the incident, and curiosity seekers may become unreasonable while attempting to obtain a better view. In some types of disaster, looting is a potential problem.

Routes to be used by ambulances and rescue vehicles must be established and kept open.

The early establishment of effective communication may be a police responsibility. In their role as first responders, it may be they who must sound the first alert. This should be done according to established procedure and through established channels of command so supervisory personnel always know what has been and needs to be done. These supervisors must assist in coordinating the rescue effort with other services and can do this only if well informed by personnel in the ranks.

Coordination of rescue effort may be a duty of the police. Often this is accomplished through cooperative effort between the police and fire departments.

Fire Department

Fire fighters share with the police the role of first responder. Depending on the type of incident, they may be first on the scene.

Besides the obvious duty of putting out fire, they will figure prominently in extrication of victims and should also be alert for dangerous situations that must be corrected for further safety of the victims. They will assist also in establishing communication and should have preestablished procedures for the transmission of information.

Triage

Originally a term meaning "to sort," triage was first applied in a medical sense during the Napoleonic wars. Today, it means the process of sorting and classifying victims into treatment priority categories and routing them to the appropriate treatment facility.

During a mass casualty incident, triage takes on different and more serious implications than during more routine situations. The most basic tenet now becomes the determination of salvageability. This can present considerable conflict for medical personnel accustomed to making all-out efforts for patients with minimal chance for survival. During a disaster, patients who are unlikely to survive despite maximal effort, as well as those whose survival would require the unreasonable deployment of limited resources, are deemed unsalvageable, and no or minimal effort is expended on them. In the field, this means they receive little or no care and are placed in low-priority categories, being transferred next to last, just ahead of the actual dead. If they survive to reach the hospital and their condition does not warrant a change in category, they receive only supportive, palliative care.

This approach can be difficult for medical and rescue personnel to adopt. But, the primary aim of the rescue effort is to salvage the greatest number possible. Spending inordinate amounts of time and resources—both of which are limited—on victims unlikely to survive, defeats this intent and deprives salvageable victims of necessary care.

Types of Triage

Triage is not a onetime activity but an ongoing process that is repeated as patients progress in the rescue and treatment operation. Primary triage occurs in the field and is the first classification effort. It is begun by the first qualified personnel on the scene. This may be police or fire personnel, or EMTs from the local EMS system. These personnel may later be relieved by an organized triage team, usually consisting of physicians and nurses. This transfer of responsibility must occur smoothly. It is essential that the team not waste time retriaging victims already prioritized by the original personnel. This temptation can be considerable when professionals take over from paraprofessional personnel. The loss of time and the repetitive effort are not justifiable.

The main aim of primary triage is the rapid classification of all victims. Victims should be seen and categorized as quickly as possible so that salvageable victims are not overlooked while time is spent on the unsalvageable or minimally injured. Minimal treatment is given during the primary triage process unless adequate backup medical personnel are on-site to provide more. Lacking this, the team should limit treatment to opening airways and controlling life-threatening blood flow.

During primary triage, a tagging system should be initiated that will be adhered to throughout the disaster operation. (See the section on triage tagging.)

Secondary triage occurs—if adequate personnel are available—

at the departure point (ambulance loading area). With the responsibility of the location and initial categorization of victims discharged, victims can be reexamined in somewhat more depth and the priority changed if indicated. Secondary triage aims for more accurate categorization and seeks to enhance survival chances by not overestimating or underestimating a victim's need.

Both primary and secondary triage seek to avoid the "load and go" approach, an experience that occurs in many actual disaster situations. In these incidents, the somewhat natural tendency to grab and transfer those victims closest to the ambulance loading area results in hospitals initially receiving large numbers of walking wounded while the transfer of the more seriously injured is unduly delayed. This can result in early overload of hospital facilities and exhaustion of medical supplies necessary for those in greatest need of care. The delayed treatment of seriously injured patients—and the resultant loss of life—is obvious.

Triage is again repeated as victims arrive at the hospital. This tertiary triage is aimed at reaffirming treatment priorities and directing victims to the appropriate treatment area within the hospital. (See the section on hospital triage and treatment areas.) Tertiary triage should not be regarded as a de novo process. It should be utilized to further the accuracy of the first two steps in the process. The tendency at the hospital may be to ignore the decisions made in the field and retag victims. This not only wastes time and is repetitive but it greatly increases the likelihood of inaccuracy.

Triage Categories

In all stages of triage, it is important to adopt and adhere to a uniform system of priorities. Confusion results if all personnel do not adopt the same terminology and utilize consistent definitions for these terms. The system used should avoid too many and too complex categories. The use of a few simple categories—applied consistently—avoids confusion and chaos. A good system being used increasingly is that of four priority categories. These might be designated first priority, second priority, walking wounded, and lowest priority.

First-priority victims are those who are seriously injured but whose chances of survival are good if treatment is adequate and prompt. These victims warrant first consideration.

Second priority is given to those with serious injury but whose treatment can be somewhat delayed without undue threat of loss of life or limb.

Walking wounded are those victims with relatively minor injuries whose treatment may consist of only first aid or whose treatment can be delayed for extended periods without deleterious effect. They need not necessarily be truly walking, as victims with minor fractures of the leg would be included in this group.

Lowest-priority victims are those not salvageable even with prompt attention and, of course, the actual dead.

Tagging

A system of triage tagging should be adopted that will be followed uniformly throughout the disaster operation. The tag itself should not be complicated yet should provide space for important notations. It should be readily identifiable and provide for prompt identification of the victim's priority.

An excellent tag has been devised by *The Journal of Civil Defense* in Starke, Florida. Called the Medical Emergency Triage Tag (METTAG), it is distinctive and provides for quick notation of important identifying factors (sex, name, address) as well as notation of treatment given, and it provides illustrations for noting location of injuries. Priority category is indicated by a series of colored bands on the bottom of the tag. The category of a particular victim is indicated by tearing off the colored bands down to the category desired. From inside out, these categories are as follows:

Black, 0, unsalvageable
Red, I, highest priority
Yellow, II, second priority
Green, III, walking wounded

All emergency vehicles should carry an extra supply of tags in case some are lost or are torn from the patient.

A backup system that adheres to the same categories may be desirable and could be used if tags are not readily available. For example, the priority category can be marked on the victim's forehead or arm with pens or markers. The tags could then be used when they became available without disturbing the categories already assigned. A suggested system is as follows:

XXX—First priority
XX—Second priority
X—Walking wounded
O—Unsalvageable

The numbers used in the METTAG system (0, I, II, III) could be substituted if that system were in use.

Triage Teams

The medical triage team has increasingly become a part of disaster planning. This resource should be drawn from a single source, preferably the major resource hospital in the area, to facilitate training and organization of the team and simplify their pickup for transportation to the scene. Traditionally, surgeons have acted in this capacity but this is a function increasingly appropriate to emergency department personnel.

Whatever the final composition of the team, it must be drawn from a single source. The members of the team must be thoroughly trained and briefed on the function they are to serve. Especially if house officers are used, attention must be paid to updating their training, and any changes in team membership caused by rotating house officers must be detected and new members trained. Emergency medicine residents are a source of house officers that is easy to keep current.

The disaster plan must provide for assembling the team at a designated place for transport to the site. The method of transportation must be worked out, as well as the assembly, storage, and pickup of any equipment the team is to carry.

The triage team must be immediately and easily identifiable at the site. Hard hats or vests of durable reflective material, clearly marked, have been used. The chief triage officer should be identified by slight variation in uniform.

The safety of the teams while on-site must also be assured. While competent medically, these personnel are largely unfamiliar with working in other than indoor environments. Instruction should be provided to the team in recognizing fire hazard and actions necessary to avoid fire or explosion, dealing with downed power lines, and precautions to take while working near toxic atmospheres.

Control

For control of the disaster effort, a central control point for the entire operation should be established. This is often located in a facility in conjunction with the police or fire department. It should be staffed by personnel from these departments and any other services vital to the operation. The control center is responsible for receiving and collating information from the scene, the hospitals, and other services involved. The center provides additional personnel and equipment to the scene as needed. The control center should also have a mechanism for gathering up-to-the-minute information on the status and supplies of individual hospitals, e.g., the availability of blood, so that accurate decisions may be made for the dispersal of victims. This information should be obtained on a daily, ready basis. Waiting until a disaster has occurred to begin gathering such information is inefficient and ineffective.

Additionally, a command post at the disaster site is vital. This post should be in close proximity to but a safe distance from the actual site. Staffed by supervisory personnel from the police and fire departments and a medical command officer, the command post is responsible for the receipt of information from the control center and the decisions in putting it to use. The on-site communications center is also located here. The command post must be readily identifiable by features such as banners and lights. Arriving ambulances should report here for instructions on dispersal.

Communications

Communications has been cited as the single largest problem in dealing with a disaster. It can almost be expected that communication will break down, so this probability must be anticipated. Telephone communication, especially with hospitals, may almost certainly be expected to fail as circuits are jammed with calls from private citizens seeking information. Radio communication, especially the hospital emergency area radio (HEAR) system, or fire and police frequencies, are commonly used.

Of equal importance with having equipment, however, is the establishment of organized procedures for its use. Communication often fails because protocols have not been established in the planning phase. This enhances the importance of channeling communication through the control center and the on-site command post so communication can be monitored. The unexpected arrival of large numbers of casualties at a hospital must be avoided.

Public Health Considerations

Because of the inherent disruption of normal services, especially when the disruption is due to the physical damage of public or private facilities, certain public health problems may result from the disaster. Water supplies may become contaminated and waste disposal services disrupted or terminated. Food supplies may become contaminated or destroyed either as a direct result of the disaster incident or because of the loss of refrigeration facilities. Shelter may be needed by huge numbers of persons left homeless. All this results in serious threat of the outbreak of disease at a time when the community is ill-prepared to deal with an epidemic.

These possibilities must be considered in the disaster planning process. In a disaster situation extensive enough to produce these disruptions, local agencies will probably be ineffective and state or federal governments will need to be called upon to provide the needed relief. However, a mechanism must be included in the local plan for recognizing the need for outside assistance, and for initiating early calls for help.

Psychiatric Considerations

The psychiatric aspects of disaster have been studied and the reactions of both victims and workers outlined elsewhere. While an in-depth discussion of this topic is beyond the scope of the present work, some useful information can be gleaned that provides practical tips on dealing with disaster victims.

Disaster workers must be prepared to meet and deal with a variety of reactions from victims. The disaster workers must not expect to use a single approach to all victims any more than they would with all patients in any other setting. Keeping victims together as much as possible provides relief from fear and also affords the opportunity for victims to ventilate feelings by discussing and reliving the incident with others involved. This is an added advantage of clearing entire hospital wards and admitting all disaster victims to the same area. Only a very disturbed victim will require isolation. This is done not only to protect the disturbed one but to diminish further emotional trauma to the other victims.

The provision of hot drinks and blankets to victims provides a sense of being looked after and a comforting feeling of shelter from the threat they have faced.

Adoption of a leadership role by disaster workers helps calm the inner turmoil the victims are experiencing. A facade of confidence on the part of these workers does much to assure the victims that they are safe. Directions given to victims should be in gentle but firm words to convey the impression that they are being helped by someone capable of taking care of them.

In the recovery period, the individual practitioner will need to be alert for signs that a particular patient may be developing emotional sequelae requiring further psychiatric intervention.

Dealing with the Dead

Provision must be made for the removal, storage, and identification of the deceased. In general, these victims are the last to be dealt with while rescue of the living is ongoing. An area at the disaster site should be designated for collecting the bodies. Depending upon numbers, a temporary morgue may have to be established in whatever facility is available. Refrigerated trucks may be useful for this function. Local funeral directors can be of invaluable assistance in this operation.

No bodies or parts of bodies should be moved before the medical examiner has taken charge. Any personal articles of victims should be left where found to assist the medical examiner in identifying bodies.

The medical examiner assumes responsibility for coordinating the identification process. The disaster site is documented with maps, diagrams, and photographs. Bodies and personal belongings are tagged with reference to their position on the map.

The Hospital Phase

Hospital preparation for disaster involves many details. An overview will be given here. An excellent treatment of the subject is included in "Disaster Planning," *Emergency Department Organization and Management*. The reader is referred to this source for more detailed discussion.

At the hospital, preparation must be made to rapidly accommodate the large influx of casualties. Since normal emergency department services may be expected to be overloaded with the arrival of the first few victims, dealing with the disaster rapidly becomes a whole-hospital operation. The disaster plan must be set up to use personnel, space, and supplies most efficiently.

Control Center

An inhospital command center must be set up to coordinate the activity. Since the operation becomes one of total hospital involvement, this center is best located elsewhere than in the emergency department, which will be busy enough treating the victims. The center should be controlled by an administrative official with the authority to command the entire operation. The official should be assisted by whatever department heads may be required. All information coming into or going out of the hospital should be channeled through this office.

Activating the Plan

Once the decision has been made to activate the disaster plan, several things need to be done rapidly. Everyone must know his or her job and be prepared to act accordingly. It is too late to consult the disaster manual when the alert is sounded. Savage has suggested that personnel carry action cards detailing individual responsibilities which can be consulted rapidly if workers are uncertain about how to proceed.

A system for calling in personnel not on duty is imperative. Since this can involve a large number of calls, a cascade or pyramid system has been suggested whereby the hospital switchboard notifies a small number of persons who each in turn notifies a certain number of others who in turn call others. In this way large numbers of personnel can be contacted without tying up operators and hospital telephone lines.

A rapid survey of the hospital must be made and arrangements begun for the discharge or transfer of patients to make room for incoming casualties. Matters are simplified if one or more nursing units are cleared of all patients and set up to receive disaster victims. This allows casualties to be admitted to a concentrated area that can be kept supplied more easily and augments keeping track of individual patients.

All support services should have provisions within their respective departments for activation of the plan. These services include radiology, laboratory, central supply, and blood bank. Each area should rapidly survey its stock and personnel, and prepare accurate current information for the control center.

A designated area of the hospital should be prepared to function as a temporary morgue should the usual morgue facilities prove inadequate.

Treatment Areas

Specific areas of the hospital should be designated for treating specific degrees of injury. In general, areas should be established

for these functions: (1) receiving and triage, (2) resuscitation and treatment of the critically injured, (3) intermediate treatment, (4) delayed treatment, and (5) palliative treatment only.

Receiving and triage. This area must obviously be established at or near the emergency entrance. The ambulance approach to the hospital should be kept clear and allow one-way approach and departure only.

The triage area should be at or adjacent to the entrance. It should be as large as possible and allow shelter for victims during the triage process. Only the functions of triage and the initiation of documentation should be done here. No treatment should be attempted.

Critical treatment area. This area is to receive those requiring the most extensive resuscitation. It is usually located in the emergency department itself as it is already equipped and staffed for such care. Once stabilized, a patient may, if condition permits, be transferred to the intermediate care area to await surgery or admission.

Intermediate treatment area. This area receives seriously injured but stable patients who require a certain amount of care and observation but not major resuscitative effort.

Delayed treatment area. This area is designated to handle those patients whose treatment may be delayed for extended periods without undue injury. The walking wounded would be directed here. The term *delayed* infers only that treatment may be delayed if necessary. As much actual treatment as allowed by the availability of personnel will be done. This includes suturing lacerations and minor orthopedic procedures.

Palliative treatment area. This is reserved for those patients deemed unsalvageable who may reach the hospital prior to death. Only supportive treatment is given here and the patients should be made as comfortable as possible. This is the only treatment area in which visitors to the patients should be allowed.

Documentation

Personnel should be in the triage area to begin documentation. It may be desirable to use the existing emergency chart since it is a record familiar to hospital personnel. Some consider this too cumbersome, however, and have opted for using special disaster tags that are, in effect, minicharts. In either event, once the patient's identification and designated treatment area are entered on the record, one copy of the record should be removed and sent to the information center so casualty lists can be begun. The rest of the record should remain with the patient throughout the treatment process. Should patient and record become separated, it can be extremely difficult to determine patient status and what has already been done or not done. Likewise, all laboratory reports and roentgenograms should remain with the patient.

Security

With activation of the disaster plan, steps should be taken to institute and maintain traffic and crowd control. All entrances to the hospital should be locked except those being used to admit or discharge victims and personnel. These open entrances should be controlled so that unauthorized persons cannot gain admission to any except designated public areas. Designated waiting areas for the public and the press should be established and maintained, preferably remote from treatment areas. Definite routes should be established for patient flow, and these corridors should be patrolled to ensure smooth flow and prevent unauthorized traffic.

Public Relations

The hospital public relations officer acts as liaison between the hospital and the public and press. This officer should be supplied with casualty lists and patient condition reports as soon as they become available. These reports should be updated as often as possible so relatives can be kept informed. All statements being issued from the hospital should be channeled through this office.

Personnel, possibly volunteers, should be assigned to this office to help assist relatives who will congregate at the hospital. Keeping them as informed as possible, supplying coffee and cold drinks, and, in general, providing as many amenities as possible will do much to prevent the restlessness that easily sets in among people in these circumstances.

Communications

The primary instrument of communication of all hospitals, the telephone, can rapidly become overloaded in a disaster situation. The switchboard can expect to become swamped with calls from relatives trying to locate or obtain information about their loved ones. Telephone circuits in general may become overloaded by the increased demand of the public.

Some relief can be gained by commandeering pay phones for hospital use. As these phones bypass the switchboard, they supplement the hospital's telephone system and can be used for both incoming and outgoing calls.

Alternative forms of communication may have to be utilized. If a hospital participates in the HEAR system of VHF radio communication, this resource can be used. However, the HEAR system is limited in the amount of traffic it can handle and it cannot be the sole backup system of communication.

Radios in emergency vehicles can be another source of communication. Since these vehicles will often be at the hospital entrance to discharge victims, they can be used to relay information to other vehicles at a distance from the hospital.

Commercial radio and television can also be used to notify hospital personnel to report to work.

BIBLIOGRAPHY

American College of Emergency Physicians: Role of the emergency physician in mass casualty/disaster management. *JACEP* 5:901–903, 1976.

Alter AJ: Environmental health experiences in disaster. *Am J Public Health* 60:475–480, 1970.

Baker FJ: Management of mass casualty disasters. *Top Emerg Med* 1:149–157, 1979.

Bohn GA, Richie CG: Learning by simulation. The validation of disaster simulation: Medical scheme planning. *J Kans Med Soc* 71:418–425, 1970.

Bouzarth WF, Mariano JP: Disaster preparedness, in Schwartz GR, Safar P, Stone JH, et al (eds): *Principles and Practice of Emergency Medicine*, vol II. Philadelphia, Saunders, 1978, pp 1422–1427.

Burt FN: Principles of on-site triage, lecture given to paramedics. Providence Hospital, Southfield, Mich, 1977.

Clark RB: Disaster drills, letter to the editor. *JACEP* 7:416, 1978.

Cross RE: The team approach to disaster care. *J Emerg Nurs* 3:17–19, November–December 1977.

DeMars ML, Buss RM, Cleland LC: The use of victim-tracking cards in a community disaster drill, paper presented at Ninth Annual Workshop of the University Association for Emergency Medicine, Orlando, Fla, May 24, 1979.

Disaster planning—Fact or fiction?, editorial. *Br Med J* 2:406–407, 1975.

Disaster planning, in Jenkins AL, van de Leuv JH (eds): *Emergency Department Organization and Management*, ed 2. St Louis, Mosby, 1978, pp 243–261.

Edwards GJ: Psychiatric aspects of civilian disasters. *Br Med J* 1:944–947, 1976.

Emergency Health/Medical Services Annex to Wayne County Basic Plan. Westland, Mich, Wayne County Health Department, 1976.

Evans D: Simulated aircraft disaster instructional exercise at Baltimore-Washington International airport. *Avia Space Environ Med* 47:445–448, 1976.

Fishel ER: Exercise 'Med-Ex' 73. *Md State Med J* 23:46–48, 1974.

Fisher CJ Jr: Mobile triage team in a community disaster plan. *JACEP* 6:10–12, 1977.

Gibson WH: Disaster planning. *J Soc Occup Med* 26:136–138, 1976.

Gierson ED, Richman LS: Valley triage: An approach to mass casualty care. *J Trauma* 15:193–196, 1975.

Hays MB, Stefanki JX, Cheu DH: Planning an airport disaster drill. *Avia Space Environ Med* 47:556–560, 1976.

Holloway RD, Steliga JF, Ryan CT: The EMS system and disaster planning: Some observations. *JACEP* 7:60–61, 1978.

Holloway RM: Medical disaster planning, I: Urban areas. *NY State J Med* 71:591–595, 1971.

Holloway RM: Medical disaster planning, II: New York City's preparations. *NY State J Med* 71:692–694, 1971.

Irving M: Major disasters: Hospital admission procedures. *Br J Med* 63:731–734, 1976.

Members of the medical staff of three London hospitals: Moorgate tube train disaster, Part I: Response of medical services. *Br Med J* 3:727–731, 1975.

Miller PJ: The management of major accidents. *Injury* 2:168–181, 1971.

Mills WJ: The exchangeable uniform stretcher, letter to the editor. *Alaska Med* 15:1–2, 1973.

Moles TM: Planning for major disasters. *Br J Anaesth* 49:643–649, 1977.

Naggan L: Medical planning for disaster in Israel: Evaluation of the military surgical experience in the October 1973 War, and implication for the organization of the civilian disaster services. *Injury* 7:279–285, 1976.

Patterson C, Rowbottom B: Explosion! A case study in disaster drills. *J Emerg Nurs* 3:9–13, November–December 1977.

Pedersen EB: Safety at disaster sites. *Aust Fam Phys* 7:25–29, 1978.

Planning for disaster, editorial. *Br Med J* 3:3–4, 1972.

Recommended Procedures for Writing Emergency Health/Medical Services Plan (Annex to County Plan). Lansing, Mich, Michigan Department of Public Health, 1979.

Rutherford WH: Surgery of violence, II: Disaster procedures. *Br Med J* 1:443–445, 1975.

Savage PEA: Disaster planning. A major accident exercise. *Br Med J* 4:168–171, 1970.

Savage PEA: Disaster planning: Protective clothing for medical teams. *Injury* 7:286–287, 1976.

Savage PEA: Disaster planning: A review. *Injury* 3:49–55, 1971.

Savage PEA: Disaster planning: The use of action cards. *Br Med J* 3:43–45, 1972.

Shamer LC: Triage: The treatment of mass casualties by fire/rescue personnel. *Int Fire Chief* 43:18–21, 1977.

Spitz WU: Medical examiner at scene of major disaster. Communication from Wayne County medical examiner, Detroit, Mich, undated.

Stalcup SA, Oscherwitz M, Cohen MS, et al: Planning for a pediatric disaster: Experience gained from caring for 1600 Vietnamese orphans. *N Engl J Med* 293:691–695, 1975.

Tarrow AB: The Philadelphia airport disaster exercise. *S Afr Med J* 52:157–158, 1977.

Theoret JJ: Exercise London: A disaster exercise involving numerous casualties. *Can Med Assoc J* 114:697–699, 1976.

Watler P, Brooks S, Orchid R: Galveston's grain elevator explosion. *Emergency* 10:32–33, 1978.

Watt J: The role of the services in accident and disaster. *Injury* 8:250–259, 1977.

Wilkins EW (ed): Disaster planning, in *MGH Textbook of Emergency Medicine*. Baltimore, Williams & Wilkins, 1978, pp 743–749.

Wilson RI: The role of the hospital in disasters. *Injury* 5:228–232, 1974.

CHAPTER 145
EMERGENCY
DEPARTMENT
ADMINISTRATION

John H. van de Leuv

INTRODUCTION

Administration of the emergency department (ED) has become a complex task. In the sixties the director of the ED—usually one of the emergency physicians elected as president—had the primary duty to schedule the physicians; second, as leader of the ED the director was responsible for its smooth function. Later, when emergency physicians began to gain acceptance, the director became part of the medical staff structure, and finally gained a seat on the executive committee of the medical staff.

Now, the complex and multifaceted duties and responsibilities of the emergency department director (EDD) are numerous (Table 145-1). In order to keep the ED functioning at full efficiency and provide the highest possible quality care in the shortest time possible, the EDD must be involved in every aspect of the function of the department.

The neophyte in emergency care is usually not the best choice for the position of EDD. It takes maturity, diplomacy, tenacity, an ulcer-resistant physique, ingenuity, and leadership. The EDD is, or must be, a highly developed, politically oriented person able to negotiate for a contract and to deal with the medical staff, administration, ancillary services, the public, and the prehospital phase of emergency care on a day-to-day basis.

How does one become an EDD? Since there is not enough taught on the subject in the emergency residency programs, it must be learned by experience. Working as an associate director or even without a title under the tutelage of an established EDD is probably the best way of getting there. Otherwise, keeping a low profile in the first year or two and not impetuously wanting to change everything immediately is another. There is no way, even with the best lecture and preceptorship, that the role of the EDD can be learned. Most of it must be experienced, which means being an EDD or being very close to one. Working as an associate EDD for a length of time and being ''put in charge'' often enough is probably the best way to learn the job.

QUALIFICATIONS OF THE EMERGENCY DEPARTMENT DIRECTOR

The EDD must be able to meet certain qualifications. Some of these are measurable; others are abstract and can be gauged only by the results of the direction. The most obvious qualifications are:

1. Dedication. The EDD must be dedicated to a career in emergency medicine, and, therefore, is presumably a full-time emergency physician.
2. Leadership.
3. Effectiveness in communications.
4. Management abilities, including both skills and style. (A manager with good skills may reach goals regardless of style, but a manager with a poor style may not.)
5. Educational acumen. The EDD must be able to teach those who work in the department, especially if residents rotate through the ED.

THE CHAIN OF COMMAND

A department with one head who has total authority is the ideal situation. However, often the hospital administration and/or medical staff are not willing to delegate all power to one person. The pictured chain of command (Fig. 145-1) is the ideal. Of course, variations will occur and are necessary to preserve a major mode of impact. The EDD (or medical director) is responsible to administration for nonclincal matters and to the leadership of the medical staff for clinical quality of care, even if the EDD has full control. However, practically speaking, the EDD usually has all the clinical control and equal if not more administrative control.

Table 145-1. Duties and Responsibilities of the Emergency Department Director

A. Interaction with the medical staff
   1. Committee structure
      a. Committee member
      b. Get staff physicians appointed to committee
   2. Department meetings
   3. Respond to complaints by medical staff members
   4. Education for medical staff (BLS, ACLS, etc.)
   5. Social
B. Interaction with administration
   1. Regular meetings with administrative officer(s)
   2. Relate to managing personnel of ancillary services
   3. Aid in public relations programs and marketing
   4. Budget process
C. Interaction with staff physicians
   1. Scheduling
   2. Meetings
   3. Hiring (and firing)
   4. Education
   5. Review of capabilities and evaluations
   6. Social
D. Interact with emergency department personnel
   1. Education
   2. Evaluation
E. Interact with EMS system
   1. Education
   2. Meetings
   3. Advisers
   4. Telecommunications
F. Developing policies, procedures, and protocols
G. Quality control
   1. Risk management
   2. Care reviews
H. Community level involvement
   1. Public relations (radio, TV)
   2. Education
I. Monthly, annual reports
J. Inspections and surveys
   1. JCAH
   2. Health department
   3. Fire department
   4. Pharmacy board, etc.
K. Patient complaints
L. Planning

RULES

The rules which govern the function of the ED are similar to those for other departments. They are:

1. Joint Commission on Accreditation of Hospitals (JCAH) standards
2. Hospital or ED policies and procedures.
3. State department of health rules.
4. Fire codes.
5. Medical staff bylaws, and rules and regulations.

JCAH Standards

Hospitals, including EDs, are accredited by the JCAH. The length of accreditation varies with the deficiencies, or their lack, discov-ered at a survey. In the past 2 or 3 years, the standards have not changed appreciably. The principle on which JCAH promulgates and bases all its standards is: "Any individual who comes to the hospital for emergency medical evaluation or initial treatment shall be properly assessed by qualified individuals, and appropriate services shall be rendered within the defined capability of the Hospital."

Standard I

A well-defined plan for emergency care, based on community need and on the capability of the hospital, shall be implemented by every hospital.

Standard I mandates that every person presenting to the ED is evaluated and then either treated or referred "to an appropriate facility" (which would include a clinic, physician's office, or other hospital). This interpretation of the standard also attempts to address the various levels of capability that a given hospital can offer the patient. Although this categorization is by no means ideal, it is the first attempt at a nationwide one. Regional variations exist and must be accepted in lieu of the JCAH interpretation. Patient transfer, appropriate identifying signs, disaster plans, and communications are discussed briefly.

Standard II

The emergency department/service shall be well organized, properly directed, and staffed according to the nature and extent of health care needs anticipated and the scope of services offered.

The interpretation of standard II describes the desired relationship between the ED and other departments in the hospital. It also relates to the direction of the department or service by a physician member of the active medical staff and alludes to the qualifications and authority of the EDD. The EDD is responsible for the "quality, safety and appropriateness" of care provided in the department, and for the evaluation of such. The JCAH allows the direction of a level III department to come from a physician or a committee. Standard II further defines the acceptable methods of physician staffing, which may be by supervised house staff, contracted physicians, or medical staff members. If the medical staff assumes care in the ED, it shall be in accordance with the clinical competence and privileges of the physicians involved. Consultation (i.e., on-call rotation) is also delineated. Nursing requirements are discussed, and the relevant training for nursing and other personnel is described. All aspects of the ED must be defined in writing.

Standard III

The emergency department/service shall be appropriately integrated with other units and departments of the hospital.

This standard deals with ancillary services, specifically laboratory, radiology, and operating suites. It specifies the needs for the different category levels and refers to other sections of the manual that have impact on emergency services.

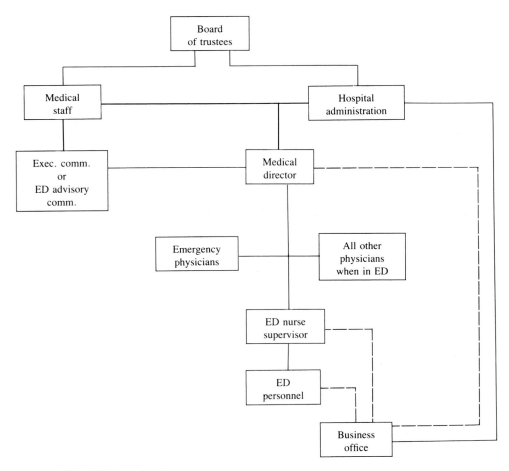

Figure 145-1. ED administration.

Standard IV

All personnel shall be prepared for their emergency care responsibilities through appropriate training and educational programs.

In standard IV the focus is on training of personnel. Included are the orientation and continuing education programs.

Standard V

Emergency patient care shall be guided by written policies and procedures.

Policies and procedures are highlighted in standard V. A list of the base minimum of policies is given in Table 145-2. It is this standard and standard VIII that probably occupy much of the time of the surveyors of the JCAH. Since the list of policies, regarded as a minimum, is growing, the EDD should be well prepared for each subsequent JCAH survey. Some of the required policies are superfluous for a large emergency service but they are checked nevertheless.

Standard VI

The emergency department/service shall be designed and equipped to facilitate the safe and effective care of patients.

Standard VI deals with the physical plant of the ED and the suggested minimal equipment and supplies. It stresses accessibility, identification of entrance, observation beds, communications in the department, special examinations, and lists partially the needed equipment, supplies, and drugs.

Standard VII

A medical record shall be maintained on every patient seeking emergency care and shall be incorporated into the patient's permanent hospital record. A control register shall adequately identify all persons seeking emergency care.

Standard VII describes the requirements for the emergency record and the log. Emergency records vary considerably from department to department. The minimum requirements for information contained in the medical record and log are outlined.

Standard VIII

The quality and appropriateness of patient care provided in the emergency department/service shall be continuously reviewed, evaluated, and assured through establishment of quality control mechanisms.

Table 145-2. JCAH Policies and Procedures: Standard V

- Location, storage, and procurement of medications, blood, supplies, and equipment at all times.
- Provision of care to an unemancipated minor not accompanied by parent or guardian, or to an unaccompanied unconscious patient.
- Circumstances under which the patient's personal physician is to be notified or given reports.
- Confidentiality of patient information and the safeguarding of records.
- Release of authorized information and materials to police or health authorities.
- Transfer and discharge of patients.
- The emergency medical record, including any consent for treatment.
- Infection control measures, including procedures designed to eliminate the possibility of contamination and cross infection.
- Procedures to be followed in the event of equipment failure.
- Pertinent safety practices.
- Control of traffic, including visitors.
- Dispensing of medications in accordance with the requirements of the Pharmaceutical Services section of this Manual.
- The handling and safekeeping of patients' valuables.
- The role of the emergency department/service in the hospital disaster plans.
- Specification of the scope of treatment allowed, including the general and specific procedures that may not be performed by medical staff members in the emergency department/service, and the use of anesthesia.
- Who, other than physicians, may perform special procedures, under what circumstances, and under what degree of supervision. Such procedures include, but are not limited to, cardiopulmonary resuscitation, including cardiac defibrillation; endotracheal intubation; tracheostomy and cricothyrotomy; respiratory care, including assisted ventilation and humidification; the administration of parenteral antiarrhythmic and other specified medications; and the obtaining of arterial and venous blood samples and other laboratory specimens.
- The use of standing orders.
- The property exchange system, when necessitated by the transportation and transfer of patients.
- Circumstances that require the patient to return to the emergency department/service for treatment.

- The emergency management of individuals who have actual or suspected exposure to radiation or who are radioactively contaminated. Such action may include radioactivity monitoring and measurement; designation and any required preparation of space for evaluation of the patient, including, as required, discontinuation of the air circulation system to prevent the spread of contamination; decontamination of the patient through an appropriate cleansing mechanism; and containment, labeling, and disposition of contaminated materials. The individual responsible for radiation safety should be notified.
- Handling of alleged or suspected rape victims, or victims of sexual molestation. Criteria for an adequate medicolegal evaluation should include examination and treatment; required patient consent; collection, retention, and safeguarding of specimens, photographs, and other evidentiary material; maintaining a detailed receipt for all material released; and, as legally required, notification of, and release of information to, the proper authorities. Examination of, and consultation with, the patient shall take place only when visual and auditory privacy are assured.
- Handling of alleged or suspected child abuse cases. Criteria for alerting emergency department/service personnel to the possibility of child abuse should be developed. Pertinent information may be obtained for the history, physical examination, laboratory and radiological tests, photographs, and observations of parent/child interactions. In addition to such information, the medical record should document the treatment given, and any required reporting to the proper authorities.
- The management of pediatric emergencies.
- Individuals dead on arrival, any legally required collection and preservation of evidence, and reporting to the proper authorities.
- The management of patients who are under the influence of drugs or alcohol, or who are emotionally ill or become difficult to manage.
- The initial management of patients with burns, hand injuries, head injuries, fractures, multiple injuries, poisoning, animal bites, gunshot and stab wounds, and other acute problems.
- Precautions to be taken in preventing the occurrence of accidents to unconscious or irrational patients.
- Tetanus and rabies prevention/prophylaxis.

Finally, standard VIII of the JCAH deals with quality review and quality control. This is the aspect of care that needs to be part of a continuous, defined process involving physicians, nursing personnel, and medical record librarians. Such processes as daily administrative tasks, complaints of physicians and nurses, death records, and other reviews occupy considerable time and require effort by all the physicians and nurses. If residents rotate through the ED, specific attention must be given to the records they produce from the standpoint of appropriateness, completion, and compliance with the department's customs. Standard VIII also mandates review of x-rays and a mechanism for handling variances. This aspect of review may need a strong policy drawn up by the ED and the radiology department since many legal actions can be avoided if these matters are handled well and expeditiously.

Policies and Procedures

Next to the JCAH standards, the policies and procedures (P&P) book is the most important set of rules by which the ED operates. Every occurrence of operational value that happens with a certain frequency—sometimes only after two or three times—should be covered with a policy or a procedural description. The EDD is

responsible for setting policies. The approval of a new policy or procedure should involve both the administration—ultimately the board of trustees—and the medical staff. There are really several types of policies:

Administrative policies. First, there is a set of administrative policies that apply to all departments of the hospital.

Departmental policies. Next there are the departmental policies and procedures which are exclusive to a department, although they may deal with the relationship between two departments. A list of common policies and procedures for the ED is given in Table 145-2. There are certain policies that are particular for a given ED but most apply to all departments.

Review. All policies have to be reviewed annually and there are different ways of doing so. The simplest, perhaps, is to list all policies and provide check-off spaces for the annual review.

Disclaimer. It is advisable to precede policies or procedures which describe a certain clinical maneuver with a disclaimer in case there is a deviation from the order or an omission of a step. This disclaimer should read approximately as follows: ''There may be a deviation from the following procedure if it is deemed necessary by the attending physician, nurse or other emergency department personnel. This deviation does not constitute a breach of the standard of care.''

Other Rules

State Department of Health

Usually the state department of health or the local government has certain rules with which EDs must comply. These may vary from the type of soap that is provided to the level of lighting. It behooves the EDD to become familiar with these rules.

Fire Department Codes

Fire department (FD) regulations play a significant part in the design of a department, and, to a degree, in its operation, directly or indirectly. For instance, the FD may object to patients on stretchers, parked in the hallways, especially those that are part of an exit route. Fire codes regulate such things as width of corridor exits, width, type, and location of doors, placement of sliding windows, maximum number of people in waiting rooms, floor covering materials, etc. These codes also must be learned, so that they might be considered in the design and/or operation of the department.

Medical Staff Bylaws, Rules, and Regulations

The medical staff bylaws, rules, and regulations, as well as "politics," impose certain control over the ED operation. There are some "golden rules" which most EDDs should follow in caring for patients in the ED. Golden rule 1: Never admit an "attached" patient without notification of the attending physician. Golden rule 2: In case of a dispute over admission of a patient, the attending physician or a designated alternate, but not a resident, must evaluate the patient and take responsibility for the decision. Golden rule 3: When the emergency physicians write orders on admitted patients, they must ascertain that these are the orders desired by the attending physician. There are several ways of doing this. One can write as the last order: "Please call Dr. _____ and read the above orders to him/her and ask for any further orders." Or one can write: "Please notify Dr. _____ that the patient has arrived on the floor and read the orders written"; or "the above orders are written at Dr._____'s request and he/she is aware of the patient's condition and admission, and he/she will see the patient at _____ a.m./p.m." Once contact has been made by the floor nurse, the assumption of responsibility is virtually completed.

EFFICIENCY

In the ED efficiency is almost synonymous with attaining the lowest possible put-through time. Efficiency is dependent on a number of factors: architectural design, patient mix, fluctuations of patient load, staffing, response by ancillary services (especially laboratory and x-ray), availability of dictation of emergency records, computerized medical records library, and adequate supplies and equipment, among others. It is not always possible to provide or control all the efficiency factors, but the EDD must always strive to attain as much efficiency as possible.

Design

Architectural design of the department is an important factor in the smoothness of the ED operation. Where it may be possible to put through as many as 60 patients in an 8-h span in one department, only 30 or 50 might be handled in another, given the same circumstances except for layout. There are several major types of design which will give maximum opportunity to deal with the patients efficiently. One essential is the number of treatment spaces. Although there is no concrete rule, one space for every 2000 patient visits is quite acceptable. When a new department is built there should be space for growth. The EDD and ED staff must be very closely involved when a new department is planned. No one else has the working knowledge of department functions.

Accessibility

Accessibility for both ambulatory and ambulance patients—preferably by separate entrances—must be easy and well identified. There should be sufficient parking adjacent to the ED. Twelve to fourteen spaces for every 20,000 annual patient visits seems adequate. The parking area should be well lit. Access must be easily controlled by security personnel.

Triage, Registration, and Waiting Areas

The triage area must be situated so that both ambulatory and ambulance patients can be easily attended. Registration must be located next to triage so that the patient does not have to guess where to go next. In the registration area attention must be given to privacy. If the patient is not immediately taken to a treatment area, there must be a pleasant waiting area for both the patient and accompanying persons. Toilets, pay phones, television, magazines, and possibly a children's corner and beverage machines should be part of the waiting area.

Treatment Areas

The entrance into the treatment area must be through automatically activated sliding or swinging doors, preferably visible from the control center (i.e., nurse's station). If triage is not performed at the front entrance, ambulance patients must be quickly assessed, upon entrance, to ascertain the treatment space proper for the patient. Individual treatment spaces should not be less than 8 by 10 feet, although the size may be predetermined by the health department. They should be curtained to afford privacy, yet open enough to allow adequate observation when needed. All treatment spaces should be equipped with a good adjustable source of light, and oxygen, suction, and electrical outlets. A wall-mounted sphygmomanometer, ophthalmoscope, and otoscope may be useful. Each treatment space should be prewired for monitoring at the bedside, at the nurse's station, or both.

Separate rooms should be available for the following: eye, ear, nose, and throat; obstetrics and gynecology; cardiac; major trauma; orthopedics; and psychiatry. A separate room should be provided for police and rescue personnel. An observation room should be available to observe emergency patients and should not be used as an overflow area for admitted patients.

The major trauma and cardiac resuscitation rooms should be nearest to the rescue vehicle entrance. In smaller emergency departments, these can be one and the same.

Emergency departments that handle a large volume of patients should be equipped with an x-ray unit with dedicated personnel and dark room, and a small laboratory where the physician may perform procedures such as Gram's stain, urinalysis, and peripheral smear.

There should, of course, also be clean and dirty utility rooms and adequate storage space for the usual supplies and equipment. A space in which the stretchers and wheelchairs are stored should ideally be situated near the entrance to the emergency department.

The design must be suited to the use of the facility. If separate treatment areas are needed for ambulatory (nonurgent) and reclining (urgent) patients, there must be variations in essential space and equipment to suit need. Emergency departments with large and frequent fluctuating patient populations may use a modular design in which one or more parts can be closed or opened according to need.

Control Station

The control station should be centrally located to eliminate unnecessary walking, and so that all patients can be observed from this area. Central monitors must be placed here.

Equipment

Equipment for each of the treatment areas must include sturdy carts that can be manipulated to raise the head or foot and are equipped with side rails and space for the patient's clothing, intravenous poles, and oxygen tanks.

A Mayo table, and a shelf for materials such as tongue blades, ear specula, dressings, lubricant, gloves, thermometers, and oral airways should be provided.

In addition to the general equipment and supplies, the cardiac treatment area must have a monitor-defibrillator unit; a crash cart with emergency medications and intravenous solutions; an intubation box with a laryngoscope and selection of blades, nasal and endotracheal tubes and guidewires, lubricating jelly, and suction tips; oxygen masks; and airways. It is advisable to store equipment in the cardiac area in such a way that it is readily visible to all the staff. Hanging the equipment on a pegboard is one way to solve the problem. In the resuscitation area, it is essential to have various sizes of equipment available to accommodate patients of all ages, unless a separate pediatric crash care is available. Portable oxygen and suction units should be available. A separate portable monitor unit that can be used during transport or in other treatment areas, when indicated, should be available. The resuscitation area should have a portable x-ray unit dedicated to that area or, if possible, an overhead x-ray unit.

The eye, ear, nose, and throat room should have all the basic equipment plus the following: a slit lamp; an instrument tray for eye treatments; a tray with instruments and supplies for nose and ear problems; ophthalmic and otic medications; a special ear, nose, and throat (Ritter) chair; a light source or head mirror, or a telescopic light on a headband; and a double loupe.

More and more hospitals are being equiped with communication and telemetry equipment to provide rescue personnel access to the emergency physician and for interhospital communication. This equipment should be centrally located for easy accessibility by trained personnel yet should afford privacy during the communication process.

Offices

The emergency department must have an office for the medical director, the head nurse or supervisor, the unit manager if the department has one, and space where the department secretaries can work. Offices of the director and head nurse must be adjacent to but not necessarily in the department.

Specialized Emergency Departments

There are special considerations for EDs which are "specialized." Children's hospitals, where virtually no adults are seen, may need a special design. In many of the busy EDs there would be an advantage to separating children from adults for obvious reasons. There is also a trend to alter the methods for seeing patients with minimal complaints, in order to expedite the care and be able to effect a minimal charge.

Trauma centers may have a different orientation to the design of the ED because of the more intensive treatment provided in the ED.

Patient Mix and Load

The patient mix is a variable that cannot be predicted. However, staffing must be such that a sudden appearance of one or more critical patients can be handled without the need for additional personnel, unless disaster proportions are reached. The patient load is quite predictable and usually subject to daily ups and downs as well as seasonal fluctuations. This makes it possible to staff the department accordingly with physicians, nurses, and other personnel.

Ancillary Services

The location and the efficient handling of services provided by the ancillary departments (especially radiology and laboratory) are essential to overall efficiency. All studies ordered by the ED should be given priority status. There must be, however, a distinction between those that have absolute first priority (as in resuscitations) and those that are "stat" requests. Routine studies should also be separately labeled. This affords the possibility of assuring that first-priority services are dealt with expeditiously. If there is a question about the time it takes for services to be provided, a time study can be undertaken to show the department involved where the problem lies.

Other Efficiency Factors

Other factors affecting the efficiency in the department range from the responsiveness of the consultants to the availability of supplies and equipment. With regard to the consultant's response, a reasonable policy is one which states that a response time of less than 1 h is obligatory. Difficulties occur when the consultant is in surgery at the time of the initial call. There is not much that can be done about this situation, except to find another consultant, if this is possible.

Some modes of record keeping can vastly improve turnaround time. The use of a scribe, dictating the record with instant transcription and/or the use of a computer are methods to improve recording time and thus shorten waiting time. Having all the usually needed supplies and equipment in the ED saves time. Transportation of patients (to and from the radiology department, for instance) is another factor in efficiency.

RECORD KEEPING

Proper recording is one of the surest means of avoiding possible lawsuits. This includes all aspects of the ED records—the main record, instructions, consents, etc. There is no substitute for a well-documented patient encounter, especially in court.

ED Record

The ED record serves as the basis of the documented care provided. At least three copies—the original for medical records, a copy for the treating physician (i.e., ED group), the attending physician, or the clinic, and a copy for the billing office—must be provided. If the attending physician is not on the hospital staff and the patient is released to be followed by this physician, a decision must be made about whether to send a copy to this physician. If the medical record copy is not easily retrievable, especially at night, consideration should be given to an extra copy which could be filed in the ED for 3 to 4 months.

Instructions

The next most useful document is the instruction sheet or booklet given to the patient on dismissal. Instructions to patients should be specific, written or printed, and individualized when needed, and a copy should be kept for the medical record. The instructions should be in simple language and multilingual in areas where a significant sector of the population does not speak English. The patient or patient's representative should sign the instructions and this signature should be witnessed.

ED Log

In the absence of a computer-produced log, the ED should keep a log which contains the following information: time of arrival; mode of arrival (include rescue squad name if applicable); the patient's last name, first name, age; diagnostic impressions; description of treatment provided; name of treating physician; family physician or clinic ancillary studies done; time of discharge; mode of discharge; if the patient was admitted, the room number; if transfer took place, the destination. The log (and/or computer bank) may also list useful additional information, such as motor vehicle accidents; motorcycle accidents; pediatric, surgical, or medical cases; medications; orthopedic appliances. Such information is mainly useful for statistics and studies.

Other Forms

There are other forms routinely used in EDs. Most significant are those used for recording data on critically ill or injured patients: ACLS records, neurological check records, and records for diabetic complications. The ED also must have a supply of absence from work or school forms, incident reports, transfer forms, various insurance forms, telemetry report forms, and laboratory and radiology procedure request forms.

LEGAL CONSIDERATIONS

Although most of the administrative aspects that have legal implications have been dealt with in other sections of this chapter, it is important to point out some areas that may cause problems. Here is a list of the nine most common reasons for legal action:

1. Things taken for granted
2. Not calling proper consultants
3. Lack of communications
4. Prescribing indiscriminately
5. Providing inadequate coverage
6. Wrong things said at the wrong time
7. Problems not discussed with patients
8. Exceeding medical skills
9. Billing injudiciously

As far as the emergency record is concerned there are ways to protect oneself:

1. Document the patient's complaint in his or her own words. Also document the lack of a complaint. Significant remarks should be put in quotation marks.
2. Document all findings, even significant negative ones.
3. Recommendations and instructions from consultants should be recorded (and signed by the physicians).
4. Exact discharge instructions to a patient should be recorded and transmitted to the patient. If printed instructions are used, additional verbal instructions should be recorded as well.

Additional legal concerns are reports to authorities, coroner's cases, treatment of intoxicated and substance abuse patients, drawing laboratory studies (especially blood alcohol) in prisoners or other alleged intoxicated persons, alleged sexual assault, alleged child abuse, treatment of minors. The scope of this chapter is not wide enough to discuss all of these; Chapter 141 contains more in-depth discussion.

REVIEW OF CARE

Care review used to be calling *auditing*. The audits required by the JCAH have changed. The JCAH mandates the review process but limits its requirements to a reasonable level of review. The proper review necessitates correction of deficiencies and ascertaining that the deficiencies have been corrected or decreased. Basically, the need is for daily administrative reviews encompassing no more than 10 percent of the daily charts. A combined physician/nursing review on a regular basis (e.g., 15 to 20 records per month) is also a good habit. There are of course other reviews. A review of a particular physician's records for a period of time, a monthly review of one day's records or more, a complaint-oriented review, and other such reviews are all valid. The JCAH stipulates an antibiotic usage review. This is fairly hard to comply with unless measures can be taken to assure follow up of the patients involved. A mandatory review is the monthly death review, which includes all patients who died in the ED and within 24 h after admission to the hospital. The medical staff audit committee should receive copies of all reviews to be included in the agenda of the meetings. The essentials for record review are:

- The process must be kept simple.
- The review must be limited to the aspect of emergency care selected by the ED review committee.
- A record must be kept of every review.
- The review results must be conveyed with the least delay to those reviewed in order to effect a change in behavior.
- A repeat review in the areas found deficient must be done in a 6- to 12-month time span.

STAFFING THE ED

Physicians

The number of physicians needed to staff a given department depends on the total number of annual visits, the design of the department, the mix of conditions seen, seasonal fluctuations, and the availability of residents on rotation.

It has been said that a physician can deal quite comfortably with an average of four patients an hour. Perhaps this is the best gauge for the number of physicians needed and for determining the need for double coverage.

There must be one person responsible for the quality of care given and the performance of the physicians. Usually a group of physicians has a director, the chief of the department or a physician with another title who has this responsibility, which carries with it the duty of discipline, hiring, and firing. In a corporate setting these duties may fall on a board of directors, who nevertheless will usually charge a president of the group with the administration of the department.

Nurses and Other Personnel

The management of the nursing team usually does not fall on the shoulders of the EDD. However, the EDD should have considerable input in matters pertaining to nursing personnel.

MONEY AND CONTRACTS

Reimbursement for services rendered in an ED occurs in one of several ways.

1. The hospital bills the patient for the total, without distinction between hospital and physician fees.
2. The hospital bills the patient but identifies the physician's fee.
3. The physician group bills the patient for the physician's component of the bill.

4. The individual physicians as independent contractors bill the patient.

Hospital Bills without Identification of Physician Component

There must be some agreement between the group of physicians and the hospital about how physicians are to be reimbursed. Usually, this agreement is a salary arrangement, which is most common in university settings, but not unusual in community hospitals and government-owned institutions.

Hospital Bills and Identified Physician's Fees

When the hospital bills the patient and identifies the physician's fee, there must be an understanding about how to divide the remittance. The best and most advisable arrangement is for the physician's fee to be a percentage of the gross billing, although a salaried ED physician is also possible.

Physician Group Bills the Patient

Either the group of physicians as a whole or a physician acting as head of a group bills the patient. The monies collected then can be allocated to the physicians in the group as salaries, which may or may not be dependent on hours worked, or apportioned to the independent contractors in the group on the basis of hours worked. In the corporate arrangement the physicians are employees of the group and subject to all benefits equally. The group usually pays the liability insurance fees. The group can also operate as a partnership. The main difference between the corporation and the partnership is the liability concept and the provision of benefits. When a physician is an independent contractor, he or she is responsible for benefits, liability insurance, and other amenities.

Independent Contractor Bills Patient

If an independent contractor has an arrangement where he or she is responsible for billing and collecting fees, the contractor obviously is entirely self-sufficient. This arrangement is very rare. Independent contractors must make sure that they are indeed operating as such. The IRS has stringent rules that distinguish independent contractors from employees.

Those physicians who derive their income from a fee-for-service concept, whether the fee is billed as part of the hospital-generated bill, by the emergency physician group, or by an independent contractor, are private practicing physicians just like other members of the staff who operate on a fee-for-service basis.

New Ruling

Billing, especially where the hospital is involved, will change drastically with the new federal Tax Equity and Fiscal Responsibility Act (TEFRA) rule 108. This rule states that the hospital can no longer bill for the physician's component on the hospital's bill.

Contracts with Hospitals

Contracts with hospitals vary greatly. There are a few components of the contract that must be scrutinized closely.

1. The status of the department (i.e., does it have its own chief with a seat on the medical executive committee?) should be clearly defined.
2. A set of rules and regulations supported by the medical staff and administration should be established.
3. The method of fee setting must be spelled out and it must be made clear that the leveling of the fees is the prerogative of the physician or group of physicians.
4. The respective responsibilities of the hospital and the group should be clearly delineated.
5. Other major items of the contract are the terms, the method of resolution of a controversy, the examination of books (if the hospital bills and collects), liability insurance; and the termination clause.

ESSENTIAL BACKUP SERVICES

A discussion of administration of the ED is not complete without mention of some valuable assets to the department: the backup services.

Social Services

Social services are a most worthwhile adjunct to any ED. Numerous times patients must be placed in care centers, alleged child abuse must be followed, sexual assault victims need counseling, etc. The efforts of the social service department will save the ED physician and ED personnel countless hours.

Security

Security is a must, especially in urban hospitals. There is a controversy whether the security people need to wear uniforms and be highly visible or not. Whatever the case, most EDs could not function well without some type of security.

Pastoral Care

Pastoral care is another essential service to patients and relatives. Every ED physician can recount occasions where a member of the pastoral care service has played an important role in such situations as deaths in the ED, patients with serious illnesses, etc.

Patient Representative

In those EDs where a patient representative or official is present to act as liaison between the ED personnel and those in the waiting room, there is usually a better atmosphere of understanding about delays.

BIBLIOGRAPHY

Cameron CTM: *Public Relations in the Emergency Department*. Bowie, Md. Brady, 1980.

Ciancutti AR: *Emergency Care Handbook*. Westport, Conn, Technomic, 1977.

Fleisher G, Ludwig S (eds): *Textbook of Pediatric Emergency Medicine*. Baltimore, Williams & Wilkins, 1983, sec. VI.

George JE: *Law and Emergency Care*. St Louis, Mosby, 1980.

Jenkins AL, van de Leuv JH: *Emergency Department Organization and Management*. St Louis, Mosby, 1978.

Joint Commission on Accreditation of Hospitals: *Accreditation Manual for Hospitals*. Chicago, 1983.

MacDonald MR: *Department of Emergency Medicine Guidelines, Policies and Procedures*. St Louis, Mosby, 1979.

Mancini MR, Gale AT: *Emergency Care and the Law*. Rockville, Md, Aspen Systems, 1981.

Richards EP III, Rathbun KC: *Medical Risk Management*. Rockville, Md, Aspen Systems, 1983.

Yanda, RL: *Doctors as Managers of Health Teams*. New York, Am Mgmt, 1977.

INDEX

Note: Page numbers in *italic* indicate illustrations.